MAINGOT'S
ABDOMINAL
OPERATIONS

VOLUME TWO

EIGHTH EDITION

MAINGOT'S ABDOMINAL OPERATIONS

EIGHTH EDITION

Edited by

Seymour I. Schwartz, MD
Professor of Surgery, University of Rochester, Rochester, New York

Harold Ellis, DM, MCh, FRCS
Professor of Surgery, Westminster Medical School, London, England

with
Wendy Cowles Husser, BS
Senior Information Analyst, University of Rochester, Rochester, New York

VOLUME TWO

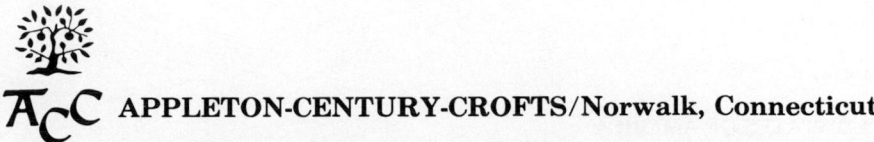 APPLETON-CENTURY-CROFTS/Norwalk, Connecticut

Copyright © 1985 by Appleton-Century-Crofts
A Publishing Division of Prentice-Hall, Inc.

Copyright 1969 by Meredith Corporation
Copyright 1961, 1955, 1948 by Appleton-Century-Crofts, Inc.
Copyright 1940 by D. Appleton-Century Company, Inc.

85 86 87 88 89 / 10 9 8 7 6 5 4 3 2 1

Prentice-Hall International, Inc., London
Prentice-Hall of Australia, Pty. Ltd., Sydney
Prentice-Hall Canada, Inc.
Prentice-Hall of India Private Limited, New Delhi
Prentice-Hall of Japan, Inc., Tokyo
Prentice-Hall of Southeast Asia (Pte.) Ltd., Singapore
Whitehall Books Ltd., Wellington, New Zealand
Editora Prentice-Hall do Brasil Ltda., Rio de Janeiro

Library of Congress Cataloging in Publication Data

Maingot, Rodney, 1893–1982
  Maingot's Abdominal operations, 8th ed.

  Rev. ed. of: Abdominal operations / Rodney Maingot and British and American contributors. 7th ed. c1980.
  Includes bibliographical references and index.
  1. Abdomen—Surgery. I. Schwartz, Seymour I.,
1928–   . II. Ellis, Harold, 1926–   . III. Husser,
Wendy Cowles. IV. Title. V. Title: Abdominal operations.
[DNLM: 1. Abdomen—surgery. WI 900 M225a]
RD540.M24 1985   617'.55   84–11034
ISBN 0–8385–6100–4 (Set)
ISBN 0–8385–6099–7 (Volume II)

Design: Jean M. Sabato-Morley

PRINTED IN THE UNITED STATES OF AMERICA

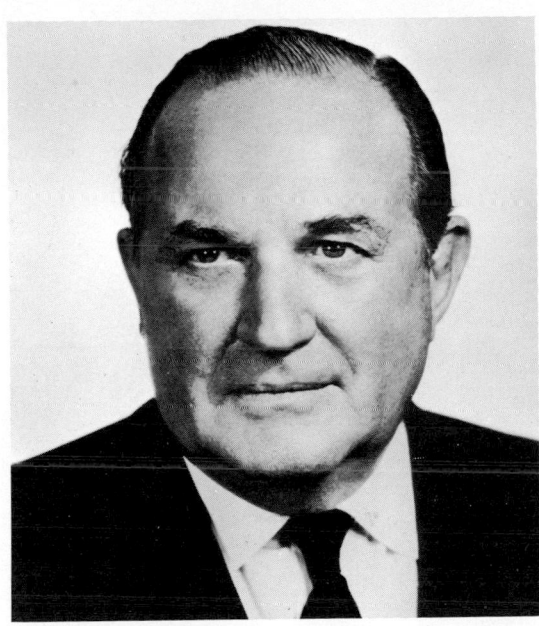

Rodney Maingot
(1893–1982)

Rodney Maingot was born in Trinidad. He spent his medical student days at St. Bartholomew's Hospital Medical School, London, and qualified in 1916. He joined the Royal Army Medical Corps and served as Captain in Egypt and Palestine, being twice mentioned in despatches. On demobilisation he returned to St. Bartholomew's to continue his surgical training and gained his FRCS in 1920. He was appointed to the Consultant staff of the Royal Free Hospital, London, which he served for many years with great distinction. In addition, he was Consultant Surgeon at the Southend General Hospital, where his Saturday clinics and operating sessions attracted visitors from all over the world. During World War II he served as Regional Consultant to the Emergency Medical Service.

Rodney Maingot's fame was as a surgical teacher and he was particularly interested in the abdominal cavity. Biliary surgery was his particular metière, but he also made great contributions to the surgery of hernia and was especially proud of his "Keel repair" for large incisional hernias. He lectured with distinction, and his clear, beautifully illustrated talks took him to many parts of the world. He was particularly well known and popular in the United States. His reputation was spread even more widely through his numerous textbooks, characterised by their clear writing, superb illustrations, meticulous production, and detailed, indeed encyclopaedic, knowledge.

Rodney was especially proud of his *Abdominal Operations*. The First Edition appeared in 1940; it boasted 1385 pages and, apart from short contributions by two internists (Dr. R.S. Johnson on postoperative chest complications and Dr. L.T. Bond on sternal puncture), the whole massive work was entirely the effort of this remarkable man. Some of the figures by Miss Pauline Larivière, a pupil of Max Brödel, live on today.

A Second Edition appeared in 1948. Now Rodney had collected eight contributors: five from the United Kingdom, two from the United States, and one from Australia. For the Third Edition, in 1955, there were now 24 contributors. Those from the United States included such famous names as Brunschwig, DeBakey, Cooley, Dragstedt, Harrington, and Pack. The United Kingdom contributors included two future Presidents of the Royal College of Surgeons—Russell Brock and Cecil Wakeley. The succeeding editions contained increasing numbers of contributors whose names formed a veritable *Who's Who* of international surgery. The Seventh Edition, published in 1980 when Rodney was in his ninth decade, found him still actively concerned with editing and writing this monumental work, as well as carrying out an extensive and personal correspondence with his numerous contributors all over the world.

The last few months of his life were passed in poor physical health but he remained in full mental vigour right until the end. Shortly before he died, I visited him with David Stires of Appleton-Century-Crofts. He fully realised that he would never live to see the Eighth Edition, nor indeed to have the strength even to undertake the task. The fact that *Abdominal Operations* was not only to continue but was to bear his name, gave him immense pleasure and satisfaction.

Maingot's introduction to the first edition had a first paragraph consisting of one sentence:

> This book is intended to present detailed consideration of the technique of modern abdominal operations.

This aim, we hope, lives on today.

Harold Ellis

v

Contributors

Maria D. Allo, MD
Assistant Professor of General Surgery and
Surgical Endocrinology
The Johns Hopkins University
Baltimore, Maryland

Frank Ashton, ChM, FRCS
Professor of Surgery
Department of Surgery
Queen Elizabeth Hospital
Birmingham, England

Arthur H. Aufses, Jr., MD
Franz W. Sichel Professor of Surgery
Chairman, Department of Surgery
Mount Sinai Medical Center
New York, New York

Richard H. Bell, Jr., MD
Assistant Professor of Surgery
University of Cincinnati
Assistant Chief, Surgical Service
Veterans Administration
Cincinnati, Ohio

Jeffrey S. Bender, MD
Surgical Resident
Wayne State University
Detroit, Michigan

Leslie H. Blumgart, MD, FRCS
Professor of Surgery
Royal Postgraduate Medical School
London, England

John W. Braasch, MD, PhD
Lahey Clinic Foundation
Assistant Clinical Professor
Harvard Medical School
Boston, Massachusetts

Cedric Bremner, ChM, FRCS
Professor of Surgery
University of the Witwatersrand
Johannesburg, South Africa

**Willem H. Brummelkamp, MD,
PhD, FRCS(Hon)**
Professor of Surgery
University of Amsterdam
Amsterdam, The Netherlands

John G. Buls, MD
Clinical Instructor of Surgery
Division of Colon and Rectal Surgery
University of Minnesota Medical School
Minneapolis, Minnesota

L. John Chalstrey, MD, FRCS
Consultant Surgeon
St. Bartholomew's Hospital
London, England

Prabir K. Chaudhuri, MD
Associate Professor of Surgery
Loyola University Medical Center
Staff Physician, Department of Surgery
Hines Veterans Administration Hospital
Maywood, Illinois

Avram M. Cooperman, MD
Professor of Surgery
New York Medical College
Valhalla, New York

Alfred Cuschieri, MD, ChM, FRCS
Professor of Surgery
Ninewells Hospital and Medical School
Dundee, Scotland

Tapas K. Das Gupta, MD, PhD
Professor of Surgery
Head, Division of Surgical Oncology
Department of Surgery
University of Illinois at Chicago
Chairman, Division of Surgical Oncology
Department of Surgery
Cook County Hospital
Chicago, Illinois
Consultant to Surgical Oncology

Surgical Service
West Side Veterans Administration Hospital
Chicago, Illinois

Michael E. DeBakey, MD, MS(Surg)
Chancellor, Baylor College of Medicine
Chairman, Department of Surgery
Baylor College of Medicine
Houston, Texas

Anthony J. Edis, MD, FACS
Associate Professor of Surgery
Royal Perth Hospital
Western Australia

F. Henry Ellis, Jr., MD, PhD
Chief of Thoracic and Cardiovascular Surgery
New England Deaconess Hospital and
Lahey Clinic Medical Center
Boston, Massachusetts

Harold Ellis, DM, MCh, FRCS
Professor of Surgery
Westminster Medical School
London, England

Kenneth Eng, MD
Associate Professor of Surgery
Department of Surgery
New York University School of Medicine
New York, New York

Stanley R. Friesen, MD, PhD
Professor of Surgery and Lecturer in the
History of Medicine
University of Kansas Medical Center
Kansas City, Kansas
Consultant, Veterans Administration
Medical Center
Kansas City, Missouri

Brian G. Gazzard, MA, MD, FRCP
Consultant Physician
Westminster Hospital
London, England

Gary D. Gill, FRACP
Consultant in Nuclear Medicine
and Ultrasound
Repatriation General Hospital
Heidelberg, Australia

Marvin L. Gliedman, MD
Professor and Chairman
Department of Surgery
Albert Einstein College of Medicine

Surgeon-in-Chief
Combined Departments of Surgery
Montefiore Medical Center/Albert Einstein
College of Medicine
New York, New York

Michael S. Gold, MD
Associate Professor of Surgery
Albert Einstein College of Medicine
Chief of Surgery
Einstein Division/Montefiore Medical Center
New York, New York

Stanley M. Goldberg, MD
Clinical Professor of Surgery
Director, Division of Colon and Rectal
Surgery
University of Minnesota Medical School
Minneapolis, Minnesota

Ward O. Griffen, Jr., MD, PhD
Executive Director
American Board of Surgery
Philadelphia, Pennsylvania

Oscar H. Gutierrez, MD
Associate Professor of Radiology
Head, Cardiovascular Radiology
Department of Radiology
University of Rochester School of Medicine
and Dentistry
Rochester, New York

Peter R. Hawley, MS, FRCS
Consultant Surgeon
St. Mark's Hospital
London, England

J. Lynwood Herrington, Jr., MD
Professor of Clinical Surgery
Vanderbilt University Medical Center
Attending Surgeon
St. Thomas Hospital
Nashville, Tennessee

Louis F. Hollender, MD
Department of Surgery
Centre Hospitaliere Universitaire de
Hautepierre
Strasbourg, France

Edward R. Howard, MD, FRCS
Consultant Surgeon
King's College Hospital
London, England

Miles Irving, MD, ChM, FRCS
Professor of Surgery
University of Manchester
Hope Hospital
Salford, England

Shunzaburo Iwatsuki, MD
Associate Professor of Surgery
Department of Surgery
University of Pittsburgh
Presbyterian University Hospital of Pittsburgh
Children's Hospital of Pittsburgh
Veterans Administration Hospital of
Pittsburgh (Oakland)
Pittsburgh, Pennsylvania

**David G. Jagelman, MS(London),
FRCS(Eng), FACS**
Department of Colorectal Surgery
Cleveland Clinic Foundation
Cleveland, Ohio

David Johnston, ChM, MD, FRCS
Professor of Surgery
University of Leeds
Leeds, England

S. Austin Jones, MD
Clinical Professor of Surgery
University of California at Irvine
Irvine, California

George L. Jordan, Jr., MD, MS(Eng), FACS
Distinguished Service Professor of Surgery
Baylor College of Medicine
Houston, Texas

D. Michael King, MB, FRCR
Consultant Radiologist
Westminster Hospital
London, England

Raymond M. Kirk, MS, FRCS
Consultant Surgeon
Royal Free Hospital Medical School
London, England

John S. Kirkham, MChir, FRCS
Consultant Surgeon
St. James' Hospital
London, England

Gabriel A. Kune, FRACS, FRCS
Professor of Surgery
University of Melbourne
Melbourne, Australia

S. Arthur Localio, MD
Professor of Surgery
New York University School of Medicine
New York, New York

Adrian Marston, DM, MCh, FRCS
Consultant Surgeon
The Middlesex Hospital
London, England

Rene Menguy, MD
Professor of Surgery
University of Rochester
School of Medicine and Dentistry
The Genesee Hospital
Rochester, New York

Christian Meyer, MD
Department of Surgery
Centre Hospitaliere Universitaire de
Hautepierre
Strasbourg, France

A.R. Moossa, MD, FRCS, FACS
U.C.S.D. Medical Center
University of California
San Diego, California

George L. Nardi, MD
Visiting Surgeon
Massachusetts General Hospital
Professor of Surgery
Harvard Medical School
Boston, Massachusetts

Mitchell J. Notaras, FRCS
Consultant Surgeon
Barnet General Hospital
London, England

Lloyd M. Nyhus, MD
Warren H. Cole Professor and
Head, Department of Surgery
University of Illinois at Chicago
Chicago, Illinois

T. George Parks, MCh, FRCS
Professor of Surgical Science
The Queen's University of Belfast
Belfast, Ireland

Raymond Pollak, MB, FRCS(Edin)
Assistant Professor of Surgery
Department of Surgery
University of Illinois at Chicago
Chicago, Illinois

John H.C. Ranson, MA, BM, BCh
Professor of Surgery
New York University School of Medicine
New York, New York

Mark M. Ravitch, MD
Surgeon-in-Chief
Montefiore Hospital
Professor of Surgery
University of Pittsburgh School of Medicine
Pittsburgh, Pennsylvania

William H. ReMine, MD, MS(Surg)
Mayo Clinic
Rochester, Minnesota

Grant V. Rodkey, MD
Visiting Surgeon, Massachusetts
General Hospital
Associate Clinical Professor of Surgery
Harvard Medical School
Boston, Massachusetts

Eric S. Rolfsmeyer, MD
Surgical Associates Ltd.
Sioux Falls, South Dakota

David A. Rothenberger, MD
Clinical Assistant Professor of Surgery
Division of Colon and Rectal Surgery
University of Minnesota Medical School
Minneapolis, Minnesota

Avni Sali, PhD, FRACS
Consultant Surgeon
Repatriation General Hospital
Heidelberg, Australia

John L. Sawyers, MD
Professor of Surgery
Chairman, Department of Surgery
Vanderbilt University Medical Center
Nashville, Tennessee

Seymour I. Schwartz, MD
Professor of Surgery
Department of Surgery
University of Rochester School of Medicine
and Dentistry
Rochester, New York

Michael H. Scott, MB, ChB, FRCS(Eng)
Fellow in Surgery
University of California
San Diego, California

Byers W. Shaw, Jr., MD
Assistant Professor of Surgery
Department of Surgery
University of Pittsburgh
Presbyterian University Hospital of Pittsburgh
Children's Hospital of Pittsburgh
Veteran's Administration Hospital of
Pittsburgh (Oakland)
Pittsburgh, Pennsylvania

G. Tom Shires, MD
Lewis Atterbury Stimson Professor
and Chairman
Department of Surgery
Cornell University Medical College
Surgeon-in-Chief
The New York Hospital–Cornell Medical Center
New York, New York

Jovitas Skucas, MD
Professor of Radiology
Department of Radiology
University of Rochester
School of Dentistry
Rochester, New York

Sir Geoffrey Slaney, ChM, FRCS
Professor of Surgery
Department of Surgery
Queen Elizabeth Hospital
Birmingham, England

Lewis Spitz, PhD, FRCS
Professor of Surgery
Hospital for Sick Children
London, England

Fritz Starer, FRCP(Edin), FRCR
Consultant Radiologist
Westminster Hospital
London, England

Thomas E. Starzl, MD, PhD
Professor of Surgery
Department of Surgery
University of Pittsburgh
Attending Physician
Presbyterian University Hospital of Pittsburgh
Children's Hospital of Pittsburgh
Veterans Administration Hospital of
Pittsburgh (Oakland)
Pittsburgh, Pennsylvania

Felicien M. Steichen, MD
Director of Surgery
Lenox Hill Hospital
New York, New York

Professor of Surgery
New York Medical College
Valhalla, New York

Norman W. Thompson, MD
Henry King Ransom Professor of Surgery
Chief, Endocrine Division of Surgery
University of Michigan Medical School
Ann Arbor, Michigan

**Alexander J. Walt, MB, ChB, MS(Minn),
FRCS(Eng), FRCS(Canada), FACS**
Penberthy Professor and Chairman
Department of Surgery
Wayne State University
Chief of Surgery
Harper-Grace Hospitals
Detroit, Michigan

Kenneth W. Warren, MD
Attending Surgeon
New England Baptist Hospital
Former Chairman
Department of Surgery
The Lahey Clinic
Burlington, Massachusetts
Former Surgeon-in-Chief
New England Baptist Hospital
Lecturer Emeritus
Harvard Medical School
Boston, Massachusetts

Claude E. Welch, MD
Senior Surgeon
Massachusetts General Hospital
Clinical Professor of Surgery Emeritus
Harvard Medical School
Boston, Massachusetts

John P. Welch, MD
Associate Surgeon
Hartford Hospital

Hartford, Connecticut
Associate Professor of Surgery
University of Connecticut School of Medicine
Farmington, Connecticut
Adjunct Assistant Professor of Surgery
Dartmouth Medical School
Consultant Surgeon
Newington Veterans Administration Hospital
Newington, Connecticut

Christopher B. Williams, FRCP
Consultant Physician
St. Mark's Hospital
London, England

George A. Wilson, MD
Associate Professor of Nuclear Medicine
Department of Radiology
University of Rochester
School of Medicine and Dentistry
Rochester, New York

**John Wong, MB, BS, PhD, BSc(Med),
FRACS, FRCS(Edin), FACS**
Department of Surgery
University of Hong Kong
Queen Mary Hospital
Hong Kong

Robert M. Zollinger, MD
Emeritus Regents Professor and Chairman
Department of Surgery
The Ohio State University College of Medicine,
Formerly Assistant Professor of Surgery
Harvard Medical School
Surgeon, Peter Bent Brigham Hospital
Boston, Massachusetts

Robert M. Zollinger, Jr., MD
Associate Professor of Surgery
Case Western Reserve University
School of Medicine and University Hospitals
Cleveland, Ohio

Contents

Preface

To walk in the steps of a master is always a difficult task. To follow Rodney Maingot, one of the greatest surgical authors, in the editorship of a leading textbook of operative surgery surely falls into this category. We feel privileged, however, to have been asked to accept the challenge and we humbly offer this revision of a surgical classic.

In order to provide an appropriate "modernization," we have selected surgeons, internists, and radiologists in active practice who are acknowledged authorities and teachers in their specialties. Some are contributors to previous editions but many are new recruits to this work. The majority are drawn, once again, from the United States of America and from the United Kingdom, but also represented are France, Holland, Australia, South Africa, and Hong Kong. We are indebted to our contributors for their splendid efforts.

Although the title remains, the book is new both in its concept and in the factual material presented. Descriptions of the techniques of the major abdominal operations within the repertoire of the general surgeon persist as the nucleus. We have not, however, directed our efforts toward the production of an atlas; rather, we have attempted to synthesize a complete expression of the science and art of abdominal surgery. We have included concise accounts of modern diagnostic procedures, including radiology and endoscopy, relevant pathologic anatomy, preoperative assessment, indications for and choice of operation, postoperative care, and complications. The majority of the text and illustrative material has been carefully revised. Where possible, overlap and repetition have been minimized. To satisfy this desideratum, what had previously been considered as individual chapters have been fused into broader topics with a cohesion that parallels the surgeon's interests.

It is to sophisticated students of surgery, either in training or in practice where the learning process continues, that this edition is directed. As editors we can only hope that we have satisfied the desires and needs of our audience.

Harold Ellis
Seymour I. Schwartz

Acknowledgments

We would like to thank our co-authors for their enthusiasm, care, and dedication in providing new chapters or in revising their previous contributions.

Our Publisher, Appleton-Century-Crofts, has worked with concern and efficiency in producing the extensive changes necessary for this new edition. We would particularly like to thank David Stires, Executive Vice-President and Publisher, and Joanne Jay, Director, Production Services.

Finally, we must express our very deepest appreciation to Gill Baker in London for her skilled, dedicated, and cheerful help.

Harold Ellis
Seymour I. Schwartz

MAINGOT'S
ABDOMINAL OPERATIONS

VOLUME TWO

EIGHTH EDITION

SECTION VII
Small Intestine

40. Neonatal Intestinal Obstruction and Intussusception in Childhood

Lewis Spitz

Intestinal obstruction, from a wide variety of causes (Table 40–1), comprises the major proportion of all infants admitted within the first 28 days of life to a neonatal surgical unit. There can be no doubt that the management of these lesions, the incidence of which individually is rare, is best undertaken by paediatric surgeons in specifically designated neonatal surgical centres. It is only in such centres that the expertise from the various supportive services such as anaesthesia, radiology, pathology, paediatrics, and nursing is readily available. The combined efforts of all these disciplines is reflected in the greatly improved survival rates achieved in these centres over the individual surgeon operating in relative isolation on the occasional newborn infant. The surgical neonate can be safely transported over long distances provided the infant is well prepared and cared for during the transfer.

GENERAL PRINCIPLES

The cardinal feature of intestinal obstruction in the newborn infant is the presence of bile-stained vomiting. A truly bile-stained vomit is green in colour. It occurs in all obstructive lesions situated below the ampulla of Vater. Many infants produce the occasional yellow vomit, resulting from the concentration of carotene pigments from the colostrum. This is of little significance unless it is persistent, at which point an obstructive lesion proximal to the ampulla of Vater should be suspected. All infants with bilious or persistent vomiting should be promptly transferred to the neonatal surgical centre where appropriate investigations will be undertaken to elucidate the cause and where treatment can be instituted without undue delay. Procrastination increases the risk of complications, such as gangrene, perforation and septicaemia, and adversely affects the ultimate prognosis.

The extent of abdominal distension is related to the level of the obstruction. In duodenal and high jejunal obstruction the distension is restricted to the upper abdomen, whereas in low ileal and colonic obstruction there may be massive distension, severe enough to cause elevation and splinting of the diaphragm with resultant respiratory embarrassment (Fig. 40–1). Distension evident at birth is usually due to either meconium ileus or meconium peritonitis. Oedema of the abdominal wall or periumbilical erythema is an ominous physical sign, indicating the presence of a gangrenous obstruction or of peritonitis (Fig. 40–2).

Ninety eight percent of normal infants will pass meconium in the first 24 hours of life. Depending upon the stage of gestation when the intestinal lesion develops, the infant may pass either normal-appearing meconium, which was already present in the colon at the time when the obstruction developed or, more commonly, small quantities of greyish mucus may be evacuated per rectum. Delayed passage of meconium should always raise the suspicion of Hirschsprung's disease especially when it occurs in the otherwise healthy full-term infant.

Waves of peristaltic activity may be visible through the thin abdominal wall of the newborn infant. Despite obvious hyperperistalsis, the in-

TABLE 40–1. CLASSIFICATION OF NEONATAL INTESTINAL OBSTRUCTION

I. Mechanical
  A. Intraluminal
    1. Meconium ileus
    2. Inspissated milk syndrome
  B. Conditions affecting the bowel wall
    1. Atresia/stenosis
    2. Hirschsprung's disease
    3. Anorectal agenesis
  C. Lesions compressing the bowel
    1. Malrotation and/or volvulus
    2. Duplications
    3. Irreducible inguinal hernia
    4. Other lesions
II. Paralytic ileus
  A. Necrotising enterocolitis
  B. Septicaemia

fant with an uncomplicated obstruction does not appear to be in any pain. With the development of complications, it is possible to detect abdominal tenderness and eventually the infant will become septicaemic. Hypothermia, jaundice, acidosis and thrombocytopenia are the hallmarks of septicaemia in infancy.

As far as investigation of the obstructed infant is concerned, frequently the only diagnostic examination required is an erect and supine ab-

dominal x-ray. This will show dilated loops of intestine containing air–fluid levels (Fig. 40–3). In duodenal atresias the classic double-bubble appearance is seen while the rest of the abdomen is radiopaque. The further distal the obstruction, the more fluid levels develop. In infancy it is not possible with any degree of certainty to distinguish small from large intestine and a contrast enema may be the only reliable means of establishing the site of the obstruction. The presence of calcification is evidence of an intrauterine perforation. (Intraperitoneal meconium becomes calcified in a very short space of time.) The admixture of air and meconium gives a mottled "ground-glass" appearance, which is commonly found in meconium ileus but may be seen in any low intestinal obstruction. Intramural gas (pneumotosis intestinalis) is diagnostic of necrotising enterocolitis. Pneumoperitoneum, due to intestinal perforation, is best seen in the subdiaphragmatic area on the erect abdominal x-ray. In selected cases where the infant is critically ill and especially in infants requiring mechanical ventilation, free peritoneal air may be seen on the lateral decubitus x-ray.

It is particularly in incomplete or intermittent obstructions such as malrotation, meconium ileus, and Hirschsprung's disease, that

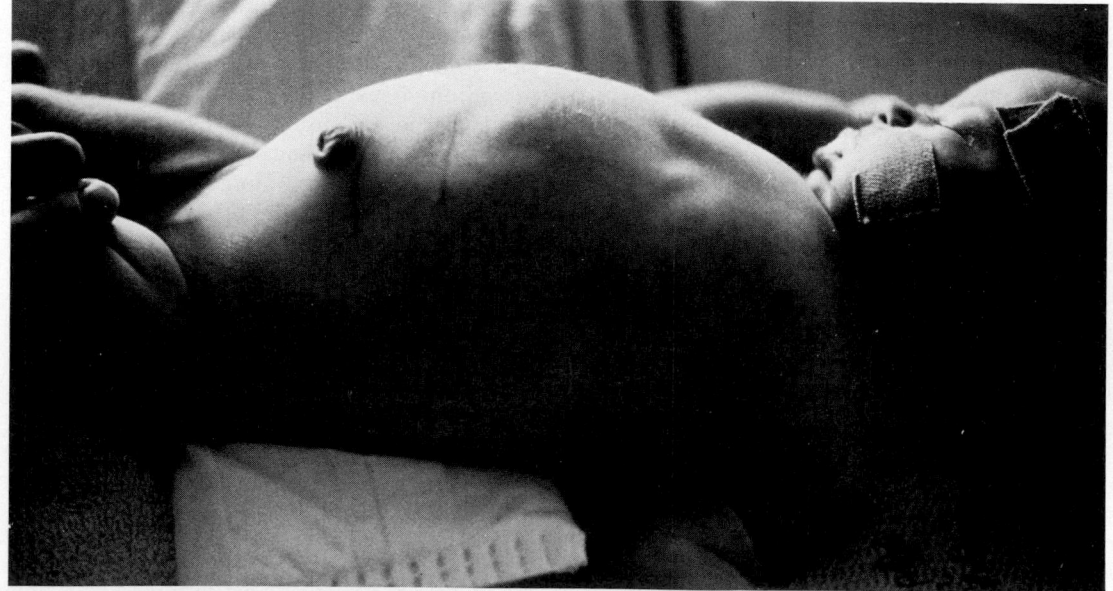

Figure 40–1. Abdominal distension in an infant with a distal intestinal obstruction. Note the "ladder pattern" of distended loops of bowel in the upper abdomen.

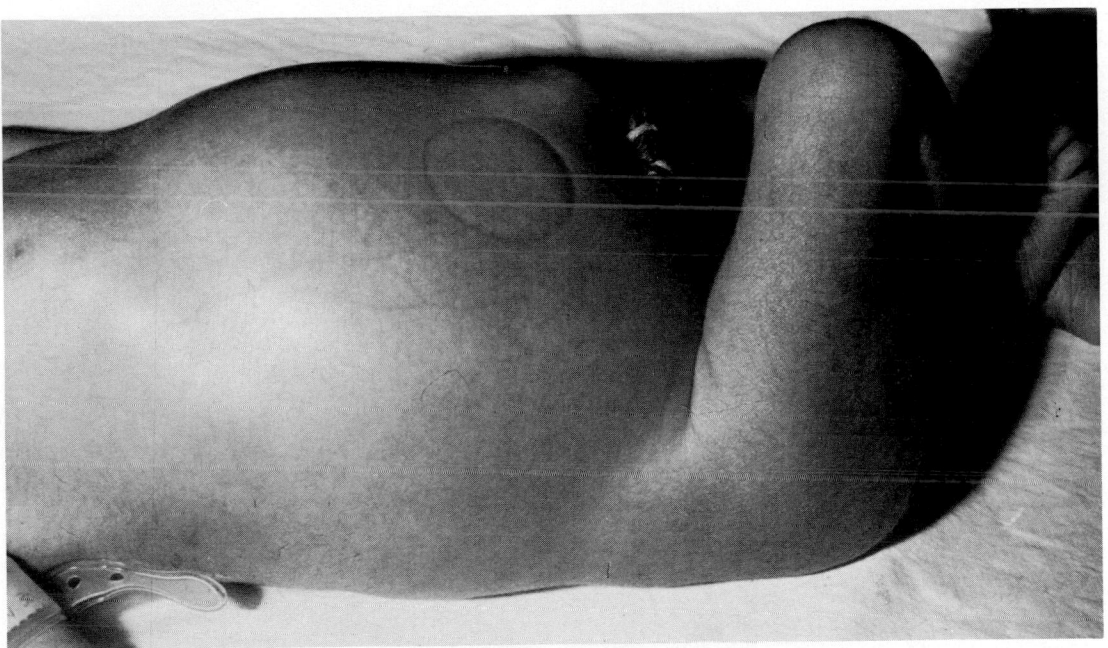

Figure 40–2. Oedema of the anterior abdominal wall in a newborn infant with an intestinal perforation. The ring to the right of the umbilicus is the impression left by the bell of the stethoscope. Note also the shiny appearance of the skin. Abdominal distension is also prominant.

further radiologic investigations are required. The barium meal examination has been found to be more valuable than the barium enema in the diagnosis of malrotation, while contrast enemas are used in the diagnosis of the latter two conditions.

Transport. The most vital requirements for safe transportation are protection against hypothermia and aspiration pneumonia. A simple transport incubator is sufficient to prevent hypothermia in most cases, but additional precautions to maintain body temperature may be required, especially in temperate climates. Wrapping the head and limbs of the infant in silver foil is an effective method of reducing heat loss. All infants with suspected intestinal obstruction require nasogastric decompression. A large-calibre nasogastric tube (size 8 to 10 gauge for full-term infants and size 6 gauge for premature infants), kept patent on free drainage and aspirated at frequent intervals, will prevent vomiting and possible inhalation of vomitus during transfer. Mechanical ventilation may be required for the infant with concomitant respiratory distress syndrome. This particularly applies in the very premature infant with necrotising enterocolitis.

Preoperative Assessment and Management. Urgent resuscitation is required for the severely dehydrated, shocked, and septicaemic infant. Intravenous plasma (20 ml/kg) may be infused as rapidly as possible and broad-spectrum antibiotic cover (penicillin, gentamicin and metronidazole) commenced. Resuscitation should be initiated at the referral hospital but should not be allowed to delay transfer, as all the resuscitative measures can be continued during transportation. Prolonged resuscitation may be detrimental, as there is a relatively short period of stabilisation, which develops within a few hours of commencement of therapy, during which surgery should be performed. Gross electrolyte imbalance and disturbance of acid–base equilibrium should be corrected as far as possible prior to surgery. Close monitoring of plasma glucose and calcium levels is important. Hypoglycaemia may cause cerebral damage, whereas hypocalcaemia is a potent cause of convulsions at this age.

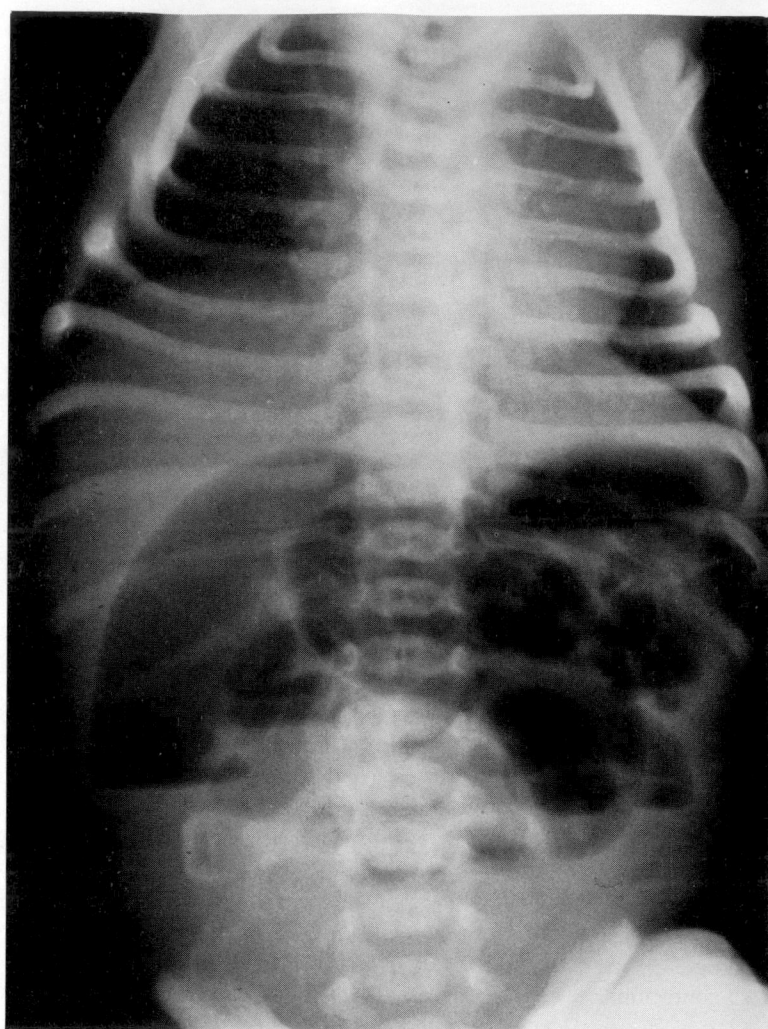

Figure 40–3. Abdominal radiograph in an infant with intestinal obstruction. There are numerous air–fluid levels and distended intestinal loops of varying calibre. It is impossible at this age to distinguish small from large intestine on the plain abdominal radiograph.

Anaesthesia. General endotracheal anaesthesia is generally recommended. It relieves the infant of the effort of respiration while supplying full requirements for oxygenation. Blood for transfusion should be available at the time of surgery. The amount of infant serum required for compatibility studies can be minimised by having available a 10-ml sample of maternal blood, which should accompany the infant at the time of transfer. Close monitoring of the infant's temperature, blood pressure, and pulse rate and accurate replacement of operative blood loss will ensure safe anaesthesia. The newborn infant's blood volume measures 85 ml/kg body weight so that any loss exceeding 8 to 10 ml/kg should be immediately replaced. Maintenance intravenous fluids during abdominal surgery requires the administration of 0.18 percent saline in 4 percent dextrose at a rate of 6 ml/kg per hour.

Postoperative Care. Monitoring of the infant's temperature and vital functions should continue as required in the postoperative period. Temperature is maintained in an incubator or under a radiant heat cradle. By keeping the infant in a thermoneutral environment with high humidity, metabolic requirements are kept to a minimum. Blood sugar levels are monitored every 6 hours by the dextrostix method for the first 48 hours postoperatively. Additional glucose over and above that supplied by maintenance intravenous fluids may be provided by boluses of 1 ml/kg body weight of 50 percent dextrose solution. Serial determinations of serum bilirubin are essential, especially in the ill premature infant. Phototherapy, which utilises fluorescent light to break down unconjugated bilirubin to a more water-soluble form, which can then be excreted in the bile and in the urine, has virtually replaced exchange transfusion for indirect hyperbilirubinaemia. The latter method may still be required for rapidly rising bilirubin levels.

Maintenance fluid requirements are given in the form of a 10 percent glucose in 0.18 percent saline; potassium chloride (20 mmol/L) is added once urine flow is established. All fluid losses, e.g., nasogastric aspirate, ileostomy losses etc., are replaced with normal saline with potassium chloride (20 mmol/L). The fluid requirements for the neonate may be calculated according to the following scheme:

Birth Weight (g)	Maintenance Fluid
<1500	180 ml/kg per 24 hours
1500–2500	150 ml/kg per 24 hours
>2500	120 ml/kg per 24 hours

Fluid requirements in the first 24 hours after surgery are minimal, and as the renal function is restricted in the first 4 weeks of life, it is customary to limit the volume of maintenance fluid during the first week as follows:

- First 48 hours postoperatively: 1/3 of maintenance fluid
- 48–96 hours postoperatively: 2/3 of maintenance fluid
- > 96 hours postoperatively: full requirements

The above are merely guidelines and each individual infant must be carefully assessed and fluid requirements modified according to its needs, which may vary in each 6-hourly period.

After extensive bowel resections or the establishment of a high enterostomy or in conditions where return of bowel function is expected to be unduly delayed, for example, duodenal atresia, exomphalos, necrotising enterocolitis, prolonged administration of intravenous fluids may be necessary. In these circumstances, all the nutrient requirements, fluid, electrolytes, calories, trace elements, and vitamins are supplied by parenteral nutrition. It is possible, by regular resiting of the infusion site, to be able to administer total parenteral nutrition to infants over a period of many weeks by peripheral route without having to resort to a central venous catheter. The advantages of the peripheral route is a much lower incidence of major sepsis and thrombosis, but it does expose the infant to the trauma of repeat venipuncture and, more importantly, to the risk of tissue necrosis should extravasation of the hyperosmotic fluid occur.

In infancy and childhood, the regimen for full parenteral nutrition is introduced gradually over 6 days in order to minimise hypoglycaemia, glucosuria and hypophosphataemia.

The full regimen consists of:

- Intralipid 20 percent: 1 ml/kg/hr for 20 hours (plus vitlipid infant 1 ml/kg to maximum of 4 ml)
- Vamin glucose (plus Ped. El 5 ml/kg): 6 ml/kg/hr for 8 hours
- Dextrose 10 percent (plus potassium phosphate (K_2HPO^4 17.42 percent): 5 ml/kg/hr for 16 hours plus solivito 1 ml/kg (maximum 4 ml) per 500 ml

This regimen delivers a total 103 Kcal in a volume of 154 ml/kg per 24 hours. Higher concentrations of glucose may be administered when a central venous catheter is available. In these circumstances it is possible to achieve a caloric intake of 100 to 120 cal/kg per 24 hours without increasing the total fluid volume. Infants receiving parenteral nutrition require careful regular biochemical monitoring to avoid gross imbalances of electrolytes and blood sugars. Serial liver function tests to permit early detection of cholestasis are also important.

Oral feeding is commenced as soon as normal gastrointestinal (GI) peristaltic function has returned. Breast milk is ideal but formula preparations are entirely satisfactory. It is customary to commence with half-strength milk in small quantities at frequent intervals and gradually to increase the volume of each feed while lengthening the period between feeds. The development of unexpected diarrhoea following milk feeds may be due to a temporary lactose intolerance, which commonly occurs after GI surgery in the neonatal period. The diagnosis is established by detecting reducing sugars in both the urine and stools. The diarrhoea resolves promptly on changing to a lactose-free milk formula. In other situations, particularly following major intestinal resections or high enterostomies, considerable difficulty may be experienced in establishing the infants on oral nutrition. The feeds commonly recommended in these situations are lactose-free, medium-chain triglyceride formulae or comminuted chicken mixtures.

MECONIUM ILEUS

Cystic fibrosis is a genetic disorder of exocrine functions, characterised by obstructive lesions throughout multiple-organ systems and disturbances of mucus and electrolyte secretions. It is more common in Caucasians and is inherited in an autosomal recessive fashion. Chronic obstructive pulmonary disease eventually affects all patients and is responsible for the majority of the morbidity and almost all of the mortality beyond the neonatal period. GI symptoms occur in 85 to 90 percent of patients with cystic fibrosis, the most common problem being malabsorption due to exocrine pancreatic deficiency.

Meconium ileus occurs in 10 to 15 percent of infants with cystic fibrosis. In this condition the meconium is extremely viscid, sticky, and tenacious. There is a significant decrease in water and electrolyte content while the concentration of calcium is increased.

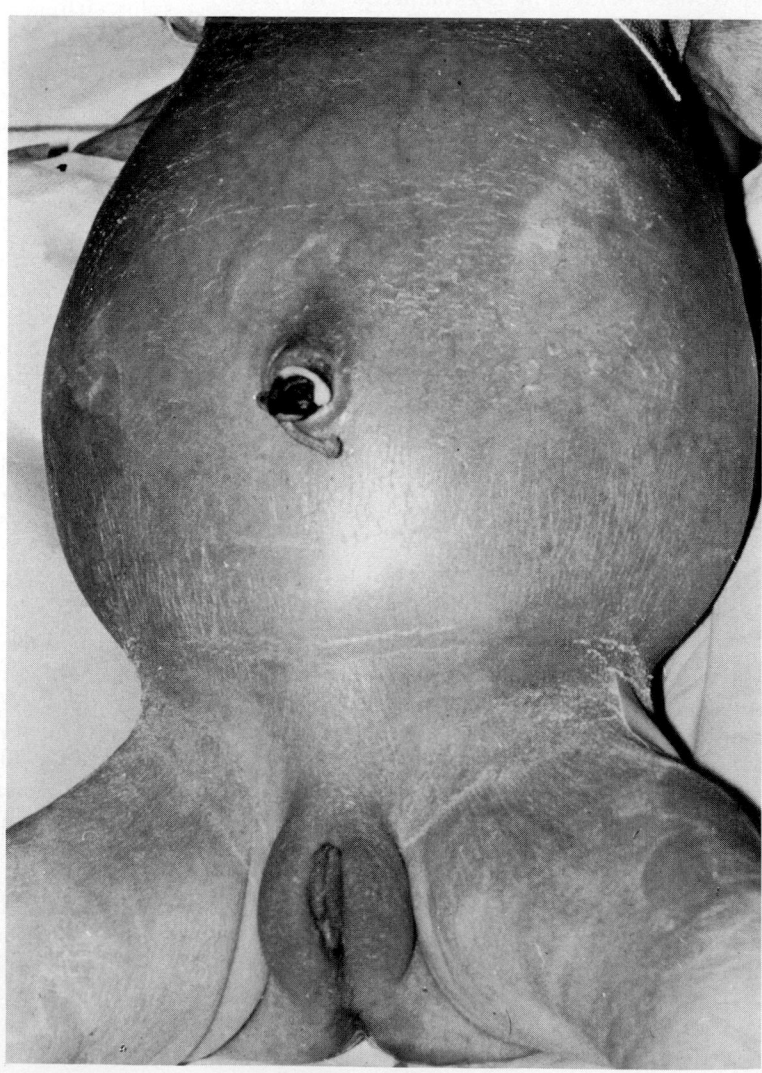

Figure 40–4. Abdominal distension present at birth in a female infant with meconium ileus.

Pathology

In uncomplicated meconium ileus the proximal ileum is enormously distended with thick, sticky, tenacious dark-green to black meconium. The wall of this part of the intestine is greatly hypertrophied. The dilatation decreases further proximally in the upper ileum and jejunum, where the contents are semifluid due to the action of intestinal bacteria introduced postnatally. The distal ileum and colon are contracted and narrow and usually contain small greyish pellets of inspissated meconium. The immediate cause of the obstruction is the viscid tenacious meconium which cannot be propelled through the alimentary canal even by the greatly hypertrophied small intestine.

As many as half the cases of meconium ileus are complicated by gangrene and perforation, volvulus, atresia, or meconium peritonitis. Volvulus, gangrene, or perforation may occur as perinatal or postnatal complications; atresias and meconium peritonitis are due to similar events occurring during intrauterine life. Extravasation of meconium into the fetal peritoneal cavity causes an intense inflammatory reaction. Calcification of the meconium can occur very rapidly. The meconium peritonitis may either resolve completely, leaving only intraabdominal calcification as evidence of its occurrence, or it may result in dense, adhesive meconium peritonitis or meconium pseudocyst with intestinal obstruction. The meconium peritonitis will remain sterile, provided the perforation has completely sealed prior to birth.

Clinical Manifestations

Meconium ileus classically presents with signs of intestinal obstruction within 48 hours of birth. Abdominal distension (Fig. 40–4) is often noted to be already present at birth. In uncomplicated cases the infant is otherwise well,

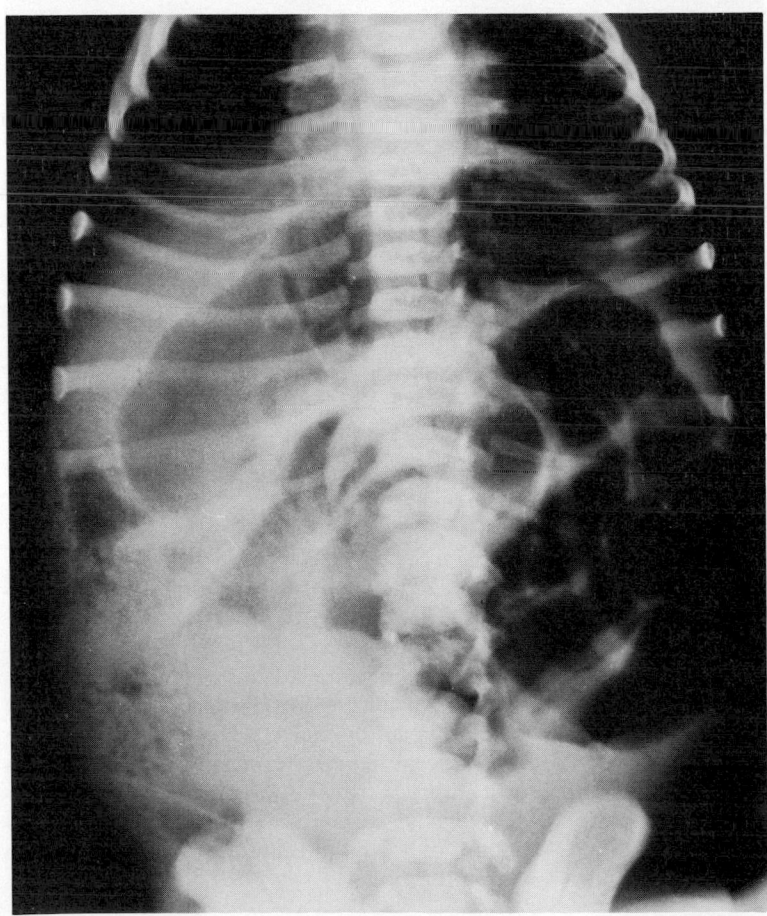

Figure 40–5. Plain abdominal radiograph showing dilated loops of intestine of varying calibre. There are no obvious air–fluid levels. Note the "ground-glass" appearance of air admixed with meconium in the right lower quadrant.

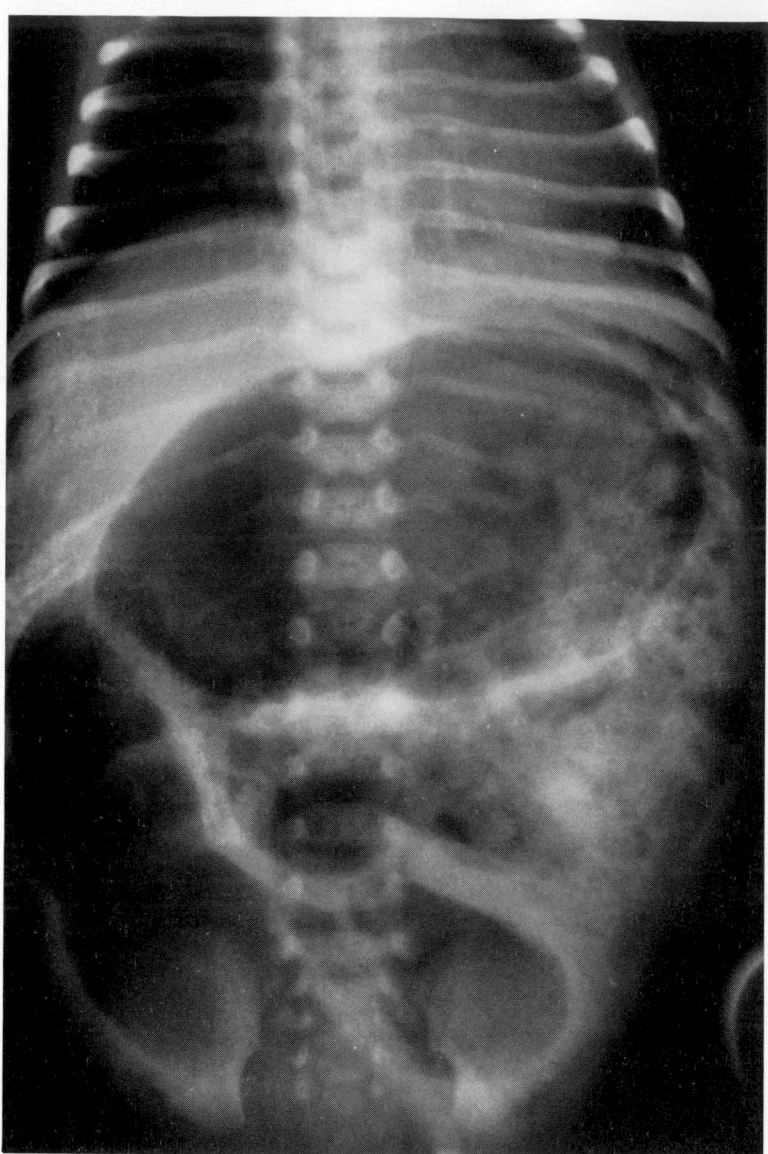

Figure 40–6. Abdominal radiograph in an infant with meconium peritonitis. The walls of the dilated loops of intestine are separated by intraperitoneal fluid. Note the calcification in the right upper quadrant due to escape of meconium from the lumen of the intestine.

whereas in the complicated case, presentation occurs earlier and the infant is severely distressed. Polyhydramnios occurs in up to 20 percent of cases. A positive family history is helpful in establishing a diagnosis.

Abdominal examination reveals the presence of dilated, thickened, firm loops of intestine. Active peristaltic waves are often visible. The presence of oedema of the anterior abdominal wall or periumbilical erythema signifies the development of a complication such as volvulus

and gangrene or perforation and secondary bacterial peritonitis.

The majority of infants fail to pass any meconium per rectum. A few infants will evacuate small plugs of mucus and the occasional patient will pass a single, normal-appearing meconium stool. Rectal examination may either reveal a tight empty rectum or a rectum containing greyish plugs of meconium. Very rarely, a small amount of normal meconium will appear on the examining finger.

Diagnostic Studies

Radiologic Examination

The plain abdominal x-ray typically reveals dilated loops of intestine of varying calibre with an absence or scarcity of air–fluid levels. Small bubbles of air may be seen within the sticky meconium mass, giving the appearance of "ground glass" (Fig. 40–5). This sign is not pathognomonic of meconium ileus and may occur in any condition where large quantities of meconium are present, such as distal ileal atresia or total colonic aganglionosis. The presence of calcification in the peritoneal cavity is indicative of meconium peritonitis (Fig. 40–6). A contrast enema will demonstrate a microcolon containing pellets of inspissated mucus plugs (Fig. 40–7).

Laboratory Investigations

The diagnosis of cystic fibrosis is established by the finding of high concentrations of sodium and chloride in the sweat. This is generally attributed to a failure of ductal reabsorption. The basis of the test is the iontophoresis of the choli-nergic drug, pilocarpine, into the skin. The drug stimulates the sweat glands to secrete sweat, which is collected and the concentrations of sodium and chloride are determined. To obtain reliable measurements at least 100 μg of sweat is necessary. This is usually difficult to obtain in the infant less than 3 to 4 weeks of age. Concentrations of sodium and chloride greater than 60 mmol/L are diagnostic. Other laboratory tests that have been used include the measurement of albumin levels in the meconium by the BM teststrip test (albumin is elevated due to the absence of proteolytic enzymes in the meconium), measurement of sodium concentration in nail clippings, and estimate of immune reactive tryptic activity (IRT) in the serum.

Treatment

Before embarking on a plan of treatment it is mandatory to distinguish the complicated form of meconium ileus from the simple form of the condition. Operative intervention is required for the complicated form whereas relief of the obstruction may be achieved by nonoperative measures in the uncomplicated variety.

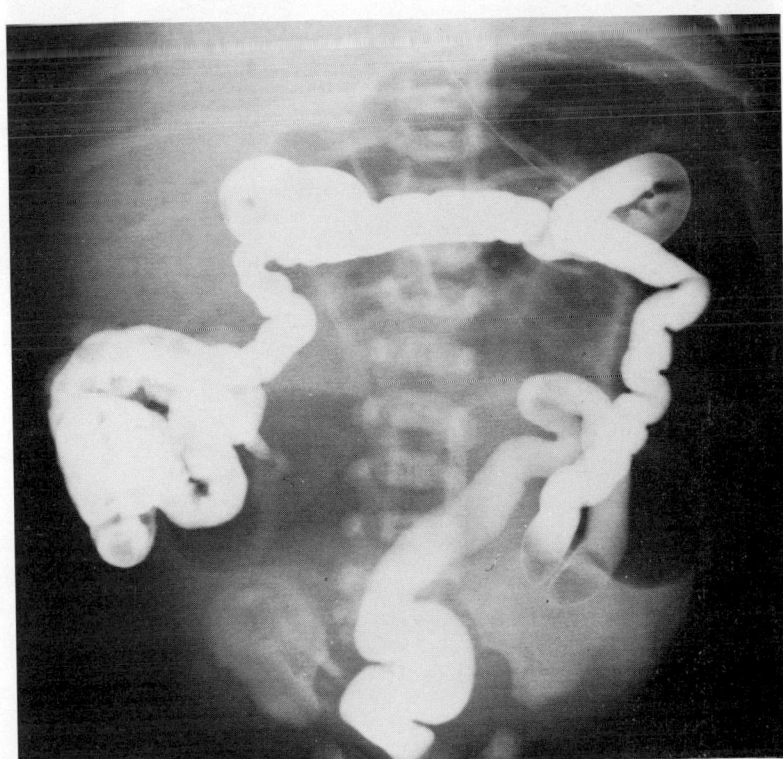

Figure 40–7. Gastrografin enema in uncomplicated meconium ileus showing the small calibre "unused" colon containing filling defects of inspissated mucus plugs.

Nonoperative Management

This method of treatment should only be considered in uncomplicated meconium ileus. Clinically or radiologically, signs of volvulus, gangrene, perforation, peritonitis, or atresia of the small intestine are absolute contraindications for this form of treatment. The infant should be adequately prepared for the procedure by prior correction of any fluid and electrolyte imbalances and by ensuring that the infant's temperature remains normothermic throughout the procedure. The procedure should be performed under full fluoroscopic control and conducted by an experienced radiologist. Close supervision by the surgical team should be maintained.

Noblett (1961) recommends an initial diagnostic barium enema to exclude any possible distal bowel obstruction. This is followed by the gentle instillation of warm, full-strength diatrizoate meglamine (Gastrografin) via a small Foley catheter inserted into the distal rectum. The balloon of the Foley catheter is slowly distended and the buttocks of the infant are strapped together to prevent leakage of the contrast material. Gastrografin has two unique properties: (1) it is hyperosmolar (osmolality 1900 mOsm/L) and (2) it contains an emulsifying agent (Tween 80). The former property causes fluid to be drawn into the lumen of the intestine while the latter property reduces the surface tension of the meconium, thereby facilitating its expulsion. The Gastrografin is instilled into the large intestine and its progress proximally is carefully monitored by fluoroscopy. The colon is generally narrow and collapsed and the procedure

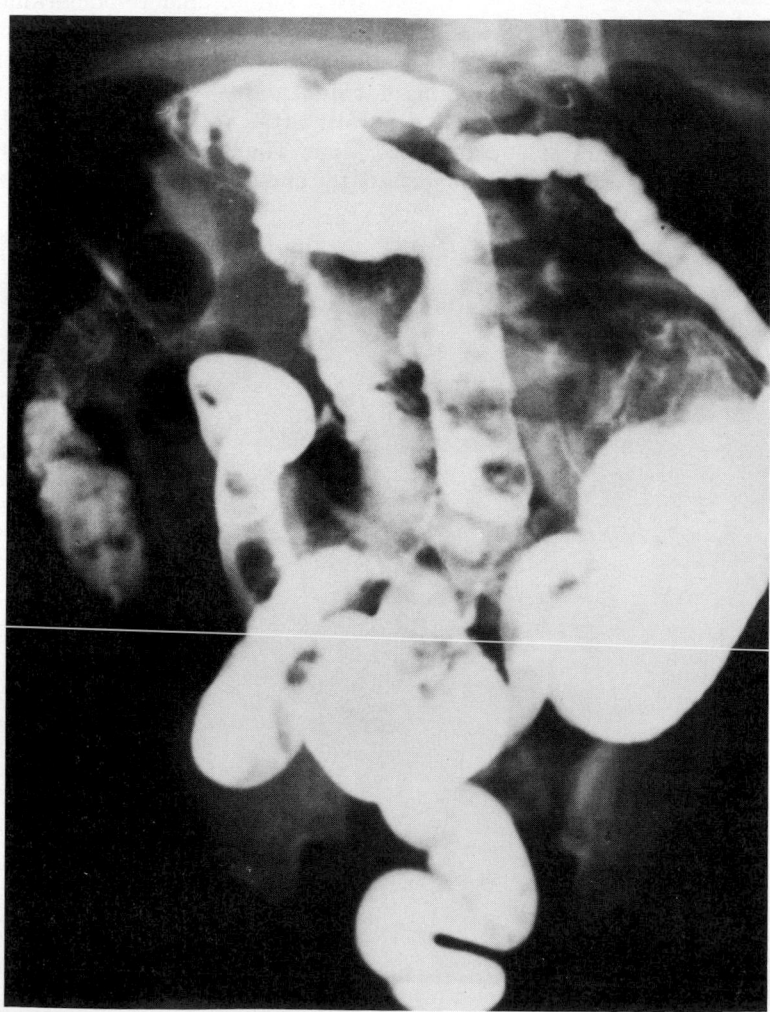

Figure 40–8. Successful therapeutic Gastrografin enema showing the contrast medium entering numerous dilated loops of small intestine.

can only be judged to have succeeded if the Gastrografin can be demonstrated to have entered the proximally dilated meconium-filled ileum. Once this has been achieved the catheter is deflated and withdrawn without attempting to drain off the Gastrografin (Fig. 40–8).

The infant is returned to the ward while intravenous fluid therapy is maintained. The evacuation of semifluid meconium usually commences soon after completion of the therapeutic enema and continues for 24 to 48 hours. A second enema may be required for retained meconium, but failure to evacuate a substantial amount of meconium after the first investigation should be regarded as a failure of this method of management and should not be an indication for a second enema. In such cases, surgery is necessary to relieve the obstruction.

Operative Management

Surgical intervention is indicated for patients with complicated meconium ileus and for those patients who fail to respond to nonoperative treatment. The aim of surgical treatment is to relieve the intestinal obstruction (Fig. 40–9) by evacuating the meconium mass from the distal

ileum (Figs. 40–10 and 40–11). The dilated bowel may be resected (Fig. 40–12A) and an end-to-end anastomosis performed (Fig. 40–12B). The method that has achieved most popularity is an end-to-side enterostomy. In the procedure, devised by Bishop and Koop (Fig. 40–12C), the maximally dilated proximally placed ileum is resected and an anastomosis is fashioned between the end of the proximal ileum and the side of the distal collapsed ileum in such a manner that the end of the distal intestine is brought out onto the anterior abdominal wall as an ostomy that functions as a safety valve. Liquid bowel content and intestinal gas are able to escape through this enterostomy until the distal bowel becomes disimpacted, at which point the preferred route through the intestine can be taken.

An alternative approach, the Santulli enterostomy, is to anastomose the end of the distal intestine to the side of the proximal bowel, fashioning an enterostomy out of the end of the dilated proximal ileum (Fig. 40–12D). A catheter, secured in position in the distal bowel at surgery in the case of the Santulli enterostomy or introduced intermittently into the enterostomy in

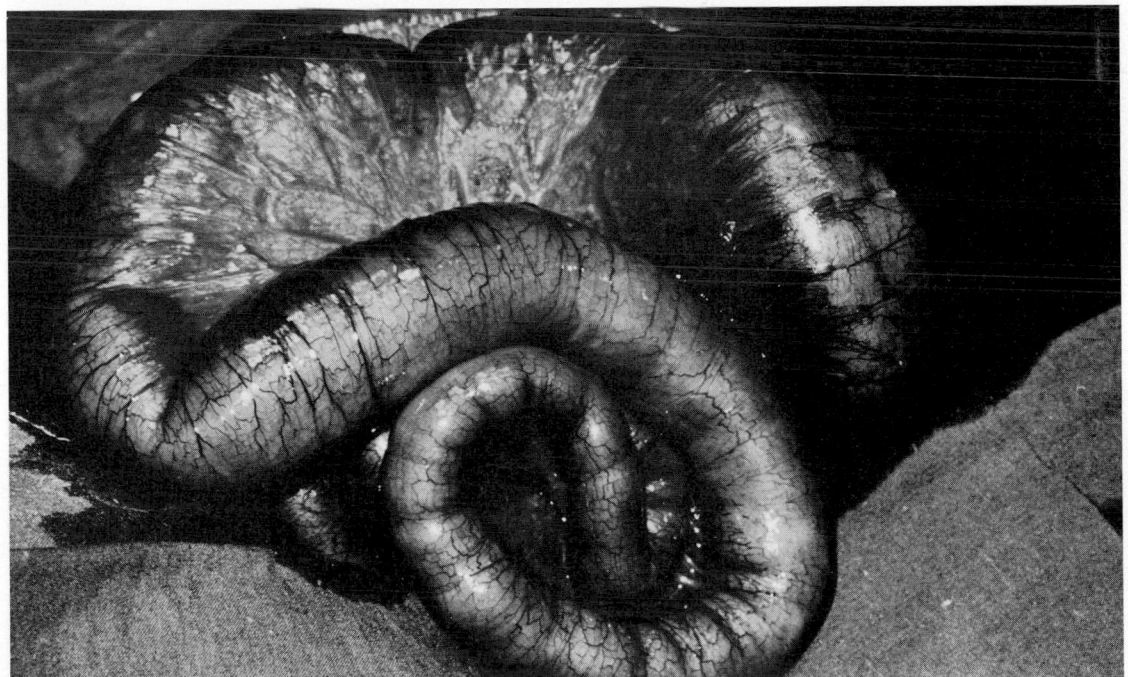

Figure 40–9. Operative appearance of the dilated meconium-filled loops of ileum in meconium ileus.

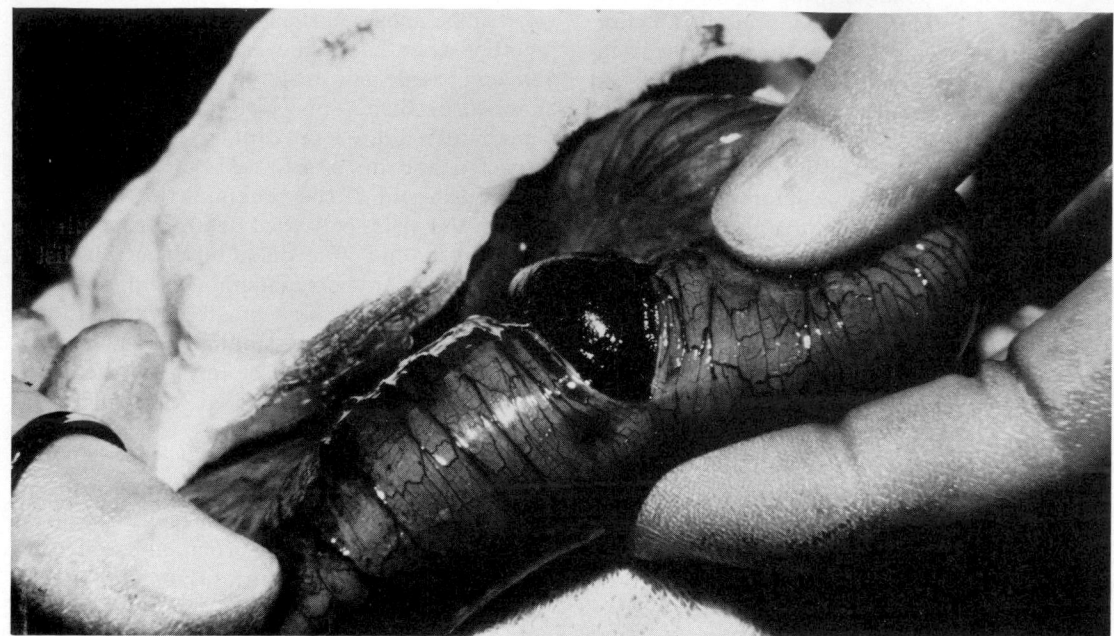

Figure 40–10. The ileum has been opened to reveal the thick, sticky meconium mass adherent to the mucosal surface of the intestine.

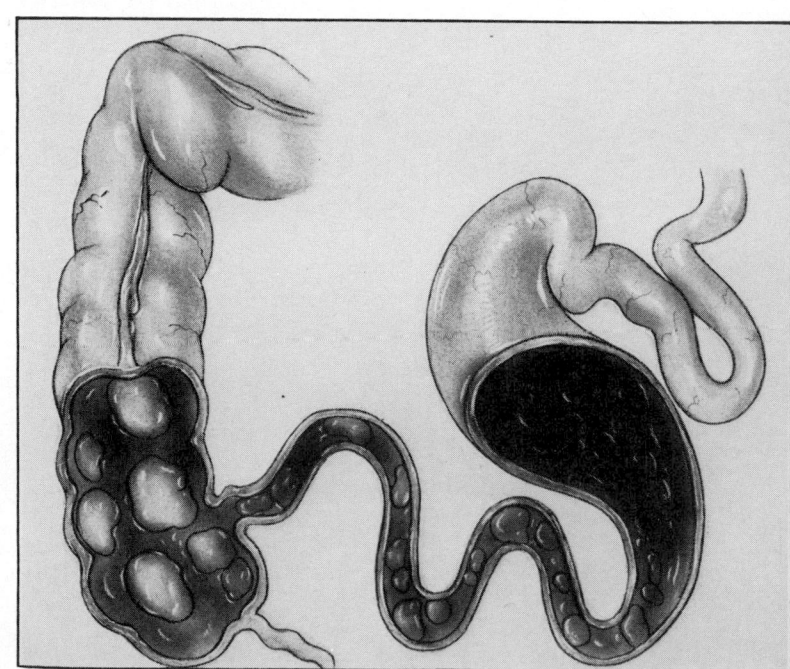

Figure 40–11. Diagrammatic appearance of the bowel in meconium ileus. The mid-ileum is distended with thick tenacious meconium while whitish-grey mucus plugs are present in the terminal ileum and colon.

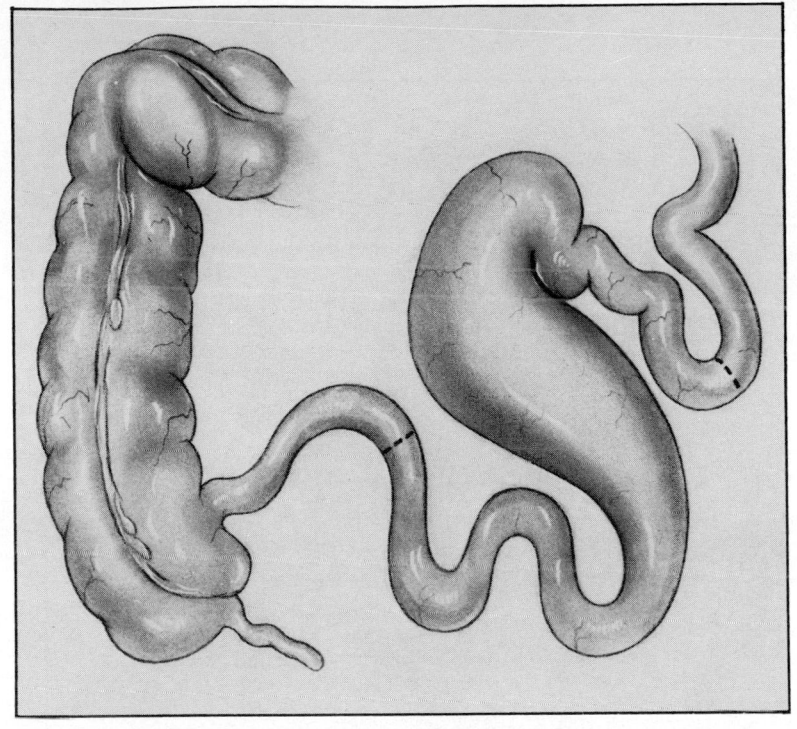

Figure 40–12. The operative correction of meconium ileus. **A.** Extent of resection including the grossly dilated ileum.

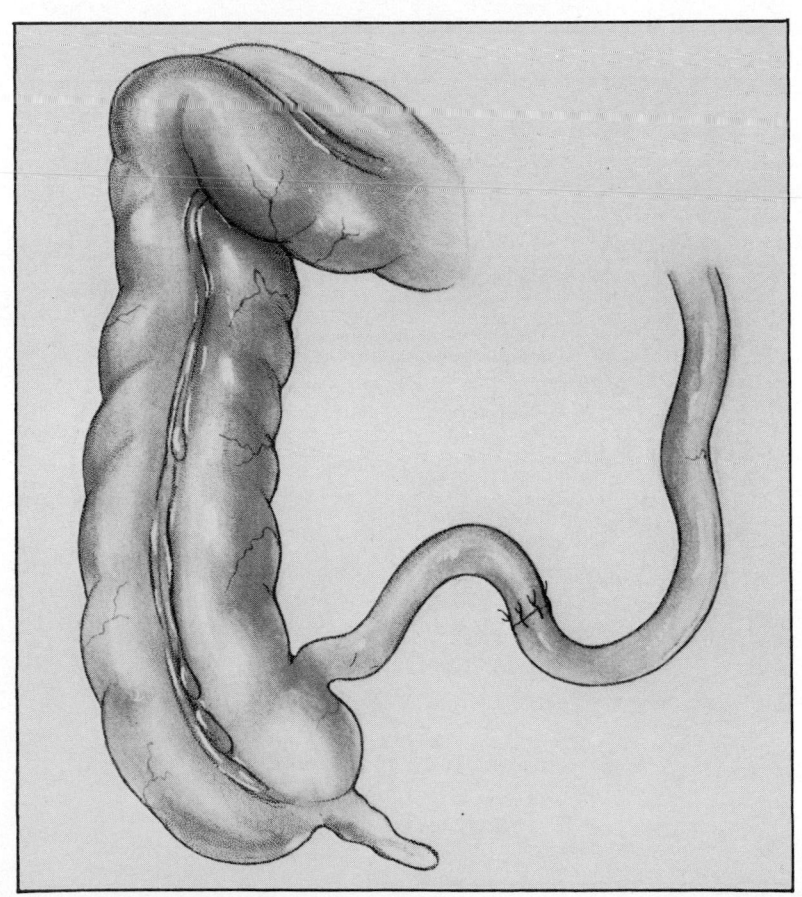

Figure 40–12. B. End-to-end reconstitution of intestinal continuity.

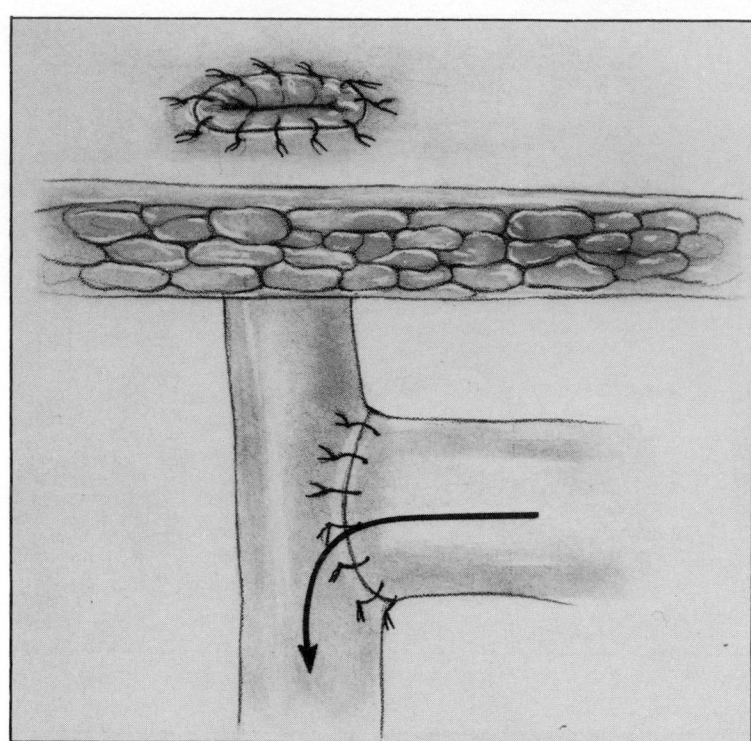

Figure 40–12. C. Bishop–Koop anastomosis. The proximal bowel is anastomosed end-to-side to the distal bowel, the proximal end of which forms the ileostomy.

C

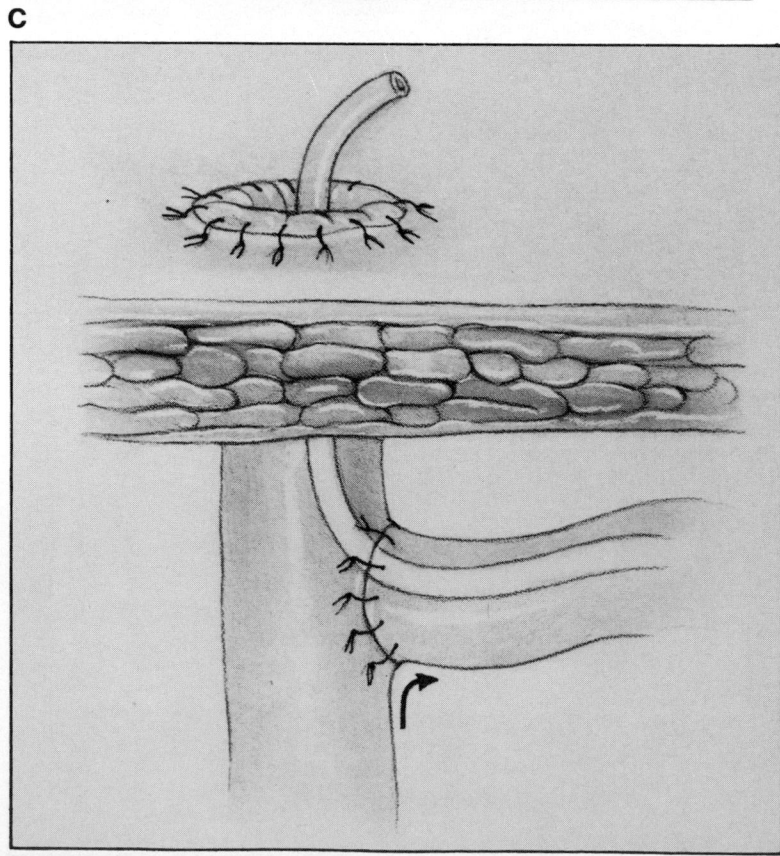

Figure 40–12. D. Santulli ileostomy. The end of the proximal bowel forms the enterostomy while the proximal end of the distal bowel is anastomosed to the side of the proximal bowel. A tube is placed through the ileostomy into the distal bowel for irrigation purposes.

D

the Bishop–Koop procedure, is used to instill saline or Gastrografin to clear out the content from the distal ileum and colon. A simple double-barrel enterostomy with minimal resection has also been advocated.

In all the enterostomy procedures, a second operative procedure is required once satisfactory function of the distal intestine has been achieved. In order to circumvent the necessity for a two-stage procedure, we have preferred a primary end-to-end anastomosis after resection of any bowel with questionable viability and only after total clearance of all content from the proximal and distal bowel. This is achieved by gentle irrigation with a warm saline solution with or without Gastrografin or Tween 80 of the intestine at laparotomy via a catheter introduced into the open bowel. Excessive trauma to the bowel should be avoided and the washout fluid should be shown to have passed through the rectum before the anastomosis is performed. The anastomosis is performed with a single layer of interrupted seromuscular sutures.

Postoperative Care. The infant is nursed in an incubator with high humidity. Prophylactic broad-spectrum antibiotics and regular chest physiotherapy will help to prevent pulmonary infections from which patients with cystic fibrosis are prone to suffer. The definitive diagnosis is dependent upon the results of a sweat test performed at around the age of 4 weeks.

Oral feeds are commenced as soon as the ileus has resolved.

Pancreatic exocrine replacement therapy (pancreatin) is commenced as soon as regular formula feeds are tolerated. The dosage of replacement therapy is adjusted according to the individual patient's response.

Prognosis

It is rare for the infant with uncomplicated meconium ileus to succumb to the effects of the intestinal problem. This statement applies equally to those infants treated nonoperatively and operatively. The mortality rate for the complicated variety of meconium ileus is entirely dependent upon the extent of the pathology and the delay in effecting appropriate treatment. There does not appear to be any evidence to suggest that the infant presenting with meconium ileus is any more severely affected than

the infant presenting with pure pulmonary manifestation of cystic fibrosis.

Chronic obstructive pulmonary disease eventually occurs in all cases and is responsible for the majority of the morbidity and for almost all of the mortality. GI manifestations include rectal prolapse (20 percent), intussusception (less than 5 percent), gallstones, and pancreatitis (Park and Grand, 1981; Schwachman, 1975).

Meconium Ileus Equivalent

This term, coined by Jensen in 1962, refers to an intraluminal obstruction due to the presence of ingested food particles in the distal intestine. It is almost always associated with the cessation of pancreatic enzyme replacement or appears to coincide with a respiratory tract infection. The occurrence of abdominal colic, in association with palpable rubbery firm masses on abdominal examination, and the radiologic picture of dilated loops of intestine filled with bubbly faecal content, is diagnostic. The obstruction generally responds to conservative measures, including distal bowel washouts with Gastrografin. The incidence of this complication ranges from 10 to 20 percent.

Inspissated Milk Syndrome

This is a rare condition, occurring exclusively in formula-fed infants. The infant presents with the clinical features of intestinal obstruction between the 5th and 14th day of life. The obstruction is caused by the impaction of inspissated milk curds in the distal ileum. The precise cause for the inspissation is uncertain but a minor deficit of amino acid absorption has been identified in some of the patients. The condition, if diagnosed early enough, responds to nonoperative measures, such as Gastrografin enemas, but surgery may be required for impending perforation. It is essential to perform a rectal biopsy to exclude Hirschsprung's disease as a possible cause for the obstruction.

ATRESIA AND STENOSIS

Historical Review

The first report of an intestinal atresia is credited to Benninger in 1673. The part of the intestine affected was the colon. Goeller documented the first ileal atresia in 1684, duodenal atresia was first recorded by Calder in 1733, and annular pancreas by Von Ecker in 1862. In 1812, Meckel reviewed the subject and discussed the aetiology and pathology of the condition. In 1889, Bland-Sutton proposed a classification of the various types of intestinal atresia. This classification, aside from the incorporation of multiple atresias and the "Christmas tree" ("apple-peel") deformity, remains applicable to the present time. In 1900, Tandler postulated that atresia resulted from a failure of recanalisation of the solid phase of bowel development. In 1911, Fockens performed the first successful correction of an intestinal atresia. In an extensive review of cases in London, Spriggs, in 1912, proposed that mechanical accidents, including vascular occlusions, may be responsible for the development of an atresia.

The fundamental differences in the aetiology, pathogenesis, and associated anomalies in artesias involving the duodenum and those affecting the rest of the intestine, merit separate discussion of each of the areas affected.

Duodenal Atresia and Stenosis

Incidence

The incidence of duodenal atresia is estimated at about 1 per 10,000 live births. A familial incidence is not a feature of duodenal atresia, but the occurrence of the anomaly in more than one sibling in a family has been recorded (Hyde, 1965).

Anatomy (Fig. 40–13)

In 50 percent of cases there is a true atresia present in the second part of the duodenum. Complete separation of the two segments is present in a quarter of these cases. The remaining anomalies are composed of duodenal diaphragm with or without a central aperture in 40 percent of cases and duodenal stenosis in 10 percent of cases. The duodenal diaphragm with a central aperture may progress as a result of chronic distension into the classical "wind-sock" deformity. In these cases the level of the obstruction appears to be more distal than the actual site of attachment of the duodenal diaphragm. Duodenal stenosis is frequently associated with the so-called annular pancreas, in which the head of the pancreas overlies the narrowing in the second part of the duodenum (Fig. 40–14). Isolated annular pancreas in the absence of an

intrinsic duodenal lesion is a rare phenomenon. The second part of the duodenum is affected in well over 80 percent of cases, the obstruction being preampullary in one third and postampullary in two thirds of the patients (Bill and Pope, 1954; Gourevitch, 1971).

Associated Anomalies

Over half the patients with duodenal atresia have other congenital anomalies. Down's syndrome is present in up to 30 percent of cases and requires accurate preoperative assessment and full parental consultation prior to surgical correction of the atretic or stenotic duodenum. The frequency of associated anomalies is as follows:

Down's syndrome	30 percent
Incomplete rotation of the midgut	30 percent
Congenital cardiac disease	20 percent
Genitourinary anomalies	10 percent
Oesophageal atresia	8 percent
Anorectal malformations	7 percent
Skeletal anomalies	6 percent

Embryology

The frequent association of other anomalies in conjunction with duodenal atresia appears to be indicative of a developmental rather than an acquired lesion in utero. Tandler (1900) proposed a failure of recanalisation after a temporary solid state as the embryologic explanation for duodenal atresia. He observed an epithelial occlusion of the duodenum during the sixth and seventh weeks of intrauterine life. Lynn and Espinas (1959) produced evidence for a duodenal occlusion in 20 of 68 apparently normal human embryos examined between 5 and 8 weeks of gestational age. Boyden (1967) has made the most extensive embryologic study of the duodenum. He has demonstrated that vacuoles develop in the duodenum as the occluding epithelium begins to break up. At the 15-mm stage these vacuoles coalesce to form two channels separately, into each of which drains a division of the hepatopancreatic duct. This state is transitory and, as fusion of the two vacuoles occurs, the lumen of the duodenum is reestablished. Failure of the final stage of fusion results in an atresia or stenosis at the level of the papilla of Vater. Others have challenged this hypothesis, showing that the epithelial proliferation

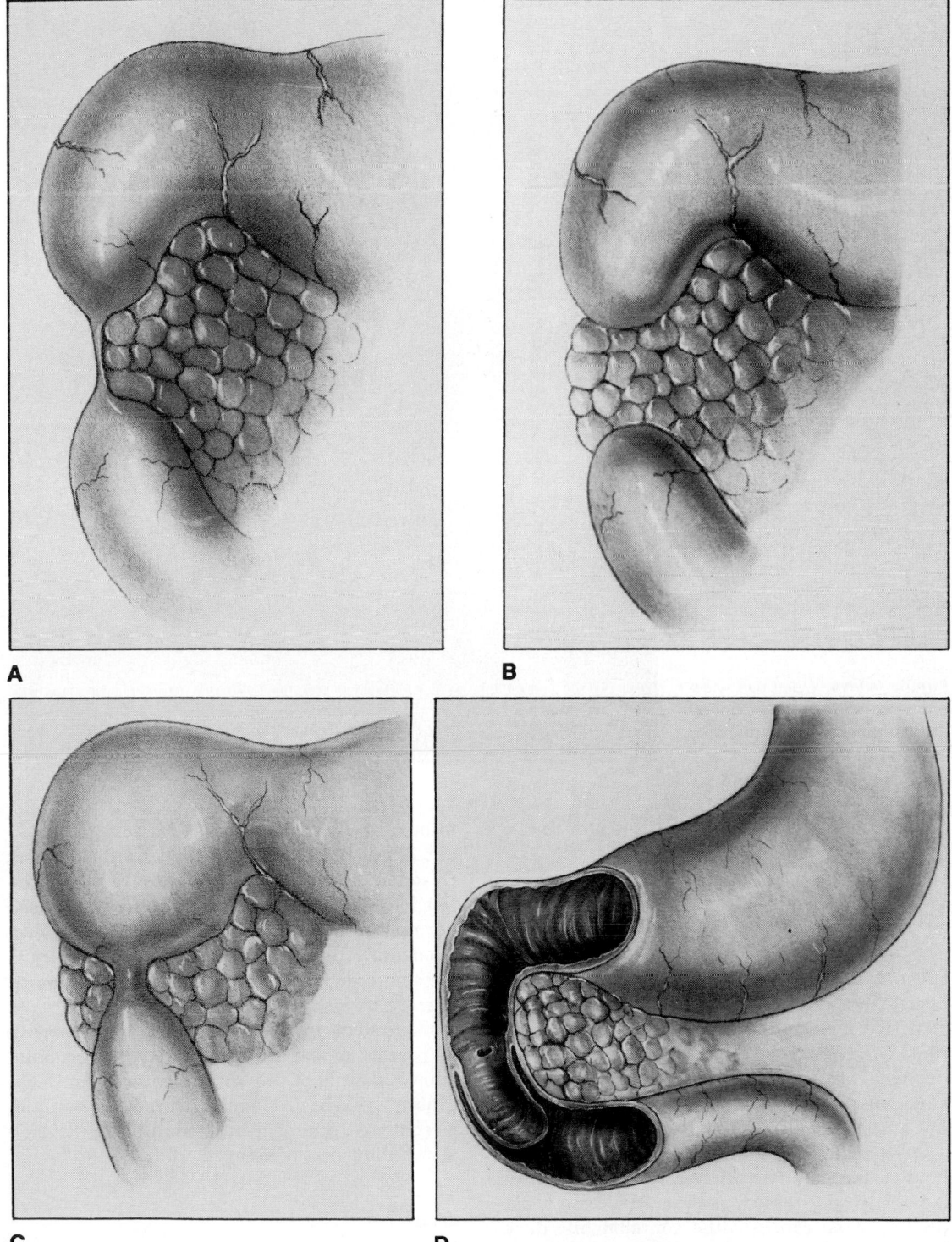

Figure 40–13. Diagrammatic representation of the various types of intrinsic duodenal obstructions. **A.** Duodenal atresia with fibrous connection. **B.** Duodenal atresia with complete separation. **C.** Duodenal stenosis. **D.** Duodenal diaphragm with "windsock" deformity.

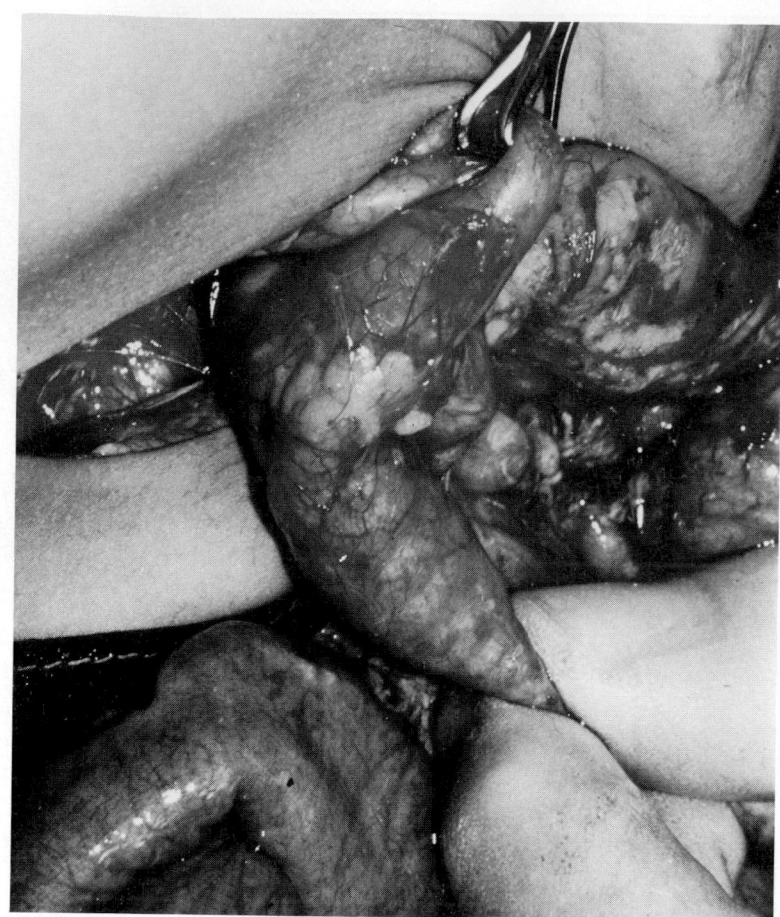

Figure 40–14. Operative view of partial annular pancreas overlying the anterior wall of the second part of the duodenum.

never completely occludes the lumen of the intestine.

Clinical Manifestations

The presence of polyhydramnios during the third stage of gestation should alert the clinician to the possibility of a high intestinal obstructive lesion. Although the majority of infants will be affected by an oesophageal atresia, duodenal atresia features next on the list of possible causes. Almost half the infants with duodenal atresia are born prematurely.

Vomiting usually commences within a few hours of birth. In two thirds of cases the vomitus is heavily bile-stained, as the obstruction is distal to the entrance of the common bile duct. In the one third of patients where the obstruction is in the supraampullary region of the duodenum, the vomitus will be clear but persistent. As the obstruction is located high in the alimentary tract, abdominal distension, if present at all, is confined to the upper abdomen. Gastric peristaltic waves may be visible in the left hypochondrium. Meconium may be passed per rectum in as many as half the infants with duodenal atresia. In general, the consistency of the small amounts of meconium that are passed is more inspissated than normal.

Jaundice has been noted on admission in 30 percent of the infants. The hyperbilirubinaemia is mainly of the unconjugated type. Dehydration, weight loss and disturbances of fluid, electrolytes, and acid–base equilibrium develop as the diagnosis is delayed.

Diagnostic Studies

The straight erect abdominal x-ray reveals the classical "double-bubble" appearance in complete duodenal atresia (Fig. 40–15). A large air–fluid level is present in the left upper quadrant,

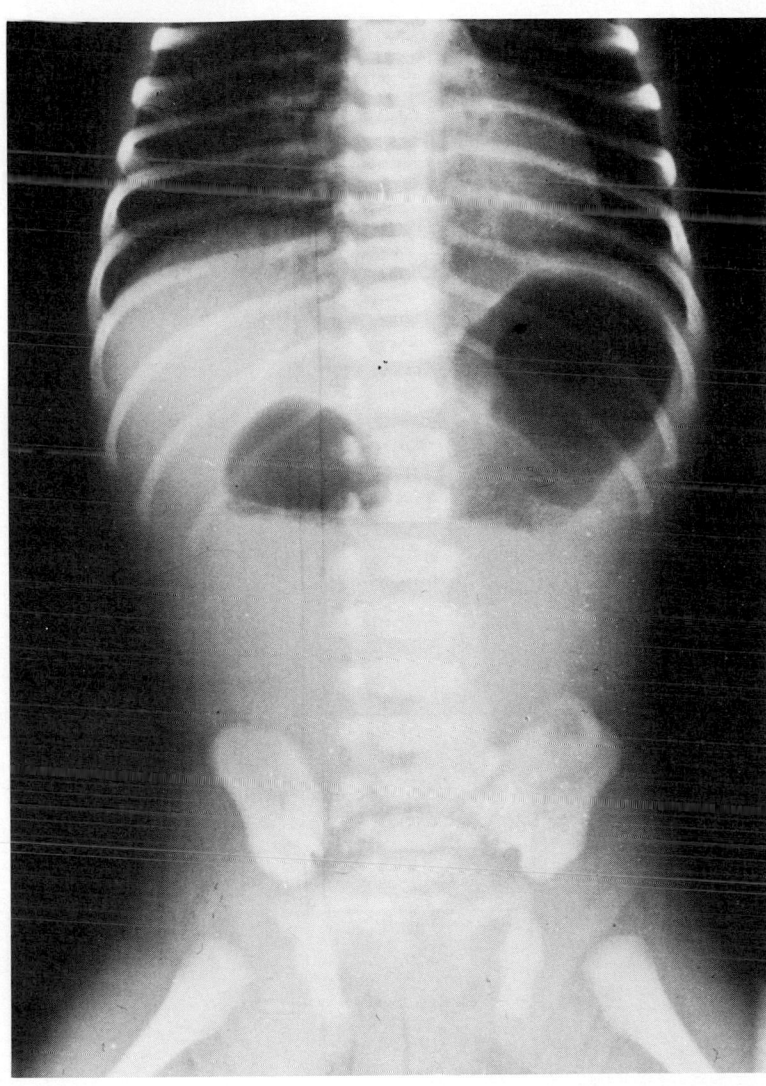

Figure 40–15. Straight, erect abdominal radiograph showing the classical "double-bubble" appearance of duodenal atresia.

representing the dilated stomach, whereas a smaller air–fluid level to the right of the midline indicates the position of the dilated proximal duodenum. Contrast studies in the typical case are superfluous. Small amounts of gas may be seen in the distal intestine even in complete atresias (Astley, 1969). It is claimed that the air reaches the small intestine via a bifid biliary tree, with one limb of the common bile duct draining into the proximal duodenum and the other limb draining into the distal duodenum. Contrast studies are necessary in cases of incomplete duodenal obstruction, where it is important to differentiate duodenal stenosis or other intrinsic duodenal obstruction from extrinsic compression due to malrotation.

Treatment

Preoperative Preparation. Infants presenting within the first 24 hours of life are generally in a satisfactory condition. Correction of dehydration and acid–base imbalance is required for infants in whom the diagnosis has been delayed beyond the first day of life.

Operative Procedure. With the exception of the duodenal web, the procedure of choice for the correction of intrinsic duodenal obstruction is a bypass operation. The proximity of the biliary–pancreatic systems renders more direct procedures hazardous. Of the bypass procedures, duodenoduodenostomy (Fig. 40–16) is the most physiologic. Duodenojejunostomy is reserved for high duodenal atresias with a long gap between the segments. Gastrojejunostomy is mentioned only to be condemned, as there is an unacceptable high incidence of stomal ulceration and afferent loop stasis (Girran and Stephens, 1974).

The duodenoduodenostomy is performed via a right upper quadrant, transverse muscle-cutting incision. The hepatic flexure of the colon is mobilised and the duodenum is widely exposed. Intestinal malrotation, if present, is corrected by the standard Ladd's procedure. The duodenum is mobilised by the Kocher manoeuvre. The proximal segment of the duodenum is generally grossly dilated and its muscle wall greatly hypertrophied. The distal duodenum is narrow and collapsed. The adjacent walls of the proximal and distal duodenal segments are approximated over a distance of 1.0 to 1.5 cm, with interrupted seromuscular sutures (4/0 or 5/0 polyglycolic acid sutures). Two parallel incisions approximately 1.0 cm in length are made in the proximal and distal duodenum immediately adjacent to the previously inserted seromuscular sutures. The anastomosis (side-to-side) is performed using interrupted 4/0 or 5/0 gauge sutures (Prolene or polyglycolic acid sutures). A transanastomotic tube is invaluable in providing postoperative enteral nutrition without

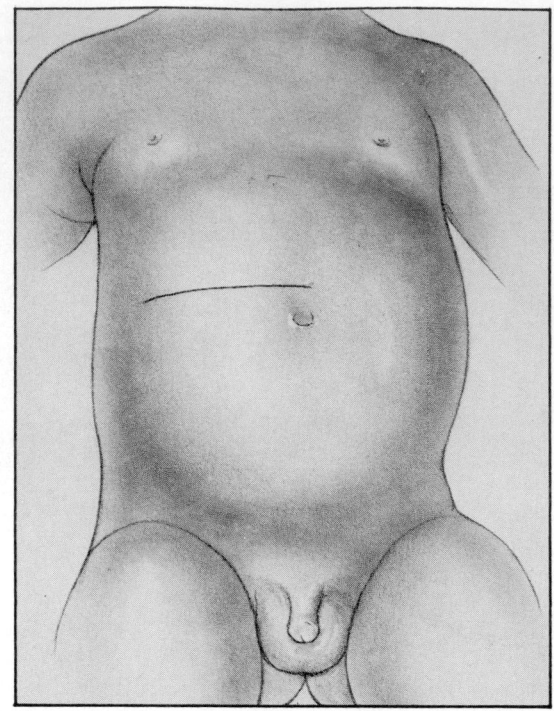

A

Figure 40–16. Operative correction of a duodenal atresia. **A.** Incision.

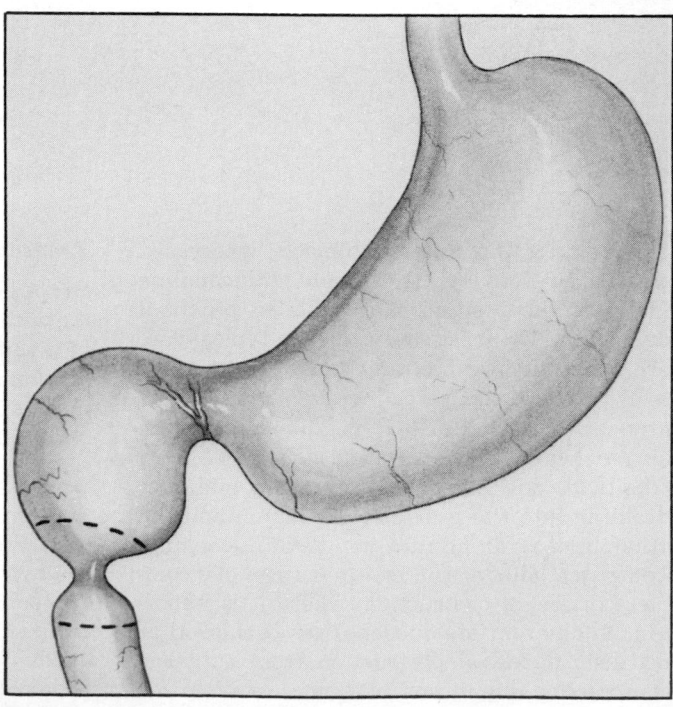

Figure 40–16. B. Anatomy of the anomaly.

B

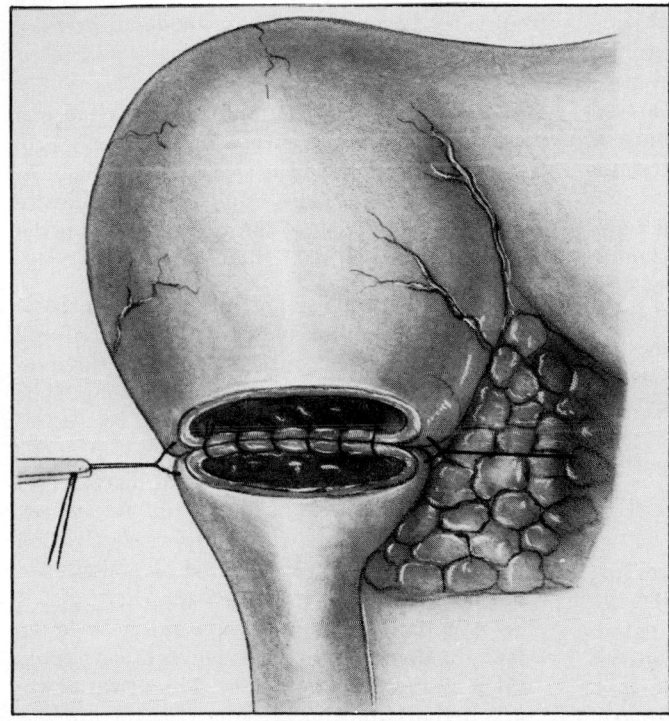

Figure 40–16. C. Side-to-side duodenoduo-denostomy.

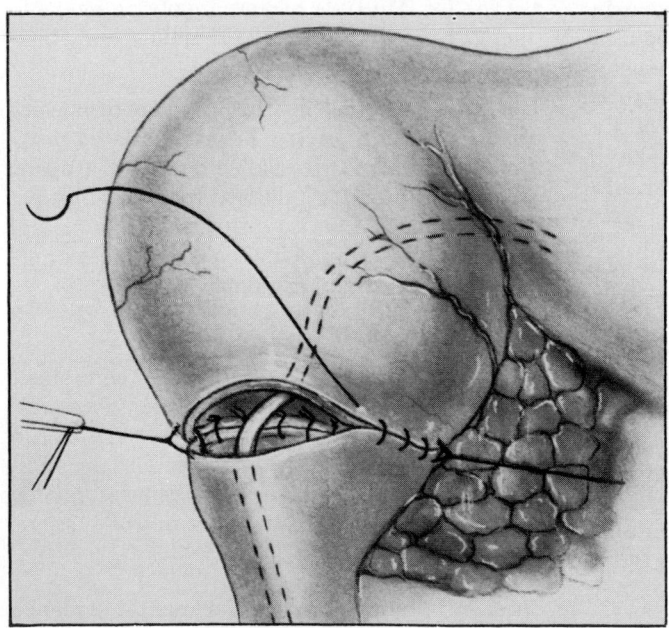

Figure 40–16. D. Transanastomotic feeding tube in position.

having to resort to parenteral feeding. A thin Silastic tube is introduced into the stomach via a Stamm gastrostomy and is manipulated through the anastomosis into the proximal jejunum. Passing the tube through the duodenum can be a difficult procedure and is best performed before completing the anterior part of the anastomosis. The duodenoduodenostomy is completed by inserting a few anterior seromuscular sutures.

Duodenal webs or diaphragms are best approached via a longitudinal lateral duodenotomy sited at the level of attachment of the membrane. The membrane is excised only after the ampulla of Vater has been identified. The raw edges of the membrane following excision are oversewn with 4/0 or 5/0 polyglycolic acid sutures.

Before closing the abdomen it is essential to exclude additional intestinal anomalies, particularly distal atresias.

Postoperative Care. Fluid and electrolyte homeostasis is maintained by "maintenance" intravenous fluid administration supplemented by replacement of nasogastric or gastrostomy aspirate. Characteristically, there is a prolonged period of duodenal ileus due to impaired peristalsis of the hypertrophied and dilated proximal duodenum and to anastomotic oedema. During this phase, when normal nutrition obviously cannot be tolerated, feeds may be introduced into the distal intestine via the transanastomotic tube. The use of a transanastomotic tube is not without complications. Perforation of the jejunum and disruption of the anastomosis have been described and retraction of the tube into the stomach is a common occurrence.

Results. Mortality in intrinsic duodenal obstructive lesions is directly related to the severity of any associated congenital anomalies and to the degree of prematurity of the infant. The overall mortality rate ranges from 25 to 33 percent. Infants with Down's syndrome are at greater risk, due to the frequent occurrence of congenital cardiac anomalies and to their increased susceptibility to overwhelming infection (Perrelli and Wilkinson, 1975; Stauffer and Irving, 1977; Young and Wilkinson, 1966).

Atresias of the Small Intestine

Incidence

Although an incidence of 1 in 1500 live births is generally quoted in the literature, experience at the Hospital for Sick Children, London, appears to indicate that the lesion is rarer than quoted, and, in contrast to other centres, is less frequently encountered than duodenal atresia.

Anatomy

The classification of the jejunoileal atresia has been modified only slightly since the early proposals of Bland-Sutton in 1889 and Spriggs in 1912 (Martin and Zerella, 1976). A diagrammatic representation of the various types is depicted in Figure 40–17.

- *Type I:* Mucosal (septal, diaphragm) atresia with the muscular coats of the proximal and distal segments in contact. Defects in the mesentery have not been observed in this type of atresia. (*20 percent*)
- *Type II:* Atresia involving one segment of the intestine with the proximal and distal blind ends connected by a fibrous cord. (*40 percent*)
- *Type III:* (a) Atresia with complete separation of the blind ends accompanied by a V-shaped defect in the mesentery. (*35 percent*)
  (b) Atresia with an extensive mesenteric defect, the distal ileum receiving its blood supply via a single ileocolic artery. The distal bowel is coiled around this vessel giving the appearance of a "Christmas tree" "apple-peel" deformity (Dickson, 1970).
- *Type IV:* Multiple atresia involving variable lengths of the intestine (El Shafie and Rickham, 1970). (*5 percent*)

The gross pathologic features of an atresia comprise a greatly hypertrophied and dilated proximal segment of variable length and a small collapsed intestine distal to the atresia. Histopathologically, the villi in the distal segment are hypertrophied while they appear normal in the proximal segment.

Associated Anomalies

Although 20 percent of infants with jejunoileal atresias have additional associated anomalies, the majority of these involve other parts of the GI tract. The most common anomalies are malrotation, with or without volvulus, exomphalos or gastroschisis, and meconium ileus.

Aetiology

Substantial clinical and experimental evidence has accumulated to support the hypothesis that intestinal atresia results from an intrauterine vascular occlusion to the involved segment of intestine (Earlam, 1972; Guttman et al, 1975).

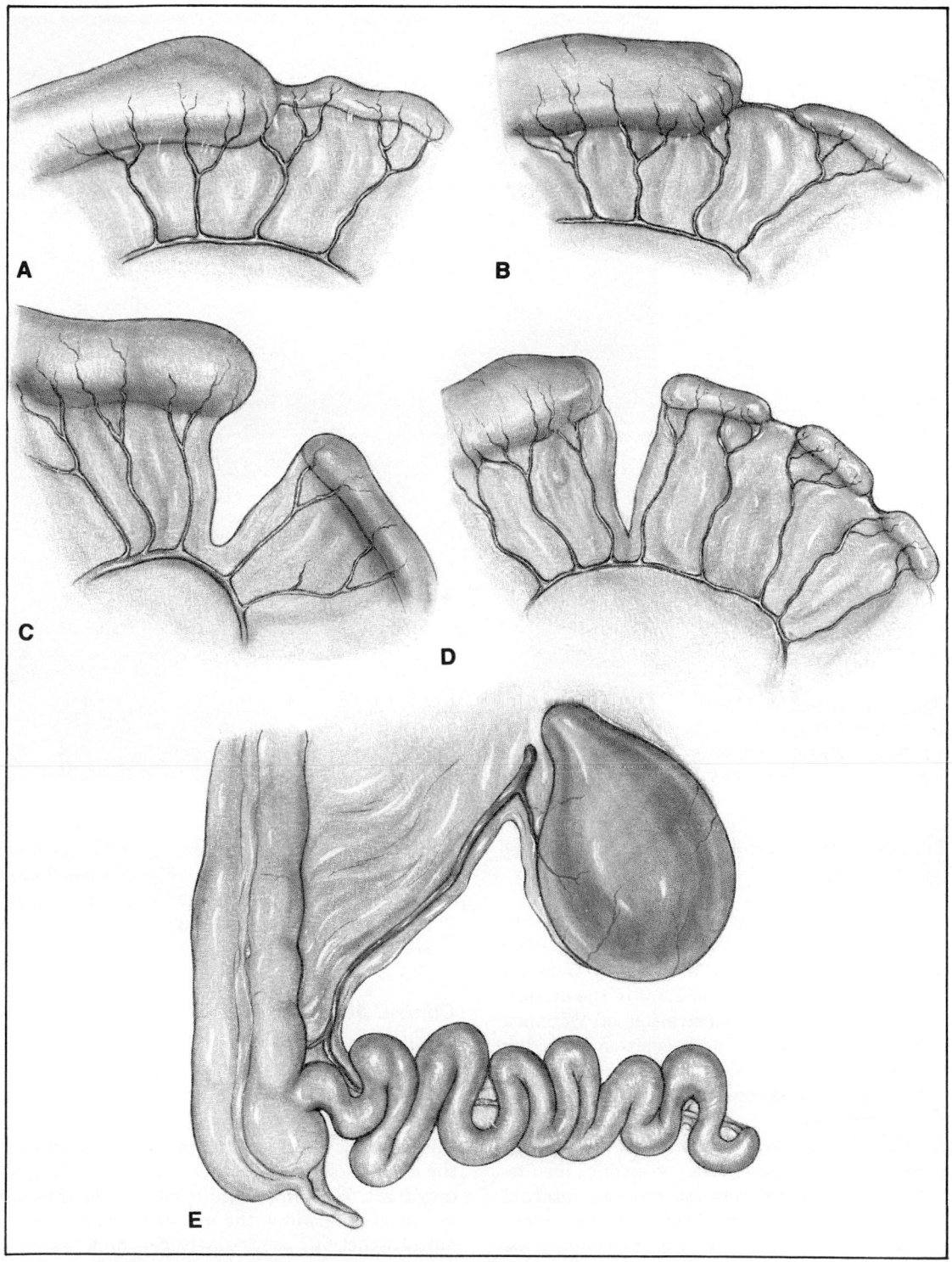

Figure 40–17. Types of atresia (classified by Louw, modified by Grosfeld): **A.** Mucosal occlusion; ends in continuity. **B.** Ends joined by solid cord. **C.** Ends separated; gap in mesentery. **D.** Multiple atresias. **E.** Wider gap; ''apple peel'' deformity of distal ileum. (*Source: From Ellis H: Intestinal Obstruction. New York: Appleton-Century-Crofts, 1982, p 110, with permission.*)

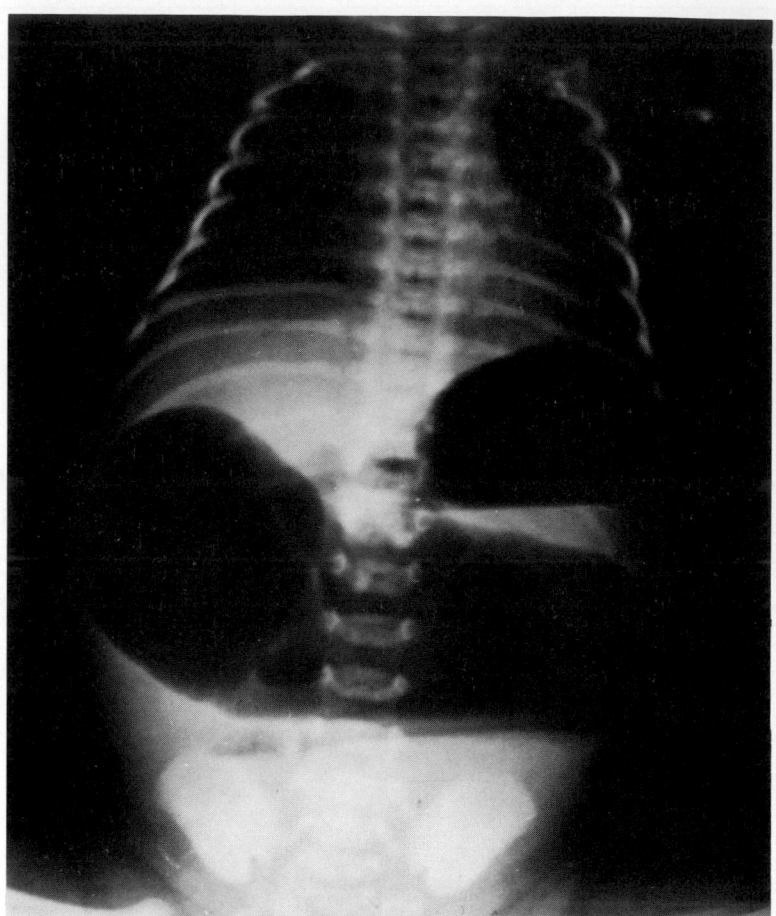

Figure 40–18. Straight abdominal radiograph in a proximal jejunal atresia showing the massive dilatation of the proximal bowel.

The accumulated evidence may be summarised as follows:

1. Bile pigments, squames, and lanugo hairs are often found in the distal intestine, suggesting that continuity of the alimentary tract existed prior to the development of the atresia.
2. The pathologic demonstration of V-shaped mesenteric defects in association with the atresia indicates that the mesenteric vascular occlusion affected a defined segment of arterial supply.
3. Clinical evidence of atresia as a result of late intrauterine mesenteric vascular insults, such as volvulus, intussusception, internal hernia, strangulation of bowel in the umbilical ring, or perforation, can occasionally be found on careful histopathologic examination.
4. Experimental creation of intestinal atresias by devascularising segments of foetal intestine. This experiment was originally reported by Barnard and Louw in 1956 and was later confirmed by Courtois (1959), Santulli and Blanc (1961), Abrams (1968), and many others.

Clinical Manifestations

Polyhydramnios occurs in approximately one third of infants with high jejunal obstruction (Lloyd and Clatworthy, 1958). As the amniotic fluid is normally absorbed in the distal ileum, the frequency of polyhydramnios decreases as the level of obstruction descends in the alimentary tract. With improved resolution of antenatal ultrasonography, the presence of an intestinal obstruction, particularly the high lesions, can be detected on routine scans. Males and females appear to be equally affected. One third of the infants are of low birth weight.

The clinical features are similar to those

discussed under the section on neonatal intestinal obstruction in general. Bile-stained vomiting occurs in over 80 percent of cases. Abdominal distension may be restricted to the upper abdomen in high jejunal atresias, but in most other cases abdominal distension is a prominent feature and may occasionally be severe enough to cause respiratory distress. Although the majority of infants will fail to pass meconium, small amounts of apparently normal meconium are evacuated in 20 percent of cases with jejunoileal atresia. The passage of one or two normal meconium stools should not divert attention from the diagnosis of an intestinal obstruction. Jaundice is frequently associated with high intestinal obstruction lesions during the neonatal period. The unconjugated hyperbilirubinaemia results from an increased enterohepatic circulation of bilirubin as a consequence of the deconjugating action of β-glucuronidase in the proximal bowel.

Diagnostic Studies

The plain erect and supine abdominal x-rays will reveal the presence of air–fluid levels in dilated bowel and an absence of gas beyond the level of the obstruction. In high jejunal atresias there are only a few gas-filled loops, while the rest of the abdomen appears opaque. The number of air–fluid levels increases proportional to the level of the obstruction. Differentiation between low small bowel and colon obstruction on plain abdominal radiography is often impossible during the neonatal period (Figs. 40–18 and 40–19). A diagnostic barium enema in these circumstances may be of considerable value. A

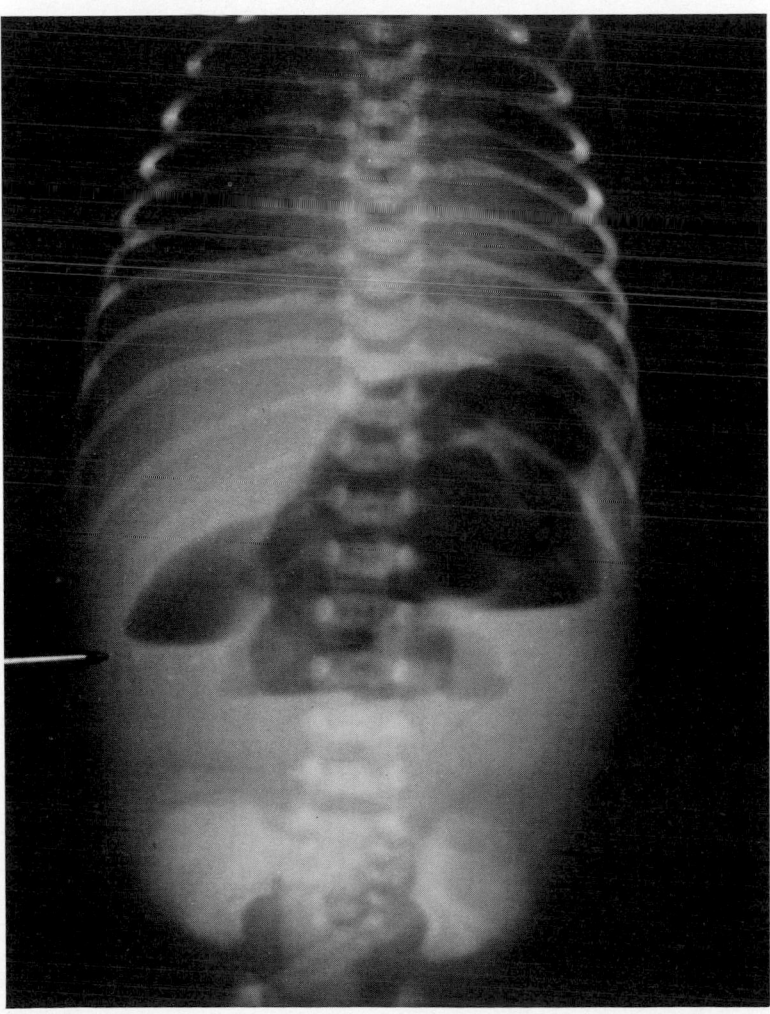

Figure 40–19. Straight, erect abdominal radiograph in a mid–small bowel atresia.

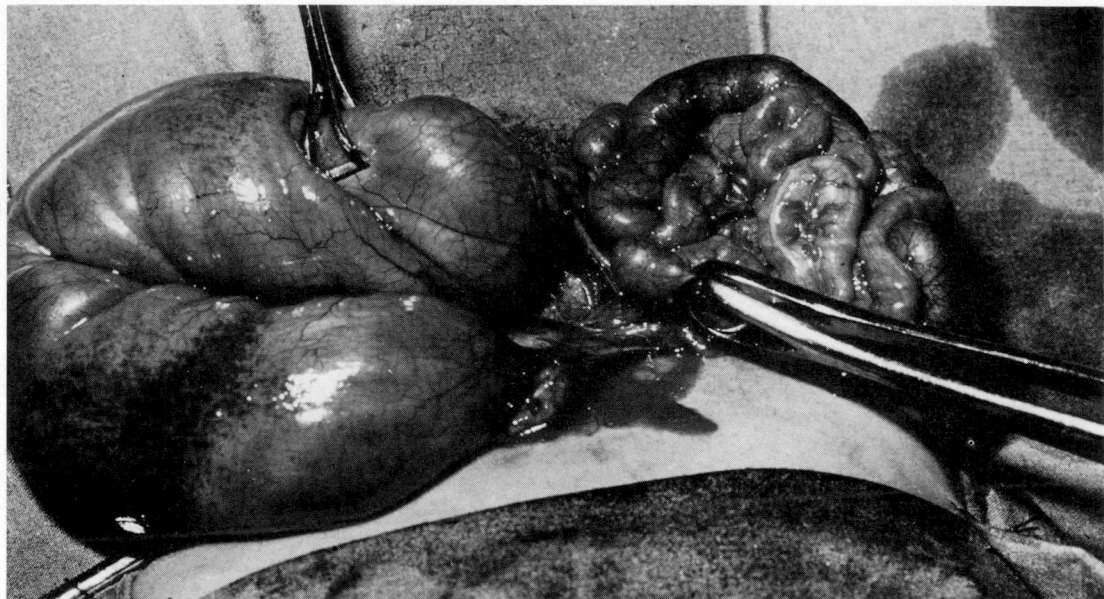

Figure 40–20. Operative picture of intestinal atresia showing the massively dilated proximal bowel and the fibrous connection with the narrow collapsed distal bowel.

narrow collapsed large bowel (microcolon) is indicative of a more proximal obstruction. The position of the caecum will provide useful information with regard to the rotation of the intestine. Calcification indicative of the occurrence of an antenatal perforation occurs in 10 percent of cases.

Treatment

The general principles regarding transportation, preoperative assessment, and resuscitation and anaesthesia are discussed in the section on neonatal intestinal obstruction.

Operative Procedure. Laparotomy is performed via an upper abdominal, transverse muscle-cutting incision. The bowel is inspected and the proximal and distal ends of the atresia identified (Figs. 40–20 and 40–21). Any associated malrotation is corrected by means of a standard Ladd's procedure. Approximately 1 to 2 cm of the distal bowel is resected and a warm saline solution is gently injected into the lumen of the distal bowel to exclude the presence of an unsuspected distal atretic mucosal membrane. If the total length of bowel is sufficient

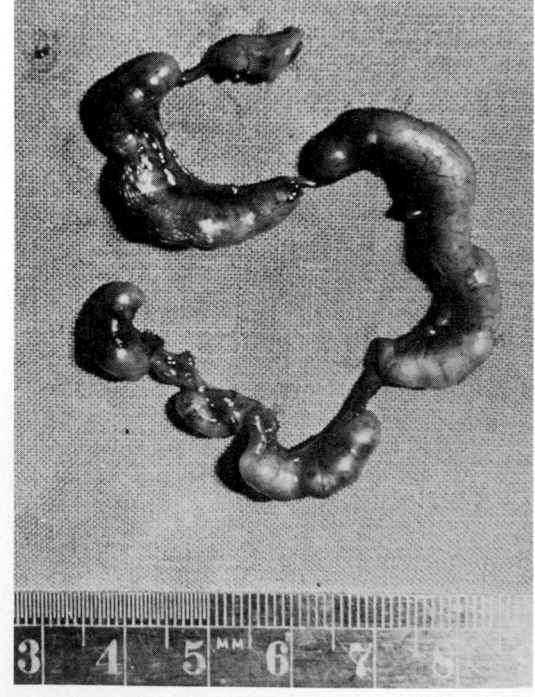

Figure 40–21. Resected specimen in a case of multiple atresias.

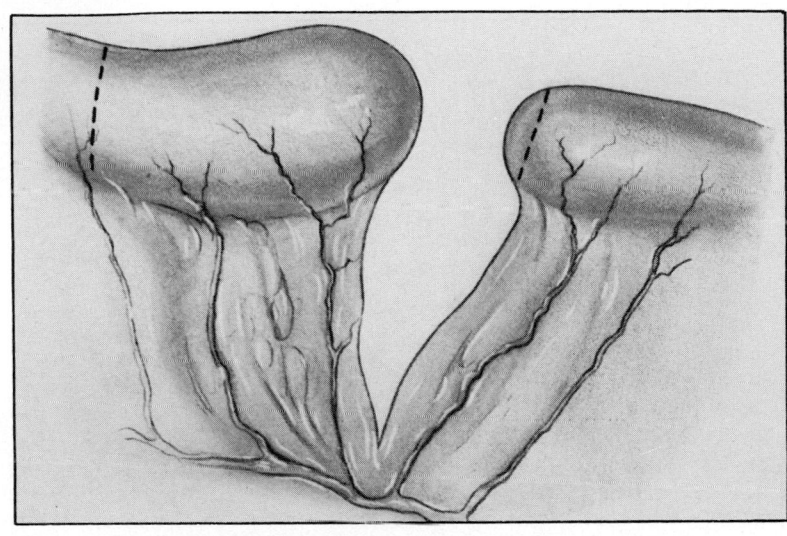

Figure 40–22. Technique for correction of an intestinal atresia. **A.** Resection of the proximal and distal segments.

A

and the distance between the duodenojejunal flexure and the atresia is adequate, resection of the proximal bowel should be extended back until the diameter of the bowel approaches 1.0 to 1.5 cm. This will permit the construction of an end-to-end anastomosis (Fig. 40–22). In high jejunal atresia or in cases with considerable loss of small intestine, a tapering procedure of the proximal segment will result in an end-lumen of 1.0 cm in diameter. The tapering is performed by excising a long, triangular segment of the antimesenteric border of the proximal bowel (Fig. 40–23).

The anastomosis between the proximal and distal intestine is carried out in an end-to-end fashion using a single layer of 5/0 gauge polyglycolic acid or Prolene seromuscular sutures. Using the seromuscular technique, it is possible to achieve an end-to-end anastomosis even in the presence of great discrepancies between the

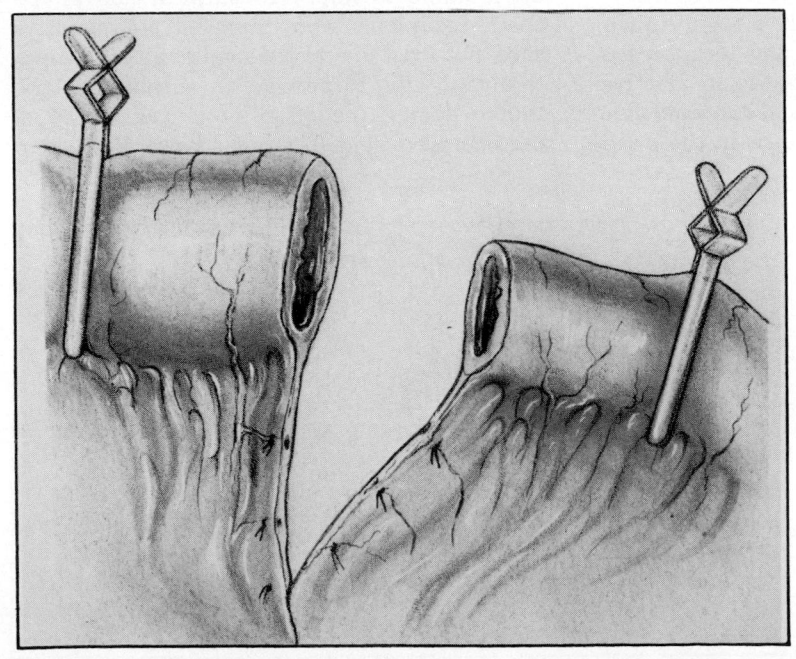

Figure 40–22. B. End-to-end anastomosis.

B

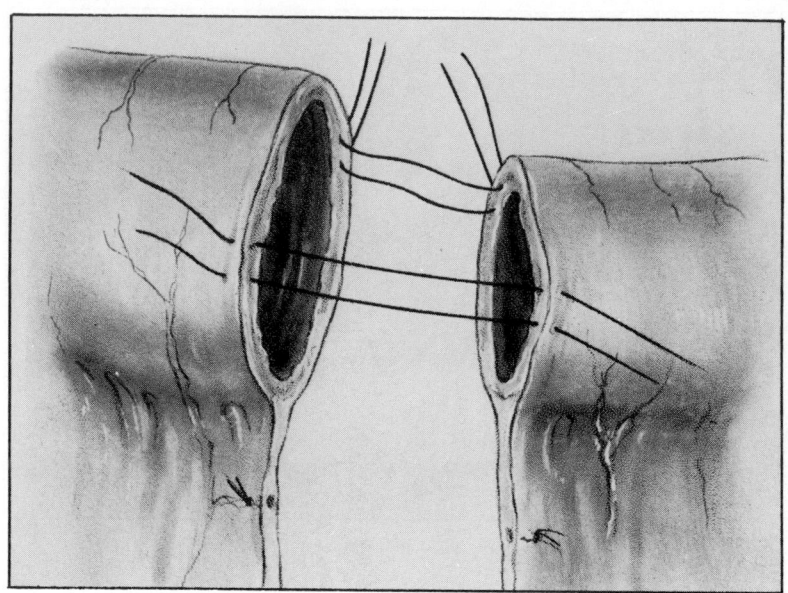

Figure 40–22. C. Seromuscular technique of anastomosis.

C

bowel lumens. The mesenteric defect is approximated and the abdominal incision closed either en masse or by layered closure. The skin edges are approximated using a subcuticular suture. The peritoneal cavity is not usually drained, but careful peritoneal toilet with a dilute solution of povidone iodine is carried out prior to closure of the abdomen. This applies particularly where gross peritoneal contamination has occurred, either pre- or intraoperatively.

In high jejunal atresias it is useful to perform a Stamm gastrostomy and insert a fine Silastic transanastomotic tube via the gastrostomy into the distal bowel. As in duodenal atresia, return of effective peristalsis in the proximal jejunum may be considerably delayed and the transanastomotic tube for feeding purposes greatly simplifies the postoperative management.

Results

The survival rate for intestinal atresias has steadily improved since the first successful correction in 1911. Improved survival is directly attributable to improved surgical and anaesthetic techniques and improved postoperative care, not least due to the availability of parenteral nutrition to provide an adequate caloric intake during the often prolonged period of postoperative ileus. The importance of resection

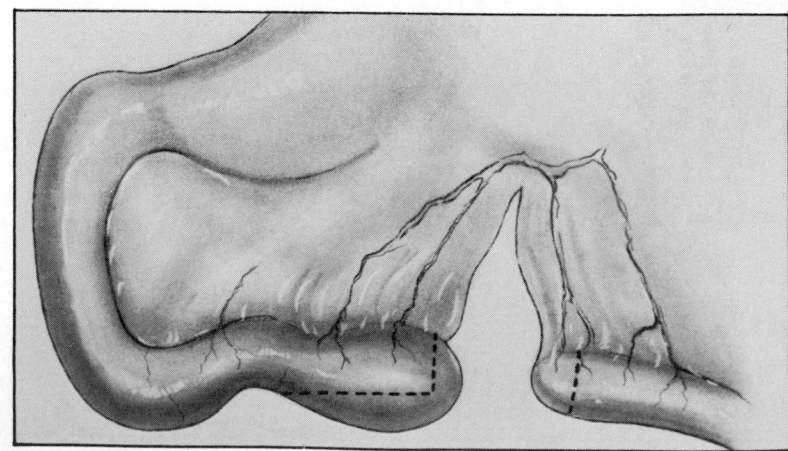

Figure 40–23. Tapering proximal jejunoplasty for high intestinal atresia. **A.** Method of resection of proximal loop on antimesenteric border.

A

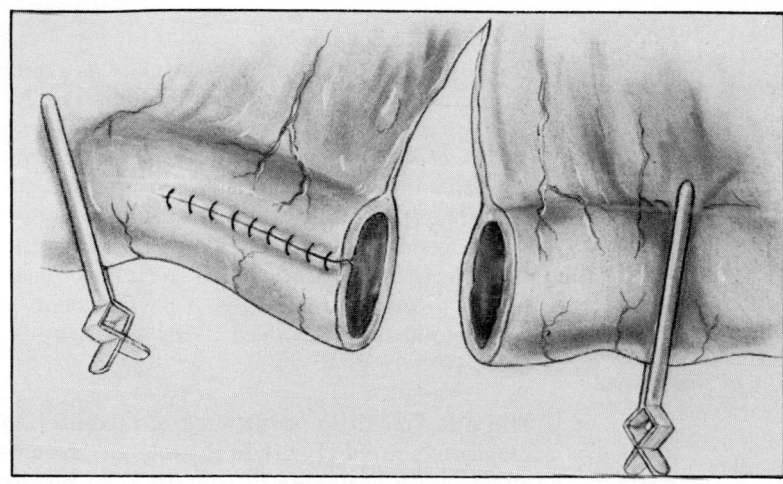

Figure 40–23. B. Proximal jejunoplasty.

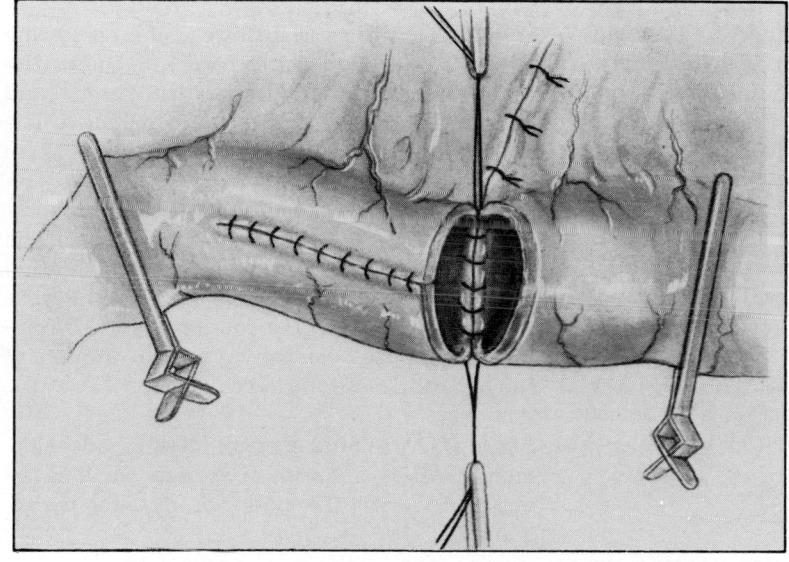

Figure 40–23. C. End-to-end anastomosis.

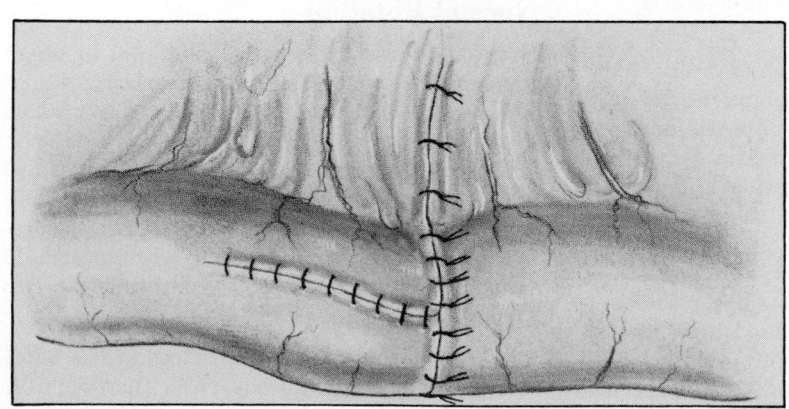

Figure 40–23. D. End-to-end anastomosis completed.

of the dilated proximal bowel and a short length of the distal segment in achieving a usefully functional anastomosis has been demonstrated by Nixon (1960) and Louw (1966). The mortality rate is related to: (1) the level of the atresia (the higher the obstruction the greater the mortality), (2) the extent of intestinal resection, and (3) the presence of additional congenital anomalies and/or the degree of prematurity.

Although the provision of parenteral nutrition has improved survival in patients previously considered to be hopeless, a useful guide to prognosis is that at least 15 cm of small intestine with an intact ileocaecal valve of 25 to 30 cm without an ileocaecal valve is necessary for the establishment of adequate oral nutrition.

Atresias of the Colon

These are much less common than small intestinal atresias and comprise around 1 to 5 percent of all GI atresias. The aetiology and clinical presentation is similar to that of small intestinal atresias except that the onset of bilious vomiting may be delayed for a few days and the abdominal distension is much more pronounced. In the presence of a competent ileocaecal valve, distension of the proximal colon may reach enormous proportions or may result in caecal perforation. The operative approach is similar to that of small bowel atresias. In atresias involving the right colon, resection, and end-to-end anastomosis is recommended. In other sites a temporary colostomy with later reconstruction is the safest course of action (Benson et al, 1968).

MALROTATION

Malrotation refers to any interference with the process of orderly fetal rotation of the midgut and the normal fixation of the mesenteries.

Historical Review

The studies of Frazer and Robbins in 1915 and Dott in 1923 helped to formulate the embryologic anatomy of normal intestinal development. The genesis of malrotation is based on errors that may occur during the normal process. In 1936, William Ladd published his classic article on malrotation, in which emphasis was placed on the importance of dividing peritoneal bands which cross over the duodenum and of placing the caecum in the left upper quadrant. The principles of the operation have remained unchanged ever since.

Embryology

The alimentary tract initially develops as a tube extending down the midline of the embryo. As it lengthens it extends into the extraembryonic coelom of the umbilical cord and later returns from this into the peritoneal cavity as the abdominal cavity enlarges. The foregut is supplied by the coeliac artery, the midgut by the superior mesenteric, and the hindgut by the inferior mesenteric artery. Three stages of development of the midgut are recognised (Gray and Skandalakis, 1972) (Fig. 40–24).

Stage I. Fourth to tenth week of intrauterine life. Due to rapid growth of the midgut, the coelomic cavity is unable to contain it within its confines. The midgut is forced out into the physiologic hernia within the umbilical cord.

Stage II. Tenth to twelfth week of intrauterine life. The midgut migrates back into the peritoneal cavity. The small intestine returns first and lies mainly on the left side of the abdomen. The caecocolic loop returns last, entering the abdomen in the left lower quadrant, but rapidly rotating through 270 degrees in a counterclockwise direction to attain its final position in the right iliac fossa. Simultaneous with the rotation of the midgut, the duodenojejunal loop likewise undergoes a 270 degree counterclockwise rotation, coming to rest behind and to the left of the superior mesenteric vessels.

Stage III. The final stage of intestinal development consists of fusion of various parts of the mesentery with the posterior parietal peritoneum.

Consequences of Errors of Normal Rotation

Stage I. Arrest of development at this stage results in the occurrence of an *exomphalos* (omphalocoele). There is persistence to a greater or lesser extent of the physiologic hernia in the umbilicus. The contents of the exomphalos are visible through a thin transparent membrane consisting of amnion on the exterior, peritoneum on the internal surface, with a variable amount of Wharton's jelly separating the two layers.

1. *Exomphalos Major.* The defect in the anterior abdominal wall is greater than 5 cm in diameter. It contains a large proportion of

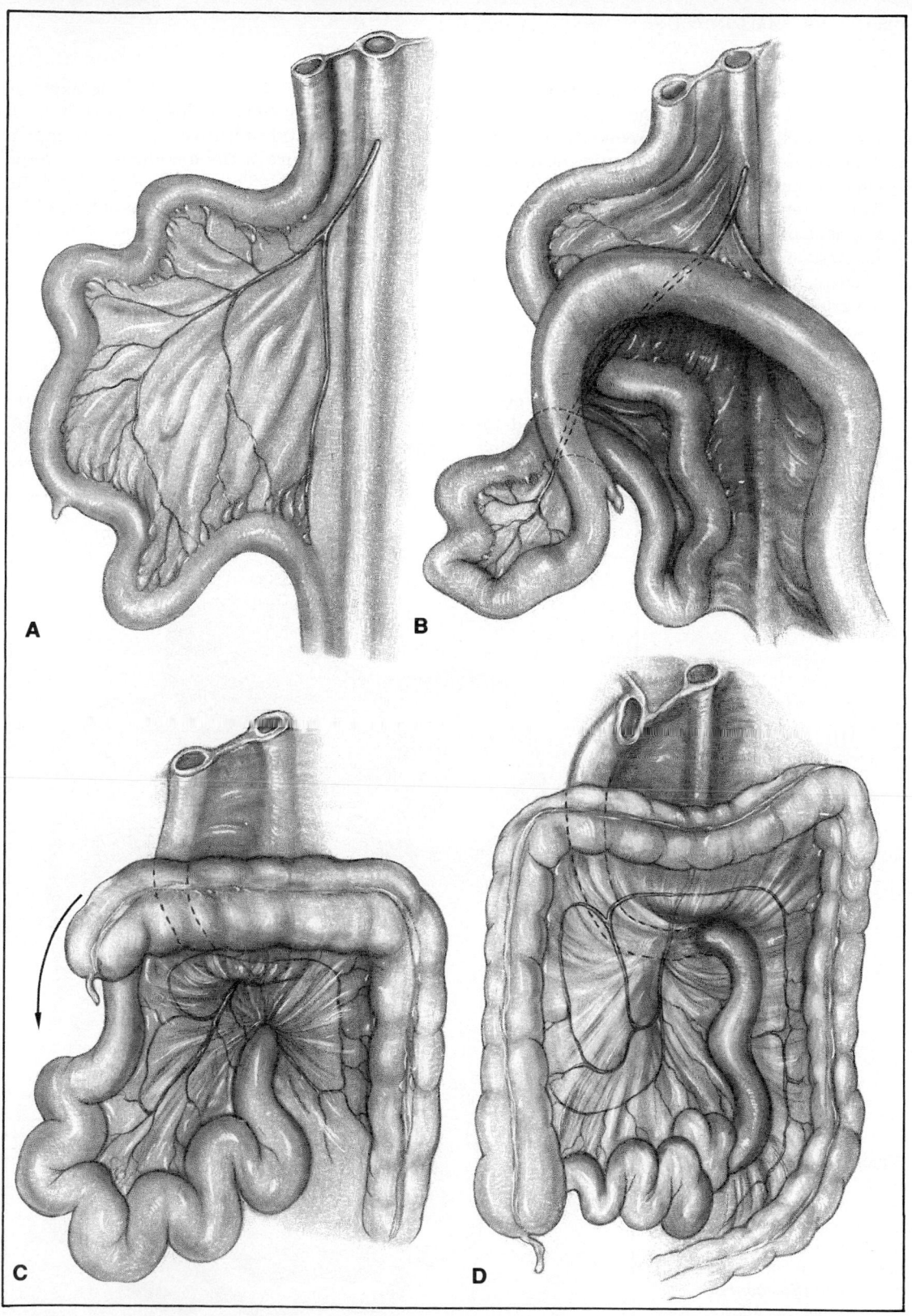

Figure 40–24. Stages in fetal midgut rotation. (*Source: From Ellis H: Intestinal Obstruction. New York: Appleton-Century-Crofts, 1982, p 224, with permission.*)

the intestines and usually part of the liver. Associated congenital anomalies, particularly cardiac defects, are frequently present.

2. *Exomphalos Minor*. The defect in the umbilical ring measures less than 5 cm in diameter. The contents are usually confined to a short segment of small intestine. Additional malformations are rare.

3. *Gastroschisis*. This refers to the extrusion of a variable amount of intestine, which may even extend to involve the stomach, through a defect located immediately to the right of a normally formed umbilical cord. The bowel itself is foreshortened, thickened, and oedematous and adjacent loops are matted together. There is no evidence of a covering

sac. The most logical embryologic explanation is that the gastroschisis results from an early antenatal rupture of a minor exomphalos with closure of the umbilicus around the extruded bowel. This would account for the constant site of the defect, the absence of a covering sac and the infrequent occurrence of associated anomalies.

In all these anomalies involving arrest in the first stage of intestinal development, errors of midgut rotation form an integral part.

Stage II. Errors occurring during this stage result in a variety of abnormalities, the most frequent of which is the incomplete rotation.

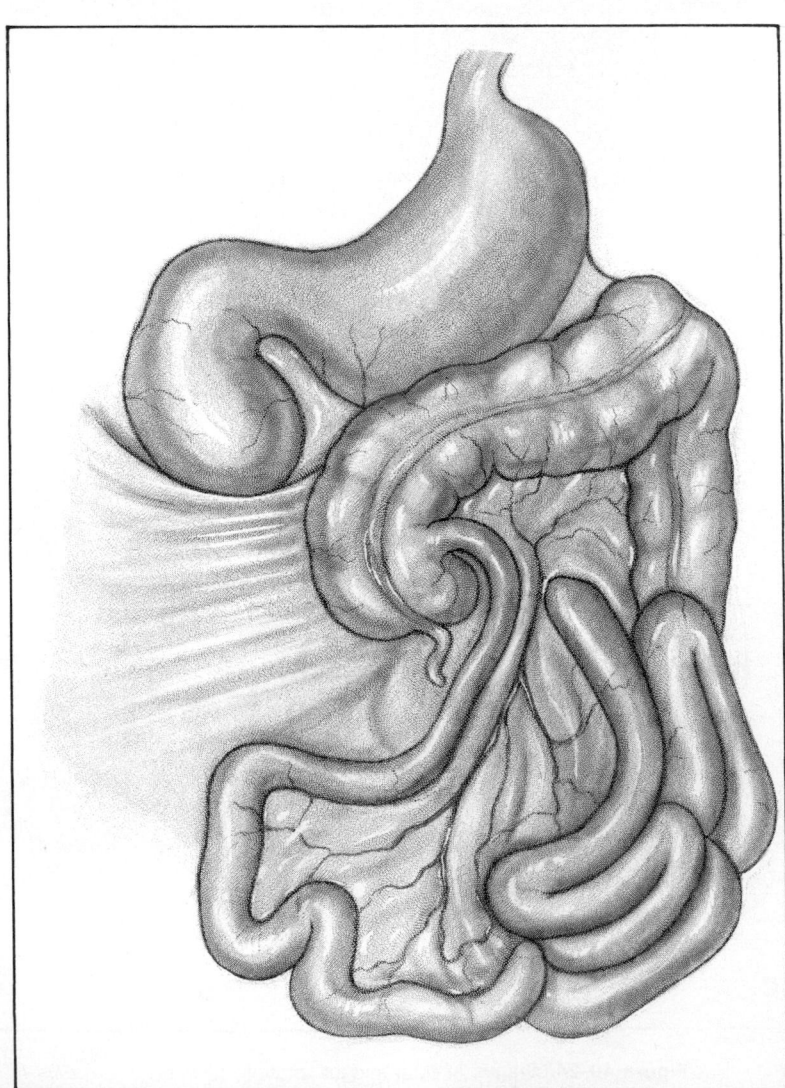

Figure 40–25. Anatomy of the most common variety of malrotation, with the caecum lying in the subhepatic position and Ladd's bands crossing the second part of the nonrotated duodenum. (*Source: From Ellis H: Intestinal Obstruction. New York: Appleton-Century-Crofts, 1982, p 120, with permission.*)

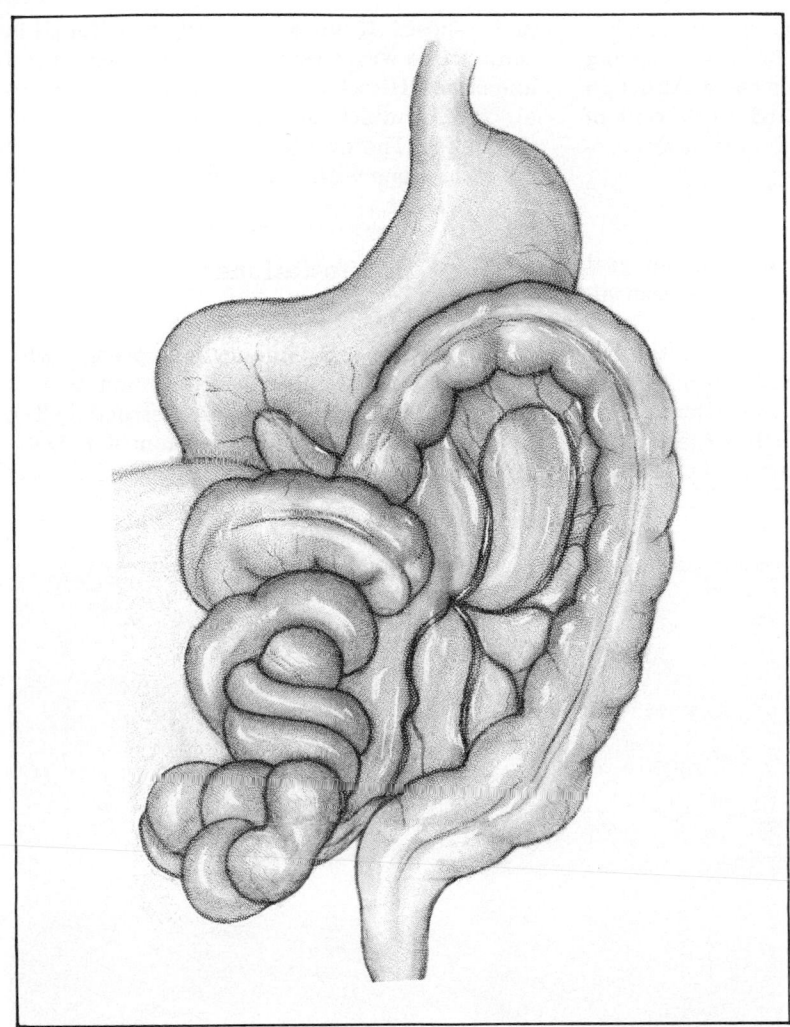

Figure 40–26. Anatomy of midgut volvulus revealing the extent of bowel involved in the twist. (*Source: From Ellis H: Intestinal Obstruction. New York: Appleton-Century-Crofts, 1982, p 119, with permission.*)

1. *Nonrotation.* Failure of rotation following reentry into the peritoneal cavity leaves the major part of the colon on the left side of the abdomen, the small intestine to the right, and the caecum suspended in the midline.
2. *Incomplete Rotation.* The caecum is situated in a subhepatic portion in the right hypochondrium. Peritoneal bands (Ladd's bands), which cross and may compress the second part of the duodenum, attach the caecocolic loop to the posterior abdominal wall (Fig. 40–25). A second and potentially more dangerous consequence of this incomplete rotation is that the entire midgut hangs suspended on the superior mesenteric vessels by a narrow stalk. It is this narrow base mesentery that is prone to undergo volvulus, forming a strangulating closed-loop type of obstruction (Fig. 40–26).
3. *Reversed Rotation.* The final 180 degree rotation occurs in a clockwise direction rather than counterclockwise so that the colon comes to lie posterior to the duodenum and the superior mesenteric vessels.
4. *Hyperrotation.* Instead of rotation stopping at 270 degrees it continues through 360 degrees or even 450 degrees so that the caecum comes to rest in the region of the splenic flexure of the colon in the left upper quadrant.
5. *Encapsulated Small Intestine.* This rare anomaly arises when the avascular sac that forms the lining of the extraembryonic coelom returns en masse into the abdomen together with the intestine.

Stage III. Rotation has occurred normally, but the final stage of fixation is defective, leaving a mobile caecum and ascending colon. Although this is present in an estimated 10 percent of asymptomatic individuals, volvulus of the caecum may occur.

Associated Anomalies

The occurrence of malrotation as an integral part of exomphalos/gastroschisis has been alluded to earlier. Malrotation also occurs as a constant associated problem in congenital diaphragmatic hernia (Bochdalek hernia) and prune-belly syndrome, and in the latter is especially frequently associated with congenital intrinsic obstructions of the duodenum (atresia and stenosis). It has occasionally been found in conjunction with oesophageal atresia, anorectal anomalies, Hirschsprung's disease (de Bruyn et al, 1982), biliary atresia, and urinary tract anomalies. The overall incidence of additional malformations with malrotation is between 10 to 20 percent.

Clinical Manifestations

Neonatal Period

Malrotation in early infancy may present with either acute strangulating obstruction or with recurrent episodes of subacute obstruction. The first, and at times the only, symptom of malrotation is bile-stained vomiting, the significance of

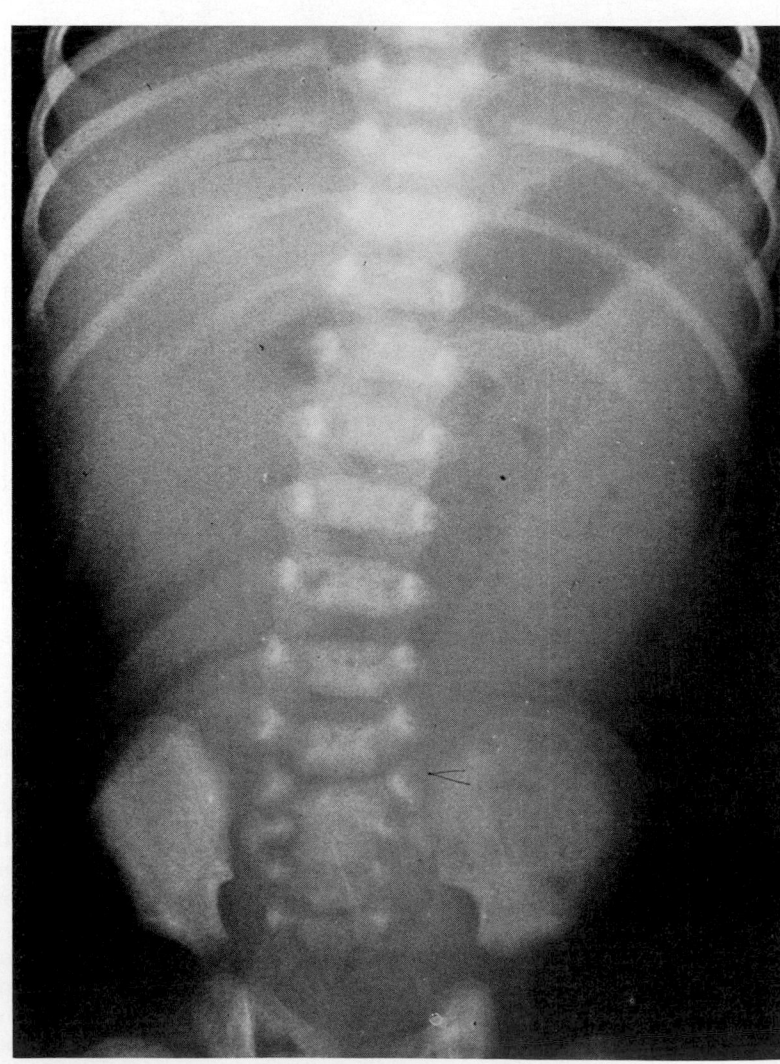

Figure 40–27. Plain abdominal radiograph in a malrotation with volvulus revealing the paucity of gas beyond the stomach and duodenum.

which has already been discussed. The importance of urgent investigation to determine the cause of bilious vomiting cannot be over emphasised.

Acute strangulating obstruction results from midgut volvulus and is almost, but not exclusively, confined to infants in the first month of life. The clinical features of volvulus include shock, abdominal distension, and tenderness and the passage of dark red blood per rectum. Oedema and erythema of the anterior abdominal wall develop as the volvulus progresses to intestinal gangrene, perforation, and peritonitis.

Older Infants and Childhood

A wide spectrum of clinical symptoms have been ascribed to malrotation. The most common is intermittent or cyclic vomiting, which may on occasion be bile-stained. Failure to thrive and malnutrition in association with malrotation may be due either to an inherent intestinal malabsorption problem or to chronic decreased oral intake. Early satiety associated with the intake of food results in the reluctance to eat. Recurrent abdominal pain is extremely prevalent among school children. An organic cause for the pain can be identified in less than 10 percent of cases. Where the pain is particularly severe or accompanied by episodes of bilious vomiting, further GI studies are necessary to exclude an organic cause. Other symptoms ascribed to malrotation include malabsorption and diarrhoea, chronic abdominal distension and constipation, chylous ascites from chronic lymphatic obstruction and obstructive jaundice from compression of the common bile duct.

Radiologic Examinations

The features suggestive of volvulus on plain abdominal x-ray include fluid levels in the stomach and duodenum giving a "double-bubble" appearance on the erect film and a relative paucity of gas in the rest of the intestine (Fig. 40–27). Contrast studies are unnecessary where these radiologic features are accompanied by the clinical signs of acute strangulating obstruction. Urgent resuscitation and emergency laparotomy is the best course of action.

Both upper and lower GI contrast studies have been advocated for the diagnosis of malrotation (Berdon et al, 1970; Simpson et al, 1972). The barium enema examination only gives information about the position of the caecum (Fig.

40–28). The barium meal and follow-through examination is the procedure of choice, as it provides details not only of the configuration of the duodenum but also on the degree and nature of a possible co-existing intrinsic duodenal obstruction (Fig. 40–29). The hazards of such an investigation have been overstressed in the past—provided sufficient care is exercised by the radiologist to avoid vomiting and aspiration of contrast, the infant should come to no harm. Thin barium is preferable to Gastrografin as it provides superior definition while avoiding the dangers of dehydration as a result of the hypertonicity of the Gastrografin solution. The newer water-soluble contrast agents, e.g., metrozamide, are isotonic and do not have the disadvantages of Gastrografin.

Treatment

Patients presenting with acute strangulating obstruction and volvulus require rapid resuscitation before proceeding to surgery. This comprises an intravenous infusion of plasma (20 ml/kg of body weight), correction of electrolyte and acid–base imbalance, cross-matching of blood, broad-spectrum antibiotic cover (penicillin, gentamicin, and metronidazole), and attempts to maintain body temperature. The period of resuscitation should be long enough to ensure maximum therapeutic response. This is generally achieved in 1 to 2 hours of intensive therapy. Prolonging the resuscitation beyond this point exposes the intestine to further irreversible damage from ischaemia.

The operative approach consists of an upper abdominal transverse muscle-cutting incision. The incision should be long enough to enable thorough examination of all the abdominal viscera. A small volume of yellow peritoneal fluid is almost invariably present in any early intestinal obstruction. Blood-stained fluid is indicative of intestinal necrosis.

The twist in established volvulus usually occurs in a clockwise direction and the involved bowel, if not frankly gangrenous, is congested and cyanotic (Fig. 40–30). The intestine is delivered into the wound and the volvulus untwisted by carefully rotating the involved mass of intestine in a counterclockwise direction. Once the volvulus has been reduced, the bowel is covered with warm moist swabs. It may be necessary to leave the bowel undisturbed for up to 10 minutes before being able to assess the extent of

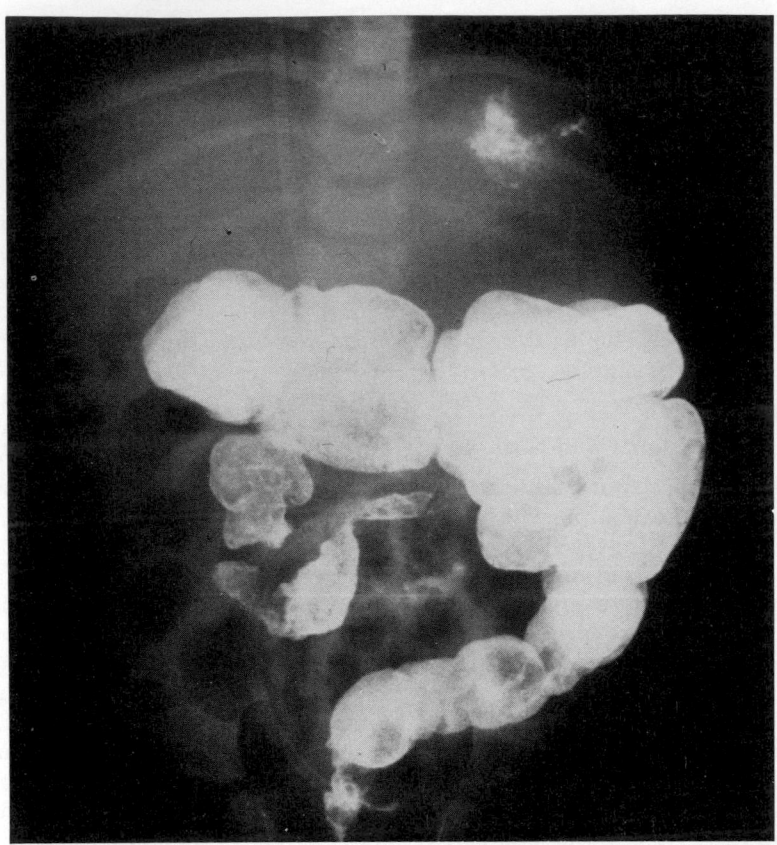

Figure 40–28. Barium enema in malrotation showing the subhepatic portion of the caecum.

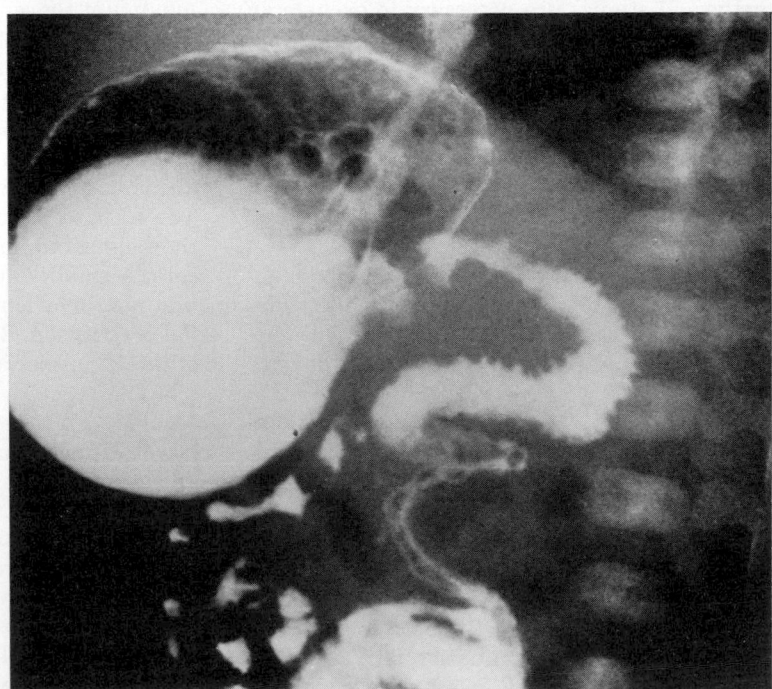

Figure 40–29. Contrast meal in malrotation revealing the "twisted ribbon" or "corkscrew" appearance of the duodenum involved in the volvulus.

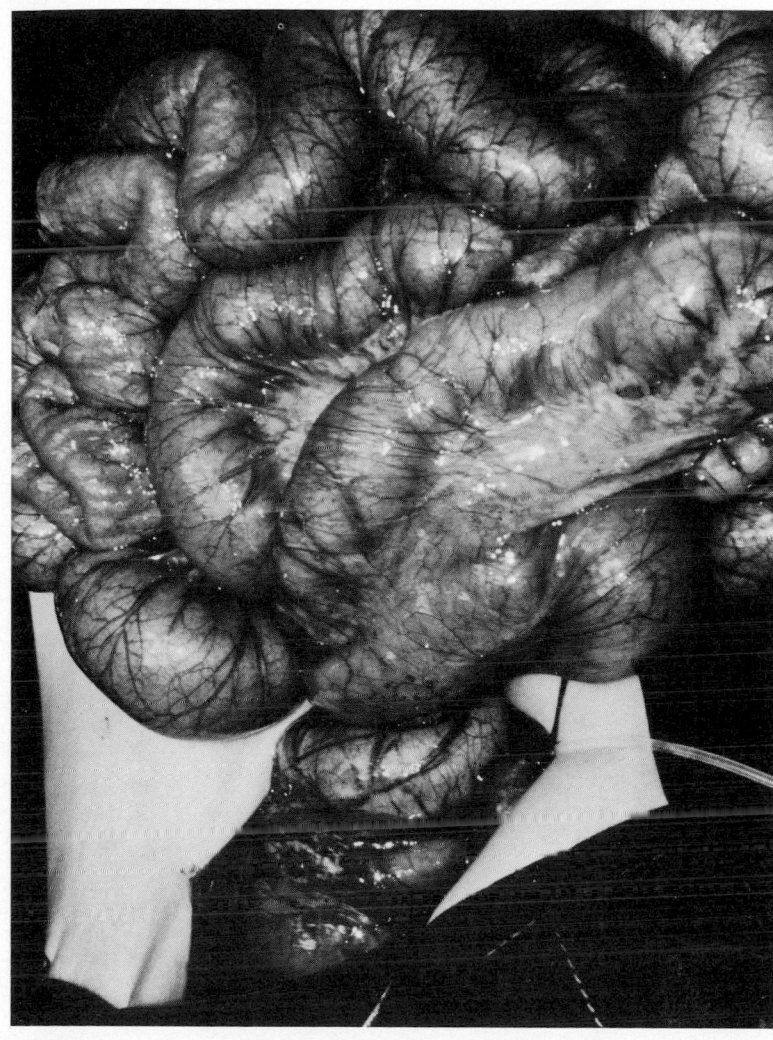

Figure 40–30. Operative view of malrotation with volvulus showing the 360 degree twist in the base of the mesentery.

ischaemic damage. In cases of apparent total midgut gangrene, obviously necrotic intestine should be excised and enterostomies fashioned in bowel of doubtful viability. A "second-look" laparotomy is performed 24 hours later when the full extent of gangrene can be accurately defined and either a direct anastomosis between viable intestine performed or further resection and temporary enterostomies reestablished. Shorter sections of necrotic intestine should be excised and an end-to-end anastomosis constructed.

In all cases of malrotation, with or without necrosis, the tendency towards volvulus can be effectively prevented by the classic Ladd's procedure (Fig. 40–31). This consists of full mobilisation of the caecum and ascending colon by divid-

ing the Ladd's bands that cross the second part of the duodenum and attach to the posterior abdominal wall and the gallbladder. The duodenum is Kocherised and duodenojejunal junction freed by dividing the ligament of Treitz. The effect of this procedure is to straighten the course of the duodenum so that, instead of the normal C-curvature, the duodenum courses directly downwards to the right of the vertebral column. Adhesions in the base of the mesentery, which compress the venous and lymphatic return and narrow the base of the mesentery, making it more prone to twist, are divided, thereby widening the attachment of the midgut to the posterior abdominal wall. The small intestine is placed on the right of the peritoneal cavity while the large bowel lies on the left, with

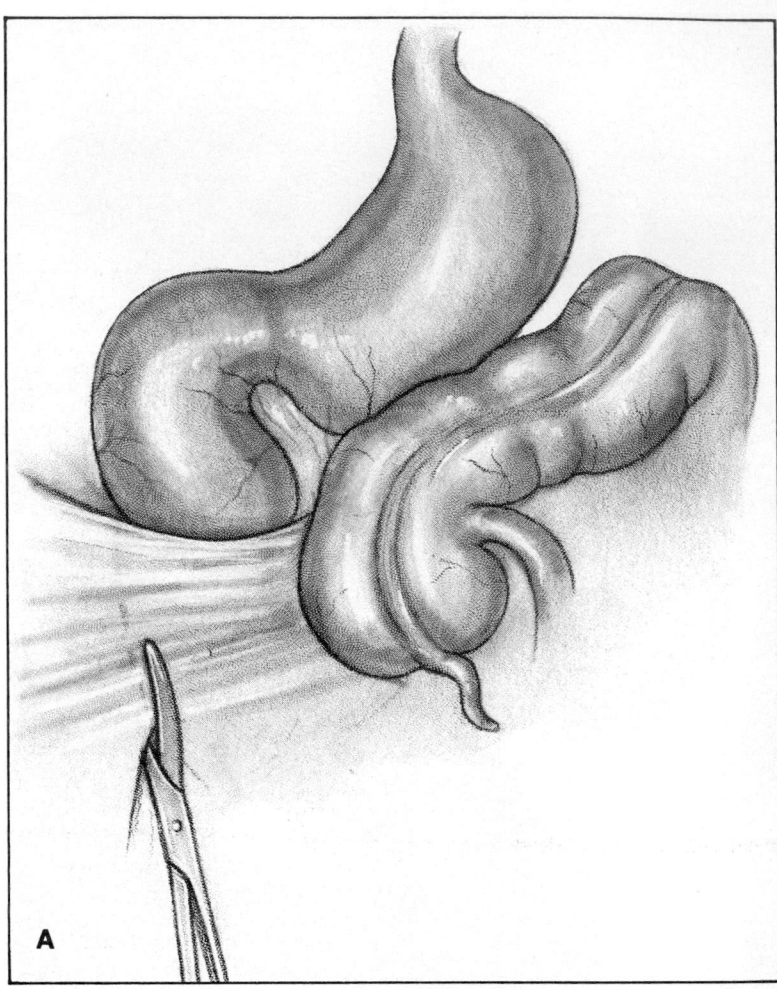

Figure 40–31. Principles of the Ladd's procedure for correction of malrotation. **A.** Division of Ladd's bands and splaying of the mesentery at its base.

the caecum in the left hypochondrium. Some authors advocate fixing the intestine in this, the foetal position, but, in general, most surgeons rely on postoperative adhesions to accomplish fixation. If circumstances permit, the appendix is removed or invaginated in order to prevent the confusion that may arise should appendicitis subsequently develop in the abnormally sited organ.

DUPLICATIONS OF THE INTESTINE

Duplications can occur anywhere in the alimentary tract from the mouth to the anus. They may be spherical or tubular in shape and are almost invariably located on the mesenteric as-

pect of the bowel or between the leaves of the mesentery. The tubular duplications usually communicate with the adjacent intestine whereas the cystic duplications tend to be completely separate. The wall of the duplication contains one or several layers of muscle, part of which may be shared with the adjacent intestine. The mucosal lining is always representative of some part of the alimentary tract, however remote from the site of attachment of the duplication. The presence of ectopic gastric mucosa, particularly in tubular duplications having a communication with the normal intestine, exposes the mucosa at the neck of the duplication to the risk of peptic ulceration with the possible complications of haemorrhage and/or perforation.

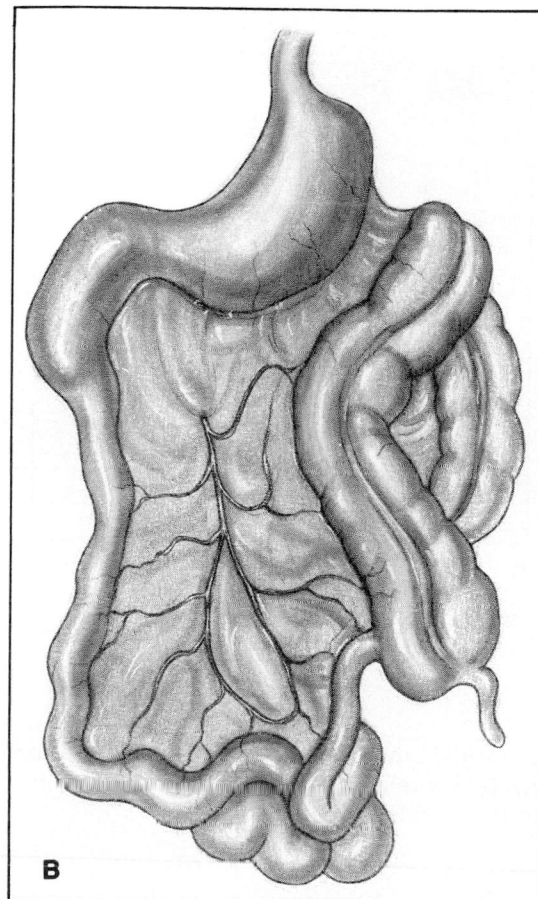

B

Figure 40–31. B. Repositioning of the bowel into the nonrotated position with the duodenum running straight downward on the right of the abdomen and the caecum lying in the left hypochondrium. Note the wide-base of mesentery. (*Source: From Ellis H: Intestinal Obstruction. New York: Appleton-Century-Crofts, 1982, p 122, with permission.*)

Embryology

Three theories regarding the embryogenesis of intestinal diverticuli have attracted the most attention (Vaage and Knutrud, 1974).

Persistence of Transitory Diverticuli. Lewis and Thyng, in 1907, observed outpouchings of the developing foetal intestine between the sixth and eighth weeks of intrauterine life. They postulated that remnants of these diverticuli may persist between the leaves of the mes-

entery or in the bowel wall itself and give rise to duplication cysts.

Errors of Recanalisation of Epithelial Plugs. This theory is based on the hypothesis that various portions of the alimentary tract, chiefly the duodenum, become completely occluded by epithelial proliferation between the fifth and eighth weeks of foetal development (Bremer, 1944). Failure of the normal process of recanalisation by coalescence of vacuoles could conceivably result in the formation of duplication cysts. There is no convincing evidence to support the occlusion theory in any part of the GI tract; even if this theory were operative it fails to explain why duplications are virtually restricted to the mesenteric aspect of the intestine.

Traction Between Adhering Neural Tube Ectoderm and Gut Endoderm. In 1954, Fallon et al proposed that duplications may result from failure of normal separation, during the fourth week of development, of the gut endoderm and the neural tube ectoderm. These two germ cell layers are normally separated by the intervening notochordal mesoderm layer which will eventually form the vertebral column. Should complete separation of these two germ cell layers fail to occur, a cord of cells from the dorsal aspect of the developing gut will be pulled backward toward the developing vertebral column. If the attachment breaks at both ends, a duplication cyst will develop. If the attachment only separates at the notochordal end but remains patent at the gut end, a tubular duplication forms (Fig. 40–32). Persistence of the attachment at both ends results in an anterior spina bifida or split vertebra, in association with either type of duplication (Bentley and Smith, 1960). The frequency of vertebral anomalies with all types of duplications was first recognised by Beardmore and Wiglesworth in 1958.

Clinical Manifestations

The main presenting symptoms consist of vomiting, abdominal pain, and rectal bleeding. An abdominal mass may be palpable, especially in the cystic type. The range of symptoms will vary according to the site of the attachment and the nature of the diverticulum.

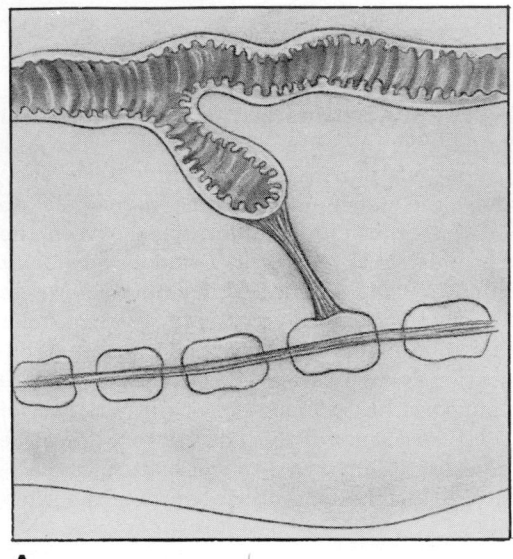 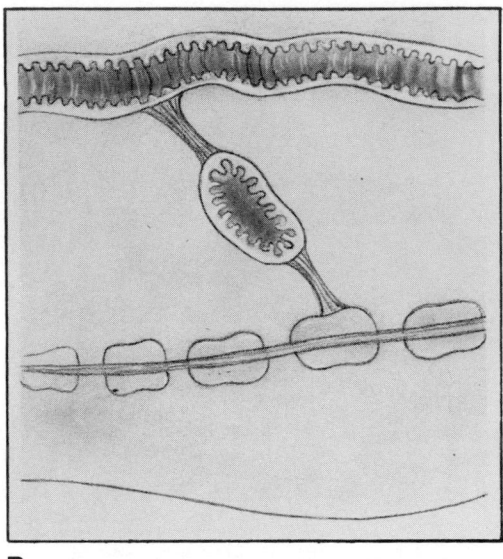

A   **B**

Figure 40–32. Neurenteric theory for the development of duplications. **A.** Posterior traction without separation resulting in tubular duplication. **B.** Separation from the developing intestine forming a cystic duplication.

Site. The frequency with which the different parts of the intestine are affected are as follows:

Stomach	6 percent
Duodenum	7 percent
Small bowel	63 percent
Colon	17 percent
Rectum	7 percent

With reference to the small bowel, ileal duplications are far more common than lesions in the jejunum.

Age. The majority of duplications present before 2 years of age and many occur within the neonatal period.

Type. Cystic duplications outnumber tubular lesions by approximately 9 to 1. Symptoms most often associated with the former type result from intestinal obstruction due to compression of the adjacent bowel. Pain, haemorrhage, and perforation secondary to peptic ulceration due to heterotopic gastric mucosa constitute the chief clinical presentation of the tubular duplications.

Rare Presentations. Volvulus with gangrene, intussusception, especially in the small intra-mural ileal duplication, and entrapment of an ingested foreign body in a tubular lesion are unusual presentations.

Variation of Symptoms According to Location

STOMACH. Large cystic duplications may remain asymptomatic or may be discovered as a result of abdominal distension and a palpable mass. (Bartels, 1967; Parker et al, 1972; Pruksapong, 1979). Smaller cysts located near the pylorus cause gastric outlet obstruction and may mimic the syndrome of hypertrophic pyloric stenosis.

DUODENUM. The lesions are invariably cystic and are situated within the convexity of the C-loop of duodenum partially embedded in the pancreas. Obstruction of the duodenum is the most common presentation, but perforation may occur occasionally (Soper and Selke, 1970).

SMALL INTESTINE. Large cystic duplications tend to obstruct the lumen of the adjacent intestine and produce symptoms of intestinal obstruction. These lesions usually present in early infancy, with an associated palpable abdominal mass (Grosfeld et al, 1970). Occasionally, large cysts

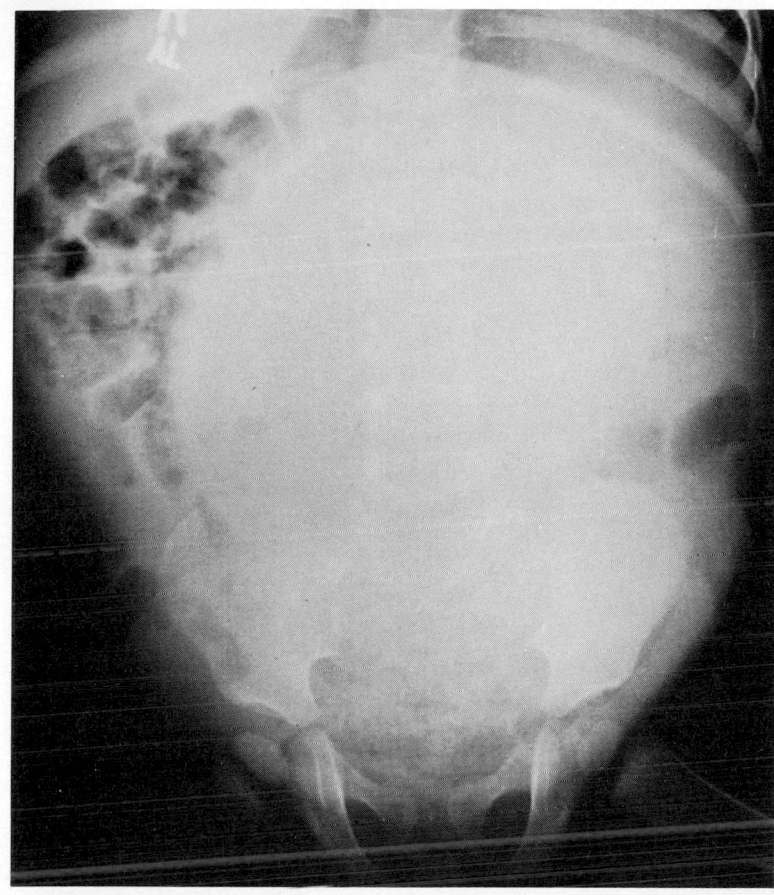

Figure 40–33. Plain abdominal radiograph in a large cystic duplication showing displacement of the intestine by a large radiopaque mass.

may remain asymptomatic and may only be discovered on routine physical examination. Smaller cysts may produce an intussusception or cause a volvulus.

The extent of tubular duplications varies from a few millimetres to over 100 cm or more. Communication may be at both ends but a single caudal opening is most common. Symptoms result from peptic ulceration, similar to that found in Meckel's diverticula, due to the presence of ectopic gastric mucosa. The ulcer is situated at the interface between the gastric and small intestinal mucosa and causes pain, haemorrhage, or may perforate, resulting in generalised peritonitis.

COLON AND RECTUM. Cystic duplications in this part of the intestine are most commonly located in the retrorectal or presacral space and produce symptoms by partially occluding the rectum. These cysts must be differentiated from sacrococcygeal teratomas and anterior menin-

gocoeles. Tubular duplications are more common and can occur anywhere along the length of the colon, but most often occur as duplications of the hindgut, including the anus, and may be associated with double external genitalia (Ravitch, 1953; Smith, 1969; Soper, 1968).

Diagnostic Studies

In addition to the features of intestinal obstruction, the plain abdominal x-ray in large cystic duplications will reveal a radiolucent, space-occupying lesion (Fig. 40–33). Barium contrast studies may also reveal partial obstruction of the involved segment of intestine, particularly the duodenum and retrorectal areas (Fig. 40–34). Ultrasound scan is invaluable in the diagnosis of cystic lesions (Fig. 40–35). Radioisotope scans using technetium-99 may assist in localising ectopic gastric mucosa (Fig. 40–36).

The detection of vertebral anomalies, such as split vertebra, missing hemivertebra, espe-

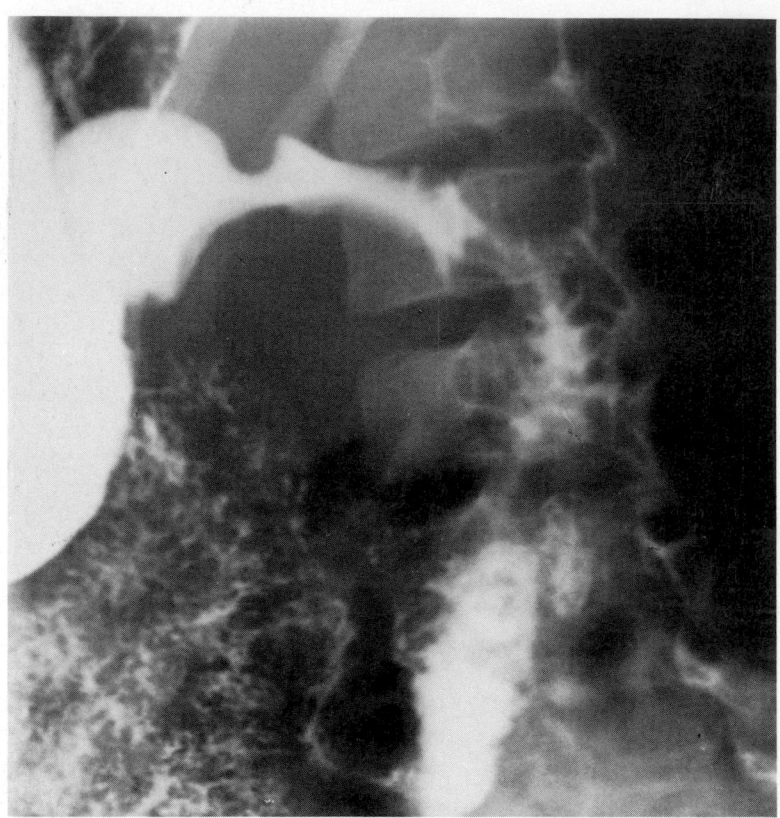

Figure 40–34. Barium contrast study of a duodenal duplication cyst showing widening and posterior displacement of the duodenal C-loop.

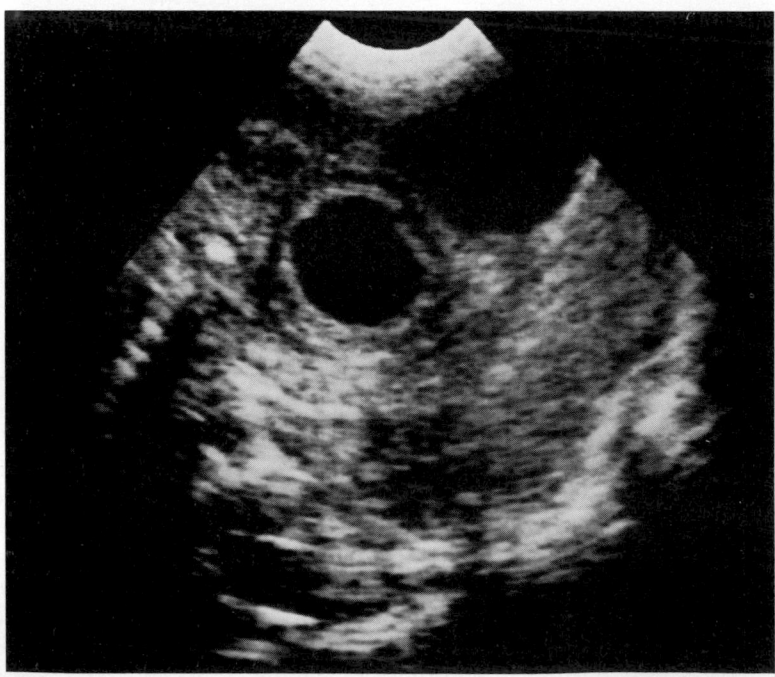

Figure 40–35. Ultrasound scan of a gastric duplication cyst showing a cystic lesion with a well-developed muscular wall.

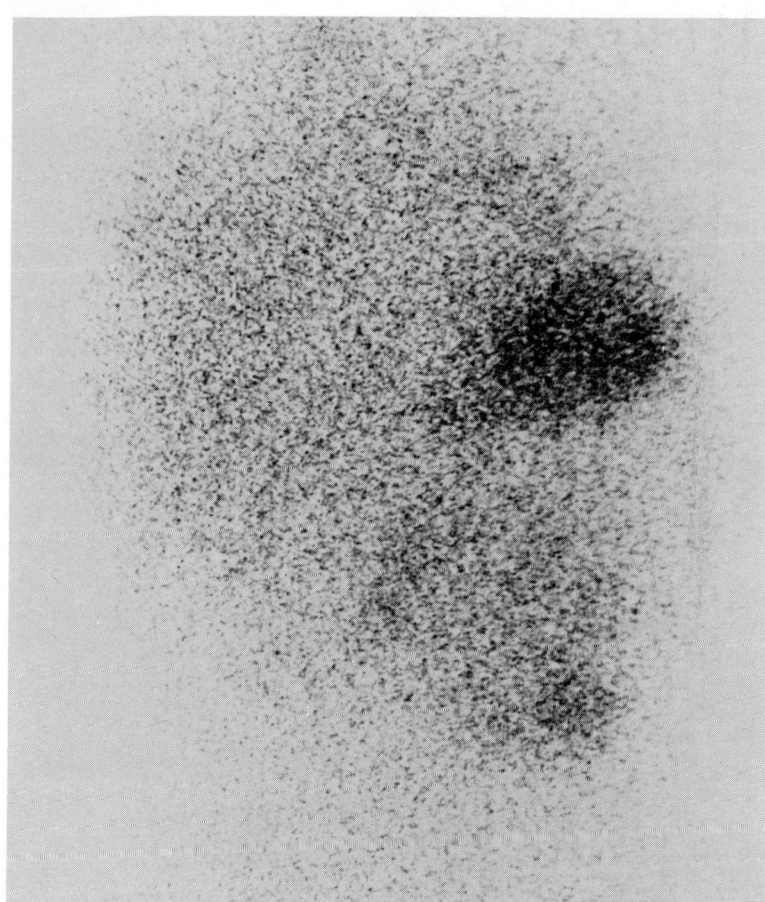

Figure 40–36. Technetium-99 scan showing abnormal uptake of radioactive material in the ectopic gastric mucosa of a duplication situated inferior to the well-defined gastric uptake.

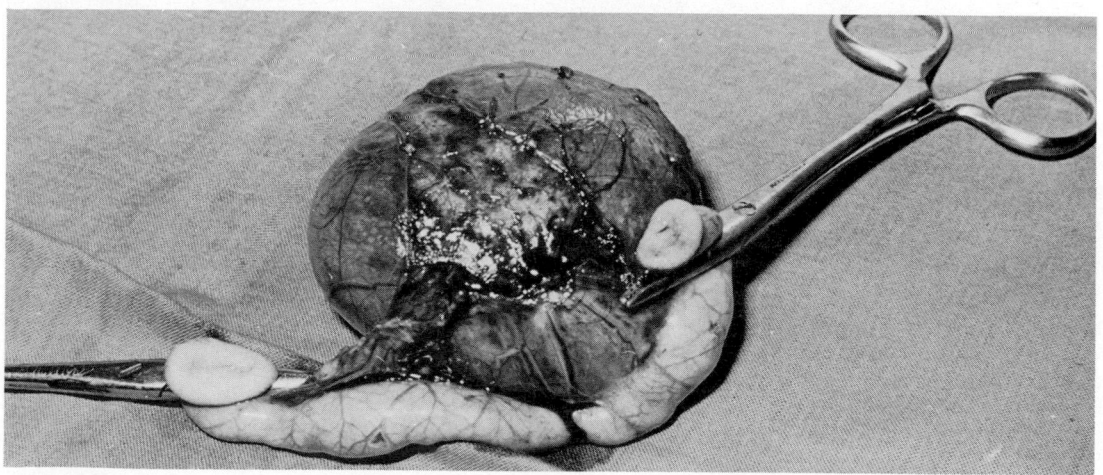

Figure 40–37. Resected specimen in a case of cystic duplication of the small intestine.

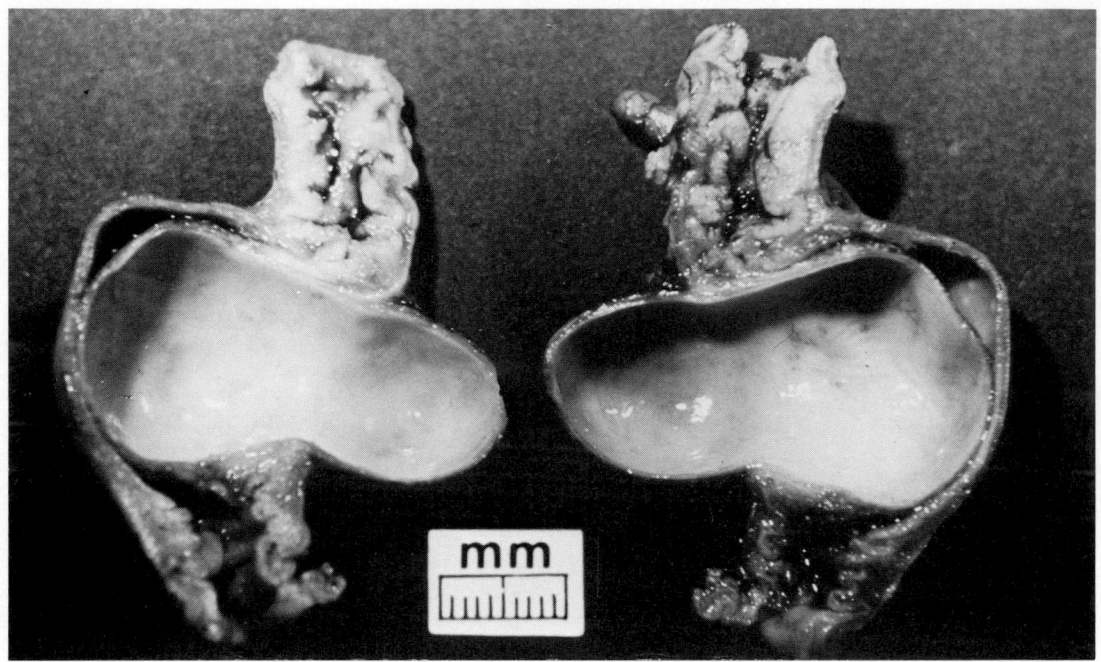

Figure 40–38. Duplication cyst of the small intestine impinging upon the lumen of the adjacent intestine.

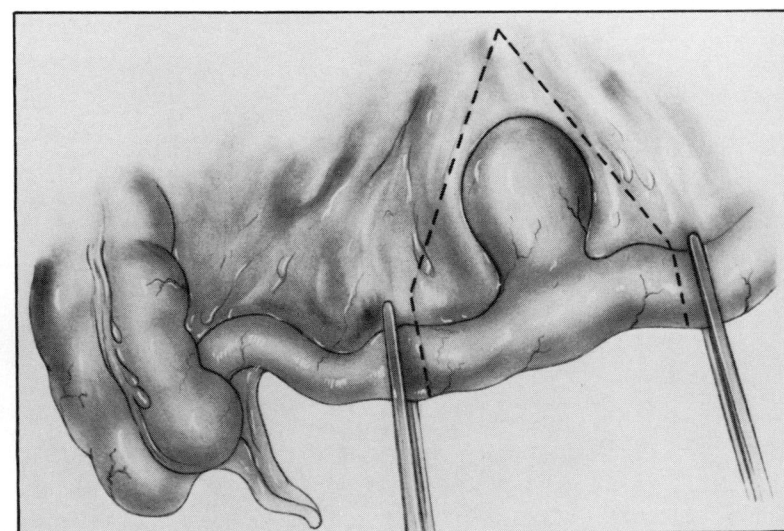

Figure 40–39. Operative technique for correction of duplications. **A.** Resection of cyst en bloc with adjacent intestine.

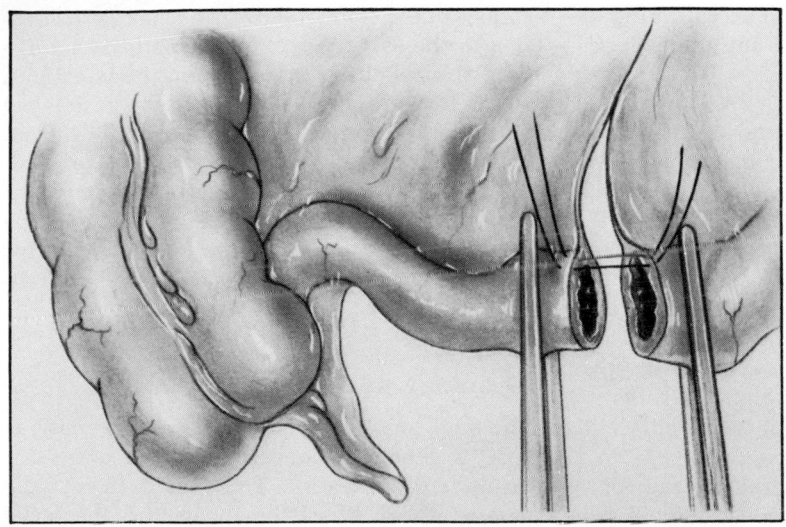

Figure 40–39. B. End-to-end seromuscular anastomosis with interrupted sutures.

cially in the thoracic region, should alert the clinician to the possibility of an intestinal or thoracic duplication.

Treatment

Cystic Duplications

In most cases these can be totally excised together with the involved segment of intestine and a wedge of the mesentery (Figs. 40–37 and 40–38). Bowel continuity is restored by an end-to-end single layer seromuscular anastomosis (Fig. 40–39). This procedure is not applicable in situations in which excision would endanger adjacent structures, for example, the duodenum. The most widely practiced treatment of duodenal cysts is to marsupialise the cyst into the duodenum via an anastomosis in the com-

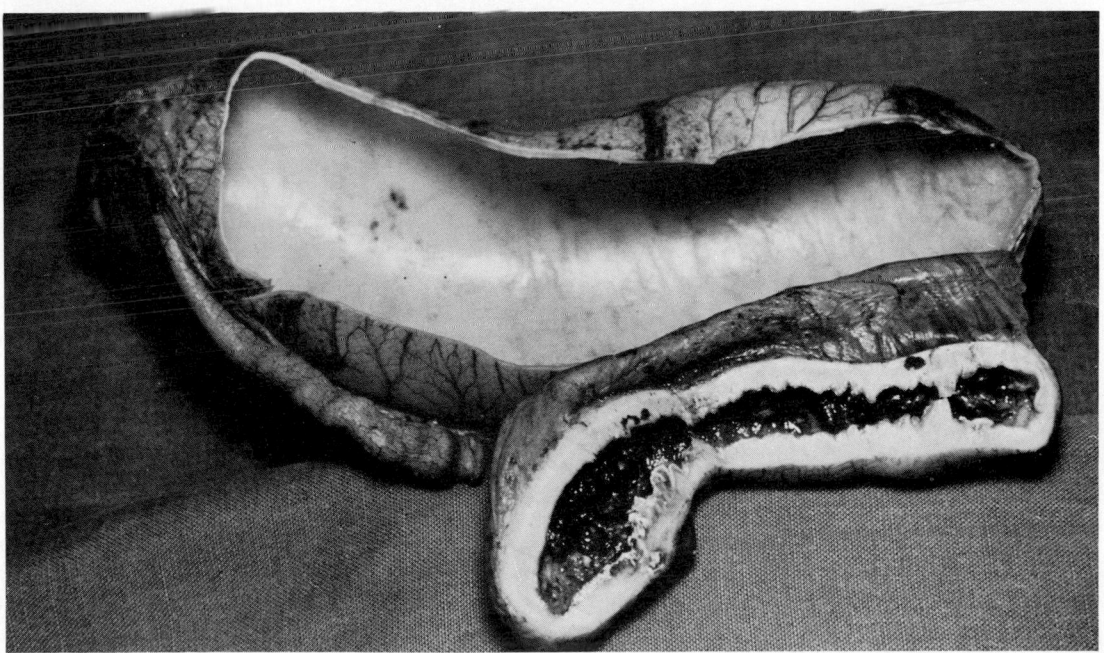

Figure 40–40. Operative specimen of a tubular duplication of the ileum.

mon wall. Alternatively, the mucosal lining of the cyst wall may be stripped out and excised.

Tubular Duplications

If the attached segment of intestine is not too extensive, the best method of management is total excision of the tubular duplication and end-to-end anastomosis of the bowel ends (Fig. 40–40). An alternative method of treatment, especially where long segments of bowel are involved, is to strip out the mucosal lining of the duplication, leaving the seromuscular layer intact. It is essential to ensure that all ectopic gastric mucosa is excised and that the remaining duplication drains freely into the adjacent intestine.

Special attention is required for the combined thoracoabdominal duplications. These consist of cystic or tubular posterior mediastinal thoracic duplications that are separate from the oesophagus or share a common wall with the oesophagus but do not communicate with its lumen. They may communicate via a narrow tube-like extension passing through the diaphragm or the oesophageal hiatus and continuing posterior to the stomach and pancreas with the duodenum or upper jejunum. Complete excision of these cysts requires a combined thoracoabdominal approach.

NECROTISING ENTEROCOLITIS

This is a relatively recently documented entity, affecting mainly premature infants or term infants who have experienced severe perinatal stress. It has emerged as the most common surgical emergency in the neonatal period, affecting between 2 and 5 percent of all neonates admitted to intensive or special care units.

Historical Review

Although the disease remained unnamed until the late 1950s, the description by Siebold in 1825 of a premature infant who died on the second day of life of a perforation of the stomach is probably the first recorded case of necrotising enterocolitis (NEC). In 1931, Thelander reviewed the literature of perforation involving the GI tract. A total of 84 of 85 recorded infants died, surgery having only occasionally been attempted. The first lead on the trail towards the recognition of NEC was the description of perfo-

rations of the colon following exchange transfusion in the early 1950s. NEC emerged as a distinct clinical entity in Europe in the late 1950s but its appearance in the Americas was delayed for a further decade. As recently as 1967 (Touloukian et al), it carried a mortality rate exceeding 70 percent, but with a better appreciation of the pathogenesis, early recognition, and the prompt institution of effective conservative treatment, the mortality has decreased dramatically.

Aetiology and Pathogenesis

The final common event in the pathogenesis of NEC is generally thought to be an ischaemic insult to the intestine. This results in mucosal damage that allows the invasion of bacterial flora that normally colonises the lumen of the intestines. Lloyd (1969) postulated that the normal response to hypoxia in the newborn was similar to the diving response of certain mammals in whom the cerebral circulation was protected at the expense of less vital organs such as the intestine. Touloukian et al (1972) confirmed a dramatic reduction in mesenteric blood flow in response to asphyxia in the newborn piglet. Barlow and Santulli (1975) were able to provoke bloody diarrhoea in neonatal rats subjected to profound asphyxia and in addition showed a protective effect of breast milk. The protective effect, originally thought to be due to immunoglobulin A (IgA), was eventually ascribed to macrophages present in breast milk (Barlow et al, 1974).

A wide variety of predisposing risk factors have been implicated in the aetiology of NEC. These include birth asphyxia, polycythaemia, catheterisation of the umbilical artery, respiratory distress syndrome, exchange transfusion (Corkery et al, 1968), and congenital cardiac disease. In a large prospective study, Kliegman et al (1982) were unable to demonstrate statistical significance to any of the perinatal risk factors listed above in a series of 48 infants with NEC compared with 553 low-birth-weight controls.

Clustering of cases of NEC and outbreaks of the condition in epidemic proportion in some institutions have suggested a primary infectious origin. Lawrence et al (1982) proposed that the environment in the neonatal intensive care unit delays normal colonisation of the intestine and allows colonisation with one or a few bacterial strains to occur without competitive inhibition from other strains. The immature intestine is able to absorb macromolecules intact, especially in the distal ileum, and toxic products from proliferating bacteria are able to produce mucosal damage following absorption. Numerous bacteria have received attention but the clostridial species has been most extensively studied. As yet, no direct evidence exists to implicate *Clostridia* infection with NEC. Other bacteria that have been implicated include *Escherichia coli,* streptococci, staphylococci, *Pseudomonas, Salmonella, Klebsiella,* and *Aerobacter.*

Pathology

This condition may affect any part of the GI tract, but the most frequently affected sites are the terminal ileum and the colon. The lesions in the affected part vary from a mild inflammatory reaction to frank gangrene with full-thickness necrosis and perforation. Subserosal gas bubbles involving long segments of intestine may be visible. Occasionally, the entire small and large intestine is affected. The antimesenteric borders of the intestine are the most severely affected (Benirschke, 1975).

Microscopically, there is an ischaemic necrosis of the mucosa with ulceration, haemorrhage, and oedema. The degree of inflammatory cell infiltrate is variable. Gas bubbles in the submucosa and subserosa may be strikingly evident and these are responsible for the classical pneumatosis intestinalis, which is the hallmark of the radiologic diagnosis of the condition.

Clinical Manifestations

The condition most commonly affects the stressed premature infant (Mizrahi et al, 1965; Rossier et al, 1959), but the healthy full-term infant is not immune. The condition is well documented in the postoperative period in neonates undergoing cardiac or abdominal surgery. Symptoms most frequently develop between the second and tenth day of life. The majority of infants have received oral feeds prior to the onset of NEC, formula feeds more often than breast feeds, but a small proportion of affected infants had never been fed prior to the onset of NEC.

The clinical features comprise one or a combination of the following:

1. Reluctance to feed. This is the earliest sign of NEC and should lead to prompt investigation and treatment.
2. Abdominal distension due to paralytic ileus develops in 90 percent of patients.
3. Passage of blood and mucus in the stool occurs in over 50 percent of cases but the blood may only be detected by chemical or microscopic examination.
4. Vomiting occurs in over 70 percent of patients. Initially the vomitus contains ingested food only, but as the condition progresses, bilious vomiting develops.
5. Hypothermia.
6. Apnoeic attacks.

Physical examination of the abdomen reveals the presence of the abdominal distension (Fig. 40–41); as the disease process progresses, erythema and oedema of the abdominal wall, initially confined to the periumbilical region, develop. These signs signify the presence of imminent gangrene of the intestine with or without perforation and peritonitis. Abdominal tenderness is usually a late feature. Where the disease process is confined to a specific area, usually the ileocaecal or sigmoid regions, a palpable mass representing matted loops of intestine or local abscess formation, may be detected.

Diagnostic Studies

Laboratory Investigations

The occurrence of leucocytosis is variable; a low absolute granulocyte count is a poor prognostic indicator. Serial platelet counts are most informative. Thrombocytopenia is due to a combination of increased peripheral destruction and disseminated intravascular coagulation secondary to gram-negative septicaemia. Acid–base disturbances consist of a metabolic acidosis combined with a respiratory component due either to preexisting respiratory distress syndrome, or to respiratory embarrassment developing secondary to the NEC. The infants are also prone to develop hypoglycaemia.

Radiologic Examinations

Pneumatosis intestinalis in the form of intramural gas bubbles or of linear outline of the bowel wall is diagnostic of NEC (Fig. 40–42). It occurs in 70 to 80 percent of cases. Gas in the portal venous system (Fig. 40–43) is an omi-

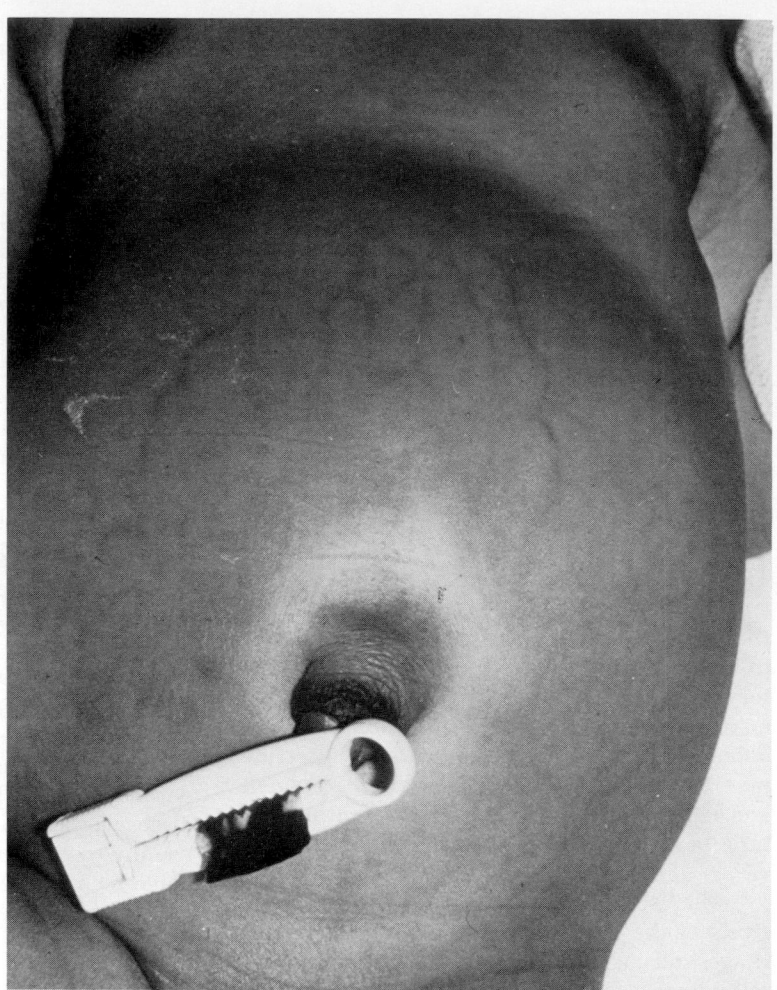

Figure 40–41. Abdominal distension with erythema and oedema of the anterior abdominal wall in an infant with established necrotising enterocolitis.

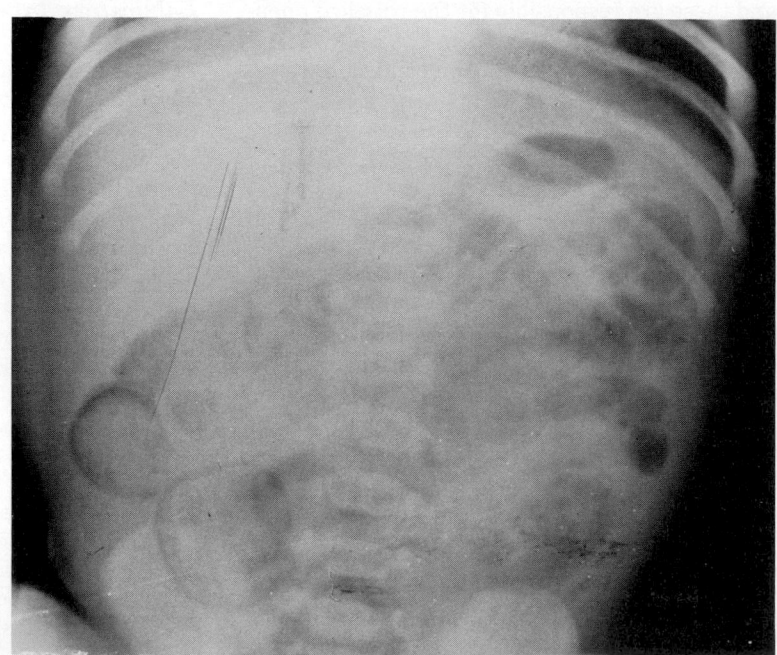

Figure 40–42. Plain abdominal radiograph in necrotising enterocolitis showing classical pneumatosis intestinalis most obvious in the right lower quadrant.

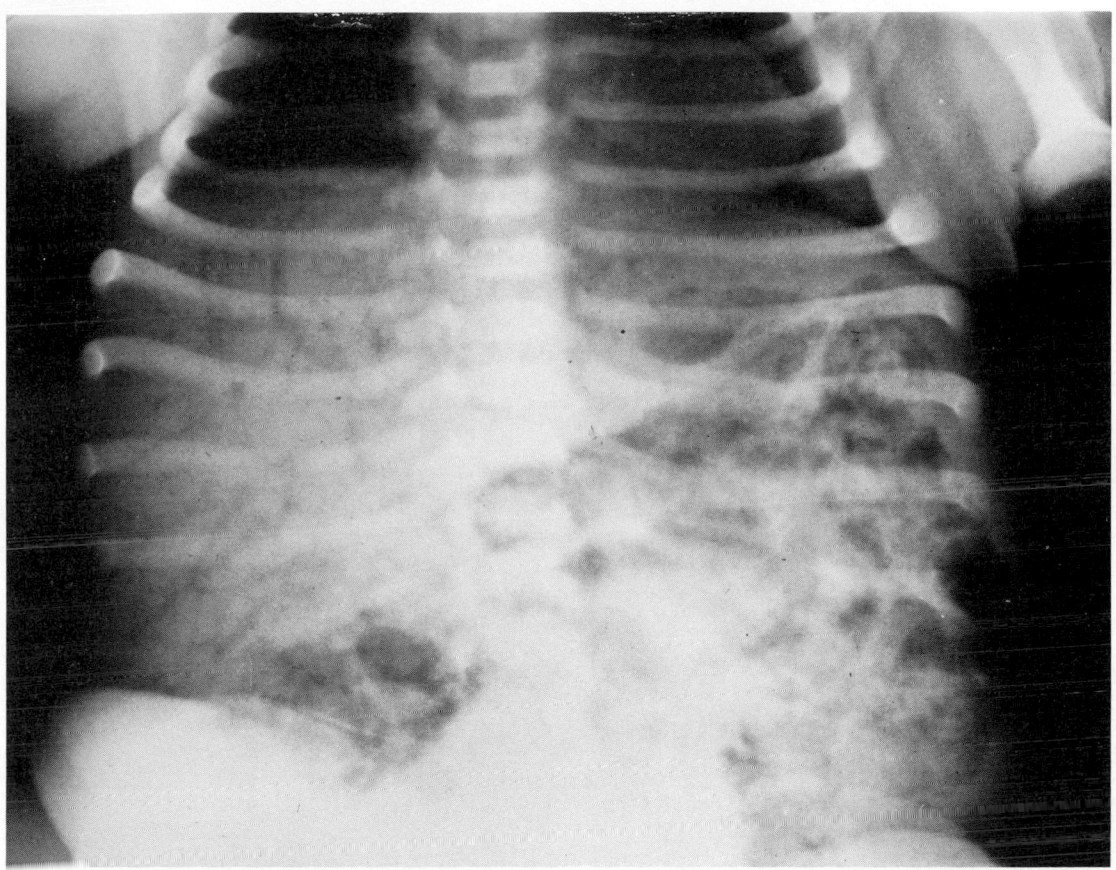

Figure 40–43. Abdominal radiograph showing extensive gas in the portal venous system in an infant with advanced necrotising enterocolitis.

nous sign, formerly considered to be associated with an invariably fatal outcome, but with early intensive treatment this is no longer the case. Pneumoperitoneum signifies an intestinal perforation (Fig. 40–44). Other nonspecific radiologic signs include dilated loops of intestine with air–fluid levels, separation of bowel loops, indicating the presence of intramural oedema or free peritoneal fluid and toxic dilatation of the colon and the static intestinal loop.

Treatment

The improved prognosis of infants with NEC is directly attributable to early diagnosis and prompt aggressive medical therapy. The importance of repeated clinical examinations and serial laboratory investigations (haemoglobin, leucocyte and platelet counts, serum electrolytes, and acid–base status) and serial plain erect and supine abdominal radiographs in as-

sessing the progress of the disease cannot be overemphasised. Improvement of these parameters indicates a good response to medical therapy, whereas deterioration signifies the failure of medical management and progression of the disease process.

Medical Management

1. Complete cessation of oral intake for a minimum of 10 to 14 days. Too early reintroduction of oral feeds may result in a recurrence of the NEC.
2. Nasogastric decompression with intravenous replacement of aspirated content with 0.9 percent saline plus potassium chloride 20 mmol/L volume for volume.
3. Total parenteral nutrition for at least 10 to 14 days, that is, during the period of no oral feeding.
4. Parenteral antibiotics—penicillin, gentamicin, and metronidazole. The results of bacte-

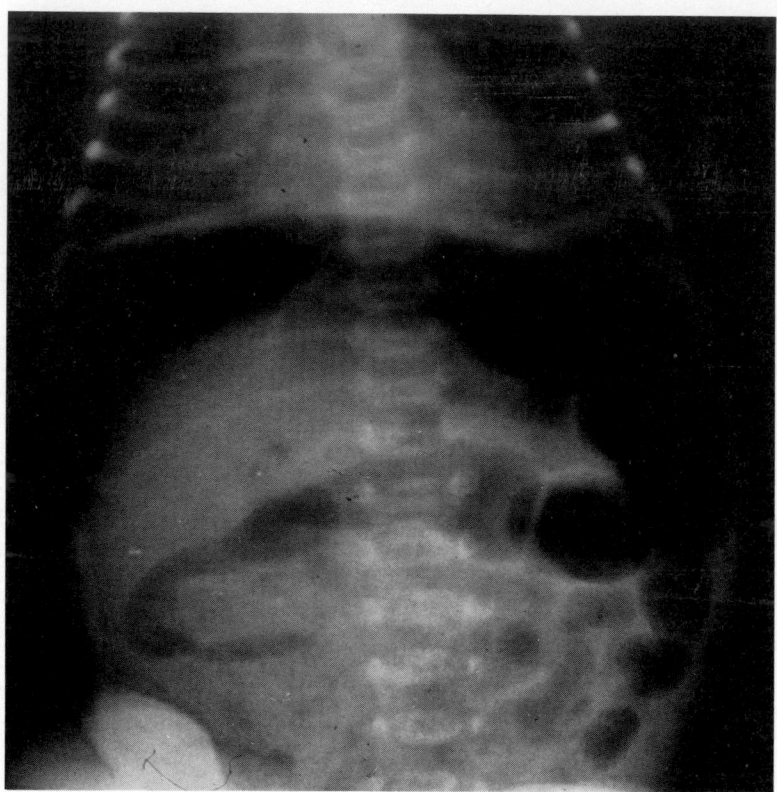

Figure 40–44. Erect abdominal radiograph showing marked pneumoperitoneum indicating perforation in an infant with necrotising enterocolitis.

riologic investigations of blood, stool, and gastric aspirate may dictate a change in antibiotic regimen.

Indications for Surgical Intervention

Absolute Indications

1. Pneumoperitoneum indicates a free perforation of the intestine. Unfortunately this radiologic sign is only present in 50 to 60 percent of cases with established perforations.
2. Intestinal obstruction usually develops as a result of stricture formation in those infants responding to conservative treatment. These ischaemic strictures develop in 15 to 20 percent of infants treated medically (Fig. 40–45).
3. Profuse lower intestinal haemorrhage.

Relative Indications

1. Failure to respond to conservative measures or frank clinical deterioration.
2. Persistent abdominal tenderness.
3. Oedema or erythema of the anterior abdominal wall.

4. The presence of a palpable abdominal mass.
5. A "static loop" on abdominal radiograph.
6. Persistent acidosis.
7. Deteriorating thrombocytopenia.

It is the combination of the relative parameters rather than one individual feature that indicates a surgical approach to the problem (Kosloske et al, 1980).

Abdominal paracentesis has been recommended to establish the diagnosis of intestinal gangrene in the critically ill infant who may fail to demonstrate the clinical features of peritonitis and where pneumoperitoneum is not present. A positive tap is where brown fluid and/or bacteria on Gram smear are obtained with a volume of fluid in excess of 0.5 ml.

Surgical Management

Rapid intensive resuscitation should be carried out to restore the circulating blood volume, correct acid–base and electrolyte imbalances, and improve hypothermia and hypoglycaemia.

At laparotomy via a generous upper abdominal, transverse muscle-cutting incision, the en-

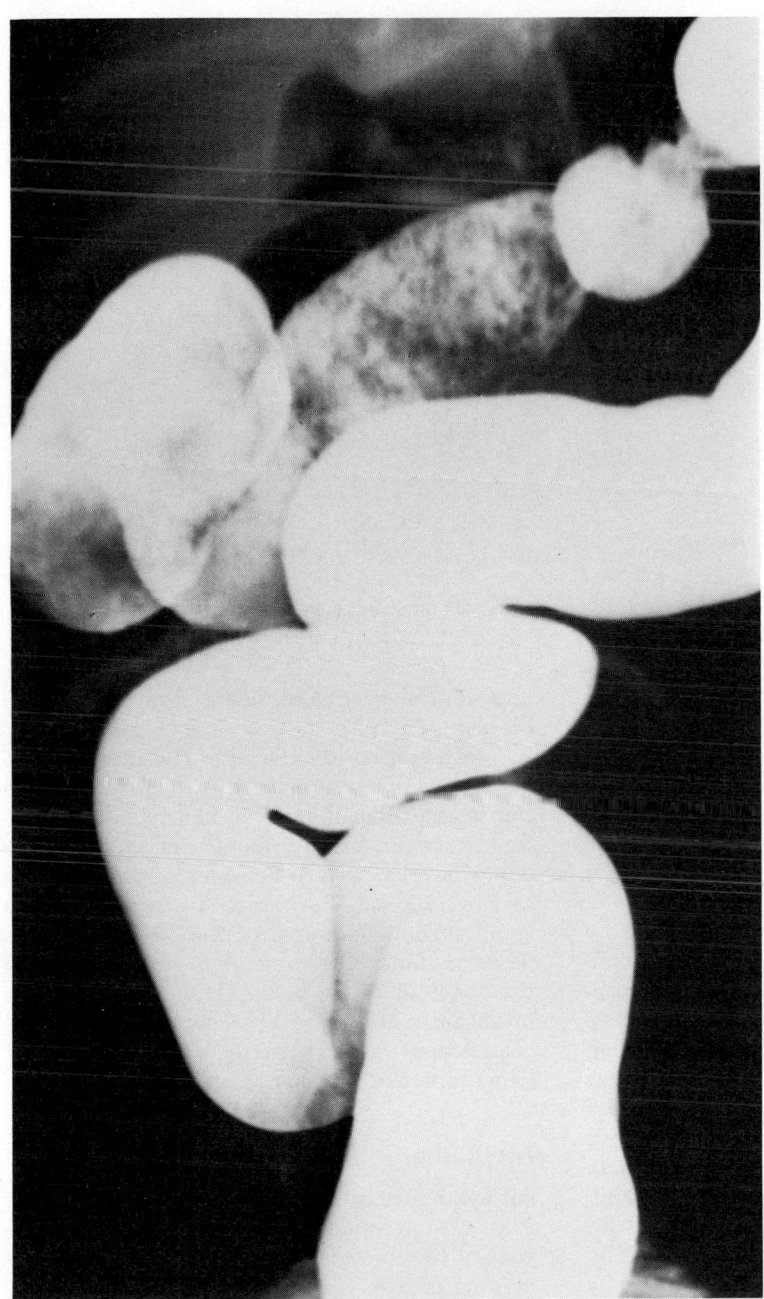

Figure 40–45. Barium enema examination performed in the recovery phase of necrotising enterocolitis showing stricture formation in the left transverse colon.

tire intestine must be thoroughly assessed. All frankly gangrenous or perforated intestine is resected and the bowel ends are exteriorised, either separately or as a double-barrel enterostomy (Fig. 40–46). No attempt is made to restore intestinal continuity by primary anastomosis in the acute phase of the disease, as there is an appreciable incidence of anastomotic leaks or

stricture formation. Where very extensive involvement is present, it may be necessary after resection of obviously necrotic intestine to resort to a second-look laparotomy 24 hours after the primary procedure in an attempt to conserve the maximum length of viable intestine.

Restoration of bowel continuity is delayed until the infant has fully recovered and is in

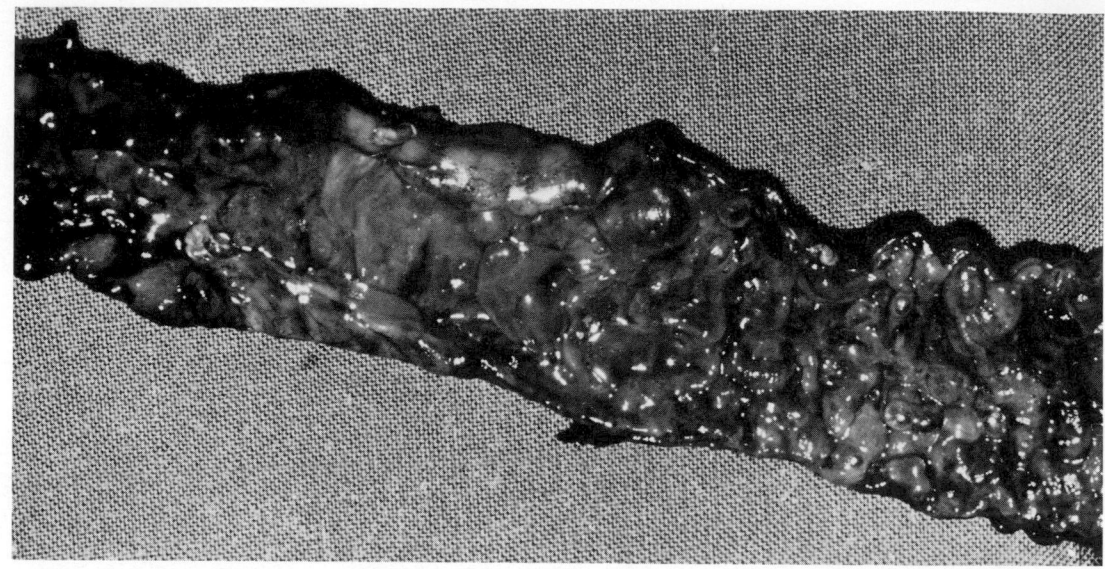

Figure 40–46. Resected colon in necrotising enterocolitis showing extensive ulceration and oedema of the mucosa surface.

positive nitrogen balance. This may vary in individual cases from 6 weeks to 6 months.

INTUSSUSCEPTION IN CHILDHOOD

Historical Review

Intestinal invagination was first described by Barbette in 1692. In 1789, John Hunter demonstrated the pathologic specimen from a 9-month-old infant who died of an intussusception. Up to the mid-nineteenth century, intussusception was almost always fatal, operative therapy was rarely employed, and the main methods of treatment consisted of insufflating the rectum with air introduced by bellows or by attempting to reposition the intestine by means of a wand. The first successful operative reduction of an intussusception in an infant was carried out by Jonathan Hutchinson in 1871. Disillusioned by the high operative mortality rate, Hirschsprung introduced a plan of controlled hydrostatic pressure reduction of intussusception in 1876. By 1905, he was able to publish the results of 107 personally treated cases; the overall success rate was 65 percent. The use of radiology in the diagnosis of intussusception was first suggested by Ladd in 1913. The use of contrast enema to effect reduction of an intussusception was reported simultaneously by Paeliquen in France, Olsson

and Pallin in Scandinavia, and Retan and Stephens in 1927.

Intussusception refers to the invagination of one part of the intestine into itself. The condition classically affects well-nourished male infants between 6 and 9 months of age who suddenly develop severe episodes of excruciating abdominal colic. The clinical picture progresses rapidly from abdominal pain to vomiting to the passage of blood and mucus in the stool within the space of a few hours. Left untreated, the infant ultimately develops a complete intestinal obstruction that eventually leads to intestinal gangrene, perforation, peritonitis, and death.

Incidence

Although intussusception may occur at any age, it is most frequently encountered in the first year of life, more specifically between 6 and 9 months of age. It is known to occur in utero, where it has been shown to be the cause of an intestinal atresia. It occasionally presents in the neonatal period, when it is almost invariably caused by an identifiable leading point, for example, duplication, Meckel's diverticulum, tumour, and so on. Postoperative intussusception most frequently affects the small intestine and occurs more often than can be accounted for by mere chance. It has been described after resection of abdominal tumours, operations for

Hirschsprung's disease, anorectal anomalies, and liver tumours.

The overall incidence of intussusception in childhood ranges from 1.49 (MacMahon, 1955) cases per 1000 live births to 2.27 per 1000 live births (Ross et al, 1962).

Sex. A male preponderance in the order of 3:2 is a constant feature in most series.

Race. Although some studies indicate that intussusception may be more common in Caucasians, this has not been substantiated in the large series.

Season. Two peaks have been found, one in spring and summer, coinciding with a high incidence of gastroenteritis, and the other in midwinter during the high period of respiratory infections. There appears to be so much variation in peak periods in the reported series that no consistent pattern can be identified.

Nutrition. Although reputed to occur predominantly in overweight infants, recent series have shown that infants with intussusception are no better nourished than the general population and a significant number (25 percent) are frankly malnourished.

Aetiology

In approximately 5 percent of cases an identifiable leading point has been documented. This may consist of Meckel's diverticulum, polyp, small duplication cyst, ectopic pancreatic nodule, malignant tumour, or submucosal haemorrhage of Henoch–Schonlein purpura. In the remainder no leading point can be identified. In all patients undergoing operative intervention for intussusception, marked lymphadenopathy and hypertrophy of Peyer's patches in the distal ileum is found. Possible aetiologic factors incriminated as causing the lymphadenopathy include viral infections (adenovirus, Echo virus, enterovirus, etc.) (Ross et al, 1962) and allergic reactions to changes in diet. A history of a recent upper respiratory tract infection or diarrhoeal episodes has been elicited in about 20 percent of cases.

Pathogenesis

The intussusception is composed of two parts: (1) *the intussusceptum*—the invaginating por-

tion of the intestine; and (2) *the intussuscipiens*—the part of intestine containing the intussusceptum. The effects arising from the intussusception are two-fold:

1. Incomplete intestinal obstruction due to compression of the lumen of the intussusceptum by the surrounding intussuscipiens. This is directly responsible for the colicky abdominal pain so classic in intussusception.
2. Obstruction to the vascular supply to the intussusception as a result of the acute angulation of the vessels at the site of the invagination. This causes immediate congestion of the venous and lymphatic return and results in swelling of tissues. The mucosal cells become engorged with blood and mucus, produced by the goblet cells. Blood and mucus escape into the lumen of the intestine from the swollen engorged bowel and give rise to the so-called "red-currant jelly" content that may be evacuated per rectum or may be found on the examining finger after rectal examination. As venous congestion increases and arterial inflow continues, the tissue pressure builds up to a stage when further arterial inflow is impeded and necrosis and gangrene occurs.

Clinical Manifestations

Symptomatology

Abdominal Pain. The pain is classically colicky in nature, appears in paroxysms, and is particularly severe in intensity. The infant draws up the legs and becomes profoundly pallid during the episodes. Between attacks the infant may either be listless from exhaustion or behave entirely normally. Pain is a dominant feature in over 75 percent of cases.

Vomiting. Almost all patients with intussusception experience vomiting. Initially, the vomiting is reflex in nature and consists of gastric content. Later, the vomitus becomes bile-tinged as the effects of the intestinal obstructive element of the intussusception develop.

Blood in the Stool. At least two thirds of all patients pass blood and mucus in the stools. In some cases the blood appears early whereas in others it may be delayed for 1 or 2 days. The admixture of blood and mucus gives rise to the characteristic "red-currant jelly" appearance in the stools.

Defecation. No clear pattern is present. Most frequently the infant will have evacuated stool already present in the rectum at the onset of the intussusception. Occasionally, normal stools continue to be passed in the presence of an established intussusception, but in a small proportion of cases diarrhoea is present even after the onset of the intussusception.

Physical Findings

Between attacks of abdominal colic the patient may be quiet and apathetic, allowing examination to proceed unconcernedly. At other times the child is restless and irritable and will not lie still during examination.

Abdominal Mass. A mass, classically described as "sausage-shaped," is palpable in 85 percent of cases. Occasionally, the mass is only discovered on rectal examination. The abdomen is generally flat, flaccid, and nontender. The position of the mass will vary with the site and extent of the intussusception but in most cases it lies across the upper abdomen. An intussusception confined to the hepatic flexure of the colon may be difficult or impossible to palpate due to the overlying liver.

Rectal Examination. A mass previously undetected on abdominal palpation may be found in rectal examination, but generally those intussusceptions palpable on rectal examination are also palpable per abdomen. Blood and mucus will often be present on the examining finger following the the digital examination.

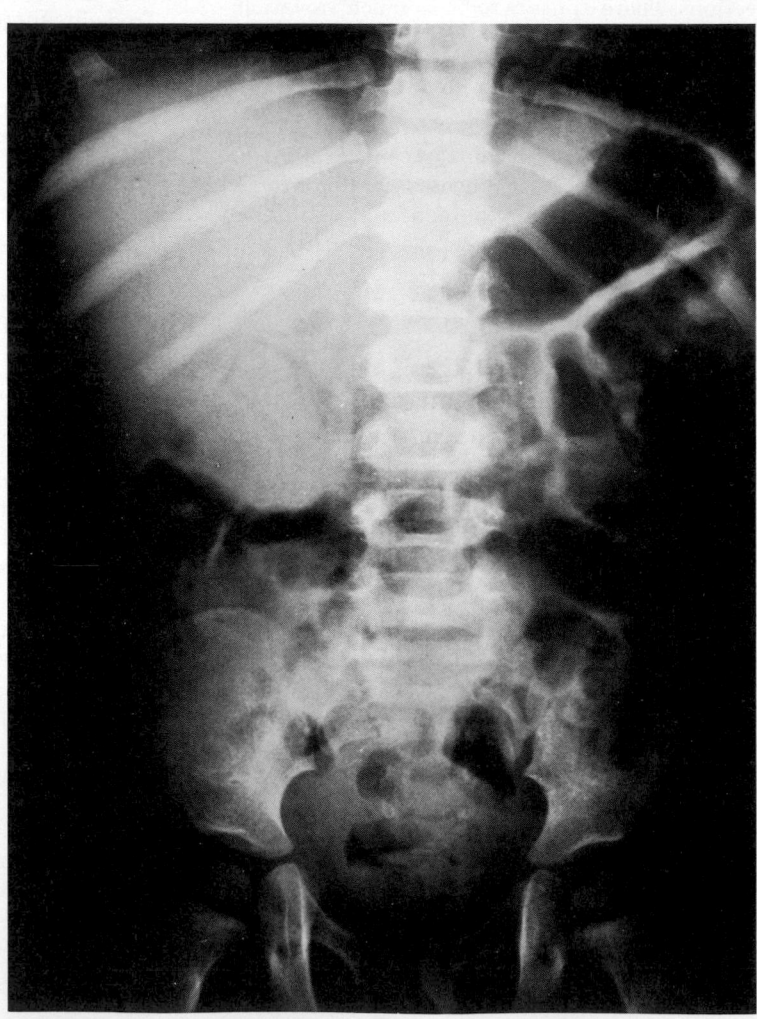

Figure 40–47. Plain abdominal radiograph showing the soft tissue mass in the right hypochondrium representing the head of the intussusception.

Other Physical Signs. These include pyrexia and dehydration, especially where there has been excessive vomiting or shock where the intussusception has become gangrenous. Overt signs of intestinal obstruction or peritonitis are features of delayed diagnosis and treatment.

Diagnostic Studies

In the majority (over 80 percent) of cases, the diagnosis is established on clinical examination by palpating the "sausage-shaped" abdominal mass. The diagnosis in the remaining cases may be made on radiologic examination. A soft-tissue mass may be seen on the plain abdominal x-ray (Fig. 40–47). The diagnostic features on barium enema examination include (1) obstruction to the free flow of barium proximally by the head of the intussusception, (2) a meniscus sign produced by barium outlining the smooth head of the intussusception, and (3) a "coiled-spring" appearance of barium diffusing between the two apposing layers of the intussusception within the intussuscipiens (Fig. 40–48).

Where the intussusception is confined to the small intestine, diagnosis by contrast enema is impossible. In these cases, and in particular in those developing in the postoperative period, diagnosis may only be established at laparotomy for prolonged postoperative "ileus."

Treatment

Irrespective of the method of treatment, all patients should be prepared as follows:

1. A nasogastric tube should be passed and the stomach evacuated of its content. The tube should be left on free drainage and aspirated at least hourly.
2. An intravenous infusion should be commenced and any fluid and electrolyte imbalance corrected.
3. A sample of blood should be sent for compatibility studies.

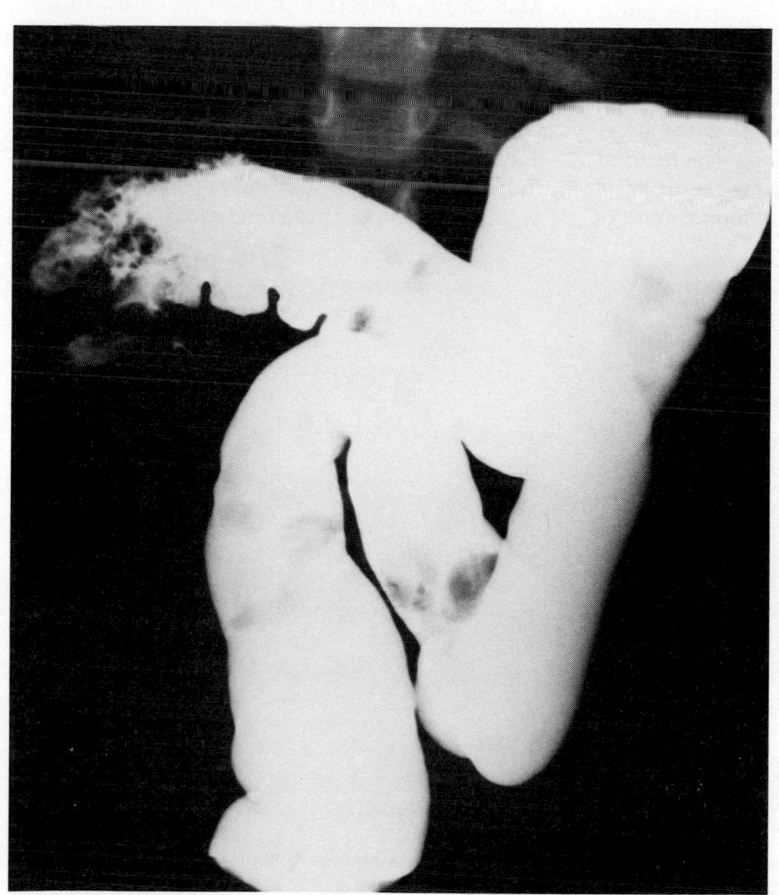

Figure 40–48. Barium enema examination showing hold-up of barium in the region of the hepatic flexure indicating the apex of the intussusception.

4. The operating theatre should be alerted. This will avoid unnecessary delay should hydrostatic reduction fail.

Hydrostatic Reduction

This is undoubtedly the treatment of choice for the uncomplicated case. The chief contraindications are the presence of peritonitis, complete intestinal obstruction, or a severely ill and shocked patient (Levick, 1970). Relative contraindications include those infants less than 1 month of age when a primary cause is very likely, a prolonged history, and repeated recurrences.

Technique. The hydrostatic reduction is more likely to succeed if the infant is well sedated and is not straining and evacuating the barium before a reasonable head of pressure can be achieved. A 1:3 barium sulphate in warm isotonic saline solution is used. A large-calibre rectal tube is inserted into the anal canal and the buttocks of the infant are firmly held together to prevent leakage of barium out of the anus. The reservoir of barium is raised to 90 to 120 cm above the patient and barium is allowed to flow freely into the distal bowel, screening the patient at frequent intervals to follow the progress of the contrast material. Once the head of the intussusception is reached, progress of the hydrostatic reduction is carefully monitored. As long as reduction is proceeding, pressure may be maintained, but failure of progress for longer than 5 minutes should be regarded as a danger sign. The pressure should be released and the barium syphoned off. After a short interval, a further attempt at hydrostatic reduction may be attempted.

Signs of successful hydrostatic reduction are:

1. Free reflux of contrast into a number of small-bowel loops after reduction of the intussusception.
2. Expulsion of faeces and flatus with the barium.
3. Disappearance of symptoms and of the palpable abdominal mass.
4. Postevacuation films confirming the disappearance of the intussusception.

Failure to achieve successful hydrostatic reduction is an absolute indication for urgent operative treatment. The success rate for hydrostatic reduction varies in different centres, but with careful selection of suitable cases, success rates of 60 to 70 percent should be achieved.

Operative Management

Laparotomy is performed via a right transverse abdominal muscle-cutting incision located either just above or just below the level of the umbilicus. Two or three fingers are inserted into

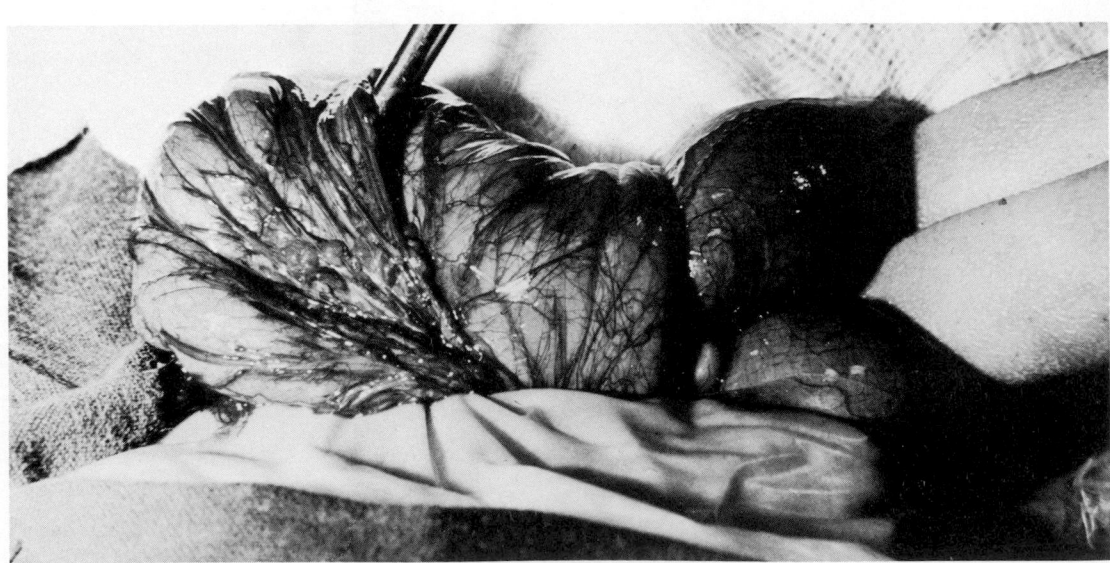

Figure 40–49. Operative appearance of an intussusception showing invagination of the small intestine into the colon (on the left in the photograph).

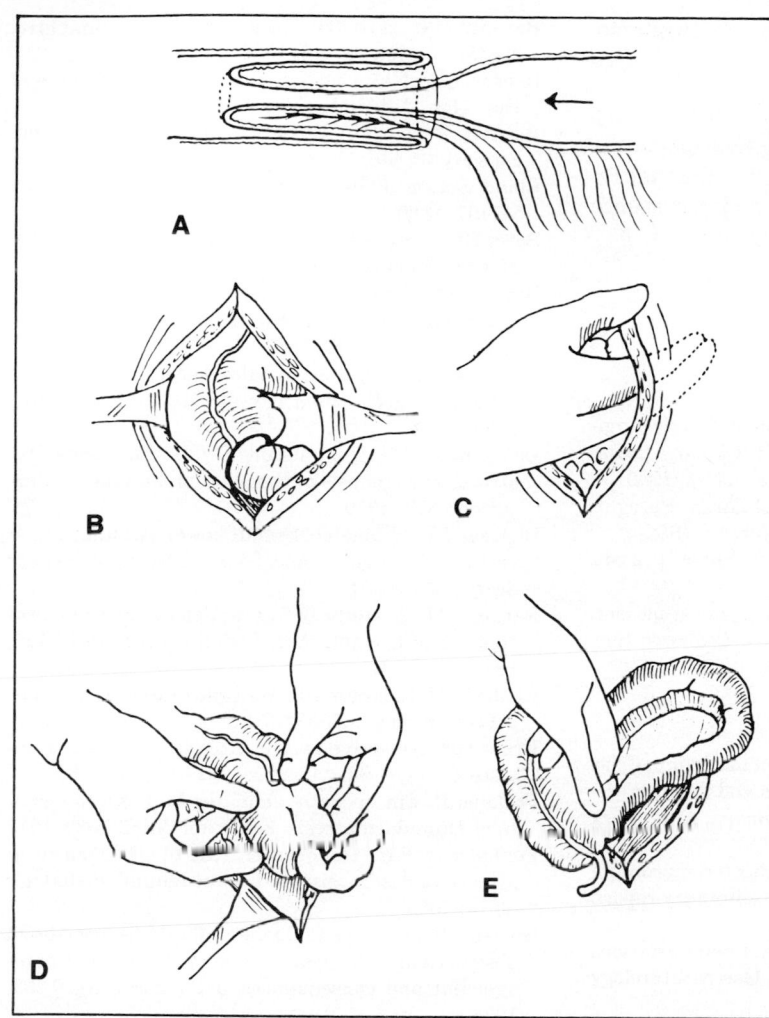

Figure 40–50. Manual reduction of an intussusception. **A.** Diagrammatic representation of intussusception. **B.** Laparotomy findings of the invagination of ileum into the colon. **C.** Manual reduction commencing inside the abdomen. **D.** Delivery of the intussusception into the incision. **E.** Final reduction of the intussusception.

the peritoneal cavity and the head of the intussusception is identified (Fig. 40–49). By gently squeezing the bowel immediately distal to the intussusception, the head of the intussusception is gradually reduced (Fig. 40–50) until a stage is reached when the involved bowel can be lifted into the wound without traumatising the intestine. For the usual ileocolic intussusception this manoeuvre can be achieved when the intussusception has been reduced back into the ascending colon or caecum. The residual few centimetres of the intussusception can now be fully reduced under direct vision. Warm moist swabs are placed over the exposed intestine and the vascularity assessed.

Manual reduction should be discontinued if there is failure of progress or when splitting of the serosal surface of the intussuscipiens occurs. The procedure is clearly not applicable in cases with a frankly gangrenous intussusception. Marked mesenteric lymphadenopathy is invariably present and should not be regarded as being the result of an infective aetiology. The appendix may be removed following manual reduction if the vascularity of the caecum is beyond doubt and if the involved bowel is not excessively oedematous.

Resection is necessary for the gangrenous intussusception, for the intussusception that cannot be reduced manually, and for definitive treatment of local primary lesions. Formal hemicolectomy is unnecessary, the least amount of bowel compatible with a safe anastomosis should be excised. Enterostomies are rarely required and a single layer end-to-end anastomosis should be performed.

Recurrence Rate

The risk of recurrence following hydrostatic reduction is 7 to 10 percent, that for manual reduction is less than 2 percent, and recurrence following resection is excessively rare.

BIBLIOGRAPHY

Neonatal Intestinal Obstruction

Coran AG: Nutritional support of the pediatric surgical patient, in Holder TM, Aschraft KW (eds): Pediatric Surgery. Philadelphia: WB Saunders, 1980

Filston HC: Surgical Problems in Children: Recognition and Referral. St. Louis: CV Mosby, 1982

Rickham PP, Lister J, et al: Neonatal Surgery, 2 edt. London: Butterworths, 1978

Rowe MI: Physiology of the pediatric surgical patient, in Holder TM, Aschraft KW (eds): Pediatric Surgery, Philadelphia: WB Saunders, 1980

Meconium Ileus

Bishop HC, Koop CE: Management of meconium ileus: Resection, Roux-en-Y anastomosis and ileostomy irrigation with pancreatic enzymes. Ann Surg 145:410, 1957

Noblett HR: Treatment of uncomplicated meconium ileus by Gastrografin enema: A preliminary report. J Pediatr Surg 4:190, 1961

Park RW, Grand RJ: Gastrointestinal manifestations of cystic fibrosis: A review. Gastroenterology 81:1143, 1981

Santulli TV, Blanc WA: Congenital atresia of the intestine: Pathogenesis and treatment. Ann Surg 154:939, 1961

Shwachman H: Gastrointestinal manifestations of cystic fibrosis. Ped Clin North Am 22:787, 1975

Inspissated Milk Syndrome

Cook RCM, Rickham PP: Neonatal intestinal obstruction due to milk curds. J Pediatr Surg 4:599, 1969

Cremin BJ, Smythe PM, et al: The radiological appearance of the "inspissated milk syndrome": A cause of intestinal obstruction in infants. Br J Radiol 43:856, 1970

Atresia and Stenosis

Abrams JS: Experimental intestinal atresia. Surgery 64:185, 1968

Astley R: Duodenal atresia with gas below the obstruction. Br J Radiol 42:351, 1969

Barnard CN, Louw JH: The genesis of intestinal atresia. Minn Med 39:745, 1956

Benson CD et al: Congenital atresia and stenosis of the colon. J Pediatr Surg 3:253, 1968

Bill AH, Pope WH: Congenital duodenal diaphragm. Surgery 35:486, 1954

Bland Sutton J: Imperforate ileum. Am J Med Sci 98:457, 1889

Boles ET, Vassy LE, et al: Atresia of the colon. J Pediatr Surg 11:69, 1976

Boyden EA, Cope JG, et al: Anatomy and embryology of congenital intrinsic obstruction of the duodenum. Am J Surg 114:190, 1967

Courtois B: Les origines foetales des occlusions congénitales du grêle dites par atrésie. J Chir 78:405, 1959

DeLorimier AA, Fonkalsrud EW, et al: Congenital atresia and stenosis of the jejunum and ileum. Surgery 65:819, 1969

Dickson JAS: Apple peel small bowel: An uncommon variant of duodenal and jejunal atresia. J Pediatr Surg 5:595, 1970

Earlam RJ: A study of the aetiology of congenital stenosis of the gut. Ann R Coll Surg Engl 51:126, 1972

El Shafie M, Rickham PP: Multiple intestinal atresias. J Pediatr Surg 5:655, 1970

Evans CH: Collective review. Atresias of the gastrointestinal tract. Surg Gynecol Obstet 92:1, 1951

Fockens P: Ein operativ geheilter Fall von kongenitaler Dünndarmatresie. Zentralbl Chir 15:532, 1911

Fonkalsrud EW, DeLorimier AA, et al: Congenital atresia and stenosis of the duodenum. Pediatrics 43:79, 1969

Girvan DP, Stephens C: Congenital intrinsic duodenal obstruction: A 20-year review of its surgical management and consequences. J Pediatr Surg 9:833, 1974

Gourevitch A: Duodenal atresia in the newborn. Ann R Coll Surg Engl 48:141, 1971

Guttman FM, Braun P, et al: The pathogenesis of intestinal atresia. Surg Gynecol Obstet 141:203, 1975

Hays DM: Intestinal atresia and stenosis. Current Problems in Surgery. Chicago: Year Book, 1969

Howard ER, Biemann H, et al: Proximal jejunoplasty in the treatment of jejunal atresia. J Pediatr Surg 8:685, 1973

Hyde JS: Congenital duodenal atresia in four sibs. JAMA 191:51, 1965

Kullendorff CM: Atresia of the small bowel. Ann Chir Gynecol 72:192, 1983

Lloyd JR, Clatworthy HW: Hydramnios as an aid to the early diagnosis of congenital obstruction of the alimentary tract: A study of maternal and fetal factors. Pediatrics 21:903, 1958

Louw JH: Jejunoileal atresia and stenosis. J Pediatr Surg 1:8, 1966

Lynn HB, Espinas EE: Intestinal atresia. Arch Surg 79:357, 1959

Martin LW, Zerella JT: Jejunoileal atresia: A proposed classification. J Pediatr Surg 11:399, 1976

Meckel JF: Hanbuch der Pathologischen Anatomie, vol 1. Leipzig: CH Reclam, 1812

Nixon HH: An experimental study of propulsion in isolated small intestine, and applications to surgery in the newborn. Ann R Coll Surg Engl 27:105, 1960

Perrelli L, Wilkinson AW: Mortality and neonatal duodenal obstruction. J R Coll Surg Edinb 20:365, 1975

Rickham PP: Intramural intestinal obstruction. Prog Pediatr Surg 2:73, 1971

Santulli TV, Blanc WA: Congenital atresia of the intestine. Pathogenesis and treatment. Ann Surg 154:939, 1961

Spriggs NI: Congenital intestinal occlusion. Guy's Hosp Rep 66:143, 1912

Stauffer UG, Irving IM: Duodenal atresia and stenosis—Longterm results. Progr Pediatr Surg 10:49, 1977

Tandler J: Zur Entwicklungsgeschichte des menschlichen Duodenum in frühen Embryonalstadien. Morphol Jb 29:187, 1900

Touloukian RJ: Composition of amniotic fluid with experimental jejuno-ileal atresia. J Pediatr Surg 12:397, 1977

Young DG, Wilkinson AW: Mortality in neonatal duodenal obstruction. Lancet ii:18, 1966

Malrotation

Andrassy RF, Mahour GH: Malrotation of the midgut in infants and children. A 25-year review. Arch Surg 116:158, 1981

Berdon WE, Baker DH, et al: Midgut malrotation and volvulus. Which films are most helpful? Radiology 96:375, 1970

Bill AH: Malrotation of the intestine, in Ravitch MM, Welch KJ, et al (eds): Pediatric Surgery, 3 edt. Chicago: Year Book, 1979, p 912

Brennon WS, Bill AH: Prophylactic fixation of the intestine for midgut non-rotation. Surg Gynecol Obstet 138:181, 1974

de Bruyn R, Hall CM, et al: Hirschsprung's disease and malrotation of the midgut. An uncommon association. Br J Radiol 55:554, 1982

Filston HC, Kirks DR: Malrotation—The ubiquitous anomaly. J Pediatr Surg 16:614, 1981

Gray SW, Skandalakis JE: Embryology for surgeons. The embryological basis for the treatment of congenital defects. Philadelphia: WB Saunders, 1972, p 135

Howell CG, Vozza F, et al: Malrotation, malnutrition and ischaemic bowel disease. J Pediatr Surg 17:469, 1982

Janik JS, Ein SH: Normal intestinal rotation with non-fixation: A cause of chronic abdominal pain. J Pediatr Surg 14:670, 1979

Kieswetter WB, Smith JW: Malrotation of the midgut in infancy and childhood. Arch Surg 77:483, 1958

Simpson AJ, Leonides JC, et al: Roentgen diagnosis of midgut malrotation: Value of upper gastrointestinal radiographic study. J Pediatr Surg 7:243, 1972

Steward DR, Colodny AL, et al: Malrotation of the bowel in infants and children: A 15-year review. Surgery 79:716, 1976

Duplications of the Intestine

Bartels RJ: Duplication of the stomach. Am Surg 33:747, 1967

Beardmore HE, Wiglesworth FW: Vertebral anomalies and alimentary duplications. Ped Clin North Am 5:457, 1958

Bentley JFR, Smith JR: Developmental posterior enteric remnants and spinal malformations: The split notochord syndrome. Arch Dis Child 35:76, 1960

Bremer JL: Diverticula and duplications of the intestinal tract. Arch Pathol 38:132, 1944

Fallon M, Gordon ARG, et al: Mediastinal cysts of foregut origin associated with vertebral abnormalities. Br J Surg 41:520, 1954

Grosfeld JL, O'Neill JA Jr, et al: Enteric duplications in infancy and childhood. Ann Surg 172:83, 1970

Gross RE, Holcomb GW: Duplications of the alimentary tract. Pediatrics 9:449, 1952

Gross RE, Neuhauser EBD, et al: Thoracic duplications which originate from the intestine. Ann Surg 131:363, 1950

Lewis FT, Thyng FW: The regular occurrence of intestinal diverticula in embryos of the pig, rabbit and man. Am J Anat 7:505, 1907

Parker BC, Guthrie J, et al: Gastric duplications in infancy. J Pediatr Surg 7:294, 1972

Pruksapong C, Donovan RJ, et al: Gastric duplications. J Pediatr Surg 14:83, 1979

Ravitch MM: Hindgut duplications, doubling of colon and genital urinary tracts. Ann Surg 137:588, 1953

Schwesinger WH, Croom RD III, et al: Diagnosis of an enteric duplication with pertechnetate. Ann Surg 181:428, 1975

Smith ED: Duplication of the anus and genitourinary tract. Surgery 66:909, 1969

Soper RT: Tubular duplication of colon and distal ileum. Surgery 63:998, 1968

Soper RT, Selke AC: Duplication cyst of the duodenum. Surgery 68:562, 1970

Vaage S, Knutrud O: Congenital duplications of the alimentary tract with special regard to their embryogenesis. Prog Ped Surg 7:103, 1974

Wrenn EL Jr: Tubular duplication of the small intestine. Surgery 52:494, 1962

Pyloric Mucosal Diaphragm

Bell MJ, Ternberg JL, et al: Prepyloric gastric antral web. A puzzling epidemic. J Pediatr Surg 13:307, 1978

Bronsther B, Nadeau MR, et al: Congenital pyloric atresia: A report of three cases and a review of the literature. Surgery 69:130, 1971

Gerber BD, Aberdene SD: Prepyloric diaphragm: An unusual abnormality. Arch Surg 90:472, 1965

Ghent CN, Denton MD: Mucosal diaphragm of the gastric antrum: A case report and review of the literature. Can J Surg 17:247, 1974

Necrotising Enterocolitis

Barlow B, Santulli TV: Importance of multiple episodes of hypoxia or cold stress on the development of enterocolitis in an animal model. Surgery 77:687, 1975

Barlow B, Santulli TV, et al: An experimental study of acute necrotizing enterocolitis: The importance of breast milk. J Pediatr Surg 9:587, 1974

Benirschke K: Pathology of neonatal enterocolitis, in Necrotizing Enterocolitis in the Newborn Infant. Sixty-eighth Ross Conference on Pediatric Research. Columbus, Ohio: Ross Laboratories, 1975, p 29

Berdon WE, Grossman H, et al: Necrotizing enterocolitis in the premature infant. Radiology 83:879, 1964

Corkery JJ, Dubowitz V, et al: A colonic perforation after exchange transfusion. Br Med J 4:345, 1968

Kliegman RM, Hack K, et al: Epidemiologic study of necrotizing enterocolitis among low-birth-weight infants. J Pediatr 100:440, 1982

Kosloske AM: Necrotizing enterocolitis in the neonate. Surg Gynecol Obstet 148:259, 1979

Kosloske AM, Papile LA, et al: Indications for operation in acute necrotizing enterocolitis of the neonate. Surgery 87:504, 1980

Lawrence G, Bates J, et al: Pathogenesis of neonatal necrotizing enterocolitis. Lancet i:137, 1982

Lloyd JR. The etiology of gastrointestinal perforations in the newborn. J Pediatr Surg 4:77, 1969

Mizrahi A, Barlow O, et al: Necrotizing enterocolitis in premature infants. J Pediatr 66:697, 1965

Rossier A, Sarrut S, et al: L'entercolite ulcero-necrotique du premature. Semin Hop Paris 35:1428, 1959

Rotimi VO, Duerden BI: The development of the bacterial flora in normal neonates. J Med Microbiol 14:51, 1981

Santulli, TV, Schullinger JN, et al.: Acute necrotizing enterocolitis in infancy: A review of 64 cases. Pediatrics 55:376, 1975

Schmid KO, Quaiser K: Uber eine besonders schwer verlaufene Form von Enteritis beim saugling. Osterr Z Kinderh 8:114, 1953

Siebold JF: Gerburtshulfe, Frauenzimmer und Kinderkrankheiten. Heft I Leipzig 5:3, 1825

Thelander HE: Perforation of the gastrointestinal tract of the newborn infant. Am J Dis Child 58:371, 1939

Thomas DFM: Pathogenesis of neonatal necrotising enterocolitis. J R Soc Med 75:838, 1982

Touloukian RJ, Berdon WG, et al: Surgical experience with necrotizing enterocolitis in the infant. J Pediatr Surg 2:389, 1967

Intussusception

Ein SH, Stephens CA: Intussusception: 354 cases in 10 years. J Pediatr Surg 6:16, 1971

Gierup J, Jorulf H, et al: Management of intussusception in infants and children. A survey based on 288 consecutive cases. Pediatrics 50:535, 1972

Janik JS, Cranford J, et al: The well-nourished infant with intussusception. Fact or fallacy? Am J Dis Child 135:600, 1981

Levick RK: Management of intussusception: Barium enema versus surgery: Clin Pediat 9:457, 1970

MacMahon B: Data on the etiology of acute intussusception in childhood. Am J Hum Genet 7:430, 1955

Ravitch MM: Intussusception in Infants and Children. Springfield, Illinois: Charles C. Thomas, 1959

Ross JG, Potter CW, et al: Adenovirus infection in association with intussusception in infancy. Lancet ii:221, 1962

Suita A: Intussusception in infants and children. Z Kinderchir 9:193, 1970

41. Meckel's Diverticulum; Diverticulosis of the Small Intestine; Umbilical Fistulae and Tumours

Harold Ellis

MECKEL'S DIVERTICULUM

Historical Note

Soderlund (1959) gives an interesting account of the early history of this most common congenital abnormality of the gastrointestinal (GI) canal. From the end of the seventeenth century, diverticula were observed as contents of hernial sacs—by Lavater in 1672, Littré in 1770, and Mery in 1701. To this day, a hernial sac containing a Meckel's diverticulum is termed Littré's hernia, although there is some debate as to whether the three cases he described where a portion of the intestinal circumference was strangulated in a hernial sac were, rather, examples of Richter's hernia implicating a portion of the circumference of the small intestine, as described by Richter in 1777. Ruysch published a drawing of a diverticulum of the small intestine which he observed at autopsy and added two additional cases in 1701.

In 1808, Johann Friedrich Meckel, Professor of Anatomy at Halle, stated that the diverticulum comprised a remnant of the duct between the intestinal tract and the yolk sac. As evidence he put forward the observations that more than one diverticulum with the same structure as the small intestine is never found in the same embryo, that the diverticulum is always situated on the distal part of the small intestine and on its outer circumference, and that coincidental malformations are often present. Meckel gave a more detailed account of his observations the following year. He pointed out that although the duct generally disappears in the tenth week of fetal life, he had seen it to persist after this time in two cases, and he described a case in which the duct persisted in its entirety as far as the umbilicus. His account of the origin of the diverticulum was so clear that his name has become eponymously and permanently attached to this abnormality.

In 1898, Kuttner described intussusception of a Meckel's diverticulum. In 1904, Salzer described ectopic gastric mucosa in the diverticulum and, in 1907, Deetz noted the association of this aberrant gastric mucosa with ulceration of the adjacent ileum.

Incidence

Meckel's diverticulum has been reported in various autopsy series to have an incidence varying from 0.3 to 2.5 percent (Mackey and Dineen, 1983; Soderlund, 1959). This quite wide difference in the incidence figures is probably due to the fact that pathologists vary in the enthusiasm with which they study the distal ileum. Soderlund reports the very careful study carried out in a series of 1954 children undergoing appendicectomy in which at least the terminal 100 cm of the ileum was explored. Meckel's diverticulum was then found in 63 of the children, (3.2 percent). In most reported series there is a male-to-female preponderance of approximately 3 to 2.

Anatomy

Developmentally, the vitelline duct connects the yolk sac and the midgut of the embryo at an early stage in foetal life. Thus, in the 3-week-old embryo, the yolk sac forms the ventral aspect of the gut and communicates through a wide short vitelline duct, which gradually elongates and narrows. During the fifth week (at the 7-mm stage) the midgut normally closes off completely by atrophy of the vitelline duct to form a fibrous cord, which subsequently becomes absorbed. The blood supply to the vitelline duct comes from paired ventral branches of the abdominal aorta, the vitelline arteries. Normally, the left artery involutes while the right persists to form the superior mesenteric artery. Meckel's diverticulum receives its blood supply from a remnant of the right vitelline artery, usually as an end branch of the superior mesenteric. Occasionally, as stressed by Rutherford and Akers (1966), the Meckel's diverticulum may be associated with a mesodiverticular band, which may represent an accentuation of the normal end artery that supplies the diverticulum and that comes to run in the separate mesentery or may represent the persistence of the left vitelline artery. The importance of this band, as will be discussed later, is that it creates a triangular hiatus under which a loop of intestine can become strangulated.

Failure of all or a portion of the vitelline duct to become obliterated accounts for the various forms of this anomaly (Figs. 41–1 through 41–3):

1. There may be a completely obliterated duct persisting as a band between the umbilicus and the small intestine, or the cord may extend from the diverticulum to the umbilicus.
2. The vitelline duct remains patent throughout (persistent omphaloenteric fistula).
3. The duct may persist in part of its course as a sinus opening at the umbilicus without attachment to the small intestine or with the band passing to the ileum or as an enterocystoma—an intermediate cyst attached by a fibrous cord to both the umbilicus and the small intestine.
4. Most commonly, a persistence of the proximal portion of the duct results in the formation of a Meckel's diverticulum (at least 90 percent of cases).

The size and shape of the diverticulum varies greatly, between 1 and 26 cm in length, although usually the diverticulum is between 3 and 5 cm long. Soderlund (1959) found that the diverticulum was situated from 10 to 150 cm from the ileocaecal valve. In children it usually lay about 40 cm from the valve, whereas the distance was about 50 cm in adults. The diameter is somewhat less than that of the ileum but it may occasionally be a narrow appendix-like protrusion.

It possesses a mesentery and it has an independent arterial supply from an arcade of the ileal vessels, except in those cases in which the diverticulum is unusually small. It may fold over on itself and lie by the side of the gut, and it may be covered by a filmy membrane when it lies flat on the mesentery of the intestine. Outpouchings or diverticula may be present on the diverticulum itself (Fig. 41–4).

Associated Congenital Malformations

Meckel's diverticulum occurs more commonly in individuals born with other congenital malformations, especially exomphalos, oesophageal atresia, anorectal atresia, and gross malformations of the central nervous system or the cardiovascular system (Simms and Corkery, 1980). In Soderlund's study of 413 clinical cases, there were 22 congenital malformations in 19 of them. Recently, Hemingway and Allison (1982) have reported an interesting association between angiodysplasia of the caecum and ascending colon and Meckel's diverticulum in five patients aged 13 to 21. Angiodysplasia had previously only been reported in patients over the age of 35.

Although isolated cases of Meckel's diverticulum among relatives have been described, there is no evidence for believing that Meckel's diverticulum is an inherited trait.

Heterotopic Mucosa

The lining of the diverticulum is the same as that of the ileum in the majority of cases. However, heterotopic gastric, duodenal, colonic, or pancreatic tissue may occur, either singly or in combination. Mackey and Dineen (1983) carried out microscopic examination of 140 symptomless Meckel's diverticula removed incidentally at operation. In 23 (16.4 percent), heterotopic mucosa was identified—gastric mucosa was present in 15, pancreatic tissue was found in 3, another 3 had colonic mucosa, 1 con-

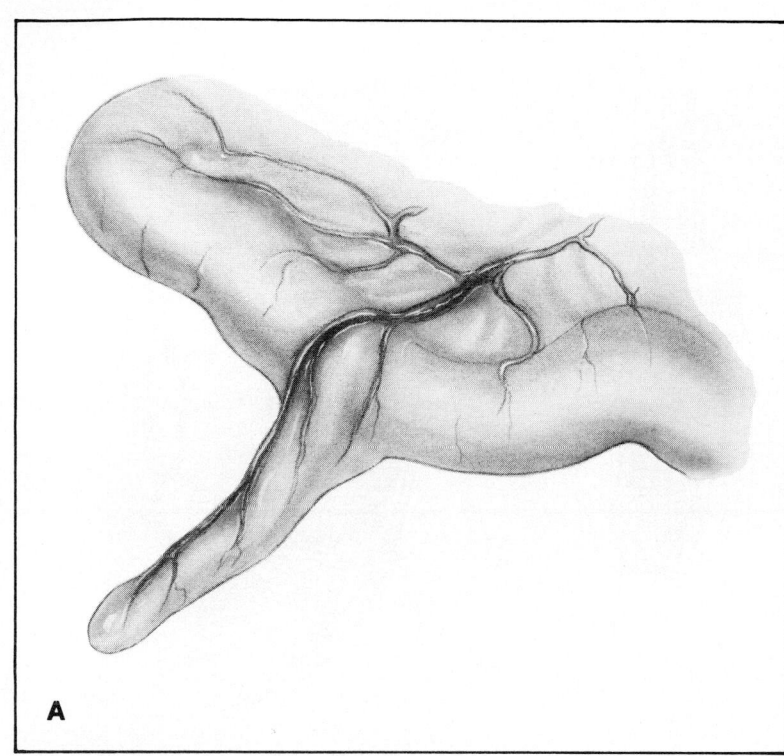

Figure 41-1. Meckel's diverticulum and its associated anomalies. **A.** The usual type. Persistence of the proximal portion of the duct results in the formation of a Meckel's diverticulum (about 90 percent of cases).

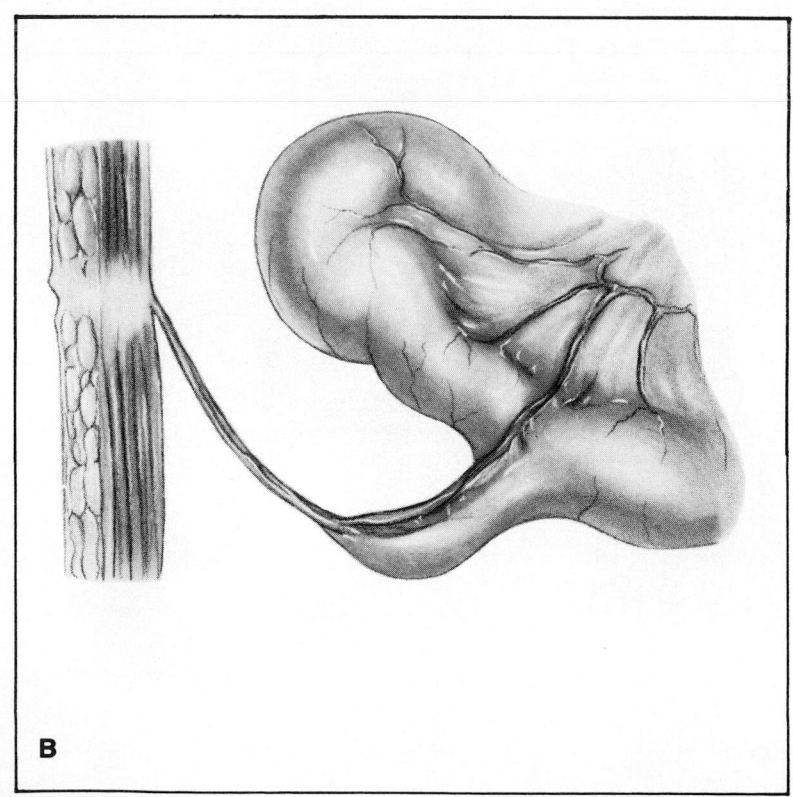

Figure 41-1. B. A fibrous cord extends from the diverticulum to the umbilicus.

1088

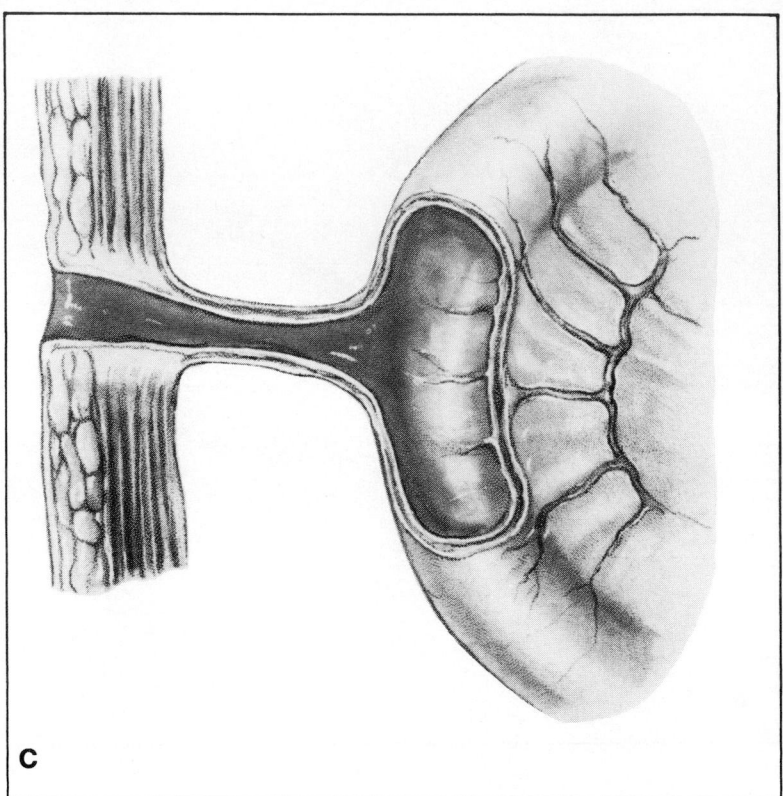

Figure 41–1. C. The vitelline duct remains patent throughout (persistent omphaloenteric fistula).

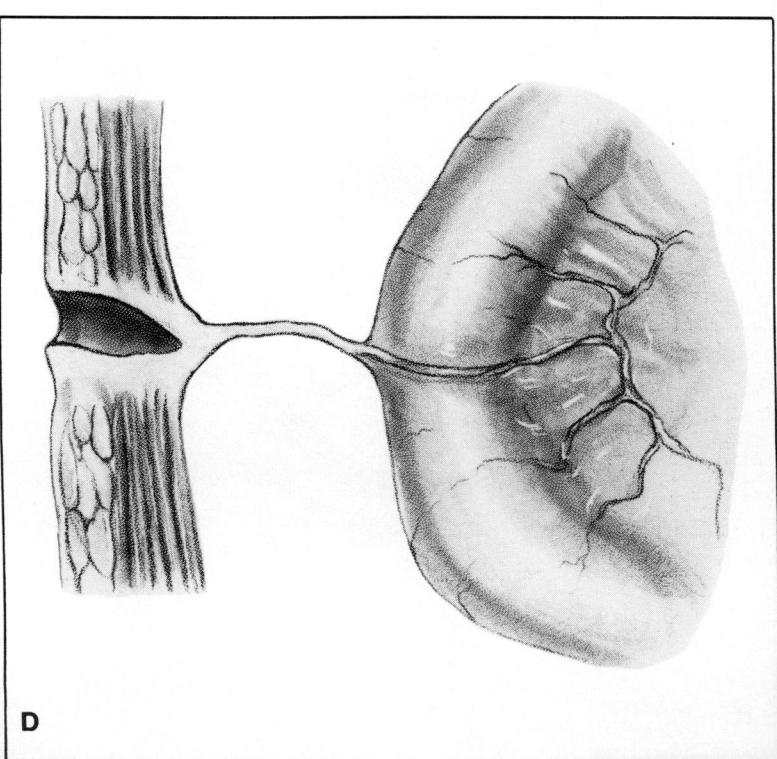

Figure 41–1. D. The duct persists in the distal part of its course.

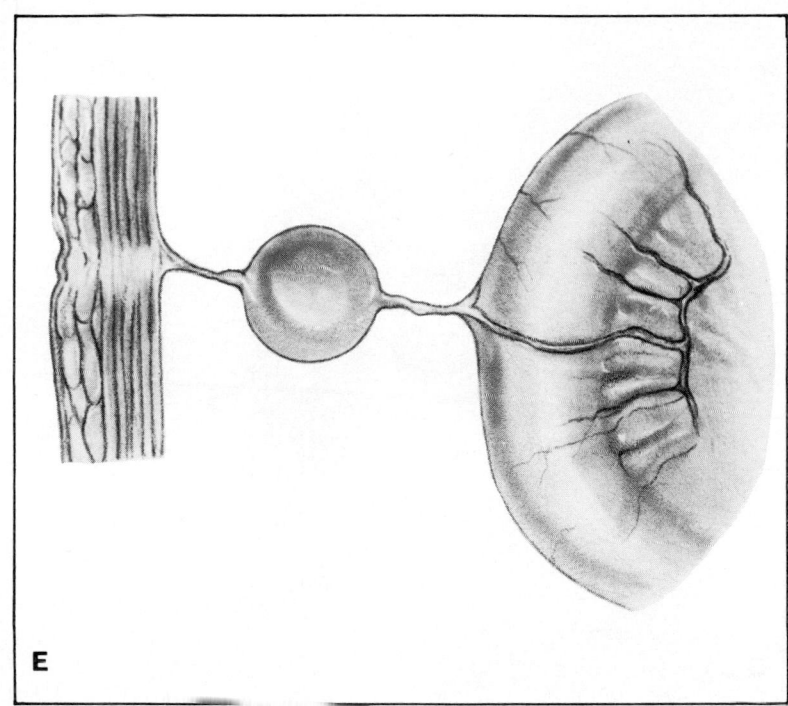

Figure 41–1. E. Enterocystoma. An intermediate cyst attached by a fibrous cord both to the umbilicus and to the ileum.

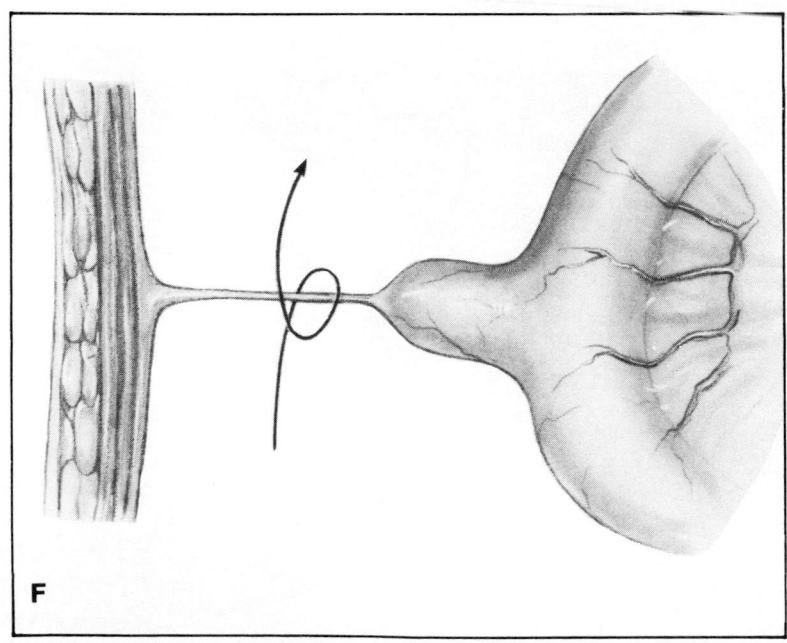

Figure 41–1. F. Torsion.

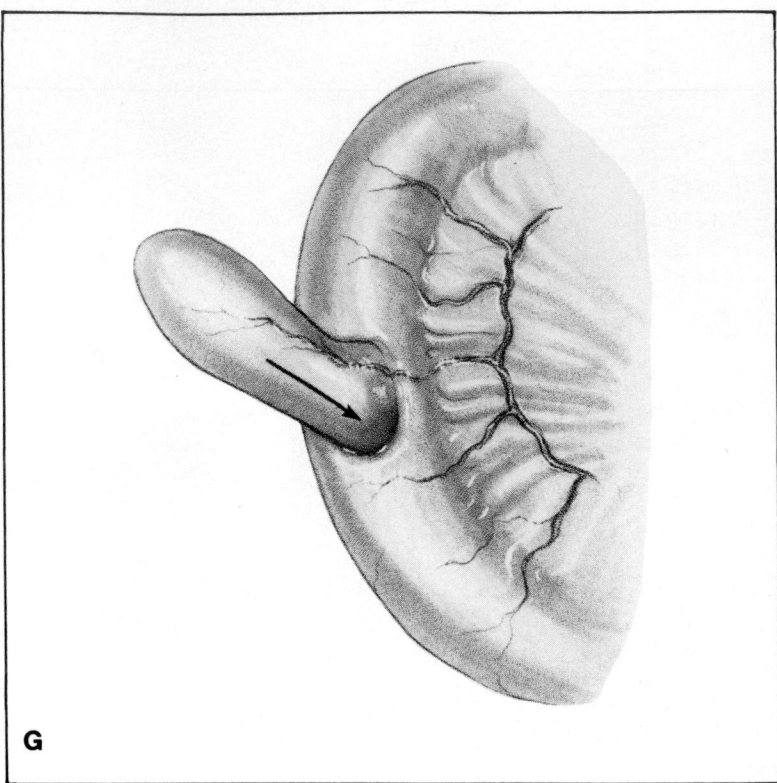

Figure 41–1. G. Intussusception.

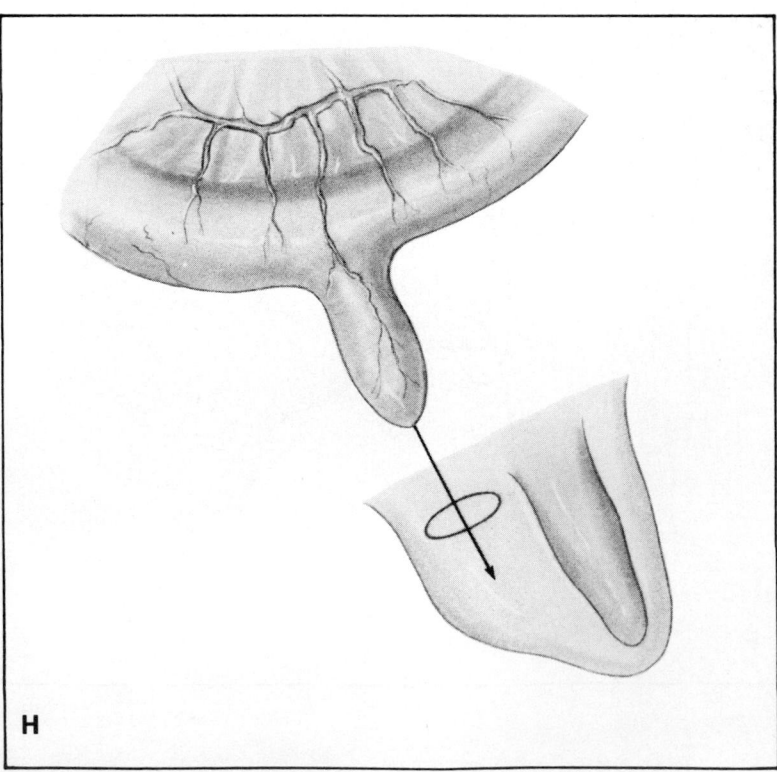

Figure 41–1. H. Littré's hernia.

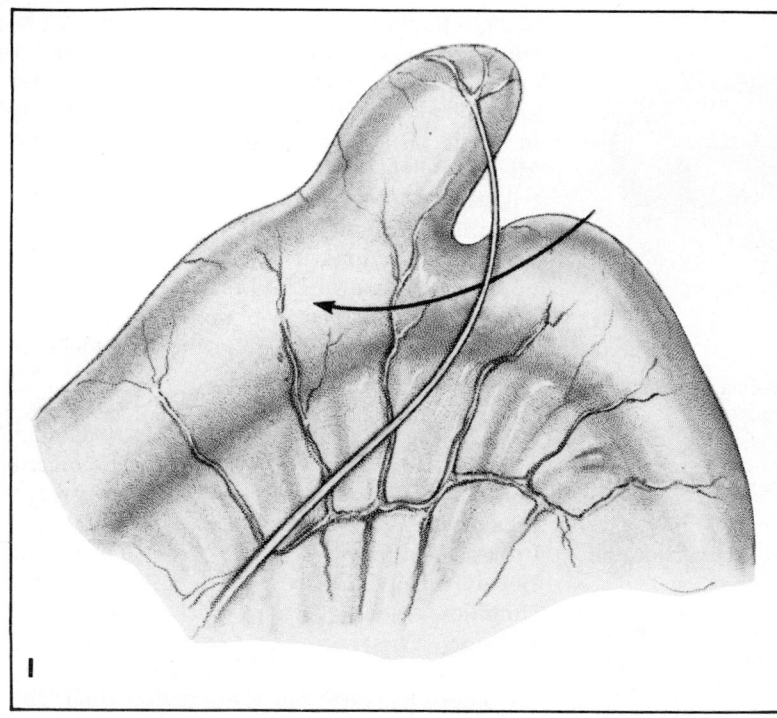

Figure 41–1. I. Obstruction due to mesodiverticular band.

tained jejunal mucosa, and 1 had both gastric and duodenal tissue. In a further 62 instances in which the Meckel's diverticulum was removed because of symptoms, the incidence of heterotopic mucosa was higher, identified in 21 patients (34 percent). Of these, 19 had gastric mucosa, 1 pancreatic tissue and 1 colonic mucosa.

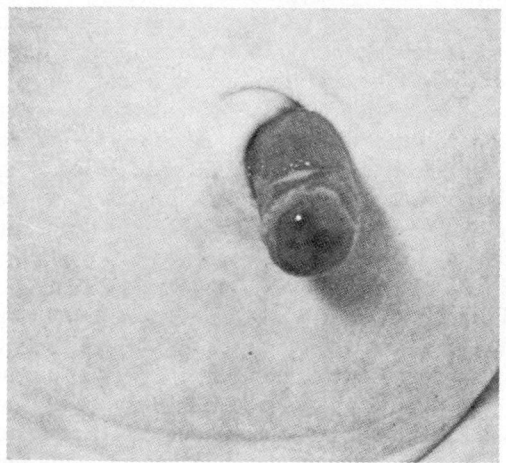

Figure 41–2. Enteric umbilical fistula. (*Source: From Gracey LRH, Williams JA: Meckel's diverticulum in children. Br J Clin Pract 17:315, 1963, with permission.*)

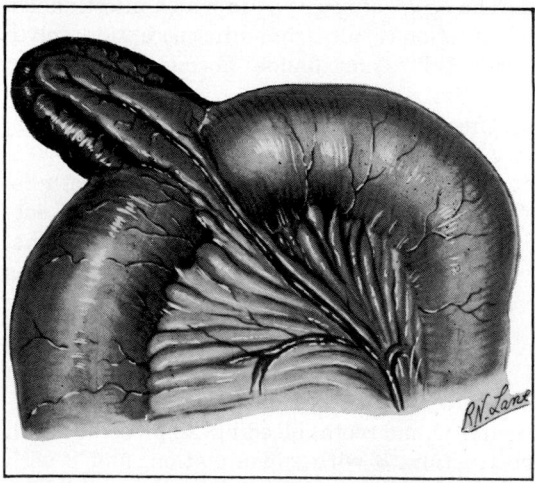

Figure 41–3. Meckel's diverticulum. Note blood supply to the diverticulum.

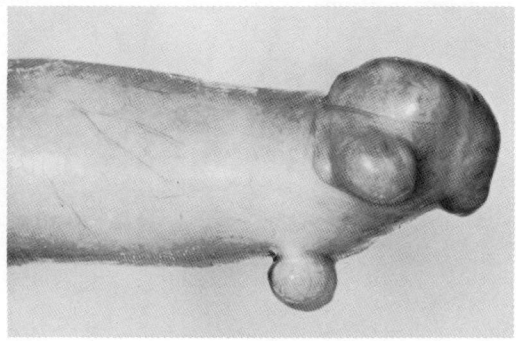

Figure 41–4. Outpouchings or diverticula of a Meckel's diverticulum. (*Courtesy of Mr. L. Gracey.*)

Complications

The complications of Meckel's diverticulum may be classified as follows:

1. The *peptic group,* in which the heterotopic gastric mucosa results in the development of a chronic peptic ulcer in the diverticulum itself or adjacent to its stoma. This may present with haemorrhage or, less frequently, acute perforation.
2. The *inflammatory group,* in which acute inflammatory changes take place which may result in gangrene and perforation. Perforation may also result from penetration by foreign bodies. In this group the signs and symptoms closely mimic those of acute appendicitis.
3. The *obstructive group,* in which intestinal obstruction results from intussusception, volvulus, adhesions, bands, fibrous cord, foreign bodies, or concretions.
4. The *umbilical group,* which includes fistula, cyst, and granuloma.
5. The *tumour group,* which includes both benign (myoma, lipoma, neuroma, and adenoma) and malignant (adenocarcinoma, leiomyosarcoma, and carcinoid tumour), as well as cysts.

Rutherford and Akers (1966) found the following incidence of complications in a series of 80 children with symptomatic Meckel's diverticula: 43 had rectal bleeding, 26 presented with obstruction, 8 with inflammation, and 3 with perforation (2 from peptic ulceration and 1 from a pin). Mackey and Dineen (1983) list the complications of 68 patients with symptomatic Meckel's (1983) diverticulum as follows: obstruction

in 23, inflammation in 21, haemorrhage 17, Littré's hernia in 8, umbilical fistula in 3, and 1 example each of multiple calculi, torsion, and an abdominal wall abscess. Soderlund (1959), in series of 142 patients with symptomatic Meckel's diverticulum found the following distribution: peptic ulceration in 40, bands, volvulus, and obstruction in 40, intrussusception in 19, acute inflammation in 24, umbilical fistula in 15, and Littré's hernia in 4.

Williams (1981), in a review of 1806 collected cases, found the following incidence of complications:

Haemorrhage	31 percent
Inflammation	25 percent
Bowel obstruction due to band, etc.	16 percent
Intussusception	11 percent
Hernial involvement	11 percent
Umbilical sinus or fistula	4 percent
Tumour	2 percent

There has been much discussion about the risk of a Meckel's diverticulum undergoing one or another of these complications. Soltero and Bill (1976) have carried out an estimation of this possibility by studying a stable population of over a million people over a 15-year period. During this time 202 examples of complications of Meckel's diverticulum were encountered. They assume a 2 percent incidence of diverticulum in the population, and, from life table calculations, they estimate that in infancy a child with a Meckel's diverticulum runs a 4.2 percent risk of developing symptoms, dropping to 3 percent in adults and almost zero in old age.

The presentation of Meckel's diverticulum in hospital practice is well reviewed by Mackey and Dineen (1983). Over a 50-year period at the Cornell Medical Center in New York, a total of 402 examples of Meckel's diverticulum were recorded. Of these, 45 percent were incidental findings at postmortem, 35 percent incidental findings at laparotomy, and 1.5 percent were incidental at radiologic examination. Definite symptoms attributable to the diverticulum accounted for 17 percent of the patients; another 1.5 percent had possible symptoms. In this study, patients most likely to develop symptoms from the diverticulum are those under the age of 40, with a diverticulum 2 cm or more in length and probably also if the patient is male. The presence of heterotopic mucosa makes the diverticulum more likely to undergo complications, but in many cases cannot be detected by gross findings. Indirect evidence is the presence of submucosal or mucosal nodularity, scarring, or inflammatory adhesions.

Clinical Manifestations

In most cases a Meckel's diverticulum is an incidental finding at postmortem or laparotomy. When symptoms occur, the clinical manifestations vary with the type of complication present, and in most cases the diagnosis can only be made with certainty at operation.

Haemorrhage. The passage of blood per rectum in a child should always raise the possibility of haemorrhage from peptic ulceration of a Meckel's diverticulum. Bleeding can also occur in young adults; in Soderlund's series there were 24 such cases, with an age range of from 6 months to 22 years (3 were adults). Rutherford and Akers reviewed the nature of the rectal bleeding in 43 children. Bright red bleeding was recorded by history or direct observation in 47 percent. Dark red or "maroon" stools were observed in 58 percent, and there was some overlap between the two. Tarry stools as the only evidence of bleeding were reported in only three

patients (7 percent) and none presented with anaemia or occult blood in the stools. A history of previous bleeding was elicited in 40 percent of the patients. Occult bleeding is, in fact, extremely rare. Farthing and colleagues (1981) report an example of this in a girl aged 14 and state that an extensive search of previous publications failed to produce any other examples.

Inflammation. This closely simulates the clinical features of acute appendicitis and its complications. Therefore, the diverticulum should always be sought in a patient undergoing operation for appendicitis but who is found to have a normal appendix, especially in children. The acutely inflamed diverticulum may proceed to perforation with localised abscess or general peritonitis (Fig. 41–5). Peritonitis may also follow perforation of a peptic ulcer of the diverticulum or foreign body perforation. Rosswick (1965) reviewed 50 case reports of foreign body perforation of Meckel's diverticulum and no less than 28 of these were due to fish bones. Other foreign bodies included a cherry stone, a knitting needle, a gramophone needle, a wooden splinter, and a chicken bone. Six of these patients were younger than 10 and three were older than 70. I have records of three patients that I have operated upon with this complication, the foreign

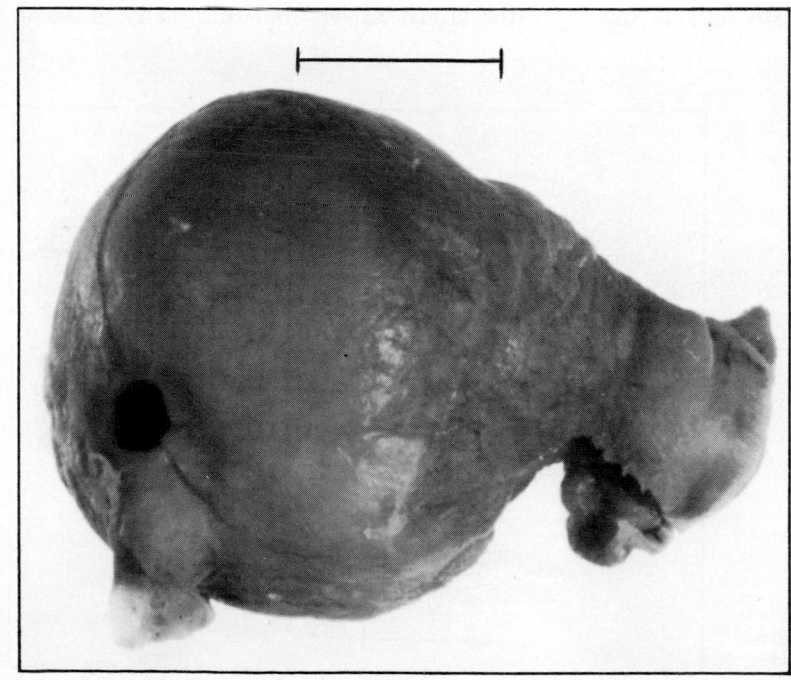

Figure 41–5. Perforated Meckel's diverticulum. (Bar equals 1 cm.)

body being a fish bone in two cases and a rolled up piece of apple peel in the third (Fig. 41–6); in this case, the 13-year-old boy had eaten an apple 33 hours previously. Three examples of gangrene of a Meckel's diverticulum due to impaction of slow-release iron tablets also have been recorded.

Intestinal Obstruction. This may result from intussusception (Fig. 41–7), torsion, a band, or obstruction within a hernia.

Rutherford and Akers (1965) reviewed 26 instances of this complication in children and found that volvulus around a vitelloumbilical cord occurred 7 times (with infarction in 5 instances), intussusception in 7, obstruction in an inguinal hernia in 2, and obstruction following inflammation with adhesions in 4. In 6 patients a segment of intestine had become trapped under a cord or band coursing between the diverticulum and the base of the mesentery and half of these had progressed to infarction at the time of laparotomy. They observed such a band as an incidental finding in 6 other patients (Fig. 41–8). They suggest that this mesodiverticular band represents a persistence of the vitelline arterial system; this author has observed this in one nonobstructed case.

Vellacott (1981) reports what appears to be a unique case of haemoperitoneum resulting from haemorrhage from the midpoint of such a mesodiverticular band, the Meckel's having the appearances of having undergone torsion. There have been three case reports of obstruction due to impacted food material in the ileum above the Meckel's diverticulum, due to coconut, orange pulp, and sauerkraut (Lawrence, 1982).

Umbilical Fistula. The presence of a fistula at the umbilicus suggests the presence of a patent vitelline duct. The diagnosis of fistula is certain when ileal contents ooze through the umbilicus.

Littré's Hernia. The presence of a Meckel's diverticulum in a hernia sac is rare and has perhaps received more attention in surgical publications than it deserves. I have personally never seen a case. It may occur as an incidental finding in a nonstrangulated case or, an exceedingly rare phenomenon, as the content of a strangulated hernia. Castleden (1970) gives the incidence of the various hernias containing a Meckel's diverticulum as inguinal 50 percent, femoral 20 percent, umbilical 20 percent, and incisional and other hernias 10 percent. A Meckel's diverticulum within an umbilical hernia is a particularly rare finding. The possibility of a coincidental Meckel's diverticulum should be borne in mind, however, in newborn infants with omphalocele. Soderlund (1959) notes that a diverticulum was present in 4 of 24 such cases in the study. Apart from this rarity, it is, of

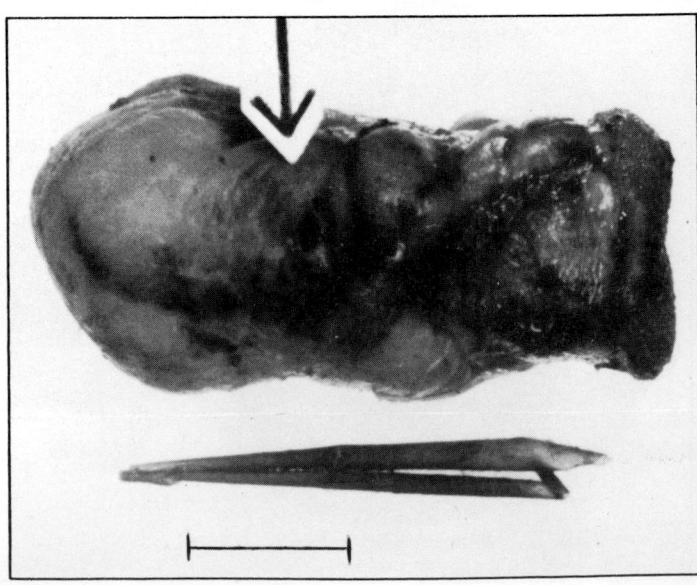

Figure 41–6. Meckel's diverticulum perforated by a rolled piece of apple peel. (Bar equals 1 cm.)

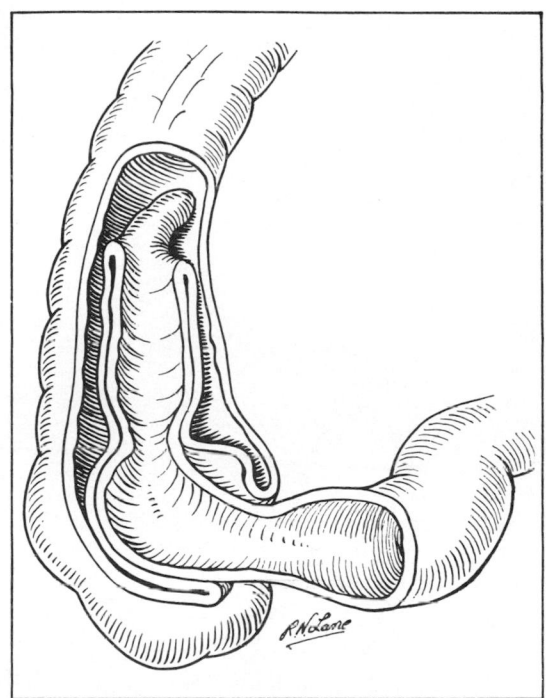

Figure 41-7. Intussusception of a Meckel's diverticulum.

course, impossible to diagnose the presence of a Meckel's diverticulum, preoperatively in either a simple or strangulated hernia.

Further information can be found in a monograph by Watson (1948) who presents a series of 259 examples of Littré's hernia, and in an interesting account by Leslie and colleagues (1983) of a unique case of a small bowel fistula complicating a strangulated Meckel's diverticulum within a femoral hernia. Perlman and colleagues (1980) review the 43 published cases in the English language of femoral hernia containing a strangulated Meckel's diverticulum.

Neoplasm. Weinstein et al (1963) review this rarity. In a collected series of 106 cases, 26 were benign; the most common was leiomyoma, followed by fibroma, haemangioendothelioma, neuroma, and lipoma. Of the 80 malignant cases, 35 were sarcomas, 29 were carcinoids, and 16 were adenocarcinomas. Ewerth and colleagues (1979) report a highly malignant adenocarcinoma arising from a Meckel's diverticulum and review 20 other recorded examples of such a lesion. Tumour formation appears to be the least common pathologic condition to which

Meckel's diverticulum is prone. For example, there was not a single example in the extensive series reported by Soderlund (1959) of 413 clinical cases in adults and children.

Diagnostic Studies

Rather surprisingly, a Meckel's diverticulum is rarely demonstrated on a routine barium meal and follow through; the reason for this is not obvious since jejunal diverticula show readily (Bartram and Amess, 1980). However, a small bowel enema, carried out by an infusion of dilute barium through a nasogastric tube guided into the duodenum will demonstrate the diverticulum in about 0.7 percent of all examinations. The injection of contrast material into an umbilical fistula differentiates a patent vitelline duct communicating with the ileum from a patent urachus communicating with the urinary bladder.

In 1970, Jewett et al, demonstrated that the ectopic gastric mucosa in a Meckel's diverticulum could be visualised by a technetium scan of the abdomen, using Tc-99m-pertechnetate. They reported two examples in children, both of whom presented with rectal bleeding. By 1982, this same group at the Children's Hospital in Buffalo were able to report a series of 270 such scans carried out in children with a calculated accuracy of some 90 percent. This is certainly a technique that is valuable in the investigation of obscure lower GI bleeding in children and young adults. Figure 41-9 (author's case) demonstrates such a scan; this was a young man aged 30 who had experienced central abdominal pains since a schoolboy. In the few months before admission to Westminster he had had two episodes of melaena, each requiring transfusion with four units of blood. A barium meal and follow-through, gastroscopy, barium enema, and colonoscopy were all negative. The technetium scan showed a takeup in the lower left abdomen and a diagnosis of a Meckel's diverticulum was made. At operation there was indeed a large Meckel's diverticulum that contained no less than three ulcers. Following its resection in 1979 he has remained free from further symptoms.

Treatment

Resection of a Meckel's diverticulum is, of course, performed when it is the site of any of

1096

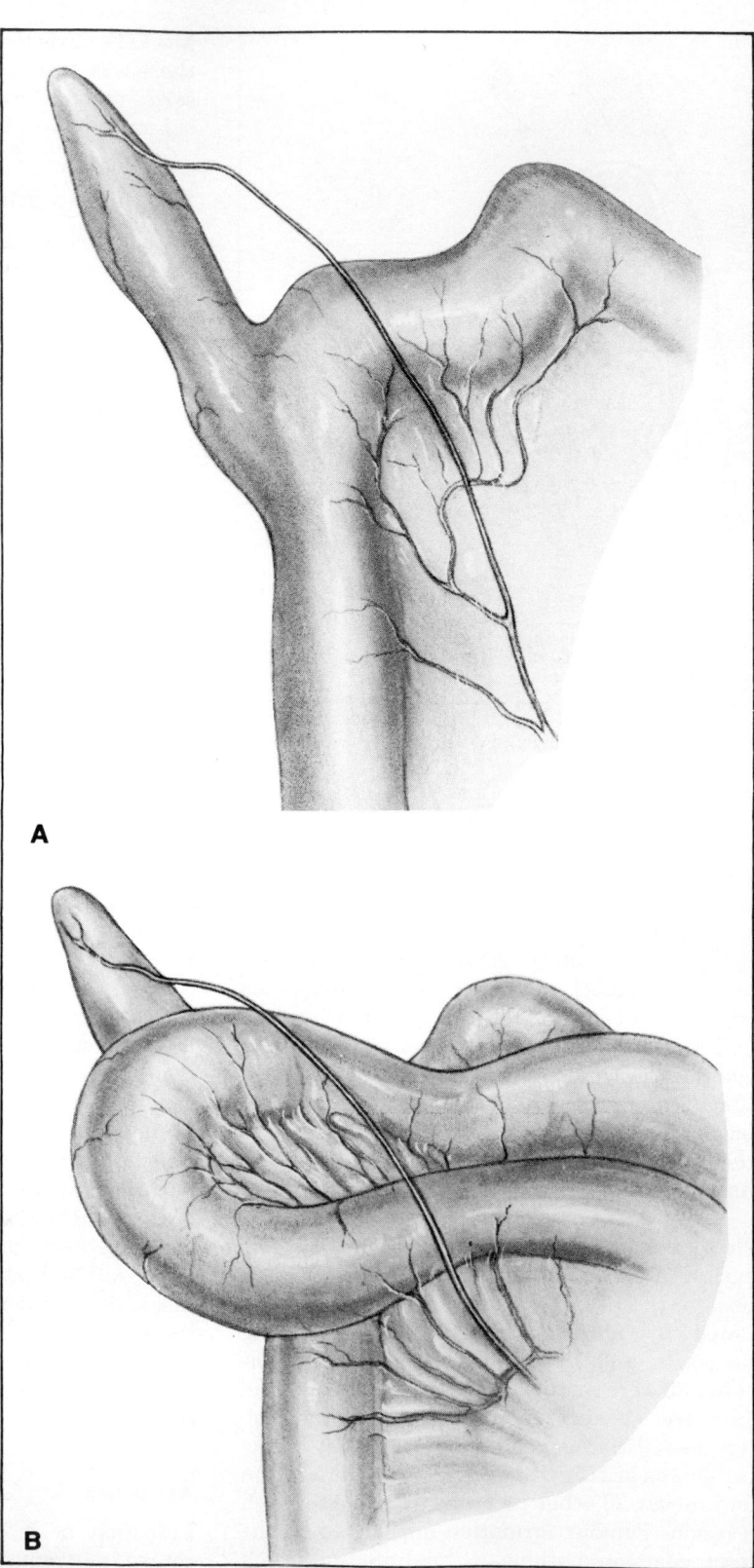

Figure 41–8. A and **B.** Intestinal obstruction resulting from volvulus around a vitelloumbilical cord (or mesodiverticular band).

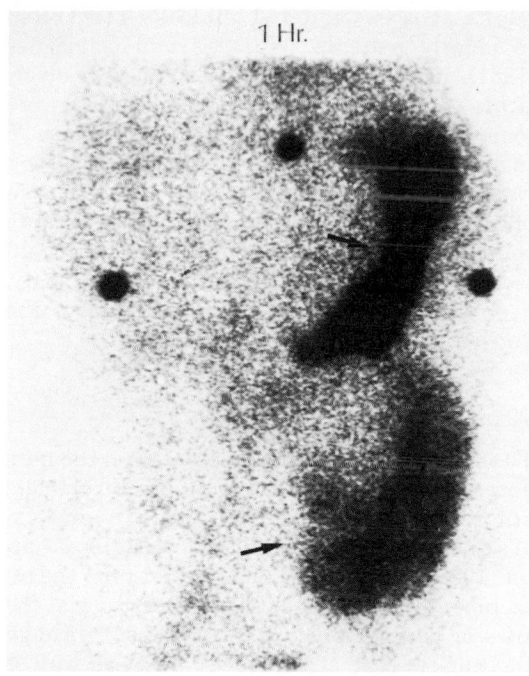

Simple excision is satisfactory in most cases. The diverticulum is clamped in the transverse axis of the ileum in order to avoid narrowing of the lumen when the defect is closed by means of two layers of 2/0 continuous catgut (Fig. 41–10). It is important to divide the supplying artery on the ileal mesentery and to excise the distal segment that crosses the ileum. This will avoid the possibility of later band obstruction from fibrosis of the distal arterial segment.

Resection of a segment of the ileum containing the diverticulum, followed by end-to-end anastomosis, is reserved for patients with peptic ulceration (which may involve the adjacent ileum), a gangrenous diverticulitis affecting the base of the diverticulum, or in those rare cases of malignant disease. When the diverticulum has a mesentery, this should be isolated,

Figure 41–9. One-hour technetium scan demonstrating a Meckel's diverticulum. The upper arrow points to the stomach image, the lower arrow to the visualised diverticulum.

the complications already described. Most surgeons would advise the removal of an asymptomatic pouch when found incidentally at laparotomy in infants, children, or young adults, if there is attachment by bands either to the umbilicus or by a mesodiverticular vascular strand, or if there is any palpable thickening or adhesions suggestive of ectopic tissue. A wide-mouthed, thin-walled unattached diverticulum in an adult patient can probably be quite safely left alone (Williams, 1981). In exploring the right iliac fossa for a suspected acute appendicitis, a normal appendix is, of course, an indication for searching for an inflamed Meckel's diverticulum. However, most surgeons would agree that if an acutely inflamed appendix is found there is no need to search for a Meckel's diverticulum (Lang-Stevenson, 1983). Indeed, the association of acute appendicitis with an acute Meckel's diverticulitis, although recorded, is extremely rare (Moore and Johnston, 1976).

There are two techniques for excision of the diverticulum—simple excision or resection with the segment of ileum containing the diverticulum.

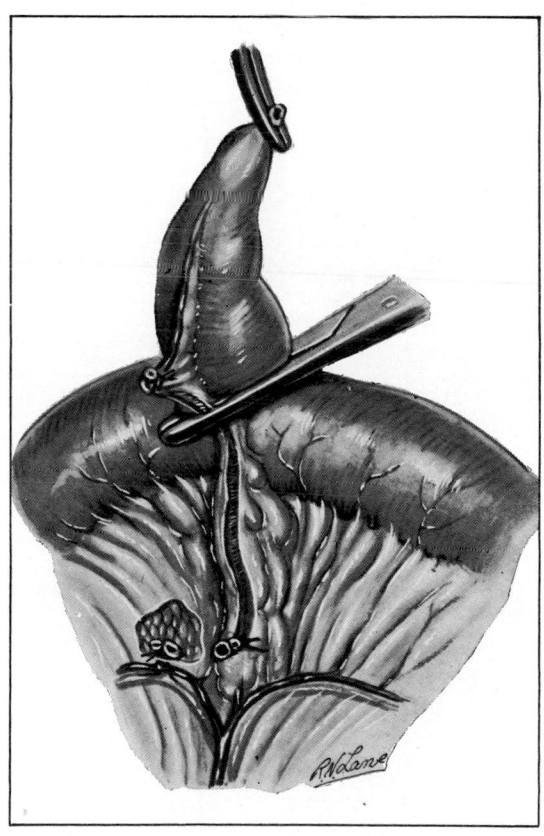

Figure 41–10. Excision of a Meckel's diverticulum. (*Source: Adapted from Gross RE: Meckel's diverticulum: Diverticulectomy, in Gross RE (ed): An Atlas of Children's Surgery. Philadelphia: WB Saunders, 1970, with permission.*)

clamped, divided, and ligated first. Following resection of the bowel containing the diverticulum, intestinal continuity is restored by a two-layer catgut anastomosis.

DIVERTICULOSIS OF THE SMALL INTESTINE

Incidence

Solitary or multiple diverticula may occasionally be found in the jejunum or, much less commonly, in the ileum (Fig. 41–11). Simultaneous involvement of both jejunum and ileum is rare. Rosedale and Lawrence (1976) carried out careful autopsies with air distension of the bowel and detected four examples of jejunal diverticulosis in 300 autopsies (1.3 percent), while Shackelford and Marcus (1960) found only 1 example in 750 upper GI barium studies. Males are affected rather more often than females, and, although the condition can be seen in young

adults, it is encountered clinically most often in elderly patients. Williams and colleagues (1981), in a review of 34 patients with diverticula of the small intestine, found that 18 were male and 16 female. The ages ranged from 26 to 87 years, with a mean of 67. The distribution was as follows: 4 had a solitary diverticulum of the jejunum, 19 were multiple jejunal, 5 were solitary ileal, 5 were multiple ileal, and 1 affected the entire small intestine. Interestingly, 8 of the patients also had diverticula of the duodenum.

Anatomy

The diverticula are usually situated on the mesenteric border of the intestine but diverticula of the antimesenteric border (apart from Meckel's diverticulum) have also been described (Carter, 1959). The diverticula arise between the attachments of the leaves of the mesentery at the sites of perforations of the vasa recta through the muscle coat of the bowel. The sac wall is

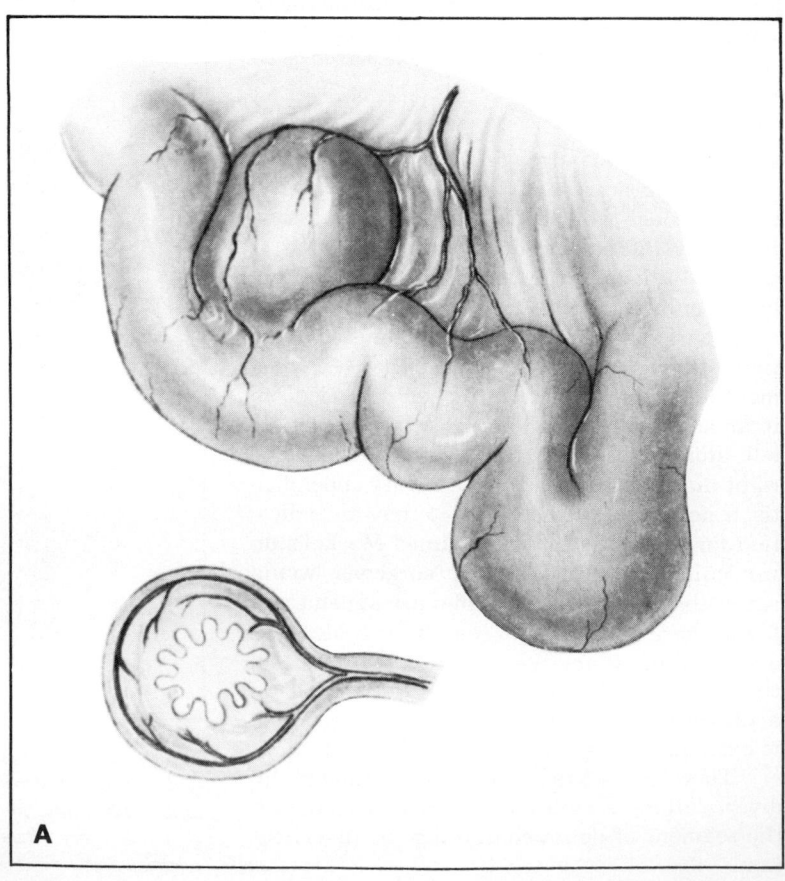

Figure 41–11. Solitary **(A)** and multiple **(B)** diverticula of the jejunum. Inset demonstrates the normal blood supply of the jejunum in transverse section.

A

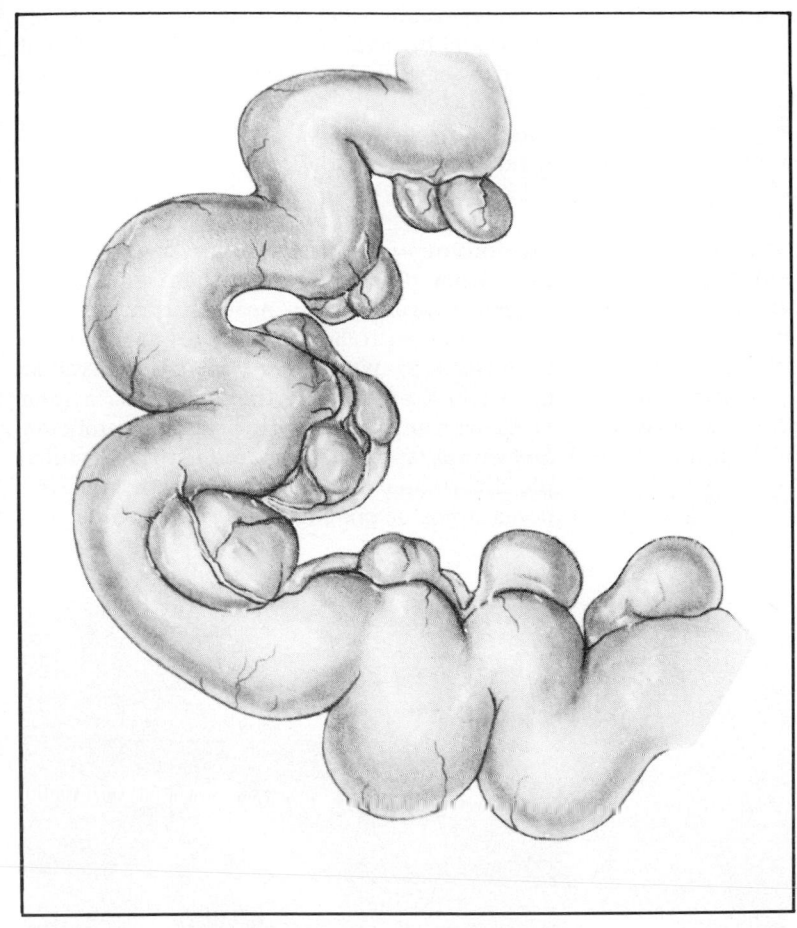

Figure 41–11. B.

thin and composed largely of mucosa with sub-mucosal fibrous tissue. It lacks a well-developed muscle layer. Heterotopic tissue is not found in these diverticula, unlike its common occurrence in Meckel's diverticulum.

The incidence in the elderly implies that the condition is usually acquired and that the diverticula are due to pulsion of mucosa through the weakest part of the intestinal wall, as was originally suggested by Sir Astley Cooper in 1807 when he gave the first description of this condition as a postmortem finding.

Complications

Diverticula of the small intestine are symptomless in the majority of cases. Eckhauser et al (1979) estimate that complications occur only in 6 to 10 percent of cases. These may be classified as follows:

Diverticulitis and Perforation. Inflammation in a diverticulum is usually due to foreign body inspissation or the presence of an enterolith (Bewes et al, 1966). When perforation occurs, it may result in a generalised peritonitis, a localised abscess, or intestinal fistula formation between adjacent loops of bowel. The perforated diverticulum may be partly hidden by the mesenteric fat and may be difficult to detect (Kveim, 1981).

Haemorrhage. Haemorrhage from small bowel diverticula is a rare cause of melaena, which may be massive and repeated. A diverticulum should always be sought in a severely bleeding patient who, at laparotomy, has no other obvious source. Its presence may be indicated by arteriography (Donald, 1979).

Obstruction. An intestinal diverticulum may produce obstruction by postinflammatory adhesions or by volvulus of the diverticulum-bearing loop of intestine.

Metabolic. Jejunal diverticulosis may result in the so-called blind-loop syndrome, which is better termed "the small intestine stasis syndrome" (Ellis and Smith, 1967), comprising some or all of the following features: diarrhoea, steatorrhoea, abdominal pain, and anaemia due to vitamin B_{12} deficiency. In 1930, Taylor noted an example of "pernicious anaemia" in this condition. Montuschi in 1949 first reported the association of steatorrhoea with jejunal diverticulosis. A classic account of the jejunal diverticulosis syndrome, including the development of frank subacute combined degeneration of the cord, was given by Badenoch and colleagues in 1955 and Watkinson et al gave the first report, in 1959, of improvement both in stools and B_{12} level after resection of the affected segment of jejunal diverticulosis. Cooke and colleagues (1963) give an extensive review of this interesting metabolic association with jejunal diverticula.

Miscellaneous. Various other complications have been described. Infestation with round worms or thread worms, neoplastic change, and association with pneumatosis cystoides have been reported. We recorded what is believed to be the first example of the latter, i.e., a man of 63 who presented with pneumoperitoneum and who at laparotomy was found to have multiple diverticula of the jejunum with superimposed areas of pneumatosis. He recovered fol-

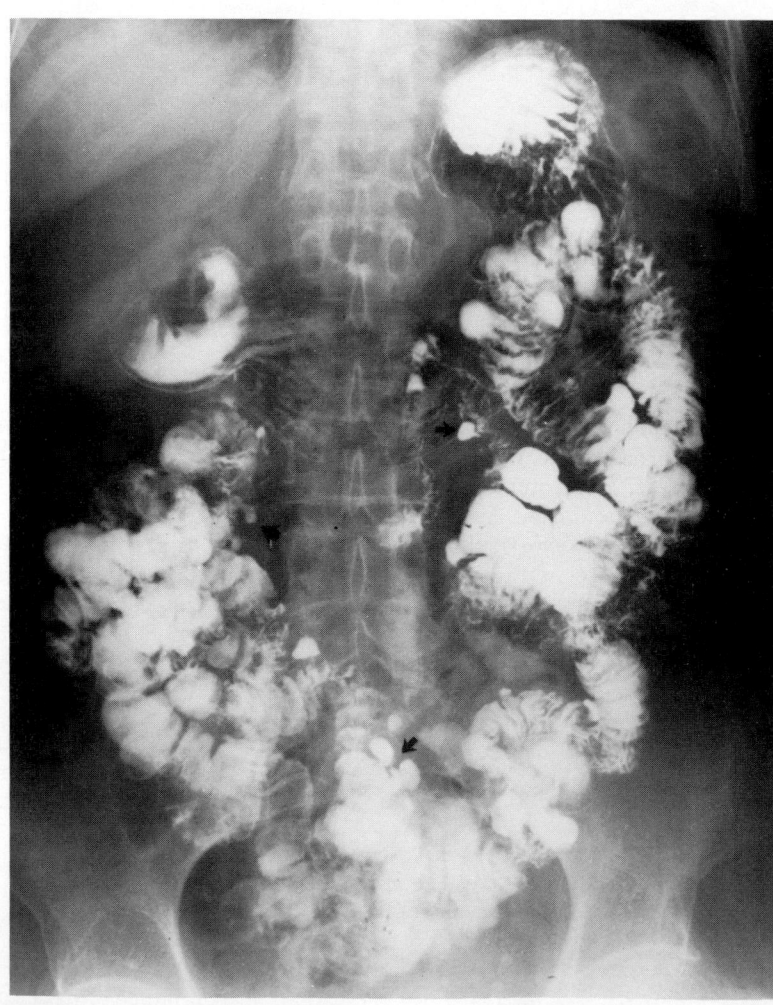

Figure 41–12. Barium follow-through examination demonstrating multiple jejunal diverticula (*arrows*).

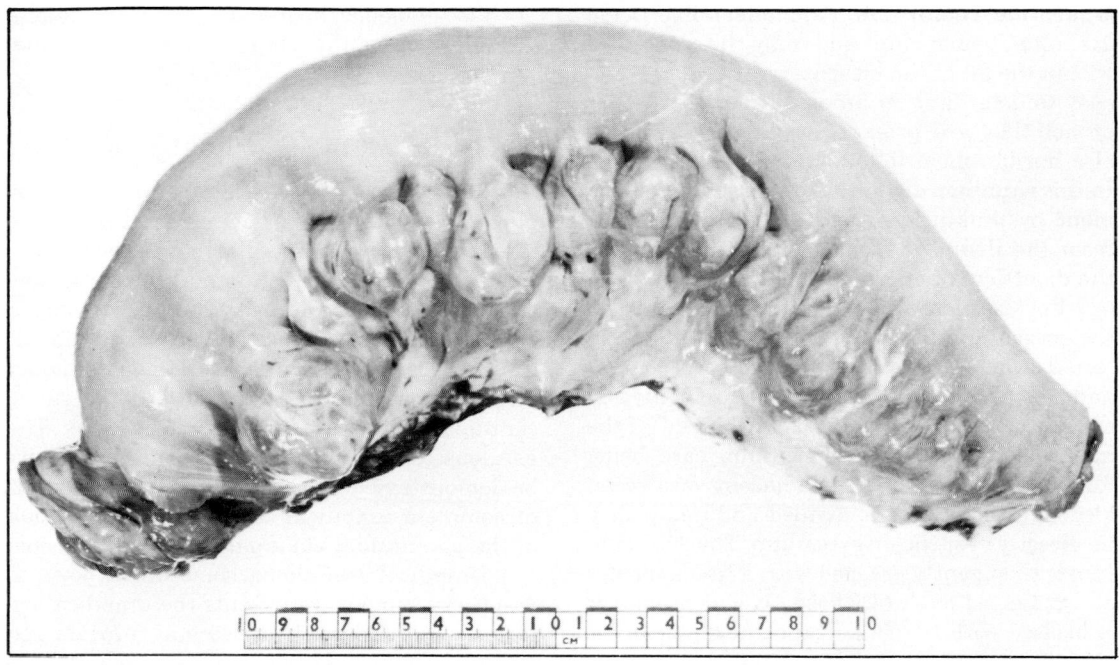

Figure 41–13. Resected specimen of localised segment of jejunal diverticulosis.

lowing resection of the affected segment (Craft and Ellis, 1967).

Diagnosis

Jejunal diverticula are symptomless in the great majority of cases. Vague abdominal discomfort may occur or there may be recurrent attacks of colicky abdominal pain, indicating a subacute obstruction. The symptoms are rather nonspecific and it may only be the onset of an unmistakable event such as haemorrhage or perforation that leads to the establishment of the correct diagnosis. Jejunal diverticula should also be suspected in patients presenting with megaloblastic anaemia, steatorrhoea, and the other features of the "blind loop syndrome."

Sometimes the diagnosis is suggested by a plain film of the abdomen that shows scattered pockets of air, but a careful barium meal and follow-through examination of the small intestine will confirm the diagnosis in the majority of cases (Fig. 41–12).

Treatment

As in the duodenum, the mere presence of a small intestinal diverticulum is not sufficient reason for its removal. A thorough search should be made for all other possible causes of symptoms, and treatment should be deferred until they have been excluded.

In patients presenting with steatorrhoea or megaloblastic anaemia, a sustained course of an intestinal antibiotic such as neomycin, together with vitamin B_{12} replacement, may keep the condition in check. When medical treatment fails, however, or in the presence of serious complications, operation must be considered the treatment of choice.

Severe haemorrhage, perforation, or obstruction are, of course, indications for urgent laparotomy.

In the case of a solitary diverticulum, simple diverticulectomy will suffice. Inversion of the diverticulum should not be carried out because of the possibility of subsequent intussusception. When the diverticula are confined to a small segment of the bowel, resection and end-to-end anastomosis should be undertaken (Fig. 41–13). When the diverticula are scattered throughout the whole length of the small intestine, resection should be limited to the segments containing the largest diverticula. In an emergency situation resection should be confined to the segment bearing the affected diverticulum.

Operative Technique. Jejunoileal diverticula are often paper-thin and may lie concealed within the fat of the mesentery. It is not always easy to determine in an empty bowel whether or not they are present, despite the evidence of a barium meal follow-through examination. In this situation, distension of the suspected segment by milking gas and fluid content along from the ileum or stomach helps to blow out the diverticula and make them evident.

For excision of a solitary diverticulum on the mesenteric border of the intestine, the affected segment should be emptied of its content and noncrushing clamps applied proximally and distally. An incision is made in the leaf of the mesentery over the diverticulum, care being taken to avoid cutting the adjacent vasa recta, although these may be divided and tied if they lie directly over the diverticulum. The diverticulum is then gently grasped with a tissue forceps and dissected out to its base, at which point it is excised with scissors. The resulting defect is closed transversely in two layers of 2/0 chromic catgut and further sutures repair the leaf of the mesentery.

For diverticula of the antimesenteric border, the technique of excision is exactly similar to that described for Meckel's diverticulum.

UMBILICAL FISTULAE AND TUMOURS

Umbilical abnormalities (apart from hernia) may be classified as follows:

1. Anomalies of the vitellointestinal duct
   a. Patent duct (umbilical fistula)
   b. Umbilical granuloma
2. Anomalies of the urachus
   a. Urachal cyst
   b. Patent urachus
3. Tumours of the umbilicus

4. Miscellaneous, including "umbolith," pilonidal sinus of the umbilicus, endometrioma, etc.

Anomalies of the Vitellointestinal Duct

As already stated, the vitellointestinal duct may persist in whole or in part. Complete persistence is extremely rare and results in an external umbilical fistula. Such a fistula may discharge faeces, but more commonly it discharges only a small amount of mucus. The absence of faecal discharge is due to peristalsis in the patent duct passing from the umbilicus toward the subjacent ileum and preventing any ileal reflux. The fistulous connection with the bowel may easily be demonstrated by sinography. The treatment of complete umbilical fistula is total excision of the patent duct via a paraumbilical incision.

Umbilical granuloma, sometimes known as raspberry tumour, represents the umbilical extremity of the duct. It appears as a bright red granulomatous swelling, and the persistent mucoid discharge from it may produce a considerable degree of umbilical dermatitis. Most commonly there is no connection between the umbilical granuloma and the underlying ileum, but in about one third of cases a fibrous cord or narrow fistula connects the ileum to the umbilicus (Fig. 41–14). Because of the danger of such a band causing acute intestinal obstruction, laparotomy is advised in all cases of umbilical granuloma.

Anomalies of the Urachus

The allantois may very rarely persist between the fundus of the bladder and the umbilicus, forming a completely patent urachus. This produces a congenital urinary fistula and may occasionally be associated with membranous obstruction of the urethra. Equally rarely, the

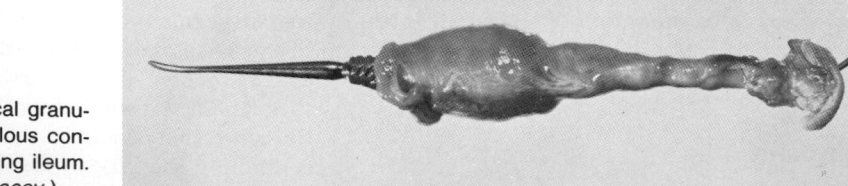

Figure 41–14. Umbilical granuloma with narrow fistulous connection to the underlying ileum. (*Courtesy of Mr. L. Gracey.*)

umbilical end may persist as an umbilical abscess. Effective treatment involves drainage of the abscess in the acute stage, followed by complete excision of all the urachal remnants when the infection has subsided.

Tumours of the Umbilicus

Such tumours are rare. Endometrioma may occur and occasionally a squamous cell carcinoma is found. Lymphatic spread from such a tumour may involve inguinal nodes in both groins. The primary tumour is best treated by wide local excision and the secondary nodes by block dissection. Secondary carcinoma of the umbilicus may occur by transcoelomic spread. The primary tumour is almost always in some abdominal organ, e.g., the stomach.

Miscellaneous

Sebaceous material may collect in the umbilicus, then inspissate and form a sebaceous horn or "umbolith." These accretions may be easily lifted out intact, and this should be done preoperatively while the abdomen is being shaved and prepared for operation.

Very rarely, in patients with cirrhosis of the liver and severe portal hypertension, a mass of veins may form at the umbilicus, resembling a tumour—the so-called Cruveilhier–Baumgarten syndrome (Fig. 41–15).

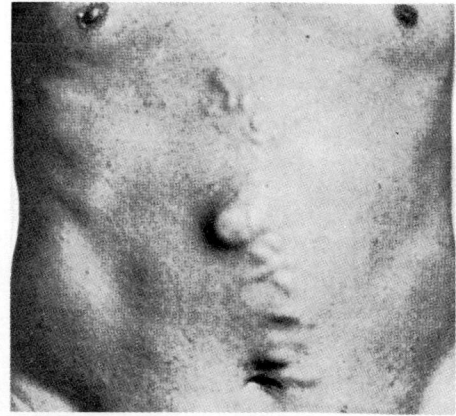

Figure 41–15. Distended umbilical veins in hepatic cirrhosis. (*Source: From Sherlock S, Brit J Clin Pract, with permission.*)

BIBLIOGRAPHY

Meckel's Diverticulum

Bartram CI, Amess JA: The diagnosis of Meckel's diverticulum by small bowel enema in the investigation of obscure intestinal bleeding. Br J Surg 67:417, 1980

Castleden WM: Meckel's diverticulum in an umbilical hernia. Br J Surg 57:932, 1970

Cooney DR, Duszynski DO, et al: The abdominal technetium scan (a decade of experience). J Pediatr Surg 17:611, 1982

Deetz E: Perforationsperitonitis von einem Darmdivertikel mit Magenschleimhautbau ausgehend. Dtsch Z Chir 88:482, 1907

Ewerth S, Hellers G, et al: Carcinoma of Meckel's diverticulum. Acta Chir Scand 145:203, 1979

Farthing MG, Griffiths NJ, et al: Occult bleeding from Meckel's diverticulum. Br J Surg 68:176, 1981

Hemingway AP, Allison AJ: Angiodysplasia and Meckel's diverticulum: A congenital association? Br J Surg 69:493, 1982

Jewett TC, Duszynski DO, Allen JE: The visualization of Meckel's diverticulum with ^{99m}Tc-pertechnetate. Surgery 68:567, 1970

Kuttner H: Ileus durch Intussusception eines Meckelschen Divertikel. Beitr Klin Chir 21:298, 1898

Lang-Stevenson A: Meckel's diverticulum: To look or not to look; To resect or not to resect. Ann R Coll Surg Engl 65:218, 1983

Lawrence RE: A case of coconut bezoar and Meckel's diverticulum. Postgrad Med J 58:119, 1982

Leslie MD, Slater ND, et al: Small bowel fistula from a Littré's hernia. Br J Surg 70:244, 1983

Mackey WC, Dineen P: A fifty year experience with Meckel's diverticulum. Surg Gynecol Obstet 156:56, 1983

Meckel JF: Beyträge zur vergleichenden Anatomie. Leipzig: Carl Heinrich Reclam, 1808, p 91

Meckel JF: Ueber die Divertikel am Darmkanal. Arch Physiol 9:421, 1809

Moore T, Johnston AOB: Complications of Meckel's diverticulum. Br J Surg 63:453, 1976

Perlman JA, Hoover HC, et al: Femoral hernia with strangulated Meckel's diverticulum (Littré's hernia). Am J Surg 139:286, 1980

Rosswick RP: Perforation of Meckel's diverticulum by foreign bodies. Postrad Med J 41:105, 1965

Rutherford RB, Akers DR: Meckel's diverticulum: A review of 148 pediatric patients, with reference to the pattern of bleeding and to mesodiverticular vascular bands. Surgery 59:618, 1966

Salzer H: Ueber das offene Meckelsche Divertikel. Wien Klin Wschr 17:614, 1904

Sellink JL: Meckel's diverticulum, in Sellink JL (ed): Radiological Atlas of Common Diseases of the Small Bowel. Leiden: Stenfert Kroese BV, 1976, p 338

Simms MH, Corkery JJ: Meckel's diverticulum: Its association with congenital malformation and the significance of atypical morphology. Br J Surg 67:216, 1980

Soderlund S: Meckel's diverticulum; a clinical and histologic study. Acta Chir Scand (suppl)248:1, 1959

Soltero MJ, Bill AH: The natural history of Meckel's diverticulum and its relation to incidental removal. Am J Surg 132:168, 1976

Vellacott KD: Haemoperitoneum due to Meckel's diverticulum. J R Coll Surg Edinb 26:89, 1981

Walsh PV: Slow-release iron tablet and gangrene of Meckel's diverticulum. Br J Clin Pract 34:258, 1980

Watson LF: Hernia, 3 edt. St. Louis: CV Mosby, 1948, p 547

Weinstein EC, Dockerty MB, et al: Neoplasms of Meckel's diverticulum. Surg Gynecol Obstet 116:103, 1963

Williams RS: Management of Meckel's diverticulum. Br J Surg 68:477, 1981

Jejunal Diverticula

Badenoch J, Bedford PD, et al: Massive diverticulosis of the small intestine with steatorrhoea and megaloblastic anaemia. Q J Med 24:321, 1955

Bewes PC, Haslewood GAD, et al: Bile acid enteroliths and jejunal diverticulosis. Br J Surg 53:709, 1966

Carter RA: Multiple congenital diverticula of the jejunum. Br J Surg 46:586, 1959

Cooke WT, Cox EV, et al: The clinical and metabolic significance of jejunal diverticula. Gut 4:115, 1963

Cooper AP: The anatomy and surgical treatment of crural and umbilical hernia. London: Cox, 1807

Craft I, Ellis H: Pneumatosis cystoides intestinalis associated with jejunal diverticula, presenting as pneumoperitoneum. Proc R Soc Med 60:141, 1967

Donald JW: Major complications of small bowel diverticula. Ann Surg 190:183, 1979

Eckhauser FE, Zelenock GB, et al: Acute complications of jejunal-ileal pseudodiverticulosis: Surgical implications and management. Am J Surg 138:320, 1979

Ellis H, Smith ADM: The blind-loop syndrome. Monogr Surg Sci 4:193, 1967

Kveim MHR: Jejunal diverticulosis with perforation and peritonitis. Acta Chir Scand 147:305, 1981

Montuschi E: Jejunal insufficiency with hypoproteinaemic oedema. Proc R Soc Med 42:868, 1949

Rosedale RS, Lawrence HR: Jejunal diverticulosis. Am J Surg 34:369, 1936

Shackleford RT, Marcus WY: Jejunal diverticula—a cause of gastrointestinal haemorrhage. Ann Surg 151:930, 1960

Taylor GW: Intestinal diverticulosis, pernicious anemia, bilateral suprarenal apoplexy: Report of a case. N Engl J Med 202:269, 1930

Watkinson G, Feather DB, et al: Jejunal diverticulosis with steatorrhoea and megaloblastic anaemia improved by excision of diverticula. Br Med J 2:58, 1959

Williams RA, Davidson DD, et al: Surgical problems of diverticula of the small intestine. Surg Gynecol Obstet 152:621, 1981

42. Surgery of Crohn's Disease

Rene Menguy

Dr. Burrill B. Crohn died on July 28, 1983 at the age of 99, during preparation of this chapter. He contributed much to his profession and the honors that he received during his long and active life were rightly deserved. May these pages be a homage to his memory.

INTRODUCTION

Crohn's disease is a relatively new condition. It was only in 1932 that Crohn, Ginzburg, and Oppenheimer based the description of this disease on a series of 14 cases. Before this publication, a few sporadic papers had appeared with descriptions of what could have been cases of Crohn's disease. Their now classic paper clearly distinguished Crohn's disease from hyperplastic ileocecal tuberculosis and, since then, reported cases of intestinal tuberculosis have become rare, at least in most developed countries.

In their original report, Crohn et al described this condition as affecting only the distal small bowel and therefore coined the term of "terminal ileitis." Because of the perjorative connotation attached to this term, it was later replaced by that of "regional enteritis." It later became apparent that, although the terminal ileum is indeed the most frequently involved segment of intestine, other segments of small intestine may also be affected. Moreover, subsequent reports indicated that this disease may affect the duodenum, the stomach, the esophagus, and the mouth. In 1960, much confusion surrounding inflammatory bowel disease of the colon was eliminated when Lockhart–Mummery and Morson showed that Crohn's disease also involves the colon, establishing a basis for differentiation of Crohn's disease of the colon (transmural colitis, granulomatous colitis) from chronic ulcerative colitis (mucosal colitis).

During the years following the original report by Crohn et al, the frequency of this condition, wherever reported, increased dramatically. At present, the prevalence in the United States is about 3 cases per 100,000 persons per year. It appears now that the incidence may have slowed or stopped altogether. The incidence is higher in Jews, particularly Ashkenazim, among whom the prevalence may be as high as 10 per 100,000 persons per year. Black persons are affected only rarely and, in this author's experience, only those with mixed black and Caucasian ancestry appear liable to this disease. Men and women are affected equally.

With the very first reports of this condition, a genetic factor became apparent. The occurrence of first-degree relatives with Crohn's disease, according to various reports, ranges from 3 to 18 percent. This increased familial incidence probably is not due to environmental factors since it is uncommon for the condition to affect both spouses.

One of the more interesting features of Crohn's disease is its uneven global distribution. Its incidence is highest in industrialized areas of the world. This factor is modified by climactic conditions: areas with a cooler climate have a higher incidence. The incidence of Crohn's disease is high in Scandinavia, the British Isles, Germany, and the United States, where the incidence is higher in the North than in the South.

The etiology remains unknown. From time to time, interest in a transmissable factor flares for a while and then dies; no one has ever brought forth any convincing evidence for such a factor. Epidemiologic studies based on "time–space clustering" have failed to demonstrate this condition as contagious.

Crohn's disease affects mainly young adults. The peak age distribution lies between

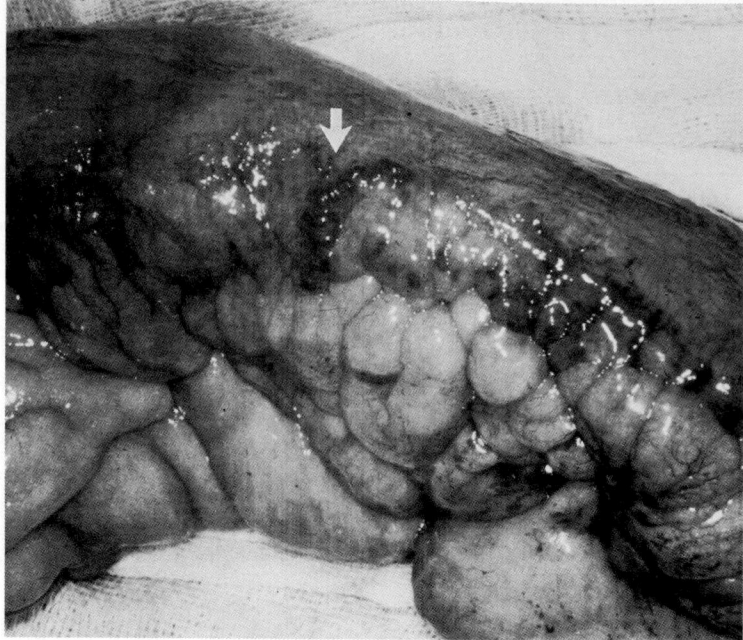

Figure 42–1. This illustrates the peculiar, and very characteristic, corkscrew appearance of the serosal vessels in Crohn's disease. This is a skip lesion in the mid-small bowel. Notice that, in addition to the abnormal appearance of the blood vessels, the mesenteric fat is encroaching on the antimesenteric border of the intestine. The mesentery is markedly thickened and edematous and contains large lymph nodes.

the second and fourth decades. It is common in children. In Van Patter's classic paper, 14 percent of 600 patients had developed symptoms before they were fifteen.

Patients with Crohn's disease may be classified into different groups according to the intestinal segments involved:

Ileocolic involvement, small and large intestine	40 percent
Small intestinal involvement, without involvement of the colon	30 percent
Colon involvement, without involvement of the small bowel	25 percent
Anorectal involvement (disease limited to the distal large intestine)	5 percent

The age distribution of patients among the different groups is similar. This chapter is devoted to Crohn's disease of the intestine, exclusive of the colon.

PATHOLOGIC ANATOMY

Gross Changes

The changes produced by this condition are very characteristic and, with rare exceptions, unmistakable. Involvement is segmental and, in most patients with small-bowel pattern of disease, is limited to the distal ileum, with a sharp cutoff at the ileocecal junction. The affected segment is thickened and less pliable than normal intestine. The serosa feels rough and has an inflamed, violaceous appearance. The mesenteric fat encroaches on the antimesenteric border of the bowel, so that, where the disease is most severe, the gut may be completely surrounded by mesenteric fat. The mesentery of the diseased segment is thickened, edematous, and contains enlarged lymph nodes. Vessels running from the mesentery to the diseased segment have a corkscrew appearance (Fig. 42–1). Proximally, there is a transition zone, several inches in length, over which the disease gradually tapers off and the bowel assumes a normal appearance. Frequently the diseased segment of intestine is densely adherent to other tissues: ileac fossa, omentum, sigmoid, bladder, and healthy loops of small bowel. In patients with long-standing disease, the proximal intestine is often dilated from chronic obstruction. Dilated small bowel proximal to strictured intestine may contain grossly diseased mucosa. The only condition capable of mimicking the florid changes of Crohn's disease is hypertrophic ileocecal tuberculosis, which has become very rare. Both illnesses are chronic and are associated with fever and

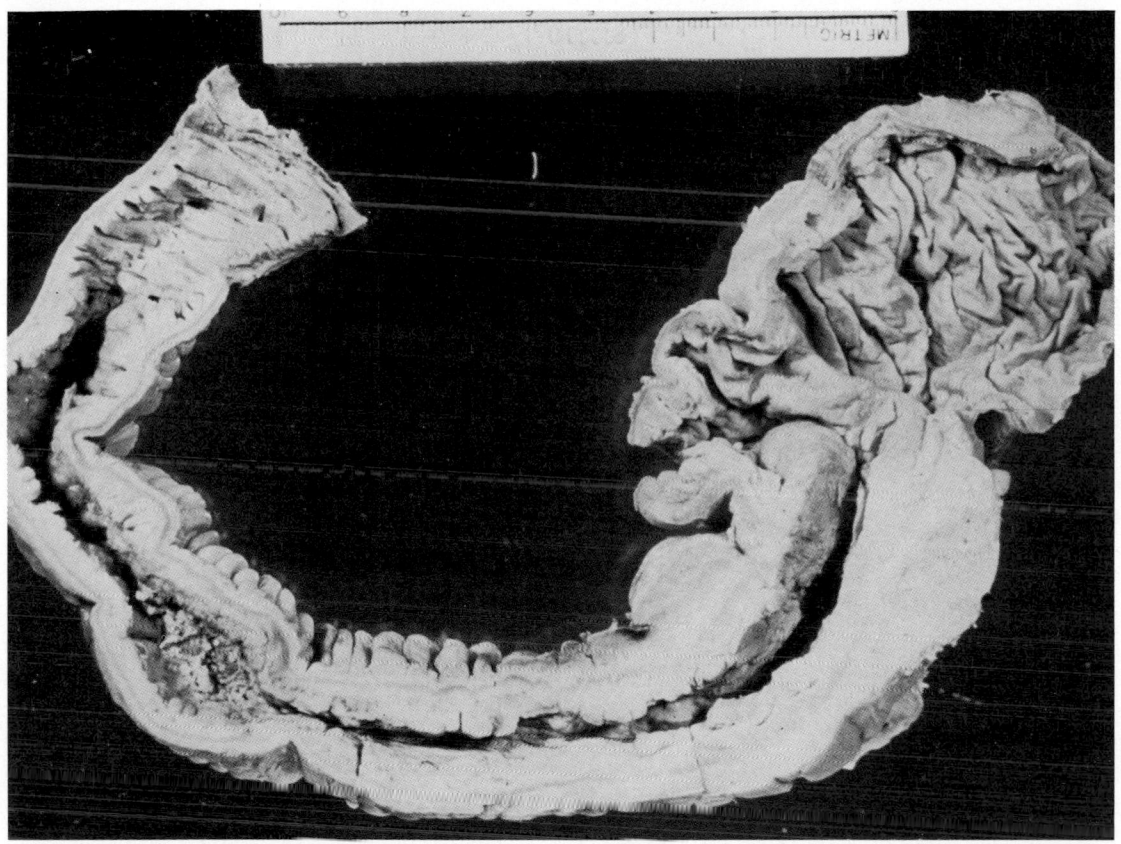

Figure 42–2. Example of unusually severe thickening of the bowel wall in a patient with far-advanced regional enteritis. Cases of this degree of severity are no longer seen today, since most patients would undergo surgery before reaching this stage. (*Source: From the collection of The Armed Forces Institute of Pathology, courtesy of Dr. Henry Rappaport.*)

weight loss, and are capable of producing a mass lesion in the ileocecal area along with a stricture of the terminal ileum. The strictures produced by ileocecal tuberculosis are shorter than those caused by Crohn's disease and there are always nodules (having the appearance of grains of rice) on the serosa. In Crohn's disease, the finding of an intraabdominal mass represents not only the thickened, diseased terminal ileum but also healthy tissues, such as the omentum and loops of small bowel adherent to it. In tuberculosis, the mass results primarily from the remarkable thickening of the cecum.

There are instances when, during an exploratory laparotomy for acute appendicitis, one finds an acutely inflamed violaceous terminal ileum with enlarged mesenteric nodes in its mesentery. Experience has shown that the ma-jority of patients presenting in this manner will not develop Crohn's disease and, in all probability, many of them represent cases of infection by *Yersinia enterolytica*, which is being recognized more frequently in the United States.

When operating on a patient who has Crohn's disease of the terminal ileum, it is important to explore the entire small bowel in search of other affected segments. Separate diseased segments are very characteristic of Crohn's disease. They are known as "skip lesions" and the intervening healthy bowel is known as a "skip area." In patients with primary disease in the terminal ileum, skip lesions are usually also in the ileum and often are situated close to the main lesion. Approximately 5 percent of patients with Crohn's disease have a diffuse jejunoileitis. In the author's experi-

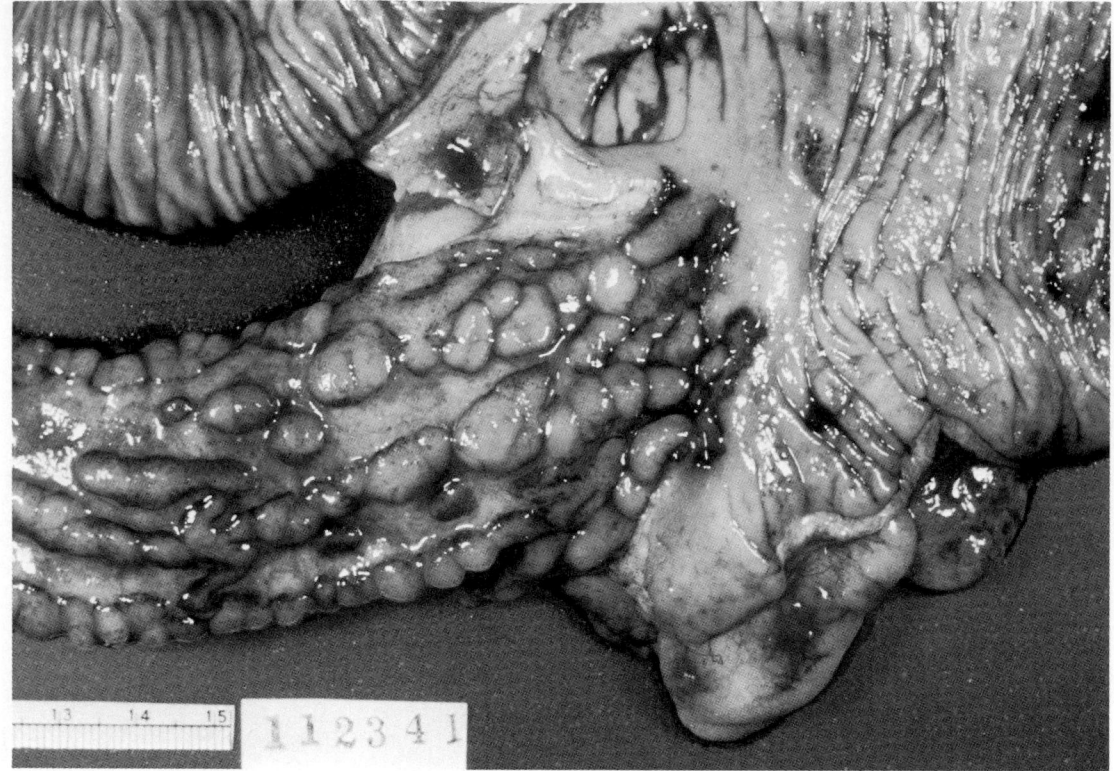

Figure 42–3. Characteristic appearance of the terminal ileum and ileocecal junction in a patient with regional enteritis. Notice the characteristic "cobblestone" appearance of the mucosa. Also note that, although the florid disease ceases abruptly at the ileocecal junction, there are some aphthous ulcers in the mucosa of the cecum.

ence, these patients also have colonic involvement. Long segments of jejunum and ileum are diseased with short skip areas. Before the introduction of parenteral hyperalimentation, this form of inflammatory bowel disease had a deadly prognosis. Approximately 1 to 2 percent of patients with Crohn's disease have gastroduodenal involvement. Disease in this segment of the gut is better diagnosed by means of x-ray and endoscopy. In the author's experience, gross changes on the outside of the duodenum are not always easy to recognize and they are particularly discrete on the outside of the stomach. Gastroduodenal involvement is always associated with disease in the small intestine and in the colon.

The opened intestine shows the characteristic long narrowing of the lumen due to thickening of the bowel wall—thickening that in extreme cases, although rarely seen today, can be truly enormous (Fig. 42–2). The mucosa in the most severely affected portion of the surgical specimen is ulcerated. The ulcers have the appearance of long furrows ("rake ulcers") running along the longitudinal axis of the bowel. The intervening islands of mucosa appear raised, which gives to the mucosal surface its characteristic "cobblestone" appearance (Fig. 42–3). When Crohn's disease involves only the small intestine, the changes cease abruptly at the ileocecal valve. At the proximal margin of the diseased segment, there is a more gradual transition into healthy mucosa, with the deep longitudinal ulcers becoming more shallow and shorter and gradually giving way to discrete pinhead-size "aphthous" ulcers. Fistulous tracts may be found penetrating deep into, or through, the wall of the diseased segment of intestine.

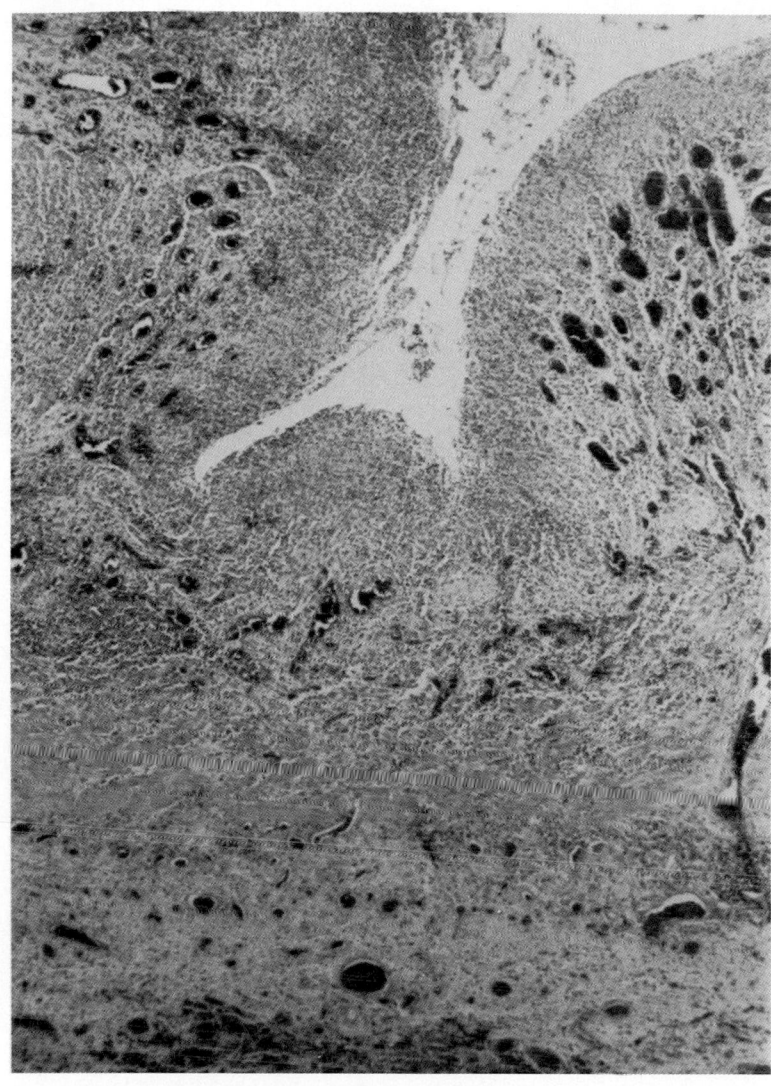

Figure 42-4. Low-power view of a cross-section of the mucosa of the terminal ileum in a patient with regional enteritis, showing a characteristic ulceration.

Microscopic Changes

Microscopic examination of the diseased intestine reveals a number of changes that, taken together, are highly diagnostic.

Ulcerations. On longitudinal sections, these have the appearance of fissures that extend more or less deeply into the wall of the intestine (Figs. 42–4 and 42–5). The deep ones tend to form fistulas. The latter become lined by surface epithelium, which explains their extraordinary chronicity.

Fibrosis. The bowel wall is thickened due to edema or fibrosis in the submucosa (Fig. 42–6).

Lymphangiectasia. Lymphatic channels are dilated (Fig. 42–7).

Nodular Lymphoid Hyperplasia. Lymphoid hyperplasia may lead to follicle formation in the mucosa (Fig. 42–8). Giant cells may be found in some follicles. Caseation is never seen. Lymphoid hyperplasia is not always present but, when found, is absolutely diagnostic (Fig. 42–9).

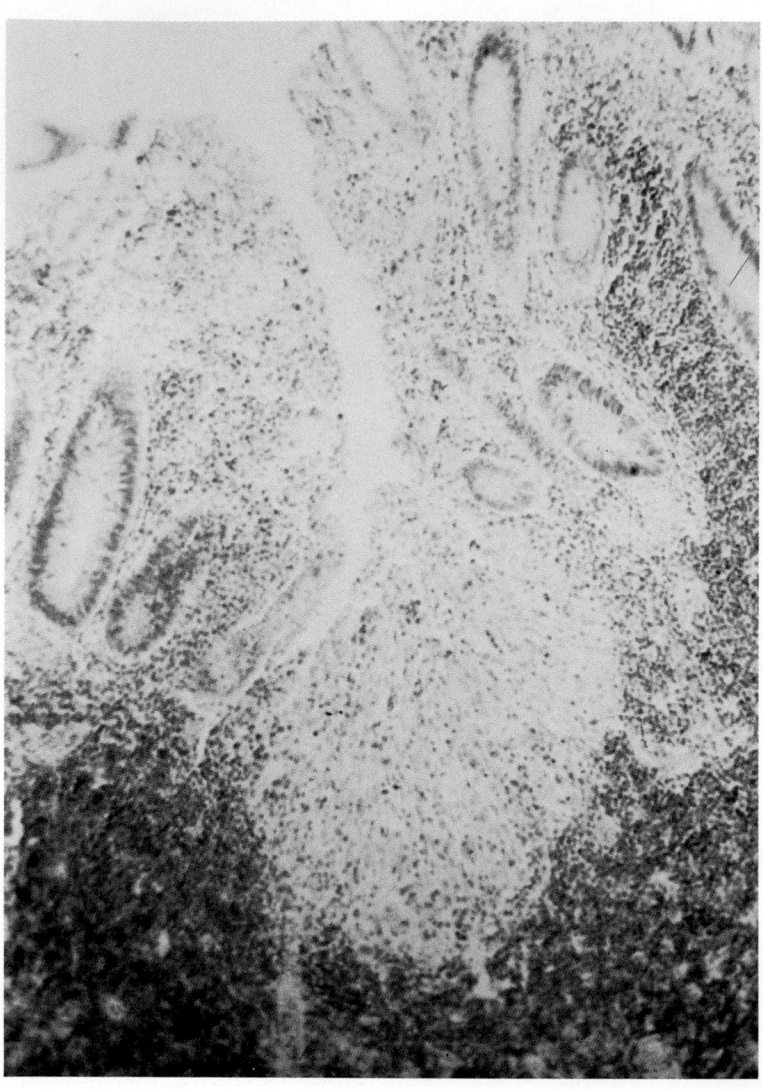

Figure 42–5. Example of a deep ulcer or "fissure" in the terminal ileum of a patient with regional enteritis. The fissure, which almost looks like a cutting artefact, is surrounded by considerable inflammation and necrosis.

CLINICAL MANIFESTATIONS

Typically, the onset of Crohn's disease is insidious, although in some cases patients present with a picture evoking acute appendicitis and the correct diagnosis is made only at laparotomy. More often, patients experience a combination of systemic and gastrointestinal (GI) symptoms. The former are due to the chronic inflammatory process. The latter result from the impairment of intestinal transport in the diseased loop of bowel by narrowing of the bowel and altered peristalsis.

Systemic manifestations consist of loss of appetite, lassitude, low-grade fever, and night sweats. An insidious weight loss is common. The most frequent digestive symptom is diarrhea, which almost all patients with Crohn's disease experience at one time or another. The diarrhea may be intermittent or continuous. Steatorrhea and hematochezia are often present. The diagnosis is rarely made at this stage. With progression of the disease, symptoms of low-grade small bowel obstruction appear and patients begin to experience colicky abdominal pain 1 to 3 hours after eating. The discomfort is often associated

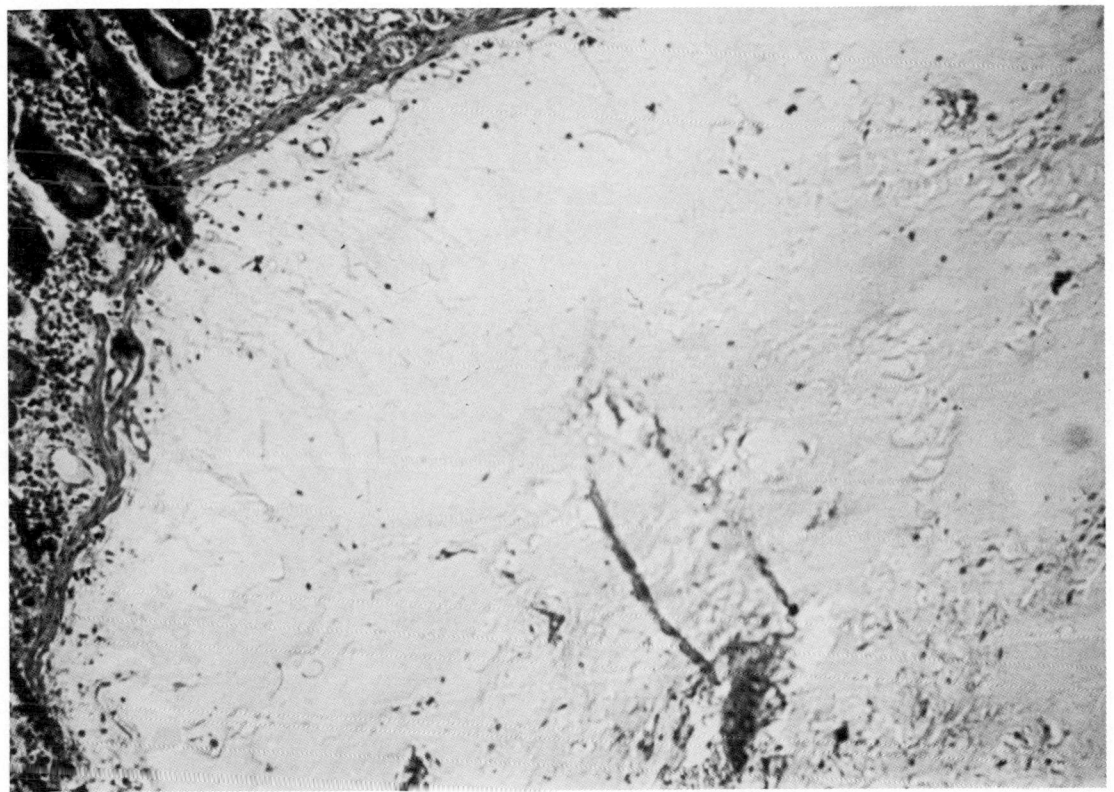

Figure 42–6. Low-power view of a section of the terminal ileum in a patient with regional enteritis, demonstrating very marked edema in the submucosa.

with borborygmi and is usually followed by diarrhea. A continuous dull ache in the right lower quadrant may develop. This suggests that the parietal peritoneum in the right iliac fossa is becoming inflamed. At this stage, a doughy, ill-defined mass in the right lower quadrant may be palpable. The mass consists of the diseased segment of terminal ileum to which other tissues, such as the omentum, the sigmoid, the urinary bladder, and healthy loops of small intestine, have become adherent (Fig. 42–10). A walled-off abscess is frequently contained within the mass in which one or more fistulous tracts going from the diseased intestine to other viscera or tissues is often found.

In addition to the more general signs and symptoms already described, there are some manifestations of a more specific nature that are very typical of this disease.

Urologic Manifestations

Enterovesical fistulae occur in from 5 to 10 percent of patients with Crohn's disease of the terminal ileum. Symptoms consist of recurrent episodes of lower urinary tract infection with dysuria and increased urinary frequency. Pyuria, pneumaturia, and fecaluria may occur. Long-standing enterovesical fistulas may cause contracture of the bladder and urinary incontinence. The opening on the bladder side is usually too small to be seen at cystoscopy. The finding of a zone of bullous cystitis in a patient with lower urinary tract symptoms and known Crohn's disease should suffice to make the diagnosis. An x-ray of a centrifuged urine sample after a barium study of the small bowel may give vivid, albeit indirect, proof of the fistula (Fig. 42–11).

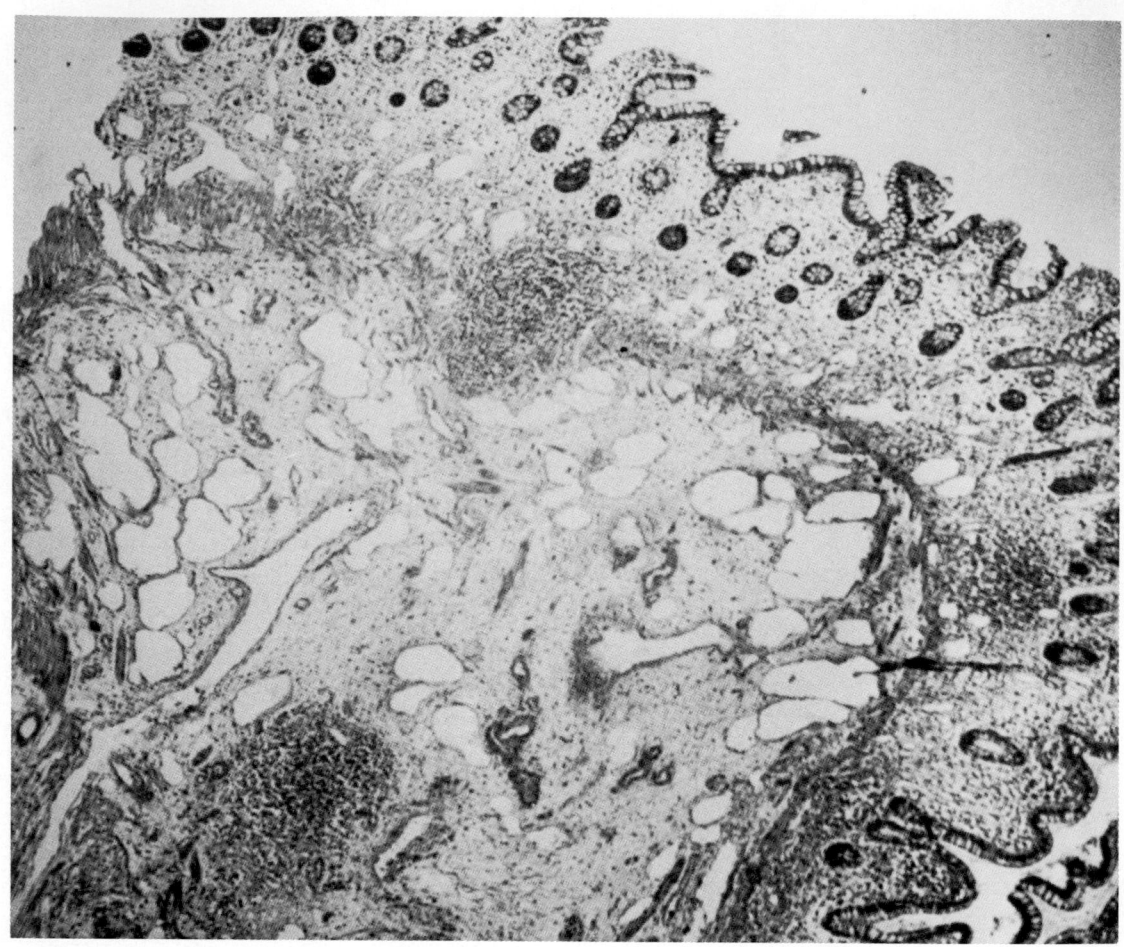

Figure 42–7. A good example of dilated lymphatic channels—lymphangiectasia—in the submucosa in a patient with regional enteritis.

Figure 42–9. Section taken from the terminal ileum with regional enteritis showing epitheliod giant cells in a noncaseating granuloma.

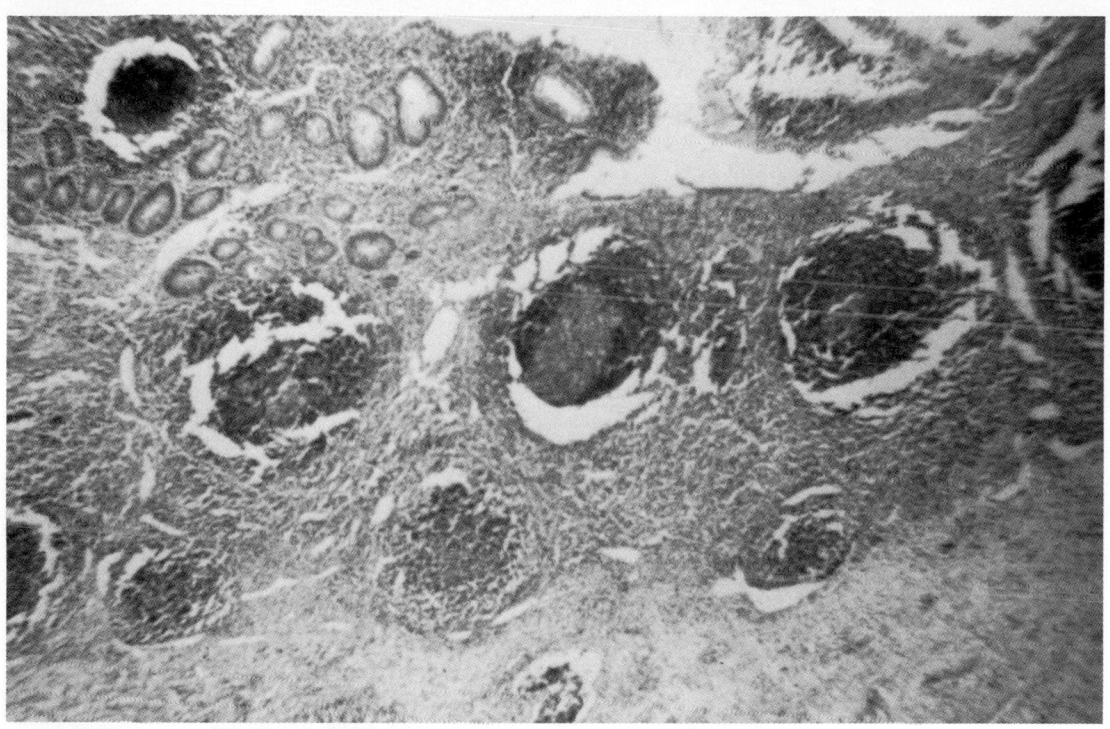

Figure 42–8. This low-power view of a section of the mucosa of the terminal ileum in a patient with regional enteritis shows numerous noncaseating granulomas.

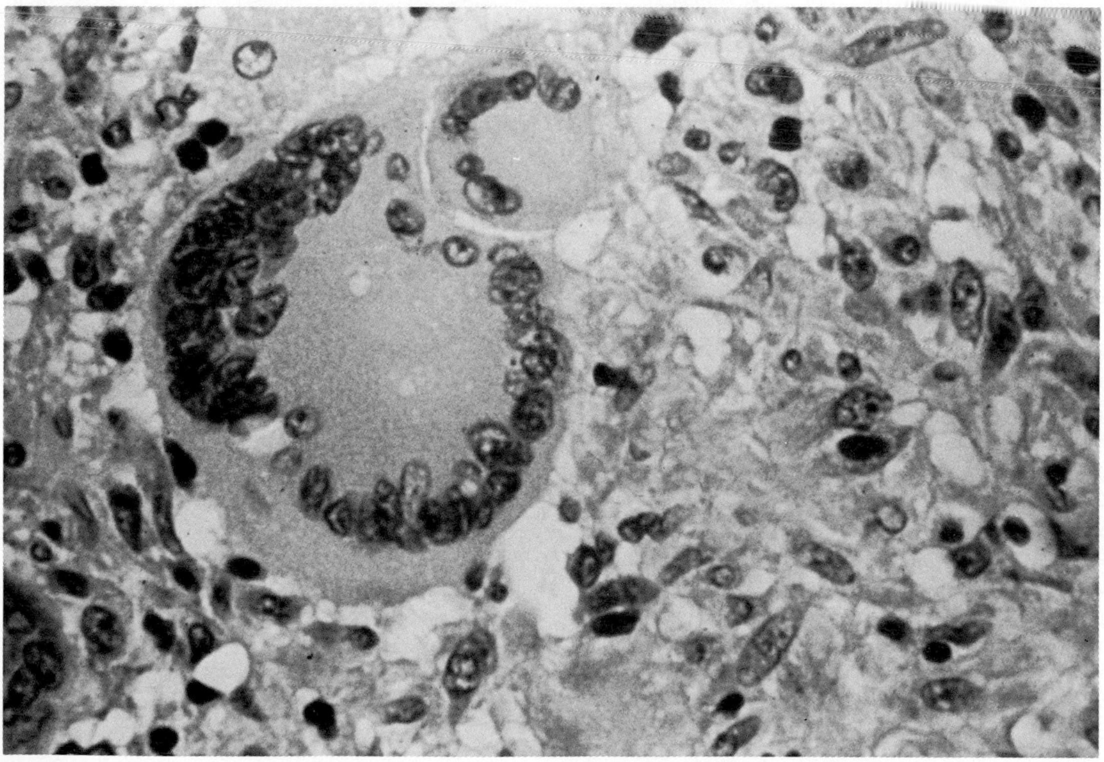

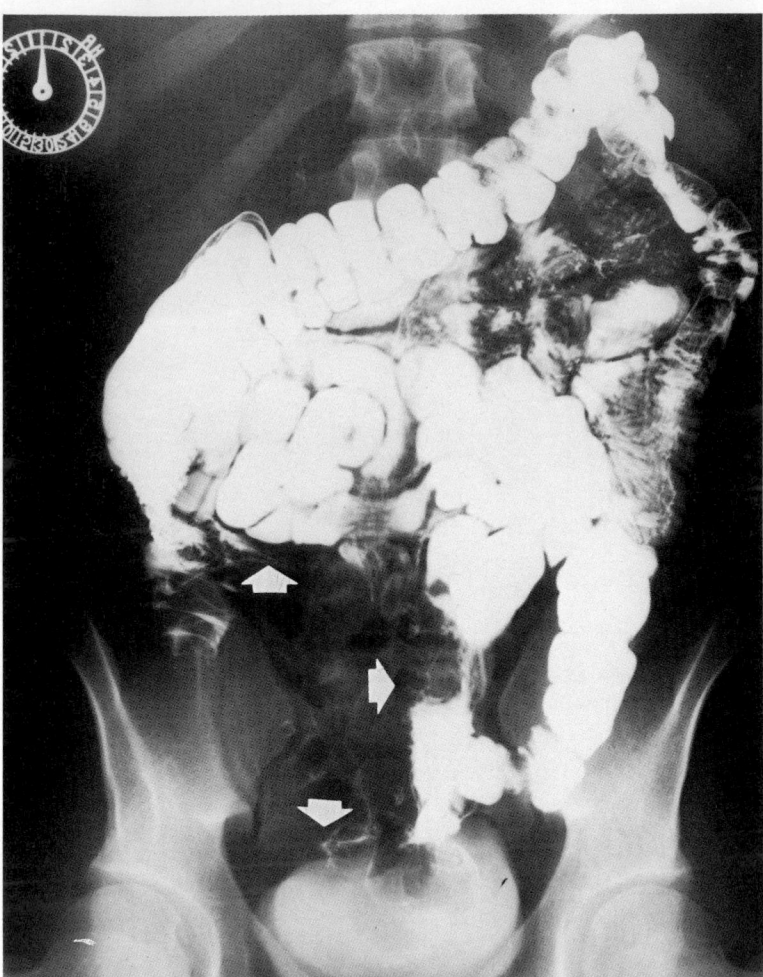

Figure 42–10. This patient has extensive regional enteritis of the terminal ileum complicated by an ileovesical fistula. Note the mass effect, with displacement of healthy bowel (*arrows*). The lower arrow points to a segment of diseased terminal ileum adherent to the urinary bladder.

Another important urologic complication of Crohn's disease is compression of the right ureter by periureteral fibrosis as it crosses over the pelvic brim behind the diseased terminal ileum (Fig. 42–12). Hydronephrosis occurs, although obstructive renal injury on this basis is rare. It is important to be aware of this possible complication and order an intravenous pyelogram at some point in the workup of the patient with disease in the terminal ileum, particularly if there is a mass in the right lower quadrant. This study is particularly important in patients about to undergo surgery for involvement of the terminal ileum, because ureteral compression, if present, can be corrected at the time of surgery by ureterolysis. From simple compression and partial obstruction of the right ureter, the problem may evolve toward the development of the rare complication of an ileoureteral fistula.

Patients with disease involving the terminal ileum have an increased incidence of nephrolithiasis related to hyperoxaluria. This, in turn, occurs because patients with ileal disease may have steatorrhea. The latter reduces the concentration of calcium in the lumen of the intestine. The reduced availability of calcium for the formation of insoluble calcium oxalate complexes increases the absorption of oxalate. Thus, the prevention of nephrolithiasis in patients with extensive ileal disease consists in the prescription of a low-fat, low-oxalate diet.

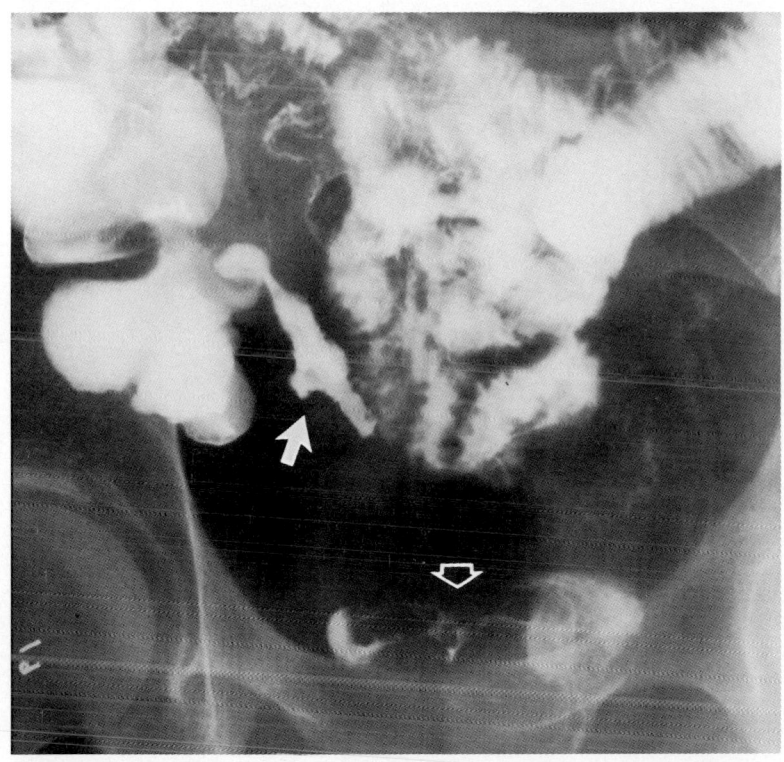

A

Figure 42–11. A. Small bowel study in a patient with Crohn's disease of the terminal ileum. *Solid Arrow:* Rigid, narrow terminal ileum proximal to the cecum. *Open Arrow:* A segment of terminal ileum "stuck" to the bladder. There is a faint outline of a fistulous tract at this level.

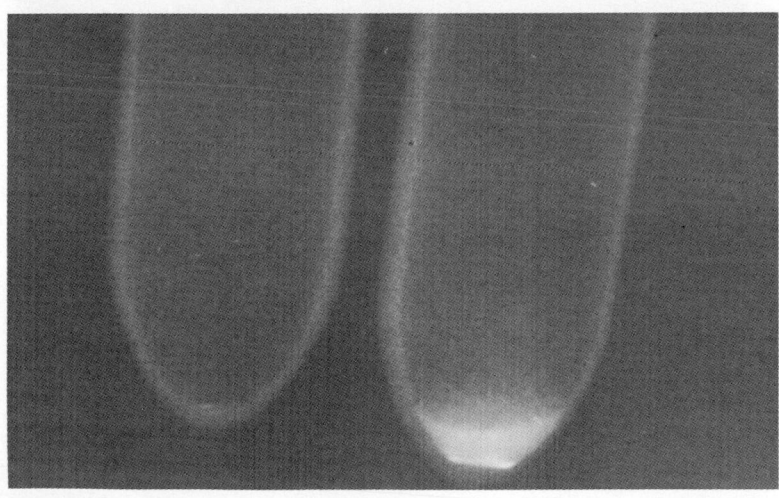

B

Figure 42–11. B. After this study was done, a urine sample was taken and centrifuged. The x-ray of the urine sample shows that it contains barium, thus confirming the presence of an ileovesical fistula.

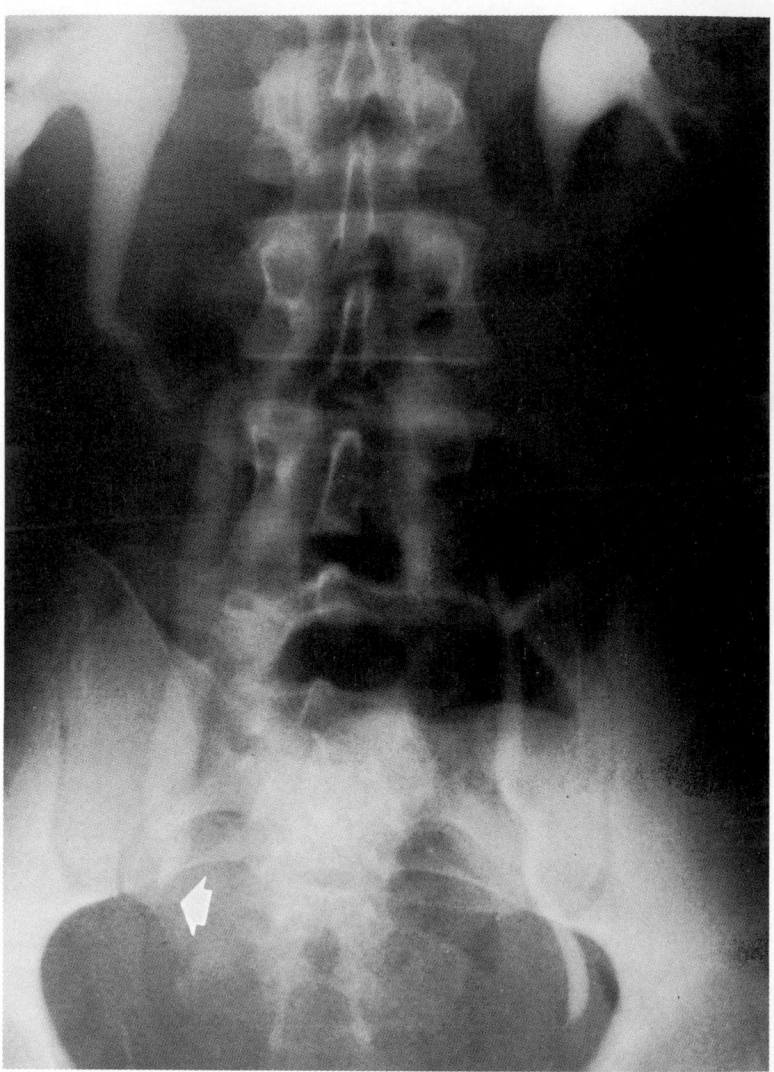

Figure 42–12. A. Intravenous pyelogram in a patient with regional enteritis of the terminal ileum. Note that the right ureter is narrowed at the point where it crosses over the rim of the pelvis. Proximally, there is moderate hydronephrosis.

A

Another mechanism for urinary stone formation in patients with Crohn's disease is dehydration associated with severe diarrhea. This is a particularly serious problem in patients with diffuse jejunoileitis or in patients with an extensive ileocolitis who have lost their colon, along with important lengths of small bowel, and have a permanent ileostomy. Extrarenal fluid losses from the ileostomy may be large enough to make it difficult for the patient to stay ahead of losses with enteral fluid intake. The highly concentrated urine increases the risk of stone formation.

Fistula Formation

The development of a fistulous tract between the diseased small bowel and other organs or tissues or the abdominal skin (Fig. 42–13) is so typical of this disease that special comment is warranted. Several decades ago, when surgery was performed at a much later stage in the evolution of the disease, the incidence of fistulous tracts was much higher than it is today. In Van Patter's series, the incidence of external and internal fistulas was 21 and 45 percent, respectively. In a more recent study, the incidence

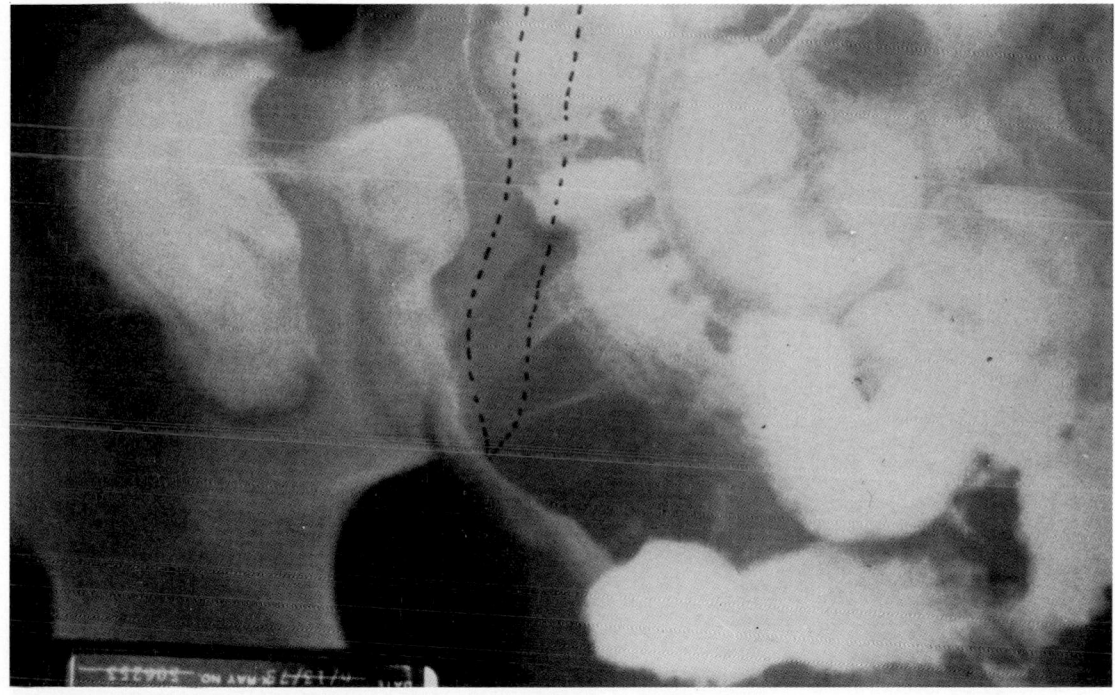

B

Figure 42-12. B. Spot view of the terminal ileum in the same patient. The outline of the right ureter, taken from the intravenous pyelogram, was traced onto the film to demonstrate the relationship between the diseased terminal ileum and the point where the ureter is obstructed.

of both internal and external fistulous tracts in patients with disease limited to the small bowel was 17 percent. Fistulas are more common in patients with ileocolitis.

External fistulas often occur after surgery and are a result of a spontaneous perforation walled off by the tissues of the abdominal wall adjacent to a surgical incision, or of a leaking anastomosis after ileal resection. The cutaneous opening of the fistula communicates with the intestine by an often complicated tract. The latter often communicates with an abscess that may be deep to the psoas iliac muscles (Fig. 42-14) or in the right flank. This author has seen two patients with tracts going around the iliac crest and presenting in the right buttock. The more common internal fistulas are as follows: ileo-ascending colon, ileoileal (Fig. 42-15), ileosigmoid, ileovesical, ileovaginal.

Ileosigmoid fistulas present important problems when surgery for disease of the terminal ileum is being considered. The sigmoid joined to the ileum by a fistulous tract may be diseased or it may be normal. If it is diseased, this has to be determined prior to surgery, as closure of the opening in the sigmoid will not suffice. The diseased colon will have to be resected as well.

For these reasons, these fistulous tracts have little tendency to heal spontaneously. Several years ago, there was considerable interest in using parenteral hyperalimentation to heal fistulous tracts. Although this modality is capable of reducing fluid and electrolyte losses from enterocutaneous fistulas, the latter almost never heal permanently. Drainage reappears with resumption of oral feeding.

Perianal Disease

Patients with Crohn's disease are prone to perianal disease in the form of fistulas-in-ano and

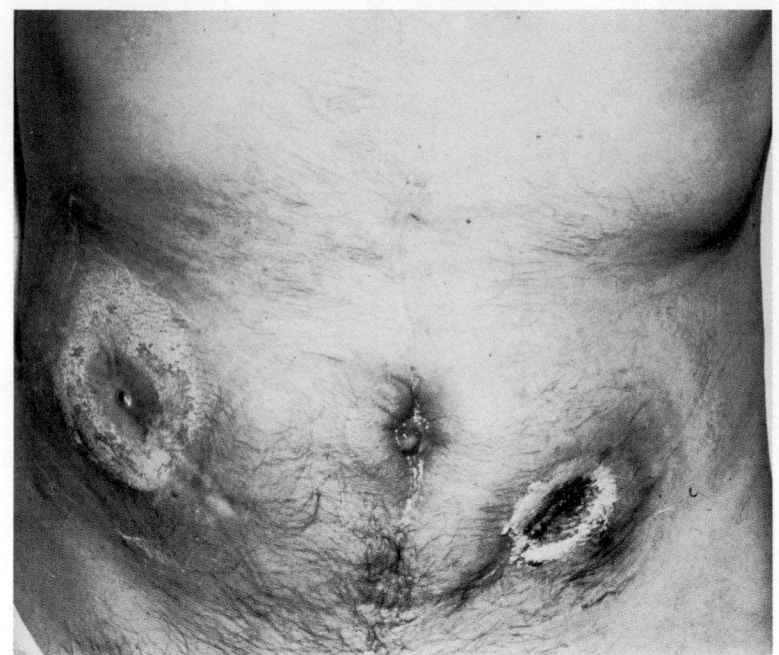

Figure 42–13. Example of multiple enterocutaneous fistulas in a patient with extensive jejunoileitis. Note that all of the fistulous openings are located in old scars.

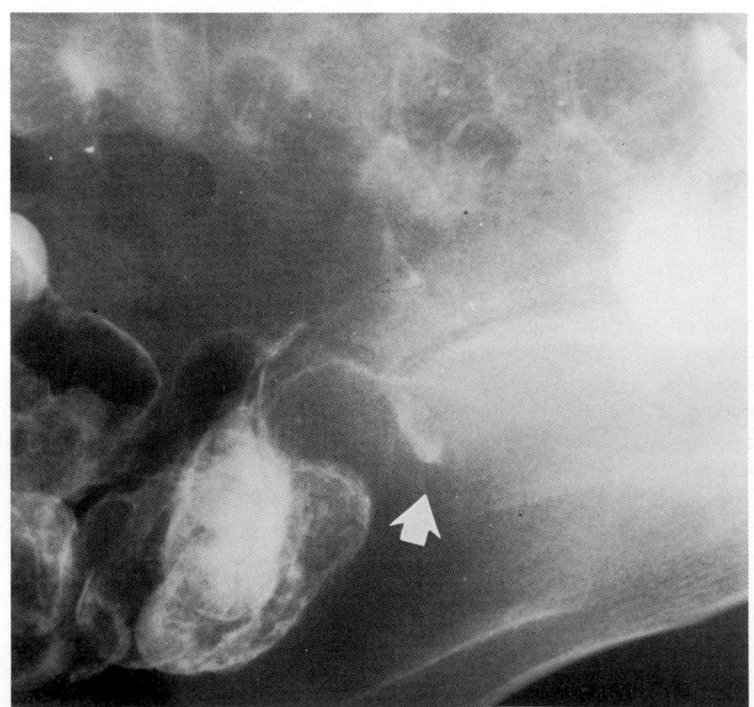

Figure 42–14. Crohn's disease of the terminal ileum. The arrow points to a deep fistulous tract in the terminal ileum proximal to the ileocecal valve and communicating with a psoas abscess.

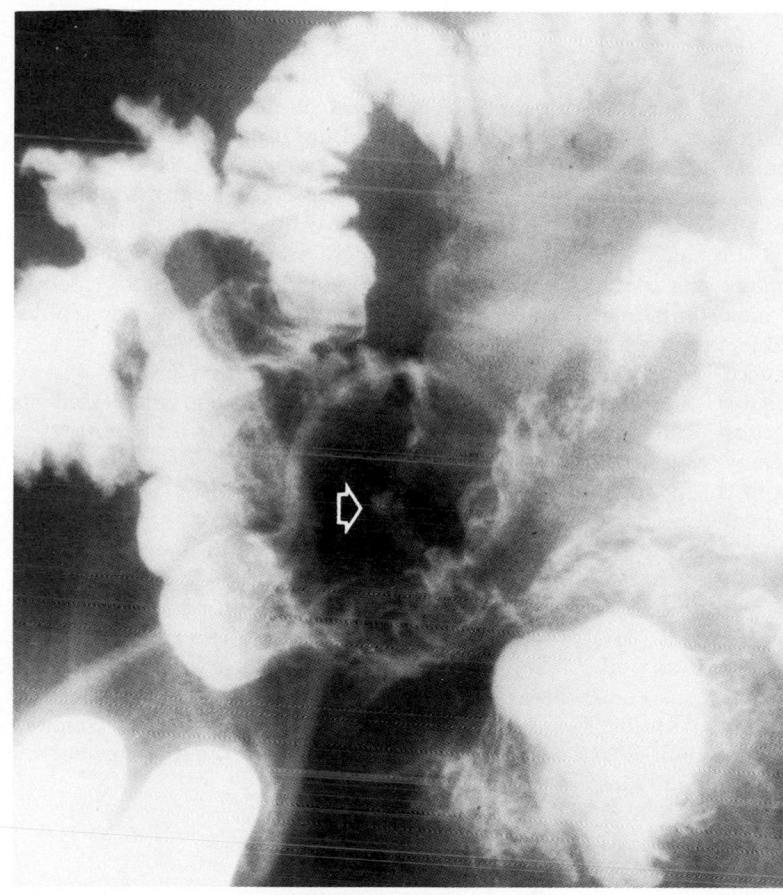

Figure 42–15. Excellent definition of the terminal ileum obtained by the technique of enteroclysis. A fistulous tract joining two loops of diseased terminal ileum is very clearly defined (*arrow*).

perianal abscesses. The perianal skin takes on a characteristic violaceous discoloration. Edematous skin tags, often mistaken for hemorrhoids, surround the anal canal. When the process is severe and of long standing, gradual destruction of the external and internal sphincters and of the perineal body, with fecal incontinence, may occur. This process can be hastened by inappropriate perianal surgery.

Mild perianal disease may occur, albeit infrequently, in patients with disease limited to the small intestine. The finding of severe and florid perianal disease signifies rectal involvement.

Gynecologic Manifestations

The diseased terminal ileum often becomes adherent to pelvic structures. In women, dyspareunia may occur as a result of this. A fistula may extend from the terminal ileum to the vagina. In patients with rectal involvement, a rectovaginal fistula is a common occurrence. It may be the first manifestation of rectal disease. The vaginal opening is sometimes hard to locate.

Gallbladder Disease

The prevalence of cholelithiasis (32 to 34 percent) is higher in patients with Crohn's disease of the terminal ileum than in the general population. The impaired absorption of bile acids from the diseased terminal ileum reduces the bile acid pool and lithogenicity of bile increases. It has been shown that this already high prevalence of gallstones in patients with Crohn's disease is further increased by parenteral hyperalimentation, an important observation in view of the fact that many patients with severe Crohn's require parenteral hyperalimentation at one time or another to manage complications.

Malnutrition and Systemic Manifestations

Varying degrees of malnutrition are found in almost all cases of Crohn's disease. The severity of these changes is proportional to the extent of small bowel involved and is most severe in patients with extensive jejunoileitis and with extensive ileocolitis. The metabolic deficit results from several factors. A major one is the impairment by disease of two important functions of the terminal ileum: absorption of vitamin B_{12} and of bile acids. Reduced absorption of bile acids increases the concentration of bile acids in the colon. This, in turn, causes diarrhea. Increased fecal loss of bile acids may tax hepatic synthesis of these compounds to the point of lowering the bile acid pool and reducing the postprandial duodenal bile acid concentration. This, in turn, causes impaired micelle formation and fat malabsorption. Reduced absorption of vitamin B_{12} may result in lower serum B_{12} levels. Lower folate levels may be present as well.

Anemia and hypoalbuminemia are common and are more severe in patients with ileocolitis than in patients with disease limited to the terminal ileum. The anemia results in part from moderate occult bleeding, but mostly from vitamin B_{12} and particularly folate deficiencies. Hypoalbuminemia is common to many conditions whose dominant manifestation is diarrhea, and Crohn's disease is no exception. A large amount of protein is lost from the inflamed mucosa. When this increased loss is accompanied by a reduction in caloric intake due to loss of appetite, discomfort with meals, etc., hepatic synthesis of albumin may not be able to stay ahead of fecal losses, and hypoalbuminemia, sometimes severe enough to cause edema, may occur.

The erythrocyte sedimentation rate is almost always elevated.

One of the more distressing consequences of the malnutrition brought about by this condition is impairment of growth and development in patients with onset of the disease during the first two decades of life. This problem is common to all types of inflammatory bowel disease. The combination of chronic malnutrition, vitamin deficiency, fecal caloric and protein loss, and deficiency in trace elements such as zinc result in growth retardation and impairment of sexual maturation. The effects of the disease per se may be compounded by the metabolic effects of steroids when these are used to control complications. It is well known that steroids retard bone growth. The delayed physical and sexual maturation may lead to indelible emotional scarring. Surgical eradication of the disease is always followed by a spurt of "catch-up" growth. In our experience this occurs even after puberty but not after epiphyseal closure. It is essential that, in growing children afflicted with Crohn's disease, surgery, if indicated, be performed in time to allow the child to complete normal physical development.

The peculiar inflammatory process operating in Crohn's disease characteristically affects tissues other than those in the intestinal tract.

Ocular Involvement

Ocular disorders are found in approximately 3 percent of patients with small bowel disease. The incidence is the same in patients with disease of the large intestine. The risk of developing ocular complications is greatest during the early course of the bowel disease and when the disease is clinically active. The most common ocular manifestations are uveitis, corneal ulcers, and blepharitis.

Joint Manifestations

A migratory polyarthritis, usually involving the large joints, is seen in about 5 percent of patients with small bowel disease. Crippling deformities rarely occur. The joint manifestations are more common in patients who also have ocular complications.

Skin Involvement

Skin lesions taking the form of erythema nodosum occur in about 5 percent of patients. Pyoderma gangrenosa no longer occurs as frequently as previously (Fig. 42–16). It is probable that this lesion is secondary to the malnutrition caused by Crohn's disease rather than to the inflammatory process per se. It is therefore less common because of the improved treatment that these patients receive today.

Fluid and Electrolyte Disturbances

Exacerbation of the diarrhea during periods of activity of the disease may result in clinically significant dehydration and reduced urine out-

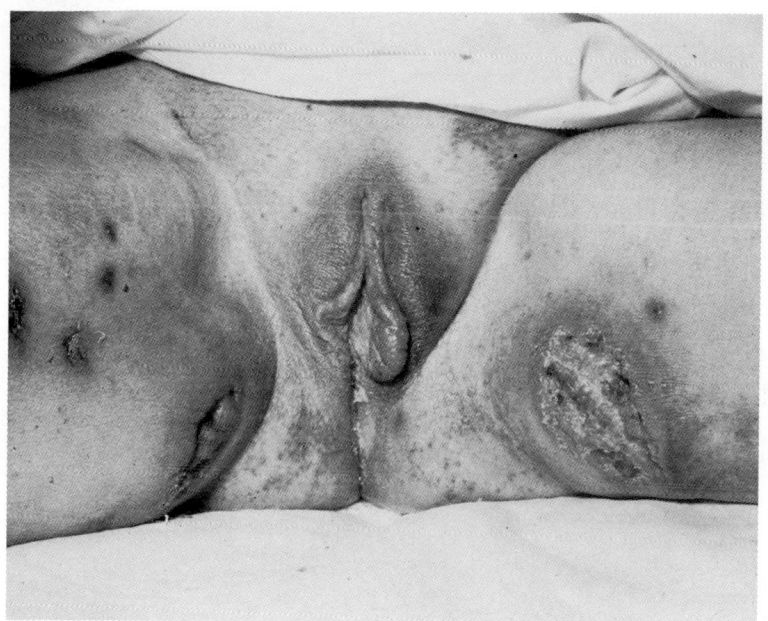

Figure 42–16. This is an example of moderately severe pyoderma gangrenosa in a patient with extensive Crohn's ileocolitis. Actually, the lesions seen here are in a stage of rapid healing, as this picture was taken 5 days after surgery. In the author's experience, the incidence of this very distressing complication of inflammatory bowel disease has decreased dramatically during the past decade, probably due to better nutritional care of these patients.

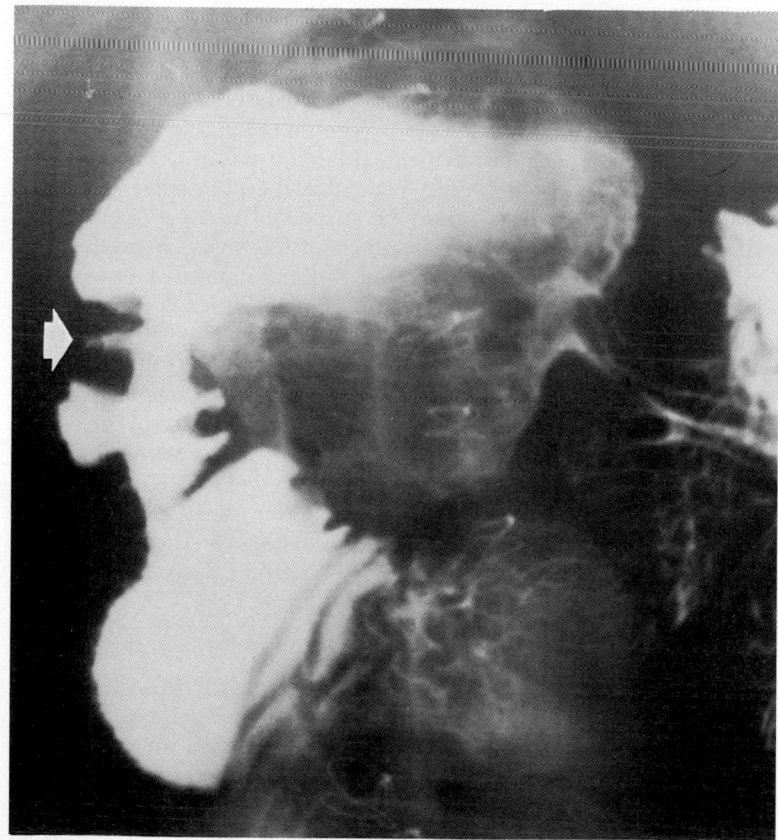

Figure 42–17. Upper GI series in a patient with extensive Crohn's ileocolitis. Duodenal involvement is present, as shown by the segmental narrowing of the second portion of the duodenum and the deep ulcerations (*arrow*).

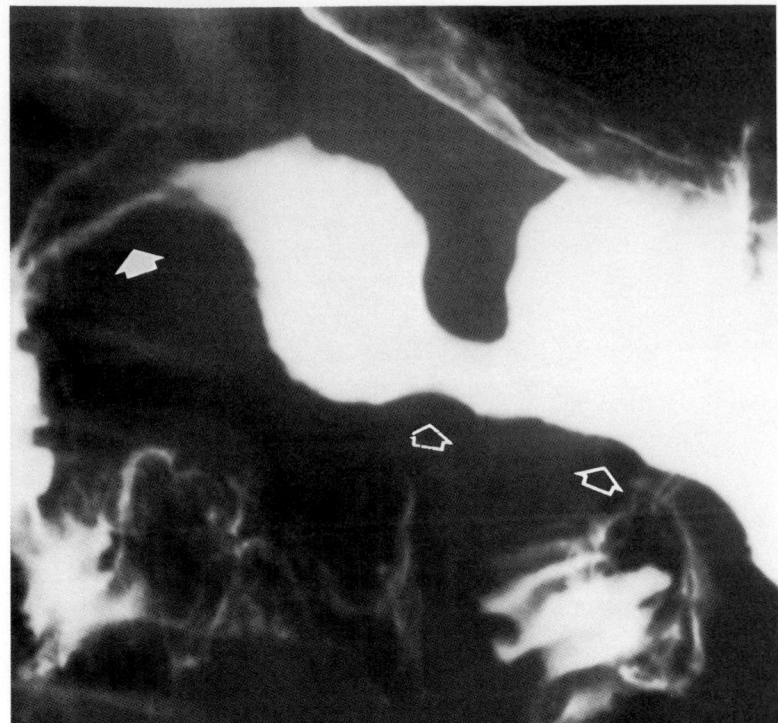

Figure 42–18. Gastroduodenal involvement in a patient with Crohn's ileocolitis. *Solid Arrow:* The narrowed first and second portions of the duodenum. *Open Arrows:* The greater curvature of the antrum, which has the rigid, scalloped contour characteristic of gastric involvement.

put. The frequent recurrence of such episodes may precipitate nephrolithiasis. Fecal losses of potassium and magnesium may cause lowered serum levels of these elements. Although fecal losses of calcium may be high, particularly in patients with steatorrhea, hypocalcemia is found only in the presence of vitamin D deficiency. The latter is rare, but it may occur if the steatorrhea is very severe. This tends to be a problem in patients with diffuse jejunoileitis.

Unusual Anatomic Locations of Crohn's Disease

Diffuse Jejunoileitis

Extensive involvement of the entire small bowel occurs in 3 to 10 percent of patients with Crohn's disease. In this author's experience, these patients also have colonic involvement.

Duodenal Disease

Duodenal involvement occurs in approximately 1.5 percent of patients with Crohn's disease. It is always associated with involvement of other intestinal segments, usually of the small bowel and the colon. When duodenal involvement becomes evident, the diagnosis of Crohn's disease has usually been already established. Duodenal disease may be suspected when a patient with a known diagnosis of Crohn's disease develops early satiety as well as nausea and vomiting after meals. An upper GI series is usually diagnostic. Deep ulcers with a cobblestone pattern in the mucosa are readily seen (Fig. 42–17). At endoscopy, aphthous ulcers are visualized in the duodenal mucosa. Free perforation of the duodenum may occur (one case in the author's experience). More typically, however, a fistula will extend from the duodenum into a neighboring organ, usually the colon. (On the other hand, a fistula may extend from diseased colon into nondiseased duodenum.)

Gastric Disease

Involvement of the stomach is rare. In the author's experience, it is never isolated, but is always found in association with involvement of the duodenum, and always in patients with ileocolitis. The manifestations are those of early satiety and gastric outlet obstruction. Bleeding, sometimes massive, may occur (Fig. 42–18).

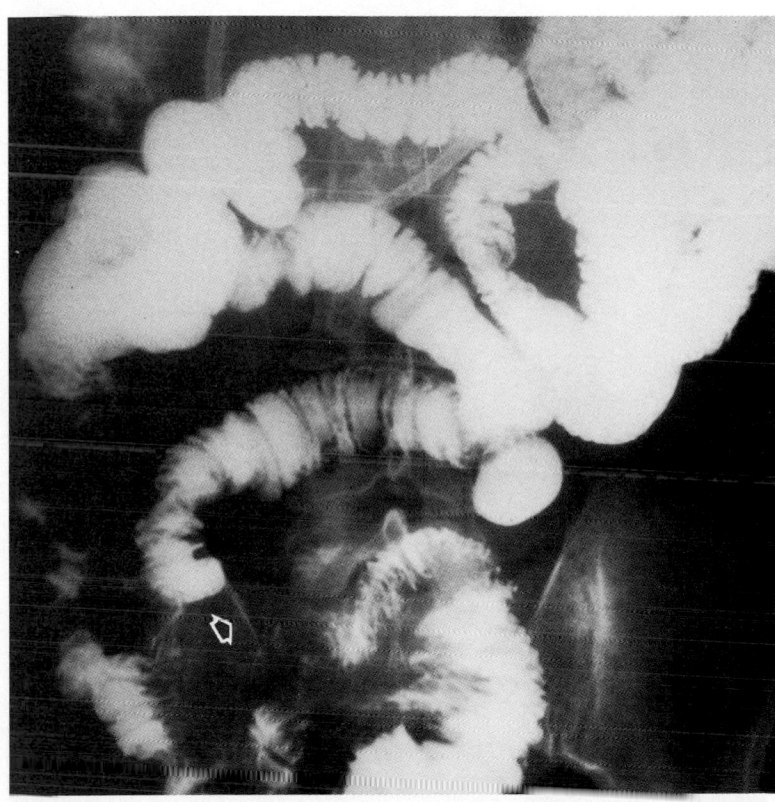

Figure 42-19. This is an illustration of the use of enteroclysis to outline the terminal ileum, which is demonstrated here with excellent mucosal detail. Several loops of terminal ileum are matted together and at least two of the loops are joined by a fistula, to which the arrow is pointing.

Esophageal Disease

Involvement of the esophagus has been reported, but it must be very rare. The author has seen only one patient with documented inflammatory bowel disease of the terminal ileum who had a severe esophageal stricture. The histology was not specific for Crohn's disease and the patient had a long-standing hiatal hernia with a shortened esophagus.

Buccal Disease

Granulomatous and nongranulomatous ulcers are occasionally found on the tongue and in the mouth of patients with extensive and active disease in the intestine. The oral ulcers usually heal after removal of the diseased intestine.

DIAGNOSIS

The most important step in reaching a diagnosis of Crohn's disease is suspecting the possibility of this diagnosis when confronted by such early manifestations as a fistula-in-ano, weight loss

and failure to thrive, night sweats, and vague abdominal pain. In its typical location in the terminal ileum, one can usually elicit some tenderness to deep palpation of the right lower quadrant and in cooperative thin patients, an ill-defined mass is often palpable.

The next step in reaching a diagnosis is a contrast radiologic study of the small intestine. As an initial screening procedure, a conventional small bowel follow-through as part of an upper GI series suffices. If the study is positive, a separate examination is undertaken in the form of a small bowel enema or enteroclysis. This study consists of a double-contrast examination of the small bowel done by injecting a mixture of barium and methylcellulose into the duodenum via an appropriate nasogastric tube. Excellent mucosal detail can be obtained using the multiple spot technique (Figs. 42-15 and 42-19). Mucosal detail in the terminal ileum and cecum can be enhanced by air insufflation into the colon.

When small bowel disease is demonstrated by these measures, one must then use a barium enema to assess the condition of the colon. Re-

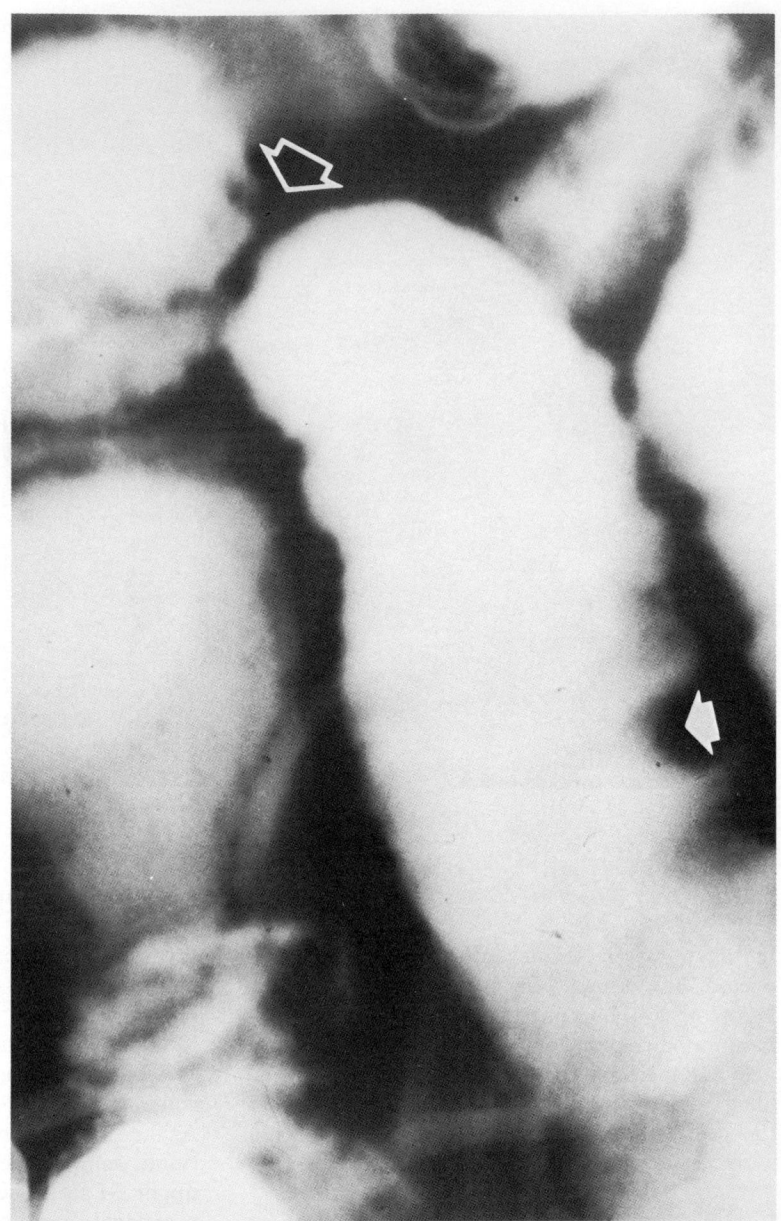

Figure 42–20. This is an example of very early Crohn's disease. This young woman, age 32, had had diarrhea for approximately 6 months. The spot-view of the terminal ileum shows only thickening of the mucosal folds with "thumb-printing" (*solid arrow*).

flux of barium into the ileum provides good imaging of the contour of the terminal ileum.

The radiologic findings depend on the stage of the inflammatory disease. At the prestenotic stage, one may see nonspecific changes of inflammation such as thickening of mucosal folds, "thumb-printing" of the contour of the terminal ileum (Fig. 42–20). These changes can be produced by other types of enteritis such as *Yersinia enterolytica*.

With progression of the disease, the typical linear ulcers that break up the mucosal surface into islands—"cobblestone pattern"—can be easily demonstrated (Fig. 42–21). In addition, one looks for deep ulcers or fissures and sinus tracts. The affected segment appears rigid (Fig. 42–22), and thickening of its walls separates it from adjacent loops of small bowel. One also looks for skip lesions in the proximal intestine.

At the stenotic stage, the cobblestone pat-

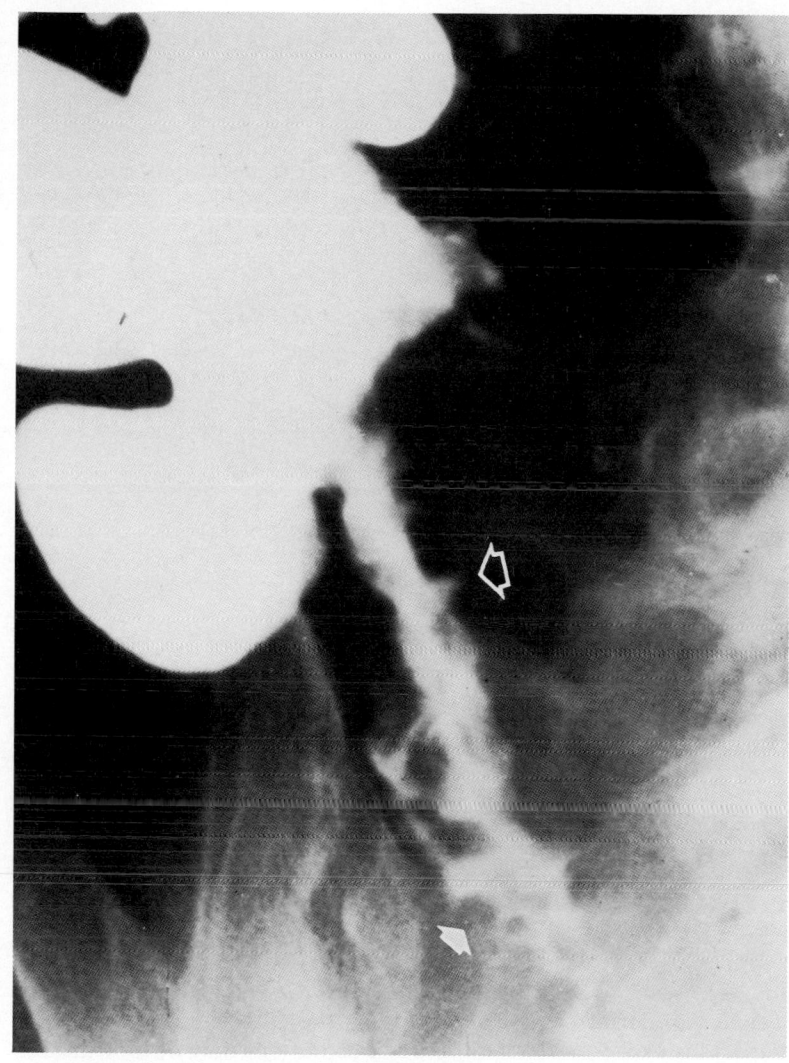

Figure 42–21. The terminal ileum is rigid and narrowed. Deep ulcers—"rose-thorn ulcers"—can be seen (*open arrow*) and the mucosal pattern is follicular, reflecting the "cobblestone" surface of the mucosa (*solid arrow*).

tern disappears. The affected segment of terminal ileum takes on the appearance of a narrow, rigid tube to which the term of "string sign" has been applied (Fig. 42–23). The proximal intestine is dilated, sometimes markedly.

Fistulous tracts are a hallmark of Crohn's disease and, when found, are diagnostic. Early filling of the colon indicates an ileosigmoid fistula, a common complication of disease in the terminal ileum. When the terminal ileum appears "stuck" to the region of the urinary bladder, one should suspect an ileovesical fistula (Figs. 42–10 and 42–11A).

Duodenal involvement is suggested by the finding of a cobblestone pattern, thickness of the mucosal folds, deep ulcers, narrowing of the lumen, particularly in the postbulbar region, and sometimes by fistula formation (Fig. 42–17). Rigidity and scalloping of the contour of the greater curvature of the antrum indicate gastric disease (Fig. 42–18). Sometimes a double-contrast radiologic technique is capable of demonstrating aphthous ulcers in the gastric mucosa.

Unlike inflammatory bowel disease in the colon, where one often faces a diagnostic dilemma between Crohn's disease and chronic ulcerative colitis, the differential diagnosis in small bowel disease is a relatively simple matter since there is no condition, with the exception of the now rare ileocecal tuberculosis, capable

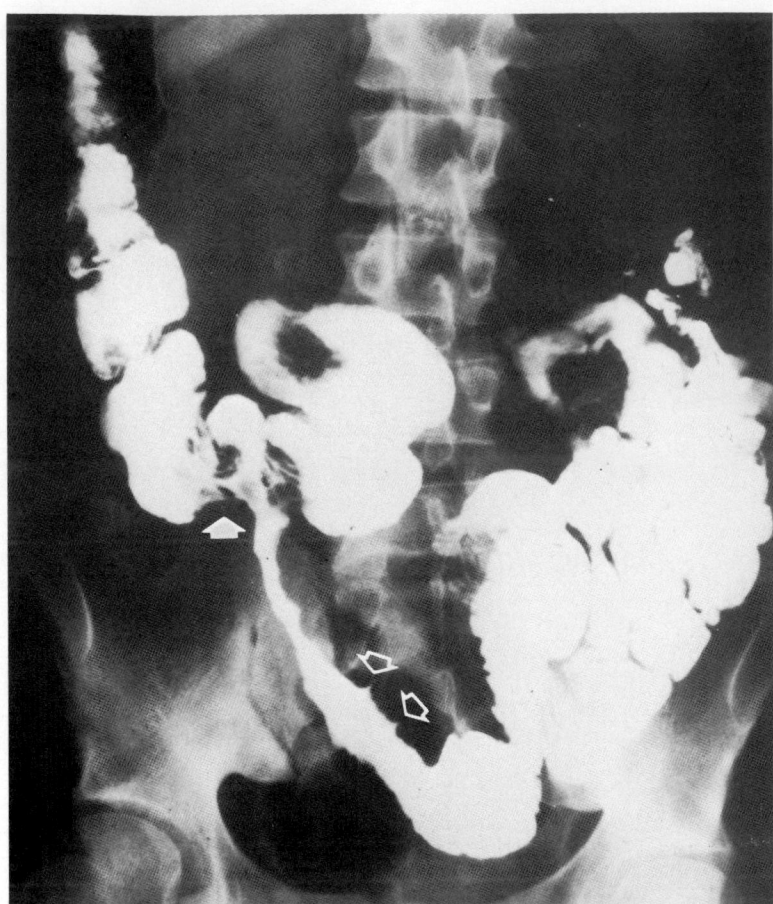

Figure 42–22. This patient had an ileocolectomy for regional enteritis 4 years previously. There is definite recurrent disease in the neoterminal ileum, which is rigid and narrowed. On the medial side, thumb-printing, giving a scalloped appearance to the contour of the terminal ileum, can be seen. *Open Arrows:* Deep ulcerations. *Solid Arrow:* The anastomosis between the neoterminal ileum and the ascending colon.

of mimicking the radiologic signs of florid Crohn's disease. The one and important exception to this is the occasional difficulty in differentiating between Crohn's disease of the terminal ileum and intestinal lymphoma. Although the radiologic findings in intestinal lymphoma are usually diagnostic, they may be difficult to differentiate from those of Crohn's disease in some patients. Under these conditions, colonoscopy with mucosal biopsy of varying segments of the colon, including the ileocecal valve and the terminal ileum, if possible, should be performed to document the diagnosis of Crohn's disease. If the biopsies are negative, an exploratory laparotomy should be the next step.

DIFFERENTIAL DIAGNOSIS

In certain areas of the world, such as South Africa, where both amoebiasis and Crohn's disease are common, the differential diagnosis between these two conditions may be difficult. Examination of stools for trophozoites should be part of the initial workup. Amoebiasis does not produce radiologic changes in the small bowel. Mass lesions in the colon—amoeboma—are rare, even in areas where amoebiasis is endemic, and are radiologically different from the lesions produced by Crohn's disease.

The differentiation from hyperplastic ileocecal tuberculosis may be difficult. The diagnosis is helped by a history of exposure to other patients with tuberculosis. Chest x-ray and tuberculin skin tests are important, since a negative skin test rules out tuberculosis. Primary intestinal tuberculosis, however, may occur in the absence of pulmonary involvement. Strictures are common in both conditions but are usually short, less than 3 cm, in tuberculosis and considerably longer in Crohn's disease. In intestinal tuberculosis, fistulas are uncommon.

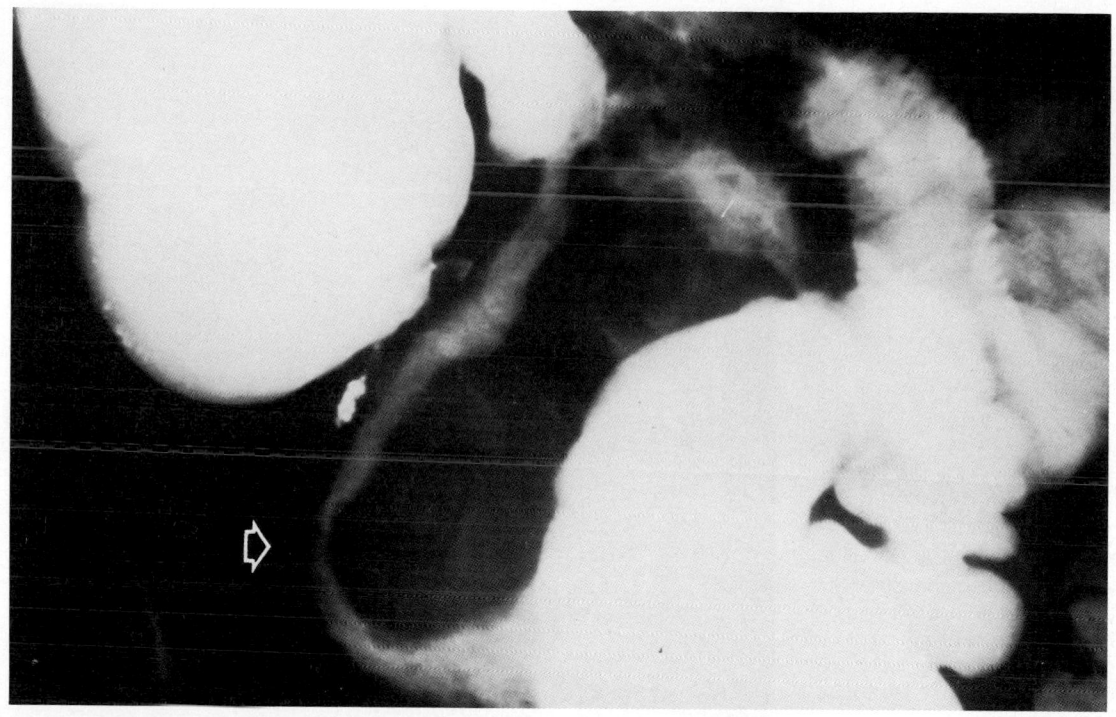

Figure 42–23. Regional enteritis of the terminal ileum at the final stage. All mucosal pattern has been destroyed. The diseased bowel has been reduced to a narrow, rigid tube, giving the classical "string sign."

Tuberculosis enteritis tends to leave the ileocecal valve fixed and widened instead of stenotic, as in Crohn's disease. The diagnosis may require laparoscopy, which will show serosal nodules characteristic of intestinal tuberculosis, or colonoscopy with biopsy of the cecal mucosa and a search for bacilli in histologic sections as well as appropriate cultures of biopsy material.

As mentioned above, the differential diagnosis from intestinal lymphoma in the terminal ileum may be very difficult and, at times, impossible. One point to remember is that Crohn's disease tends to narrow the lumen of the affected segment and cause obstruction, whereas the latter is uncommon with lymphomas (Fig. 42–24). At times the differential diagnosis may require an exploratory laparotomy.

One of the more difficult diagnostic problems is presented by the patient with only a short history of diarrhea and nonspecific general symptoms such as night sweats, fever, weight loss, and the like, and in whom the x-rays of the small intestine show only equivocal findings, such as widening of mucosal folds (Fig.

42–20). A very helpful diagnostic procedure in these patients is to attempt to take mucosal biopsies from the terminal ileum via the colonoscope (Fig. 42–25). In patients who are at such an early stage in the evolution of Crohn's disease, random biopsies of the colonic mucosa are unlikely to be positive.

COMPLICATIONS

Bowel Obstruction

Acute small bowel obstruction is the most common complication of Crohn's disease of the small intestine. It usually takes the course of "acute or chronic" obstruction, with the acute event occurring against a background of months or years of symptoms of partial small bowel obstruction: postprandial colicky pain with radiologic evidence of dilatation of the small intestine above the stenotic and diseased terminal ileum. Complete obstruction of the lumen rarely occurs. Obstruction, when it develops, results from

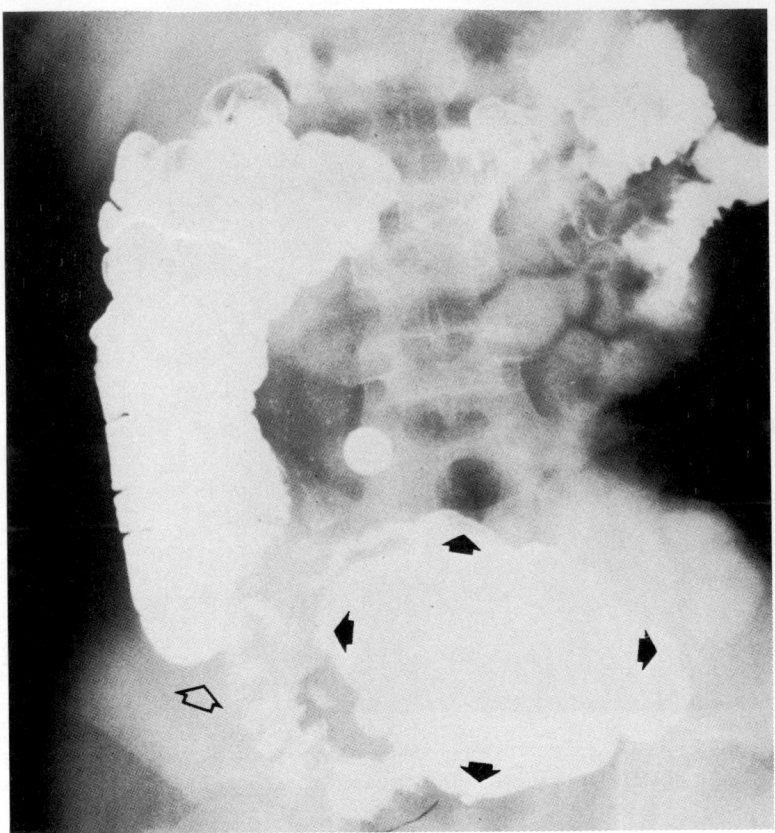

Figure 42–24. Example of intestinal lymphoma involving the terminal ileum in a 12-year-old boy. The open arrow points to the ileocecal valve; note that there is no evidence of obstruction. The solid arrows outline a large abscess cavity. This patient had been treated for almost 1 year with a mistaken diagnosis of Crohn's disease.

the combination of severe narrowing of the lumen and impaction of nondigestible fiber in the strictured bowel and impaired peristalsis in the diseased segment. Obstruction is the most common indication for surgical intervention in the treatment of intestinal Crohn's disease and, ideally, should be carried out before complete bowel obstruction has developed.

Fistula Formation

Fistula formation is both a complication of Crohn's disease and a feature of the illness so characteristic as to have major diagnostic importance. Fistulous tracts in this condition take on a peculiar chronicity due in large part to the fact that the tracts are lined by columnar epithelia that prevent their healing, similar to timber shoring up a tunnel to prevent it from collapsing. Fistulous tracts are often associated with abscesses, particularly when they end blindly in the peritoneal cavity or in the retro-

peritoneal tissues. When the effects of sepsis are added to those of the disease, the impact on the patient's general condition can be quite devastating. For this reason, the development of fistulas and abdominal masses (which are simply walled-off abscesses) are an important indication for surgical intervention.

Perianal Disease

Perianal disease, because of the intense discomfort that it causes, is an important complication of Crohn's disease. In its most severe form, it occurs mainly in patients with colorectal involvement.

Free Perforation

Because the process of fissure formation in Crohn's disease is slow, it tends to lead to the development of fistulous tracts rather than to free perforation into the peritoneal cavity. By

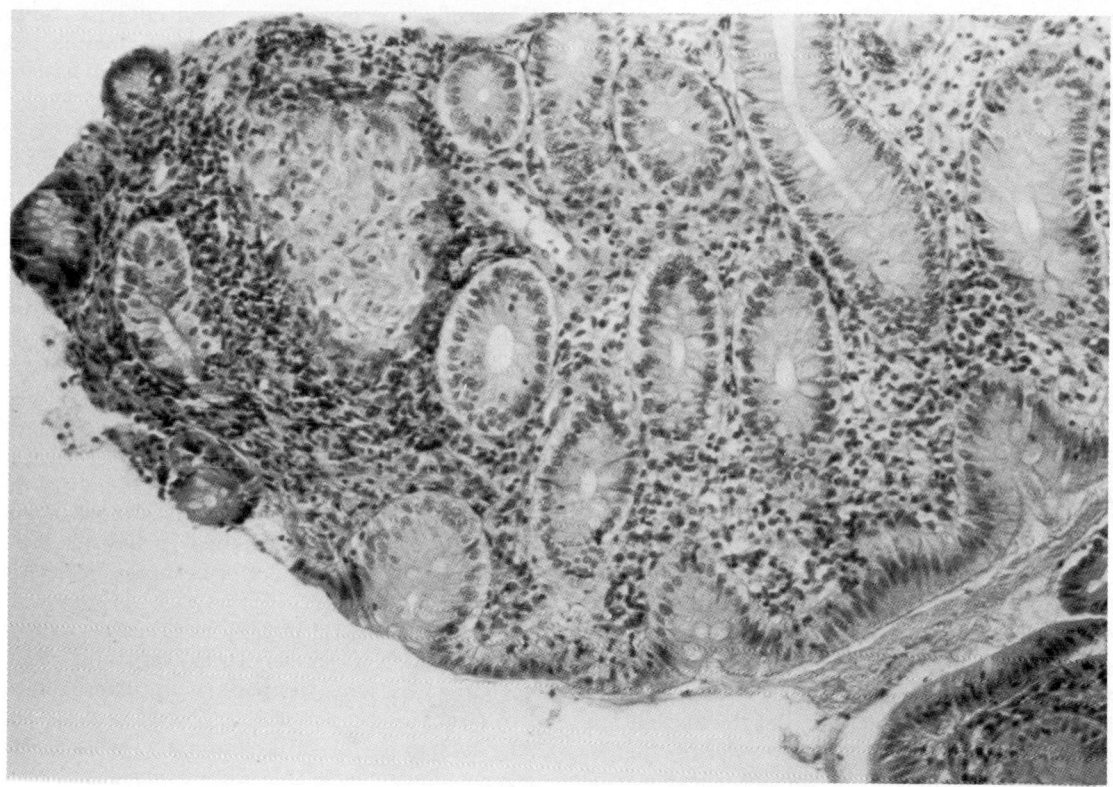

Figure 42–25. A patient with very early disease in the terminal ileum (see Fig. 42–20) was colonoscoped and a mucosal biopsy was taken from the terminal ileum through the ileocecal valve. One of the sections shows a noncaseating granuloma, thus establishing the diagnosis of Crohn's disease.

the time these deep ulcers or fissures reach the serosa of the diseased segment of intestine, the latter has become adherent to neighboring viscera or tissues into which the fistula penetrates. For many years, it was believed that free perforation does not occur in this condition. Although it is rare, a total of over 100 cases of free perforation from Crohn's disease of the small intestine had been reported by 1972. The author has personally managed eight patients with this complication: one with duodenal perforation, one with colonic perforation, and six with ileal perforations. Naturally, free perforation is a formal indication for immediate surgical intervention.

Hemorrhage

Bleeding in patients with disease limited to the small intestine is usually occult. Gross lower GI bleeding is common only in patients with colonic involvement.

Intractable Disease

Intractable disease, or failure of medical management, is the third most common indication for surgery. Poor response to treatment describes a variety of situations.

It most commonly represents patients with a stenotic terminal ileum whose symptoms of partial small bowel obstruction after each meal have caused a reduction in caloric intake and weight loss. It would also include patients with duodenal involvement and gastric outlet obstruction who are losing weight because of frequent nausea and vomiting.

In this category, one would also include children who, although they may not have a specific complication of Crohn's disease, are failing to show normal growth. Fifteen to twenty percent of patients with Crohn's disease have symptoms before the age of fifteen. At least one third of these children experience problems with growth and development. The majority of patients with childhood onset have localized disease, which lends itself very well to local resection and reestablishment of continuity. The matter of a recurrence in the future is far less important than the opportunity of giving the child a chance to grow.

Systemic complications that often develop in patients who do not respond to treatment have already been described.

Development of Intestinal Carcinoma

The possibility that Crohn's disease, like chronic ulcerative colitis, may predispose to malignant degeneration was first raised in 1953, when Ginzburg et al reported a case of adenocarcinoma in a patient with regional enteritis. Since then, over 50 such cases have been reported and it is now generally accepted that the association of the two conditions is not a matter of chance. A figure of 0.08 percent for the incidence of small bowel carcinoma in patients with Crohn's disease has been given. This figure is greater than the incidence of de novo adenocarcinoma in the small intestine. It is interesting to note that 27 percent of the reported cases of adenocarcinoma complicating Crohn's disease have developed in segments of diseased small intestine that were left in situ and bypassed, a now obsolete method of surgical treatment. In a Mt. Sinai Hospital of New York series, the overall incidence of carcinoma in patients with Crohn's disease was 4.8 percent, by comparison with an incidence of 11.2 percent in patients with chronic ulcerative colitis. Approximately 57 percent of cases of carcinoma in patients with Crohn's disease appeared in the intestine. The remainder were extraintestinal. Seventy percent of the tumors develop in the terminal ileum. There is usually an interval of many years between the first symptoms of inflammatory bowel disease and the onset of cancer. The latter is often "invisible" and difficult to detect, either by the surgeon or the pathologist. Five-year survival rates are less than 4 percent. A small number of patients with intestinal lymphoma developing in the diseased terminal ileum of patients with regional enteritis have been reported. At present, the number is too small to determine whether this is a real association or a random occurrence.

TREATMENT

Because the cause of Crohn's disease is unknown, the treatment is supportive and symptomatic, with the empiric use of agents such as steroids and immunosuppressive drugs. Surgical intervention is indicated mainly for complications.

The most important aspect of long-term management is the maintenance of adequate nutrition and the symptomatic treatment of the dominant symptom of diarrhea. In addition, palliative medical treatment of perianal disease is frequently necessary.

The diet should be high in calories and low in fiber, such as citrus fruits, vegetable skin, corn and nuts, etc., particularly in patients with symptoms of partial small bowel obstruction. The avoidance of milk and milk products is purely empirical, as this often seems to improve the patient's diarrhea. This may be explained by a lactase deficiency in some patients. Often diarrhea is relieved by the administration of psyllium compounds such as Metamucil. Another effective approach to the treatment of diarrhea, although it is unfortunately an expensive one, consists of the administration of the bile-salt-binding resin, cholestyramine, 3 times daily. The most commonly used antidiarrheal agents are Lomotil and Imodium. Because they tend to make the patient sleepy, they can interfere with work and should not be used for maintenance management.

Antibiotics have not been very helpful in the treatment of perianal disease. Small collections of pus, such as perianal abscesses, should be drained, using the minimal amount of surgery required to provide adequate drainage. Sitz baths and perianal hygiene help to relieve the patient's distress. Recently, short series, 10 days or so, of metronidazole reduce, sometimes dramatically, drainage from fistulae-in-ano although permanent healing cannot be expected to occur. Antibiotics should not be used for the definitive management of intraabdominal abscesses. These require surgery, and the administration of antibiotics should only be used to prepare patients for an operation.

Both sulfasalazine and steroids are prescribed for the treatment of acute exacerbations. Steroids are very useful, particularly when they are administered judiciously. Their chief usefulness lies in their ability to induce a remission. They should therefore be given during acute flare-ups. An example would be a patient with duodenal involvement without marked stenosis, but with enough edema and acute inflammation of the duodenum to impair peristalsis and cause gastric stasis. To be effective, the treatment must begin with high doses, i.e., 60 mg of prednisone daily. The doses are tapered off as soon as the desired effect is attained. Sulfasalazine is also useful for the treatment of acute exacerbations. Some use it for long-term maintenance treatment. However, there is no evidence that either sulfasalazine or steroids reduce the rate of recurrence of the disease after surgery, or prevent acute attacks.

Immunosuppressive agents have been used in the treatment of Crohn's disease for about 15 years. Azathioprine (Imuran) has received the longest trial. It takes about 3 months, on average, before the beneficial action of this drug can be demonstrated. Therefore, in patients with active, severe disease, a remission must be brought on with steroids before Imuran in prescribed. A major drawback to the use of Imuran is its toxicity: 4 percent of patients treated with Imuran have developed acute pancreatitis. An analogous drug, 6-mercaptopurine, has been introduced more recently, with apparent good results. However, if anything, it is more toxic than Imuran.

When evaluating the effects of any drug treatment of patients with Crohn's disease, one must remember that spontaneous remissions occur in this condition. Therefore, the effects of any drug must be compared with those of a placebo given concurrently to a control group of patients.

Acute attacks are often associated with a marked deterioration of the patient's nutritional status due to a reduction in caloric intake and also to fecal losses of protein as the diarrhea becomes more severe. In recent years, the more frequent use of parenteral hyperalimentation for the treatment of severe flare-ups of inflammatory bowel disease has dramatically benefited patients with very severe disease. One of the main achievements of parenteral hyperalimentation is to improve the general condition of patients who are candidates for surgery. At one time it was hoped that long-term parenteral hyperalimentation would lead to permanent healing of enterocutaneous fistulas. Although it is true that fluid and electrolyte losses from fistulous tracts diminish dramatically during parenteral hyperalimentation, discharge from the tracts recurs after oral feeding is resumed. It is therefore inappropriate, in addition to becoming prohibitively expensive, to attempt to cure established fistulous tracts in Crohn's disease with parenteral hyperalimentation. However, as a method of preparing a severely malnourished patient for surgery, this modality is an extraordinarily valuable adjunct to the surgical armamentarium.

Indications for Surgery

In recent years, there has been a trend to earlier surgery for this condition, largely because of the failure of medical management. For many years, the awareness of the very high recurrence rates dampened enthusiasm for surgery. In the late 1950s, steroids seemed to offer hope that has since faded as it became evident that the long-term course of regional enteritis was not significantly ameliorated. Similar disappointments followed the introduction of immunosuppressive agents and parenteral hyperalimentation. It is now generally appreciated that a given rate of recurrence after surgery is a less important consideration than providing patients with a better quality of life during the symptom-free intervals between operations, for those who do have recurrences. A decade or two ago, few physicians recognized growth retardation as an indication for surgery in children with Crohn's disease.

In the United States, the cumulative probability of abdominal surgery 5 years after the onset of symptoms is approximately 30 percent if only the colon is involved. By 10 years, it is about 60 percent if only the small bowel is involved, but rises to about 80 percent in patients with ileocolitis.

The indications for surgery vary according to the anatomic locations of the disease. In patients with ileocolitis, the major indications for surgery are, in order of decreasing frequency: internal fistulas and sepsis, intestinal obstruction, perianal disease, and poor response to medical management. In patients whose disease involves only the colon, the indications are as follows: poor response to medical management, internal fistulas and sepsis, toxic megacolon, perianal disease and intestinal obstruction. In patients with involvement limited to the small intestine, the indications for surgery are as follows:

- Partial or complete small bowel obstruction (50 to 70 percent)
- Abdominal mass
- Enteric fistulas, sepsis
- Poor response to medical management, anemia, weight loss
- Growth retardation
- Right hydroureter, and
- Free perforation and peritonitis.

Perianal disease is rarely severe enough in patients with disease limited to the small bowel to require surgery, by contrast with patients with colorectal involvement, in whom chronic perineal sepsis frequently causes complete loss of anal continence. It must be recognized that when these patients finally are operated on, they often have several complications, some of which may have been present for a long time. Obstruction becomes the most common indication for surgery in many series because, by virtue of its compelling nature, it forces the hand of the patient's physician in the direction of surgery.

Surgical Treatment

As has been repeatedly emphasized in this chapter, many patients with Crohn's disease are in a severe state of malnutrition with anemia and hypoproteinemia by the time the need for surgery presents. Whenever the surgery is not urgent, patients who are malnourished should be prepared for surgery by a 1- to 2-week course of parenteral hyperalimentation. Nutritionally depleted patients become immunodeficient and have a higher risk of postoperative septic complications. This situation can be reversed by hyperalimentation.

Because the terminal ileum remains by far the most common site of involvement in patients with the small bowel pattern of disease, this discussion will revolve around the treatment of patients with involvement of the distal small bowel.

Preoperative evaluation of the patient should include a barium enema and colonoscopy, with random biopsies of the colonic mucosa at all levels of the colon. This serves to determine whether or not the colon is involved. Patients with florid disease in the ileum may have mild disease in the cecum. This is not always obvious at surgery and prior knowledge of the extent of the disease helps in planning the resection lines.

Because of the frequency with which patients with regional enteritis involving the terminal ileum have right-sided hydronephrosis, it is useful to obtain an intravenous pyelogram at some point during the workup of the patient, certainly before surgery. Prior knowledge of the proximity of the right ureter to the diseased terminal ileum helps to avoid operative injury to the ureter. Also, it suggests the necessity of ureterolysis when diseased bowel is removed. Although some find it useful to place a ureteral catheter on that side before the operation, this author has not found it necessary to do so.

Patients with partial small bowel obstruction should be given a liquid diet for several days prior to surgery to ensure decompression of the healthy intestine. During the 24 hours preceding the operation, this author orders the following antibiotic combination: neomycin, erythromycin, and metronidazole. In addition, cephazolin is administered on call to the operating room and for 24 hours after the operation. Enemas are administered on the evening before surgery until returns are clear. In this author's experience it is unnecessary to subject these patients to a formal bowel prep with cathartics and enemas for several days because of the additional fluid and electrolyte and protein depletion that this regimen can cause.

Patients previously treated with steroids should be covered with steroids throughout the operative and postoperative recovery phase, unless the last dose of prednisone was given more than 6 months before surgery. Personal preference is to give 150 mg of Solu-Cortef intravenously in the operating room immediately before the induction of anesthesia (assurance that the patient has received the medication). The evening of surgery, the patient receives 150 mg of cortisone acetate intramuscularly. The dose of cortisone acetate is reduced by 100 mg a day over the next 2 days, after which oral prednisone can be resumed.

A Foley catheter must always be positioned in the bladder before surgery because of the frequency with which diseased terminal ileum is densely adherent to pelvic structures.

The author's preference is for vertical incisions because of the better exposure and the ease of extending the incision up or down. The incision should always be slightly to the left of the umbilicus. In this way, the scar will not interfere with the subsequent siting of an ileostomy, should one become necessary in the future.

The abdomen is then thoroughly explored to assess the severity of the disease and to look for skip lesions. The exploration must include a careful examination of the colon.

In patients with involvement limited to the terminal ileum, the distal line of resection is at the level of the proximal ascending colon. The line of resection should be placed 8 to 10 cm proximal to the point where a transition can be seen between diseased bowel and normal-appearing intestine. It is good practice to examine the resected specimen immediately to make sure that the bowel is free of disease, both grossly and microscopically, at the lines of resection. One must not excise large segments of healthy intestine in attempts to forestall a recurrence. Such a practice does not reduce the recurrence rate and, when more surgery is required later, it increases the risk of a short-bowel syndrome. The mesentery is divided in the most convenient manner without attempting to excise the mesenteric nodes. The anastomosis between the neoterminal ileum and the ascending colon is constructed, according to one's preference, with a manual or a stapled technique. The diseased segment is often densely adherent to pelvic structures from which the bowel is dissected methodically and with sharp dissection. Before beginning the dissection, one should identify the right ureter and retract it out of harm's way over a traction tape after following its course down to the pelvis. Any fibrous tissue surrounding the ureter is carefully dissected away. Above all, one should resist any temptation to perform a simple bypass; this author has never found this to be necessary. A now completely outdated approach, it leaves a focus of disease in the abdomen, fails to relieve the patient of some of the systemic manifestations of the disease, and, more importantly, exposes the patient to the risk of cancer developing in the bypassed segment.

During the dissection, it is not unusual to uncover sinus tracts. These are dealt with ap-

propriately. When they extend into a healthy loop of a small bowel or the sigmoid, the opening must be closed carefully. In dealing with an ileovesical fistula, it is not necessary to remove a cuff of bladder along with the diseased terminal ileum. The latter is simply dissected off the bladder, and the defect in the bladder is then closed with absorbable sutures placed in the muscle wall of the bladder. One should not attempt to find the opening in the mucosa. It is always very small. The Foley catheter must be left in the bladder for 7 or 8 days after the operation.

Sinus tracts extending into the lateral wall of the pelvis or the right flank or behind the psoas (Fig. 42–14) are very treacherous, since they often communicate with a deep abscess. The opening into the abscess is enlarged, its contents are thoroughly curetted and it is drained externally via a stab-wound, placed as far lateral as possible, in the right flank.

Skip lesions, when present, occasionally pose difficult judgmental problems. When a short segment of healthy intestine separates a skip lesion from the main disease in the terminal ileum, it is tempting to excise the two segments together so as to have only one anastomosis. If the skip segment is short, that is, 6 inches or less, it does not make sense to construct two anastomoses to save such a short segment of intestine. However, when it is possible to save more than one foot of intestine, one should by all means remove the diseased segments separately. Skip lesions in the ileum must be removed, as they are certain to cause trouble in short order. Jejunal skip lesions may be left alone, particularly when they have not been identified with any symptoms, unless it is apparent that they are about to cause obstruction. When one does so, however, it is with the realization that the patient is being exposed to the risk of a complication from the skip lesion, even though it may not have been causing symptoms previously.

When extensive dissection leaves oozing, raw peritoneal surfaces, these must be drained externally with appropriate suction catheters. Routine drainage after an ileocolectomy for disease in the terminal ileum is a matter of individual judgment.

The usual indication for surgery in patients with gastroduodenal involvement is duodenal narrowing severe enough to cause gastric retention (Fig. 42–26). If the symptoms do not remit with an increase in the dosage of steroids, it

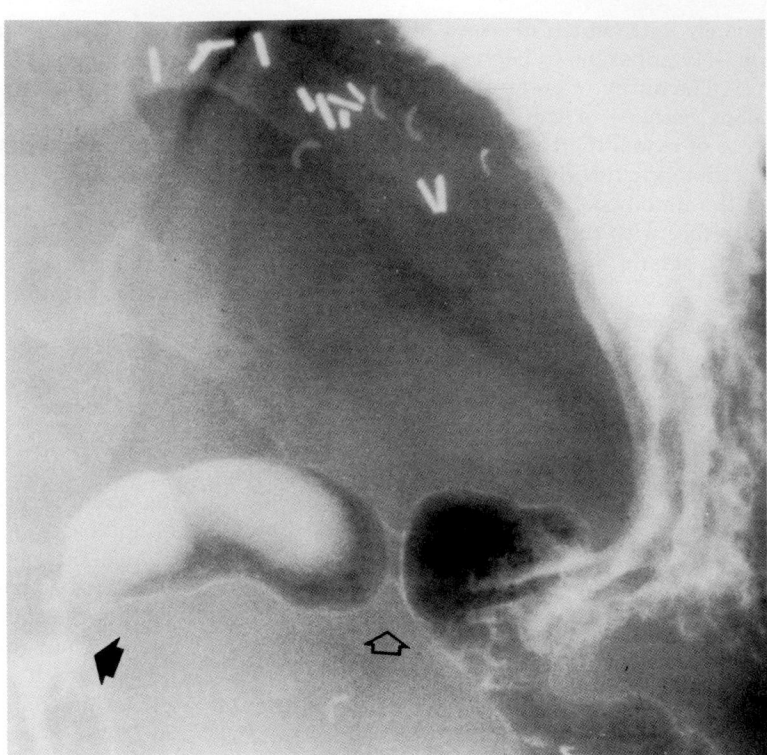

Figure 42–26. This is a good example of duodenal involvement eventually producing a near-complete stricture of the second portion of the duodenum (*solid arrow*). The open arrow points to the pyloric canal.

is obvious that one is dealing with cicatricial stenosis and surgery becomes necessary. The safest procedure is a gastrojejunostomy sited on the posterior wall of the antrum, as close to the pylorus as the gastric involvement, when present, will permit. A complementary vagotomy is done unless there is an associated gastric motor disorder, in which case reliance on administration of H_2 blockers postoperatively to prevent the development of marginal ulceration is my preference.

Closure of the abdominal incision deserves a special consideration. It has been my experience that patients with inflammatory bowel disease, and particularly those with Crohn's disease, tolerate nonabsorbable suture materials poorly. Suture granulomas, abscesses, and sinus tracts in the wound are common. Therefore, this author has made it a practice always to use absorbable suture material for wound closure in all of these patients.

The Appendix and Undiagnosed Crohn's Disease

A question raised frequently involves dealing with the appendix when exploring a patient with a clinical diagnosis of acute appendicitis and finding a normal appendix but an edematous, purple terminal ileum with a thickened mesentery containing enlarged lymph nodes. Under these circumstances, one may actually be dealing with early Crohn's disease, or one may be faced with a patient having ileitis due to *Yersinia enterolytica.* The appendix should be removed. This will at least ensure that any symptoms developing later in the right lower quadrant will not be attributable to appendicitis. This approach has been associated in everyone's experience with an only minimal risk of enterocutaneous fistula. Many patients who fit this picture remain healthy, and thus represent obvious cases of ileitis due to causes other than Crohn's disease. Some patients develop symptoms of florid inflammatory bowel disease and are managed appropriately.

Free Perforation

As mentioned above, free perforation with spreading peritonitis is a rare complication of Crohn's disease. A surgeon, encountering this problem for the first time, may be uncertain about its management. Most general surgeons

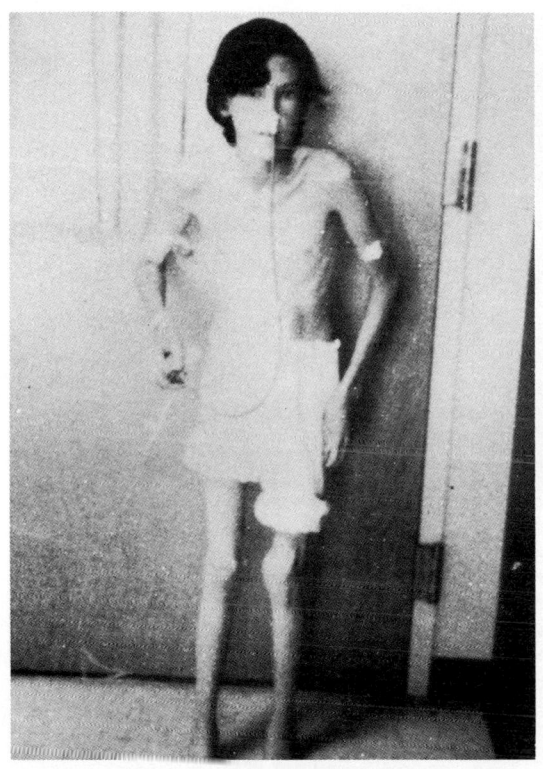
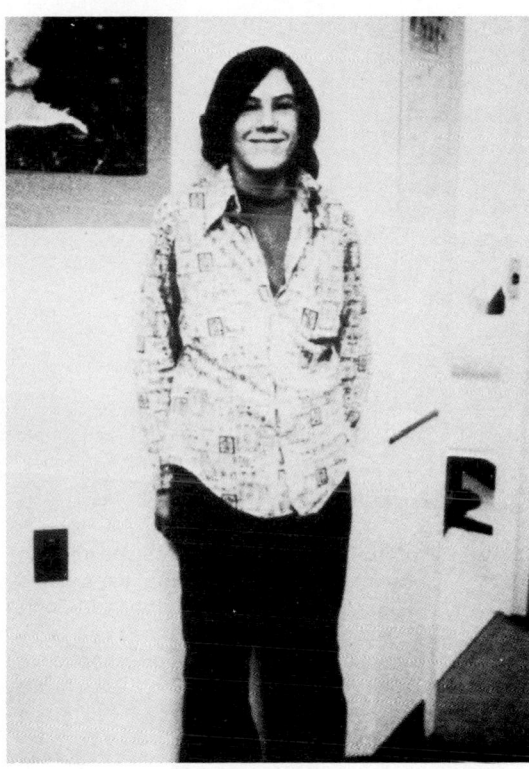

A   D

Figure 42–27. A. This 17-year-old boy had a 6-year history of regional enteritis. When this photograph was taken, he had developed complete small bowel obstruction and underwent surgery several days later. **B.** The same boy, 6 months later, after a remarkable spurt of ponderal and linear growth.

are accustomed to treating free perforations of closed intraabdominal viscera by suture plication. Indeed, a review of the literature of 10 years ago indicates that many of the reported cases of free perforation of Crohn's disease of the small intestine had been dealt with in this manner and with disastrous consequences. As anyone familiar with Crohn's disease would expect, sutures placed in diseased bowel do not hold and reperforation may be expected to occur. The only safe way to deal with this problem is to excise the diseased bowel as if the case were elective. Reestablishment of continuity is delayed. Either the anastomosis is constructed and protected by a temporary ileostomy, or a double-barreled cutaneous ileocolostomy is constructed and closed 6 to 8 weeks later. Naturally, as one would in any case of peritonitis, the peritoneal cavity is liberally irrigated and drained in addition to starting triple antibiotic therapy as soon as the diagnosis is known.

POSTOPERATIVE COMPLICATIONS

After surgery for regional enteritis posteroperative complications are those common to all abdominal operations.

It has been said that there is a higher rate of anastomotic failure after ileocolostomy for Crohn's disease than after a similar operation for another condition, such as cancer; this has not been my experience. It must be stressed, however, that the proximal and distal margins of resection must be free, at least of gross disease such as aphthous ulcers.

Postoperative intraabdominal abscesses, not directly related to perforation or anastomotic failure, may develop in anatomic locations such as the pelvis, the paracolic gutter, the right paracolic gutter, and the subphrenic spaces, where collected blood and serous exudate form an ideal culture medium for microorganisms. In my own practice, these compli-

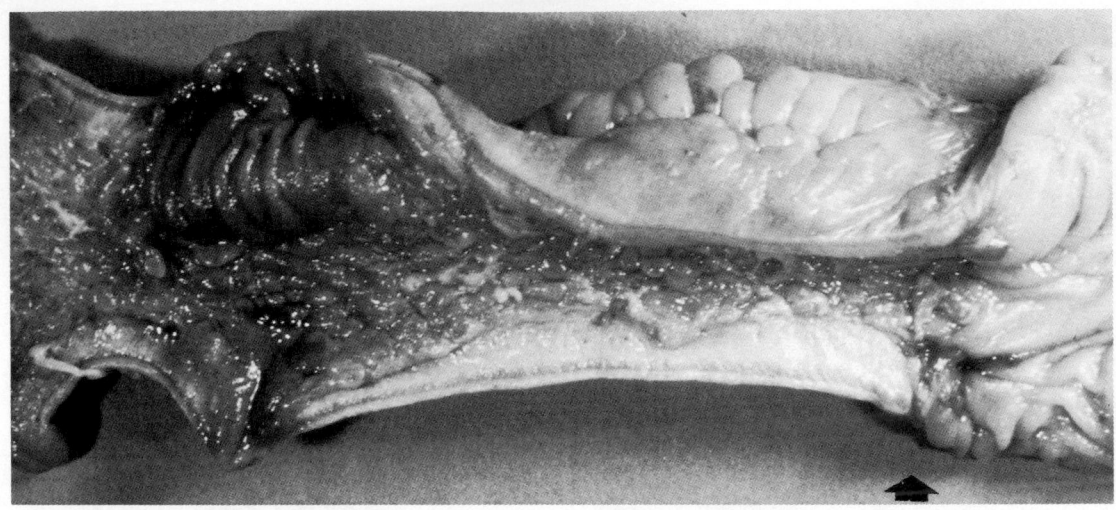

Figure 42–28. Characteristic appearance of recurrent disease in the neoterminal ileum. The anastomotic line is defined by the arrow and the ascending colon is to the right. Note that the length of diseased bowel is short—in this case, approximately 3 to 4 inches. As expected, the main symptoms experienced by this patient were those of high-grade partial small bowel obstruction. This segment of diseased bowel is not accomplishing any useful function. Moreover, it is interfering with the function of the healthy intestine above it; therefore, it must be removed.

cations have been eliminated by systematic postoperative drainage, as described earlier.

Many patients with inflammatory bowel disease undergo multiple intraabdominal operations and are liable, as would anyone else, to form adhesions and develop bowel obstruction on this basis. This possibility must be kept in mind whenever patients present with recurrent symptoms of obstruction. There is a tendency to attribute such symptoms to recurrent inflammatory bowel disease and therefore defer appropriate surgery, which, in many cases, is extremely simple. Fortunately, it is possible, with modern radiologic techniques, to differentiate obstruction caused by adhesions from that due to recurrent inflammatory bowel disease.

Results of Surgery

Because most patients with this condition are young, the surgical mortality rate is low. Hellers reported a surgical mortality rate of 1.2 percent in 431 patients operated for involvement of the terminal ileum. This figure is representative of most other series. As previously mentioned, the mortality rate has been lowered in recent years by the addition of hyperalimentation to the preoperative preparation.

Surgery is characteristically followed by a marked improvement in most aspects of body metabolism. Nowhere is this more dramatic than in children who exhibit a spurt in linear and ponderal growth after surgery (Fig. 42–27). Adults usually experience weight gain. Diarrhea is improved, although it rarely disappears completely. In some patients, removal of the ileocecal valve leads to a continuation of the diarrhea. These patients derive some relief from the administration of cholestyramine, which can then be tapered off as the diarrhea improves.

In keeping with the weight gain, the serum albumin rises, as does blood hemoglobin. The erythrocyte sedimentation rate returns to normal. Serum iron increases.

In general, there is a remarkable improvement in the patient's general health and sensation of well-being.

Recurrence After Surgery for Crohn's Disease

It is a well-accepted fact that surgery for Crohn's disease is associated with a high recurrence rate. When all operations for Crohn's disease were considered, the annual recurrence rate was 3.9 percent at 8 years, by which time 85 percent of the recurrences had taken place. At 15 years, the cumulative risk of recurrence was 42 percent. There were almost no recurrences after 15 years. The recurrence rate was lower in patients with disease limited to the small bowel. There, a cumulative recurrence rate at 14 years was 38 percent. Highest rates of recurrence were found in patients with ileocolic distribution of disease. These rates were estimated for patients requiring reoperation for their recurrence. Hellers found an overall recurrence rate of 42 percent 9 years after surgery. The figure is close to the ones given above and is higher only because all recurrences were considered.

After surgery for involvement of the terminal ileum, recurrences almost always appear in the neoterminal ileum immediately proximal to the anastomosis. The segment involved is often short (Fig. 42–28). Occasionally, the recurrence appears in a new site remote from the anastomosis.

After a second ileocolic resection for a first recurrence, one should expect a second recurrence rate that is slightly higher than the first cumulative recurrence rate: 40 percent after 5 years and 65 percent after 10 years.

Although these figures paint a gloomy picture, it must be remembered that when a segment of small bowel is diseased, it has lost any useful function and, by obstructing the intestinal stream, it impairs the function of the remaining healthy intestine above it. In most cases, therefore, the patient is helped by removal of the diseased segment.

With appropriate medical and surgical care, and despite the high incidence of recurrent disease, the majority of patients with inflammatory bowel disease can be maintained in a state of health that allows them to function as useful members of society.

BIBLIOGRAPHY

Andersson H, Filipsson S, et al: Urinary oxalate excretion related to ileocolic surgery in patients with Crohn's disease. Scand J Gastroenterol 13:465, 1978

Atwell JD, Duthie HL, et al: The outcome of Crohn's disease. Br J Surg 52:966, 1965

Blumgart LH, Thakur: Ureter-oileal fistula due to Crohn's disease. Br J Surg 58:469, 1971

Collins WJ: Malignant lymphoma complicating regional enteritis. Am J Gastroenterol 68:177, 1977

Cooke WT, Swan CHJ: Diffuse jejuno-ileitis of Crohn's disease. Quart J Med 172:583, 1974

Crohn BB, Ginzburg L, et al: Regional enteritis: A pathological and clinical entity. JAMA 99:1323, 1932

Donnelly GJ, Delaney PV, et al: Evidence for a transmissible factor in Crohn's disease. Gut 18:360, 1977

Dyet JF, Pratt AE, et al: The small bowel enema: Description and experience of a technique. Br J Radiol 49:1039, 1976

Farmer RG: Studies of family history among patients with inflammatory bowel disease. VI World Congress of Gastroenterology, abstracts, 1978, p 56

Farmer RG, Hawk WA, et al: Clinical patterns in Crohn's disease: A statistical study of 615 cases. Gastroenterology 68:627, 1975

Farmer RG, Hawk WA, et al: Indications for surgery in Crohn's disease. Analysis of 500 cases. Gastroenterology 71:245, 1976

Floch HF, Slattery LR, et al: Carcinoma of the small intestine in regional enteritis. Am J Gastroenterol 70:520, 1978

Fonkalsrud EW, Ament ME, et al: Surgical management of Crohn's disease in children. Am J Surg 138:15, 1979

Ginzburg L, Schneider KM, et al: Carcinoma of the jejunum occurring in a case of regional enteritis. Surgery 39:347, 1956

Greenstein AJ, Sachar DB, et al: Patterns of neoplasia in Crohn's disease and ulcerative colitis. Cancer 46:403, 1980

Heaton KW, Read AE: Gall stones in patients with disorders of the terminal ileum and disturbed bile salt metabolism. Br Med J 3:494, 1969

Hellers G: Crohn's disease in Stockholm county 1955–1974. A study of epidemiology, results of surgical treatment and long-term prognosis. Acta Chir Scand (suppl):490, 1979

Hopkins DJ, Horan E, et al: Ocular disorders in a series of 332 patients with Crohn's disease. Br J Opthalmol 58:732, 1974

Janowitz HD: Crohn's disease—50 years later. N Engl J Med 304:1600, 1981

Koch TR, Cave DR, et al: Crohn's ileitis and ileocolitis: A study of the anatomical distribution of recurrence. Dig Dis Sci 26:528, 1981

Krog E, Krog B: Regional ileitis (Crohn's disease). I. Kinetics of bile acid absorption in the perfused ileum. Scand J Gastroenterol 11:481, 1976

Kyle J: An epidemiological study of Crohn's disease in northeast Scotland. Gastroenterology 61:826, 1971

Kyle J, Stark G: Fall in the incidence of Crohn's disease. Gut 21:340, 1980

Lock MR, Farmer RG, et al: Recurrence and reoperation for Crohn's disease. The role of disease location in prognosis. N Engl J Med 304:1586, 1981

Lockhart-Mummery HE, Morson BC: Crohn's disease (regional enteritis) of the large intestine and its distinction from ulcerative colitis. Gut 1:87, 1960

Mekhjian HS, Switz DM, et al: Clinical features and natural history of Crohn's disease. Gastroenterology 77:898, 1979

Menguy R: Surgical management of free perforation of the small intestine complicating regional enteritis. Ann Surg 175:178, 1972

Miller DS, Keighley A, et al: Crohn's disease in Nottingham: A search for time-space clustering. Gut 16:454, 1975

Miller LJ, Thistle JL, et al: Crohn's disease involving the esophagus and colon. Case Report. Mayo Clin Proc 52:35, 1977

Monk M, Mendeloff AI, et al: An epidemiological study of ulcerative colitis and regional enteritis among adults in Baltimore. I. Hospital incidence and prevalence, 1960–1963. Gastroenterology 53:198, 1967

The National Cooperative Crohn's Disease Study. Gastroenterology 77:825, 1979

Pitt HA, King W, et al: Increased risk of cholelithiasis with prolonged total parenteral nutrition. Am J Surg 145:106, 1983

Present DH, Korelitz, BI, et al: Treatment of Crohn's disease with 6-mercaptopurine. A long-term, randomized, double-blind study. N Engl J Med 302:981, 1980

Present DH, Rabinowitz JG, et al: Obstructive hydronephrosis. A frequent but seldom recognized complication of granulomatous disease of the bowel. N Engl J Med 280:523, 1969

Rozen P, Zonis J, et al: Crohn's disease in the Jewish population of Tel-Aviv-Yafo. Epidemiology and clinical aspects. Gastroenterology 76:25, 1979

Tootla F, Lucas RJ, et al: Gastroduodenal Crohn disease. Arch Surg 111:855, 1976

Van Patter WN, Bargen JA, et al: Regional enteritis. Gastroenterology 26:347, 1954

43. Tumours of the Small Intestine

Peter R. Hawley

INTRODUCTION

Tumours of the small intestine are uncommon but are seen from time to time by every practicing surgeon and can present difficult problems of diagnosis. It is strange that the upper and lower gastrointestinal (GI) tract together should be responsible for more than 40 percent of all neoplasms and yet there are so few in the intervening small bowel. The majority are found in the duodenum, upper jejunum, and terminal ileum, whereas the distal jejunum and proximal ileum are relatively immune. Perhaps the rapidity with which ingested carcinogenic agents are transported through the small bowel prevents their action.

Symptoms can be insidious in onset and vague in presentation. To make the diagnosis at an early stage in the disease, the surgeon must be "small bowel conscious." The long delay between the onset of symptoms and the diagnosis and the frequency with which they present as acute obstruction or perforation contribute to the poor prognosis. Perhaps this is because the undergraduate and the surgeon have been taught that such tumours are a pathologic curiosity and only of academic interest.

It is highly desirable, for statistical and other reasons, that the exact position of the tumour in the small intestine be determined. The length of the small bowel is variable and in life is considerably shorter than the average 22 feet found at autopsy. If measured at laparotomy, it is found to be only from 11 to 13 feet long; a 3 metre aspirating tube will often pass from the mouth into the caecum or ascending colon. The length is continually changing due to muscular activity.

The position of the tumour can be estimated by inspecting the mesenteric vascular arcades and fat. The vasa recta become shorter, the arcades increase in number, and the fat is more prominent from proximal jejunum to terminal ileum. It is desirable to measure the length of the small bowel and the position of the tumour before resection.

PRIMARY BENIGN TUMOURS

Primary tumours of the small intestine are rare, both in clinical medicine and at autopsy, with an incidence of approximately 0.1 percent. Raiford (1932) found 88 cases among 56,500 subjects, one third of whom were discovered at autopsy and the remainder at laparotomy. Good (1963) stated in 1963 that in a 20-year period at the Mayo Clinic, 659 tumours of the small intestine were diagnosed, 304 at necropsy and 355 at operation. Approximately half were benign and half were malignant. However, an accurate classification of small bowel tumours from these earlier reports is often impossible as some articles classify them simply as polyps without further description. In a comprehensive review, River et al (1956) reported 1399 cases of benign small bowel tumours. This must represent only part of the true incidence of such tumours, because only a proportion of those discovered are reported and many are symptomless. Of the 1399 cases, there were 198 in the duodenum, 272 in the jejunum, and 606 in the ileum whereas 17 occurred at the ileocaecal junction. Of the remainder, the site of 113 was unspecified and 193 were multiple. Clinical and autopsy series that include benign and small bowel tumours usually list adenomas, leiomyomas, lipomas, vascular tumours, and fibromas (inflammatory pseudotumours) in varying orders of frequency. In the autopsy and surgical series from the Mayo Clinic, however, leiomyoma was almost twice as common as any benign tumour, followed by lipoma and adenoma in equal numbers. Haemangiomas were less common. In many articles Peutz–Jegher polyps had been included with a diagnosis as adenomas. Most investigators would now agree that the polyps in the Peutz–Jegher syndrome should be considered as hamartomas and not adenomas.

Adenomas

Adenomas of the small intestine are rare. In a 1981 study by Perzin and Bridge, 51 small bowel tumours containing adenomatous tissue were found among 392,000 surgical pathology cases studied between 1971 and 1978 at Columbia University and the Presbyterian Hospital in New York; 13 of their cases were pure adenomas, 33 had adenomatous and carcinomatous tissue co-existing, and 5 were adenomas with separate carcinomas in the same specimen. When the tumours cause symptoms and are excised, it is common to find that they have already undergone malignant change. It seems that they behave in a way similar to that of adenomas in the large bowel, and show an increased propensity to undergo malignant change as their size increases. They are often single but may be multiple and are found more commonly in the duodenum and terminal ileum than in the intervening part of the small intestine. The one exception to the small incidence of adenomatous polyps in the duodenum is in association with familial polyposis coli (Yao et al, 1977). In the last 10 years it has become apparent that adenomas and adenocarcinomas occur frequently in this condition, adenomas being found in approximately 50 percent of 60 patients with familial polyposis who have been subject to upper GI endoscopy at St. Mark's Hospital.

Leiomyoma

Skandalakis et al (1962) reviewed 713 collected cases, of which just over half were benign and the rest malignant. The lesions are very rarely multiple, they occur as commonly in males as in females, and, although they can occur at any age (one has been reported present at birth),

they are observed most commonly in the sixth decade. They are found more frequently at autopsy than at operation, the incidence being between 1 and 2 per 10,000 examinations.

The jejunum and ileum are the most common sites of these tumours, but if the relative lengths of the bowel are taken into consideration, the muscle most frequently involved is situated first in a Meckel's diverticulum, second in the duodenum, and last in the jejunum and ileum. These tumours can grow into the lumen of the bowel or extramurally or both, forming a "dumb-bell" tumour. As they grow larger, they undergo haemorrhagic necrosis and, if intraluminal, become typically ulcerated at the apex. In a large extramural myoma, the necrotic centre becomes honeycombed with blood-filled cavities until finally there is only a shell of tumour tissue, which may perforate into the peritoneal cavity.

It is difficult for the pathologist to tell when early malignant change occurs, for the muscle fibres blend with the surrounding tissues and infiltration cannot be defined. Pleomorphism, the number of mitoses, and the presence of abnormal mitotic figures may be the only clues to a malignant transformation.

Lipoma

Lipomas are the third most common type of benign small bowel tumour. Of 219 cases collected by River et al (1956), 113 were found in the ileum, 35 in the duodenum, 34 in the jejunum, and 13 at the ileocaecal valve. In 22 cases, the site was not specified. Such tumours are usually single but can be multiple and are commonly small and symptomless; more than 80 percent occur as intraluminal growths. Very occasionally, they grow large and cause symptoms of obstruction or bleeding.

Haemangioma

Haemangiomas of the small bowel can involve the mucosa, submucosa, or muscle layer. Of the 127 collected cases of River et al (1956), 36 were in the ileum, 32 in the jejunum, and 8 in the duodenum. The site was not specified in 26 cases. In this series, 51 patients had multiple tumours, and of these, 11 were in different parts of the small intestine. Intestinal haemangiomas are sometimes associated with similar lesions in the skin or buccal cavity. They vary from minute capillary haemangiomas to large cavernous tumours sometimes involving the entire GI tract.

Tumours of neurogenic origin, such as the neurofibroma (sometimes as part of von Recklinghausen's neurofibromatosis) occur, but they represent only occasional cases in collected series.

The clinical presentation and treatment of benign tumours are not discussed separately, because, in practice, it is often impossible to differentiate between benign and malignant lesions until laparotomy has been performed.

Polyposis

Peutz–Jeghers Syndrome

In 1921, Peutz described seven cases of intestinal polyposis with abnormal pigmentation that had occurred in three generations of a Dutch family. It was not until Jeghers et al (1949) published an account of ten cases and reviewed the literature of generalised intestinal polyposis with melanin spots of the oral mucosa, lips, and digits that the diagnostic significance of the syndrome became recognised. From that time, it became gradually known as the Peutz–Jeghers syndrome.

This syndrome appears to have a genetic basis, as it has a high familial incidence. It is thought to be caused by a Mendelian-dominant gene of high penetrance. The sex incidence is equal and the average age of the patients at the time of diagnosis is in the third decade, with extremes of 2 and 77 years. No race appears to have a particular predisposition or immunity to this disease.

The characteristic pigmentation (Fig. 43–1) consists of sharply defined macules 1 to 2 mm in diameter, black or dark brown in colour, which are found around the lips and on the buccal mucosa. Less commonly, these macules ap-

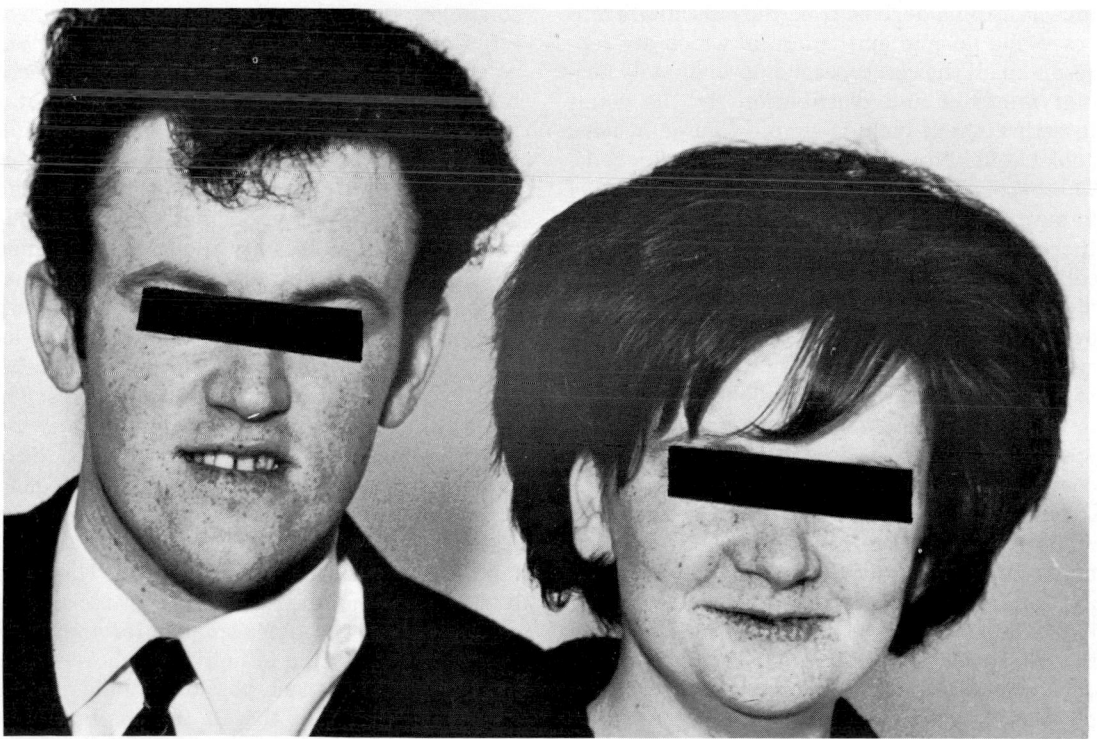

Figure 43–1. Peutz–Jeghers syndrome. A brother and sister who both show typical pigmentation on the lips and around the mouth. Both have had operations to remove all large polyps from the whole of the GI tract. (*Courtesy of Mr. Norman Machie of St. Mark's Hospital, London, and Mr. O.V. Lloyd-Davies.*)

pear around the eyes, ears, and nostrils and on the fingers and toes. The number can vary between a single spot on the buccal mucosa to a multitude on the face and periphery. They are noted in early childhood, and although the buccal lesions persist, the others tend to fade with age. They have been shown to consist of multiple melanin pigment cells in the deepest layers of the epithelium with collections of melanophores in the underlying dermis.

The intestinal polyps are found most frequently in the small intestine, particularly in the jejunum and less commonly in the stomach and large bowel. They can also vary in number between a solitary polyp, which is exceptional, and a very large number. The polyps are slow growing and range in size from small sessile nodules a few millimetres across to large pedunculated polyps 7 cm in diameter. Macroscopically they do not look very different from adenomatous polyps of the colon, but their histologic appearance is characteristic. The polyps are never pigmented. On microscopic examination they are found to consist of a branching smooth muscle stroma derived from the muscularis mucosae and normal epithelium in which are represented all the cell types in approximately normal numbers and distribution. In the small intestine, these include simple columnar cells, goblet cells, Paneth cells, and argentaffin cells. These polyps must, therefore, be regarded as hamartomas and not neoplasms, in which case there is one predominant type of proliferating cell. This concept is now generally accepted, but difficulties in histologic interpretation previously led to confusion, as the polyps were regarded by some as neoplastic, the appearances of tubules penetrating the stalk being mistaken for invasive carcinoma. As hamartomas, the polyps, unlike the true adenomas of familial polyposis of the colon, cannot be regarded as premalignant lesions. However, an increasing number of case reports have been published in which malignant degeneration has occurred in genuine Peutz–Jeghers polyps. These arise mainly in the duodenum but also have been described in the stomach, jejunum, and colon. The incidence of carcinoma is greater than can be explained on a chance association, but the true relationship of the condition to malignant disease remains uncertain (Linos et al, 1981).

The severity of the pigmentation is not proportional to the number of polyps present. Pigmentation without polyps occurs in 15 percent of the relatives of those with the full syndrome.

Other abnormalities have been reported in association with the syndrome in sufficient numbers to suggest that the connection is more than fortuitous. Ovarian cysts and tumours have been found in a large number of cases. These include multiple small cysts, solitary cystadenomas, and a variety of malignant tumours. Bladder, bronchial, and nasal polyps have also been recorded in affected families and clubbing seems to be a real—although inconsistent—association.

The majority of patients are diagnosed because of GI symptoms or are found as symptomless relatives. GI haemorrhage and attacks of intermittent small bowel obstruction are the most common presentation, but the polyps may be seen on rectal examination and one patient vomited gastric polyps (Ellis, 1967). The haemorrhage may be an acute haematemesis or melaena or an iron-deficiency anaemia caused by repeated microscopic blood loss. The small intestinal polyps cause abdominal pain because of recurrent intussusception, which usually reduces spontaneously but sometimes progresses to gangrene of a long segment.

Fifty percent of patients have rectal and colonic polyps, and they may present with rectal bleeding. A polyp should be removed and care taken to differentiate it histologically from an adenomatous polyp, particularly if there are several present within view of the sigmoidoscope and familial adenomatosis coli is suspected. The buccal cavity should be examined, as this may be the only site of abnormal pigmentation. Full radiographic examination and upper and lower GI endoscopy should be carried out in order to estimate as accurately as possible the size and position of the larger polyps. The disease may be suspected for the first time when a barium meal examination is performed in the investigation of haematemesis. The more usual presentation, however, is at laparotomy for intussusception in a patient who has had a previous operation for a similar condition. The intussusception should be reduced if possible and the polyp removed through a small enterotomy incision. If the intestine is nonviable, however, as limited a resection as possible should be performed. The rest of the GI tract is examined for polyps, but these are notoriously difficult to palpate and are better left in situ at the emergency operation (Fig. 43–2).

A conservative policy has generally been advocated and operation indicated only for continuous haemorrhage or obstructive episodes.

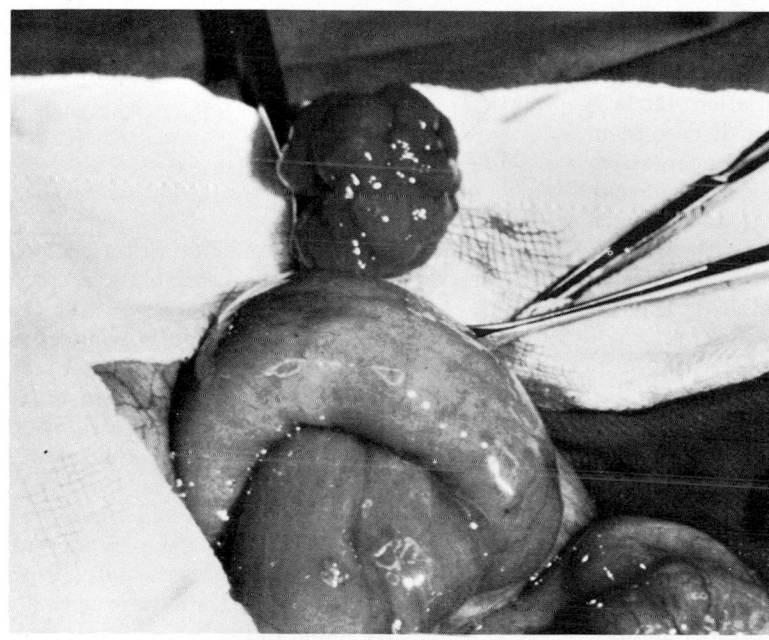

Figure 43-2. Peutz–Jeghers polyp exposed and about to be removed. (*Courtesy of Mr. Norman Machie of St. Mark's Hospital, London, and Mr. O.V. Lloyd-Davies.*)

As the growth rate of these tumours is not known and they seem to have periods of quiescence and activity, the prognosis is uncertain. In the established case, most episodes of abdominal pain and obstruction can be managed by intravenous infusion and gastric aspiration, further laparotomy being undertaken only if the obstruction fails to resolve. This approach in patients who have had at least one laparotomy previously and continuing symptoms would seem to have much to recommend it. At St. Mark's Hospital, this type of procedure has been performed on six patients after careful preoperative mapping of tumours radiologically. All the large tumours have been excised by gastrotomy and multiple enterotomies; small ones are diathermied. The operations have been accomplished without complication and with complete relief of symptoms. The patients remain well for up to 10 years, and one patient required a second operation to remove multiple polyps about 10 years after the primary procedure, but it is too early to know the true success of this procedure. In view of the incidence of ovarian tumours, the ovary should always be carefully examined at laparotomy.

Cronkhite–Canada Syndrome

Cronkhite and Canada in 1965 reported two patients with generalised GI polyposis, alopecia, and atrophy of the fingernails. More cases have since been described. The "polyposis" is due to a polypoid irregularity of the mucosa, which shows stromal oedema and cystic dilatation of the crypts when examined microscopically. The rest of the bowel wall is normal. The change is probably due to a deficiency state and is not neoplastic.

Heterotopic Tissues

Heterotopic pancreas presents as a small submucosal tumour. Endometriosis of the small intestine is rare and presents as a mass, usually in the terminal ileum, and can cause intestinal obstruction. There is puckering of the mucosa over a hard nodule. Endometriosis may also be found in the sigmoid colon and pelvis. The diagnosis is suspected from the history and the presence of chocolate cysts in the ovary at laparotomy.

MALIGNANT TUMOURS

Malignant tumours of the small intestine, like their benign counterparts, are uncommon (Awrich et al, 1980). Of 121,278 patients registered between 1944 and 1976 at the M.D. Anderson Hospital and Tumor Institute, there were 204 patients coded as having a primary malignant neoplasm of the small intestine. Arthaud and

Guinee (1979), excluding secondary and concurrent tumours, found 1.2 percent of GI malignant lesions situated in the small intestine, an incidence of 0.49 per 100,000 population. Little is known of any aetiologic factors. It does seem surprising, however, that with such a large area of mucosa at risk the incidence is so small compared with that of neoplasms in the stomach and large bowel. It is of interest that in the small intestine itself the majority of lesions are found close to the proximal and distal ends.

Carcinoma

Adenocarcinoma is the most common malignant tumour of the small bowel (Figs. 43–3 and 43–4). In Arthaud and Guinee's series, 32 patients had jejunal or ileal adenocarcinoma. The sex incidence was equal and the average age just under 50 years. In most series there is a slight male predominance, and the average age is about 60 years. The lesions are usually annular or ulcerative tumours. As the contents of the small bowel are fluid, obstruction does not normally occur until the stricture is so advanced that stenosis is almost complete. On microscopic examination most tumours prove to be well differentiated adenocarcinomas. By the time the diagnosis is made, lymph node metastases have usually occurred. The average survival rate in the Mayo Clinic series was 22 percent at 5 years.

There is speculation concerning the possibility of long-standing Crohn's disease of the small bowel predisposing to carcinoma (Hoffman et al, 1977).

Carcinoid Tumours

Carcinoid is perhaps an unfortunate term which implies a benign tumour resembling a carcinoma. Carcinoid of the appendix, which is the most common site, very frequently behaves in an entirely benign manner (see Chapter 48). Carcinoids elsewhere in the GI tract metastasise by both the lymphatics and the bloodstream and have all the characteristics of a rather slowly growing malignant tumour (Marks, 1979).

The life history of the carcinoid tumour has been well documented, particularly by Moertel et al (1961) in a Mayo Clinic series of 209 patients. These tumours arise from the argentaffin cells, which are found in the bases of the crypts of Lieberkuhn. These cells are often termed Kultschitzsky cells, to commemorate that histologist's original morphologic description, or more commonly argentaffin cells because of the presence of cytoplasmic granules that stain black with Masson ammoniacal silver solution—hence the term argentaffinoma, which is sometimes used to describe the tumour.

Carcinoids occur throughout the GI tract,

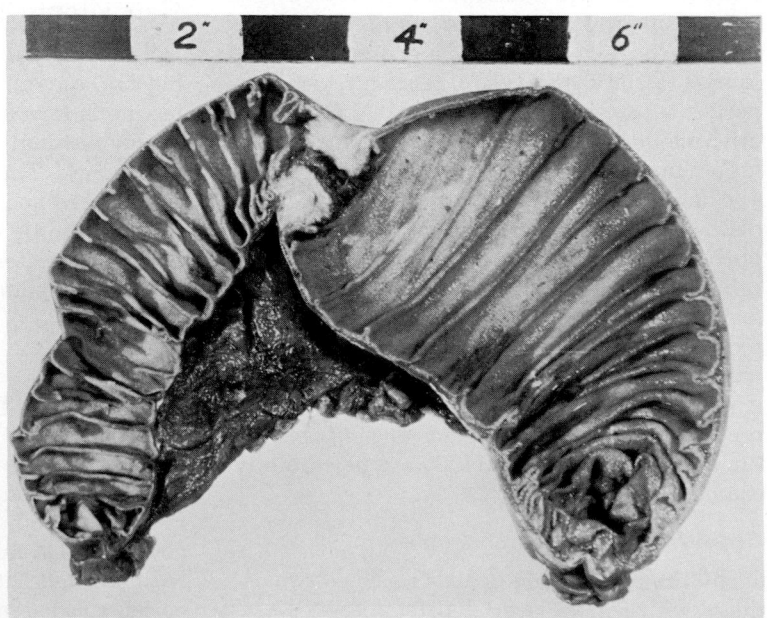

Figure 43–3. Annular carcinoma of the jejunum with proximal obstruction. (*Courtesy of Mr. Norman Machie of St. Mark's Hospital, London, and Mr. O.V. Lloyd-Davies.*)

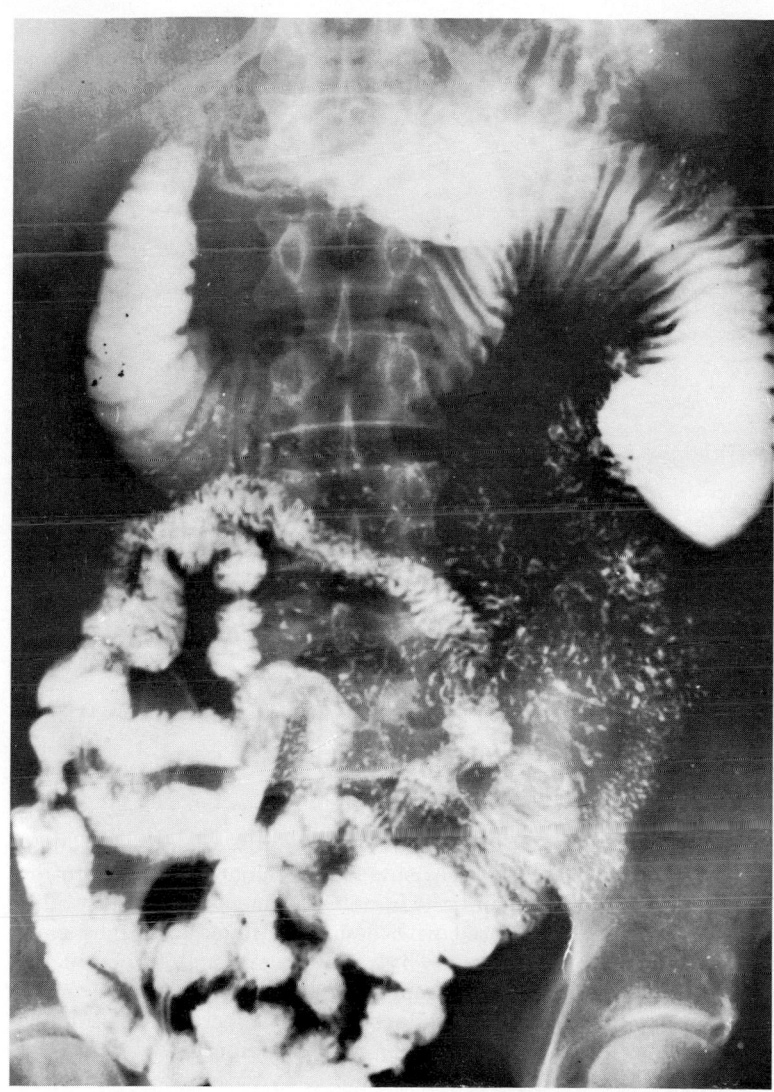

Figure 43–4. Barium meal and follow-up examination showing dilated proximal jejunum and site of annular carcinoma shown in Figure 43–3. (*Courtesy of Mr. Norman Machie of St. Mark's Hospital, London, and Mr. O.V. Lloyd-Davies.*)

more especially in the appendix and ileum, all those occurring at the latter site usually arising in the terminal 2 or 3 feet; they are also found at the ileocaecal valve. The lesions are hard, white nodules that arise in the deep aspect of the mucosa, and the primary tumour is small, varying between 0.5 and 3.5 cm in diameter. On fixing the freshly removed specimen in formaldehyde, the tumour assumes a typical bright yellow colour. A multifocal origin occurs more commonly than with any other tumour. In the Mayo Clinic series, one third of the patients had more than one tumour; some of them had two, but the majority had three or more, and a few had dozens distributed throughout the length

of the small intestine. Possibly because of their relatively benign course, argentaffinomas are frequently found in association with other malignant neoplasms of the GI tract. They metastasise to the regional lymph nodes and to the liver; distant metastases rarely occur (Fig. 43–5). The growth rate of these tumours is extremely slow, and it is therefore not surprising that twice as many are found incidentally at autopsy as are found at operation.

Although argentaffinomas have been described at all ages from childhood to extreme old age, the majority of patients are in the sixth or seventh decades whether the diagnosis is made at operation or postmortem. The sex ratio

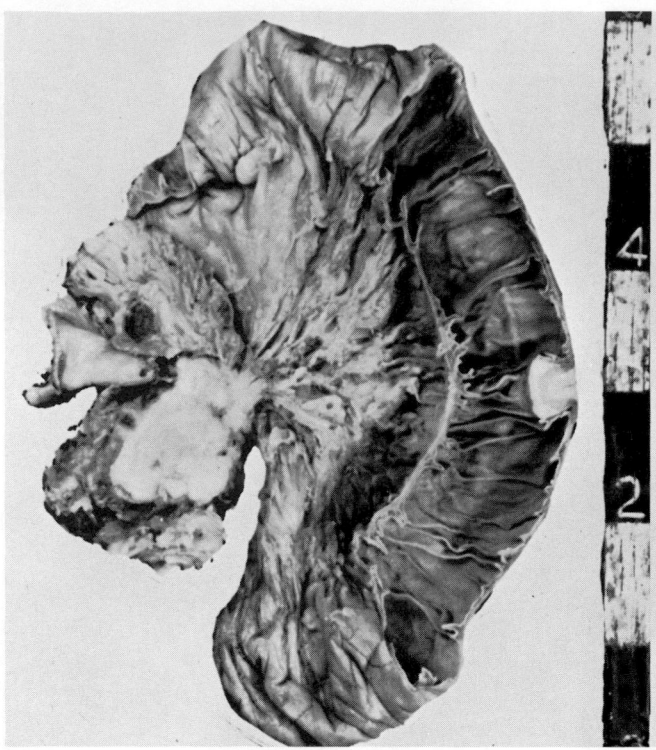

Figure 43–5. Carcinoid tumour of ileum showing small primary tumour that has not ulcerated the mucosa, and a much larger mass of secondary carcinoid in the mesenteric nodes. (*Courtesy of Mr. Norman Machie of St. Mark's Hospital, London, and Mr. O.V. Lloyd-Davies.*)

is similar to that of adenocarcinoma, being two males to one female.

The histology of carcinoid tumour is characteristic—even when the somewhat "fickle" special staining techniques have failed to show the typical granules. The tumours consist of collections of small, closely packed uniform cells that are arranged in well-defined solid clumps or strands with, here and there, small glandular lumina or distinct acini. The cells at the periphery of the clumps are often arranged in a palisade-like way; in these areas, the characteristic cytoplasmic granules are most numerous. The nuclei of the cells are small, round and stain very darkly; mitotic figures are difficult to find. The granules are an artefact owing to the reaction between 5-hydroxytryptamine in the cytoplasm and the formaldehyde fixative. The longer fixation by formalin is delayed, the fewer granules that can be demonstrated.

Carcinoid tumours may occur elsewhere in the GI tract. Those in the colon tend to be the most malignant and about 60 percent have metastases; the most common site throughout the large bowel is the caecum. Rarely, they may be found in the rectum, the biliary tract, and

the pancreas. Occasionally a carcinoid tumour is found arising from a major bronchus, protruding into the lumen as a smooth rounded swelling covered with a normal mucosa. It may cause symptoms by producing bronchial obstruction with an audible wheeze on respiration or may lead to collapse of the affected lobe. Interestingly, the bronchial carcinoid may produce features of the carcinoid syndrome because venous drainage passes, of course, into the systemic circulation.

Carcinoid Syndrome

Malignant carcinoids secrete 5-hydroxytryptamine (5-HT), or serotonin, into the portal circulation. Normally this is inactivated by the liver. However, when extensive hepatic metastases occur, the 5-HT they secrete enters the systemic circulation and results in the carcinoid syndrome (Beatson et al, 1981; Marks, 1979). Carcinoids have been reported in sites draining directly into the bloodstream (for example, ovary or deposits in the abdominal wall) and these will produce the syndrome in the absence of hepatic deposits (Feldman and Jones, 1982).

Other substances which may be secreted by

the carcinoid cells include insulin, ACTH, prostaglandins, bradykinin, histamine, kalikrein and calcitonin.

The carcinoid syndrome comprises one or more of the following features:

1. An enlarged liver or abdominal mass produced by the tumour and its secondaries
2. Flushing with attacks of cyanosis
3. Diarrhoea with noisy borborygmi
4. Bronchospasm
5. Pulmonary or tricuspid stenosis with congestive cardiac failure

Special Investigations. As already mentioned, carcinoid of the appendix is nearly always an incidental finding at examination of a removed appendix.

If the carcinoid syndrome is suspected, the diagnosis is confirmed by measurement of the urinary excretion of 5-hydroxyindole acetic acid (5-HIAA), which is the major metabolite of 5-HT. The normal value is 2 to 9 mg in a 24-hour urine specimen, but in patients with the carcinoid syndrome it may reach 1000 mg or more.

Secondaries in the liver are confirmed by liver scanning or imaging and the GI location of the tumour may require barium studies and fibre-optic endoscopy.

Treatment of Malignant Carcinoid Tumours

Carcinoid tumours of the small and large bowel, if operable, are treated in exactly the same way as carcinomas, by wide resection of the tumour and involved lymph nodes. A careful search is made for tumours elsewhere in the bowel because multiple carcinoids are not uncommon. A small carcinoid tumour of the rectum, if less than 2 cm in diameter and confined to the mucosa, may be treated by local excision but large tumours require radical resection.

The 5-year survival when "curative" resection is possible is in the region of 70 percent.

When the features of the carcinoid syndrome are present, it is likely that there will be extensive hepatic metastases. Even here, surgery may play a part because it is worthwhile resecting as much tumour as possible to reduce the bulk of secreting carcinoid. If possible, the primary itself should also be resected, since this may progress to produce obstructive symptoms. It may be possible to carry out a partial hepatectomy for localised liver deposits. More often, the deposits are scattered through the liver but even

here worthwhile regression has occurred following enucleation of these deposits. It must be remembered that the carcinoid tumour tends to grow more slowly than carcinoma, so that even with liver metastases the 5-year survival is in the region of 20 percent.

Nonsurgical Management of Metastases. Even when the tumour is beyond surgical cure, there is still much to be offered to the patient with carcinoid syndrome. The nonsurgical modalities include:

1. Embolisation of hepatic metastases
2. Cytotoxic chemotherapy
3. Pharmacologic therapy

Hepatic artery ligation has been used for the management of inoperable hepatic metastases but more recently the less invasive technique of hepatic artery embolisation, using material such as absorbable gelatine sponge, has yielded excellent results, with reduction in the size of the liver and disappearance of the carcinoid syndrome features (Matson et al, 1982).

Cytotoxic drugs may produce useful remissions in the carcinoid syndrome. Those most often used are 5-fluorouracil, cyclophosphamide and streptozotocin, alone or in combination.

A wide variety of pharmacologic agents may be used as antagonists to the humoral agents responsible for the carcinoid syndrome. These include serotonin antagonists such as methysergide, kinin inhibitors, including chlorpromazine and phenoxybenzamine, and codeine phosphate or diphenoxylate hydrochloride (Lomotil) for nonspecific treatment of the diarrhoea.

Lymphoma

These tumours are the third most common form of malignant neoplasm of the small intestine. They are most frequent in the ileum, coinciding with the large number of normal lymphoid follicles in this region (Gray et al, 1982). Dawson et al in their 1961 review of 126 cases considered the tumours to be primarily situated in the intestine if there was no palpable superficial lymphadenopathy, the chest radiographs showed no mediastinal node involvement, the leucocyte counts (total and differential) were within normal limits, and, at laparotomy, the bowel lesion predominated—the only lymph nodes obviously affected being those in the immediate neigh-

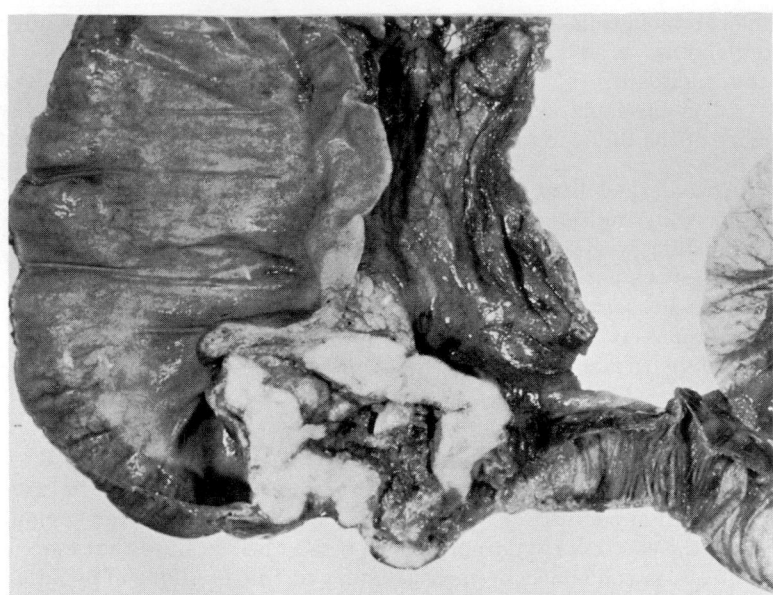

Figure 43–6. Reticulum cell sarcoma of the terminal ileum. (*Courtesy of Mr. Norman Machie of St. Mark's Hospital, London, and Mr. O.V. Lloyd-Davies.*)

bourhood, and, finally, when the liver and spleen were free of tumour.

Intestinal lymphomas occur three times more frequently in men and, under the age of 20 years, they are twice as common. The average age of presentation is less than with other malignant tumours, being in the fifth decade. This is due to more cases occurring in patients under 20 years of age. The tumours present as ulcerating or infiltrative types, polypoid tumours being least common. They sometimes become bulky and involve a long segment of intestine which becomes rigid (Fig. 43–6). The regional lymph nodes are usually enlarged—but not always by tumour deposits—but some show changes of reactive hyperplasia only.

The frequency with which lymphomas perforate must also be mentioned. Their true nature can be unrecognised, as there may be a ragged hole in the bowel with slightly thickened oedematous edges and nothing else to suggest that a tumour is the underlying cause. A lymphoma must always be suspected as the origin of a perforation at an unusual site that has occurred for no obvious reason. A fistula between one piece of bowel and another may develop. In addition, the diagnosis must be suspected in any ulcerated plaque-like lesion—particularly in the terminal ileum—when considerable necrosis is present. The histologic picture can be very difficult to interpret and, therefore, the pa-

thologist may be uncertain whether or not an inflammatory or a neoplastic condition exists.

The association of malabsorption with lymphoma was recognised more than 40 years ago by Fairley and Mackie (1939). In 1965, Ramot and colleagues described a group of patients, all of whom were Oriental Jews or Arabs, with primary small bowel lymphoma, malabsorption, and abdominal pain. In 1968, Seijffers et al coined the term Mediterranean-type lymphoma. However, this condition has since been described in patients of a low socioeconomic standard beyond the Mediterranean, and the term "Western-type lymphoma" is used. The different morphologic features of these types have been described by Lewin et al (1976). An abnormality of protein synthesis has been described in a number of patients with this disease. An IgA abnormality, consisting of a portion of the α-heavy chain without light chains, is synthesised and the condition termed α-chain disease. A familial incidence of lymphoma of the small intestine in association with immunologic deficiency has also been described.

Sarcoma

Of the malignant connective tissue tumours of the small intestine, the leiomyosarcoma is the most common. The review of these malignant tumours by Skandalakis (1962) shows that, as is the case with their benign counterparts, leiomyosarcomas are fairly evenly distributed throughout the small intestine, being slightly more common in the jejunum than the ileum. The sex incidence is equal, and although widely distributed through the age groups, the tumours are most commonly found in the sixth decade. They are often smaller in size (less than 5 cm) than the leiomyomas at the time of diagnosis, particularly in the younger age group. As with benign tumours, they undergo central necrosis as they increase in size, and often the middle of the tumour consists of a series of blood-filled cavities which may rupture into the bowel lumen with severe or fatal haemorrhage, or else perforate into the peritoneal cavity. Histologically, it is difficult to differentiate between benign and malignant tumours (Fig. 43–7). Leiomyosarcomas spread by direct infiltration of the surrounding structures or of the abdominal wall, and metastasise via the bloodstream to the liver, lungs, and bones. Widespread peritoneal and mesenteric implants may be found. One third of tumours will have metastasised by the time laparotomy is performed.

Secondary Tumours

Secondary involvement of the small intestine in malignant disease is common, but this is almost always part of a generalised spread with multiple seedlings in the peritoneal cavity and, frequently, ascites. Rarely, however, a secondary tumour may be a discrete nodule, and this diagnosis must be considered in the differentiation of tumours of the small bowel. The most common site of the primary tumour is the cervix uteri, followed by cutaneous melanoma, other parts of the GI tract, and kidney. The tumours occur months or years after the primary tumour has been excised and sometimes, in the case of melanoma, present before the primary tumour has been located. There may be no other sign of secondary neoplasm. The metastases are blood-borne and are more commonly situated in the upper part of the ileum. The melanomas have a typical appearance, being umbilicated initially and later having a rolled, scalloped margin with an ulcerated centre.

DUODENAL TUMOURS

The tumours of the duodenum are considered separately from the remainder of those of the small intestine, because the position of the neoplasm to some extent alters the clinical presentation and makes treatment much more formidable.

The classification of tumours at this site will be similar to that of tumours of the small intestine in general, except that the frequency

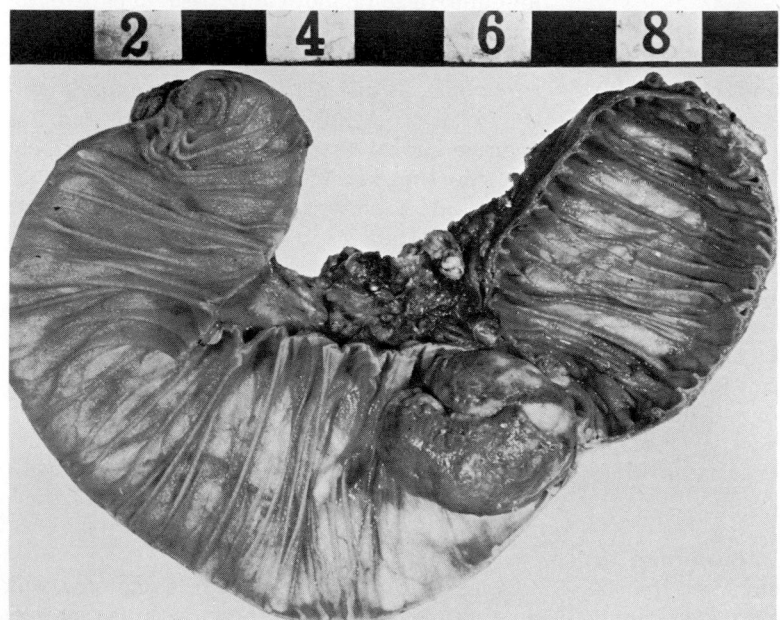

Figure 43–7. Leiomyosarcoma of the jejunum predominantly of the intramural type. (*Courtesy of Mr. Norman Machie of St. Mark's Hospital, London, and Mr. O.V. Lloyd-Davies.*)

with which each variety occurs is different and the histologic characteristics of some tumours are modified by the structure of the duodenum.

There are no independent aetiologic factors. Although duodenal tumours are rare, this site is exceeded only by the terminal ileum as the most common seat of both benign and malignant growths of the small intestine.

Benign Tumours

Benign tumours are rare and represent 16 percent of all neoplasms of the small intestine.

Adenomas

Adenomas are alleged to be the most common type of benign tumour to be found in the duodenum. In a collected series by River et al (1956) there were 73 adenomas, 35 lipomas, 32 myomas, and 8 haemangiomas. They tend to be in the proximal part of the duodenum, whereas malignant tumours are more distally placed. They usually occur in the second and third portions of the duodenum, where they are easily removed. Occasionally, they are multiple, and then some of the polyps are located in the third and fourth portions of the duodenum.

Adenomas are usually small, pedunculated tumours and are found incidentally on radiologic or endoscopic examination of the upper GI tract or at operation or autopsy. Occasionally, they grow large—up to 7 or 9 cm in diameter.

The Brunner gland "adenoma" is really a hamartoma and is not precancerous. It is commonly confused with adenoma and this probably accounts for the relatively high incidence mentioned above.

Until recently, patients with familial polyposis coli were thought to have adenomas confined to the colon. Recent studies have shown that these adenomas may occur in the small bowel and stomach, particularly in the periampullary region of the duodenum. The incidence is possibly as high as 50 percent of all patients with polyps. These adenomas can undergo malignant change and deaths from periampullary carcinoma have occurred in a number of patients with familial polyposis (Yao et al, 1977).

Mesodermal Tumours

There are many varieties of mesodermal tumours occurring in the duodenum. More than 30 types have been listed, but the only commonly described ones are the lipoma, myoma, and haemangioma. Fibromas, myxomas, lymphangiomas, and neurogenic tumours are reported occasionally. They do not differ from those found elsewhere in the small intestine.

The symptoms are epigastric pain with proximal lesions and melaena and subsequent anaemia in those placed distally. If the tumour arises from the papilla of Vater, however, jaundice can occur, even with benign lesions.

Malignant Tumours

Carcinoma

Of all the duodenal tumours, a little more than one third are found to be malignant, and of these, carcinoma is by far the most common type (Alwark et al, 1980; Lillemoe and Imbambo, 1980; Spira et al, 1977).

Pathology. Carcinoma of the duodenum is classified according to its relationship to the ampulla of Vater, as the situation will alter the symptoms and signs, the treatment, and the prognosis. The high incidence of ampullary tumours is of interest. This site marks the junction of the foregut and midgut, and the mucosa of the dodenum, ampulla, common bile duct, and pancreatic duct are in close association.

Carcinoma is rarely found in the first part of the duodenum, and most supraampullary tumours will arise in the second part above the ampulla. In 253 Lahey Clinic cases of pancreatoduodenectomy for periampullary cancer, Warren et al (1967) found the incidence of duodenal carcinoma, as distinct from periampullary cancer, to be equal in men and women, and the average age to be 52 years. In periampullary growths, three males to every female were affected, and the average age was 56 years, with a range of from 12 to 78 years.

The growths are either papilliferous or ulcerative in form, the latter sometimes growing around the circumference of the lumen and occluding it. The majority are fairly well-differentiated adenocarcinomas, but some are anaplastic.

The tumours spread by direct infiltration and relatively late by the lymphatics, as compared with other sites in the gastrointestinal tract.

Clinical Manifestations. The symptoms will depend upon the site of the growth. In the periampullary group, 83 percent developed obstructive jaundice; this is initially fluctuating, unlike that from carcinoma of the head of the pancreas or common bile duct. More than 80 percent of the patients had faecal occult blood present. The combination of fluctuating jaundice and blood loss is very suggestive of the diagnosis and is unlike the picture of stones occluding the common bile duct (when bleeding is quite uncommon). A little less than half of the patients had dull aching pain in the right upper quadrant of the abdomen. The average weight loss was a little less than 14 pounds. In the group of patients with duodenal tumours, pain was the most common symptom. This pain was an aching discomfort in the right upper quadrant radiating to the back, but not so severe as the pain of carcinoma of the pancreas. It can easily be mistaken for a manifestation of duodenal ulcer, except that it is relieved by vomiting and made worse by food intake. Jaundice is not such a common feature, occurring only in one third of patients, and is the result of the tumour infiltrating through the duodenal wall and compressing the common bile duct. These patients progress to duodenal obstruction more commonly than do those in the ampullary group, owing to the absence of, or late onset of jaundice, which might alert the surgeon to the diagnosis. Vomiting is more common, and the vomitus may not contain bile if the carcinoma is supraampullary; these patients can mimic those with pyloric stenosis. There is a more profound weight loss than in the ampullary group. In the Lahey Clinic series, all the patients with duodenal carcinomas had positive occult blood in the stools.

The physical signs include a palpable tumour in about 25 percent of cases, and there may be evidence of obstruction, with a dilated stomach and visible peristalsis. Investigations should include a full blood count and faecal occult blood test. A glucose tolerance curve will be abnormal in about 30 percent of those with ampullary tumours and in 10 percent of those with duodenal tumours.

Diagnostic Studies. A barium meal x-ray examination will show obstruction or a filling defect in the duodenum. A diagnosis based on x-ray findings is reached more commonly than in tumours more distally placed in the small bowel; also, approximately two thirds of duodenal lesions and one third of ampullary lesions can be located by x-ray examination. The efficacy of radiologic means of diagnosis is increased if a duodenal tube is passed and barium instilled directly into a paralysed duodenum. Upper GI endoscopy will play a vital role with respect to earlier detection of duodenal neoplasms. Whenever symptoms suggest a duodenal lesion, investigation is not complete without endoscopy of the entire duodenum. Any lesion should be biopsied but remember that many tumours will show areas of co-existing benign and malignant growth.

Treatment. The interval between the onset of symptoms and operation commonly varies between 3 and 6 months and is, again, considerably less than with more distally placed tumours.

There may be considerable doubt about the preoperative diagnosis, but it is essential that the exact type of lesion be identified when the abdomen is opened. The procedure necessary will vary, depending upon the site and the nature of the tumour. Pancreatoduodenectomy carries such a high morbidity and mortality rate that it should be done only for a definite malignant lesion, when cure is possible.

GENERAL CONSIDERATIONS

Clinical Manifestations

Patients with a tumour of the small intestine present with a variety of symptoms. The most constant of these are weight loss, intermittent colicky abdominal pain, and GI haemorrhage and anaemia. Vomiting, diarrhoea, and general malaise and weakness are also commonly found. The symptoms are initially vague and the time taken to establish the diagnosis is usually long, sometimes a few weeks but usually between 6 and 18 months and, occasionally with carcinoid or benign tumours, many years.

The symptoms are caused by obstruction and profound weight loss in malignant tumours and by blood loss in benign tumours. Owing to the intermittent and nonspecific nature of the symptoms, a wrong diagnosis of functional illness may be made. This error will be avoided if the possibility of a small intestinal tumour is considered.

The physical signs most commonly found are a palpable lump, distension of the abdomen and tenderness, which is usually in the epigastrium or around the umbilicus if the lesion is jejunal or in the right iliac fossa or midline below the umbilicus if it is ileal. There may be a fluid splash, borborygmi, and visible peristalsis in patients with subacute obstruction. Other signs include anaemia and wasting.

All too frequently, no diagnosis is reached until the patient develops either acute intestinal obstruction or a perforation.

Diagnostic Studies

The investigations that contribute toward the diagnosis are a full blood count to show if there is a hypochromic anaemia, faecal occult blood tests, and radiologic studies of the GI tract.

A plain abdominal x-ray may show evidence of subacute intestinal obstruction with a dilated stomach, duodenum, or intestinal loops. A barium meal and follow-up examination should be carried out, and if these are negative and the diagnosis still in doubt, a "small bowel enema" should be performed. Whatever method is employed, the accuracy of the diagnosis falls as the lesion is placed more distally. Some tumours situated in the terminal ileum show up on retrograde filling of the bowel in a barium enema examination. The radiologic presentation of these tumours may be as an acutely obstructed intestine caused by an intussusception or an annular carcinoma. If the patient has recurrent attacks of subacute obstruction, every attempt should be made to perform an x-ray study of the abdomen during an attack.

Gastrointestinal Haemorrhage

The tumour presenting with bleeding, usually in the form of melaena or with anaemia and a continually positive faecal occult blood test, can be very difficult to locate. The problem is complicated by the presence of colonic diverticular disease, small adenomatous polyps in the colon, or peptic ulceration. The site of the bleeding is often uncertain; unfortunately sometimes the small intestinal tumour remains undiagnosed until after a colonic or gastric resection has been performed. If the responsible lesion could be in the small intestine, every effort should be made to locate it prior to laparotomy, as it may be such a small tumour as to be almost impossible to find by sight and touch.

Following the finding of a normal bleeding and clotting time, prothrombin time, and a negative Hess test, together with negative upper GI endoscopy, sigmoidoscopy, and colonoscopy, radiologic examination of the small bowel should be undertaken. If all these investigations yield negative results and the bleeding continues, technetium scanning should be carried out. This will not show the site of bleeding but will indicate in which quadrant of the abdomen it occurs. Selective superior mesenteric angiography may show the site of the lesion, particularly if an angiomatous malformation is responsible, but if there are no marked blood vessel abnormalities, the site of bleeding will only be detected if the bleeding is brisk.

Laparotomy

Following investigation, with or without a definitive diagnosis in the case of a suspected tumour of the small intestine, laparotomy is carried out. The findings at operation may give a good idea of the pathologic changes and will influence the procedure. If an intussusception is present, it should be reduced, if possible, unless the viability of the gut is obviously impaired. If a pedunculated tumour is found, it is almost certainly an adenoma and can be removed by simple enterotomy and excision. If the lesion is sessile, a segment of bowel should always be excised with the tumour, as it is impossible to tell in most cases whether it is benign or malignant. If situated in the terminal ileum, the tumour is likely to be a carcinoid or a lymphoma, and if in the jejunum, a carcinoma, or a smooth muscle tumour. The small, tight annular stricture with dilatation of the proximal gut is a carcinoma, and, by the time laparotomy takes place, there will usually be involvement of the lymph nodes in the mesentery. This tumour should be resected together with a V-resection of the mesentery with all the nodes that can be removed, the continuity of the intestine being restored by end-to-end anastomosis. If the operation is palliative, better results will be obtained by removing the primary tumour than by doing a simple bypass operation.

The carcinoid tumour will be recognised as a flat button-like plaque in the terminal ileum, usually without involvement of the serosal layer. The primary tumour is always small, rarely being more than 3.5 cm in maximum diameter and more commonly being 0.5 to 1.5 cm in diameter. If it has metastasised to the mesenteric lymph nodes, these structures will be white and hard and often larger than the primary tumour. Obstructive symptoms are caused not by occlusion of the lumen of the bowel by the primary growth, but by kinking of it by the mass of nodes in the mesentery or by the mesentery itself being fixed. The rest of the small intestine and the appendix should be very carefully examined, as these tumours are commonly multifocal and often very small. In most cases, these will lie in the same segment of ileum, and if none more proximally or distally can be felt, a wide resection of bowel on each side of the primary tumour and a V-resection of the mesentery are wise precautions. If the tumour is within 20 cm of the ileocaecal valve, a right hemicolectomy should be performed. A radical operation is advisable in the presence of a moderate number of liver metastases, as these are very slow growing.

Lymphomas originating in the small bowel will often present as ulcerated, thickened, greyish plaques in the ileum causing stenosis of the lumen. The main differential diagnosis is Crohn's disease; it may be difficult to differentiate the disorders at the time of operation, particularly as the regional lymph nodes are large in both conditions. The serosa may be involved in lymphoma, and in Crohn's disease the fat is oedematous and tends to grow around the circumference of the ileum. The lesion should be resected with a reasonable margin of intestine on each side and the obviously involved nodes removed. The fact that the nodes are enlarged and possibly cannot all be excised should not prevent a radical operation, as many such nodes will show only signs of reactive hyperplasia. If a lymphoma is suspected, the paraaortic nodes, liver, and spleen must be carefully examined to exclude a generalised disease of the reticuloendothelial system; if there is any doubt, a biopsy specimen of the liver and lymph nodes should be taken. As for frozen sections, it is asking too much of the pathologist to differentiate between a lymphoma and an inflammatory condition on a small fragment of tissue.

The smooth muscle tumour will be found as a small intraluminal nodule, a dumbbell tumour, or a large mass (often the size of a fetal head) protruding from the wall of the small intestine. It is dark red in colour and may have undergone cystic degeneration. It is impossible, in the absence of obvious metastases, to ascertain if the tumour is malignant or benign. If malignant, it may be fixed to the abdominal wall

and other loops of intestine. Metastases tend to occur later with sarcomas than with other malignant tumours, and therefore, even if a large mass that has infiltrated surrounding structures is found, the condition may still be potentially curable. The other reason for doing a radical excision—even if removal of part of the abdominal wall and several loops of bowel is necessary—is because a simple bypass procedure is of little value to the patient and does not prevent the complications of massive haemorrhage and perforation causing death from fulminating peritonitis.

Tumours of the jejunum within 20 cm of the ligament of Treitz are difficult to resect with an adequate margin. It is better in such cases to excise the segment of jejunum, mobilising the fourth part of the duodenum if necessary, and then securely to close the upper and lower ends of the bowel. The continuity of the alimentary tract is reconstructed by mobilising the third part of the duodenum, making an incision in the mesocolon, and swinging the distal jejunum to the right and bringing it up through the mesocolon to lie adjacent to the mobilised duodenum. A side-to-side anastomosis is then carried out in the usual manner, and when this has been completed, the upper edge of the incised mesocolon is sutured to the duodenum anteriorly and the cut edge of the mesentery of the jejunum stitched to the peritoneum of the posterior abdominal wall.

Persistent Gastrointestinal Haemorrhage

The underlying cause of haemorrhage will usually be a haemangioma or a small intraluminal smooth muscle tumour. Persistent haemorrhage without other signs or symptoms is often more caused by a benign rather than a malignant tumour if the origin is found to be in the small intestine. If, after exhaustive investigation of the whole of the GI tract, no cause for the bleeding has been found, laparotomy will often be fruitless and the aetiology of the haemorrhage will remain obscure.

The laparotomy should be carried out if possible when the patient is known to be bleeding. The whole of the GI tract must be carefully examined, especially in the absence of an obvious cause for the blood loss. This procedure includes mobilisation of the stomach and a wide gastrotomy, as well as mobilisation of the whole of the duodenum, including the third and fourth parts. The latter cannot be examined without complete mobilisation from under the superior mesenteric pedicle, and it is surprising how large a tumour at this site can be missed on successive laparotomies unless this manoeuvre is carried out. It will prevent some patients from having a blind gastrectomy with no alteration in symptoms. Small leiomyomas or haemangiomas can sometimes be found by making enterotomies at two or three sites in the small intestine and introducing a light inside the lumen; a small sigmoidoscope is a convenient method of doing this. The wall is then transilluminated, and in a darkened theatre, the vascular pattern is clearly demonstrated and tiny abnormalities may be observed. An alternative method is to manipulate a long fibre-optic endoscope through the stomach and into the small intestine at laparotomy.

Acute Abdominal Emergency

An emergency will arise when acute intestinal obstruction or perforation of the tumour occurs. Unfortunately, almost one third of patients remain "undiagnosed" until one of these situations has arisen, and in many, metastases will have already developed. The annular carcinoma is the tumour that most commonly defies diagnosis until an episode of acute obstruction arises. Any polypoid neoplasm, however, benign or malignant, can present in this way either by directly occluding the lumen or, more usually, by producing an intussusception. This defect is reduced if possible, and if not, a resection is undertaken. Unless the tumour is a pedunculated adenoma, a radical excision must be performed.

The tumours that present as an acute perforation are usually the smooth muscle tumour and the lymphomas. If the tumour is large, it is likely to be the former and if small, the latter. As already stated, the lymphomas occasionally present as a ragged perforation with little evidence of underlying tumour. In these cases, resection of the segment of bowel should always be undertaken, as simple closure of the perforation may result in the diagnosis being missed and also invite the recurrence of perforation at the same site.

BIBLIOGRAPHY

Alwmark A, Anderson A, et al: Primary carcinoma of the duodenum. Ann Surg 191:13, 1980
Arthaud JB, Guinee VF: Jejunal and ileal adenocarci-noma: Epidemiological considerations. Am J Gastroenterol 72:638, 1979
Awrich AE, Irish CE, et al: A twenty-five-year experience with primary malignant tumours of the small intestine. Surg Gynecol Obstet 151:9, 1980
Beatson H, Homan W, et al: Gastrointestinal carcinoids and the malignant carcinoid syndrome. Surg Gynecol Obstet 152:268, 1981
Cronkhite LW, Canada WJ: Generalised gastrointestinal polyposis: An unusual syndrome of polyposis, pigmentation, alopecia and onychotrophia. N Engl J Med 252:1011, 1955
Dawson IMP, Cornes JS, et al: Primary malignant lymphoid tumours of the intestinal tract. Report of 37 cases with a study of factors influencing prognosis. Br J Surg 49:80, 1961
Ellis H: The Peutz–Jegher syndrome. Hosp Med 1:730, 1967
Fairley NH, Mackie, FP: The clinical and biochemical syndrome in lymphoadenoma and allied diseases invading the mesenteric lymph glands. Br Med J 1:375, 1939
Feldman JM, Jones RS: Carcinoid syndrome from gastrointestinal carcinoids without liver metastases. Ann Surg 196:33, 1982
Good CA: Tumours of the small intestine. AJR 89:685, 1963
Gray GM, Rosenberg SA, et al: Lymphomas involving the gastrointestinal tract. Gastroenterology 82:143, 1982
Hoffman JP, Taft DA, et al: Adenocarcinoma in regional enteritis of the small intestine. Arch Surg 112:606, 1977
Jeghers H, McKusick VA, et al: Generalised intestinal polyposis and melanin spots of the oral mucosa, lips and digits. N Engl J Med 241:993, 1031, 1949
Lewin KJ, Kahn LB, et al: Primary intestinal lymphoma of "Western" and "Mediterranean" type, alpha-chain disease and massive plasma cell infiltration. Cancer 38:2511, 1976
Lillemoe K, Imbambo AL: Malignant neoplasma of the duodenum. Surg Gynecol Obstet 150:822, 1980
Linos D, Dozois R, et al: Does Peutz–Jegher's syndrome predispose to gastrointestinal malignancy? Arch Surg 116:1182, 1981
Marks C: Carcinoid Tumours. A Clinicopathological Study. Boston: GK Hall, 1979
Maton PN, Camilleri M, et al: Role of hepatic embolisation in advanced carcinoma tumours. Gut 23:917, 1982
Moertel CG, Sauer WG, et al: Life history of the carcinoid tumor of the small intestine. Cancer 14:901, 1961
Norberg K-A, Emas S: Primary tumours of the small intestine. Am J Surg 142:569, 1981
Perzin KH, Bridge MF: Adenomas of the small intestine. A clinicopathological review of 51 cases and a study of their relationship to carcinoma. Cancer 48:799, 1981
Peutz JLA: Obereen zeer merkwaardige, geocombi-

neerde familiaire Polyposis van de Slijmvliezen van den Tractus intestinalis met die van de Neuskeelholte en Gepaard met eigen aardige Pigmentaties van Huiden Slijmvliezen. Nederl. Maands Chr. Geneesk 10:134, 1921

Raiford TS: Tumors of the small intestine. Arch Surg 25:122, 321, 1932

Ramot B, Shahin N, et al: Malabsorption syndrome in lymphoma of the small bowel. Isr J Med Sci 1:221, 1965

Reddy RR, Schuman BM, et al: Duodenal polyps: Diagnosis and management. J Clin Gastroenterol 3:139, 1981

River L, Silverstein J, et al: Collective review: Benign neoplasms of the small intestine. A critical comprehensive review with reports of 20 new cases. Int

Abst Surg (Surg Gynecol Obstet) 102:1, 1956

Seijffers MJ, Levy M, et al: Intractable watery diarrhoea, hypokalemia and malabsorption in a patient with Mediterranean type of abdominal lymphoma. Gastroenterology 55:118, 1968

Skandalakis JE, Gray SW, et al: Smooth muscle tumors of the alimentary tract. Springfield, Illinois: Thomas, 1962

Spira IA, Ohazi A, et al: Primary adenocarcinoma of the duodenum. Cancer 39:1721, 1977

Warren KW, Veidenheimer, MD, et al: Pancreaticoduodenectomy for periampullary cancer. Surg Clin North Am 47:639, 1967

Yao T, Iida M, et al: Duodenal lesions in familial polyposis of the colon. Gastroenterology 73:1086, 1977

44. Acute Intestinal Obstruction

Harold Ellis

GENERAL CONSIDERATIONS

Introduction

There is no better way to introduce this section than to quote the opening paragraph of the chapter on intestinal obstruction in Berkeley Moynihan's textbook on abdominal operations published in 1926:

> When called upon to deal with a case of acute intestinal obstruction the surgeon is confronted with one of the gravest and most disastrous emergencies. The patient may be, and often is, a man or woman in the prime of life, in full enjoyment of vigorous health, who, without warning, is suddenly seized with the most intolerable pain in the abdomen, followed by collapse and vomiting, at first slight, but later unremitting. The abdomen distends, intestinal action ceases, and the bowel above the block, loaded with retained and septic contents, becomes a vehicle for the absorption of products whose intensely poisonous action hastens the patient to his end.

Success in the treatment of acute intestinal obstruction depends largely upon early diagnosis, skillful management, and an appreciation of the importance of treating the pathologic effects of the obstruction just as much as the cause itself. When obstruction is recognised and treated efficiently in its earliest stages, the immediate and late results are extremely gratifying in the great majority of patients. Unfortunately, there is often delay, which sometimes can be attributed to tardiness on the part of the patient but all too often is the fault of the surgeon. As a result of this delay, distended or strangulated bowel becomes seriously or irreparably damaged, and the picture changes to one of extreme danger, so that relief of the obstruction may not be sufficient to prevent a fatal issue.

Classification

Acute intestinal obstruction is divided into two main types—mechanical and neurogenic. In *mechanical obstruction* the intestinal contents are prevented from passing along the bowel by an acute obstruction of the lumen of the gut. Mechanical obstruction, in turn, is subdivided into simple and strangulated. In the first there is purely obstruction to the passage of intestinal contents, but in the second there is, in addition, obstruction of the blood supply of the involved segment of the gut. Although it is true that as progressive distension of the bowel occurs, the blood supply of the intestine even in a simple obstruction may become compromised.

In *neurogenic obstruction* (paralytic ileus) the intestinal contents do not traverse the bowel because of intestinal paralysis.

Mechanical obstruction is classified not only according to whether it is simple or strangulated, but also according to its aetiology, its site, and its speed of onset.

The aetiology is considered conveniently under the three headings that apply to any occluded tube within the body:

1. *Causes in the lumen:* gallstone ileus, food bolus obstruction, faecal impaction, etc.
2. *Causes in the wall:* congenital atresia, bowel neoplasms, inflammatory strictures, etc.
3. *Causes outside the wall:* strangulated internal or external hernia, obstruction due to adhesions or bands, volvulus, and intussusception.

The site of the obstruction is classified into high or low in the small intestine or as a large bowel obstruction.

The speed of onset determines whether the obstruction is acute, chronic, or acute superimposed on chronic. In acute obstruction, the onset

TABLE 44–1. COMMON CAUSES OF OBSTRUCTION AND OVERALL MORTALITY RATE IN 1890s, 1920s, 1940s—1950s, AND 1960s—1970s

	Study (Years)				
	Gibson (1888–98)	Vick (1925–30)	Wangensteen (1942–52)	Waldron & Hampton (1944–56)	Ellis (1962–80)
Type of Obstruction (%):					
Adhesions	18	7	31	40	26
Hernia	35	49	10	12	21
Intussusception	19	12	3	4	2
Tumour	—	13	27	14	30
Volvulus	12	0.2	3	6	6
Mortality	43	26	11	14	6
Total Cases	1000	6892	1252	493	253

(*Source: From Ellis H, 1982, with permission.*)

is sudden and the symptoms severe. In chronic obstruction, the symptoms are insidious and slowly progressive, as for example in most cases of carcinoma of the large bowel. Acute symptoms may supervene as a chronic occlusion suddenly becomes complete.

MECHANICAL OBSTRUCTION

Aetiology

The picture of acute obstruction has changed quite remarkably in the active life-time of surgeons today. Until the 1920s and 1930s, strangulated external hernias accounted for a high percentage of the total cases of intestinal obstruction. In 1900, Gibson collected 1000 examples of intestinal obstruction in papers published between 1888 and 1898, and 35 percent of these were due to strangulated hernias; bands accounted for 18.6 percent of the cases. In 1932, Vick reviewed 6892 patients with acute obstruction dealt with between 1925 and 1930 in 21 hospitals in Great Britain. No less than 49 percent were due to strangulated external hernias; adhesions were responsible for 7 percent. In more recent times, strangulated hernias have become much less frequent, no doubt because of the considerable enthusiasm with which hernias are repaired electively, even in the relatively old and feeble. Adhesions, in contrast, have become more and more common, and this, in turn, can be attributed to the enormous increase in the frequency of abdominal surgery. Thus, in 1955, Wangensteen, surveying 1252 cases of obstruction, reported only a 10.4 per-

cent incidence of strangulated hernia, compared with 37 percent due to adhesions. Waldron and Hampton (1961) reported 40 percent of their 493 cases due to adhesions and 12 percent to strangulated hernias. These same authors reviewed five large series of cases published between 1905 and 1931 and noted that 7.5 percent were due to adhesions compared with 58.2 percent produced by strangulated hernias. However, an analysis of five more large series of cases be-

TABLE 44–2. COMMON CAUSES OF OBSTRUCTION AT EACH AGE GROUP

Neonate	Congenital atresia
	Volvulus neonatorum
	Meconium ileus
	Hirschsprung's disease
	Imperforate anus
Infant	Strangulated inguinal hernia
	Intussusception
	Complications of Meckel's diverticulum
	Hirschsprung's disease
Young adult	Adhesions and bands
	Strangulated inguinal hernia
Middle age	Adhesions and bands
	Strangulated inguinal hernia
	Strangulated femoral hernia (in women)
	Carcinoma of the colon
Elderly	Adhesions and bands
	Strangulated inguinal hernia
	Strangulated femoral hernia (in women)
	Carcinoma of the large bowel
	Diverticulitis
	Impacted faeces

(*Source: From Ellis H, 1982, with permission.*)

tween 1940 and 1953 showed that the incidence of adhesions had risen to 38.2 percent with strangulated hernias falling to 24.1 percent. The more extended figures of these authors, together with those from this author's unit, are of some interest when placed side-by-side for comparison (Table 44–1). Our series of 253 patients operated on between 1962 and 1980 is biased by two factors. First, these were all adult patients and second, ours is a referral unit with particular interest in malignant disease, which accounts for the high proportion of patients with obstruction due to tumours.

Incidence

Age and Sex. Intestinal obstruction may occur at any age. Although it is comparatively rare in children and in young adults, its incidence rises in middle age and reaches a plateau in those over 50. The most common causes vary widely at each age group, and it is important for the clinician to bear in mind the frequencies according to age.

The common causes of obstruction at each age group are presented in Table 44–2.

A strangulated hernia is, it will be noted, an important cause of intestinal obstruction from infancy to old age. One therefore need not apologise for emphasising that the hernial orifices must be carefully examined in every case. It is a wise clinician who goes to the bedside of every elderly and obese patient with acute abdominal pain firmly resolved to search for a

small strangulated femoral hernia beneath the abdominal fat.

The sex incidence of obstruction is roughly equal, although the Registrar General's returns do demonstrate a slightly higher death rate in females than in males.

Site. About 80 percent of intestinal obstructions occur in the small bowel and about 20 percent in the large. In 1953, Becker, reviewing 1007 cases of acute intestinal obstruction in New Orleans, found 20.4 percent were situated in the large bowel. Michel, Knapp, and Davidson in 1950 found that 16 percent of 580 cases involved the colon. In our own series at Westminster 32.8 percent of our 253 patients had large bowel obstruction, but this reflects our particular interest in neoplastic disease; 58 of the patients had malignant obstruction of the large intestine.

Demography. Wide variations occur in the common causes of intestinal obstruction among different races and communities. These variations probably depend on many factors, which include anatomic differences, variations in life expectancy, dietary habits, and genetic differences. They form a fascinating field for future clinical research. Some statistics from India, East and West Africa, and the West Indies are presented in Table 44–3.

In less developed communities, strangulated hernia remains, as it once was in the United Kingdom, the most common cause of

TABLE 44–3. CAUSES OF OBSTRUCTION IN INDIA, AFRICA, AND THE WEST INDIES

	Study (Locale)						
	Gill & Eggleston (Punjab)	McAdam (Kampala, Uganda)	White (Bulawayo, Zimbabwe)	Chiedozi (Benin City, Nigeria)	Cole (Ibadan, Nigeria)	Badoe (Accra, Ghana)	Brooks & Butler (Jamaica)
Type of Obstruction (%):							
Adhesion	15	4	17	10.8	10	10	23
Hernia	27	75	36	65	35	77.6	25
Intussusception	12	4	7	11.4	27	4	19
Malignancy	—	1	—	0.3	1	0.6	5
Tuberculosis	3	—	—	—	0.7	—	—
Volvulus:							
Large bowel	9	13	11		0.7	4	6
Small bowel	16	0.4	8	8	3	1	0.4
Total Cases	147	794	172	316	436	782	250

(*Source: From Ellis H, 1982, with permission.*)

strangulation—35 percent in Nigeria, 36 percent in the Rhodesian black, 27 percent in the Punjab, 25 percent in Jamaica, and no less than 75 percent in Uganda. In Malaysia, Ti and Yong (1976) found that the sophisticated local Chinese population had adhesions as the most common cause of obstruction, whereas the Malay, Indian, and Ceylonese patients presented most frequently with strangulated hernias.

Perhaps more remarkable is the marked frequency of volvulus in many population groups and strange differences in the incidence of involvement of the small or large intestine in this condition. Thus in Uganda, McAdam (1961) reported a 13 percent incidence of sigmoid volvulus and in Rhodesia nearly 20 percent of 112 obstructions were caused by sigmoid volvulus, but there, volvulus of the small intestine is also remarkably common (11.6 percent). This is attributed to the short mesentery and highly mobile small bowel in the Bantu. In the Punjab, both volvulus of the small and large intestine are common, accounting for nearly a quarter of 147 cases reported by Gill and Eggleston (1965). Andersen (1956) in West India, had 33 cases of volvulus (19 of the large and 14 of the small intestine) in 161 obstructions, while in Iran, Saidi (1969) reported that, of 286 obstructions, 13.6 percent had sigmoid, 5.7 percent caecal, and 22.7 percent small intestinal volvulus. Taha and Suleiman (1980) report that volvulus of the sigmoid colon accounted for 33 percent of all emergency admissions with intestinal obstruction to their hospital in Khartoum in the Sudan, and 70 percent of all cases of colonic obstruction. Kaltiala et al (1972) report that small bowel volvulus is also surprisingly common in Finland.

In India, tuberculosis of the intestine is relatively common although nowadays in the West it is practically nonexistent. There was, for example, a 3 percent incidence in the Punjab series. Tandon and Prakash (1972) studied 212 patients with chronic or subacute intestinal obstruction in Delhi. No less than 159 of these were diagnosed as tuberculosis, compared with only 10 examples of Crohn's disease.

A quite remarkable incidence of intussusception is reported from Ibadan, in West Nigeria, by Cole (1965). Here, in a band about 100 miles across, intussusception, mainly the caecocolic type, accounted for no less than 27 percent of 436 admissions with obstruction and was second only to hernia in frequency. It occurs in both children and young adults in this particular community, where volvulus in contrast is much rarer than in Ghana or East Africa. Kark and Rundle (1960) have similarly commented on the comparative frequency of idiopathic intussusception in the adult black population of Natal.

The low incidence of carcinoma in less developed countries is also demonstrated in Table 44-3, which may reflect the lower life expectancy in these communities, with a comparatively small proportion of the population entering the cancer age group. Dietary and genetic factors may also have important roles in this respect.

Physiologic and Pathologic Derangements

Fluid and Electrolyte Disturbances. Between 8 and 10 L of fluid are secreted daily into the alimentary canal from stomach, small intestine, biliary tract, and the pancreas; all but a very small amount is subsequently reabsorbed from the colon. This vast fluid shift is equivalent to about a quarter of the entire body water, or three times the total plasma volume.

An obstruction in the small intestine will cut off this fluid from the absorptive surface of the colon, and the accumulated intestinal juices will be lost to the body's economy, either in the vomitus, the gastric aspirates, or merely by sequestration within the dilated loops of obstructed bowel. Apart from loss of water, there will be accompanying losses of electrolytes, especially sodium, chloride, and bicarbonate, the exact concentrations depending on the particular site of the intestinal obstruction (Table 44-4).

The fluid loss becomes aggravated as the intestine dilates and becomes venously congested. There is then an increase in fluid and

TABLE 44-4. APPROXIMATE ELECTROLYTE CONTENT OF GI TRACT

Fluid	mmol/L		
	Sodium	*Potassium*	*Chloride*
Gastric juice	60	10	100
Bile	145	5	100
Pancreatic juice	140	5	75
Small bowel contents	110	5	100

electrolyte loss into the bowel lumen. The elegant experimental studies of Shields (1965) have shown that not only does the ileum above the obstruction fail to absorb water and sodium but, as time passes, their rate of secretion into the gut lumen, together with that of potassium, is actually increased. With this there is considerable protein leakage from the engorged capillaries. Strangulation of the bowel will be accompanied by accumulation of protein and electrolyte-rich exudate into the peritoneal cavity, and infarction of an extensive length of intestine will be associated with marked sequestration of blood into the bowel wall itself.

Bacteriology. The normal upper small intestinal contents are virtually sterile; the distal small gut fluid may yield a scanty growth of faecal flora. The situation is quite different in the presence of obstruction. Bishop and Allcock (1960) aspirated samples of small bowel contents in 27 cases of obstruction and found profuse bacterial colonies, predominantly faecal in type, above the point of occlusion. The longer the period of obstruction, the higher up the bowel did this contamination extend. The small gut below the obstruction was sterile or contained only scanty transient flora. Sykes et al (1976), using modern culture techniques, have demonstrated a considerable increase in the anaerobic organisms above the obstruction, especially *Bacteroides*. This was particularly evident in patients with large bowel obstruction.

These investigations indicate that bacterial contamination in the obstructed gut is derived from ingested organisms. Normally, these organisms traverse the small intestine so rapidly that significant growth is impossible. In the presence of stasis obstruction, however, proliferation by geometric progression results in rapid colonisation of the gut lumen.

The faeculent fluid within the obstructed small gut represents bacterial breakdown of what are normally sterile contents.

Pathology. Acute intestinal obstruction in its simple form consists of an interruption to the lumen of the bowel. Even in the absence of strangulation, ischaemic changes progressing to necrosis and perforation may occur. Pressure necrosis may take place at the site at which a tight band passes across a loop of gut or where a foreign body or impacted faeces may produce stercoral ulceration of the bowel wall with resul-

tant perforation and peritonitis. In many cases of acute obstruction of the colon by a stenosing carcinoma, the ileocaecal valve remains competent with gross distension of the proximal colon, more particularly the caecum, which may, in advanced cases, literally burst (Fig. 44–1A,B).

Every abdominal surgeon is perfectly familiar with the sight of heavy, oedematous, cyanosed loops of intestine above a simple occlusion that has been present for some time and also with the marked intraperitoneal exudation, occasionally already infected, encountered in such cases. In advanced examples, there may be serosal tears along the antimesenteric border of the distended loops with, fortunately, infrequent actual perforation with flooding of the peritoneal cavity with intestinal contents. The dramatic return of bowel colour to normal after decompression of the gut demonstrates that these changes are caused by the effects of high intraluminal pressure upon the bowel wall circulation.

Changes in Strangulation Obstruction. Strangulated intestinal obstruction represents a considerably more complex problem than simple occlusion of the gut. In addition to all the physiologic disturbances associated with simple obstruction discussed earlier, the body must cope also with blood loss in the infarcted bowel, impending or actual death of tissue within the strangulated segment, the transudation of toxic material across the wall of the bowel into the peritoneal cavity, and, in late cases, the toxaemia produced by frank perforation of the gangrenous segment.

As the pressure within the obstructed loop exceeds the venous pressure in the bowel wall and adjacent mesentery, there is venous engorgement of these vessels, followed by capillary rupture with haemorrhagic infiltration. This occurs first in the submucosa, then the mucosa, and then throughout all the layers of the wall of the intestine. Thrombosis in the intramural and mesenteric veins hastens this ischaemic process. Necrosis first appears in the mucosal surface, as discussed by Bussemaker and Lindeman (1972), because of the relative vulnerability of intestinal epithelium to anoxia. Indeed, it is not rare to see in the resected specimen of ischaemic bowel a fairly healthy external appearance accompanied by a surprising degree of mucosal damage. Eventually perforation of the necrotic segment takes place.

Apart from this risk and the actual blood

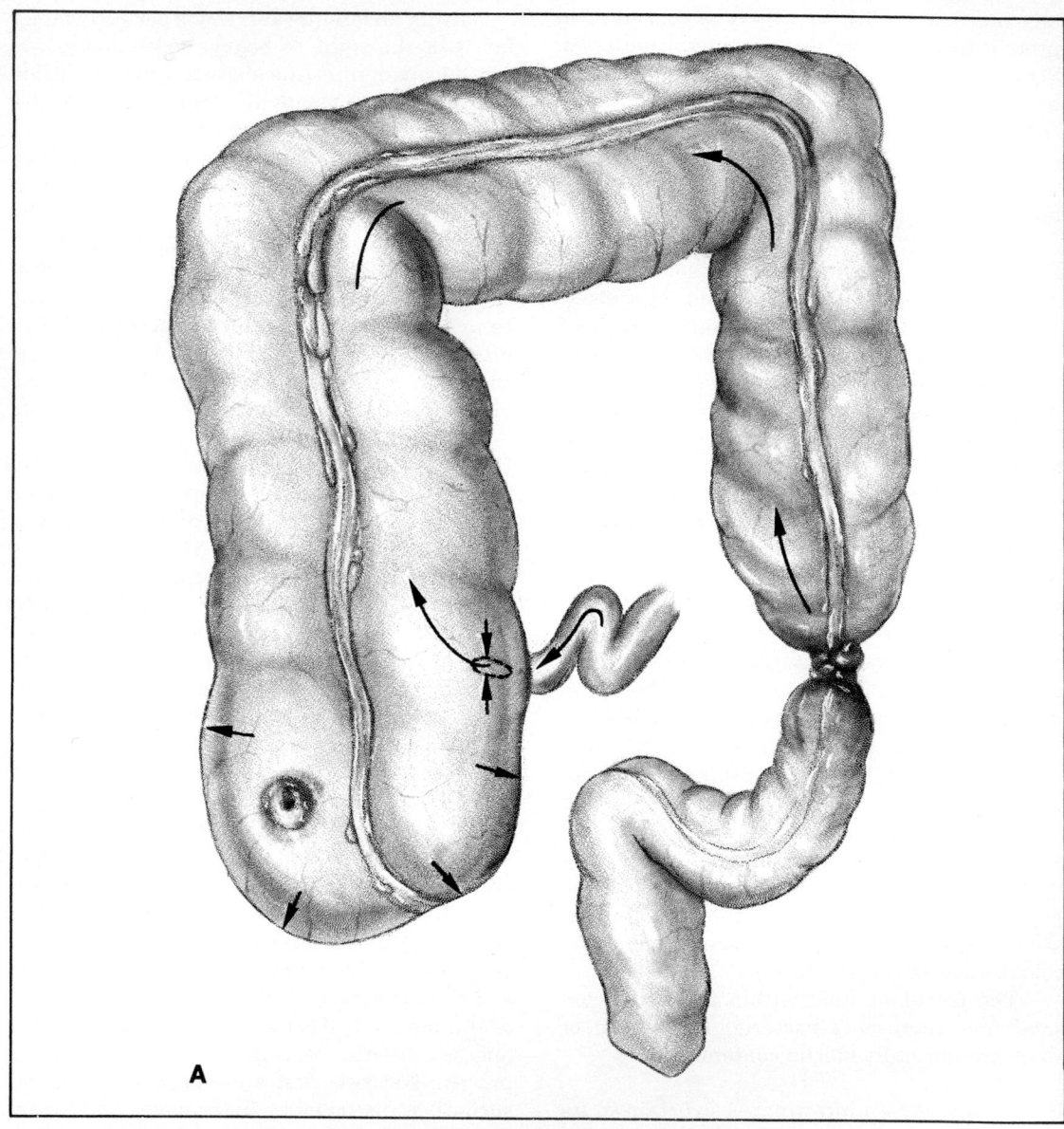

A

Figure 44–1. A. A competent ileocecal valve results in gross distension of the large bowel, especially of the caecum, which may necrose and perforate.

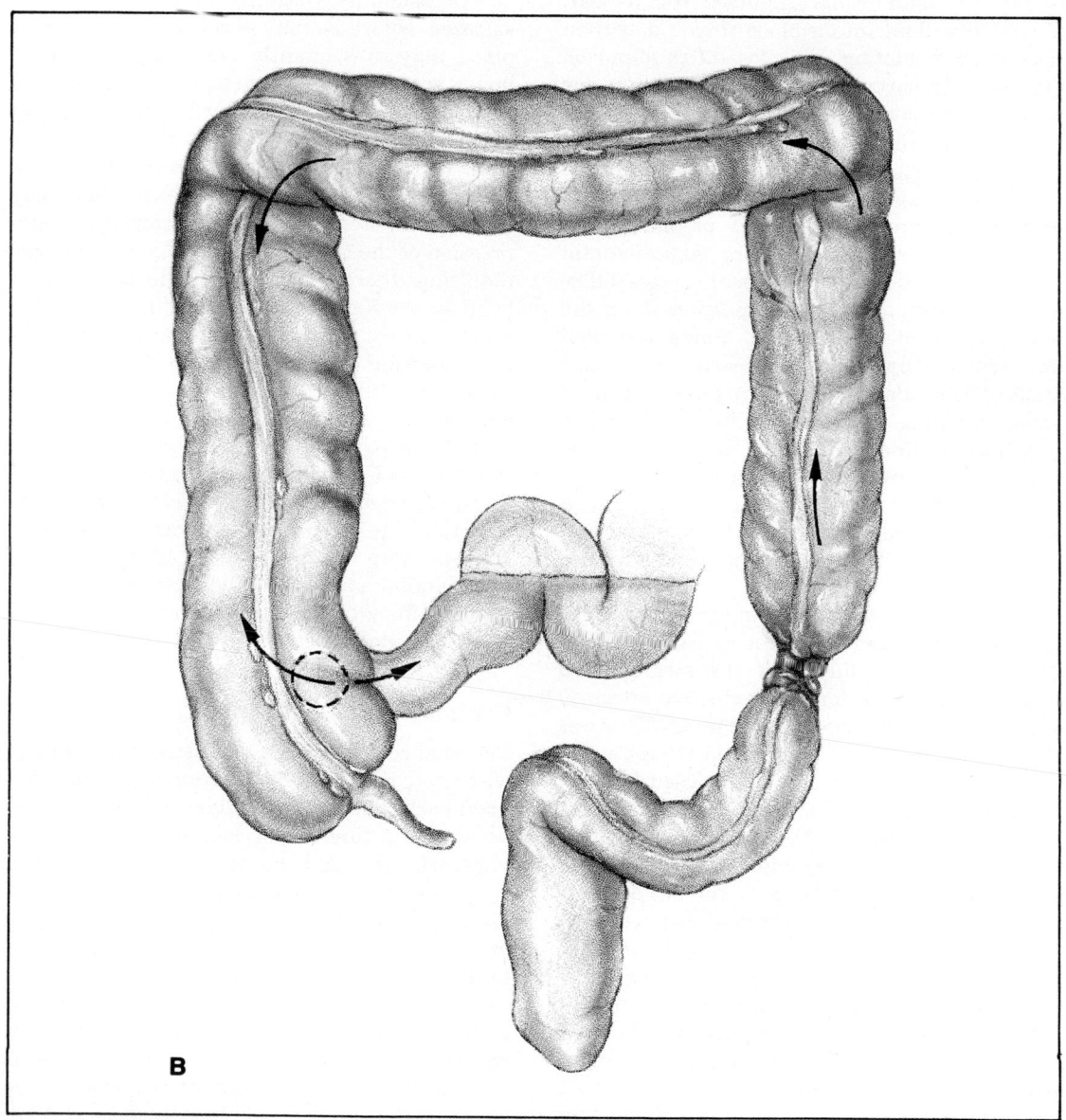

Figure 44–1. B. An incompetent valve allows ileal reflux and small bowel distension. (*Source: From Ellis H, 1982, with permission.*)

loss to the wall of the infarcted bowel, perhaps the most important factor in the lethal consequences of strangulation is the toxic transudation into the peritoneal cavity across the damaged bowel wall from organisms within the gut lumen. The fluid exudate changes from a clear, plasma-like fluid into a blood-tinged and then foul, dark exudation. This loss of protein-rich fluid is an important contributing factor to the hypovolemic shock. The exact nature of this toxic factor remains the subject of debate. Gram-positive and gram-negative organisms have their proponents, either as a direct effect or from the production of exo- or endotoxins. Much of the rather conflicting experimental studies in this field may represent species differences. However, there is no question about the toxic nature of this exudate, which was well demonstrated by the classic experiments of Aird (1936). Transudate from a strangulated loop of small intestine was collected in a rubber bag and injected into guinea pigs. Up to 24 hours, the cultures were sterile and the fluid was without effect. After this, however, the fluid grew both aerobic and anaerobic organisms and animals injected with this material died within a few hours.

It has been known for many years that antibiotics given systemically, intraperitoneally, or directly into the lumen of the strangulated bowel have a considerable protective effect on survival in the experimental situation. This was first shown by Harper and Blain (1945), using penicillin in dogs with isolated closed loops of small intestine, and the work was considerably extended by Cohn (1961).

As well as throwing interesting light on the importance of gut bacteria in the aetiology of the toxaemia of strangulation, these experiments also underline the value of systemic antibiotic therapy in the management of strangulation obstruction. Not only will this counteract the toxaemia, but will also support bowel of borderline viability while revascularisation takes place.

Interesting confirmation of the importance of bacterial toxins in the morbid effects of strangulation obstruction have been demonstrated by studies on strangulated empty or sterile intestine and investigations on germ-free animals. Yale and Balish (1979), for example, demonstrated that germ-free dogs survived infarction of isolated segments of small intestine that were uniformly lethal in conventional dogs and also in germ-free animals contaminated with *Clostridium perfringens* or with *B. fragilis*. In dogs contaminated with a pure culture of *Escherichia coli*, however, only one third of the animals died.

Occasionally a strangulated loop of bowel, released before actual perforation has taken place, may subsequently undergo ischaemic fibrosis with resultant stricture formation. This condition was seen particularly when reduction by taxis was carried out for strangulated hernias. The site of obstruction has three variants of essentially the same type of lesion. There may be a double stenotic ring, resulting from compression of the two limbs of the loop at the hernial ring, there may be a single constricting band in those cases where one limb has made a satisfactory recovery, or the entire strangulated segment may undergo fibrotic changes resulting in a tubular stenosis. This condition has been well reviewed by Barry (1942), who gives an interesting historical account of this condition, and by Cherney (1958) who reviews a total of 83 reported cases. The development of obstruction due to the stenosis varied from 7 to 10 days to up to several years after strangulation. Similar strictures have also occurred following injury to the intestine and as a sequel of mesenteric embolism.

Clinical Manifestations

The chances of a successful issue in a patient with acute intestinal obstruction depend largely upon early and accurate diagnosis. The importance of the time factor has already been emphasised, and this is borne out by all statistics.

Accurate clinical diagnosis involves the following steps: (1) the discovery of the presence of an intestinal obstruction, (2) an attempt to locate its level, that is to say, where it is situated in the bowel, (3) an attempt to differentiate between simple and strangulating obstruction, although, as we shall see, is often little more than an inspired guess, and (4) diagnosis of the cause of the obstruction. It is surprising that a diagnosis that one would think so simple as obstruction of the bowel is so often missed.

Simple mechanical obstruction may be confused with (1) acute gastroenteritis, (2) pancreatitis, (3) appendicitis, (4) perforated peptic ulcer, (5) renal or biliary colic, (6) torsion of an ovarian cyst, or (7) rare medical causes, e.g., diabetic precoma. Special forms of obstruction and their differential diagnoses are discussed in another chapter.

There are four common complaints of patients with acute obstruction: (1) pain, (2) vomiting, (3) constipation, and (4) distension. They may all exist in a particular case or occur in any combination. The typically colic pain—cramp-like and intermittent—may have been disguised by morphia; vomiting is delayed in low-gut obstruction and may indeed be completely absent in colonic occlusions; distension may be imperceptible in a high small-bowel obstruction. If the obstruction is incomplete, flatus may still pass and, in any case, a loaded colon below an obstruction may still provide one or two bowel actions before constipation becomes total.

Symptoms

Pain. Pain is the most common symptom in obstruction of the small intestine. The onset may be insidious or abrupt in the simple obstructions, but with strangulation, the onset is usually sudden and severe. The pain is colicky in nature and occurs in spasms lasting from 1 to 3 minutes. It increases in intensity, often to an agonising peak, and then ceases, only to recur again and again. In the intervals between the bouts of colic, the patient may experience complete relief, or there may be a continued ache as a result of the intestinal distension.

Synchronous with the pain, it is often possible to hear borborygmi, and on auscultation loud splashing, rushing, or tinkling sounds may be heard. If there are large amounts of free fluid in the peritoneal cavity, transmitted heart and breath sounds may be detected through the stethoscope.

Vomiting. Vomiting may be reflex, such as may accompany any acute abdominal pain, but it is then followed by persistent regurgitant vomiting. A high, small-gut obstruction is characterised by copious vomiting from the start. At an early stage, the vomitus consists of semi-digested food and opalescent gastric chyme. Later on, watery fluid laden with bile is voided in large amounts, and, finally, the stage is reached when the vomit is composed of dark brown, foul-smelling fluid, the so-called faeculent vomiting. This fluid results from profuse bacterial growth in the stagnant and obstructed intestinal contents. Because of the copious fluid loss, dehydration rapidly becomes clinically ob-

vious and is characterised by the dry shrunken skin, the sunken eyes, the extreme thirst, and scanty urine output of the patient.

If the obstruction is situated in the distal ileum, vomiting is not such a prominent feature; dehydration, too, is a more tardy process. Cases of large-bowel obstruction may proceed to a fatal issue without vomiting during any stage of the disease.

To sum up: First, the higher the level of the block in the bowel, the more copious the vomiting; second, the more turbid and faeculent the vomitus, the more grave and late the obstruction.

Absolute Constipation (the Passage of Neither Flatus nor Faeces). This condition is a common although unreliable symptom of obstruction. Thus, a patient may be constipated for a week or more without having obstruction, yet another patient with a strangulated loop of small intestine may have just had the bowels opened. In Richter's hernia and in intussusception, there may be normal movements; again, in a large-bowel obstruction owing to a stenosing carcinoma, there may be natural or enema-produced evacuation of faecal contents distal to the occlusion.

It was once the practice to administer an enema or to give two diagnostic enemas in order to determine whether the patient was capable of passing flatus or faeces. If no flatus was passed even after the administration of the second enema, it was usually assumed that complete intestinal obstruction was present. This test is unreliable and exhausting to the patient; plain films of the abdomen will give much more reliable evidence of the true state of affairs, and the two-enema test for intestinal obstruction should be relegated to the shelves of surgical history.

Distension. The degree of distension depends on the site of the obstruction and upon the time factor. Thus, when the proximal jejunum is occluded, the stomach becomes distended with gas and accumulated secretions so that the epigastric region may, in the later stages, be more prominent and tense. When the ileum is involved, the central portion of the abdomen is moderately blown out, and when the distal colon is blocked, there is considerable universal distension of the abdomen with well-marked bulging in the flanks. Volvulus of the sigmoid may be accompanied by distension of stupendous proportions.

Inspection may reveal distended coils of intestine or visible peristalsis. The latter is not of itself pathognomonic of obstruction and may be present in a nonobstructed individual who has a thin abdominal wall or ventral hernia. Nevertheless, visible peristalsis associated with colicky pain at once suggests the presence of an obstructive lesion of the gut.

Signs

In addition to the classic quartet of pain, vomiting, absolute constipation, and distension, a number of features are valuable in the diagnosis of acute obstruction.

Scars. The presence of an abdominal scar, whether recent or old, always suggests an underlying band or adhesions.

Vital Signs. In the early stages of simple acute intestinal obstruction, the temperature, pulse, respiration, and blood pressure are usually within normal limits. At a late stage in obstruction, the patient becomes anxious and pale, with a feeble rapid pulse, falling temperature and blood pressure, and typical features of dehydration. Shock may be more marked in the strangulated case.

Palpation. Palpation usually reveals tenderness and release tenderness. This, together with muscle guarding, tends to be more marked in the strangulated case but is by no means invariably so. A mass may be detected on palpation, such as a carcinoma of the colon, diverticulitis of the sigmoid loop, or an intussusception. The hernial orifices should, of course, be methodically palpated, and a rectal examination should be performed. Typically, in an intestinal obstruction, the rectum is ballooned. Occasionally a low-lying obstructive tumour or an impacted mass of faeces may be found. At other times, a pelvic tumour may be palpable through the rectal mucosa, or there may be tell-tale blood or slime on the examining finger.

Abdominal Auscultation. Abdominal auscultation should never be omitted, and findings are particularly characteristic when noisy sounds accompany each wave of colicky pain.

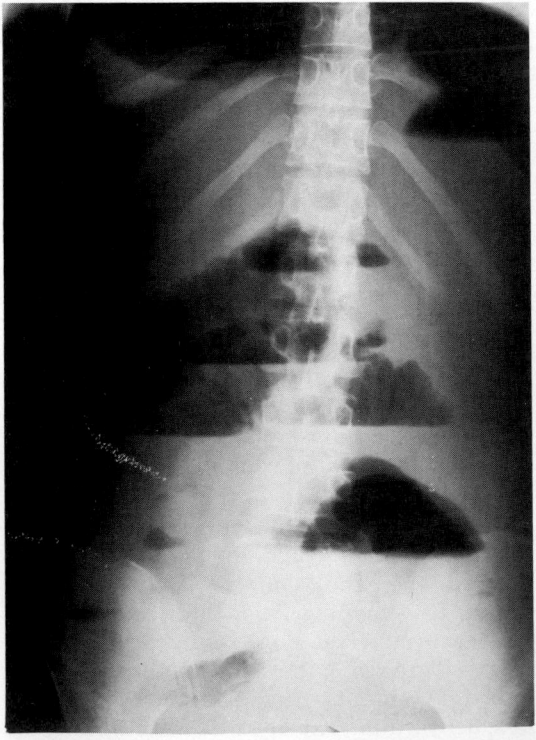

Figure 44–2. Plain x-ray of the abdomen in a patient with intestinal obstruction due to an adhesion. In the erect position the typical fluid levels can be seen. (*Source: From Ellis H, 1982, with permission.*)

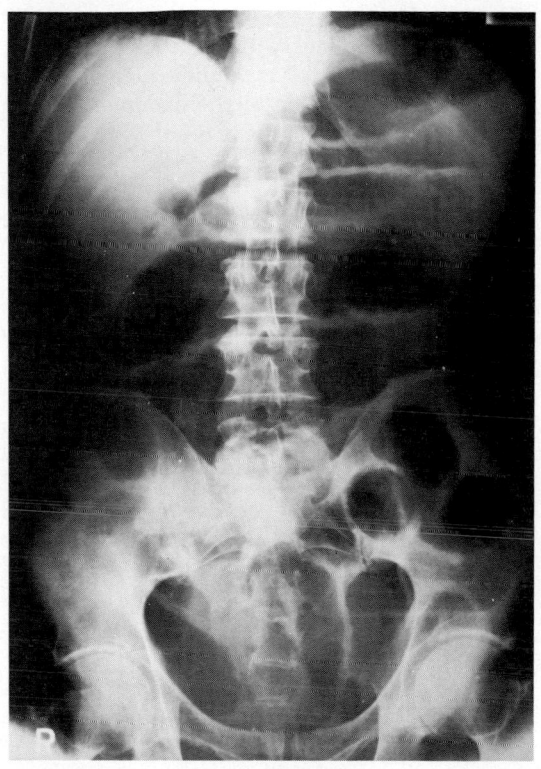

Figure 44–3. The same patient supine. X-ray shows the distribution of distended loops of small intestine. (*Source: From Ellis H, 1982, with permission.*)

Diagnostic Studies

Laboratory Tests. A full blood count, packed cell volume, serum electrolyte determination, and blood urea level should be estimated as soon as possible after the patient's admission. Leucocytosis is suggestive of strangulation but is not at all a reliable sign. Elevation of the haemoglobin and of the packed cell volume is an important indicator of haemoconcentration and a valuable guide to fluid replacement. Severe electrolyte depletion owing to loss of gastrointestinal (GI) fluid will be reflected by lowered serum sodium, potassium, chloride, and bicarbonate with a raised blood urea.

X-ray Examination. X-ray investigation is by far the most important of all the special methods of enquiry, but some 5 percent of those with acute intestinal obstructions have normal x-ray findings. Methods include:

1. Plain x-ray films taken in the erect and lying positions (Figs. 44–2 and 44–3).
2. Follow-through studies after ingestion of a radiopaque meal. Although iodinated aqueous media such as Gastrografin are popular,

they rapidly lose density in transit owing to imbibition of water. A micropaque barium sulphate suspension maintains its opacity, and there is little danger of its impaction above a small-bowel obstruction because of the considerable fluid accumulation above the block, which rapidly dilutes the medium. Figures 44–4 and 44–5 are good examples of small-bowel obstruction demonstrated by this means.

3. X-ray studies of the suspected site of the lesion after introduction of the opaque medium through an indwelling intestinal tube.
4. Barium-enema x-ray investigation is particularly helpful in cases of obstructing lesions of the colon caused by carcinoma or diverticulitis. Reflux of barium through the ileocaecal valve may demonstrate a small-bowel obstruction accurately.

Plain x-ray films of the abdomen should be performed routinely in all cases of intestinal obstruction. The physical basis of the radiologic signs is that gas and fluid accumulate in the bowel above the blockage. With the patient in the erect position, the association of gas and fluid gives rise to a series of fluid levels. With

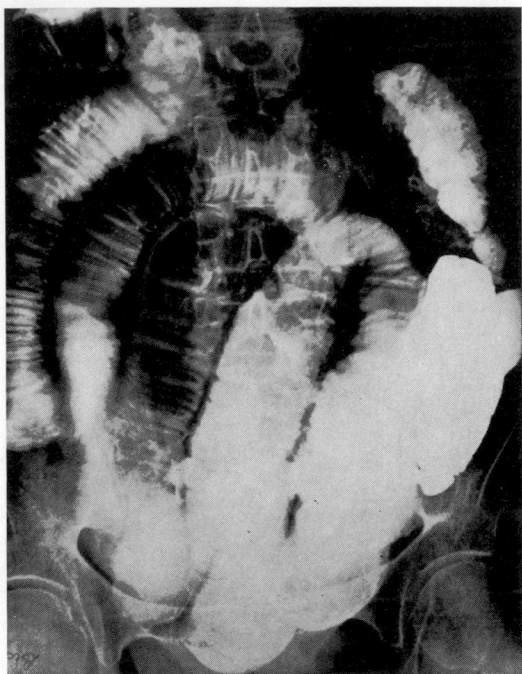

Figure 44–4. Barium meal x-ray examination showing acute small-gut obstruction.

the patient in the supine position, the x-ray picture shows the amount and distribution of gas in the gut. The distended loops of small intestine generally lie transversely in a step-ladder fashion across the central abdomen. Typically, the shadows of the valvulae conniventes traverse the complete width of the bowel shadow and are spaced at regular intervals. In some 5 percent of cases, the obstructed bowel is entirely fluid-filled, and the absence of air–fluid levels may delay diagnosis if this is not realised, as shown by Kingsnorth (1976).

The gas shadows of the large intestine tend to locate peripherally and typically show haustral folds that do not completely traverse the width of the gut and are irregularly spaced. The distended caecum is smooth walled and is usually easily recognised in the right iliac fossa. In total obstruction, gas shadows within the rectum are absent.

Two specific forms of intestinal obstruction may give quite typical appearances on plain x-ray films. A gallstone ileus may show air in the biliary system (as a result of a cholecystoduodenal fistula) together with direct visualisation of the stone and x-ray evidence of small-bowel ob-

struction. Volvulus of the sigmoid colon usually reveals a tremendously distended sigmoid loop, which may extend up to the diaphragm and may even fill the right side of the abdomen. It has been aptly termed the bent inner tube sign.

Location of the Obstruction

The following recapitulates the features that suggest the level of obstruction:

- *High small-gut obstruction* is suggested by early profuse and frequent vomiting with rapid development of dehydration due to excessive fluid loss. Oliguria, insatiable thirst, a rising blood urea level, early collapse, and sunken facial features may be present—all characteristic of an excessive loss of fluid and electrolytes. Distension may be absent in the early stages, but later on it becomes manifest, although tending to be limited to the epigastrium. Flatus and faeces may be passed, with or without the aid of enemas.

- *In low small-gut obstruction,* the onset tends to be more gradual and the case pursues a less urgent course. There is severe and frequent colicky pain. The vomiting is later and less profuse than that which accompanies high lesions. Distension involves the central abdomen.

- *In acute large-gut obstruction,* there is often little or no vomiting, no shock, and no dehydration. There is absolute constipation and considerable abdominal distension. In early cases, the caecum bears the brunt of the distension and becomes ballooned, while at a later stage the whole abdomen and flanks are blown out. At times, a mass or tumour may be felt per abdomen or per rectum. The final picture shows a huge barrel-shaped abdomen.

Differentiation Between Simple and Strangulated Obstruction

Many thousands of pages have been written by experienced surgeons on the means of differentiating between a simple and strangulated obstruction. Various authorities stress a variety of factors in the history, examination, and special investigations. A sudden onset of pain that is continuous rather than colicky, the early appearance of shock, and the presence of pyrexia, tachycardia, marked abdominal tenderness, release tenderness, guarding, a tender abdominal

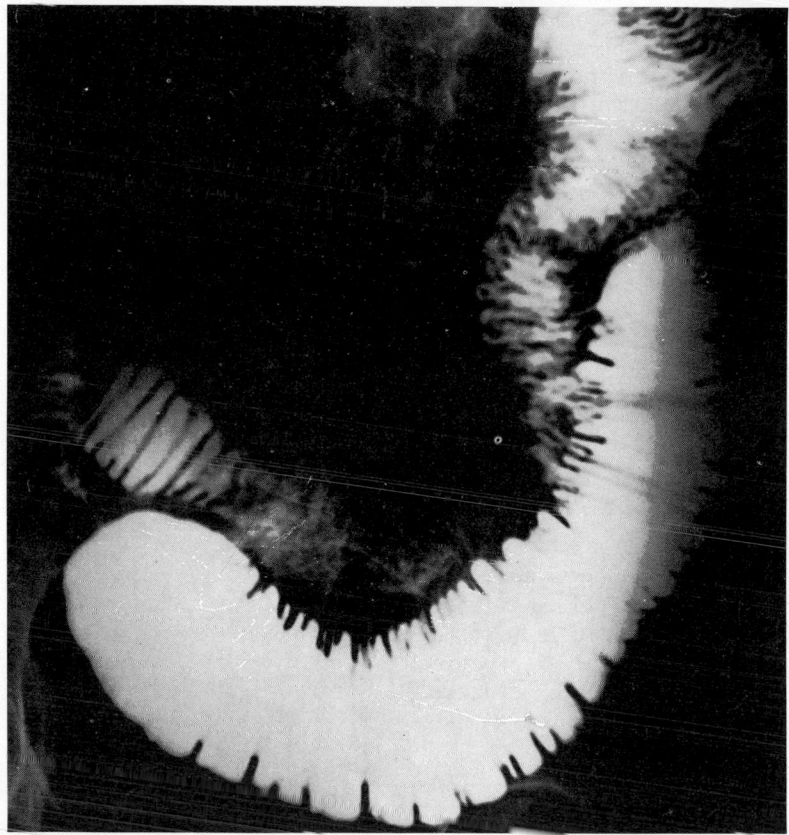

Figure 44–5. Barium meal x-ray examination showing obstruction of the efferent limb of the jejunum following partial gastrectomy by the Billroth II method. The obstruction was caused by a band.

mass, and an elevated leucocyte count are all said to favour strangulation. Yet close analysis of any series of cases or, indeed, a critical examination of one's own experience will soon reveal that attempts at such a differential diagnosis are little more than an academic exercise.

Savage (1955) quotes 3 of his series of 115 patients with small bowel obstruction who were relatively fit, had a long history of obstructive bowel sounds and a lack of abdominal tenderness and rigidity, yet in whom, at operation, a gangrenous and disintegrated strangulated loop of bowel was found. Cooke (1958) carried out an extensive enquiry among senior surgical registrars in Great Britain and found that nearly all felt unable to distinguish with any certainty between simple and strangulated obstruction. Silen et al (1962) found that only 17 out of 112 cases of strangulated obstruction (15 percent) were correctly diagnosed as such on initial hos-

pital admission. Indeed, in 37 percent of the cases the presence of intestinal obstruction, with or without strangulation, was not even suspected at this stage, the diagnoses included acute cholecystitis, pancreatitis, appendicitis, diverticulitis, gastroenteritis, and various gynaecologic emergencies. Simple obstruction of the small bowel was the admitting diagnosis in the remaining 48 percent of the cases. Interestingly, no less than 18 percent of the x-rays of the abdomen were interpreted as being normal.

When the matter is put to the close analysis of a series of cases, it is obvious that although trends undoubtedly exist, no criteria are infallible. Shatila et al (1976) compared 50 patients with strangulation with 53 simple occlusions. The two groups proved to be comparable regarding pain, vomiting, distension, elevation of pulse and temperature, and the presence of tenderness and rebound. A mass was more common in strangulation (including strangulated hernia), however, and rigidity, shock, a depressed temperature, and rectal bleeding occurred in a few cases of *late* strangulation. The white cell count, deemed a definitive differential sign by many authors, was elevated above 11,000 in 45 percent of the simple and 62 percent of the strangulated cases.

Careful studies of the clinical features of simple and strangulated obstructions carried out by Becker (1952) and by Zollinger and Kinsey (1964) demonstrate the same lesson; their interesting comparative figures are presented in Table 44-5. Plain x-rays of the abdomen are not of help in differentiating between the two conditions (Nadrowski, 1974).

Perhaps the single most vitally important fact that a surgeon must bear in mind in dealing with a case of acute intestinal obstruction is the realisation that no matter how well the patient and how relatively innocent the local signs may be, there are no clinical means or any accurate laboratory tests that will indicate whether a strangulated loop of intestine, with all its potential for destroying the patient, may or may not be present.

Treatment

With only few exceptions, intestinal obstruction requires urgent surgical intervention, principally because of the difficulty of differentiating between a simple and a strangulated obstruction. The exceptions to this rule are early postoperative or later recurrent obstructions owing to adhesions and partial large-bowel obstruction.

Where the obstruction is caused by adhesions, a trial of conservative treatment with nasogastric suction coupled with intravenous fluid replacement can be attempted, but it must be abandoned at once at any sign of deterioration in the patient's condition. An incomplete large-bowel obstruction owing, for example, to a stenosing carcinoma of the colon, may be relieved by an enema, allowing later elective operation to be performed. Here, too, any failure of conservative treatment must be followed without delay by surgical intervention.

Preparation for operation comprises the institution of gastric suction, administration of intravenous fluids and antibiotic therapy. Gentamicin or a cephalosporin, together with metronidazole, provide a suitable broad-spectrum

TABLE 44-5. CLINICAL FEATURES OF SIMPLE AND STRANGULATED OBSTRUCTIONS

Becker (1952) (New Orleans)	324 Simple Cases (%)	88 Strangulated Cases (%)
T 37.7 C+	16	23
P 100+	15	23
Abdominal or pelvic tenderness	73	82
Mass	5	10
Leucocytosis	44	50
All these signs absent	12	7

Zollinger & Kinsey (1964) (Columbus, Ohio)	387 Simple Cases (%)	45 Strangulated Cases (%)
T 37.2 C+	38	45
P 100+	38	52
Mass	22	32
Constant pain	18	20
WBC 15,000+	27	38

(*Source: From Ellis H, 1982, with permission.*)

cover in this situation. The patient's serum electrolytes and haemoglobin percentage are checked. Blood is grouped and cross-matched, and a blood transfusion is given if shock is obvious.

Operation must not be delayed for the many hours that it would take to restore normality to a grossly dehydrated patient; transfusion is commenced, continued during the operation, and carried on in the postoperative period.

Specific Operations

In the treatment of acute intestinal obstruction, the following operations may be employed:

1. Exploratory laparotomy for obstruction of uncertain origin.
2. External drainage of the intestine (enterostomy, caecostomy, or colostomy) proximal to the obstruction.
3. Short-circuiting operations, e.g., enteroanastomosis or ileocolic anastomosis.
4. Resection of bowel either to remove the obstructing lesion, e.g., a carcinoma of the colon, or because a strangulated segment of bowel has undergone irreversible ischaemic change.
5. Lysis of bands or adhesions.
6. Planned operations for specific obstructive le-

sions, i.e., a strangulated external hernia or laparotomy for intussusception in a child.

Exploratory Laparotomy. Operations should be performed with the primary objective of saving life by the simplest procedure consistent with ultimate recovery. The two essential steps in the operation are to discover and deal with the obstructing agent and to determine the state of viability of the liberated segment of gut. Special attention must be paid, from this point of view, to the intestine at the exact site of obstruction, as it is there that necrosis is likely to commence.

When the obstruction is of uncertain origin, the abdomen is best explored through a right paramedian paraumbilical incision, one third being above and two thirds being below the level of the umbilicus. The incision should be small in the first instance, about 10 cm in length, but it should be enlarged without hesitation either upward or downward if the operative findings necessitate it.

The surgeon should conduct the exploration on definite, set lines. When the peritoneal cavity is opened, the caecum should first be palpated and then inspected. If it is distended, the obstruction must be in the colon. The large bowel is then further explored and the lesion either resected, short-circuited, or a caecostomy or a colostomy performed.

If the caecum is collapsed, the obstruction must be in the small intestine, where a search for the obstructing agent should accordingly be made. The last loop of the ileum is picked up and the collapsed gut run through the fingers, loop by loop, until, eventually, distended bowel is met. At this point, where collapsed gut meets distended gut, lies the site of the blockage. The actual lesion will therefore be seen and can, in the majority of cases, be dealt with immediately. When, however, it is considered inadvisable to remove the cause of the obstruction at once, it may be bypassed by a short-circuiting operation, or, in grave cases, the dilated intestine situated above the blockage, may be drained by an enterostomy. Whatever procedure is decided upon, it is wise first to decompress the small intestine. In many cases, this can be achieved by retrograde "milking" of the distended intestine, emptying the loops backwards into the duodenal loop by running them between the index and the middle fingers. The fluid contents regurgitate into the stomach,

from whence the anaesthetist is able to aspirate them via a large-bore stomach tube (Jones and Matheson, 1968). If this fails, a long sucker tube needs to be introduced through a small enterotomy. The instrument devised by Savage is especially useful.

Enterostomy. A distended loop of intestine near the obstruction is brought out through the abdominal wound, emptied by milking with the fingers, and noncrushing rubber-covered clamps are applied to each end. The abdominal wound is then packed off, great care being taken to prevent contamination from the highly infective contents of the bowel when it is opened.

The best technique is the Witzel method, in which a 14 French rubber catheter is buried in a 3-cm serous tunnel on the antimesenteric border of the bowel wall using a running suture of 00 chromic catgut. The tip of the catheter is passed into a small stab incision into the lumen of the bowel, which is first thoroughly cleaned out by means of a suction tube. The catheter should be placed with its tip pointing upward against the intestinal stream, as near to the obstruction as possible. The catheter is stitched to the margins of this incision, and the burying suture is then continued over the site and beyond it for an additional 5 cm. The loop is returned to the abdomen and the tube is brought out through a small stab incision, except in the case of a "blind" enterostomy, in which case the tube is led out through the lower end of a small abdominal wound. The catheter may be wrapped in omentum, and it is advisable to anchor the intestine to the parietal peritoneum with a few catgut stitches around the point where the tube is drawn through the abdominal wall. It should also be securely fastened to the skin by an encircling stitch and by adhesive tape in order to prevent its becoming kinked, twisted, or dragged upon; its end is directed into a plastic bag at the side of the bed.

In the postoperative period, care is taken to keep the lumen of the catheter clear by an occasional injection of saline. The catheter should be left in situ until it works loose; this may take a week or a fortnight, after which time the small serous line tunnel will be found to heal rapidly and usually without leakage.

An intestinal fistula is likely to result if too large a catheter is used or of the lumen of the gut is too much narrowed by the infolding suture.

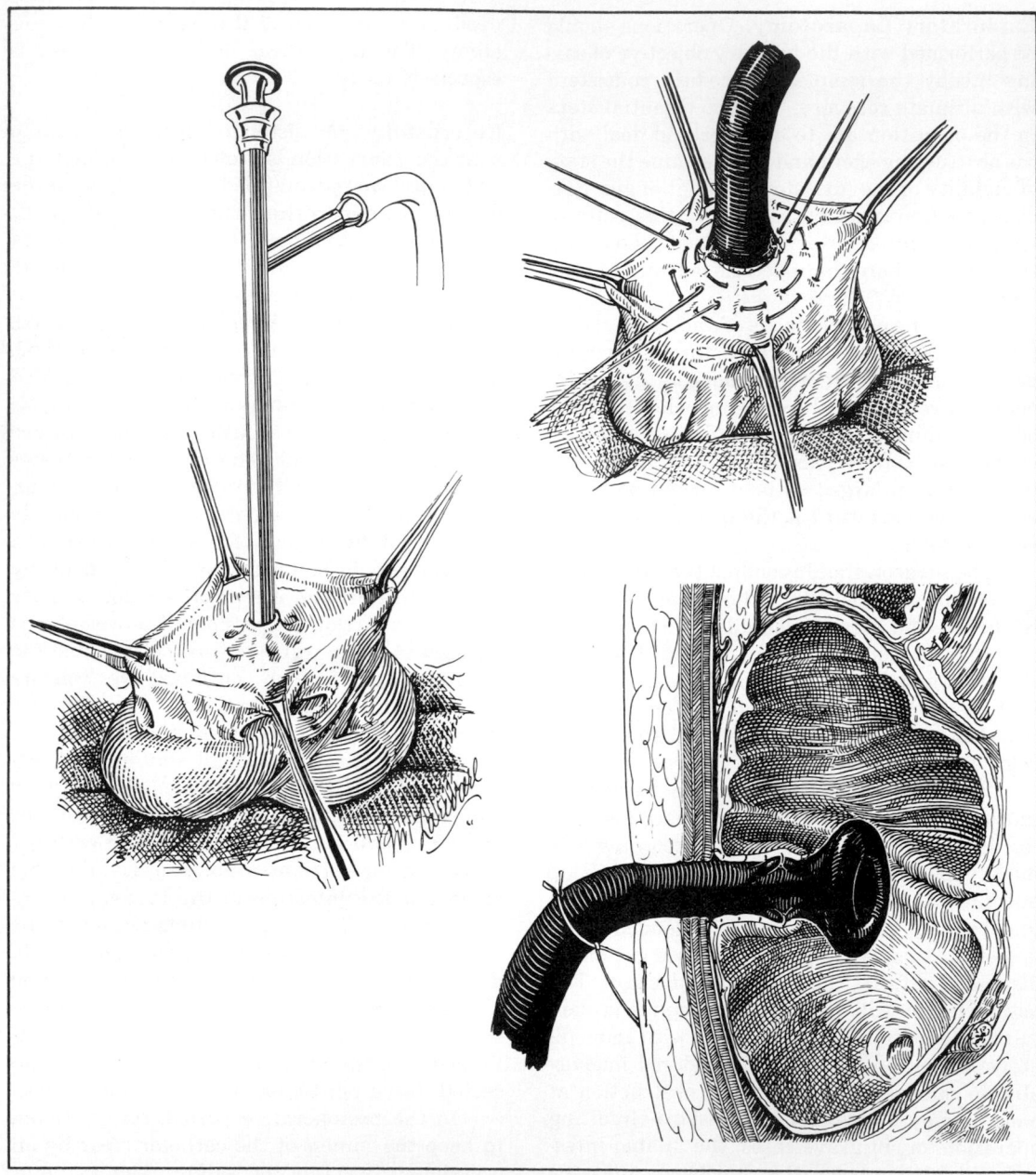

Figure 44–6. Valvular caecostomy. This is the Stamms or the "inverted inkpot" method. A Foley or other type of balloon catheter is preferred to the one illustrated. This method of replacing the caecum (with its inlying catheter) in the abdominal cavity and anchoring the bowel wall to the parietes has found general favour. Some surgeons prefer to exteriorise the caecum and to anchor the gut to the surface of the abdominal wall.

Caecostomy. A portion of the caecum is drawn gently through the incision, with the greatest care being taken not to tear the friable gut (Fig. 44–6). Steadying the caecum with the fingers, the point of a trocar and cannula (connected to suction apparatus) is inserted into the capacious lumen of the bowel, and the pent-up gas and faecal fluid are rapidly removed by suction.

As soon as its contents have been withdrawn, the walls of the caecum collapse and become thicker and more vascular. The caecum is then steadied and lifted upward with tissue forceps, and its base grasped either by the assistant's fingers or by a soft bowel clamp. A purse string suture of thread or catgut is introduced around the punctured area, which is enlarged with the diathermy needle to accommodate a medium-sized Foley catheter or a Winsbury–White catheter. The tube is pushed into the lumen of the caecum by means of a haemostat and the purse string pulled tight and tied. Two or three more purse string sutures are then inserted, applying the Stamm valvular method to the caecum.

The tube requires frequent syringing with saline to prevent its blockage. In most cases, the fistula rapidly dries up when the catheter is withdrawn about postoperative day 14, but in some instances formal closure will be necessary.

The whole topic of caecostomy is reviewed by Jackson and Baird (1967).

Transverse Colostomy. In most cases of acute large-gut obstruction calling for drainage of the faecal stream onto the surface, a transverse colostomy is preferable to caecostomy, as it produces complete defunctioning of the distal colon.

Treating Acute Large-Gut Obstruction

Some 80 percent of large-gut obstructions are simple, the most common causes being cancer and diverticulitis. In Great Britain, internal strangulation of the colon is rare, volvulus of the sigmoid being the chief cause.

Obstruction of the left colon owing to carcinoma may be chronic or acute in roughly equal numbers. In the chronic form, it is sometimes possible to relieve the obstruction by enemas and colonic wash-outs, but in other cases, one must plan a staged operation with preliminary colostomy.

The majority of patients give a history of flatulence, alteration of bowel habit, and the passage of blood and mucus for weeks or months before the onset of acute colonic obstruction. In a few, acute obstruction is precipitated by barium enema. Occasionally, symptoms have been present only for a short time, or indeed, are nonexistent before a sudden blockage occurs in the large intestine. In this group, accurate diagnosis is often difficult.

Plain x-ray films of the abdomen and sigmoidoscopy may help to locate the site of the obstruction.

The treatment of acute obstruction of the left colon will vary according to the condition of the patient, the degree of distension present, the nature of the obstructing agent, and the site of the obstruction in the presence or absence of other conditions of disease in these often elderly patients.

In cases of colonic obstruction due to carcinoma or diverticulitis situated distal to the splenic flexure, it is advisable to perform a formal laparotomy rather than to carry out a blind caecostomy or colostomy. It is important to determine the exact nature of the obstruction; furthermore, especially in diverticulitis, it is far from unusual to find a co-existing small-bowel obstruction from an adherent loop of ileum that has become firmly stuck to the inflammatory colonic mass.

The abdomen is best explored through a lower right paramedian incision. The caecum is first inspected; if it is distended, the diagnosis of large-gut obstruction is immediately confirmed. It is best to decompress the large bowel by means of trocar and cannula inserted through the caecal wall and attached to the suction apparatus. The small aperture in the caecum is then closed by means of a purse string suture (Fig. 44–7). Deflation of the colon renders exploration of the abdomen safe and easy. The site and characteristics of the obstruction are determined, and a colostomy is constructed. The colostomy of choice for obstructing lesions of the left colon is in the right half of the transverse colon, and it is fashioned through a small transverse rectus muscle-splitting incision. The portion of colon selected for colostomy is freed of omentum and drawn through the separate small incision by means of a sling of rubber tubing. The main abdominal incision is then sutured and sealed off. No stitches are used to anchor the colon to the abdominal wall, and the colostomy is opened immediately by means of the diathermy knife. The colostomy is re-

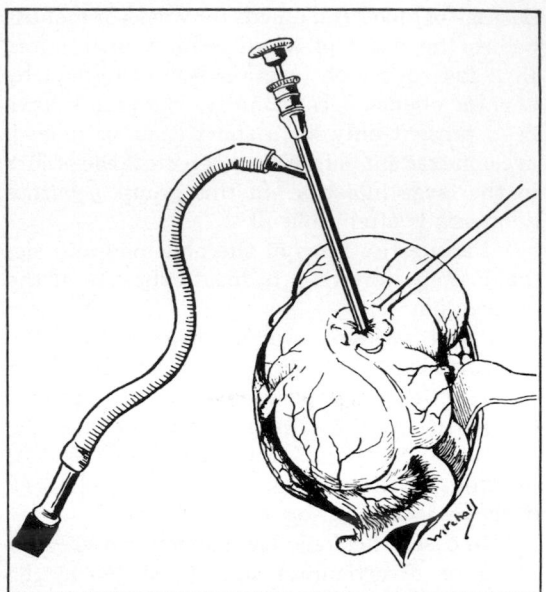

Figure 44–7. Aspirating gas and fluid contents with a Mayo–Ochsner trocar and cannula from proximal colon before exploring the abdomen in acute large-bowel obstruction. (*Courtesy of Mr. Henry Thompson.*)

tained in position either by means of a plastic rod passed through its mesocolon or by suturing the cut edge of the bowel mucosa to the lips of the skin incision by means of a continuous 00 catgut suture; the latter is my invariable practice.

After an interval of 2 to 3 weeks, when the incision has healed and when the patient and the colon have both been rendered fit for operation, the abdomen is once again explored.

At this second-stage operation, a left paramedian incision is fashioned, allowing resection of the left colon with end-to-end anastomosis. After complete recovery of the patient, from 4 to 6 weeks later, the third-stage operation—closure of the colostomy—is performed. It is wise practice to check the integrity of the colonic anastomosis before so doing by means of a limited barium enema examination. Any evidence of local leakage indicates that the closure of the colostomy should be deferred. The steps of this three-stage procedure are shown in Figures 44–8, 44–9, and 44–10.

For obstructing carcinoma of the right colon, the treatment of choice is immediate right hemicolectomy after decompression of the bowel. If the tumour is unresectable, an ileo-

transverse short circuit should be performed. If the general condition of the patient is extremely poor, a caecostomy may be indicated as a first-stage procedure.

Mortality

The statistics of the Registrar General for England and Wales provide accurate records of the mortality rate for intestinal obstruction. These are recorded under two headings: "intestinal obstruction without mention of hernia" and "hernias of the abdominal cavity with obstruction." Although the death rate per million for intestinal obstruction without mention of hernia fell from 50 in 1940 to 30 in 1950, the figures have declined rather less sharply since then. In 1959 there were 21 deaths per million in men and 18 in women; a decade later the figures were 21 and 24, respectively. In the latest returns, for 1980, there were 17 deaths per million in males and 26 per million in females. In 1955, there was a total of 2603 deaths from intestinal obstruction, of which 1253 were due to strangulated hernias. By 1980 the total had fallen to 1561, of which 510 were strangulated hernias. These figures are shown in more detail in Table 44–6.

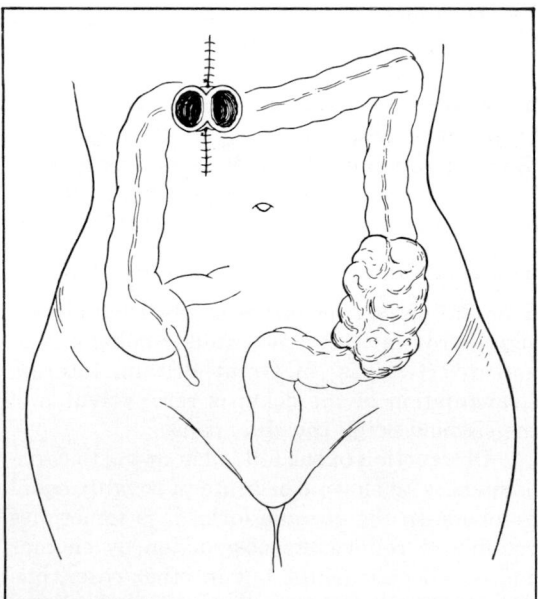

Figure 44–8. Obstructing carcinoma of the pelvic colon. Loop colostomy opened to relieve obstruction. First stage.

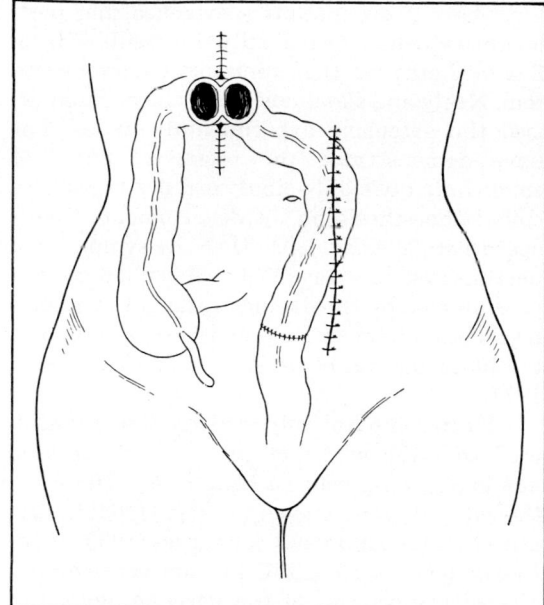

Figure 44–9. Second stage. Left paramedian incision, resection of growth together with extensive margin of colon and related mesentery, end-to-end anastomosis.

This rather minor decline in death rate is in contrast to the figures for acute appendicitis, which have shown a steady and progressive fall over the past 40 years and now amount to about 4 deaths per million compared with 60 per million in 1940. Published mortality figures for large series of cases demonstrate that the very high mortality, in the region of 25 percent of all cases, which were typical of publications in the 1920s and 1930s, have now come down to the region of 5 to 10 percent. A selection of such figures is presented in Table 44–7.

The improvement in prognosis that has occurred in recent years is no doubt due to a combination of improved anaesthesia, better knowledge of fluid and electrolyte replacement, efficient blood transfusion services, and the introduction of antibiotics.

The major factors having a negative influence on survival rate of intestinal obstruction are: strangulation of the bowel with gangrene or, worse still, perforation; delay in treatment with severe distension and gross electrolyte and fluid imbalance; and extremes of age (mortality is especially high in childhood and in the elderly).

The effect of strangulation on the mortality rate is striking and can be seen in comparisons

between mortality figures of patients with simple obstruction and those with strangulation (Table 44–8).

ILEUS

Intestinal obstruction may result, not from any of the numerous mechanical causes previously listed, but from loss of the normal propulsive activity in all or part of the alimentary canal. This is a state of affairs that may be just as dangerous, indeed as lethal, as mechanical obstruction. To this situation of functional obstruction have been applied the terms *paralytic ileus* or *adynamic ileus*. In many instances the bowel is not paralysed but is reflexly inhibited, and the term *neurogenic ileus* is more appropriate and more accurate in such cases.

A number of widely differing aetiologies may produce the same clinical picture:

1. Postoperative (by far the most common)
2. Peritonitis
3. Reflex ("the retroperitoneal syndrome")
4. Spinal injuries
5. Metabolic disturbances (uraemia, diabetic coma, myxoedema, and potassium depletion)
6. Ganglion-blocking agents

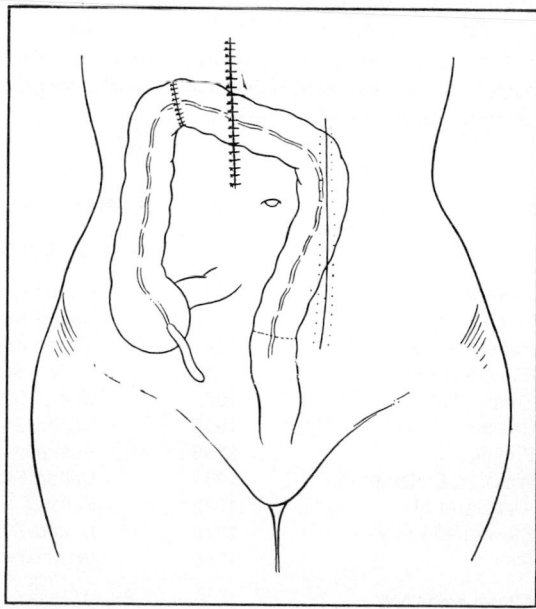

Figure 44–10. Third stage. Closure of colostomy.

	Total Deaths	Without Hernia	With Hernia
1955	2603	1350	1253
1965	2377	1454	923
1975	1909	1146	763
1977	1851	1099	752
1978	1794	1022	772
1980	1561	1051	510

[a] England and Wales.
(*Source: From Ellis H, 1982, with permission.*)

Clinical Manifestations

Postoperative Ileus. This is certainly the most common cause of ileus and, indeed, some degree of this is inevitable even after the most trivial of intraabdominal procedures. Its exact mechanism is not yet completely understood. In many cases the origin is probably multifactorial, including sympathetic stimulation, associated peritonitis or peritonism from extravasated blood, serum, or other fluids (whose effects themselves are poorly understood) and postoperative potassium depletion. In prolonged and serious cases, there is the complicating factor that a mechanical element may be introduced by the matting together of loops of intestine by postoperative fibrinous adhesions.

The myogenic contractility of the intestine following laparotomy is unimpaired, and the bowel retains its responsiveness to both electrical and chemical stimulation.

There is accumulating evidence that postoperative ileus is principally the result of a reflex mediated via the sympathetic nervous system. Neely and Catchpole (1971) have summarised the extensive experimental studies that have demonstrated the protective effect of splanchnic division, spinal cord destruction or spinal anaesthesia on the development of postoperative ileus. Evidence that the sympathetic nervous system is involved in this phenomenon is reinforced by the demonstration of increased levels of both adrenaline and noradrenaline in the blood plasma of patients with ileus (Petri, 1977).

Until comparatively recently, it was considered that the whole of the intestine became atonic following routine laparotomy. However, the work of Wells and co-workers (1964) in Liverpool and Rothnie and colleagues (1963) at St. Bartholomew's Hospital, London considerably altered the concept of the pathophysiology of this syndrome. Employing x-ray studies with contrast material, serial plain x-rays of the postoperative abdomen, prolonged auscultation using a microphone, and kymography, these investigators have been able to show that gastric stasis occurs after any operation, especially when the peritoneal cavity is opened. In the latter group this lasts from 18 hours to approximately 4 days. Contractions of the small intestine, however, in the absence of any complicating factors, return within a few hours, so that contrast material placed in the duodenum spreads through the small intestine and reaches the caecum within about 24 hours. The large bowel, by contrast, shows stasis that persists

TABLE 44–7. MORTALITY FIGURES IN INTESTINAL OBSTRUCTION (ALL CAUSES) 1920s–1970s

Authors	Year	Locale	Total	Mortality (%)
Souttar	1925	United Kingdom	3064	26
Vick	1932	United Kingdom	6892	26
Hudson et al	1941	United Kingdom	670	22
Eliason & Welty	1947	United States	292	11
Smith et al	1955	United States	1252	14.5
Becker	1955	United States	1007	18.7
Barling	1956	Australia	355	20
Waldron & Hampton	1961	United States	493	14
Kaltiala et al	1972	Finland	558	8
Stewardson et al	1978	United States	238[a]	5.5
Ellis	1980	Westminster	253[b]	6

[a] Small bowel only.
[b] Adults.
(*Source: From Ellis H, 1982, with permission.*)

TABLE 44–8. EFFECT OF STRANGULATION ON MORTALITY RATE

Authors	Year	Locale	Total Patients	Mortality rate (%)	
				Simple	*Strangulated*
Hudson et al	1941	London	670	15	77.4
Becker	1955	New Orleans	1007	14	30.5
Savage	1960	London	179	12	21
Waldron & Hampton	1961	Houston	493	11.3	28.8
Leffall et al	1965	Washington	1700	3	30.7
Kaltiala et al	1972	Finland	558	5	30

(*Source: From Ellis II, 1982, with permission.*)

for one or two days following laparotomy. In the normal subject, swallowed air is passed per rectum after about 30 minutes, but the situation is quite different in the postoperative patient. Air-swallowing is often marked in such cases, particularly in those who are apprehensive, retching or in pain. The atonic stomach distends with swallowed air, a good deal of which passes through the pylorus, whence it is passed on rapidly to distend the atonic colon. The usual cause of postoperative distension is, in fact, gas in the paralysed colon. This appears to be a simple explanation of the meteorism that is so often a feature of the first and second postoperative days, especially in tense and anxious patients. The absence of bowel sounds in the postoperative period appears to equate with the empty small intestine. When fluid and air are injected into the duodenum through a nasogastric tube, bowel sounds are heard at once. The return of borborygmi indicates not, as was previously thought, the return of small intestinal function, but rather the restoration of normal gastric and colonic motility (Fig. 44–11).

Further clinical and experimental studies, using more sophisticated techniques, have confirmed these classically simple observations. Wilson (1975) studied postoperative colonic motility in man using radiotelemetering capsules and radiopaque markers. He confirmed that colonic activity returned within about 16 hours following extraabdominal procedures but was delayed on average for 40 to 48 hours after laparotomy. The length of the operation had little or no effect on the duration of colonic stasis and he failed to demonstrate any influence of the amount of postoperative analgesia upon the duration of colonic inactivity. In this context it is interesting that Ingram and Sheiner (1981), in a study of gastric emptying following cholecystectomy, found that delay in this respect was

significantly proportional to the administration of opiates.

Woods and colleagues (1978) suggest that postoperative ileus is primarily a colonic problem. They studied postoperative electromechanical activity of the gastric antrum, small intestine, right colon, and sigmoid colon in monkeys in response to retroperitoneal dissection and temporary clamping of the renal pedicle. After operation, myoelectrical activity was decreased transiently in the antrum and for only a few hours in the small bowel. Right colon contractile activity was decreased significantly for 24 hours and that of the sigmoid colon for 72 hours. Similar findings were reported by Graber and colleagues in 1982 using both strain gauges and electrodes. Interestingly, they found no difference in the extent of the ileus in comparing minimal laparotomy and extensive dissections of the bowel.

Peritonitis. Ileus is an invariable accompaniment of peritonitis. It is often stated that this is due to some direct toxic effect of the purulent peritoneal exudate upon the intestine itself, but this is not confirmed by either experimental or clinical observations. The mechanism is no doubt a complex one, compounding sympathetic stimulation, metabolic disturbances (including potassium depletion), gaseous distension, and operative handling in those cases that have been submitted to laparotomy.

The Retroperitoneal Syndrome. Neurogenic ileus may follow any condition that disturbs the retroperitoneal tissues, presumably as a result of reflex stimulation of the sympathetic outflow. Thus, it may follow extensive retroperitoneal dissection, such as a bilateral lumbar sympathectomy or nephrectomy, and may be found in retroperitoneal haemorrhage as a result of

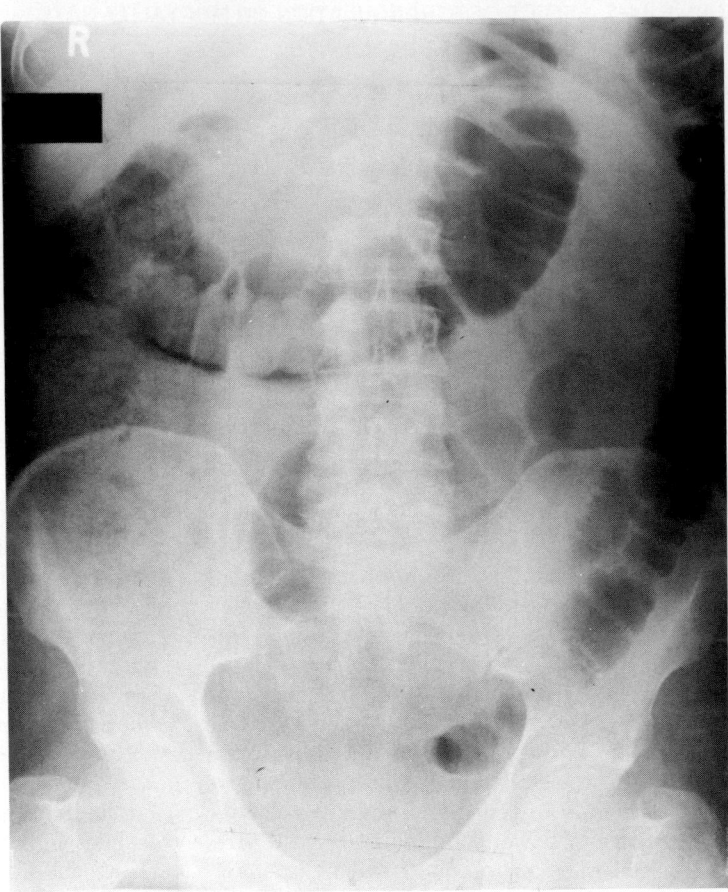

Figure 44–11. Plain x-ray of the abdomen (supine) in postoperative ileus. Note the dilatation of the entire large intestine with gas. (*Source: From Ellis H, 1982, with permission.*)

trauma or rupture of an aortic aneurysm.

The "retroperitoneal syndrome" became well recognised in World War II when a gunshot wound producing retroperitoneal haemorrhage would frequently result in an ileus that closely simulated the features of an intraperitoneal injury and might lead to laparotomy.

The silent, distended abdomen associated with acute pancreatitis represents a variant of this syndrome.

Spinal Injuries. It is well recognised that spinal trauma, fractures and cord transection result in functional intestinal obstruction. Indeed, in an extensive review of this subject in 1970, Watkin used the term *spinal ileus*.

These cases should be distinguished carefully from the acute duodenal ileus that may follow the application of a plaster spica, the so-called "cast syndrome." Here the acute lordosis results in obstruction of the third part of the duodenum between the superior mesenteric vessels and the lumbar spine.

Metabolic Disturbances. Ileus may complicate the severe metabolic disturbances of uraemia and diabetic coma. It has been reported by Boruchow et al (1966) in severe myxoedema, where the clinical picture may lead to ill-advised surgical intervention.

Potassium depletion is well known to be associated with ileus. It is important, therefore, to replace potassium in patients with severe postoperative ileus in which loss of potassium in the gastric aspirate aggravates the obligatory urinary loss of potassium in the postoperative catabolic phase.

Ganglion-blocking Agents. The full picture of ileus may be seen in patients receiving heavy doses of ganglion-blocking agents such as Probanthine or hexamethonium bromide.

Pathologic Changes

At autopsy examination of the patient who has died of ileus, the stomach and the whole of the bowel are found to be thin walled and distended. The gut is cyanosed and will contain considerable amounts of gas and a watery brown faeculent fluid. The peritoneal cavity in such an advanced case will usually contain purulent fluid, and the loops of bowel may well be kinked and tethered together with fibrinous adhesions. There are three important morbid effects of ileus:

1. Severe fluid, electrolyte, and protein depletion. Congestion and increased permeability of the capillaries in the wall of the distended bowel enable free transudation of plasma into the lumen and into the peritoneal cavity. Neither the plasma that oozes into the gut nor the gastric and intestinal digestive juices that are poured into it can be reabsorbed, so they are lost whether they are vomited, aspirated, or left in situ. The result is a fall in blood volume and of the essential electrolytes (particularly sodium, potassium, and chloride). Eventually, the patient passes into oligaemic shock, with resultant renal and circulatory failure.
2. Gross gaseous distension of the intestine impairs its blood supply and allows toxic absorption to occur from the gut lumen in a manner exactly similar to that described under the section on morbid effects of intestinal obstruction.
3. The gross abdominal distension impairs both respiratory and cardiac function. Pressure on the great veins may lead to venous thrombosis in the caval, portal, or peripheral venous systems.

Diagnosis

The typical clinical features of ileus are abdominal distension, effortless vomiting (which in the postoperative patient will occur during the first 2 or 3 days following surgery), or, if nasogastric aspiration is being used, copious aspirate, together with absolute constipation. The patient complains only of the discomfort commensurate with abdominal distension and the laparotomy wound. The patient is anxious and uncomfortable. The pulse is elevated and the temperature usually normal unless there is the complicating factor of a pyrexia from, for example, a postoper-

ative atelectasis. The abdomen is distended, with generalised tenderness. The mixture of gas and fluid within distended bowel loops may enable a splash to be elicited. The abdomen is silent on prolonged auscultation.

X-ray pictures of the abdomen, taken with the patient in the erect position, show the presence of scattered fluid levels; with the subject in the supine position, typically gas is distributed throughout the small and large intestine.

The important and often difficult but vital differential diagnosis is between neurogenic ileus and a postoperative mechanical obstruction produced by fibrinous bands or adhesions between the loops of intestine, or to the abdominal wall, or to the pelvic floor after an abdominoperineal excision of rectum or by protrusion of a loop of bowel through a partial dehiscence of the abdominal wound in its deeper layers.

Accurate diagnosis is of great importance, because neurogenic ileus is treated conservatively and is aggravated by unnecessary laparotomy, whereas mechanical obstruction in these circumstances usually requires urgent surgical relief. A further complicating factor that makes clinical differentiation so difficult is that the stage of neurogenic ileus may pass insidiously into that of mechanical obstruction.

Careful consideration of the following criteria will suggest mechanical rather than neurogenic obstruction in the postoperative period:

1. Persistence of the clinical picture of ileus for 4 or more days following operation or the onset of obstruction after this time.
2. The patient has passed flatus or has even had the bowels open and this then ceases.
3. The presence of noisy peristaltic rushes on abdominal auscultation in the absence of the passage of flatus. It is important to notice that in gross ileus, splashing sounds may occasionally be heard in the fluid-filled distended loops of intestine and that, moreover, there may be transmitted breath and heart sounds in such circumstances.
4. The presence of colicky abdominal pain.
5. X-ray films of the abdomen demonstrate a local loop of distended small intestine in the absence of gas shadows in the large bowel.

Gammill and Nice in 1972 gave an extremely comprehensive review of the radiology of the abdomen in this situation. They note that more than two air–fluid levels in dilated small intestine is associated with either dynamic or adynamic ileus. Dilated small intestine in the absence of colonic gas is strongly suggestive of obstruction of the small intestine. Distended small bowel together with gas in the undistended colon suggests either partial or resolving small intestinal obstruction or adynamic ileus. A follow-up film 2 to 4 hours later is useful in these circumstances because an unchanged pattern in likely due to an adynamic obstruction. Dilatation of the small intestine with associated gas in the distended colon signifies either an adynamic ileus or a large bowel organic obstruction. In such instances, a barium enema can demonstrate the presence of a mechanical blockage in the large bowel. These authors could not confirm the suggestion that the presence of two air–fluid levels in the same loop at different heights with relation to the vertical axis is useful in distinguishing between dynamic and adynamic ileus. In spite of this careful study, these authors must confess that occasionally plain x-rays give completely confusing findings and under such circumstances the only safe rule is to rely on clinical judgement.

Quatromoni and colleagues (1980) reviewed 41 patients with early postoperative small bowel obstruction, of which 30 resolved without operation and 11 required laparotomy. They found that clinical signs and symptoms could not be relied upon to distinguish between mechanical and neurogenic ileus and the plain films, even when subsequently reviewed by a senior radiologist, failed as accurate discriminants between the two groups of patients.

Differential diagnosis is indeed difficult and requires the highest degree of clinical judgement. It is aided by most meticulous and often-repeated examination of the patient. Noisy bowel sounds and cramping pains may indeed represent mechanical obstruction, but they also occur quite frequently just as the ileus is about to relieve itself and flatus is passed. If differential diagnosis seems quite impossible, it is then better to explore the abdomen; although reexploration in a case of neurogenic ileus is harmful, failure to open a mechanical obstruction—particularly in the presence of intestinal strangulation—is likely to prove lethal.

Treatment

Prophylaxis is important. The surgeon should ensure, if at all possible, that the patient is in normal fluid and electrolytic balance before operation. At laparotomy, gentle handling of tissues and a sound technique that reduces the possibility of leakage of intestinal contents or of blood into the peritoneal cavity are essential. Attention to such details is of much greater value to the patient than an impressive speed in operating. To quote Moynihan:

> In all the movements of a surgeon, there should be neither haste nor waste. It matters less how quickly an operation is done than how accurately it is done. Speed should result from the method and the practised facility of the operator and should not be his first and formal intention. It should be an accomplishment, not an aim. And every movement should tell, every action should achieve something. A manipulation, if it requires to be carried out, should not be half done and hesitatingly done. It should be deliberate, firm, intentional and final. Infinite gentleness, scrupulous care, light handling, and purposeful, effective, quiet movements which are not more than a caress are all necessary if an operation is to be the work of an artist and not merely a hewer of flesh. For every operation, even those procedures which are now quite commonplace, should be executed not in the spirit of an artisan who has a job to get through, but in the spirit of an artist who has something to interpret or create.

In the postoperative period, anxiety is relieved by reassurance and the judicious use of opiates. Air-swallowing should be discouraged, and the early use of gastric suction is instituted if vomiting or excessive belching occurs.

In the established case, gastric suction is instituted to remove swallowed air and thus prevent further gaseous distension. The aspiration of gastric contents also produces relief of nausea and deals with the concomitant gastric dilatation. Intestinal intubation by means of the Miller–Abbott or similar tube, theoretically so attractive, is difficult in practice because of failure to pass into the atonic alimentary tract; thus, most surgeons in Great Britain appear to have abandoned use of this tube in cases of paralytic ileus.

Fluid and electrolyte balance are maintained by means of an intravenous drip; the amounts given are estimated by a combination of sound clinical assessment, scrupulously kept fluid balance charts, and daily serum and urine biochemical estimations.

Once efficient nasogastric suction has been instituted, there is no contraindication to giving the patient small quantities of flavoured water to drink at regular intervals; they help to keep the mouth clean and are good for morale.

Pethidine (meperidine) or morphine and chlorpromazine are prescribed regularly.

Strict, repeated, clinical observations, together with x-ray films of the abdomen, are essential in order to detect whether or not a mechanical obstruction may be supervening.

During the anxious waiting period, most surgeons adopt a completely conservative approach. Cathartics, enemas, and rectal washouts have no effect on established ileus. Electrical stimulating devices for the gut, pantothenic acid, and posterior pituitary extract have had only short periods of popularity. Based on the theory of reflex sympathetic inhibition of the bowel, Neely and Catchpole (1971) have advocated the pharmacologic sympathetic blockade of the intestine followed by parasympathetic stimulation. Guanethidine (20 mg) is given intravenously in the drip over approximately 40 minutes while the blood pressure and the pulse are monitored. When bowel sounds have been established, a subcutaneous injection of bethanecol chloride (2.5 mg) is given and may be repeated after 30 minutes if flatus has not passed in that time. If motility is lost after the effect of the drugs has worn off, the presence of some other basic pathology is suggested, such as a large retroperitoneal haematoma. It is important, of course, to exclude by all means a coexisting organic lesion, which would completely veto this pharmacologic therapy. Although this treatment is largely empirical, it is in keeping with considerable experimental information on this important topic, and further work is awaited with interest.

BIBLIOGRAPHY

Aird I: Discussion on intestinal strangulation. Proc R Soc Med 29:991, 1936

Andersen DA: Volvulus in Western India. Br J Surg 44:132, 1956

Badoe EA: Patterns of acute intestinal obstruction in Ghana. West Afr Med J 17:194, 1968

Barry HC: Fibrous stricture of the small intestine following strangulated hernia. Br J Surg 30:64, 1942

Becker WF: Acute adhesive ileus: A study of 412 cases with particular reference to the abuse of tube decompression in treatment. Surg Gynecol Obstet 95:472, 1952

Becker WF: Acute obstruction of the colon. An analysis of 205 cases. Surg Gynecol Obstet 96:677, 1953

Becker WF: Intestinal obstruction. An analysis of 1007 cases. South Med J 48:41, 1955

Boruchow IB, Miller LD, et al: Paralytic ileus in myxedema. Arch Surg 92:960, 1966

Bishop RF, Allcock EA: Bacterial flora in the small intestine in intestinal obstruction. Br Med J 1:766, 1960

Brooks VEH, Butler A: Acute intestinal obstruction in Jamaica. Surg Gynecol Obstet 122:261, 1966

Bussemaker JB, Lindeman J: Comparison of methods to determine viability of small intestine. Ann Surg 176:97, 1972

Cherney LS: Intestinal stenosis following strangulated hernia; review of the literature and report of a case. Ann Surg 148:991, 1958

Chiedozi LC, Aboh IO, et al: Mechanical bowel obstruction. Review of 316 cases in Benin city. Am J Surg 139:389, 1980

Cohn I: Strangulation Obstruction. Springfield, Illinois: Charles C Thomas, 1961

Cole GJ: A review of 436 cases of intestinal obstruction in Ibadan. Gut 6:151, 1965

Coletti L, Bossart PA: Intestinal obstruction during the early post-operative period. Arch Surg 88:774, 1964

Cooke RV: Discussion on small bowel obstruction. Proc R Soc Med 51:503, 1958

Eliason EL, Welty RF: A ten-year survey of intestinal obstruction. Ann Surg 125:57, 1947

Ellis H: Intestinal Obstruction. New York: Appleton-Century-Crofts, 1982

Gammill SL, Nice CM: Air fluid levels; their occurrence in normal patients and their role in the analysis of ileus. Surgery 71:771, 1972

Gibson CL: A study of 1000 operations for acute intestinal obstruction. Ann Surg 32:486, 1900

Gill SS, Eggleston FC: Acute intestinal obstruction. Arch Surg 91:589, 1965

Graber JN, Schulte WJ, et al: Relationship of duration of post-operative ileus to extent and site of operative dissection. Surgery 92:87, 1982

Harper WH, Blain A: The effect of penicillin in experimental intestinal obstruction: A preliminary report on closed loop studies. Bull Johns Hopkins Hosp 76:221, 1945

Hudson RV, Smith R, et al: The prognosis of acute intestinal obstruction—experiments with intraperitoneal sulphanilamide. Lancet 1:438, 1941

Ingram DM, Sheiner HJ: Post-operative gastric emptying. Br J Surg 68:572, 1981

Jackson PP, Baird RM: Cecostomy. An analysis of 102 cases. Am J Surg 114:297, 1967

Jones PF, Matheson NA: Operative decompression in intestinal obstruction. Lancet 1:1197, 1968

Kaltiala EH, Lenkkeri H, et al: Mechanical intestinal obstruction. An analysis of 577 cases. Ann Chir Gynaecol Fenniae 61:87, 1972

Kark AE, Rundle WJ: The pattern of intussusception in Africans in Natal. Br J Surg 48:296, 1960

Kingsnorth AN: Fluid-filled intestinal obstruction. Br J Surg 63:289, 1976

Leffall LD, Quander J, et al: Strangulation intestinal obstruction: A clinical appraisal. Arch Surg 91:592, 1965

McAdam IWJ: A three year review of intestinal obstruction: Mulago Hospital, Kampala, Uganda. East Afr Med J 38:536, 1961

Michel ML, Knapp L, et al: Acute intestinal obstruction. Comparative studies of small intestinal and colic obstruction. Surgery 28:90, 1950

Mortality Statistics England and Wales. London: Her Majesty's Stationary Office, 1980

Moynihan B: Abdominal Operations, vol 1. London: WB Saunders, 1926

Moynihan B: Abdominal Operations, vol 2. London: WB Saunders, 1926

Nadrowski LF: Pathophysiology and current treatment of intestinal obstruction. Rev Surg 31:381, 1974

Neely J, Catchpole B: Ileus; the restoration of alimentary motility by pharmacological means. Br J Surg 58:21, 1971

Petri G: Invited commentary on the use of chlorpromazine in the treatment of adynamic ileus. World J Surg 1:659, 1977

Quatromoni JC, Rosoff L, et al: Early post-operative small bowel obstruction. Ann Surg 191:72, 1980

Rothnie NG, Harper RAK, et al: Early post-operative gastrointestinal activity. Lancet 2:64, 1963

Saidi F: The high incidence of intestinal volvulus in Iran. Gut 10:838, 1969

Savage PT: Discussion on small bowel obstruction. Proc R Soc Med 51:507, 1955

Savage PT: The management of acute intestinal obstruction. A critical review of 179 personal cases. Br J Surg 47:643, 1960

Shatila AH, Chamberlain BE, et al: Current status of diagnosis and management of strangulation obstruction of the small bowel. Am J Surg 132:299, 1976

Shields R: The absorption and secretion of fluid and electrolytes by the obstructed bowel. Br J Surg 52:774, 1965

Silen W, Hein MF, et al: Strangulation obstruction of the small intestine. Arch Surg 85:121, 1962

Smith GA, Perry JF, et al: Mechanical intestinal obstructions. A study of 1252 cases. Surg Gynecol Obstet 100:651, 1955

Stewardson RH, Bombeck T, et al: Critical operative management of small bowel obstruction. Ann Surg 187:189, 1978

Sykes PA, Boulter KH, et al: The microflora of the obstructed bowel. Br J Surg 63:721, 1976

Taha SE, Suleiman SI: Volvulus of the sigmoid colon in the Gezira. Br J Surg 67:433, 1980

Tandon HD, Prakash A: Pathology of intestinal tuberculosis and its distinction from Crohns disease. Gut 13:260, 1972

Ti TK, Yong NK: The pattern of intestinal obstruction in Malaysia. Br J Surg 63:963, 1976

Vick RH: Statistics of acute intestinal obstruction. Br Med J 2:546, 1932

Waldron GW, Hampton JM: Intestinal obstruction: A half century comparative analysis. Ann Surg 153:839, 1961

Wangensteen OH: Intestinal Obstructions, 3 edt. Springfield, Illinois: Charles C Thomas, 1955

Watkin DFL: Spinal ileus. Br J Surg 57:142, 1970

Wells C, Tinkler L, et al: Post-operative gastrointestinal motility. Lancet 1:4, 1964

White A: Intestinal obstruction in the Rhodesian African: A review of 112 cases. East Afr Med J 38:525, 1961

Wilson JP: Post-operative motility of the large intestine in man. Gut 16:689, 1975

Woods JH, Erickson LW, et al: Post-operative ileus; a colonic problem. Surgery 84:527, 1978

Yale CE, Balish E: Intestinal obstruction in germ free and mono-contaminated dogs. Arch Surg 114:445, 1979

Zollinger RM, Kinsey DL: Diagnosis and management of intestinal obstruction. Am Surg 30:1, 1964

45. Special Forms of Intestinal Obstruction

Harold Ellis

ADULT INTUSSUSCEPTION

Introduction. Intussusception can occur at any age. Although there is a good deal of overlap, it is convenient from the aetiologic, pathologic, and clinical points of view to divide the cases into those occurring in children, where the peak incidence is under 2 years of age, and those found in adult patients. Childhood intussusception (see Chapter 40) accounts for approximately 80 to 90 percent of all cases of infantile obstruction. In about 90 percent of these cases no obvious aetiologic factor can be found at operation. In contrast, in the adult, intussusception is comparatively rare, accounting for about 5 percent of all obstructions, and in the great majority of instances has some obvious causation. This is usually a tumour forming the apex of the intussusception, which tends to be a benign lesion in small bowel intussusceptions and a malignant tumour in intussusceptions of the colon (Table 45–1).

Among the benign tumours, submucous lipoma, most frequently found in the caecum and ascending colon, is a frequently reported cause of intussusception (Fig. 45–1); Wychulis et al give an excellent review of the extensive experience of the Mayo Clinic in this respect. The benign pedunculated tumour of the small intestine associated with the Peutz–Jegher syndrome, although unusual, has a strong association with intussusception so that acute abdominal pain in a patient with the typical pigment spots on the face, lips, and oral mucosa should be suspected of this condition (Fig. 45–2). Leiomyoma and leiomyosarcoma may be responsible, as well as the more common adenomas and adenocarcinomas of the bowel.

Das Gupta and Brasfield (1964), in an extensive experience at the Memorial Sloan-Kettering Hospital, New York, note that intussusception is the most common finding in patients with metastatic melanoma who have gastrointestinal (GI) obstructive symptoms. They point out that the metastasis may not uncommonly be solitary and, under such circumstances, resection should certainly be performed.

Among the nontumourous causes reported are granuloma of the appendix stump (Hanson et al, 1967), an inverted Meckel's diverticulum (Harkins, 1933), and the excluded small bowel segment following jejunoileal bypass for morbid obesity (Lavery and Fazio, 1978). Goodall (1963) has reviewed 38 cases associated with typhoid or with bacillary or amoebic dysentery.

Adult intussusception is surprisingly common in some African communities. Cole (1965), for example, found that caecocolic intussusception occurs in a small area of western Nigeria in greater numbers than anywhere else in the world. He recorded no less than 76 such cases out of a total of 119 intussusceptions in a review of 436 cases of intestinal obstruction in Ibadan. Kark and Rundle (1960) note the high frequency of adult intussusception in the Natal Africans. In 8 years, they collected 67 cases of intussusception, of which only 16 were under 5 years of age. Eight cases occurred between 5 and 14 years and no less than 43 were in adults. Apical pathology was found in only six of the adult patients—two amoebomas, and one each of a simple tumour, a tuberculous ulcer, acute nonspecific ulcer of the terminal ileum, and an appendix stump—three more of the patients, however, had worm infestations and three had amoebic dysentery.

1183

TABLE 45–1. ADULT INTUSSUSCEPTION—ASSOCIATED BENIGN AND MALIGNANT TUMOURS

	Donhauser & Kelly (1950)	Roper (1956)	Brayton & Norris (1954)	Weilbaecher et al (1971)
Number of cases	593	134	80	160
Type (%)				
Enteric	64	50	46	48
Colic	36	50	54	52
Tumours (%)				
Benign				
Enteric	40	45	49	28
Colic	22	18	35	24
Malignant				
Enteric	13	19	19	24
Colic	33	54	56	54
Overall malignancy (%)	19	37	38	42

(*Source: From Ellis H, 1982, with permission.*)

Clinical Manifestations. The clinical picture of intussusception in the adult is usually dominated by the general signs and symptoms of intestinal obstruction. Intussusception is suggested by the presence of an abdominal mass and the passage of blood per rectum. Because intussusception in the adult is often a chronic or relapsing affair, the diagnosis may be suggested by repeated incidents of subacute obstruction and by variability of abdominal signs. Thus, during the height of an attack, an obvious mass may be present but may disappear completely when the patient is reexamined just a few hours later, by which time the symptoms have subsided. Rarely, an intussuscepting carcinoma of the sigmoid colon may prolapse per rectum or be seen through the sigmoidoscope (Edna, 1978). The useful clue of the typical facies of the Peutz–Jegher syndrome have already been mentioned.

Radiologic Examination. A plain x-ray of the abdomen demonstrates dilated loops of small intestine with fluid levels. A chronic small bowel

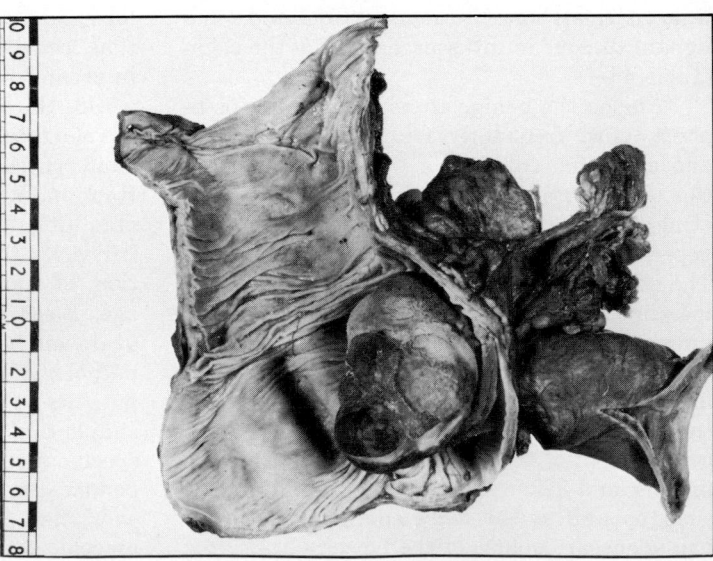

Figure 45–1. An intussuscepting lipoma of the ileum prolapsing into the caecum, removed by right hemicolectomy. (*Source: From Ellis H, 1982, with permission.*)

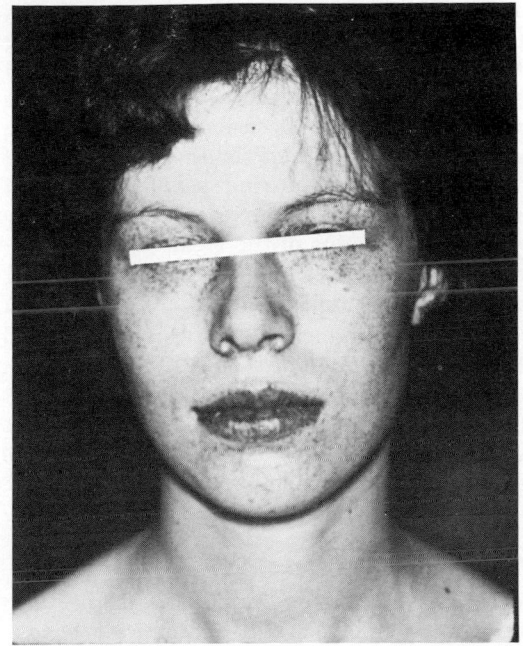

Figure 45–2. The characteristic pigment spots of the Peutz–Jegher syndrome. Notice that the "freckles" also involve the lips. (*Source: From Ellis H, 1982, with permission.*)

intussusception may be demonstrated by a barium follow-through examination and an intussuscepting large bowel tumour is readily visualised on barium enema. Indeed, this may produce at least temporary reduction of the intussusception (Fig. 45–3).

Treatment. Treatment of adult intussusception is invariably surgical. The diagnosis at operation is not difficult to make. With large bowel intussusception, the risk of a malignancy as the cause is high and therefore, the surgeon is best advised to proceed to resection without any attempt at reduction. With intussusception of the small intestine, a cautious attempt at reduction should be made. If it is found that the lesion is necrotic, reduction should not be pursued and resection carried out at once. In the idiopathic case, nothing further than reduction need be performed (Aston and Machleder, 1975). A benign tumour should be removed locally but if there is any question of malignancy, then adequate resection should be effected. In cases of the Peutz–Jegher syndrome, where further epi-

sodes of intussusception are to be anticipated, it is important to preserve as much bowel as possible; here, a simple enterotomy with removal of the offending polyp is all that is required provided that the bowel is perfectly viable.

VOLVULUS

Volvulus, or twisting of the intestine, occurs in the small bowel, the caecum, and, especially, the sigmoid colon. Only a few examples of volvulus of the transverse colon have been recorded, and that of the splenic flexure is still rarer. Volvulus is comparatively unusual in Western Europe, North America, Australia, and among the white population of Africa, but it is one of the most common causes of acute intestinal obstruction in Eastern Europe and the Soviet Union (Peterson, 1934), Scandinavia (Kaltiala et al,

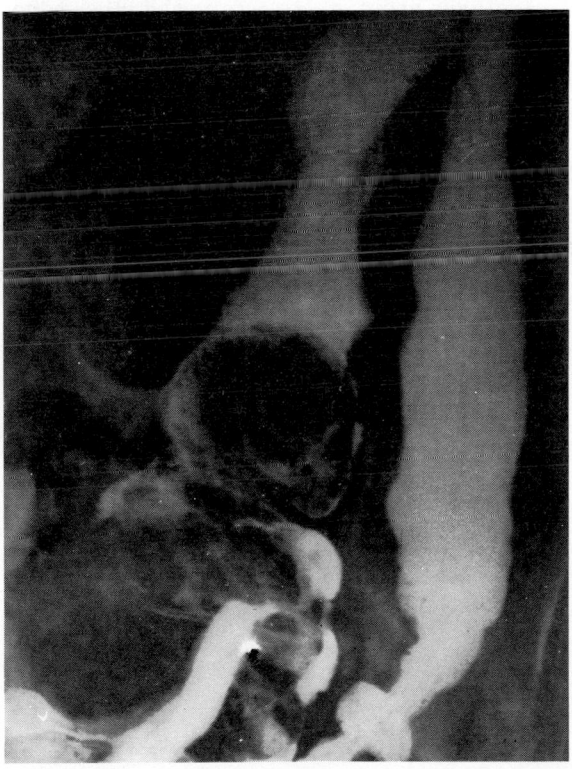

Figure 45–3. Ileocaecal intussusception due to a polypoid malignant growth situated near the ileocaecal valve. Right hemicolectomy with end-to-side anastomosis by the open method. (*R. Maingot's patient.*)

1972), Iran (Boulvin et al, 1969; Saidi, 1969), India, and among the black population of Eastern Africa (Shepherd, 1969). Table 45–2 summarises the incidence of volvulus in published figures from various parts of the world. In our own series of 253 adult obstructions, volvulus accounted for 6 percent of the cases.

Aetiology. The various aetiologic factors can be classified as follows.

CONGENITAL ABNORMALITIES. Bowel that is firmly tethered to the posterior abdominal wall cannot undergo torsion. In contrast, a loop of bowel hanging on an unduly long and mobile mesentery or mesocolon with a short base is at risk of torsion. It is probable that racial anatomic variations of this nature may be at least one factor in the wide geographic variation noted. A special example is the faulty rotation of the intestine in foetal life that may result in volvulus neonatorum.

ACQUIRED FACTORS. Mesenteric and other adhesions may produce narrowing of the base of attachment of a loop of intestine. Alternatively, a loop of free gut may be fixed at its apex to the parietes by postoperative adhesions.

It is often said that a bulky vegetable diet may lead to overloading of the sigmoid colon and certainly the geographic distribution of volvulus corresponds closely to populations living on a mainly bulky vegetarian diet. Although an enormously distended pelvic colon is a constant finding in sigmoid volvulus, it usually contains only gas with some liquid faeces. Sinha (1969) did not find a single case of overloading of the colon with a faecal mass in his personal series of 211 patients with volvulus of the sigmoid colon in India. Occasionally, acute volvulus may be precipitated in the late stages of pregnancy or even during parturition. Kohn and colleagues (1944) reported a patient who underwent volvulus of the sigmoid in two consecutive pregnancies and collected a total of 41 examples of sigmoid volvulus associated with pregnancy. Donhauser and Atwell (1955) found that no less than 10 of their 100 patients with caecal volvulus were pregnant. Diagnosis, not unnaturally, is particularly difficult if volvulus occurs at the time of delivery (Simons, 1950) or during the puerperium (Rose, 1941).

Volvulus of the Caecum

Although volvulus of the caecum is the term commonly employed, it is anatomically a misnomer. Halvorsen and Semb (1975), in their review of 30 examples of this emergency, point out that the adjacent terminal ileum and ascending colon are usually involved and, occasionally, that torsion may even implicate the transverse colon. Other terms employed include volvulus of the ileocolic segment, ileocaecal volvulus, and volvulus of the right colon (Fig. 45–4).

The volvulus usually occurs in a clockwise direction, the caecum passing upward and then to the left. The twist varies from 90 degrees to as many as three complete twists. Obviously

TABLE 45–2. GEOGRAPHIC VARIATIONS IN THE INCIDENCE OF VOLVULUS

Reference	Region	No. of Cases of Obstruction	Incidence (%) of Volvulus
Agarwal & Mistra (1970)	Northern India	? (excluding hernias)	40
Andersen (1956)	Western India	168 (excluding hernias)	24
Ellis (1981)	London	253	6
McIver (1933)	Boston	335	4
Osime (1980)	Nigeria	142 (excluding hernias)	9
Saidi (1969)	Iran	286	32
Sinha (1969)	India	710	29
White (1961)	Zimbabwe	172	31

(*Source: From Ellis H, 1982, with permission.*)

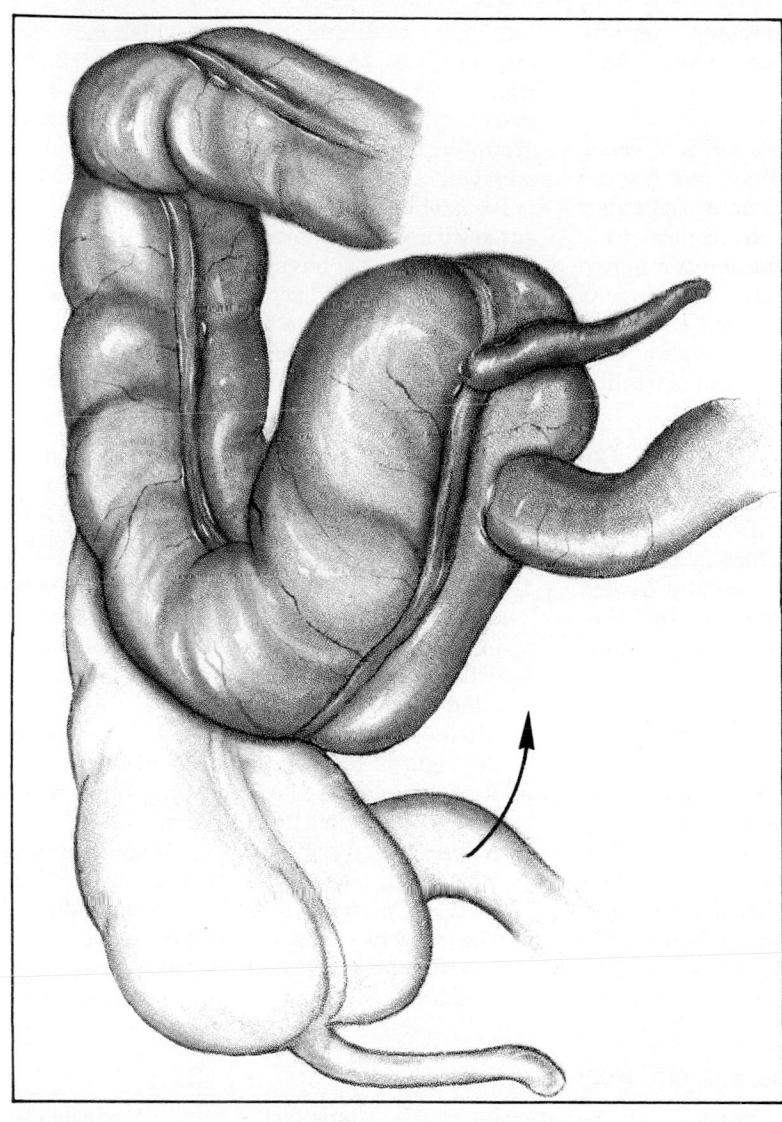

Figure 45–4. Caecal volvulus. The mobile peritonealised caecum and ascending colon enable torsion to occur.

torsion cannot occur if the caecum is firmly fixed to the posterior abdominal wall and volvulus depends on abnormal motility of both the caecum and ascending colon. This may take the form of a complete malrotation, a common ileocaecal mesentery or imperfect fixation. Wolfer et al (1942) found that 14 out of 125 cadavers had a caecum sufficiently mobile to allow the possibility of volvulus. Donhauser and Atwell (1949) found in their necropsy study that there was sufficient mobility of the caecum to permit pathologic rotation in 20 percent of their subjects. One might wonder, therefore, why caecal volvulus is relatively uncommon in Western Europe and the United States, whereas a higher

incidence has been reported in Iran, India, and Scandinavia.

Predisposing factors include extremes of dietary intake, previous abdominal operations, or history of previous inflammation in the peritoneal cavity with resultant adhesion formation. Pregnancy, pelvic tumours, or cysts may result in upward displacement of the caecum. Jordan and Beahrs (1953) suggest that withdrawal of abdominal packs or undue manipulation of the ileocaecal region at operation might precipitate volvulus and they report six cases of caecal volvulus occurring between 2 and 15 days after laparotomy. Krippaehne et al (1967) implicate gaseous distension of the bowel. No less than

4 of their 22 patients were undergoing intermittent positive pressure respiration when caecal volvulus occurred.

Clinical Manifestations. Most series of cases that have been reported are small, and few include more than 30 patients from a particular institution. When these cases are collected together, however, the sex distribution is roughly equal and the ages range from the teens to 100 years, with the majority in the fifth and sixth decades. A selection of the major reviews with sex distribution, age distribution, and mortality is shown in Table 45–3.

As with the more common volvulus of the sigmoid, caecal volvulus may manifest itself either as an acute or a chronic obstruction. Even when the patient presents in the acute condition, there is often a previous history of recurrent subacute attacks as Donhauser and Atwell found in 73 of the 100 patients reviewed.

The patient presents with colicky abdominal pain, usually in the right lower quadrant. Distension is a marked feature, but with a symmetry of the abdomen, the grossly dilated right colon producing a tympanitic mass which may be situated in the right iliac fossa but which may flop over onto the left side of the abdomen. Nausea or vomiting and absolute constipation are accompanying features. Anderson and Lee (1980) give a careful analysis of their 41 patients admitted to the Surgical Units in Edinburgh.

Hinshaw et al (1959) have suggested that cases of volvulus of the caecum can be divided into an acute fulminating type which may rapidly progress to gangrene, often requiring a right hemicolectomy and accompanied by high mortality, compared with an acute obstructive group with a slower onset, a lower mortality, and where detorsion and caecostomy usually prove adequate treatment. Most authors do not agree with this categorisation but rather regard the condition as having a spectrum ranging from patients who complain of mild episodes of recurrent pain due to repeated episodes of volvulus to the acute fulminating form described above.

Radiologic Examination. Although the diagnosis may be suspected clinically, it can usually be clinched by radiography (Fig. 45–5). McGraw et al (1948) list the following radiologic signs:

1. Great distension of the caecum, which is often ectopically placed and frequently located in the left upper quadrant of the abdomen (where it may even be mistaken for the dilated stomach).
2. Distended loops of small intestine located to the right of the caecal gas shadow.
3. Visualisation of the ileocaecal valve when the caecum is outlined by gas.
4. A spiral distortion of the mucous membrane folds in the colon at the point of obstruction.
5. Evidence of small intestinal obstruction.
6. The presence of a single fluid level in the caecum compared with the usual two large fluid levels in cases of volvulus of the sigmoid.

TABLE 45–3. CAECAL VOLVULUS: AGE, SEX, MORTALITY

Reference	Total	Male:Female	Age (Yr)	Mortality (%)
Anderson & Lee (1980) Edinburgh	41	10:31	20–90	14.6
Brystrom et al (1972) Stockholm	40	13:27	20–90	17.5
Dowling & Gunning (1969) Oxford	11	6:5	23–84 (mean 57)	0
Halvorsen & Semb (1975) Norway	30	11:19	20–100 (peak 50–80)	17
O'Mara et al (1979) Baltimore	50	18:32	14–88 (mean 53)	12
Smith & Goodwin (1973) California	24	9:15	21–94 (mean 60)	13
Wilson (1965) Vancouver	20	9:11	mean 60	10

(*Source: From Ellis H, 1982, with permission.*)

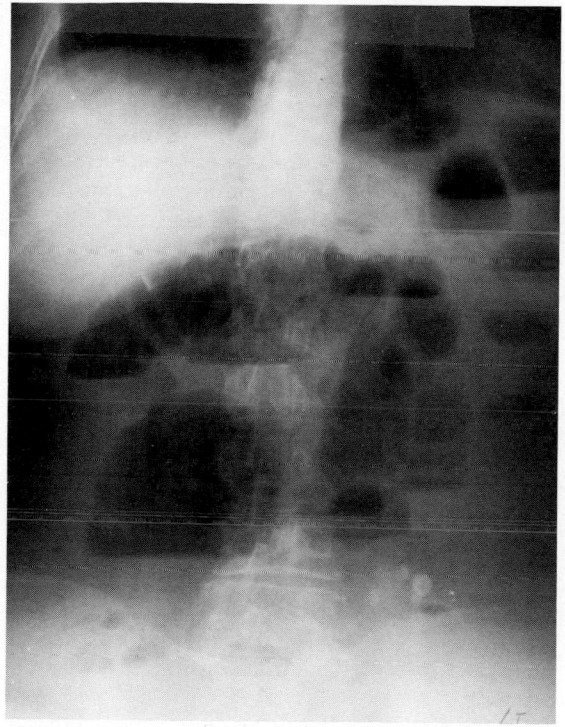

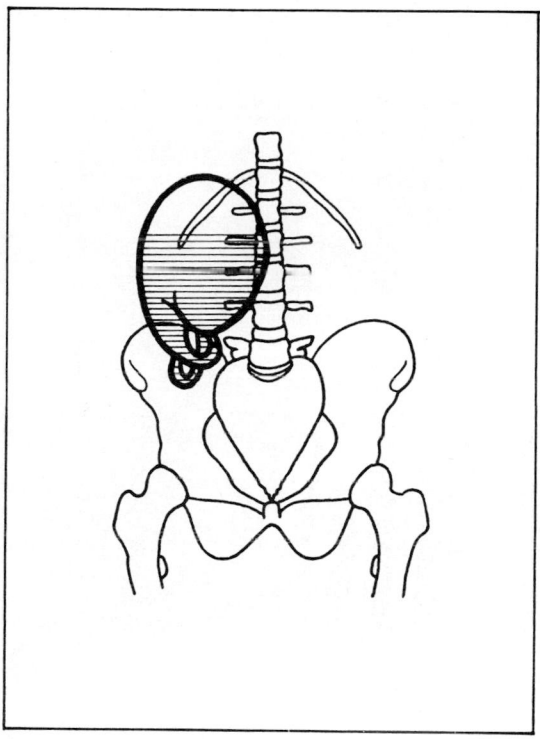

A   **B**

Figure 45–5. A. Plain abdominal x-ray of caecal volvulus. (*Courtesy of P. Bevan, Dudley Road Hospital, Birmingham.*) **B.** Diagram of radiologic appearance. (*Source: From Ellis H, 1982, with permission.*)

A barium enema may be useful in chronic cases and demonstrates the opaque medium cut off at the transverse colon or at the hepatic flexure, beyond which is seen the gas-filled right colon. In the acute form, the patient's condition is usually too grave to allow this radiologic examination.

Treatment. For practical purposes, operative treatment is mandatory. Colonoscopic detorsion, so successful in sigmoid volvulus, has been attempted but with less effect. Anderson et al (1978) report one success in three patients in which it was attempted.

The abdomen is explored through a generous right paramedian or midline incision. When detorsion is possible and the gut is viable, reduction is carried out with the utmost gentleness, because the bowel wall is extremely thin and may have partial tears already present. In the majority, the twist is clockwise, but cases of counterclockwise torsion have been reported. If the bowel is viable, most surgeons consider that

a caecopexy is sufficient, tacking the caecum to the parietal wall with a series of interrupted nonabsorbable sutures. In the author's practice, this technique suffices in patients with recurrent mild episodes but in the acute attack, preference is both to decompress the caecum and to prevent further volvulus by the same manoeuvre to establish a temporary caecostomy (Fig. 45–6).

Resection is indicated when reduction proves to be impossible or when the involved segment of intestine is frankly gangrenous. Here, the choice lies between primary right hemicolectomy, which can be performed in the majority of cases, or the exteriorisation–resection operation of Mikulicz, which is the wiser undertaking in the advanced case and the seriously ill patient.

In some cases a small patch of gangrene on the caecal wall can be used as the site of the caecostomy, thus avoiding resection.

With regard to risk of further volvulus, this may certainly occur if surgery comprises merely

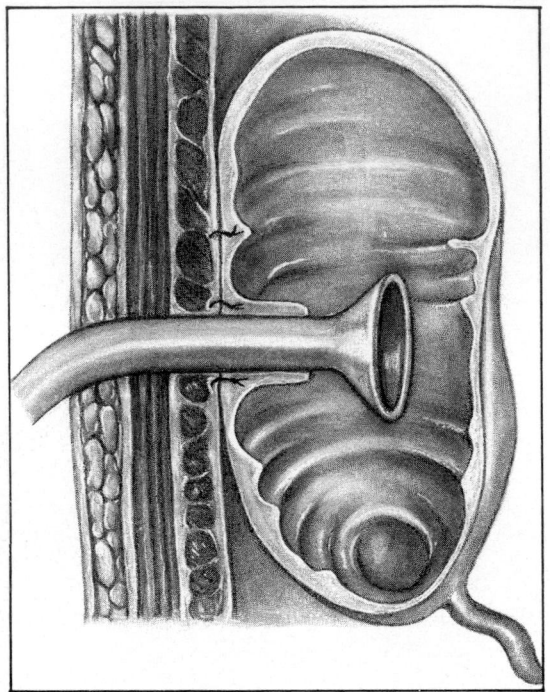

Figure 45–6. Caecostomy. This combines the virtues of both decompression and fixation of the distended and mobile caecum. (*Source: From Ellis H, 1982, with permission.*)

simple detorsion. As reported by Halvorsen and Semb (1975), of seven patients undergoing this procedure who survived the operation, two had occasional symptoms of pain and one developed a definite recurrence. Recurrent attacks have also been reported after caecopexy but are very rare after caecostomy and, not surprisingly, unknown after right hemicolectomy.

SIGMOID VOLVULUS

Volvulus of the sigmoid colon is a fascinating condition with wide geographic variations, a peculiar association with mental deficiency and with the possibility, in the majority of cases, for treating the immediate emergency by nonoperative means.

Geographic Distribution. Sigmoid volvulus is a relatively unusual emergency in Western Europe and North America, yet it is extremely common in Eastern Europe, parts of Eastern and Central Africa, and India. Peterson (1934)

provided details of the wide variation of the incidence of this emergency in Europe (Table 45–4). Shepherd (1969) reviews the wide variations throughout Africa—from extreme rarity in some parts of Western Africa to a reported incidence of 54 percent of all cases of intestinal obstruction in Ethiopia. Taha and Suleiman (1980) reported that 33 percent of all obstructions they treated in the Sudan were due to this cause. Andersen (1956) points out the great variations in India between east and west and among various religious and social groups.

Although it would be of the greatest interest, this author finds no satisfactory figures which compare the incidence of volvulus in the black and white populations in the United States living under roughly comparable social and dietetic conditions.

Pathology. In most cases of sigmoid volvulus, the upper limb of the loop descends in front of the lower, twisting on its mesenteric axis from one half to two turns in a counterclockwise direction.

Predisposing conditions are always quoted as a long and freely movable sigmoid loop on a long and freely movable mesosigmoid, adhesions either tethering the base of the two limbs close together or fixing the apex, loading of the colon with faecal material, or gross distension and thickening of the sigmoid colon as occurs in acquired megacolon. However, Hughes (1980) points out that there may be an important difference in the type of volvulus seen in "high-risk" countries, comprising a long thin-walled sigmoid loop with a narrow mesentery at its neck and prone to gangrene, compared with that usually seen in Western countries, where the

TABLE 45–4. GEOGRAPHIC DISTRIBUTION OF THE INCIDENCE OF SIGMOID VOLVULUS

	(%)
Soviet Union	19.4
Finland	11.9
Japan	10.2
Sweden	7.5
United States	4.5
Germany	3.7

(*Source: From Peterson L: Beitrag zur Kenntnis des ileum terminale fixatum und ileus ilei terminalis fixati. Acta Chir Scand (suppl):32, 1934, with permission.*)

bowel is often enormously hypertrophied, the changes persisting beyond the neck of the volvulus well into the rectum, which suggests that the twist is merely a mechanical complication of some specific colonic abnormality.

Another interesting difference between cases of volvulus seen in the Western world and in developing countries is that in the former group the affected bowel is principally distended with gas whereas in the latter there may be faecal overloading of the sigmoid loop. Osime, (1980) in a recent report of 13 cases of sigmoid volvulus from Benin in Central Nigeria, noted that all the cases were male, the diet comprised large amounts of vegetable material, and the sigmoid was loaded with faeces. In contrast, however, Sinha (1969) did not find faecal loading in any of his 211 cases in Patna, India. (Certainly there would be great interest in a detailed pathologic comparison of specimens of sigmoid volvulus obtained from different parts of the world to confirm or refute these suggested differences.)

There is a well-documented association between sigmoid volvulus and mental disease (Johnston and Gibson, 1960; Khoury et al, 1977; String and DeCosse, 1971). This association may well be due to the high incidence of gross constipation and long continued neglect of bowel habit in these predominantly elderly, mentally disturbed, and institutionalised patients.

Clinical Manifestations. Volvulus of the sigmoid colon in the Western world usually occurs in middle-aged or elderly patients. Reports from the developing world usually record younger patients. Sigmoid volvulus can occur in young adults and has even been reported in childhood. The first account of this was by Carter and Hinshaw (1961) who recorded a case in a 14-day-old infant and another in a 10-year-old child.

Western series usually show a male preponderance but in the developing communities male patients form 90 percent or more of most published series (Shepherd, 1969).

The condition has a wide range of presentation, from grumbling attacks of recurrent subacute obstruction to fulminating strangulation with gangrene perforation. Hinshaw and Carter (1957), in a detailed study of 55 cases, divide their patients into two major clinical types:

The acute fulminating form occurs in the younger individual, with sudden onset, a rapid course, early vomiting, diffuse abdominal pain, marked tenderness and collapse, and with rapid development of gangrene.

A subacute progressive form occurs typically in older patients, with a gradual onset, often with a history of previous attacks, which run a benign course and in which gangrene develops more slowly. There is tremendous distension of the abdomen in contrast to the more acute type. Vomiting is a late feature.

This contrast is summarised in Table 45–5.

Although this is a convenient clinical classification, it must be stressed that the clinical features, in fact, form a spectrum rather than occurring in two clearly defined groups.

The striking clinical feature of sigmoid volvulus is the rapid and extreme inflation of the abdomen. Certainly the most extreme examples of gross gaseous distension are found in this condition.

Radiologic Examination. Plain x-ray films of the abdomen usually reveal a tremendously distended sigmoid loop, which may extend up to, and even elevate, the diaphragm (Fig. 45–7). The huge gas shadow may be looped on itself, giving the typical "bent inner tube sign" and there may be two fluid levels on the erect film, one in the proximal and one in the distal limb of the obstructed loop. In late cases, the right colon then becomes progressively distended with gas and, if the ileocaecal valve is incompetent, small intestinal fluid levels then become manifest.

The plain film is usually sufficient for diagnosis but in subacute cases, a limited barium enema examination reveals the sigmoid twist at the base of the mesocolon, above which is seen the grossly gas-dilated loop of obstructed sigmoid.

Differential Diagnosis. This falls into three main categories:

1. The gross distension and the radiologic appearance may suggest the less common caecal volvulus.
2. A diagnosis of large bowel obstruction may be made without considering sigmoid volvulus and the surgeon diagnoses the more common obstructing carcinoma of the sigmoid or diverticular disease. This is unfortunate, because it may detract the surgeon from attempting conservative reduction which, in such a subacute case, might have a high chance of success.

TABLE 45–5. ACUTE VOLVULUS OF THE SIGMOID COLON

Features	Acute Fulminating	Subacute Progressive
Previous attack	Infrequent	Frequent
Onset	Sudden	Gradual
Clinical course	Rapid, often catastrophic	Slow, but progressive
Pain	Diffuse, severe, often steady	Less marked, occasional cramps
Vomiting	Early	Late, may be negligible
General appearance	Prostration, shock common	Shock, uncommon or late
Distension	Less marked, may be none	Usually extreme
Signs of peritoneal irritation	Usually definite, rebound tenderness or rigidity	Usually not present
Peristalsis	Violent hyperactivity, later silent	Usual pattern in colonic obstruction
Leucocytosis	Frequent	Infrequent
Roentgenologic findings	Frequently not distinctive	Frequently diagnostic
Presence of strangulation	Frequent and early	Infrequent and late
Differential diagnosis	Perforated viscus or strangulated bowel	Obstruction of left colon

(*Source: Adapted from Hinshaw DB, Carter R, et al, 1957, with permission.*)

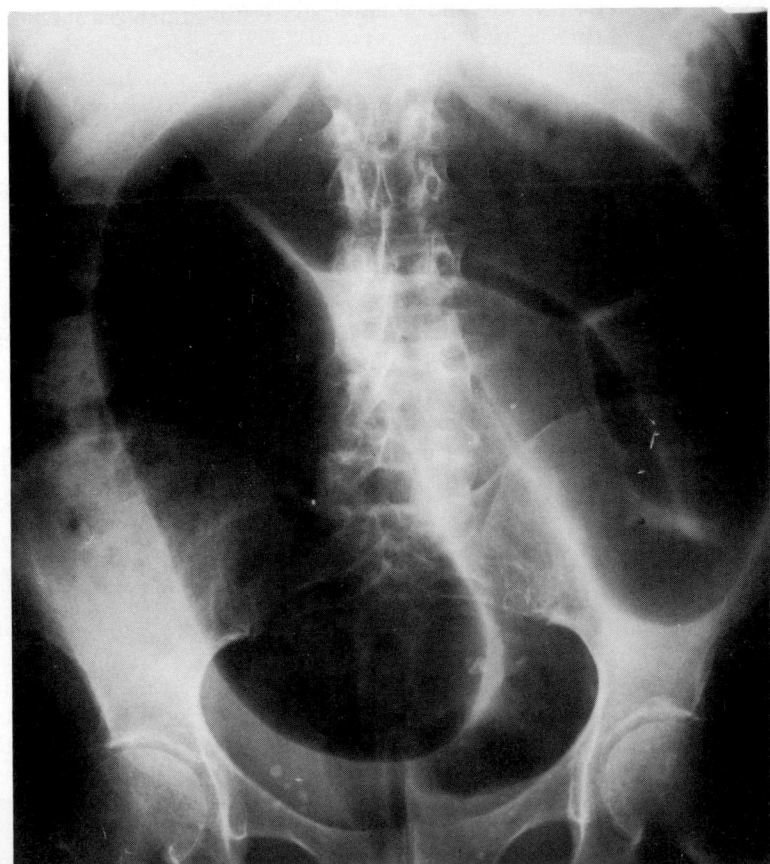

Figure 45–7. Plain abdominal x-ray showing the "bent inner tube sign" of a sigmoid volvulus.

3. The more fulminating cases complicated by gangrene or perforation mimic other abdominal catastrophies, including mesenteric vascular occlusion, peritonitis from a perforated diverticulitis, appendix or peptic ulcer, or acute pancreatitis.

Treatment. The aims of treatment are twofold—first, to relieve the torsion and second, to prevent recurrence. The latter is an important consideration because the risk of recurrent volvulus after either conservative or operative detorsion is high. Initial treatment can be either conservative or operative.

CONSERVATIVE TREATMENT. Spontaneous untwisting of a sigmoid volvulus or its relief by a simple enema or by a barium enema may occur. Nonoperative reduction is attempted by passing a well-lubricated soft rubber flatus tube through a sigmoidoscope inserted as high as possible into the rectum with the patient lying in the left lateral position under a general anaesthetic. By gentle manipulation, the tube frequently passes into the twisted area and this is followed by a dramatic gush of flatus and liquid faeces with immediate decompression of the abdomen. The tube is left in place, if possible, for 48 hours. Hughes (1980) points out that the enormous hypertrophy of the muscle in the volved sigmoid makes tight twisting almost impossible and this, together with the fact that the vessels to the sigmoid loop in this condition are large and thick-walled, makes gangrene a relatively rare and relatively late affair. All these factors render sigmoidoscopic evacuation a safe procedure.

If reduction cannot be effected, the tube is left in place so that it can be manipulated into the sigmoid loop at the operative detorsion that must be proceeded with if this conservative method fails.

Bruusgaard (1947) did much to popularise this method and reported an extensive experience in Oslo of no less than 136 patients. In 123, the volvulus was fully relieved with the recovery of the patients. Three died in spite of having the volvulus untwisted but at autopsy the colon was found to be viable. There was one perforation of the colon with death, despite immediate operation, and only nine patients could not be relieved conservatively and required immediate operative treatment. More recently

Prather and Bowers (1962) confirmed the value of conservative treatment with 17 successes in 18 episodes of sigmoid volvulus.

There have been recent reports of successful detorsion of sigmoid volvulus using the colonoscope without even using an anaesthetic. The technique has the additional advantage that the mucosa within the volvulus can be inspected and the viability of the segment can be checked (O'Connor, 1979; Starling, 1979).

OPERATIVE TREATMENT. Operative intervention is necessary in early cases if conservative measures fail, in advanced cases that suggest that strangulation may have supervened, and electively in order to prevent recurrence.

With a rectal tube in place, the abdomen is opened through a generous left paramedian or midline incision. The twisted sigmoid loop is gently reduced and the rectal tube threaded up into it in order to facilitate decompression. If a rectal tube has not been passed, it may be necessary to deflate the enormously distended loop by means of a trocar attached to a suction pump. Resection is then performed with end-to-end anastomosis. If the bowel is already gangrenous, a Mikulicz exteriorisation resection is performed or, if the distal extent of the gangrene makes it impossible to bring the distal limb to the skin surface, a Hartmann operation, with a proximal terminal colostomy and closure of the rectal stump, is carried out.

Elective resection should be performed in patients who have been treated conservatively or who have been previously treated by simple operative detorsion in order to prevent the risk of recurrence of the volvulus. The dilated and rather thickened large bowel makes this a relatively easy procedure (Fig. 45–8).

Prognosis. Conservative management or simple intraabdominal detorsion is associated with an excellent immediate prognosis although the risk of subsequent recurrence of the volvulus, unless definitive treatment is carried out, must be stressed. The mortality rate becomes high in the presence of gangrene, associated medical disease, delay in treatment, or inappropriate therapy—for example, failure to proceed to laparotomy if intubation fails.

Thus, in an extensive study of 425 episodes of volvulus in Uganda, Shepherd (1969) noted

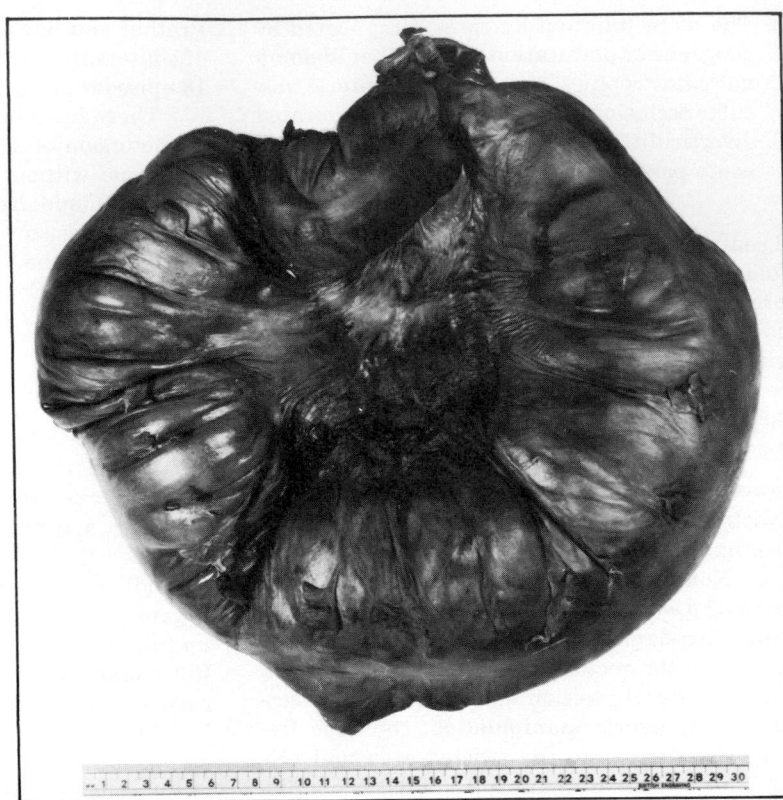

Figure 45–8. Sigmoid volvulus. Elective resection after successful detorsion via the sigmoidoscope. (*Source: From Ellis H, 1982, with permission.*)

an 8 percent incidence of gangrene. When this occurred, the mortality was 47 percent compared with 8 percent in the nongangrenous group.

Wertkin and Aufses (1978) have published a valuable collective review concerning prognosis following sigmoid volvulus. In 389 reports of nonoperative treatment, 14.7 percent were unsuccessful. There were 2 percent deaths and 55.7 percent recurrences. In 178 primary resections with immediate anastomosis, the death rate was 7 percent and recurrences occurred in only 0.1 percent. Ninety eight patients who underwent a Mikulicz or Hartmann procedure were associated with a 24 percent death rate, presumably because gangrene was often present, but there were no recurrences. Of 124 operative detorsions alone, 18 percent resulted in death with a 13 percent recurrence. Of 220 patients subjected to detorsion and attempts at fixation of the bowel, deaths occurred in 9 percent and no less than 38 percent recurred, showing the difficulty of any attempt at fixation of the redundant sigmoid loop and the importance of its resection.

Volvulus of the Small Intestine and Intestinal Knotting

Volvulus neonatorum is a well-recognised paediatric emergency (see Chapter 40). Volvulus of the small intestine in adults is very uncommon in the Western world. When it does occur, it is usually due to tethering of a loop of bowel at its apex, usually as a result of a postoperative adhesion.

However, in some parts of the world the emergency is far less rare. Agarwal and Misra (1970) reported no fewer than 29 examples seen in 1 year in their hospital in Northern India. These accounted for 20 percent of all cases of intestinal obstruction excluding strangulated hernias. Interestingly, in the same period, a similar number of examples of volvulus of the sigmoid was encountered. Wapnick (1973), in a review of 136 patients with volvulus treated in Zimbabwe, noted that no fewer than 51 had volvulus of the small intestine. In addition, there were 2 examples of caecal volvulus, 56 of sigmoid volvulus, and 27 of ileosigmoid knotting. Vaez-Zadeh and colleagues (1969) in Iran found that no less than 41 of 205 cases of small intestine obstruction in adults in Iran were due to small bowel volvulus (19.6 percent). This emergency occurred especially in male farmers on a bulky diet. Duke and Yar (1977) noted a high incidence of small bowel volvulus in Afghanistan and have noted that the patients are male farmers or nomads on a high fibre diet. The emergency is particularly likely to occur during the period of Ramadan when the population fasts throughout the day, eating only one large meal in the evening.

The aetiology of this condition is poorly understood and its rarity in Europe and North America unexplained.

Knotting of the bowel (compound volvulus) is likely to occur in regions where sigmoid volvulus is common. In the ileosigmoid form, a loop of ileum knots around the base of the sigmoid volvulus in a complex manner, often resulting in gangrene both of the ileal and the sigmoid loop (Fig. 45–9). Less commonly, a true knot forms between two loops of ileum. Shepherd

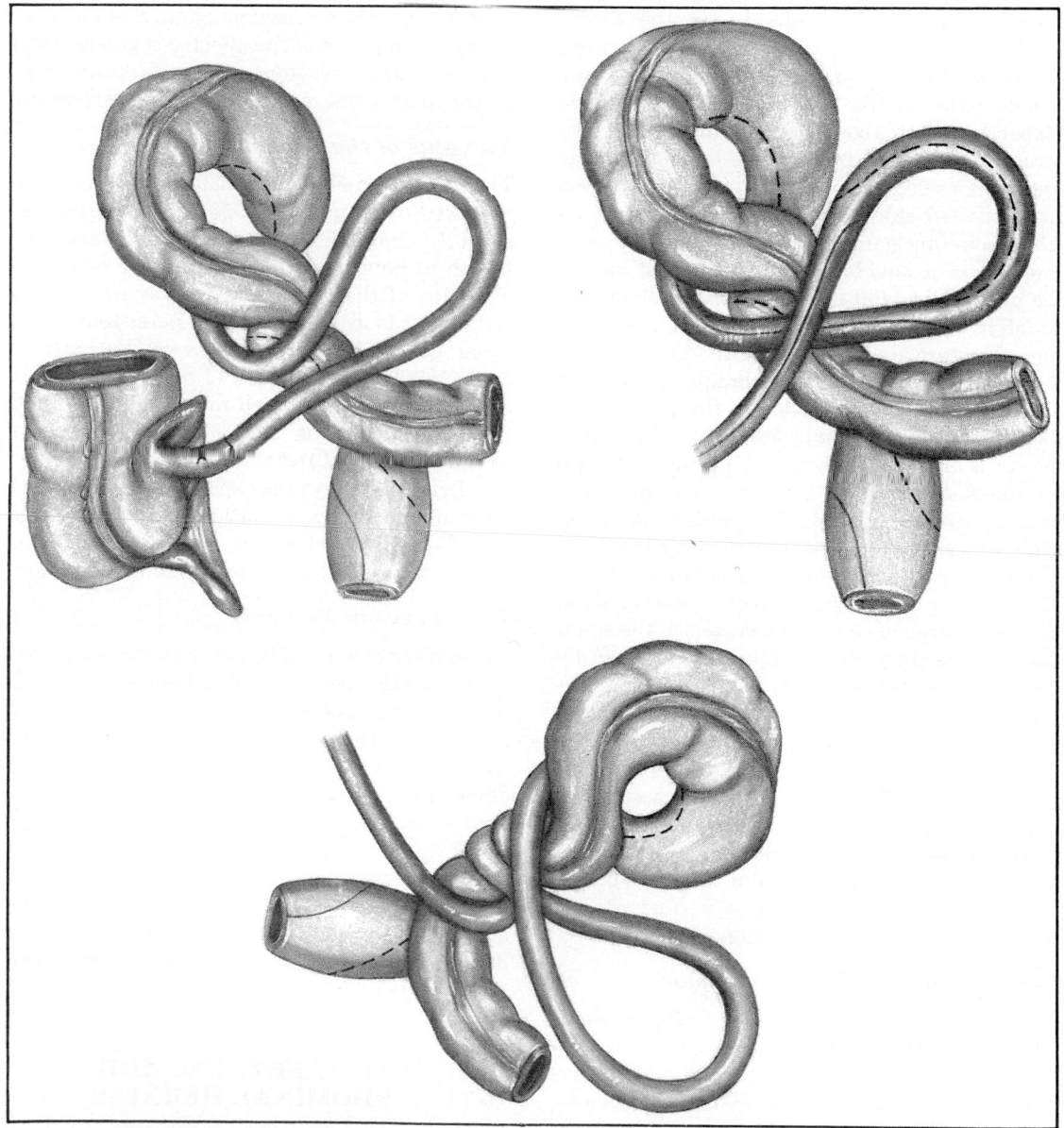

Figure 45–9. These three diagrams demonstrate the complex steps of ileosigmoid knotting. (*Source: From Ellis H, 1982, with permission.*)

(1969), in his classic article from Uganda, noted that intertwining of two loops of bowel accounted for nearly one fifth of all cases of volvulus seen; gangrene was present in 80 percent and the mortality rate was 50 percent.

Surgery for Ileosigmoid Knotting

This author has no direct or indirect experience with a case of ileosigmoid knotting in the United Kingdom. Ver Steeg and Whithead (1980), in reporting a case, could find only one other report in the United States. Surprisingly, it is comparatively common in Finland and the Soviet Union (Kallio, 1932). One can do no better, therefore, than to paraphrase the excellent article by Grave (1976) who has had an extensive experience of this condition in Zimbabwe: A generous abdominal incision is employed. The gangrenous sigmoid is drawn to the right to expose the left side of its mesentery. This shows the encircling gangrenous small bowel tightly applied in a double layer. No attempt should be made to try and undo the knot or divide the small bowel. The descending colon, sigmoid, and upper rectum are mobilised by dividing the parietal peritoneum. Crushing clamps are applied to the descending colon and to the rectum just below the rectosigmoid junction. The large bowel is then divided, thus allowing elevation of the knotted small intestine. The proximal ileum is divided between clamps above the knot. The ileocaecal junction is now inspected and the distal end of the involved ileum identified. The ileum is divided between clamps 5 cm distal to the gangrenous area. The vessels of the small bowel mesentery are clamped and divided by incising the mesentery on its right-facing surface close to the involved small bowel. A direct small bowel anastomosis may be possible when 5 to 10 cm of terminal ileum is present and clearly viable. When such is not the case, Grave advises closure of the terminal ileum with ileocaecal anastomosis. The Hartmann procedure disposes of the divided ends of the large bowel. Colorectal anastomosis can be performed 3 to 6 weeks later as a second stage procedure.

Volvulus of the Transverse Colon

This is an unusual emergency. Zinkin et al (1979) note that only 44 cases have been published in the English language since Kallio reported 2 examples and reviewed 16 previous reports in 1932. Seven further examples have recently been reported from Edinburgh by Anderson and colleagues (1981).

Aetiologically, there may be nothing more to find than a redundant loop of transverse colon. Patients may present either with repeated episodes of abdominal pain due to recurrent or chronic torsion, or with acute large bowel obstruction. Not surprisingly, the exact location is rarely thought of preoperatively.

Early or recurrent problems are easily managed by transverse colectomy. The more acute case can be dealt with very adequately by means of a temporary transverse colostomy, which not only decompresses the bowel but adequately fixes the transverse colon. Should there be frank gangrene of the affected segment, then exteriorisation colostomy of the Mikulicz type of the transverse colon should be performed.

Volvulus of the Splenic Flexure

This, is extremely unusual but has been well reviewed by Blumberg (1958) who reported the seventh example of this condition and the fourth to have undergone successful resection. Volvulus of the splenic flexure occurs when a redundant loop is present on a persistent mesocolon. Of the 16 patients reviewed by Lantieri et al (1979) no fewer than 11 had had previous abdominal surgery which may have interfered with the supporting ligamentous attachments of the splenic flexure.

Detorsion may occur spontaneously, during a barium enema examination or by the passage of a flatus tube. However, resection should be advised to prevent recurrent episodes of torsion.

Rare Types of Volvulus

Appendiceal knotting has been described on two occasions (Hughes, 1949; Mikal and Byers, 1956) and there has been one example of knotting of a Meckel's diverticulum around the adjacent loop of ileum (Dowse, 1961). A man-made cause of volvulus is reported by Wapnick et al (1979)—torsion of a Kock reservoir at its attachment to the anterior abdominal wall. Volvulus of the small intestine has been reported in two cases after jejunoileal bypass for obesity—yet another of the multitudinous complications of this accident-prone operation (Ackerman and Abou-Mourad, 1979).

INTERNAL APERTURES AND INTRAABDOMINAL HERNIAS

Introduction. By far the most common cause of an intraabdominal aperture is an adhesive band through which a loop of small intestine may prolapse and become strangulated. There are, however, a large variety of internal apertures and intraabdominal hernias which are rare causes of intestinal obstruction and strangulation. The majority of these are congenital in origin, but they may result from inflammation, trauma, or previous abdominal surgery. A good example of the last is the defect in the transverse mesocolon at the time of performance of a retrocolic partial gastrectomy or posterior gastroenterostomy; another is the paracolic or paraileal space that may result from the fashioning of a terminal colostomy or ileostomy. A loop of intestine slipping through one of these apertures is likely to become strangulated by its fibrous margins.

The various internal orifices can be classified as follows:

1. Mesenteric and mesocolic defects
2. Retroperitoneal hernias related to
   a. duodenum
   b. appendix and caecum
   c. sigmoid colon
3. The foramen of Winslow
4. Rare hernias of the abdominal wall and the pelvis
   a. obturator
   b. sciatic
   c. lumbar
   d. supravesical

Mesenteric and Mesocolic Defects. Apertures in the mesentery or in the mesocolon may allow protrusion of a loop of intestine through the defect with consequent strangulation. Janin et al (1980), in a masterly review of this subject, could collect only 57 examples among 7 large series of intestinal obstructions amounting in all to over 3000 patients.

Strangulation may occur through a defect in the terminal ileal mesentery. Although this may occur as a result of previous surgery, it is likely that the majority of these defects are congenital in origin (Garden et al, 1980). Defects may also occur in the transverse mesocolon and in the mesentery of a Meckel's diverticulum.

Rarely, there may be a defect in the greater omentum, which is usually considered congenital (it has been found in the foetus at term), but it may follow inflammation or previous surgery. The great majority of defects are situated at the free edge of the omentum. The most up-to-date article, with a report of two personal cases, is by Jamart and colleagues (1980). It is nearly always the small intestine that is involved, herniating through the orifice from behind forward. Figure 45–10 is the sketch made of an operation performed by this author on a patient with this condition in 1954. The patient, a 58-year-old male, made an uneventful recovery; there was no history of previous surgery or of abdominal trauma.

Defects producing intestinal obstruction have been reported in the left paracolic gutter (Orr, 1966), the sigmoid mesocolon (Fiddian, 1961), and the falciform ligament of the liver (Werbin et al, 1969).

Clinical Manifestations. The presenting features of strangulation through these defects is acute intestinal obstruction. In some instances, a palpable abdominal mass may be present. Not surprisingly, a preoperative accurate diagnosis of the exact cause of the occlusion is rarely made.

Treatment is, of course, surgical. If the bowel is viable, it is reduced and the defect repaired. Gangrene of the bowel is treated by appropriate resection.

The only other way in which these mesenteric and mesocolic defects may present is as an incidental finding during a laparotomy for another condition. If thus found, certainly the

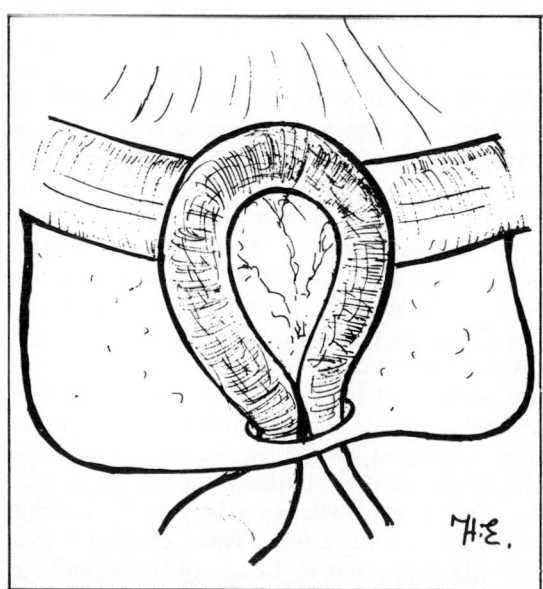

Figure 45–10. Transomental hernia. Sketch made by the author in his operative notes. (*Source: From Ellis H, 1982, with permission.*)

defect should be repaired and this is illustrated by an instructive case report by Meade (1942). His patient was found to have an ileocaecal mesenteric defect at appendicectomy. The defect was not closed, the patient developed intestinal obstruction 7 days postoperatively and was found to have 6 feet of gangrenous intestine herniating through the defect at the second operation.

Retroperitoneal Hernias

There are a number of fossas related to the duodenum, the ileocaecal region, and the sigmoid colon. In an extensive review of 467 cases of intraabdominal hernias by Hansmann and Morton (1939), 53 percent occurred in the paraduodenal region, 13 percent were associated with the caecum and terminal ileum, and 6 percent were in the sigmoid region. Early studies considered that a loop of bowel could enter into any of the numerous retroperitoneal fossas, perhaps when of rather greater than usual size. It was then thought that progressive stretching of the recess would allow more and more intestine to enter the fossa until this contained almost the whole of the small bowel. However, it was Andrews, in 1923, who demonstrated the impossibility of this classic concept. He pointed out that there was no differential pressure between these pouches and the general peritoneal cavity and that, therefore, there is no propulsive force to account for the formation of such hernias. Moreover, he noted the following objections to the classic theory. First, almost invariably all, or almost all, of the small intestine is incorporated into these hernias; second, cases have been observed in newborn infants; third, only the small bowel is involved, never the omentum or other viscera; and finally, often the loops of small intestine within the hernia are adherent to one another by filmy fibrous tissue that represents retroperitoneal connective tissue. Andrews put forward the hypothesis that the duodenal types of hernias, and probably also the paracaecal hernias, are in fact anomalies of intestinal rotation in which the small intestine is trapped behind the transverse mesocolon as the caecum rotates from the left to the right side of the abdomen to become fixed to the posterior peritoneum. This concept was strongly supported by Longacre (1934) and by Zimmerman and Anson (1967).

Willwerth et al (1974), in an important contribution to this difficult subject, suggest the following classification of paraduodenal hernias:

- *Type 1, left mesocolic hernia,* resulting from invagination of the left mesocolon in the avascular area behind the inferior mesenteric vessels—a left paraduodenal hernia (Fig. 45–11).
- *Type 2, right mesocolic hernia,* resulting from nonrotation of the small intestine and subsequent entrapment by rotation and fixation of the caecum and ascending colon—the right paraduodenal hernia (Fig. 45–12).
- *Type 3, transverse mesocolic hernia,* resulting from reversed rotation of the midgut with invagination of the transverse colon and portion of the right colon. This last type of hernia is extremely rare.

Clinical Manifestations. Many paraduodenal hernias are asymptomatic and are simply detected incidentally at laparotomy or autopsy. Rarely, they may present with acute intestinal obstruction and under these circumstances it is unusual for the diagnosis to be made correctly before operation.

Plain x-rays of the abdomen, by showing an agglomeration of small bowel loops into one portion of the abdominal cavity, may suggest the diagnosis, as may a barium meal and follow-through examination in the subacute case, which may demonstrate a conglomeration of small bowel loops (Thoren, 1978).

Surgical Management. This depends on a clear understanding of the congenital defect (Willwerth et al, 1974). The right paraduodenal hernia is mobilised by freeing the lateral peritoneal margin of the right colon over to the left side. Thereafter, the hernial sac can be opened, allowing free access to its contents. The left paraduodenal hernia can usually be reduced without too much of a problem and the neck of the sac sutured, but the neck of the sac may require preliminary dilatation and adhesions of the small bowel may require lysis.

Paracaecal Hernias

The fossas in relationship to the ileocaecal region are less common sites of hernias than the paraduodenal region. Hansmann and Morton (1939) found only 61 cases reported in this region, of which 31 were labelled paracaecal, 16 ileoappendicular, and 14 ileocolic. These have been accepted as herniations into preformed pouches, although, once again, Andrews (1923) suggests that these are of developmental origin. Their genesis is easily explained on the basis of a minor error of rotation of the midgut with

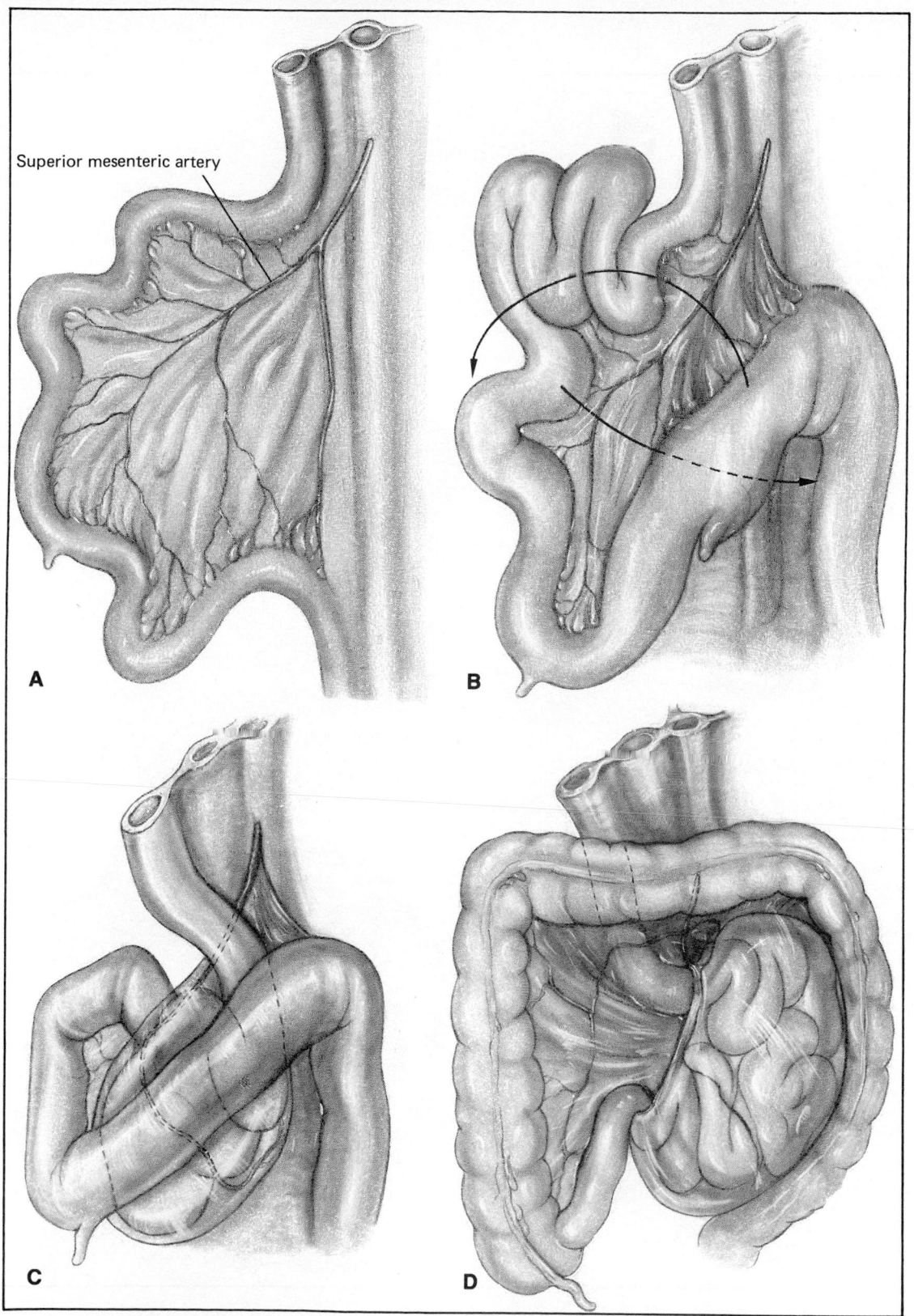

Figure 45–11. Stages in the development of a left paraduodenal hernia. (*Source: From Ellis H, 1982, with permission.*)

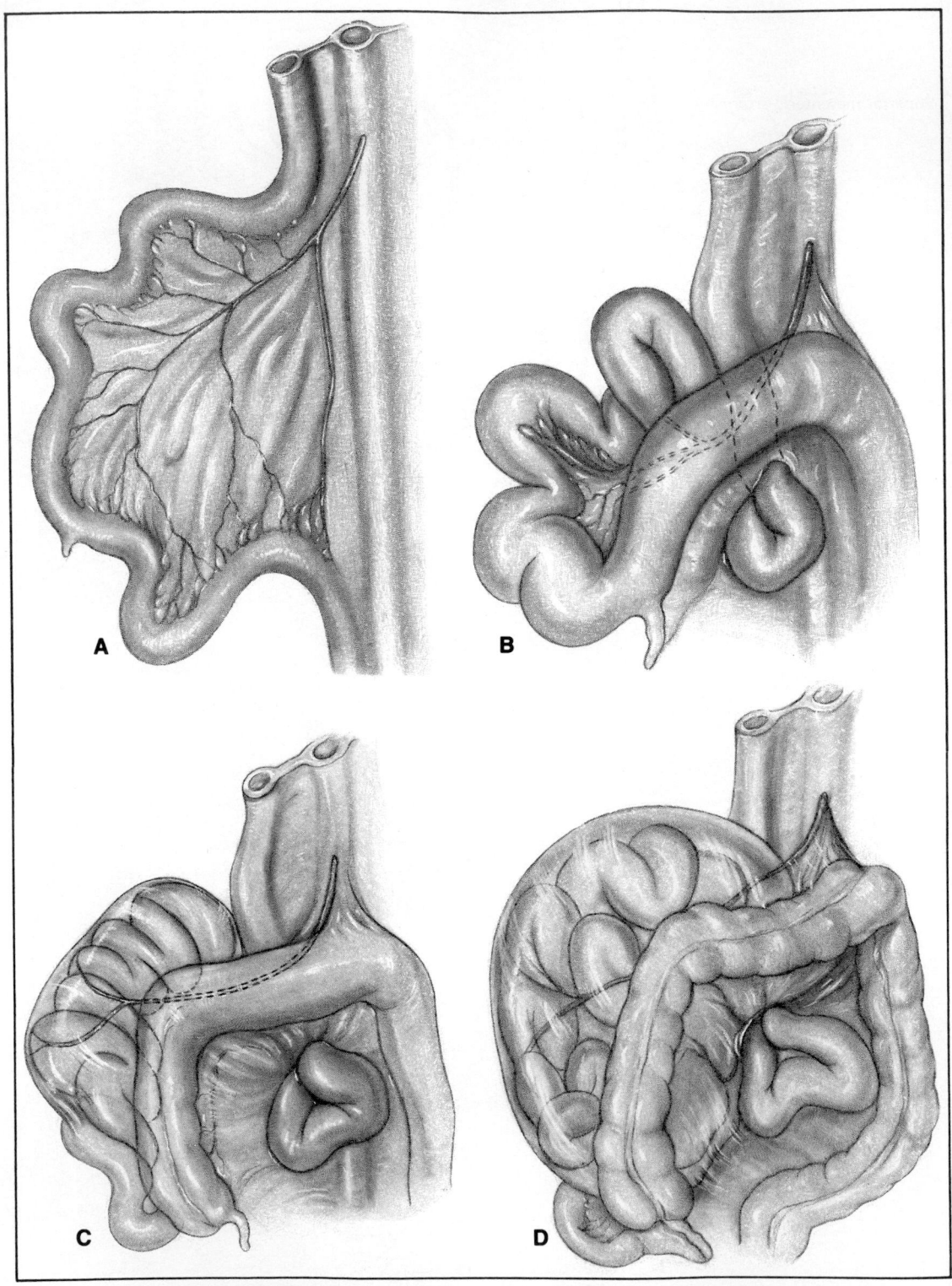

Figure 45–12. Stages in the development of a right paraduodenal hernia. (*Source: From Ellis H, 1982, with permission.*)

incarceration behind the caecum during the final stages of descent and fixation of the right colon. One may note that the much more common retrocaecal or retroperitoneal appendix is an example of the same phenomenon in which the appendix is trapped behind the mesentery of the ileocaecal region during this phase of rotation.

Intersigmoid Hernias

These are rare and constituted only 28 of the 467 cases of intraabdominal hernia collected by Hansmann and Morton (1939). Here, a portion of small bowel becomes trapped in a fossa between the two loops of sigmoid colon.

Hernia of the Foramen of Winslow

Hernias through the foramen of Winslow have been reported on rare occasions, either as incidental findings at autopsy or laparotomy, or presenting with intestinal obstruction.

Blandin, in 1834, gave the first postmortem description of a case and here, the whole small intestine had herniated through the foramen into the lesser sac. Treves (1888) reported the first laparotomy, but to Neve (1892) goes the distinction of recording the first successful surgical cure for this condition. By 1939, Hansmann and Morton were able to collect 37 cases in their collective review of 467 examples of intraabdominal hernias and by 1977, the numbers had reached the 90s (Schwartz, 1977).

Occasionally the preoperative diagnosis has been made, or at least suggested, by barium enema (Zinken and Moore, 1980) or by barium meal and follow-through examination. The majority of patients present with intestinal obstruction and there may be a history of previous intermittent attacks of pain. The only suggestive physical sign is a palpable tender mass in the epigastrium.

In some cases, the herniated bowel may rupture through the gastrohepatic omentum and thus return into the main peritoneal cavity.

Surgical treatment comprises gentle stretching of the opening with the index finger; blind division with the knife or scissors must be avoided. If the obstruction cannot thus be released, the bowel loop should be emptied completely by means of a trocar and cannula connected to a suction apparatus. After the strangulated loop of intestine has been withdrawn, the foramen of Winslow should be closed by means of an omental plug. Naturally, if the bowel is of doubtful viability or frankly necrotic, resection is required.

ADHESIONS AND BANDS

Introduction. Adhesions or solitary bands are the most common cause of intestinal obstruction in the Western world. Table 45–6 presents a series of figures drawn from publications in Europe and North America over the last 60 years which demonstrate that one in every three cases of intestinal obstruction might be due to this cause. In interpreting published figures, one should note that some series exclude strangulated external hernias and others confine their analysis to small bowel obstruction; in the latter instance, the figure rises to some 60 percent of the total cases.

We have already noted that obstruction due to adhesions has become more common in proportion to the epidemic nature of abdominal operations throughout the technically advanced world. In contrast, in developing communities, where laparotomies are a rarity, obstruction due to adhesions is uncommon (see Chapter 44).

Classification. Adhesions can be classified into congenital and acquired. Congenital adhesions, although common, only occasionally cause trouble and indeed adhesions that give rise to intestinal obstruction are nearly always preceded either by an operation or by a local or diffuse severe intraperitoneal inflammation.

Perry et al (1955) analysed 1252 obstructions at the University of Minnesota and found that 31 percent were due to adhesions. Of these, 79 percent were postoperative, 18 percent inflammatory, and 3 percent congenital. Of the inflammatory causes it was interesting that 42 percent followed acute appendicitis, 14.5 percent diverticulitis, and others resulted from pelvic infection, Crohn's disease, and cholecystitis. Festen (1982) reported 36 postoperative small bowel obstructions requiring surgery in a series of 1476 laparotomies in neonates and children. Of these, one was an intussusception, one an internal hernia, and the remaining 33 were due to postoperative adhesions. Eighty percent of these occurred within 3 months of surgery. Appendicectomy and gynaecologic operations always figure prominently in statistical analyses of postoperative adhesions. Although much less

TABLE 45–6. ADHESIONS AND BANDS AS CAUSES OF OBSTRUCTION

Author (Year)	Place	Total No.	Adhesions (%)	Notes
Flesch-Thebesius (1920)	Frankfurt	368	31	Excludes strangulated hernias
Souttar (1925)	United Kingdom	3064	11	
Vick (1932)	United Kingdom	6892	6	
McIver (1932)	Boston, Massachusetts	335	30	
Moss & McFetridge (1934)	New Orleans, Louisiana	511	27	
Nemir (1952)	Philadelphia, Pennsylvania	430	33	
Perry et al (1955)	Minneapolis, Minnesota	1252	31	
Raf (1969a)	Stockholm	2295	64	Small intestine only (excludes hernias, neoplasms, and Crohn's)
Playforth et al (1970)	Lexington, Kentucky	111	54	Small intestine only
Stewardson et al (1978)	Chicago, Illinois	238	64	Small intestine only
Ellis (1981)	London	253	26	

(*Source: From Ellis H, 1982, with permission.*)

common, abdominoperineal excision of the rectum and total colectomy have a high incidence of postoperative adhesions; the explanation for this could be that the removal of the whole colon and omentum leaves only the small intestine to become adherent to the long abdominal scar.

Although postoperative adhesions may involve any of the intraabdominal viscera, obstruction from this cause usually implicates small intestine, especially the ileum. Thus, Miller and Winfield (1959) documented the site of obstruction in a series of 43 postoperative cases of obstruction due to adhesions. Thirty two involved ileum, four jejunum, six "small intestine" not specifically designated, and only one involved the large bowel—the sigmoid colon which was obstructed by a fibrous band.

Aetiology. From the earliest days of abdominal surgery, surgeons were familiar with the fibrinous adhesions that develop within a few hours of operational trauma. This fibrin can either be reabsorbed completely or become orga-

nised by the ingrowth of fibroblasts to develop into established fibrous adhesions. As this author has pointed out in several essays on the subject (Ellis, 1962, 1982A,B), some surgeons and pathologists, through armchair reasoning rather than experimental observations and basing their analogy on the healing of cutaneous wounds, assumed that the factor that decides whether adhesions are absorbed or become organised depends on whether or not the peritoneal endothelium is intact. It has been assumed that anything which damages the endothelium—rough handling, retraction, surgical denudation and so on—necessarily results in fibrous adhesions. This led to the surgical principle that peritoneal injury must be avoided at all costs, that raw damaged serosal surfaces must be eliminated within the peritoneal cavity, and that peritoneal defects must be oversewn or patched wherever possible.

However, when the armchair theory was put to the test, both by experiment and by careful clinical observation (Ellis, 1962), the results were very different. It is now well established that large peritoneal defects which are left open and bleeding heal within a few days into a smooth glistening new serosa. However, if the injury is accompanied by vascular damage (for example if the tissues are crushed, sutured, or ligated), then indeed adhesions develop, and injection studies show that these comprise active vascular ingrowths of newly formed vessels into ischaemic tissue.

In many instances, these vascular grafts are undoubtedly lifesaving, preserving the viability of an anastomosis, reinforcing the integrity of a traumatised segment of intestine, or preventing an ischaemic appendix or gallbladder from rupturing into the general peritoneal cavity. Experimentally, if adhesions are prevented from developing to a segment of intestine deprived of its blood supply by wrapping the segment in a sheet of polythene film, then gangrene of the segment invariably takes place. If, however, adhesions are allowed to develop, the bowel segment, up to a certain critical level, remains viable (Ellis, 1962).

Buckman and colleagues (1976A,B) have shown that peritoneal defects have a high plasminogen activity which is lost in peritoneum that has been rendered ischaemic by grafting or by tight suturing and, moreover, such ischaemic tissue may actively inhibit fibrinolysis by normal tissues. This phenomenon also explains the failure of intact peritoneum to lyse fibrinous adhesions to adjacent ischaemic tissue. This work has been elegantly confirmed by Raftery (1981).

This thesis, that fibrous adhesions develop in relation to areas of ischaemia and represent vascular grafts into such tissues (Fig. 45–13), explains the great majority of instances in which acquired adhesions are found within the peritoneal cavity. Thus, a pelvic tumour which has undergone avascular degeneration or torsion will become wrapped in dense adhesions; fragments of ruptured spleen, completely deprived of their anatomic blood supply, are found adherent and revascularised from adjacent tissues. Adhesions form to the line of a bowel anastomosis or to a laparotomy scar as a result of the strangulating effects of sutures on the local tissues in such situations. It is well-recognised that a laparotomy performed some time after an episode of general peritonitis, when the whole of the abdominal cavity would have been coated with fibrinous exudate, usually reveals

very little in the way of widespread adhesions, yet the strands that are present are localised to those areas where intense tissue anoxia have occurred, for example, to the appendix after an attack of acute appendicitis or to the gallbladder after an episode of gangrenous cholecystitis. Moreover, it is well known that large defects in the pelvic peritoneum after radical pelvic clearance operations heal smoothly and without adhesions, as demonstrated many years ago by Robbins et al (1949).

The peritoneum reacts in a similar manner to foreign material as it does to ischaemic tissue, therefore granulomas and adhesions may result from fragments of gauze, unabsorbed suture material or talc or starch glove powder introduced at the time of laparotomy. The starch can be demonstrated by viewing a biopsy of the adhesion under polarised light which reveals typical Maltese crosses.

Attempts to Prevent Adhesions. The present century has witnessed an enormous amount of work on attempts to prevent adhesions and the enormous corpus of experimental and laboratory studies has been reviewed by Boys (1942), Connolly and Smith (1960), and more recently by this author (Ellis, 1971). The various methods may be divided into:

1. *Attempts to prevent fibrin deposition* in the postoperative peritoneal exudate. This has involved the use of anticoagulants such as sodium citrate, heparin, dicoumarol and dextran, and aprotinin (Trasylol).
2. *Attempts to remove the fibrin exudate* by means of intraperitoneal lavage, enzymes such as pepsin, trypsin, and papain, and fibrinolytic agents such as streptokinase, actase, and urokinase.
3. *Attempts to separate bowel surfaces* have included distension of the abdominal cavity with oxygen, stimulation of peristalsis with prostigmine, and the use of substances such as olive oil, liquid paraffin, amniotic fluid, and membranes such as oiled silk, silver or gold foil, free grafts of omentum and silicones to separate damaged loops of bowel.
4. *Attempts to inhibit fibroblast proliferation* have included the use of antihistamines, steroids, and even cytotoxic drugs.

The story for all these substances has been very much the same; initial enthusiasm, often actual employment in clinical cases, then fur-

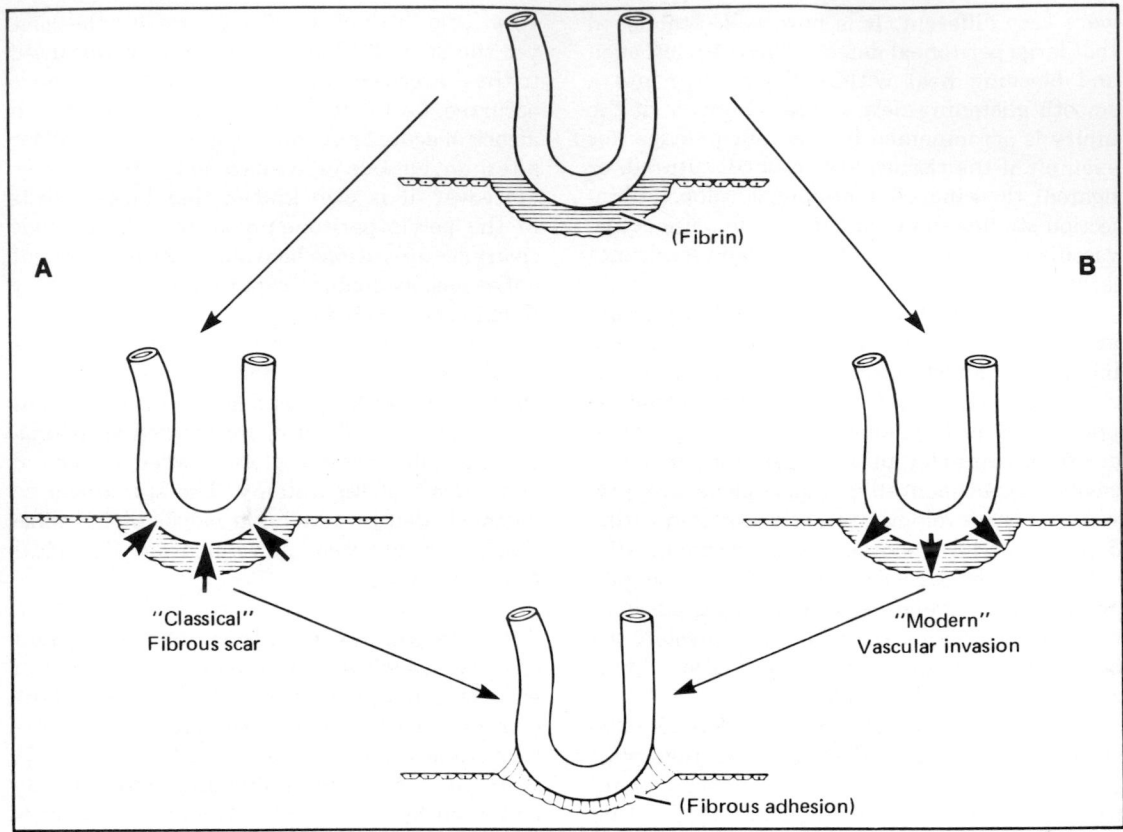

A

B

(Fibrin)

"Classical"
Fibrous scar

"Modern"
Vascular invasion

(Fibrous adhesion)

Figure 45–13. The aetiology of adhesions. At the top of the diagram is the damaged serosa. A loop of intestine adheres to it by fibrinous exudation. At the bottom of the diagram is the end result, the fibrous permanent adhesion. Pathway A is the "classic" concept; the serosal injury was said to heal as fibrous scar. Pathway B is the modern concept; vascular ingrowth occurs into the ischaemic tissue. When the ischaemic crisis is over, the vascular collateral channels resorb, leaving a fibrous matrix. (*Source: From Ellis H, 1982, with permission.*)

ther investigations which showed either no effect at all or an actual increase in adhesion formation compared with controls, followed finally by the abandonment of that particular technique.

A RATIONAL APPROACH TOWARD ADHESIONS. It is this author's belief that the surgeon's attitude towards intraabdominal adhesions must change. These have been considered as things to be avoided or prevented at all costs, to be destroyed and divided wherever and whenever encountered. Undoubtedly intestinal obstruction from adhesions is a relatively common surgical emergency as already noted, but this must be put against the fact that nearly all patients who have undergone a major laparotomy have adhesions, which in the very great majority of instances are, and remain, completely symp-

tomless. Weibel and Majno (1973) studied 298 subjects at autopsy who had had previous laparotomies and 67 percent of these showed adhesions. After multiple operations, the incidence rose to 93 percent. In a study by this author of 50 consecutive patients submitted to laparotomy after previous abdominal surgery, no less than 44 had developed adhesions. Indeed, in many cases, adhesions may well have been protective or even lifesaving to the patient, preventing leakage of suture lines, protecting devascularised damaged intestine, and walling off inflammatory collections.

Armed with the knowledge of how adhesions develop, the surgeon must prevent unnecessary adhesions from developing, control those adhesions which must inevitably form in order to obtain their beneficial effects but avoid, where possible, the risk of subsequent obstruction, and finally, in those patients who suffer from repeated episodes of obstruction, try to devise the best possible management following lysis of the adhesions.

Unnecessary adhesion formation can be reduced by meticulous surgical technique, and this must include the prevention of granuloma formation from foreign material such as gauze, glove powder, or long and redundant ends of nonabsorbable sutures. Wherever possible, peritoneal defects should be left open rather than be pulled together under tension. For example, this author never reperitonealises the gallbladder bed after cholecystectomy or the pelvic floor after an anterior resection of the rectum.

When adhesion formation is almost certain to occur as a result of local tissue ischaemia, for example to the under surface of the abdominal laparotomy incision or to an anastomotic line, measures should be taken to ensure that such adhesions will develop to any structure other than small intestine because, as already noted, the great majority of episodes of intestinal obstruction due to adhesions implicate the small bowel. For this reason, it is this author's practice to draw the omentum down over other abdominal organs before closing the abdominal incision and to wrap it over any anastomotic line. It is important, where possible, to preserve the omentum; this should be first step in carrying out a total colectomy. The reported high incidence of intestinal obstruction due to adhesions following this particular operation is, in this surgeon's view, due to the fact that so many surgeons remove the omentum along with the colon, thus leaving only the small intestine available to adhere to the laparotomy wound along the line of closure. If for any reason the omentum has to be removed or is unavailable, this author occasionally uses a flap of falciform ligament or the broad ligament in the female patient.

Diagnosis. Intestinal obstruction due to adhesions may present in the early postoperative period or may occur at any time—months or many years—after abdominal surgery or an intraabdominal inflammatory episode.

When symptoms arise shortly after an abdominal operation, it is not only a matter of considerable importance but also often one of great difficulty to decide whether the situation is due to mechanical causes or to postoperative ileus (see Chapter 44). We can summarise here

that the differential diagnosis depends upon first, a meticulous analysis of the symptoms, second, on abdominal auscultation and third, on a careful study of x-rays of the abdomen, which may need to be repeated after several hours.

The patient with late adhesive obstruction may give a history of a number of previous episodes of subacute obstruction. The clinical features are those of classic low, small gut obstruction with severe central colicky abdominal pain, nausea, vomiting (at first bile stained but later becoming faeculent), and abdominal distension. Examination reveals central distension of the abdomen, nearly always with an abdominal scar from previous surgery, with diffuse and often rebound tenderness, and with markedly increased bowel sounds. Plain x-rays of the abdomen usually (but not invariably) demonstrate multiple fluid levels.

The features of obstruction in conjunction with the scar on the abdomen combine to produce the classic clinical picture of intestinal obstruction caused by adhesions.

Treatment. It is a very good general rule that acute small bowel mechanical obstruction is a mandatory indication for urgent surgery. Obstruction due to adhesions, however, provides two common examples of reserved qualifications to this rule.

First, it is not uncommon to see a patient a few days after a major abdominal operation which has been complicated by a severe ileus who complains of abdominal pains and whose previously silent abdomen now reveals peristaltic noises. In such circumstances, a period of doubt exists with uncertainty whether these signs represent a recovering ileus, soon to be rewarded by the passage of flatus, or the first stages of development of a mechanical obstruction. Under these conditions, obviously one must continue conservative treatment and to keep a watchful eye on the situation. Fresh x-rays of the abdomen at this stage are also helpful; gas extending through the large bowel suggests a recovering ileus, whereas loops of distended small intestine with multiple fluid levels would indicate mechanical obstruction. Certainly, if the patient has already passed flatus or has had a bowel action and then becomes distended with colicky pain, the diagnosis must be one of adhesive obstruction and surgery is indicated.

There is a tendency to delay reoperating

on the abdomen in these circumstances and certainly no surgeon relishes reoperating on a patient in the early postoperative period. However, delay may prejudice the viability of a strangulated loop of bowel or may force the surgeon into the position of operating on a patient already exhausted by prolonged and fruitless conservative treatment.

The second indication for a trial of conservatism is in the patient who has suffered repeated previous episodes of intestinal obstruction with several previous operations for lysis of adhesions. Not uncommonly, the operation notes on such patients bear warnings of the masses of adhesions encountered within the abdomen and admonitions to stay out if possible. Under these circumstances, one is encouraged by the fact that matted loops of intestine which are stuck to one another are unlikely to be strangulated. Here certainly a trial period of nasogastric aspiration and intravenous fluid replacement is completely justified in the hope that the obstruction is incomplete and that spontaneous remission will occur—indeed, this may well have already happened in previous episodes. The most careful observation must be carried out in such a case and any deterioration in the patient's condition, such as increase in distension, tenderness or guarding, or a rise in pulse or temperature, or increase in the gaseous distension on repeated x-rays of the abdomen, indicate that immediate operative intervention must be advised.

When operation is indicated in the early postoperative period, laparotomy is carried out through the recent abdominal wound. A loop of bowel may be found to have become adherent to the serosal aspect of the wound and, not infrequently, this occurs at the site of a partial dehiscence of the wound. More frequently, the adhesive obstruction is found at the site of the operative area itself; for example, a loop of small intestine may be found adherent to the pelvic floor after an abdominoperineal excision of the rectum, or herniation may have occurred through a mesenteric or mesocolic defect which has been imperfectly sutured. On other occasions, loops of bowel are found matted to each other as a result of fibrinous adhesions, particularly after an acute inflammatory episode such as peritonitis. Having freed the obstruction, the bowel is decompressed, preferably by retrograde milking of the intestine back into the stomach, where the fluid can be aspirated via a nasogas-

tric tube. Any anatomic defect, if present, is repaired.

In late cases, it is usually possible to open the abdomen through the old abdominal incision. However, if the former operation had been carried out through a gridiron appendix incision, a median or paramedian paraumbilical incision is employed. Great care must be taken in opening the peritoneum because so frequently a loop of bowel is adherent to the under surface of the scar.

The operation for late intestinal obstruction due to adhesions can be one of the simplest or one of the most testing in surgery. At one end of the spectrum, there may be a solitary band that yields to a single snip of the scissors; at the other, the surgeon encounters a matted mass of intestines that requires the greatest care and patience to free by sharp dissection. In some cases it may be judicious to resect or bypass an inextricably fused clump of obstructed bowel.

In cases of recurrent widespread adhesions, a number of plication procedures have been advocated, designed to avoid acute kinks of matted bowel. The operation was first reported by the Finnish surgeon, Wichmann in 1934, but was popularised by Noble in 1937. More recently, transmesenteric plication of loops of small intestine in a serpentine pattern has been advocated (Childs and Phillips, 1960). These procedures are illustrated in Figure 45–14 and 45–15. Certainly the Childs technique appears to be safer than the Noble plication, but several reports of series of patients show that there is a significant mortality with both these procedures, and follow-up shows that further episodes of obstruction may still, unfortunately, occur (Hollender et al, 1971).

This author has no personal experience of these plication procedures and is not convinced from reading of published results that the incidence of recurrent intestinal obstruction is any lower following these operations than when simple division of the adhesive bands is performed.

In 1959, Baker described an ingenious technique of threading a tube down the whole length of the small intestine via a jejunostomy which, by its intrinsic stiffness, would prevent kinking while adhesions develop. Munro and Jones (1978) give a good technical account of this procedure in the treatment of complicated small bowel obstruction (Fig. 45–16).

Obviously, where there is a single band or

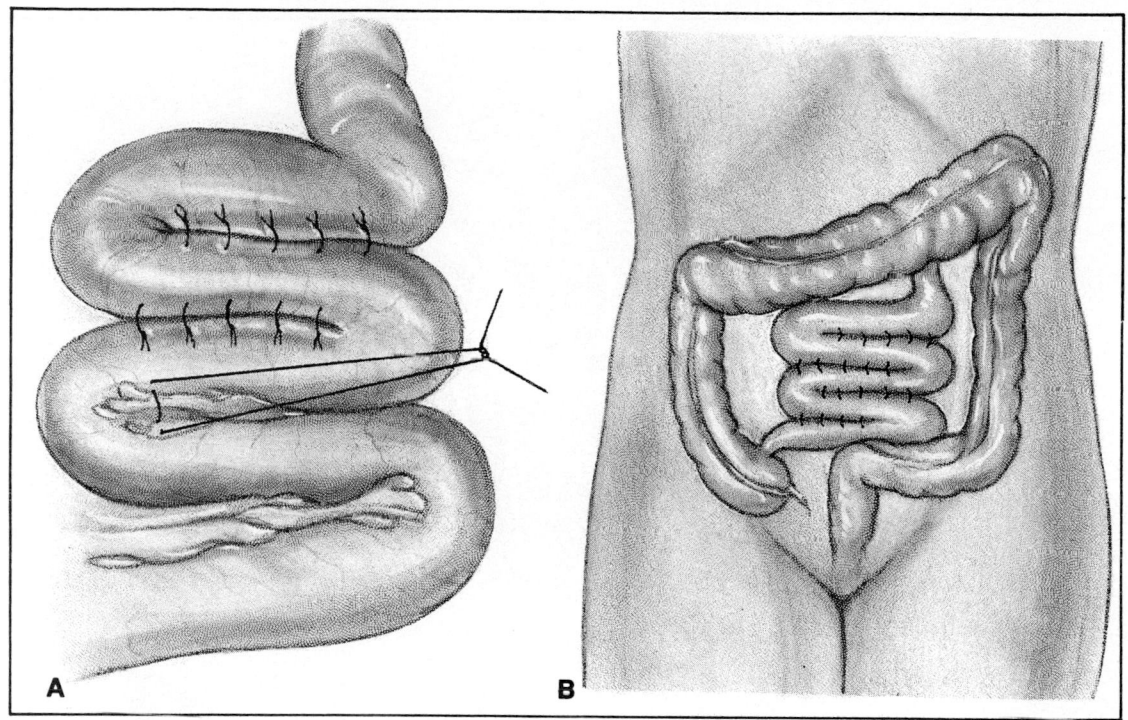

Figure 45–14. Plication of the intestine. **A.** The operation in progress. **B.** The procedure completed. (*Source: From Ellis H, 1982, with permission.*)

a few adhesions, simple division alone is all that is indicated. Where multiple severe adhesions are present, particularly in recurrent cases, more information is required regarding the wisest procedure to adopt—plication, intubation, or simply lysis.

GALLSTONE ILEUS

Obstruction of the bowel by an impacted gallstone is an unusual but well-recognised entity, first described by Bartholin in 1654. Indeed, even in the nineteenth century, it was well known that small gallstones could be extruded via the common bile duct into the duodenum, accompanied by severe abdominal colic, and might then pass per rectum, but that large gallstones could ulcerate insidiously into the adjacent gut and impact lower down the intestine to produce acute obstruction. By 1892 Naunyn could give a full description of the pathology of this entity and describe no less than 127 collected cases.

In most large series of intestinal obstruc-

tions, gallstones account for 1 to 2 percent of all cases. McLaughlin and Raines (1951), in a collected series of 19,692 cases of intestinal obstruction, found the incidence of gallstone obturation to be 1.9 percent, whereas Stitt and colleagues (1967), in a 5-year review of 265 cases of complete small intestinal obstruction, found that 11 were caused by gallstones (2.4 percent.) In Japan, the phenomenon appears less common; only 112 cases have been reported between 1903 and 1978 (Kasahara et al, 1980).

The majority of cases occur in people between the ages of 60 and 80. Kirkland and Croce (1961), reviewing 145 published cases, found that 70 percent occurred over the age of 60; these authors also noted in their own experience of 2500 admissions for gallbladder disease that gallstone ileus accounted for 0.5 percent of the cases. Females heavily outnumber males in all published series; thus, Brockis and Gilbert (1957) found a relationship of 7:1 in a review of 179 cases, and Stitt and colleagues (1967) put the ratio as 8:1. Anderson and Zederfeldt (1969) in their series of 44 cases, noted that 38 (86 percent) were females; the average age was 75

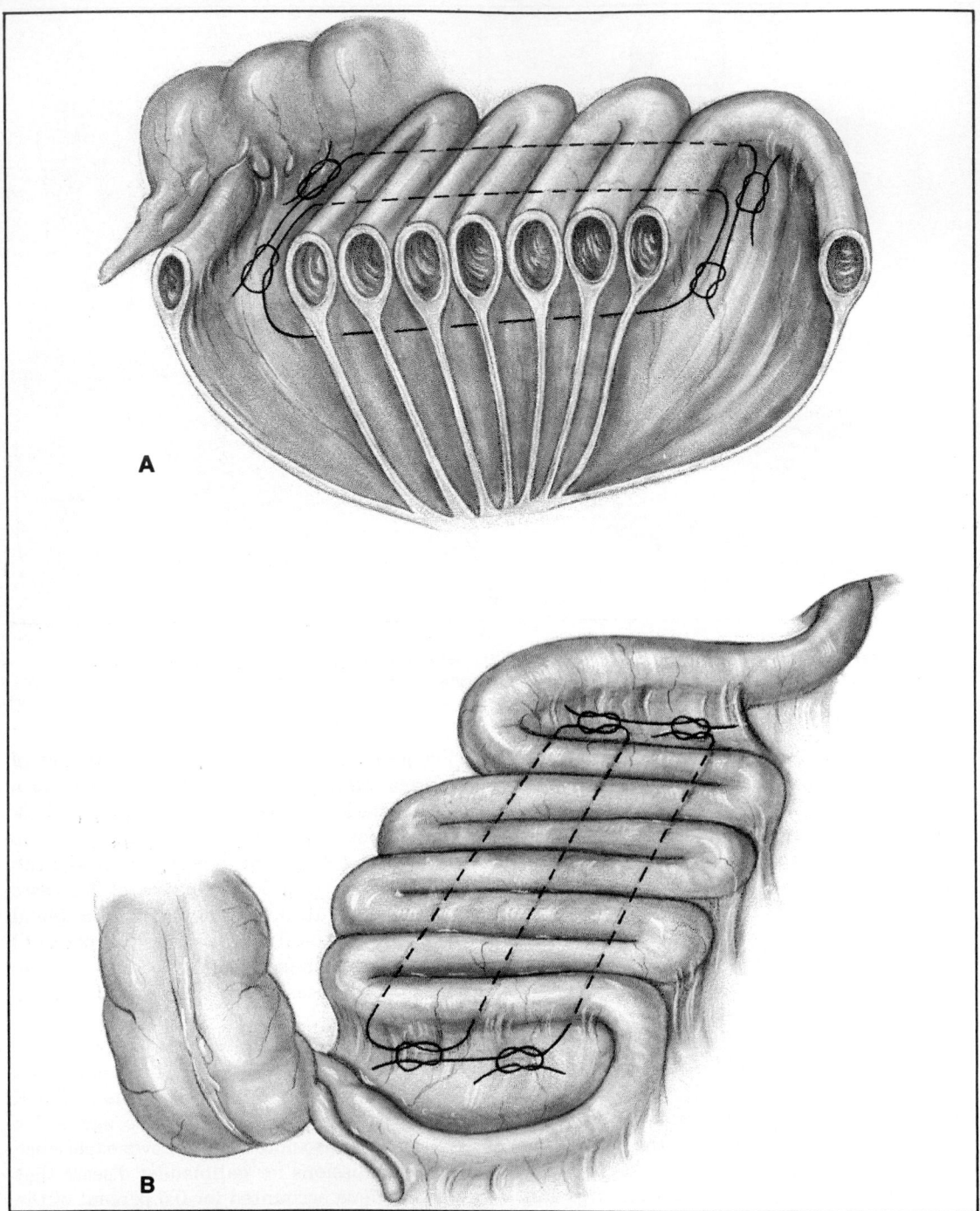

Figure 45–15. Two diagrammatic views of transmesenteric plication. (*Source: From Ellis H, 1982, with permission.*)

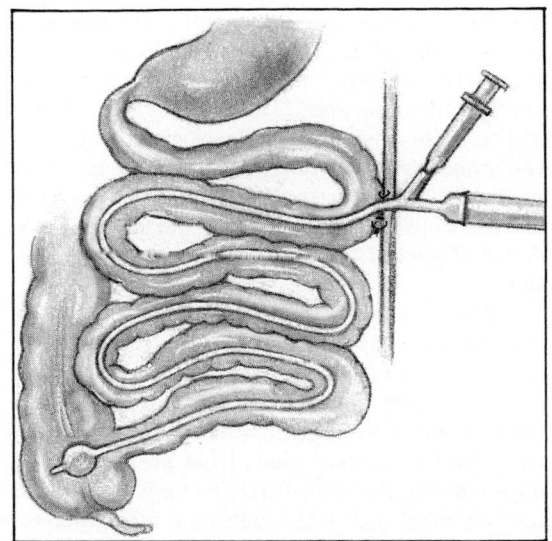

Figure 45–16. Intestinal intubation via a jejunostomy. (*Source: From Ellis H, 1982, with permission.*)

years. A collected review from six Swedish hospitals (Svartholm et al, 1982) reports on 83 cases, 56 of which were female. They ranged in age from 41 to 100, with an average of 75 years.

The incidence of carcinoma of the gallbladder is allegedly higher in the presence of a biliary enteric fistula; Day and Marks (1975) note two examples in their 34 cases of gallstone ileus.

In order to occlude the lumen of the intestine, the gallstone must necessarily be large— 2.5 cm or more in diameter. It is, of course, well recognised that small stones are often passed via the common bile duct into the duodenum and traverse the alimentary canal without further symptoms (Gardner et al, 1966). A minute percentage of such stones may, in fact, form the nucleus of an enterolith that reaches proportions sufficient to obstruct the bowel lumen. The vast majority of gallstones producing ileus, however, are of such size that they can enter the intestinal tract only by a process of ulceration. Most enter via a cholecyst–duodenal fistula, but the stone may ulcerate through the gallbladder wall into the jejunum, ileum, colon, or, rarely, stomach, and, in addition, a large stone impacted in the lower end of the common bile duct may fistulate through the ampulla into the duodenum; an example of this is presented by Wakeley and Willway (1935). Courvoisier (1890) carried out autopsies on 36 cases of gallstone

ileus and located fistula into the duodenum in 25, into the small intestine in 1, into the colon in 1, into both duodenum and colon in 2, and into the common bile duct in 7 of the patients. Wright and Trafford (1953) state that the gallbladder fistula communicates with the duodenum in about 85 percent of cases.

The most common site for impaction of the gallstone is in the lower ileum, but the stone may lodge anywhere along the alimentary canal. Brockis and Gilbert (1957), reviewing 179 cases, found that impaction occurred in the ileum in 72 percent and the jejunum in 17 percent; the remaining 11 percent lodged in the stomach, duodenum, colon, or rectum. The percentage of stones impacted in the colon is small, and instructive cases have been reported by Lloyd Williamson (1952) and by Pryor (1959), who found that a co-existing diverticulitis of the sigmoid loop was the cause for a gallstone obstructing at that level. Middleton and Muscroft (1980) describe impaction of a calculus in the duodenal cap.

A point of considerable practical importance is the relative frequency of recurrent gallstone ileus. Although Rogers and Carter (1958) found only seven reports of recurrence, Fiddian (1959) found that, of 13 cases, two had recurrent obstruction and 3 further patients were found to have two stones contained within the small intestine at the time of the original operation. By 1963, Buetow and colleagues were able to collect 44 published cases of recurrent gallstone ileus and add two more of their own, so that this type appears to constitute approximately 5 percent of all cases. The mortality rate of the second obstruction is 20 percent. Almost 60 percent of the recurrent cases occurred within 30 days of the original obstruction. Examples occurring very soon after the initial obstruction suggest that more than one stone is already present within the alimentary canal, and this is especially likely if the obstructing stone is barrel-shaped with one end concave. Later recurrences are presumably caused by the passage of further stones from the gallbladder reservoir through the fistulous tract into the gut lumen.

Armitage and colleagues (1950) point out that a bile acid enterolith may be difficult to differentiate with the naked eye from a gallstone within the bowel lumen. Such enteroliths may be deposited around a nucleus of a fruit stone or some other foreign material and often form above some obstruction in the bowel—for example, in cases of duodenal or jejunal diverticula. For accurate differentiation, chemical analysis is necessary. The bile enterolith consists mainly of bile acid, whereas gallstones contain considerable amounts of pigment and cholesterol. Gallstones are often radiopaque, whereas the bileacid enteroliths are translucent to x-rays.

Clinical Manifestations. The signs and symptoms are those of intermittent or complete intestinal obstruction. Often there is a history of calculous cholecystitis with recurrent attacks of biliary colic (60 percent of the patients reviewed by Kirkland and Croce in 1961) while in others there is no recognised antecedent. In many cases, the obstruction that results is at first a partial one and may remain relatively mild or intermittent for hours or days, probably as the stone pushes its way along the alimentary canal; but finally, the clinical picture usually becomes that of acute, low smallgut obstruction.

A combination of circumstances results in a delay in diagnosis in a surprisingly high proportion of patients. The present attack may delude the victim into believing that it is merely another episode of biliary colic, which has been experienced in the past and which will probably pass again; the delusion is heightened because the attack is, in fact, often intermittent in nature. The patient is usually elderly and therefore, often neither a good witness nor an especially complaining one. Brown et al (1966) found that of their 13 cases at the Western Infirmary, Glasgow, no less than 6 patients had delays of from 5 to 14 days before admission to hospital. Stitt and colleagues (1967) noted in their 11 cases at St. Michael's Hospital, Toronto, a time lag of 1 to 7 days (with an average of 3) before definitive treatment; in the 28 cases at Cook County Hospital, Chicago (reviewed by Anderson et al, 1967), the average duration was 6.7 days, with a range of 24 hours to 21 days.

The diagnosis should certainly be considered when an elderly female patient, with a previous history of gallbladder disease, presents with features of intestinal obstruction. An extremely rare sign reported by Done and colleagues (1962) is the presence of gallstones in the vomitus; one is not surprised to find that the authors could discover no other published report of this phenomenon.

Radiologic Examination. Rigler et al (1941) consider that preoperative diagnosis can and

should be made more frequently by the help of x-ray investigation. The radiologic criteria that, when present, lead to a positive diagnosis of gallstone ileus are: (1) air or contrast medium in the biliary system, (2) direct visualisation of the stone, or indirect visualisation by contrast media in the intestine, (3) change in position of a previously observed stone, and (4) x-ray evidence of partial or complete intestinal obstruction.

They reviewed 14 known cases of gallstone ileus and, no doubt assisted by hindsight, found positive evidence in 13 patients. All 13 showed gas or contrast medium in the biliary tree; four showed the presence of a stone (in two of them there had been movement from previous x-ray appearance); and one further stone showed on barium meal follow-through as a filling defect. In two additional cases, stones were seen in the gallbladder. Haffner et al (1969), in 20 cases, found pneumobilia in 15 patients and visualised the stone itself in 10.

The presence of air in the biliary tree in a patient with intestinal obstruction is all but pathognomonic. Other causes of gas in the bile passages on radiographic examination are the recent passage of the stone through the common bile duct, a previously performed choledochoenterostomy, a previous wide sphincterotomy, or an emphysematous cholecystitis (Stitt et al, 1967). Figure 45–17 is a reproduction of a plain x-ray photograph of a patient with gallstone ileus.

Treatment. The usual preoperative care is instituted, including suction through a nasogastric tube, fluid and electrolyte replacement by intravenous drip, and blood transfusion if shock is present.

The abdomen should be opened through an adequate right paramedian paraumbilical incision. The distended small intestine is followed down and the diagnosis of gallstone obstruction becomes obvious when a hard mass is encountered at the junction of dilated and collapsed gut. In the majority of instances, the stone is lying surprisingly loosely within the gut lumen and is easily removed through a longitudinal incision, which is then sutured transversely. Naturally, before one opens the bowel, noncrushing clamps are applied above and below and the whole area is carefully packed off.

The stone may be firmly impacted with threatened gangrene or even perforation, both

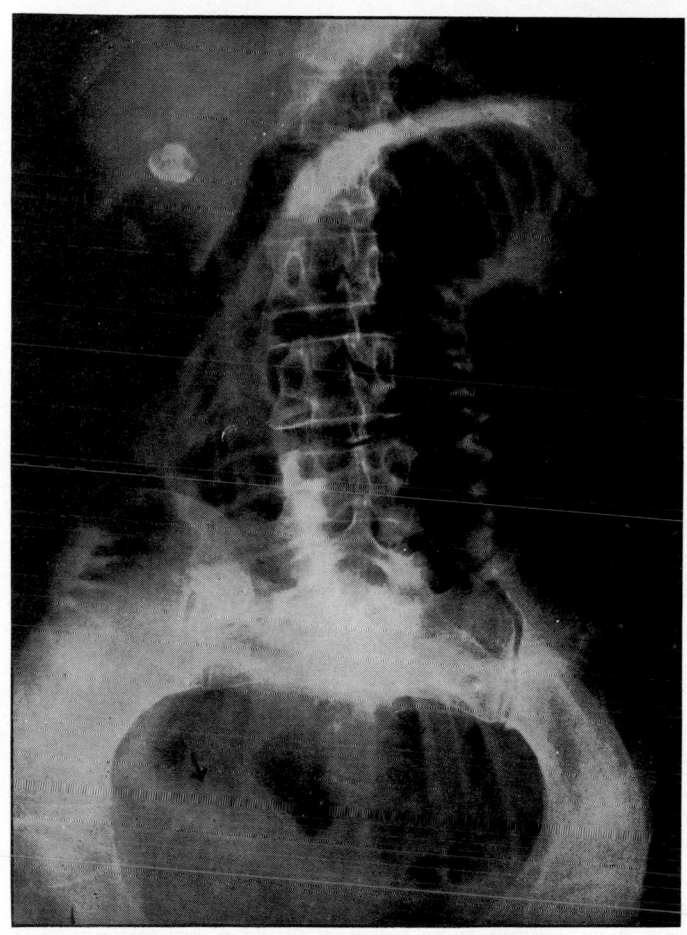

Figure 45–17. Gallstone obstruction. Plain x-ray. Note distended coils of small intestine and the site of the obstruction (*arrow*) caused by large circular gallstone. There is a fairly large gallstone in the gallbladder. The impacted stone in the lower ileum was removed, and the gallbladder was excised 6 weeks later. The 79 year-old female patient made a good recovery. (*R. Maingot's case.*)

fortunately uncommon; resection of the affected portion of the intestine must then be carried out and intestinal continuity restored by end-to-end anastomosis. If the proximal bowel is grossly distended, it should be decompressed by means of a Savage decompressor passed through a separate stab incision.

A gentle but purposeful search of the small and large bowel for other stones should be made, especially if the stone that has been removed is faceted, has a concave surface, or has obviously fragmented.

The gallbladder area should then be palpated. If a large stone is felt, it should be removed by cholecystostomy—unless the general condition of the patient precludes this procedure. The incision in the gallbladder can be sutured tightly, as the gallbladder will be decompressed through its fistula.

Before the patient is discharged from hospital, x-ray investigation of the stomach, duode-num, and gallbladder should be carried out. If a stone or stones cannot be demonstrated on radiologic examination, it is wise to adopt a conservative attitude. If, however, one or more large stones are displayed, or if the patient suffers from recurrent attacks of colic, the correct treatment is elective cholecystectomy.

Buetow and colleagues (1963) advised correction of the fistula and removal of the gallbladder as early as possible after the original emergency exploration because of the risk (already discussed) of recurrent gallstone ileus; indeed, Berliner and Burson (1965) advocate immediate cholecystectomy with repair of the cholecystduodenal fistula at the time of the initial operation for gallstone ileus—providing the patient does not present a prohibitive operative risk. They report three such cases and they are supported by Day and Marks who successfully treated three patients with immediate entero-lithotomy, fistula repair, and cholecystectomy.

These authors stress that this procedure should be reserved for selected low-risk cases.

Although I have treated one of my five patients with gallstone ileus by such an extensive one-stage repair procedure, it could be said that there is little to defend the operation. Most of the patients are old and feeble, often with obstruction that has been present for some days. Providing that the bowel is carefully examined for a second stone and that any remaining massive stone within the gallbladder is removed by cholecystotomy, it is rather unlikely that further stones will fistulate from the gallbladder into the gut lumen, as the majority of fistulae rapidly shrink down once the stone has passed. Certainly, then, a later elective cholecystectomy for persistent biliary symptoms should be carried out, but the added risk of mortality and morbidity precipitated by cholecystectomy and fistula repair at the time of the initial emergency procedure should be avoided.

It is of interest that, on occasions at least, an impacted gallstone may be released by a simple enema or a barium enema. Whitcomb et al (1963) record two cases in which a barium enema refluxing into the terminal ileum disimpacted a gallstone that was subsequently passed per rectum.

Prognosis. The mortality rate of gallstone obstruction is high, for reasons already discussed—the age of the usual patient and delays in diagnosis. As with other forms of intestinal obstruction, however, the picture is becoming slightly less gloomy. Kirkland and Croce (1961) found that before 1940 the mortality rate ranged between 50 and 60 percent in published series, whereas in reviewing cases since 1940 they found a mortality rate of 25 percent. In the patients reported from Scandinavia by Fjermeros (1964) the overall death rate from 1884 has been 45 percent—but in the period 1942 to 1962, it was 34 percent. More recently, Hesselfeldt and Jess (1982) noted 7 deaths in 39 cases in Copenhagen; two of these were in moribund patients. Ferry et al (1982) from Lyon, recorded only one death in 13 gallstone obstructions. In this author's series of five cases, there was one death—this in a patient admitted moribund with advanced obstruction; he died shortly after a "forlorn-hope" enterostomy had been performed under a local anaesthetic.

UNCOMMON AND MISCELLANEOUS CAUSES OF INTESTINAL OBSTRUCTION

One of the fascinations of the acute abdomen is the wide variety of unusual conditions that may be encountered at operation; it is surprising how often rarities seem to occur. The surgeon must be fully aware of these possibilities and fully able to cope with any situation that may be found at laparotomy.

Intraluminal Foreign Bodies

An extraordinarily wide variety of foreign bodies may be introduced into the upper and lower parts of the alimentary tract. Fortunately, the majority pass spontaneously per rectum but occasionally perforation, ulceration, or obstruction may occur. It is the last of these complications that is the main interest here.

Foreign bodies in the bowel may be classified as follows:

1. Swallowed foreign bodies, food, foreign bodies introduced per rectum
2. Bezoars—trichobezoars, phytobezoars, and concretions
3. Worms
4. Transmural migration

Swallowed foreign bodies are particularly likely to be found in children, but other special categories include mental defectives, psychiatric cases, prisoners, and circus side-show performers. Among the wide variety of swallowed objects, two modern variants deserve mention. Dassel and Punjabi (1979) described the ingestion of balloons filled with marijuana by convicts attempting to smuggle this drug into prison. Of their three patients, two presented with obstruction. (The third developed an overdose when the swallowed balloon came undone.) Muhletaler et al (1980) report two cases of partial obstruction due to the packing of a desiccant in bottles of capsules. This may be swallowed inadvertently by partially sighted persons instead of their pills.

Fortunately, if the swallowed object can traverse the oesophagogastric junction then, in the great majority of cases, it is likely to pass through the alimentary canal without causing further harm.

Intestinal obstruction due to impacted food

is rare but has been superbly reviewed by Ward-McQuaid (1950) who collected 178 cases with no fewer than 45 different obstructing agents. Stephens (1966) later raised this to 63 foodstuffs. Heading the list was the persimmon. The skin of this fruit contains shiboul, a cement substance that is precipitated by the acid in the stomach and agglutinates the seeds and fibres into a type of bezoar. The majority of obstructing food materials are those rich in fibre, dessicated fruits that swell when they take up water, or substances resistant to the digestive enzymes.

There are two other important predisposing factors. Mastication is often absent or inefficient, either because the patient is edentulous or because the food was bolted. The other factor is that the patient has had a previous partial gastrectomy or a gastroenterostomy. In these instances, the stoma allows the bolus to pass easily into the upper small intestine. Norberg (1961) has reviewed 28 examples of intestinal obstruction in 26 patients (2 having had 2 episodes of obstruction). The causative agents were orange in 25 cases, and 1 example each of apple, grapefruit, and some fruit-like material. Every one of these patients had undergone a previous partial gastrectomy.

Clinical Manifestations. Large numbers of cases probably never come to the surgeon or indeed hospital. They settle down after an attack of acute central abdominal pain followed by passage of the offending material. The signs and symptoms are typical of intestinal obstruction but unless there is a clear-cut history, the diagnosis of food impaction is unlikely to be made. It should certainly be suspected in an edentulous patient who has undergone a previous partial gastrectomy and who admits to ingestion of a large amount of fruit material.

Treatment. If the condition is suspected, a short period of conservative treatment is indicated. In most cases coming to surgery, the specific diagnosis is not made until laparotomy. The site of impaction is usually the lower ileum and the affected loop is swollen, reddened, and oedematous. Once it is obvious that the obstruction is due to an intraluminal bolus, this can frequently be broken up and milked into the caecum, from whence spontaneous passage takes place. If this cannot be done easily, or if the viability of the bowel is jeopardised, then

enterostomy and removal of the occluding material or even a localised resection may be needed.

Personal Cases. This author has dealt with eight patients with food bolus obstruction while at Westminster, six of whom required laparotomy. In four, the material had impacted into the terminal ileum and could be milked into the caecum. In three of these, the food material was not identified, but in the fourth, it was a mass of chestnuts. One patient, with two segments of orange caught in a loop of intestine tethered by adhesions from a previous laparotomy, required an enterotomy. A further patient with inspissated mushrooms in the terminal ileum required resection because the distended segment of bowel perforated during delivery. Two patients were treated conservatively; one was a child with "tiger" nuts impacted in the rectum and the second was a patient who had swallowed half an orange the evening following total dental extraction. Fortunately the offending object was passed naturally.

Bezoars

Bezoars are concretions found in the stomach and intestine, both in man and other animals, particularly in goats and sheep.

Trichobezoars consist of matted masses of hair and are usually encountered in young girls who get into the habit of trichophagy (hair swallowing).

Phytobezoars are made up of vegetable material. About 75 percent of reported cases are due to ingestion of persimmon but other fruits and vegetables with a high fibre and cellulose content may be responsible.

Concretions are unusual but have been reported in workers using furniture polish made up of a strong alcoholic solution of shellac, as well as in patients taking large amounts of magnesium, sodium carbonate, or aluminium hydroxide gel.

Bezoars may produce ulceration (resulting in GI haemorrhage), perforation, and intestinal obstruction. In their classic review of bezoars, DeBakey and Ochsner (1938, 1939) found that trichobezoars were complicated by obstruction in 10 percent of cases and phytobezoars in 25 percent.

Worms

Intestinal obstruction due to masses of round worms (*Ascaris lumbricoides*) is common in Africa and in the Far East, but now, with international travel so common, surgeons in temperate countries should not ignore this possibility.

Obstruction is particularly likely to occur in children and young adults (Ihekwaba, 1980). Louw (1966) found that this amounted to the second most common cause of acute abdominal emergency admission to the Children's Hospital in Cape Town, next only to appendicitis. Impaction may occur anywhere along the small intestine but is particularly common in the terminal ileum. Obstruction may be precipitated by a recently taken vermifuge, which may result in a solid mass of tightly packed dead worms in the intestine.

The diagnosis of ascariasis as the causative agent of obstruction is based on a previous history of worms, vomiting of worms, the presence of worms or ova in the stools, and a palpable mass, which was present in 63 percent of Louw's 68 cases. Characteristically this is putty-like in consistency and commonly below and to the right or to the left of the umbilicus.

Treatment. In mild cases, conservative treatment is initiated, but antihelminthics or purgatives should be avoided until the attack has settled because dead or dying worms tend to convert a partial into a complete obstruction.

In the more acute cases, or when the diagnosis is in doubt, laparotomy is performed. The mass of worms should, if possible, be milked through the ileocaecal valve into the colon. If fragmentation is not possible or if the bowel is not viable, then Louw recommends resection as being safer and more satisfactory than enterotomy.

Transmural Migration

A rare cause of intestinal obstruction is the migration of a foreign body into the stomach, duodenum, or bowel with subsequent impaction. Such incidents have been reported in gunshot wounds in which the missile had not been removed from the peritoneal cavity and subsequently ulcerated into the gut lumen. Laparotomy packs and surgical instruments may also behave in such a manner, but not unnaturally such accidents are rarely reported.

Intraluminal Obstruction of the Rectum

The rectum, a storage organ, is well adapted to its function and in consequence it is unusually obstructed by its contents. Even when this does happen, the obstruction is rarely total.

Faecal impaction is particularly likely to occur in elderly debilitated bed-bound patients. Impaction may occur as a result of inspissation of barium sulphate after a barium enema examination or if the patient had undergone a barium meal examination immediately before laparotomy and the contrast has not been eliminated from the bowel.

Faecal impaction may occur in patients who are receiving large doses of codeine, anticholinergic drugs, or other constipating agents. Spira et al (1975) have reported five examples of faecal impaction presenting with acute obstruction in drug addicts following methadone ingestion.

For size and variety of foreign objects placed within the orifices of the human body, pride of place goes to the rectum. Although requiring great ingenuity on the part of the surgeon for their removal, they rarely produce intestinal obstruction.

Drugs Causing Intestinal Obstruction

Potassium chloride strictures of the small bowel are perhaps the best example of drug-induced intestinal obstruction. However, a large variety of drugs may induce this emergency and, although uncommon, it is never less important, because failure to recognise this condition may in some cases lead to unnecessary operation. In addition, a wide knowledge of these problems could reduce the incidence of this situation.

George (1980) has given a masterly brief review of this subject. He classifies the drug induced causes as follows:

1. Within the lumen:
   a. inspissated barium sulphate following radiologic investigation (see the section on Foreign Bodies)
   b. potassium salts producing mucosal ulceration and stricture
2. Within the wall:
   a. anticoagulants producing intramural haematoma of the small intestine
   b. drugs affecting smooth muscle—antihistamines, opiates, clonidine

c. drugs interfering with parasympathetic nerve transmission—autonomic ganglion blockers, muscarinic antagonists. The tricyclic antidepressants also have powerful anticholinergic action and may cause ileus

3. Outside the wall:
  a. drugs causing mesenteric vascular occlusion—contraceptive pill, steroids
  b. practolol
  c. irradiation from thorum and radioactive gold

Potassium chloride stricture and practolol-induced peritonitis are of particular interest and require further consideration.

Potassium Chloride Stricture

In the 1960s, a number of reports noted a surprising increase in the incidence of small bowel ulcers and then their probable iatrogenic origin. Thus Baker et al reported in 1964 12 patients with primary ulceration and stenosis of the small intestine, 11 of whom had received enteric-coated preparations containing potassium chloride.

Lawrason et al (1965) confirmed this association in an extensive survey of hospitals in the United States. Dogs and monkeys were then given diuretics and potassium chloride alone or in combination, either in the ordinary form or in enteric-coated capsules. Ulcerative lesions were easily produced in the intestine of monkeys, but only rarely in dogs, when the animals were given thiazide–potassium chloride tablets, but were not found when the diuretic was given alone. A rash of reports of strictures of the small intestine following thiazide and potassium chloride combined therapy soon followed. Abbruzzese and Gooding (1965) stressed the importance of early recognition of this syndrome since the symptoms might resolve after discontinuation of medication. I have personally dealt with two cases of potassium chloride stricture presenting with intestinal obstruction (Fig. 45–18).

Enteric-coated potassium chloride tablets are no longer being used but cases still occur from time to time, as shown by a report by Tresadern et al (1977) where a child accidentally ingested enteric-coated potassium chloride tablets and developed multiple small bowel strictures.

Ideally, potassium supplements should be given in the diet or in liquid form, but potassium chloride solution is unpalatable. This led to the

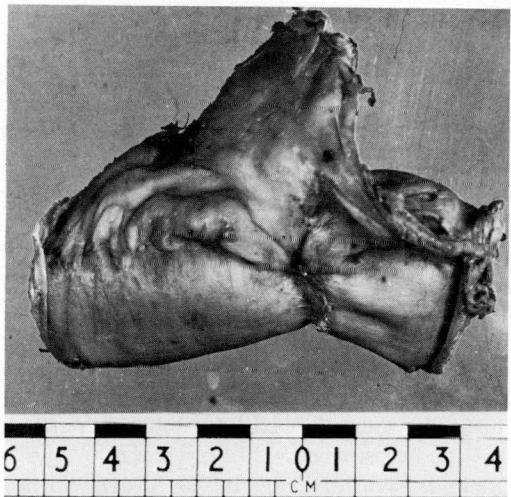

Figure 45–18. A stricture at the jejunoileal junction due to potassium chloride ingestion. (*Source: From Ellis H, 1982, with permission.*)

formulation of potassium chloride in a wax spongy matrix (slow-K). However, if intestinal transit time is delayed by general debility, immobility, drug therapy, or a low volume high calorie liquid diet, then even this preparation can produce ulceration and stricture formation in the small intestine (Farquharson Roberts et al, 1975).

Practolol-Induced Sclerosing Peritonitis

Practolol-induced sclerosing peritonitis was first described by Brown and colleagues in 1974. By 1977, Jackson noted that 60 additional cases were now known and reported 6 more patients with this condition. The pathology is quite extraordinary; the entire small intestine is surrounded by a membrane of fibrous material which causes shortening and angulation of the bowel and which, in turn, results in subacute intestinal obstruction. The membrane may also extend over the large intestine, stomach, and liver but does not normally cause compression of these organs.

The patient presents with symptoms and signs of subacute obstruction and there is often a palpable mobile mass within the abdomen. At operation, the small intestine is found matted together and encased in a white fibrous membrane, which represents the mobile mass which is so often palpable. It is necessary to strip this membrane away completely, thus exposing the normal serosa of the intestine from the duodenum to the terminal ileum. Fortunately, a plane of cleavage exists between the membrane and the underlying intestine, which is avascular and enables the surgeon to dissect and strip the membrane from the wall.

Eltringham and colleagues (1977), reporting an additional nine patients from Bristol, found that subsequent progress following this stripping operation was entirely satisfactory with a period of follow-up of a maximum of 20 months.

Although this drug (a β-adrenergic blocking agent) has now been withdrawn in the United Kingdom, it is still possible that patients may inadvertently be taking practolol and it may be that other drugs in the future will produce this mysterious phenomenon. Marigold et al (1982) note that two patients have been described who might have sclerosing peritonitis and had been treated with propranolol, another two who have been on oxyprenolol, and an additional patient treated with tenolol. The mechanism for this condition appears to be entirely unknown. Myllarniemi and Leppaniemi (1981) have carried out electron microscopy in three cases and have found no evidence of mesothelial cells with their characteristic microvilli. They suggest that the process is one of destruction of the mesothelium with progressive connective tissue formation.

Patients developing this peculiar membrane have been reported in whom there has been no question of ingestion of any drug. In a fascinating report from Singapore, Foo and colleagues (1978) record 10 cases of this condition in young women within the narrow age range of 13 to 18 years in which the obstruction was due to a membrane encasing the small bowel in the manner of a cocoon. In none was there any previous history of abdominal surgery, peritonitis, or drug ingestion. A further case has been reported from Israel by Sayfan et al (1979) in a girl aged 12.

Radiotherapy Stricture

Abdominal or pelvic radiotherapy may produce severe pathologic changes in both small and large bowel, resulting in ulceration, fistula formation, dense adhesions, and stricture. Irradiation injury to the bowel is particularly likely to follow radiotherapy in the treatment of uterine carcinoma. Joelsson and Raf (1973) collected 24 cases of small intestine stricture following radiotherapy for carcinoma of the uterus out of an estimated 3000 patients treated in Stockholm, an incidence of about 0.7 percent. They pointed out that this is particularly likely to occur if a loop of small intestine has become adherent in the pelvis as a result of previous surgery or inflammatory disease. Of their 24 cases, 15 had previous abdominal surgery and 5 more had adhesions to the genital organs. Jackson (1976) has carried out an important study of irradiation damage to the bowel. Of his 52 patients, 25 followed radiotherapy for cervical carcinoma and another 13 had radiotherapy for bladder cancer. The time interval ranged from a few months to 5 years or more. Small bowel stricture occurred in 14 of his cases and colorectal stricture in an additional 21 cases.

The treatment of postirradiation stricture of either the small or the large intestine may be both technically extremely difficult and also hazardous for the patient. The pelvis may be frozen with dense fibrosis as a result of the radiotherapy so that dissection in this situation with obliteration of the normal anatomic planes is difficult with a high risk of damage to the bowel itself, to the bladder, and to the lower ends of the ureters. Although there is often no clinical evidence of intestinal damage a few centimetres away from the strictured area of the bowel, the microscopic extent of radiation damage may be much greater than is detected by naked eye, and this particularly applies to the blood vessels. Jackson, therefore, advises wide resection of lesions of the small intestine with temporary loop ileostomy. For large bowel strictures, he recommends resection and restoration of continuity with a covering colostomy when the pelvis is free from fibrosis. If the lesion is low in the rectum and dissection is difficult, however, a Hartmann-type operation is used. In this way anastomotic breakdown is prevented and poor healing of the irradiated perineum, which may be seen after abdominoperineal resection, is avoided.

BIBLIOGRAPHY

Adult Intussusception

Aston SJ, Machleder HI: Intussusception in the adult. Am Surg 41:576, 1975

Brayton D, Norris WJ: Intussusception in adults. Am J Surg 88:32, 1954

Cole GJ: A review of 436 cases of intestinal obstruction in Ibadan. Gut 6:151, 1965

Das Gupta TK, Brasfield RD: Metastatic melanoma of the gastrointestinal tract. Arch Surg 88:969, 1964

Donhauser JL, Kelly EC: Intussusception in the adult. Am J Surg 79:673, 1950

Edna TH: Colo rectal intussusception due to leiomyoma. Acta Chir Scand 144:409, 1978

Goodall P: Intussusception in adults complicating specific inflammatory diseases of the intestine. Gut 4:132, 1963

Hanson EL, Goodkin L, et al: Ileocolic intussusception in an adult caused by a granuloma of the appendix stump: Report of a case. Ann Surg 166:150, 1967

Harkins HN: Intussusception due to invaginated Meckel's diverticulum. Report of two cases with a study of 160 cases collected from the literature. Ann Surg 98:1070, 1933

Kark AE, Rundle WJ: The pattern of intussusception in Africans in Natal. Br J Surg 48: 296, 1960

Lavery IC, Fazio VW: Intussusception following jejunoileal bypass for morbid obesity. Report of a case. Dis Colon Rectum 21:128, 1978

Roper A: Intussusception in adults. Surg Gynecol Obstet 103:267, 1956

Weilbaecher D, Bolin JA, et al: Intussusception in adults. Am J Surg 121:531, 1971

Wychulis AR, Jackman RJ, et al: Submucous lipomas of the colon and rectum. Surg Gynecol Obstet 118:337, 1964

Volvulus

Ackerman NB, Abou-Mourad NN: Obstructive, pseudo-obstructive and enteropathic syndromes after jejunoileal bypass. Surg Gynecol Obstet 148:168, 1979

Agarwal RL, Misra MK: Volvulus of the small intestine in northern India. Am J Surg 120:366, 1970

Andersen DA: Volvulus in western India. A clinical study of forty cases with particular reference to the conservative treatment of pelvic colon volvulus. Br J Surg 44:132, 1956

Anderson JR, Lee D: Acute caecal volvulus. Br J Surg 67:39, 1980

Anderson JR, Lee D, et al: Volvulus of the transverse colon. Br J Surg 68:179, 1981

Anderson MJ, Okike N, et al: The colonoscope in cecal volvulus. Report of three cases. Dis Colon Rectum 21:71, 1978

Blumberg NA: Volvulus of the splenic flexure: Report of a case with a review of the literature. Br J Surg 46:292, 1958

Boulvin R, Esphahani A, et al: 494 cas de volvulus aigu du colon. Mem Acad Chirurgie (Paris) 95:467, 1969

Bruusgaard C: Volvulus of the sigmoid colon. Surgery 22:466, 1947

Bystrom J, Backman L, et al: Volvulus of the caecum. An analysis of 40 cases and the value of various surgical methods. Acta Chir Scand 138:624, 1972

Carter R, Hinshaw DB: Acute sigmoid volvulus in children. Am J Dis Child 101:631, 1961

Donhauser JL, Atwell S: Volvulus of the caecum. A review of 100 cases in the literature and a report of six new cases. Arch Surg 58:129, 1949

Dowling BL, Gunning AJ: Caecal volvulus. Br J Surg 56:124, 1969

Dowse JLA: Meckel's diverticulum. Br J Surg 48:392, 1961

Duke JH, Yar MS: Primary small bowel volvulus. Arch Surg 112:685, 1977

Grave GF: Large bowel volvulus. Br J Hosp Med 15:66, 1976

Halvorsen JF, Semb BHK: Volvulus of the right colon. A review of thirty cases with special reference to the late results of various surgical procedures. Acta Chir Scand 141:804, 1975

Hinshaw DB, Carter R: Surgical management of acute volvulus of the sigmoid colon. A study of 55 cases. Ann Surg 146:52, 1957

Hinshaw DB, Carter R, et al: Volvulus of the cecum or right colon. A study of 14 cases. Am J Surg 98:175, 1959

Hughes LE: Sigmoid volvulus. J Roy Soc Med 73:78, 1980

Hughes M: A case of Bilharzia of the appendix with strangulation of ileum. Br J Surg 36:428, 1949

Johnston IDA, Gibson JB: Megacolon and volvulus in psychotics. Br J Surg 47: 394, 1960

Jordan GL, Beahrs OH: Volvulus of cecum as a postoperative complication: Report of six cases. Ann Surg 137:245, 1953

Kallio KE: Knotenbildungen des darmes. Acta Chir Scand (suppl)70:21, 1932

Kaltiala EH, Lenkkeri H, et al: Mechanical intestinal obstruction (an analysis of 577 cases). Ann Chir Gynaecol 61:87, 1972

Khoury GA, Pickard R, et al: Volvulus of the sigmoid colon. Br J Surg 64:587, 1977

Kohn SG, Briele HA, et al: Volvulus complicating pregnancy. Am J Obstet Gynecol 48:398, 1944

Krippaehne WW, Vetto M, et al: Volvulus of the ascending colon. A report of 22 patients. Am J Surg 114:323, 1967

Lantieri R, Teplock SK, et al: Splenic flexure volvulus: Two case reports and review. AJR 132:463, 1979

McGraw JP, Kremen AJ, et al: The roentgen diagnosis of volvulus of the cecum. Surgery 24:793, 1948

McIver MA: Acute intestinal obstruction—General considerations. Am J Surg 19:172, 1933

Mikal S, Byers JA: Closed loop obstruction of the ileum due to an appendiceal knot. JAMA 160:49, 1956

O'Connor JL: Reduction of sigmoid volvulus by flexible sigmoidoscopy. Arch Surg 114:1092, 1979

O'Mara CS, Wilson TH, et al: Cecal volvulus. Analysis

of fifty patients with long-term follow-up. Ann Surg 189:724, 1979

Osime U: Volvulus of the sigmoid colon. J Roy Coll Surg (Edinburgh) 25:32, 1980

Peterson L: Beitrag zur Kenntnis des ileum terminale fixatum und ileus ilei terminalis fixati. Acta Chir Scand (suppl):32, 1934

Prather JR, Bowers RF: Surgical management of volvulus of the sigmoid. Arch Surg 85:869, 1962

Rose I: Volvulus of caecum, associated with putrid puerperial endometritis and gangrenous vulvitis. Br Med J 2:577, 1941

Saidi F: The high incidence of intestinal volvulus in Iran. Gut 10:838, 1969

Shepherd JL: The epidemiology and clinical presentation of sigmoid volvulus. Br J Surg 56:353, 1969

Simons P: Volvulus of the caecum and pre-eclampsia complicating labour. Am J Obstet Gynecol 57:448, 1950

Sinha RS: A clinical appraisal of volvulus of the pelvic colon. Br J Surg 56:838, 1969

Smith WR, Goodwin JN: Cecal volvulus. Am J Surg 126:215, 1973

Startling JR: Initial treatment of sigmoid volvulus by colonoscopy. Ann Surg 190:36, 1979

String ST, De Cosse JJ: Sigmoid volvulus. An examination of the mortality. Am J Surg 121:293, 1971

Taha SE, Suleiman SI: Volvulus of the sigmoid colon in the Gezira. Br J Surg 67:433, 1980

Vaez-Zadeh K, Dutz W, et al: Volvulus of the small intestine in adults. A study of predisposing factors. Ann Surg 169:265, 1969

Ver Steeg KR, Whithead WA: Ileosigmoid knot. Arch Surg 115:761, 1980

Wapnick S: Treatment of intestinal volvulus. Ann R Coll Surg 53:57, 1973

Wapnick S, Grosberg S, et al: Volvulus of the Kock reservoir. Dis Colon Rectum 22:55, 1979

Wertkin MG, Aufses AH: Management of volvulus of the colon. Dis Colon Rectum 21:40, 1978

White A: Intestinal obstruction in the Rhodesian African. East Afr Med J 38:525, 1961

Wilson R: Volvulus of the cecum. Can J Surg 8:363, 1965

Wolfer JA, Beaton LE, et al: Volvulus of the cecum. Anatomical factors in its etiology: Report of a case. Surg Gynecol Obstet 74:882, 1942

Zinkin LD, Katz LD, et al: Volvulus of the transverse colon. Report of a case and review of the literature. Dis Colon Rectum 22:492, 1979

Apertures and Intraabdominal Hernias

Andrews E: Duodenal hernias—A misnomer. Surg Gynecol Obstet 37:740, 1923

Blandin PF: Traite D'Anatomie Topographique, 2 edt. Paris: Germer-Bailliere, 1834

Fiddian RV: Herniation through mesenteric and mesocolic defects. Br J Surg 49:186, 1961

Garden OJ, Kahn JS, et al: Internal strangulation through a terminal ileal mesenteric defect. J R Coll Surg (Edinburgh) 25:198, 1980

Hansmann GH, Morton SA: Intra-abdominal hernia. Report of a case and review of the literature. Arch Surg 39:933, 1939

Jamart J, Guillemin F, et al: Hernies transepiploiques. Lyon Chirurgical 76:49, 1980

Janin Y, Stone AM, et al: Mesenteric hernia. Surg Gynecol Obstet 150:747, 1980

Longacre JJ: Mesentericoparietal hernia. Duodenal hernias of Treitz. Surg Gynecol Obstet 59:165, 1934

Meade HS: Hernias through the mesentery of the ileocaecal junction. Irish J Med Sci 6:103, 1942

Neve A: Hernia into the foramen of Winslow; laparotomy; recovery. Lancet 1:1172, 1892

Orr KB: Strangulated internal hernia: An unusual case. Med J Austral 1:1025, 1966

Schwartz HF: Herniation through the foramen of Winslow. Report of a case. Dis Colon Rectum 20:521, 1977

Thoren L: Right para-duodenal mesocolic hernia. Acta Chir Scand 144:267, 1978

Treves F: The anatomy of the intestinal canal and peritoneum in man. Br Med J 1:470, 1885

Werbin N, Mazor A, et al: Incarceration of the small bowel within congenital hernia in the falciform ligament. Harefua 96:193, 1979 (in Hebrew with an English summary)

Willwerth BM, Zollinger RM, et al: Congenital mesocolic (paraduodenal) hernia. Embryological basis of repair. Am J Surg 128:358, 1974

Zimmerman LM, Anson BJ: Anatomy and Surgery of Hernia, 2 edt. Baltimore: Williams and Wilkins, 1967

Zinkin LD, Moore D: Herniation of the cecum through the foramen of Winslow. Dis Colon Rectum 23:276, 1980

Adhesions

Baker JW: A long jejunostomy tube for decompressing intestinal obstruction. Surg Gynecol Obstet 109:519, 1959

Boys F: The prophylaxis of peritoneal adhesions. A review of the literature. Surgery 11:118, 1942

Buckman RF, Buckman PD, et al: A physiological basis for the adhesion-free healing of deperitonealized surfaces. J Surg Res 21:67, 1976

Buckman R, Woods M, et al: A unifying mechanism in the etiology of intraperitoneal adhesions. J Surg Res 20:1, 1976

Childs WA, Phillips RB: Experience with intestinal plication and a proposed modification. Ann Surg 152:258, 1960

Connoly JE, Smith JW: The prevention and treatment of intestinal adhesions. Surg Gynecol Obstet 110:417, 1960

Ellis H: The aetiology of post-operative abdominal adhesions. Br J Surg 50:10, 1962

Ellis H: The cause and prevention of post-operative intraperitoneal adhesions. Surg Gynecol Obstet 133:497, 1971

Ellis H: Intestinal Obstruction. New York: Appleton-Century Crofts, 1982

Ellis H: The causes and prevention of intestinal adhesions. Br J Surg 69:241, 1982

Festen C: Post-operative small bowel obstruction in infants and children. Ann Surg 196:580, 1982

Fleschn: Thebesius Über ileus durch Verwachsungen und Stränge. Deutsche Zeitschrift fur Chirurgie 157:60, 1920

Hollender LF, Otten F, et al: La plicature mesenterique selon Childs et Phillips. Lyon Chirurgical 67:24, 1971

McIver MA: Acute intestinal obstruction: General considerations. Arch Surg 25:1098, 1932

Miller EM, Winfield JM: Acute intestinal obstruction secondary to post-operative adhesions. Arch Surg 78:952, 1959

Moss N, McFetridge EM: Acute intestinal obstruction. A comparative study of 511 cases. Ann Surg 100:158, 1934

Munro A, Jones PF: Operative intubation in the treatment of complicated small bowel obstruction. Br J Surg 65:123, 1978

Noble TB: Plication of small intestine as prophylaxis against adhesions. Am J Surg 05:41, 1937

Perry JF, Smith GA, et al: Intestinal obstruction caused by adhesions: A review of 388 cases. Ann Surg 142:810, 1955

Playforth RH, Holloway JB, et al: Mechanical small bowel obstruction: A plea for earlier surgical intervention. Ann Surg 171:783, 1970

Raf LE: Causes of small intestinal obstruction. A study covering the Stockholm area. Acta Chir Scand 135:67, 1969

Raftery AT: Effect of peritoneal trauma on peritoneal fibrinolytic activity and intraperitoneal adhesion formation. An experimental study in the rat. Eur Surg Res 13:397, 1981

Robbins GF, Brunschwig A, et al: Deperitonealization: A clinical and experimetnal observation. Ann Surg 130:466, 1949

Souttar HS: Contribution in: Discussion on acute intestinal obstruction. Br Med J 2:1000, 1925

Stewardson RH, Bombeck T, et al: Critical operative management of small bowel obstruction. Ann Surg 187:189, 1978

Vick RM: Statistics of acute intestinal obstruction. Br Med J 2:546, 1932

Weibel MA, Majno G: Peritoneal adhesions and their relation to abdominal surgery. Am J Surg 126:345, 1973

Wichmann SE: Uber die Peritonisierung von Wundflachen am Dunndarm. Langenbeck Archiv fur Klinische Chirurgie 179:589, 1934

Gallstone Ileus

Anderson RE, Woodward N, et al: Gallstone obstruction of the intestine. Surg Gynecol Obstet 125:540, 1967

Andersson A, Zederfeldt B: Gallstone ileus. Acta Chir Scand 135:713, 1969

Armitage G, Gowweather FS, et al: Observations on bileacid enteroliths with an account of a recent case. Br J Surg 38:21, 1950

Berliner SD, Burson LC: One stage repair for cholecystduodenal fistula and gallstone ileus. Arch Surg 90:313, 1965

Brockis JG, Gilbert MC: Intestinal obstruction by gallstones. A record of 179 cases. Br J Surg 44:461, 1957

Brown DB, Kerr IF, et al: Gallstone obstruction. Br J Surg 53:672, 1966

Beutow GW, Glaubitz JP, et al: Recurrent gallstone ileus. Surgery 54:716, 1963

Courvoiser LG: Beitrage zu Pathologie und Chirurgie der Gallenwage, Leipzig: FCW Vogel, 1980

Day EA, Marks C: Gallstone ileus. Review of the literature and presentation of thirty-four new cases. Am J Surg 129:552, 1975

Ferry C, Godard J, et al: L'ileus biliare. 13 cas chez 12 malades. Lyon Chirurgical 78:233, 1982

Fiddian RV: Gallstone ileus—Recurrences, multiple stones. Postgrad Med J 35:673, 1959

Fjermeros HF: Gallstone ileus. Acta Chir Scand 128:186, 1964

Gardner AMN, Holden WS, et al: Disappearing gallstones. Br J Surg 53:114, 1966

Haffner JFW, Semb LS, et al: Gallstone ileus. A report of 22 cases. Acta Chir Scand 135:707, 1969

Hesselfeldt P, Jess P: Gallstone ileus. A review of 39 cases with emphasis on surgical treatment. Acta Chir Scand 148:431, 1982

Hudspeth AS, McGuirt WF: Gallstone ileus. A continuing surgical problem. Arch Surg 100:668, 1970

Kasahara Y, Umemura H, et al: Gallstone ileus. Review of 112 patients in the Japanese literature. Am J Surg 140:437, 1980

Kirkland KC, Croce EJ: Gallstone intestinal obstruction. A review of the literature and presentation of 12 cases including 3 recurrences. JAMA 176:494, 1961

Lloyd Williamson JCF: Obstruction of the colon by gallstone. Br J Surg 39:339, 1952

McLaughlin CW, Raines M: Obstruction of the alimentary tract from gallstones. Am J Surg 81:424, 1951

Middleton MD, Muscroft TJ: Duodenal obstruction due to gallstones. J R Coll Surg Edinburgh 25:41, 1980

Naunyn B: A Treatise on Cholelithiasis. London: New Sydenham Society, 1892

Pryor JH: Gallstone obstruction of the sigmoid colon with particular reference to aetiology. Br J Surg 47:259, 1959

Rigler LG, Borman CW, et al: Gallstone obstruction.

Pathogenesis and roentgen manifestations. JAMA 117:1753, 1941

Rogers FA, Carter R: Recurrent gallstone ileus. Am J Surg 96:379, 1958

Stitt RB, Heslin DJ, et al: Gallstone ileus. Br J Surg 54:673, 1967

Svartholm E, Andren-Sandberg A, et al: Diagnosis and treatment of gallstone ileus. Acta Chir Scand 148:435, 1982

Wakeley CPG, Willway FW: Intestinal obstruction by gallstones. Br J Surg 23:377, 1935

Whitcomb JG, Broome DA, et al: Barium enema reduction of gallstone ileus. Am J Surg 106:592, 1963

Wright PJM, Trafford PA: Gallstone ileus. Br J Surg 41:6, 1953

Miscellaneous

Abbruzzese AA, Gooding CA: Reversal of small bowel obstruction: Withdrawal of hydrochlorthiazide potassium chloride therapy. JAMA 192:781, 1965

Baker DR, Schrader WH, et al: Small bowel ulceration apparently associated with thiazide and potassium therapy. JAMA 190:586, 1964

Brown P, Baddeley H, et al: Sclerosing peritonitis, an unusual reaction to a β-adrenergic blocking drug (practolol). Lancet 2:1477, 1974

Dassel PM, Punjabi E: Ingested marijuana-filled balloons. Gastroenterology 76:166, 1979

DeBakey M, Ochsner A: Bezoars and concretions. A comprehensive review of the literature with analysis of 303 collected cases and presentation of 8 additional cases. Surgery 4,5:934, 132, 1938, 1939

Eltringham WK, Espiner HJ, et al: Sclerosing peritonitis due to practolol: A report on nine cases and their surgical management. Br J Surg 64:229, 1977

Farquhason-Roberts MA, Giddings AEB, et al: Perforation of small bowel due to slow release of potassium chloride (Slow-K). Br Med J 3:206, 1975

Foo KT, Ng KC, et al: Unusual small intestinal obstruction in adolescent girls: The abdominal cocoon. Br J Surg 65:427, 1978

George CF: Drugs causing intestinal obstruction: A review. J R Soc Med 73:200, 1980

Ihekwaba FN: Intestinal ascariasis and the acute abdomen in the tropics. J R Coll Surg Edinburgh 25:452, 1980

Jackson BT: Bowel damage from irradiation. Proc R Soc Med 69:683, 1976

Jackson BT: Surgical treatment of sclerosing peritonitis due to practolol. Br J Surg 64:255, 1977

Joelsson I, Raf L: Late injuries of the small intestine following radiotherapy for uterine carcinoma. Acta Chir Scand 139:194, 1973

Lawrason FD, Alpert E, et al: Ulcerative–obstructive lesions of the small intestine. JAMA 191:105, 1965

Louw JH: Abdominal complications of Ascaris lumbricoides infestation in children. Br J Surg 53:510, 1966

Marigold JH, Pounder RE, et al: Propranolol, oxyprenolol and sclerosing peritonitis. Br Med J 284:870, 1982

Muhletaler CA, Gerlock AJ, et al: The pill bottle dessicant. A cause of partial gastrointestinal obstruction. JAMA 243:1921, 1980

Myllarniemi H, Leppaniemi A: Peritoneal fibrosis due to practolol. Scanning electron microscopical and histological observations. Acta Chir Scand 147:137, 1981

Norberg PB: Intestinal obstruction due to food. Surg Gynecol Obstet 113:149, 1961

Sayfan J, Adam YG, et al: Peritoneal encapsulation in childhood. Am J Surg 138:725, 1979

Spira IA, Rubenstein R, et al: Fecal impaction following methadone ingestion simulating acute intestinal obstruction. Ann Surg 181:15, 1975

Stephens FO: Intestinal colic caused by food. Gut 7:581, 1966

Tresadern J, Rickwood AMK, et al: Multiple small bowel strictures in a child and accidental potassium chloride ingestion. Br Med J 2:1124, 1977

Ward-McQuaid N: Intestinal obstruction due to food. Br Med J 2:1106, 1950

46. Intestinal Resection and Anastomosis

Seymour I. Schwartz

Several techniques are available for resection and anastomosis of the small intestine and the colon. The choice of the procedure should be determined by a consideration of the following factors: (1) age and general condition of the patient, (2) nature of the pathologic lesion, (3) location of the lesion, (4) presence or absence of obstruction, and (5) familiarity of the surgeon with a particular technique.

INDICATIONS FOR RESECTION AND BYPASS OF THE INTESTINE

Resection of a portion of the bowel, followed by immediate or delayed anastomosis, is necessary for a variety of pathologic states: (1) congenital atresia or stenosis of the small intestine or colon, (2) certain traumatic lesions of the intestine and/or colon resulting in perforation or destruction of the bowel, or extensive lacerations of the mesentery with compromised blood supply to a segment of the intestine, (3) benign and malignant lesions of the intestine, (4) inflammatory processes of the small intestine, such as Crohn's disease, or of the large intestine, such as Crohn's colitis, ulcerative colitis, and diverticulitis, (5) chronic fecal fistula, (6) gangrene of the intestine caused by strangulation, either within an external hernia, within an internal hernia sac, or a consequence of torsion around adhesive bands, (7) irreducible intussusception, frequently associated with tumors, (8) some cases of meconium ileus, (9) some forms of duplication, and (10) removal of tumors of the mesentery that will result in compromise of vascular supply to the segment of bowel.

Intestinal bypass is indicated to decompress the proximal intestine when resection of the obstructing lesion would be difficult or would compromise the patient.

GENERAL PRINCIPLES

In all instances the intestine should be handled gently. With the advent of antibiotic coverage, almost all anastomoses are carried out as open anastomoses. Closed anastomoses essentially are only of historical interest. The amount of spillage into the peritoneal cavity can be controlled by atraumatic intestinal clamps or occlusive tapes placed proximal or distal to the resection.

The extent of resection is determined by the nature and size of the lesion. In the case of malignant tumor, generally 5 to 6 cm of normal intestine are resected on either side of the grossly involved segment. The extent of resection in these patients is also dependent upon the lymphatic drainage in the mesentery and mesocolon. Adequate resection of this lymphatic drainage and associated blood vessels may sufficiently divorce larger segments of the intestine from their blood supply, thereby necessitating a more extensive resection, e.g., right colectomy and distal ilectomy, coupled with ileotransverse colostomy for cecal carcinoma. In the case of Crohn's disease, the resection is carried out just beyond the limits of grossly involved intestine, and frozen sections are not used to determine the presence of microscopic involvement.

Healthy and supple segments of intestine with good blood supply should be anastomosed.

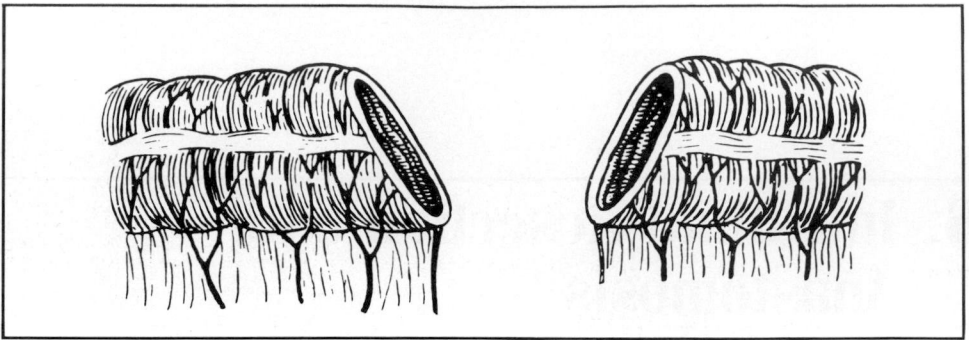

Figure 46–1. Oblique section of the colon ends ensures a good blood supply to all parts of the cut edge. (*Source: From Goligher JC, 1980, with permission.*)

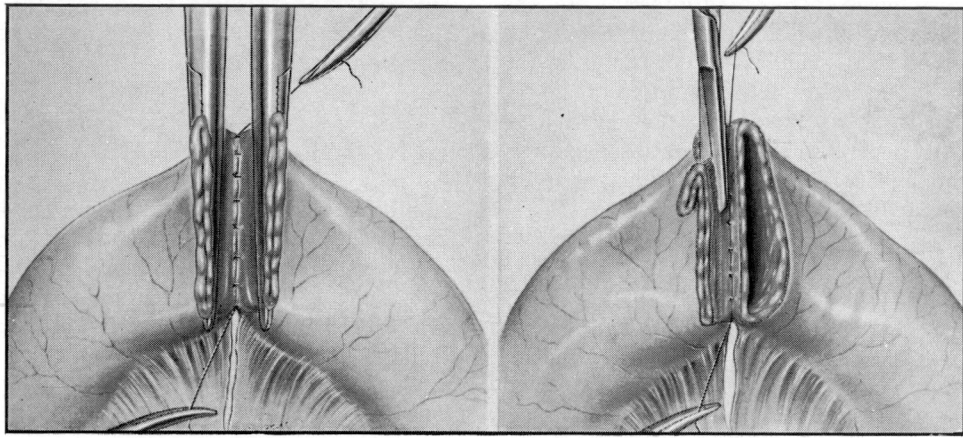

Figure 46–2. Enterectomy followed by end-to-end anastomosis.

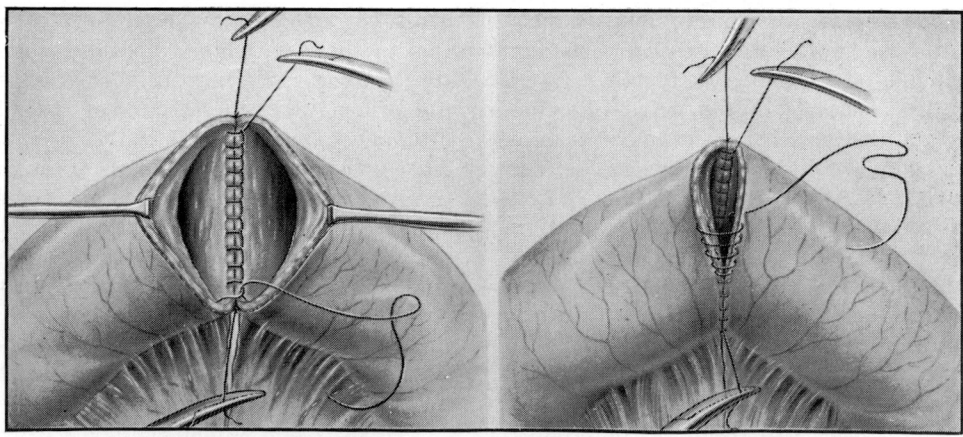

Figure 46–3. Enterectomy followed by end-to-end anastomosis.

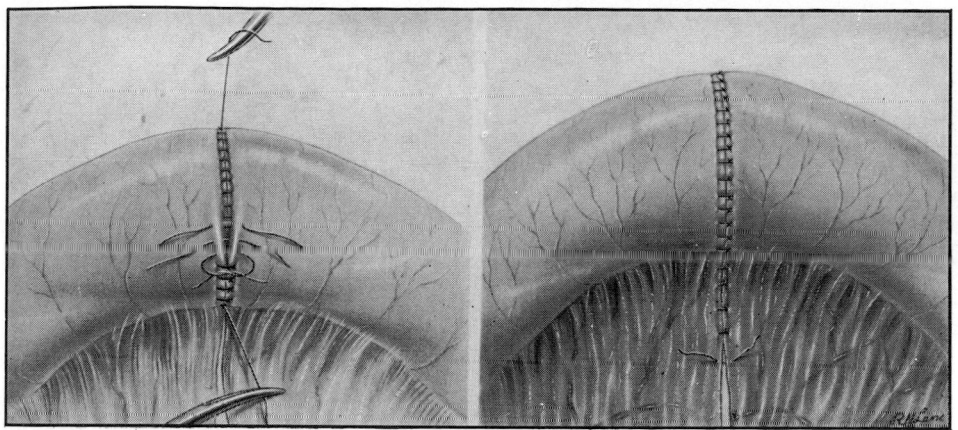

Figure 46–4. Enterectomy with end-to-end anastomosis. Operation completed by closing defect in the mesentery.

The anastomosis itself should be watertight, with an adequate stoma, and the suture line should be free from any tension. Closure of the intestine is carried out accurately, taking care to avoid interruption of significant vascular supply. In the case of marginal supply, the portion of the intestine to be anastomosed should be obliqued, so that a greater portion is removed from the antimesenteric side to ensure adequate vascularization of the anastomosis (Fig. 46–1). The mesentery also should be closed in a precise fashion to avoid internal herniation. This closure can be facilitated by placement of the initial sutures in the angle prior to performing the intestinal anastomosis per se.

TYPES OF ANASTOMOSES

The types of anastomoses used to reestablish intestinal continuity include: (1) end-to-end anastomosis, (2) functional end-to-end anastomosis, (3) end-to-side anastomosis, (4) side-to-side anastomosis, and (5) side-to-end anastomosis.

End-to-End Anastomosis. This is the type most frequently used for reestablishment of small intestinal continuity (Figs. 46–2 through 46–4) and also for colocolostomy. Minimal to moderate disparity between the two limbs of the intestine, such as ileum and colon, can be compensated for by enlargement of smaller lumen either obliquing that limb with the smaller lumen, or by longitudinally dividing the intestine along the antimesenteric border (Fig. 46–5). The end-to-end anastomosis can be established either by sutures or by staple technique, using triangulation with three TA staplers, or using the end-to-end stapler.

In the case of disparate lumens, a functional end-to-end anastomosis may be accomplished by closing the two ends of the intestine

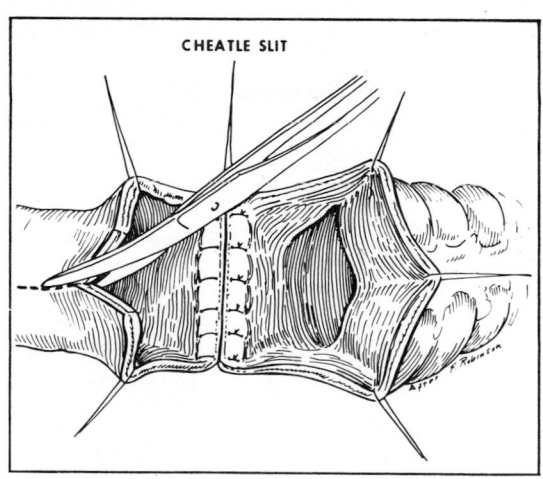

Figure 46–5. Ileocolostomy. The cheatle cut. (*Courtesy of Dr. R. Turnbull.*)

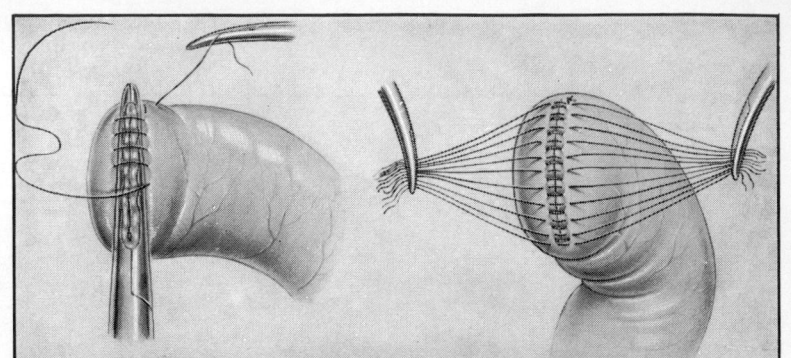

Figure 46–6. Lateral or side-to-side anastomosis. Closure of the end of the bowel with continuous Mikulicz stitch and series of interrupted sutures of fine silk.

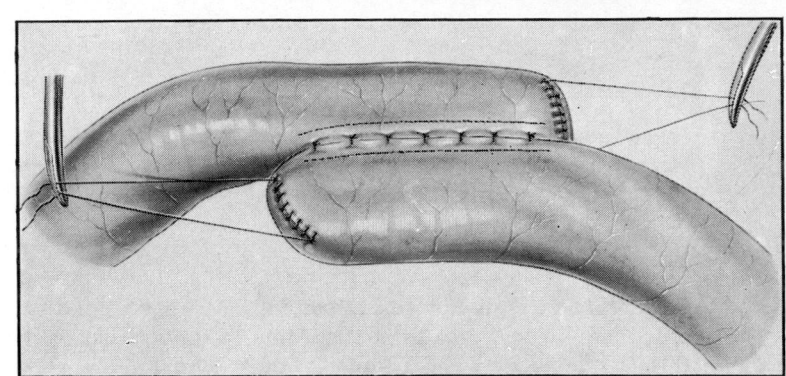

Figure 46–7. Lateral or side-to-side anastomosis.

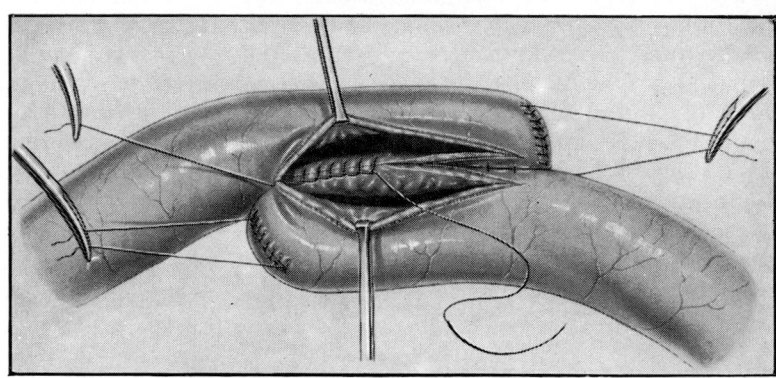

Figure 46–8. Lateral or side-to-side anastomosis.

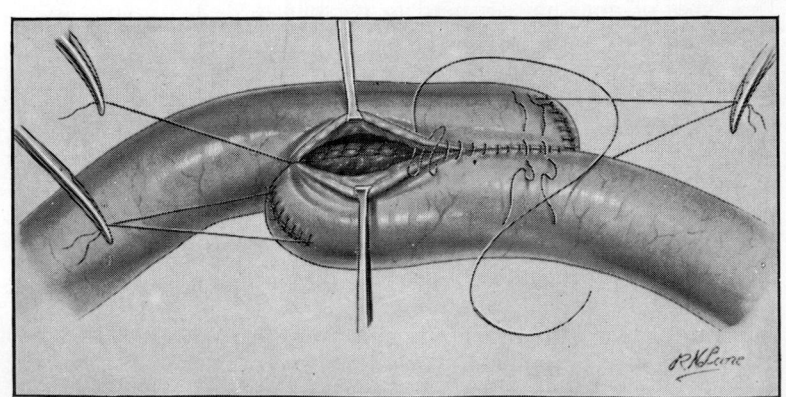

Figure 46–9. Lateral or side-to-side anastomosis.

and carrying out a side-to-side anastomosis in immediate proximity to the closed ends. This may be performed by suture technique (Figs. 46–6 through 46–9) or using staples to close the two ends, creating the anastomosis with a GIA stapler.

End-to-Side Anastomosis. The end-to-side anastomosis is used in the creation of a Roux-Y limb (Fig. 46–10), or, for anastomosis of two segments with disparate lumens (Fig. 46–11). The sizes of the lateral opening in the intestine should be equivalent to that of the lumen of the intestine to be anastomosed. This stoma should be made at a distance from the mesenteric resection to avoid injury of the mesenteric vascular supply. This anastomosis may be accomplished with a suture or staple technique.

Side-to-Side Anastomosis. This is used most commonly to bypass an obstructed segment of the intestine, leaving that segment in place. An adequate stoma is ensured, and there is no problem about the disproportionate diameters of the proximal and distal bowel. The anastomosis should be effected in the antimesenteric portion, employing either a suture technique or the GIA stapler. When side-to-side or end-to-side anasto-

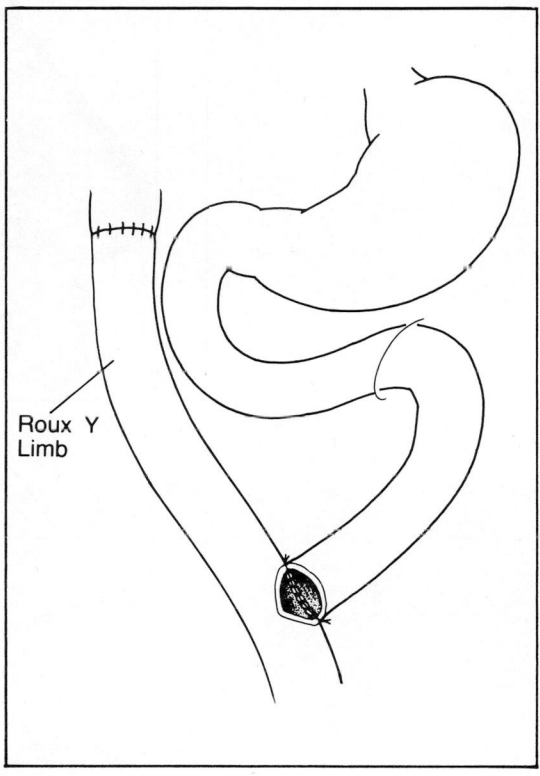

Figure 46–10. Jejunojejunostomy Roux-Y anastomosis.

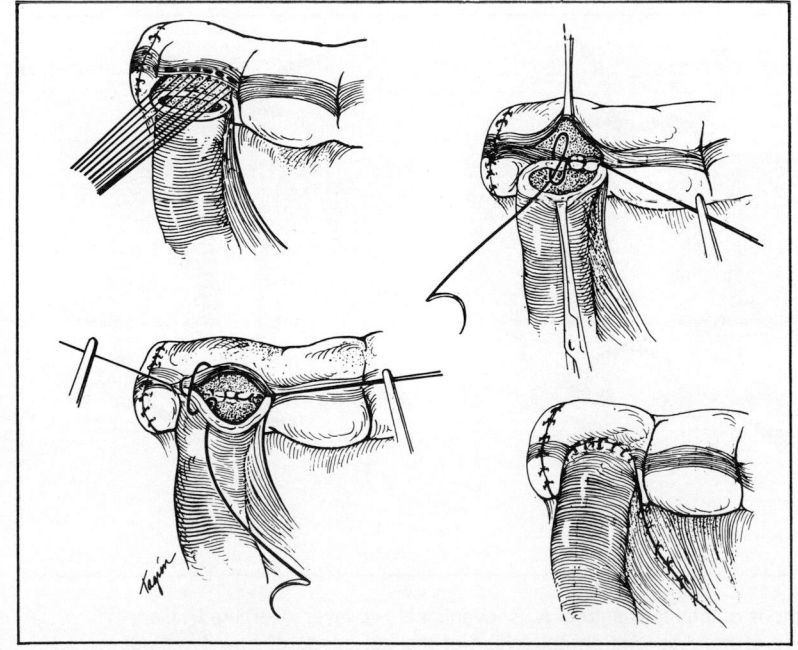

Figure 46–11. End-to-side ileocolostomy. (*Source: From Donaldson GA, Welch JP: Management of cancer of the colon. Surg Clin North Am 54:713, 1974, with permission.*)

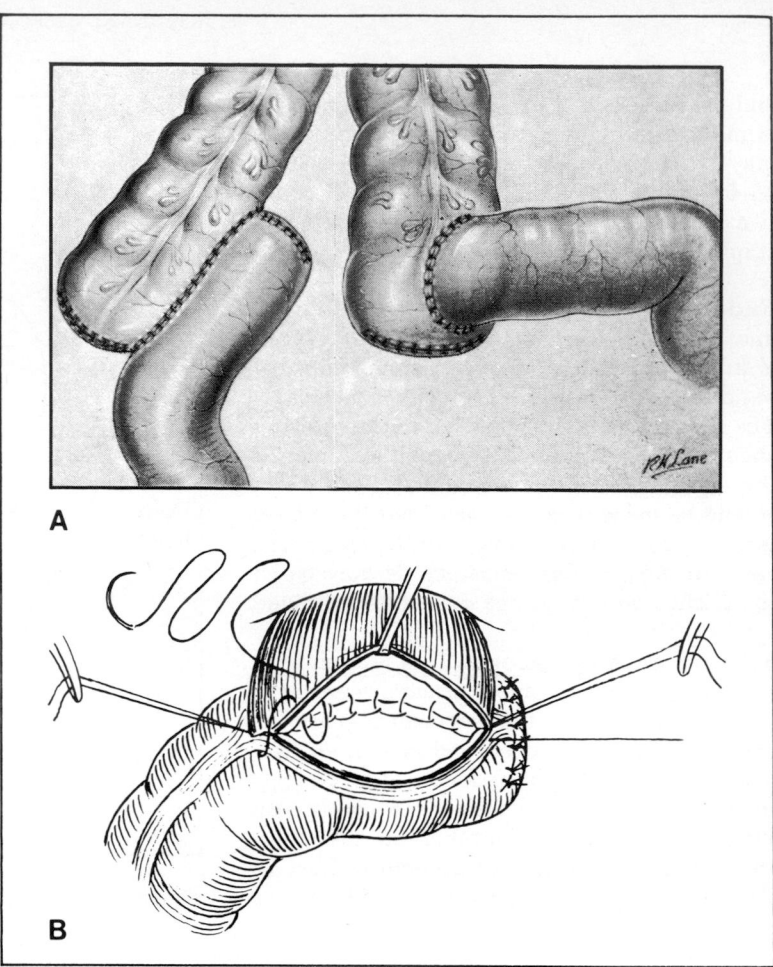

Figure 46–12. A. Side-to-end anastomosis and end-to-side ileocolostomy. B. Side-to-end rectocolostomy.

A

B

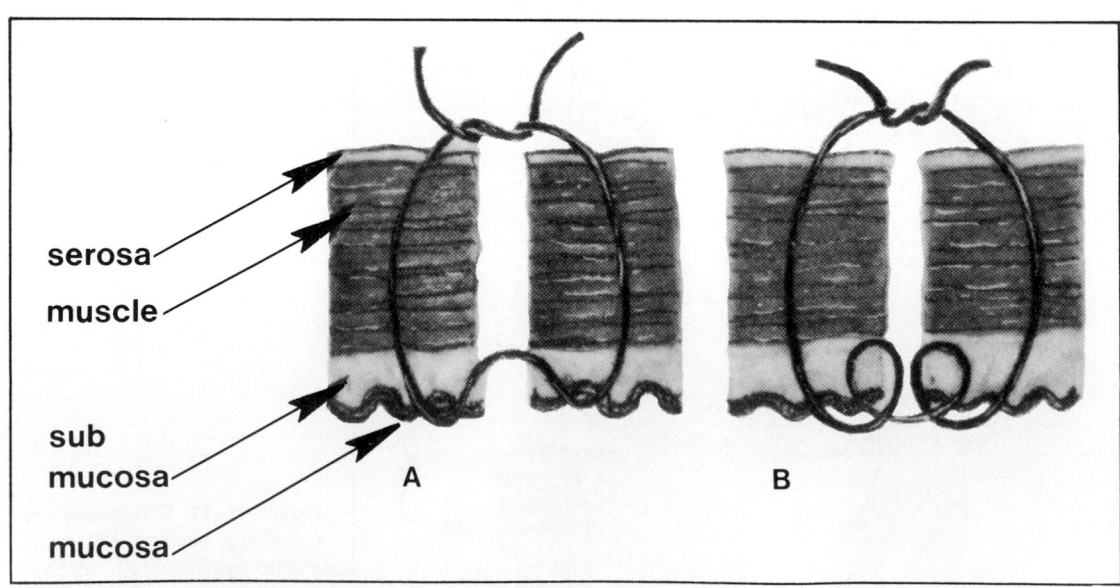

serosa

muscle

sub
mucosa

mucosa

A   B

Figure 46–13. Two methods of intestinal suture. A. Conventional two-layer inverting. B. Gambee single layer designed to produce end-on apposition of the cut edges of bowel without mucosa pouting. (*Source: Adapted from Goligher JC, 1980, with permission.*)

mosis is carried out with the proximal segment transected, it is important that no more than 1.5 cm of proximal jejunum, ileum, or colon be allowed to extend beyond the anastomosis because the pouch may perforate or become gradually enlarged and balloon to produce symptoms of indigestion, abdominal pain, distention, and even recurrent intestinal obstruction. This is termed the "blind loop" syndrome, which may cause malnutrition, a sprue-like state, and microcytic or macrocytic anemia.

Side-to-End Anastomosis. This may result in a functional end-to-end anastomosis, particularly when employed to reestablish continuity between the descending colon and rectum (Fig. 46–12). The end of the proximal limb is closed and an opening is made along the antimesocolic portion of the colon. This ensures good vascularity and definition of the serosal surface for the posterior layer of the anastomosis. A small, blind loop fills the presacral space in the immediate posterior period and later becomes incorporated in the stoma as it stretches.

TECHNIQUES OF ANASTOMOSIS

It has been generally considered important to achieve serosal aposition when anastomosing intestine. This is most readily effected by a two-layer technique using interrupted, nonabsorbable sutures in the seromuscular layer in an inverting fashion (Lembert), and an inner layer of sutures placed through-and-through the entire thickness, using either interrupted nonabsorbable or continuous absorbable material. When a continuous, absorbable suture is used in this fashion, the posterior layer is usually placed as a locked suture, and continued anteriorly as an inverting Connell stitch. An alternative approach employs two layers of continuous suture, with an outer seromuscular layer and an inner mucosal, or through-and-through layer.

As Goligher has pointed out, following a decade of debate, the principle of avoiding mucosal eversion has been firmly reestablished. But whether the two-layer technique is preferable is still a question. A single-layer interrupted nonabsorbable technique that avoids eversion was introduced by Gambee (Fig. 46–13A), and modified by DeAlmelda (Fig. 46–13B) in order to facilitate insertion of the needle. Irvin and Edwards compared the one-layer inverting tech-

nique, using silk sutures, with the two-layer technique for intraperitoneal colon anastomoses, and noted no significant difference in anastomotic leaks. In a controlled trial, Everett reported similar results but, with lower anterior rectosigmoid anastomoses, the incidence of anastomotic dehiscence was significantly less with a one-layer technique. By contrast, Goligher et al reported a higher incidence of anastomotic leak with the one-layer technique for both high and low colon anastomoses.

Suture Material

The choice of suture is dictated by individual preference. There is suggestion that polyglycolic acid is superior to catgut for the inner layer of the conventional two-layer colonic and rectal anastomoses. Silk, Prolene, and fine wire all have been used as nonabsorbable sutures for either the interrupted single-layer anastomosis, or for the outer layer of the two-layer anastomosis.

SPECIFIC PROCEDURES

Enteroenterostomy

After the lines of resection of the small intestine have been established, an opening is made with the tip of a small curved hemostat in an avascular portion of the mesentery immediately subjacent to the bowel wall at the site elected for transection. Through this opening, a portion of rubber tubing or umbilical tape is inserted. A second piece of rubber tubing or tape is used to encircle the bowel distally, and direction lines for transection of the mesentery are made through the thin peritoneal layer with a knife.

The mesentery, with its contained blood vessels, is serially clamped and divided between forceps and complete hemostasis is secured by means of fine ligatures. The blood vessels should be ligated individually. In the case of extremely fatty areolar tissue, transfixion suture ligatures are preferable. After the mesentery has been divided along an appropriate line, and the points selected for division of the bowel are cleared of mesenteric vessels, the operative field is isolated with packs. Paired clamps are applied to the two areas of small intestine that have been prepared for transection, and the intestine is divided with cautery or knife and the segment containing the lesion is removed (Figs. 46–14 and 46–15).

1228

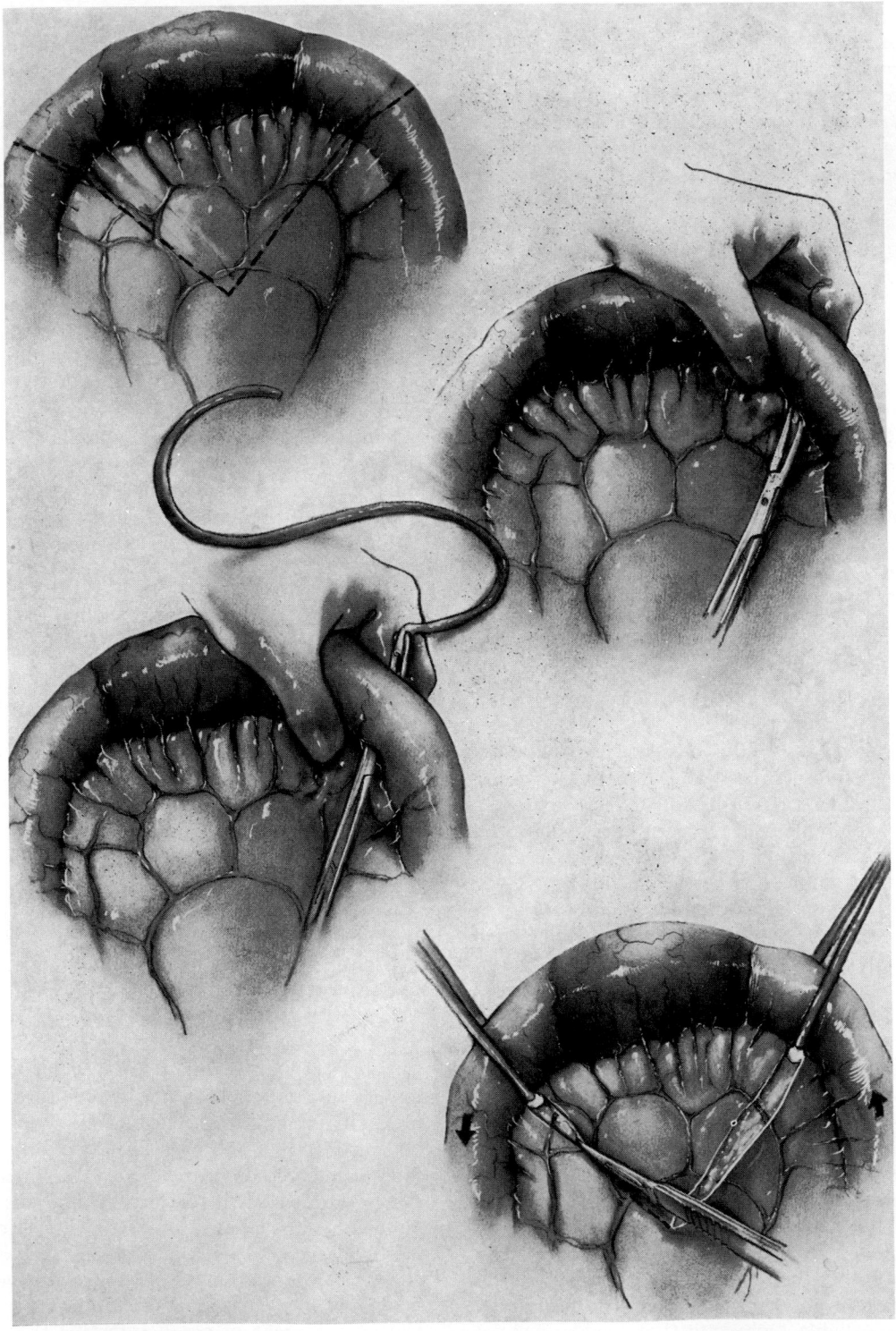

Figure 46–14. Enterectomy with end-to-end anastomosis—the open method. (*Source: From Madden JL, 1964, with permission.*)

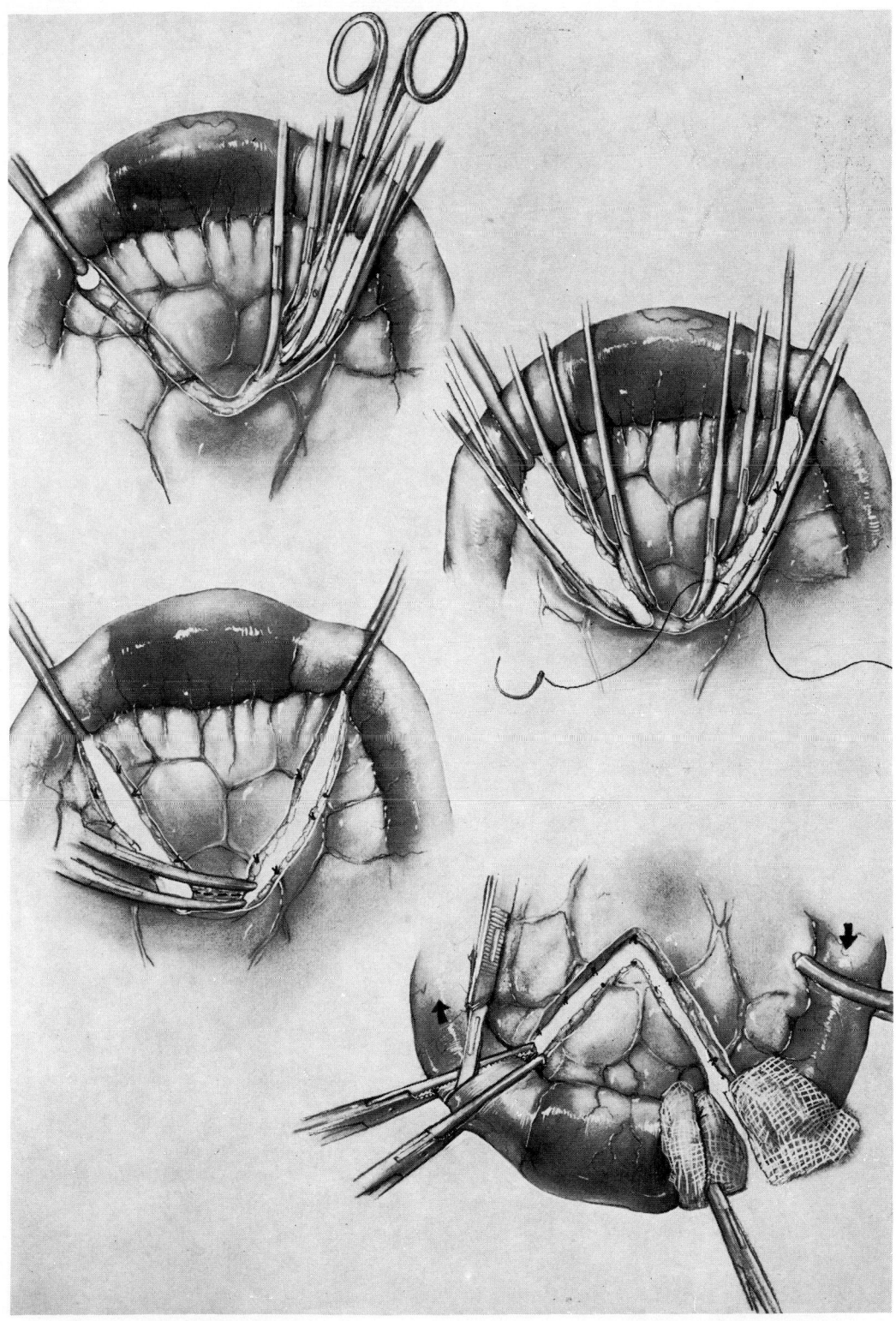

Figure 46–15. Enterectomy with end-to-end anastomosis—the open method. (*Source: From Madden JL, 1964, with permission.*)

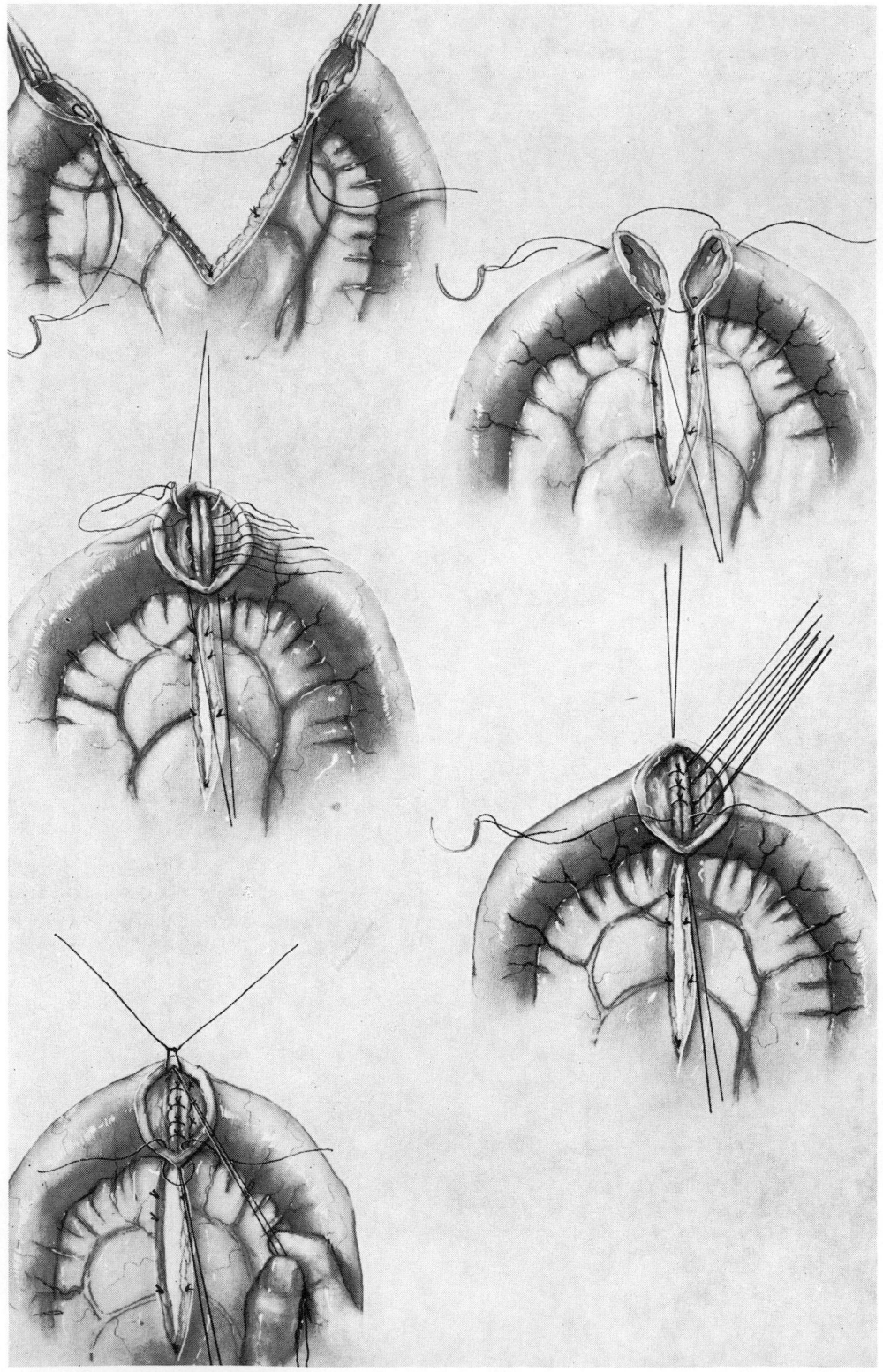

Figure 46–16. Enterectomy with end-to-end anastomosis—the open method. (*Source: From Madden JL, 1964, with permission.*)

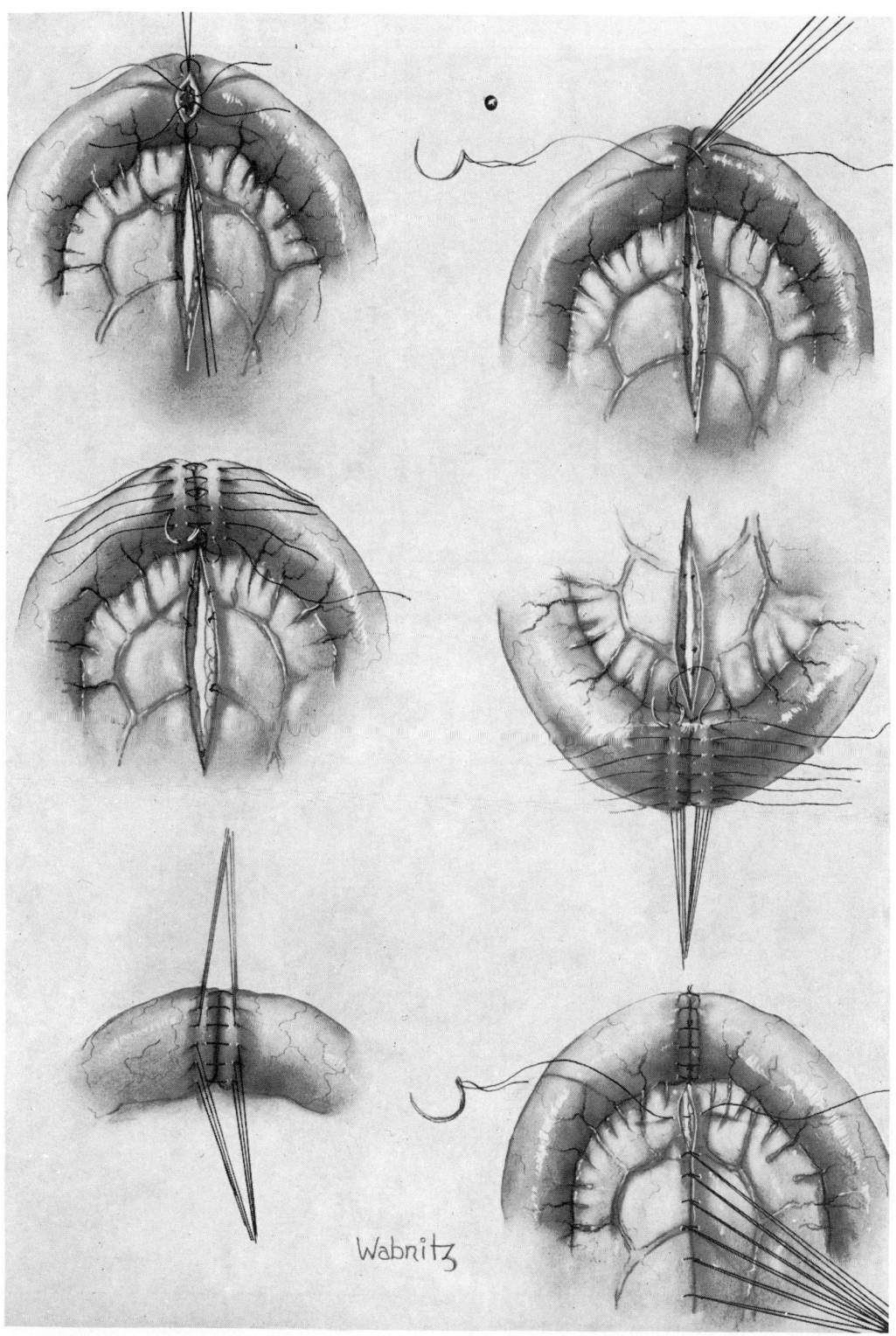

Figure 46–17. Enterectomy with end-to-end anastomosis—the open method. (*Source: From Madden JL, 1964, with permission.*)

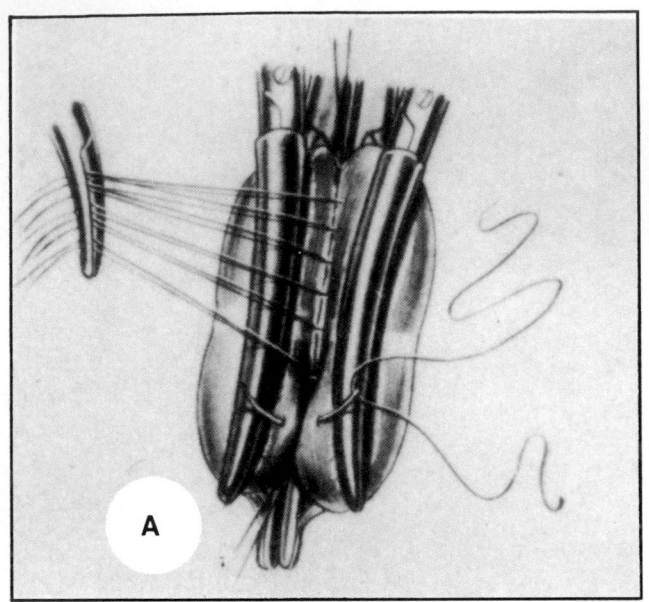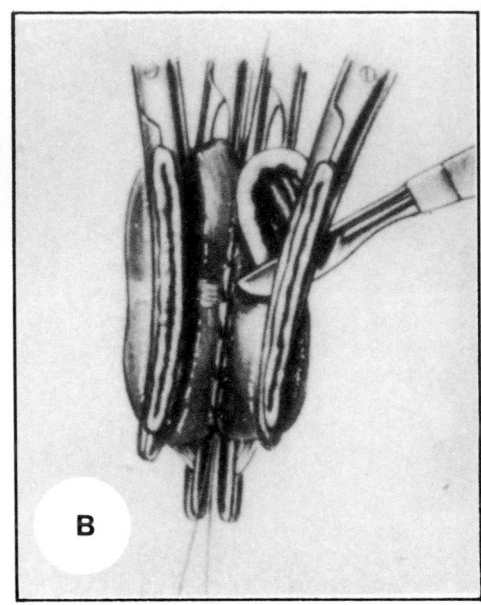

Figure 46–18. A. Insertion of posterior row of Lembert sutures of interrupted fine serum-proof silk. **B.** Excising crushing clamp together with the fringe of crushed bowel wall. (*Source: Goligher JC, 1980, with permission.*)

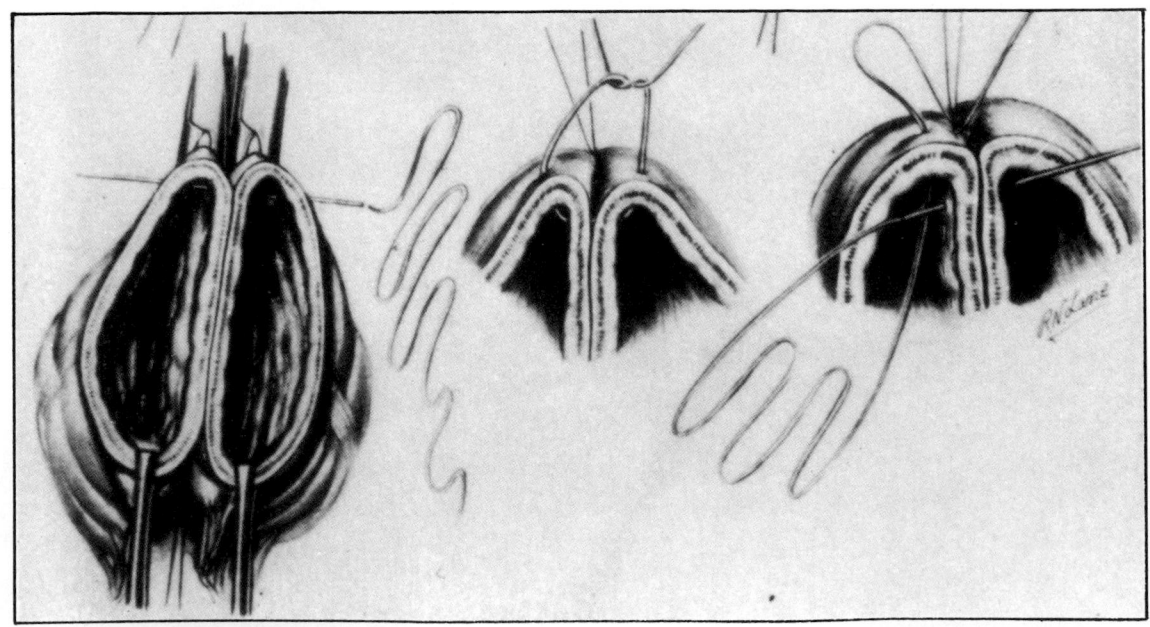

Figure 46–19. Commencement of through-and-through stitch of continuous catgut. (*Source: From Goligher JC, 1980, with permission.*)

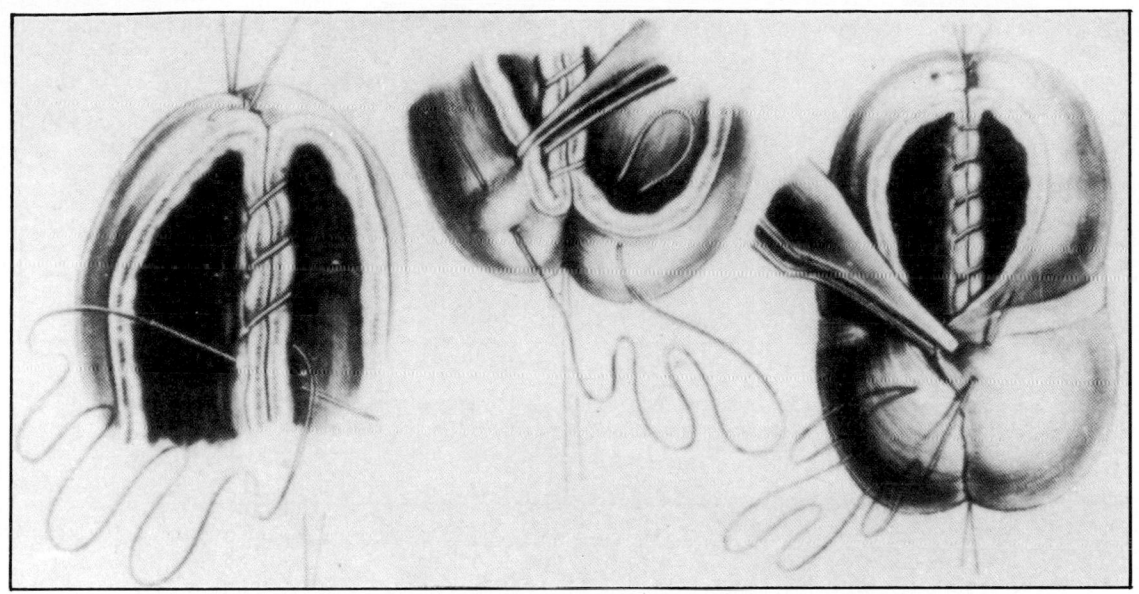

Figure 46–20. Further steps in the insertion of the through-and-through suture. Note that the stitch returns along the anterior wall as a Connell stitch. (*Source: From Goligher JC, 1980, with permission.*)

The anastomosis may be carried out according to the technique already described in Figures 46–2 through 46–4. The proximal and distal segments to be united are held together, the clamps are rotated outward and the posterior surfaces are joined together with a series of closely applied interrupted sutures of fine silk. Interrupted Lembert or Halsted sutures may be used. The clamps are removed, the devitalized margins of intestine resulting from the crushing clamps are trimmed away, and the second posterior row of sutures consisting of a continuous interlocking stitch of 000 chromic catgut or Dexon is introduced through all the layers. This suture is continued anteriorly as a Connell suture, producing a watertight inversion of the anterior margin of the intestine. The anastomosis is completed by introducing a row of Lembert sutures of fine silk that inverts the anterior suture line. Some surgeons prefer to perform this axial union with a series of fine interrupted silk sutures for the anterior and posterior rows (Figs. 46–16 and 46–17). After the posterior row has been placed, it is continued anteriorly with a series of closely applied in-out-out-in sutures, with the knots lying inside the lumen of the gut. An inverting effect is achieved by maintaining traction on the previously placed suture while tying. The first layer is then reinforced with interrupted sutures placed seromuscularly in a Lembert inverting fashion. The mesentery is then closed.

End-to-End Colocolostomy and End-to-End Rectal Colostomy

The standard method detailed by Goligher (Figs. 46–18 through 46–22) is preferred by many surgeons. It is a two-layer inverting technique using nonabsorbable material such as silk as an outer seromuscular stitch, and polyglycolic suture as an inner through-and-through suture. An alternative one-layer inverting technique may be used (Figs. 46–23 through 46–25). Nonabsorbable sutures such as silk, linen, cotton, Prolene, and fine wires are used. A posterior row of sutures is placed before tying them, and the two segments of bowel are brought into juxtaposition while these sutures are made taut. The first suture is placed at the mesenteric poles of the two stumps, passed from the mucosal aspect of the colon through the serosa and then through the rectal wall from without inward.

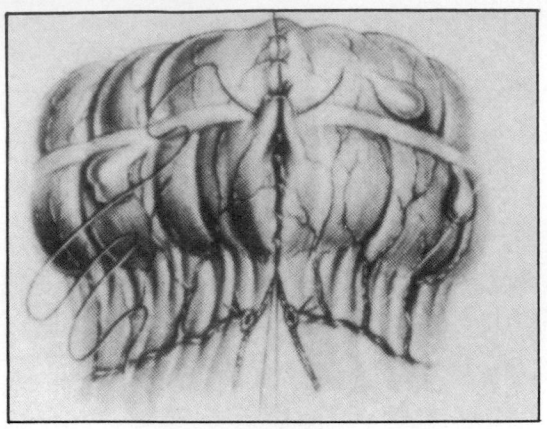 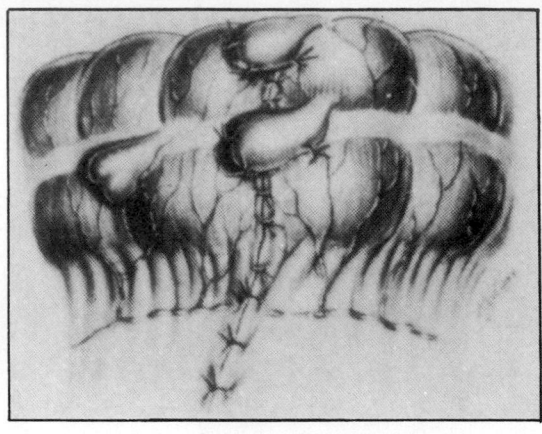

A   B

Figure 46–21. A. Insertion of anterior row of Lembert sutures of silk. **B.** Suture of appendices epiploicae over the anastomosis for additional security. (*Source: From Goligher JC, 1980, with permission.*)

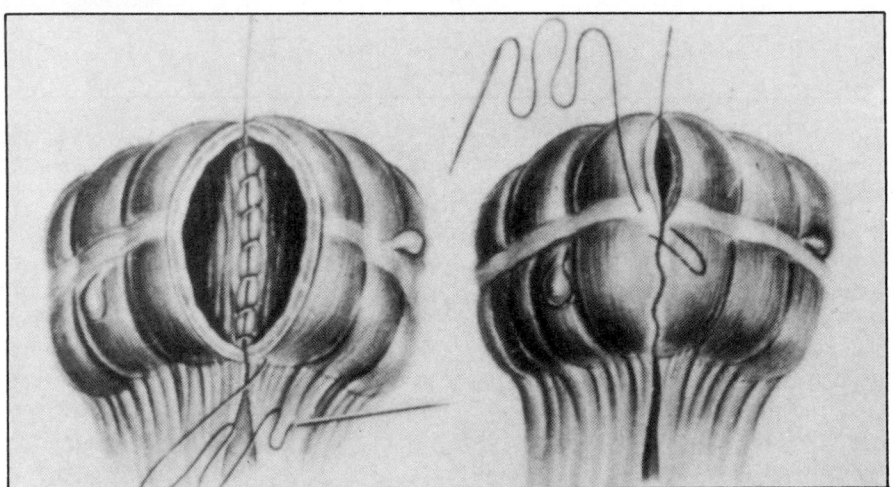

A   B

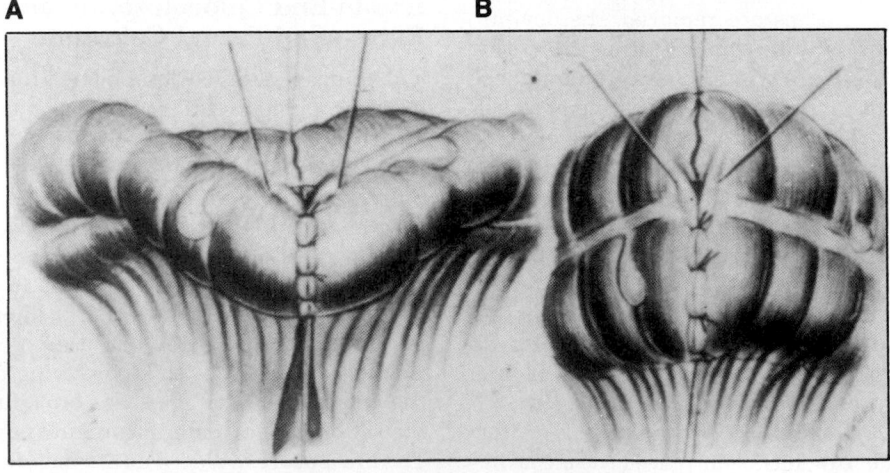

C   D

Figure 46–22. Alternative preferred technique of suture, suitable when the colon stumps can be freely rotated, as is usually possible. The through-and-through suture is inserted first (**A** and **B**); this suture line is then buried by Lembert stitches, first posteriorly (**C**) and then anteriorly (**D**), and these sutures are inserted very deeply, usually through all coats and often embracing the catgut suture. (*Source: From Goligher JC, 1980, with permission.*)

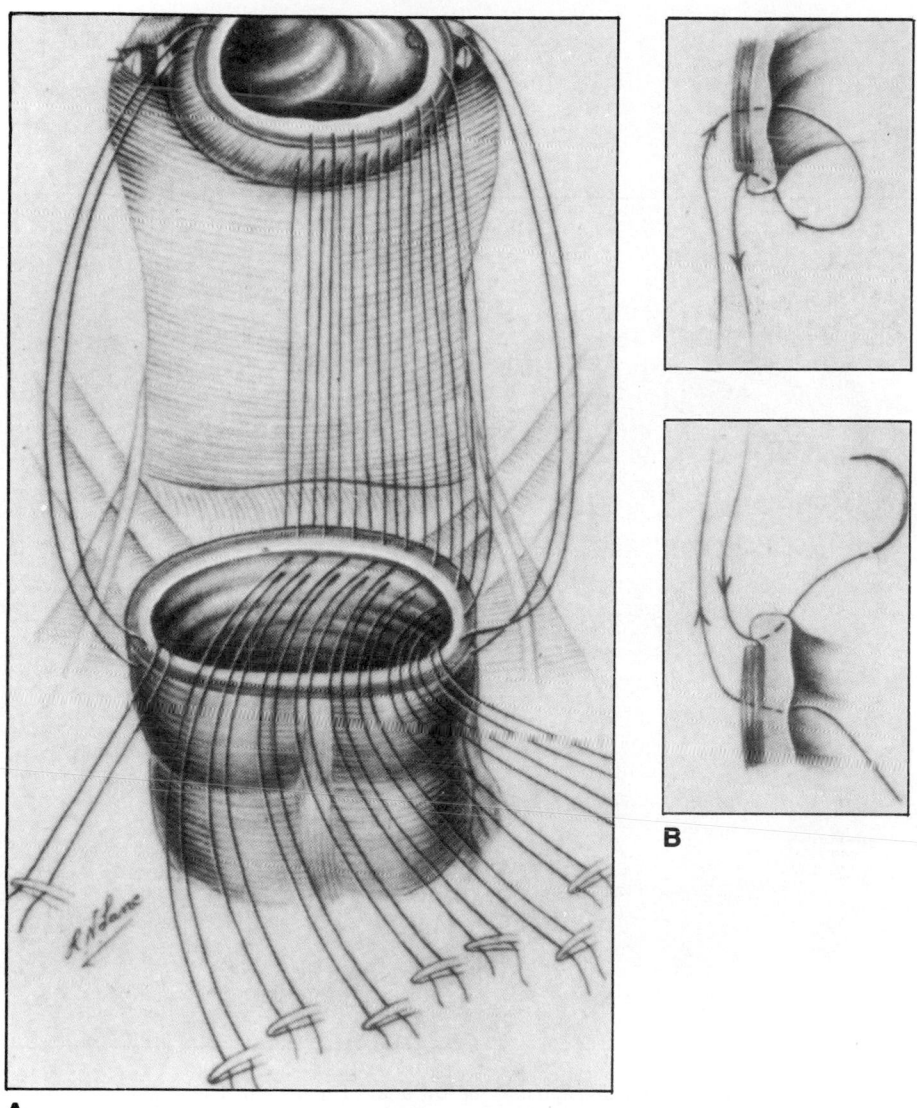

A

B

Figure 46–23. The one-layer anastomosis for low anterior resection. **A.** With open colon and rectal stumps separated by 12 to 15 cm, interrupted vertical mattress sutures of 3-0 silk are placed in the posterior two thirds of the bowel circumference; the first one in the midline posteriorly, the next two on either side one third of the circumference from the posterior midline, and the remainder at intervals of 4 mm to fill these two gaps. **B.** The exact course of the vertical mattress suture, which starts and finishes at the colonic mucosa. (*Source: From Goligher JC, 1980, with permission.*)

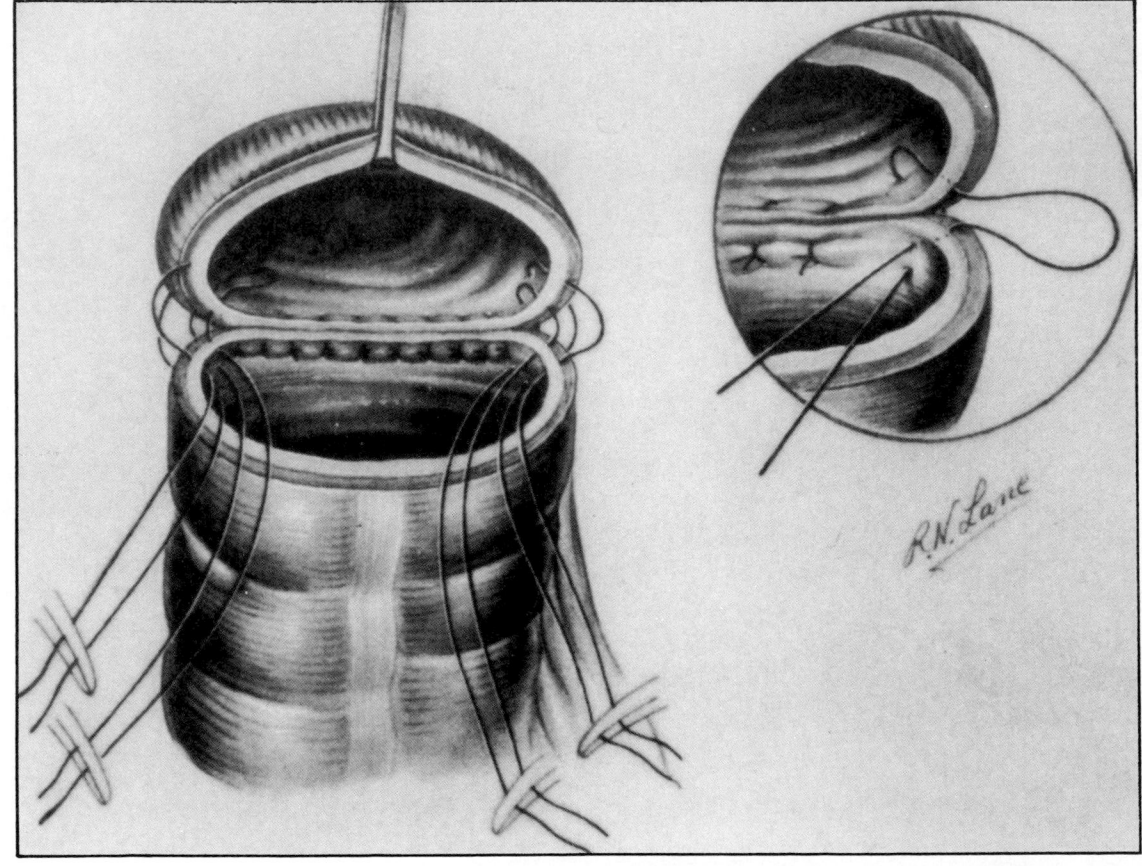

Figure 46–24. The one-layer anastomosis for low anterior resection. The colonic stump has been slid down on the tautly held untied silk sutures to make contact with the rectal stump and the silks are then tied with their knots on the colonic mucosa. *Inset:* When the most lateral sutures are tied, they coapt and turn in the lateral corners very effectively. (*Source: From Goligher JC, 1980, with permission.*)

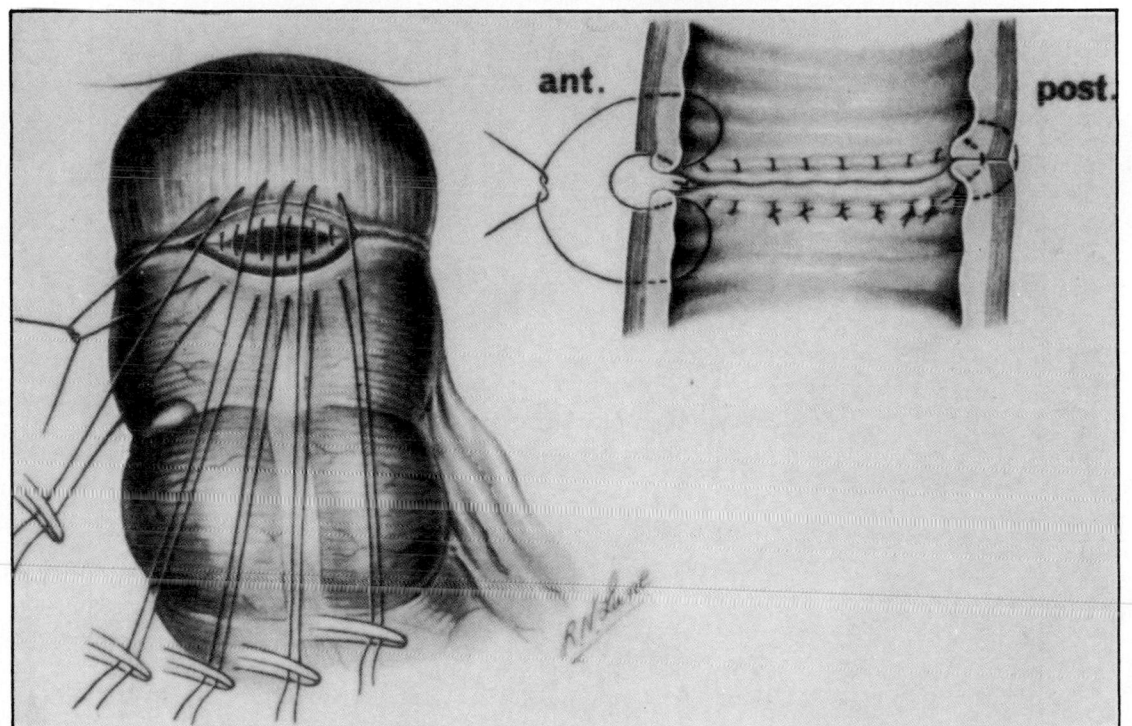

Figure 46–25. The one-layer anastomosis for low anterior resection. The anterior third of the bowel circumference, which remains unsutured, can be closed by a small series of Gambee sutures of 3-0 silk, if the anastomosis is not too low in the pelvis for this type of stitch to be feasible. *Inset:* The course of the anterior Gambee sutures compared with that of the posterior vertical mattress stitches. (*Source: From Goligher JC, 1980, with permission.*)

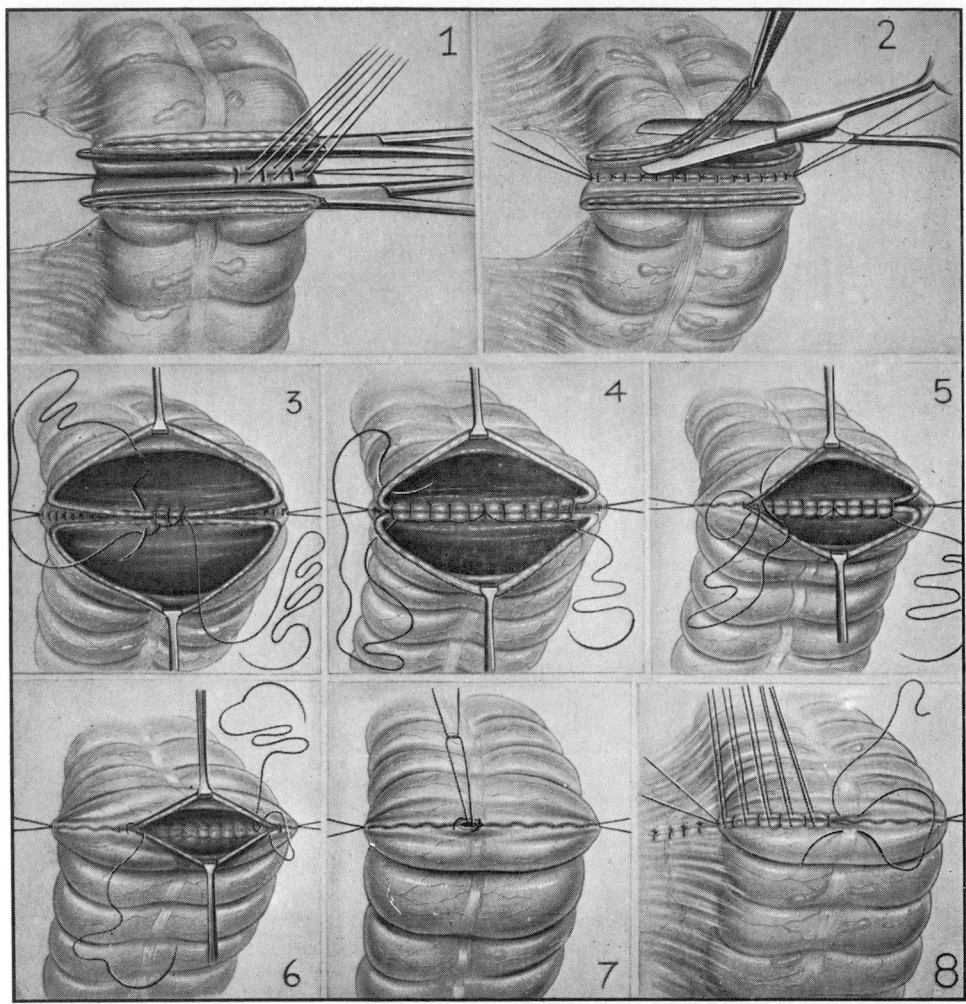

Figure 46–26. End-to-end colocolostomy—the open operation using two rows of sutures: An outer interrupted and an inner continuous layer.

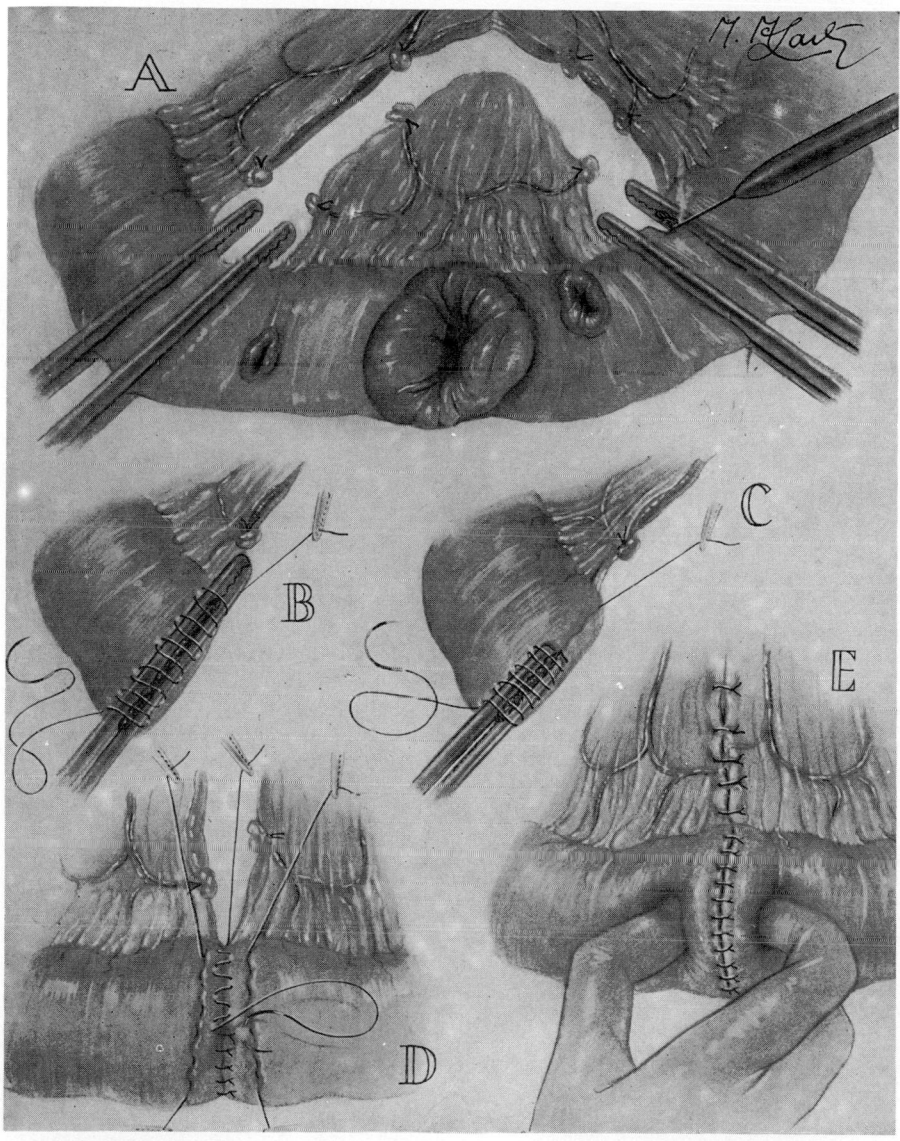

Figure 46–27. Segmental resection of small intestine with end-to-end (closed) anastomosis by Parker–Kerr basting stitch method. **A.** Damaged and perforated segment of intestine is resected. **B** and **C.** Introduction of the basting stitches. **D.** End basting stitches held with hemostats. Posterior continuous suture of 000 (m.3) chromic catgut is introduced. It is better to insert Lembert seromuscular silk sutures after posterior and anterior continuous sutures have been inserted and tied and after nylon basting stitches have been pulled out. **E.** Fingers break down agglutinated ends.

It is then brought back from the mucosa through the entire wall of the rectum and the entire wall of the colon from without inward. The anterior sutures may be placed as Gambee stitches or Lembert sutures of the horizontal mattress type. The completed anastomosis is inspected from the outside, and mattress sutures are used to reinforce any apparent defects.

An alternative approach is shown in Figure 46–26, in which an end-to-end colocolostomy is carried out using interrupted seromuscular sutures followed by continuous locked catgut sutures posteriorly, and continued anteriorly as a Connell suture. The anterior row is then enforced with interrupted Lembert sutures placed in a mattress fashion.

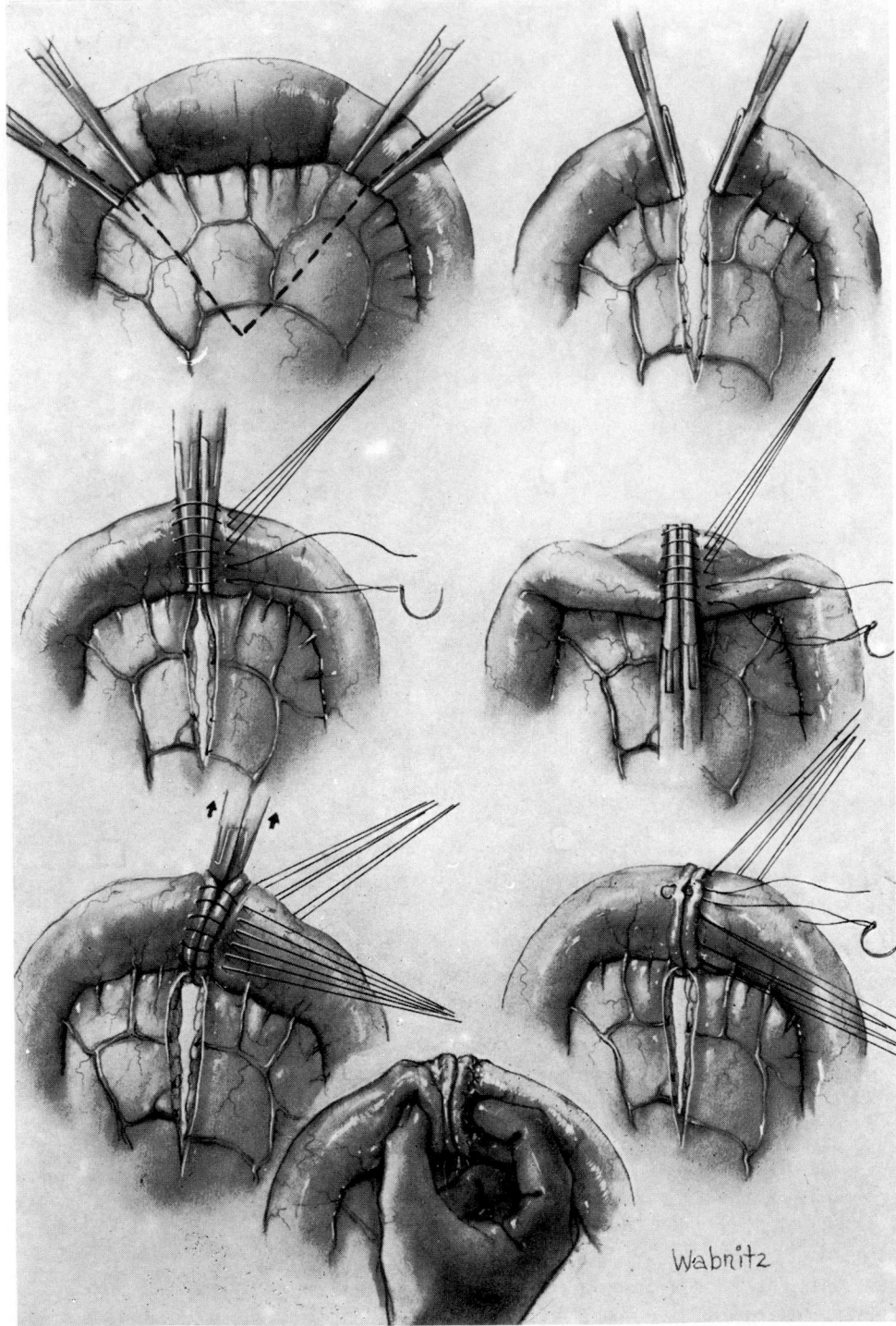

Figure 46–28. Axial union by the closed method as practiced by Dennis. (*Source: From Madden JL, 1964, with permission.*)

Closed or Aseptic Methods of Anastomosis

Techniques of aseptic anastomosis are never truly aseptic, but they do minimize spillage; they had their place in history prior to the use of antibiotics effective against intestinal bacteria. The Parker–Kerr technique, introduced in 1908, employs basting stitches to close the intestine and, following conventional anastomosis, the basting stitches are removed (Fig. 46–27). The technique of Dennis (Fig. 46–28) can also be performed with conventional clamps.

Monro stated that, in all methods of closed anastomosis, certain points require special attention:

1. To avoid the necessity of putting the final sutures at the mesenteric border into the mesentery itself, the bowel must be cleaned of its mesentery for 5 mm. This allows sufficient room for the final sutures to be placed in the bowel wall itself and not in the mesentery, where they might give rise to a hematoma or might endanger the blood supply of the anastomosis.
2. The line of transection of the bowel must be oblique, removing more of the antimesenteric border. This not only ensures a good blood supply but also enables the surgeon to allow for inequality in size of the two bowel ends.
3. In all these anastomoses, the points at either end of the clamps require special attention. Thus, sutures are inserted at each of the two points, but they are tied only after removal of the clamps. Inturning and approximation of the points are thereby ensured.
4. In all closed anastomoses, the sutures on which the anastomosis depends must be inserted from outside the bowel. These sutures must include the submucosa, which is the strongest layer.
5. The anastomosis may be fashioned with one or two layers of sutures. The addition of an outer layer of interrupted silk sutures adds to the safety of the operation.

Criticisms advanced against the aseptic technique are the following:

1. hemostasis might be incomplete
2. the method is not completely aseptic

3. the inturned flange subsequently may produce obstruction
4. a stricture subsequently may develop because mucous membrane is not approximated precisely to mucous membrane
5. all suturing has to be done from outside the bowel and the layers cannot be seen

BIBLIOGRAPHY

Connell FG: Intestinal sutures. Phil Monthly Med J 1:37, 1899

DeAlmelda AC: A modified single layer suture for use in the gastrointestinal tract. Surg Gynecol Obstet 132:985, 1971

Dennis C: Resection and primary anastomosis in the treatment of gangrenous or non-reducible intussusceptions in children. Ann Surg 126:788, 1947

Everett WG: A comparison of one layer and two layer techniques for colorectal anastomosis. Br J Surg 62:135, 1975

Gambee LP: Single-layer open intestinal anastomosis applicable to small as well as large intestine. West J Surg 59:1, 1951

Goligher JC: Treatment of carcinoma of the colon, in Goligher JC (ed): Surgery of the Anus, Rectum and Colon, 5 edt. London: Cassell Ltd, 1984, p 424

Goligher JC: Treatment of carcinoma of the rectum, in Goligher JC (ed): Surgery of the Anus, Rectum and Colon, 5 edt. London: Cassell Ltd, 1984, p 502

Goligher JC, Lee PWG, et al: A controlled comparison of one- and two-layer techniques of suture for high and low colorectal anastomosis. Br J Surg 64:49, 1977

Irvin TT, Edwards JP: Comparison of single-layer inverting, two-layer inverting, and everting anastomoses in the rabbit colon. Br J Surg 60:453, 1973

Madden JL: Atlas of Technics in Surgery, 2 edt. New York: Appleton-Century-Crofts, 1964

Parker EM, Kerr HH: Intestinal anastomosis without open incisions by means of basting stitches. Johns Hopkins Hosp Bull 19:132, 1908

Ravitch MM: Sewing with staples. Clin Med 81:17, 1974

Steichen FM: The use of staples in anatomical side-to-side and functional end-to-end enteroanastomoses. Surgery 64:948, 1968

Welch JP, Donaldson GA: Recent experience in the management of cancer of the colon and rectum. Am J Surg 127:258, 1974

Zollinger RM: Atlas of Surgical Operations, 5 edt. New York: Macmillan, 1983

47. Serosal Patch for Intestinal Perforation or Enterocutaneous Fistula

S. Austin Jones

INTRODUCTION

The modern trend in the treatment of intestinal perforations and enterocutaneous fistulas is to emphasize the use of hyperalimentation (total parenteral nutrition, TPN) and general supportive measures, hoping for spontaneous closure. Should an operation prove unavoidable, primary resection and anastomosis are generally recommended. This approach is associated with a definite morbidity and mortality. Also, the cost for the basic 2-week support has averaged about $225 per day, and if this figure is multiplied by the average of 60.8 treatment days, a cost of $13,680 is arrived at for the nutritional solutions alone for each patient treated.

A direct attack on the source of the fistula in patients who fail to heal promptly on conservative therapy will result in a significant saving of time, expense, and morbidity. It is to this purpose the serosal patch has been applied based on a remarkable ability of the bowel serosa to seal visceral perforations, recent or chronic, relatively clean or grossly infected. Although the use of a serosal patch is rarely needed, when it is, nothing else will take its place.

HISTORICAL BACKGROUND

In 1959 we resected a large hepatic flexure carcinoma that was adherent to the second portion of the duodenum. An en bloc dissection removed the majority of the lateral wall of the descending duodenum. This large defect was closed without difficulty by fashioning an open side-to-side anastomosis between the remaining duodenum and a loop of jejunum. Turnbull had used this open technique successfully in treating duodonal fistulas due to Crohn's disease.

In 1963 Kobald and Thal reported the experimental closure of clean duodenal defects in dogs using a patch of jejunal serosa to seal the opening they had created. At that time we were searching for a satisfactory method of closing a perforated duodenal stump; we had been motivated by a patient with this complication who failed to respond to prompt tube duodenostomy and feeding jejunostomy. It was our feeling that an open duodenojejunostomy would be less than ideal because it would divert the alkaline juices from the gastrojejunostomy and set the stage for marginal ulceration. We therefore carried out a series of experiments to evaluate the ability of intact bowel wall to close "clean" perforations with the hope that this approach could be applied to infected defects. Our own experiments in dogs demonstrated that the serosal patch was effective as a method of closing the duodenal stump primarily or in the presence of infection. Subsequently, we have applied the technique to a series of diverse clinical circumstances.

GENERAL CONSIDERATIONS

Because the great majority of intestinal defects can be managed by simple suture repair or exteriorization, and a trial of TPN and other supportive measures may be successful, the number

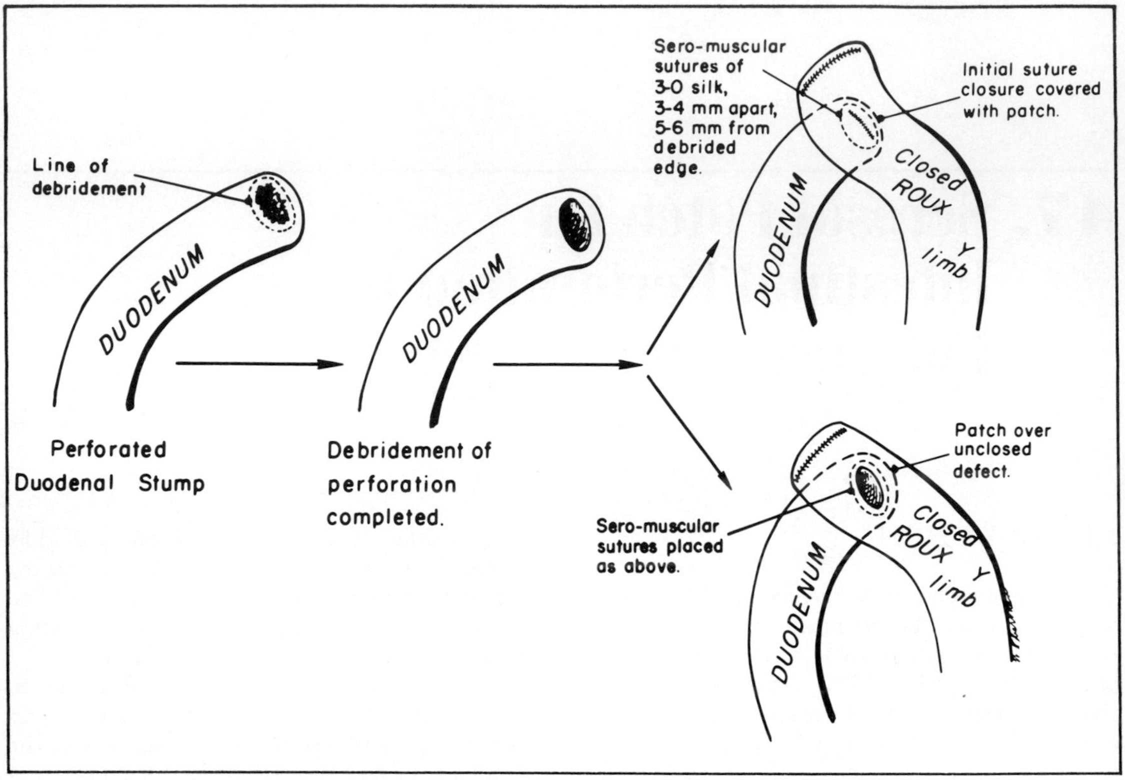

Line of
debridement

DUODENUM

Perforated
Duodenal Stump

Debridement of
perforation
completed.

DUODENUM

Sero-muscular
sutures of
3-0 silk,
3-4 mm apart,
5-6 mm from
debrided
edge.

Initial suture
closure covered
with patch.

DUODENUM

Closed
ROUX
Y
limb

Sero-muscular
sutures placed
as above.

Patch over
unclosed
defect.

DUODENUM

Closed
ROUX
Y
limb

Figure 47–1. After debriding the defect, the patch may be used to buttress a sutured closure (*top right*) or to close the unsutured opening (*bottom right*).

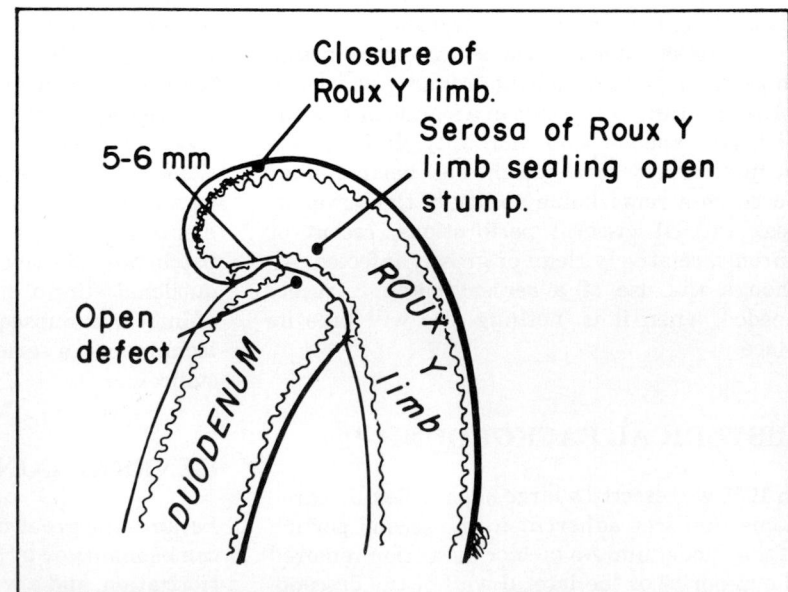

Closure of
Roux Y limb.

Serosa of Roux Y
limb sealing open
stump.

5-6 mm

Open
defect

DUODENUM

ROUX Y
limb

Figure 47–2. A closed Roux-Y limb patches the open end of the duodenum. Note that seromuscular sutures holding the patch are not in the margin of the defect but are some distance away in relatively healthy tissue.

of reported series in which the serosal patch has been applied is limited. Our initial report of the use of a serosal patch in 28 patients has been endorsed by the experiences of other surgeons. The cumulative experiences have demonstrated that the serosal patch method of closure for visceral defects functions in the presence of gross infection. Also, it has been shown that the serosal patch provides temporary closure of a perforated carcinoma. It has been demonstrated to be more effective than omentum as a sealing agent. The applicability of the serosal patch technique is limited only by the ingenuity of the surgeon, as is best evidenced by the variety of patients in whom we have applied the procedure.

TECHNIQUE

Although the basic concept of the serosal patch is simple, its success depends upon precise technique. The serosa must be approximated to serosa if optimal results are to be achieved. As a corollary, suturing small bowel over a defect in the esophagus is less likely to succeed than is covering an opening in the stomach that has a serosal layer. In reference to healing potential, it makes little difference whether a simple loop of bowel or a Roux-Y limb is employed as long as the resultant anatomic configuration is physiologically satisfactory. In some cases a simple side-to-side patch employing adjacent intestinal or even gastric serosa may be used.

The bowel to be patched must be gently cleared of fat and adjacent inflammatory tissue until a layer of serosa with a good blood supply is visible for at least 6 to 7 mm from the edge of perforation (Fig. 47–1). After debriding the defect, the edges of the perforation should be approximated with a single layer of absorbable suture if this can be accomplished without tension. A limb of intestine used to provide the serosal patch is then sutured in place over this temporary closure. If the defect cannot be approximated without tension, a limb of intestine, that providing the serosal patch, is sewn in position directly over the debrided opening. Interrupted sutures of 3-0 silk positioned 3 to 4 mm apart, 5 to 6 mm from the debrided edge, and including the seromuscular layers of both the bowel being patched and the bowel used for patching are to be employed. It is essential that the patch not be sewn directly to the edges of the defect whether the patch is used to buttress the suture line or as the sole method of closure (Fig. 47–2).

CLINICAL APPLICATIONS

Categories of patients in whom the serosal patch technique has been applied include: (1) chronic intestinal perforations, (2) acute intestinal perforations, (3) trauma, (4) prophylaxis, and (5) iatrogenic defects.

Chronic Intestinal Perforations

Seven patients with chronic intestinal perforations are presented in Table 47–1. These include patients with duodenal cutaneous fistula, perforated chronic gastric ulcer, enterocutaneous fistula, fistulas consequent to breakdown of Billroth I and Billroth II anastomoses. In two of the patients, Case 4 and Case 6, perforations were present within an abscess cavity. Serosal patch closure of a perforated duodenal stump is shown in Figure 47–3. The application of the technique to breakdown of a Billroth I anastomosis is shown in Figure 47–4. The adjacent limb of the small intestine has been used to close a chronic enterocutaneous fistula, as shown in Figure 47–5. Serosal patch closure of perforated duodenal ulcer located within an abscess cavity is shown in Figure 47–6. Closure of a disrupted Finney pyloroplasty by a serosal patch is depicted in Figure 47–7. In Cases 2 and 7 the serosal patch succeeded after a previously applied omental patch failed. In two other patients, Cases 4 and 6, the serosal patch was effective in the face of an adjacent abscess.

Acute Intestinal Perforations

Eight patients had acute intestinal perforations closed with the serosal patch technique (Table 47–2). These included: leaking esophagogastric anastomosis, leaking gastrostomy, leaking pyloroplasty, perforated gastric ulcer, perforated duodenal stump, and disrupted gastroduodenostomies. The one failure in the series of 28 patients occurred in Case 10; this was a leaking esophagogastrostomy in which the patch failed to achieve primary closure.

TABLE 47–1. CHRONIC INTESTINAL PERFORATIONS

Case No. and Pathology	Duration of Perforation	Supportive Treatment	Technique of Serosal Patch Closure	Result
Case 1 Caucasian male, age 57; perforated duodenal stump; enterocutaneous fistula	1 year	Hyperalimentation for 3 months, no improvement	Roux-Y serosal patch to perforated duodenal stump	Well; home on 11th PO day
Case 2 Caucasian male, age 51; breakdown of Billroth I anastomosis; enterocutaneous fistula	2.5 months	1st repair 13 days PO using omental patch which failed; fistula persisted after hyperalimentation and tube jejunostomy for 2 months	Roux-Y serosal patch to close leak at anastomosis	Well; home on 7th PO day
Case 3 Caucasian male, age 57; small bowel enterocutaneous fistula	"Many years" followed appendectomy in 1943	Numerous unsuccessful surgical repairs at outside hospitals	Fistula excised; lateral serosal jejunal patch	Well; home on 17th PO day
Case 4 Caucasian male, age 48; chronic perforated duodenal ulcer; subhepatic abscess cavity	Several months (history unreliable)	Routine preparation for surgery	Serosal patch over perforation using jejunal loop	No abdominal problems; transfered to psychiatric ward
Case 5 Caucasian female, age 53; chronic duodenocutaneous fistula following Billroth II, perforated stump	9 months	Three drainage procedures at outside hospital	Suspected proximal limb hypertension corrected and rigid open duodenal stump closed with a Roux-Y serosal patch	Benign course; home on 11th PO day
Case 6 Caucasian male, age 62; chronic perforated gastric ulcer; large rigid walled subhepatic cavity	31 days	Routine preparation for surgery	Gastric biopsies benign; defect closed with Roux-Y serosal patch	Benign course; home on 15th PO day
Case 7 Caucasian female, age 59; gastroduodenocutaneous fistula from breakdown of Finney pyloroplasty	10 weeks	Wound dehisence 9 days PO, pyloroplasty noted to be leaking; closed by suture and omental patch; unsuccessful. Fistula developed in 3 days. Hyperalimentation for 2 months.	6 × 8 cm defect closed with Roux-Y serosal patch; could not completely close abdominal wall; patch could be observed and showed no leakage	Benign course; home as soon as abdominal wound healed

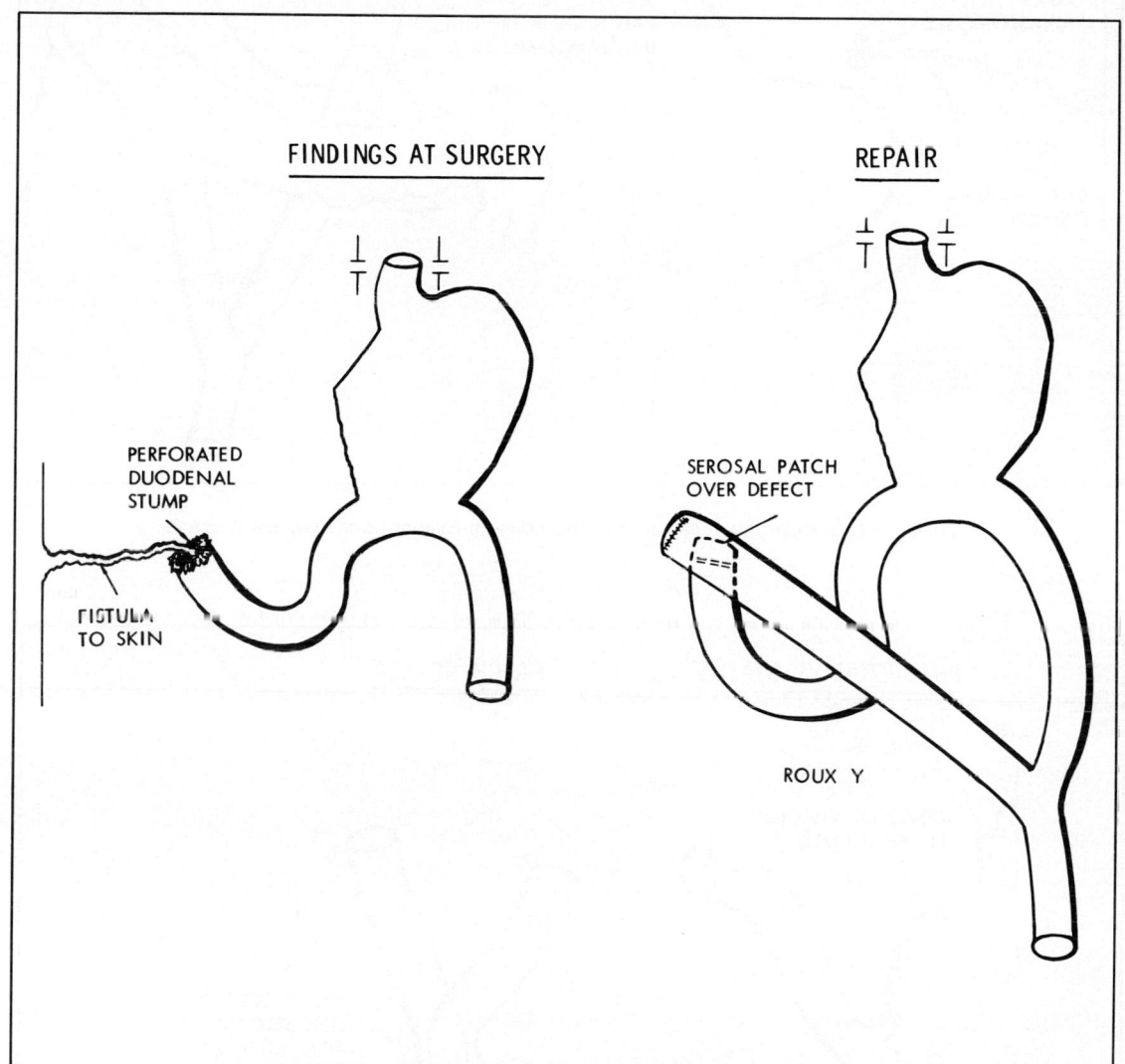

Figure 47–3. Serosal patching of perforated duodenal stump (Case 1).

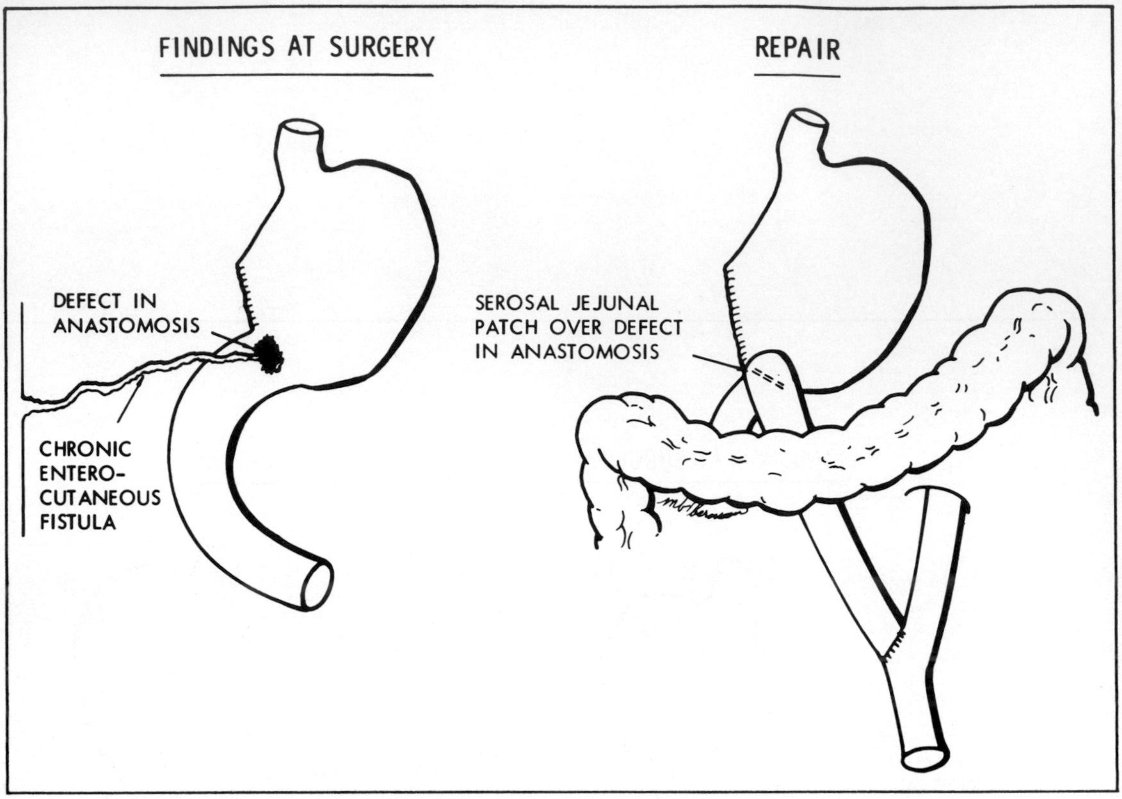

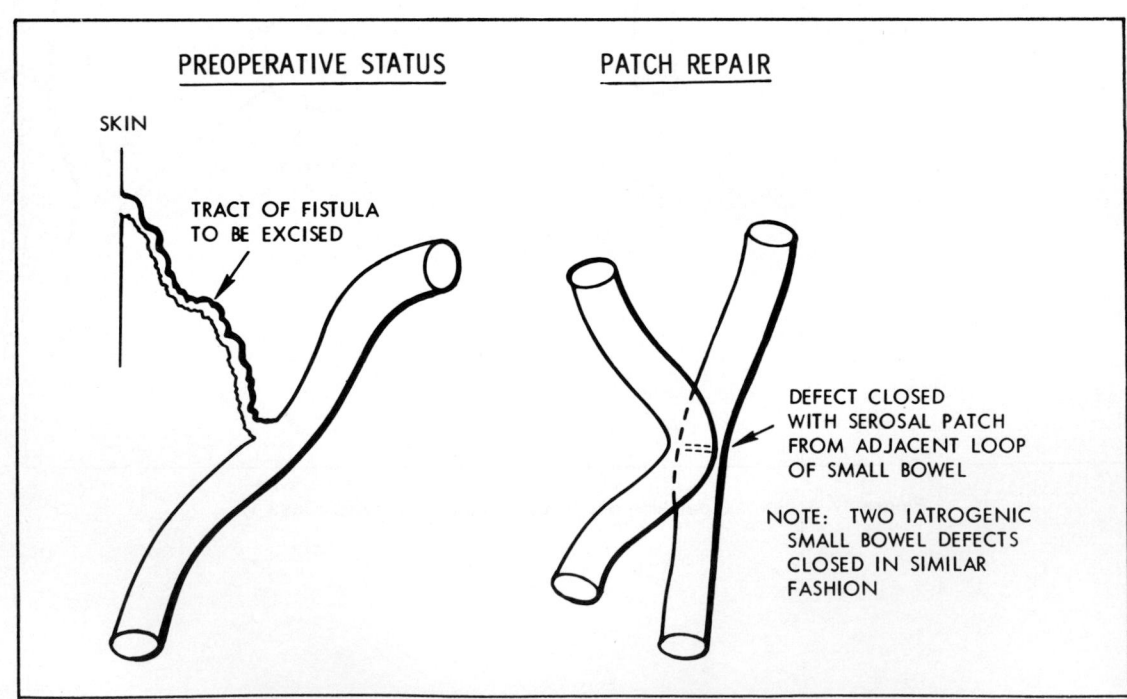

Figure 47–4. Serosal patch closure of breakdown of Billroth I anastomosis (Case 2).

FINDINGS AT SURGERY

REPAIR

DEFECT IN ANASTOMOSIS

CHRONIC ENTERO-CUTANEOUS FISTULA

SEROSAL JEJUNAL PATCH OVER DEFECT IN ANASTOMOSIS

PREOPERATIVE STATUS

PATCH REPAIR

SKIN

TRACT OF FISTULA TO BE EXCISED

DEFECT CLOSED WITH SEROSAL PATCH FROM ADJACENT LOOP OF SMALL BOWEL

NOTE: TWO IATROGENIC SMALL BOWEL DEFECTS CLOSED IN SIMILAR FASHION

Figure 47–5. Serosal patch of chronic enterocutaneous fistula (Case 3).

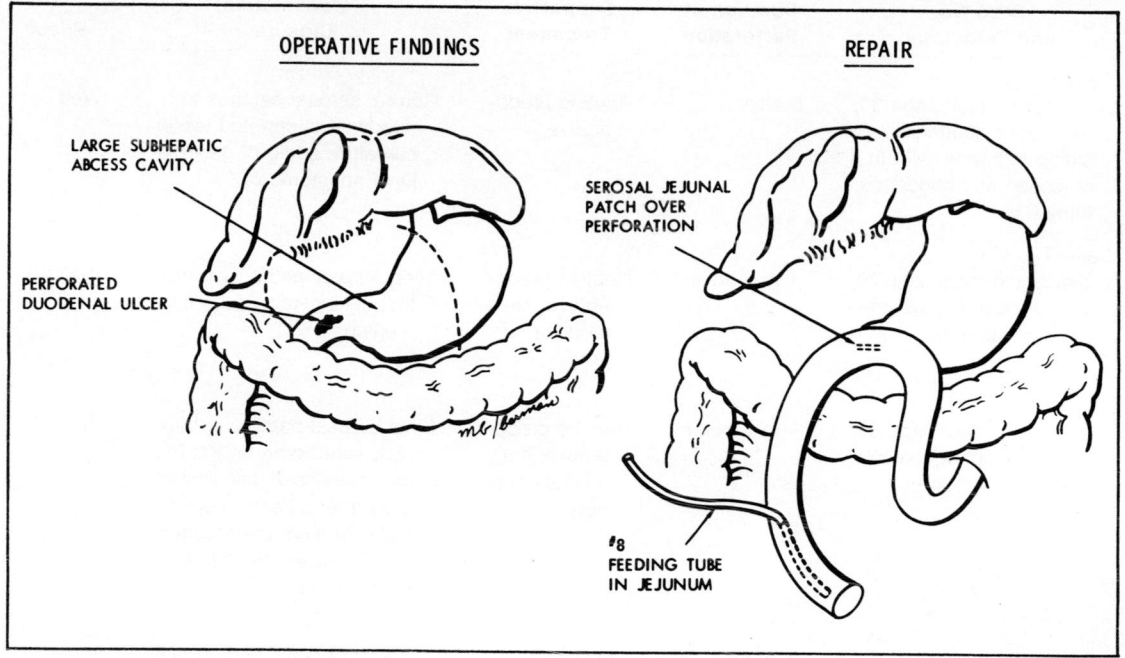

Figure 47–6. Serosal patch closure of perforated duodenal ulcer within abscess (Case 4).

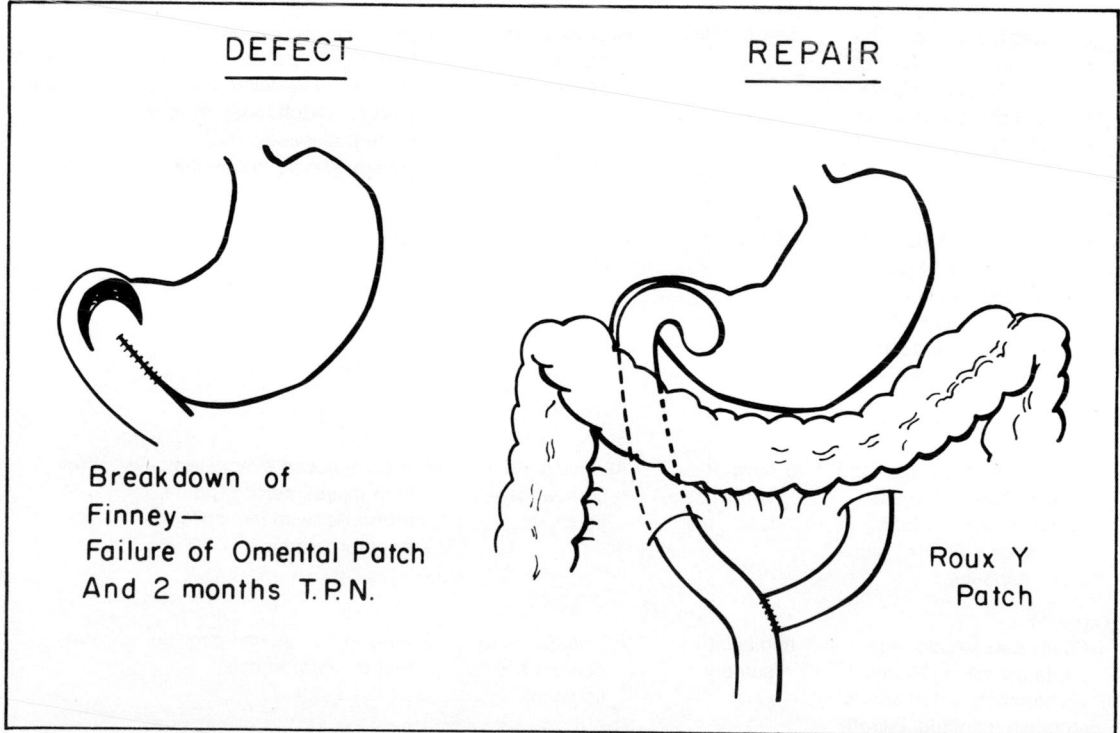

Figure 47–7. Serosal patch closure of disrupted Finney pyloroplasty (Case 7).

TABLE 47-2. ACUTE INTESTINAL PERFORATIONS

Case No. and Pathology	Duration of Perforation	Supportive Treatment	Technique of Serosal Patch Closure	Result
Case 8 Caucasian male, age 55; perforated duodenal stump following Billroth II resection and duodenostomy tube	8 days	Routine preoperative	Roux-Y serosal patches to duodenal stump and lesser curvature angle of gastrojejunal anastomosis	Well
Case 9 Caucasian male, age 79; leak of esophagogastrostomy anastomosis	4 to 5 hours	Routine preoperative; immediate surgery	Loop serosal patch over defect; jejunostomy tube for feeding	Well
Case 10 Caucasian male, age 69; leak of esophagogastrostomy anastomosis	4 to 5 hours	Routine preoperative; immediate surgery	Loop serosal patch over defect; sent home on 8th PO day; developed pain immediately after a heavy meal that night; formed enterocutaneous fistula which sealed spontaneously	Well
Case 11 Caucasian male, age 29; leak of gastrostomy	4 to 5 hours	Routine preoperative; immediate surgery	8 × 8 cm breakdown of gastrostomy patched with Roux-Y limb; serosal patch held despite gross sepsis and severe PO upper GI bleeding	Well
Case 12 Caucasian male, age 70; perforated DU treated by Heineke–Mikulicz pyloroplasty which broke down on PO day 7	4 to 5 hours	Routine preoperative; immediate surgery	Jejunal loop serosal patch over perforation; *permanent sections showed duodenal carcinoma;* patch held; multiple system diseases made definitive surgery impossible	"Well" as regards patch
Case 13 Black male, age 62; excision of pancreatic pseudocyst, distal pancreas, spleen and greater curvature of stomach; gastric closure leaked 1 week later	24 hours	Routine preoperative	Jejunal loop serosal patch over very tenuous closure of old gastrostomy; V and P added	Died of terminal renal failure
Case 14 Caucasian male, age 52; leaking Billroth I anastomosis; *S. aureus* infection; septic shock, jaundice; moribund	5 days of known leak	All measures to combat septic shock	350 cc abscess evacuated; loop jejunal serosal patch, retrocolic, with infracolic entroenterostomy	Well
Case 15 Caucasian female, age 73; large colon CA invading stomach; colon and ½ stomach resected; Billroth I anastomosis leaked on PO 5, and developed severe septic shock	Immediate surgery	All measures to combat septic shock	Roux-Y patch sewed over defect in anastomosis	Well

Trauma

Serosal patches were applied to traumatized organs on five occasions (Table 47–3). In two patients, a transected tail of the pancreas was buttressed with serosa of the stomach. In another patient the duct of Santorini was implanted into the second portion of the duodenum, and the anastomosis was patched. In the remaining two patients a serosal patch was applied to a duodenal injury (Fig. 47–8).

Prophylaxis

In two patients serosal patches were applied prophylactically anticipating the potential for a leak related to inflammation in the region of a suture line (Table 47–4).

Iatrogenic Defects

Six patients developed intestinal defects related to surgical procedures, either immediately or several days after the injury (Table 47–5). These included five duodenal leaks and one small bowel disruption. One patient who died had demonstrated failure of the patch to control the leak; the other five patients all had autopsy confirmation that the patch had sealed.

Acknowledgment. Gratitude is expressed to George L. Juler, M.D., Alan B. Gazzaniga, M.D., and Byron Wood, M.D. for permission to use their cases in compiling this series.

TABLE 47–3. PATCHES FOR TRAUMA

Case No. and Pathology	Duration of Perforation	Supportive Treatment	Technique of Serosal Patch Closure	Result
Case 16 Caucasian male, age 15; traumatic performation posterior wall, 3rd portion of duodenum, blunt trauma	24 hours	Routine preoperative	Roux-Y serosal patch	Well
Case 17 Caucasian male, age 24; GSW of anterior and posterior duodenal walls "terribly lacerated and contused"; multiple other injuries	6 hours	Routine and treatment of shock	Both duodenal defects closed by serosal patch Roux-Y limb	Uneventful recovery; home well
Case 18 Caucasian male, age 22; GSW shattered tail of pancreas—also involved adrenal, kidney, spleen, stomach	7 hours	Routine and treatment of shock	Pancreatic tail resected, over-sewed; serosa of stomach used as a buttress patch	Home well
Case 19 Caucasian male, age 48; 90% traumatic pancreatectomy; large gastric laceration; gallbladder avulsed	5 hours	Routine and treatment of shock	Duct of Wirsung ligated; Santorini implanted and anastomosis patched; cholecystectomy and Billroth II	Benign course PO; home well
Case 20 Caucasian female, age 21; laceration of tail of pancreas	6 hours	Routine and treatment of shock	Tail of pancreas resected, over-sewed, and buttressed with serosa of stomach; multiple other injuries repaired	Uneventful PO course; home well

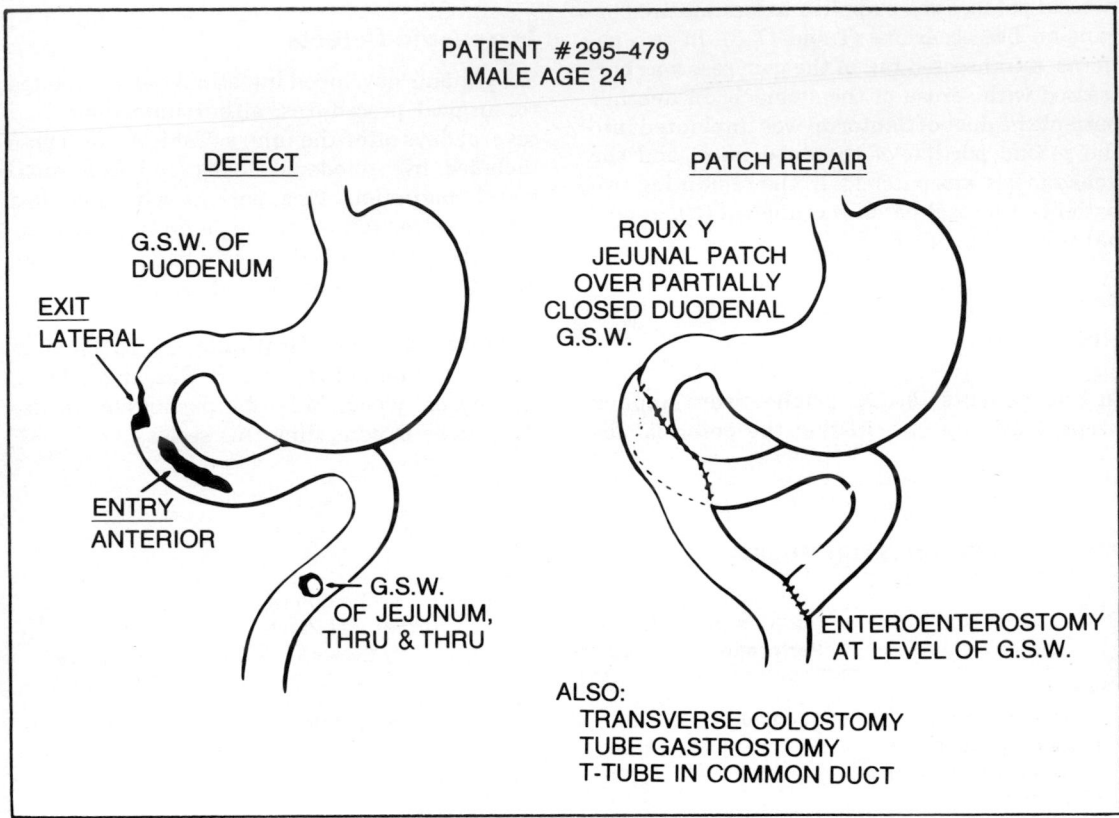

Figure 47–8. Closure of two duodenal defects using a Roux-Y jejunal serosal patch.

TABLE 47–4. PROPHYLACTIC PATCHES

Case No. and Pathology	Duration of Perforation	Supportive Treatment	Technique of Serosal Patch Closure	Result
Case 21 Caucasian male, age 29; previous vagotomy and Jaboulay; latter changed to Billroth II	Immediate (at surgery)	Gastric suction because of slow empty-ing	Jaboulay changed to Billroth II; duode-nal stump closure insecure; opening produced by the takedown of Jabou-lay inflamed; both suture lines but-tressed by serosal patches using the efferent jejunal limb	Well
Case 22 Black male, age 45; 3-cm mass in pancreatic head; duodenum thick-walled, resembling Crohn's; all biopsies benign	Immediate (at surgery)	Routine preop-erative or-ders	Diagnostic duodenostomy closed with protective patch; cholecystojejunos-tomy and posterior gastroenteros-tomy performed	Well

TABLE 47–5. IATROGENIC DEFECTS

Case No. and Pathology	Duration of Perforation	Supportive Treatment	Technique of Serosal Patch Closure	Result
Case 23 Caucasian female, age 62; perforation of duodenum in passage of Baker tube at surgery	Immediate		Fourth portion duodenum perforated; immediate transverse suture closure patched with adjacent jejunum	Died of pancreatic atrophy and congestive heart failure *one month after patching*
Case 24 Caucasian male, age 66; one-year post abdominal colectomy and ileoproctostomy; entered septic, moribund, large horseshoe abscesses from anastomotic leak; treated by Hartmann's procedure, ileostomy; iatrogenic small bowel defect patched. Operated 1 week later for enterocutaneous fistula produced by retention suture; patched; both serosal patches remained firmly sealed	a. Immediate b. 1 week	Antibiotics, fluid imbalance	In each instance leak closed with serosal patch of adjacent jejunum	Expired with sepsis and renal failure, 17 days after admission
Case 25 Caucasian female, age 66; V and P for supposed DU found on permanent section to be duodenal CA; Whipple done; abscess drained, limb used to patch jejunal defect	Immediate	Defect produced when abscess drained	Inflamed and friable tissue; tenuous suture line covered with serosal patch	Expired from metastatic disease *60 days after patching*
Case 26 Caucasian male, age 79; right transabdominal nephrectomy for staghorn calculus; moribund	7 days	Treatment of septic shock	1 cm posterior duodenal defect patched; gross peritonitis; extensive drainage instituted	Expired from overwhelming sepsis 6 days after patching
Case 27 Caucasian male, age 52; outside hospital; attempt to remove distal common duct stone reportedly injured duodenum and pancreas; Billroth II performed; developed perforated duodenal stump PO day 13; not seen in consultation until PO day 26; on PO day 30 was operated upon as a last resort; moribund	17 days	Treatment of septic shock	Both wide open duodenostomy site and duodenal stump covered with serosal patches; loop with enteroenterostomy below	Expired from overwhelming sepsis 6 days after patching

(continued)

TABLE 47–5. (CONTINUED)

Case No. and Pathology	Duration of Perforation	Supportive Treatment	Technique of Serosal Patch Closure	Result
Case 28 Caucasian female, age 27; Auto vs auto-; transection of ⅔ of 2nd part of duodenum; sutured and protected with a serosal patch; 6 days later a RLQ abscess was drained, the patch inadvertently pulled away from the closure, *and not replaced as it "looked secure";* bile drainage appeared 4 days later but no further aggressive therapy was used	On entry	Routine preoperative workup	Roux-Y patch to duodenal defect; sealed duodenal area completely until disrupted by surgeon at second procedure	Initial patch was completely sealed at 6 days; died from peritonitis from perforated duodenal stump 58 days after patch was disrupted

BIBLIOGRAPHY

Ballinger WF, McLaughlin ED, et al: Jejunal overlay closure of the duodenum in the newborn: Lateral duodenal tear caused by gastrostomy tube. Surgery 59:450, 1966.

Barber WF: Discussion of Jones SA, Gazzaniga AB, et al: The serosal patch—A surgical parachute. Am J Surg 126:187, 1973

Boyden AM: Discussion of Jones SA, Gazzaniga AB, et al: The serosal patch—A surgical parachute. Am J Surg 126:187, 1973

Critselis AN, Papaioannou AN: Serosal patch vs. duodenojejunostomy in duodenal stump closure. Letter to the Editor. Arch Surg 112:670, 1977

Jones SA, Gazzaniga AB, et al: The serosal patch—A surgical parachute. Am J Surg 126:187, 1973

Jones SA, Gregory G, et al: Surgical management of the difficult and perforated duodenal stump. Am J Surg 108:257, 1964

Jones SA, Steedman RA: Management of chronic infected intestinal perforations by the serosal patch technique. Am J Surg 117:731, 1969

Kobald EE, Thal AP: A simple method for the management of experimental wounds of the duodenum. Surg Gynecol Obstet 116:340, 1963

McKittrick JE: Use of a serosal patch in repair of duodenal fistula. Calif Med 103:433, 1965

Webster MW Jr, Carey LC: Fistulas of the intestinal tract. Curr Probl Surg Vol 13(6), 1976

Wolfman EF Jr, Trevino G, et al: An operative technique for the management of acute and chronic latero-duodenal fistulas. Ann Surg 159:563, 1964

SECTION VIII
Appendix and Colon

48. Appendix
Harold Ellis

HISTORICAL NOTE*

The first appendicectomy was performed by Amyand, surgeon to Westminster and St. George's Hospitals and Sergeant Surgeon to George II. In 1736, he operated on a boy aged 11 suffering from a right scrotal hernia accompanied by a fistula. Within the scrotum was found the appendix, perforated by a pin. The appendix was ligated and all or, more likely, part of it, removed with recovery.

In 1755, Heister recognised that the appendix might be the site of acute primary inflammation. He described an autopsy on the body of a criminal who had been executed and wrote:

> When about to demonstrate the large bowel, I found the vermiform appendix of the caecum preternaturally black. As I was about to separate it, its membranes parted and discharged two to three spoonfuls of matter. It is probable that this person might have had some pain in the part.

In 1824, Loyer-Villermay gave a presentation to the Royal Academy of Medicine in Paris entitled "Observations of Use in the Inflammatory Conditions of the Caecal Appendix," in which he described two examples of acute appendicitis leading to death. In both cases at autopsy the appendix was found to be black and gangrenous, while the caecum was scarcely involved. Three years later these observations were confirmed by Melier. Unfortunately, at this stage the pathologic picture became obscured. The writings of Husson and Dance in 1827, Goldbeck in 1830 and, most powerfully of all, Dupuytren in 1835 developed the concept of inflammation arising in the cellular tissue

surrounding the caecum; it was Goldbeck who invented the term "perityphlitis," which did much to delay the progress of the understanding of this disease.

The first textbook to give a description of the symptoms that accompanied inflammation and perforation of the appendix was published by Bright and Addison in 1839. The terms "typhlitis" and "perityphlitis" remained in use until the end of the nineteenth century. It was Fitz, Professor of Medicine at Harvard, who in 1886 gave a lucid and logical description of the clinical features and described in detail the pathologic changes of the disease; he was as well the first to use the term "appendicitis." He wrote:

> In most fatal cases of typhlitis, the caecum is intact whilst the appendix is ulcerated and perforated. The question should be entertained of immediate opening. If any good result is to arise from such treatment it must be applied early.

Turning now to the evolution of the operative treatment of appendicitis, Hancock in London successfully drained an appendix abscess in a female patient aged 30 who was in her eighth month of pregnancy. In 1848, he wrote:

> It may be premature to argue from the result of one case, but I trust that the time will come when this plan will be successfully employed in other cases of peritonitis terminating in effusion, which usually end fatally.

Parker of New York advocated earlier incision of appendix abscesses in 1867; following the publication of his paper many similar accounts were published.

From the priority point of view, Shepherd has shown that, in 1880, Tait of Birmingham operated upon a patient suffering from a gangrenous appendicitis and removed the appendix,

---

* For detailed accounts of the history of appendicitis, the reader is referred to the fascinating books by Sir Zachary Cope (1965) and Dr. Ralph Major (1945).

1255

with recovery of the patient. However, Tait did not record this case until 1890. Credit for the first published account of appendicectomy must go to Kronlein in 1886, although the patient, aged 17, died 2 days later. In 1887, Morton of Philadelphia successfully diagnosed and excised an acutely inflamed appendix lying within an abscess cavity. Two years later, McBurney in New York pioneered early diagnosis and early operative intervention and also devised the muscle-splitting incision named after him. Early intervention was still further popularised by the teaching of Murphy of Chicago. Both these surgeons pioneered the removal of the appendix before perforation had been allowed to take place.

It soon became evident that while the results of appendicectomy for the acutely inflamed unperforated appendix were satisfactory, the operative death rate for the later perforated cases with peritonitis was distressingly high. Ochsner in Chicago and Sherren at The London Hospital were both advocates in the early years of the twentieth century of conservative treatment in late cases. The discovery of antibiotics, fortunately, resolved the controversy between the schools of conservative and active surgery in such cases.

ANATOMY

The appendix arises from the posteromedial aspect of the caecum, about 2.5 cm below the ileocaecal valve. It is the only organ in the body that has no constant anatomic position; in fact its only constant feature is its mode of origin from the caecum, where it arises from the site at which the three taeniae coli coalesce. It varies considerably in length, from 1 to 25 cm, but it averages 5 to 10 cm. The various positions of the appendix are: paracolic (the appendix lies in the sulcus on the outer side of the caecum), retrocaecal (the organ lies behind the caecum and may even be totally or partially extraperitoneal), preileal, postileal, promontoric (the tip of the organ pointing toward the promontory of the sacrum), pelvic (here the appendix dips into the pelvic cavity), and midinguinal (subcaecal). The retrocaecal position is the most common. Wakeley (1933), in an analysis of 10,000 cases at postmortem, gives the location of the appendix as follows: retrocaecal, 65.28 percent; pelvic, 31.01 percent; subcaecal, 2.26 percent; preileal,

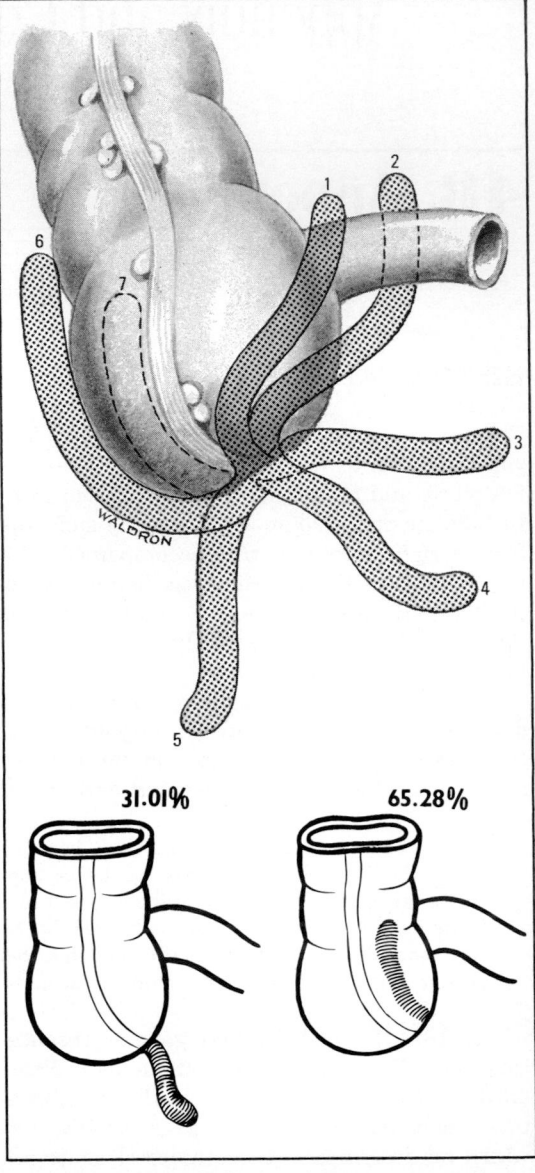

Figure 48–1. *Top:* Various positions that the appendix can occupy: (1) preileal; (2) postileal; (3) promontoric; (4) pelvic; (5) subcaecal; (6) paracolic or precaecal; (7) retrocaecal. *Bottom Left:* Location of the appendix in Wakeley's series of 10,000 cases (pelvic or descending position). *Bottom Right:* Location of the appendix in Wakeley's series of 10,000 cases (postcaecal and retrocaecal). (*Source: Adapted from Wakeley C, 1933, with permission.*)

1 percent and right paracolic and postileal, 0.4 percent (Fig. 48–1).

Williamson et al (1981) found that of 105 retrocaecal appendices removed at operation, 12 (11.4 percent) extended retroperitoneally. In this position the appendix may extend upward as far as the kidney and indeed in 2 of these 12 cases, the patient experienced pain in the right flank.

The appendix may be situated in the left lower quadrant of the abdomen in cases of transposition of the viscera. Here the clue may be the observation that the patient has dextrocardia; this author has correctly diagnosed and operated on such a case. A particularly long appendix may also extend over into the left side of the abdomen and, if inflamed, produce left iliac fossa pain. In cases of malrotation of the bowel, where the caecum fails to descend to its normal position, the appendix may be found in the epigastrium, abutting against the stomach or beneath the right lobe of the liver.

Robinson (1952), in reporting a case of congenital absence of the appendix, was able to collect only 68 other examples, a figure sufficiently indicative of the great rarity of this condition.

Duplication of the appendix is an anomaly of extreme rarity and fewer than 100 cases have been reported (Khanna, 1983). Wallbridge (1962) classified duplication of the appendix into three types. Type A comprises partial duplica-

tion of the appendix on a single caecum. Type B has a single caecum with two completely separate appendices. This is further subdivided into B1, which is also called "bird-like appendix" due to its resemblence to the normal arrangement in birds, where there are two appendices symmetrically placed on either side of the ileocaecal valve, and Type B2, where one appendix arises from the usual site on the caecum, with another rudimentary appendix arising from the caecum along the line of a taenia coli. In Type C there is a double caecum, each of which bears an appendix. Tinckler (1968) has described a unique case of a triple appendix, associated with a double penis and ectopia vesicae.

Embryologically, the appendix is part of the caecum, of which it forms the distal end and which histologically it closely resembles, with the exception that it contains an excess of lymphoid tissue in the submucous layer. The mesentery of the appendix is contiguous with the lower leaf of the mesentery of the small intestine, and it passes behind the terminal ileum. The appendicular artery runs in the free border of the mesentery of the appendix and is a branch of the ileocolic artery (Fig. 48–2). This repre-

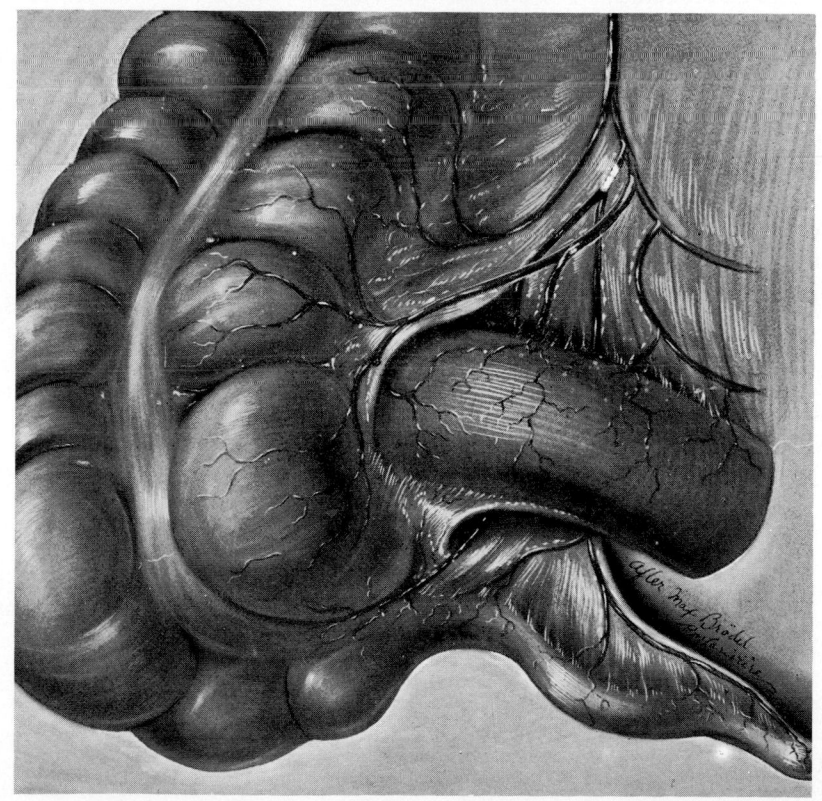

Figure 48–2. The appendix and its blood supply.

sents the entire arterial supply of the organ and thrombosis of this artery in acute appendicitis inevitably results in gangrene and subsequent perforation. This is in contrast to acute cholecystitis, where the rich collateral blood supply of the gallbladder, from its bed in the liver, accounts for the comparative rarity of gangrene.

The veins from the appendix drain into the ileocolic vein which in turn empties into the superior mesenteric vein. A variable number of slender lymphatic channels traverse the mesoappendix to empty into the ileocaecal nodes.

ACUTE APPENDICITIS

Incidence

Acute appendicitis is the most common cause of the "acute surgical abdomen" in the United Kingdom but since the disease is not notifiable, its exact incidence is not known.

The Hospital Inpatient Enquiry (1976), which estimates the total hospital inpatient discharges in England and Wales, gives the annual estimated total of acute appendicitis based on a one tenth sample at 62,060, a figure that had remained relatively stable over the past 5 years.

Pieper and Kager (1982), in a careful study from Sweden, estimate a yearly incidence of 1.33 cases of appendicitis per thousand of the population in males and 0.99 per thousand in females (this difference is statistically significant, $p = 0.002$). In this study, of 971 cases, the ages of the patients ranged from 1 year to 89 years with a median of 22. Twenty five percent of the patients were younger than 14 years and 75 percent younger than 33. Although these authors could find no evidence of a fall in the incidence of acute appendicitis, other studies indicate a steady decline in appendicitis and appendicectomy. Noer (1975) reported a decrease in the incidence of acute appendicitis from 1.3 per thousand to 0.5 per thousand over a 30-year period from 1943 to 1972 in a study of a well-defined population in Norway.

Castleton et al (1959) reviewed 19 major hospitals in the United States and found the total number of acute appendicectomies had dropped when 1941 figures were compared with 1956. This was not attributed to the increase in admittance at rural or community hospitals, since a study of 20 such hospitals also showed a decline in the number of appendicectomies. Palumbo (1959) also noted a decline in the number of cases of appendicitis at his Veteran's Administration hospital from 1947 to 1958.

Such figures need cautious interpretation, since many studies do not differentiate between all cases of appendicectomy and those in which the diagnosis of acute appendicitis was confirmed.

Geographic Distribution

Appendicitis is most frequently observed in North America, the British Isles, Australia, and New Zealand and among white South Africans. It is rare in most of Asia, Central Africa, and among the Eskimos. When people from these areas migrate to the Western world or change to a Western diet, appendicitis becomes prevalent, suggesting that the distribution of this disease is determined environmentally rather than genetically. It is undoubtedly much more common among the meat-eating white races and relatively rare in those who habitually live on a bulk cellulose diet. Quite unexplained variations in incidence in various parts of England were found by Baker and Liggins (1981)—14.6 per 10,000 cases of acute appendicitis in the North compared with 10.4 and 10.6 in Central and Southern England, with no consistent socioeconomic variations. Again, these authors suggest dietary differences might be contributory factors.

Many surgeons believe that there is a familial tendency in this disease that could be explained by an inherited malformation of the organ. However, the incidence of a large number of cases in the same family can equally be explained by the common nature of this disease. Andersson and colleagues (1979) compared 29 children between the ages of 5 and 15 suffering from acute appendicitis with 29 controls. Twenty in the study group compared with four in the controls gave a history of appendicitis in parents or siblings.

Pathology

Cases of appendicitis are best classified as follows:

1. Acute appendicitis without perforation
2. Acute appendicitis with perforation
   a. With local peritonitis
   b. With local abscess (appendix mass)

Acute appendicitis is not associated with any specific bacterial, viral or protozoal invader.

The bacteriology of the inflamed organ is that of the normal bowel flora, suggesting secondary invasion of damaged tissue from the lumen of the bowel. A detailed study by Pieper and colleagues (1982) of the bacteriology of 50 inflamed appendices gave both aerobic and anaerobic isolates from all cases. Anaerobic bacteria were found more frequently than aerobic (141 versus 96 isolates). *Escherchia coli* was the most common aerobic bacterium (47 out of 50 patients). Ten patients also harboured other aerobic gram-negative rods, including *Klebsiella, Proteus,* and *Pseudomonas.* Enterococci (*Streptococcus faecalis* and *S. faecium*) were found in 15 patients and streptococci (*S. mitior, S. milleri,* and *S. salivarius*) in 21 patients. Of the anaerobic strains, *Bacteroides fragilis* predominated. Anaerobic gram-positive cocci were next in frequency, while *Clostridium perfringens* was cultivated from nine patients.

Examination of a series of fresh specimens of acutely inflamed appendices will show that these fall into two groups. The first demonstrate a "catarrhal" inflammation of the whole organ, while the second group demonstrate an obstruction of the appendix beyond which there is acute inflammation, distension with pus, and in later cases progression to gangrene and eventually perforation.

Catarrhal appendicitis is initially a mucosal and submucosal inflammation. In early cases, the appendix may appear quite normal externally or may merely show hyperaemia. On slitting it open, however, the mucosa will be seen to be thickened, oedematous, and reddened; later it becomes studded with dark brown haemorrhagic infarcts, patches of grey-green gangrene or small ulcers. Eventually the whole appendix becomes swollen and turgid and the serosa becomes roughened, loses its healthy sheen and is coated with a fibrinous exudate. The probable aetiology of this condition is bacterial invasion of the lymphoid tissue in the appendix wall and indeed some cases are probably localised manifestations of a generalised enteritis. Because the lumen of the appendix is not obstructed, these cases rarely progress to gangrene, and in many instances the acute inflammatory attack will resolve spontaneously. In other cases, however, swelling of the lymphoid tissue in the appendix wall may lead to obstruction of the lumen and the condition may then proceed to obstructive appendicitis and gangrene. Even when the acute inflammatory process subsides, the appendix probably never regains its pristine state; adhesion formation and kinking of the appendix may lead to a final episode of acute obstructive appendicitis. It is interesting that an episode of gangrenous appendicitis may well be preceded by several milder and resolving attacks (Fig. 48-3).

Obstructive appendicitis is the dangerous type, for the appendix becomes a closed loop of bowel containing decomposing faecal matter. The changes following the sudden blocking of the lumen of the appendix depend on the amount and the character of the content distal to the obstruction. If the lumen is empty, the appendix distends with mucus to form a mucocele (Fig. 48-4). When the appendix becomes obstructed, the process of events is accumulation of normal mucus secretion, proliferation of the contained bacteria, pressure atrophy of the mucosa, which allows bacterial access to the deeper tissue planes, inflammation of the walls of the appendix with vessel thrombosis which, since the blood supply is an end-artery system, leads inevitably to gangrene and then perforation of the necrotic appendix wall. On other occasions, bacterial invasion occurs through pressure erosion of a contained faecolith, which may discharge into the peritoneal cavity through the perforation.

The relationship between obstruction of the appendix and gangrenous appendicitis was demonstrated in 1914 by Wilkie, who showed that acute appendicitis followed ligation of the appendix in the rabbit. Wangensteen and colleagues documented in 1937 and 1940 that combined obstruction and bacterial infection resulted in acute appendicitis, whereas, if the appendix was first washed free of faecal material and then ligated, a mucocele developed as mucus continued to be secreted within the bacteria-free lumen of the appendix. These classic studies have recently been elegantly extended by Pieper et al (1983) who showed that obstruction of the appendix in the rabbit using a balloon catheter introduced via a caecostomy resulted in 12 hours in the inflammatory changes that histologically in all respects were similar to appendicitis in man.

The obstruction may be due to a large number of possible causes—inflammatory swelling of the lymphoid tissue in the appendix wall may, as we have noted, occlude the lumen. Kinks and adhesions may result from congenital bands or from previous episodes of inflammation. One or

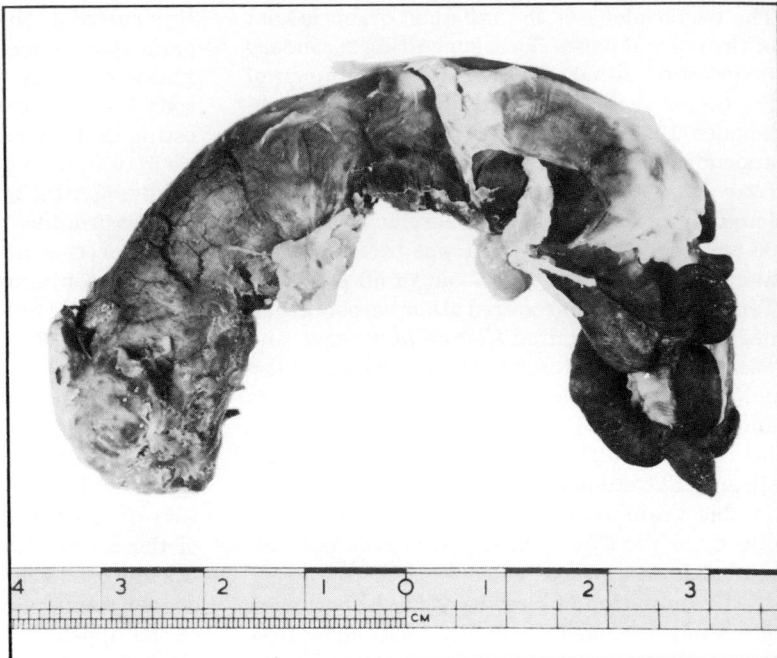

Figure 48–3. An acutely inflamed appendix; the distal half is gangrenous.

more faecoliths are commonly found within the appendix lumen in the normal organ; it is a frequent finding in about two thirds of all gangrenous appendices to find a faecolith firmly impacted at the junction between the uninflamed proximal and the gangrenous distal part of the appendix. Other foreign bodies, such as food debris, worms, or even a gallstone, have been found to obstruct the appendix lumen.

Perhaps the rarest cause of obstructive ap-

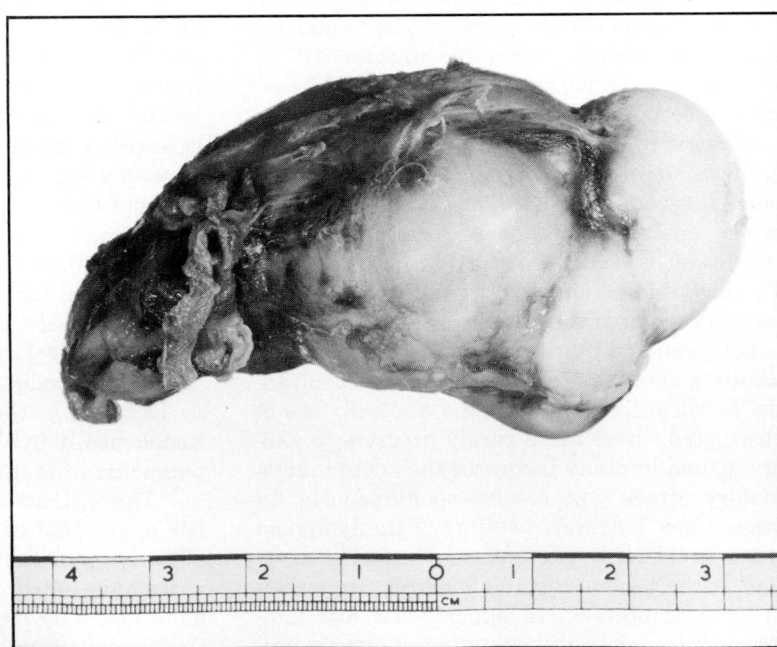

Figure 48–4. Mucocele of the appendix.

pendicitis is the appendix becoming strangulated within a hernial sac. Thomas et al (1982) report seven such cases. The most common hernia to be involved is the right femoral, then the right inguinal, but cases have been reported of acute appendicitis within a left inguinal, an umbilical, an incisional, and an obturator hernia. The usual diagnosis is, of course, a strangulated hernia and the correct diagnosis virtually has never been made before operation.

The Appendiceal Faecolith

Faecal material is commonly present in both the normal and the inflamed appendix and this should be differentiated from the true faecolith, which is ovoid, about 1 to 2 cm in length, and faecal coloured. Unlike ordinary faeces, the true faecolith shows a well-ordered lamination in section. Shaw (1965) showed that the great majority of these faecoliths are radiopaque and in 10 percent of cases of acute appendicitis contain sufficient calcium to be demonstrated on a plain x-ray of the abdomen. In a study of 240 cases of acute appendicitis, in which the appendix specimen was x-rayed, faecoliths were demonstrated in 33 percent of cases. When a faecolith was present, 77 percent of the specimens were gangrenous, compared with 42 percent when there was no evidence of a stone (Fig. 48–5).

Effects of Perforation

The appendix may rupture at any spot, but most frequently the site of perforation is along the antimesenteric border. Following perforation, a localised abscess may form in the right iliac fossa or the pelvis, or diffuse peritonitis may ensue. Whether the peritonitis remains localised or becomes generalised depends on many factors, including the age of the patient, the virulence of the invading bacteria, the rate at which the inflammatory condition has progressed within the appendix, and the position of the appendix.

It is usually stated that poorer localisation of the infection occurs in infants, due to the fact that the omentum of the child is filmy and less able to form a protective sheath around the inflamed appendix. A more likely explanation is that delays in diagnosis are more prone to occur in infants. A similar state of affairs occurs in the elderly. In the nonobstructed type of acute appendicitis, the disease is comparatively

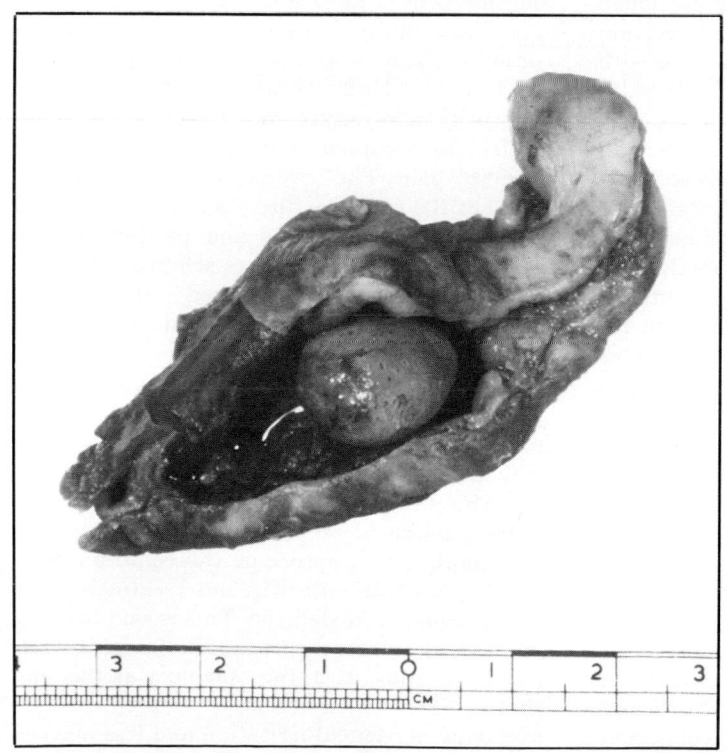

Figure 48–5. Gangrenous appendix containing a large faecolith.

limited in its course and the peritoneum has ample time for inflammatory adhesions to form. In contrast, in the acute obstructive form, the rapidity of the process gives little time for defensive adhesions to develop before the sudden flood of infected contents. An appendix situated in the retrocaecal or pelvic location is probably more likely to form a local abscess than one in the preileal or subcaecal position.

Clinical Manifestations

The patient with acute abdominal pain remains one of the last bastions of clinical medicine. There is no other common situation where clinical features, accurate diagnosis, and immediate decision are of such importance (Ellis, 1968). In most other fields, an initially tentative or even incorrect clinical diagnosis is not necessarily harmful; we can wait until it is confirmed or refuted by laboratory investigations or by the clinical progress of the case. In an acute abdominal emergency, however, delays of even a few hours in initiating the correct line of treatment may make the difference between a smooth or a stormy course or even place the patient in lethal danger. For example, to leave an early case of acute appendicitis undiagnosed overnight and well sedated with morphia may mean missing the opportunity of almost certain smooth recovery for this patient. In dealing with the patient with acute abdominal pain, the surgeon must realise that reliance is almost entirely on clinical features rather than on laboratory and radiologic investigation. Surgeons have become so accustomed, in recent years, to being able to skimp on history and examination in other situations that it comes as something of a shock to realise, in dealing with an acute abdominal emergency, that dependence is on the five senses for diagnosis. It is a very good aphorism that, in the diagnosis of the acute abdomen, special investigations can be used only to reinforce a clinical diagnosis; seldom, if ever, can they establish or refute it. This aphorism is particularly apt in the case of acute appendicitis.

It is important to remember that abdominal pain may result from disease of almost any organ of the body. Apart from the abdominal and retroperitoneal viscera themselves, including, of course, the pelvic organs, one must also consider diseases of the chest, the central nervous system, and even of the ears and the throat. Metabolic disorders, particularly diabetes, may give acute abdominal symptoms and finally the psychologic disturbance of the "Munchausen syndrome" provides us with an occasional diagnostic difficulty. The novice may well smile at the long list of differential diagnoses for acute appendicitis given in textbooks until, as personal experience grows, the chagrin of slowly ticking off mistakes one by one from the list comes to pass. It has been said that nothing can be so simple nor yet so difficult as the diagnosis of acute appendicitis.

The classic story of acute appendicitis is the onset of central, colicky, abdominal pain followed by nausea or one or more episodes of vomiting, with the pain, after several hours, shifting to the lower right abdomen. The pain is now continuous and severe, so that the patient finds movement uncomfortable and wishes to lie still, often with the legs flexed. Sleep is impossible. With progression of the disease process, the pain spreads diffusely over the abdomen.

The explanation of the pain distribution is that the central colicky pain is the result of stretching of the inflamed appendix wall. When the inflammatory process extends to the serosa, the parietal peritoneum is involved and the pain now shifts to the site of the appendix. Later diffuse spread of the pain corresponds with the development of generalised peritonitis.

Occasionally there is no history of this classic shift of pain. The onset of central pain might have occurred during sleep or, because of its relatively mild nature, may be forgotten by the patient preoccupied by the much more intense parietal pain. The severity and time relationships of the pain are also very variable—rapid progression to gangrene and peritonitis may take place within 12 hours whereas in other instances an acutely inflamed but nonperforated appendix may be removed after 3 or 4 days.

The patient may give a history of several previous mild attacks of what undoubtedly must have been appendicitis but which were overlooked as a mild "stomach ache."

The bowels are usually constipated but there may be accompanying diarrhoea, which is a confusing symptom as the condition may be diagnosed as enteritis and treatment may in consequence be delayed. This is said to occur particularly when the appendix lies in the retroileal position. It is the appendix at this site that is likely to be deceptive. It produces less overlying peritoneal irritation and less marked shift of pain than acute appendicitis occurring in one or other of the more usual positions of the appendix.

Examination commences with a careful inspection of the patient; the patient is usually flushed and in obvious pain, which is aggravated by movement. The pain becomes progressively worse as the disease progresses. Movement is avoided and the knees are often flexed. The tongue is at first lightly furred, then becomes progressively coated and the breath foul, although there is no absolute finding in acute appendicitis so one should not be surprised to find a patient with a perfectly clean moist tongue in this condition. The temperature and pulse are both usually raised and the rise progresses during the course of the disease. In adults, the usual finding is a temperature elevated about 1°C above normal; higher temperatures can be expected in children but a very high pyrexia, although occasionally seen in acute appendicitis, suggests some other diagnosis such as a pyelitis or respiratory infection.

An interesting study of 100 consecutive patients with acute appendicitis by Smith (1965) showed that only 60 had a temperature of 37.2°C or more and only 75 had a coated tongue.

The abdomen is now systematically and gently palpated with the warmed hand. In early cases this reveals localised tenderness, slight guarding, and release tenderness over the region of the appendix. Classically, this coincides with McBurney's point, but if the appendix is lying in one of its less common positions, this localised tenderness may be in the right flank, low down in the abdomen, towards the umbilicus, or even in the left iliac fossa. When the unperforated appendix is hanging over the brim of the pelvis or is lying wholly within the pelvis, abdominal rigidity and tenderness may be absent but rectal examination reveals definite tenderness anteriorly on the right side. In late cases with generalised peritonitis, the abdomen is diffusely tender, rigid, and silent on auscultation and the patient is obviously extremely ill. Later still, the abdomen is distended and the patient shows all the features of advanced peritonitis.

If the perforated appendix has become walled-off by surrounding structures into an appendix abscess, palpation reveals the tender swelling in the right iliac fossa and there may also be a boggy mass on rectal examination. There may be mucous diarrhoea due to irritation of the rectum and frequency of micturition

caused by congestion of the wall of the bladder by the pelvic abscess. However, the rest of the abdomen is soft, with no evidence of generalised peritonitis, and bowel sounds are present.

It should be stressed, of course, that the physical signs of acute appendicitis are not specific but are merely those produced by local peritoneal irritation in the right iliac fossa—the most common cause of which is acute inflammation of the appendix. Exactly the same clinical features are seen in other causes of lower right sided inflammatory disease—for example an acute Meckel's diverticulitis or an acute terminal ileitis. The most constant and reliable signs of local peritoneal irritation are local tenderness and guarding; a completely soft abdomen is most unlikely to harbour any serious surgical intraabdominal catastrophe.

Difficulties in Diagnosis

Difficulties in diagnosis are likely to be encountered in patients who present with diarrhoea, and who mimic an enteritis, or who have an appendix in the pelvic position, so that abdominal signs are minimal in the early hours and the diagnosis may be missed if a rectal examination is not performed. Patients who are obese disguise the physical signs of localised tenderness and guarding under their body fat and poor historians are their own worst enemies. However, any experienced surgeon would say that the greatest difficulties lie with young children, the elderly, and the pregnant.

Appendicitis in Children. In the infant the appendix has a relatively wide lumen and appendicitis is rare under the age of 2 years. However, it has been recorded in babies but a few days old (Coetzee, 1958; Fields et al, 1957) and even in premature babies. Ayalon et al (1979) report an example in a 31-week-old premature infant and have collected 23 previous published cases. From the age of 2, the incidence rises to a peak at about 11 years of age and then declines gradually at 15 before dropping rapidly thereafter (Leffall et al, 1967).

Both the mortality and morbidity of appendicitis are higher in preschool children than in those over the age of 5. The most likely explanation is that delays in diagnosis are more prone to occur in infants, so that a higher proportion are admitted to hospital with established peritonitis. Jackson (1963) studied 313 children up to the age of 12 years with acute appendicitis in Newcastle. Almost 50 percent had a perforated appendix at the time of admission. Perforation could be closely correlated with delay in parents sending for the doctor. Details were available in 285 of these cases; in 73 the delay was up to 12 hours and 24 percent had perforated. In 80, the delay was up to 24 hours and 42 percent had perforated. No less than 80 of the children did not reach hospital until the second day and 60 percent were perforated. A further 52 had delays of more than 48 hours, and of these no less than 83 percent had perforated. One third of the children had been given purgatives by the parents and 62 percent of these had a perforated appendix compared with 42 percent of the unpurged group. Fortunately, there was only one death in this series (0.3 percent). Fields and Cole (1967), in a study of 7000 patients with acute appendicitis at all ages in Los Angeles, found that 22 percent had perforated by the time of admission and there was a 2.4 percent overall mortality. In this series, 30 cases occurred in infants aged 3 years or less. Eighteen of these had perforated and four more were gangrenous but not yet ruptured. There were 2 deaths among these 30 children.

It is important to recognise that the clinical picture of acute appendicitis in young children is often atypical. Rather than a story of a shift of pain, there is frequently only the complaint of generalised abdominal pain. It is a good rule that if there is localised tenderness and muscle guarding in the right iliac fossa in a previously healthy child, then the chances are very strong indeed that the diagnosis is one of acute appendicitis. Thus, in a group of 153 children in Aberdeen subjected to surgery for acute abdominal pain, no less than 114 had confirmed acute appendicitis. A further 21 operated upon with this diagnosis were found to have a normal appendix and most of these had acute mesenteric adenitis. Of the remaining 18 children, 11 had intestinal obstruction (mostly intussusception) and 7 had visceral injuries (Jones, 1974; Winsey and Jones, 1967).

Appendicitis in the Elderly. Appendicitis is undoubtedly a more serious situation in the elderly than in younger patients. Peltokallio and Jauhiainen (1970) have shown that the clinical features of patients with acute appendicitis over the age of 60 are quite similar to younger age groups as regards pattern and duration of symptoms, the temperature changes and the white

cell responses. However, at operation both gangrenous changes and perforation occurred five times as often in the older age group. These findings suggest that poorer localisation of the infection and diminished blood supply of the appendix are important factors in allowing rapid progression of the disease. Similar findings have been reported by other investigators. For example, Andersson and Bergdahl (1978) found that half of their 68 patients with acute appendicitis over the age of 60 had perforations, and postoperative complications occurred in one third of these patients. Owens and Hamit (1978) reviewed 68 appendicectomies in patients between the ages of 65 and 99. Four of these were normal but, of the remainder, three quarters had ruptured at the time of surgery. Six of the patients died, all with perforated appendices. Interestingly, 21 of the cases had delays of 48 hours or more before surgical consultation took place.

There are other problems that face the surgeon dealing with an elderly patient with suspected acute appendicitis—there is inevitably a higher incidence of associated diseases that affect the general condition of the patient. The number of alternative causes of intraabdominal emergencies is greater, so that the differential diagnosis poses wider problems. Finally, there is little doubt that most elderly patients are less likely to complain of pain than younger people, and their stoic attitude is probably a powerful component in delay in seeking surgical treatment.

Appendicitis in Pregnancy. This is not an infrequent occurrence, since the pregnant woman is neither more nor less prone to appendicitis than a nonpregnant young adult. Block (1960) analyses 373 such cases and notes that the incidence is equally distributed through the three trimesters. Punnonen and colleagues (1979) estimate the incidence of appendicitis as 1 in 1455 pregnancies. They review 24 appendicectomies during pregnancy with only 1 fetal death, which was due to immaturity. The remaining pregnancies proceeded uneventfully to term. Diagnosis is undoubtedly more difficult in the pregnant woman. In the first trimester, the history of amenorrhoea and the local physical signs may lead to the diagnosis of a ruptured ectopic pregnancy. The nausea and vomiting may be put down to physiologic "morning sickness," with consequent delay in diagnosis. As the pregnancy progresses, the uterus enlarges and the appendix is pushed upward and more laterally so that the pain, tenderness, and guarding are situated in the mid or upper abdomen and may lead to confusion with pyelitis or cholecystitis. Moreover, the stretched abdominal muscles in the later stages of pregnancy make the detection of guarding or rigidity difficult.

Appendicitis in the Appendiceal Stump. Francis (1979) points out that not even a clear history of a previous appendicectomy invariably rules out the diagnosis of acute appendicitis. He describes a female of 44 who had undergone a previous appendicectomy for acute appendicitis and who presented with a perforated appendix stump 1 cm in length. It is possible to carry out a subtotal appendicectomy, overlooking the stump if the appendix is kinked, bound to the caecum by adhesions, or obscured by oedema of the adjacent caecum.

Diagnostic Studies

Acute appendicitis, it must be stressed, is essentially a clinical diagnosis; there is no laboratory or radiologic test yet devised that is diagnostic of this condition.

White Blood Count. A polymorph leucocytosis is stressed by American authors as an important feature of acute appendicitis. Certainly the white cell count is raised above 12,000 in about three quarters of patients with acute appendicitis. However, it is only slightly raised or entirely normal in the remainder, and one must not discount the diagnosis under these circumstances. In a detailed study of 493 patients with acute appendicitis, Pieper et al in 1982 noted that only 66.7 percent had a white cell count of 11,000 or more and in only 5.5 percent was it raised above 20,000. Doraiswamy (1979) points out that a combination of a raised white cell count combined with neutrophilia is useful in children, particularly when these figures are age-adjusted. He found that in 225 children with acute appendicitis 96 percent had neutrophilia and 42 percent a raised white count. This compared with 50 children submitted to operation in whom a normal appendix was found, where the figures were 30 and 4 percent, respectively, and in a 100 children whose acute abdominal pain resolved without surgery, where the corresponding percentages were 32 and 3 percent. Bower et al (1981) found that only 15 out of 382 children with histologically inflamed appendices had both a normal white cell count and a normal differential count.

Urine Examination. This, of course, should be a routine in every patient with acute abdominal pain. The presence of haematuria or pus cells in the urine point to a urinary tract infection but by no means exclude acute appendicitis. In an important study, Graham (1965) quantitatively analysed midstream urine specimens in 71 patients operated upon with a diagnosis of acute appendicitis. Of these, 62 had an acutely inflamed appendix removed and in the remaining 9 the organ was normal (3 of these had mesenteric adenitis and the other 6 had no abnormality found at operation). In the whole group of patients, microscopic pyuria was found in nine, all of whom were female and one of whom also had haematuria. One male with acute appendicitis had microscopic haematuria. Graham notes that the distribution of microscopic pyuria was about that to be expected in the normal population. If pus cells or red cells are found in the urine, certainly the clinical features should be carefully reviewed. If the surgeon is satisfied that appendicitis cannot be ruled out, operation under such circumstances is entirely justified; often the inflamed appendix will be found to be adherent to the right ureter or to the bladder.

Radiography (Figs. 48–6 and 48–7). Plain films of the abdomen in the erect and supine position are of value in the differential diagnosis of acute abdominal pain, but the radiologic features are often nonspecific and must be interpreted with caution. Thus free intraperitoneal gas may be demonstrated, suggesting a perforated peptic ulcer, but, as is mentioned later, this radiologic sign is occasionally seen in cases of perforated appendicitis.

There are a number of radiologic signs that have been described in plain x-rays of the abdomen in patients with acute appendicitis. Brooks and Killen (1965) list these as follows:

1. Fluid levels localised to the caecum and to the terminal ileum, indicating local inflammation in the right lower quadrant of the abdomen
2. Localised ileus, with gas in the caecum, ascending colon, or terminal ileum

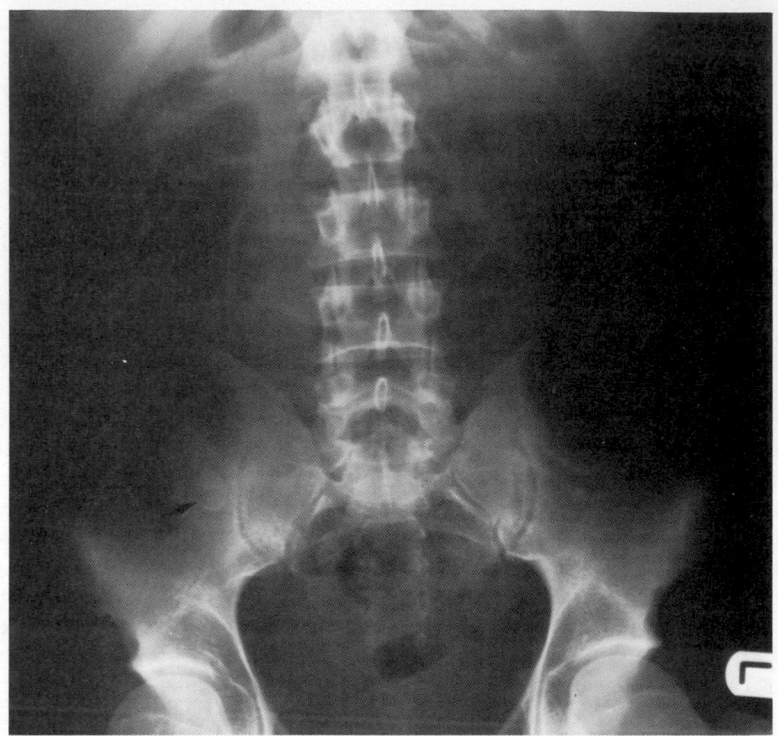

Figure 48–6. An unusually large faecolith in the appendix (*arrow*). The patient had a gangrenous appendicitis.

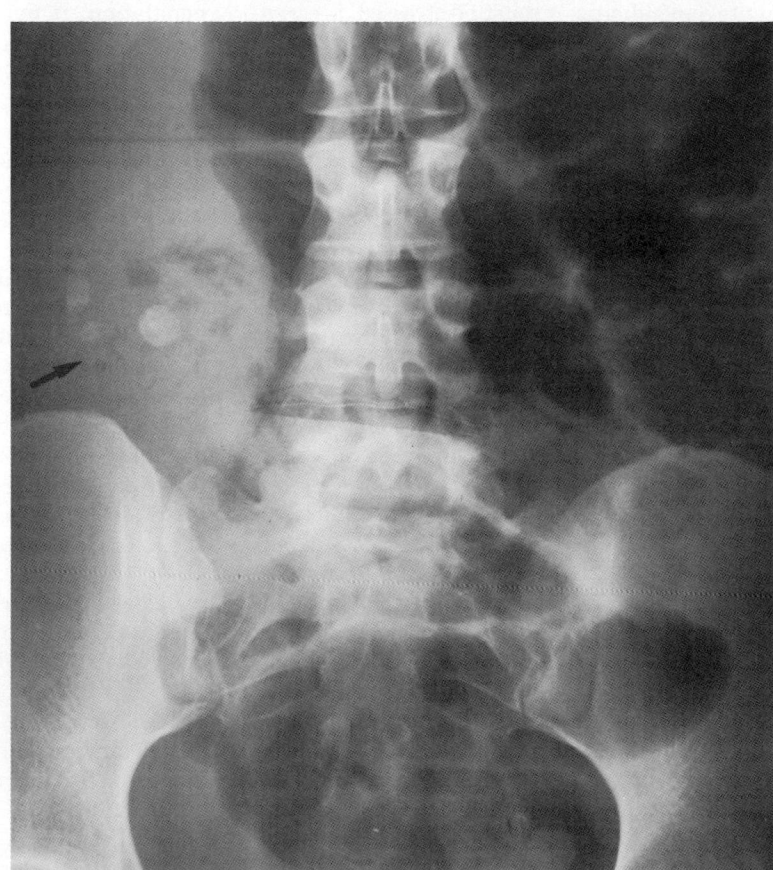

Figure 48–7. Plain x-ray of the abdomen—appendix abscess. There is a large soft-tissue mass (*arrow*) that displaces the large bowel medially and contains faecoliths and free gas.

3. Increased soft tissue density in the right lower quadrant
4. Blurring of the right flank stripe, the radiolucent line produced by fat between the peritoneum and transversus abdominis
5. A faecolith in the right iliac fossa (which may be confused with a ureteric stone, a gallstone, or a calcified mesenteric lymph node)
6. Blurring of the psoas shadow on the right side
7. A gas-filled appendix
8. Free intraperitoneal gas
9. Deformity of the caecal gas shadow due to an adjacent inflammatory mass. This is difficult to interpret because there may be disturbance of caecal gas from intraluminal fluid or faeces

Brooks and Kellen reviewed the x-rays of 200 patients undergoing laparotomy for acute appendicitis without knowing the diagnosis. Fifty four percent of the cases of acute nonperforated appendicitis were positive for one or more of these signs and the figure rose to 80 percent in advanced cases. However, 14 of 41 cases in which the appendix was not acutely inflamed (37 percent) had similar x-ray findings—12 of these had another acute lesion, including ruptured ovarian follicle or intestinal obstruction, but 3 had no abnormal findings at surgery.

Saebo (1978) has reported three examples of pneumoperitoneum associated with perforated appendicitis and found about 40 published reports of this condition. He points out that often appendicectomy is performed without x-raying the abdomen, so that more cases may occur than appear in published reports. (A recent example was the first time the present author personally encountered such a case.)

It is extremely rare for gas to be seen in a normal appendix or in the appendix distended as a part of large bowel obstruction. Killen and Brooks (1965) add five examples of a gas-filled appendix in gangrenous appendicitis to the four cases previously reported.

The use of an emergency barium enema examination is almost confined to practice in the United States and is rarely, if ever, ordered in the United Kingdom. Smith et al (1979) enumerate the radiologic signs of appendicitis on barium enema as:

1. Persistent nonvisualisation of the appendix (although this occurs in 5 to 10 percent of normal barium enema examinations)
2. Partial visualisation of the appendix
3. Pressure defect on the caecum
4. Irritability of the caecum and terminal ileum on screening

Rare cases have been reported of even the acutely inflamed appendix being filled on radiologic examination. These authors point out that perforation of the inflamed appendix due to the x-ray examination is unlikely and also stress that they would only advise a barium enema in equivocal cases.

Differential Diagnosis

Already stated is that nothing can be so easy, nor so difficult, as the diagnosis of acute appendicitis. The clinical features and special investigations are all nonspecific and the list of differential diagnoses is long indeed.

In many instances, a diagnosis of acute appendicitis is made but at laparotomy some other acute abdominal condition, which itself requires urgent surgery, is discovered; for example, an acute Meckel's diverticulitis or a perforated peptic ulcer. A small proportion of cases will be found to have a normal appendix and the exact diagnosis of the cause of the pain may never be found. Provided the proportion of such cases is kept low, the surgeon must accept a number of such negative laparotomies, placing them against the risk of leaving a possibly early acutely inflamed appendix within the abdomen. In children, some of these patients will have acute mesenteric adenitis and the differential diagnosis between the two conditions is, in the author's opinion, impossible to make with any accuracy. The tragedy comes when an appendicectomy is performed in a patient who has some medical condition such as diabetes or pleurisy that is responsible for the pain and where operation can only aggravate the condition.

The differential diagnosis can be considered under the following headings:

1. Other intraabdominal causes of acute pain
2. Acute pain of gynaecologic origin
3. Urinary tract conditions
4. Chest conditions
5. Diseases of the central nervous system
6. Other medical conditions

Other intraabdominal diseases that commonly mimic acute appendicitis are perforated peptic ulcer, acute cholecystitis, acute intestinal obstruction, gastroenteritis, acute sigmoid diverticulitis, acute regional ileitis, and, in children, intussusception, acute Meckel's diverticulitis, and mesenteric adenitis. In women, acute salpingitis, a ruptured ectopic pregnancy, ruptured cyst of the corpus luteum, and a twisted ovarian cyst need to be considered.

Colic from a right-sided ureteric calculus or acute pyelonephritis usually has radiation of the pain from loin to the groin. A calculus may be seen on a plain x-ray of the abdomen and confirmed on an emergency pyelogram. The urine must be tested for blood and pus cells in every case of acute abdominal pain but, as already noted, the presence of either of these abnormalities does not exclude acute appendicitis.

A basal pneumonia and pleurisy may give referred abdominal pain that may be surprisingly difficult to differentiate from an acute abdomen, especially in children. Jona and Belin in 1976 noted that 12 of 250 children presenting with acute abdominal pain had basal pneumonia as the only cause and only 2 of these had abnormal physical findings when the chest was examined. However, the abdominal pain was severe, associated with abdominal tenderness and even, on occasion, with absent bowel sounds. These authors stress that a chest x-ray is invaluable and should include a lateral film because the basal consolidation may be hidden by the diaphragm in the posteroanterior film.

A coronary thrombosis may be accompanied by marked epigastric pain but generalised abdominal pain and rigidity are rare and the condition is only occasionally confused with appendicitis.

Diseases of the central nervous system should be kept in mind in the differential diagnosis. The lightning pains of tabes dorsalis have all but disappeared from clinical practice but abdominal pain and local tenderness may occur in the 2 or 3 days before the rash of herpes zoster appears. In this group simulated abdominal pain, the so-called Munchausen syndrome, may be included, which is suggested by the presence of multiple abdominal scars, a bizarre history, no fixed address, and occasionally the telltale scars over the veins of the antecubital fossae of the drug addict.

Medical conditions that may be confused with acute appendicitis include infective hepatitis in the preicteric phase, gastroenteritis, sickle cell crisis (which should always be considered in black children) and, very rarely, acute porphyria. In young children, tonsillitis, acute respiratory tract infection, otitis media, and meningitis can all present with acute abdominal pain. Undiagnosed diabetes can undoubtedly mimic an acute abdominal emergency, especially in children. Valerio (1976) stresses three important clinical clues—a history of polyuria, polydipsia, and anorexia that precede the abdominal pain; deep sighing and rapid respirations; and severe dehydration. The abdominal pain is usually generalised, in contrast to the localised tenderness and pain of acute appendicitis. It may be difficult to get a urine specimen to test for sugar because of the dehydration; an immediate blood sugar estimation should be performed. The abdomen will become pain-free and soft within a few hours of appropriate treatment for the diabetes, but obviously very close observation is required during this critical period.

The accuracy of diagnosis of acute appendicitis has been carefully studied by Pieper et al (1982). They reviewed 1018 appendicectomies carried out in Stockholm in patients whose ages ranged from 1 to 89 years. The diagnosis was correct in 67.6 percent of the cases, in 77.7 percent of the males and 58 percent of the females. The diagnostic accuracy was low in the female group aged 10 to 39 years, where it fell to 52.7 percent. In this group, gynaecologic disorders were found in 15.5 percent of cases. Below the age of 10, appendicitis was confirmed in 72.9 percent of cases and above the age of 60 in 66.7 percent. Surgical diseases that mimic acute appendicitis accounted for 4.1 percent of patients in this study. Of the patients on review, 28.3 percent did not require surgery. Of these 288 patients, 149 had no disease at all at operation. The remaining 139 had a variety of conditions, including mesenteric adenitis (63 patients), gynaecologic disorders (26 patients), gastroenteritis (24 patients), and urinary tract infection or stones (12 patients).

Treatment

The correct treatment of appendicitis in all its aspects is one of the most important subjects in abdominal surgery because it is the most common major abdominal condition calling for emergency operation.

The treatment of acute appendicitis is appendicectomy—and the sooner done the better. There are four exceptions to this excellent rule:

1. The patient is moribund with advanced peritonitis; here the only hope is to improve the condition by intravenous fluids, nasogastric suction, antibiotics, and blood transfusion in an attempt to get the patient fit for operation.
2. The attack has already resolved; in such a case appendicectomy can be advised as an elective procedure to prevent recurrence, but there is no immediate emergency.
3. Where circumstances make operation difficult or impossible, for example in a small boat at sea. Here reliance must be placed on a conservative regime in the hope that resolution will occur or a local appendix mass may form. If available, morphia, antibiotic therapy, and intravenous fluids are given; this is preferable to attempting surgery in less than optimal conditions.
4. An appendix mass has formed without evidence of general peritonitis (see the following).

Preoperative Preparation. If the diagnosis is one of a straightforward acute appendicitis, no special steps need be taken apart from those of any routine abdominal operation. Broad-spectrum antibiotic therapy is commenced to cover both aerobic and anaerobic organisms. This author's current practice is to use cephuroxime and metronidazole, discussed later in the chapter.

   If the diagnosis of a generalised peritonitis is made, intravenous fluid therapy is commenced and nasogastric aspiration commenced.

Choice of Incision

Experience should enable the surgeon to determine with a fair degree of accuracy the position and the pathologic changes in the appendix before operation. When the patient is fully anaesthetised, the surgeon should once again systematically palpate the abdomen in an endeavour to locate the position of the appendix. A circumscribed lump may be felt or a diffuse thickening may be made out or a movable tumour may be identified. The incision can then be carefully planned to give adequate exposure without being excessive.

   A right iliac fossa skin crease muscle-split incision is used (Fig. 48–8), commencing just above and medial to the anterior superior iliac spine. It is a mistake to place the incision too medially; this brings the surgeon down onto the anterior rectus sheath and not over the oblique

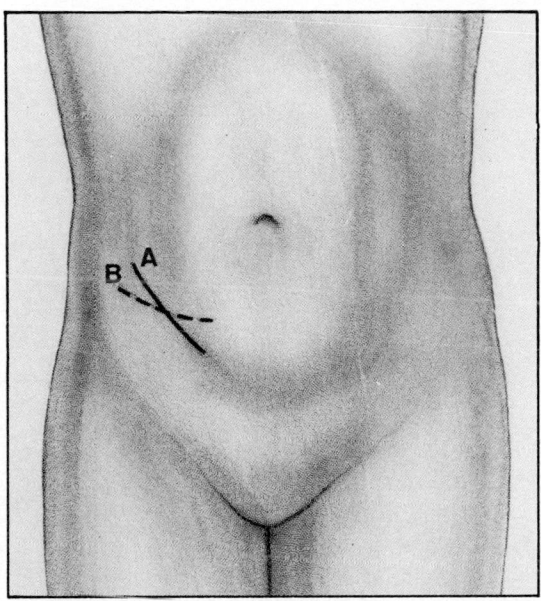

Figure 48–8. The appendicectomy incision. The classic oblique McBurney incision (A) is usually replaced by the cosmetically better skin crease incision (B).

muscles. After splitting the oblique muscles in the lines of their fibres (Fig. 48–9) the muscles are retracted and the peritoneum exposed. Moist packs are placed around the wound and the peritoneum opened cautiously. In a true case there is usually at least a serous exudate in the peritoneal cavity or frank pus may be present. A swab is taken and the fluid sucked away.

   A well-placed incision should bring the surgeon immediately onto the caecum. This is picked up with the fingers and slowly and carefully withdrawn through the incision. The index finger may be used to lift the appendix and coax it onto the surface, but whenever this manoeuvre is necessary it must be performed with the greatest gentleness. There is nothing more dangerous than the so-called hooking out or blind dissection with the fingers of a friable gangrenous appendix, especially when it happens to be fixed to the lateral wall of the pelvis or embedded in coils of small intestine. In such cases the appendix is not uncommonly ruptured or torn in half by clumsy manipulations. If any difficulty is encountered in localising the appendix, it can be found by tracing the taeniae coli along the caecum to their junction at the appendix base.

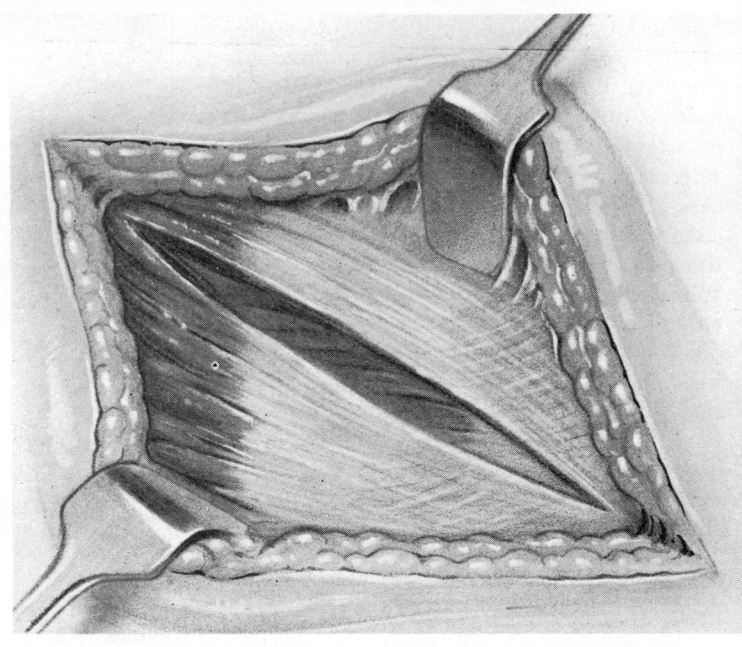

Figure 48–9. A. A gridiron incision. The aponeurosis of the external oblique muscle has been divided in line with its fibres.

A

If careful palpation indicates that the delivery of the appendix is going to be difficult, the surgeon ascertains whether further access is needed medially or laterally. In the former case, the incision may be extended inward through the sheath of the rectus muscle or in the latter the oblique muscles are divided transversely or obliquely in line with the incision; the transverse division affords an excellent approach to an appendix lying far out in the loin above the

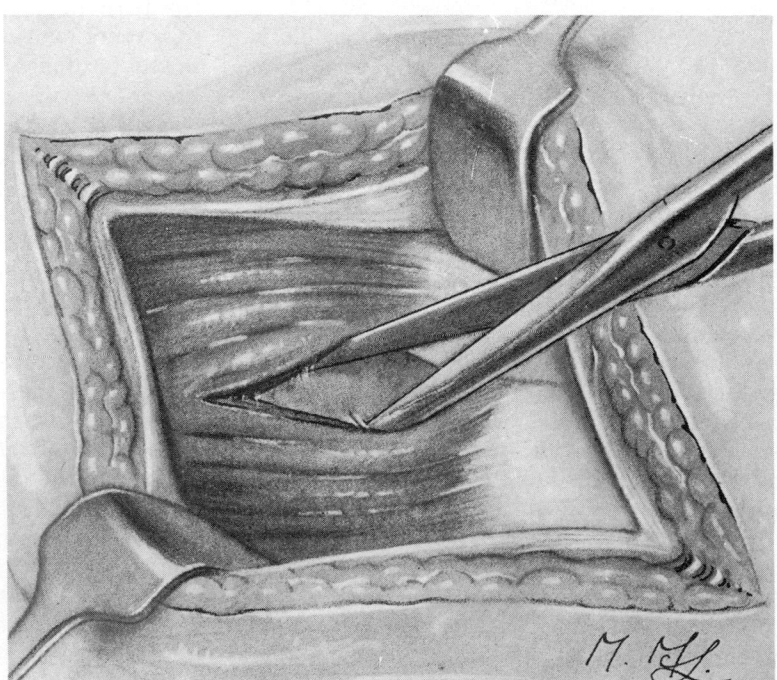

Figure 48–9. B. McBurney incision. Internal oblique and transversus muscles are split. The skin incision should be placed transversely or obliquely to lie in one of Langer lines.

B

level of the anterior superior iliac spine even in the most hidden, adherent retrocaecal situation in an obese subject.

While mentioning extension of the incision in this way, it is worth noting that there are some who advise a lower right paramedian incision for appendicectomy, particularly if the diagnosis is in some doubt or, in female patients, if there is a question of a gynaecologic cause for the acute abdominal pain. However, there is no doubt that the right iliac fossa incision gives the most direct access to the appendix even in the most difficult cases. Even if the diagnosis proves to be incorrect, most other local pathologies can be dealt with through this incision, especially if it is extended as described above. On numerous occasions this author has dealt with

a ruptured ectopic pregnancy, acute Meckel's diverticulitis, acute caecal diverticulitis, and even, in one case, a mucocele of the gallbladder through this approach. If, however, it is found that the cause of the acute abdominal condition is out of reach of this incision, for example, a perforated duodenal ulcer, then the incision is left open, the appropriate vertical incision performed, the emergency is dealt with appropriately, and then both incisions closed at the end of the laparotomy.

Having delivered the appendix, it is removed under direct vision and all intraabdominal manipulations must be reduced to a minimum. The appendix is held up by tissue forceps applied around the appendix in such a manner as to encircle the organ and yet not inflict any

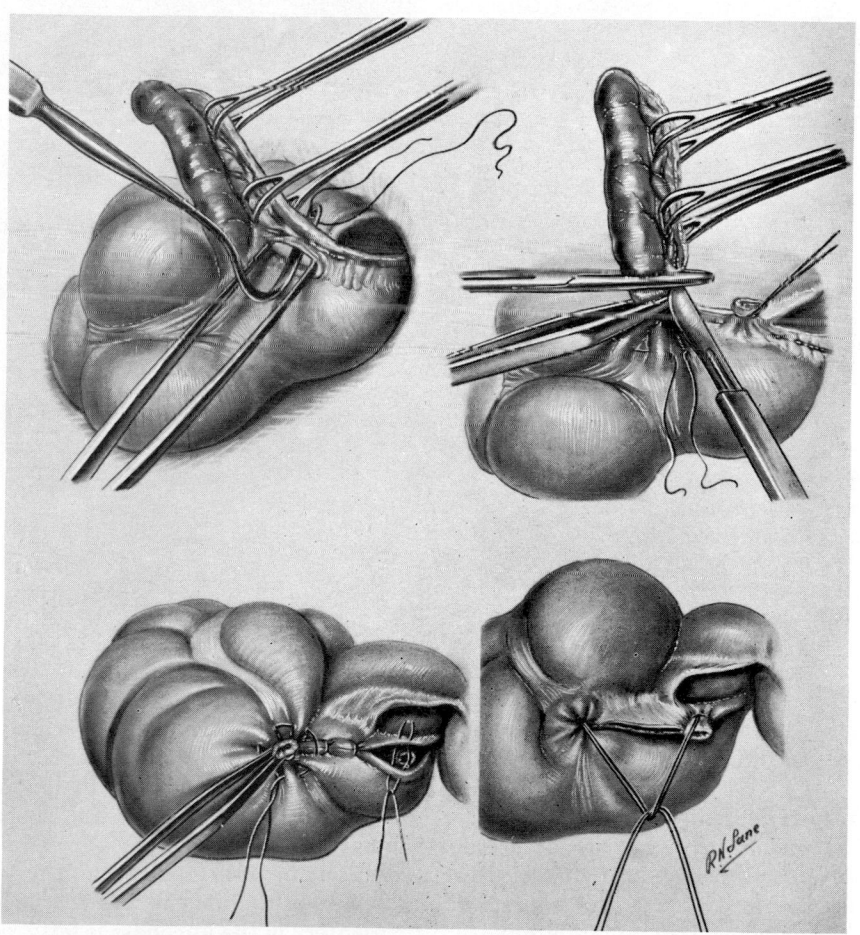

Figure 48–10. Appendicectomy. The purse string method. Note how the Babcock forceps are applied to the mesoappendix to avoid any damage to the acutely inflamed appendix.

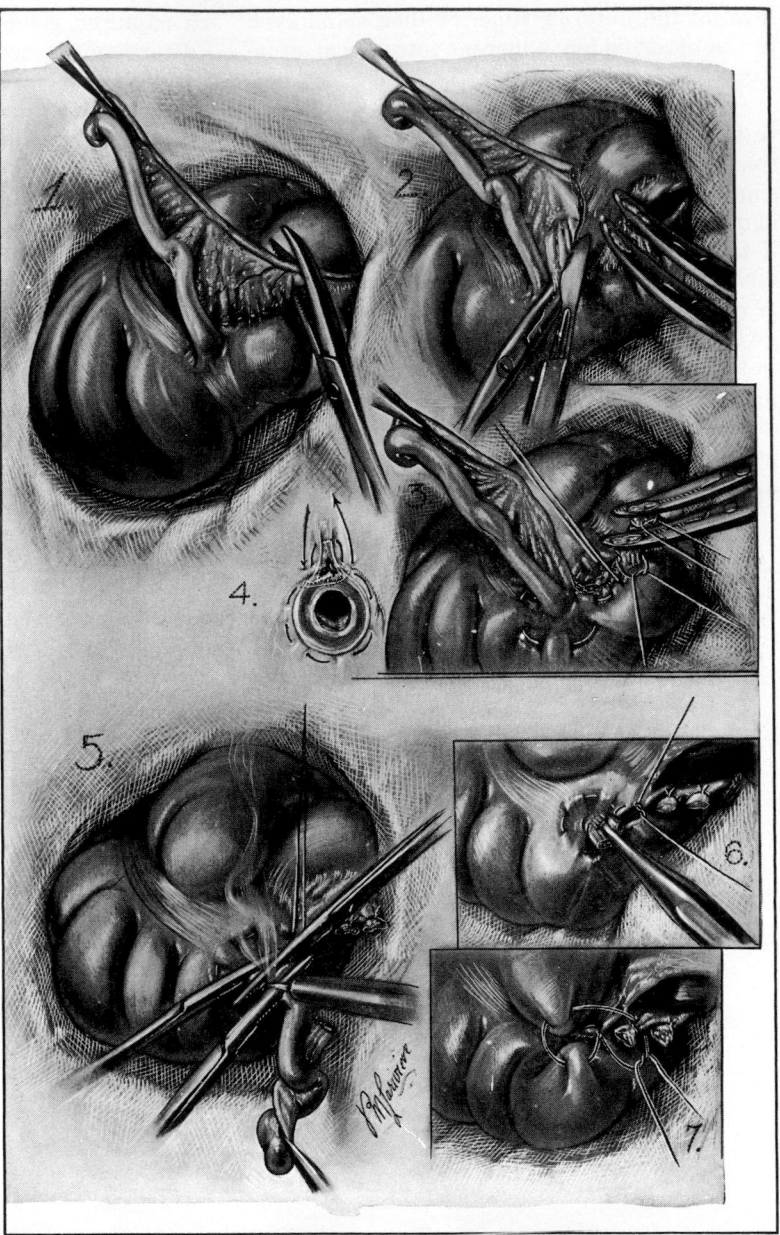

Figure 48–11. Appendicectomy. Intraluminal invagination of the stump. (*Source: From Ochsner A, Lilly G: The technique of appendectomy. Surgery 2:532, 1937, with permission.*)

damage to it. In some instances it may be preferable to grasp the mesoappendix with the forceps.

The appendix mesentery may be long, in which case appendicectomy is a simple procedure, or the appendix may be found closely bound to the caecum by congenital adhesions or inflammatory bands that require preliminary mobilisation before dealing with the vessels in the mesoappendix. If the mesoappendix is long,

thin, and rather redundant, it may be simply transfixed and ligatured with thread, after which it is divided close to the appendix at the base of the organ (Fig. 48–10). It is more usual to have to divide the mesoappendix by clipping and dividing it seriatim, section by section, until the base of the appendix is reached. When the mesentery of the appendix is fatty, oedematous, or frankly gangrenous, the ligatures have to be applied with special care, as they are very likely to cut through this friable and buttery structure. If there is any difficulty, the vessels should be cautiously oversewn with interrupted atraumatic thread sutures.

The mobilised appendix is held upward and its base crushed with two artery forceps. After removal of the first (close to the caecal wall), the crushed appendix area is ligated with thread, the ends of which are cut short. A purse string suture of 2/0 chromic catgut is next inserted about 1 cm from the appendix. This suture passes through the seromuscular coat, especially at the longitudinal bands, and great care is taken to avoid puncturing the gut or pricking a blood vessel.

The appendix is divided close to the artery forceps (Fig. 48–11) and the stump invaginated by the purse string suture. This is reinforced by a second purse string or a Z stitch to secure even further inversion of the stump.

When the caecal wall is sodden with oedema, it may be impossible to invaginate the stump. In such a case, two thread ligatures are applied to the base of the appendix and the ligature may with advantage be left long in order to anchor a portion of the mesoappendix over the vulnerable spot (Fig. 48–12).

It is tempting to draw the handy, bloodless fold of Treves and to stitch it over the appendix stump; to do so, however, may lead to angulation and subsequent obstruction of the last inch or so of the ileum. Care must also be taken not to hitch up the terminal ileum with one or other of the purse string sutures.

Retrograde Appendicectomy

Occasionally the inflamed appendix in the retrocolic position is firmly bound down along the length of the ascending colon and cannot be delivered into the wound. It is of the utmost importance to have the whole length of the appendix in view during the operation; otherwise the tip of the appendix may be overlooked. Under such circumstances, retrograde appendicectomy is performed. The base of appendix is freed until the whole circumference of the organ near its caecal junction can be visualised. Tissue forceps are applied around the appendix base and the first inch or so of the appendix freed. It is then a simple matter to ligature the base of the appendix, insert a purse string suture, clamp and divide the appendix, and invaginate its stump. We then proceed to define the remainder of the mesoappendix and to clip, cut, and tie small portions of it at a time until the entire mesoappendix is divided and the organ is removed in toto (Fig. 48–13).

Occasionally the appendix will be found firmly wrapped in adherent omentum. In such a case, the appendix should be removed together

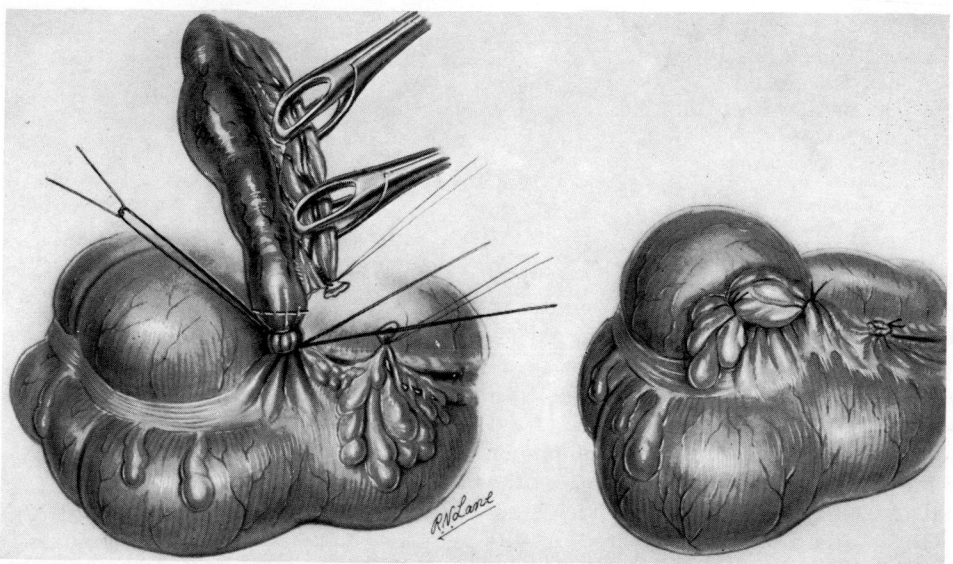

Figure 48–12. Appendicectomy. Simple double ligation of the crushed area of the stump without inversion of the stump.

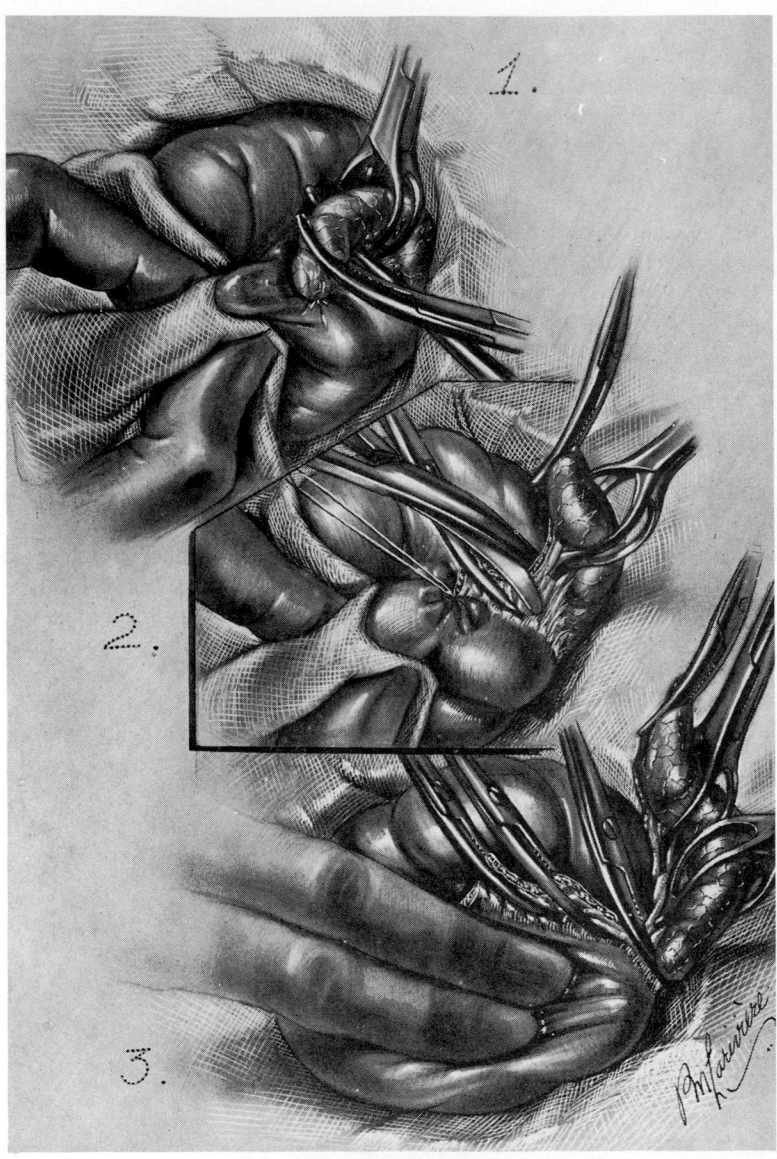

Figure 48–13. Retrograde appendicectomy. (*Source: From Maingot R: The Management of Abdominal Operations, 2 edt. HK Lewis, 1957, with permission.*)

with its protective omental sheath. Attempts to free the omentum may result in spillage of a collection of pus into the peritoneal cavity.

Closure of the muscle split incision is simplicity itself. The peritoneum is closed with chromic catgut, the transversus and internal oblique muscles are left unsutured and one or two catgut sutures are employed to appose the external oblique aponeurosis. The skin is sutured with interrupted nylon stitches (Fig. 48–14).

Drainage is not generally advised following appendicectomy but a corrugated drain should be passed down to the appendix base and brought out through the lateral extremity of the wound where there has been a local abscess, leaving behind a shaggy, granulating cavity, or where difficulty has been encountered in dealing with the appendix stump.

The Appendiceal Mass

Occasionally a patient will present with a walled-off perforated appendix that has formed an inflammatory mass. Usually there is a history of 4 or 5 days of preceding pain. The condition is probably being seen less commonly nowa-

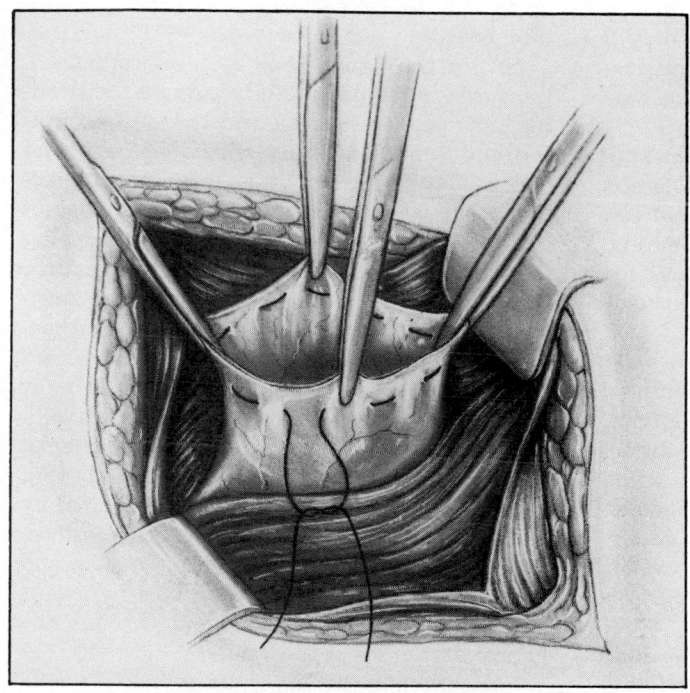

A

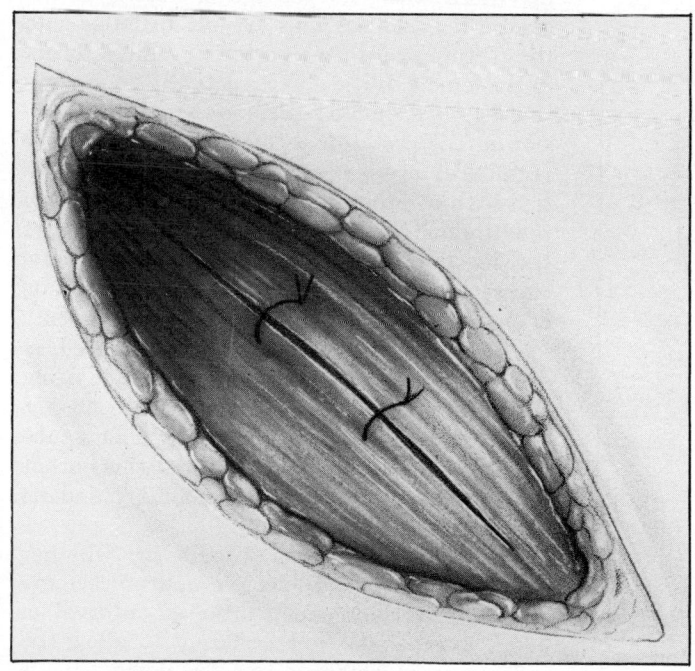

B

Figure 48–14. Closure of the muscle split incision. **A.** The peritoneum is closed with a purse string suture. **B.** One or two catgut sutures close the external oblique.

days as a result of improved health education. Thus, Bradley and Isaacs, in a 1978 review of 2621 cases of acute appendicitis treated between 1962 and 1976 in Atlanta, found that only 2 percent had an appendix abscess on admission, and here the average duration of symptoms was 9 days.

The clinical features are a swinging temperature with an elevated pulse rate. There is a tender mass in the right iliac fossa that can often also be palpated on rectal examination. However, there is no evidence of a generalised peritonitis in that the rest of the abdomen is soft and bowel sounds are present.

In such instances, the initial treatment should be conservative. The patient is placed on bedrest and maintained on fluids only. A careful watch is kept on the general condition, temperature, pulse, and, above all, on the size of the mass, which is marked out on the abdominal wall with a skin pencil. Systemic antibiotics are avoided at this stage because they merely result in a honeycomb of chronic abscess cavities (Stammers, 1957).

On this regime, the majority of appendix masses resolve but if the swelling is obviously enlarging over the next day or two or if the pyrexia becomes more elevated, the appendix

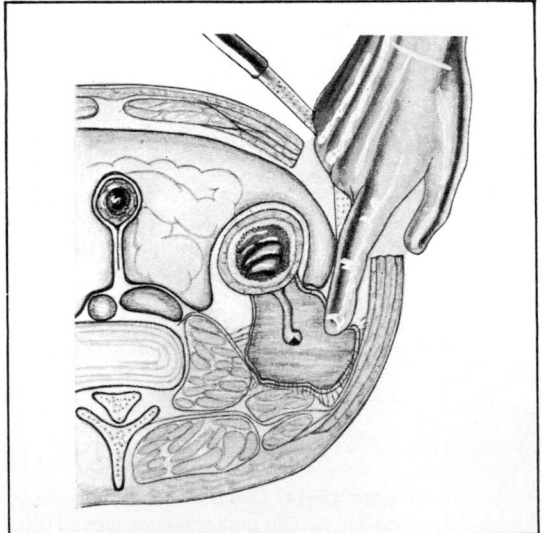

Figure 48–15. Drainage of appendix abscess employing the extraperitoneal route. (*Source: From Fitzgerald P: Appendix Abscess, in Rob C, Smith R (eds): Operative Surgery, 2 edt. Philadelphia: JB Lippincott, 1969, with permission.*)

should be drained through a small incision over the apex of the mass; the surrounding adhesions allow this to be performed extraperitoneally (Fig. 48–15).

After the patient has been anaesthetised, the surgeon should carefully palpate the swelling and make an incision over the most projecting and superficial part of the abscess. The oblique muscles are split, as in an appendicectomy approach. If possible, the lateral edge of the peritoneum is exposed and, by stripping it medially with the finger, the mass is reached retroperitoneally. If this is impossible, the peritoneum is gently opened and the peritoneal cavity is cautiously packed off with gauze before inserting the index finger down to the most prominent and cystic portion of the abscess wall. This gives free vent to the abscess contents, which are rapidly aspirated. If the appendix readily comes to hand, it should be excised by one of the techniques previously described. More often, appendicectomy is impossible and the abscess cavity should be drained by means of a perforated tube brought out through the lateral extremity of the wound.

Occasionally the appendix abscess presents in the pelvis. The characteristic features are diarrhoea with the passage of mucus in the stools. The abscess may be felt to bulge into the rectum or into the posterior vaginal fornix in the female. If the abscess actually points into the vagina, it should be drained through an incision in the posterior fornix, but in most cases rectal drainage is prefered. The bladder is emptied with a catheter, and the patient placed in the lithotomy position. The index finger locates the site of maximum point softening in the anterior rectal wall and through this area the points of a closed artery forceps are gently and evenly forced in an upward direction. This procedure can also be performed under direct vision using a lighted proctoscope (Figs. 48–16 and 48–17). Some surgeons attempt keeping a drainage tube within the pelvic abscess cavity but this author finds it dislodges almost immediately and its use has been abandoned.

Whether resolution occurs or whether drainage is required, elective appendicectomy should be recommended after an interval of about 8 weeks—a time sufficient to allow the inflammatory condition to settle down. This is because of the significant risk of further episodes of acute appendicitis if the damaged appendix is not removed. Useful accounts of series

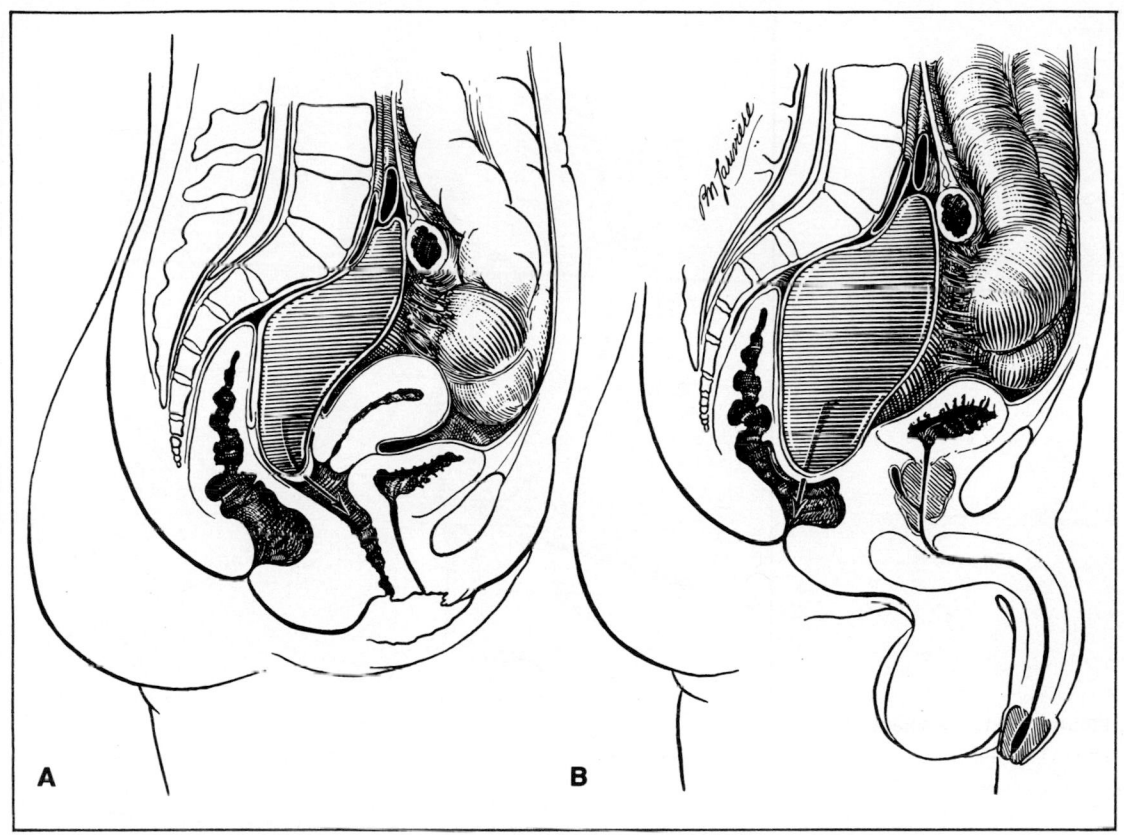

Figure 48-16. Pelvic abscess. **A.** The abscess is bulging into the posterior vaginal fornix. **B.** The abscess is pointing into the rectum.

of cases have been published by Foran et al in 43 adult patients and by Gastrin and Josephson in 59 children. Skoubo-Kristensen and Hvid (1982) review 193 patients treated conservatively for an appendix mass over a 10-year period in Aarhus, Denmark. One hundred and seventy (88 percent) settled. Of the 23 who required early operation, 6 had small bowel obstruction, 14 had unresolved abscesses, and 3 were suspected of having a perforated abscess; 1 of these was confirmed at operation. There was one death and this was in a female patient aged 86. Of the 170 patients discharged after conservative treatment, 12 were readmitted within 3 months with either a further abscess or an attack of appendicitis and an elective appendicectomy was carried out at 3 months on the rest of the patients. These authors note that there are wide variations in the recurrence rate following conservative treatment of appendix ab-

scess, varying from 7 to 46 percent in different series, but the majority of recurrences are likely to occur in the early months after resolution of the mass.

Rarely the appendix abscess may rupture into the bladder, producing an appendicovesical fistula into the intestine or onto the skin to produce an appendicocutaneous fistula (Fig. 48–18). Hedner et al in a 1978 review of such fistulae, report a case that presented with a faecal fistula in the right buttock.

Antibiotic Therapy

Before the antibiotic era, sepsis was a common complication following appendicectomy. Wound infection rates would vary from about 5 percent in cases of early inflammation to 75 percent if the appendix was gangrenous or perforated. Other septic complications—pelvic abscess, subphrenic abscess, portal pyaemia, and septicae-

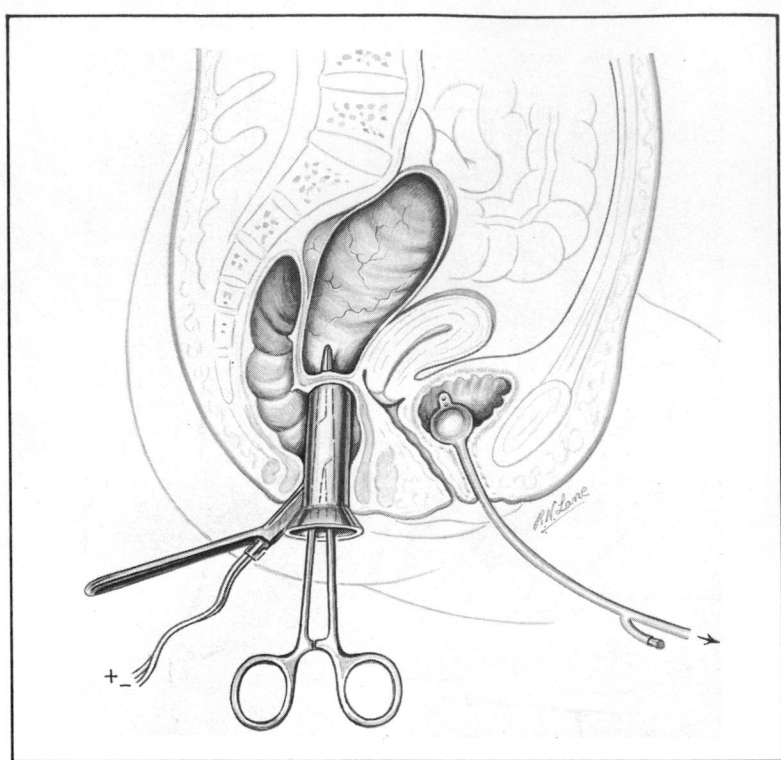

Figure 48–17. Drainage of a pelvic abscess.

mia—were not uncommon in advanced cases and accounted for much of the mortality of this disease.

Controlled studies have demonstrated the undoubted value of antibiotics, whether given systemically or topically, in greatly reducing this state of affairs. Everson and colleagues found the incidence of wound infection in gangrenous or perforated appendices to drop from 16 out of 19 cases in a control group to 9 out of 30 cases receiving systemic cephaloridine. Bates and colleagues, in a 1974 study of 200 patients randomised between controls and those receiving topical ampicillin powder, showed that wound infection fell from 16 percent to 3 percent. In those cases with peritonitis, 9 of 14 controlled cases (64 percent) became infected, compared with 2 of 15 patients (13 percent) receiving topical ampicillin.

In the section earlier in this chapter describing the bacteriology of acute appendicitis it was pointed out that the infection is produced by a mixed inoculum of aerobic and anaerobic organisms and there is good evidence that synergy exists between these two groups (Kelly, 1980). Dealing with the anaerobic organisms

alone is highly effective in preventing the development of postoperative sepsis (Gottrup, 1980; Pinto and Sanderson, 1980; Rodgers et al, 1979; Willis et al, 1976). Metronidazole alone, given either as a suppository or intravenously, is probably sufficient prophylaxis in cases of early appendicitis, but when the appendix is gangrenous or perforated, best results are obtained by using a broad-spectrum antibiotic against the aerobic organisms combined with metronidazole. In a controlled study, Saario et al (1983) could demonstrate no difference between cefuroxime and gentamicin in combination with metronidazole; in 42 patients with peritonitis due to perforation of the appendix randomised between the two regimes there were 4 wound infections in each group. Since cefuroxime avoids the nephrotoxic and ototoxic risks of gentamicin, this antibiotic, in combination with metronidazole, is this author's choice.

Postoperative Complications

The enormous difference between the usually smooth postoperative course following appendicectomy in a case of early acute appendicitis and the stormy recovery that so often accompanies the removal of the gangrenous perforated appendix with generalised peritonitis emphasises the importance of early diagnosis and treatment.

Paralytic Ileus. The invariable accompaniment of general peritonitis, it is treated by means of regular doses of morphia, gastric aspiration, careful fluid and electrolyte replacement by intravenous drip, and antibiotic therapy using metronidazole and cefuroxime, although guided by the bacteriologic study of the peritoneal exudate. Careful watch must be maintained to differentiate mechanical obstruction as a result of early postoperative adhesions, since continued ileus requires conservative therapy while mechanical obstruction calls for urgent laparotomy.

Septic Complications. These include *local wound abscess,* which is dealt with by removal of a suture and gentle probing of the wound to release the pus. A *pelvic abscess* is particularly likely to occur after removal of a perforated pelvic appendix. As well as fever there is often diarrhoea with mucus discharge per rectum. Rectal examination reveals a tender pelvic mass which, in most cases, drains spontaneously either into the vagina or the rectum. Occasionally drainage needs to be performed through the rectum or the posterior fornix of the vagina under a general anaesthetic (Figs. 48–16 and 48–17). *Subphrenic abscess* is now much less common after a perforated gangrenous appendix than it was in the pre-antibiotic era. Wang and Wilson, for example, reviewing 93 cases occurring between 1955 and 1975, found that only 8 percent followed appendicitis.

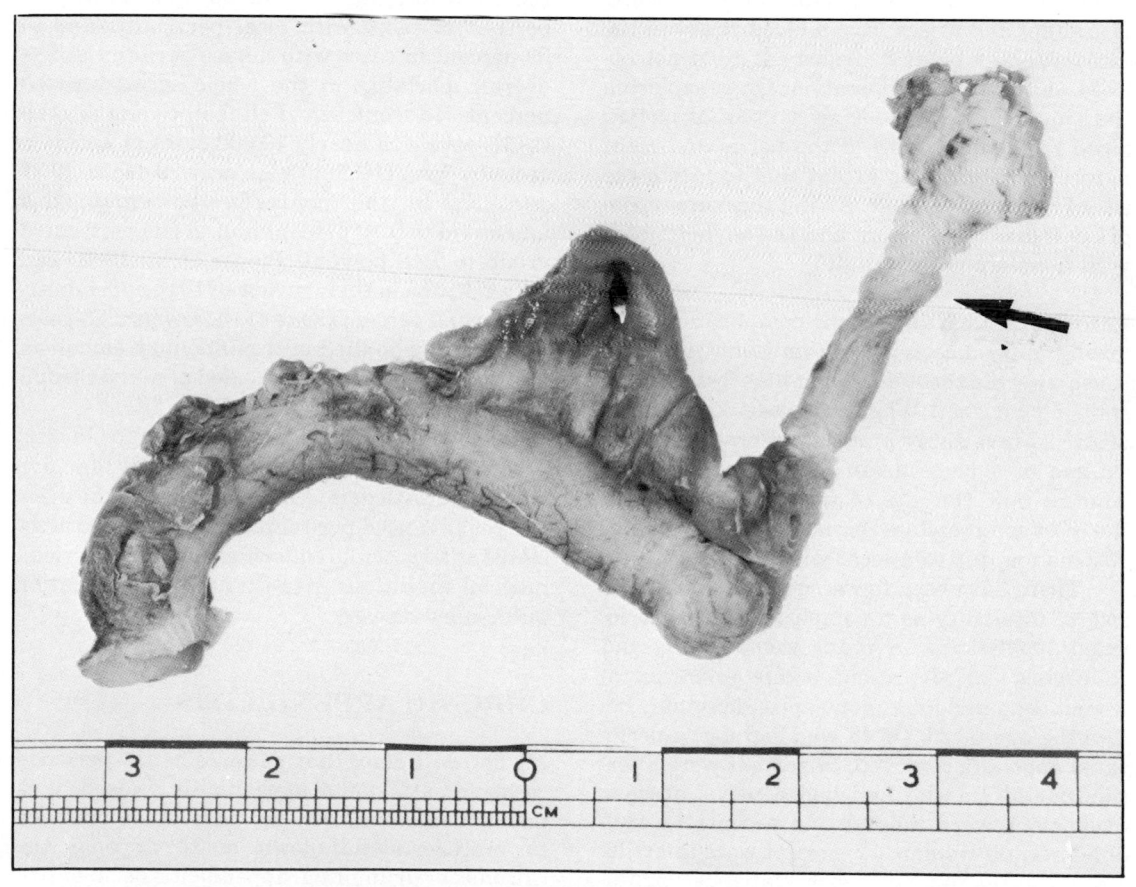

Figure 48–18. Appendicocutaneous fistula cured by appendicectomy. The fistulous tract, which led to the skin surface, is arrowed.

Rupture of the Stump or Caecal Wall. This tragedy is rare but it occurs when a portion of the caecal wall or the appendix stump gives way in the first few days after appendicectomy. Probably the most common cause is administration of an enema, which unduly distends the gut and causes it to rupture at some weakened spot. Enemas should, of course, never be prescribed postoperatively in bowel surgery; the general peritoneal cavity at once becomes flooded with faecal contents and enema fluid.

The only hope of saving the patient's life is immediate laparotomy and the performance of a caecostomy.

Metronidazole and cefuroxime are administered by the intravenous route.

Haemorrhage. Sudden abdominal pain and shock at any time during the first 72 hours after appendicectomy may mean either leakage from the stump or a slipped arterial ligature, both of which are rare today. More often bleeding is gradual and arises from a blood vessel in the mesoappendix or in a divided adhesion not noticed at the time of operation. On reexploring the wound, after removing a mass of clotted blood from the hollow of the pelvis and right paracolic gutter, it is exceptional to locate the site of the haemorrhage. At best the mesoappendix is ligated once more and the wound closed with a generous tube drain.

Late Complications. Late complications following appendicectomy are unusual. It is rare to see a hernia through a right iliac fossa muscle splitting incision. When this does occur, there is almost invariably a history of prolonged sepsis and of a large drain having been used at what is now the site of the hernia. Probably the most common late complication is intestinal obstruction due to a local adhesive band.

There have been few accurate studies of the risk of infertility as a complication of a perforated appendicitis in young women. Wiig and colleagues (1979) present a late follow-up of women who had undergone appendicectomy before the age of 25. Of 48 who had had a perforated appendix removed, 19 percent were infertile, but of 16 who had had a pelvic abscess, 31 percent were infertile. In a control group of 58 normal women, 12 percent were infertile. These figures did not reach statistical significance but at least suggest that only a pouch of Douglas abscess might be important in producing tubal occlusion. Obviously this is a subject worthy of more intensive study.

Mortality Rate

The dramatic effect of antibiotics on the mortality rate from sepsis is well illustrated by the statistics related to appendicitis. Until 1938, more than 3000 deaths from acute appendicitis took place in England and Wales each year; by 1945 the number had fallen to 1774, to 498 in 1964, and 375 in 1969. By 1980, the annual deaths amounted to only 179 cases, of which 10 were in children between 1 and 9 years of age (four male and three female deaths per million of the population). The statistics quoted by one of the most expert surgeons of his day, when antibiotics were not available, are of great interest; Grey Turner (1955), reviewing over 2500 personal appendicectomies, found a mortality of 0.68 percent in cases of early acute appendicitis. However, this shot up to approaching 10 percent in cases with local peritonitis and to 29 percent in cases with diffuse peritonitis. The overall mortality in the whole series was 3.5 percent. In contrast, Peltokallio and Tykka (1981) reviewed nearly 10,000 cases of appendicectomy from Helsinki with only 29 deaths (0.27 percent). In the nonperforated group, this amounted to 0.12 percent and in the perforated group to 1.18 percent. Pieper et al (1982) had only 2 deaths in their review of 1018 appendicectomies (0.2 percent). One of these was a 73-year-old female who died of a pulmonary embolism and the other, a lady of 84, died of a myocardial infarction.

The deaths that do occur in appendicitis are usually in infants or in the elderly, and are associated with delays in diagnosis and the presence of advanced peritonitis. They are also associated with patients suffering from other serious medical conditions, particularly myocardial or pulmonary disease.

CHRONIC APPENDICITIS

No one will deny that patients can experience *recurrent* attacks of appendicitis. Indeed, it is not unusual for one or more such episodes to precede a full-blown acute appendicitis. Chronic, or grumbling, appendicitis as an entity is still the subject of controversy. Today there are many more sceptics than believers and, personally, this author is quite convinced that there is no such organic entity. It has been well said that "the appendix does not grumble—it either screams or remains silent."

It was once fashionable to blame many of the psychosomatic conditions that beset the abdomen (of which the irritable bowel syndrome is the most common) to chronic appendicitis and to remove the offending organ. The results, however, are not at all good. An interesting study by Ingram and Evans (1965) reviewed 118 young women who had undergone appendicectomy a year previously. Of those treated for acute appendicitis, 90 percent were perfectly well and satisfied at review but 55 percent of those whose appendix was normal at operation were still experiencing symptoms at the time of follow-up.

UNUSUAL CONDITIONS OF THE APPENDIX

Diverticulum. This condition, or diverticulosis, is occasionally found (Fig. 48–19) and is documented in detail by Wilson (1950).

Intussusception. This is a rare condition and about 160 cases have been reported since McKidd described the first example in 1858. Fraser (1943) reported 7 new cases and reviewed 75 previously published examples. The disease may occur at any age, although the majority are seen in the first two decades of life. Occasionally a mucocele of the appendix, an adenomatous polyp, a carcinoid tumour, or foreign body may precipitate the condition.

The intussusception may start either at the tip or at the base of the appendix, complete inversion into the caecum being the final result in either case. In most of the collected cases, the insussusception was of the simple form, i.e., inversion into the caecum, but in some instances the appendicular inversion was associated with caecocolic or ileocolic intussusception. Rarely the intussuscepted appendix has presented on rectal examination.

Cleland (1953) notes that six cases have been reported in which the stump of the recently amputated appendix formed the apex of a colic intussusception. The main symptom is colic and the outstanding physical sign is a palpable mass in the right iliac fossa that is slightly tender but freely movable. The intussusception can be visualised on barium enema examination

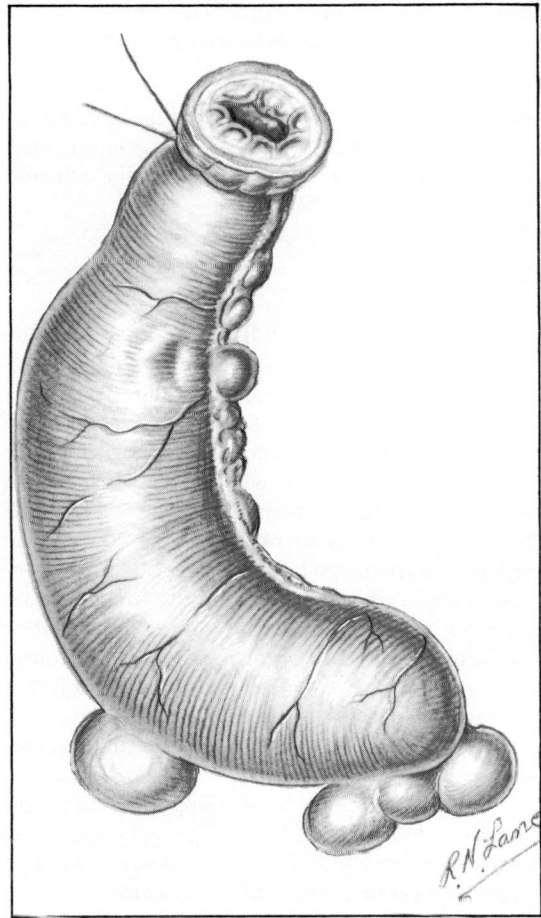

Figure 48–19. Diverticulosis of the appendix.

but, of course, the exact nature of the intussusception is rarely guessed at.

It is usually possible to reduce the intussusception by operative manipulation. When reduction is complete the appendix is excised in the usual way. If it is not possible to effect reduction, a local resection with ileocolic anastomosis is performed.

Torsion. This unusual condition was first described by Payne (1918). Since then but a few cases have been described, the latest by Petersen in 1982. In the majority of cases the appendix was in the pelvic position and had undergone torsion in an anticlockwise direction. The aetiologic factors are unknown but a lax, fan-shaped mesoappendix and the presence of foreign bodies in the appendix have both received attention. The signs and symptoms are those of acute appendicitis and the treatment is expeditious appendicectomy.

Endometriosis. The appendix is affected in less than 1 percent of cases of pelvic endometriosis. Rarely is only the appendix affected (Longman et al, 1981).

TUMOURS

Tumours of the appendix are unusual. This probably reflects merely the small surface area of mucosa that is available for malignant change and, pro rata, it is probably just as liable to the development of cancer as any other part of the large bowel, of which it represents an adnexa. It is true, however, that the distribution of tumour type is in rather sharp contrast to the rest of the large bowel. By far the most common neoplasm of the appendix is the carcinoid tumour, which accounts for some 85 percent of all tumours of this organ and which is found in about 0.1 percent of all appendices subjected to careful histologic examination. As with the rest of the large bowel, villous tumours and carcinomas may also occur.

Benign tumours of the appendix are rare but include adenomatous polyps, mucous cystadenoma, leiomyoma, fibroma, and neuroma. The mucous cystadenoma, while uncommon, may obstruct the lumen of the appendix and distend the organ with mucus to form a mucocele. The other benign lesions, since they develop in the wall of the appendix, do not obstruct its lumen, are rarely of clinical significance, and are usually only detected as an incidental observation in an appendicectomy specimen or at postmortem.

The malignant tumours comprise carcinoid, villous adenocarcinoma and what has been termed the colonic type of adenocarcinoma.

Carcinoid Tumour

As already mentioned, this is the most common of all tumours of the appendix and the only one likely to be encountered by a general surgeon in routine practice. It is usually a solitary finding, although occasionally may be associated with carcinoids of the ileum. In the detailed study by Moertel and colleagues in 1968 at the Mayo Clinic, 71 percent occurred in the tip, 22 percent in the body, and 7 percent at the base of the appendix from a total of 144 specimens. The tumour may occur at any age, including children, although it tends to affect patients in their thirties and forties. When the tumour occurs in the tip of the appendix, it is usually easily identified by the surgeon at laparotomy, but those in the body or at the base may mimic a faecolith.

Pathology. Carcinoid tumours arise from the argentaffin cells, which are situated in the bases of the crypts of the intestinal mucosa. These cells are often termed Kulchitsky cells, in honour of the histologist who gave the original description. Characteristically, the cells contain silver-staining granules in their cytoplasm; hence the alternative name of argentaffinoma.

To the naked eye, the tumour in the appendix forms a hard greyish-yellow nodule arising in the deep aspect of the mucosa with a diameter varying between 0.5 and 3.5 cm. On microscopic examination, the muscle wall is invaded and in many cases the overlying peritoneum is involved. Metastatic spread, however, is very rare. In the study by Moertel, metastases were present in 1.4 percent of cases and was practically confined to lesions that were larger than 2 cm in diameter. Such tumours account for only 1 percent of carcinoids of the appendix. In the study by Svendsen and Bulow (1980) in 64 patients with carcinoid tumours of the appendix under the age of 40, only 1 patient had local metastases and in this case the tumour was 2 cm in diameter.

The majority of carcinoids are found incidentally on routine histologic study of appendices removed during the course of laparotomies for other procedures. Acute appendicitis is not commonly caused because of the usual location at the tip of the organ. However, the lumen may be occluded by a tumour at the base or in the body of the appendix, and the carcinoid may then present as a case of acute appendicitis or even as an appendix abscess (Fig. 48–20).

The carcinoid syndrome, resulting from the secretion of 5-hydroxytryptamine into the portal circulation is seen only in examples of extensive malignant carcinoids, nearly always associated with hepatic metastases. In these instances the appendix is rarely the primary site and the tumour is usually situated in the terminal ileum.

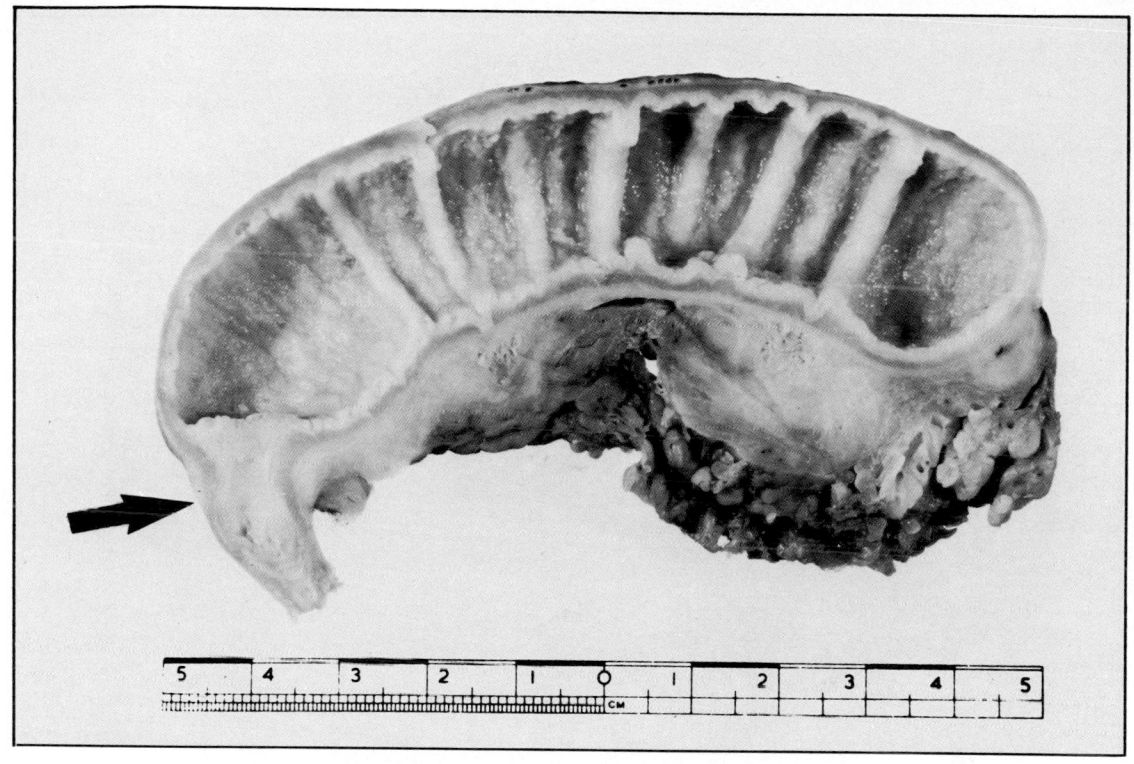

Figure 48–20. Carcinoid tumour (*arrow*) at the base of the appendix producing acute appendicitis.

Villous Tumours

Villous tumours of the appendix may be papillary or adenomatous. The majority are noninvasive but have a propensity to fill the appendix with mucus and to make a differentiation from a benign mucocele of the appendix difficult. If unruptured, the tumour will rarely metastasise, but perforation of a malignant mucocele may result in the development of pseudomyxoma peritonei.

Adenocarcinoma

The first case of carcinoma of the appendix was described by Berger in 1882. Menon in a 1980 report of two cases presenting as appendicular masses was able to collect fewer than 200 examples in English language publications and presents a valuable clinical review of the subject.

The adenocarcinoma of the appendix resembles the histologic appearance of similar tumours elsewhere in the large bowel, except that mucus secretion is rather more prominent. The lesion may be polypoid or ulcerative and may cause haemorrhage or obstruction of the appendix. Typically the tumour arises at the base of the appendix in patients over the age of 50. It may be an incidental finding or may present as acute appendicitis or as an appendix abscess. If the tumour invades the caecum it may be difficult to differentiate it from a primary carcinoma of caecal origin. Hesketh (1963), in a study of a collected series of 95 cases, found that the majority presented as acute appendicitis, an appendix abscess, or with chronic right iliac fossa pain. In 14 percent the tumour was detected as an incidental finding at laparotomy and in another 11 percent widespread metastases were found at presentation.

Management

It would be rare indeed for a surgeon to make a diagnosis of a tumour of the appendix before operation. If the tumour is discovered at laparotomy, either in dealing with an acutely inflamed

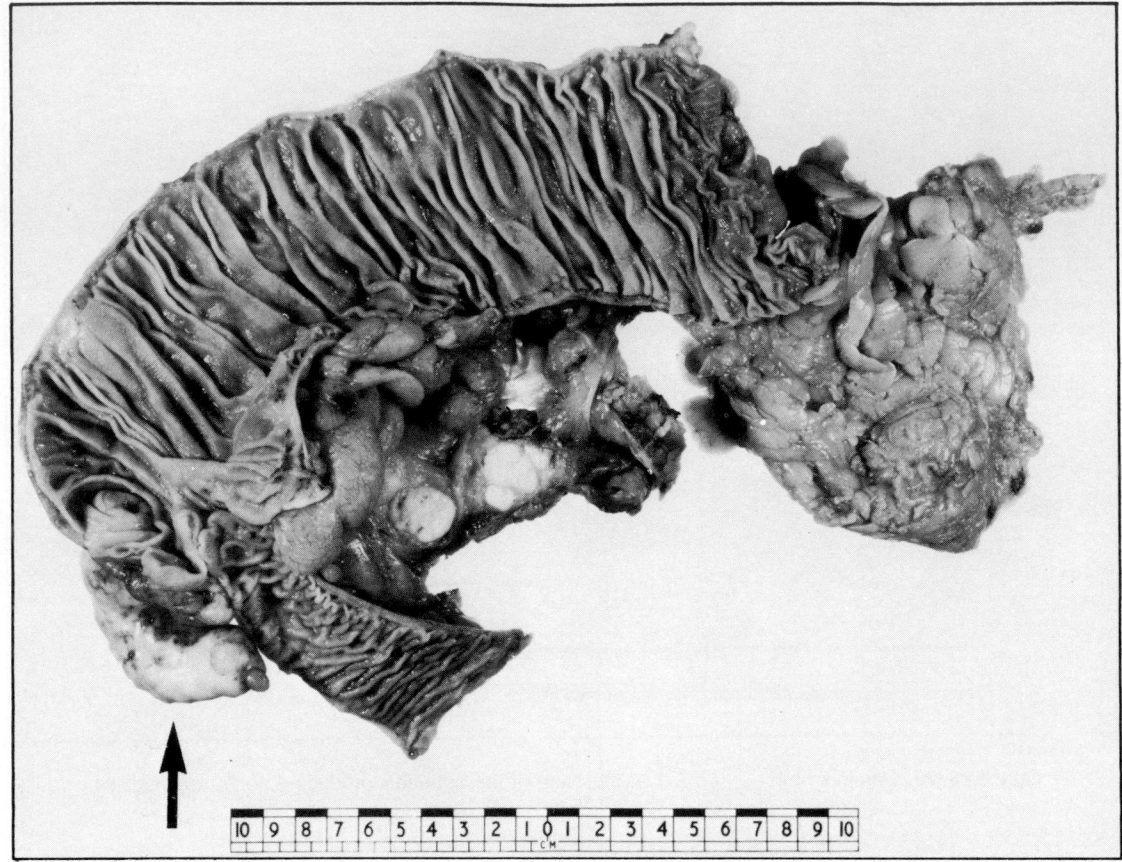

Figure 48–21. Adenocarcinoma of the appendix (*arrow*) removed by right hemicolectomy. Note enlarged and involved lymph nodes in the mesocolon.

appendix or as an incidental finding, then fine judgement is required in its management. If a confident diagnosis of a carcinoid tumour is made, the rest of the small intestine should be carefully examined for other carcinoid tumours, since occasionally these may be multiple. The mesoappendix and right mesocolon are examined carefully for lymph node involvement and the liver accurately palpated. In the vast majority of cases, the findings will be completely negative and under such circumstances, particularly if the carcinoid tumour is less than 2 cm in diameter, nothing more needs to be done but to carry out appendicectomy. If, however, involved nodes are found, then a right hemicolectomy is the treatment of choice and this is indicated also in the rare instances when the carcinoid tumour is more than 2 cm in diameter.

Where the tumour of the appendix is obviously malignant, then a right hemicolectomy is performed (Fig. 48–21).

There will be circumstances where the diagnosis is not established until the postoperative examination of the specimen. If this proves to be a carcinoid tumour and the resection has been adequate, no further procedure need be contemplated. If by chance the carcinoid involved the bases of the appendix and histologic examination showed that the resection had been incomplete, then there is certainly a case for reoperation, with excision of an adequate cuff of surrounding caecal wall. If the specimen were to show the presence of an undoubted adenocarcinoma, then even if resection had been adequate, the patient should be advised to submit to a formal right hemicolectomy.

Prognosis

With rate exceptions, carcinoid tumour of the appendix is cured by appendicectomy. The only exceptions are those unusual cases where the tumour is more than 2 cm in diameter or where there is evidence of lymphatic or hepatic spread at the time of operation.

With regard to the prognosis of carcinoma of the appendix, it is difficult to give accurate figures when the total number of cases reported is in the region of 200. Andersson et al (1976), in a well-documented paper, point out that the prognosis of malignant mucocele of the appendix is excellent following appendicectomy provided that the mucocele had not perforated, had not invaded the submucosa, and was confined to the tip. In 6 cases submitted to appendicectomy, all 6 achieved 5-year survival. In a review of 51 cases of primary adenocarcinoma of the appendix of the colonic type, these authors noted that of 26 patients treated by appendicectomy alone, 12 (46 percent) were still alive 5 years after the operation compared with 15 (60 percent) of 25 subjected to right hemicolectomy.

BIBLIOGRAPHY

Andersson A, Bergdahl L, et al: Primary carcinoma of the appendix. Ann Surg 183:53, 1976

Andersson N, Griffiths H, et al: Is appendicitis familial? Br Med J 2:697, 1979

Andersson A, Bergdahl L: Acute appendicitis in patients over sixty. Am Surg 44:445, 1978

Ayalon A, Mogilner M, et al: Acute appendicitis in a premature baby. Acta Chir Scand 145:285, 1979

Barker DJP, Liggins A: Acute appendicitis in nine British towns. Br Med J 283:1083, 1981

Bates T, Down RHL, et al: Topical ampicillin in the prevention of wound infection after appendicectomy. Br J Surg 61:489, 1974

Berger A: Ein Fall von Krebs des Wurmfortsatzes. Berl Klin Wschr 19:616, 1882

Bower RJ, Bell MJ, et al: Diagnostic value of the white blood count and neutrophil percentage in the evaluation of abdominal pain in children. Surg Gynecol Obstet 152:424, 1981

Black WP: Acute appendicitis in pregnancy. Br Med J 1:1938, 1960

Bradley EL, Isaacs J: Appendiceal abcesses revisited. Arch Surg 113:130, 1978

Brooks DW, Killen DA: Roentgenographic findings in acute appendicitis. Surgery 57:377, 1965

Burge RE, Dennis C, et al: Histology of experimental appendiceal obstruction (rabbit, ape and man). Arch Pathol 30:481, 1940

Castleton KB, Puestow CB, et al: Is appendicitis decreasing in frequency? Arch Surg 78:794, 1959

Cleland G: Caecocolic intussusception following appendicectomy. Br J Surg 41:108, 1953

Coetzee T: Acute appendicitis in an infant. S Afr Med J 32:890, 1958

Cope Z: A History of the Acute Abdomen. London: Oxford University Press, 1965

Doraiswamy NV: Leucocyte counts in the diagnosis and prognosis of acute appendicitis in children. Br J Surg 66:782, 1979

Ellis H: Diagnosis of the acute abdomen. Br Med J 1:491, 1968

Everson NW, Fossard DP, et al: Wound infection following appendicectomy: The effect of extraperitoneal wound drainage and systemic antibiotic prophylaxis. Br J Surg 64:236, 1977

Fields IA, Cole NM: Acute appendicitis in infants thirty-six months of age or younger. Ten year survey at the Los Angeles County Hospital. Am J Surg 113:269, 1967

Fields IA, Naiditch MJ, et al: Acute appendicitis in infants: Ten year survey at the Los Angeles County Hospital. Am J Dis Child 93:287, 1957

Fitz RH: Perforating inflammation of the verniform appendix with special reference to its early diagnosis and treatment. Trans Assoc Am Physicians 1:107, 1886

Foran B, Berne TV, et al: Management of the appendiceal mass. Arch Surg 113:1144, 1978

Francis D: The grumbling appendix. Br Med J 2:936, 1979

Fraser K: Intussusception of the appendix. Br J Surg 31:23, 1943

Gästrin U, Josephson S: Appendiceal abcess—acute appendicectomy or conservative treatment? Acta Chir Scand 135:539, 1969

Gottrup F: Prophylactic metronidazole in prevention of infection after appendicectomy: Report of a double-blind trial. Acta Chir Scand 146:133, 1980

Graham JA: Urinary cell counts in appendicitis. Scot Med J 10:126, 1965

Hedner J, Jansson R, et al: Appendico-cutaneous fistula. A case report. Acta Chir Scand 144:123, 1978

Hesketh KT: The management of primary adenocarcinoma of the vermiform appendix. Gut 4:158, 1963

Ingram PW, Evans G: Right iliac fossa pain in young women. Br Med J 2:149, 1965

Jackson RH: Parents, family doctors and acute appendicitis in childhood. Br Med J 2:277, 1963

Jona JZ: Basilar pneumonia simulating acute appendicitis in children. Arch Surg 111:552, 1976

Jones PF: Abdominal emergencies in infancy and childhood, in Jones PF (ed): Emergency Abdominal Surgery. Oxford: Blackwell, 1974, p 135

Kelly MJ: Wound infection: A controlled clinical and experimental demonstration of synergy between aerobic (*Escherichia coli*) and anaerobic (*Bacteroides fragilis*) bacteria. Ann R Coll Surg Engl 62:52, 1980

Khanna AK: Appendix vermiformis duplex. Postgrad Med J 59:69, 1983

Killen DA, Brooks DW: Gas-filled appendix: A roentgenographic sign of acute appendicitis. Ann Surg 161:474, 1965

Langman J, Rowland R, et al: Endometriosis of the appendix. Br J Surg 68:121, 1981

Leffall LD, Cooperman A, et al: Appendicitis. A continuing surgical challenge. Am J Surg 113:654, 1967

McBurney C: Experience with early operative interference in cases of disease of the vermiform appendix. N Y Med J 50:676, 1889

Major RH: Classic Descriptions of Disease, 3 edt. Springfield, Illinois: Charles C Thomas, 1944

Menon NK: Primary adenocarcinoma of the appendix. Postgrad Med J 56:448, 1980

M'Kidd J: Case of invagination of caecum and appendix. Edinb Med J 4:793, 1858

Moertel GC, Dockerty MB, et al: Carcinoid tumours of the vermiform appendix. Cancer 21:270, 1968

Noer T: Decreasing incidence of acute peritonitis. Acta Chir Scand 141:431, 1975

Office of Population Censuses and Surveys: Hospital In-patient Inquiry 1976. Series MB4 No. 7. London: Her Majesty's Stationery Office, 1976, p 61

Owens BJ, Hamit HF: Appendicitis in the elderly. Ann Surg 187:392, 1978

Palumbo LT: Appendicitis—is it on the wane? Am J Surg 98:702, 1959

Parton LI: Appendico-vesical fistula: Report of a case and survey of the literature. Br J Surg 45:583, 1958

Payne JE: A case of torsion of the appendix. Br J Surg 6:327, 1918

Peltokallio P, Jauhianen K: Acute appendicitis in the aged patient. Study of 300 cases after the age of 60. Arch Surg 100:140, 1970

Peltokallio P, Tykka H: Evolution of the age distribution and mortality of acute appendicitis. Arch Surg 116:153, 1981

Petersen KR, Brooks L, et al: Torsio appendicis veriformis. Report of an unusual case. Acta Chir Scand 148:383, 1982

Pieper R, Kager L: The incidence of acute appendicitis and appendectomy. An epidemiological study of 971 cases. Acta Chir Scand 148:45, 1982

Pieper R, Kager L, et al: Acute appendicitis: A clinical study of 1,018 cases of emergency appendectomy. Acta Chir Scand 148:51, 1982

Pieper R, Kager L, et al: Obstruction of the appendix vermiformis causing acute appendicitis. An experimental study in the rabbit. Acta Chir Scand 148:63, 1982

Pieper R, Kager L, et al: The role of Bacteroides fragilis in the pathogenesis of acute appendicitis. Acta Chir Scand 148:39, 1982

Pinto DJ, Sanderson PJ: Rational use of antibiotic therapy after appendicectomy. Br Med J 280:275, 1980

Punnonen R, Aho AJ, et al: Appendicectomy during pregnancy. Acta Chir Scand 145:555, 1979

Robinson JO: Congenital absence of vermiform appendix. Br J Surg 39:344, 1952

Rodgers J, Ross D, et al: Intrarectal metronidazole in the prevention of anaerobic infections after emergency appendicectomy: A controlled clinical trial. Br J Surg 66:425, 1979

Saario I, Arvilommi H, et al: Comparison of cefuroxime and gentamicin in combination with metronidazole in the treatment of peritonitis due to perforation of the appendix. Acta Chir Scand 149:423, 1983

Saebø A: Pneumoperitoneum associated with perforated appendicitis. Acta Chir Scand 144:115, 1978

Shaw RE: Appendix calculi and acute appendicitis. Br J Surg 52:451, 1965

Skoubo-Kristensen E, Hvid I: The appendiceal mass. Results of conservation management. Ann Surg 196:584, 1982

Smith DE, Kirchmer NA, et al: Use of the barium enema in the diagnosis of acute appendicitis and its complications. Am J Surg 138:829, 1979

Smith PH: The diagnosis of appendicitis. Postgrad Med J 41:2, 1965

Stammers FAR: Treatment of acute appendicitis. Br Med J 1:225, 1957

Svendsen LB, Bülow S: Carcinoid tumours of the appendix in young patients. Acta Chir Scand 146:137, 1980

Thomas WEG, Vowles KDJ, et al: Appendicitis in external herniae. Ann R Coll Surg Engl 64:121, 1982

Tinckler LF: Triple appendix verniformis—a unique case. Br J Surg 55:79, 1968

Turner GG, Rogers LC (eds): Modern Operative Surgery, 4 edt. London: Cassell, 1956, vol 1, p 1142

Valerio D: Acute diabetic abdomen in childhood. Lancet 1:66, 1976

Wakeley CP: The position of the vermiform appendix as ascertained by an analysis of 10,000 cases. J Anat 67:277, 1933

Wallbridge PH: Double appendix. Br J Surg 50:346, 1962

Wang SMS, Wilson SE: Subphrenic abscess. The new epidemiology. Arch Surg 112:934, 1977

Wangensteen OH, Bowers WF: Significance of the obstructive factor in the genesis of acute appendicitis. An experimental study. Arch Surg 34:496, 1937

Wiig JN, Janssen CW, et al: Infertility as a complication of perforated appendicitis. Late follow-up of a clinical series. Acta Chir Scand 145:409, 1979

Wilkie DPD: Acute appendicitis and acute appendicular obstruction. Br Med J 2:959, 1914

Williamson WA, Bush RD, et al: Retrocecal appendicitis. Am J Surg 141:507, 1981

Willis AT, Ferguson IR, et al: Metronidazole in prevention and treatment of *Bacteroides* infections after appendicectomy. Br Med J 1:318, 1976

Wilson RR: Diverticula of appendix and certain factors in their development. Br J Surg 38:65, 1950

Winsey HS, Jones PF: Acute abdominal pain in childhood: Analysis of a year's admissions. Br Med J 1:653, 1967

49. Hirschsprung's Disease and Anorectal Anomalies

Lewis Spitz

HIRSCHSPRUNG'S DISEASE

Historical Background

The first recorded report of intestinal aganglionosis is attributed to Ruysch who, in 1691, described the necropsy features of a megacolon in a 5-year-old girl. Although sporadic reports appeared during the next two centuries, it was Hirschsprung in 1886 who clearly defined the clinicopathologic features of the condition that now bears his name. Hirschsprung focused his attention on the dilated segment, which he believed to be a true congenital malformation. Marfan in 1895 questioned his interpretation and proposed that the dilatation occurred secondarily in response to a distal obstruction. Klingman (1938) believed the disease was due to an overactive parasympathetic innervation and used an atropine derivative with some degree of success. Some surgeons, believing that normal colonic innervation could be restored by dividing the sympathetic nerve supply, claimed successes after lumbar sympathectomy (Wade and Royle, 1927). In 1946, Ehrenpreis demonstrated in neonates that although a motility disturbance was present at birth, the dilatation developed secondarily over a period of weeks or months. Swenson in 1948 reported a significant breakthrough in the knowledge of the pathophysiology of Hirschsprung's disease. Confronted with a 4-year-old boy in cardiorespiratory failure from massive abdominal distension, in desperation he fashioned a sigmoid colostomy. The child made a spectacular recovery, only to relapse later when the colostomy was closed. Radiologic studies revealed the narrow irregular distal colonic segment with massive proximal dilatation. Resection of the abnormal distal segment resulted in return of normal intestinal function. The true nature of the abnormality in colonic innervation was finally unravelled by Zuelzer (1948), Whitehouse (1948), and Bodian (1949).

Pathology

The basic pathologic defect in Hirschsprung's disease is an abnormality of the innervation of the distal intestine. The deficit always involves the internal anal sphincter and extends proximally for varying distances. In 75 percent of cases the abnormal segment is restricted to the rectosigmoid area, while in less than 5 percent of patients the entire colon and a variable amount of small intestine is involved. The abnormal innervation results in a functional obstruction due to failure of distal propagation of intestinal peristaltic waves.

The gross pathologic changes consist of a fairly normal calibre aganglionic rectum, which extends proximally into the grossly dilated, thickened and hypertrophied normally innervated but functionally obstructed colon. The cone-shaped area between the dilated and collapsed intestine is referred to as the "transitional" zone.

The classic histologic feature of Hirschsprung's disease consists of a total absence of ganglion cells in the intermuscular plexus of Auerbach as well as in the submucosal plexus of Meissner. This is associated with an increase in large nerve trunks in the affected bowel and an increase in the number and diameter of nerve cells in the mesenteric plexus. Acetylcholinesterase staining techniques reveal an increase in acetylcholinesterase activity in the parasympathetic nerve fibres in the lamina propria mucosae, the muscularis mucosae, and in the circular muscle fibres (Lake et al, 1978; Meier-Ruge et al, 1972). The variability of cholinergic activity in the aganglionic bowel is thought to be responsible for the differing clinical features in patients with the same extent of involvement. Fluorescent histochemical studies for the localisation of monoamines show that adrenergic fibres, which are normally distributed in close association with the parasympathetic ganglion cells, are directed towards the muscle layers in Hirschsprung's disease. Both cholinergic and adrenergic fibres are greatly increased in the distal aganglionic segment while their distribution gradually decreases in the more proximally affected intestine.

The pathophysiologic effects of the abnormal innervation responsible for the changes in Hirschsprung's disease varies in the different sections of the involved bowel:

1. The most severely affected aganglionic distal rectum contains variable amounts of cholinergic and adrenergic fibres. The bowel activity is uncoordinated, irregular, and prone to mass contractions. It is unable to relax, probably due to the absence of synaptic influences of ganglion cells. Direct action of adrenergic fibres on the smooth muscle is thought by some to be responsible for the tonic contractions.
2. The proximal aganglionic segment possesses no ganglion cells and a decreased number of intermuscular nerve fibres. The absence of ganglion cells reduces coordinated peristalsis, the decrease in cholinergic fibres results in contractions and the absence of adrenergic fibres prevents relaxation.
3. The transitional segment contains few ganglion cells and also few postganglionic cholinergic nerve fibres. The propulsive force is reduced but the segment is dilated.

Clinical Manifestations

Incidence. Approximately 1 in 5000 newborn infants is affected by Hirschsprung's disease. The condition affects all racial groups but is thought to occur less often in the American black. The overall sex incidence reveals a male preponderance of 4:1. This male preponderance gradually fades as the length of involved colon increases, so that the sex incidence in cases with total colonic involvement amounts to a ratio of 2:1 in favour of the males.

Hereditary Factors. There is a definite increased predisposition in siblings and offspring of index cases. Carter has shown a 2 percent risk for offspring of short-segment index patients but the risk increases to 12.5 percent in the case of long-segment disease.

Associated Anomalies. Although Hirschsprung's disease has been found in combination with almost every known congenital anomaly, only two conditions appear to concur to a significant degree. Down's syndrome occurs in 5 to 10 percent of patients and urologic anomalies are present in approximately 3 percent of patients. Other conditions that have been noted to be present more often than by mere chance are pyloric stenosis, malrotation, Meckel's diverticulum, and anorectal anomalies. In addition to associated genitourinary anomalies, urinary abnormalities arising secondary to the obstruction caused by Hirschsprung's disease itself are found in up to one third of cases. These include vesicoureteric reflux, hydronephrosis, and bladder function disorders that develop as a consequence of faecal impaction.

Presentation in the Neonatal Period

Complete Intestinal Obstruction. There is bilious vomiting, complete obstipation, and abdominal distension (Fig. 49–1).

Delayed Passage of Meconium. Spontaneous evacuation of meconium normally occurs within the first 24 hours of birth in 98 percent of healthy infants. Failure to pass meconium on the first day of life should alert the clinician to the possibility of Hirschsprung's disease. This feature was present in 94 percent of patients in Swenson's (1973) series of 501 cases. It is generally accompanied by vomiting, which may be bilious in nature, and by abdominal distension. These symptoms may instantly resolve once evacuation of meconium is stimulated, either by digital rectal examination or by saline rectal washouts. The constipation, abdominal distension, and vomiting recur within a few days and the infant fails to thrive.

Enterocolitis. This is characterised by the presence of profuse diarrhoea containing blood

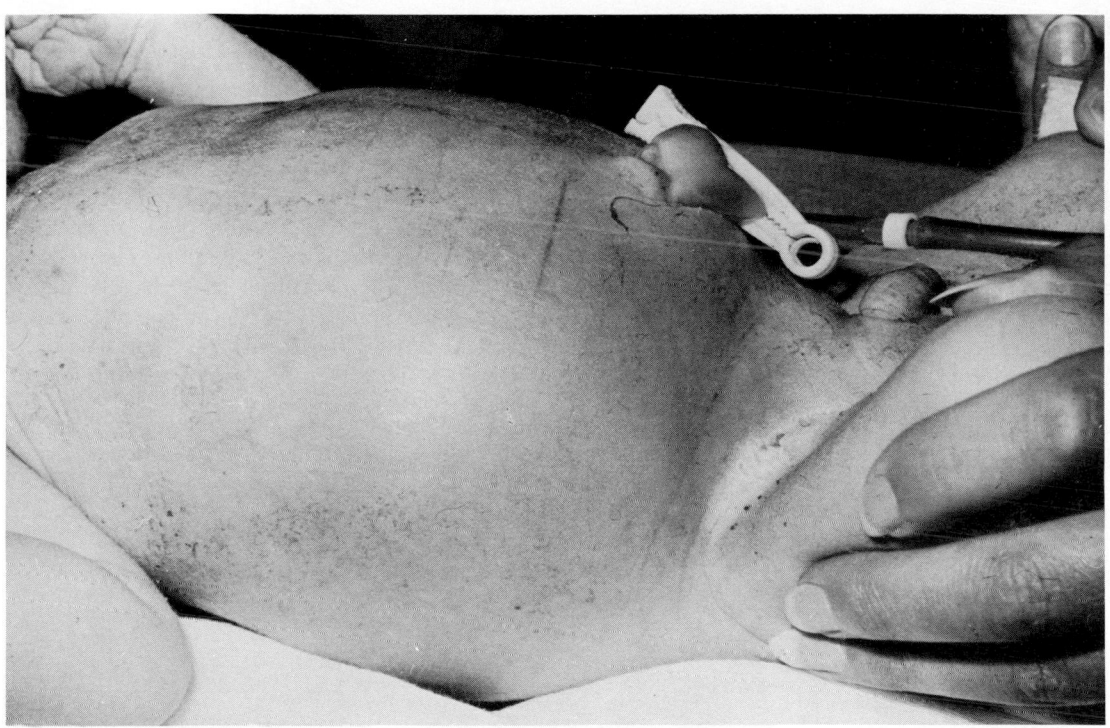

Figure 49–1. Abdominal distension in an infant with Hirschsprung's disease. The infant classically fails to pass meconium within the first 24 hours of life.

and mucus associated with abdominal distension and vomiting. The fluid and electrolyte losses may be so severe and occur so rapidly that the infant presents in hypovolaemic shock. Although most cases of enterocolitis develop during the second to fourth weeks, it has been diagnosed within the first week of life and may present at any age, even many years after successful surgical correction. Formerly, up to one third of infants and children manifested enterocolitis at the initial presentation, but with increased awareness of the significance of delayed passage of meconium, this complication of delayed diagnosis, is becoming a less common method of presentation (Bill and Chapman, 1962).

Presentation in the Older Infant and Child

Chronic intractable constipation, unresponsive to dietary measures, is the hallmark of Hirschsprung's disease presenting in the older infant or child. Stool is evacuated at irregular inter-

vals, often many days apart and only with great effort. The consistency of the stool varies from hard and pellet-like to voluminous, extremely foul-smelling, and pasty-liquid in consistency. Soiling, not generally recognised as occurring in Hirschsprung's disease, was a feature in 3 percent of patients in Swenson's series. Meteorism contributes to the abdominal distension. Failure to thrive is a constant feature and malnutrition to a greater or lesser extent is commonly encountered in late presenting cases.

Visible peristaltic waves may be seen on abdominal inspection. Rectal examination reveals an empty rectum and a taut anal sphincter. Withdrawal of the examining finger may precipitate an explosive evacuation of foul-smelling semiliquid faeces, especially in the young infant.

The severity of the symptomatology varies, not only with the age of the patient at presentation, but also with the extent of involvement. In general, the greater the extent of involvement the more severe the clinical picture but it should be appreciated that patients with similar lengths of aganglionic bowel may present with quite disparate clinical features.

Diagnostic Studies

A high index of clinical suspicion and an acute awareness of the significance of delayed passage of meconium will undoubtedly lead to earlier diagnosis, particularly within the neonatal period, and will help to decrease complications that arise as a consequence of delayed diagnosis. Confirmation of the diagnosis may be achieved by one or more of the following investigations: radiologic, manometric, histopathologic, or histochemical.

Radiology. The plain erect and supine abdominal radiographs show dilated loop of bowel of varying extent, length, and distribution (Fig. 49–2). Although the anatomic distribution of bowel gas may suggest a low colonic obstruction, it is generally recognised that the distinction of small from large intestine on the plain radiograph is unreliable in early infancy. The erect radiograph shows fluid levels of varying length.

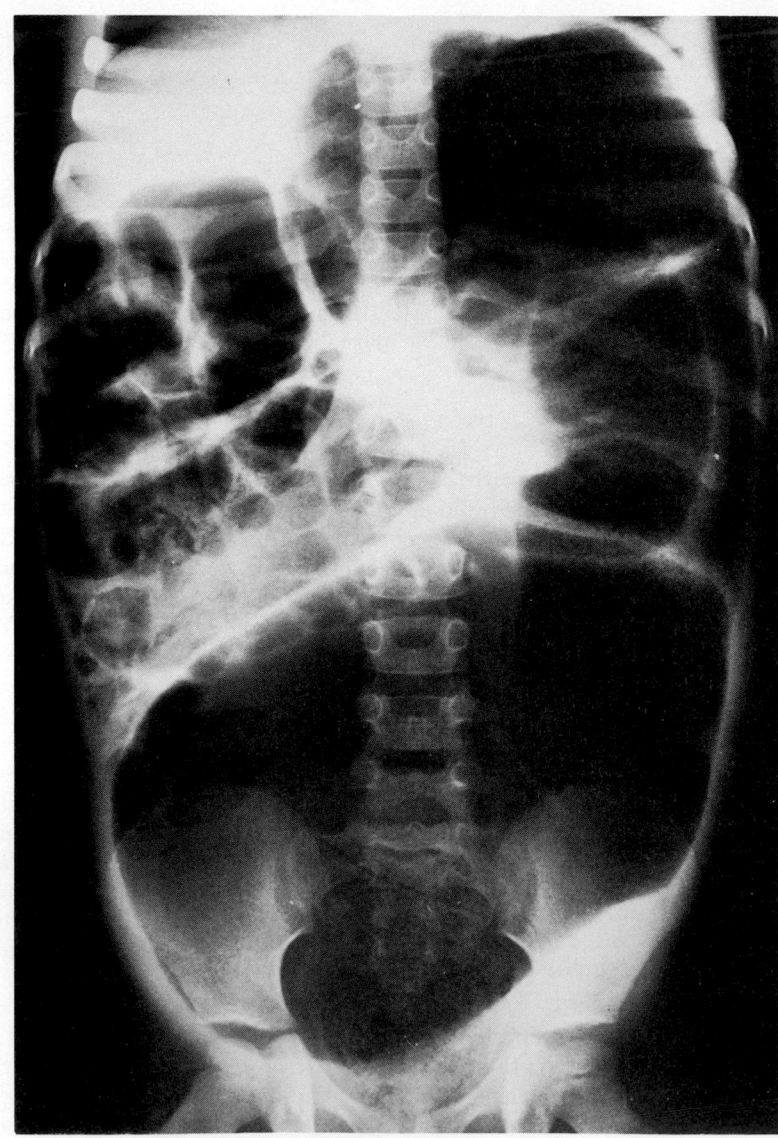

Figure 49–2. Abdominal radiograph in an infant with Hirschsprung's disease showing massive distension of the rectum and sigmoid region of the colon.

A dilated sigmoid loop may be recognised as arising from the pelvis. The pelvis is usually devoid of gas shadows. The main value of the plain radiographs is to alert the radiologist to the need for further investigation by means of contrast studies.

Barium is the contrast medium of choice for the diagnosis of Hirschsprung's disease. A 30 percent w/v solution is used. Prior preparation of the colon with enemas or cathartics should be avoided as they may deflate the megacolon or distend the aganglionic segment and result in a false-negative study. Digital rectal examination, especially in the neonate, may obliterate the narrow distal aganglionic segment and should be specifically excluded from the physical examination of the newborn with suspected Hirschsprung's disease if a diagnostic enema is to be carried out.

A small soft rubber catheter is inserted just within the anal canal and the buttocks are strapped together to avoid leakage of contrast.

With the infant in the lateral position, the barium solution is slowly injected into the rectum. Filling of bowel is continued until an obviously dilated area is visible. At this stage the instillation of contrast is stopped and the catheter withdrawn. Further radiographs in the supine, oblique, and prone position are taken. In cases where the diagnosis remains doubtful, delayed films are taken 12 to 24 hours later.

The diagnostic criteria on barium examination are as follows (Berdon and Baker, 1965):

- *Disparity in Size (Fig. 49–3).* The funnel-shaped transition between the narrow aganglionic segment and the dilated proximal bowel is diagnostic of Hirschsprung's disease. This feature may only be appreciated on the delayed films. It is often stated that the disparity in size is unreliable in the neonatal period because there has been insufficient time for the dilatation to develop. This is fallacious, as experienced radiologists will achieve a posi-

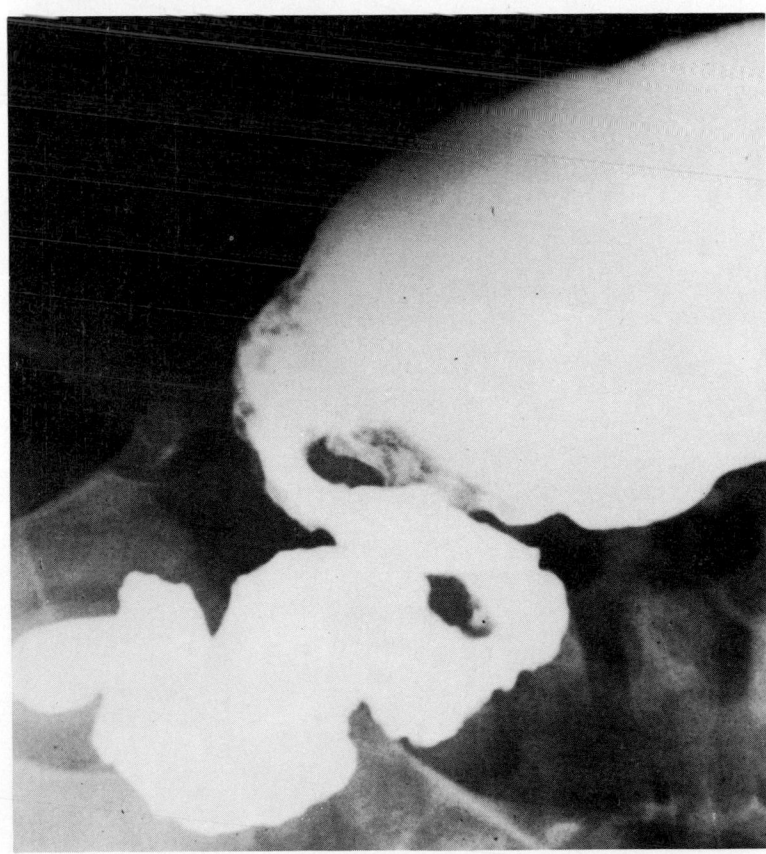

Figure 49–3. Barium enema examination showing the narrow irritable spastic aganglionic lower rectum with contrast material entering the proximally dilated ganglionic colon.

tive diagnosis in over 80 percent of patients.
• *Irregularity in Contour.* The aganglionic segment reveals irregular contractions which
manifest as deep sawtooth filling defects or
as fine marginal serrations. The irritability
and irregular contraction waves of the aganglionic segment are best visible during fluoroscopic examination.

The radiographic appearance of total colonic aganglionosis varies from a uniformly narrow contracted colon to a virtually normal-appearing large intestine. In the latter case,
failure to achieve any significant evacuation of
contrast on the delayed 24-hour film should be
regarded as highly suspicious of Hirschsprung's
disease (Fig. 49–4).

Manometry. The purpose of electromanome-
try is to study the motility of the bowel by measuring intraluminal pressures (Aaronson and
Nixon, 1972; Lawson and Nixon, 1967). Particular attention is given to the propagation of propulsive peristaltic waves and to the function of
the internal anal sphincter, with special emphasis on the presence or absence of the relaxation
reflex.

The basic equipment necessary for anorectal manometry consists of a probe, comprising
a rectal balloon and one or more pressure transducers, sited in the anal canal at the level of
the internal sphincter. A recording device will
document the pressures during the various
stages of the investigation. A normal response
consists of a relaxation wave in the internal

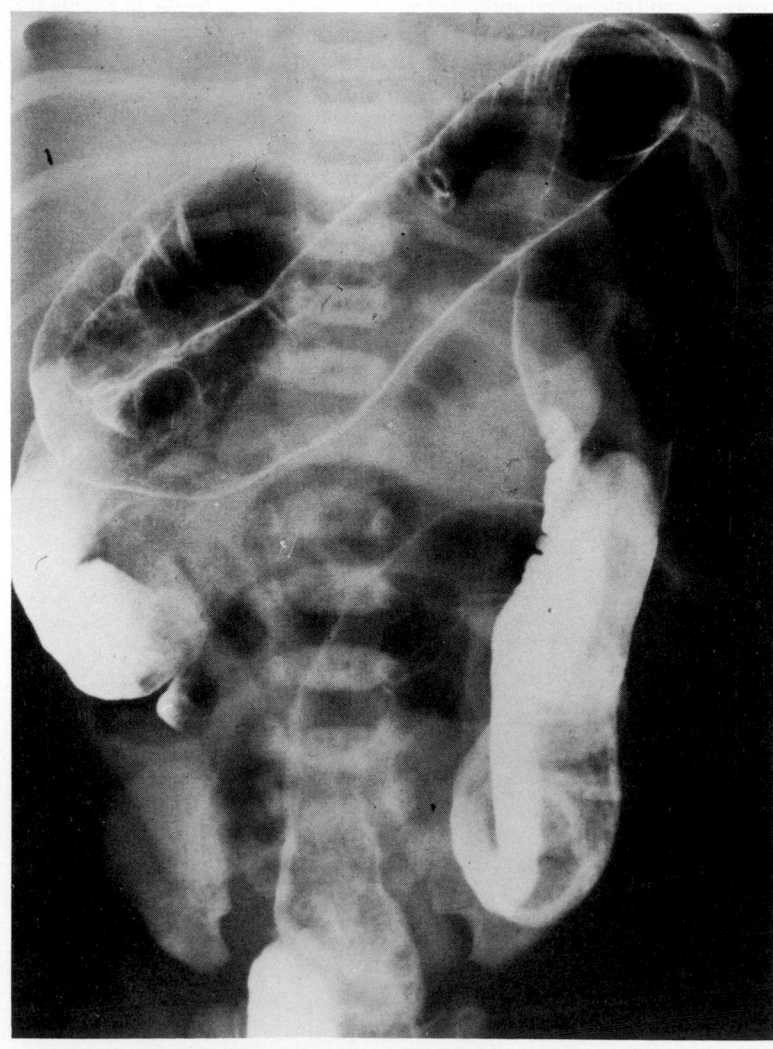

Figure 49–4. Barium enema in long-segment Hirschsprung's disease showing a virtually normal calibre colon but there is considerable retention of contrast in the 24-hour postevacuation film.

sphincter zone in response to distension of the rectal balloon. Failure of internal sphincter relaxation in association with spontaneous multisegmental mass contractions in the rectum is diagnostic of Hirschsprung's disease.

Although the demonstration of genuine internal sphincter relaxation excludes the diagnosis of Hirschsprung's disease, the absence of relaxation waves cannot be accepted as reliable evidence for the diagnosis. It is especially in the early newborn period when this reflex may be physiologically absent that false-positives may be obtained in the manometric evaluation. Nevertheless, Holschneider (1980) has reported a diagnostic accuracy of 96 percent using this method of diagnosis.

Morphology. The histopathologic diagnosis of Hirschsprung's disease relies upon the absence of ganglion cells in the myenteric (Auerbach) as well as the submucosal (Meissner) nerve plexuses. In addition, there are large nerve trunks and a greatly increased presence of parasympathetic nerve fibres. The accuracy of diagnosis has been facilitated by the advent of histochemical techniques that specifically stain acetylcholinesterase, an enzyme found in large quantities in parasympathetic nerve fibres.

Until relatively recently a full-thickness biopsy of the rectal wall was required for accurate histopathologic diagnosis. The technique, which involves a transanal approach, is a difficult procedure in the small infant and requires the administration of a general anaesthetic. It was attended by a significant morbidity from haemorrhage and/or infection and resulted in scarring, which made subsequent definitive treatment difficult. The suction biopsy technique introduced by Noblett in 1969 has virtually totally superceded the full-thickness biopsy. Suction biopsy specimens consist of mucosa and submucosa and can be obtained without resorting to anaesthesia or sedation (Fig. 49–5).

Suction biopsies are performed at three levels from the anal verge—2, 3, and 5 cm—although in the neonate only one biopsy at 2 to 3 cm may be sufficient for diagnostic purposes. It is our practice to submit the 2- and 5-cm biopsy specimens for histochemical stains, while the 3-cm biopsy is examined by conventional haematoxylin and eosin stains. The latter speci-

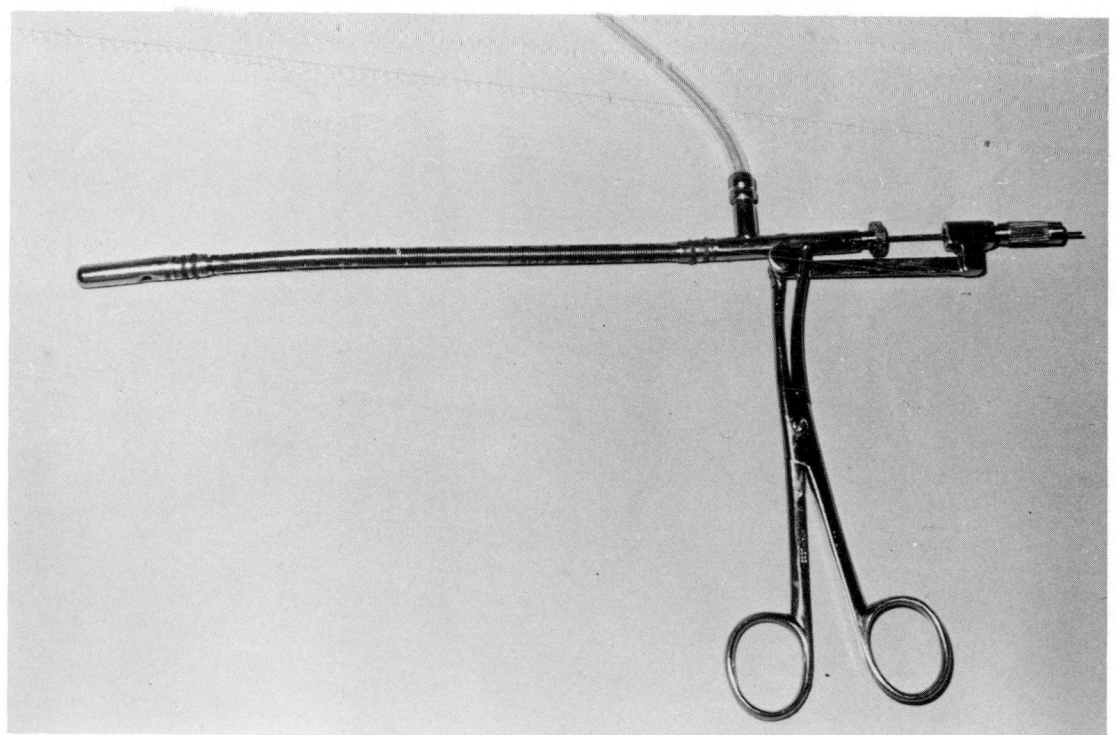

Figure 49–5. Noblett suction biopsy instrument.

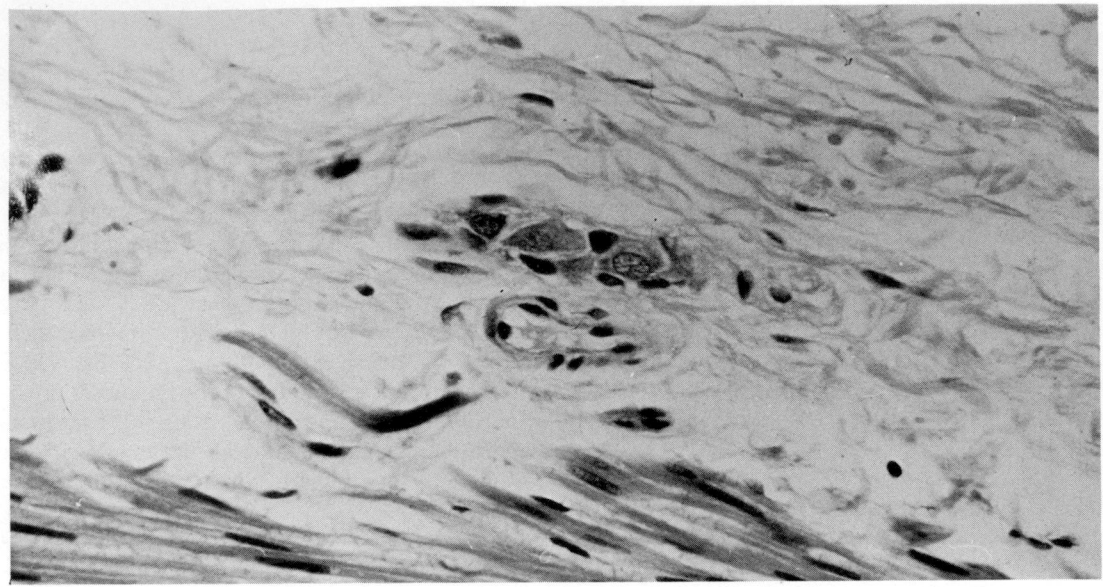

Figure 49–6. Rectal biopsy showing normal ganglion cells with characteristic vacuolated cytoplasm and prominent nucleoli.

men may be submitted for frozen section if a rapid diagnosis is required. Multiple serial sections of all specimens are examined. The criteria of the morphologic diagnosis (demonstrated in Figs. 49–6 through 49–8) are:

1. Absence of ganglion cells in the submucosa
2. The presence of large nerve trunks in the submucosa
3. An increase in acetylcholinesterase activity in the parasympathetic nerve fibres in the

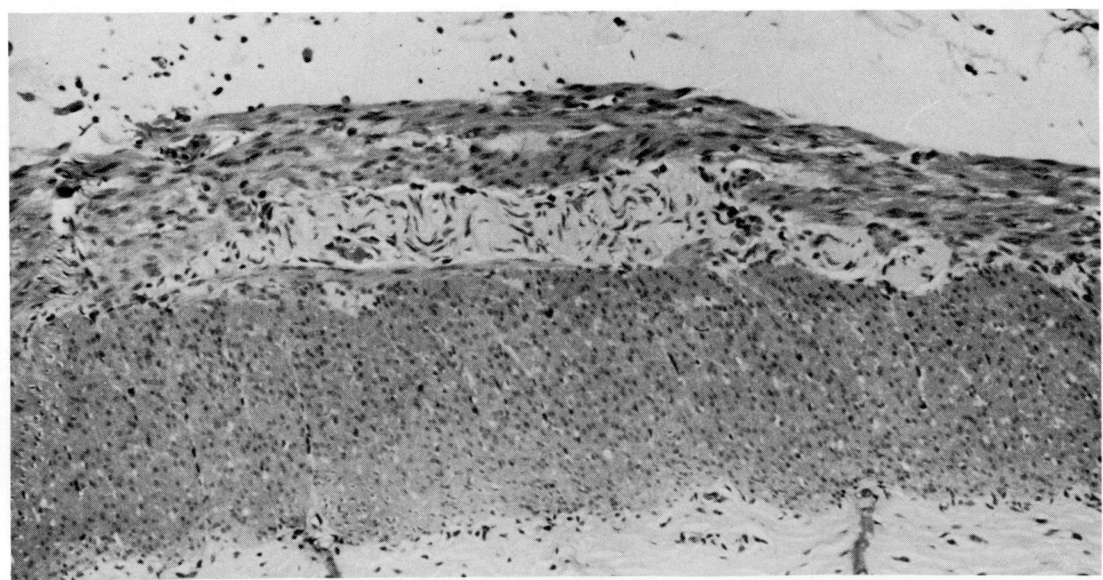

Figure 49–7. Full-thickness rectal biopsy in Hirschsprung's disease showing the hypertrophied nerve trunks in the intermuscular plexus. No ganglion cells are present.

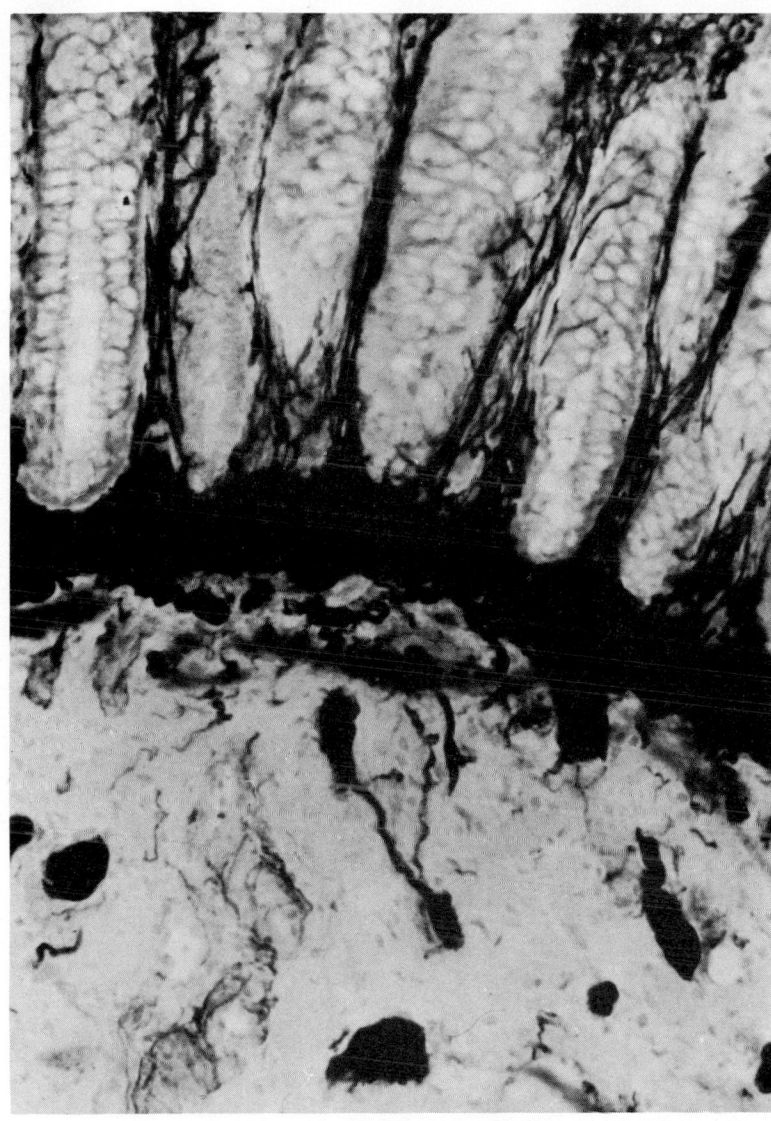

Figure 49–8. Acetylcholinesterase staining technique in Hirschsprung's disease showing a greatly increased nerve complement in the submucosa and in the lamina propria of the rectal suction biopsy specimen.

muscularis mucosae and in the lamina propria

Complications from suction biopsy are rare and consist mainly of transient haemorrhage and infection. Failure to adhere to a meticulous technique may result in full-thickness biopsy, particularly when excessive pressure is applied to the biopsy instrument. In approximately 5 percent of cases, the biopsy specimen is inadequate for accurate diagnosis, but even in these patients the demonstration of increased acetylcholinesterase activity in the lamina propria may be sufficient to allow a diagnosis.

Treatment

The aim of treatment is to relieve the intestinal obstruction by either resecting or bypassing the aganglionic bowel. Temporary relief of the obstruction pending the results of investigations to establish the definitive diagnosis may be obtained by gentle warm saline rectal washouts. Where these manouevres are unsuccessful in causing evacuation of the obstructed bowel, emergency colostomy may be necessary. Although definitive treatment may be undertaken in the neonatal period, most surgeons would prefer to perform a defunctioning colostomy while delaying definitive treatment until the infant is 6 to 9 months of age or at least 3 months have elapsed since establishing the colostomy in order to allow the dilated bowel to return to a normal calibre.

Infants presenting with enterocolitis are often critically ill due to massive fluid and electrolyte losses, and emergency colostomy under these circumstances could prove fatal. These infants require intensive resuscitative measures, including circulatory fluid volume expansion (plasma 20 ml/kg intravenously as rapidly as possible), and correction of acid–base imbalance and fluid and electrolyte deficiencies. In addition, gentle rectal washouts with small volumes of warm isotonic saline will achieve decompression of the obstructed bowel and will reduce the danger of perforation. One or two litres of isotonic saline may be required before adequate decompression is achieved and clear returns of infused saline are obtained. Tap water for the washouts should never be used, as absorption of the hypotonic water from the rectum may lead to circulatory overload and water intoxication.

Infants in good general condition with short segment aganglionosis in whom rectal washouts produce effective decompression may be maintained on regular washouts until the definitive treatment can be safely performed.

Temporary Colostomy

Unless the extent of aganglionosis has been accurately established by barium enema examination, frozen section histopathology should be considered mandatory to determine the siting of the colostomy. A laparotomy is performed via a lower left paramedian incision. Seromuscular biopsies from the dilated and collapsed bowel are submitted for frozen section examination. Where there is no clear-cut transition between dilated and collapsed bowel, seromuscular biopsies are taken at progressively proximal intervals until normally ganglionic intestine is identified. In total colonic aganglionosis the entire colon may appear narrow and collapsed. The appendix submitted for frozen section examination will reveal an absence of ganglion cells; in this situation serial biopsies of the small intestine will eventually determine the site at which the enterostomy should be established.

Siting of the Colostomy. For the usual type of rectosigmoid aganglionosis (Fig. 49–9), a right

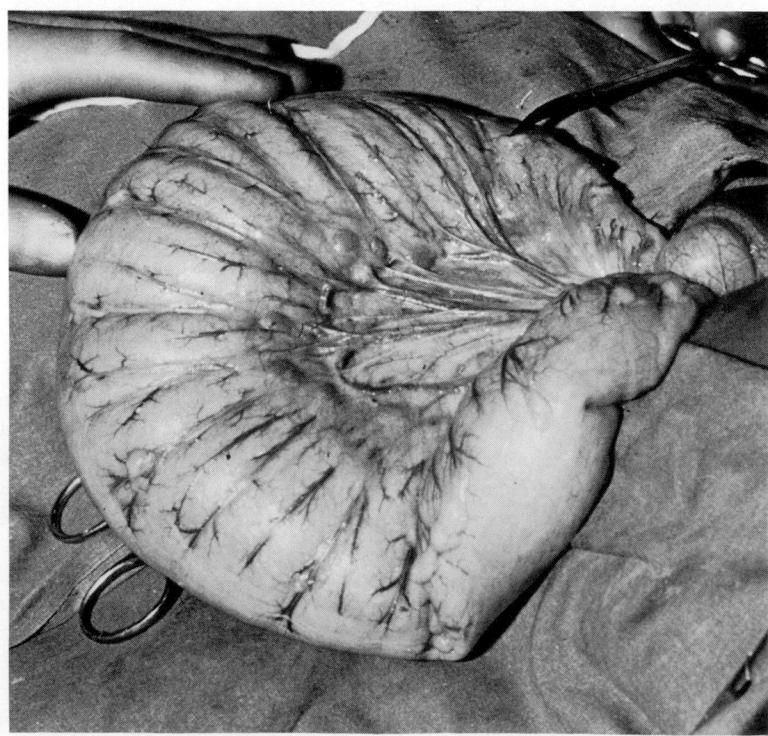

Figure 49–9. Operative appearance of the dilated and hypertrophied proximal colon in Hirschsprung's disease.

transverse colostomy will provide proximal decompression while allowing the definitive treatment to be performed in the distal defunctioned bowel. Where the aganglionic segment extends beyond the sigmoid colon, the colostomy is fashioned in the most distally ganglionate bowel in order to conserve the maximum amount of intestine. The precise location of the colostomy under these circumstances can only be determined on the basis of accurate frozen-section histopathologic examination.

Technique of Colostomy. The technique for the fashioning of a right transverse colostomy, being the most common site for colostomy formation, is described in detail (Fig. 49–10). The technique is equally applicable to any other site in the colon. The Nixon (1976) skin-bridge colostomy is most appropriate for infants and children, as it dispenses with the need for a glass rod to prevent retraction of the bowel.

A wide-based V-incision is made in the right upper abdominal quadrant. The apex of the V is directed caudally and the length of the incisions should measure 2 to 3 cm. The full thickness of the flap is elevated proximally to expose the underlying fascia. Shallow elipses of skin are excised on either side of the incision, in order to prevent compression of the bowel when the skin bridge is sutured in position. A transverse incision is made in the centre of the exposed fascia through the full thickness of the

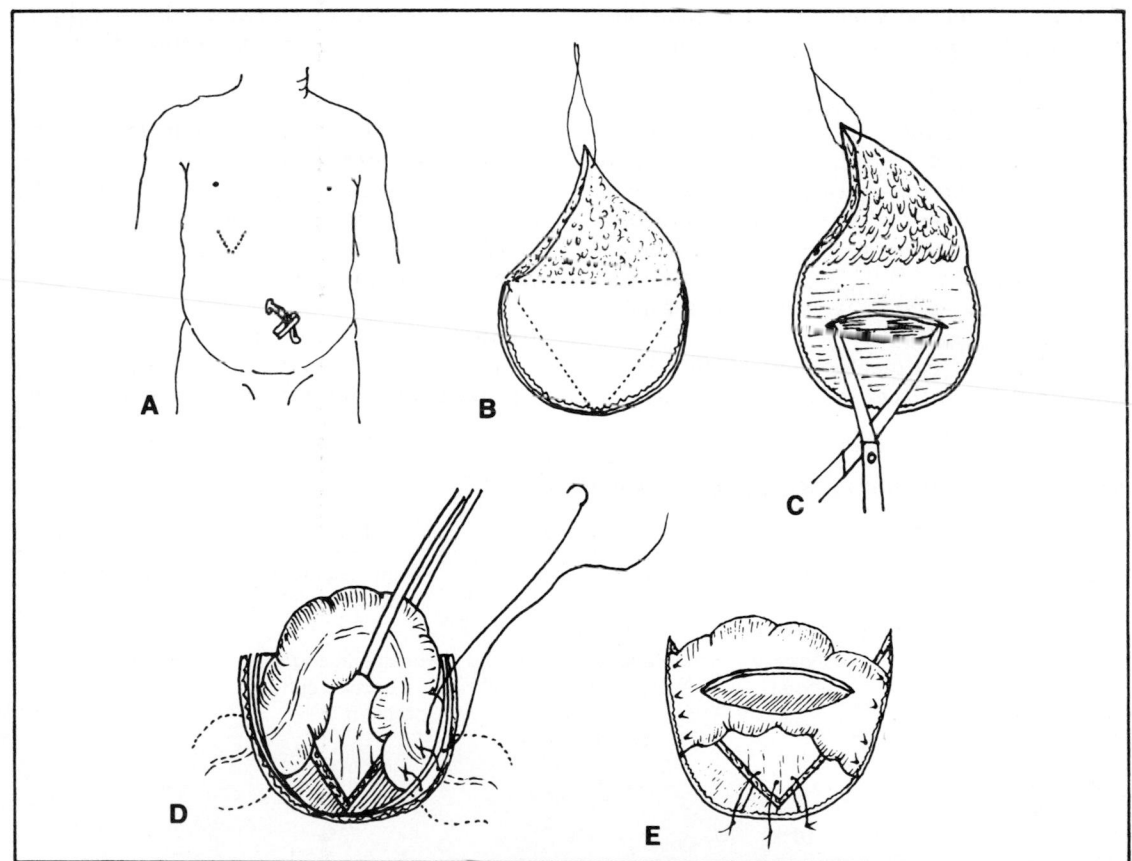

Figure 49–10. Principles of the skin-bridge technique for fashioning a right transverse colostomy: **A.** V-shaped incision in right hypochondrium. **B.** Excision of ellipses of skin on either side of the V to allow free passage of the colon without compression. **C.** Division of muscle fibres and peritoneum transversely. **D.** Delivery of right transverse colon and seromuscular sutures attaching colon to the peritoneal layer circumferentially. **E.** Securing the skin bridge in position. Colostomy opened and full thickness of bowel wall sutured to edges of skin.

abdominal musculature. After opening the peritoneum, the segment of transverse colon immediately to the left of the hepatic flexure is lifted out of the wound and a vascular arcade in the mesocolon adjacent to the bowel wall is ligated and divided to allow free passage of the skin bridge through the defect. The incised edges of the peritoneum are now sutured circumferentially to the seromuscular layer of the colon with interrupted fine sutures to prevent small bowel from prolapsing alongside the colostomy. Particular care should be exercised to avoid entering the bowel lumen, as this may result in fistula formation. The skin bridge is directed through the mesenteric defect and the apex sutured to the anterior abdominal wall. The colostomy is opened and the full thickness of the bowel wall is sutured to the cut edges of the skin. A full-thickness biopsy at the colostomy site should be submitted for further histologic examination.

Intravenous fluid therapy is maintained until the colostomy is functioning adequately enough to permit oral nutrition. Approximately 7 to 10 days postoperatively, saline washouts of the distal limb are carried out to evacuate the content of the defunctioned bowel. The patient is discharged from the hospital when the mother is competent to carry out efficient colostomy care.

Definitive treatment is delayed until the infant is 6 to 9 months of age or at least 3 months have elapsed since the colostomy has been established. This allows maximum contraction of the dilated hypertrophied bowel and facilitates the pull-through procedures.

Complications of colostomy in infancy and children are unfortunately not uncommon. Minor complications include excoriation of the surrounding skin and ulceration and bleeding of the exposed mucosa, which may cause an iron-deficiency anaemia and retraction of the colostomy. Excessive colostomy actions may be due to either stenosis of the proximal stoma, to massive saline losses in the colostomy fluid, or to recurrent enterocolitis. Prolapse of the colostomy is also common and may affect either the proximal or more commonly the distal limb.

Definitive Treatment

There are at least four recognised surgical procedures that may be recommended. Each has its own advantages and disadvantages but the overall results are roughly equivalent (Table 49–1). The most important factor in determining the eventual outcome is the expertise and experience of the surgeon concerned. There can be no justification for a surgeon performing the occasional operation for Hirschsprung's disease when paediatric surgical expertise is available.

Preoperative Preparation. The patient is admitted to hospital 3 days before surgery for colonic washouts. These are performed with saline

TABLE 49–1. COMPARISON OF SURGICAL TECHNIQUES

	Swenson	Duhamel	Soave	Rehbein
Advantages	Eliminates aganglionic segment	Technical ease avoiding pelvic dissection	Avoids extensive pelvic dissection	Purely abdominal approach
Disadvantages	Technically difficult	Retained anterior aganglionic wall; potential pouch impaction	Retains aganglionic muscular cuff of rectum	Retains a long rectal stump
Complications				
1. *Early*				
a. Anastomotic leak	10%	7%	5%	3%
b. Stenosis	8%	9%	12%	3%
2. *Late*				
a. Constipation	10%	7%	10%	8%
b. Incontinence	12%	7%	3%	0%
c. Diarrhoea/ entercolitis	12%	6%	6%	6%

solution until the bowel to be used for the pull-through procedure is completely cleared of all content. Only clear fluids orally are permitted on the day prior to surgery. Metronidazole is administered for 48 hours preoperatively and an aminoglycoside is given parenterally with the premedication and once again 6 hours postoperatively.

The patient is placed in the lithotomy position on the operating table. This position will permit simultaneous access to the abdomen and perineum. An indwelling urethral catheter is used to decompress the bladder during the operation and for the first 3 to 5 postoperative days. The anal sphincter is forcibly dilated to facilitate the operative approach and to paralyse the sphincter during the early postoperative period. The abdomen, perineum, and upper thighs are prepared with an antiseptic solution, e.g., povidone–iodine.

The originators of the four procedures most commonly performed for Hirschsprung's disease have recently described the technical details of their operations in Holschneider's monograph (1982) on the subject. An outline of each procedure with reference to various modifications is presented.

For practical purposes it should be assumed that the infant had previously had a right transverse colostomy with histopathologic determination of the extent of the aganglionic segment. Where an end colostomy had been fashioned for longer segment disease, the colostomy will have to be mobilised and utilised as the definitive level for the pull-through procedure. Failure to have previously defined the precise extent aganglionic segment, will necessitate the availability of frozen section histopathology at the definitive procedure in order to select the optimal site of proximal resection. The macroscopic appearance of the bowel is notoriously unreliable in determining the level of resection. This applies even when there is a clearly defined cone present between the proximally dilated ganglionic and distally collapsed aganglionic colon.

Swenson's Procedure (Fig. 49–11). The operative approach is via a left paramedian rectus retracting or rectus splitting incision. The incision extends from the symphysis pubis to just above the level of the umbilicus. The proximal site for resection is identified on the basis of histopathologic examination. The proximal colon and mesentery are freed to provide a suffi-

cient length for reconstruction without interfering with the blood supply. This is accomplished by dividing sufficient sigmoid vessels close to their origin that adequate blood flow is provided to the colon via arcades in the attached mesentery.

Attention is now directed towards the pelvis. The peritoneal reflection from the rectosigmoid and rectum on both sides and around the rectum anteriorly is divided. The ureters and vasa deferentia are identified to protect them from injury during the pelvic dissection. The superior haemorrhoidal artery is divided to reduce blood loss during the pelvic dissection. In order to preserve pelvic autonomic nerve supply, the dissection to free the rectum is made directly on the muscular wall. Numerous short vessels supplying the rectum are identified, doubly ligated, and divided. The vessels on the rectal side may be cauterised if ligation appears difficult. As the dissecting proceeds deeper into the pelvis, individual vascular control becomes impossible but, as the dissection is now beyond the area of supply of the middle haemorrhoid vessels, bleeding is easily controlled by a short period of packing. The dissection should continue through the levator ani muscle right down to the perineal floor. This part of the procedure is tedious and time consuming and requires a patient and meticulous technique.

The surgeon now leaves the abdominal field and turns to the perineum, which has been previously prepared and the anus forcibly dilated. A long, curved clamp is inserted into the anal canal and, with the help of an assistant, the inside of the rectosigmoid is grasped within the clamp. The rectum is now everted and prolapsed (intussuscepted) through the anal canal to reveal the mucocutaneous line laterally and posteriorly. Failure to identify this line of demarcation clearly indicates that the pelvic dissection is inadequate. The rectum should be returned to the pelvic cavity and further dissection performed. Anteriorly, the extent of the dissection stops short of the pelvic floor so that the mucocutaneous line is obscured in this part of the bowel.

The prolapsed everted rectum is cleaned with povidone–iodine solution and an incision 1.5 cm proximal to the mucocutaneous line is made through the full thickness of the anterior rectal wall for half the circumference of the bowel. Through this incision a long curved forceps is inserted either into the pelvis, when a section of rectum had been previously excised,

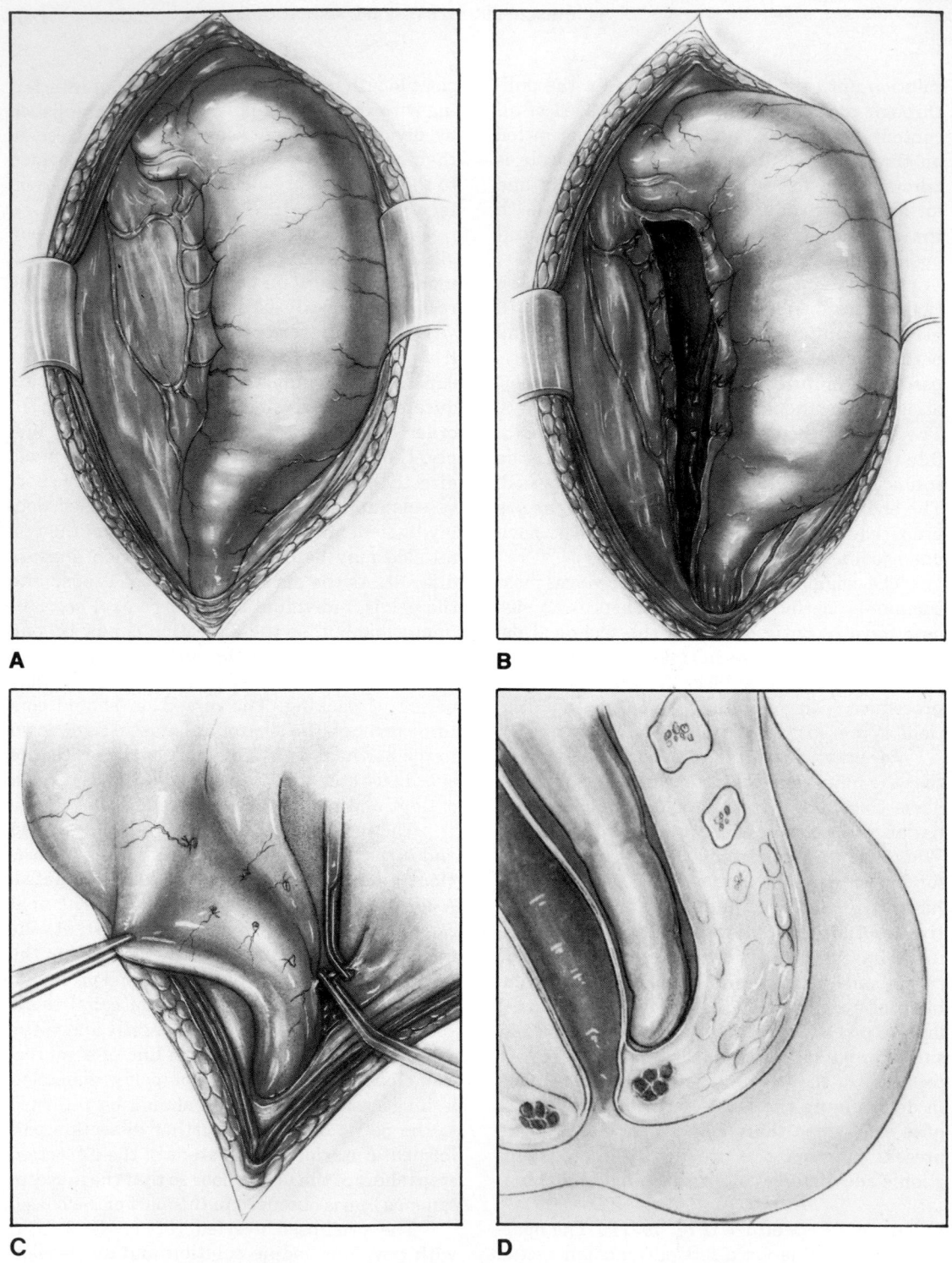

Figure 49–11. A through **J.** Technical principles of the Swenson's procedure for Hirschsprung's disease: **A.** Appearance of the dilated proximal colon contrasted with the narrow spastic aganglionic rectum. **B.** Dissection of the rectum toward the pelvic floor. **C.** Plane of dissection of the rectum in the pelvis keeping as close as possible to the muscular wall of the rectum. **D.** Rectal dissection is completed circumferentially down to the level of the dentate line.

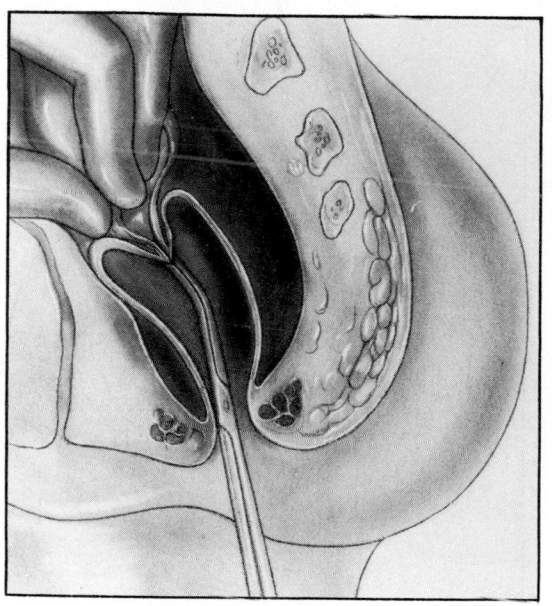

E

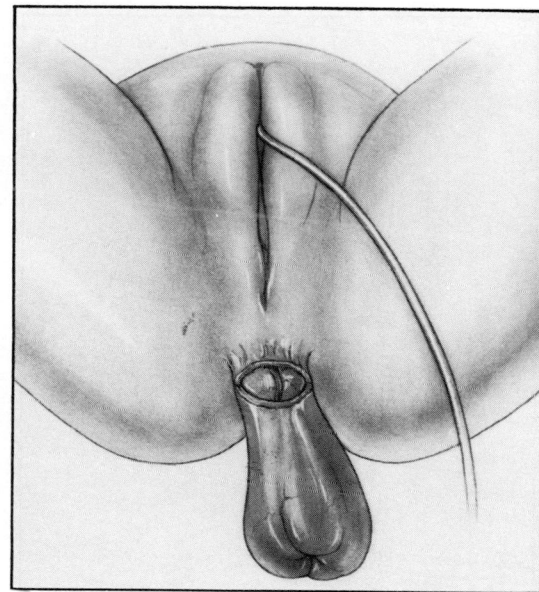

F

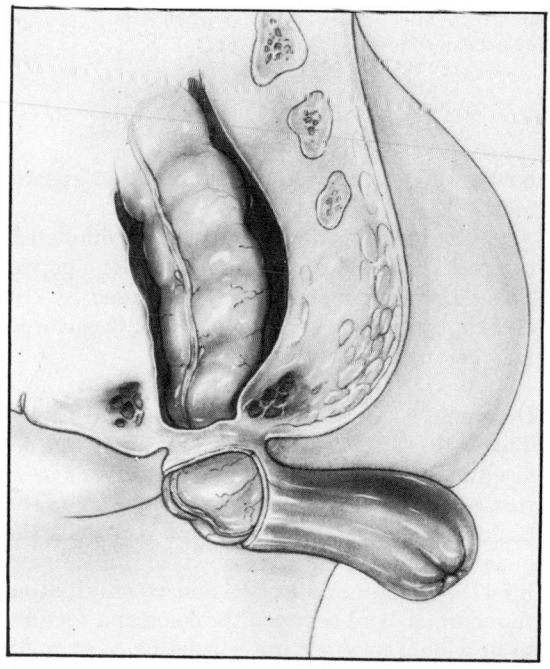

G

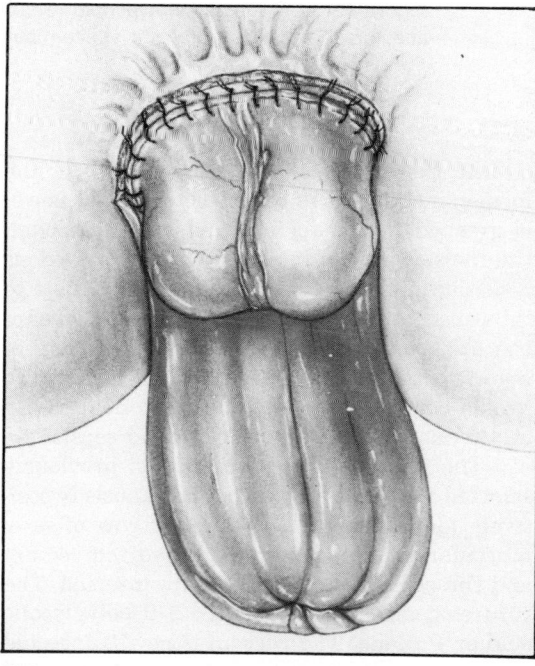

H

Figure 49–11. E. The proximal colon is intussuscepted into the rectum and prolapsed out of the anus everting the anal mucosa. **F.** Incision in the anterior wall of the everted anus—1.5 cm from the anal verge. **G.** The proximal colon is pulled through the incision in the anterior rectal wall until the predetermined site of resection (ganglionic bowel) is reached. **H.** Seromuscular anastomosis between the anterior wall of the rectum and the ganglionic colon.

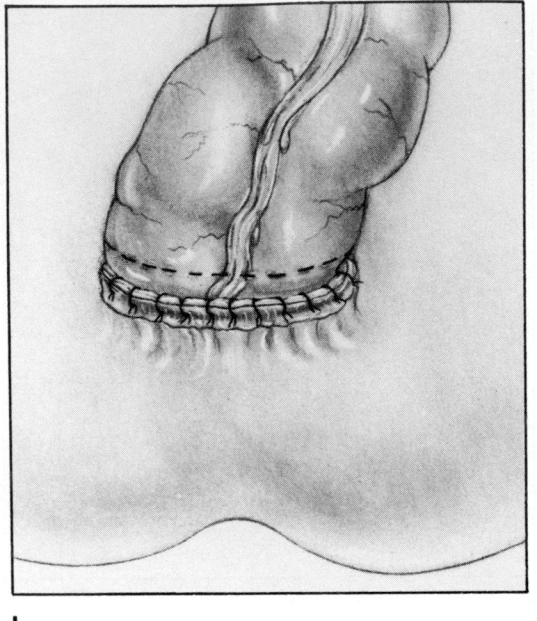
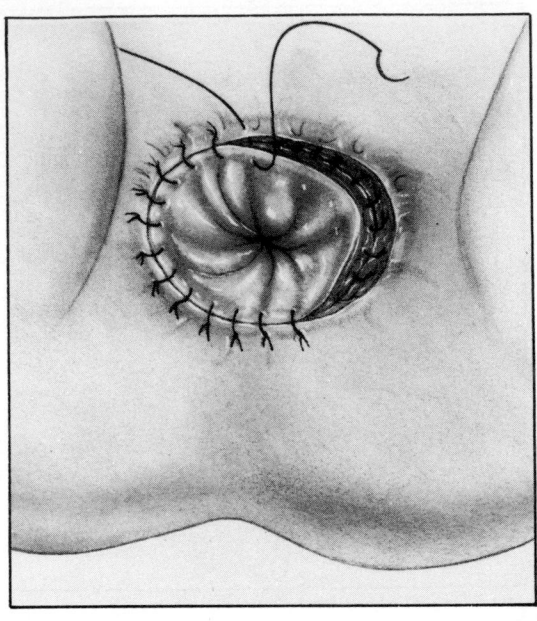

I   J

Figure 49–11. **I.** Posterior level of the anastomosis 0.5 cm from the anal verge. **J.** Completed anastomosis with second layer of interrupted full-thickness sutures.

or into the lumen of the rectosigmoid. In the former instance, the closed-off proximal bowel is grasped in the forceps and pulled through the incision in the rectum. Where no previous resection had been carried out, it is possible to intussuscept the proximal bowel to the level of the site selected for anastomosis without opening the lumen of the intestine. This manoeuvre avoids contamination of the peritoneal cavity and reduces the incidence of wound sepsis.

The site on the proximal colon previously selected for the level of the anastomosis is positively identified and the anterior row of seromuscular sutures between the everted rectum and the pulled-through colon are inserted. The sutures consist of interrupted 5/0 polyglycolic acid or Prolene. The rectum is now transected by extending the anterior incision to within 0.5 cm of the mucocutaneous line posteriorly. The posterior layer of seromuscular sutures are now inserted. The redundant pulled-through colon is excised, leaving a small cuff distal to the seromuscular row of sutures. A second layer of 5/0 sutures, including the full thickness of the

bowel wall, is inserted to complete the anastomosis.

When the anastomosis has been completed, the rectum is allowed to return into the pelvis. The abdominal incision may be closed by the assistant while the perineal operator is performing the anastomosis.

Duhamel's Procedure (Retrorectal Pull-Through) (Fig. 49–12). This procedure was devised in 1956 to avoid the tedious pelvic dissection required in the Swenson's procedure. The basic principle of the operation is to pull the ganglionic proximal colon down to the anus behind the aganglionic rectum and, by eliminating the common wall between the colon and rectum, to provide a new rectum consisting of aganglionic rectum anteriorly and ganglionic colon or ileum posteriorly.

The operative approach is via a left paramedian incision. The rectum is mobilised and divided at or just below the peritoneal reflection in the pouch of Douglas. The end of the proximal colon is closed off to prevent faecal contamina-

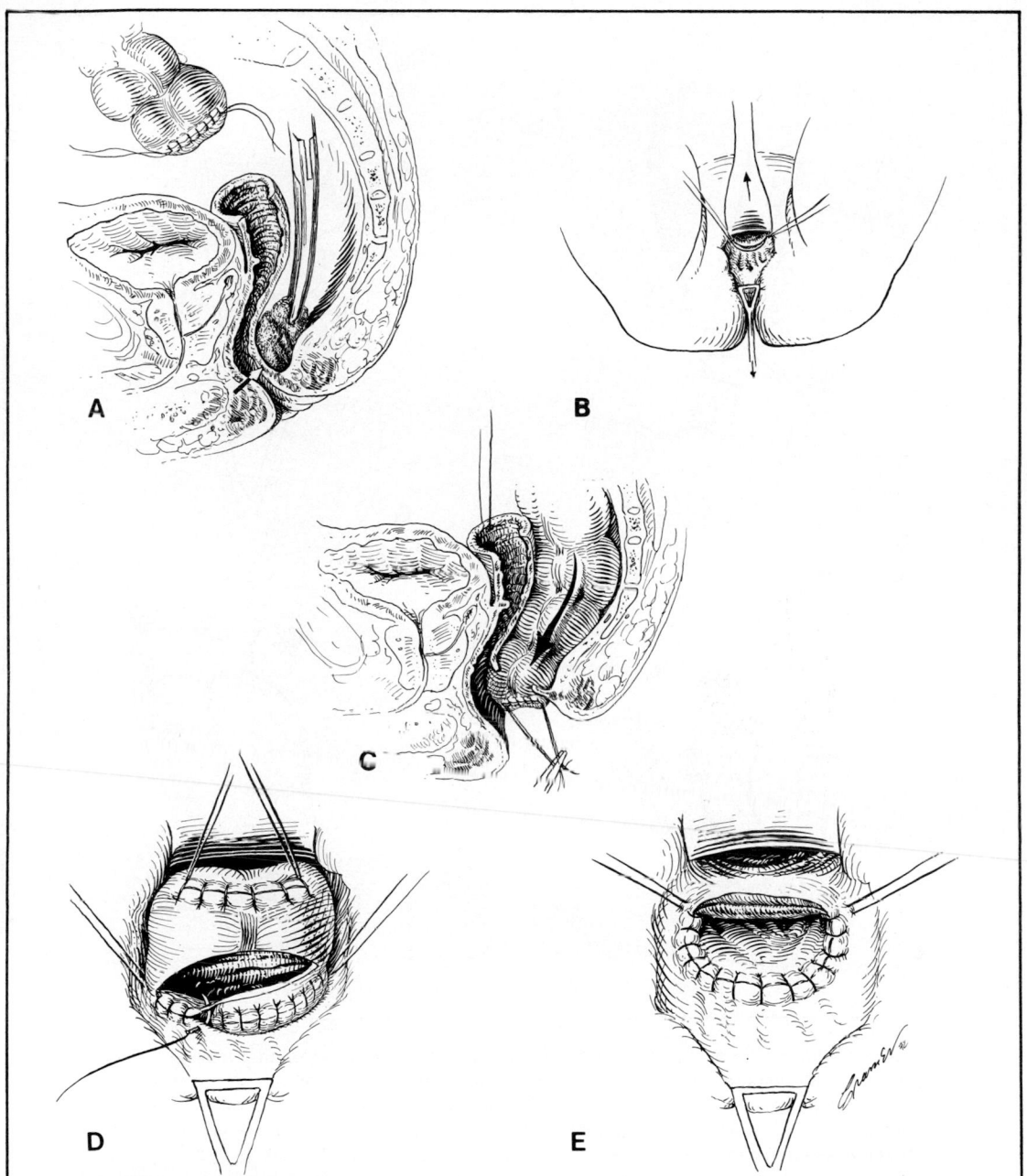

Figure 49–12. A through I. Technique of modified Duhamel operation: The aganglionic bowel above the rectum has been resected and the end of the colon closed. **A.** The open end of the rectum is seen. The retrorectal tunnel is developed by blunt dissection down to the level of the dentate line. **B.** A transverse incision is made in the posterior rectal wall at the level of the dentate line for a distance of 180 degrees. **C.** The presacral space has been entered from below and a clamp is used to draw the proximal colon down through the incision in the posterior rectal wall. **D.** A one-layer anastomosis between the inferior margin of the rectal incision and the apposing colonic wall is performed. The end of the colon beyond the suture line is then amputated. **E.** A posterior anastomosis is seen with an anterior wall consisting of approximated anterior wall of colon and posterior wall of rectum.

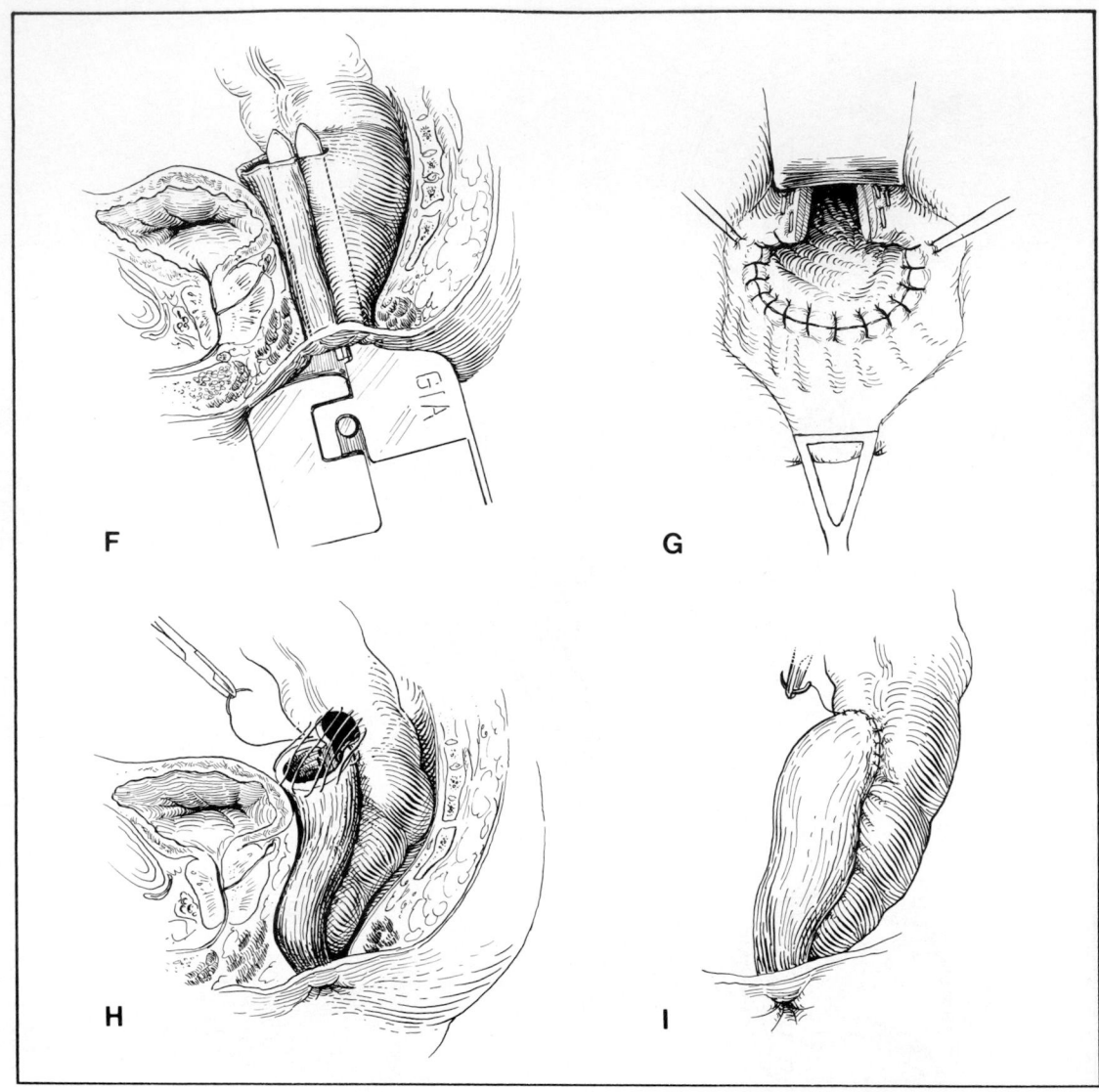

Figure 49–12. F. GIA anastomotic stapler has been inserted from below after making a small incision in the colon at the level of the upper end of the rectum. One arm of the stapler is in the rectum and the other in the colon. **G.** The spur between the rectum and colon has been stapled and divided, creating a long side-to-side anastomosis. **H.** The upper end of the rectum is anastomosed end-to-side to the colon. **I.** The anastomosis is completed.

tion. The plane of cleavage in the midline of the retrorectal space is entered and developed down to the pelvic floor. A pledget on a long curved forceps is inserted into the retrorectal tunnel and gently pushed caudally until the posterior wall of the anal canal is everted through the previously dilated anal canal.

A transverse incision is made through the posterior half of the anal canal at the level of

the dentate line. This incision extends through the full thickness of the rectal wall. A second long curved forceps is passed through this incision and the pledget on the forceps inserted into the retrorectal space from above is grasped. Using the pledget as a guide, the second forceps is drawn retrogradely through the retrorectal space into the peritoneal cavity. The proximal colon is grasped with the forceps and drawn into the retrorectal space until it emerges through the posterior rectal opening. Care must be exercised to ensure that the mesentery of the pulled-through colon is correctly oriented and lax enough to permit the proximal ganglionic colon to be brought down to the anus without compromising its blood supply. The end of the proximal bowel is opened and sutured circumferentially to the edges of the posterior rectal incision using a single layer of interrupted full-thickness 4/0 sutures (polyglycolic acid or silk).

Using the GIA stapling instrument, with one limb inserted into the rectum and the other into the lumen of the pulled-through colon, the common wall (i.e., the posterior wall of the rectum and the anterior wall of the proximal colon) is mechanically anastomosed and divided. It is important to ensure that the ends of the GIA stapler extend at least 1 cm beyond the open rectum in order to divide the common wall completely and to avoid the retention of a spur. If the division of the common wall has been incomplete, the remaining spur can be eliminated by using the stapling devices a second time or by dividing and suturing the remaining septum. The open end of the rectum is closed end-to-side to the colon with a single layer of 4/0 interrupted seromuscular sutures.

The abdominal incision is closed without the use of peritoneal drainage.

For long-segment Hirschsprung's disease, the Martin (1968) modification of the Duhamel operation has been advocated. This modification provides a much longer side-to-side anastomosis between the ganglionic ileum and the retained

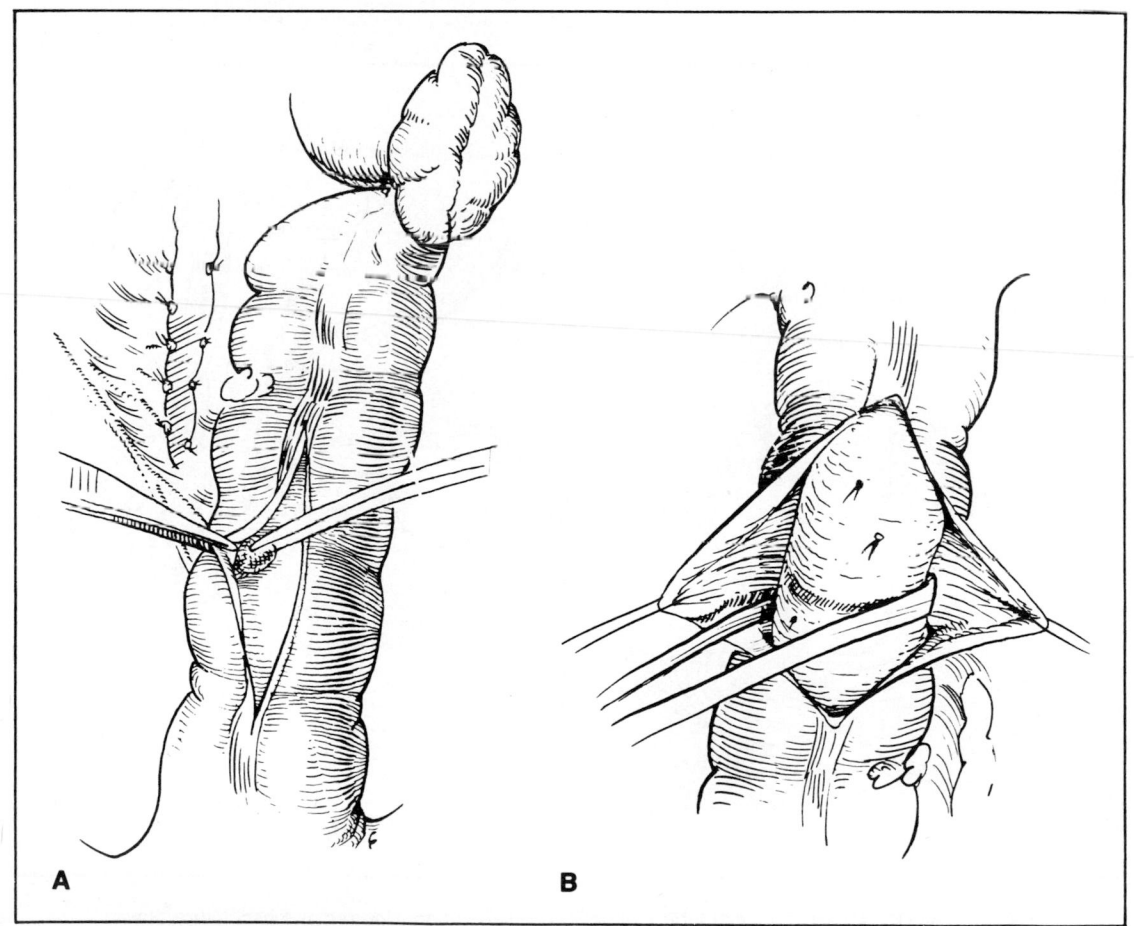

Figure 49–13. A through **E.** Principles of the Soave (endorectal) procedure: **A.** Incision through the muscular wall of the rectum or proximal colon. **B.** Development of the mucosal tube.

distal colon, which extends to the level of the splenic flexure. The long side-to-side anastomosis is constructed using the GIA stapling instrument inserted through a series of incisions in the sigmoid and descending colon. The aim of the procedure is to retain a significant length of aganglionic colon to provide an effective absorptive area while the ganglionate ileum acts as an effective peristaltic mechanism. In our experience, the excessively long Martin modification is unnecessary and an anastomosis 10 to 15 cm long is sufficient for nutritive purposes and to ensure a reasonably well-formed stool.

Soave's Procedure (Extramucosal Endorectal Pull-Through) (Fig. 49–13). The technique of extramucosal dissection of the rectosigmoid was originally described by Rehbein (1959) for use in high-level anorectal malformations. Its application for the treatment of Hirschsprung's disease was later described by Soave (1966).

The initial separation of the seromuscular from the mucosal layer is facilitated by injecting a 0.5 percent procaine hydrochloride or 1:400,000 adrenaline in saline solution between the layers. The infiltration should be performed in the rectal wall, 4 to 5 cm above the pelvic peritoneal reflection. A long longitudinal incision is made through a taenia in this area. The mobilised mucosal tube is freed circumferentially from the outer muscular layers and the muscular tube transected. With traction applied to the distal edges of the muscular tube, the mobilisation of the mucosal tube is carried distally to within 2 to 3 cm of the dentate line by a combination of sharp and blunt dissection.

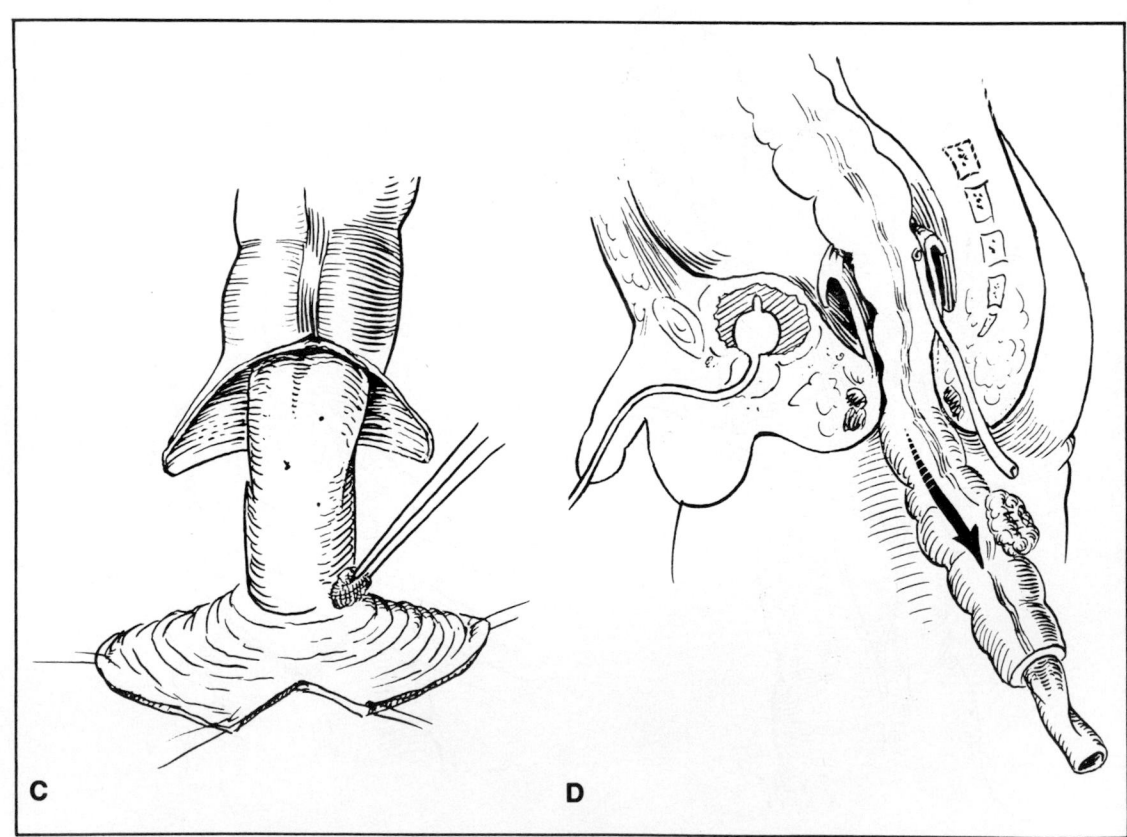

Figure 49–13. C. The mucosal tube is mobilised off the underlying rectal musculature down to the level of the dentate line. **D.** The mucosal tube has been transected at the level of the dentate line and the colon is pulled through the seromuscular cuff of the rectum until the determined site of anastomosis has been reached.

anastomosis to be performed with a two-layer technique, consisting of an inner seromuscular to rectal muscular cuff and an outer full-thickness colon to anal mucosa anastomosis using interrupted 4/0 polyglycolic acid sutures. Before closing the abdominal incision, the muscular cuff of the rectum is loosely sutured to the seromuscular layer of the pulled-through colon. The rectal cuff should be drained to prevent the formation of a haematoma which is liable to become infected.

Rehbein's Procedure (Deep Anterior Resection). This procedure is carried out at 3 to 4 months of age without the prior routine fashioning of a colostomy. Before commencing the abdominal approach the anus is vigorously dilated with a spreading instrument or, in older children, digitally. An indwelling urinary catheter is used to drain the bladder. Traction sutures are inserted into the peritoneum on either side of the rectum. The operative field in the small pelvis is made more accessible by drawing the traction sutures cranially.

The superior haemorrhoidal vessels are ligated and divided and the peritoneal reflection around the rectum is divided. The perirectal tissues are carefully separated until the external longitudinal muscle layer is exposed. Further dissection on this layer is carried progressively distally to the level of the levator ani muscle, i.e., 2 to 3 cm from the peritoneal reflection in infants and 4 to 5 cm in older children. The rectum is transected at this level and the lumen cleaned with a povidone–iodine solution.

The proximal colon is now mobilised and the dilated hypertrophied segment resected. An end-to-end anastomosis is performed using a single layer of interrupted 4/0 or 5/0 polyglycolic acid sutures. When the large bowel is greatly dilated, a tapering procedure is carried out in the descending colon to create a lumen approximately equivalent to that of the transected rectum. This is used for the colorectal anastomosis.

Postoperatively, it is important to carry out regular rectal bougienage to prevent anastomotic stenosis. This may involve digital dilatations in the infant, while Hegar's dilators are used in the older child.

An outline of the advantages and disadvantages of the four techniques, together with the incidence of postoperative complications associated with the procedures, are shown in Table 49–1.

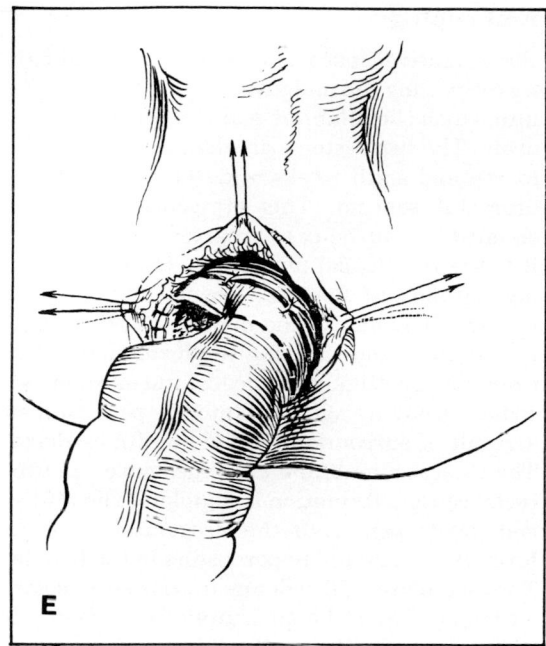

Figure 49–13. E. Resection of the aganglionic bowel and primary anastomosis between the full thickness of the colon and the mucosal cuff at the level of the dentate line.

The site of the anastomosis on the proximal colon is identified for the presence of ganglion cells and the colon is mobilised to obtain sufficient length for the pull-through to be performed without tension.

Attention is now directed to the anus which is dilated and, with the aid of retractors or traction sutures, the dentate line is brought into the operative field. The procaine or adrenaline solution is instilled into the wall just above the dentate line and an incision 1 cm proximal to the line is made. The submucosal plane is carefully developed until it joins with the mucosal tube mobilised from above. At this point the mucosal tube is free to be pulled through the muscular cuff to the level in the proximal colon selected for the anastomosis.

In Soave's original procedure the seromuscular coat of the pulled-through colon is sutured to the everted rectal mucous membrane. A rectal tube is inserted into the lumen of the colon and the excess colon excised, leaving the everted bowel to protrude through the anus for 10 days when a delayed anastomosis is performed. Boley's (1964) modification consists of a primary

ANORECTAL ANOMALIES

Although not strictly within the purview of this text on abdominal surgery, a short section on anorectal anomalies, one of the most common causes of neonatal intestinal obstruction, should prove valuable to the general surgeon confronted with a newborn infant with an "imperforate anus." The crucial factor in the management of such an infant is the distinction between the high or supralevator anomalies and the low or translevator anomalies. The former requires a temporary colostomy followed by the rerouting of the rectum to a newly fashioned anal orifice, while a local perineal procedure will correct the latter anomaly.

Historical Background

Although the treatment of anorectal anomalies has been punctuated by numerous events through many centuries, the operation of proctoplasty, devised by Amussat in 1835, marked the transition from earlier efforts at blunt puncture of the blind rectum with trocar or bistoury to modern attempts to preserve function of the anorectal sphincter mechanism. In 1856, Chassaignac proposed the construction of a preliminary iliac colostomy, with a view to later passing a probe into the terminal rectum to act as a guide for the perineal procedure. In 1880, McLeod suggested a combined abdominal exploration with perineal dissection. A one-stage abdominoperineal procedure in the neonatal period was proposed by Rhoads et al in 1948 in order to avoid the necessity for a preliminary colostomy.

One of the major advances in determining the level of the blind rectal pouch was the demonstration by Wangensteen and Rice in 1930 that, by holding the infant's head down, gas in the distal intestine would rise to outline the rectal pouch. A plain x-ray with the infant in this inverted position would demonstrate the terminal gas shadow, and by orientating this to certain bony landmarks, the type of anomaly could be diagnosed.

The importance of the puborectalis muscle in maintaining continence and its preservation and utilisation during abdominoperineal pullthrough procedures was first recognised by Stephens in 1953. This observation formed the basis of modern techniques in the treatment of high anorectal anomalies.

Embryology

The primitive cloaca consists of a posterior cavity containing the midgut and an anterior cavity into which the allantois and mesonephric ducts drain. The two systems are divided between the fourth and sixth weeks of development by the urorectal septum. This crescentic spur was claimed by Tourneux to progress caudally until it meets the cloacal membrane. Others, including Rathke and Rettener, consider the septum to form by fusion in the midline of two lateral mesodermal folds. During the formation of the urorectal septum, the cloacal membrane becomes deeply invaginated into the perineum as a result of surrounding build-up of mesoderm. The cloacal membrane atrophies once the urorectal septum formation is complete. The Müllerian ducts penetrate the urogenital sinus to form the uterus and upper vagina in the female. The final phase of development consists of posterior migration of the anus away from the developing urogenital tract by an ingrowth of mesoderm derived from the genital folds.

Failure of complete development of urorectal septum results in the high or supralevator anomalies, while low or translevator anomalies arise from defects in the development of the proctodeum and genital folds.

Classification of Anorectal Anomalies (Fig. 49–14)

In 1970 an international classification of anorectal anomalies was agreed by an ad hoc committee of internationally recognised experts in the field. This classification was devised in an attempt to promote an understanding and to unify reporting into a complex array of anorectal deformities. The reader is referred to this classification for further information regarding the 27 different types of anomalies which have been listed. Basically, the classification is as follows:

I. *MALE*
  A. Low (translevator)
    1. At normal anal site
      a. Anal stenosis
      b. Covered anus—complete
    2. At perineal site
      a. Anocutaneous fistula (covered anus—incomplete)
      b. Anterior perineal anus
  B. Intermediate
    1. Anal agenesis

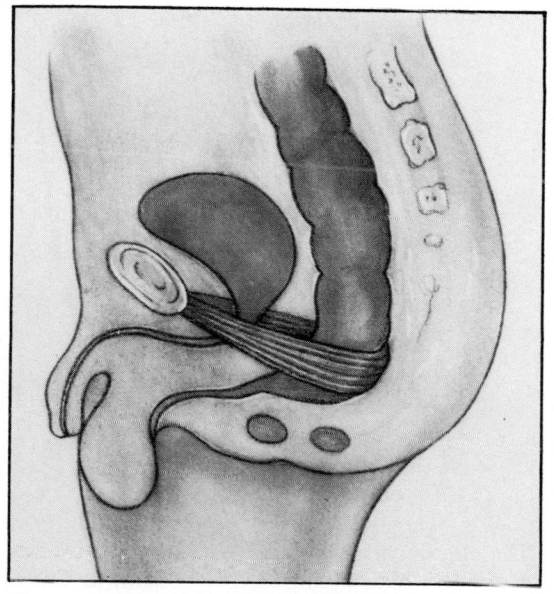
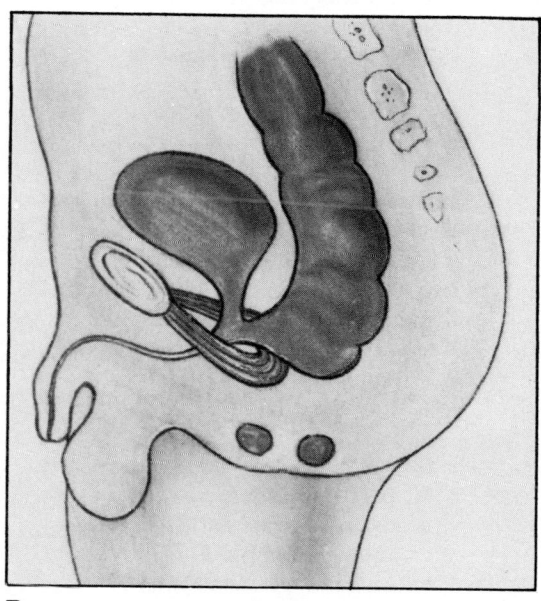

A

B

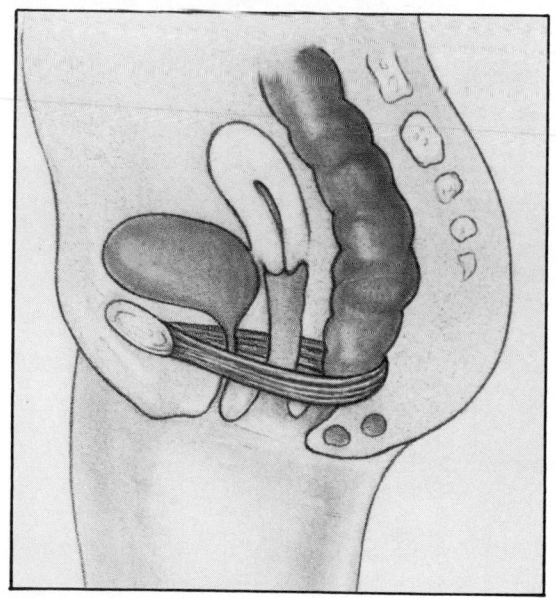
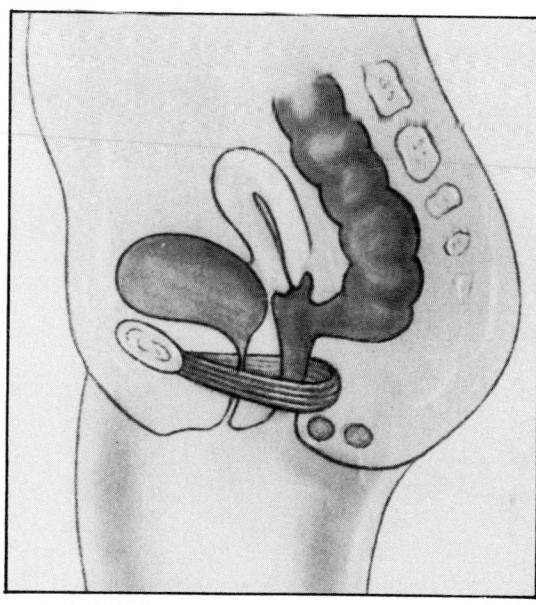

C

D

Figure 49–14. Common types of anorectal anomalies: **A.** Low lesion in the male—covered anus with or without anocutaneous fistula. **B.** High lesion in the male—anorectal agenesis with rectourethral fistula. **C.** Low lesion in the female—ectopic anus with anovulvar or anovestibular fistula. **D.** High lesion in the female—anorectal agenesis with rectovaginal fistula.

a. Without fistula
b. With fistula, rectobulbar
C. High (supralevator)
  1. Anorectal agenesis
  a. Without fistula
  b. With fistula
    i. Rectourethral
    ii. Rectovesical
  2. Rectal atresia
D. Miscellaneous
  1. Imperforate anal membrane
  2. Cloacal exstrophy
  3. Others
II. *FEMALE*
  A. Low (translevator)
    1. At normal anal site
    a. Anal stenous
    b. Covered anus—complete
    2. At perineal site
    a. Anocutaneous fistula (covered anus—incomplete)
    b. Anterior perineal anus

3. At vulvar site
  a. Anovulvar fistula
  b. Anovestibular fistula
  c. Vestibular anus
B. Intermediate
  1. Anal agenesis
  a. Without fistula
  b. With fistula
    i. Rectovestibular
    ii. Rectovaginal—low
C. High (supralevator)
  1. Anorectal agenesis
  a. Without fistula
  b. With fistula
    i. Rectovaginal—high
    ii. Rectocloacal
    iii. Rectovesical
  2. Rectal atresia
D. Miscellaneous (as in males)

The classification is complex and takes into account the relationship of the rectum and anus

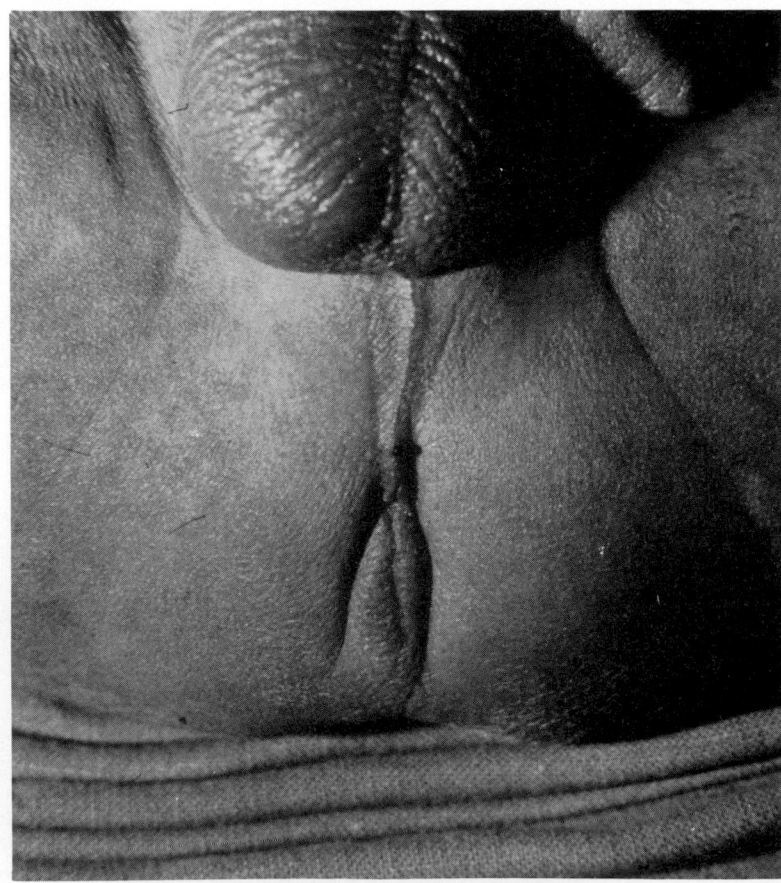

Figure 49–15. Male infant with a low anorectal anomaly. The presence of meconium on the perineum determines that the lesion is a low variety, that is, covered anus with anocutaneous fistula.

to the levator ani musculature. The high lesions terminate above the levator ani and require complex surgery for correction, while the low lesions terminate below the levator and can be repaired by local perineal procedures.

Statistically, there are a few lesions that predominate in the area of anorectal anomalies. In the male, these comprise the covered anus (low anomaly) and rectal agenesis with rectourethral fistula (high anomaly). The equivalent lesions in the female are the ectopic anus (perineal, vestibular or vulvar orifice) and the rectal agenesis with rectovaginal (high) or rectocloacal fistula.

Diagnosis

A careful clinical examination will elucidate the diagnosis in the vast majority of cases (Figs. 49–15 through 49–17). The scheme of investigation for the male and female infant is as fol-

lows. Meticulous examination of the perineum forms the keystone of the clinical diagnosis (Table 49–2).

Radiologic Studies

Invertogram (Figs. 49–18 and 49–19). The upside down x-ray originally described by Wagensteen and Rice in 1930 is used to determine the distance between the blind rectal pouch and a marker placed on the anal dimple. Gas normally reaches the distal rectum 18 hours after birth, so that there is little point in taking this x-ray before the infant is 24 hours of age. The preferred method of obtaining a satisfactory invertogram is as follows. A smear of barium paste is placed on the anal dimple to outline the natal cleft. The infant is held upside down for 3 to 5 minutes to allow meconium in the distal pouch to be displaced by gas present in the lumen of the bowel. A true lateral x-ray of the pelvis is taken with the x-ray beam centred on the

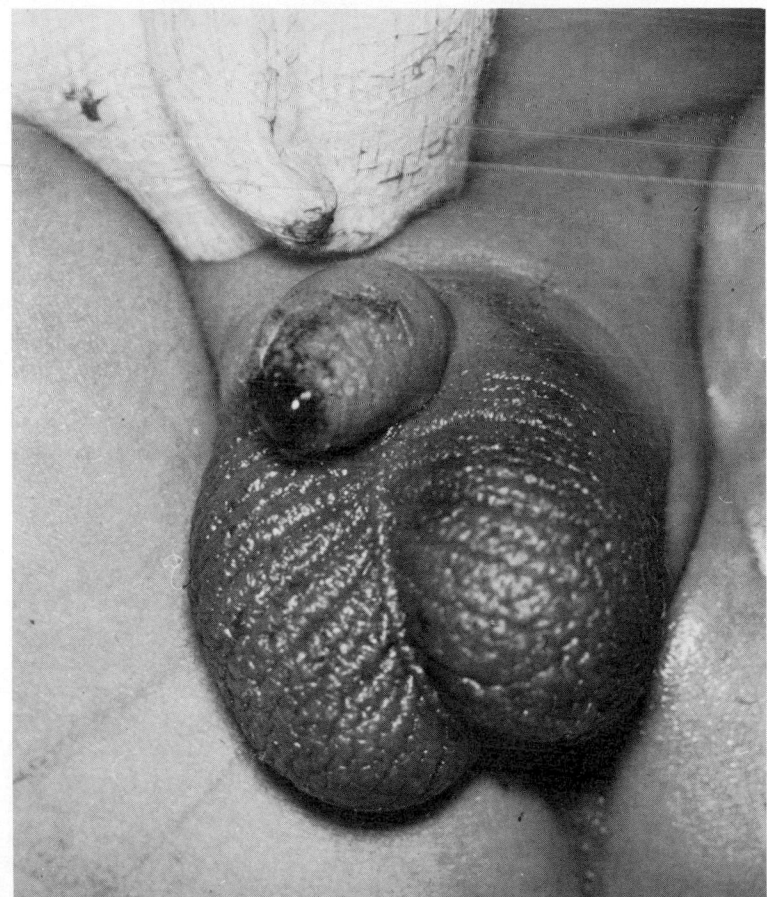

Figure 49–16. Male infant with an imperforate anus. The presence of meconium in the urine signifies a high lesion with either rectourethral or rectovesical fistula.

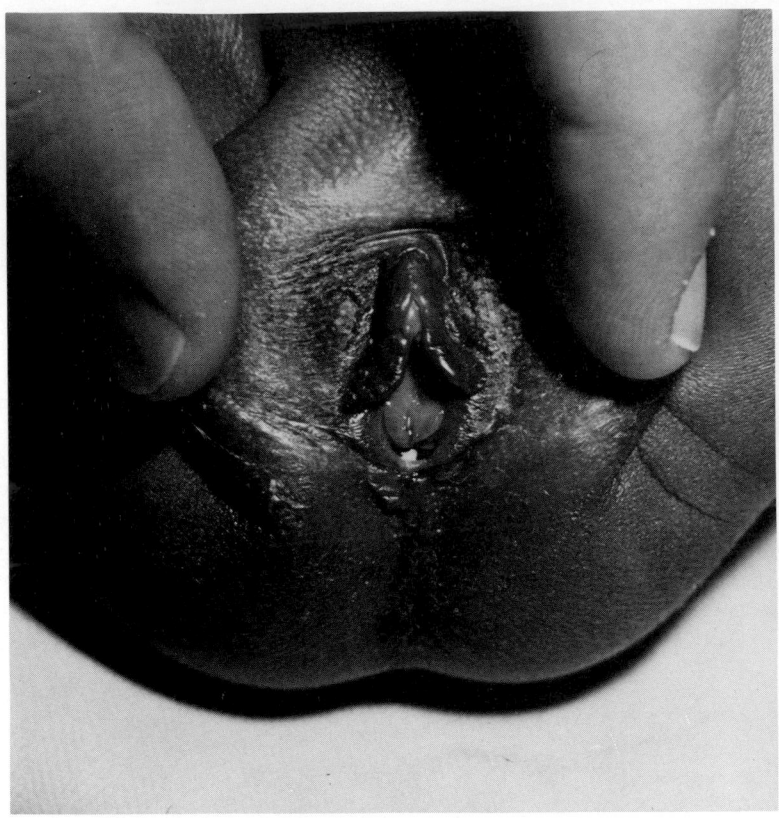

Figure 49–17. Female infant with an ectopic anus and anovulvar fistula, a low lesion.

greater trochanter of the femur and with the hips of the infant only slightly flexed. It is generally recognised that the distance between the air shadow in the rectal pouch and the anal dimple can be very misleading in assessing the level of the lesion and that it is far more reliable to relate the air shadow to bony points on the pelvis that indicate the level of the puborectalis muscle. The puborectalis lies just below a line drawn from the middle of the symphysis pubis to the sacrococcygeal junction. Cremin et al (1973) prefer to relate the gas shadow to the ischium. The level of the levator muscle is at the junction of the body and tail of the comma-shaped ischial shadow. A terminal gas shadow ending above the level of the levator muscle signifies a high lesion, while in low lesions the gas shadow projects well beyond bony landmarks and extends almost to the anal dimple.

Cystourethrography. The demonstration of a rectourinary fistula on cystourethrography in male infants may be very useful when the level of the lesion is in doubt (Fig. 49–20).

Contrast Radiography. Murugasu in 1970 advocated the injection of water-soluble contrast material into the distal pouch via a needle inserted into the perineum and advanced under fluoroscopic control until the blind pouch is punctured and meconium aspirated.

Ultrasonography. The distance between the anal dimple and blind pouch can be accurately determined by ultrasound scan but, as previously stated, this measurement is unreliable in assessing the level of the lesion.

It is our policy to perform a colostomy for all lesions that are obviously not low on careful clinical examination and on the inverted lateral radiograph. The precise anatomy of the anomaly can then be determined by distal loop contrast studies. This policy may result in a small number of unnecessary colostomies being carried out for low lesions but is preferable to blind surgical exploration of the perineum, which may result in irreversible damage to the levator ani muscle.

TABLE 49–2. DIAGNOSTIC APPROACH TO ANORECTAL ANOMALY

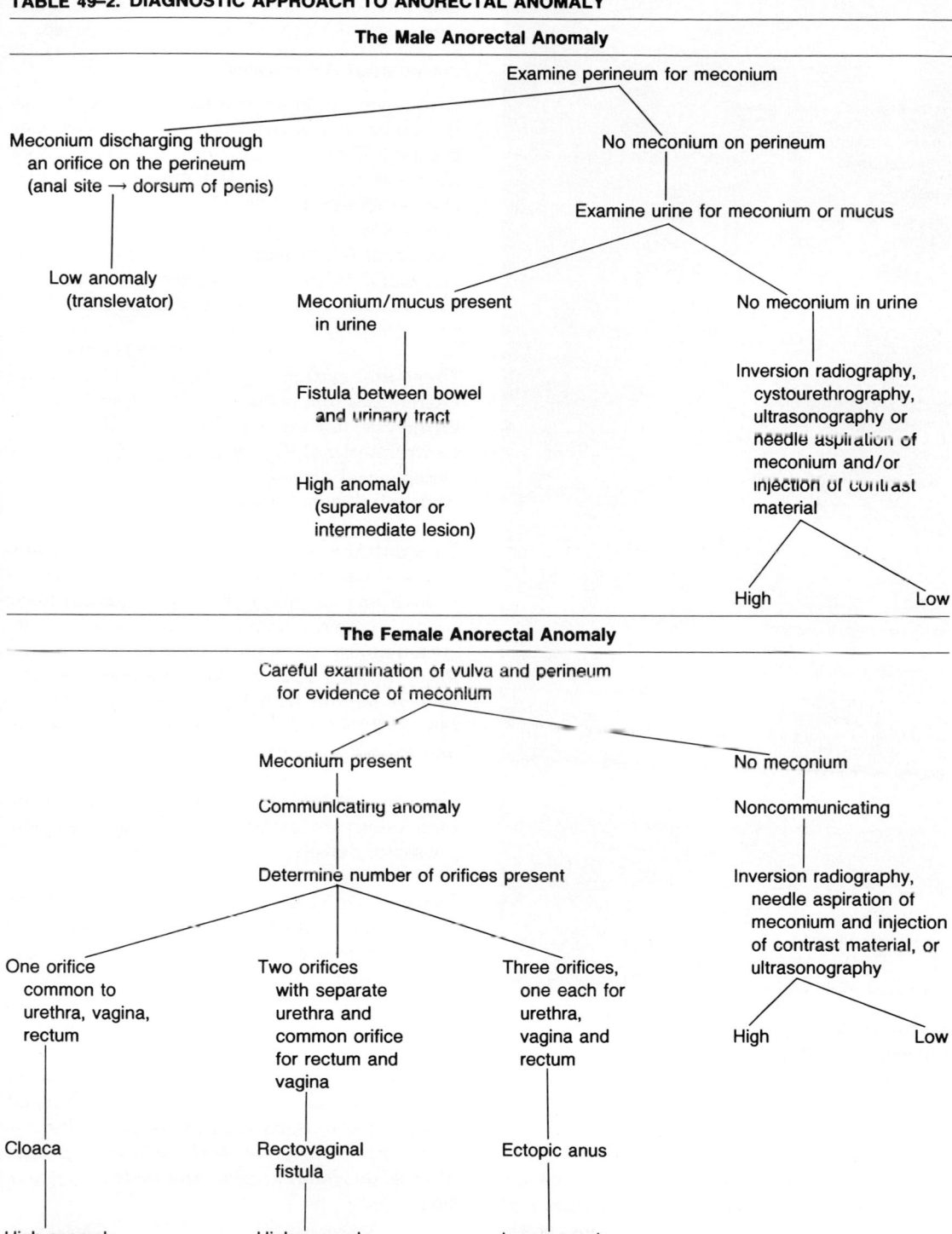

The Male Anorectal Anomaly

Examine perineum for meconium

Meconium discharging through an orifice on the perineum (anal site → dorsum of penis)

No meconium on perineum

Low anomaly (translevator)

Examine urine for meconium or mucus

Meconium/mucus present in urine

No meconium in urine

Fistula between bowel and urinary tract

Inversion radiography, cystourethrography, ultrasonography or needle aspiration of meconium and/or injection of contrast material

High anomaly (supralevator or intermediate lesion)

High   Low

The Female Anorectal Anomaly

Careful examination of vulva and perineum for evidence of meconium

Meconium present

No meconium

Communicating anomaly

Noncommunicating

Determine number of orifices present

Inversion radiography, needle aspiration of meconium and injection of contrast material, or ultrasonography

One orifice common to urethra, vagina, rectum

Two orifices with separate urethra and common orifice for rectum and vagina

Three orifices, one each for urethra, vagina and rectum

High   Low

Cloaca

Rectovaginal fistula

Ectopic anus

High anomaly (supralevator)

High anomaly (supralevator)

Low anomaly (translevator)

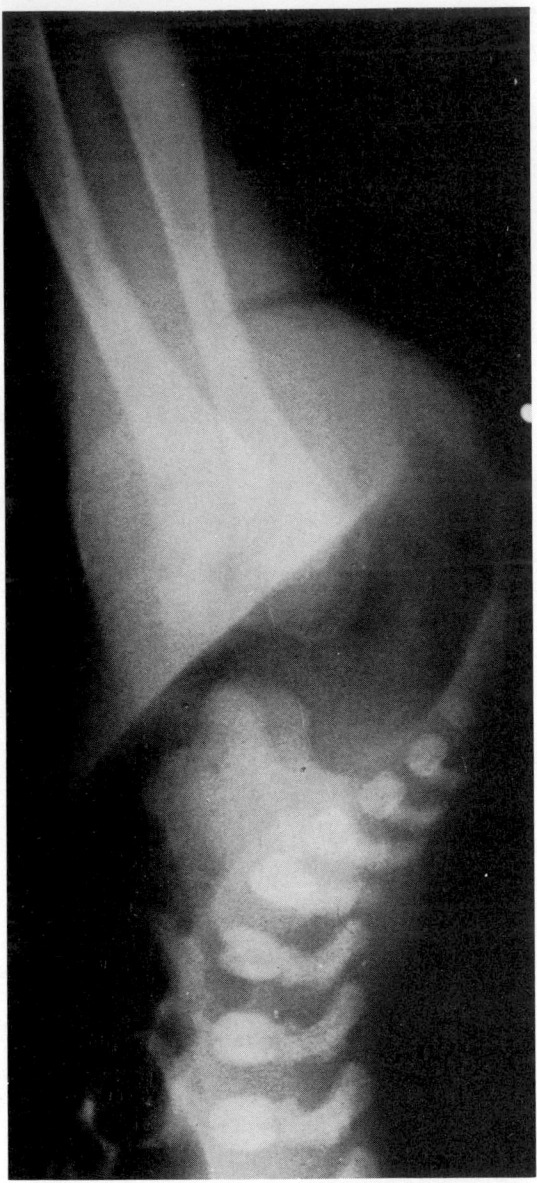

Figure 49–18. Inverted lateral radiograph showing air in the rectum well below the pelvic diaphragm and ending just below the skin of the perineum. A low lesion.

Additional Investigations. The high association of urologic anomalies with anorectal malformations demands full investigation of the urinary system by ultrasonography, micturating cystourethrography, and, in selected cases, excretory urography. X-rays of the sacral vertebra should always be taken. An absence or

deformity of three or more sacral vertebra carries a poor outlook for eventual continence.

Associated Anomalies

A wide variety of associated congenital anomalies occur with anorectal anomalies. The combination of anomalies forms the VATER association—V = vertebral, A = anorectal, T = tracheooesophageal, E = (o)esophageal, and R = radial and renal. Hasse in 1976 analysed the additional malformations among 1420 patients and found an overall incidence of 41.6 percent. The various systems were affected as follows:

	Percent
Urogenital system	19.7
Extremities and spine	13.1
Cardiovascular system	7.9
Gastrointestinal (GI) system	6.0
Oesophageal atresia	5.6
Abdominal wall defects	1.9

Urogenital System. Anomalies consist of unilateral renal agenesis, renal dysplasia, hydronephrosis and horseshoe kidneys. Vesicoureteric reflux, ectopic ureters and vesicoureteric obstruction are the main anomalies affecting the lower urinary system. Approximately 50 percent of infants with high lesions and 20 percent with low lesions have associated urogenital anomalies.

Cardiovascular Anomalies. The most common lesions are tetralogy of Fallot and ventricular septal defects.

Skeletal Defects. The significance of absence or deformity of the sacral vertebrae has already been discussed under the section on radiologic investigation. Other vertebral defects include missing vertebra and hemivertebrae, which may result in subsequent scoliosis in later life.

GI System. Oesophageal atresia, with or without tracheooesophageal fistula, occurs in about 5 percent of infants with anorectal malformations. Other anomalies include Hirschsprung's disease, duodenal atresia, and midgut malrotation.

Treatment

Normal Continence. "A properly functioning anus is an unappreciated gift of the greatest

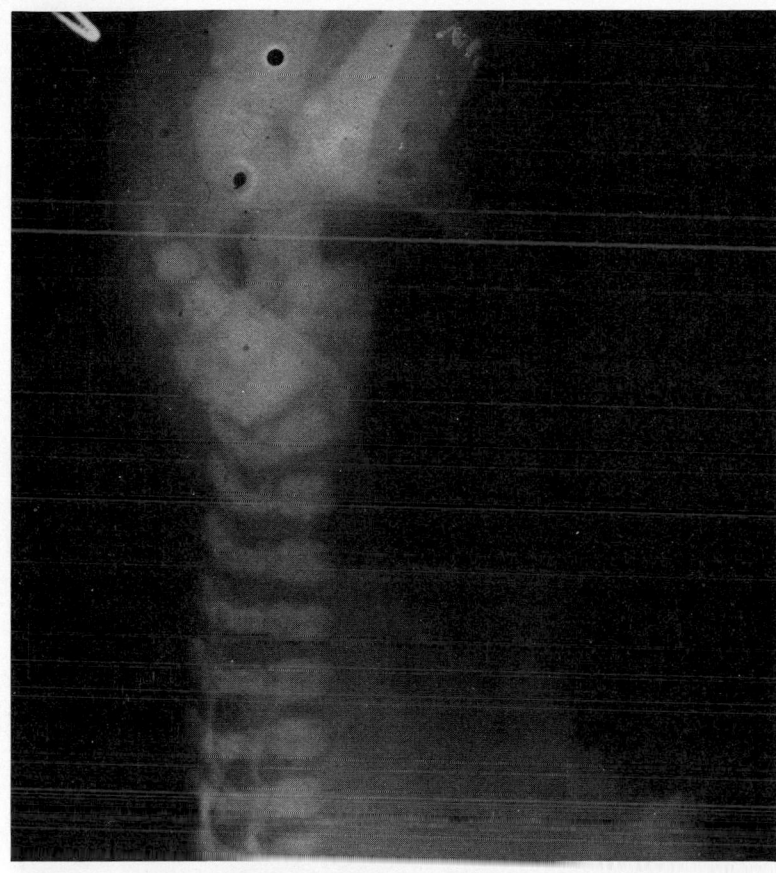

Figure 49–19. Inverted lateral radiograph in a high anorectal anomaly. The gas shadow in terminal rectum ends above the puborectalis line.

price." These words were written in 1959 by Willis Potts who, at the time, commented that atresia of the rectum was more poorly handled than any other congenital anomaly of the newborn.

The main concern in treating anorectal malformations is to preserve as far as possible normal control. In order to achieve this goal it is necessary to understand the mechanism by which normal control is maintained. Four basic mechanisms are involved:

1. Internal sphincter. This is a continuation and thickening of the inner circular layer of the bowel wall. This smooth muscle is capable of tonicity and is probably the most important factor in anorectal resistance.
2. Levator ani muscle and particularly the puborectalis component. Fibres from the puborectalis interlace with the deepest fibres of the internal sphincter. In high anorectal malformations, this is the only muscle available for control.

3. Intact nervous arc, consisting of sensory receptors in the anal canal and pelvic musculature, the pelvic sympathetic and parasympathetic plexuses and an intact central nervous system.
4. Perineal cutaneous sensation.

On the basis of the clinical and radiologic investigations the distinction between low (translevator) and high (supralevator and intermediate) lesions will have been established. If there is any doubt after full investigations performed at the appropriate time, the lesion should preferably be initially managed as a high lesion. Subsequent loopogram and/or micturating cystourethrography will define the precise anatomy of the lesion. The aim of treatment is to create an orifice for the intestine in an appropriate position in the perineum while attempting to achieve the maximum possible functional continence. For low lesions a local perineal procedure will satisfy the above criteria, while high lesions require an initial colos-

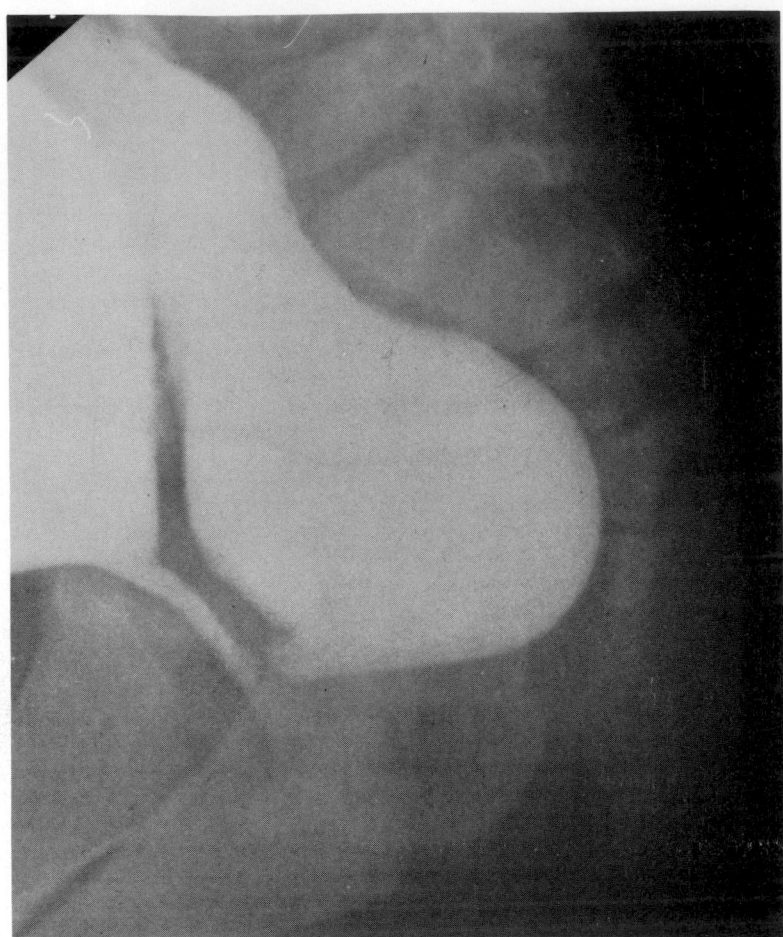

Figure 49–20. Contrast study in a male infant with an anorectal anomaly. Simultaneous injection of contrast into the bladder and into the distal limb of the colostomy shows the blind-ending rectal pouch and the fistulous connection with the urethra.

tomy followed by an appropriate pull-through procedure that utilises all the remaining structures involved in maintaining continence. These include the levator ani muscle and in particular the puborectalis sling, the pelvic neural pathways, and the perineal skin for sensory purposes.

Low Lesions

Male. A perineal anoplasty is performed in male newborn infants when a definitive diagnosis of a covered anus has been made. The procedure should ideally be carried out under general endotracheal anaesthesia, with the infant supported in the lithotomy position. The fistula between the bowel and perineum is isolated and probed. The fistulous opening is widened into the anal canal by means of a V–Y plasty procedure (Fig. 49–21). The V-incision is based posteriorly while the Y-incision extends superiorly

in the posterior wall of the anal canal. The procedure is completed by loosely suturing the flap of skin into the posterior wall of the anal canal with 4/0 or 5/0 polyglycolic acid or chromic catgut sutures. Any anterior extension of the fistulous tract should be laid open widely. Severe anal stenosis or a completely covered anus is managed on a similar basis with the fashioning of an anal orifice by a cruciate incision centred over the anal dimple. The skin flaps are secured up in the anal canal with loosely approximating sutures.

Female. Minor degrees of anterior displacement of the anus may require no formal treatment except for possible dilatation. Anovestibular fistula may be treated either by a cutback (Fig. 49–22), popularised by Browne (1951) and Nixon (1964), or by a V–Y anoplasty similar to the procedure described above for male infants.

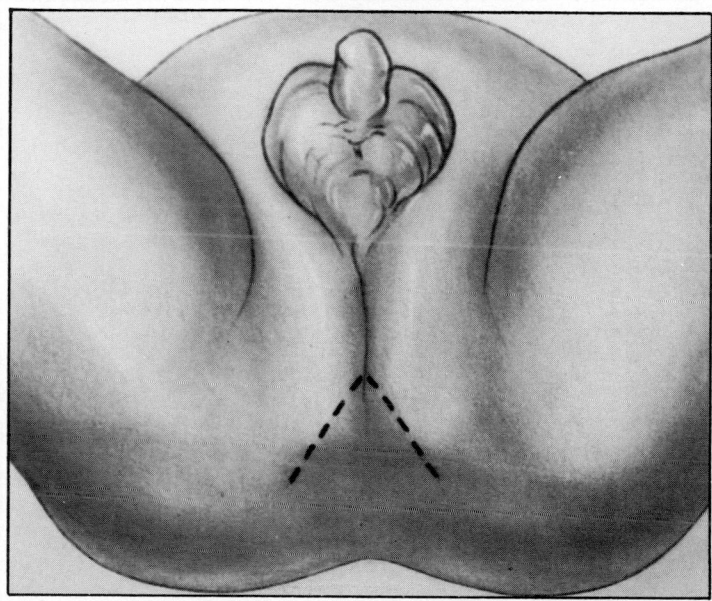

A

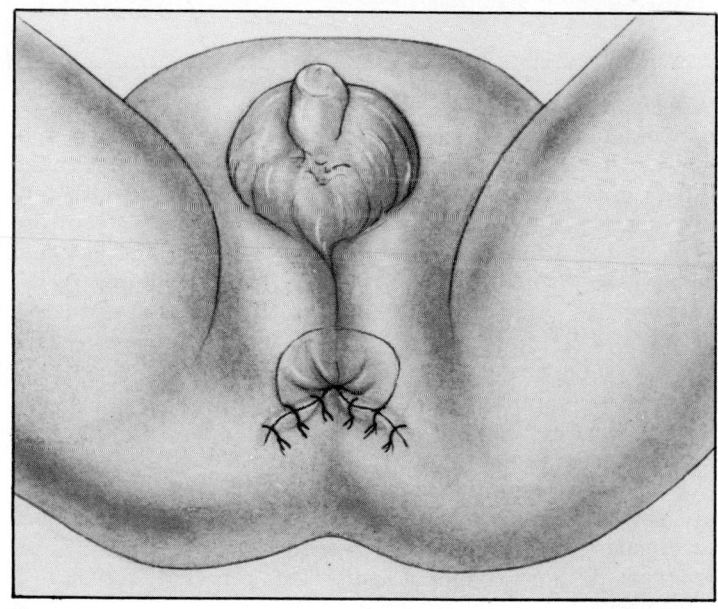

Figure 49–21. A and **B.** Technical details of the V–Y plasty for correction of a covered anus with an anocutaneous fistula in a male infant.

B

The advantage of the V–Y plasty is that the muscle fibres of the external sphincter are visualised and deliberately pushed backward while the V-incision extends through the mucosa of the anal canal only. The skin flap is sutured into the defect in the anal wall. It is claimed that the skin-lined anal canal avoids the necessity for regular postoperative dilatations.

The cutback procedure is simply performed by placing one blade of a pair of scissors into the fistulous tract and passing it backward as far as possible under the skin without allowing the blade to migrate deeply, where it may endanger the puborectalis muscle sling. The other blade of the scissors lies outside on the perineum in the midline. The intervening skin is divided in the midline by closing the blades of the scis-

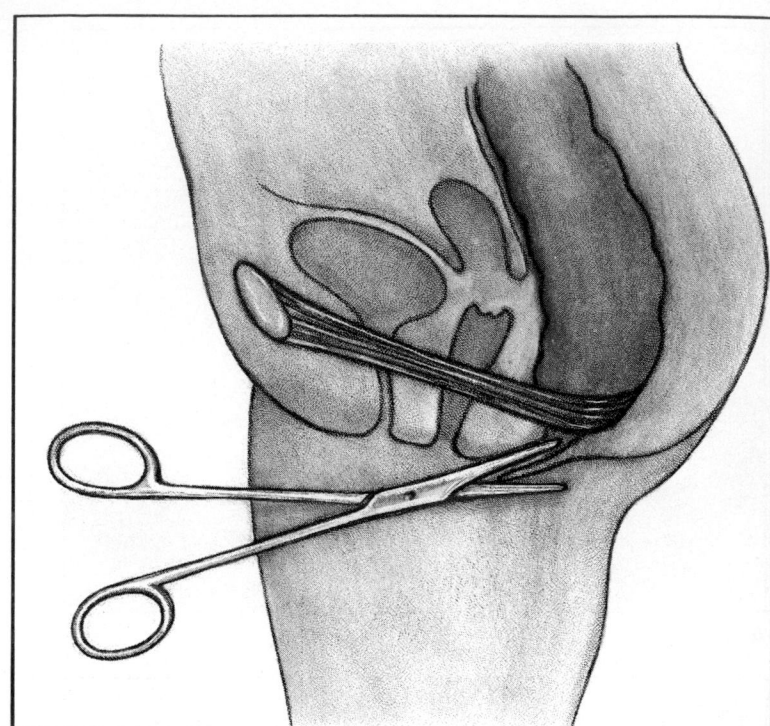

Figure 49–22. Diagrammatic representation of the cutback procedure for an anovulvar or anovestibular fistula.

sors. A few sutures are inserted to approximate the perineal skin and the anal mucosa and to achieve haemostasis. following the cutback procedure, the anal orifice should readily accept a size 10–12 Hegar's dilator.

In the case of anovestibular fistula where the fistulous tract runs upward parallel with the posterior wall of the vagina, a short cutback procedure only should be performed. This is followed by regular postoperative dilatations and it may be necessary to carry out a subsequent anal transposition for hygienic purposes at around the age of 4 years.

The perineal anoplasty is carried out with the child in the lithotomy position. A cruciate incision is made over the site of the external sphincter previously determined with the nerve stimulator. The skin flaps are elevated and the external sphincter again identified by means of the nerve stimulator. The anovestibular fistula is circumscribed with sharp dissection. Using multiple stay-sutures on the ectopic orifice, the bowel wall is dissected proximally, freeing it anteriorly from the posterior vaginal wall and laterally and posteriorly from the levator muscles. When 3 to 4 cm of bowel has been mobilised, the external sphincter zone is entered in its centre and a tunnel created to the site of

dissection of the anovestibular fistula. The mobilised bowel is then pulled through the tunnel, rerouted through the centre of the external sphincter zone, and seromuscular sutures are inserted to anchor the bowel to the external sphincter musculature. The procedure is terminated by suturing into the bowel the cruciate skin flaps fashioned at the anal dimple site. This results in the formation of a skin-lined neo-anal canal.

AFTERCARE OF LOW ANOMALIES. It is absolutely essential to carry out regular anal dilatations, not only until healing of the perineal procedure has occurred but until the entire area has become supple again. This process takes up to 3 months to occur. Strict adherence to this rigid programme will result in the attainment of normal continence in 90 to 95 percent of cases. Failure to carry out regular dilatations may allow the newly fashioned orifice to become stenosed, resulting in chronic faecal retention and secondary megacolon, which is extremely refractory to treatment.

High Lesions

Once the diagnosis of a supralevator or intermediate lesion has been established, immediate colostomy should be fashioned and definitive procedure delayed until the infant is 9 to 12 months of age. The author's preference is for a right transverse skin-bridge colostomy according to the method described in the section on Hirschsprung's disease. The advantage of the right transverse colostomy is that it leaves the entire left colon free and uncontaminated for the definitive pull-through procedure. A theoretic disadvantage of a transverse colostomy is the possible increased incidence of hyperchloraemic acidosis. It may be safely stated that this complication is virtually unknown in the absence of a significant renal abnormality and the role of the length of defunctioned colon may be incidental.

Definitive Pull-Through Procedure. The requirements for the ideal procedure are:

1. The rerouted intestine should lie within the entire puborectalis sling.
2. The puborectalis sling should remain undamaged by the procedure.
3. There should be minimal interference with the nerve supply to the bladder and bowel.
4. The anal orifice should be of adequate size and lined by perineal skin capable of providing sensory function.
5. Any fistulous connection should be securely divided close to the organ of attachment.

The author's preference is for the sacroabdominoperineal endorectal pull-through procedure as variously described by Stephens (1971), Kieswetter (1967), and Rehbein (1959) (Fig. 49–23). The sacroperineal procedure is performed solely for the purpose of identifying and dilating the puborectalis muscle sling. The endorectal abdominal dissection satisfies the requirement for minimal interference with the nerve supply to the pelvic viscera and allows safe and secure closure of the fistulous connection with the genitourinary system.

Preoperative preparation consists of mechanical clearance of the distal colon for a period of 3 days prior to surgery. Prophylactic antibiotic chemotherapy consists of metronidazole (7.5 mg/kg body weight) instilled into the colon after each washout and parenteral gentamicin (2 mg/kg) with the premedication and once again 6 hours postoperatively.

The operative procedure is performed under general endotracheal anaesthesia. An indwelling urethral catheter is inserted into the bladder, or alternatively a gum-elastic bougie may be used to aid with the identification of the urethra during the mobilisation of the puborectalis muscle and again when the rectourinary fistula is divided.

Sacroperineal Procedure. The infant is placed in the prone position with the pelvis elevated by sandbags or rolled-up sheets. The external sphincter zone is located by means of a nerve stimulator and a cruciate incision made over this area. The full-thickness skin flaps are undermined to reveal the muscle fibres of the external sphincter. A vertical incision, 3 to 4 cm long, is made with its centre placed at the sacrococcygeal joint. The sacrococcygeal joint is disarticulared and the coccyx may either be excised or retained and retracted caudally. Haemostasis is secured by cauterising the median and lateral sacral vessels. The dissection is deepened anteriorly on the superior aspect of the levator muscle until the posterior wall of the rectum is reached. The posterior wall of the rectum is traced caudally until the V-shaped opening of the puborectalis sling is identified. The dissection continues in this plane just posterior to the urethra using a curved forceps (Lahey-type) until the tip of the forceps can be felt through the perineal incision. The forceps is directed through the centre of the external sphincter zone to complete the tunnel within the puborectalis sling. A Penrose drain is drawn through the tunnel and the puborectalis sling is gently and progressively dilated with Hegar's dilators within the Penrose drain to a size 10 to 12 calibre dilator. The Penrose drain is secured to the perineal incision and an excess of 10 to 15 cm of drain is left in the pelvis above the levator muscle for later identification during the abdominal procedure. The drain will eventually act as a guide for the rerouting of the bowel to the perineum. The sacral incision is closed in layers with a subcuticular suture to the skin.

Abdominoperineal Procedure. The infant is placed supine in the lithotomy position for this part of the procedure. The approach is either via a Pfannenstiel suprapubic or left lower paramedian incision. The rectum is mobilised just above the pelvic peritoneal reflection, taking care not to damage the ureters. A 1:200,000 solution of epinephrine in normal saline is injected into the submucosal layer of the rectum circumferential at the level of the peritoneal

1322

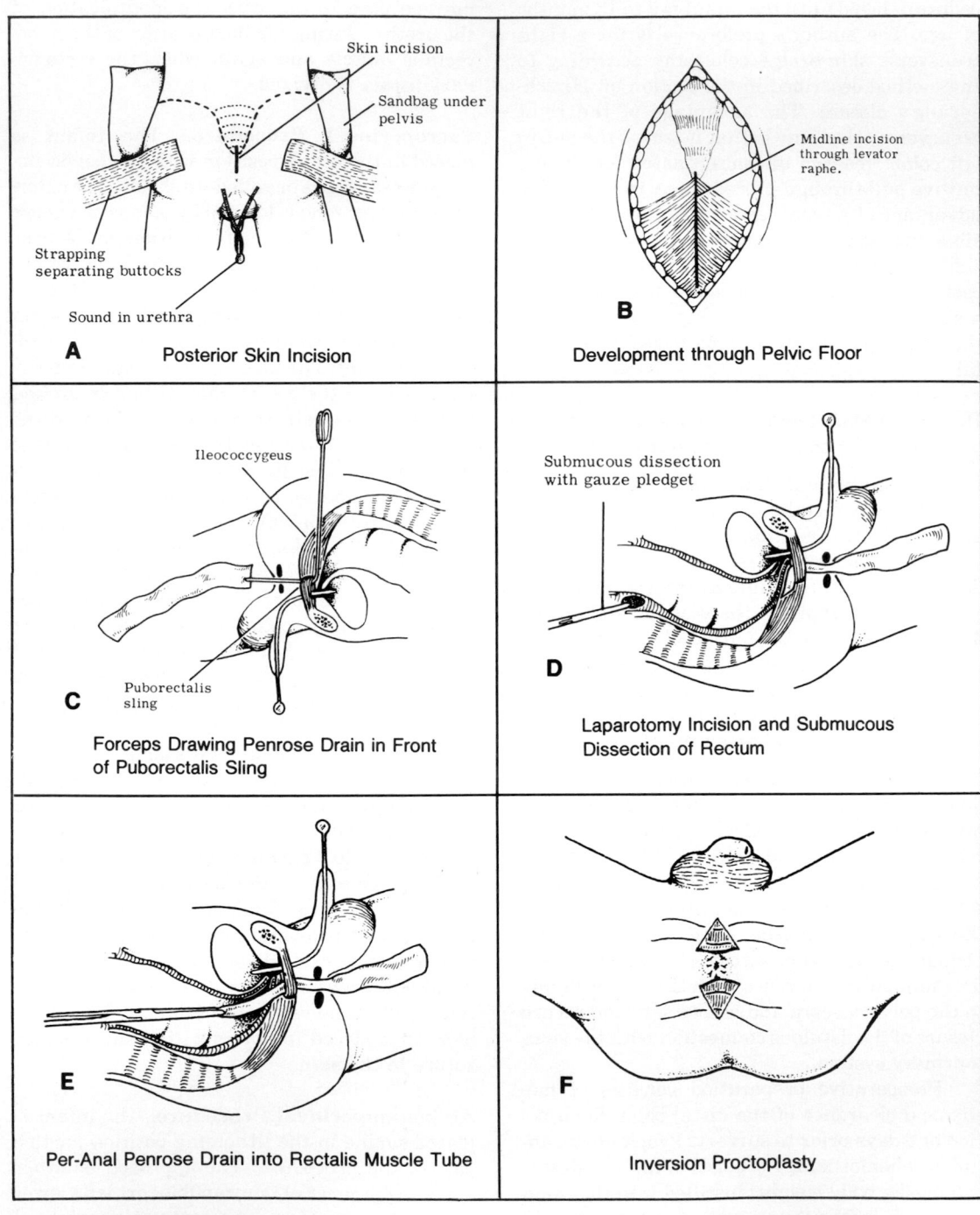

Figure 49–23. Kiesewetter-type operation for rectal agenesis. **A,B,** and **C.** Sacral phase to develop a track in front of the puborectalis sling. **D** and **E.** Abdominal phase to complete the track through the rectal muscle cuff to enable the colon to be pulled through to the anal site. **F.** Perineal phase to form and invert an anus.

reflection. This has the effect of reducing haemorrhage during the extramucosal dissection. The seromuscular coat is incised circumferentially at this level without entering the lumen of the rectum. Stripping of the mucosa from the seromuscular tube proceeds easily once the correct plane of dissection has been established. Numerous small blood vessels passing from the seromuscular layer to the mucosa require coagulation. The fistulous connection with the genitourinary system is reached when the mucosal tube arches forward, leaving muscle fibres in the base of the blind pouch visible. The fistula is transfixed, ligated, and divided as close as possible to the organ of attachment (urethra, vagina, or bladder).

An incision is made in the base of the blind seromuscular pouch and the redundant Penrose tubing left in the pelvis above the levator muscle during the seroperineal procedure is located. Identification of the tubing may be aided by passing a small Hegar's dilator upward through the tubing from the perineal route. The proximal rectum and colon is mobilised to provide sufficient length for bowel to reach the perineum without any tension. This invariably necessitates ligation and division of the inferior mesenteric vessels. The rectum is now pulled through the seromuscular cuff to the perineum, utilising the pathway previously created within the puborectalis sling. Care should be taken to ensure that the mesentery of the pulled-through bowel is correctly oriented and under no undue tension. The abdominal incision may now be closed while the anocutaneous anastomosis is fashioned.

PERINEAL PROCEDURE. Interrupted seromuscular sutures are inserted to attach the rectum to the external sphincter. The perineal skin flaps are sutured into the pulled-through colon to fashion an interdigitating type of anastomosis. Inversion of the anastomosis may be achieved by excising anteriorly and posteriorly based triangles of perineal skin in front of and behind the newly created anal canal and suturing the defects together in the midline.

Postoperative management consists of routine intravenous therapy. The urethral catheter may be removed after 3 to 5 days. Anal dilatations are permitted after 10 to 14 days, and when the anastomosis has completely healed, closure of the colostomy may be performed.

There are a number of alternative procedures for correcting high anorectal anomalies. These include neonatal pull-through procedures, the sacroperineal pull-through procedure, the Mollard (1978) perineoabdominal procedure, and the de Vries and (1982) Pena operation. The latter procedure involves a vertical posterior approach through the posterior rectal wall to the fistula. The fistula is isolated and divided from within the rectal lumen and the puborectalis and external sphincter mechanisms are reconstructed around the pulled-through rectum. This is a relatively recent development and proper evaluation requires long-term follow-up studies.

Results. Approximately 50 percent of patients attain full continence following a properly performed pull-through procedure. Half of the remainder achieve socially acceptable but not normal control and mainly have difficulty during bouts of diarrhoea. The final 25 percent have unacceptable results as far as control is concerned. Many of these have intrinsic neurologic deficits as evidenced by deformity or absence of more than three sacral vertebrae. A curious feature of anorectal anomalies is the total unexpected attainment of continence around the age of puberty in patients formerly classified as having poor control. There is no doubt that motivation plays an extremely important role in this reversal of events. It is thus axiomatic that final assessment of continence should await developments at the age of puberty and the various salvage procedures for continence should be delayed until the patient has passed through puberty.

BIBLIOGRAPHY

Hirschsprung's Disease

Aaronson I, Nixon HH: A clinical evaluation of anorectal pressure studies in the diagnosis of Hirschsprung's disease. Gut 13:138, 1972

Berdon WE, Baker DH: The roentgenographic diagnosis of Hirschsprung's disease in infancy. AJR 93:432, 1965

Berdon WE, Koontz P, et al: The diagnosis of colonic and terminal ileal aganglionosis. AJR 91:680, 1964

Bill AH, Chapman ND: The enterocolitis of Hirschsprung's disease. Its natural history and treatment. Am J Surg 103:70, 1962

Bodian M, Stephens FD, et al: Hirschsprung's disease and idiopathic megacolon. Lancet i:6, 1949

Boley SJ: New modification of the surgical treatment of Hirschsprung's disease. Surgery 56:1015, 1964

Boley SJ, Lafer DJ, et al: Endorectal pull-through procedure for Hirschsprung's disease with and without primary anastomosis. J Pediatr Surg 3:258, 1968

Duhamel B: Une nouvelle opération pour le mégacôlon congénital. L'abaissement rétrorectal et transanal du côlon et son application possible au traitement de quelques autres malformations. Presse Méd 64:2249, 1956

Duhamel B: A new operation for the treatment of Hirschsprung's disease. Arch Dis Child 35:38, 1960

Ehrenpreis Th: Megacolon in the newborn. Acta Chir Scand 94:112, 87, 1946

Ehrenpreis Th: Megacolon in the newborn. A clinical and roentgenological study with special regard to the pathogenesis. Acta Chir Scand 94:112, 1946

Garrett JR, Howard FR, et al: Autonomic nerves in rectum and colon in Hirschsprung's disease. A cholinesterase and catecholamine histochemical study. Arch Dis Child 44:406, 1969

Grob M: In Ehrenpreis Th (ed): Hirschsprung's Disease. Chicago: Year Book, 1970

Hirschsprung H: Stuhltragheit Neugebornener infolge Dilatation und Hypertrophie des Colons. Jahresbericht Kinderheilkd 27:1, 1888

Holschneider AM, et al: Clinical and electromanometrical investigations of postoperative continence in Hirschsprung's disease Z Kinderchir 29:39, 1980

Holschneider AM (ed): Hirschsprung's Disease. Stuttgart: Hippokrates Verlag, 1982

Howard ER, Garrett JR: Histochemistry and electron microscopy of rectum and colon in Hirschsprung's disease. Proc R Soc Med 63:1264, 1970

Klingman WO: The treatment of neurogenic megacolon with selective drugs. J Pediatr 13:805, 1938

Lake BD, Puri P, et al: Hirschsprung's disease: An appraisal of histochemically demonstrated acetylcholinesterase activity in suction rectal biopsies as an aid to diagnosis. Arch Pathol Lab Med 102:244, 1978

Lawson JON, Nixon HH: Anal canal pressures in the diagnosis of Hirschsprung's disease. J Pediatr Surg 2:544, 1967

Lillie JG, Crispin AR: Hirschsprung's disease in the newborn. Ann Radiol 14:265, 1971

Martin LW: Surgical management of Hirschsprung's disease involving the small intestine. Arch Surg 97:183, 1968

Martin LW, Caudill DR: A method for elimination of the blind rectal pouch in the Duhamel operation for Hirschsprung's disease. Surgery 62:951, 1967

Meier-Ruge W, Lutterbeck PM, et al: Acetylcholinesterase activity in suction biopsies of the rectum in the diagnosis of Hirschsprung's disease. J Pediatr Surg 7:11, 1972

Meunier P, Marechal JM, et al: Accuracy of the manometric diagnosis of Hirschsprung's disease. J Pediatr Surg 13:411, 1978

Nixon HH: Megacolon and other congenital anomalies of the colon, in Goligher JC (ed): Surgery of the Anus, Rectum, and Colon. London: Bailière Tindall, 1976

Noblett HR: A rectal suction biopsy tube for use in the diagnosis of Hirschsprung's disease. J Pediatr Surg 4:406, 1969

Rehbein F: Intraabdominelle Resektion oder Rektosigmoidektomie bei der Hirschsprung'schen Krankheit. Chirurgie 29:366, 1958

Rehbein F, Morger R, et al: Surgical problems in congenital megacolon. J Pediatr Surg 1:526, 1966

Schnaufer L, Talbert JL, et al: Differential sphincteric studies in the diagnosis of anorectal disorders of childhood. J Pediatr Surg 2:538, 1967

Shandling B, Auldist AW: Punch biopsy of the rectum for the diagnosis of Hirschsprung's disease. J Pediatr Surg 7:546, 1972

Soave F: Hirschsprung's disease: Technique and results of Soave's operation. Br J Surg 53:1023, 1966

Sulamaa M: Clamp à anastomose pour l'abaissement rétrorectal et trans-anal dans la maladies de Hirschsprung. Ann Chir Inf 9:63, 1968

Swenson O, Bill AH: Resection of rectum and rectosigmoid with preservation of sphincter for benign spastic lesions producing megacolon. Surgery 24:212, 1948

Swenson O, Sherman JO, et al: Diagnosis of congenital megacolon: An analysis of 501 patients. J Pediatr Surg 8:581, 1973

Swenson O, Sherman JO, et al: The treatment and postoperative complications of congenital megacolon: A 25-year follow-up. Ann Surg 182:266, 1975

Wade RB, Royle ND: Operative treatment of Hirschsprung's disease. A new method with explanation of technique and results of operation. Med J Aust 1:137, 1927

Whitehouse F, Kernohan JW: Myenteric plexus in congenital megacolon. Arch Intern Med 82:75, 1948

Zuelzer WW, Wilson JL: Functional intestinal obstruction on a congenital neurogenic basis in infancy. Am J Dis Child 75:40, 1948

Anorectal Anomalies

Amussat JJ: Observation sur une opération d'anus artificiel pratiquee avec succès par un nouveau procédé. Gaz Med (Paris) 1835

Berdon WE, Baker DH, et al: The radiologic evaluation of imperforate anus. Radiology 90:466, 1968

Bill AH Jr: Pathology and surgical treatment of imperforate anus. JAMA 166:1429, 1958

Bill AH Jr, Johnson RJ: Failure of migration of the rectal opening as the cause for most cases of imperforate anus. Surg Gynecol Obstet 106:643, 1958

Browne D: Some congenital deformities of the rectum, anus vagina and urethra. Ann R Coll Surg Engl 8:173, 1951

Browne D: Congenital deformities of the anus and rectum. Arch Dis Child 30:42, 1955

Cremin BJ, Cywes S, et al: Radiological diagnosis of

digestive tract disorders in the newborn. London: Butterworths, 1973, p 120

de Vries PA, Pena A: Posterior sagittal anorectoplasty. J Pediatr Surg 17:638, 1982

Hasse W: Associated malformations with anal and rectal atresia. Prog Ped Surg 9:100, 1976

Kiesewetter WB, Nixon HH: Imperforate anus. I. Its surgical anatomy. J Pediatr Surg 2:60, 1967

Kiesewetter WB: Imperforate anus. II. The rationale and technique of the sacro-abdomino-perineal operation. J Pediatr Surg 2:106, 1967

Ladd WE, Gross RE: Congenital malformations of anus and rectum. Am J Surg 23:167, 1934

Mollard P, Marechal JM, et al: Surgical treatment of high imperforate anus with definition of the pubo rectalis sling by an anterior perineal approach. J Pediatr Surg 13:499, 1978

Murugasu JJ: A new method of roentgenological demonstration of anorectal anomalies. Surgery 68:706, 1970

Nixon HH, Callaghan RP: Ano-rectal anomalies: Physiological considerations. Arch Dis Childhood 39:158, 1964

Ravitch MM: Anal ileostomy with sphincter preservation in patients requiring total colectomy for benign conditions. Surgery 24:170, 1948

Rehbein F: Operation for anal and rectal atresia with recto-urethral fistula. Chirurgie 30:417, 1959

Rehbein F: Imperforate anus: Experiences with abdomino-perineal and abdomino-sacro-perineal pull through procedures. J Pediatr Surg 2:99, 1967

Rhoads JE, Piper RL, et al: A simultaneous abdominal and perineal approach in operations for imperforate anus with atresia of the rectum and rectosigmoid. Ann Surg 127:552, 1948

Santulli TV, Schullinger JN, et al: Malformations of the anus and rectum. Surg Clin North Am 45:1253, 1965

Santulli TV, Kieswetter WB, et al: Anorectal anomalies: A suggested international classification. J Pediatr Surg 5:281, 1970

Smith ED: Urinary anomalies and complications in imperforate anus and rectum. J Pediatr Surg 3:337, 1968

Stephens FD, Smith ED: Ano-Rectal Malformations in Children. Chicago: Year Book, 1971

Stephens FD: Malformations of the anus. Aust NZ J Surg 23:9, 1953

Stephens FD: Imperforate rectum. A new surgical technique. Med J Aust 1:202, 1953

Swenson O, Donnellan WL: Preservation of the puborectalis sling in imperforate anus repair. Surg Clin North Am 47:173, 1967

Wangensteen OH, Rice CO: Imperforate anus. A method of determining the surgical approach. Ann Surg 92:77, 1930

50. Diverticular Disease of the Colon

T. George Parks

HISTORICAL BACKGROUND

Credit for the earliest detailed description of diverticular disease of the colon is usually ascribed to Cruveilhier (1849) in *Traité d'Anatomie Pathologique Générale*. Virchow in 1853 described a condition of "isolated circumscribed adhesive peritonitis" and, although he also described colonic diverticula, he did not associate the two lesions. Habershon, in 1857, a physician at Guy's Hospital, London, is given the credit of having published the first account of colonic diverticula in the English language. Two years later Jones reported a case of diverticulitis complicated by fistulisation into the urinary bladder.

Toward the end of the nineteenth century, Graser in Germany emphasised the pathologic significance of the condition, when he described the hyperplastic stenosing form of the disease known as peridiverticulitis and emphasised its simulation to carcinoma of the sigmoid colon. Moynihan (1907) reported a case of peridiverticulitis under the title "A Mimicry of Carcinoma" and underlined the difficulties in the differential diagnosis. Wilson in 1911, after careful pathologic study, suggested that chronic inflammation could be responsible for the segregation of colonic epithelium from which carcinoma might subsequently develop. Although this view was held for a time by Mayo (1917) and others, little concrete evidence was put forward to support it.

Spriggs and Marxer (1927) stressed the importance of radiology in establishing a diagnosis and assessing the extent and degree of involvement. They described in detail what they called "the prediverticular state," although Marxer (1923) had earlier introduced the term in his writings.

The place of surgery in the treatment of diverticular disease was emphasised by Mayo et al (1907) who recommended the use of a temporary colostomy followed by resection for the treatment of obstruction associated with inflammation. However, it was not until Smithwick showed in 1942 that surgery could be carried out with an acceptable mortality that resection of the diseased segment was frequently undertaken as a planned procedure.

The term "diverticulosis" was proposed independently in 1914 by Case and de Quervain to describe the condition characterised by the presence of uncomplicated and noninflamed colonic mucosal pouches (Fig. 50–1). The terms "diverticulitis" and "peridiverticulitis" indicate inflammation in and around diverticula. The distinction between diverticulosis and diverticulitis is not always clear and thus it is helpful to adopt the nomenclature "diverticular disease" to encompass the complicated as well as the uncomplicated state.

INCIDENCE

It is difficult to assess accurately the frequency with which diverticular disease occurs in the community as it often remains symptomless and many patients with the disorder do not present for investigation at hospital.

The prevalence of diverticular disease of the colon varies considerably in different parts of the world. In rural Africa and Latin America and certain areas of Asia, the incidence is very low compared with that in the Western countries. Wells (1949) pointed out that in West Africa, the native who ingests a bulky diet rarely suffers from diverticular disease. On the other hand, volvulus of the excessively large colon is relatively common. Interestingly, colonic

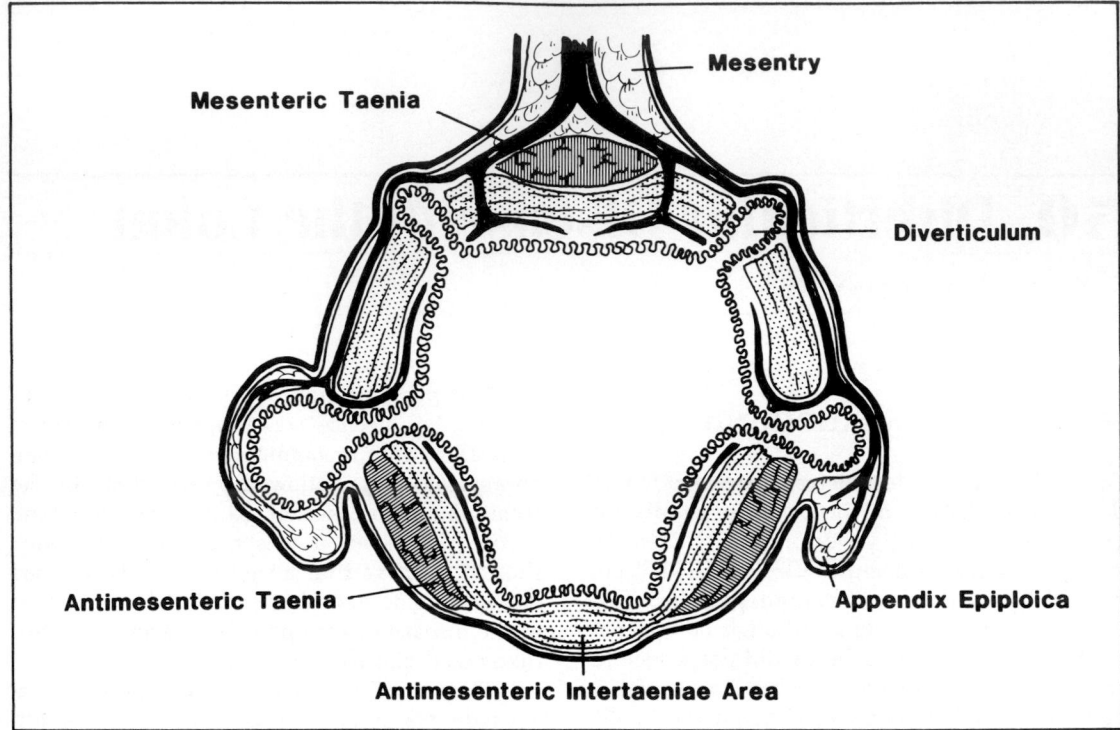

Figure 50–1. Diagrammatic representation of the relationship of diverticula and blood vessels to the taeniae coli.

diverticula are not uncommon among those of African extraction who are resident in North America.

There is a considerable weight of evidence relating the dietary fibre intake to the prevalence of diverticular disease of the colon (Painter and Burkitt, 1971). When more refined techniques for milling of grain were introduced in Great Britain about 100 years ago, the fibre content of flour dropped to about one tenth of its former level. Subsequently, the incidence of diverticula began to rise in the community in which the intake of fibre was markedly reduced. It is now widely accepted that an adequate intake of dietary fibre in the form of wholemeal bread, fruit and vegetables, and a reduced intake of refined carbohydrates considerably reduces the tendency to develop colonic diverticula.

Colonic diverticula are uncommon in patients under 40 years of age. In this country about 5 percent of patients in the fifth decade of life have colonic diverticula and by the eighth or ninth decade up to 50 percent of individuals are affected.

Diverticular Disease in the Elderly. The incidence of diverticular disease increases with longevity. Furthermore, if complications develop in elderly patients, the associated mortality is higher than for those of a younger age group. Older patients also suffer from a higher incidence of concurrent disease and if inflammatory complications ensue, the sufferers are less likely to withstand their adverse effects. Colonic haemorrhage in the elderly hypertensive subject is not infrequently associated with diverticulosis.

Diverticular Disease in Young Subjects. Diverticular disease presenting in younger individuals tends to be a more aggressive form of disease and associated with more troublesome recurrent episodes of inflammation. Hannan et al (1961) reported that an operative procedure was required in more than 60 percent of younger patients with symptomatic diverticular disease compared with only 20 or 30 percent of all patients with diverticular disease who came under their care. A high complication rate and

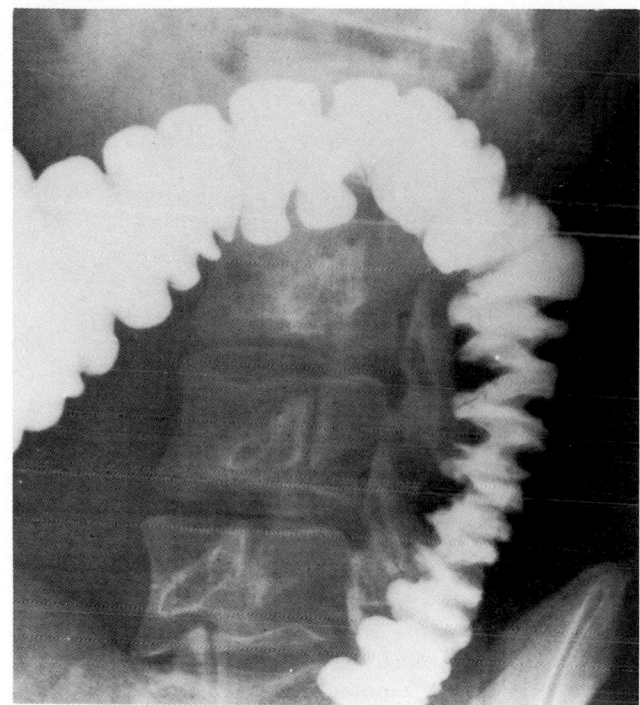

Figure 50–2. Barium enema of a male patient aged 25 years who had had a previous pelvic abscess secondary to acute peridiverticulitis confirmed at laparotomy and treated by drainage alone. A few diverticula were present and marked zig-zag deformity due to muscle thickening and shortening was demonstrable in the sigmoid and descending colon.

a high readmission rate was reported by Ouriel and Schwartz (1983) in patients under the age of 40 years suffering from diverticular disease of the colon. Figure 50–2 demonstrates marked muscle abnormality in a patient who had perforated diverticular disease when 25 years old whereas Figure 50–3 shows considerable diverticular formation by the age of 33 years.

PATHOLOGY

Morphologic Features

Although the circular muscle fibres of the colon form a complete layer, the outer longitudinal fibres are concentrated into three bands or taeniae leaving much of the colonic wall devoid of a distinct longitudinal coat. Thus, when diverticula develop, they occur in the areas between the taeniae (Fig. 50–1), i.e., in the lateral intertaeniae areas and much less commonly in the antimesenteric intertaeniae area. The herniations of the mucous membrane tend to occur alongside arteries which penetrate the muscle wall en route to the submucosa and mucosa. Vessels larger than those that reach the antimesenteric region penetrate the muscle wall in

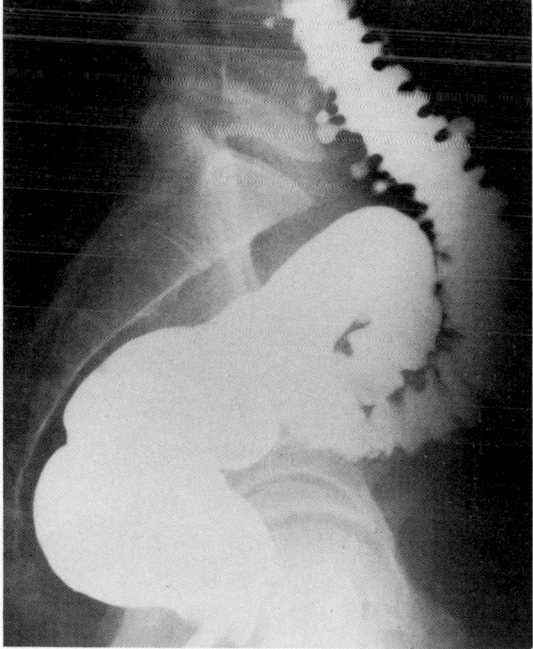

Figure 50–3. Radiograph of the same patient as illustrated in Figure 50–2, taken after an interval of 8 years when the patient was age 33. Considerable progress of the disease process with marked diverticular formation.

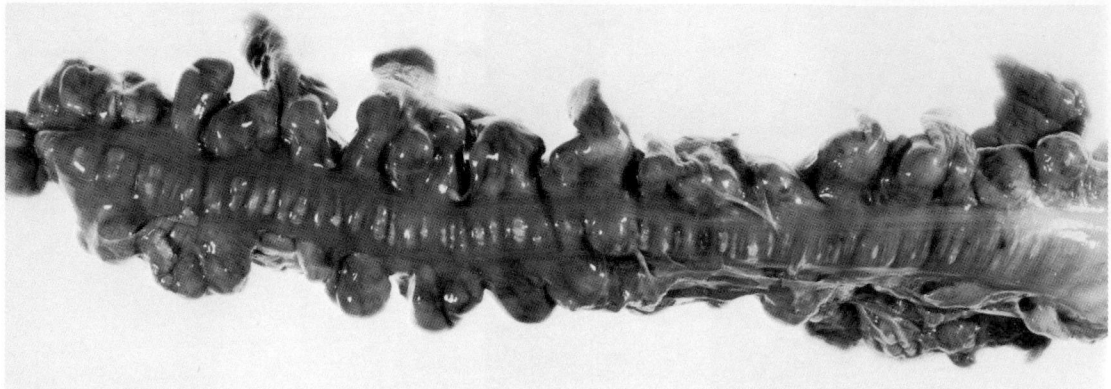

Figure 50–4. Specimen showing numerous large diverticula in the lateral intertaeniae areas. Early diverticular formation between the antimesenteric taeniae.

the lateral areas. Figure 50–4 shows a segment of sigmoid colon in which large diverticula are present in the lateral areas whereas small pouches at an early stage of development are seen in the area between the two antimesenteric taeniae.

Colonic diverticula are for the most part false diverticula, the wall being made up of mucosa and muscularis mucosae covered by serosa. Initially the diverticula are covered by muscle but as they enlarge, the investing muscle thins and atrophies and virtually disappears except perhaps for an area around the neck. Early lesions are small protrusions into which and from which faecal material can pass readily. As they enlarge they become flask-like in shape with a

relatively narrow neck. It is inevitable that faecal stasis will occur in these diverticula, particularly because there is a lack of muscle in the wall (Fig. 50–5)

It was pointed out by Morson (1963) that one of the most consistent features of the diverticular colon is the thickening of the muscle coats (Fig. 50–6). As a result of thickening and shortening, the colonic wall is concertinaed. This leads to the formation of thick circular muscle folds which project into the lumen of the bowel causing considerable narrowing (Fig. 50–2). The mucosa and submucosa are also heaped up, thus causing further encroachment on the lumen. The mesocolon of the diverticular colon also tends to be shortened. Although the

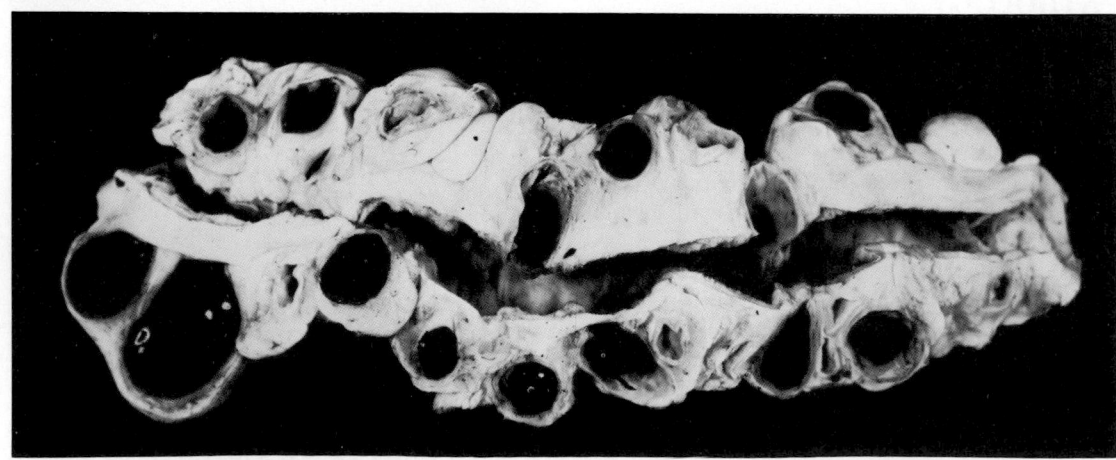

Figure 50–5. Specimen demonstrating numerous faecoliths in sigmoid diverticula.

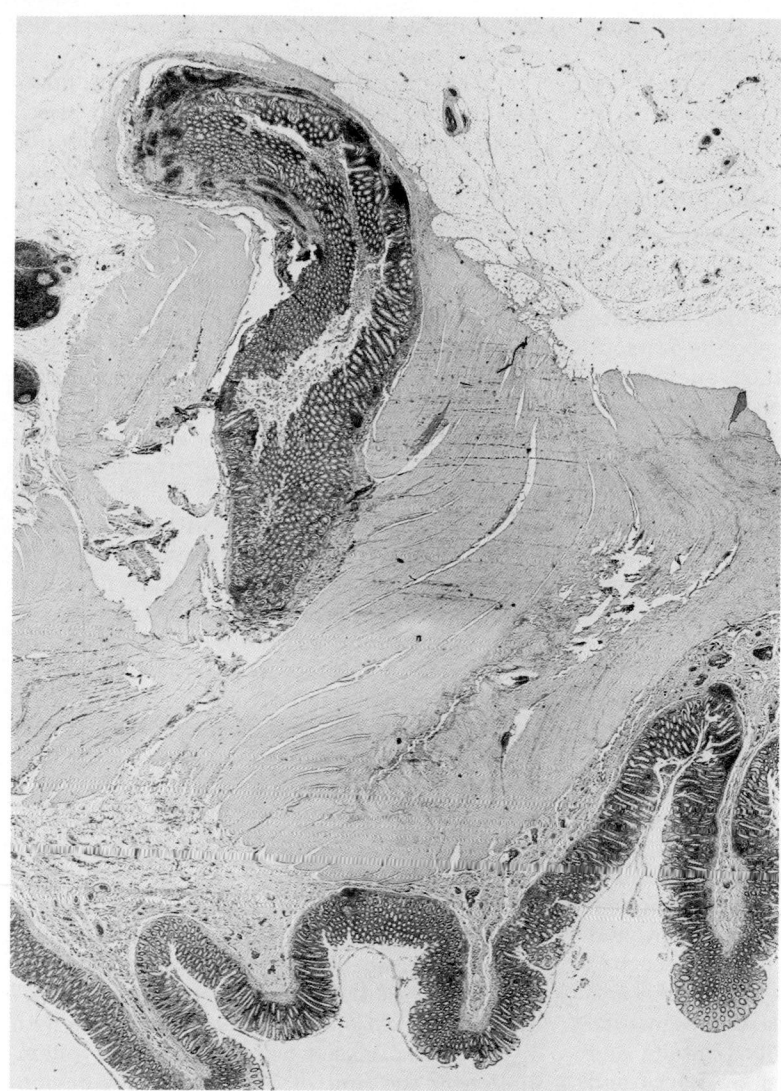

Figure 50–6. Photomicrograph demonstrating marked thickening of the colonic muscle. A diverticulum is shown in the upper part of the section.

majority of patients with diverticular disease have this muscle abnormality as a main feature, there are some patients who have diverticula widely scattered and densely concentrated along the colon and who have no evidence of muscular thickening.

Inflammatory Aspects

The earliest signs of inflammation often occur in lymphoid tissue at the apex of a diverticulum. This may result from abrasion of the mucosal lining of the pouch by inspissated faeces which forms a faecolith (Fig. 50–5).

Low grade inflammation extends readily to involve adjacent peritoneum, pericolic fat, and mesenteric fat because the diverticula are thin walled and lie mainly outside the muscular wall of the colon.

The inflammation commonly spreads for a considerable distance from a single diverticulum along the outer aspect of the colonic muscular tube so that the bowel becomes encased and involved in an acute inflammatory reaction, culminating in the development of a large and often palpable tender mass.

Because the peritoneum is usually involved in the inflammatory process, adhesion of the involved segment to the parietes or to other organs is common. This may help to wall off infection and localise an abscess on the one hand or allow the development of an internal fistula on the other. If prior adherence of colonic visceral peritoneum to parietal peritoneum or other viscera has not occurred, then an open breach in the diverticular wall will lead to free communication between the colonic lumen and the peritoneal cavity, and hence generalised peritonitis.

In some instances, spread of inflammation occurs between the mesenteric leaves or into the retroperitoneal area. If an abscess develops and subsequently ruptures, then an indirect communication with the colonic lumen may establish itself.

Resolution of pericolic inflammation results in fibrosis but residual walled-off chronic abscesses may occur. Recurrent episodes of acute inflammation are common. Narrowing of the lumen of the bowel due to a combination of muscular hypertrophy and fibrosis is inevitable.

COLONIC MOTILITY

Arfwidsson (1964) reported significant increases in intraluminal pressure activity in patients with colonic diverticular disease, compared with control subjects under resting conditions, after food intake, and following cholinergic stimulation. Painter and Truelove (1964) found no major difference in diverticular disease and normal colons during basal motility recordings, but they noted an enhanced response to morphine and prostigmine in diverticula-bearing segments. An exaggerated response to food intake and prostigmine was demonstrated by Parks and Connell in 1972 and, in addition, fast wave activity similar to that recorded in some patients with irritable bowel syndrome. Although such pharmacologic stimuli are relatively uncommon in normal life, the frequently recurring physiologic stimulus of eating may be relevant in the pathogenesis of colonic diverticula.

Following simultaneous manometric and cineradiographic studies, Painter et al (1965) postulated that contraction of interhaustral rings, which can effectively occlude the bowel lumen, leads to the formation of multiple isolated short segments along the colon. The tendency to develop temporary occlusion of the lumen is accentuated by the prominence of the crescentic folds of circular muscle and the folds of redundant mucosa. It is evident that further contraction of the walls of the closed segments

thus formed, sets the scene for considerable rise in intraluminal pressure.

When motility was assessed in colons manifesting the prediverticular state, Arfwidsson (1964) claimed that the pressures generated were higher than normal and suggested that these findings supported the view that an abnormality in the muscle is the primary defect in diverticular disease. Furthermore, the fact that the motility index is reduced after eating bran lends support to the hypothesis that narrowing of the colonic lumen associated with a low food residue may predispose to diverticular formation. Hodgson, in 1972, demonstrated that administration of methylcellulose leads to a reduction of rectal and colonic pressures in patients with diverticular disease and the author has demonstrated similar effects with ispaghula.

Following resection of the sigmoid colon for diverticular disease, Parks showed in 1970 that the apparently normal segments that remain may exhibit abnormal motility response to stimuli, similar to, but less in degree, than regions of established disease. These findings suggest that there is a primary muscular abnormality which exists in segments of the colon which are free from diverticula.

Compliance Studies of the Colonic Wall

Although increased intracolonic pressure may be important in the aetiology of diverticular disease, it does not appear to be the only factor. Compliance of the sigmoid colon was assessed by Parks and Connell (1969) in patients with diverticular disease who had no signs of inflammation at the time of the study. They demonstrated that the colonic muscle, in spite of its thickness, is unable to resist pressure as well as normal colonic muscle in control subjects. It was also demonstrated that a lower threshold for distension type pain exists in diverticular disease, indicating an increased sensitivity of the colonic muscle to stretch. This weakness or loss of compliance of the wall could be relevant in the aetiology of diverticular disease.

CLINICAL MANIFESTATIONS

It is estimated that only 10 to 20 percent of persons with colonic diverticula develop symptoms related to their presence. Diverticular disease of the colon may be associated with quite troublesome symptoms even in the absence of inflammation. Recurring episodes of lower abdominal cramps can result from a degree of functional obstruction secondary to the narrowing and excessive segmentation of the sigmoid. In clinical practice, the clinician may find it difficult to differentiate between painful noninflammatory and inflammatory diverticular disease. In some patients with a presumptive diagnosis of diverticulitis who have undergone operation, the resected specimens have shown multiple diverticula, thickening of the wall, and narrowing of the lumen but without microscopic evidence of inflammation.

Abdominal pain, especially in the left lower quadrant, is a cardinal feature and is the most common symptom requiring hospital admission. Persistent pain is suggestive of an inflammatory origin. Central and lower abdominal cramp may signify a degree of obstruction.

Intermittent diarrhoea or alternating constipation and diarrhoea are common symptoms. Constipation may become troublesome in patients with a significant degree of narrowing in the sigmoid segment due to either the muscular abnormality or fibrosis.

Nausea and vomiting of a reflex nature may be associated with an acute inflammatory reaction. Alternatively, these symptoms may be mechanical in nature due to large or small bowel obstruction. Urinary symptoms due to irritation of the ureter or bladder are not infrequent.

On physical examination the abdomen may be tender in the left lower quadrant. Guarding and rebound tenderness may be present. A palpable mass is not uncommon in the left iliac fossa. Occasionally rectal examination may reveal a tender mass or even a pelvic abscess. Abdominal distension may also be present.

Sigmoidoscopy will help to rule out other conditions, particularly neoplasm of the rectum. Hyperaemic, oedematous mucosa is sometimes visible in the rectosigmoid region. Straight and erect x-ray of the abdomen may reveal a soft tissue mass in the left iliac fossa, air under the diaphragm, or dilatation of the colon, indicating obstruction.

Extent of Colonic Involvement. In approximately 65 percent of cases the sigmoid colon alone is affected. However, in combination with other segments it is involved in about 95 percent of cases (Fig. 50–7). Although there are some

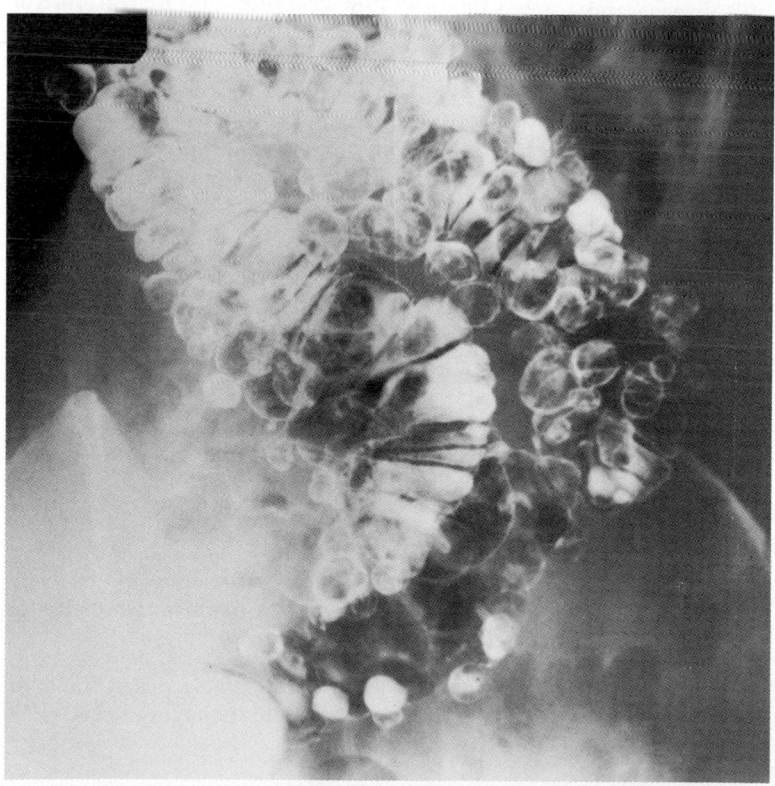

Figure 50–7. Barium enema showing the colon studded with numerous large diverticula.

patients in whom only the sigmoid is affected initially and in whom other regions subsequently become involved, this does not necessarily occur. It would seem that if a segment of colon is prone to be affected this is often determined early on in the course of the disease and progression is more often within the segment or segments initially involved rather than occurring in a stepwise fashion, segment by segment, along the length of the colon. The majority of patients with disease initially localised to the distal colon are generally not destined for the relentless progression of the disorder to involve additional segments. In a 1958 series, Horner demonstrated that two thirds of patients with colonic diverticula did not have relentless advance of the disease along the colon.

In the author's experience, severe inflammatory complications occur as commonly in patients with distal disease as in patients with total colonic involvement.

DIFFERENTIAL DIAGNOSIS

Diverticular disease of the colon may simulate many other abdominal conditions, including carcinoma of the colon, irritable bowel syndrome, acute appendicitis, Crohn's disease and ulcerative colitis, ischaemic colitis, urinary tract disorders, and pelvic inflammatory disease.

Carcinoma of the Colon. Of all the conditions which may simulate diverticular disease, one of the most important and, on occasion, one of the most difficult to differentiate is carcinoma of the colon. Within the colon itself both conditions have a predilection for the sigmoid segment. Furthermore, both conditions can occur coincidentally in the same area. Clinical features associated with the two disorders are often remarkably similar. Symptoms such as alteration of bowel habit, lower abdominal pain, and rectal bleeding readily occur in either condition. However, the typical patient with inflammatory diverticular disease is more likely to have severe abdominal pain, tenderness, fever, and leucocytosis. With carcinoma, bleeding is often occult or mild, whereas in diverticular disease it may be mild, moderate, or severe. Hughes (1975) reckoned that up to one fifth of cases of so-called perforated diverticulitis were eventually diagnosed as carcinoma.

The prognosis in patients with carcinoma is diminished by the co-existence of diverticular disease. Not infrequently definitive surgery is delayed to allow the inflammatory process to settle on the premise that the clinician is dealing with benign disease alone. If the segment of colon harbours carcinoma then the opportunity for cure of that patient may be considerably lessened by the delay (Fig. 50–8).

Furthermore, when carcinoma arises in a patient who has already been diagnosed as having symptomatic diverticular disease, malignancy may go unrecognised as it is all too often assumed that the symptoms are due to diverticular disease. Careful double-contrast barium enema and, if necessary, colonoscopy are of prime importance in reaching an accurate diagnosis.

The following points help in the radiologic differentiation of diverticular disease from colonic cancer.

1. Typically the stricture due to diverticular disease is longer and more tapered at both ends than carcinoma (Fig. 50–9).
2. The colonic mucosa remains intact in diverticular strictures whereas it is eroded in carcinoma.
3. Propantheline bromide administration during barium enema examination may help to relieve spasm associated with diverticular disease but has no effect in carcinomatous strictures.
4. A repeat radiologic examination after a short interval to allow resolution to occur may help clarify the situation in doubtful cases.

Irritable Bowel Syndrome. The patient with irritable bowel syndrome is usually younger than the diverticular patient and typically presents with a longer history of abdominal pain and alteration in bowel habit. The pain tends to be more diffuse and is often referred to the upper or right side of the abdomen. Pellet-type stools and mucus may be passed. Passage of stool or flatus may relieve symptoms.

Acute Appendicitis. Diverticular disease is liable to be confused with acute appendicitis in the following circumstances:

1. When acute inflammation occurs at the apex of a redundant sigmoid loop lying to the right of the midline

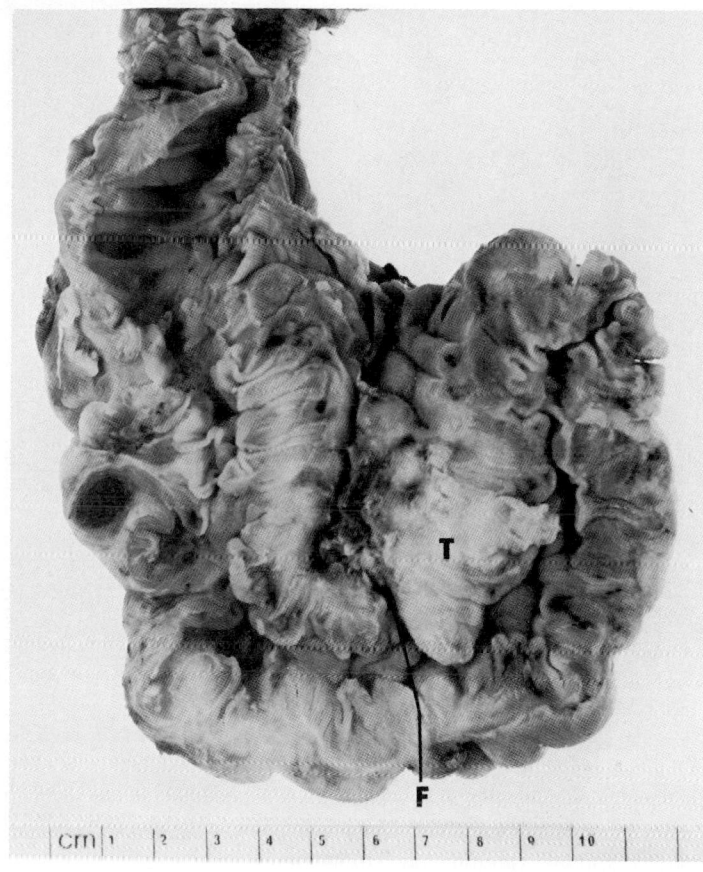

Figure 50–8. Resected specimen of sigmoid colon showing gross muscle thickening with narrowing of the lumen and concertinaed effect of advanced diverticular disease. A co-existing tumour (T) was confirmed as a moderately well differentiated invasive adenocarcinoma, and a colovesical fistula was also present; the colonic component is shown by arrow F.

2. When acute inflammation occurs in a caecal diverticulum
3. Or when a patient presents with a pelvic abscess and it is feasible that the lesion could have arisen from either a pelvic appendix or from an inflamed diverticulum in a sigmoid loop lying in the pelvis

Ulcerative Colitis. The persistence and the severity of the diarrhoea typical of ulcerative colitis is noteworthy. Bleeding per rectum is greater and abdominal pain much less in ulcerative colitis compared to diverticular disease. Sigmoidoscopy and biopsy readily establish the diagnosis of inflammatory bowel disease because the rectum is almost always involved.

Crohn's Disease. Crohn's disease of the colon may simulate the symptoms of diverticular disease in that left lower quadrant pain and tenderness associated with altered bowel habit may be present in either condition. In Crohn's disease, however, the diarrhoea tends to be unremitting over a longer period of time. Moreover, patients with the disease tend to be younger, although older persons are sometimes affected. The co-existence of anorectal disease or perianal inflammation points towards the correct diagnosis.

Errors in diagnosis are more likely to occur when the two diseases co-exist. Schmidt et al in 1968 reported 26 cases of co-existence of diverticular and Crohn's disease of the colon. The combined disease abnormalities were usually present in the rectal mucosa on sigmoidoscopy. The incidence of postoperative complications was much higher in patients with combined disease than in those with diverticular disease alone.

Ischaemic Disease of the Colon. Ischaemic colitis and diverticular disease affect similar age groups. However, the sudden onset of acute diarrhoea and haemorrhage associated with left-

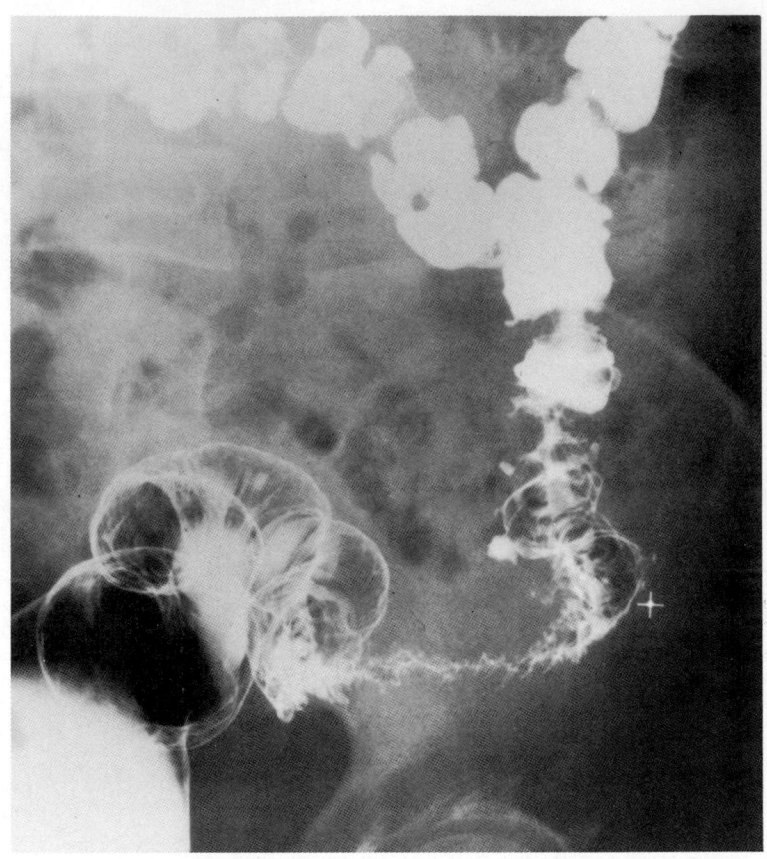

Figure 50–9. A long sigmoid stricture with tapered ends and intact mucosa associated with diverticular disease.

sided abdominal pain and tenderness in elderly patients is suggestive of colonic ischaemia. An early barium enema will help to clarify the diagnosis. The more severe forms of colonic ischaemia presenting with acute peritoneal signs may progress to gangrene. Efforts should be made to differentiate these cases from perforated diverticular disease.

DIETARY AND MEDICAL MANAGEMENT OF UNCOMPLICATED DIVERTICULAR DISEASE

It is now generally accepted that increasing the amount of fibre in the diet is beneficial to patients suffering from uncomplicated diverticular disease (Painter et al, 1972; Brodribb, 1977; Parks, 1980; Hyland and Taylor, 1980). The additional fibre ingested leads to the passage of a softer and bulkier stool. The increased volume of faeces is partly due to the additional residue of indigestible fibre and partly to the entrapment of water in the stool. The changes in the volume and consistency of the stool helps to maintain a greater diameter of colonic lumen and leads to a reduction in segmental activity, a lower intraluminal colonic pressure, and an increase in the transit rate through the intestine.

Fruit and vegetables vary considerably in the proportion of indigestible fibre that they contain and hence in the amount of water retained by the fibrous material. Each gram of fibre from fruit and vegetables, such as apples, oranges, carrots, and brussels sprouts retains 2 to 3 g of water.

The addition of bran to the diet helps to ensure that the faecal residue is more voluminous and that the stools are softer and passed more easily without straining. The fibre derived from wheat bran has also a laxative effect, which is greater than fibre derived from fruit and vegetables. Each gram of unprocessed bran binds with approximately four times its own weight of water. Because of its bulking properties it is not unusual for patients who commence taking bran to develop a bloated sensation in the abdomen. For a time they may complain of the passage of excess gas and also complain of flatulence. When adaptation to the new regimen takes place over the ensuing weeks, these symptoms gradually settle.

Initially an intake of about 5 or 10 g of bran daily is advised, the amount being increased to 20 g over a 3- or 4-week period. Coarse bran has been shown to be more effective than fine bran in increasing the stool weight, regulating the transit time, and reducing the motility index (Findlay et al, 1974). There seems little doubt that patients with diverticular disease are helped symptomatically by the ingestion of a high fibre diet although the efficacy of this moiety in the diet has been questioned by some authors (Ornstein et al, 1981). A high fibre diet also seems to afford some protection against the development of further complications after acute inflammatory attacks (Hyland and Taylor, 1980). Findlay et al (1974) have shown that although basal motility remains unchanged during bran therapy, the colonic response to food and prostigmine is reduced.

One of the disadvantages of unprocessed bran is that it lacks palatability for some patients who prefer to take other vegetable fibre. It should be remembered that wholemeal bread and several palatable breakfast cereals can provide a good complement of dietary fibre. Several pharmaceutical bulk additive preparations have an important hydrophylic property thereby maintaining an increased volume of faecal residue. For example, methylcellulose (Celevac) absorbs about 25 times its own weight in water. Ispaghula husk (Isogel, Fybogel, or Regulan) retains about 40 times its own weight in water. Sterculia (Normacol or Movicol) and psyllium seed powders (Metamucil) act in a similar fashion.

Patients who suffer from the pain of colonic spasm may be relieved by mebeverine hydrochloride (Colofac). This drug acts directly on the smooth muscle of the colonic wall and is preferable to anticholinergic drugs, such as probantheline bromide (Probanthine), which act through the autonomic nervous system. Anticholinergic drugs have the drawback that they cause dry-

ness of the mouth and mucous membranes, blurring of vision, and even urinary retention.

COMPLICATIONS

The complications of diverticular disease fall broadly under two headings, inflammatory complications and haemorrhage. Inflammation around diverticula may lead to peridiverticulitis and pericolitis which may progress to the formation of an inflammatory mass, particularly in the sigmoid region. The inflammation may gradually subside but in some cases it progresses to form a localised paracolic abscess. Alternatively, sepsis may spread to cause a generalised peritonitis of a purulent or faecal nature depending on whether or not there is a direct breach in the colonic wall. Inflammation may culminate in the formation of an internal or external fistula. It can also lead to obstruction of the large intestine or even of the small intestine if the latter becomes involved in the inflammatory mass.

Haemorrhage related to colonic diverticula may be mild, moderate, or severe. In the majority of cases the bleeding ceases spontaneously but occasionally persistent bleeding may require intensive investigation and emergency surgery.

Management

Acute Diverticulitis, Localised Peritonitis, and Pericolic Abscess

Persistent and severe pain in the lower abdomen, especially in the left lower quadrant but sometimes also in the hypogastrium extending to the right of the midline is accompanied by acute tenderness. Localised guarding and rigidity are present and, not uncommonly, a mass is palpable in the left iliac fossa. Tachycardia, pyrexia, and leucocytosis are to be expected.

Initial Management. Bedrest is advised. Depending on the severity of the inflammatory process, intravenous fluids may be required. In addition, in more acute cases nasogastric suction may have to be instituted. Antibiotic therapy, such as metronidazole, together with a cephalosporin is recommended. An analgesic, e.g., pethidine, is given for the relief of pain. Morphine is best avoided in view of its tendency to increase intracolonic pressures. Purgatives, wash-outs, and barium enema examinations are avoided early in the course of management of patients with these complications.

On a conservative regimen as outlined, subsidence of the symptoms and signs may be expected in a high percentage of cases after which the colon may be examined by barium enema to confirm the diagnosis of diverticular disease and to exclude other large bowel pathology (Fig. 50–10). Careful sigmoidoscopy should also be undertaken when the acute phase has passed.

During the period of observation, careful watch is kept for evidence of spreading peritonitis or adverse changes in the vital signs which would indicate the need for surgical intervention.

A patient with a phlegmonous mass or a small paracolic abscess may improve symptomatically with concomitant subsidence of inflammation while on a conservative regimen. Likewise, a small abscess situated between the leaves of the mesentery may remain confined and gradually resolve. However, the majority of patients with paracolic abscesses will require surgical drainage. If the lesion is well walled-off then simple incision and drainage alone may be satisfactory but often a proximal transverse colostomy is added. In recent years, many surgeons believe that a more aggressive approach is indicated and there have been an increasing number of encouraging reports in which excision of the perforated segment has been undertaken at the initial operation.

Perforation with Generalised Peritonitis

When a colonic diverticulum ruptures directly into the peritoneal cavity, widespread contamination ensues with resultant faecal peritonitis. Rupture of paracolic abscess may lead to widespread purulent peritonitis.

Initial Management. If the patient is seriously ill and in a state of shock, the initial aim is to institute resuscitative measures and seek to reestablish and maintain an adequate circulation. Patients suffering from faecal peritonitis are often in profound shock and it may be diffi-

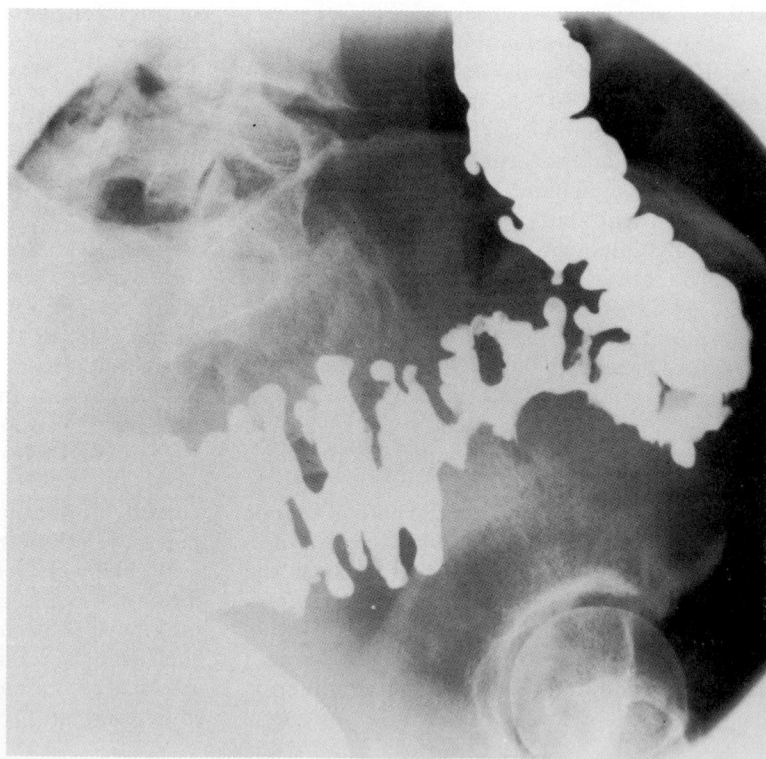

Figure 50–10. A large paracolic abscess associated with severe diverticular disease of the sigmoid colon.

cult or impossible to obtain optimal circulatory stability prior to surgery. Intravenous fluids and intravenous antibiotics against aerobic and anaerobic bacteria are commenced.

Operative Approaches. A wide range of surgical procedures have been tried in an effort to cope with this highly lethal complication. The prognosis is related to the age and state of the patient. Elderly patients and those with concomitant disorders have a worse prognosis.

In the past decade there have been gradual changes in the operative policy at many centres, the emphasis nowadays on more radical procedures for treatment of perforation associated with localised or generalised peritonitis. The initial surgical procedures fall broadly into two groups: those in which the diseased segment is left in situ at the time of the first operation and those in which the diseased segment is removed from the peritoneal cavity at the time of the original surgery (Fig. 50–11).

OPERATIONS IN WHICH THE DISEASED SEGMENT IS LEFT IN SITU AT THE INITIAL OPERATION

Peritoneal Toilet and Drainage Plus Colostomy. For many years this procedure had wide acceptance for patients with generalised peritonitis. The peritoneal cavity is thoroughly irrigated with warm saline, adequate drainage is established in the left lower quadrant, and a right transverse colostomy performed. However, this procedure is associated with a high mortality, particularly if the peritonitis is of the faecal variety. A distinct disadvantage is that the septic focus still remains within the peritoneal cavity and this seat of inflammation may continue to cause toxicity. Furthermore, it may lead to further contamination of the peritoneal cavity.

Suture of Perforation; Peritoneal Toilet and Drainage; Proximal Colostomy. Attempts to suture an oedematous, inflamed, friable, and perforated colon is an unsatisfactory procedure. The wall surrounding the perforation is unyield-

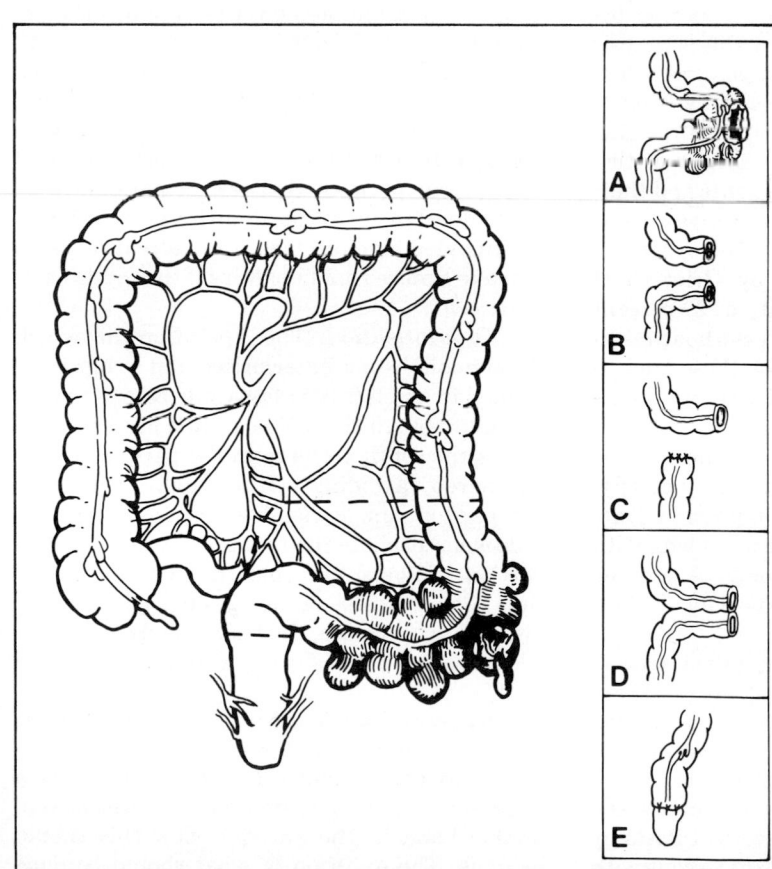

Figure 50–11. A diagrammatic representation of operations in which the perforated segment is removed from the peritoneal cavity. **A.** exteriorisation, **B.** surgical excision, end colostomy, mucous fistula, **C.** Hartmann's operation, **D.** Paul Mickulicz's procedure, **E.** primary resection and anastomosis.

ing and lacks pliability. The risk of subsequent breakdown is high. The formation of a proximal colostomy, although beneficial, is no guarantee against further leakage at the site of the original perforation because it is apparent that there is often considerable faecal loading between the site of the closed perforation and the site of the transverse colostomy.

The above operations are only the first phase of the classical three-stage procedure, the second stage being resection of the involved segment and the third stage, the closure of the colostomy. There are considerable drawbacks to the three-stage approach, which for many years held a foremost place in the management of acute complications of diverticular disease.

Some valid criticisms of the three-stage approach are worthy of consideration. Of prime concern is the high mortality and morbidity. In a collective survey of 15 groups of reputable surgeons who treated patients suffering from perforated diverticulitis by laparotomy and drainage with or without proximal colostomy, the overall mortality was 37.7 percent (Painter, 1975). These reports relate to the period between 1957 and 1971. Although the prognosis has improved considerably today because of better resuscitative measures and much more effective antibiotic regimens, particularly relating to gram-negative infection, the results of this policy are still not as good as patients and their surgeons would desire. A retrospective review of 1353 cases with acute perforated diverticulitis treated surgically was made by Grief et al (1980). They reported a mortality of 29 percent in patients treated by colostomy without resection, compared to 12 percent for those treated by primary resection or exteriorisation of the diseased segment.

The fistula rate following proximal colostomy with drainage varies from 5 to 20 percent in different series and is equally high in patients who have closure of the perforation along with concomitant transverse colostomy. A chronic colocutaneous fistula is likely to prolong the hospital stay considerably.

In some patients the inflammatory process is slow to subside after the first phase. There is also the added risk of leaving the perforated sigmoid carcinoma in situ for an unduly long period before the second stage. A further disadvantage of the three-stage procedure is the length of time for which transverse colostomy may be present and for the patient to cope with

a malodourous fluid effluent from the proximal stoma. In fact, a significant number of patients do not proceed to the second and third stages. It is clear that the three-stage approach necessitates considerable hospitalisation and each operation carries with it a potential morbidity and mortality.

Suture of Perforation; Peritoneal Toilet and Drainage Without Colostomy. This is an unsatisfactory method and mentioned only to be condemned. It is too much to expect a friable, inflamed, and loaded colon, which perforated in the first instance, to regularly remain soundly sealed after closure. The risks are too high to be acceptable.

OPERATIONS DESIGNED TO REMOVE THE PERFORATED SEGMENT. Surgical procedures to remove the diseased or perforated segment of bowel from the peritoneal cavity have found a distinct place and today play an increasingly important role in the management of perforated diverticulitis. First, they minimise continuing toxaemia that would otherwise result from the continuing inflammation and second, they remove the potential hazard of further leakage and contamination of the peritoneal cavity by colonic content. There can be little argument that excisional surgery is the procedure of choice in coping with a direct open perforation associated with faecal peritonitis. Even in patients with generalised purulent peritonitis associated with an inflamed sigmoid loop, the patient is likely to make a more rapid recovery if the septic focus is removed.

Exteriorisation. The operation in which the sigmoid loop is exteriorised and a colostomy formed in the left iliac fossa was recommended by Staunton (1962). Although this procedure removes the septic focus from the peritoneal cavity thereby avoiding further contamination of the peritoneum, it has the disadvantage that it does not exclude the toxins from the inflamed portion of bowel entering the circulation and thus adversely affects the patient's general condition. Furthermore, the lesion tends to be malodourous and not easily cared for by the nursing staff.

Surgical Excision; End Colostomy; Mucous Fistula. When the inflamed or perforated segment has been mobilised, it takes little extra time to excise it compared with exteriorisation method, and in the author's view this should be done. The question of what should be done with the proximal and distal ends of the colon is a separate issue. Various alternatives exist. If there is a reasonable length of sigmoid colon it may be possible to bring the distal end out as a mucous fistula while the proximal end of the colon is used in the formation of an end colostomy.

This procedure has gained a distinct place in the management of complicated diverticular disease (Roxburgh et al, 1968; Taggart, 1974; Eng et al, 1977; Liebert and De Weese, 1981). This operation requires more expertise than is required for the first stage of a classical three-stage approach. It involves mobilisation and resection of an inflamed colon in a potentially haemorrhagic field.

Concern has often been expressed about the technical problems associated with the procedure. The inflamed colon may be adherent to other pelvic organs but with care it can usually be safely separated. Oedema may facilitate dissection of the tissue planes and mobilisation of the colon.

Segmental Excision; End Colostomy; Closure of Distal Stump (Hartmann's Operation). Because the mesentery of patients with diverticular disease tends to be short, it is often not possible to bring out the distal end to the surface of the abdomen as described above. This is especially true if the patient is obese or if the perforation is low down in the sigmoid colon. In such circumstances, the distal end can be oversewn as in the Hartmann operation and the proximal colon brought out as an end colostomy. In all of these procedures it is best to avoid opening up the retrorectal space in an attempt to achieve extra length as this mobilisation predisposes to the potential hazard of sepsis spreading to the retrorectal area.

Recently Einenstat et al (1983) reported their experience of the use of the Hartmann procedure in the surgical management of complicated diverticular disease (perforation, abscess formation, obstruction, and fistula formation). The mortality rate in 44 patients treated by this method was 4.5 percent.

Paul Mikulicz Procedure. Although in a minority of cases this procedure might be feasible, it is not usually possible in patients with diverticular disease to have sufficient length of colon to achieve a double-barrelled colostomy after excision of the inflamed and perforated segment.

The primary aim of the four procedures

mentioned, is to save the life of an ill and often elderly patient in the midst of an emergency situation. A further aim is to achieve a satisfactory state of health to allow restoration of the bowel continuity at a subsequent date. A bonus associated with these methods is that the number of stages is reduced to two. The operations, especially surgical excision, end colostomy, and mucous fistula and Hartmann's operation continue to gain popularity as alternatives to the classical three-stage procedure.

Primary Resection and Anastomosis. Numerous surgeons have advocated this approach on the premise that it not only eradicates the septic focus but achieves bowel continuity at the time of the initial operation. It is true that in some series reasonable results have been achieved by experienced surgeons who have been operating on well-selected cases. This procedure has a limited place in the management of perforated diverticular disease, for example, where there is a small localised abscess between the leaves of the mesentery.

It cannot, however, be too strongly emphasised that the risk of anastomotic breakdown and leakage is considerable if primary anastomosis, unprotected by a proximal colostomy is undertaken in the presence of frank sepsis in a shocked and hypotensive patient. Mortality rates in patients who developed an anastomotic leak after a single-stage resection and anastomosis has been as high as 80 percent.

In view of the clinical and experimental evidence confirming that an anastomosis undertaken in a septic field has a greatly increased risk of dehiscence, most surgeons avoid single-stage resection and anastomosis in these circumstances. Furthermore, lack of mechanical bowel preparation preoperatively adversely affects the anastomosis in the postoperative phase.

It is true that concomitant transverse colostomy gives a measure of protection to the anastomosis but it does not eliminate the risk of anastomotic leak as considerable faecal material may be present between the site of anastomosis and the colostomy. The operation of primary resection and anastomosis also takes longer than the surgical options mentioned above.

In order to acquire adequate lengths of residual bowel to achieve a join-up without tension it may be necessary to mobilise the splenic flexure, thus increasing the risk of further subphrenic contamination. Opening up the presacral space during mobilisation of the rectum is liable to increase the incidence of sepsis in that region. In addition, if a protective colostomy is included, the procedure can no longer be classified as one-stage and thus has little advantage to claim over a policy of immediate resection but delayed anastomosis until the time of the second operation.

SUGGESTED POLICY. The author's recommendation, applicable in most cases, is to excise the perforated segment as expeditiously as possible, bringing out the proximal colon as an end colostomy. The distal transection is made just below the rectosigmoid junction and oversewn, the closed end of the rectum being hitched to the sacral promontory. If faecal material is present it should be removed from the peritoneal cavity using moist sponges. Any friable necrotic material is excised and the peritoneal cavity thoroughly irrigated with copious amounts of warm saline. Antibiotics, which were commenced preoperatively as soon as the diagnosis was made, are continued for at least 1 week.

When the time comes to reestablish bowel continuity, this is most readily achieved using a circular stapling device from which the anvil has been removed to allow the passage of the shaft through the top of the rectal stump, elimi-

nating the need for a purse string suture at the rectal end. After passage through the top of the end of the stump, the anvil is reattached for its insertion into the mobilised descending colon in which a purse string suture has been inserted. This approach simplifies the restoration of bowel continuity after the Hartmann procedure, which admittedly is not always the most straightforward of operations.

Fistula

Fistulae associated with diverticular disease of the colon may communicate with internal organs or the external body surface. They may arise spontaneously as a result of the inflammatory complications of the disease itself or they may result from operative intervention in the disease process.

Colocutaneous Fistula

An external fistula may arise spontaneously on those extremely rare occasions when a paracolic abscess points and ruptures in the left iliac fossa. More often the fistula occurs after incision and drainage of a left lower quadrant abscess which is itself in communication with the colonic lumen via a ruptured diverticulum. A rare variety of colocutaneous fistula may arise when a paracolic abscess spreads downward and rup-

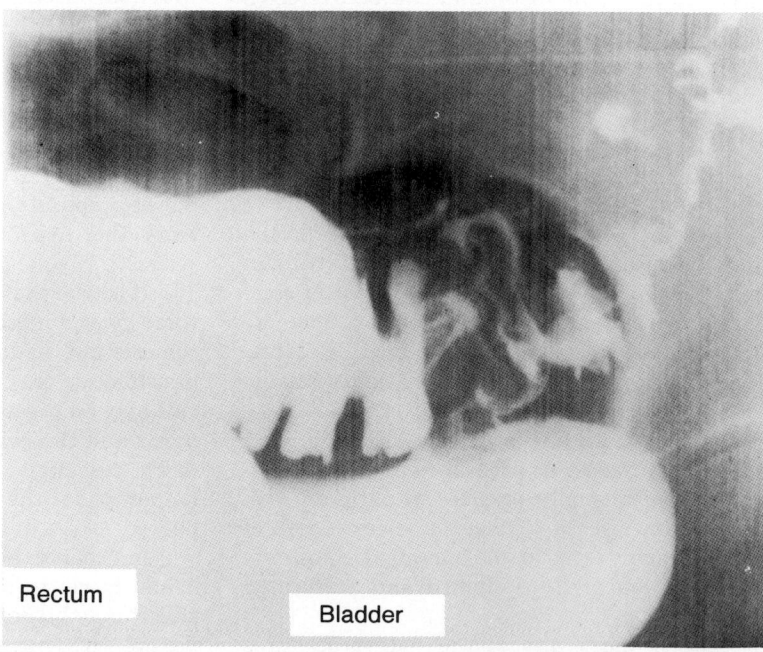

Figure 50–12. Colovesical fistula. Barium has passed from the sigmoid colon through a distinct tract into the urinary bladder.

Rectum

Bladder

tures through the levator ani into the ischiorectal fossa, necessitating drainage. In patients who have had resection of the colon for diverticular disease, a colocutaneous fistula may result from the breakdown of the anastomotic line.

The management of a colocutaneous fistula depends on the nature of the circumstances under which it has arisen. If the leakage is slight and there is no evidence of spreading peritonitis then a conservative approach is desirable. If, however, the leakage is considerable then a transverse colostomy should be established without delay. Most fistulae will heal if there is no distal obstruction. When the inflammatory reaction has settled, examination by barium enema will clarify whether or not there is narrowing at the site of the defect. It is important to determine if an adequate colonic lumen has been maintained before considering colostomy closure.

Colovesical Fistula

The most common internal fistula associated with diverticular disease is the colovesical variety (Fig. 50–12). The patient is usually male, in whom interconnection has occurred between the apex of an inflamed fairly mobile sigmoid loop and the bladder. In women, interposition of the uterus between the sigmoid colon and the bladder has a protective role. The patient may present with symptoms suggestive of urinary trace infection or, in more advanced cases, may describe the actual passage of air or faeces per urethra.

Cystoscopy usually reveals an inflamed area in the upper part of the bladder but a fistula is not always seen. Occasionally, a large intercommunication between the colon and the bladder may be visualised.

A barium enema will confirm the presence of diverticular disease and in some cases will demonstrate the passage of contrast medium into the bladder. If the fistula is small, contrast may not pass into the bladder. Likewise, contrast medium may fail to pass from the bladder into the colon during cystographic examination but in some instances contrast medium may outline the large intestine (Fig. 50–13). Because

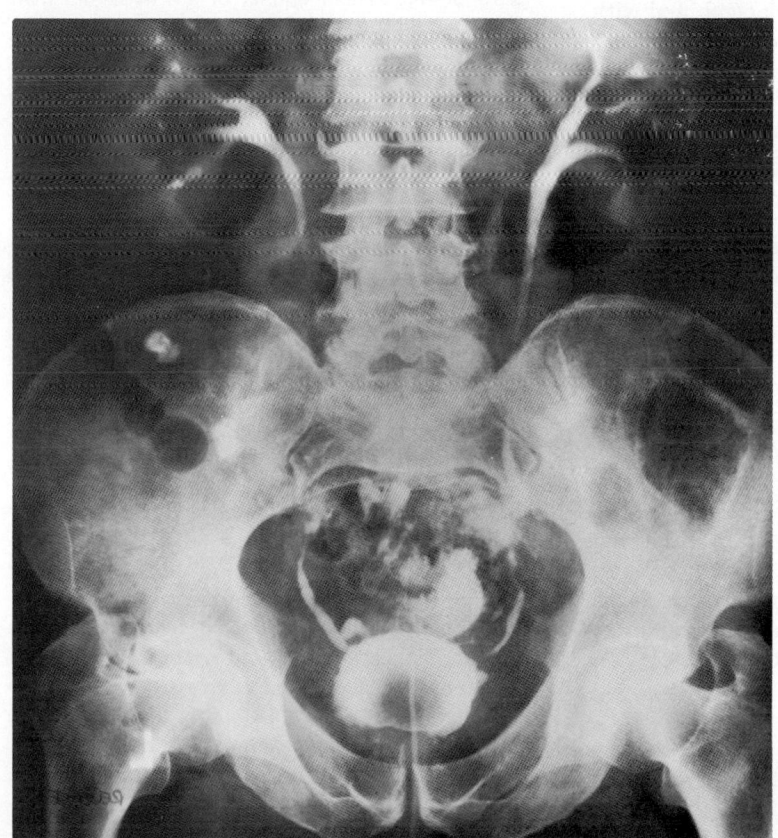

Figure 50–13. Intravenous urogram demonstrating a communication between the urinary bladder and the large intestine in a patient with diverticular disease of the colon.

these fistulae rarely heal spontaneously, surgical correction is usually advisable in all cases that are fit for major surgical intervention. It is often possible to undertake a one-stage resection, particularly if the inflammatory reaction is limited and noninflamed, pliable bowel is available proximally and distally for the formation of a colonic anastomosis. After mobilisation of the colon from the bladder, the latter is sutured with chromic catgut and urethral catheter drainage maintained for 10 days.

In some cases the inflammatory reaction in the pelvis is too advanced to proceed to one-stage resection and anastomosis. In such circumstances a preliminary proximal colostomy is carried out and a period of 2 or 3 months allowed to elapse before proceeding to resection. Although the preliminary operation does facilitate the resolution of associated pelvic inflammation, the fistula rarely heals until resection has been undertaken.

In the treatment of colovesical fistulae it is vitally important to excise the affected segment of the colon with reanastomosis of healthy colonic tissue because lesser procedures, such as division of the fistulous track combined with simple closure of the bladder and colon, are almost certain to fail.

Coloenteric Fistulae

When the colon becomes inflamed with diverticular disease it is not uncommon for a loop of the small bowel to become adherent and to become part of an inflammatory mass, particularly if a paracolic abscess has developed. In these circumstances an intercommunication may develop between the large and small intestines (Fig. 50–14).

In the surgical management of such fistulae, an en bloc resection of the segments of affected colon and small bowel is undertaken and anastomosis of both the enteric and colonic components completed. It is only in cases of advanced sepsis and gross abscess formation that one might judge it prudent to delay the colonic anastomosis until a later date. However, even in these circumstances it is evident that the small bowel continuity should be restored at the initial operation.

Colovaginal Fistula

This rare variety of fistula may arise spontaneously following sepsis in the pelvis secondary

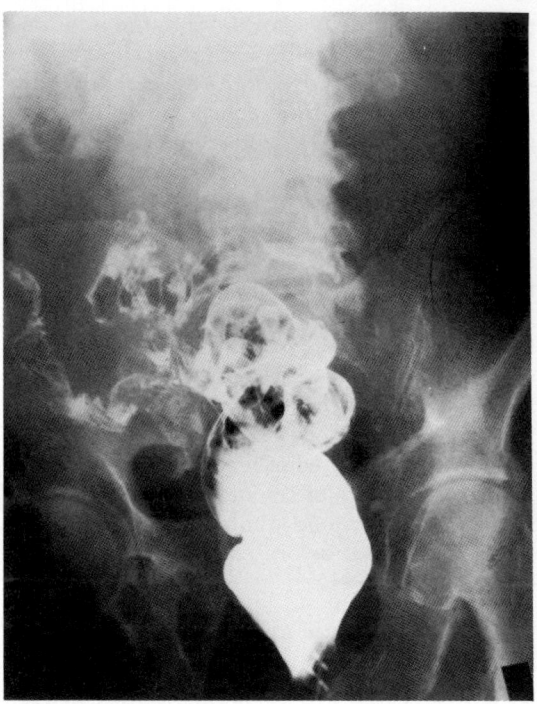

Figure 50–14. Barium enema of a 79-year-old man showing a fistula between the pelvic colon and the ileum, about 15 cm from the ileocaecal junction. Multiple diverticula are present in the pelvic colon. There is considerable stenosis at the site of the fistula and little barium passed into the colon proximal to it.

to diverticular disease or alternatively it may be the sequel to operative procedures. Depending on the circumstances it may be possible to resect the diverticular segment and perform an end-to-end anastomosis as an initial procedure with or without a temporary transverse colostomy.

Intestinal Obstruction

Intestinal obstruction associated with diverticular disease of the colon may be partial or complete and may involve either the colon or the small bowel. It is not uncommon for an acute inflammatory stenosing type of lesion or a large paracolic abscess associated with mural inflammation to lead to marked narrowing or complete occlusion of the sigmoid colon. Alternatively, an enteric loop may become adherent to or incorporated in a diverticular inflammatory mass, resulting in small bowel obstruction.

Patients with complete intestinal obstruction will require surgery when electrolyte correction and fluid replacement have been achieved. The choice of surgical procedure depends on the operative findings. The most widely practiced initial procedure has been formation of a right transverse loop colostomy with a view to resection of the stenosed diverticular segment as a second stage and colostomy closure usually as a third stage. In recent years there has been a move by numerous surgeons to proceed at the time of the initial operation to the excision of an obstructing inflammatory sigmoid mass. This having been achieved, it is the usual practice to delay an anastomosis until a subsequent date. Dudley et al (1980) have described a method of on-table orthograde irrigation of the proximal colon following resection, in order to clear it of faeces and hence proceed to primary anastomosis.

At the time of laparotomy when a mass is found in the sigmoid region it may be difficult to determine whether the lesion is due to diverticular disease alone or to carcinoma of the colon or even to co-existent carcinoma in a diverticular segment. Sometimes it is not possible to make the distinction with confidence until the lesion has been resected and the excised segment of colon opened up.

If a decision has been made to perform a transverse colostomy as the initial step in the management of an obstructing mass in the distal colon and doubt remains as to the exact nature of the lesion, then an early barium enema when the patient has recovered sufficiently may help to clarify the problem. Further information may be obtained by colonoscopy in the postoperative period. If there is still lingering doubt about the differential diagnosis then undue delay before the second stage should be avoided.

Haemorrhage

Acute massive haemorrhage may be alarming for the patient and family. A large amount of blood varying in colour from a fairly bright red to dark maroon may be passed. In older patients massive haemorrhage of colonic origin is likely to be due to either diverticular disease or angiodysplasia. Acute bleeding may also occur in ischaemic colitis but the blood loss is seldom massive. Less severe degrees of blood loss may be due to infective or inflammatory causes, internal haemorrhoids, polypi, or solitary rectal ulceration. The possibility of blood collecting in the rectum above a competent anal sphincter should be borne in mind. The presence of diverticula in a patient presenting with rectal bleeding may be coincidental and not necessarily the actual cause of the haemorrhage. Hence, care must be taken to make a correct diagnosis, including in the differential diagnosis, the possibility of the upper gastrointestinal (GI) source. Patients with severe colonic bleeding require blood replacement by intravenous transfusion.

Proctoscopy and sigmoidoscopy will aid in the elimination of other acutely bleeding lesions in the distal large bowel. A good functioning sucker may be necessary if a reasonably adequate view is to be obtained. If these investigations do not reveal a source of haemorrhage and severe colonic bleeding continues, then emergency angiography is indicated. In those cases in whom blood loss is continuing at a rate of more than 0.5 ml/min it is usually possible to demonstrate intraluminal extravasation of blood. Angiography aids in the differentiation from angiodysplasia in which vascular tufts may be seen, particularly in the caecal region or right colon during the capillary phase and premature filling of veins may be demonstrable during the venous phase. A barium enema undertaken subsequent to arteriography may be expected to demonstrate the colonic diverticula when present. However, they may not be the source of bleeding. Diverticula are present in about 25 percent of the patients who have angiodysplasia as a cause of the colonic bleeding. In patients with bleeding due to diverticular disease the haemorrhage is as likely to come from the right colon as from the left and it frequently occurs in the absence of inflammation.

Control of Haemorrhage

The intraarterial infusion of vasopressin into the appropriate mesenteric vessel via the angiographic catheter is often effective in controlling, at least temporarily, the bleeding associated with diverticular disease (Athanasoulis et al, 1975; Welch et al, 1978). Administration is continued for 24 to 48 hours. Alternatively, transcatheter embolisation using Gelfoam or Oxycel has been advocated by Goldberger and Bookstein (1977) but this procedure is not without risk in that it may cause intestinal ischaemia.

Surgery is indicated in cases of continuing

or recurrent severe haemorrhage. The procedure undertaken depends on the general condition of the patient and whether or not the site of bleeding has been accurately determined during preoperative investigations.

If the bleeding site has been clearly identified preoperatively an operation to resect the appropriate segment is the procedure usually undertaken. If the exact site of origin within the colon has not been determined then subtotal colectomy is recommended. However, a more radical approach in good risk patients has been advised by Welch et al in 1980 who recommend subtotal colectomy in the following circumstances: (1) diverticular bleeding in which the diverticula are scattered throughout the colon, (2) angiodysplasia of the right colon and extensive diverticulosis on the left colon, and (3) massive bleeding from an undertermined site within the colon.

A mortality of 11 percent among 43 patients who underwent subtotal colectomy with massive rectal bleeding was reported by Drapanas et al (1973) and death rates of up to 50 percent have been recorded in some series. Although this extensive procedure is necessary for bleeding from an undetermined colonic site, it seems preferable to undertake a more limited procedure with a lower mortality and morbidity where localisation has been possible. Patients who have had considerable blood loss and blood replacement and who undergo emergency resection of unprepared bowel loaded with faecal material are prone to a higher than usual complication rate in any event.

ELECTIVE SURGERY

Resection

When acute complications occur, there may be no reasonable alternative to urgent surgical intervention. In nonacute circumstances the indications for surgery may also be clear cut, but sometimes they are less well defined and, indeed, may be relative rather than absolute. Numerous factors such as the patient's general state of health, age, as well as the local clinical features and radiologic findings may dictate the best policy.

Some surgeons advocate surgical resection of the diseased segment after one episode of acute diverticulitis. However, it must be stressed that many patients make an excellent recovery following an acute attack of diverticulitis and they may have few symptoms or even remain completely asymptomatic for several years afterward (Parks, 1969).

Those patients who have two or more inflammatory attacks within the space of a few years should normally be considered for surgery unless there are clear contraindications on other grounds.

Patients who develop a palpable phlegmonous mass in the left lower quadrant or in the left side of the pelvis often require surgery. Although this type of lesion may respond to conservative regime it is not uncommon for such patients to require subsequent removal of the affected segment. Gross deformity of the sigmoid on radiologic examination, especially if associated with significant clinical features, weigh in favour of a surgical extirpation.

Most patients with internal fistulae are dealt with electively. A high proportion are suitable for one-stage resection but as described earlier, a minority of cases require preliminary diversionary colostomy.

The development of urinary symptoms in a patient with diverticular disease may indicate irritation of the bladder or of the ureter by an inflamed sigmoid colon and may be a premonitory warning that a colovesical fistula is developing.

Resection should be considered in those cases with repeated episodes of mild to moderate haemorrhage, especially if co-existing with other symptoms such as left lower quadrant pain or altered bowel habit.

Specific consideration should also be given to the patient who presents earlier in life, i.e., under the age of 55 years with signs of acute inflammation. Most of these individuals will require operation.

A clear indication for surgery exists in those patients in whom it has not been possible to exclude with certainty the possibility of a carcinoma in the diverticular segment. With improved radiology and the aid of colonoscopy such cases are less numerous nowadays but where doubt exists surgical intervention must be undertaken. Initially a decision is made as to whether the lesion found at laparotomy is due to diverticular disease alone or whether the segment could also be the seat of a carcinoma. When the case evidently is one of diverticular disease then a less radical dissection of the mesentery and lymphatic drainage field is undertaken. If doubt exists as to the possibility of carcinoma, this can be clearly assessed when the specimen has been removed and opened up so that the mucosal aspect can be inspected. If there is any indication of malignancy then the operative field can be reexamined and if necessary a wider excision may be undertaken.

Morbidity Following Operations for Diverticular Disease. The postoperative morbidity following resection for diverticular disease tends to be higher than that of a comparable group of patients with carcinoma. This may be accounted for by a number of factors. First, the diverticula may be associated with considerable inflammation, adherence, and chronic fibrosis and there may even by an existing paracolic abscess. Second, shortening of the colon and mesocolon means that there is less remaining colon for anastomosis following resection unless the splenic flexure is mobilised. It is important to avoid tension on the anastomosis. Third, the muscle abnormality associated with diverticular disease leads to narrowing of the lumen and friability of the wall. Hence, attempts to anastomose the abnormal thickened segment is fraught with danger. The importance of the proper choice of the proximal and distal lines of section cannot be overemphasised. Fourth, it is evident that in many instances diverticula are present in the proximal portion of the colon and the presence of one of these at the level of the line of anastomosis may compromise the safety of the junction. Finally, leakage after resection for diverticular disease is more hazardous than dehiscence after resection for carcinoma. This may be due in part to the inherent muscle abnormality or alternatively to the prior existence of sepsis.

Sigmoid Colomyotomy

The colomyotomy operation was introduced by Reilly in 1964 in an effort to relieve symptoms mainly of muscular origin in poor risk patients. It was not designed to replace resection as the treatment of choice for the vast majority of patients who require definitive surgery for complicated diverticular disease.

The technique in which a longitudinal incision through one of the antimesenteric taenia is deepened so that the circular fibres are divided and the submucosa is allowed to bulge into the myotomy wound is analogous to the Heller operation used in the treatment of achalasia. The colomyotomy incision is continued along the entire length of the narrowed segment caused by the thickened and contracted muscle wall. This usually measures at least 20 to 30 cm and may be as much as 60 cm in length. At the distal extremity, the myotomy extends beyond the rectosigmoid junction onto the upper rectum.

The operation is relatively bloodless, any small bleeders being controlled by pressure. Diathermy and ligation are best avoided because these are more liable to lead to small areas of tissue necrosis. After initial longitudinal incision using a scalpel, Reilly preferred to deepen the wound by carefully snipping with fine scissors. He stressed the importance of being conservative rather than drastic as fine submucosal blood vessels traversely are readily mistaken for muscle fibres. The mucosa itself, which is often thrown into corrugations in diverticular disease, is easily penetrated. Should the mucosa be breached it is claimed that the defect may be safely closed with catgut sutures. Some surgeons also recommend that omentum or appendix epiploicae is sewn over the areas.

It must be stressed that the colomyotomy is by no means a minor operation. Penetration of the mucosa at the time of surgery especially if it is goes unrecognised, may have catastrophic consequences. Another concern relates to the possibility of subsequent necrosis, even though the mucosa and submucosa may appear satisfactory at the time of operation. Mucosal breakdown leads to septic complications and faecal fistula formation.

Some early reports were reasonably encouraging (Reilly, 1971; Smith et al, 1971). There have been no well-designed clinical trials in which colomyotomy has been compared with surgical resection in a comparable group of patients requiring definitive surgery. On the other hand there have been discouraging features related to the operation in that the reduction of intraluminal pressure achieved initially by division of the circular fibres is not maintained and within 3 years, pressures tend to revert to preoperative levels (Smith et al, 1971; Prasan and Daniel, 1971).

The author does not advocate colomyotomy for the following reasons:

1. If the symptoms are mainly of muscular origin, considerable relief can usually be

achieved by dietary and medical measures without surgery.

2. Experimental evidence indicates that the initial reduction of intraluminal pressure achieved by the operation of colomyotomy is not maintained in the long term.

3. The main problems in diverticular patients are usually inflammatory in nature for which colomyotomy has little to offer in that the diverticular bearing segments remain in situ and complications are still liable to occur.

4. Colomyotomy does not have a convincing role in the management of bleeding diverticular disease.

5. The morbidity and mortality associated with resection would probably not be all that dissimilar from sigmoid myotomy if comparable noncomplicated cases were to be operated upon.

Transverse Taeniamyotomy

On account of the shortening of the taeniae coli, Hodgson (1974) carried out a series of transverse incisions at intervals of 2 cm on the thickened antimesenteric taeniae. As the incision does not expose the mucosa, the operation is safer than longitudinal myotomy. However, because it is not readily possible to divide the mesenteric taenia in similar fashion, lengthening of the colon by the procedure must be limited.

Pescatori and Castiglioni (1978) reported reduced motility indices and clinical improvement following transverse taeniamyotomy. However, the operation has not found a clearly established place in the surgical treatment of diverticular disease.

CAECAL DIVERTICULA

Diverticula of the caecum may occur in association with widespread colonic diverticulosis, as part of it as well, and, therefore, as an acquired lesion. Alternatively, a distinct entity of congenital origin known as solitary diverticulum of the caecum may be encountered. The pouch, which has smooth muscle in its wall, is usually situated medially near the ileocaecal valve. It is usually symptomless unless diverticulitis occurs (Anderson, 1947; Tagart, 1953; Anscombe et al, 1967).

The differential diagnosis of caecal diverticulitis include appendicitis, right-sided colonic carcinoma, solitary caecal ulcer, Crohn's dis-

ease, actinomycosis, carcinoid, tuberculosis, and chronic cholecystitis.

Right-sided diverticulitis may closely mimic appendicitis. Patients with diverticulitis tend to have a longer symptomatic period and they may have intermittent or chronic symptoms. The pain of caecal diverticulitis begins and remains in the right side of the abdomen or the right lower quadrant rather than commencing in the periumbilical region. Vomiting is uncommon in acute right-sided diverticulitis. Massive haemorrhage may occur. If a mass is present the differential diagnosis includes carcinoma, appendix abscess, Crohn's disease, and actinomycosis.

Schapira et al (1958) emphasised the features essential to making a diagnosis of caecal or right-sided diverticulitis on barium contrast examination:

1. Discrete extramural or intramural filling defect
2. Limited distensibility of the bowel wall
3. Spasm, oedema, and fixation of the bowel wall
4. Demonstration of a diverticulum or diverticula
5. An intact mucosal pattern without intraluminal filling defect
6. Absence of a constant intraluminal filling defect

The correct diagnosis of caecal diverticulitis is not often made preoperatively. If at laparotomy a mass is present it may be difficult or impossible to exclude malignancy until resection has been undertaken.

If an uncomplicated solitary diverticulum is discovered at the time of operation for some other condition, then it may be simply invaginated and buried using a purse string suture inserted in the caecal wall.

BIBLIOGRAPHY

Anderson L: Acute diverticulitis of the caecum. Surgery 22:479, 1947

Anscombe AR, Keddie NC, et al: Solitary ulcers and diverticulitis of the caecum. Br J Surg 54:553, 1967

Arfwidsson S: Pathogenesis of multiple diverticula of the sigmoid colon in diverticular disease. Acta Chir Scand (suppl):342, 1964

Athanasoulis CA, Baum S, et al: Mesenteric arterial infusion of vasopressin for haemorrhage from colonic diverticulosis. Am J Surg 129:212, 1975

Botsford TW, Zollinger RM Jr, et al: Mortality of the surgical treatment of diverticulitis. Am J Surg 121:702, 1971

Brodribb AJM: Treatment of symptomatic diverticular disease with a high fibre diet. Lancet 1:664, 1977

Case JT: The roentgen demonstration of multiple diverticula of the colon. AJR 2:654, 1914

Cruveilhier J: Traité d'Anatomie Pathologique Générale, vol 1. Paris: Bailliére, 1849, p 593

de Quervain F: Zur Diagnose der erworbenen Dickdarmdivertikel und der sigmoiditis diverticularis. Deutsche Ztschr f chir 128:67, 1914

Drapanas T, Pennington DG, et al: Emergency subtotal colectomy: Preferred approach to management of massively bleeding diverticular disease. Am Surg 177:519, 1973

Dudley HA, Racliffe AG, et al: Intra-operative irrigation of the colon to permit primary anastomosis. Br J Surg 67:80, 1980

Einenstat TE, Rubin RJ, et al: Surgical management of diverticulitis: The role of the Hartmann procedure. Dis Colon Rectum 26:429, 1983

Eng K, Ranson JHC, et al: Resection of the perforated segment: A significant advance in treatment of diverticulitis with free perforation or abscess. Am J Surg 133:67, 1977

Findlay JM, Smith AN, et al: Effects of unprocessed bran on colon function in normal subjects and in diverticular disease. Lancet 1:146, 1974

Goldberger LE, Bookstein JJ: Transcatheter embolisation for the treatment of diverticular haemorrhage. Radiology 122:613, 1977

Graser E: Über multiple falschi Darmdivertikel in der Flexina Sigmoidea. Munch med Wschr 46:721, 1899

Greif JM, Fried G, et al: Surgical treatment of perforated diverticulitis of the sigmoid colon. Dis Colon Rectum 23:483, 1980

Habershon SO: Observations on diseases of the alimentary canal. Philadelphia: Blanchard and Lea, 1857

Hannan CE, Knightly JJ, et al: Diverticular disease of the colon in younger age group. Dis Colon Rectum 4:419, 1961

Hodgson J: Effect of methyl cellulose on rectal and colonic pressures in treatment of diverticular disease. Br Med J 3:729, 1972

Hodgson J: Transverse taenia myotomy: A new surgical approach for diverticular disease. Ann R Coll Surg Engl 55:80, 1974

Horner JL: Natural history of diverticulosis of the colon. Am J Dig Dis 3:343, 1958

Hughes LE: Complications of diverticular disease: Inflammation, destruction and bleeding. Clin Gastroenterol 4:147, 1975

Hyland JMP, Taylor I: Does a high fibre diet prevent the complications of diverticular disease? Br J Surg 67:77, 1980

Jones S: Transactions of the Pathological Society of London. 10:131, 1859

Liebert CW Jr, De Weese BM: Reconstructing colonic continuity after the Hartmann operation. South Med J 13:1576, 1980

Liebert CW, De Weese BM: Primary resection without anastomosis for perforation of acute diverticulitis. Surg Gynecol Obstet 152:30, 1981

Madden JL: Primary resection and anastomosis in the treatment of preforated lesions of the colon. Am Surg 31:781, 1965

Marxer OA: Duff House Papers, vol 1. London: O.U.P., 1923, p 165

Mayo WJ: Diverticulitis of the large intestine. JAMA 69:781, 1917

Mayo WJ, Wilson LB, et al: Acquired diverticulitis of the large intestine. Surg Gynecol Obstet 5:8, 1907

Morson BC: The muscular abnormality in diverticular disease of the sigmoid colon. Br J Radiol 36:385, 1963

Moynihan BFA: The mimicry of malignant disease in the large intestine. Edinb Med J 21:228, 1907

Ornstein MH, Littlewood ER, et al: Are fibre supplements really necessary in diverticular disease of the colon? A controlled clinical trial. Br J Surg 282:1353, 1981

Ouriel K, Schwartz SI: Diverticular disease in the young patient. Surg Gynecol Obstet 156:1, 1983

Painter NS: Diverticular Disease of the Colon. London: Heinemann Medical Books, 1975

Painter NS, Almeida AZ, et al: Unprocessed bran in the treatment of diverticular disease of the colon. Br Med J 2:137, 1972

Painter NS, Burkitt DP: Diverticular disease of the colon: A deficiency disease of Western civilisation. Br Med J 2:450, 1971

Painter NS, Truelove SC: The intraluminal pressure patterns in diverticulosis of the colon. Gut 5:365, 1964

Painter NS, Truelove SC, et al: Segmentation and localisation of intraluminal pressures in the human colon with special reference to the pathogenesis of colonic diverticula. Gastroenterol 49:169, 1965

Parks TG: Post-mortem studies on the colon with special reference to diverticular disease. Proc Roy Soc Med 61:932, 1968

Parks TG: Natural history of diverticular disease of the colon. A review of 521 cases. Br Med J 4:639, 1969

Parks TG: Rectal and colonic studies after resection of the sigmoid for diverticular disease. Gut 11:121, 1970

Parks TG: Effects of indigestible fibre on colonic activity in diverticular disease, in Pichlmaier H, Grundmann R (eds): Surgery of the Colon and Rectum. Stuttgart: Springer-Verlag, 1980, p 63

Parks TG, Connell AM: Motility studies in diverticular disease of the colon. II. Effect of colonic and rectal distension. Gut 10:538, 1969

Parks TG, Connell AM: A comparison of the motility in the irritable colon syndrome and diverticular disease of the colon. Rendic di Gastroenterol 4:12, 1972

Pemberton J de J, Black BM, et al: Progress in the surgical management of diverticulitis of the sigmoid colon. Surg Gynecol Obstet 85:523, 1947

Pescatori M, Castiglioni GC: Sigmoid motility and clinical results after transverse taeniamyotomy for diverticular disease. Br J Surg 65:666, 1978

Prasad JK, Daniel O: Recurrence of high intracolonic pressure following sigmoid myotomy. Br J Surg 58:304, 1971

Rankin FW, Brown PW: Diverticulitis of the colon. Surg Gynecol Obstet 50:836, 1930

Reilly M: Sigmoid myotomy. Proc Roy Soc Med 57:556, 1964

Reilly M: Sigmoid myotomy for diverticular disease of the colon. Modern Trends in Surgery, vol 3. London: Butterworths, 1971, p 109

Roxburgh RA, Dawson JL, et al: Emergency resection in treatment of diverticular disease of the colon complicated by peritonitis. Br Med J 3:465, 1968

Ryan P: Emergency resection and anastomosis for perforated sigmoid diverticulitis. Br J Surg 45:611, 1958

Schapira A, Leichtling JJ, et al: Diverticulitis of the caecum and right colon: Clinical and radiographic features. Am J Dig Dis 3:351, 1958

Schmidt GT, Lennard-Jones JE, et al: Crohn's disease of the colon and its distinction from diverticulitis. Gut 9:7, 1968

Smith AN, Giannokos V, et al: Late results of colomy-otomy. J Roy Coll Surg Edinb 16:276, 1971

Smithwick RH: Experience with surgical management of diverticulitis of the sigmoid. Ann Surg 115:969, 1942

Spriggs EI, Marxer OA: Multiple diverticula of the colon. Lancet 1:1067, 1927

Staunton MDM: Treatment of perforated diverticulitis. Br Med J 1:916, 1962

Tagart REB: Acute phlegmonous caecitis. Br J Surg 40:437, 1953

Tagart REB: General peritonitis and haemorrhage complicating colonic diverticular disease. Ann R Coll Surg Engl 55:175, 1974

Virchow R: Virchows Archiv für Pathologische Anatomie und Physiologie und für. Klinische Medizin 5:335, 1853

Welch CE, Athanasoulis CA, et al: Haemorrhage from the large bowel with special reference to angiodysplasia and diverticular disease. World J Surg 2:73, 1978

Welch CE, Ottinger LW, et al: Haemorrhage from the colon and rectum, in Manual of Lower Gastrointestinal Surgery. New York: Springer-Verlag, 1980, p 204

Wells C: Diverticula of the colon. Br J Radiol 22:449, 1949

Wilson LB: Diverticula of the lower bowel: Their development and relationship to carcinoma. Ann Surg 53:223, 1911

51. Granulomatous Colitis and Ulcerative Colitis

Arthur H. Aufses, Jr.

GRANULOMATOUS COLITIS

Introduction

Granulomatous inflammatory bowel disease (IBD) was established as a distinct entity in 1932 with the publication of the classic paper by Crohn et al, from the Mount Sinai Hospital. In that report, 14 patients were presented, all of whom had disease limited to the terminal ileum. It was to take almost 30 years for the recognition that this illness, now known as Crohn's disease, could affect the colon without involvement of the small bowel, and to separate granulomatous colitis from ulcerative colitis, a disease first described by Wilks and Moxon in 1875.

By the late 1920s ulcerative colitis was a well-recognized disease. It was known to start in the rectum and then extend proximally. In retrospect granulomatous colitis had probably been described by Bargen and Weber prior to the Crohn et al paper. In 1930, the former authors reported 23 patients in a paper entitled "Regional Migratory Chronic Ulcerative Colitis." Seventeen of their patients had a normal rectum and three had perianal fistulas, both features now known to be typical of granulomatous colitis. The authors termed this illness "segmental colitis." In 1934 Colp, also from the Mount Sinai Hospital, described regional ileitis with involvement of the cecum (ileocolitis), but for many years Crohn and colleagues felt that those patients who had involvement of both the ileum and colon had both granulomatous ileitis and ulcerative colitis.

It remained for Wells in 1952 to point out that segmental colitis was probably a form of Crohn's disease rather than a variant of ulcer-ative colitis. He stated "this segmental colitis is a colonic form of Crohn's disease." Finally, in 1960, the classic paper of Lockhart-Mummery and Morson separated granulomatous from ulcerative colitis and firmly established the pathologic criteria necessary for the definitive diagnosis of each. They stated "we have never seen Crohn's disease and ulcerative colitis in the same patient."

Crohn's disease is now recognized as an illness that can affect all parts of the gastrointestinal (GI) tract from mouth to anus. In the past 25 years there has been a marked increase in the number of patients with this illness with involvement of the colon. At the present time approximately 70 percent of all Crohn's disease patients have involvement of some portion of the colon. Granulomatous colitis without other obvious intestinal involvement afflicts approximately 15 percent of all patients with Crohn's disease. New cases of granulomatous colitis now equal or outnumber new cases of ulcerative colitis. Since the incidence of ulcerative colitis has remained relatively static and since better pathologic recognition alone cannot account for the difference, there has been an absolute increase in the number of patients afflicted with granulomatous colitis.

Pathology

The pathology of granulomatous colitis is similar to that of Crohn's disease anywhere in the GI tract. The earliest macroscopic lesion is the apthoid ulcer. This ulcer, 1 to 2 mm in diameter, is a sharply punched out area surrounded by edematous but otherwise normal appearing mucosa. These lesions may disappear or coalesce

1351

to form the larger irregular longitudinal ulcers characteristic of Crohn's disease. There is a chronic inflammatory reaction most marked in the edematous submucosa which extends through the entire bowel wall. The colonic wall becomes thickened and rigid with narrowing of the lumen but usually not to the same extent as in small bowel Crohn's disease. As a consequence, obstruction is not as common in colonic Crohn's disease as it is in cases with ileal or jejunal involvement.

The linear ulcers intersect with transverse fissures, leading to the typical cobblestoning of the mucosa, as is seen elsewhere in the GI tract. Fistulas can develop and are most numerous in the perianal area and may involve the bladder, vagina, adjacent loops of bowel, and the abdominal wall. Skip areas (areas of involvement separated by normal bowel) are common and help to distinguish this from ulcerative colitis. In contrast to ulcerative colitis, Crohn's colitis appears to begin in most patients on the right side of the colon with the rectum spared in about 20 percent of patients. The regional lymph nodes are markedly enlarged and the creeping fat is also a characteristic of Crohn's colitis.

The gross pathologic findings of Crohn's colitis include its segmental nature, with rectal sparing, involvement of the terminal ileum with Crohn's disease, the cobblestone appearance of the mucosal surface, the marked thickening and fibrosis of the bowel wall, and the marked lymph node enlargement and the "creeping fat," as well as internal fistulas between loops of bowel and other organs.

Histologically, Crohn's colitis shows a transmural involvement with an increased submucosa and the presence of granulomata in any of the bowel wall layers or the lymph nodes are characteristic and pathognomonic of the disease. Ulcerative colitis has an inflammatory process that is limited to the mucosa and submucosa (except in toxic megacolon); the submucosa is normal in thickness and vascularity in the prominant feature. Crypt abscesses occur in over 70 percent of the patients, granulomata are very rare, and fissures and fistulas are also very rare.

Utilizing the above criteria approximately 90 percent of cases will be correctly diagnosed as either Crohn's colitis or ulcerative colitis. There will remain, however, a small group (about 10 percent) in whom a definitive diagno-sis cannot be made. These cases will be labeled "indeterminate colitis."

The characteristic microscopic feature is the presence of the epithelioid granuloma with giant cells. However, it must be pointed out that granulomas are only found in about 50 percent of patients and then only after a careful microscopic search of many sections. On the other hand, the granulomas may be found in rectal and sigmoidoscopic biopsies from apparently normal appearing mucosa.

Clinical Manifestations

The symptomatology of granulomatous colitis may be similar to that of Crohn's disease of the distal ileum or may mimic ulcerative colitis or any of the other colitidies. Fever, crampy abdominal pain, and intermittant diarrhea are the usual manifestations of the illness. On the other hand, perianal disease or growth retardation in children may precede the onset of intestinal symptoms by months or years. In Crohn's colitis, pain is usually colicky, especially when obstructive phenomena are present, and fever is present in a large percentage of patients, especially with involvement of the distal small bowel. A mass is frequently present in the right lower quadrant. Diarrhea is not usually a major problem, the clinical course is usually slowly progressive, and the disease rarely spreads in the absence of operative intervention. Crohn's colitis usually starts in the right colon, skip areas are common, and the rectum is spared and appears normal in a substantial number of patients. Occult bleeding is not infrequent, but massive bleeding is rare.

Ulcerative colitis on the other hand is characterized by urgency and tenesmus, with frequent small diarrheal stools usually containing blood. This disease tends to start in the rectum and slowly progresses proximally to involve the entire colon. Fever is unusual and a mass is rarely palpable unless a carcinoma has developed. Clinically ulcerative colitis is characterized by relapses and remissions in the majority of patients. About one quarter of the patients with ulcerative colitis will have a chronic continuous disease. Acute fulminating disease occurs in from 5 to 8 percent of patients.

Some form of perianal disease will be found in the vast majority of patients with Crohn's colitis, reaching almost 100 percent when the rectum is involved. Perianal disease may occur in ulcerative colitis but is less likely to be a major complication of the disease. Toxic megacolon is a complication of both diseases, but occurs approximately twice as frequently in ulcerative colitis as in Crohn's disease. Although cholelithiasis and nephrolithiasis occur in both illnesses they are more common in Crohn's colitis.

Diagnostic Studies

Sigmoidoscopy. Sigmoidoscopy in Crohn's colitis will reveal areas of normal mucosa, discrete apthoid ulceration or the irregular ulcers so characteristic of this illness. Ulcerative colitis, on the other hand, shows continuous change, with pinpoint ulcerations, friability, and a diffuse, hyperemic, ulcerated mucosa. Biopsy in Crohn's disease is more likely to show edema and fibrosis especially in the submucosa and the findings of granuloma confirm the diagnosis. Rectal biopsy in ulcerative colitis is more likely to show only diffuse mucosal inflammatory change.

Radiology. Once the diagnosis of colitis is suspected, confirmation can usually be obtained by appropriate roentgen examination. Marshak et al have pointed out that the conventional filled colon examination with barium should be done first. This will define the nature of the lesion in the vast majority of instances. However, should the initial examination be normal then the double air-contrast barium enema is necessary since this will identify the small apthous ulcers when they are the only manifestation of the colonic process. Using the two techniques, the roentgen examination diagnosis of inflammatory bowel disease is highly accurate. If the rectum is involved, confirmation can be obtained by sigmoidoscopic examination and biopsy. If the rectum appears normal and biopsies of the rectum are negative, colonoscopy is indicated.

Radiographically, the features characteristic of granulomatous bowel disease are similar in the small bowel and the colon. These findings include aphthoid ulcers, larger punched-out ulcers, small nodular defects, skipped lesions, contour defects, longitudinal ulcers, transverse fissures, eccentric involvement of the bowel wall, pseudodiverticula, narrowing and stricture for-

mation, cobblestone-like mucosal pattern, and sinus tracts and fistulas. Segmental involvement is typical of Crohn's colitis and the rectum is often normal. Internal fistulas and strictures are frequent. If the terminal ileum is involved in the classic changes of Crohn's disease then the colitis is Crohn's colitis.

Radiologic features of ulcerative colitis include shallow mucosal ulceration and pseudopolyp formation. The disease is generally symmetric and continuous with the rectum, which is involved in almost every instance. Fistulas are rare and strictures are uncommon. A stricture developing in a patient with ulcerative colitis must be considered to be a carcinoma until proven otherwise. Involvement of the terminal ileum may occur, but this is primarily "backwash ileitis," which is characterized by a dilated bowel with diffuse inflammatory change.

Differential Diagnosis

By far the most important disease requiring differentiation from granulomatous colitis is ulcerative colitis. Lockhart-Mummery and Morson, Korelitz et al, and Cook and Dixon have elaborated the criteria necessary to separate the two diseases, and Roth has clearly and concisely summarized the differential features. Differential features may be found in the clinical course, the radiographic appearance, and both the macroscopic and histologic appearance of the specimens.

Both granulomatous colitis and ulcerative colitis must be distinguished from other colitidies, most of which are infectious. Amebiasis may closely mimic inflammatory bowel disease but can usually be diagnosed by stool examination, colonic mucosal biopsy, and serologic testing. The "gay bowel syndrome" of venereally transmitted intestinal infection may be responsible for proctitis in various forms—straightforward rectal gonorrhea, traumatic and gonorrheal proctitis, herpes virus proctitis, and *Chlamydia proctitis*. Tuberculosis and typhoid fever have long been known to produce lesions that resemble Crohn's disease and must be considered in the differential diagnosis. Recently new infectious agents have been recognized as an etiologic agent for enterocolitis. The first of these, campylobacter fetus subspecies jejunum, may produce endoscopic, radiologic, and histologic features indistinguishable from ulcerative or granulomatous colitis. Clostridium difficile has been shown to be the agent responsible for most cases of antibiotic-induced pseudomembranous colitis. Finally, and especially in children with an acute inflammatory disease involving the terminal ileum and the colon, *Yersinia* may be the causative agent.

In the older patient with inflammatory disease of the colon, ischemic colitis, diverticulitis, and lymphoma of the colon may produce changes difficult to distinguish from Crohn's disease.

Treatment

Differentiation between granulomatous colitis and ulcerative colitis is crucial to patient management. The clinical course, susceptibility to complications, the need for surgery, operative procedures available, and prognosis for long-term health are dependent upon the correct diagnosis.

Medical Management

With the rare exception of a patient who presents with a catastrophic emergency, almost all patients referred for surgery for Crohn's colitis will have been on medical therapy, usually for a prolonged period of time. This therapy will probably have included trials of sulphasalazine, steroids, antibiotics, including metronidazole and possibly immunosuppressive agents. Any or all of these may have been effectual at one point or another. The National Cooperative Crohn's Disease Study concluded that prednisone was of significant value especially in patients with small bowel involvement, and that sulphasalazine was also effective in the treatment of active symptomatic Crohn's disease, especially with predominant colonic involvement.

Surgical Management

Patients coming to operation for granulomatous colitis have the same indications for operation as patients with primary small bowel disease but the incidence of the complications varies with the location of the inflammatory disease. Whereas obstruction, fistula, and abscess formation account for approximately 80 percent of the indications for surgery in small bowel disease, obstruction is much less common in colitis. With primary colon involvement, chronic dis-

ability, failure of medical management, and growth retardation in children and adolescents become important indications for operation. Severe perianal disease may necessitate colonic surgery as well as the occasional severe hemorrhage. Perforation is rare but when diagnosed requires emergency laparotomy. Toxic megacolon is managed nonoperatively with surgery reserved for those who do not respond to nonoperative therapy.

Preoperative Diagnosis. Preoperative preparation is important, as many of these patients will be in a moderately to severely debilitated condition. If the patient is 10 percent or more below ideal body weight, he or she may well benefit from a period of enteral or parenteral nutritional repletion prior to operation. Laxatives must be used with caution. Immunosuppressive agents should be stopped and patients on immunosuppressives should not be operated upon if there is any depression of leukocytes. Patients on steroids must have the steroids continued through the operative period.

General Principles. The principles of operative management in Crohn's disease with colonic involvement are the same as with primary small bowel involvement. Whenever feasible the diseased bowel should be resected. When the rectum has been spared, colectomy and ileoproctostomy is the procedure of choice. If the rectum is involved in addition to the rest of the colon then total proctocolectomy is required. In the rare instance where the rectum is the only site of colonic involvement, abdominoperineal resection with colostomy may be employed. If the patient has severe perianal disease, removal of the rectum will probably be required. If the disease is primarily right sided, right hemicolectomy may be sufficient. When proctocolectomy is required a standard Brooke's everting ileostomy should be performed. Because of the high incidence of recurrence in the small bowel, continent ileostomy is not indicated and because of the transmural nature of the disease, mucosal stripping with ileoanal anastomosis is not feasible.

In those instances where resection is not feasible because of the severe illness of the patient or because of severe local disease in the form of large abscesses or extensive retroperitoneal involvement, preliminary diversion is an effective means of causing subsidence of the inflammatory reaction to allow for later, easier resection.

The potential use of ileostomy to "put the bowel at rest" and allow healing was proposed by Truelove et al in England in 1965 and shortly later by Oberhelman et al. The latter subsequently gave up the procedure but a recent favorable report by Harper et al from the Oxford group suggests that ileostomy alone may have a significant role to play in the management of Crohn's colitis.

Toxic Megacolon. Although more common in ulcerative colitis, toxic megacolon certainly occurs in granulomatous colitis. It probably represents a reaction to extensive transmural inflammation and is usually accompanied by a sealed-off perforation of the bowel. This perforation is most commonly seen in the splenic flexure or in the sigmoid. Toxic megacolon is usually seen in the course of a fulminating exacerbation of the disease and is the presenting complaint in a small number of patients. The immediate management should be nonsurgical. Decompression of the distended bowel can usually be accomplished with a combination of intestinal intubation, parenteral antibiotics and steroids, intravenous alimentation, and frequent turning of the patient to reposition the colonic gas. If this fails, then urgent or emergent surgery will be required and will usually consist of diversion and/or resection of the involved bowel.

Associated Carcinoma. In recent years much attention has been focused upon the increased risk of patients with Crohn's disease to develop carcinoma. Although less than 50 cases of colorectal cancer have been reported in association with granulomatous colitis, there is no doubt that the patient suffering from Crohn's disease is at increased risk. Although the first case of carcinoma in conjunction with ulcerative colitis was not recognized and published until 50 years after the description of ulcerative colitis, the first case of carcinoma of the colon in granulomatous disease was reported in 1948, just 16 years after the Crohn, Ginzburg, and Oppenheimer paper. A recent study concludes that carcinoma of the colon and rectum in association with Crohn's disease is six times that of the average population. This incidence is still less than one half of the incidence seen in universal ulcerative colitis. In Crohn's disease, as in ulcerative colitis, the carcinomas may be multiple. In addition there appears to be a propensity for the malignancy to develop at the site of a fistula. These patients also appear to be at risk for the development of squamous cell or cloacogenic anal carcinoma. As in small bowel Crohn's disease, the bypassed loop is also at risk and cases have been reported of rectal cancer developing in patients with a rectal stump.

Recurrence. By far the most serious concern for the physician in caring for a patient with Crohn's disease is the propensity for the disease to recur following operation. Although the disease affects the entire GI tract from mouth to anus, it is rare for new areas of disease to appear clinically or radiographically in the absence of surgical intervention.

As one reads reports of recurrences of Crohn's disease, one must be aware of the definition employed by the author of the report. These definitions have ranged from clinical recurrence, to radiographic recurrence, to pathologically proven recurrence at a second operation. Clearly if proctocolectomy is performed, then a recurrence must be the development of Crohn's disease in or proximal to an ileostomy stoma. Even here the recurrence rates have ranged from 3 to 45 percent. One must be certain that the "recurrence" in the prestomal area is actually Crohn's disease and not secondary to stricture formation at the site of the stoma. If the granulomatous colitis is segmental and only a segmental resection is performed, or if the rectum has been spared and a colectomy and ileoproctostomy have been performed, then the recurrence rates in the remaining rectum colon have been reported to be as high as 90 percent after 15 to 20 years of follow-up. Despite these high rates of recurrence, however, almost all surgeons today would agree that if the rectum has been spared, ileoproctostomy should be performed. Recurrence is not certain and, should one occur, the patient will have been spared a number of years without an ileostomy.

In conclusion, one can state that despite the fact that the patient with granulomatous colitis may present as a formidable clinical problem, a combination of judicious medical and surgical management can restore that patient to good health with a life of good quality.

ULCERATIVE COLITIS

Introduction

Ulcerative colitis remains a disease of unknown etiology primarily afflicting thousands of young people every year. The disease, which may also have its onset in the older years, almost always begins in the rectum and may occasionally remain localized as an ulcerative proctitis. Most often, however the disease extends proximally and either remains limited to the rectum and sigmoid (proctosigmoiditis) or extends proximally to the left transverse colon (left-sided colitis). The most common presentation of the disease involves the entire colon (universal colitis). The ileum may be involved by "backwash ileitis" in a small percentage of cases but the findings in the ileum are not of significance and are almost always readily distinguished from Crohn's disease.

Clinical Manifestations

The symptoms are primarily diarrhea containing mucus and blood with pain that is usually predefecatory in nature and associated with urgency and tenesmus. The illness is characterized by remissions and exacerbations, but about 25 percent of cases are of a chronic continuous nature. On occasion, an acute fulminating course may bring a patient to surgery within a month of the onset of symptoms.

Perianal disease does occur, but this is not anywhere near the problem that it is in granulomatous colitis. Other extraintestinal complications include rheumatoid spondylitis and rheumatoid arthritis, erythema nodosum, and pyoderma gangrenosum. Abnormalities of liver function are seen in a fair percentage of patients, and a significant number of cases of sclerosing cholangitis have been reported in patients with ulcerative colitis.

Carcinoma of the colon in association with ulcerative colitis was first described in 1925 by Crohn and Rosenberg and is now recognized as one of the most feared complications of the illness. The major risk factors in the genesis of carcinoma are the length of time that the disease has been present and universal disease. Other risk factors that have been identified are early onset and continuous symptoms. Carcinoma rarely develops before 10 years of colitis but by the twenty fifth year of illness will have affected one third of those at risk. Unfortunately, carcinoma will frequently develop in a patient who appears to have "burnt out" disease and is essentially asymptomatic. Carcinoma does occur in left-sided disease but with only one half the incidence seen in universal disease and after a longer time interval.

Pathology

The pathology is that of an acute inflammatory reaction primarily of the mucosa, with degeneration of crypt epithelium and infiltration of the lamina propria. Crypt abscesses are characteristic but may be seen in other inflammatory disorders of the bowel. There is marked vascular congestion accounting for the reddened, inflamed, friable mucosa that is seen on endoscopic examination. The submucosa is involved, but except for the devastating complication of toxic megacolon, the inflammation spares the muscularis and serosal aspect of the bowel. With improvement in symptoms the inflammatory process resolves, and attempts at mucosal regeneration lead to the development of pseudopolyps, and mucosal bridging.

In time the mucosa becomes atropic and hypertrophy of the muscularis leads to shortening of the bowel. Fibrotic strictures may develop, but any stricture must be viewed with grave suspicion because of the possibility of the development of carcinoma. The differential diagnosis includes Crohn's colitis, ischemic colitis when the disease has its onset in the later years of life, amebiasis, and the other specific infectious colitides.

Treatment

The management of this disease remains primarily medical. The medications usually employed are antidiarrheals, azulfadine, and steroids given orally or rectally. As in Crohn's colitis, surgery is reserved for those patients who either cannot be managed successfully with nonoperative therapy or suffer one of the serious complications that occur in this illness. These complications include acute fulminating disease, hemorrhage, perforation, toxic megacolon, and carcinoma. Unlike granulomatous colitis, one can speak of surgical cure in ulcerative colitis. Once the entire colonic mucosa has been removed, the patient cannot suffer a recurrence and is cured of the illness.

When the ulcers penetrate through the muscularis mucosa into the muscular layers, the condition may become fulminating, and toxic megacolon may develop. If this complication does not respond to intubation, intravenous alimentation, and intravenous steroid therapy, surgery may be required as an emergency. Perforation can occur but this complication is fortunately rare.

The evolution of the surgical therapy of chronic ulcerative colitis provides a unique window through which to view the problems of patients with this illness. In looking at the historical aspect of any segment of abdominal surgery, one must bear in mind that our knowledge of intestinal intubation, and fluid and electrolyte management started to evolve in the late 1930s and 1940s. The early sulfa drugs became available in the late 1930s and, although introduced to the armed forces during World War II, penicillin did not become generally available to the civilian population until 1945. Streptomycin, the first of the antibiotics with any effect against gram-negative organisms, was introduced in the 1950s and our current antibiotics are phenomena of the past decade.

In 1913, Brown of St. Louis was the first to perform an ileostomy for a patient with ulcerative colitis. Unfortunately this procedure alone was insufficient to stem the tide of the colonic disease, since in most instances the inflammatory response continued even after fecal diversion. In addition the problems associated with an ileostomy created a disease unto itself.

Over the succeeding years surgeons began to add colectomy to the operation of ileostomy but it was usually performed in multiple stages because of the severe debility of the patient population requiring surgery and the inability of the surgeon to deal with hypovolemia and infection.

With the development of our understanding of fluid and electrolyte management, mortality rates began to fall; with the advent of antibiotics, sepsis and wound infection became more managable. However, the problems associated with the management of the ileostomy remained and skin excoration and stricture of the stoma were extremely common problems.

In 1951, Warren and McKittrick published their landmark paper in which they pointed out that "ileostomy dysfunction" was due to the serositis which developed when the ileostomy merely was left extending beyond the abdominal wall and allowed to mature by the gradual downgrowth of mucosa to meet the skin. Within a year Brooke published his paper on the technique of eversion and immediate maturation of the ileostomy stoma. This technique has enabled surgeons to *create* an ileostomy, which in most patients allows them to lead a normal life free of stoma problems.

At the same time Ripstein et al published their series of 72 patients who underwent simultaneous subtotal colectomy and ileostomy, with only 3 deaths. This operation became the standard for therapy of the usual case of ulcerative colitis. Abdominal perineal resection was then performed at a second operation. Today total proctocolectomy is usually performed as a single-stage procedure.

In 1966, in an attempt to eliminate permanent ileostomy, Aylett reported 300 patients who had total abdominal colectomy and ileoproctostomy performed for ulcerative colitis. This operation had the advantage of eliminating ileostomy but the disadvantage of anastomosing ileum to diseased rectum. In Aylett's hands this proved to be a successful procedure for the vast majority of his patients but most other surgeons could not duplicate his results. The concerns were the continued large number of stools, the development of progressive disease in the rectal segment, and the subsequent development of carcinoma in the remaining rectum.

Despite the fact that the Brooke ileostomy provides a very satisfactory stoma, easily cared for and with few late problems requiring reoperation, surgeons have continued to search for a method to eliminate the need of an appliance. In 1969 Kock, in the first of a series of papers, described the development of a continent reservoir that was created immediately proximal to the ileostomy stoma. This reservoir, with a nipple valve constructed in the outflow tract, allows for total continence in the vast majority of patients. The ileostomy stoma is sewn flush with the abdominal wall, it does not protrude, and the patient need not wear an appliance. The patient catheterizes the reservoir with a plastic tube at regular intervals and remains continent for the remainder of the day and night. The procedure can be fraught with technical difficulties, and revisions are necessary in a high percentage of cases.

The latest procedure to achieve good results in ulcerative colitis (and also in patients with familial polyposis) is total abdominal colectomy with mucosal stripping of the rectum and ileo-anal anastomosis. This procedure takes its origin from the pioneer work of Ravitch and Sabiston in 1947. The operation was performed primarily for polyposis and Hirschsprung's disease, but in 1977 Martin reported its use in 17 patients with ulcerative colitis. The procedure as performed today includes a reservoir constructed proximal to the ileoanal anastomosis. A temporary ileostomy is advisable to protect the anastomosis.

This operation provides the ideal solution for the patient with ulcerative colitis. It includes total removal of the colon and the mucosa that is at risk for the development of carcinoma, evacuation by the normal route through the anal canal, and the elimination of the need to wear an external appliance.

Despite effective medical management, the majority of patients with ulcerative colitis will eventually come to surgery because of continuous disease, frequent relapses, occasional fulminating complications, or the development of dysplasia or frank carcinoma. For the patient requiring surgery, there are now several procedures available that will enable that individual to lead an essentially normal life.

Associated Carcinomas

The carcinomas are often multifocal and are distributed throughout the colon. They are frequently at an advanced stage when diagnosed. Treatment consists of total proctocolectomy and ileostomy. The prognosis was always considered bleak, but the reports of Hughes et al, Greenstein et al, and Ritchie et al note a survival similar to colon cancer arising in otherwise normal bowel.

A most notable advance in the management of ulcerative colitis was the recognition of "dysplasia" or "precancer" in colonic biopsies by Morson and Pang. These epithelial changes, found in random biopsies of the colon taken at multiple sites, are often associated with unsuspected carcinoma which may be at a distance from the biopsy site.

It is now possible to establish a reasonable, cost-effective, surveillance program to detect early cancer in ulcerative colitis patients. Starting at about the eighth year of disease, colonoscopy with multiple biopsies is performed. If the biopsies are all normal colonoscopy should be repeated every 2 years. If mild or moderate dysplasia is found at any time, then repeat endo-scopy is indicated in 6 to 12 months. Should the biopsies then be normal, the patient can return to a 12- to 24-month cycle. If dysplasia continues to be present consideration must be given to proctocolectomy. If high-grade dysplasia is found at any time, surgery should be recommended. It is hoped that by such a program cancers will be detected at an earlier stage, with a resultant higher cure rate.

BIBLIOGRAPHY

Granulomatous Colitis

Bargen JA, Weber HM: Regional migratory chronic ulcerative colitis. Surg Gynecol Obstet 50:964, 1930

Colp R: A case of non-specific granuloma of the terminal ileum and cecum. Surg Clin North Am 14:443, 1934

Cook MD, Dixon MD: An analysis of the reliability of detection and diagnostic value of various pathologic features in Crohn's disease and ulcerative colitis. Gut 14:255, 1973

Crohn BB, Ginzburg L, et al: Regional ileitis; A pathologic and clinical entity. JAMA 99:1323, 1932

Crohn BB, Rosenberg H: The sigmoidoscopic picture of chronic ulcerative colitis (non-specific). Am J Med Sci 170:220, 1925

Harper PH, Truelove SC, et al: Split ileostomy and ileocolostomy for Crohn's disease of the colon and ulcerative colitis: A 20 year survey. Gut 24:106, 1983

Korelitz BI: Carcinoma of the intestinal tract in Crohn's disease: Results of a survey conducted by the National Foundation for Ileitis and Colitis. Am J Gastroenterol 78:44, 1983

Korelitz BI: Present DH, et al: Recurrent regional ileitis after ileostomy and colectomy for granulomatous colitis. N Engl J Med 287:110, 1972

Lockhart-Mummery HE, Morson BC: Crohn's disease (regional enteritis) of the large intestine and its distinction from ulcerative colitis. Gut 1:87, 1960

Marshak RH, Lindner AE, et al: Granulomatous colitis. Mt Sinai J Med 46:431, 1979

Mekhjian HS, Switz DM, et al: Clinical features and natural history of Crohn's disease. Gastroenterology 77:898, 1979

Nugent FW, Veidenheimer MC, et al: Prognosis after colonic resection for Crohn's disease of the colon. Gastroenterology 65:398, 1973

Oberhelman HA, Kohatsu S, et al: Diverting ileostomy in the surgical management of Crohn's disease of the colon. Am J Surg 115:231, 1968

Roth JLA: Diagnosis and differential diagnosis of chronic ulcerative colitis and Crohn's colitis, in Kirsner JB, Shorter RG (eds): Inflammatory Bowel Disease, 2 edt. Philadelphia: Lea and Febiger 1980, p 166

Sachar DB, Walfish JS: Crohn's disease and ulcerative colitis, in Gitnick GL (ed): Current Gastroenterology, vol 2. New York: John Wiley, 1982

Summers RW, Switz DM, et al: National cooperative Crohn's disease study: Results of drug treatment. Gastroenterology 77:847, 1979

Truelove SC, Ellis H, et al: Place of a double-barrelled ileostomy in ulcerative colitis and Crohn's disease of the colon: A preliminary report. Br Med J 1:150, 1965

Warren S, Sommers SC: Cicatrising enteritis (regional ileitis) as a pathologic entity. Am J Pathol 24:475, 1948

Wells C: Ulcerative colitis and Crohn's disease. Ann R Coll Surg Engl 11:105, 1952

Wilks S, Moxon W: Lectures on Pathological Anatomy. London: Churchill Livingstone, 1895

Ulcerative Colitis

Aylett SO: Three hundred cases of diffuse ulcerative colitis treated by total colectomy and ileo-rectal anastomosis. Br Med J 1:1001, 1966

Brooke BN: The management of an ileostomy including its complications. Lancet 2:102, 1952

Brown JY: The value of complete physiological rest of the large bowel in the treatment of certain ulcerative and obstructive lesions of this organ, with descriptions of operative technique and report of cases. Surg Gynecol Obstet 16:610, 1913

Crohn BB, Rosenberg H: The sigmoidoscopic picture of chronic ulcerative colitis (non-specific). Am J Med Sci 170:220, 1925

Greenstein AJ, Janowitz HD, et al: The extraintestinal complications of Crohn's disease and ulcerative colitis: A study of 700 cases. Medicine 55:401, 1976

Greenstein AJ, Sachar DB, et al: Cancer in universal and left-sided ulcerative colitis: Factors determining risk. Gastroenterology 77:290, 1979

Greenstein AJ, Sachar DB, et al: Patterns of neoplasia in Crohn's disease and ulcerative colitis. Cancer 46:403, 1980

Grundrest SF, Fazio V, et al: The risk of cancer following colectomy and ileorectal anastomosis for extensive mucosal ulcerative colitis. Ann Surg 193:9, 1981

Hughes RG, Hall TJ, et al: Prognosis of carcinoma of the colon and rectum complicating ulcerative colitis. Surg Gynecol Obstet 146:46, 1978

Kewenter J, Ahlman H, et al: Cancer risk in ulcerative colitis. Ann Surg 188:824, 1978

Kock NG: Intraabdominal "reservoir" in patients with permanent ileostomy. Preliminary observation on a procedure resulting in fecal "continence" in five patients. Arch Surg 99:223, 1969

Martin L, LeCoultre C, et al: Total colectomy and mucosal proctectomy with preservation of continence in ulcerative colitis. Ann Surg 186:477, 1977

Morson BC, Pand LSC: Rectal biopsy as an aid to cancer control in ulcerative colitis. Gut 8:423, 1967

Nugent WF: Surveillance of patients with ulcerative colitis. National Symposium on Colorectal Tumors, Washington, DC, September 19–21, 1983

Ravitch MM, Sabiston DC: Anal ileostomy with preservation of the sphincter. Surg Gynecol Obstet 84:1095, 1947

Ripstein CB, Gavin-Miller G, et al: Results of the surgical treatment of ulcerative colitis. Ann Surg 135:14, 1952

Ritchie JK, Hawley PR, et al: Prognosis of carcinoma in ulcerative colitis. Gut 22:752, 1981

Thayer WR Jr: Malignancy in inflammatory bowel disease, in Kirsner JB, Shorter RG: Inflammatory Bowel Disease, 2 edt. Philadelphia: Lea and Febiger, 1980, sect 3, no 15, p 265

Warren R, McKittrick LS: Ileostomy for ulcerative colitis: Technique, complications and management. Surg Gynecol Obstet 93:555, 1951

52. Tumours of the Colon

Peter R. Hawley

BENIGN COLORECTAL POLYPS

Polyps of the large bowel are common but the term polyp is purely descriptive, indicating a protuberance of the surface of the mucosa. It may be a flat, raised, sessile lesion or a pedunculated tumour on a stalk. Polyps in the colon may be single, multiple, or present in large numbers, when the term polyposis is used. Polyps can be classified on a histologic basis as adopted by the World Health Organisation in Table 52-1 (Morson and Sobin, 1976).

Histologic Types

Metaplastic Polyps. Metaplastic polyps or hyperplastic polyps, as they are sometimes referred to, are probably the most common mucosal polyps seen on sigmoidoscopy. They are slightly raised nodules, the same colour as the normal mucous membrane and they are usually multiple. The aetiology of these polyps is unknown but they may be viral in origin. They come and go, have no malignant potential, and require no treatment. Very occasionally, they will become larger and can be seen as pedunculated polyps up to 1 cm in diameter.

Neoplastic Polyps. These are *adenomatous polyps* and are subdivided into three categories: tubular, tubulovillous, and villous adenomas. The *tubular adenoma*, with the possible exception of metaplastic nodules, is by far the most common tumour in the large bowel. The majority of patients have one or two adenomas but a few patients will have considerably more. They are more commonly pedunculated than sessile. The *villous adenoma*, or papilloma as it used to be known, is commonly more extensive in origin, forming a soft flat tumour that can arise from a large area of mucosa. Villous adenomas are far less common than tubular adenomas and are found in the rectum, the rectosigmoid, and more rarely in the more proximal colon. The *tubulovillous adenoma* is an intermediate type showing some of the features of villous adenoma. It is usually smaller and more compact and often becomes pedunculated.

Malignant Potential Adenomas. All adenomatous polyps of the large bowel are potentially malignant. It has been shown in autopsy studies that the incidence of adenomatous polyps found in the colon increases with age to about 40 percent at the age of 80 years (Arminski and McLean, 1964). The malignant potential of any adenoma increases with its size. In those less than 1 cm in diameter, 1 percent show evidence of invasive cancer on microscopic examination. For those between 1 and 2 cm in diameter, the risk increases to about 10 percent and for those over 2 cm in diameter the risk is almost 40 percent (Muto et al, 1975). However, these findings are of polyps which have been removed from the rectum and sigmoid colon by sigmoidoscopy and large colonoscopic series of polypectomies suggest that the incidence of malignancy is rather less than this in the more proximal parts of the colon. There is also a difference in malignant potential according to the histologic type of the polyp; 5 percent of tubular adenomas removed show evidence of invasive carcinoma whereas 20 percent of villous adenomas show such changes. The intermediate type of tubulovillous adenoma shows an incidence of malignancy of about 12 percent.

Hamartomas. Juvenile polyps have a uniform smooth surface, macroscopically quite unlike the lobulated appearance of the adenoma. When

TABLE 52–1. HISTOLOGIC CLASSIFICATION OF BENIGN COLORECTAL POLYPS

Polyp	Single	Multiple (Polyposis)
Neoplastic Epithelial	Adenoma { Tubular Tubulovillous Villous	Polyposis coli (adenomatosis)
Hamartomas	Juvenile polyp Peutz–Jeghers polyp	Juvenile polyposis Peutz–Jeghers syndrome
Inflammatory	Benign lymphoid polyp	Occasionally multiple in the dysenteries, ulcerative colitis, Crohn's disease, diverticulitis, etc.
Unclassified	Metaplastic (hyperplastic) polyp	Often multiple
Miscellaneous	Leiomyoma Neurofibroma Lipoma Haemangioma	

the polyp is cut across, it contains cystic spaces lined with epithelium and containing mucus. Juvenile polyps occur in infancy and childhood but can be seen occasionally in the adult until the age of 40 years or more. They ulcerate and bleed and have a tendency to undergo autoamputation. The polyps of the Peutz–Jegher syndrome are also hamartomas but have a rather different appearance, showing branching polypoid lesions which histologically demonstrate an outgrowth of the muscularis mucosae covered with normal epithelial elements. Peutz–Jegher polyps are usually multiple and are associated with typical mucocutaneous pigmentation.

Inflammatory Polyps. The single benign lymphoid polyp presents as a submucosal nodule in the lower rectum and cannot usually be diagnosed without removal and histologic evaluation. Multiple inflammatory polyps often occur in severe forms of inflammatory bowel disease. Whenever there is inflammation and ulceration of the large bowel, remnants of oedematous mucous membrane may be left which become partly undermined and give rise to polypoid appearance. After the acute stage, when healing takes place and the underlying mucosa regenerates, these oedematous tags are distorted and often form bizarre polypoid shapes which can resemble pedunculated adenomas.

Miscellaneous Polyps. This group includes the nonepithelial tumours of the bowel which sometimes present as polyps. All are rare and present either as sessile or pedunculated polyps.

Clinical Manifestations

Hamartomatous polyps in children may cause bleeding, which can be quite severe and occasionally may cause attacks of pain and even intussusception. In adults, symptoms from adenomatous polyps depend upon the size and situation of the polyp. Bleeding is usually the only symptom, but large polyps in the rectum and sigmoid colon may prolapse through the anal canal. Polyps in the colon may cause colicky abdominal pain and an alteration of bowel habit, with blood and mucus in the stool. However, many polyps are symptomless and are found on sigmoidoscopic examination when the patient presents with symptoms arising from haemorrhoids, a fissure, or some other anal condition.

Diagnostic Studies

All patients with symptoms suggestive of anal, rectal, or colonic disease should be sigmoidoscoped. If a polyp is found on routine sigmoidoscopy, it should be removed for histologic examination to determine its nature. If several polyps are present, two or three should be removed and if the polyps are adenomas further investigation should be undertaken to exclude other polyps or tumours in the more proximal colon. The incidence of co-existing carcinoma of the large bowel is greater in those patients in whom adenomatous polyps are found. Investigation should be in the form of an air-contrast barium enema or colonoscopy. Whether the surgeon carries out a fibre-optic sigmoidoscopy at the initial

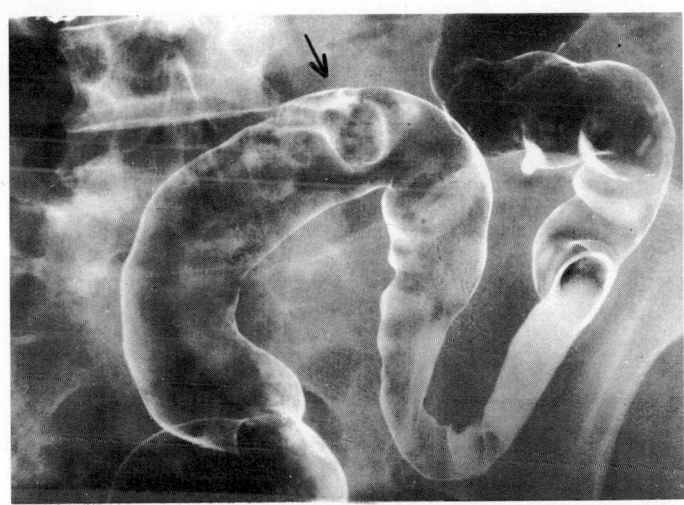

Figure 52–1. X-ray film of a polyp (double-contrast barium enema).

consultation or carries out a barium enema or a colonoscopy will depend to some extent on the facilities available and the inclinations of the surgeon (Fig. 52–1).

Treatment

In adults, polyps discovered within the large bowel should be removed because of the possible risk of malignant change being present or developing in the future. Polyps within 25 cm of the anus can usually be totally removed with biopsy forceps if they are small or by diathermy snare if larger and pedunculated. Pedunculated polyps should always be removed with as much stalk as is safely possible and submitted intact to the pathologist for histologic evaluation. Biopsies from the head of the pedunculated polyp can be misleading and are unnecessary. If a barium enema shows a polyp larger than 5 cm in diameter, colonoscopy should be carried out and the polyp removed. Colonoscopic polypectomy should always be undertaken and there is no justification for the patient to be subjected to a laparotomy and polypectomy as the former procedure is much safer for the patient.

Techniques of Endoscopic Removal

Pedunculated Polyps. Pedunculated polyps in the rectum and lower sigmoid colon may be removed through a proctoscope or sigmoidoscope in the outpatient department. Larger polyps require the use of operating proctoscopes and sigmoidoscopes and a rectal diathermy snare as shown in Figure 52–2. The lower bowel must be emptied by a hypophosphate enema and

suction must be available. Before starting the procedure, check that the wire loop on the snare is intact and can be drawn tight within the sheath when the handle is closed. After passing the proctoscope or sigmoidoscope and getting a clear view, the wire loop is passed around the polyp and then closed over the pedicle. Traction is applied to the snare to lift the pedicle away from the bowel wall and then, with repeated short bursts of diathermy using a low intensity cutting current, the wire is gradually tightened. The pedicle can then be cut through and the polyp removed from the bowel. The site of the pedicle should be carefully examined with a sigmoidoscope to ensure that there is no bleeding and that the polyp has been completely removed. If there is any bleeding, this can be controlled with a diathermy button. The patient can normally leave hospital. If the tumour is large and the pedicle broad-based or the procedure has been difficult, it is wise to keep the patient in hospital for 24 to 48 hours to make sure that there is no reactionary haemorrhage or perforation of the bowel wall.

Pedunculated polyps higher in the colon are best treated by snare removal through a fibre-optic sigmoidoscope or colonoscope. The instrument used will largely depend upon the experience and inclinations of the surgeon but large polyps in the rectum and lower sigmoid are usually best dealt with through a large operating sigmoidoscope than by removal with a fibre-optic instrument.

Large polyps on a long stalk can sometimes be prolapsed down through the anal canal and removed by transfixion and ligation of the pedi-

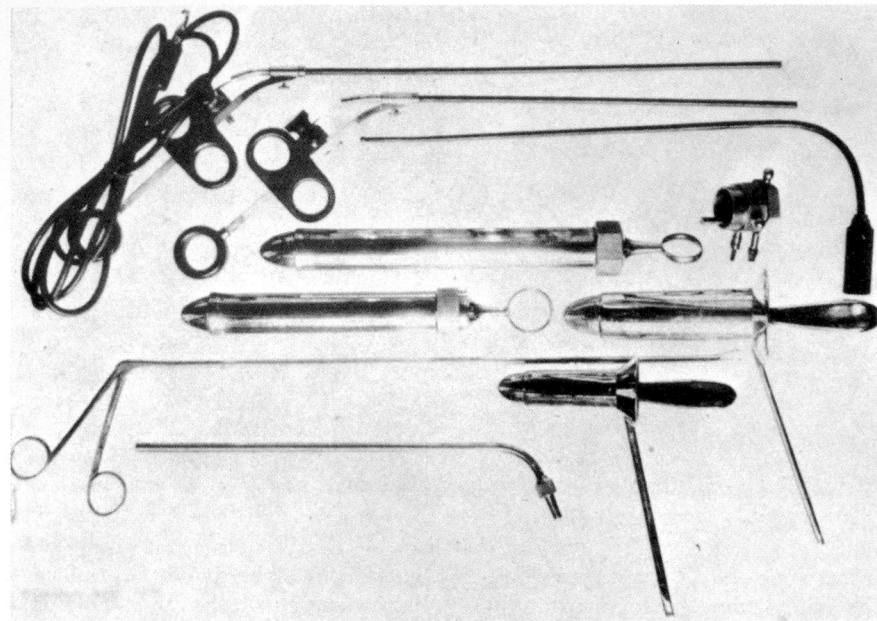

Figure 52–2. Armamentarium for snare removal of rectal polyp. *Top to bottom:* two diathermy snares, diathermy button, two operating sigmoidoscopes, operating proctoscope, swab-holding and biopsy forceps, standard proctoscope, and sucker.

cle. Occasionally, polyps as high as 25 cm will prolapse through the anus by the colon intussuscepting into the rectum. This approach is applicable when it seems inappropriate to remove a polyp with a large broad base but which can be easily snared. The colonoscope is removed, leaving the snare in situ and the polyp can then be drawn down to the rectum or even through the anal canal by the surgeon, who can then transfix and ligate the broad pedicle and remove the polyp.

Operative polypectomy for a pedunculated polyp is never carried out as a primary procedure. If resection is being performed for a carcinoma and an unsuspected polyp is found, which cannot easily be included in the resected specimen, the bowel may be incised longitudinally through the antimesenteric tenia, the polyp delivered and pedicle transfixed and ligated at its base and the polyp removed (Fig. 52–3). The incision in the colon can then be closed transversely or longitudinally (Fig. 52–4). However, it is probably better to carry out the resection and, at a later date, when the anastomosis is healed and the patient recovered from the operation to carry out a colonoscopy and snare removal.

Sessile Villous Adenomas. Sessile villous adenomas almost always occur in the rectum and distal sigmoid colon and are rare in the proximal bowel. They may present as a small tumour 1 or 2 cm in diameter but occasionally will com-

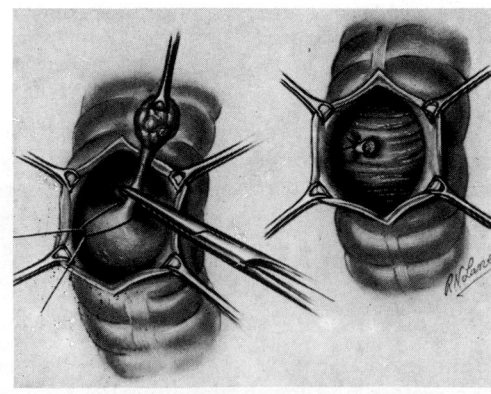

Figure 52–3. Excision of a long pedicled adenoma. (*Source: Adapted from Turell R, Brodman HR: Adenomas of the colon and rectum, in Turell R (ed): Diseases of the Colon and Anorectum, vol 1. Philadelphia: WB Saunders, 1959, p 352, with permission.*)

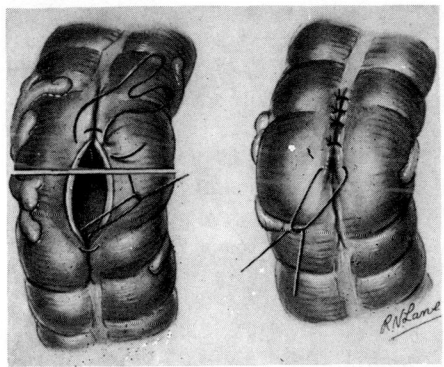

Figure 52–4. Methods of closure of the colotomy incision. Vertical closure of the bowel wall. (*Source: Adapted from Turell, R, Brodman HR: Adenomas of the colon and rectum, in Turell R* (ed): *Diseases of the Colon and Anorectum, vol 1. Philadelphia: WB Saunders, 1959, p 353, with permission.*)

pletely surround the rectum and extend from the anal canal upward for 10 or 12 cm. These sessile tumours can be treated in several ways. Traditionally, they have been biopsied and then treated by fulguration and this is still the best method if the lesion is benign and situated above 10 cm. Below this level, it is much better to remove them endoanally by infiltrating beneath the mucosa with a solution of 1:300,000 adrenaline in saline to lift the lesion off the underlying muscle and then to dissect in the submucosal space and remove the tumour, complete with a small surrounding margin of mucosa. The defect in the mucosa may be closed with a continuous catgut suture or left open to granulate and reepithelialise. In a series from St. Mark's Hospital there was a lower complication and recurrence by per-anal excision than after treatment with diathermy. The recurrence rate was 19 percent. All the recurrences were benign and most occurred within 2 years.

With a large villous adenoma of the rectum there is a high incidence of malignant change and the true nature of the tumour may not be appreciated even on multiple biopsies. The best assessment of the tumour is by careful digital palpation and if any of the tumour feels hard or fixed it is almost certainly malignant. However, excision of the rectum should not be carried out unless the presence of the carcinoma is definitely established. If the tumour on biopsy and clinical evaluation appears to be benign and encircles the rectum below 10 cm, it can usually

be excised completely by a per-anal technique. The wound needs reepithelialising to avoid stricture formation and this may be done by bringing down the upper cut edge of the mucosa to suture to the lower cut edge at the anal canal.

Malignant Polyp. What should be the attitude of the surgeon when a pedunculated polyp, which has been removed through a sigmoidoscope or colonoscope, is reported by the pathologist to contain invasive carcinoma? This implies not simply severe dysplasia in the adenoma but invasion of the cellular elements through the muscularis mucosae into the submucosa. The pathologist can only give adequate advice if all possible histologic information can be obtained. A biopsy or biopsies from the surface of the polyps do not give adequate information. The whole polyp must be carefully blocked and several sections cut through the body and the stalk (Fig. 52–5). Frozen sections are likely to be inadequate and misleading and no further action should be taken until a full report has been received from the pathologist. Necessity for fur-

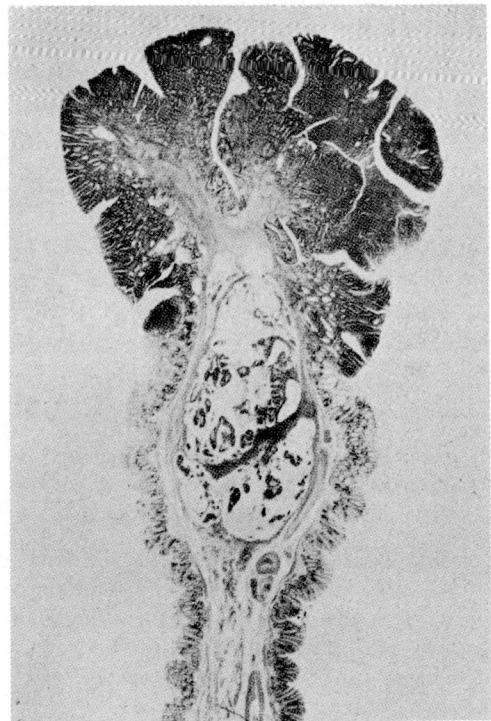

Figure 52–5. A "malignant polyp" showing mucus-secreting carcinoma invading the stalk of the polyp.

ther treatment should be determined according to the following criteria:

1. Grade of malignancy of the carcinoma. The pathologist should report whether the carcinoma is of a high grade or undifferentiated tumour, a low grade well-differentiated tumour, or of an average grade of malignancy.
2. The depth of invasion of the carcinoma into the stroma of the polyp.
3. The presence or absence of a free margin between the carcinoma and the line of excision or diathermy burn.

Experience has shown that, in pedunculated polyps, carcinoma is nearly always of a low or average grade of malignancy and the incidence of nodal metastases in such tumours is approximately 1 percent. However, very rarely the carcinoma can be of a high grade of malignancy when the incidence of lymph node metastases, even without involvement of the stalk, will be in the order of 10 percent. The surgeon will also wish to know whether the tumour is confined to the polyp and its stalk with a good free margin or whether the carcinoma extends to the level of transection. Two other factors will play a part in determining if further action should be taken:

1. The site of the polyp in the rectum or colon will determine the ease with which the patient can be kept under careful observation. If the polyp is in the rectum and the area of excision can be kept under easy view and palpation, local recurrence can be picked up at an early stage but it will be more difficult to determine this if the polyp is in the more proximal colon.
2. The age and general condition of the patient are obviously important factors, as the risk of a radical procedure must be weighed against the possibility of recurrence. Hence, there is a need for individual assessment of each patient; there are no general rules to be laid down.

Many considerations need to be taken into account in deciding the further treatment of a patient from whom a malignant polyp has been removed, and close collaboration between the pathologist and surgeon is necessary. Experience has shown that a conservative policy is justified, particularly in cases where the carcinoma is of an average grade of malignancy and confined to the stalk with a clear margin or resection. Only in those cases where the carcinoma is of a high grade of malignancy and local excision doubtful should a radical procedure be undertaken if the patient is fit for operation. Too many surgeons overreact to the pathologist reporting early invasive carcinoma and many unnecessary operations are undertaken.

After local excision of a villous tumour, the pathologist will examine the whole specimen carefully. If there are any areas of invasive carcinoma the surgeon must decide whether to carry out an anterior resection or an excision of the rectum.

INTESTINAL POLYPOSIS

General Principles

Table 52–1 shows that there are several conditions in which large numbers of polypoid tumours may be found throughout the large bowel. All of them are rare, with familial adenomatosis being the least uncommon (Bussey, 1970). It is a hereditary disease, characterised by the development within the large bowel of large numbers of adenomatous polyps (Figs. 52–6 and 52–7). There are always more than 100 polyps and commonly between 2000 and 5000. The condition is said to occur in between 1 in 11,000 and 1 in 18,000 live births. The disease is passed on by a Mendelian-dominant gene to a descendant; it is not sex-linked and every child born to an affected individual stands a 50/50 chance of contracting the disease. The affected child may in turn pass it on to a descendant, but the descendants of the unaffected children will be normal. The condition arises as a genetic mutation in a previously normal family and between 20 and 25 percent of all patients with familial polyposis arise as such.

It will be appreciated, therefore, that when any patient with familial adenomatosis is diagnosed, very careful enquiry should be made about parents and grandparents. If one parent could have been affected by polyposis and has died of what might have been bowel cancer, then all siblings of the patient should be examined; they might also have inherited the disease, even though they may be free of any bowel symptoms. The adenomas are not present at birth and are rarely found before the age of puberty or the midteens. Most carriers of the genes will have developed polyps by the age of 30. In exceptional

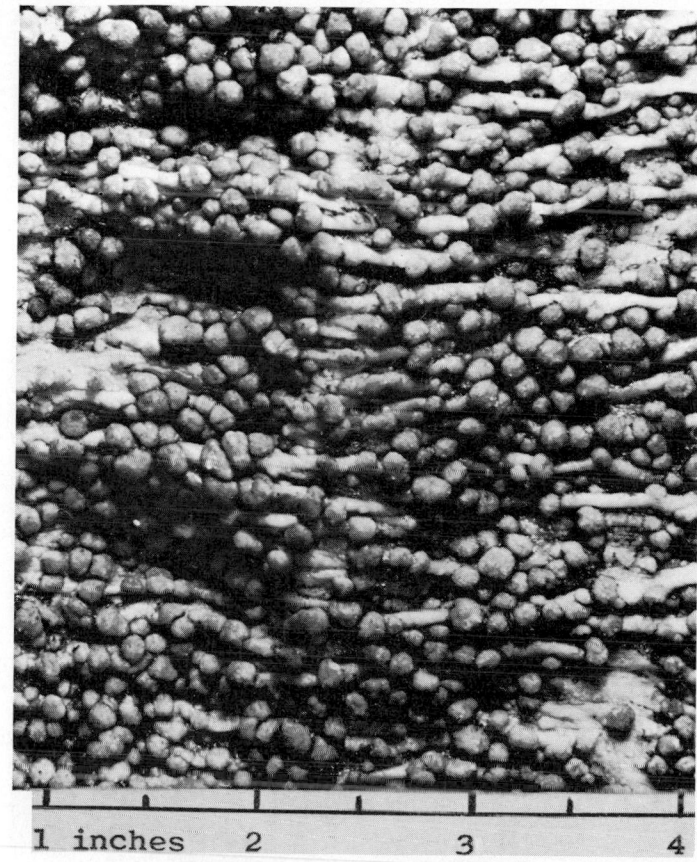

1 inches   2   3   4

Figure 52–6. Diffuse adenomatosis coli.

cases, polyps have been found for the first time in the sixth decade. It is practically unknown for carcinoma to develop under the age of 20. Most patients who have not been treated will develop carcinoma under the age of 40 and will probably die from the disease before the age of 45. Unless prophylactic measures are undertaken, every patient with familial polypsis will develop carcinoma.

Although there are clinical, sigmoidoscopic, and radiologic differences between these various forms of polyposis, final and accurate diagnosis depends on the histologic proof of the nature of the polyps concerned. It has become apparent in recent years that different kinds of polyps are occasionally found in the same patient. For example, juvenile polyps and adenomas may co-exist and no treatment should be undertaken until several of the polyps have been removed for histologic examination. Although these conditions are rare, they are of great clinical interest, for early and accurate diagnosis may lead to the prevention of carcinoma later in life.

Diagnosis

Diarrhoea and bleeding from the bowel are the two most common symptoms of polyposis but the symptoms are usually very slight and, even when extensive, there may be only a slight increase in frequency of bowel habit and a little mucus in the stool. Marked symptoms usually indicate that a carcinoma has already developed. It is important to obtain an accurate and careful family history from every patient who is seen with polyposis, to contact all members of the family and persuade those who could possibly be affected to come for sigmoidoscopic examination, even if they claim to be in perfect health and free of all symptoms.

Children at risk are examined first at about 14 or 15 years of age and are simply sigmoidoscoped. No other investigation is necessary because, if the rectum is absolutely free of polyps on careful examination they will not occur higher in the colon. However, if there are any polyps in the rectum, three or four must be re-

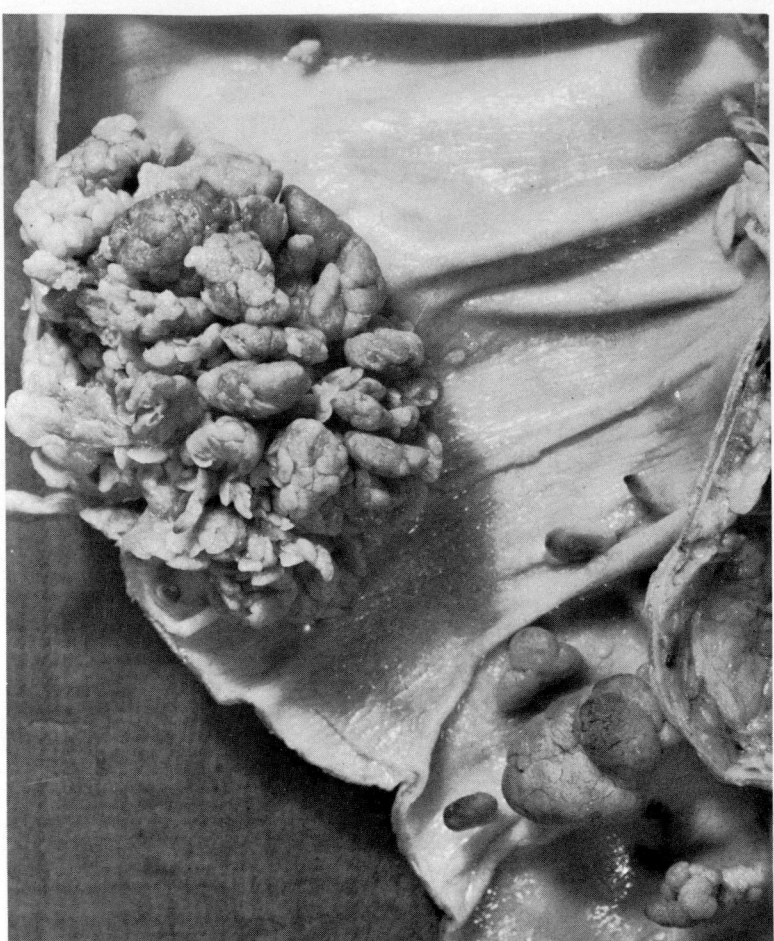

Figure 52–7. Familial polyposis coli. The large polyp proved to be benign on microscopic examination.

moved and if they prove to be adenomas on histologic examination the diagnosis is made. In such circumstances it is unwise to assume that there may be no larger polyps in the proximal colon and an air-contrast barium enema should be carried out to assess the remainder of the large bowel. It is unnecessary to submit children of affected individuals to a barium enema unless adenomas are present in the rectum. If the child has a normal rectum, repeated sigmoidoscopy is carried out every 2 years. Most children who have inherited the condition will have developed polyps by the age of 25. However, a two-year examination programme should be continued until the age of 35. It is very rare to develop polyps later than this, although it has been recorded. After the age of 35, patients should be sigmoidoscoped at 5-year intervals until the age of 60 or 65.

Gardner's Syndrome

In 1951 Gardner described a family with colonic adenomatosis associated with osteomas of the skull and mandible and multiple epidermoid cysts and fibromas of the skin. Gardner and Richards, in 1953, also described dental abnormalities, osteomas of any bone, and desmoid tumours of the abdominal wall or abdominal cavity as being associated with this condition. It was thought that Gardner's syndrome was a separate entity but it has become apparent over the last few years that there is no separation between patients with familial polyposis and Gardner's syndrome and if the features of Gardner's syndrome are looked for carefully enough some will be found in 95 percent of all cases of familial polyposis. The following manifestations may be found.

Epidermoid Cysts of the Skin. These cysts may be multiple and one or more will be present in patients with familial polypsis if sought carefully. Epidermoid cysts are very rare in children before the age of puberty but may appear in children who inherit the polyposis gene before the development of any adenomas within the large bowel.

Osteomas. Ivory osteomas usually occur in the facial bones and cranium. However, Utsunomiya and Nakamura in 1975 and later other Japanese workers reported the presence of sclerosis around the mental foramen of the mandible which they termed microosteomosis. Up to 95 percent of all patients with familial polyposis have these changes when compared with 5 percent of patients without polyposis.

Desmoid Tumours. These patients may have abnormalities of fibrous tissue. The most common manifestation is the tendency to develop desmoid tumours, which may occur in the abdominal wall, usually within the scars of abdominal operations, or within the abdominal cavity, usually in the small bowel mesentery. Approximately 10 percent of patients with familial polyposis develop some form of desmoid tumour. They seem to be made worse by operation or pregnancy. The abdominal wall tumours are unsightly but not dangerous and can be removed or partly removed for cosmetic reasons. However, the intraabdominal desmoids are a serious manifestation, leading to intestinal obstruction, retroperitoneal fibrosis, and ureteric obstruction. Although the growth rate is usually slow they can reach such a size as to cause the patient serious respiratory and cardiovascular embarrassment. The mortality is in the order of 25 percent and there is no known treatment if surgical removal proves impossible. However, they do occasionally regress spontaneously. Occasionally patients will not develop frank desmoid tumours but will develop tough fibrous tissue adhesions after operation and intestinal obstruction in a relatively common complication.

Upper Gastrointestinal Lesions. It has become apparent in the last 10 years that the adenomatous polyps in this condition are not confined to colon and rectum. Several papers from Japan reported a high incidence of gastric and duodenal adenomas and an incidence of carcinoma in the region of the ampulla of Vater (Yao et al, 1977). At St. Mark's Hospital, the incidence of duodenal adenomas is over 50 percent based on 60 duodenoscopies and biopsies in patients with familial polyposis. Most of the lesions in the stomach are hamartomas rather than adenomas. The incidence of periampullary carcinoma in 241 cases of familial polyposis operated on at St. Mark's Hospital is 11, with a further four possible cases who died elsewhere with incomplete documentation. Two thirds are adenocarcinomas of the duodenum and one third carcinomas of the biliary tree and pancreas.

Treatment

There is no cure for familial adenomatosis in that no way is known of reversing the tendency to form multiple polyps and eventually cancer. Reports (Decosse et al, 1975) that adenomas will regress with large doses of antioxidants such as vitamin C have not been substantiated. Cancer, however, can be prevented by the removal of the bowel while the polyps are still benign. Theoretically total removal of all the large bowel would be necessary to prevent cancer and, although this has been advocated in some centres, at St. Mark's Hospital it has rarely been done unless a patient is seen very late and a cancer has already developed in the rectum, or in the rare case in which the rectum is so carpeted with polyps that any other treatment is impracticable.

Colectomy with Ileorectal Anastomosis

This operation is indicated in the majority of cases of polyposis, in fact whenever there is no sign of rectal cancer or the rectum is not totally carpeted with polyps. In children picked up by screening who are found to have polyps in their early teens, if no large lesions are present in the colon or rectum, the operation can usually be left until a suitable time, for example, when school has finished and before further education or employment begins. At one time it was thought essential to clear the rectum by diathermy before ileorectal anastomosis was undertaken. This is unnecessary and in cases with complete carpeting of polyps it is unlikely that an ileorectal anastomosis would be undertaken. Colectomy is carried out and the open end of the rectum inspected. If there are any polyps which would be included in the anastomosis, these are diathermied or ligated and excised if large. The ileum is matched to the size of the rectum by carrying out a Cheatle slit if necessary. The anastomosis is marked with ligaclips. After a successful ileorectal anastomosis, rectal function is usually completely satisfactory. In most patients the bowels act between 2 and 4 times in 24 hours though in the earlier weeks movements may be more frequent. Cole and Holden believe that there is a tendency for polyps in the rectal stump to regress and even disappear following colectomy and ileorectal anastomosis. This has been observed in a number of cases at St. Mark's and no fulguration of rectal polyps should be undertaken for 2 or 3 months to see if spontaneous regression occurs. However, even if regression of rectal polyps does take place, the patient still needs careful follow-up for this abeyance is not necessarily permanent and polyps may develop again later in life.

Patients who have had an ileorectal anastomosis carried out are reviewed every 6 months. A hypophosphate enema is given and the rectum examined carefully for adenomas. It is unnecessary to fulgurate away every small polyp that arises, but polyps between 5 mm and 10 mm in diameter should be excised or fulgurated. It seems unlikely that the population of polyps remains unchanged and it is possible that spontaneous regression and formation of new polyps continually takes place.

At St. Mark's Hospital, up until December 1983, there are 293 families in the polyposis register and 960 subjects are affected members; 296 of these 960 patients have been seen at St. Mark's and 241 have undergone some form of surgery. Colectomy and ileorectal anastomosis has been undertaken in 167 of these patients with one operative death. There have been 11 subsequent cancers developing in the rectum despite follow-up and three of the patients have subsequently died. There is a cumulative risk of cancer of approximately 10 percent over a period of 25 years. A report from the Mayo Clinic (Moertel et al, 1970), however, has reported less satisfactory results with ileorectal anastomosis with a large number of patients developing carcinoma in the rectum. These authors suggest that colectomy and ileorectal anastomosis should be abandoned as the operation of choice in the treatment of this disease. At St. Mark's Hospital, however, we feel that this is still the first choice of procedure. Total proctocolectomy is indicated in all cases in

which malignant change in the rectum has already taken place and also whenever the polyps in the rectum are so numerous as to be almost confluent and it seems unlikely that the polyps could be destroyed or removed by diathermy. Proctocolectomy can be carried out with a conventional Brooke ileostomy or with a Koch reservoir ileostomy. Recently, a few patients have been treated by restorative proctocolectomy with the construction of an ileoanal pouch. This author does not believe that this should be undertaken routinely as the functional results are not as good as with an ileorectal anastomosis and the mortality and morbidity are increased. Moreover, it does not negate the necessity for continual follow-up as the incidence of upper gastrointestinal (GI) lesions means that these patients should be kept under review. At the moment, it is uncertain how often these patients should have gastroduodenal endoscopy carried out, but possibly once every 3 years is sufficient. Small duodenal adenomas can be fulgurated but large periampullary adenomas may require laparotomy and duodenotomy with removal of the polyps. Unfortunately, carcinomas often only produce symptoms late when metastases have already occurred. However, in a few patients a Whipple operation will be indicated.

Juvenile Polyposis

This is a rare form of polyposis, first described and separated from the other forms of polyposis by Veale and colleagues in 1966. There is a genetic link with adenomatosis although it is not fully understood at the present time. Juvenile polyps are hamartomas and usually arise in childhood, but they may continue to form in adults, even into middle life. They differ from adenomas in both their gross and microscopic appearances, though the differences may not be so great as to be always obvious on sigmoidoscopy. They may produce bleeding in children, sometimes prolapse through the anus, and lead to intussusception and attacks of abdominal pain. It was initially thought that treatment would only be required in order to prevent these symptoms. However, in recent years, a few cases of juvenile polyposis have been associated with colonic carcinomas. This may be because some juvenile polyps undergo metaplasia and develop into adenomas and carcinoma, or because, in fact, not all the polyps are juvenile in nature and some are adenomas from the outset. It seems at the moment that a patient with juvenile polyposis with a parent with juvenile polyposis in whom carcinoma has arisen should be treated by prophylactic colectomy and ileorectal anastomosis as though the patient had familial adenomatosis.

CARCINOMA OF THE COLON

Carcinoma is by far the most common tumour of the large intestine and the Registrar General's statistics for England and Wales show that there are approximately 16,000 deaths per year from colorectal cancer, a figure that has largely remained unchanged for the last 40 years. In 1980, there were 10,314 deaths from colonic carcinoma and 6232 deaths from rectal carcinoma, which together accounted for 12 percent of all deaths from malignant disease, second only in incidence to bronchogenic carcinoma. Although the incidence of carcinoma of the colon is greater in women than in men, the reverse is true for the rectum, although the differences are not great. There is a considerable geographic variation, which gives a clear indication of the importance of environmental factors. A review of the age adjusted death rate per 1,000,000 population, which are presumably a reflection of the incidence, in 46 nations reported in the World Health Statistics Annual (1977–78) shows a wide variation from 0.1 in Honduras to 25 in New Zealand. On both sides of the equator the incidence is much lower in tropical countries than those with a temperate climate. For example, in North America the highest rates are in Canada with a fall in incidence through the United States and Mexico to the Central American nations (Table 52–2).

Aetiology

Races who eat a bulky diet high in residue have a much lower incidence of rectal and colonic neoplasm than those who eat a highly refined low residue diet common to economically developed countries. However, when people from low incidence areas migrate to areas of high incidence, within a generation their offspring develop a high risk of colonic or rectal cancer (Stewart, 1971). For example, the Japanese and blacks in the United States have the same incidence of colonic cancer as whites. One suggestion is that fibre promotes a faster GI transit, which limits the exposure of the mucosa to carcinogens (Burkitt, 1971). Hill (1975A, 1981) considers that, although carcinogens are ingested in the diet in significant quantities, they are found in those with and without large bowel cancer and suggests that intestinal bacteria

TABLE 52–2. AGE ADJUSTED DEATH RATES PER 100,000 POPULATION FROM LARGE BOWEL CANCER FOR SELECTED NATIONS

Nation	Male		Female	
	Rank	*No.*	*Rank*	*No.*
New Zealand	1	25.6	2	24.0
Scotland	2	24.7	5	19.3
Northern Ireland	3	24.3	4	20.4
Iceland	4	23.9	3	20.6
Chile	5	23.8	1	28.4
Austria	6	23.6	11	17.4
Australia	12	21.4	10	17.5
Canada	16	20.5	6	18.5
USA	19	19.1	16	15.0
Mexico	43	2.5	43	3.3
Venezuela	40	5.0	39	5.8
Costa Rica	41	4.9	40	5.7
Dominica	44	2.2	42	3.6
Philippines	42	3.8	44	2.8
Thailand	45	1.9	45	1.2
Honduras	46	0.1	46	0.1

(*Source: From World Health Statistics Annual, 1977–78.*)

could well produce carcinogens by chemical alteration of food constituents and intestinal secretions. His own findings suggest that faecal bile acid concentration correlates with the risk of large bowel cancer in various populations. In these studies, the correlation with deoxycholic acid was better than that with total faecal bile acids. Clostridia are able to produce unsaturated bile acids and these are carried in the faeces by more than 80 percent of large bowel cancer cases compared with about only 40 percent of controls. The combination of a high faecal bile acid concentration with the carriage of clostridia characterises a high proportion of large bowel cancer cases but only a small portion of controls. This is most discriminating when the tumour is in the left colon and is a Dukes "A" case and is least effective when the tumour is a "C" case or in the right side of the colon. A decrease in dietary fat and an increase in fibre content may reduce the amount of faecal bile acid and clostridia.

Cholelithiasis is also a disease that is common in Western countries but rare in Africa and Asia. Like GI cancer, its incidence has been linked with features of diet, particularly fibre deficiency and, like colorectal cancer, is related to abnormal bile salt metabolism. It has therefore been postulated that the presence of gall stones and large bowel cancer might be associated. A number of papers examine the incidence in large bowel cancer after cholecystectomy (Castleden et al, 1978; Turnbull et al, 1981). There is no increased incidence in men, but there is a significant increase in colorectal cancer in women, the association being strongest for carcinoma of the right side of the colon. Selenium has also been implicated by Hill (1975B); the greatest incidence of colorectal carcinoma in the United States occurs where there is a low selenium level in the soil.

There are five groups of patients who are at an increased risk for developing colorectal cancer. These are patients with colorectal adenomas, those who have had one or more colorectal carcinomas resected with retention of the remaining part of the colon or rectum, families with familial polyposis, colorectal cancer families, and some patients with chronic total ulcerative colitis.

There is now ample evidence that the majority of colorectal cancers passed through the adenoma–carcinoma sequence (Morson and Day, 1981). Colorectal adenoma is a form of localised polypoid dysplasia. Most adenomas are small and remain benign but a small minority of them grow and are at risk of malignant change. There is evidence that the greater the number of colorectal adenomas in a patient the greater the risk of cancer. Patients with more than 100 adenomas are always found to have familial polypsis coli although most will have between 2000 and 5000 adenomas. Cancer risk in these patients is known to be almost inevitable.

Between 4 and 5 percent of patients who have a carcinoma of the colon or rectum will have a second synchronous carcinoma in the colon or rectum. Patients who have had a bowel resection for carcinoma are at an increased risk from a second primary metachronous tumour which is usually manifest many years after the original operation. Risk is highest in those who have had one adenoma or more as well as the carcinoma at the first operation. The magnitude of risk increases with time after about 5 years postoperatively and on average the second carcinoma is discovered 11 years after the first.

It is now recognised that there are so-called colorectal cancer families (Lovett, 1976A,B). There are no definite criteria as yet for categorising patients in this way, but in the more obvious cases several members of the family will have developed colorectal carcinoma before the age of 50 and there is a high proportion of right-sided carcinomas.

There is an increased risk of carcinoma in ulcerative colitis although the vast majority of patients with ulcerative colitis never develop this complication. Carcinoma arises in some patients with extensive colitis and a total history of 15 years or more. These patients develop dysplastic changes in colorectal biopsies and if the dysplasia is severe and persistent carcinoma results.

Incidence

Carcinoma of the colon may occur at any age, although it is usually encountered between the ages of 50 and 80, the peak age incidence being in the sixth and seventh decades. It is not uncommon to find the disease in a younger age group although it becomes rare in children and adolescents. In the Third National Cancer Survey in the United States (1975), there were only 32 children under the age of 20 with colorectal cancer, representing an incidence of 1.3 cases per million children. Twenty eight of these 32 children were between the ages of 10 and 19, representing an incidence of approximately 6.8 per million children at this age.

The frequency of carcinoma in different segments of the large bowel varies in individual statistical tables. The Registrar General's figures show that 38 percent occur in the rectum. Of the remaining large bowel, the sigmoid accounts for almost half the colonic growths, the caecum and ascending colon for approximately one quarter. The remaining frequency is transverse colon, descending colon, splenic flexure, and finally hepatic flexure. Some 4 percent are at multiple sites.

Pathology

Carcinoma of the colon has the microscopic structure of columnar cell adenocarcinoma. In about 5 percent, the tumour undergoes mucoid or colloid degeneration, and mucus secreting cells are sometimes reproduced in the metastatic deposits.

It should be remembered that, microscopically, carcinomas of the colon vary in their degree of differentiation so that tumours of high, low, and intermediate grades of malignancy are observed. Anaplastic carcinomas and those of a high degree of malignancy metastasise early, so that the size of the tumour, as a rule, is but little indication of the presence or absence of secondary deposits in the liver or elsewhere. Metastases are commonly found in the liver from venous embolism, and, in some cases, these may be encountered in the lungs. Metastases in the liver may occur without any enlargement of the related lymph nodes. Enlarged lymph nodes are usually laden with cancer cells, but at times they are inflammatory in nature, especially when the primary growth is septic and decomposing.

Macroscopic types of colonic cancer include:

1. Proliferative
2. Annular
3. Ulcerative
4. Mucoid
5. Primary linitis plastica
6. Multiple primary carcinomas of the colon

The proliferative type is most frequently seen in the caecum, the ascending colon, and the rectum. If forms a fleshy bulky polypoid mass that bulges into the lumen of the bowel.

It is a malignant adenoma of slow growth, of a low order of malignancy, and shows no eagerness to metastasise to the regional lymph nodes. The cauliflower-like swelling arises from the wall of the gut from a wide base, showing little tendency in its early stages to encircle the bowel and thus constrict it and produce obstruction.

With these right-sided growths, obstruction is usually of late occurrence—late because: (1) the proximal colon is capacious; (2) its contents are fluid; and (3) the papilliferous tumour obstructs only by virtue of its great bulk (Fig. 52–8). The surface of the neoplasm finally becomes ulcerated and this may lead to bleeding and predisposes to infection. A marked secondary anaemia of the microcytic type is frequently noticed. Frank haemorrhage is an unusual event. The proliferative (papilliferous or fungating) growths are usually well-differentiated adenocarcinomas.

The annular type of growth is seen in typical form in the pelvic colon, splenic flexure, and the upper one third of the rectum; but it may also arise in the transverse colon or even in the ascending colon a few inches above the ileocaecal valve. It is a small, densely hard, slow-growing tumour that does not project appreciably into the lumen of the bowel but rather tends to encircle the gut wall and constrict it, thus obstructing the passage of solid faecal matter. The growth leads to a purely localised constriction of the colon—as if a ring encircled the bowel (napkin-ring stricture). When the segment of bowel containing the tumour is slit open, it will be seen that the serosa is puckered, infiltrated, and drawn inward; that the growth is densely fibrotic in character; and that the mucous membrane is ulcerated. There is but minimal longitudinal spread of the growth. As a rule, with many of these ring strictures, metastases tend to occur rather late in the course of the disease (Fig. 52–9).

As already stated, these carcinomatous tumours of the colon not infrequently undergo mucoid (colloid) degeneration, and this characteristic is commonly reproduced in metastases.

Methods of Spread

In many cases, cancers of the colon grow tardily. The growth may extend by direct spread in the bowel wall, direct infiltration of adjacent tissues, invasion of the lymphatic vessels and lymph nodes, the blood stream—and thus metastasise to distant sites such as the liver,

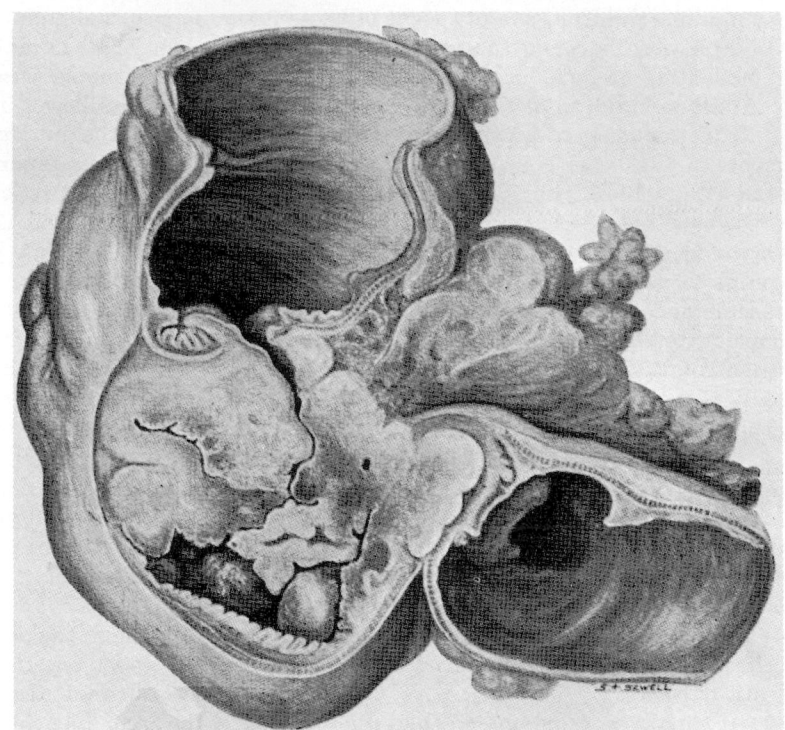

Figure 52–8. Proliferative carcinoma of the caecum causing obstruction of the ileocaecal valve.

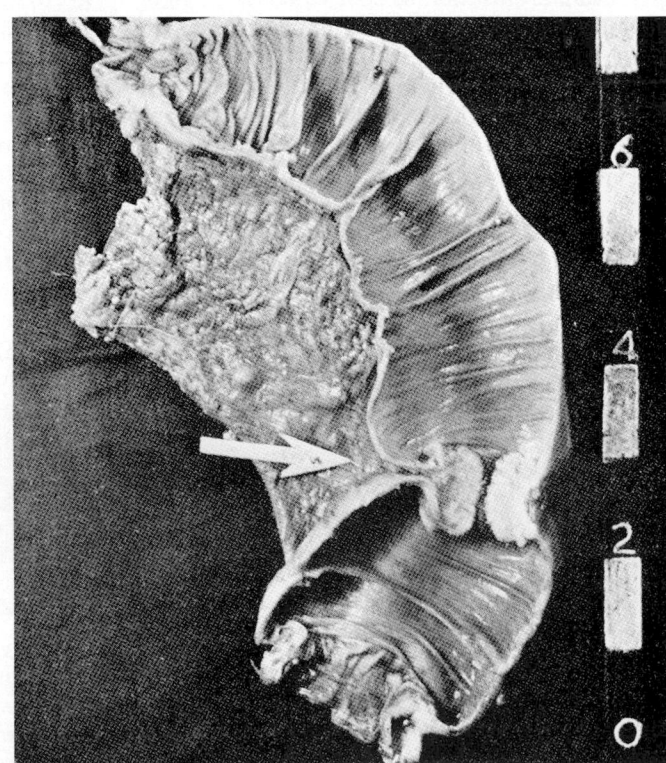

Figure 52–9. Constricting carcinoma of the descending colon. Patient had no symptoms until 9 days before admission to the hospital with intestinal obstruction. (*Source: From Maingot R: Management of Abdominal Operations, 2 edt. London: HK Lewis & Company, 1957, with permission.*)

transperitoneal implantation, and intraluminal transplantation of cancer cells.

At an early stage, the growth is limited to the mucous coat and submucosa, and shows no inclination to spread longitudinally (except in anaplastic cancers) but rather at right angles to the long axis of the bowel. It should be noted that the perineural lymph spaces may be permeated, at an early stage, by direct continuity. The tumour invades the muscularis and finally bursts through the strong unyielding serosa. The surface of the colon then becomes distorted and discoloured by greyish disc-like masses or small excrescences of pearly white growth that may shed and disseminate malignant cells throughout the peritoneal cavity.

With the onset of inflammatory changes and extramural extension of the neoplasm, the tumour becomes adherent to neighbouring structures such as a loop of intestine, the uterus, the uterine adnexa or bladder, or it becomes fused to the parietes.

It should be noted that the bulky papilliferous growths that invade adjacent organs and the tissues of the abdominal wall often show but little tendency to metastasise and that radical, and perhaps heroic, surgical intervention will often lead to spectacular results in such cases (Pittam et al, 1984). Involvement of the bladder, the uterus, a Fallopian tube, or the small intestine is no bar to radical operation. In a general way it may be stated that in the operation on the colon there are only two important factors which preclude extirpation of the growth and its attachments; these are wide peritoneal spread and massive involvement of the liver, with secondary deposits.

Peritoneal spread, when limited to a few small seedlings near the parent growth, need not deter the surgeon from performing a radical operation; the chances of early recurrence in such cases are, however, great.

It is estimated that, at the time of operation, about 40 percent of patients with colonic cancers and 55 percent of rectal cancers have lymph node involvement. The involvement of the lymph nodes is, as a rule, progressive and orderly.

There are three systems of lymphatics:

1. Intramural, which are the lymph channels in the submucous, intramuscular, and subserous coats

2. Intermediate, which are channels that transport lymph from the wall to the nodes
3. Extramural, which accompany the main blood vessels of the large bowel, e.g., epiploic, paracolic, ileocolic, right colic, middle colic, left colic, the superior and inferior mesenteric, and, finally, the paraaortic groups of lymph nodes

Venous spread, which may be local and/or distant, occurs in more than 30 percent of carcinomas of the colon.

Manipulation of the cancerous mass may pump multiple emboli of malignant cells through the portal system of the liver during the conduct of exploration and resection. For this reason, the related mesenteric blood vessels should be ligatured securely before the tumour is mobilised.

OTHER MALIGNANT TUMOURS

Malignant tumours other than carcinoma are uncommon in the colon. They comprise:

1. Carcinoid tumours
2. Malignant lymphoid tumours
3. Miscellaneous connective tissue tumours, of which the leiomyosarcoma is the only one which is not excessively rare

Carcinoid Tumours

Carcinoid tumours of the colon are rare but are more often seen in the caecum than elsewhere in the large bowel. It should be noted that the carcinoid syndrome is most unusual in connection with carcinoids of the large intestine. Carcinoids of the large bowel are single, unlike the small intestinal carcinoids which may often be multiple. They vary from a small submucous nodule or polyp, which does not recur after local excision, to a large ulcerated tumour which closely resembles a carcinoma and which metastasises to the regional nodes and to the liver.

Malignant Lymphoid Tumours

These lesions may occur in the large bowel, most commonly in association with generalised malignant lymphoma. They may also occur as a primary disease in the colon (particularly the caecum) or in the rectum in next order of frequency, with involvement of the regional lymph nodes in about 50 percent of the patients. Finally, they may present as a diffuse polyposis which may also implicate the small intestine.

It should be noticed that diffuse infiltration of the large bowel may occur in patients with leukaemia. These lesions are usually symptomless and found at postmortem examination.

Leiomyosarcoma

Leiomyosarcomas occasionally arise from the muscularis mucosae but more usually from the deeper muscle layer. They are rare, but slightly less infrequent in the rectum than the colon. They may be found as a small incidental submucous nodule but larger tumours, up to 20 cm in diameter, may occur, either within the wall of the gut, protruding into the lumen, or extramural in position. In some instances dumb-bell tumours with both intra- and extramural extensions may be found. It may be difficult to differentiate these tumours from a leiomyoma but malignant tumours tend to be larger with cystic degeneration. Malignancy is suggested by frank anaplasia, local invasion and blood-borne metastases. Lymph node spread only rarely occurs.

Screening

This depends upon the fact that all carcinomas and adenomas of a significant size bleed intermittently. Methods of detecting occult bleeding are not new but refined techniques using the haemoccult test are more reliable than the older methods. Screening should be directed initially at the groups of patients with a high risk listed earlier and there is no doubt that screening these groups is mandatory. The routine screening of the population over 45 or 50 years of age has, on the whole, resulted in poor compliance rates (Farrands et al, 1981) and a failure to attend for further investigation even when repeated occult blood tests have been positive. The pick-up rates for significant lesions has been low. Screening programmes would appear to be uneconomic at the present time as all patients with positive occult bloods should have a thorough workup which should include fibre-optic endoscopy. A far higher yield of neoplasms could be obtained by publicising the necessity to seek medical help whenever the patient has a change in bowel habit and traces of blood in the stool. Perhaps the day will not be far hence when the routine use of impregnated toilet tissue will draw attention to the person that small amounts of blood are being passed in the stool and medical advice should be sought if this persists.

Clinical Manifestations

The clinical features of cancer of the colon vary according to the type and grade of growth—proliferative, ulcerating, or annular—and its situation—in the proximal or distal part of the colon (Table 52–3).

The chief complaints of patients suffering from cancer of the colon include:

1. Abdominal pain
2. An alteration or change in bowel function
3. Rectal bleeding—bloody or tarry stools
4. Weight loss
5. Palpable mass
6. Vomiting
7. Anaemia, faintness, lassitude
8. Partial or complete obstruction
9. Melaena
10. Mucus in stools
11. Tenesmus
12. Incontinence of faeces
13. Perforation with abscess or spreading peritonitis

When dyspepsia dominates, the signs and symptoms point to an inflammatory lesion of the appendix or ileocaecal region. The most noticeable feature, however, is often a change in bowel habit. Later, there is a slight but persistent dyspepsia with some pain and tenderness felt over the caecum. Nausea, indigestion, anorexia, and loss of weight occur and simulate other abdominal diseases, such as cancer of the stomach.

In the anaemia group the patients are markedly anaemic, asthenic, lethargic, and toxic. The most striking characteristic is, of course, anaemia which may be severe. In only about 10 percent of cases of carcinoma of the caecum is macroscopic blood observed in the stools. These patients may complain of loss of weight, dyspnoea on exertion, loss of interest and extreme lassitude. On examination, there may be a suggestion of a mass in the right iliac fossa, and a barium enema x-ray examination may reveal a filling defect in the bowel. Unfortunately, a considerable number of cases of carcinoma of the caecum and ascending colon escape early detection and there may even be a "time

TABLE 52–3. CARCINOMA OF LARGE BOWEL: SITES AND SYMPTOMS

	Right Colon	Left Colon	Sigmoid	Rectum
Number of cases	109	74	114	417
Months from onset of symptoms to diagnosis	5.5	5.6	6.5	5.5
Symptoms or Signs (%)				
Pain	78	68.9	50.8	5
Bowel complaint	30	58	70.1	81
Vomiting	32	14.8	3.5	—
Bleeding	8.2	9.4	28.9	66
Weight loss	48.6	14.8	20.1	28
Faintness, lassitude	20	9.4	6.1	—
Acute obstruction	8.2	21.6	28.9	3.5
Abscess peritonitis	1	2.7	10.4	—
Mucus	—	—	6.1	22
Tenesmus	—	—	—	15
Mass	67.7	45.9	38.6	—

(*Source: Modified from Muir EG: Carcinoma of the Colon. London; Edward Arnold, 1961, with permission.*)

lag" as long as 1 to 2 years in certain instances.

Following the general examination of the patient, a thorough digital examination of the rectum and a bimanual examination of the pelvis through both the rectum and vagina should be carried out. In approximately 10 to 15 percent of left-sided growths and some 70 percent of right-sided cancers, a mass can be identified on palpation. Most rectal carcinomas are palpable with the finger and also some growths in the sigmoid colon may be felt through the rectal wall when the loop has prolapsed into the pelvis.

Diagnostic Studies

Sigmoidoscopy

There are two different views concerning the method of carrying out sigmoidoscopy. The traditional one, which this author holds, is that patients should be examined initially without any preparation of the bowel as rectal washouts or enemas can remove traces of blood and mucus in the lumen and can cause congestion of the mucosa. The patient should be examined with a rigid sigmoidoscope initially. If, from the history or the findings on examination, there is a suggestion of a lesion higher in the colon, the patient is then prepared in the outpatient department by two hypophosphate disposable enemas and then a fibre-optic sigmoidoscope passed

to view the sigmoid and the whole of the descending colon if possible. The alternative view is that no patient should be examined until the bowel has been properly prepared and a fibre-optic sigmoidoscope should be passed on every patient.

Barium Enema

The double-contrast barium enema examination, in expert hands, gives a high degree of accuracy in the diagnosis of colonic cancer. However, there are false-positive (due to faecal residue, benign polyps, diverticular disease, Crohn's disease, or even a prominent ileocaecal valve mimicking a tumour) and false-negative findings.

Colonoscopy

The examination of the colon by means of a fibre-optic endoscope has become a standard practice in colorectal surgery.

The indications for colonoscopy are becoming clearer, and it should be used as an adjunct to good radiologic examination of the colon by the double-contrast technique. Colonoscopy is of particular value in resolving difficult diagnostic problems in those areas of the bowel prone to radiologic misinterpretation, namely, the sigmoid colon and the caecum, in a patient who, with equivocal barium studies, has a possible carcinoma at this site.

Colonoscopy is also particularly useful in patients with persistent bleeding and negative findings on barium studies.

Cystoscopy and Pyelography

These examinations are called for in patients with associated urinary symptoms, e.g., enlarged prostate, when the question of ureteric (or bladder) compression is raised, when it is thought that the colonic growth has become attached to a kidney, or when the blood urea estimations are permanently raised.

Carcinoembryonic Antigen

The initial enthusiasm for carcinoembryonic antigen (CEA) as a diagnostic test has waned due to the number of false-negative and false-positive results. It has been found to give positive results in smokers, in many GI carcinomas, and also in carcinoma of the breast, bronchus, and prostate. Positive results have been found in inflammatory bowel disease, particularly Crohn's disease, in alcoholic cirrhosis, and renal disease. The CEA test can have no place in screening patients for the early detection of carcinoma (Blake et al, 1982). However, in patients with known carcinoma and a raised CEA, a rapid decline postoperatively to normal levels is a good prognostic sign. CEA is useful in the follow-up of patients and a gradually rising level months or years after an operation may be the first sign of local recurrence or metastatic disease.

Differential Diagnosis

Differential diagnosis must be made from:

1. Other diseases producing symptoms of bowel disturbance and bleeding. These include diverticular disease, ulcerative colitis, Crohn's disease of the large bowel, benign polyps, and the chronic dysenteries.
2. Pathologies producing a localised abdominal mass. On the right side, these include appendix abscess, Crohn's disease, simple ulcer of the caecum, retroperitoneal tumours, benign colonic neoplasms and, in tropical countries, ileocaecal tuberculosis and amoeboma.
3. Conditions resulting in anaemia, loss of weight, and malaise, especially carcinoma of the stomach or pancreas, uraemia, and pernicious anaemia.

Prognosis

The results of surgical treatment will depend mainly upon the grade of malignancy and its influence on local and lymphatic spread. There are now few carcinomas of the colon which the expert and determined surgeon cannot extirpate. The surgeon has learned that resection affords the maximum degree of palliation and that extensive and multiple resections may on occasion yield an unexpected cure. When there are two or three hepatic metastases that are easily accessible, these should be removed. A large single metastasis requiring a formal hemihepatectomy should be left alone at the primary operation and if it remains solitary in 3 to 6 months it should be treated surgically for possible cure. It should be remembered that in low and average grade tumours, the incidence of liver metastases is about 10 percent compared with 15 percent in high grade growths. Patients who undergo palliative resection in the presence of hepatic metastases usually survive for 1 or 2 years.

Failure to cure carcinoma of the colon is usually due to one or more of five reasons.

1. The carcinomas has invaded the blood vessels and malignant cells have been carried to the liver, giving rise to metastases.
2. The carcinoma has spread widely through the lymphatics.
3. The carcinoma cells have been caught in the suture line at the time of resection. There they proliferate and give rise to secondary spread.
4. Local recurrence develops because of incomplete removal of the tumour or implantation of tumour cells in the operative field during the operation.
5. Metastatic spread occurs not from the resected tumour but from a second undetected carcinoma.

Lymphatic metastases are less commonly found in carcinoma of the colon than in carcinoma of the rectum. In various series lymphatic metastases from colon carcinoma is present in approximately 40 percent of cases, whereas 50 percent of rectal carcinomas have already metastasised to the lymph nodes when treated.

The overall picture, however, is still rather gloomy. Results from survival of carcinoma of the colon from a national survey by the American College of Surgeons (Evans et al, 1978) showed a crude 5-year survival rate from over 38,000 cases was 36 percent and there was no statistical variation whatever the site of the carcinoma in the colon. These results are very similar to the Birmingham Region figures reported by Slaney who found that surgical excision was possible in only 71 percent of cases and that there was an overall crude 5-year survival rate of 20 percent; for those patients who had radical excision of the colon the 5-year survival rate was 42.3 percent. These overall results are in contrast with those reported from specialist centres in the United States and Britain. In St. Mark's Hospital between 1948 and 1972, of 780 patients treated for carcinoma of the colon, 66 had inoperable tumours, giving a resectability rate of 91.5 percent. This was associated with an operative mortality of 4.1 percent. Of these tumours 83.1 percent were in the left colon and splenic flexure, 11.6 percent in the caecum and ascending colon, and 5.3 percent in the transverse colon. For the 400 patients whose operations were radical, the crude 5-year survival rate was 66 percent and the corrected figure was 78.8 percent. These figures are considerably better than those obtained for rectal carcinoma and reflect the less aggressive behaviour of these tumours.

Results of surgical treatment for carcinoma of the colon have remained the same for the last 35 years. The better results from specialised centres arises because few patients with obstructive and perforated carcinomas are seen and there are many more patients with operable carcinoma. When these factors are taken into account, the true improvement in the 5-year survival rate is probably in the order of 5 percent. Under these circumstances it is doubtful if there will be any improvement in prognosis without the introduction of screening programmes, the irradication of premalignant lesions, and the pickup of tumours at an earlier stage. This will prove very costly.

BIBLIOGRAPHY

Arminski TC, McLean DW: Incidence and distribution of adenomatous polyps of the colon and rectum based on 1000 autopsy examinations. Dis Colon Rectum 7:249, 1964

Blake KE, Dalbow MH, et al: Clinical significance of preoperative plasma carcinogen embryonic antigens (CEA) level in patients with carcinoma of the large bowel. Dis Colon Rectum 25:1, 1982

Burkitt DP: Epidemiology of cancer of the colon and rectum. Cancer 28:3, 1971

Bussey HJR: Gastrointestinal polyposis. Gut 11:970, 1970

Castleden WM, Doouss TW, et al: Gallstones, carcinoma of the colon and diverticular disease. Clin Oncol 4:139, 1978

Cole JW, Holden WD: Postcolectomy regression of adenomatous polyps of the rectum. Arch Surg 79:385, 1959

DeCosse JJ, Adams MB, et al: The effect of ascorbic acid on rectal polyps of patients with familial polyposis. Surgery 78:608, 1975

Evans JT, Vana J, et al: Management and survival of carcinoma of the colon: Results of a national survey by the American College of Surgeons. Ann Surg 188:716, 1978

Farrands PA, Griffiths RL, et al: The Frome experiment—Value of screening for colorectal cancer. Lancet 1:1231, 1981

Gardner EG: A genetic and clinical study of intestinal polyposis. A predisposing factor for carcinoma of the colon and rectum. Am J Hum Genet 3:167, 1951

Gardner EG, Richards RC: Multiple cutaneous and subcutaneous lesions occurring simultaneously with hereditary polyposis and osteomatosis. Am J Hum Genet 5:139, 1953

Hill MJ: The role of colon anaerobes in the metabolism of bile acids and steroids and its relation to colon cancer. Cancer 36 (suppl):2387, 1975

Hill MJ: Metabolic epidemiology of dietary factors in large bowel cancer. Cancer Res 35:3398, 1975

Hill MJ: Bile Acids in colo-rectal carcinogenesis, in Bruce WR (ed): Gastrointestinal Cancer: Endogenous Factors, Banbury Report 7. Coldspring Harbor Laboratory, 1981

Lovett E: Family studies in cancer of the colon and rectum. Br J Surg 63:13, 1976

Lovett E: Familial cancer of the gastrointestinal tract. Br J Surg 63:19, 1976

Moertel CG, Hill JR, et al: Surgical management of multiple polyposis: The problem of cancer in the retained bowel segment. Arch Surg 100:521, 1970

Morson BC, Day D: in DeCosse JJ (ed): Pathology of adenomas and cancer of the large bowel, in Large Bowel Cancer. London: Churchill Livingstone, 1981, p 34

Morson BC, Sobin LH: Blue Book No. 15. Histological Typing of Intestinal Tumours. World Health Organisation, Geneva, 1976

Muto T, Bussey HJR, et al: The evolution of cancer of the colon and rectum. Cancer 36:2251, 1975

Pittam MR, Thornton H, et al: Survival after extended resection for locally advanced carcinomas of the colon and rectum. Ann R Coll Surg Engl 66:81, 1984

Slaney G: Results of treatment of carcinoma of the

colon and rectum, in Irvine WT (ed): Modern Trends in Surgery. London: Butterworths, 1971

Stewart HL: Geographic pathology of cancer of the colon and rectum. Cancer 28:25, 1971

Third National Cancer Survey: Incidence Data (Table 19B). Average annual age-specific incidence rates per 100,000 population, by primary site, males plus females, all races, all areas combined 1969–71; in cutler SJ, Young JL Jr (eds): Monograph No. 41, Bethesda, MD: National Cancer Institute, 1975

Turnbull PRG, Smith AH, et al: Cholecystectomy and cancer of large bowel. Br J Surg 68:551, 1981

Utsunomiya J, Nakamura T: The occult osteomatous changes in the mandible in patients with familial polyposis coli. Br J Surg 62:45, 1975

Veale AMO, McColl I, et al: Juvenile polyposis coli. J Med Genet 3:5, 1966

Yao T, Iida M, et al: Duodenal lesions in familial polyposis of the colon. Gastroenterology 73:1086, 1977

53. Resection of the Colon

Harold Ellis

HISTORICAL NOTE

Fascinating information about the early history of the operative management of large bowel cancer can be found in the textbooks of Cope (1965), Meade (1968), and Singer and Underwood (1962).

The earliest contributions were directed towards the relief of intestinal obstruction. In 1710, Littré first suggested the feasibility of opening the colon to relieve obstruction, actually in cases of children with imperforate anus. The first caecostomy was performed by Pillore in 1776 for an obstructing carcinoma and Duret in 1793 performed the first successful colostomy in a case of imperforate anus. Fine, in 1797, performed a transverse colostomy in a patient with an obstructing carcinoma at the rectosigmoid with recovery. The great danger in those days was, of course, the risk of peritonitis due to escape of the bowel contents into the peritoneal cavity. In 1839, Amussat introduced the operation of lumbar colostomy, by the extraperitoneal route, for the relief of intestinal obstruction.

The first successful resection and anastomosis of the colon for carcinoma was reported in 1844 by Reybard, and in 1879 Czerny successfully resected a growth with end-to-end anastomosis.

The risk of leakage was, of course, high, particularly in obstructed cases. In 1892, Bloch advocated extraabdominal resection of the colon obstructed by tumour; he brought out the affected loop along with the growth, opened the bowel above the tumour, waited a month, and then excised the growth, leaving two healthy ends in the wound which later he anastomosed. In 1895, Paul published his technique of extraabdominal resection of colonic cancer. He exteriorised the affected loop, sutured a glass tube into the bowel above and below the site of the growth, excised the tumour, and then crushed the spur between the two portions of the bowel, eventually closing the stoma. Three years later Mikulicz performed a similar operation, thus the procedure is usually termed the Paul–Mikulicz operation.

It was the classic studies of Miles that showed the importance of removal of regional lymph nodes in the clearing of rectal tumours and laid the basis for the modern operations of adequate wide resections.

Safe modern surgery depended on the development of efficient bowel anastomoses, dating back to the early experiments of Murphy with his button technique in 1892 and the contributions of Lembert, Halsted, the Mayo brothers, Cushing, Connell, and Moynihan, among many others.

Surgery for cancer of the large bowel could not, of course, have developed without the many ancillary measures of recent years. These include advances in anaesthesia, the development of effective broad-spectrum antibiotics, in particular those effective against bowel anaerobes, and efficient blood transfusion services.

ANATOMY OF THE COLON

The colon is about 1.5 m long, and can be easily distinguished from the small intestine by the three longitudinal bands, or taeniae coli, protruding appendages, called appendices epiploicae, and the characteristic sacculations or haustra. The caecum is the widest portion of the colon, averaging 8.5 cm in breadth, and is usually covered by peritoneum. The ascending colon is narrower, about 15 cm long, and overlies the right kidney and the iliacus and quadratus lumborum. At the hepatic flexure, the colon is closely related to the right lobe of the liver, the duodenum, and the gallbladder.

The transverse colon is not only the longest (about 0.5 m) but the most flexible section of the colon. The initial portion is closely related posteriorly to the second portion of the duodenum and the head of the pancreas. The entire transverse colon is intraperitoneal, held to the posterior abdominal wall by the transverse mesocolon. The splenic flexure forms a very sharp bend that is less accessible surgically than the hepatic flexure, since the former lies in a more superior and posterior plane (overlapped by the stomach and lower pole of the spleen) than the latter.

The descending colon is deeper and narrower than the ascending colon and is the point of the thickest muscle coat and the narrowest lumen. It crosses superficial to the psoas major muscle and becomes entirely intraperitoneal at the upper end of the sigmoid colon. The sigmoid colon forms a loop in the pelvis about 40 cm long (but quite variable in length and location) and is usually mobile on the central portion of its mesentery—the mesosigmoid. This portion of the colon is studded with appendices epiploicae, and the taeniae widen to form a completely encircling longitudinal muscle layer at the rectosigmoid junction. The sigmoid terminates at the upper end of the intraperitoneal rectum that is usually about 15 cm above the anal verge.

Blood Supply. The portion of the colon that arises from the midgut (caecum, ascending colon, and right transverse colon) is supplied by the ileocolic, right colic, and middle colic branches of the superior mesenteric artery. The left part of the transverse colon, the descending colon, and the sigmoid colon, all of which are hindgut derivatives, are supplied by the inferior mesenteric artery and its branches, including the left colic and the sigmoid arteries. The left colic artery divides into an ascending branch (that runs toward the splenic flexure, but may supply much of the transverse colon) and a descending branch (Fig. 53–1).

Anatomic studies have uncovered frequent anomalies, such as absence of the middle colic or right colic arteries, variations in the number of sigmoidal arteries, or patterns of branching of the inferior mesenteric artery. The major colic arteries divide into smaller branches that form arcades approximately 2.5 cm from the mesenteric border of the intestine. The marginal artery of Drummond is formed from these communicating vessels and allows an anastomosis of the inferior and superior mesenteric arteries via the arc of Riolan. The presence of the marginal artery should be confirmed in any operation near the splenic flexure to ensure collateral circulation. Small, straight arteries cross from the marginal artery to the mesenteric border and branch into the colon.

Ligation of the inferior mesenteric artery at the point of exit from the aorta—about 4 cm above the aortic bifurcation, opposite the third lumbar vertebra—usually does not cause ischaemia of the left colon and can allow use of the left colon for a low anastomosis. If possible, the point of division of the left colic artery is preserved, as it may serve as a second marginal artery. Rarely the middle colic and left colic branches are end arteries, and unless care is taken to ensure adequate blood supply, ligation may lead to breakdown of anastomoses after resection of tumours in the region of the splenic flexure. The ascending branch of the left colic artery does not extend as high as the splenic flexure in about one quarter of cases.

Veins generally accompany the major arteries. However, the inferior mesenteric vein runs upward in the retroperitoneum above the origin of the inferior mesenteric artery to the left of the fourth portion of the duodenum, behind the body of the pancreas, and empties into the splenic vein. The superior mesenteric vein runs to the right of the superior mesenteric artery and joins the splenic vein behind the head of the pancreas to form the portal vein.

Lymphatics. Profuse lymphatic drainage follows the major pathways of the superior and inferior mesenteric vessels, and there is abundant intercommunication between lymph channels. The epicolic nodes are small and lie immediately on the surface of the colon beneath the serous membrane. Pericolic nodes lie 1 to 2 cm from the colon along the marginal artery of Drummond. The intermediate nodes lie along the major branches of the mesenteric vessels and the principal nodes are located along the superior or inferior mesenteric vessels themselves.

PREOPERATIVE PREPARATION

Since the median age of patients with colon cancer is close to 70 years, multiple associated medi-

1383

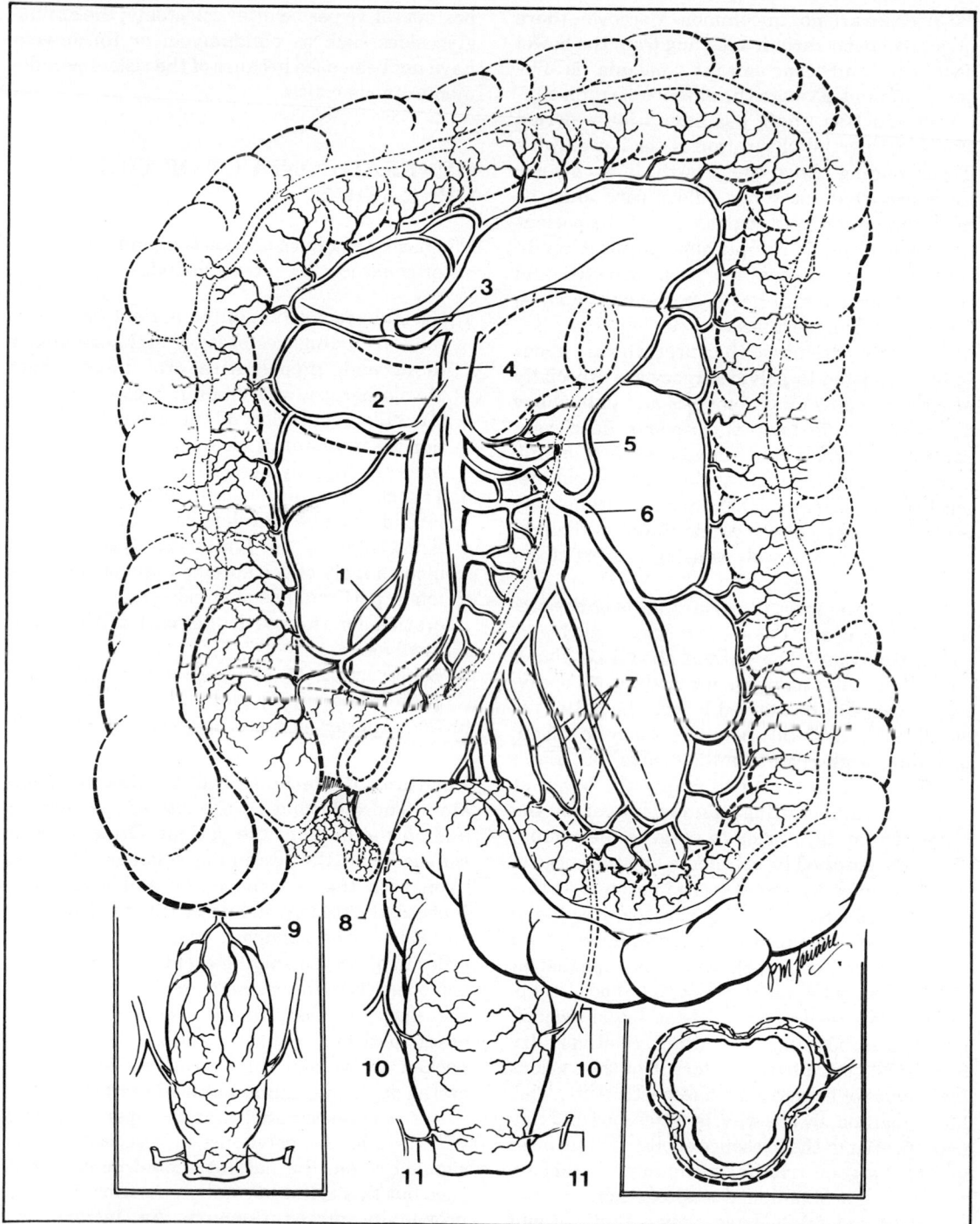

Figure 53–1. The arterial supply of the colon and rectum: (1) ileocolic, (2) ileocolic artery giving off the right colic artery, (3) middle colic artery, (4) superior mesenteric artery, (5) inferior mesenteric artery, (6) left colic artery, (7) sigmoidal branches of the inferior mesenteric artery, (8 and 9) superior haemorrhoidal artery, (10) middle haemorrhoidal artery, (11) inferior haemorrhoidal artery.

cal diseases are not uncommon. Moreover, there may have been chronic bleeding from the bowel neoplasm and concomitant anaemia is frequently found. Even in the absence of frank clinical obstruction, there has often been a period of at least partial obturation of the bowel, with faecal loading above the growth. It is obvious, therefore, that most meticulous care must be taken preoperatively to ensure that the patient has been brought to optimum physical condition, that any anaemia has been corrected, and that the large bowel has been cleansed and, as far as possible, sterilised.

Elderly patients with cancer who are about to be submitted to pelvic surgery are especially at risk of deep vein thrombosis and pulmonary embolism. A history of previous deep vein thrombosis makes this risk almost certain and, under these circumstances, low-dose subcutaneous heparin therapy (5000 units subcutaneously every 12 hours) should be instituted in the preoperative period as well as using support stockings.

One of the most important parts of the preoperative preparation is the mechanical cleansing of the colon. The patient should be placed on a fluid-only regimen for 5 days preoperatively; this can be started before the patient is admitted to hospital. Any fluids can be taken, including high-protein milk drinks, but there is little point in trying to empty the bowel at one end while putting residue into it at the other. Three days prior to surgery the rectum should be emptied by an enema and the surgeon should ensure by rectal examination that this had been effective. Two days preoperatively the patient is commenced on magnesium sulphate 4 g in 10 ml of water, which is repeated at 2-hour intervals until clear diarrhoea is obtained. This technique has been found very effective in producing a clean and relatively dry bowel and this author prefers it to the various techniques of lavage via a nasogastric tube. This latter method, by the way, is dangerous and contraindicated in the presence of obstruction; after giving it a good trial for some months this author has now abandoned it altogether.

Repeated trials have shown that without doubt prophylactic antibiotic therapy greatly reduces the incidence of postoperative sepsis. My present regimen is to use metronidazole and cefuroxime (a third-generation cephalosporin) commenced intravenously immediately before surgery and continued for 3 days into the postoperative period after colectomy; the aminoglycosides such as clindamycin or lincomycin have not been used because of the risk of pseudomembranous colitis.

GENERAL CONDUCT OF THE OPERATION

The basic principles of resection and anastomosis of the colon for cancer include:

1. Careful preparation of the patient for operation, including restoration of haemoglobin to normal, preoperative oral toilet, chest physiotherapy, and vitamin replacement.
2. Careful preparation of the colon for operation by mechanical cleansing and antibiotic cover, as already described.
3. The choice of a generous and well-planned incision to give excellent exposure.
4. Knowledge of the lymphatic drainage and blood supply of the specific regions of the colon in performance of an adequate cancer operation for the particular part of the colon involved.
5. Construction of an anastomosis with adequate blood supply and under no tension.
6. Construction of a strong wound closure.

Position of Patient and Choice of Incision. These depend on the site of the tumour and on the build of the patient. Growths from the caecum to the descending colon are operated upon with the patient supine and horizontal. If obese, the patient should be tilted to the opposite side, using sandbags or a tilting table, in order to allow the small bowel to fall away from the operative site. If the tumour is situated in the sigmoid colon, the Trendelenburg (head-down) position enables the small bowel to be packed away from the operative site and also assists with the illumination of the pelvis.

If it is anticipated that the operative field will include the pelvis, as in resection of the sigmoid colon, the patient should be catheterised, but this is not normally necessary in more proximally placed tumours. An intravenous drip is commenced, although in a patient with a normal haemoglobin blood transfusion is not usually necessary.

For tumours extending from the caecum to the midtransverse colon, a right paramedian incision gives excellent access. A left paramedian approach is used for more distally placed tumours. These incisions can be extended in either direction and, in a grossly obese patient with a lateral adherent tumour, can always be extended still further by means of a transverse limb. Although transverse or oblique muscle cutting incisions are favoured by some surgeons, these give rather more limited access and are less convenient for the placing of a colostomy or caecostomy should these be required.

Preliminary Laparotomy. Once the abdomen is opened, it should be explored carefully to assess the extent and spread of the primary tumour and possible associated pathology. It is wise to palpate the liver for secondary deposits before assessing the primary tumour. The extent of the growth and the possibility of adjacent visceral involvement are assessed. The whole of the large bowel is then carefully examined, since it is not unusual to discover a second primary tumour—indeed, the preliminary barium enema and/or colonoscopic examination may have suggested this. At the same time, careful note is made of the state of the large bowel proximal to the growth, since the presence of obstruction or of heavy faecal loading may indicate that a preliminary colostomy might be necessary before resection is attempted at a second stage. The draining lymph nodes are examined in order to determine the presence of clinically obvious lymph node deposits.

When the primary growth is mobile and there is no clinical evidence of distant spread, curative resection is indicated. A number of small scattered liver metastases should not preclude palliative resection, since this will save the patient the miseries of uncontrolled local disease. However, if the hepatic spread is extensive, then fine judgement is required to determine whether resection should or should not be attempted. Invasion of adjacent structures again requires careful assessment to determine whether en bloc resection is still feasible; this may include removal of portions of the anterior or posterior abdominal wall, omentum, stomach, duodenum, small bowel, or pelvic organs. If there is any doubt, a trial dissection is always justified, for the results of radical surgery in advanced local carcinoma in the absence of evidence of distant spread may be surprisingly good (Davies and Ellis, 1975; Pittam and Ellis, 1984).

During resection, the dissemination and implantation of tumour cells should be avoided. The growth itself should be wrapped in a gauze pack as soon as possible and packs used to protect the wound edges. Irrigation of the open ends of the bowel at the time of anastomosis should be carried out using either a 1:500 dilution of mercury perchloride or undiluted Cetavlon.

Extent of Resection for Carcinoma in Various Sites (Fig. 53–2). In good-risk patients, for curative operations, resection comprises removal of the appropriate section of bowel together with its lymphatic drainage.

Carcinoma of the caecum and proximal ascending colon should be treated by right colectomy encompassing the lymphatic drainage along the ileocolic, right colic, and right branch of the middle colic vessels.

Carcinoma of the hepatic flexure is removed preferably by right hemicolectomy, with division of the middle colic artery at its origin and anastomosis of the ileum to the distal transverse colon.

Carcinoma of the midtransverse colon requires excision of the entire transverse mesocolon, with ligation of the middle colic and preferably the right colic and the ascending branch of the left colic arteries.

Splenic flexure or descending colon carcinoma requires ligation of the left colic artery or division of the entire inferior mesenteric pedicle. In the latter, a wide mesenteric dissection is obtained, since there will be an anastomosis of the transverse colon to the rectosigmoid.

Sigmoid colon resection usually involves the preservation of the left colic branch, assuming there are no nodes high on the inferior mesenteric artery. If enlarged nodes are present, the entire inferior mesenteric pedicle is divided with anastomosis of the transverse colon or the upper descending colon to the rectosigmoid.

Multiple tumours of the colon may require subtotal colectomy with ileorectosigmoid anastomosis.

Technique of Anastomoses

There are several basic principles in the construction of a colonic anastomosis.

The blood supply to the cut margins of the bowel must be adequate. This is determined by arterial bleeding from the cut edge of the colon, the normal pink colour of the bowel right up to the anastomotic edge, and the presence of

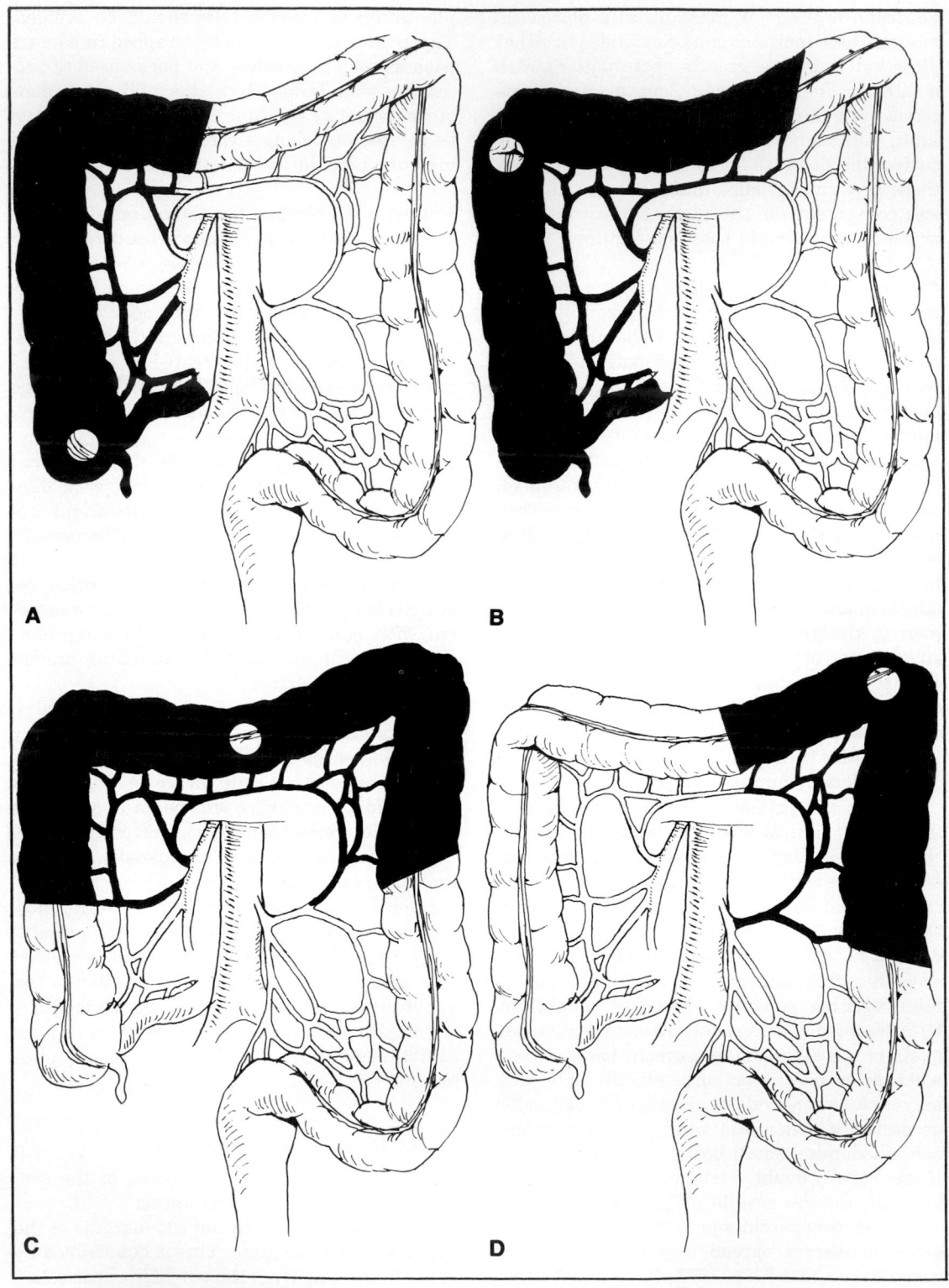

Figure 53–2. A to **G.** Extent of resection for carcinoma in various sites. **A.** Right colectomy. **B.** Right hemicolectomy with division of middle colic pedicle. **C.** Transverse colectomy. **D.** Resection of splenic flexure and ligation of left colic pedicle.

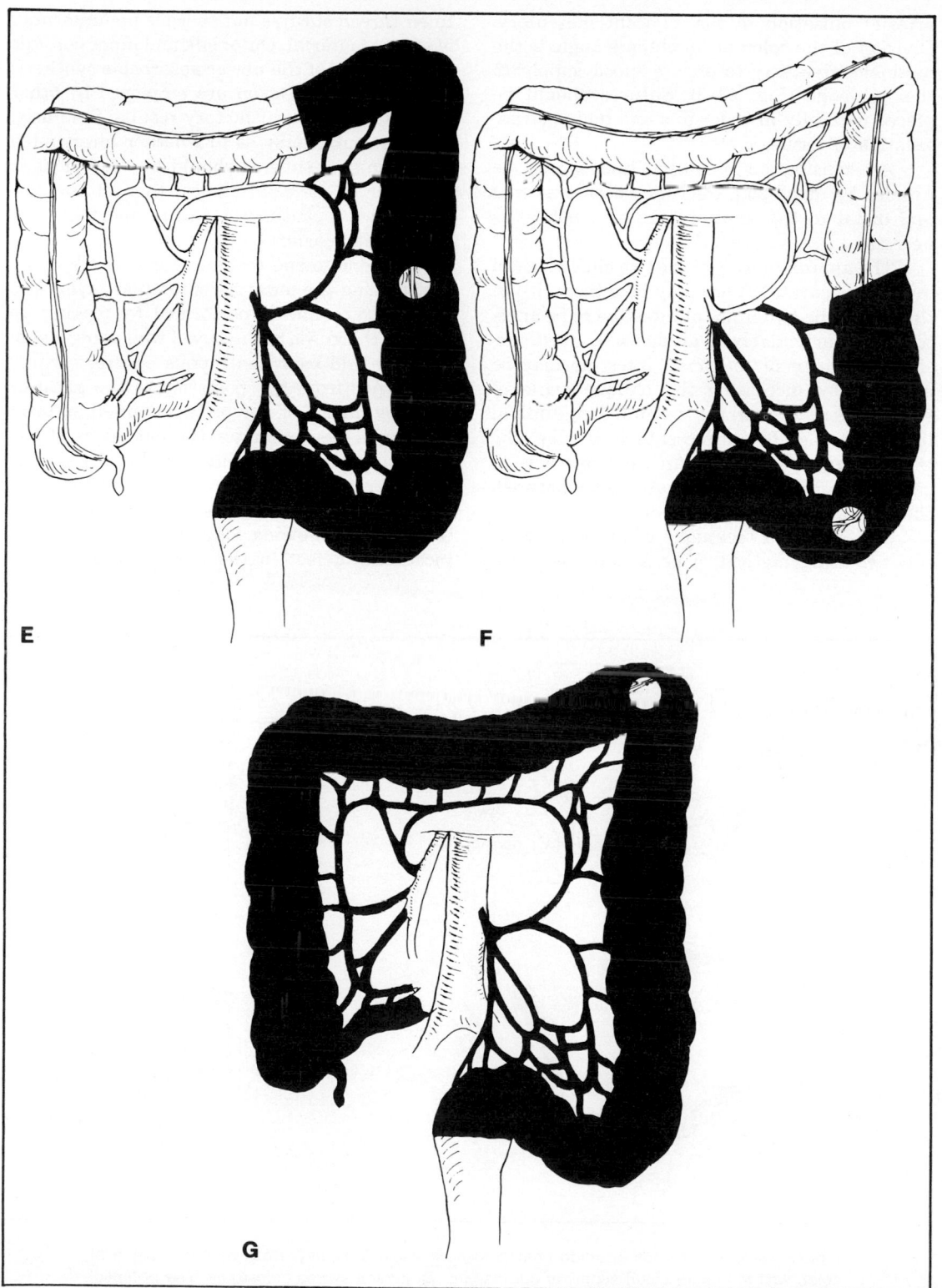

Figure 53–2. E. Left hemicolectomy. **F.** Sigmoid colectomy, sparing the left colic vessels. **G.** Subtotal colectomy.

arterial pulsation in the adjacent mesentery. Division of the colon at an oblique angle is the most effective way to ensure blood supply to the cut edge (Fig. 53–3). Sutures should be placed carefully in order to avoid undue strangulation of tissue.

All tension on a suture line should be avoided by mobilising the colon, both proximal and distal to the anastomosis, as much as is necessary.

The approximation of the two ends of bowel must be accurate. There may be a disparity in the size of the two limbs of intestine to be anastomosed, particularly in an ileocolic anastomosis. The lumen of the small intestine may be enlarged by increasing the oblique angle of sectioning or by making a small longitudinal incision along its antimesenteric border (the Cheatle cut) (Fig. 53–3). An alternative is to carry out an end-to-side anastomosis between the ileum and transverse colon.

The standard technique of anastomosis is the two-layer method. This author uses 2/0 linen thread sutures but there is no uniformity of suture material. Outer silk and inner chromic catgut or one of the newer absorbable synthetic sutures such as Dexon are employed by other authorities with satisfactory results. Similarly, there is controversy as to whether interrupted or continuous sutures should be used. This is a matter of personal choice; this author normally uses a continuous suture and finds this quicker and easier.

The end-to-end technique is carried out by first placing the outer seromuscular layer. The inner suture line is performed by picking up the full thickness of the bowel wall using a simple over and over continuous suture, turning the corner from the posterior to the anterior layer by means of one or two Connell sutures. This layer approximates the cut edges of the bowel and ensures haemostasis. Finally the anterior seromuscular layer is placed in the same fashion as was used for the posterior suture line (Fig. 53–4). Following completion of the anastomosis, the defect in the mesocolon should be

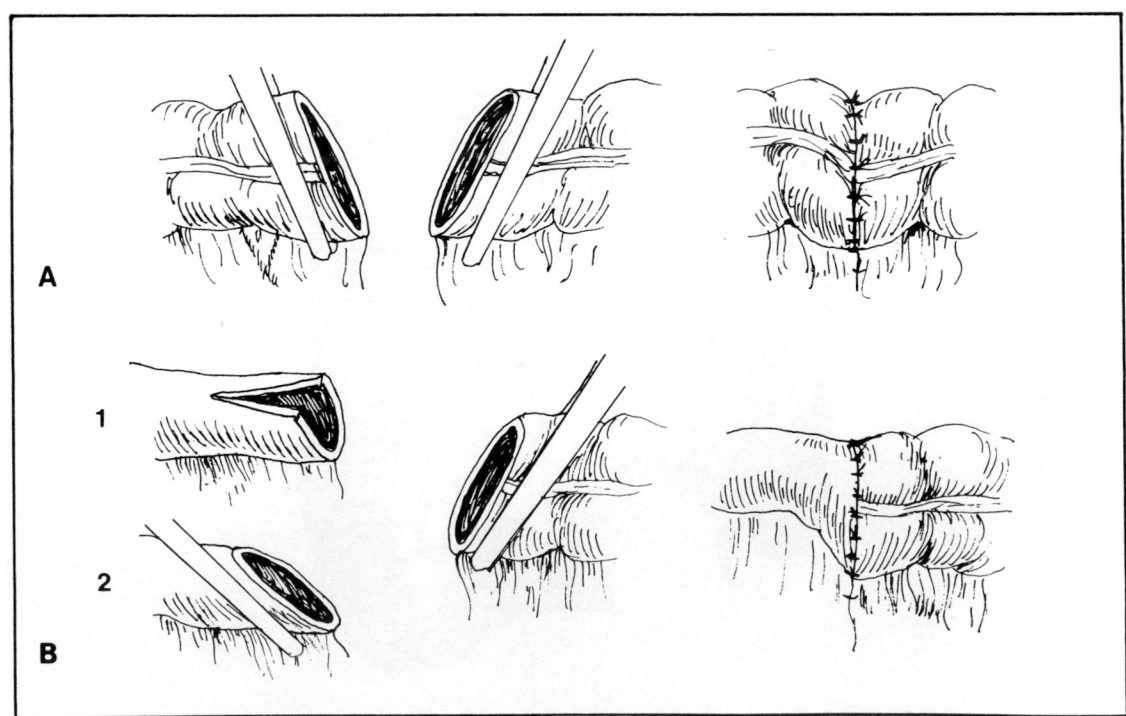

Figure 53–3. Techniques of colon anastomosis. **A.** Colocolostomy. Note oblique division of colon wall to ensure blood supply at cut margins. **B.** Ileotransverse colostomy. The potential lumen of the ileum is enlarged by (1) division on antimesenteric border (Cheatle cut) or (2) oblique division.

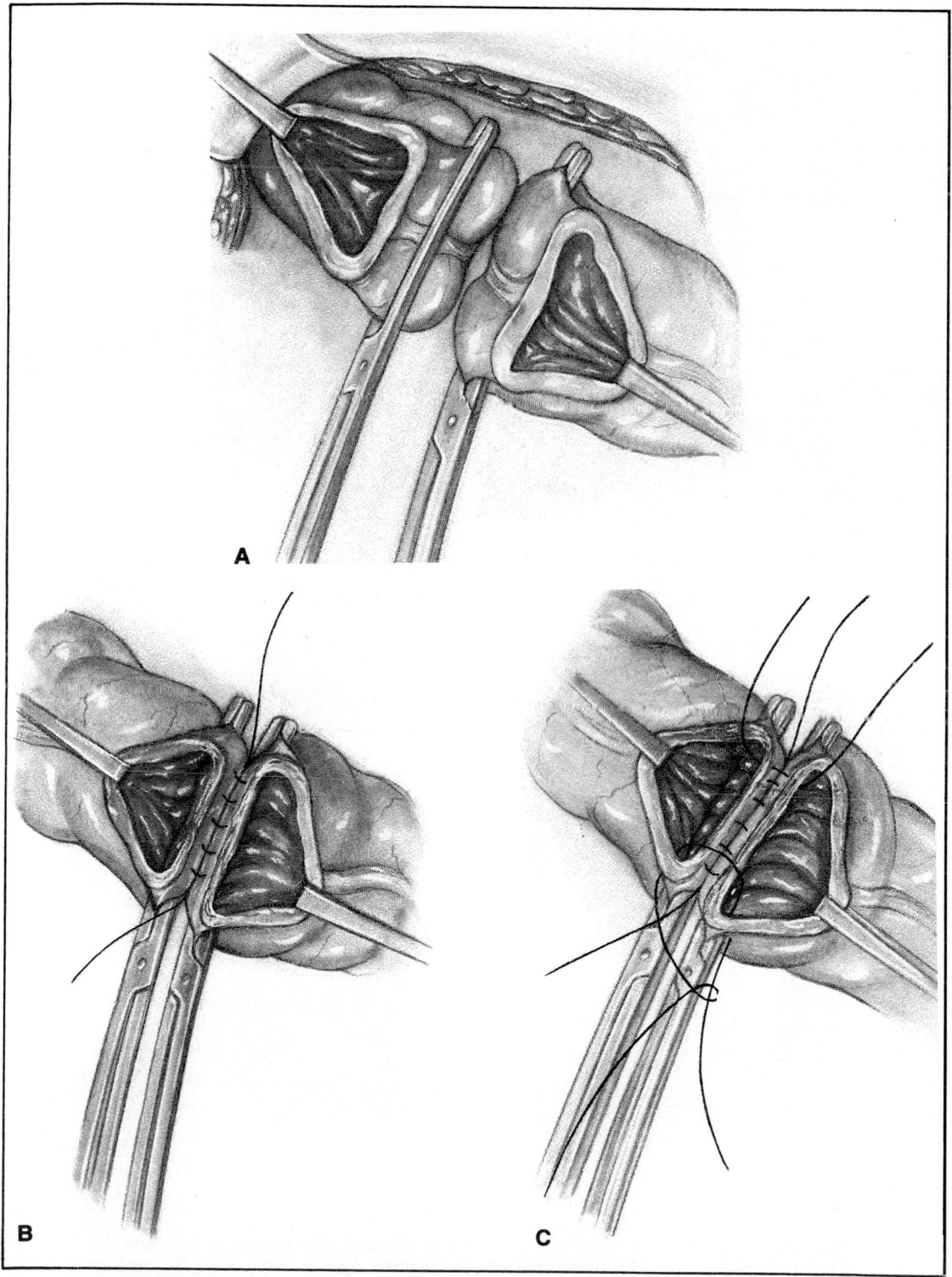

Figure 53–4. A through **G.** Colectomy: the steps in the two-layer anastomosis. **A.** The mobilised bowel ends apposed in noncrushing clamps. **B.** The posterior serosal continuous layer. **C.** The posterior all coats continuous layer.

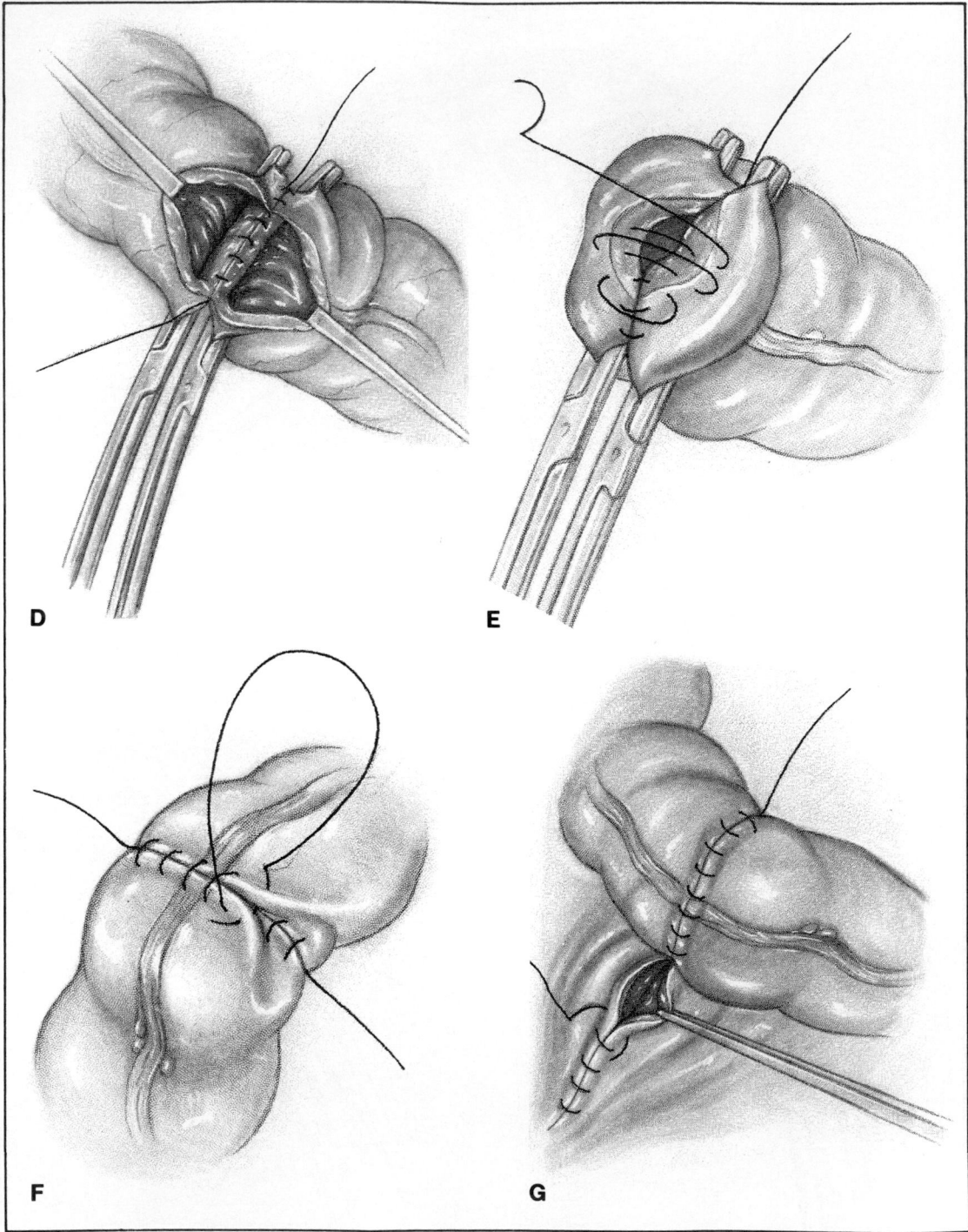

Figure 53–4. D. The corner is turned by means of a loop on the mucosa suture, and the anterior all-coats continuous layer begun. **E.** The anterior layer is inserted. **F.** The anterior serosal layer is completed. **G.** The mesocolic defect is repaired. (*Source: From Ellis H, 1982, with permission.*)

closed to prevent internal herniation of the bowel; for this a continuous thread suture is used. The omentum is then brought down and wrapped around the anastomotic line.

Several methods of one-layer anastomosis have been described (Fig. 53–5). Most surgeons use interrupted sutures. In a well-matched trial, Irvin and colleagues (1973) recorded almost identical dehiscence rates after one layer and conventional two layer inverting anastomoses (16 versus 17 percent, respectively). For low anterior resections involving the extraperitoneal rectum, there is no doubt that the single-layer interrupted technique is often easier and, perhaps, even safer (Everett, 1975).

An objection to inverting techniques is that they undoubtedly narrow the lumen of the bowel, but the trials of Goligher and colleagues (1970) have shown that everting techniques of anastomosis should not be used in colon surgery. Faecal fistulae occurred in no less than 43 percent of their patients having everting sutures compared to 8.6 percent of those treated with the inverting technique.

Use of the Stapler. All the colonic anastomoses can be carried out by means of stapling instruments. It is true to state that this technique is more popular in the US than it is in the United Kingdom, where the majority of surgeons confine the use of staplers to low rectal anastomoses.

SPECIFIC OPERATIONS

Right Hemicolectomy (Figs. 53–6 through 53–8)

The usual incision for a right hemicolectomy is a right paramedian approach. Tumour evaluation is carried out at a full laparotomy as already described. The small bowel is packed off medially. The right colon is now freed by incising the lateral peritoneal attachment from the posterior abdominal wall and the right colon is mobilised to the root of its mesocolon. It is not uncommon to find that the caecal or ascending colon tumour has already invaded the adjacent parietal abdominal wall. If so, mobilisation will require a wider excision with the removal of a section of peritoneum together with, if necessary, underlying musculature.

During mobilisation, the spermatic or ovarian vessels, the ureter, and the second part of the duodenum come into view and are carefully preserved from injury.

The hepatic flexure and the right side of the transverse colon are now mobilised. A dense ligament (the hepatocolic ligament) tethers the hepatic flexure and requires division, together with the right extremity of the gastrocolic omentum. If the tumour is in the caecum or ascending colon, the greater omentum can be separated from the right extremity of the transverse colon along what is almost a blood-

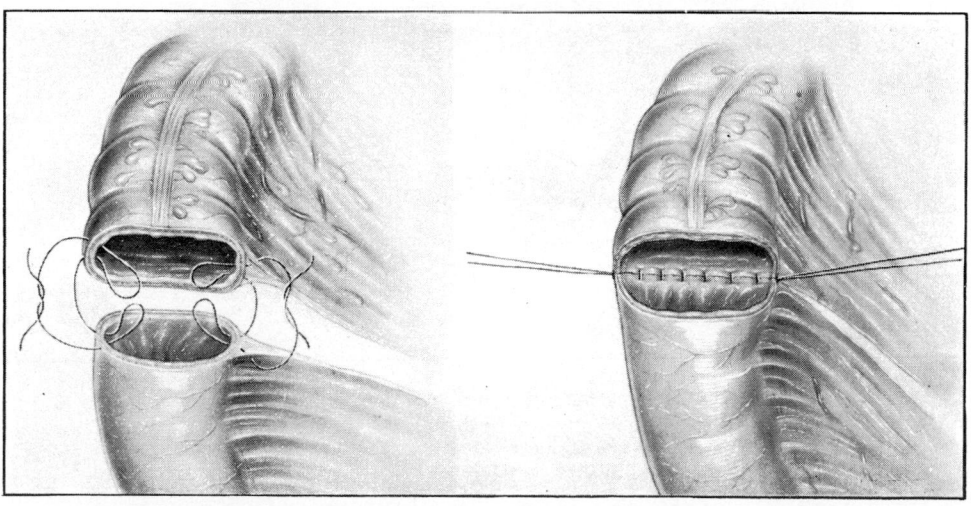

Figure 53–5. One-layer end-to-end ileotransverse colostomy. Note Connell stitches at the lateral margins.

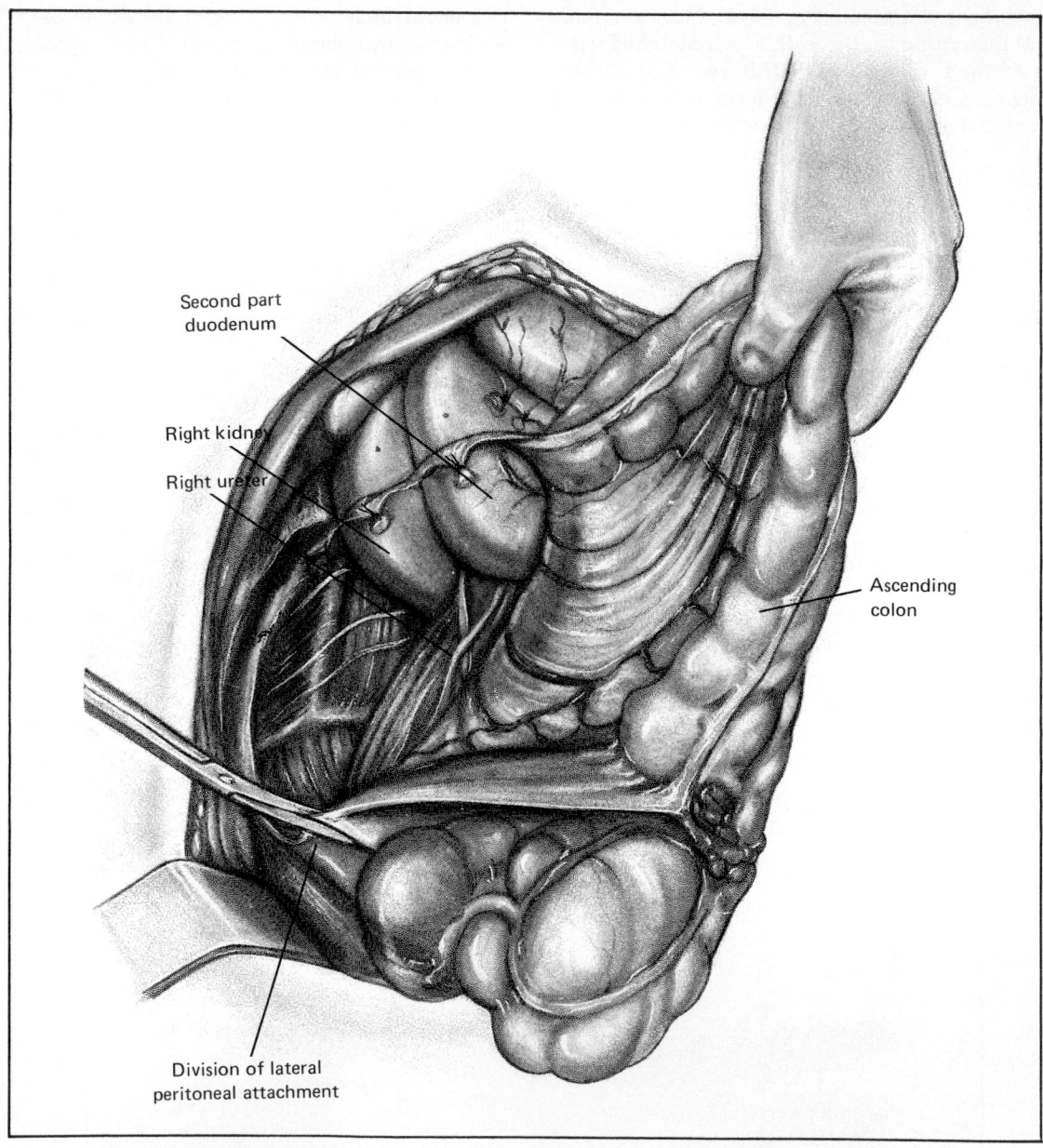

Second part
duodenum

Right kidney

Right ureter

Ascending
colon

Division of lateral
peritoneal attachment

Figure 53–6. Right hemicolectomy; mobilisation of the right colon. (*Source: From Ellis H, 1982, with permission.*)

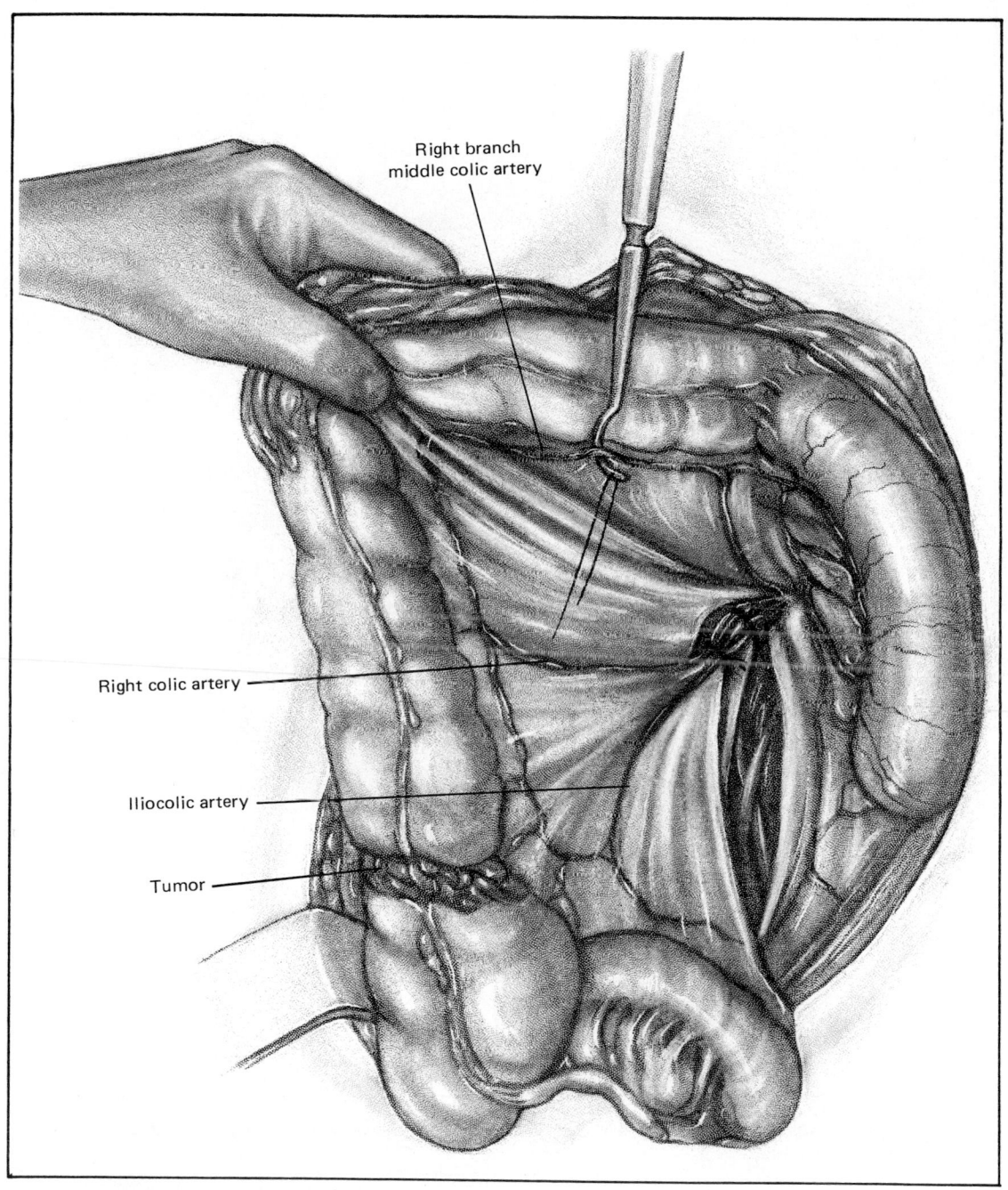

Figure 53–7. Right hemicolectomy; division of vascular pedicles. (*Source: From Ellis H, 1982, with permission.*)

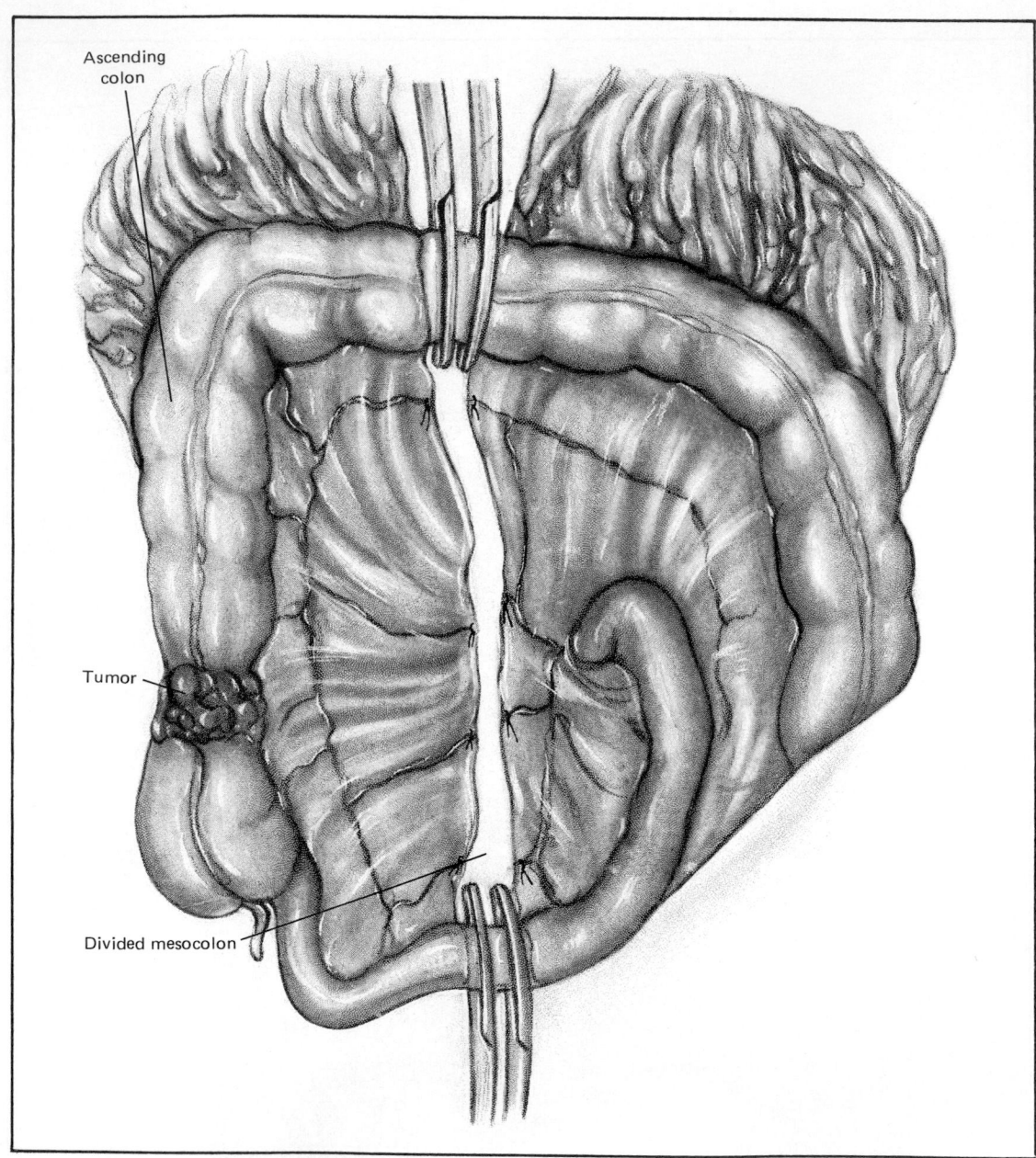

Figure 53–8. Right hemicolectomy; division of the bowel. (*Source: From Ellis H, 1982, with permission.*)

less plane. If, however, the tumour is situated in the hepatic flexure or if the omentum is actually adherent to the growth, then the adjacent omentum requires detachment and removal with the operative specimen.

Once the tumour has been mobilised, tapes are passed above and below the growth and firmly ligated to reduce intraluminal dissemination of cancer cells, and the tumour itself is wrapped in a gauze pack held by ligatures in order to minimise handling of its peritoneal surface.

Having mobilised the right half of the colon completely, the vascular pedicles are identified in its mesocolon and the ileocolic and right colic vessels are tied near their origins, using double ligation with thread. The branches of the middle colic pedicle to the right colon are similarly divided and tied. Division of the mesocolon is continued up to the edge of the transverse colon and downward across the small bowel mesentery to the wall of the terminal ileum. The exact site of division of terminal ileum and transverse

colon is chosen with particular attention to the adequacy of the blood supply at the site of the proposed anastomosis; the site of division of the ileum is usually 8 to 10 cm from the ileocaecal valve and the colon should be divided at least 8 cm clear from the macroscopic edge of the tumour. The ileum and transverse colon are now divided between clamps. The clamp placed on the ileum is angled relatively acutely, so that the diameter of the bowel wall will be comparable to that of the transverse colon.

The bowel is now ready for anastomosis. If there is little disparity in the size of the lumen of small and large bowel, an end-to-end two layer anastomosis is performed.

Quite often the colon is much wider than the terminal ileum; under these circumstances, anastomosis is performed between the end of the ileum and side of the transverse colon. The transverse colon is closed using two layers of 2/0 linen thread (Fig. 53–9). The first is passed loosely through all coats of the colon over the crushing clamp, which is then removed and the

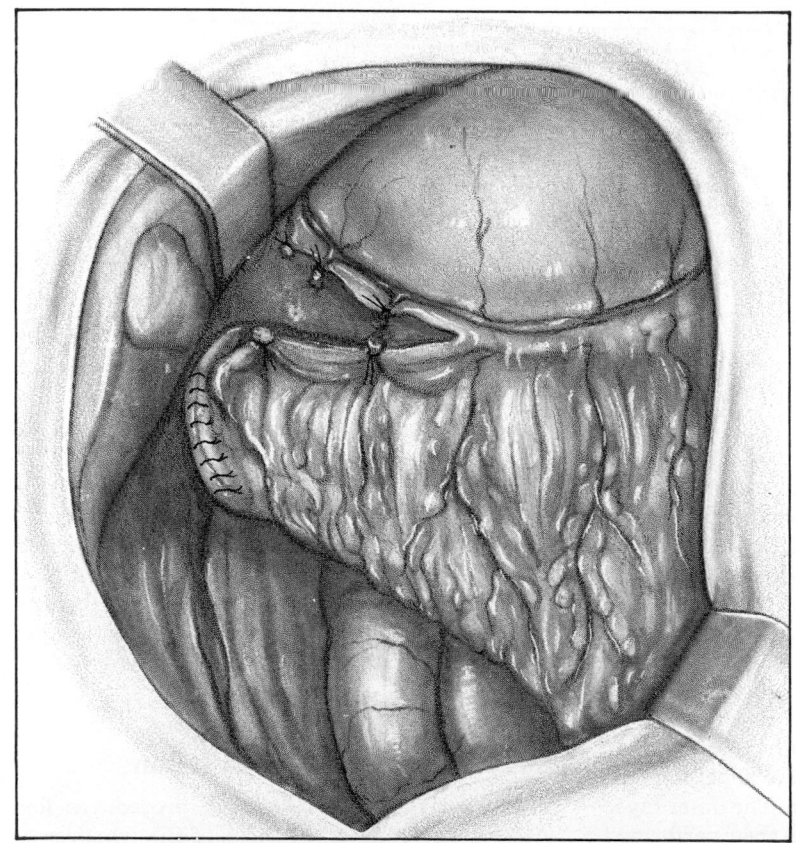

Figure 53–9. Right hemicolectomy; closure of the stump of the colon. (*Source: Ellis H, 1982, with permission.*)

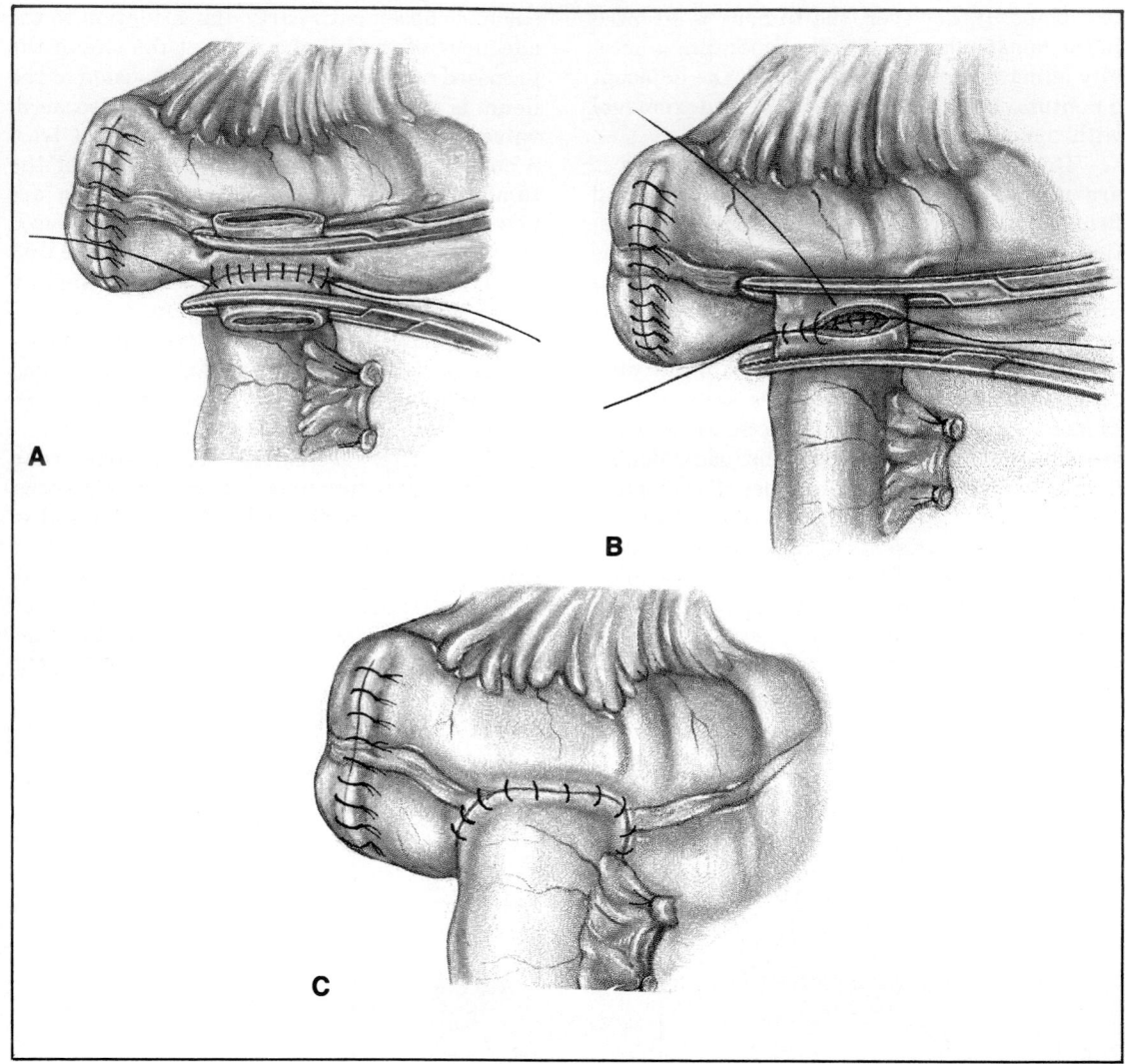

Figure 53–10. Right hemicolectomy; end-to-side ileocolic anastomosis. (*Source: From Ellis H, 1982, with permission.*)

suture line pulled tight and tied. The second layer comprises a continuous or interrupted invaginating layer of the serosal coat. The transverse colon is then picked up in a noncrushing intestinal clamp and apposed to the open end of the terminal ileum. A continuous or interrupted thread seromuscular suture apposes the peritoneal coats and the colon is then incised longitudinally to a length corresponding to the open lumen of the ileum. Any faecal material is carefully swabbed away and the open ends of the bowel washed out with 1:500 perchloride of mercury solution or Cetavlon. The inner layer of all coats 2/0 linen thread is then performed and the serosal suture then completed to cover

the anterior wall (Fig. 53–10). The noncrushing clamps are removed and the anastomosis checked, both to ensure an adequate lumen and to be certain that haemostasis has been effected. The defect in the mesocolon is closed with a continuous thread suture. The remaining omentum is then drawn over the anastomotic line and can be tacked over it with one or two interrupted sutures.

Resection of Transverse Colon

There are several alternative procedures for elective resection of a cancer of the transverse colon. The extent of the incision varies, depending on the build of the patient and the location of the primary tumour. An upper transverse incision will suffice for localised resection or for resections of either flexure. A long right or left paramedian incision is preferred if the tumour is well over to the right or left side of the transverse colon, respectively (Fig. 53–11).

If the transverse colon is redundant, simple resection of the transverse colon together with the omentum and anastomosis of the remaining portion of colon distal to the hepatic flexure and proximal to the splenic flexure is possible (Fig. 53–11). The stomach is detached from the transverse colon by serial division of the branches of the gastroepiploic arcade, which are tied with thread and then divided between ligatures. Mobilisation continues as far as the hepatic and splenic flexures. The detached transverse colon is held upward so that its

mesocolon can be inspected. The middle colic vessels are tied at their origins and divided. The transverse mesocolon is incised in an inverted V up to the bowel edge at the site selected for resection, which must be at least 8 cm from the macroscopic edge of the tumour. Here the bowel is divided between clamps and an end-to-end anastomosis performed in the manner already described. The mesocolic defect is closed.

A second alternative is an extended right hemicolectomy, if the tumour is situated in the proximal part of the transverse colon. A similar segmental resection can be carried out for tumours of the distal transverse colon, where the dissection is carried from the midportion of the transverse colon to the midportion of the descending colon. A very extensive tumour of the transverse colon may demand subtotal colec-

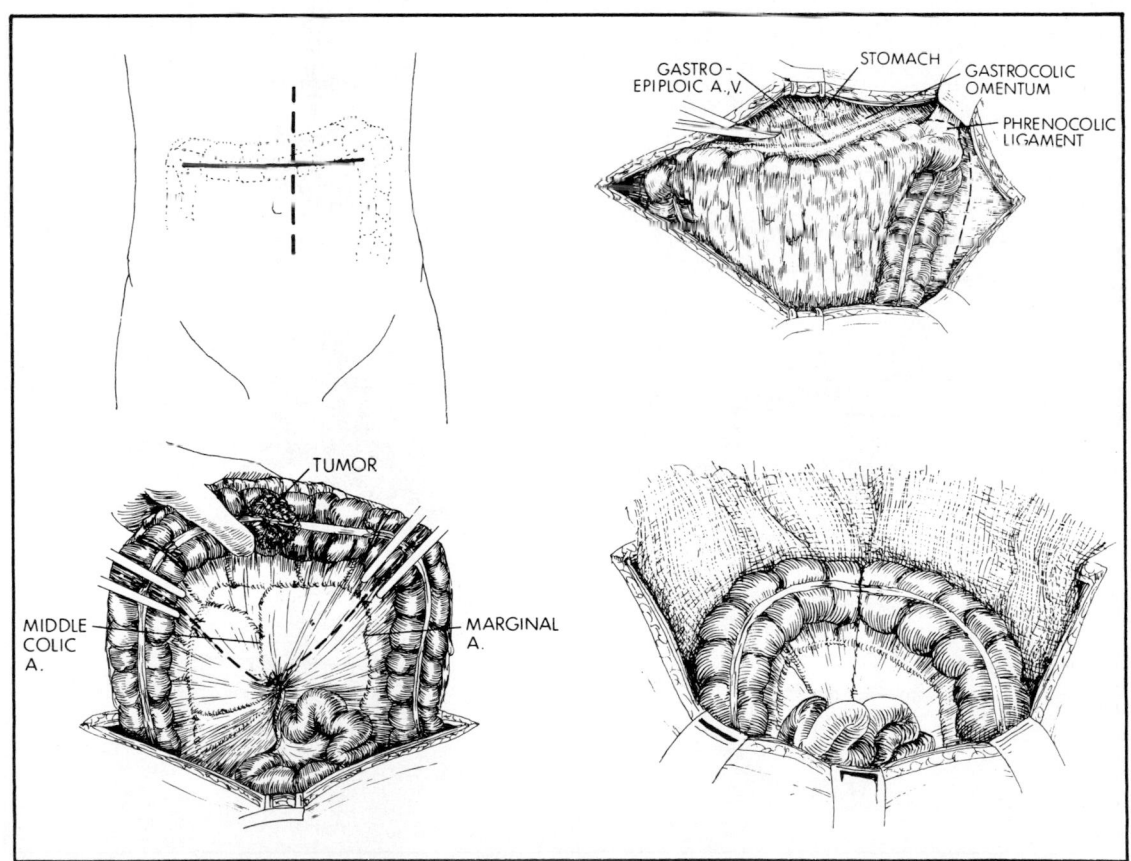

Figure 53–11. Transverse colectomy. *Top Left:* Either a transverse or vertical incision may be used. *Top Right:* Separation of the colon from the stomach by division of gastrocolic omentum above the gastroepiloic vessels. *Bottom Left:* Extent of mesenteric resection. Note redundant colon and absence of gastrocolic omentum for schematic purposes. *Bottom Right:* Final appearance of anastomosis.

tomy, with anastomosis between the ileum and the sigmoid colon.

Resection of the Splenic Flexure and Descending Colon

Cancers in this region metastasise to lymph nodes along the left colic vein and thence along the route of the inferior mesenteric vessels. If enlarged lymph nodes are palpated along the inferior mesenteric vessels, total removal of the inferior mesenteric pedicle is necessary (Fig. 53–12). The dissection will need to extend from the distal transverse colon down to the rectosigmoid where the anastomotic supply from the middle haemorrhoidal vessels is functional. However,

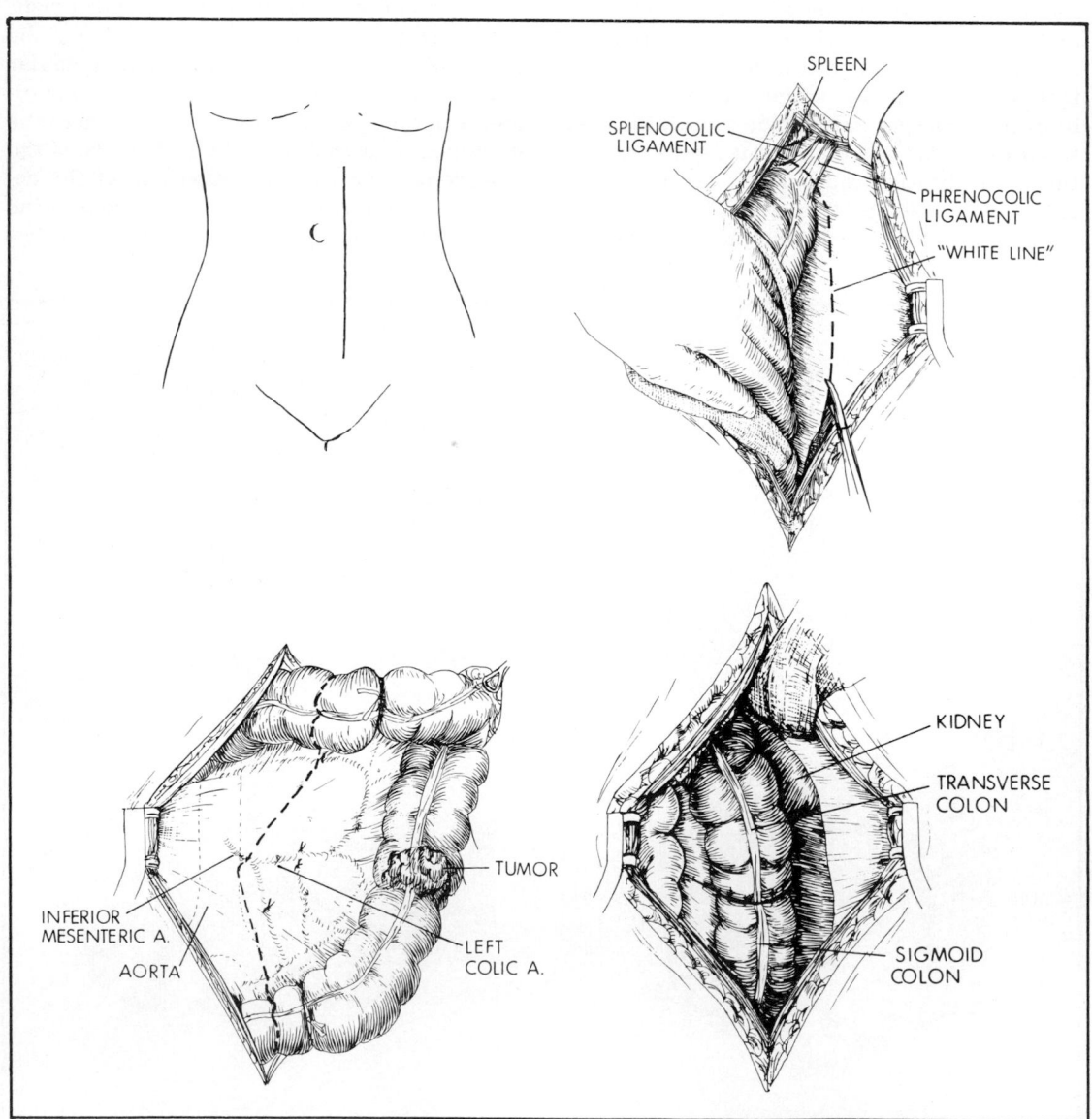

Figure 53–12. Left colectomy. *Top Left:* Left paramedian incision. *Top Right:* The lateral peritoneal reflection ("white line") is incised in an avascular plane. *Bottom Left:* Proposed mesenteric resection is carried to the inferior mesenteric artery pedicle. Note ligatures around vessels in mesentery. *Bottom Right:* End-to-end anastomosis at its completion.

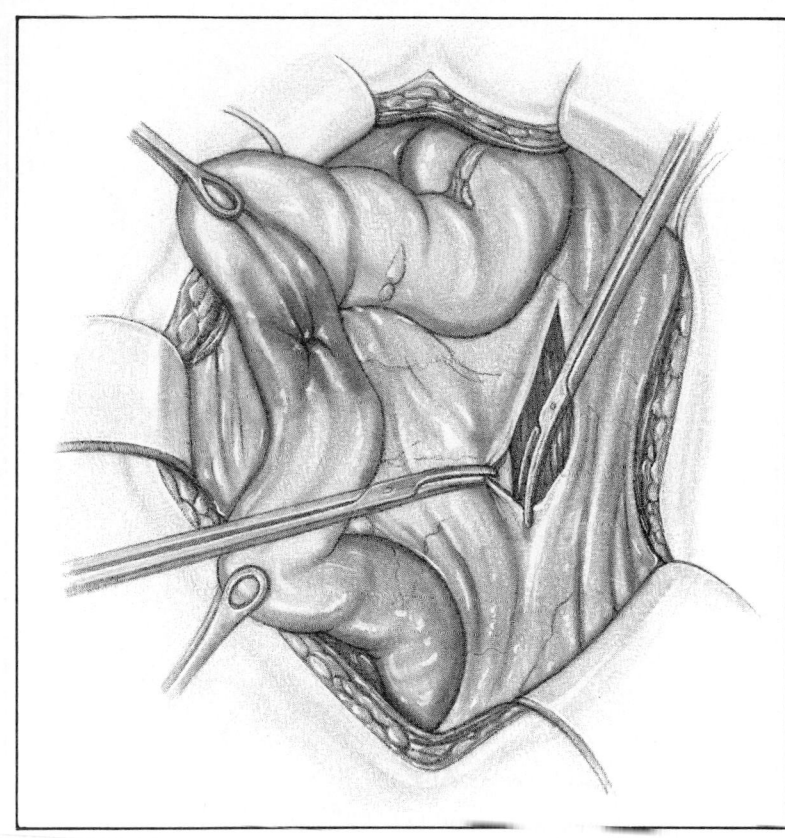

Figure 53–13. Sigmoid colectomy. Mobilisation of the sigmoid colon by division of its lateral peritoneal attachment. (*Source: From Ellis H, 1982, with permission.*)

in poor-risk patients or in those in whom no enlarged lymph nodes are found, the left colic vessels may be ligated at their base and the inferior mesenteric pedicle left intact, thus allowing an anastomosis in a more accessible area in the sigmoid colon.

The left colon is mobilised in a manner similar to the procedure on the right side but is rather more difficult on account of the higher and more inaccessible position of the splenic flexure. When this is deeply placed in an obese subject, it is better first to mobilise the transverse colon by detaching the greater omentum, then to mobilise the descending colon from its lateral peritoneal attachment and then to draw both of these downward. This allows the splenic flexure to come into view and enables division of the phrenicocolic ligament to be carried out more easily. The sigmoid colon itself is readily mobilised by division of its lateral congenital attachments, with careful preservation of the genital vessels and the left ureter.

The end-to-end anastomotic procedure is as previously described.

Sigmoid Colectomy (Figs. 53–13 through 53–16)

The sigmoid colon is the most common site for carcinomas of the colon. Where there is a relatively small tumour without evidence of wide lymphatic spread, resection of the sigmoid loop itself is performed with anastomosis of the mobilised descending colon to the rectosigmoid junction.

A long left paramedian incision provides excellent access. The sigmoid colon is mobilised by dividing its lateral peritoneal attachment along the avascular "white line," with identification and protection of the ureter and of the genital vessels. The tumour is isolated with ties placed above and below it and is surrounded by a gauze pack in the usual way. The root of the mesentery of the sigmoid is freed on the right side. The left colic and upper sigmoid vessels are now tied with thread and divided. At the lower end there is not a true mesentery and the mass of fatty tissue containing the vessels must be isolated carefully and ligated. The

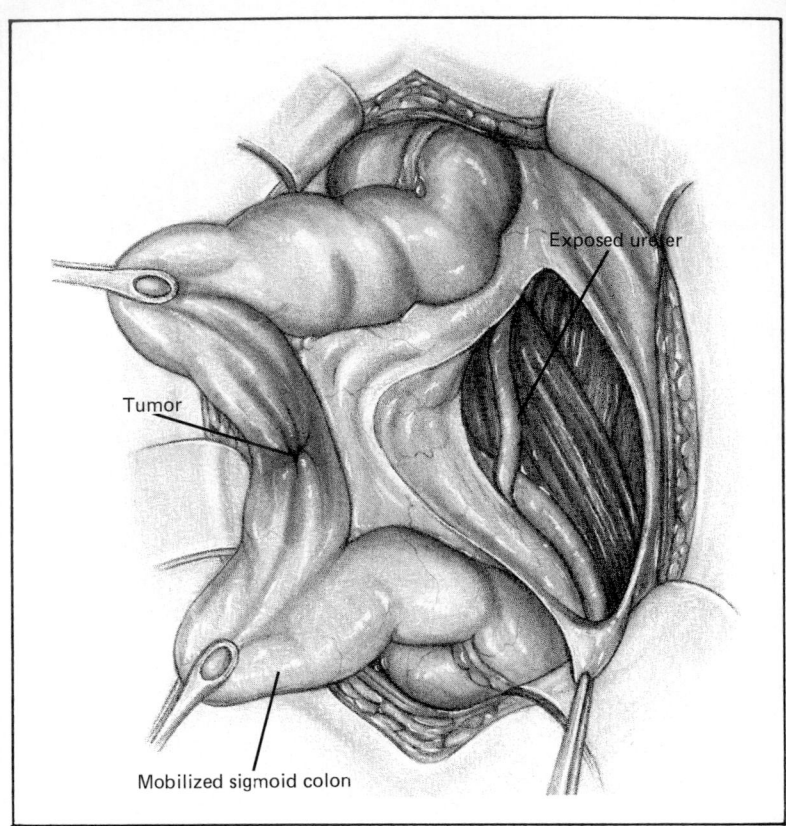

Exposed ureter

Tumor

Mobilized sigmoid colon

Figure 53–14. Sigmoid colectomy. The left ureter is visualised and carefully preserved. (*Source: Ellis H, 1982, with permission.*)

colon is divided between clamps and a two-layer end-to-end anastomosis performed as described above. The base of the mesocolic defect is closed on the medial side.

Subtotal Colectomy

Subtotal colectomy may be required when there is an extensive and complicated tumour of the colon, when there are one or more synchronous tumours, or in cases of "second look" resection of metachronous tumours.

Mobilisation of the bowel during subtotal colectomy follows the details described in previous sections. The anastomosis of the ileum to the rectosigmoid is performed by the two-layer end-to-end technique, unless there is marked disparity in size of the two sections of bowel, which dictates a side-to-end anastomosis.

POSTOPERATIVE COMPLICATIONS

Resections of the colon may be followed by any of the local and general complications that can occur after major abdominal surgery. Indeed, since the patients are often elderly and in poor general condition, it is not surprising that postoperative chest complications, deep vein thrombosis, and pulmonary embolism are far from uncommon and should be combated by appropriate prophylactic measures.

Wound Infection

Postoperative wound infection is particularly common in colonic surgery, due to the high risk of wound contamination from the opened bowel; this has been shown in very many extensive studies. Shaw and colleagues (1973), in a very extensive survey from Dundee, noted a low incidence of wound infection in clean operations such as cardiac surgery (1.1 percent) or following sympathectomy (0.8 percent), but rose to 50.4 percent in resections of the colon and rectum. Recent controlled studies have verified that meticulous bowel preparation, together with antibiotic cover that incorporates metronidazole (as described in the section on Preopera-

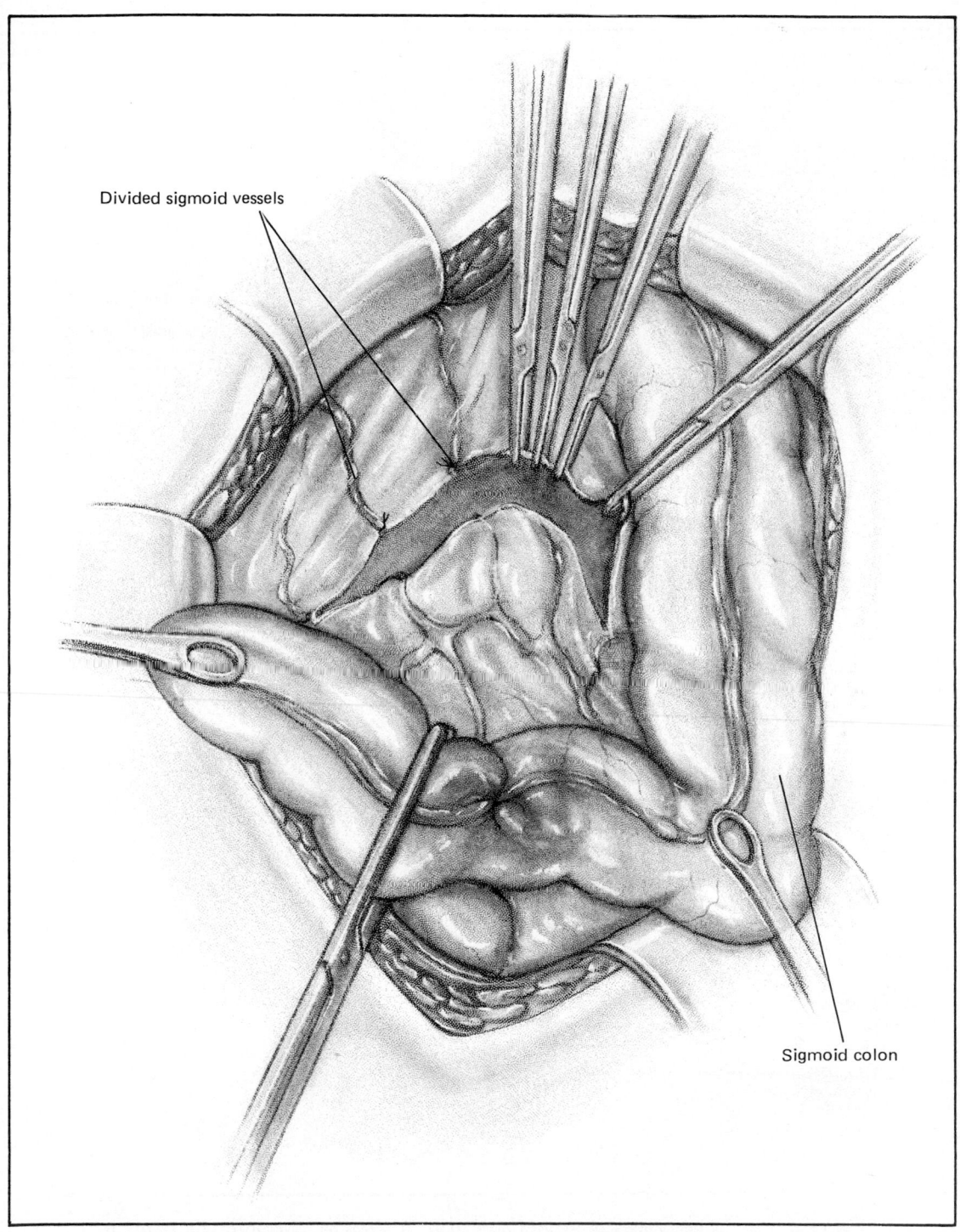

Divided sigmoid vessels

Sigmoid colon

Figure 53–15. Sigmoid colectomy. Division of the sigmoid mesocolon. (*Source: From Ellis H, 1982, with permission.*)

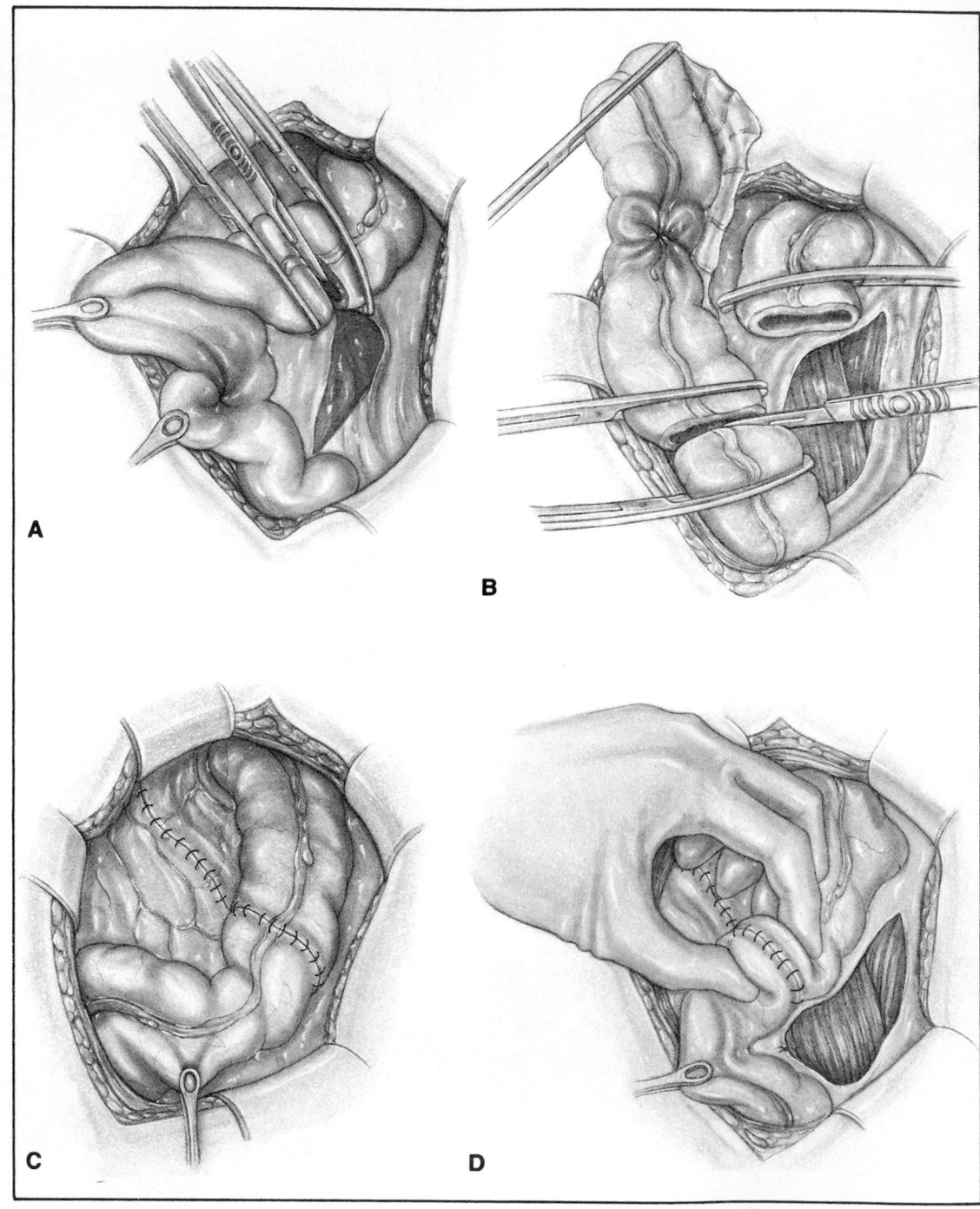

Figure 53–16. Further stages of sigmoid colectomy. **A.** Proximal division of the colon. **B.** Distal division of the colon. **C.** The anastomosis is completed. **D.** Testing the integrity of the anastomotic lumen. (*Source: From Ellis H, 1982, with permission.*)

tive Preparation), significantly reduces this risk (Keighley and Burdon, 1979; Taylor et al, 1979; Willis et al, 1977).

Anastomotic Dehiscence

The important disaster that needs a special note is leakage at the colonic anastomosis. No site is immune, but the low anterior resection, performed below the level of the pelvic peritoneal reflection, is at particular risk. It is unusual for a severe degree of leakage to take place distal to a protective colostomy.

Aetiology

This is usually complex (Khoury and Waxman, 1983). General factors include age, protein deficiency, vitamin C deficiency, jaundice, uraemia, extensive malignant disease, steroid dependence, diabetes, and anaemia. Local factors are probably even more important. These include infection in the operative field or construction of an anastomosis with inadequate blood supply, and anastomosis performed under tension or in the presence of obstruction. Local trauma and infection depresses the collagen content and tensile strength at the anastomotic site (Irvin and Hunt, 1974). Previous radiation therapy may also predispose to anastomotic disruption. If a combination of these factors is present, the surgeon may well be advised to opt for a staged operative approach.

Clinical Manifestations. Undoubtedly there are many leaks that are subclinical and require no therapy. Goligher et al (1970), for example, using sigmoidoscopy, barium enema, and digital examination, detected a 40 percent leak rate in 47 high anterior resections and no less than a 69 percent leakage rate in 26 low resections. Anastomotic leakage of clinical importance occurs in about 10 percent of all large bowel anastomoses (Fielding et al, 1980).

Unfortunately, diagnosis is often delayed. Premonitory signs that point to this complication include an untoward amount of abdominal pain, distension, toxaemia, a tender swollen reddened wound, a rising pyrexia and pulse, and abdominal tenderness with guarding and rebound. The white cell count is elevated. Unfortunately, more often it is only when frank peritonitis is obvious or when there is a discharge of faecal material through the wound or the

drain that the surgeon becomes aware that dehiscence of the colonic suture line has occurred.

Treatment. Cases of anastomotic leakage can be divided into two groups. In the first, there is a minor degree of discharge without any evidence at all of a generalised peritonitis. This may be seen occasionally after closure of a colostomy or where the anastomosis has been protected by a proximal stoma. Many of these cases are probably accounted for by the rupture of a small abscess at the suture line. In these circumstances, the patient should be carefully observed, as spontaneous closure of the fistula may be anticipated.

The second group comprises those patients with frank breakdown of the anastomosis and faecal peritonitis. Urgent operation is now required if the patient's life is to be saved. Broad-spectrum antibiotic therapy is begun, using metronidazole and either gentamicin or one of the third-generation cephalosporins. A blood transfusion should be made available.

The wound is reopened. No attempt is made to repair the leakage, but exteriorisation of the two ends of the anastomosis must be performed. Occasionally, in a low anastomosis, the distal end cannot be brought to the surface and should be sutured with interrupted nonabsorbable (cotton thread) sutures. Careful peritoneal toilet is performed and the wound closed with drainage.

Postoperative Intestinal Obstruction

Intestinal obstruction is not uncommon after colon resection. The usual cause is adhesions, either about the anastomosis or to the laparotomy wound. If the omentum can be preserved, bringing this over the anastomotic line and under the wound will reduce this risk.

TABLE 53–1. CAUSES OF LARGE BOWEL OBSTRUCTION (EDINBURGH ROYAL INFIRMARY)

Carcinoma of the colon	250(77%)
Volvulus	34(10%)
Diverticular disease	13(4%)
Adhesions	7(2%)
Intussusception	2(0.6%)
Cause unknown	8(2.5%)
Malignant—primary site unknown	10(3%)
Total	324

(*Source: From Ellis H: Intestinal Obstruction. New York: Appleton-Century-Crofts, 1982, p 236, with permission.*)

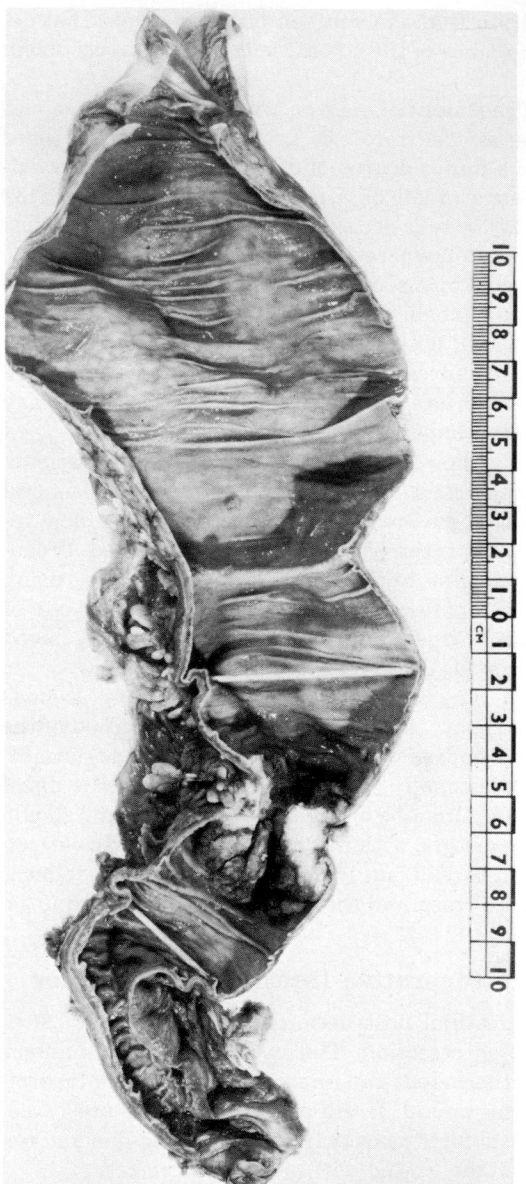

Figure 53–17. An annular constricting carcinoma of the sigmoid colon producing intestinal obstruction. Note the proximal colonic distension. (*Source: From Ellis H, 1982, with permission.*)

Another cause of postoperative obstruction is that a loop of small intestine may pass through a defect in the mesenteric suture line that has been used to close the trap between the limbs of the bowel. If there is a colostomy present, a loop of intestine may twist around it and strangulate.

OBSTRUCTED CANCER OF THE COLON

About 20 percent of intestinal obstructions are due to lesions situated in the large bowel, and by far the most common of these in the Western world is colonic carcinoma, accounting for some three quarters of the cases. As an example, Campbell et al and McLaren, in a 1956 review of 324 large bowel obstructions, found that 77 percent were due to carcinoma; volvulus and diverticular disease were second and third in frequency. Their data are given in full in Table 53–1.

Goligher (1984) estimated that about one fifth of all cases of colonic cancer developed complete obstruction, either as an acute affair or as the culmination of progressive occlusion, the so-called acute on chronic obstruction. This is more often seen in association with tumours of the left rather than the right side of the colon. This is partly accounted for by the fluid nature of faeces and the larger lumen of the colon on the right side, the tendency for right-sided tumours to be proliferative compared with the more common constricting growths on the left side and also because the most common site for cancer in the colon is the sigmoid loop (Figs. 53–17 and 53–18).

Goligher and Smiddy (1957), in a large study of 1644 consecutive cases of carcinoma of the large bowel in Leeds, found that 17.6 percent of these were obstructed; 27 percent of all tumours of the right and transverse colon and 40 percent of left-sided colonic cancers presented with obstruction. In contrast, only 4 percent of rectal cancers, which represented by far the highest proportion of the total tumours, presented with obstructive symptoms. These data are given in full in Table 53–2.

As the colonic lumen becomes narrowed by the tumour, the proximal large bowel dilates and becomes loaded with gas and faecal material. The ileocaecal valve usually remains competent, so that dilatation of the small intestine is not seen until a late stage of the disease process. In contrast, the relatively patulous and thin-walled caecum may become remarkably dilated and may, indeed, perforate. An increase

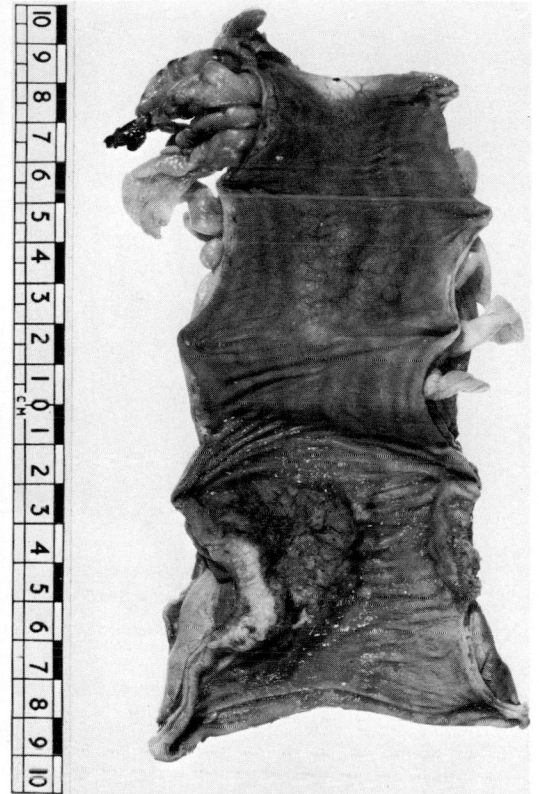

Figure 53–18. "Cauliflower" carcinoma of the ascending colon; there is no obstruction to the bowel lumen. (*Source: From Ellis H, 1982, with permission.*)

ation by impacted faeces immediately above the growth, or by perforation through the tumour itself, as well as, as already mentioned, by rupture of the tensely stretched caecum.

Preparation for Operation

In cases of subacute or partial obstruction, suggested by history of recent passage of flatus or even of stools, it is worthwhile trying to relieve the obstruction by means of a disposable enema. This is particularly likely to be effective in tumours low in the sigmoid colon or at the rectosigmoid. If this is not effective, or if the obstruction is indeed complete, there must be no hesitation in proceeding at once to surgical treatment. Precious time should not be wasted in repeated efforts at washing out the bowel, which will simply exhaust and demoralise the patient.

In most cases, the patient with large bowel obstruction due to carcinoma is in reasonably good condition because vomiting, with its associated dehydration and electrolyte loss, does not usually occur until late in the disease. In every case, the patient requires a nasogastric tube to empty the stomach before anaesthesia. An intravenous infusion is commenced and blood transfusion may be required where there has been considerable chronic loss of blood from the growth.

of caecal diameter much more than 12 cm on the abdominal plain x-ray film indicates that the risk of perforation is very great. In other instances, the ileocaecal valve is incompetent, allowing ileal reflux and small bowel distension (Fig. 53–19). Perforation of the obstructed bowel may occur either at the site of stercoral ulcer-

Choice of Operation

Fine clinical judgement is required in choosing the appropriate operation for a particular case. Factors to be considered include the general condition of the patient, the degree of obstruction, the site of the growth, whether there is

TABLE 53–2. PROPORTION OF PATIENTS WITH CARCINOMA IN DIFFERENT SITES IN LARGE INTESTINE PRESENTING WITH ACUTE OBSTRUCTION (LEEDS GENERAL INFIRMARY)

Site	No. of Growths	No. Complicated by Acute Obstruction	Incidence of Obstruction (%)
Cecum; ascending colon; hepatic flexure	178	50	28.1
Transverse colon	77	20	26.0
Splenic flexure; descending colon; sigmoid	445	180	40.4
Rectum	944	40	4.2
Total	1644	290	17.6

(*Source: From Ellis H: Intestinal Obstruction. New York: Appleton-Century-Crofts, 1982, p 237, with permission.*)

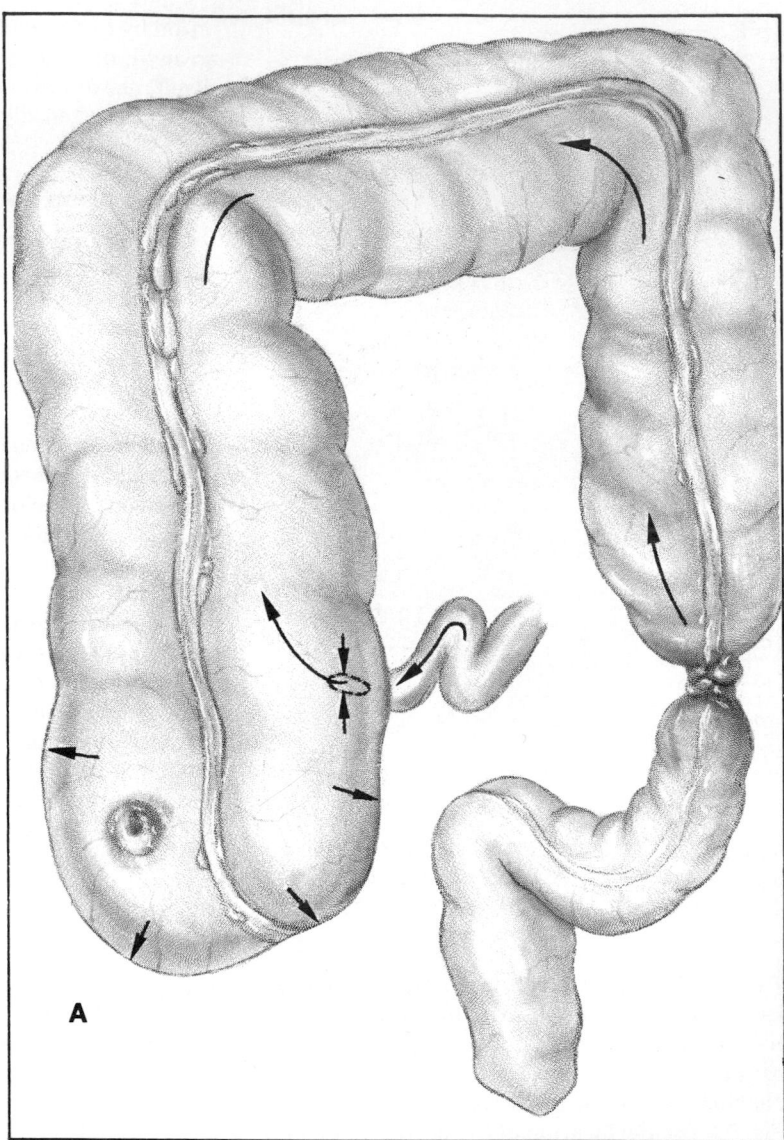

Figure 53–19. A. A competent ileocecal valve results in gross distension of the large bowel, especially of the cecum, which may necrose and perforate. (*Source: From Ellis H, 1982, with permission.*)

A

evidence of local fixation or dissemination of the tumour and, last but by no means least, the experience of the operator.

The available options are:

1. Immediate resection with restoration of continuity of the bowel (with or without proximal colostomy)
2. Resection of the tumour with exteriorisation of the divided ends (the Paul–Mikulicz or Hartmann procedures)
3. Laparotomy with preliminary decompression of the bowel by colostomy or caecostomy
4. Blind decompression

In general, resection and immediate anastomosis should not be performed in the presence of an obstructed large bowel. This is oedematous, is unprepared, with a high bacterial content above the obstruction, is difficult to manipulate and may rupture unless treated with extreme delicacy, and has an impaired blood supply. For all these reasons there is considerable risk of leakage of the anastomosis.

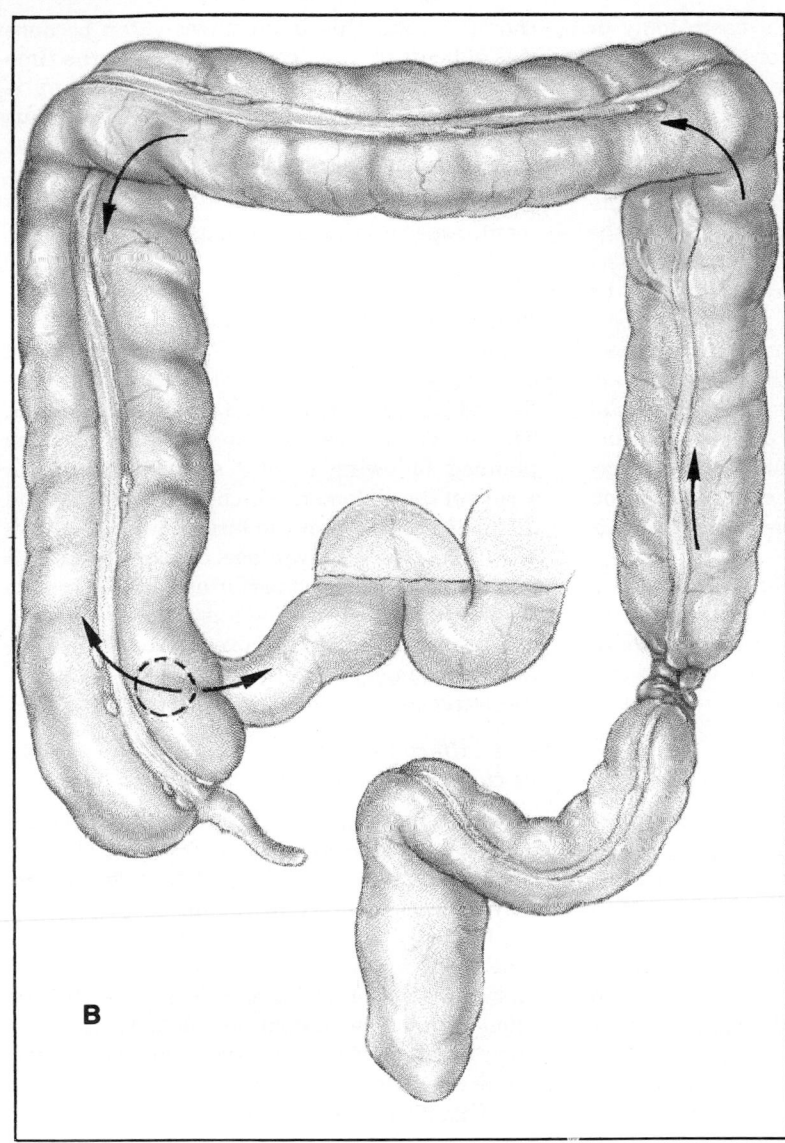

Figure 53–19. B. An incompetent valve allows ileal reflux and small bowel distension. (*Source: From Ellis H, 1982, with permission.*)

The exception to this general rule is the emergency right hemicolectomy for an obstructing carcinoma of the right colon. This is because in many instances the ileocaecal valve is competent (Fig. 53–19A), so that the small bowel is either not dilated or only moderately affected, thus allowing resection to be performed with an anastomosis of relatively normal small bowel above to collapsed colon, with its normal blood supply, distally.

It was once standard teaching that an ileotransverse short circuit should be carried out as a first stage in obstructions of this type, but this procedure carries with it all the hazards of an intestinal anastomosis and still leaves the patient requiring a second major operation to resect the growth. An ileotransverse short circuit is now only advised in those cases where there is an extensive and adherent obstructing growth in the right colon that may be considered incurable so that only a palliative short circuit can be carried out.

There may be exceptional circumstances in which the patient's general condition is extremely poor, in which case a caecostomy or even an ileostomy (in cases of obstructing carcinoma of the caecum) may be indicated as an emergency initial procedure.

Resection–Exteriorisation

The Paul–Mikulicz manoeuvre was once popular, particularly for obstructing tumours of the transverse or sigmoid colon. The involved segment of bowel is mobilised, resected, and the divided ends are brought out as a double-barrelled colostomy, which is subsequently closed. The Hartmann operation for the left colon comprises resection with either closure of the distal stump or bringing this out as a mucous fistula. The proximal bowel end is fashioned into a colostomy. This requires a major second laparotomy in order to perform subsequent reanastomosis of the divided ends.

These exteriorisation procedures have a valuable part to play in dealing with perforation or gangrene of a segment of colon, but most surgeons, in circumstances other than these, favour preliminary decompression with subsequent elective resection.

Preliminary Decompression

The majority of cases of left-sided obstructed growths are treated by laparotomy, to determine the extent of the site of the tumour, and then decompression, either by means of a transverse colostomy, which is brought out through a separate incision and immediately opened, or by a caecostomy, which is favoured when the growth implicates the transverse colon itself or when there is any technical difficulty in mobilising the transverse colon, or where the grossly distended caecum is showing signs of splitting with impending rupture.

Two or three weeks later, when the patient's condition has improved, a second-stage resection is carried out, with subsequent closure of the colostomy. The caecostomy is said to have the advantage that will close spontaneously, thus avoiding a third operation, but in practice this often fails to occur and operative closure must be performed.

Some surgeons advocate formation of the colostomy immediately proximal to the obstructing growth so that, at the second operation, the colostomy can be closed and immediate reconstitution of the bowel carried out, thus obviating a third procedure (Fig. 53–20) (Brooke, 1955; Payne and McAlpine, 1961). In this au-

thor's opinion this is an unwise step because it is difficult to avoid contamination at the time of resection and a colostomy or caecostomy is better placed above the anastomotic line, thus providing protection during its healing phase. Although the three-stage operation is time consuming to the patient, it does offer safe treatment, especially in the seriously ill patient.

"Blind" Decompression

Where the patient's condition is extremely grave or indeed moribund, a "blind" transverse colostomy or caecostomy may have to be performed, if necessary under local anaesthesia. The exact nature of the operation can be planned following careful study of the plain x-rays of the abdomen, which help to localise the distended segment of the large bowel. This procedure has the disadvantage, of course, that full laparotomy cannot be performed; a gangrenous segment of bowel may be missed or co-existing small bowel obstruction overlooked. However, in the extremely grave case, these are risks that the surgeon may feel are entirely justifiable.

Immediate Resection of the Left Colon

Although most surgeons are content to perform a right hemicolectomy for right-sided obstructive lesions, most are adamant that decompression and later resection should be carried out for left-sided lesions. Others argue, however, that meticulous surgery will often allow primary excision of obstructive lesions of the left colon without the discomforts, delays, and operative dangers of at least two, and more often three, operations in staged procedures.

This author is unaware of any prospective controlled clinical trials comparing primary against staged resection for obstructing growths of the left colon, and until such scientific evidence is available, surgeons will continue to argue the pros and cons of both techniques. Such a trial would be difficult to carry out; there are so many variables present that include such difficult things to assess as the degree of severity of the obstruction and the degree of skill of the surgeon. Until such time as a scientific answer to this problem is available, sound clinical judgement is the only basis for decision-making. There is no doubt at all in this author's mind that primary resection is perfectly sound treatment when the obstruction is not severe, when faecal loading above the occlusion is minimal,

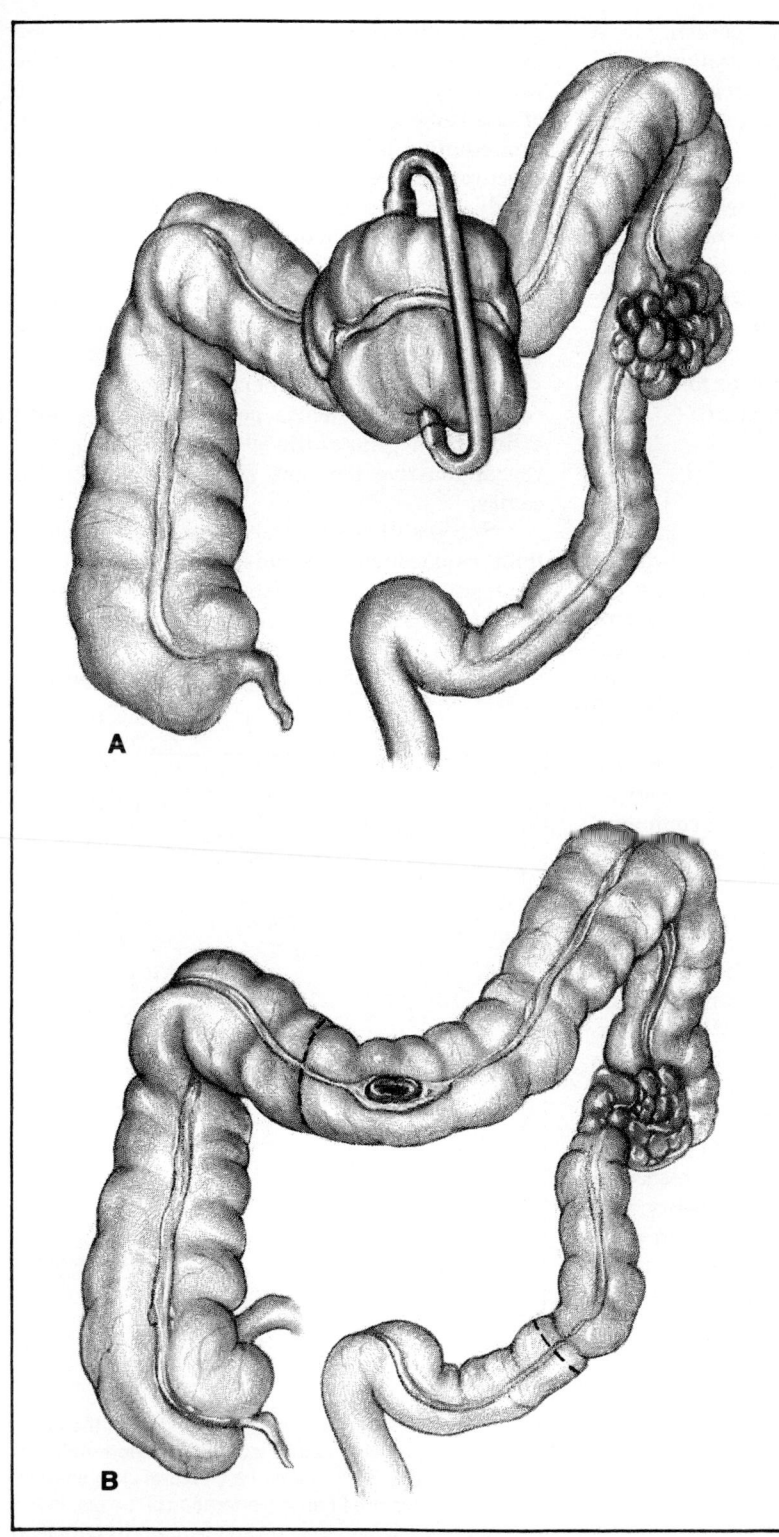

Figure 53–20. The two-stage resection advocated by Brooke. **A.** A preliminary colostomy is performed as near as possible to the site of the obstruction. **B.** At the second stage, the growth and adjacent colostomy are resected (the lines of resection are indicated). (*Source: From Ellis H, 1982, with permission.*)

and when an expert surgeon is operating on a fit patient. A limited primary resection may also be condoned when the patient's prognosis is already limited by the presence of distant, for example hepatic, metastases. In both these circumstances, however, this author's practice is to cover the anastomosis by means of a temporary loop transverse colostomy that can be closed 6 to 8 weeks later when the anastomosis has soundly healed. In the face of gross obstruction, and particularly when the surgeon is a resident in training, the safe advice is to carry out a preliminary colostomy and to follow this by resection as an elective procedure.

Prognosis

There is no doubt that the prognosis regarding immediate mortality and morbidity as well as later chances of survival is worse in the obstructed than in the electively treated patient with cancer of the large bowel. Irvin and Greaney (1977), in a review of published reports, found a postoperative mortality of between 15 and 39 percent and a 5-year survival of only 11 to 29 percent in patients operated on for colonic cancer presenting with intestinal obstruction. In their own cases, these authors compared 66 emergency resections with 176 elective operations and confirmed a higher operative mortality (37.9 compared with 11.9 percent) and a lower 5-year survival rate (22.9 compared with 41.5 percent) between the emergency and elective groups. Clark et al (1975) found that no less than 43 of their 128 patients with obstructing bowel cancer were incurable when first seen due to disseminated disease and stress the poor long-term prognosis of these patients irrespective of the surgical treatment employed. Fifty one of their cases underwent staged resection and 34 primary resection. The mortality was higher when primary resection was used than in staged procedures but at 1 and 3 years there was no significant difference in survival between the two groups.

PERFORATION

Free Perforation

Free perforation has been reported in between 0.6 and 4.7 percent of cases of colorectal cancer, with abscess formation in between 0.3 and 4

percent whereas fistulae are seen even less commonly (Welch and Donaldson, 1974). Free perforation, as already noted, may occur at the site of the tumour itself, as a stercoral perforation immediately proximal to the growth or in the caecum as a result of its gross distension. Very rarely, acute appendicitis with perforation has been reported immediately proximal to an obstructing caecal carcinoma (Fig. 53–14). In Goligher and Smiddy's series (1957), 20 of their 115 perforations occurred proximal to the obstructing lesion (Fig. 53–21).

Free perforation generally causes the clinical picture of an acute peritonitis along with a distended tympanitic abdomen. X-rays may reveal massive free gas within the peritoneal cavity.

Successful management requires adequate fluid replacement, broad-spectrum antibiotics (metronidazole with either gentamicin or a third-generation cephalosporin), and early surgery.

The most effective procedure is resection

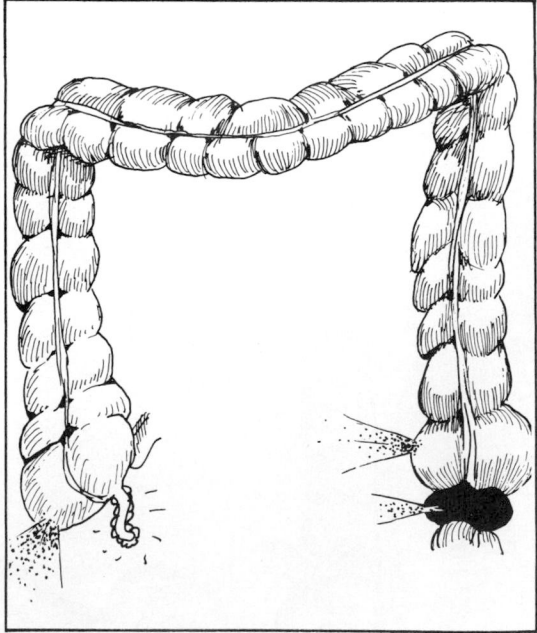

Figure 53–21. Possible sites of perforation of the colon secondary to carcinomatous obstruction: perforation of the tumour itself, perforation of a stercoral ulcer immediately proximal to the tumour, perforation of the distended caecum in a closed loop obstruction, and perforation of an acutely obstructed appendix proximal to a caecal tumour.

of the perforated colon, with exteriorisation of an end colostomy above and a mucous fistula below (Fig. 53–22), or, in the case of a rectosigmoid growth, a Hartmann procedure. Prompt removal of the source of contamination is the only effective way of reducing morbidity and mortality. In contrast, a loop transverse colostomy is unlikely to decrease the faecal contamination caused by a large perforation. As an example, Goligher and Smiddy reported a 77 percent mortality with all types of perforation treated by closure and colostomy compared to 24 percent with primary resection.

Immediate anastomosis in the presence of perforation and sepsis is not advisable because of the high risk of anastomotic breakdown in the presence of gross infection.

Caecal perforation is managed by converting the perforation into a caecostomy and then carrying out formal resection of the obstruction once the infection has settled.

Abscess

Where there has been local perforation and pericolic abscess formation, it is often extremely difficult to differentiate between a perforating carcinoma and diverticulitis.

Treatment usually necessitates preliminary abscess drainage with proximal colostomy, followed by subsequent resection, and then colostomy closure at a third stage. If the tumour is situated in the right or proximal transverse colon, a right hemicolectomy with or without immediate anastomosis is the treatment of choice. In the poor-risk patient with a large abscess, a diverting ileotransverse colon anastomosis may be elected prior to the definitive resection, although this operation is rarely performed today.

It should be noted that primary resection and anastomosis may be carried out safely under antibiotic cover in the presence of a small localised abscess in the adjacent mesocolon, which is not an unusual finding at laparotomy.

Fistula

The least common form of gross perforation is formation of a fistula to adjacent viscera, such as the small bowel, bladder, neighbouring colon, or vagina. Emergency operation is rarely neces-

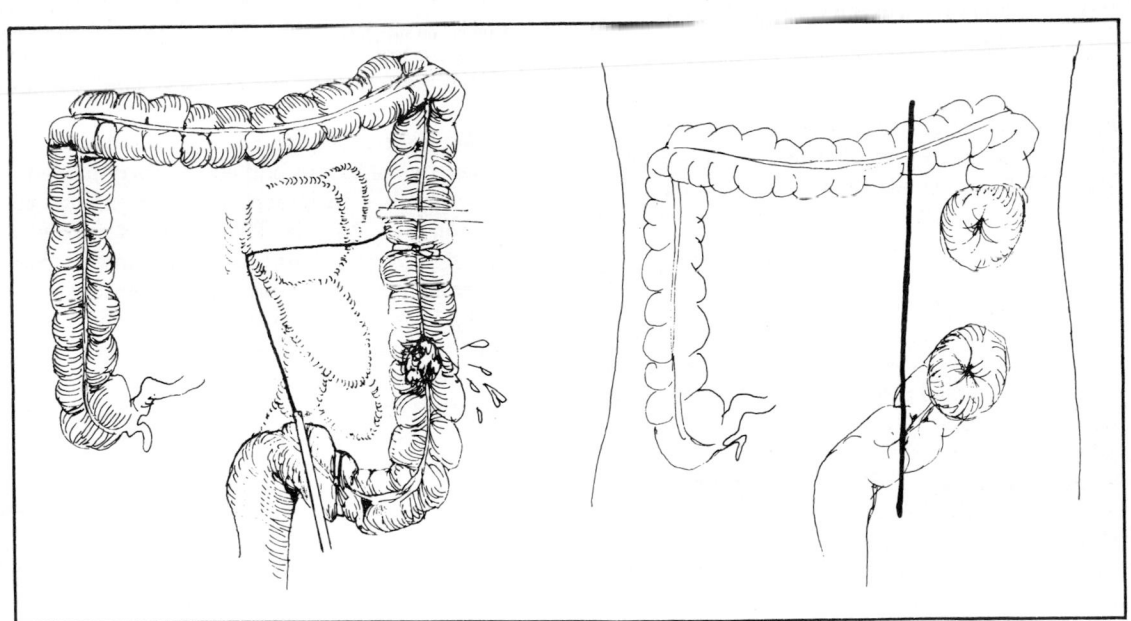

Figure 53–22. Resection–exteriorisation for a perforated carcinoma of the sigmoid colon. The left side shows the extent of the resection, the right side shows the position of the stomas on the abdominal wall at completion of the operation. Intestinal continuity can be restored electively at a second stage.

sary. After careful bowel preparation, such fistulae are not, in themselves, a bar to curative resection—a subject discussed in the following section.

RADICAL RESECTION OF COLON AND ADJACENT ORGANS

Invasion of adjacent structures by the colonic carcinoma may still be cured by extensive en bloc resection. Adjacent structures that may be found adherent to or invaded by the growth include the anterior and posterior abdominal wall, spleen, omentum, stomach, duodenum, small bowel, other areas of the large bowel, the kidney and perinephric tissues, adrenal gland, ureter, bladder, prostate, Fallopian tubes, uterus, vagina, ovary, sacrum, and iliac vessels. Moynihan (1926) advised removal of adherent abdominal wall, small intestine, or spleen should this prove necessary. Taylor (1931) reported the resection of a carcinoma of transverse colon that was invading and fistulating into the caecum and involved the stomach. Turner (1929) reported a truly remarkable series of 22 large bowel cancers that were resected en bloc with adjacent structures. There were 4 operative deaths but 8 of the patients had survived anywhere from 3 to 14 years.

More recent retrospective series have also shown that many locally advanced tumours can be cured by radical local surgery (Davies and Ellis, 1975; Kelley et al, 1981; Bonfanti et al, 1982; McGlone et al, 1982; Jensen et al, 1970). We have recently reviewed our experience of 57 large bowel carcinomas removed by extended en bloc resection (Pittam et al, 1984). Forty four of these had no clinical evidence of liver or other distant metastases but 13 had locally advanced disease with liver deposits who nevertheless underwent extended resection. In patients without liver metastases, interestingly enough, survival after extended resection was entirely similar to survival after standard resection for patients without locally invasive disease of the same Dukes' stage. The incidence of locally advanced carcinoma in our series was 22 percent, which is much higher than the 5 to 10 percent reported in other recent studies. This may represent the fact that many of these patients were tertiary referrals with advanced disease. Our operative mortality for extended resections was 13.6 percent, which is higher than the 6.7 percent operative mortality found for our standard curative excisions. We believe that this series confirms our conviction that locally advanced carcinomas of the colon or rectum that have not spread beyond the local confines, particularly to the liver, should be widely excised. Radical excision can be performed with an acceptable mortality and survival will in all probability be the same as for a similarly Dukes' stage tumour that has not spread into neighbouring organs.

A number of technical points concerning such resections are:

1. Extensive involvement of the anterior abdominal wall, or even fistulation through it, should not preclude very radical excision. Often the defect can be closed directly by adequate mobilisation but, if not, Marlex mesh is useful in closing the defect.
2. Cooke (1956) has pointed out that what at first may seem to be hopeless fixation of the tumour may be due entirely to inflammatory adhesions. In some cases it may be a wise procedure to carry out a preliminary colostomy or short circuit operation. Careful assessment of the mass over the subsequent weeks, or even months, may reveal increasing mobility of what was once a fixed mass and encourage the surgeon to reexplore the abdomen in the hope now of finding an operable situation.
3. Duodenal involvement by right-sided colonic carcinoma at first would seem to preclude resection. In fact, we have reported six such cases (two of whom had established duodenocolic fistulae) in which radical monobloc resection was possible. Two tumours were also adherent to the right kidney and another had invaded both the anterior abdominal wall and a loop of small intestine. Radical surgery was carried out in all 6 cases and three achieved long-term survival; the patient who required anterior abdominal wall and small bowel resection is, in fact, alive and well 17 years later (Ellis et al, 1972).

BIBLIOGRAPHY

Bonfanti G, Bozzetti F, et al: Results of extended surgery for cancer of the sigmoid and rectum. Br J Surg 69:305, 1982
Brooke BN: Simplified operative routine for carcinomatous obstruction of the colon. Lancet 1:945, 1955

Campbell JA, Gunn AA, et al: Acute obstruction of the colon. J R Coll Surg Edinb 1:231, 1956

Clark J, Hall AW, et al: Treatment of obstructing cancer of the colon and rectum. Surg Gynecol Obstet 141:541, 1975

Cooke RV: Advanced carcinoma of the colon with emphasis on the inflammatory factor. Proc R Soc Med 18:46, 1956

Cope Z: A History of the Acute Abdomen. London: Oxford University Press, 1965

Davies GC, Ellis H: Radical surgery in locally advanced cancer of the large bowel. Clin Oncol 1:21, 1975

Ellis H: Intestinal Obstruction. New York: Appleton-Century-Crofts, 1982

Ellis H, Naunton Morgan M, et al: Curative surgery in carcinoma of the colon involving duodenum. Br J Surg 59:932, 1972

Everett WG: A comparison of one layer and two layer techniques of colorectal anastomosis. Br J Surg 62:135, 1975

Fielding LP, Stewart-Brown S, et al: Anastomotic integrity after operations for large bowel cancer: A multi-centre study. Br Med J 2:414, 1980

Goligher JC: Surgery of the Anus, Rectum and Colon, 5 edt. London: Balliere Tindall, 1984

Goligher JC, Graham NG, et al: Anastomotic dehiscence after anterior resection of rectum and colon. Br J Surg 57:109, 1970

Goligher JC, Morris C, et al: A controlled trial of inverting versus everting suture in clinical large-bowel surgery. Br J Surg 57:817, 1970

Goligher JC, Smiddy FG: The treatment of acute obstruction or perforation with carcinoma of the colon and rectum. Br J Surg 45:270, 1957

Gordon Taylor G: Extensive carcinoma of the colon. Proc R Soc Med 24:783, 1931

Grey Turner G: Cancer of the colon. Lancet 1:1017, 1929

Irvin TT, Goligher JC, et al: A randomized prospective clinical trial of single-layer and two layer inverting intestinal anastomoses. Br J Surg 60:457, 1973

Irvin TT, Greaney MG: The treatment of colonic cancer presenting with intestinal obstruction. Br J Surg 64:741, 1977

Irvin TT, Hunt TK: The effect of trauma on colonic healing. Br J Surg 61:430, 1974

Jensen HE, Balslev I, Nielsen J: Extensive surgery in the treatment of carcinoma of the colon. Acta Chir Scand 136:431, 1970

Keighley MRB, Burdon DW: Antimicrobial Prophylaxis in Surgery. Tunbridge Wells, England: Pitman, 1979

Kelley WE, Brown PW, et al: Penetrating obstructing and perforating carcinomas of the colon and rectum. Arch Surg 116:381, 1981

Khoury GA, Waxman BP: Large bowel anastomoses. The healing process and sutured anastomoses. Br J Surg 70: 61, 1983

McGlone TP, Bernie WA, et al: Survival following extended operations for extracolonic invasion by colon cancer. Arch Surg 117:595, 1982

Meade RH: An Introduction to the History of General Surgery. Philadelphia: WB Saunders, 1968

Moynihan B: Abdominal Operations, vol 2. London: WB Saunders, 1926

Payne RL, McAlpine RE: Obstruction of the colon: Resection in two stages. Ann Surg 153:871, 1961

Pittam MR, Thornton H, Ellis H: Survival after extended resection for locally advanced carcinomas of the colon and rectum. Ann R Coll Surg Engl 66:81, 1984

Shaw D, Doig CM, Douglas D: Is airborne infection in operating theatres an important cause of infection in general surgery? Lancet 1:17, 1973

Singer S, Underwood EA: A Short History of Medicine, 2 edt. Oxford: Clarendon, 1962

Taylor SA, Cawdery HM, et al: The use of metronidazole in the preparation of the bowel for surgery. Br J Surg 66:191, 1979

Welch JP, Donaldson GA: Management of severe obstruction of the large bowel due to malignant disease. Am J Surg 127:492, 1974

Willis AT, Ferguson IR, et al: Metronidazole in prevention and treatment of bacteroides infections in elective colonic surgery. Br Med J 1:607, 1977

54. Ileoanal Pull-Through Procedures

John G. Buls
David A. Rothenberger
Eric S. Rolfsmeyer
Stanley M. Goldberg

INTRODUCTION

Patients with ulcerative colitis and multiple polyposis coli, requiring an operation, have traditionally been treated by total proctocolectomy and accompanying "Brooke" ileostomy. This operation is curative because all diseased or potentially diseased tissue is removed. It has, however, three drawbacks. First, the patients must adapt to life with a permanent ileostomy. Although the great majority of patients return to full, active, and productive lives with a stoma, some may be plagued with physical and psychologic problems. Second, there is a definite, albeit small, risk of permanent sexual or bladder dysfunction following total proctocolectomy. Finally, a persistent perineal sinus following proctectomy may be an annoying problem. Total proctocolectomy with the construction of a continent ileostomy (Kock pouch) or use of a continent ileostomy indwelling balloon device offers the patient convenience to the extent that the need for the continuous wearing of an ileostomy appliance is obviated. Nonetheless, these patients still must live with a permanent stoma and the risks of sexual and bladder dysfunction and persistent perineal sinus are unchanged. In addition, mechanical problems with the continent ileostomy, especially related to the nipple valve have occurred in a significant number of patients and often require reoperation. With refinement and modification, however, such problems are becoming less frequent.

These problems associated with total proctocolectomy have stimulated interest in sphincter-saving operations. Total colectomy and ileorectal anastomosis preserves the sphincter mechanism and thus avoids a permanent stoma. There is also no perineal wound to contend with nor is there a problem of sexual or bladder dysfunction. The patient must be subject to long-term scrutiny because of the risk of developing cancer in the retained rectum. In addition, a significant percentage of these patients have poor function or intractable proctitis. Proctectomy is ultimately required in about 20 to 25 percent of patients who undergo an ileorectal anastomosis because of the potential for cancer, the presence of a cancer, or intractable proctitis. Proponents of this alternative, however, state that when proctectomy does become necessary, the patient can then undergo an ileoanal procedure with an ileoanal reservoir. Total colectomy, rectal mucosectomy, and ileoanal anastomosis, with or without a pelvic reservoir, has recently stimulated much interest. This procedure is curative because all diseased and potentially-diseased tissue is excised but the sphincter mechanism is preserved and a permanent stoma is not required.

DEVELOPMENT OF ILEOANAL PROCEDURES

Nissen in 1933 performed a proctocolectomy and ileoanal anastomosis in a boy with familial polyposis. In 1947, Ravitch and Sabiston applied this principle to develop an experimental operation which entailed excision of the entire colon

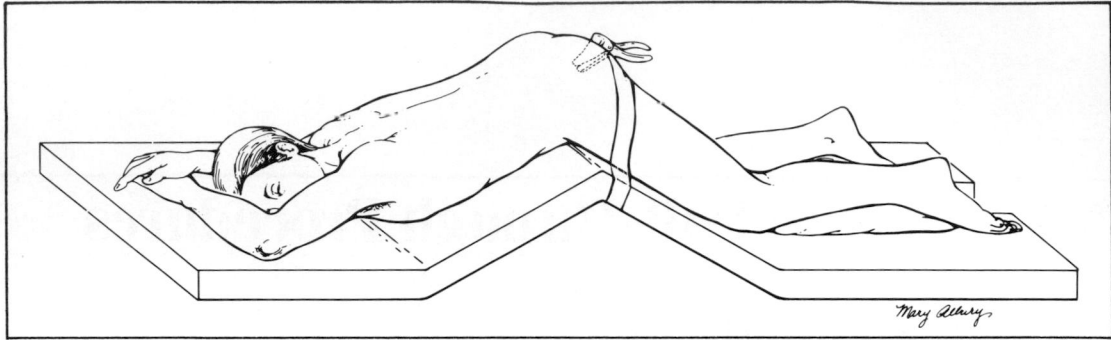

Figure 54–1. Patient in prone position to facilitate rectal mucosectomy. This allows for an easier removal of the rectal mucosa in a continuous sleeve fashion and thereby minimizes the chances of inadvertently retaining rectal mucosa.

and the mucosa of the retained rectal wall. This left the rectal muscularis, the levators, and the sphincters undisturbed while allowing for total excision of the diseased tissue. At the completion of the procedure, gastrointestinal (GI) continuity was restored by pulling the ileum through the preserved muscle sleeve and performing an ileoanal anastomosis. Ravitch in 1948, went on to apply this operation to two patients with ulcerative colitis with good success. A further small clinical experience with this operation in the early 1950s, however, revealed a successful outcome in only half of the cases. Failure was due to severe urgency, frequency, and perineal excoriation which immediately followed the operation. The enthusiasm for this procedure thus waned.

In 1964, Soave reported a similar procedure for the management of Hirschsprung's disease. Scattered reports of ileoanal pull-through procedures for ulcerative colitis or polyposis appeared in the literature over the next decade, but it was not until 1977 when Martin et al published their experience with total colectomy, rectal mucosectomy, and ileoanal anastomosis in children, that renewed interest in this procedure was stimulated. Martin's success was followed soon thereafter by Telander and Perrault, who reported success with the procedure in young adults and children. Beart et al, however, reported in 1982 less than encouraging results when this operation was performed in adults. Of their patients who had undergone total colectomy, rectal mucosectomy, and a straight ileoanal anastomosis with subsequent ileostomy

take down, 25 percent were converted to a permanent ileostomy because of stool frequency. Although there has been an improvement in the functional outcome in recent series, it is clear that at least in adults, there is still a significant rate of failure due to urgency, frequency, and a prolonged postoperative adaptation period.

Valiente and Bacon and Karlan et al had conducted animal model experiments in the 1950s in which an ileal reservoir was constructed in combination with total colectomy, rectal mucosectomy, and ileoanal anastomosis in an attempt to decrease the frequency of defecation. Since then, it has been demonstrated that a continent ileostomy pouch could act as a satisfactory reservoir. Parks and Nicholls combined all of these concepts and in 1978 published their experience with total colectomy, rectal mucosectomy, and ileoanal anastomosis in combination with a pelvic ileal reservoir. Further experience with this procedure and similar procedures with differences in pouch construction and configuration have since been reported from several centers.

PATIENT SELECTION

Patients with ulcerative colitis or familial polyposis who require colectomy and who have normal sphincter function, are potential candidates for such a "restorative" proctocolectomy. Familial polyposis, and to a lesser extent ulcerative colitis, are premalignant mucosal diseases lim-

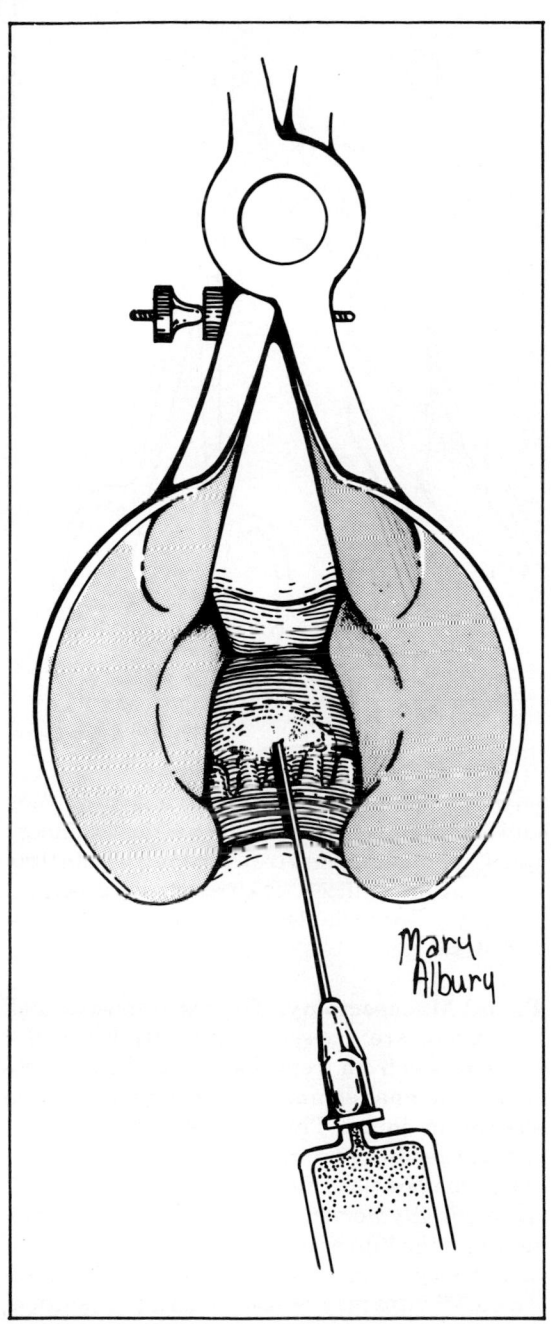

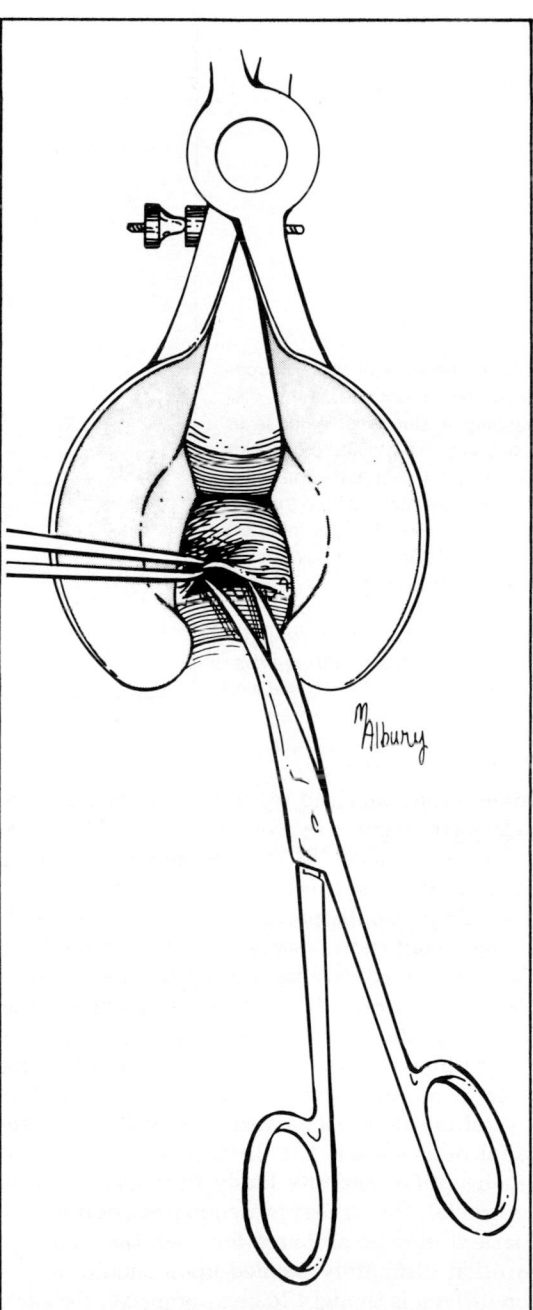

Figure 54–2. The anal canal is exposed using a Pratt bivalve anal speculum. Dilute epinephrine solution (1:200,000) is being infiltrated into the submucosal plane, commencing at the dentate line.

Figure 54–3. The rectal mucosectomy is commenced by making a circumferential incision at the level of the dentate line. Using atraumatic forceps and scissors, a dissection plane is developed between the submucosa and underlying internal sphincter muscle.

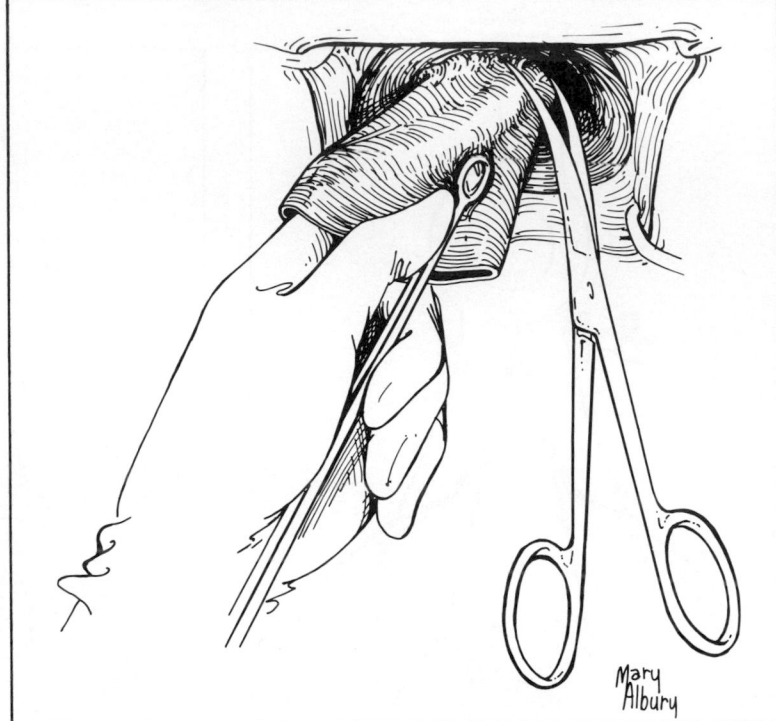

Figure 54–4. The rectal muco-sectomy is completed by dissecting a sleeve of mucosa in continuity for a distance of 4 to 6 cm from the dentate line. Ring forceps are used to hold the dissected sleeve. A finger inserted into the lumen of the developing sleeve aids in exposing the correct plane for further dissection. (*Source: From Rothenberger DA, et al, 1983, with permission.*)

ited to the colon and rectum and thus, both diseases can be cured by this procedure. This operation has no place in the treatment of Crohn's disease. Because this is a technically demanding operation, usually performed in stages and with a significant risk of postoperative complications, it should currently be limited to those considered low operative risk patients. Informed consent regarding the indications for operative intervention; the alternatives available including total proctocolectomy, continent ileostomy, ileorectal anastomosis, or ileal reservoir with ileoanal anastomosis; the pros, cons, and risks of each option; and the likely functional results is crucial. Once these prerequisites are met, the patient may be prepared for operation. The operation ultimately decided upon should be the one which is thought to be appropriate for each individual patient.

OPERATIVE PROCEDURES

Preoperative Management. A complete mechanical (clear liquids, magnesium citrate, and enemas) and intraluminal antibiotic (neomycin and erythromycin) bowel preparation is undertaken and perioperative systemic antibiotics (mefoxin) are utilized. The restorative proctocolectomy utilizing an ileal reservoir encompasses five steps.

Rectal Mucosectomy. The rectal mucosa and submucosa are excised transanally for a distance of 4 to 6 cm from the dentate line, which leaves the anal sphincters and muscle wall of the rectum intact. This phase of the procedure is more readily performed with the patient in the prone position (Fig. 54–1). In thin individuals, especially women, a modified lithotomy position with the hips and knees flexed and abducted and the legs supported by the Lloyd–Davies or Amsco stirrups may be used. This latter position provides concomitant abdominal perineal exposure and utilizes two operative teams. The anorectal canal is visualized with the aid of a Pratt bivalve anoscope and narrow Deaver or Malleable retractors. A headlight is essential. A solution of epinephrine in normal saline solution (1:200,000) is injected into the submucosal

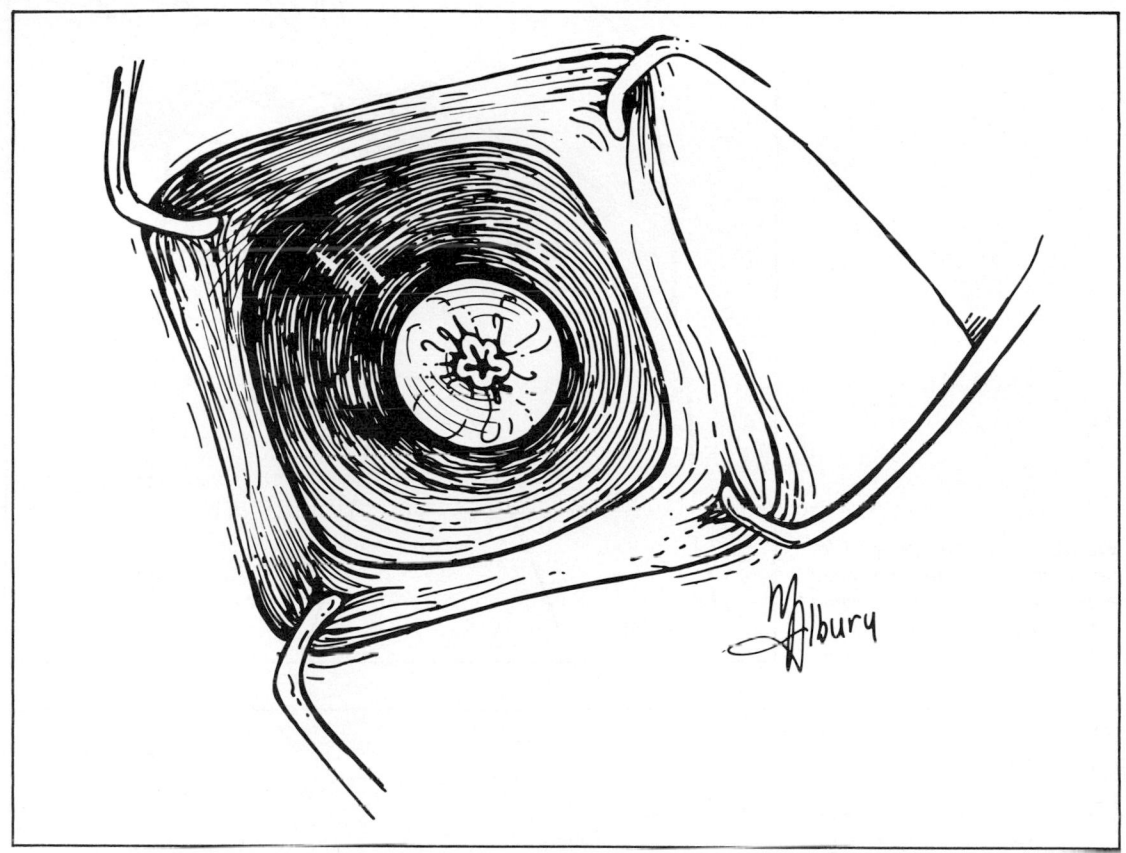

Figure 54–5. The completed rectal mucosectomy. The internal anal sphincter and circular muscle of the rectum are shown denuded of mucosa from the dentate line to a level of 4 to 6 cm proximally. The rectal mucosal sleeve has been inverted into the proximal rectum by a purse string suture. Two Gelpi retractors placed at right angles provide excellent exposure.

plane to facilitate dissection and aid in hemostasis (Fig. 54–2). A circumferential incision is made at the dentate line (Fig. 54–3). The mucosa and submucosa are elevated and dissected from the underlying muscle in a sleeve fashion (Fig. 54–4). As the dissection is carried proximally, electrocautery is used to achieve hemostasis. At the apex of the dissection, a heavy (20 Prolene) purse string suture is placed to gather together the dissected mucosa and submucosa. The tissue is inverted into the lumen of the proximal rectum and the purse string is tied (Fig. 54–5). A pack soaked in the dilute epinephrine solution is placed in the rectal muscle sleeve and retained (Fig. 54–6). If this phase of the operation has been performed with the patient in the prone position, the patient is turned and positioned supine with the legs in stirrups as described previously.

Abdominal Colectomy. Routine exploration of abdomen, placement of a nasogastric tube, and abdominal colectomy are performed through a midline abdominal incision with the patient in the modified lithotomy position. The terminal ileum is divided flush with the cecum to preserve length. A GIA-stapler is utilized to achieve this. The dissection is carried into the pelvis flush with the rectosigmoid wall, thus preserving the pelvic autonomic nerves. The previously placed purse string suture and involved rectal mucosa are palpated by the abdominal operator, who then incises the rectal wall posteriorly just distal to the purse string suture and

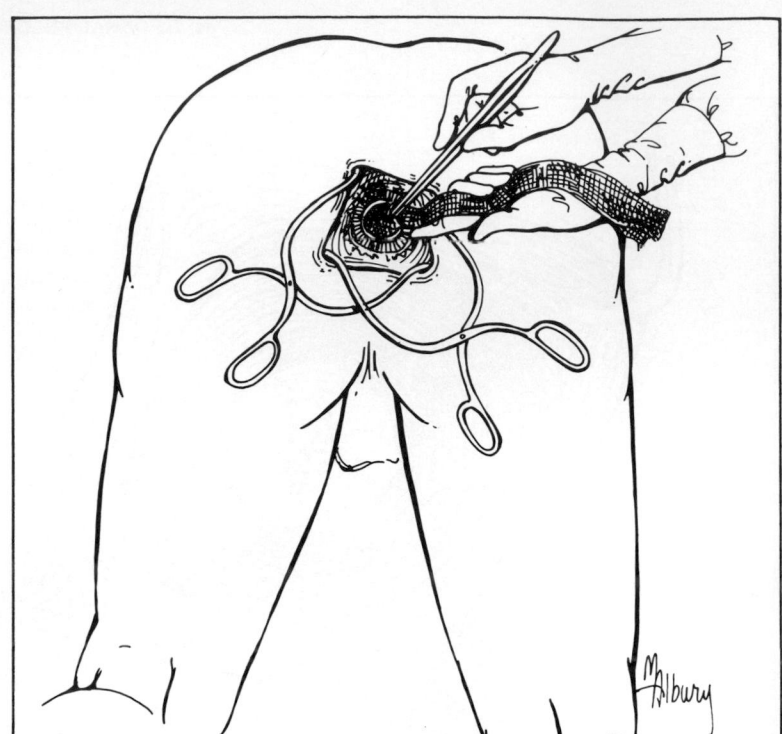

Figure 54–6. The denuded internal anal sphincter and rectal muscle cuff are lightly packed with gauze soaked in diluted epinephrine (1:200,000) solution.

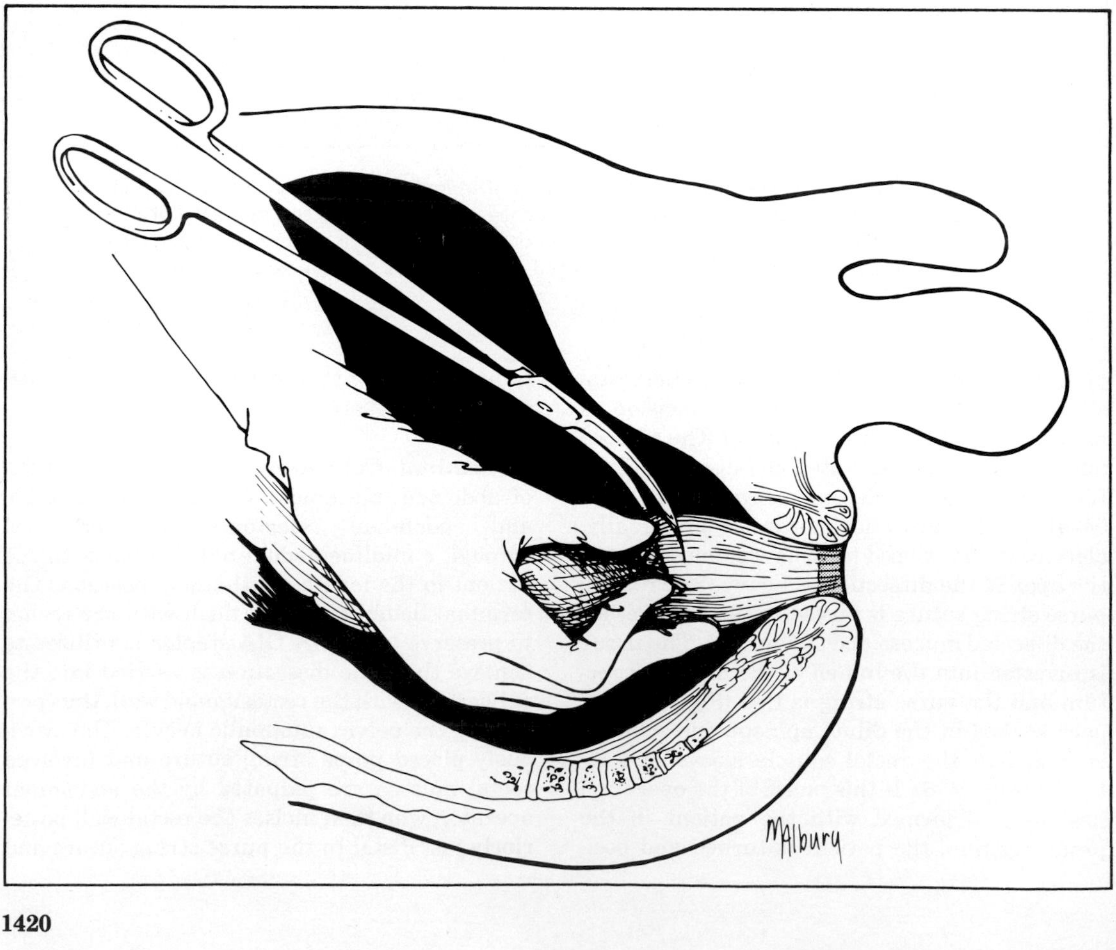

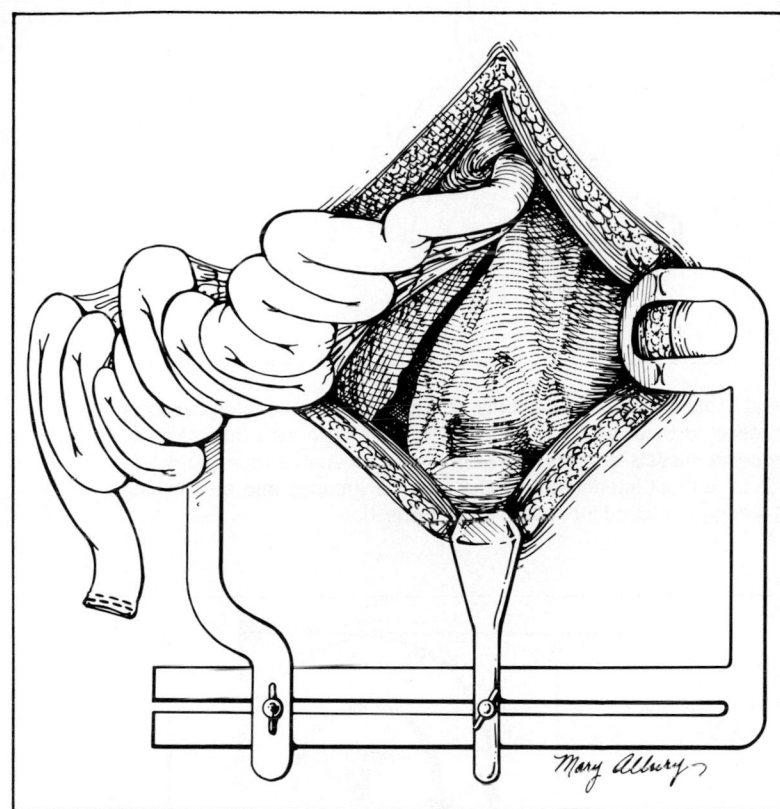

Figure 54–8. The small bowel is mobilized widely by dividing the posterior peritoneum up to the level of the duodenum, pancreas, and the superior mesenteric artery. The midline abdominal incision is shown being retracted by a self-retaining abdominal wall retractor (Balfour).

carries the incision circumferentially around the stripped rectal cuff (Fig. 54–7). The previously dissected rectal mucosal and submucosal sleeve is then resected en bloc with the colon. Thus, resection of all diseased tissue is accomplished.

Ileal Reservoir. The small bowel is mobilized widely by dividing the posterior peritoneum up to the level of the duodenum, pancreas, and the superior mesenteric artery (Fig. 54–8). The previously divided and ligated ileocolic vessels are divided again more proximally and a wedge of mesentery is excised (Fig. 54–9). Transillumination of the mesentery will demonstrate the terminal ileal branches of the superior mesenteric artery and the bridging vascular arcades. These

must be preserved to ensure vascular viability to the distal ileum. After mobilization, the distal 40 cm of the ileum is aligned in an "S" shape utilizing three 12-cm loops of bowel (Fig. 54–10). These lengths are precisely measured in the unstretched state along the antimesenteric border. Stay sutures hold the proposed pouch in position while it is placed into the pelvis. The perineal operator retrieves the spout of the aligned reservoir to make sure that it reaches the dentate line without tension prior to the actual opening of the bowel and construction of the reservoir (Fig. 54–11). If tension exists, additional mobilization is performed without sacrificing distal ileal blood flow and by careful division of the peritoneum at the base of the small bowel mesentery. The critical factor in

Figure 54–7. The patient has been turned into the supine position with the legs in stirrups. A total abdominal colectomy has been performed. The denuded rectal muscle cuff is being divided by the abdominal operator distal to the level of the muscosectomy. The right hand palpates the inverted mucosal sleeve and purse string suture to assure total removal of the diseased rectal mucosa. (*Source: From Rothenberger DA, et al, 1983, with permission.*)

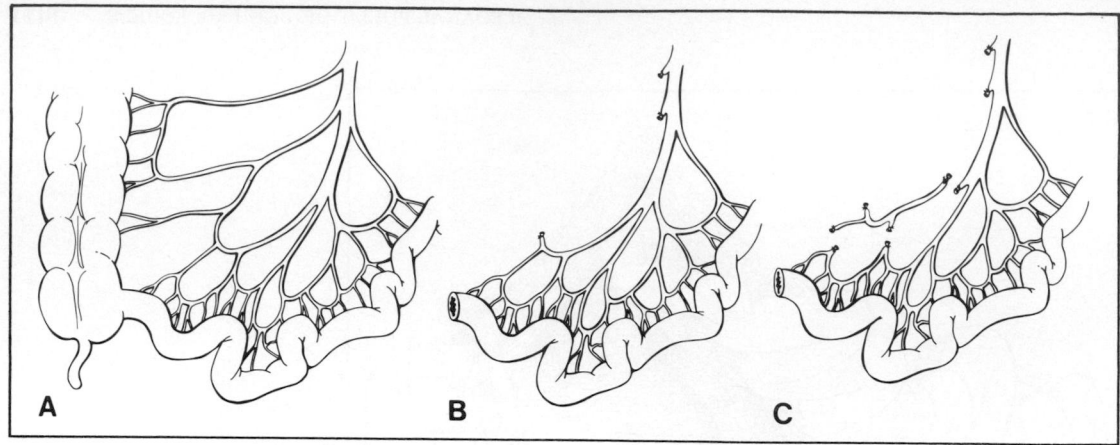

Figure 54–9. A. The normal ileocecal vascular anatomy. **B.** The residual mesenteric vessels after the colon has been resected by dividing the ileocecal vessels flush with the colon. **C.** Further division of the ileocecal vessels at a more proximal level to enable more complete mobilization of the distal ileum without interfering with the vascular arcades and so ensuring adequate blood supply. A wedge of redundant mesentery is excised.

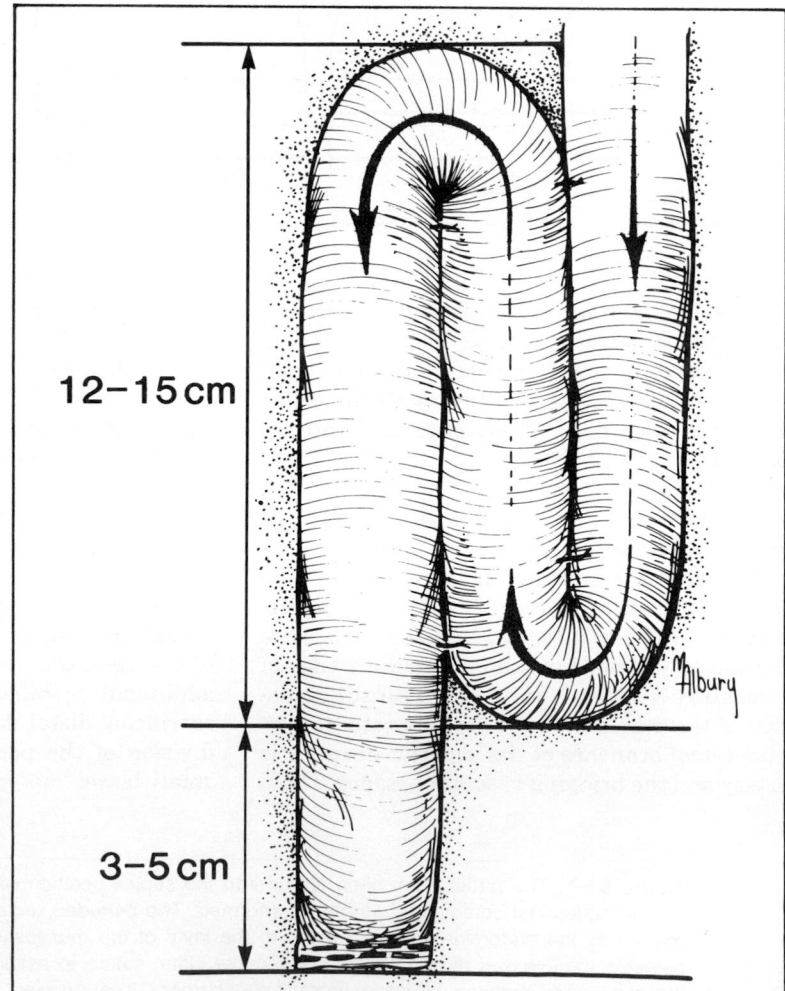

Figure 54–10. Configuration of the "S" type ileal reservoir. Three limbs of the distal ileum, each 12 to 15 cm long, are aligned side-by-side. The very distal 3 to 5 cm of the ileum will be retained as an outlet from the reservoir and will be anastomosed to the dentate line.

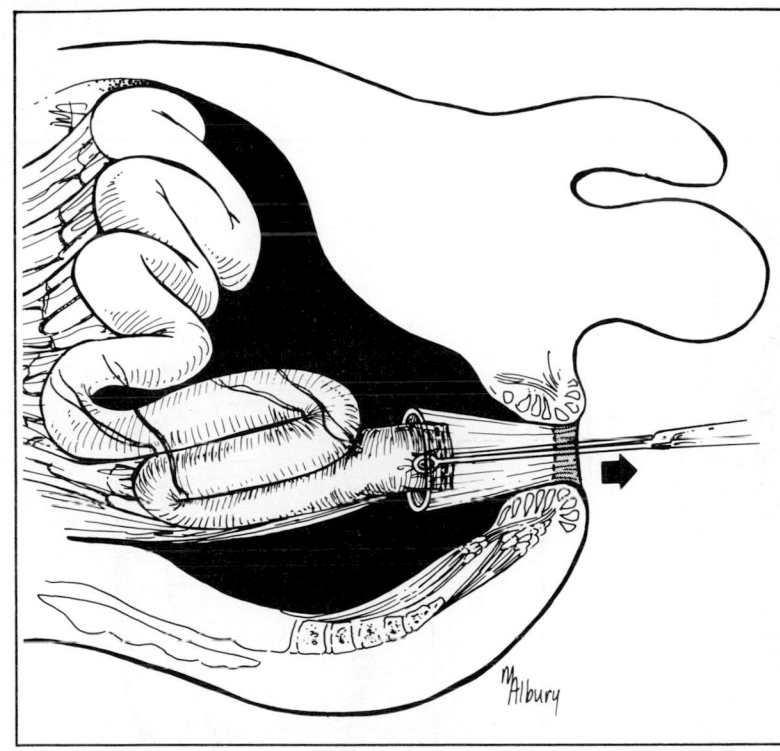

Figure 54–11. Stay sutures are holding the distal ileum in the configuration of the proposed pouch. The perineal operator retrieves the spout of the aligned reservoir by passing a ring forceps through the rectal muscle cuff. The proposed pouch is then gently manipulated into this cuff to ensure that the terminal ileum will reach the dentate line without tension.

determining if the ileum will reach the dentate line is the length of the superior mesenteric artery. This is variable. If the tip of the mobilized ileum will reach 8 cm or more beyond the symphysis pubis, it will easily reach the dentate line. The pouch is constructed by opening the bowel along the antimesenteric surface and then anastomosing adjacent walls until a triple lumen reservoir is formed. Two-layer hand-sewn anastomoses and GIA-stapled anastomoses have been tried. We currently utilize a one-layer, continuous 3-0 Vicryl or Dexon hand-sutured locked stitch. A straight, hand-held GI Keith needle facilitates the suturing (Figs. 54–12 and 54–13).

Ileoanal Anastomosis. After removing the epinephrine soaked packing from the denuded rectal muscle and anal sphincter sleeve and ensuring total hemostasis with electrocautery, pelvic drainage is achieved by placement of a soft triple lumen sump drain outside the sleeve into the pelvis and brought out through a perineal or a transabdominal stab wound (Fig. 54–14).

This will provide drainage of the pelvis postoperatively and can also be used to irrigate the cavity. Prior to manipulating the pouch into the pelvis, four anchoring sutures are placed, each into a quadrant circumferentially around the anus at the dentate line (Fig. 54–15). These are placed with deep bites and deliberately incorporate the internal anal sphincter (Fig. 54–16). In situations where tension still exists despite wide mesentery mobilization, it is advisable to anchor the ileum to the proximal anal canal by placing additional anchoring sutures into the internal anal sphincter at this level prior to final positioning of the pouch. In patients with redundant perianal skin folds, it is possible to perform an anoplasty by fashioning several broad based perianal skin flaps, undercutting them and advancing them into the proximal anal canal to allow for a more proximal mucocutaneous anastomosis (Fig. 54–17). A Babcock clamp or ring forceps is placed per anus and the pouch is guided by the abdominal operator into the pelvis through the rectal muscle sleeve to the dentate line. The small bowel mesentery can be anteriorly or posteriorly oriented but

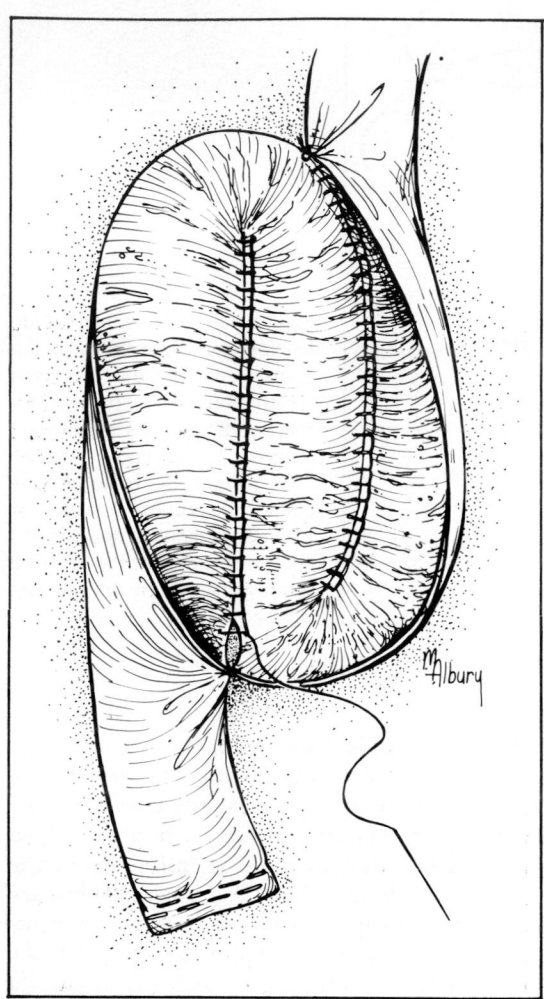

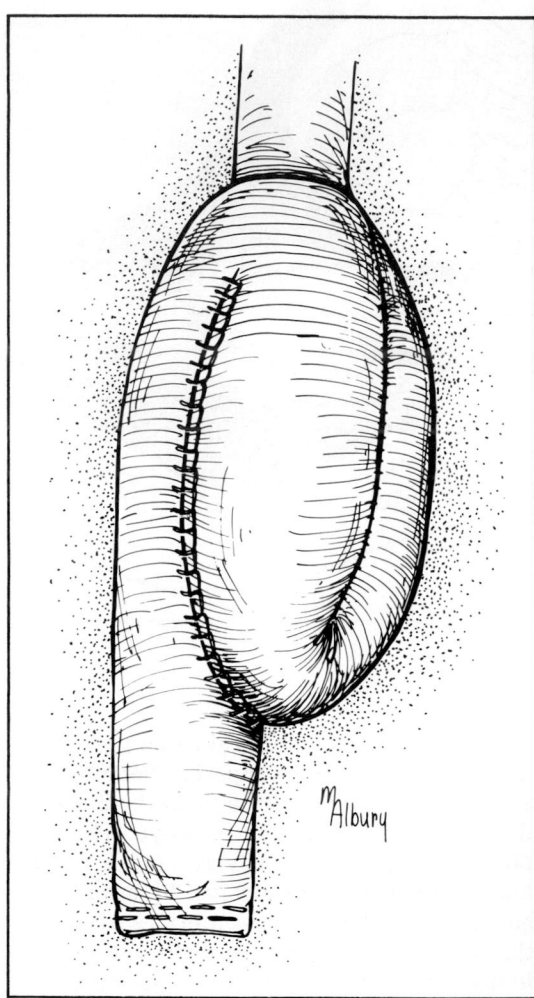

Figure 54–12. Ileal reservoir under construction. The previously measured loops of ileum have been opened along their antimesenteric borders. The adjacent loops of bowel are anastomosed using a running locking suture of 3-0 Vicryl. A hand-held straight needle facilitates the suturing. (*Source: From Rothenberger DA, et al, 1983, with permission.*)

Figure 54–13. The completed ileal reservoir of the "S" type. (*Source: From Rothenberger DA, et al, 1983, with permission.*)

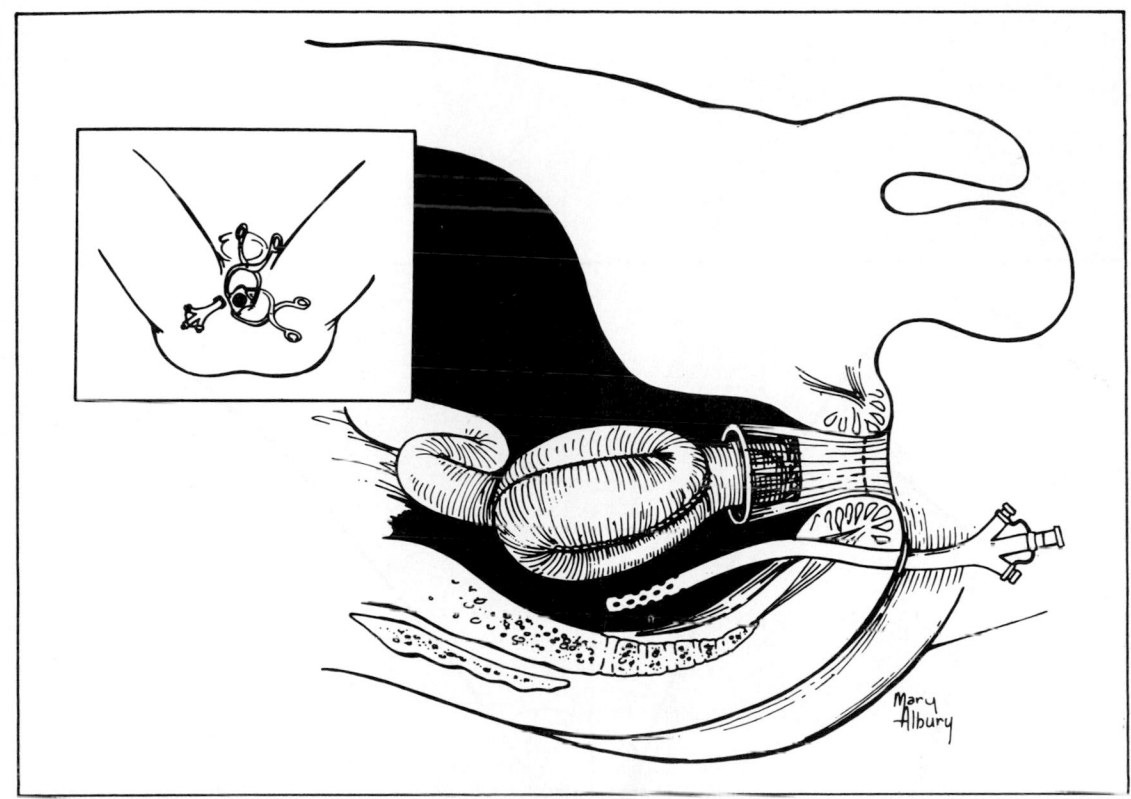

Figure 54–14. Drainage of the pelvic cavity is achieved by utilizing a soft, triple lumen sump tube. This is placed in the sacral hollow and brought out via a stab wound in the perineum (*shown*) or the anterior abdominal wall. The tube is positioned so that it lies outside the anal sphincters and rectal muscle cuff and is placed in situ before the completed ileal reservoir is finally positioned in the pelvis for the ileoanal anastomosis.

should not be under tension. Gelpi or spring retractors placed at right angles to each other provide exposure of the dentate line. A single layer anastomosis between all layers of the ileum and dentate line is performed with interrupted 3-0 Vicryl or Dexon sutures. The previously placed anchoring sutures are utilized first (Fig. 54–18). In some patients temporary drainage of the pouch is instituted at this stage by inserting a large bore (28 French 30 cc balloon) Foley catheter (Fig. 54–19). The balloon is only partly inflated.

Loop Ileostomy. The preselected stoma site is readied and a standard loop ileostomy with primary maturation of the stoma is constructed (Figs. 54–20 and 54–21).

Postoperative Management. As GI function returns, the nasogastric tube is removed and alimentation advanced to a normal diet. The pouch catheter, if utilized, and presacral drain are generally removed in 3 to 5 days when drainage is minimal. The patient is discharged from the hospital, on an average, 12 days postoperatively. Twelve weeks is usually allowed to elapse before the loop ileostomy is closed. Before this, a contrast study using a water-soluble agent is obtained to check the anatomic position of the reservoir in the pelvis and to exclude an anastomotic leak (Fig. 54–22). All patients are instructed in the proper technique of pouch intubation and irrigation in the event this is necessary after ileostomy take down. Patients are also instructed on perianal skin care to

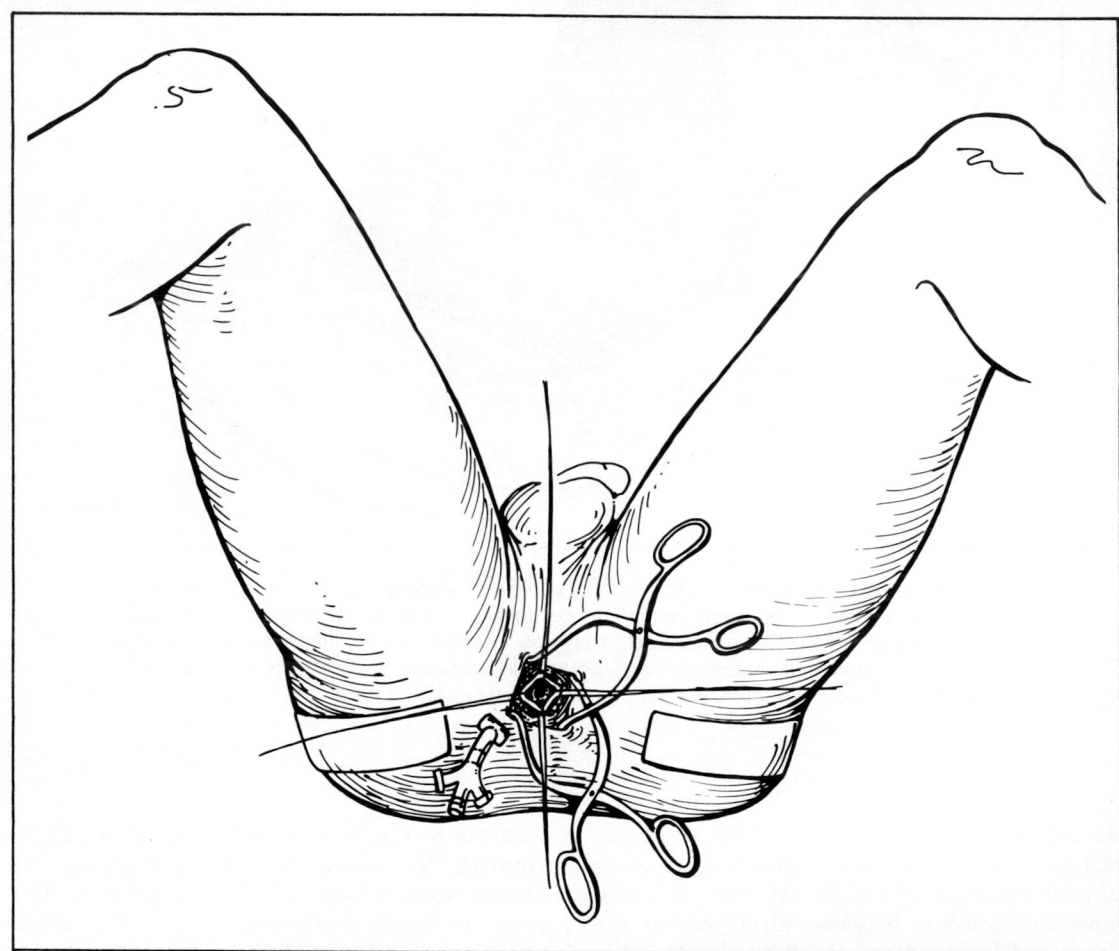

Figure 54–15. Ileoanal anastomosis is achieved by suturing the ileum to the dentate line. Four quadrant anchoring sutures of 3-0 Vicryl are placed initially. These take a deep bite of the anoderm, internal anal sphincter, and full thickness of the ileum. Gelpi retractors placed at right angles aid in the exposure.

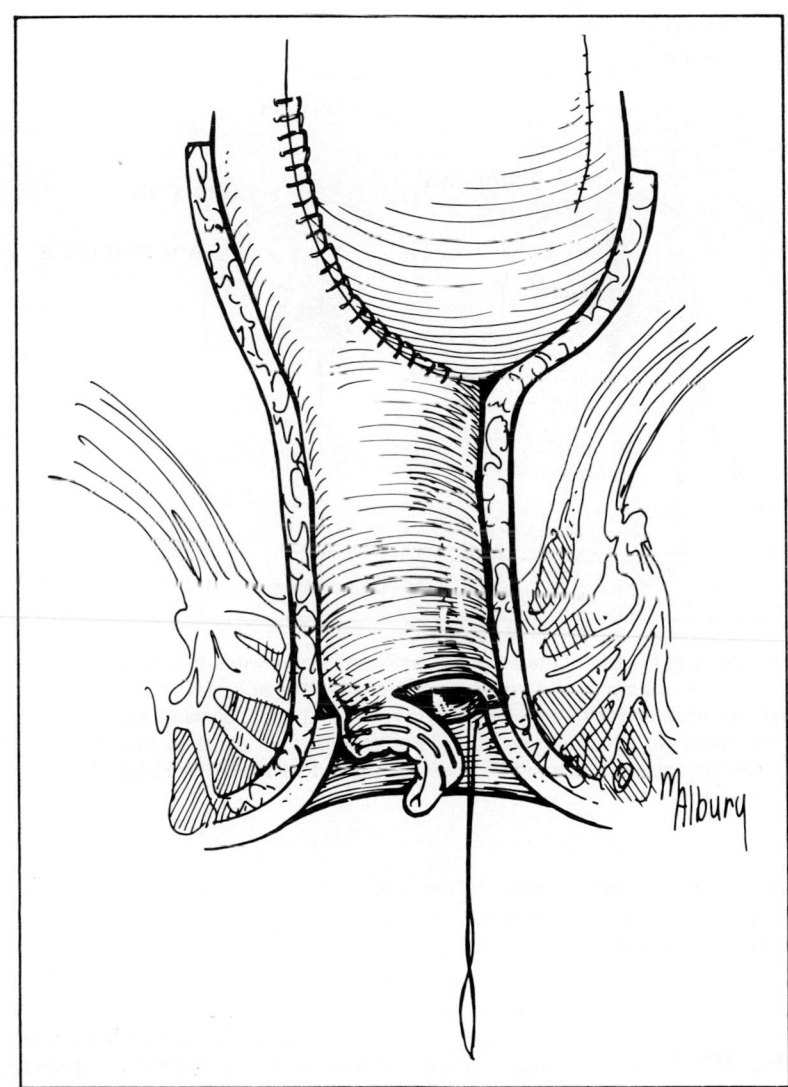

Figure 54–16. The stapled distal end of the ileum is excised to enable the anastomosis to be achieved.

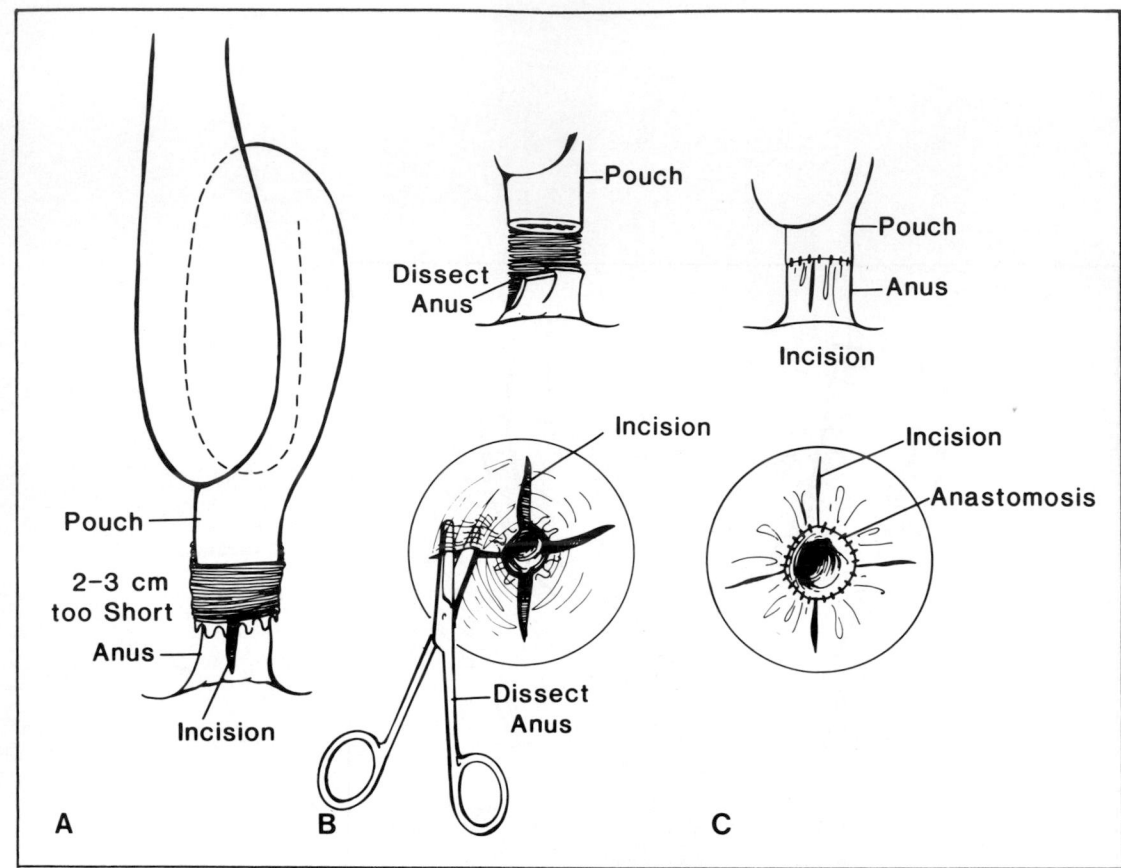

Figure 54–17. A. If tension exists at the site of the proposed anastomosis between the distal ileum and dentate line, **(B)** an anoplasty is performed by fashioning several broad based "V" flaps. Radial incisions are made and the anoderm and the redundant perianal skin flaps are undercut. **C.** These "V" flaps are advanced into the more proximal anal canal so that the ileoanal anastomosis can be achieved at a higher level but without tension. The radial incisions are left open for drainage.

avoid major problems once continuity is restored. Enterostomal therapy consultation and follow-up are essential to manage these possible problems and sequelae.

TECHNICAL CONTROVERSIES

Single versus Multiple Stage. There is some controversy regarding the necessity of performing this procedure in stages. For the patient who presents nutritionally depleted, with fulminant colitis, with sepsis, or on high doses of corticosteroids, an initial total abdominal colectomy, end ileostomy and Hartmann's pouch, or mucous fistula is advised with plans for the ileoanal procedure at a time when conditions are more optimal.

In the elective setting with a relatively healthy patient, the procedure can be performed in either one or two stages. Ravitch in his initial description of the procedure did not use a diverting ileostomy. Devine and Webb also performed the procedure as a single stage. Drobni, in 1967, reported 31 patients who had a single-stage total colectomy, rectal mucosectomy, and ileoanal anastomosis for ulcerative colitis. He described two postoperative deaths from diffuse peritonitis. Safaie-Shirazi and Soper performed the procedure in a single stage and in two out of four

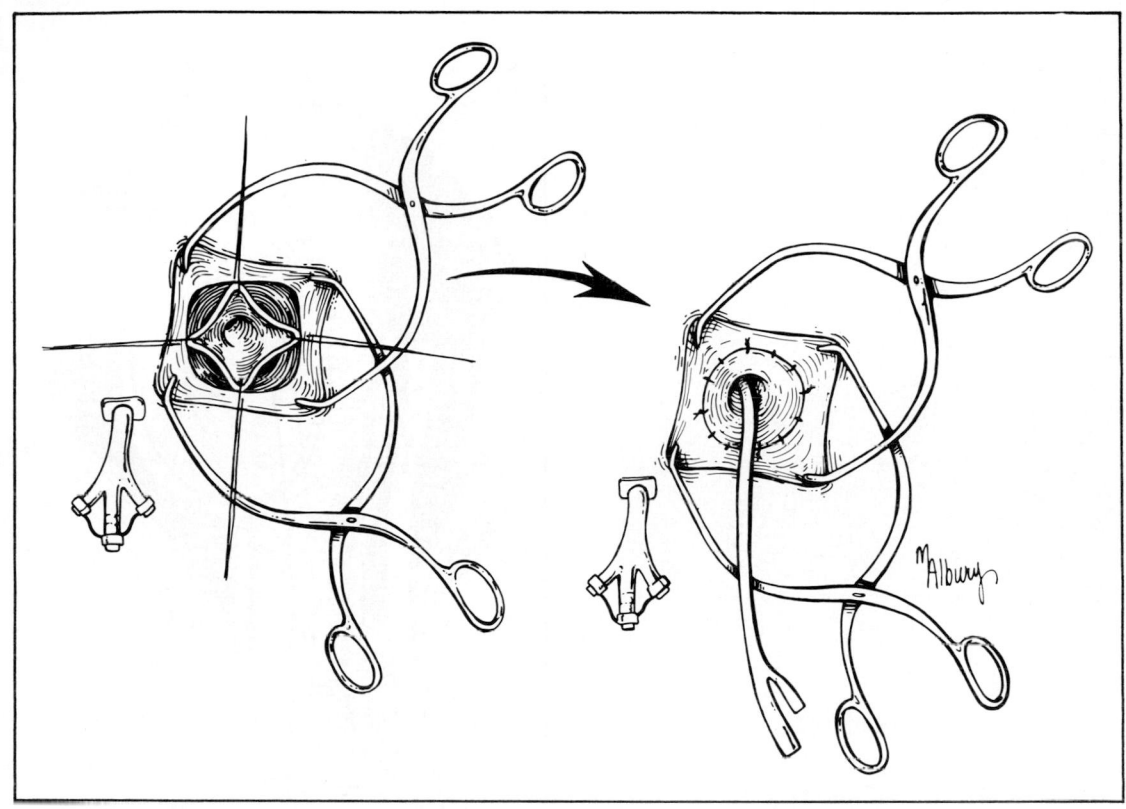

Figure 54–18. The ileoanal anastomosis is completed by placing two interrupted sutures of 3-0 Vicryl between each anchoring suture. In some patients, temporary drainage of the pouch is achieved by placing a Foley catheter into the pouch through the completed ileoanal anastomosis. The balloon of the catheter is only partly inflated.

cases described a partial anastomotic dehiscence.

Thow has successfully performed the procedure in one stage but uses a decompressing "Thow tube" passed through the small bowel to lie proximal to the reservoir. He also maintains all his patients on hyperalimentation for several weeks and thus, in essence, gives the patient a "medical ileostomy."

Our experience with the procedure performed in a single stage without temporary diversion has not been encouraging. Six patients have had a colectomy, rectal mucosectomy, and ileoanal anastomosis with an "S" reservoir performed as a single stage without a loop ileostomy. Of these, three developed pelvic sepsis with anastomotic dehiscence and one developed an ileovaginal fistula. Of the 50 patients who

have had the procedure performed with a covering loop ileostomy, however, there have been only 3 cases of significant pelvic sepsis or anastomotic dehiscence. Despite this difference in results, a covering loop ileostomy may not prevent complications of pelvic sepsis and anastomotic dehiscence but should decrease the frequency and morbidity of these two complications. In addition, performing the operation in two stages gives the patient an opportunity to live temporarily with an ileostomy, albeit, a loop ileostomy. The time spent caring for and living with a stoma gives the patient additional perspective regarding the alternative to the ileoanal procedure. A loop ileostomy correctly constructed will function in the same manner as an end ileostomy. Thus, it is not surprising that the majority of surgeons performing these procedures utilize

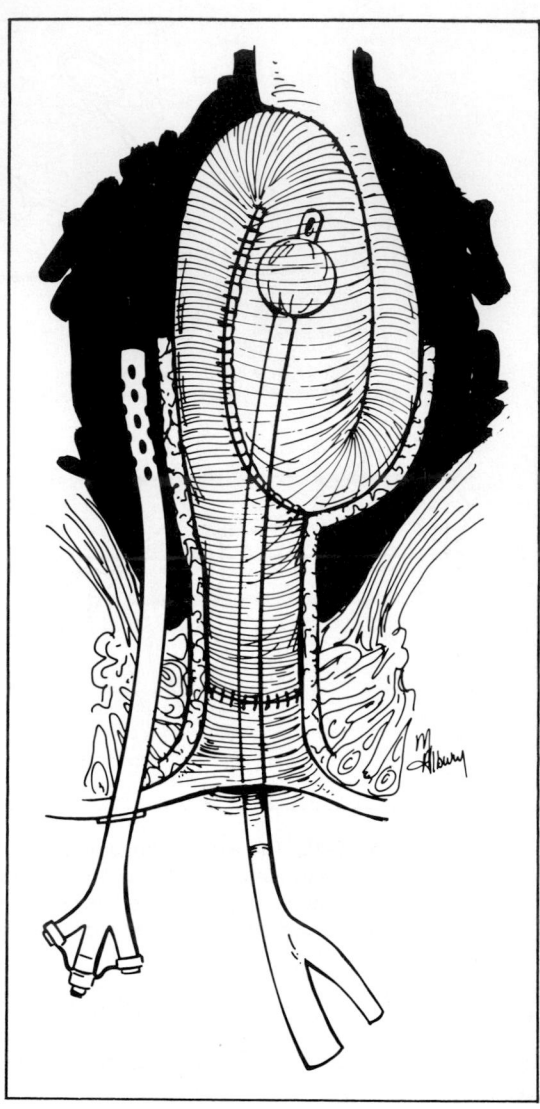

Figure 54–19. The completed operation shows the ileal reservoir resting snuggly but low in the denuded rectal muscle cuff. The efferent ileal spout is short. Foley catheter drainage of the reservoir (*shown*) is optional. Pelvic drainage, however, is essential.

a diverting loop ileostomy in hopes of avoiding or minimizing the serious complications associated with the single-stage procedure.

Rectal Mucosectomy. Contrary to original teachings that anal continence is mediated by sensory receptors in the rectal mucosa, recent clinical, physiologic, and histologic research demonstrates that the receptors necessary for the initiation of the complex anorectal reflexes needed for maintaining continence are located in the lower rectal muscularis and the levator ani. Thus, it is possible to remove all rectal mu-

cosa without interfering with the continence mechanism.

The length of rectal musculature that should be stripped of its mucosa and retained is a matter of current debate. Utsunomiya et al advocated a long mucosal stripping from the proximal rectum distally to the anus in hopes of better preserving continence. This technique had the potential added advantage of minimizing pelvic mobilization of the rectum and theoretically avoiding sexual or bladder dysfunction. More recently, Taylor et al have employed a shorter rectal mucosectomy without any func-

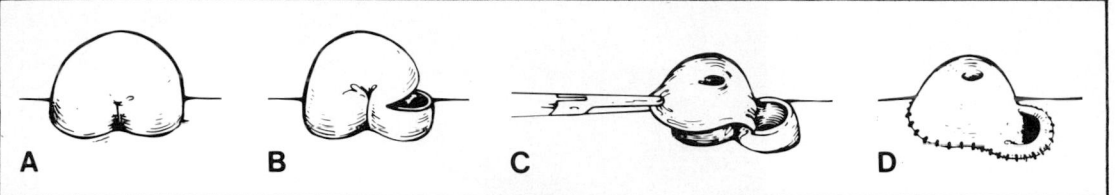

Figure 54–20. Loop ileostomy. **A.** A loop of ileum well proximal to the reservoir is brought through a previously marked stoma site in the right lower quadrant of the abdomen. If the patient had a Brooke ileostomy which has been taken down, the same site is used. **B.** The ileum is opened at skin level on the distal side. **C.** The proximal ileum is everted. **D.** Immediate mucocutaneous suture is accomplished. No rod is necessary. The ileum is anchored to the undersurface of the anterior abdominal wall with two sutures.

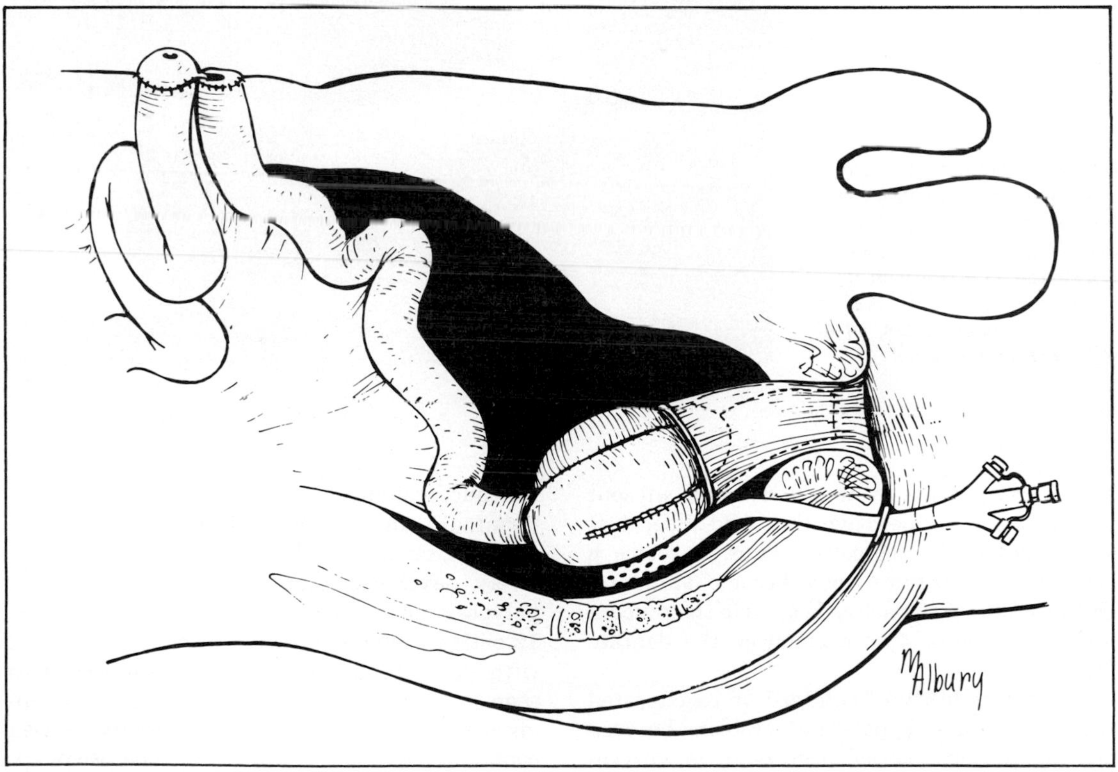

Figure 54–21. The completed procedure. The Foley catheter drain of the reservoir has not been used in this instance.

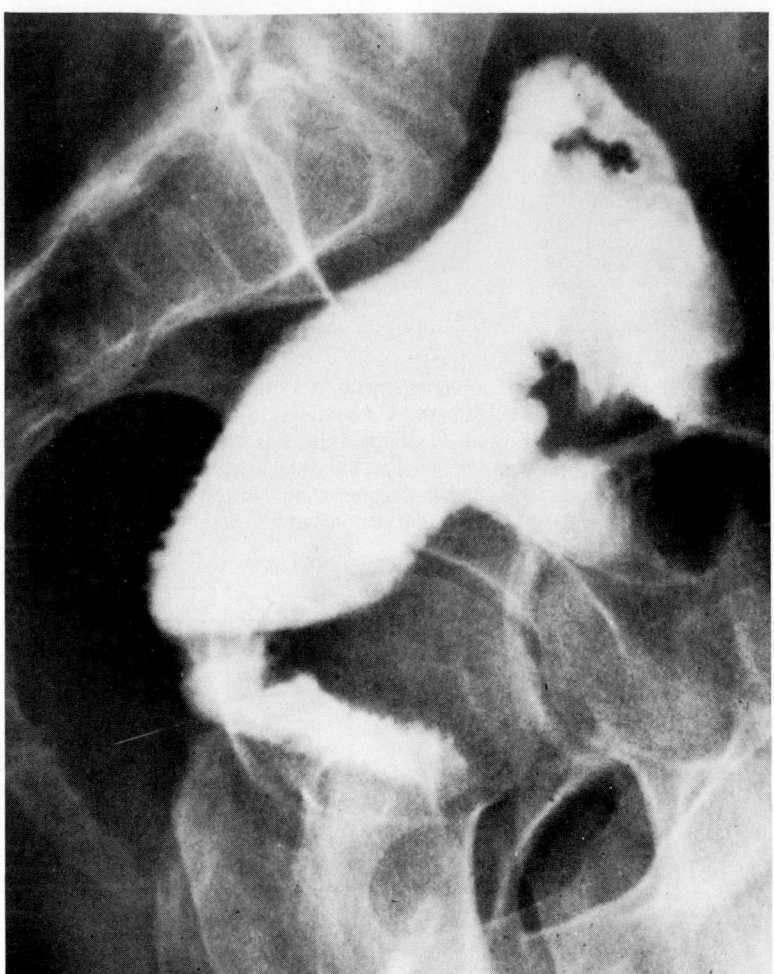

Figure 54–22. Water-soluble contrast study of the ileal reservoir, lateral view. The pouch lies within the curve of the sacrum. The ileal spout exists at an angle and is relatively short. (*Source: From Rothenberger DA, et al, 1983, with permission.*)

tional disturbance in continence and without impotence. The operative time and blood loss are considerably decreased. Thus, it seems a shorter mucosectomy may become standard. Our own current practice is to strip the mucosa for a distance of 4 to 6 cm from the dentate line.

The possibility of retained or regenerated rectal mucosa is a potential problem because any mucosa not excised from patients with ulcerative colitis or familial polyposis has the capacity to become malignant. There are two reports in the literature concerning this subject. Hampton reported two patients who underwent total colectomy, rectal mucosectomy, and ileoanal anastomosis for familial polyposis. The rec-

tal mucosectomy was complete except for the terminal 1 cm proximal to the dentate line. Both patients, one at 7 and one at 3 years postoperatively developed biopsy-proven adenomatous polyposis up to 18 cm. Wolfstein et al reported 12 patients who had the rectal mucosa removed with a curette. In 9 of 12 cases, the mucosa was seen to have regenerated. Therefore, it is advised that all the mucosa be carefully excised commencing at the dentate line. The use of curettes or corrosive solutions has been reported on an experimental basis, and is to be discouraged.

To date, there has been no report of cancer developing in the area of the mucosal proctectomy following ileoanal anastomosis but the follow-up has been relatively short. The current techniques of meticulous, complete mucosectomy will probably prove adequate but only long-term follow-up will provide a definitive answer.

Ileal Reservoir. Has the addition of an ileal pouch improved the functional results? It is clear that at least in children, the ileum can dilate and adapt to the extent that it eventually functions as an adequate reservoir after a straight ileoanal anastomosis. The period of adaptation, however, can be very difficult for the patient to tolerate. Adults fail to make the transition to adequate reservoir function in 25 to 50 percent of the cases. Taylor et al reviewed 124 patients who had undergone total colectomy, rectal mucosectomy, and ileoanal anastomosis. Seventy four patients had an ileal "J" reservoir constructed; 50 patients had a straight ileoanal anastomosis. Of the 50 patients in the group without a reservoir, 6 failed because of ongoing pelvic sepsis, 4 were satisfied with their temporary ileostomies, and 1 patient was demonstrated to have Crohn's disease. Of the remaining 39 patients who had undergone ileostomy take down, 9 failed because of excessive diarrhea and required conversion to a permanent ileostomy. In addition, 20 percent of this group suffered from major nocturnal incontinence. The complications (excessive diarrhea and major nocturnal incontinence) did not occur in the reservoir group. The group without a reservoir had an average stool frequency of 11 times in 24 hours, 18 months postoperatively compared to 7 in 24 hours at 6 months for the reservoir group. The authors concluded that the ileal pouch not only served a reservoir function, but in addition interfered with the peristalsis of the ileum. Heppell et al and Taylor in performing manometric studies have shown that good clinical results correlate with an increased capacity and compliance of the neorectum. Martin has had a similar experience. He initially performed the procedure without a reservoir resulting in a stool frequency of 18 per 24 hours, 1 week postoperatively and 8 per 24 hours, 1 year postoperatively. When the procedure was performed with a reservoir, he noted a dramatic decrease in stool frequency to 6 per 24 hours at 1 week postoperatively and 4 per 24 hours, 1 year postoperatively. It therefore, does appear that the ileum can adapt to become an adequate

reservoir in a significant percentage of patients after total colectomy, rectal mucosectomy, and ileoanal anastomosis. The addition of an ileal pouch, however, assures the patient of having a neorectum with adequate early reservoir capacity and compliance and thus, significantly improves both the early and ultimate functional results.

Pouch Types. The optimal size and configuration of the ileal reservoir is as yet unclear. Parks et al, Johnston et al, Rothenberger et al, and Martin and Fischer have utilized the "S" pouch. Utsunomiya et al and Taylor et al have used the "J" pouch. Fonkalsrud and Peck have preferred the lateral side-to-side pouch. Individualized minor modifications to these three most frequently constructed pouches continue to be described.

"S" POUCH. The "S" pouch, as described by Parks and Nicholls, is fashioned from 50 cm of ileum arranged in the configuration of a "S." At completion, the pouch consists of three 15 cm loops of ileum with a 5 cm efferent limb. This pouch is the largest of three common types. It has drawn some criticism because in Parks' initial experience, 50 percent of the patients could not evacuate the pouch spontaneously and required catherization. In more recent reports, this problem has occurred less frequently perhaps because the efferent limb and retained rectal muscle cuff were shortened. Martin and Fischer have constructed a reservoir using the "S" configuration but have made it smaller with a very short efferent limb (1 cm). Smith et al have recently demonstrated that the "S" pouch usually reaches 2 to 4 cm farther than the "J" pouch and this additional length may be valuable to avoid anastomotic tension.

"J" POUCH. This pouch consists of 24 to 40 cm of ileum doubled back on itself. A long side-to-side anastomosis is fashioned (Fig. 54–23). This pouch by virtue of the fact that there is no spout, lies lower within the rectal muscle cuff in the pelvis than the others and catheterization of the pouch has not been required.

LATERAL SIDE-TO-SIDE. This pouch involves bringing an isolated ileal segment through the denuded rectal muscularis and anastomosing it to the anal canal. Then, at a later date, a 15

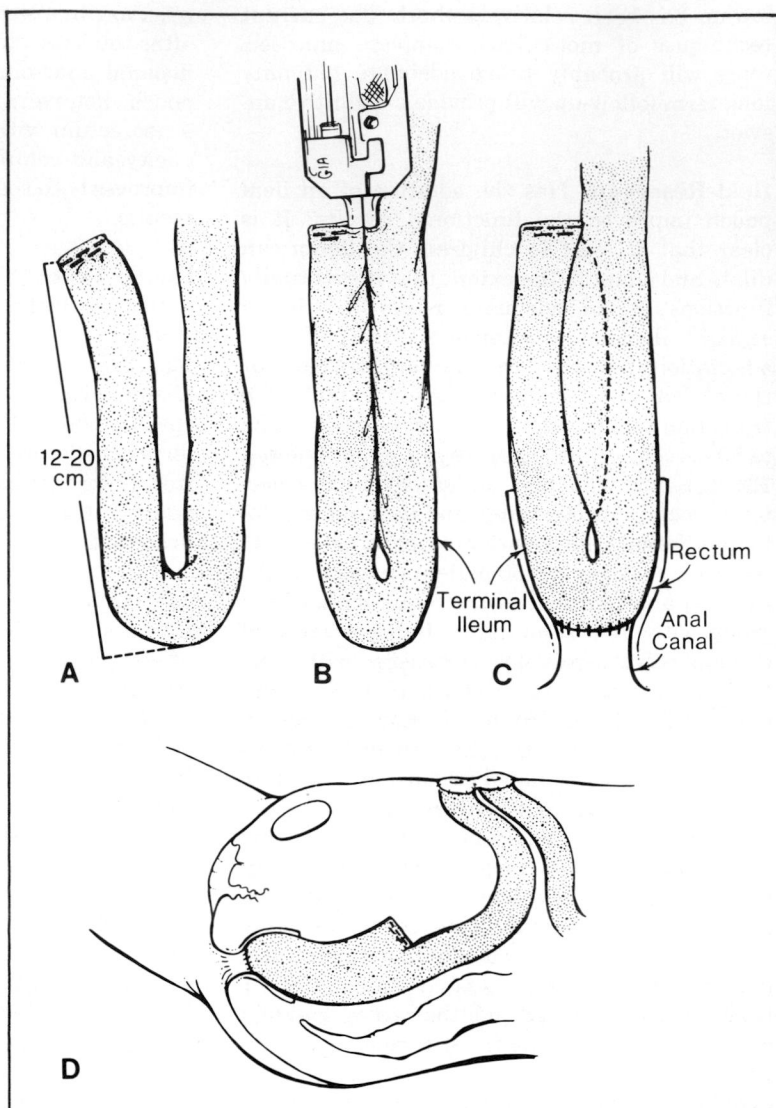

Figure 54–23. "J" Pouch. **A.** Two limbs of mobilized terminal ileum are used. The length used has varied, 12 to 20 cm. **B.** A side-to-side anastomosis is achieved using the GIA-stapler. **C.** The constructed reservoir is brought through the denuded rectal muscle cuff and a side-to-end ileoanal anastomosis is fashioned. **D.** The final configuration with a loop ileostomy.

to 20 cm side-to-side ileo–ileal anastomosis is constructed (Fig. 54–24). The pouch is thus isoperistaltic, which Fonkalsrud feels promotes peristaltic drainage. This pouch like the "S" pouch has an efferent limb, but unlike the "S" pouch, inability to evacuate the pouch spontaneously has not been a problem.

To date, no pouch configuration has proven superior to the others. Experience has suggested, however, that it is important to bring the pouch as low as possible into the pelvis to avoid a long efferent limb.

MORTALITY AND MORBIDITY

When total colectomy, rectal mucosectomy, and ileoanal anastomosis is performed in selected patients, it is a relatively safe operation. The recent literature details 265 patients having undergone an ileoanal procedure without mortality.

This operation entails several standard procedures combined into one. The patients, of course, are subject to any complication associated with an abdominal colectomy, i.e., wound

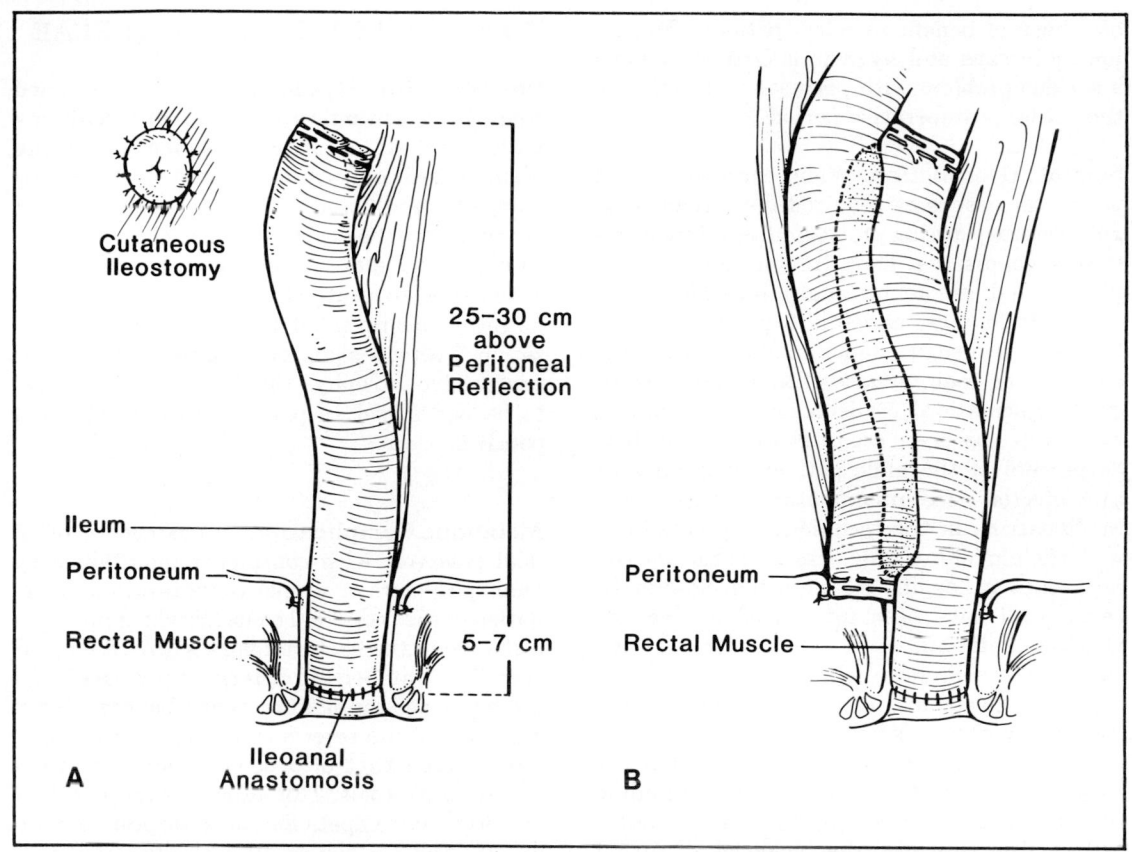

Figure 54–24. Lateral side-to-side reservoir is constructed in stages. **A.** Rectal mucosectomy with straight ileoanal anastomosis and end ileostomy. **B.** Take down of ileostomy with lateral side-to-side ileo–ileal anastomosis to create the reservoir.

infection, small bowel obstruction, and so on. There are complications, however, which although not unique to an ileoanal pull-through procedure, occur with enough frequency to warrant further discussion.

Pelvic Sepsis. The colitic patient is often on steroids and often has a suboptimal nutritional status. The reservoir with its long suture lines lies within a denuded rectal muscular tube. A certain degree of contamination during the rectal mucosal resection and with the construction of the reservoir is inevitable. These factors provide the ideal milieu for a septic process. Thus, it is not surprising that pelvic sepsis has complicated a significant percentage (13 to 24 percent) of the reported series of ileoanal procedures. In our own experience, this complication has developed in 12 percent of the cases and in some

instances, pouch removal has been required. Even if the pouch can be salvaged, manometric studies show a decreased reservoir compliance after pelvic sepsis. The decreased compliance correlates with increased fecal frequency and ultimately poor results.

Perineal Excoriation. In a recent survey of 40 patients conducted by our department, 33 patients had initially experienced some perianal skin problems. At the time of review, however, 26 described the condition of their perianal skin as excellent and stated that they rarely have problems. Ten admitted to having a skin problem about once every 2 weeks and four admitted to having chronic skin problems. Treatment consists of scrupulous perianal hygiene, which in the majority of cases, is all that is necessary. Various ointments and creams have also been of benefit in select patients. Meticulous skin care and hygiene is critical to avoid a serious problem with perineal excoriation in the initial postoperative period.

Sexual Dysfunction. Wide excision of the perirectal tissues as required for carcinoma is not necessary during proctectomy for inflammatory bowel disease. Thus, the incidence of complete sexual impotence ranges from 0 to 17 percent, but in most series is 6 percent or less. Partial loss of sexual function (decrease or difficulty in the maintenance of an erection, retrograde ejaculation, or decrease in amount of ejaculate) has been reported to occur in 5 to 34 percent of the male patients who undergo a proctectomy for inflammatory bowel disease. Modifications in the technique of proctectomy with the aim of avoiding damage to the perirectal tissues by keeping the dissection close to the rectal wall have been introduced by Lee and Dowling, Lytle and Parks, and Bauer et al. Results have been encouraging.

Total colectomy, rectal mucosectomy, and ileoanal anastomosis still require removal of the upper part of the rectum but the perirectal tissues surrounding the lower rectum containing the pelvic autonomic nerves remain undisturbed. Theoretically, the incidence of sexual dysfunction should be minimized. This seems to be the case since Taylor et al reported zero incidence of complete impotence and described only 3 male patients out of 69 with partial dysfunction (retrograde ejaculation). Parks et al, Neal et al, and Fonkalsrud reported no cases of either total or partial sexual dysfunction after rectal mucosectomy and ileoanal anastomosis in their male patients. Thirty five patients in our series are male. Two of these admitted to painful ejaculation in the early postoperative period but in both, this had resolved after 3 months. No cases of impotence were reported.

The improved results may reflect the reduction in pelvic dissection required to remove the diseased tissue but in addition, these results may be explained by the overall younger age of the patients undergoing the ileoanal procedures. The average age of our patients is 32 years (range 13 to 60 years). It appears, therefore, that rectal mucosectomy and ileoanal anastomosis can be performed with minimal risk of impotence and a very low incidence of partial sexual dysfunction, often temporary.

POSSIBLE LONG-TERM SEQUELAE

Potential for Dysplasia. Biopsies obtained from the pouch mucosa of continent ileostomy patients reveal morphologic changes suggesting an increased cell turnover. These include shortening of the villi and an increase in the number of mitoses in the crypt cells. The changes occur as early as 1 month and are still evident 1 to 2 years postoperatively. Long-term follow-up, however, has revealed a trend toward normalization with no signs of dysplasia, fibrosis, or progressive atrophy. Similar studies are yet to be performed in patients with pelvic ileal pouches.

Metabolic Complications. Construction of an ileal reservoir with continence maintained by anal sphincters or nipple valve results in stagnation of the intestinal contents which produces a change in the bacterial flora within the reservoir. The number of bacteria is increased and a greater percentage are anaerobic organisms. The flora of the reservoir effluent is intermediate between that of a conventional ileostomy and normal stools. This relative overgrowth of bacteria can compete for the absorption of vitamin B_{12} and also can result in the deconjugation of bile acids. The majority of the data regarding absorption within an ileal reservoir comes from experience gained with the Kock continent ileostomy. In 1979, Nilsson et al studied 14 patients 6 to 10 years after proctocolectomy and construction of a continent ileostomy. All patients were in excellent health and showed no outward signs of malnutrition. Absorption of vitamin B_{12} was evaluated with a Schilling test which was normal in eight patients, borderline in five, and low in one. The serum vitamin B_{12} levels, however, were normal in all 14 patients. In a 1983 update, Nilsson et al reported that serum B_{12} levels were normal in 185 patients, borderline in 14, and suboptimal in 14 patients. The latter 14 patients had undergone concomitant ileal resections. Thus, vitamin B_{12} malabsorption is a minimal problem in the absence of concomitant ileal resection. Two reports with similar findings regarding vitamin B_{12} absorption after construction of an ileal reservoir were published in 1975 by Jagenburg et al and Nicholls et al in 1981. The latter study evaluated a series of patients with a Parks "S" reservoir and ileoanal anastomosis. Nicholls et al also showed the 24-hour fecal fat excretion to be normal in all 14 patients who underwent an ileal "S" reservoir and ileoanal anastomosis. In contrast, however, back in 1979, Nilsson et al reported an increased fecal loss of bile acids in 12 of 14 patients, 2 of whom had fat malabsorption. It is possible that an increased hepatic synthesis of bile acids can compensate for the increased fecal losses. Schjonsby et al also studied patients with continent ileostomies and demonstrated vitamin B_{12} malabsorption and steatorrhea. They attributed this to a blind loop syndrome because treatment with antibiotics resulted in an increased absorption of vitamin B_{12} and a excretion of fecal fat.

Thus, it seems evident that a certain percentage of these patients develop borderline Schilling's tests and an increased loss of fecal bile acids. The clinical significance of these observations is, however, in question because the vast majority of these patients show no serious metabolic disturbance and no clinical evidence of malabsorption.

"Pouchitis." "Pouchitis" refers to inflammatory changes in the reservoir in which the mucosal surface appears reddened, edematous, and in severe cases, ulcerated. Symptomatically, there is usually a sudden increase in the number of stools with a bloody mucous discharge and occasional bouts of incontinence. The patient may experience abdominal cramps and fever. This complication has been described in 10 to 43 percent of the patients in whom an ileal reservoir has been constructed. In our own patients, 27 percent have experienced this problem. Although the exact etiology of this inflammatory reaction is unknown, it has been suggested that the condition might be secondary to an overgrowth of bacteria within the pouch. The bacterial metabolites and toxins are thus implicated in the causation of "Pouchitis." Kock et al in 1977, made the interesting observation that these inflammatory changes are seen only in patients whose initial disease was chronic ulcerative colitis and that patients with familial polyposis seem to be spared of this complication. In our experience, 10 of 50 patients with colitis have had pouchitis. One of five polyposis patients has been afflicted. It would seem that there may not be any difference. The usual treatment is with antibiotics. Azulfidine has

been used in the past and metronidazole has recently been shown to be effective. Intermittent pouch intubation with gentle irrigation may be helpful to alleviate symptoms. Usually, the problem resolves rapidly but may recur.

FUNCTIONAL RESULTS

The functional results of a given procedure are an expression of objective parameters which can be described and measured and a subjective assessment of patient satisfaction. Patient satisfaction, of course, is influenced by prior experience with the disease process being treated and expectations regarding the operative outcome.

Continence. Continence is the ability to control defecation voluntarily, to discriminate solid, gas, and liquid and to defer evacuation to a time which is socially acceptable. Taylor et al reported that 5 percent of 74 patients who had undergone a "J" pouch had major fecal incontinence while 20 percent of 50 patients who had undergone an ileoanal procedure without a reservoir had major nocturnal fecal incontinence. Heppel et al studied 12 of these 50 patients with anal manometry and found that their resting and voluntary squeeze anal pressures were essentially normal when compared with voluntary controls. This suggests that the incontinence suffered by these patients is not secondary to a sphincter injury, but rather to an inadequate reservoir capacity of the neorectum.

Although major fecal incontinence is not a frequent complication of the ileoanal procedure in which a pouch has been constructed, intermittent mucous leakage and slight fecal staining is more common. In a recent review of our own patients such minor leakage occurred in few patients during the day but in 15 percent of the patients at night. Taylor et al reported similar minor incontinence in 35 percent of their patients during the day and 65 percent of patients at night. Parks et al and Peck reported a 35 percent and 56 percent incidence, respectively. The reason why certain patients are troubled by this problem is unknown. Inability of the anal canal to completely collapse because of the ileoanal anastomosis has been suggested. Nicholls et al felt that mucous leakage could be explained by a lower resting anal canal pressure which was measured manometrically in patients with mucous leakage. Others have not confirmed these findings, although preliminary data on our own patients is suggestive that this may be the case. Whatever the reason, minor mucous leakage seems to be a frequent problem. For most patients, the treatment consists of good hygiene but often a perineal pad is required if for no other reason than to provide security to the patient especially at night. Few of our patients have altered their sleep position in order to control this problem.

Stool Frequency. The frequency of stools decreases with time as the ileal segment or pouch dilates and assumes a greater reservoir function. Peck has reported a frequency of 3.8 stools per 24 hours at 13.5 months postileostomy take down using the "S" pouch. Rothenberger et al also used the "S" pouch with resultant stool frequency of 6 per 24-hour period at 4.5 months postileostomy take down. Utsunomiya et al in a small number of patients, used three varying techniques (no pouch, later side-to-side pouch, and "J" pouch), and reported a stool frequency of 4.5 stools per 24-hour period at 4.5 months. The study suggested that the "J" pouch provided a better reservoir at least initially. Fonkalsrud, using a lateral side-to-side pouch, reported a stool frequency of 4 per 24 hours. Taylor et al, in one of the few reports comparing the ileoanal procedure done with and without a reservoir, reported a frequency of 7 stools per 24 hours at 6 months postoperative in the reservoir group, while the group without a reservoir were having 11 stools per 24 hours at 18 months postileostomy take down. Our patients state that stool frequency is influenced by social activities (i.e., work, play, and so on) and by diet. Most patients can defer defecation on an average for 8 hours if actively engaged in other activities. Then, when resting or after a meal, they may have several bowel movements over a short time period.

Habits. Urgency does not seem to be a problem for these patients. The call to stool is usually described as being similar, though not identical, to the normal urge to defecate in most of our patients. Some patients, however, have to rely on vague abdominal urges to differentiate the need to defecate. With the exception of Parks' initial experience, most series report that the vast majority of patients evacuate spontaneously without the need for intubation unrelated to the type of reservoir utilized. Five of our patients regularly intubate. These patients feel that they never completely evacuate spontaneously, thus, the need for catheterization. For most patients, defecation is completed within a matter of minutes and is not a time-consuming event.

In reviewing the recent reported series in which an ileoanal procedure has been performed, it becomes evident that the vast majority of patients do not experience major fecal incontinence. Parks et al described only 1 patient out of 20 with incontinence. Fonkalsrud reported that 92 percent of his patients could discriminate solid, liquid, and gas and that 100 percent could defer defecation. We reviewed 40 of our own patients and found only 1 patient with major fecal incontinence. This was found to be associated with "pouchitis." After therapy, continence was restored.

SUMMARY

The proper role of the procedure of total colectomy, rectal mucosectomy, and ileoanal anastomosis with an ileal reservoir for the operative treatment of ulcerative colitis and familial polyposis is currently being defined. The procedure to date has a reported mortality rate of zero and an acceptable morbidity when performed in selected patients. The majority of the patients return to their previous occupation or school within 2 to 3 months with a stool frequency of 4 to 8 per 24 hours and with adequate if not normal continence.

The functional results seem to directly correlate with the reservoir capacity of the neorectum. There seems to be little place in adults for an ileoanal procedure which brings a straight conduit of ileum to the dentate line. Rather the ileum should be fashioned into a pouch so the patient immediately starts out with a neorectum which provides a reservoir capacity. There are numerous technical variation in pouch construction, and to date, one has not been shown to be superior. The procedure is relatively new and long-term follow-up will be required in regards to possible metabolic, mechanical, or malignant problems with the reservoir.

The results of these procedures must be analyzed in the light of the alternative procedures, proctocolectomy and permanent ileostomy. It is fallacious to compare the function in patients who have had these procedures with the normal population. The early results with the procedures of total colectomy, rectal mucosectomy, ileal reservoir, and ileoanal anastomosis have, therefore, been encouraging. This operation seems to be a reasonable alternative to a permanent ileostomy in selected patients who are relatively fit, stable, reliable, and fully cognizant of the nature of this procedure and the alternatives.

The widespread use of these procedures, however, is not to be encouraged. The operation is still very much in the developmental stage and as such should only be undertaken by surgeons trained in it and should be performed in institutions capable of the specialized care, counseling, and support required for the patients pre- and postoperatively. Surgeons undertaking to perform these operations must be cognizant of all the possible variations as in some individuals it may be necessary to modify the usual routine because of unforeseen anatomic problems discovered at the time of the operation to enable a neorectum to be constructed safely.

BIBLIOGRAPHY

Adson MA, Cooperman AM, et al: Ileorectostomy for ulcerative disease of the colon. Arch Surg 104:424, 1972

Baker WNW, Glass RE, et al: Cancer of the rectum following colectomy and ileorectal anastomosis for ulcerative colitis. Br J Surg 65:862, 1978

Bauer JJ, Gelernt IM, et al: Sexual dysfunction following proctocolectomy for benign disease of the colon and rectum. Ann Surg 197:363, 1983

Bearhs OH: Present status of the continent ileostomy. Dis Colon Rectum 19:192, 1976

Beart RW, Dozois RR, et al: Ileoanal anastomosis in the adult. Surg Gynecol Obstet 154:826, 1982

Best RR: Evaluation of ileoproctostomy to avoid ileostomy in various colon lesions. JAMA 150:637, 1952

Bonello JC, Thow GB, et al: Mucosal enteritis: A complication of the continent ileostomy. Dis Colon Rectum 24:37, 1981

Brandburg A, Kock NG, et al: Bacterial flora in intraabdominal ileostomy reservoir. Gastroenterology 63:413, 1976

Burnham WR, Lennard-Jones JE, et al: Sexual problems among married ileostomates. Gut 18:673, 1977

Daly DW, Brooke BN: Ileostomy and excision of the large intestine for ulcerative colitis. Lancet 2:61, 1967

Devine J, Webb R: Resection of the rectal mucosa, colectomy, and anal ileostomy with normal continence. Surg Gynecol Obstet 92:437, 1951

Donovan JJ, O'Hara ET: Sexual function following surgery for ulcerative colitis. N Engl J Med 262:719, 1960

Drobni A: One-stage proctocolectomy and anal ileostomy: Report of 35 cases. Dis Colon Rectum 10:443, 1967

Duthie HL, Gairns FW: Sensory nerve-endings and sensation in the anal region of man. Br J Surg 47:585, 1960

Farnell MB, VanHeerden JA, et al: Rectal preservation in non-specific inflammatory diseases of the colon. Ann Surg 192:249, 1980

Flake WK, Altman MS, et al: Problems encountered with the Kock ileostomy. Am J Surg 138:851, 1979

Fonkalsrud EW: Endorectal ileal pull-through with lateral ileal reservoir for benign colorectal disease. Ann Surg 194:761, 1981

Fonkalsrud EW: Endorectal ileal pull-through with ileal reservoir for ulcerative colitis and polyposis. Am J Surg 144:81, 1982

Gerber A, Apt MK, et al: The Kock continent ileostomy. Surg Gynecol Obstet 156:345, 1983

Grundfest SF, Fazio V, et al: The risk of cancer following colectomy and ileorectal anastomosis for extensive mucosal ulcerative colitis. Ann Surg 193:9, 1981

Gruner OPN, Flatmark A, et al: Ileorectal anastomosis in ulcerative colitis: Results in 57 patients. Scand J Gastroent 10:641, 1975

Gruner OPN, Naas R, et al: Proctectomy in ulcerative colitis: Results in 143 patients. Scand J Gastroent 12:75, 1977

Hampton JM: Rectal mucosal stripping: A technique for preservation of the rectum after total colectomy for chronic ulcerative colitis. Dis Colon Rectum 19:133, 1976

Heppell J, Kelly KA, et al: Physiologic aspects of continence after colectomy, mucosal proctectomy and endo-rectal ileo–anal anastomosis. Ann Surg 195:435, 1982

Jagenburg R, Dotevall G, et al: Absorption studies in patients with "intraabdominal ileostomy reservoir" and in patients with conventional ileostomies. Gut 12:437, 1971

Jagenburg R, Kock NG, et al: Vitamin B_{12} absorption in patients with continent ileostomy. Scand J Gastroenterol 10:141, 1975

Johnston D, Williams NS, et al: The value of preserving the anal sphincter in operations for ulcerative colitis and polyposis: A review of 22 mucosal proctectomies. Br J Surg 68:874, 1981

Karlan M, McPherson RC, et al: An experimental evaluation of fecal continence sphincter and reservoir in the dog. Surg Gynecol Obstet 108:469, 1959

King SA: Enteritis and the continent ileostomy. Conn Med 41:477, 1977

Kock NG: Intra-abdominal "Reservoir" in patients with permanent ileostomy. Arch Surg 99:223, 1969

Kock NG: Present status of the continent ileostomy: Surgical revision of the malfunctioning ileostomy. Dis Colon Rectum 19:200, 1976

Kock NG, Darle N, et al: Ileostomy. Curr Probl Surg 14:1, 1977

Lane RHS, Parks AG: Function of the anal sphincters following colo-anal anastomosis. Br J Surg 64:596, 1977

Lee ECG, Dowling BL: Perimuscular excision of the rectum for Crohn's disease and ulcerative colitis. Br J Surg 59:29, 1972

Loeshcke K, Bolkert T, et al: Bacterial overgrowth in ileal reservoirs (Kock Pouch): Extended functional studies. Hepatogastroenterology 27:310, 1980

Lytle JA, Parks NG: Intersphincteric excision of the rectum. Br J Surg 64:413, 1977

Martin LW, Fischer JE: Preservation of anorectal continence following total colectomy. Ann Surg 196:700, 1982

Martin LW, LeCoultre C, et al: Total colectomy and mucosal proctectomy with preservation of continence in ulcerative colitis. Ann Surg 186:477, 1977

May RE: Sexual dysfunction following rectal excision for ulcerative colitis. Br J Surg 53:29, 1966

Neal DE, Parker AJ, et al: The long term effects of proctectomy on bladder function in patients with inflammatory bowel disease. Br J Surg 69:349, 1982

Neal DE, Williams NS, et al: Rectal, bladder and sexual function after mucosal proctectomy with and without a pelvic reservoir for colitis and polyposis. Br J Surg 69:599, 1982

Nicholls RJ, Belliveau P, et al: Restorative proctocolectomy with ileal reservoir: A pathologic assessment. Gut 22:462, 1981

Nilsson LO, Andersson L, et al: Absorption studies in patients six to ten years after construction of ileostomy reservoir. Gut 20:499, 1979

Nilsson LO, Kock NG, et al: Morphological and histochemical changes in the mucosa of the continent ileostomy reservoir 6 to 10 years after its construction. Scand J Gastroenterol 15:737, 1980

Nilsson LO, Myrvold HE, et al: Plasma levels of vitamin B_{12} in patients with continent ileostomy. Presented at American Society of Colon and Rectal Surgeons meeting, Boston, June 8, 1983

Nissen R: Demonstrationen aus de operativen Chirurgie Zunachst einige beobachtungen aus der plastischen chirurgie. Zentralbl Chir 60:883, 1933

Parks AG, Nicholls RJ: Proctocolectomy without ileostomy for ulcerative colitis. Br Med J 2:85, 1978

Parks AG, Nicholls RJ, et al: Proctocolectomy with ileal reservoir and anal anastomosis. Br J Surg 67:533, 1980

Peck DA: Rectal mucosal replacement. Ann Surg 191:294, 1980

Pemberton JH, Kelly KA, et al: Achieving ileostomy continence with an indwelling stomal device. Surgery 90:336, 1981

Philipson BR, Brandburg A, et al: Mucosal morphology, bacteriology and absorption in intra-abdominal ileostomy reservoir. Scand J Gastroenterol 10:145, 1975

Ravitch MM: Anal ileostomy with sphincter preservation in patients requiring total colectomy for benign conditions. Surgery 24:170, 1948

Ravitch MM, Sabiston DC: Anal ileostomy with preservation of the sphincter: A proposed operation in patients requiring total colectomy for benign lesions. Surg Gynecol Obstet 84:1095, 1947

Ritchie JK: Ulcerative colitis treated by ileostomy and excisional surgery—"Fifteen years" experience at St. Mark's Hospital. Br J Surg 59:345, 1972

Rolstad BS, Wilson G, et al: Sexual concerns in the patient with ileostomy. Dis Colon Rectum 26:170, 1983

Rolstad BS, Wilson G, et al: Long term sexual concerns in the patient with ileostomy. J Ent Therapy 9:10, 1982

Rothenberger DA, Vermeulen FD, et al: Restorative proctocolectomy with ileal reservoir and ileoanal anastomosis. Am J Surg 145:82, 1983

Safaie-Shirazi S, Soper RT: Endorectal pull-through procedure in the surgical treatment of familial polyposis coli. J Ped Surg 8:711, 1973

Schjonsby H, Halverson JF, et al: Stagnant loop syndrome in patients with continent ileostomy (intra-abdominal ileal reservoir). Gut 18:795, 1977

Schrock TR: Complications of continent ileostomy. Am J Surg 138:162, 1979

Smith LE, Friend WG, et al: The superior mesenteric artery: The critical technical factor in the ileal pouch pull-through operation. Presented at the American Society of Colon and Rectal Surgeons meeting, Boston, June 8, 1983

Soave F: A new technique for treatment of Hirschsprung's disease. Surgery 56:1007, 1964

Stahlgren LH, Ferguson LK: Influence on sexual function of abdomino-perineal resection for ulcerative colitis. N Engl J Med 259:873, 1958

Taylor BM: Personal communication, Mayo Clinic

Taylor BM, Beart RW, et al: Straight ileoanal anastomosis versus ileal pouch-anal anastomosis after colectomy and mucosal proctectomy. Arch Surg 118:696, 1983

Telander RL, Perrault J: Total colectomy with rectal mucosectomy and ileoanal anastomosis for chronic ulcerative colitis in children and young adults. Mayo Clinic Proc 55:420, 1980

Telander RL, Perrault J: Colectomy with rectal mucosectomy and ileoanal anastomosis in young patients. Arch Surg 116:623, 1981

Thow GB: Personal communication, Carle Clinic

Utsunomiya J, Iwama T, et al: Total colectomy, mucosal proctectomy and ileoanal anastomosis. Dis Colon Rectum 23:459, 1980

Valiente M, Bacon H: Construction of a pouch using "pantaloon" technique for pull-through of ileum following colectomy: A report of experimental work and results. Am J Surg 90:742, 1955

Watts JMcK, DeDombal FT, et al: Long term complications and prognosis following major surgery for ulcerative colitis. Br J Surg 53:1014, 1966

Wolfstein IH, Bat L, et al: Regeneration of rectal mucosa and recurrent polyposis coli after total colectomy and ileoanal anastomosis. Arch Surg 117:1241, 1982

SECTION IX
Rectosigmoid, Rectum, and Anal Canal

55. Rectal Prolapse

Mitchell J. Notaras

INTRODUCTION

The aetiology and treatment of prolapse of the rectum continues to cause controversy. It is a condition in which part or the whole of the circumference of the rectum protrudes through the anus. It may result in occasional or complete faecal incontinence. In the extreme form the rectum becomes permanently prolapsed, excoriated, and ulcerated, and bleeds, causing much distress and disablement to the patient.

Rectal prolapse is far more common in women than in men and the majority are elderly, nulliparous females. A high proportion of patients, in the author's practice, have bowel fixations or are mentally ill, and with excessive straining succeed in defaecating their rectums. Rectal prolapse may occur in children who are otherwise normal, and it is usually a mucosal type of prolapse. With advice on bowel habit and retraining, it is usually self-correcting. Mucosal prolapse also occurs in adults but is usually associated with weakened anal muscles and requires surgical treatment.

Complete prolapse of the rectum (procidentia) consists of the full thickness of the rectal wall everting through the anus so that the entire circumference of the bowel is involved. It may project externally for several centimetres. Initially, the prolapse occurs during defaecation and may be self-reducing. Later, it requires manual reduction, and finally, it reaches the stage where it protrudes when the patient is walking or may become permanently prolapsed, even when the patient is in bed.

When the anal area of these patients is examined, one may find that on separation of the buttocks, the anus gapes open, indicating a lack of tone of the external and internal sphincter muscles of the anal canal. On digital rectal examination the anus is often patulous, and the contraction of the sphincters is weakened and poorly sustained. On proctoscopic examination, the mucosa is found to be flattened and devoid of the bulging haemorrhoids and submucosal vessels that are normally present.

To complete the assessment of these patients, routine sigmoidoscopic and if possible barium enema examinations should be performed to exclude other diseases. Unfortunately most have difficulty in retaining an enema. A neurologic examination is essential and this should include serologic tests.

AETIOLOGY

The aetiology of the condition is not understood. Moschcowitz (1912) thought that complete prolapse of the rectum was the equivalent of a sliding hernia. He suggested that the increased intraabdominal pressure that followed excessive straining resulted in the peritoneum of the pouch of Douglas becoming the equivalent of a hernial sac descending onto the pelvic floor. The rectum is attached anteriorly to the peritoneum, so that eventually when the sliding hernia is pushed through the anal canal, eversion of the rectum occurs. Moschcowitz repaired such a hernia by obliteration of the peritoneal pouch using a series of circular sutures.

Broden (1968), by radiologic studies, has suggested that the prolapse begins as an intussusception, approximately at the level of the sacral promontory. Although this is an attractive theory and cineradiography has demonstrated this intussusception, it does not seem to bear with the findings on physical examination. When a patient is asked to strain, the anal margin everts and then the mucosa of the anterior wall of the rectum appears and continues everting in a rolling action. In the cineradiography of these patients, it is possible that the descent of the rectosigmoid junction is misinterpreted as an intussusception. The eversion would not appear in the film.

In recent years, attention has been focussed on the pelvic floor musculature, and Porter (1962) has shown that there is a neuromuscular deficiency in a high proportion of the patients. Another feature is that the rectal sensation is often diminished in these patients. It is not known whether these changes are primary or secondary. They are important features to be recognised in the postoperative management of patients who continue to have incontinence.

TREATMENT OF MUCOSAL PROLAPSE

Infants

In children, conservative treatment in the correction of faulty bowel habits is usually successful. Occasionally, submucosal injections of sclerosants are given. Rarely, a Thiersch type of operation, encircling the anus with a catgut ligature, may be indicated.

Adults

In adults, operative treatment is usually necessary, as conservative measures such as injection sclerotherapy and multiple rubber banding ligation have yielded poor results. In the past there have been many techniques described. In recent years, those methods that seem to give the best results have been narrowed down to mucosal excision procedures.

In mucosal prolapse, operation is aimed at excising strips of mucosa so as to produce scarring and adhesion of the mucosa to the rectal wall. This may be achieved by performing a more radical type of haemorrhoidectomy in which a larger area of rectal mucosa is excised. The author prefers to excise linear strips of mucosa from the four quadrants of the lower rectum, then to plicate the denuded area in the hope that it will fix the mucosal layers to the circular muscle.

Occasionally, the surgeon, when prepared to correct a mucosal prolapse, finds that under anaesthesia the condition proves to be a complete rectal prolapse. The patient should be forewarned and the surgeon prepared for a more radical repair in case of such an eventuality.

TREATMENT OF COMPLETE RECTAL PROLAPSE (PROCIDENTIA)

The operations used for the treatment of complete rectal prolapse may be classified as perineal or abdominal according to the approach used.

Perineal Repairs

Rectosigmoidectomy

There have been many procedures described using the perineal approach, but most, especially rectosigmoidectomy, have failed to stand the test of time because of a high recurrence rate. Rectosigmoidectomy may be indicated in the rare case of a strangulated prolapsed rectum. In principle, the operation consists of amputating the prolapsed rectum at the anal verge and at the site of amputation anastomosing the rectum and anorectum. The anastomosis is then inverted back into the pelvic cavity.

Thiersch Procedure

In this operation a wire is passed subcutaneously to encircle the anal verge, forming a ring that prevents prolapse passing through the anus. It is a procedure that is now reserved for the patient who is too ill to withstand an abdominal procedure. Other materials, such as nylon and Silastic rubber (Hopkinson and Hardman, 1973), have also been used.

The Thiersch procedure is simple, but unfortunately it has numerous disadvantages:

1. The wire ring is rigid and is situated at the anal outlet just under the perianal skin. It fails to give lateral support to the anal canal and merely acts as an obstruction to the prolapse.
2. The wire or nylon used, occasionally cuts through into the anal canal.
3. The wire may fracture.
4. Faecal impaction occurs if the wire ring is too tight.

Mesh Encirclement of the Anorectal Junction (Figs. 55–1 through 55–6)

Prior to commencement of the procedure, the patient is catheterised. A swab is inserted into the anal canal and rectum to prevent leakage of mucus and descent of the prolapse.

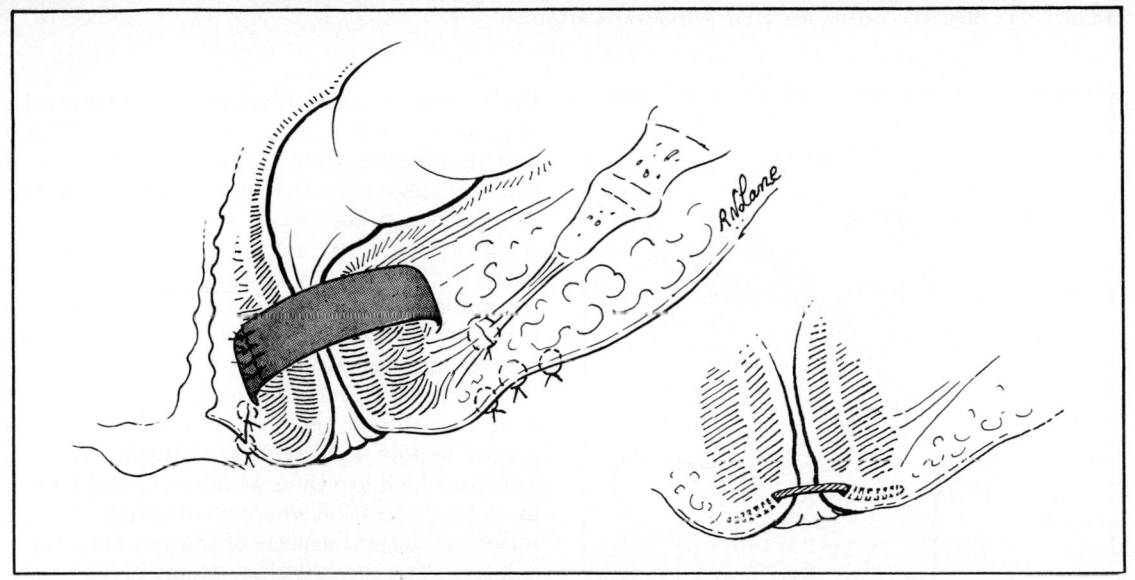

Figure 55–1. *Left:* The aim of the author's technique. A ribbon of Marlex or Mersilene mesh is placed around the anal canal and its sphincters at the level of the anorectal junction. The posterior half of the ring of mesh lies in the infralevator retrosphincteric and ischiorectal space, while the anterior half passes through the puborectalis muscles to enter the supralevator rectovaginal space. *Right:* Position of a Thiersch wire. There is no support for the anal canal, and the wire only acts as an obstruction to the intussuscepting rectal prolapse. (*Source: From Notaras MJ, 1973, with permission.*)

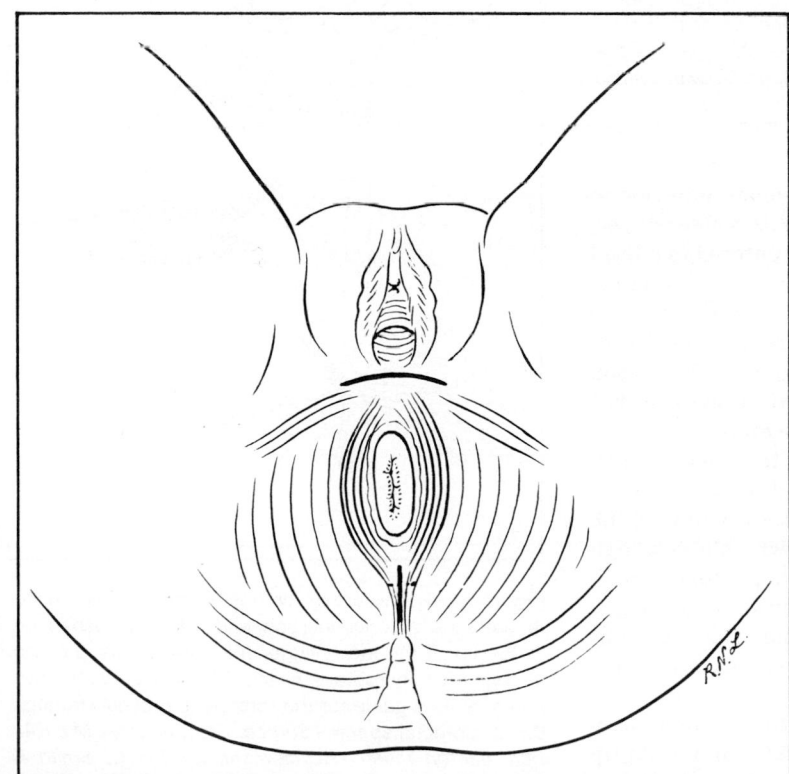

Figure 55–2. A transverse incision is made anterior to the anus for the dissection into the rectovaginal space. A sagittal incision is made posteriorly to enter the retrosphincteric space. (*Source: From Notaras MJ: Ribbon dacron mesh encirclement, in Rob C, Smith R (eds): Operative Surgery, 3 edt. London: Butterworths, 1977, with permission.*)

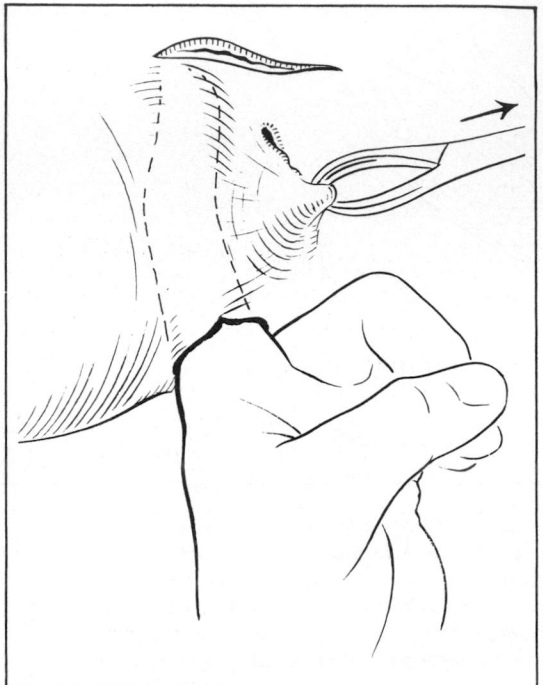

Figure 55–3. The index finger tunnels through the ischiorectal space to meet the levator muscles anteriorly. (*Source: From Notaras MJ: Ribbon dacron mesh encirclement, in Rob C, Smith R (eds): Operative Surgery, 3 edt. London: Butterworths, 1977, with permission.*)

A transverse incision is made anterior to the anus and perineal body. With scissor dissection, the rectovaginal space is entered to a level well above the pelvic floor muscle. A vertical incision is then made posterior to the anus to enter the retrosphincteric space, and the dissection is continued toward the coccyx. Thorlakson (1982) has described a similar procedure, but makes lateral incisions to the anus.

The index finger is then inserted through the posterior skin incision and by blunt dissection is pushed forward and laterally toward the ischial tuberosity. The finger, which is now high in the ischiorectal space, is then hooked medially until it meets the levator muscles, which form the roof of the space and which prevent the finger from entering the rectovaginal or supralevator space.

A large curved artery forceps is then introduced through the anterior incision and its tip directed posterolaterally toward the finger in the ischiorectal space. It is then pushed through

the levator muscles (mainly the puborectalis muscle, where it fuses with the perineal body) and thus passes from the supralevator (rectovaginal) space onto the tip of the finger in the infralevator (ischiorectal) space. The finger is withdrawn, guiding the forceps out through the posterior incision. By using this technique the rectum is safeguarded against accidental perforation by the forceps. The procedure is then repeated on the opposite side.

With the two forceps passing through both sides of the anus, the ends of a ribbon of mesh approximately 4 cm wide are attached to both forceps, which are then withdrawn, pulling the mesh into a position where it surrounds the posterior and lateral aspects of the anorectal musculature. The mesh is then double breasted anteriorly and sutured together with interrupted synthetic monofilament suture materials.

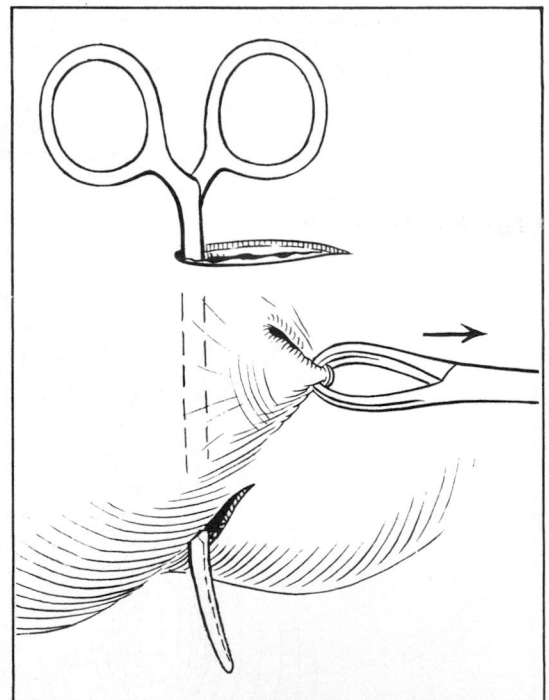

Figure 55–4. The artery forceps have been introduced through the anterior incision and the end pushed on to the tip of the index finger (Fig. 55–3) after passing through the puborectalis muscle. The finger is withdrawn and acts as a guide for the forceps to proceed through the ischiorectal space. (*Source: From Notaras MJ: Ribbon dacron mesh encirclement, in Rob C, Smith R (eds): Operative Surgery, 3 edt. London: Butterworths, 1977, with permission.*)

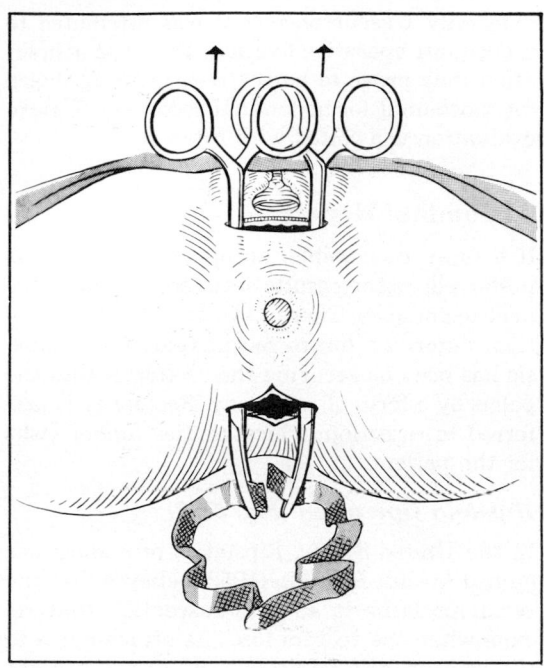

Figure 55–5. The ribbon of mesh is grasped by the forceps and pulled through. (*Source: From Notaras MJ: Ribbon dacron mesh encirclement, in Rob C, Smith R (eds): Operative Surgery, 3 edt. London: Butterworths, 1977, with permission.*)

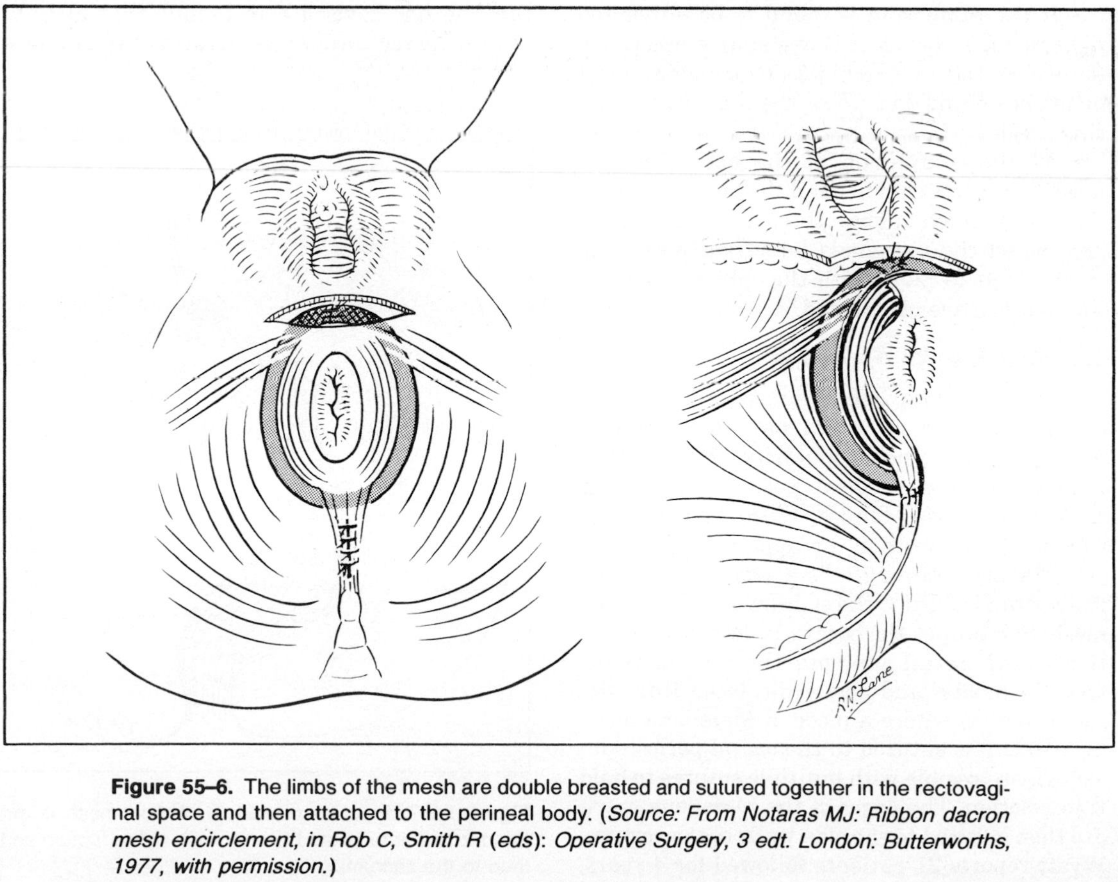

Figure 55–6. The limbs of the mesh are double breasted and sutured together in the rectovaginal space and then attached to the perineal body. (*Source: From Notaras MJ: Ribbon dacron mesh encirclement, in Rob C, Smith R (eds): Operative Surgery, 3 edt. London: Butterworths, 1977, with permission.*)

A further stitch is placed to bring together the puborectalis muscle and to include the midanterior part of the mesh of the ring in the bite. This important stitch helps to fix the mesh to the perineal body and to bury it in the muscle. 00 Dexon sutures are then used to close the subcutaneous space and to further bury the synthetic sutures. The skin is then drawn together with 00 Dexon sutures.

To assess the diameter of the circle of mesh before suturing it, various methods may be used. The mesh may be doubled breasted over a large proctoscope or, as the author prefers, two fingers are inserted into the canal and the diameter assessed digitally. This latter method requires additional gloves over the surgeon's hands and frequent changing of gloves until the diameter is assessed to be correct. Alternatively a Hegar's dilator may be used.

The postoperative management is that of establishing a suitable bowel regimen to ensure regular emptying of the rectum. Suppositories that stimulate defaecation may be necessary in addition to stool softeners.

If the mesh ring is found to be either too tight or too loose, then it is a simple procedure to reopen the anterior dissection under local anaesthesia and to correct the diameter of the ring mesh.

At the completion of the operation, the mesh is felt as a cord around the anorectal junction. It is much higher than a Thiersch wire and, when the patient is later reassessed, the mesh is felt to move with the sphincters when the muscles are contracted.

Modified Kraske Approach

Other more complicated procedures using a modified Kraske approach have been devised but have not gained popularity. Wyatt (1981) has described a perineal posterior rectopexy that shows great promise. With the patient in the jack-knife position, by approaching the retrorectal space through the anococcygeal raphe, the rectum is fixed to the sacrum with Mersilene mesh. Sometimes the coccyx is detached. In patients with rectal prolapse the rectum is extremely mobile and easily displaced from the sacral hollow where a piece of Mersilene mesh (8 × 10 cm) is sutured to the sacral periosteum as high as possible with multiple sutures to hold it in position. The edges of the Mersilene patch are then sutured to the side walls of the rectum. Wyatt reports 21 patients followed for 4 years,

with only 1 recurrence that was attributed to inadequate operative fixation. This type of operation may prove to be the treatment of choice for those unfit for abdominal rectopexy. Future evaluation is awaited with interest.

Abdominal Repair

If it is at all possible, an abdominal repair is preferred, as the results seem better than perineal techniques. There have been many operations described, but in recent years the emphasis has been on securing the rectum within the pelvis by a form of rectopexy. Rectopexy is preferred to resection, which carries higher risks for the patient.

Ripstein Operation (Fig. 55–7)

In the United States, Ripstein's procedure has gained favour. Ripstein (1952) believes that the rectal prolapse is an intussusception that results when the rectum loses its attachments to the sacrum and becomes virtually a straight tube. To prevent this straightening of the rectum, he has devised a technique that aims to retain the rectum in the sacral hollow and pre-

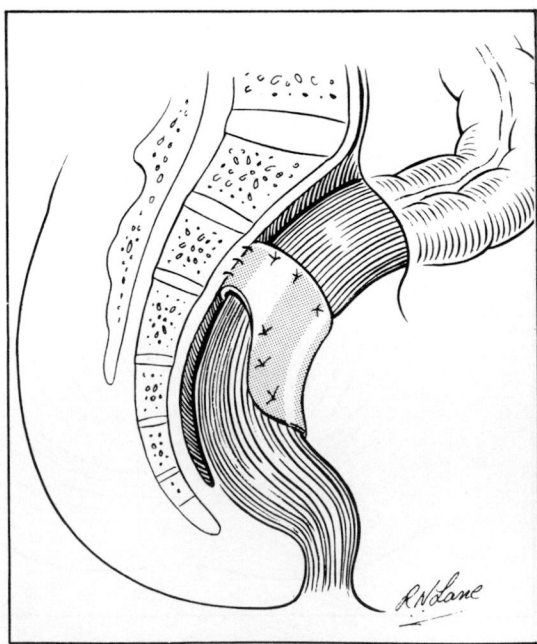

Figure 55–7. Ripstein procedure. Teflon mesh is sutured to the anterior and lateral walls of the rectum and then to the sacrum.

vent the intussusception. A pelvic floor repair is not required.

Through a lower abdominal incision the rectum is mobilised down to the levator muscles and from its attachments to the sacral hollow. A 2-inch-wide ribbon of Teflon mesh is then placed around the rectum, roughly at the level of the peritoneal reflection. The ends of the ribbon are sutured with nonabsorbable sutures to the presacral fascia and periosteum approximately 2 inches (5 cm) below the sacral promontory while carefully avoiding the presacral vessels. That part of the mesh that is against the anterior wall of the rectum is shaped like an apron, forming a sling whose edges are sutured to the rectal wall. The sling should be loose enough to allow two fingers to pass between the bowel and the sacral fascia.

Unfortunately with this method of fixation of the Teflon mesh, the rectum is completely surrounded by the mesh anteriorly and laterally and by the sacrum posteriorly. This prevents expansion of the rectum and if the mesh implant has been fixed too tightly or if there is excessive fibrous reaction, it may behave as a mechanical obstruction.

The results of several series reported show a low recurrence rate, varying from 2.3 to 12.5 percent. Launer and Fazio (1982) reported a zero operative mortality after 57 Ripstein procedures but a 26 percent morbidity. Recurrent rectal prolapse occurred in 12.5 percent and 18 percent had significant long-term obstructive symptoms. Gordon and Hoexter (1978) reviewed several series of Ripstein procedures and found a low recurrence rate (2.3 percent) but complications included faecal impaction, presacral haemorrhage, stricture, pelvic infection, small bowel obstruction and fistula due to erosion of the sling through the bowel wall.

Ivalon Sponge Rectopexy (Fig. 55–8)

The abdominal procedure for the treatment of rectal prolapse most favoured in Great Britain is the Ivalon sponge implant technique described by Wells (Ellis, 1966). The operation relies on the production of an intense fibrotic reaction generated by the Ivalon sponge when placed in the presacral space between the rectum and sacrum. The sponge is wrapped around three quarters of the circumference of the rectum leaving part of the anterior wall uncovered to allow expansion of the rectum and to prevent obstruction. The sponge is sutured to both the

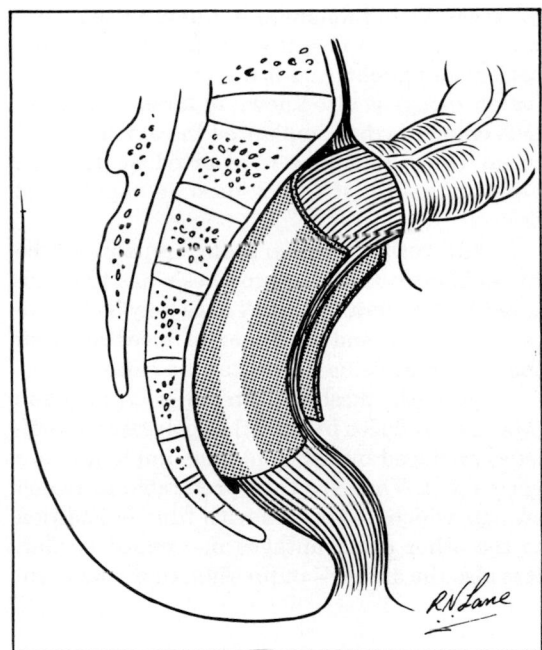

Figure 55–8. Ivalon sponge repair. The Ivalon sponge is wrapped around the rectum for most of its circumference except for a gap anteriorly. The sponge is sutured to the rectum and the hollow of the sacrum.

sacrum and rectum. It was initially thought that the rectum became adherent to the sacrum but this has not been found in reoperations and it is most likely that a thickening of the rectal wall develops that prevents the prolapse.

In this procedure the rectum is mobilised down to the levators posteriorly and the lateral ligaments are divided. A rectangular sheet of Ivalon sponge is sutured to the periosteum of the sacral hollow with nonabsorbable sutures. The rectum is elevated and the lateral edges of the sponge partially wrapped around the rectum and sutured to its anterolateral walls. The pelvic peritoneum is sutured.

Excellent results have been reported by Morgan (1972) and by Penfold (1972), but Goligher (1984) recorded a high pelvic sepsis rate of 16 percent. If the rectum or any bowel is opened during the procedure then the Ivalon sponge implant should not be used. If infection occurs the morbidity is high and the sponge should be removed rather than procrastinate, hoping that the problem will resolve on antibiotics.

Although the results have so far proved satisfactory, the Ivalon sponge has certain disadvantages when implanted in human tissue. Initial fibrosis is uncontrolled and varies from patient to patient, and it does not seem to last. Ivalon sponge is also known to induce sarcomatous changes when implanted in rats, although so far this has not been reported in humans. For this reason it is not used in the United States.

With both the Ivalon sponge repair and the Ripstein operation, the prosthesis has to be sutured to the sacral hollow. There may be technical difficulties and a danger of bleeding from the presacral veins which can be catastrophic.

Synthetic meshes such as polypropylene (Marlex, produced by Davol) or polyester (Mersilene, produced by Ethicon) once implanted are permanent. They are thus preferable to Ivalon sponge, which disappears with time in addition to the other disadvantages mentioned earlier. It is also the author's impression that when syn-

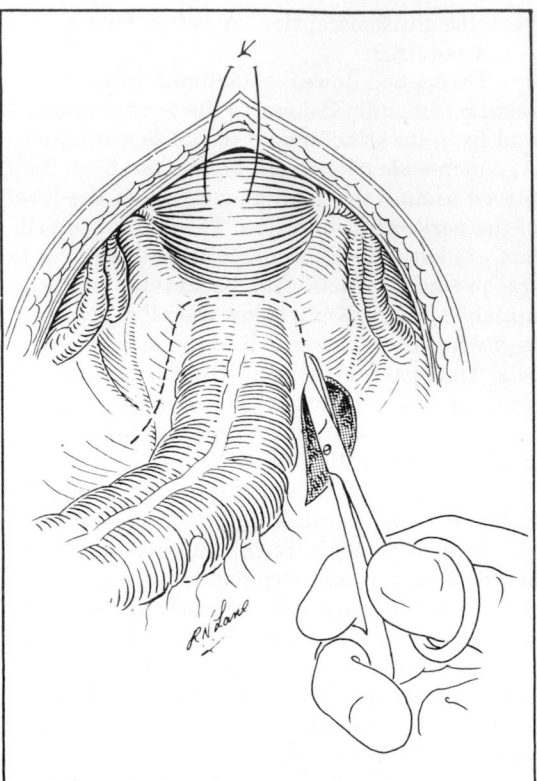

Figure 55–10. A temporary suture through the anterior abdominal wall and fundus of the uterus helps to retract the uterus in the pelvic dissection when mobilising the rectum.

thetic meshes are used, the postoperative recovery is much smoother. This is most likely due to the minimal reaction generated in the pelvis by the synthetic mesh.

Notaras Posterior Mesh Rectopexy (Figs. 55–9 Through 55–13)

To overcome some of the disadvantages of the Ripstein procedure, the author prefers to place a rectangular piece of mesh posterior to the rectum, occupying approximately a third of its circumference. This allows full expansion of the rectum, and the possible problem of obstruction as in the Ripstein procedure is overcome. The mesh, well away from the ureters, is buried in the presacral space and is hidden away from the small bowel, which might become adherent to any exposed mesh. After it has been sutured to the posterior wall of the rectum, its upper edge is then sutured to the sacral promontory. This overcomes the technical difficulties that may result in bleeding of presacral veins when

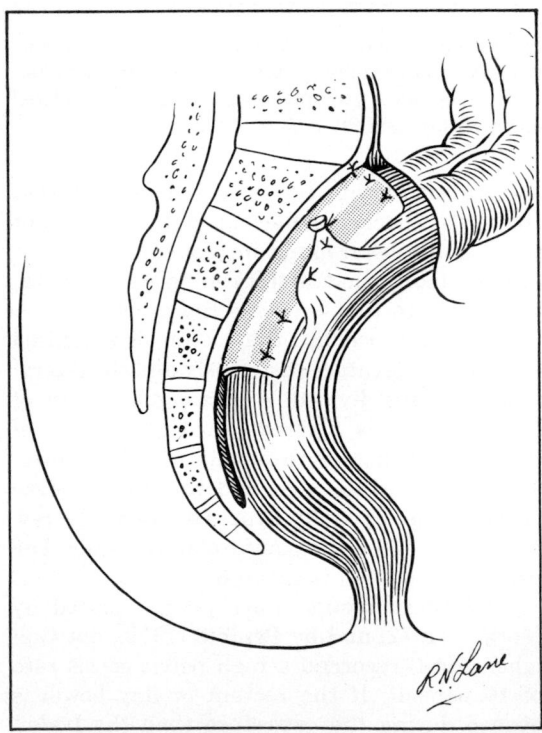

Figure 55–9. Notaras procedure. A rectangular piece of Mersilene or Marlex mesh is sutured to the mesorectum and lateral ligaments. The upper edge of the mesh is then sutured to the sacral promontory, thus avoiding the danger of bleeding of the presacral veins, which may follow when implants are sutured in the sacral hollow.

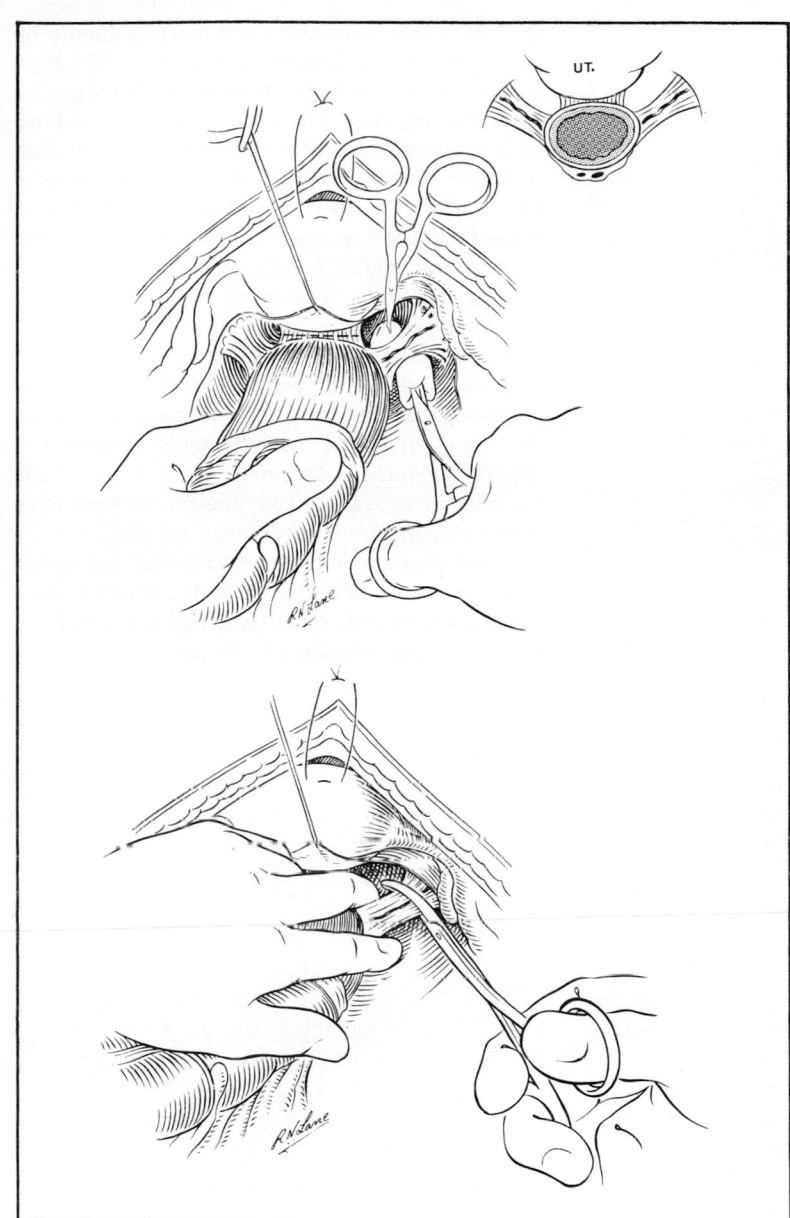

UT.

Figure 55–11. The lateral ligaments of the rectum are divided to allow full mobilisation. The only contraindication to this manoeuvre is when dealing with young males because of the risk of impotence.

attaching the Ivalon sponge or the mesh in the Ripstein procedure to the sacral hollow. The author has found this technique to be a more rapid and simple operation compared with other procedures.

Prior to operation, the patient's bowels are cleared of faeces by aperients and enemas. Forty eight hours before operation, the patient is started on a course of metronidazole (Flagyl). This is continued after the operation in the intravenous form.

Before commencement of the operation, an indwelling catheter is placed in the bladder. The patient is then placed in the Trendelenburg position. A lower midline incision from the umbilicus is made. On entering the abdominal cavity, a full laparotomy is carried out. In the female the uterus is temporarily sutured to the lower end of the incision so as to provide greater access to the pelvis. The rectum is then mobilised down to the levator muscles. The lateral ligaments are divided in a manner similar to preparing

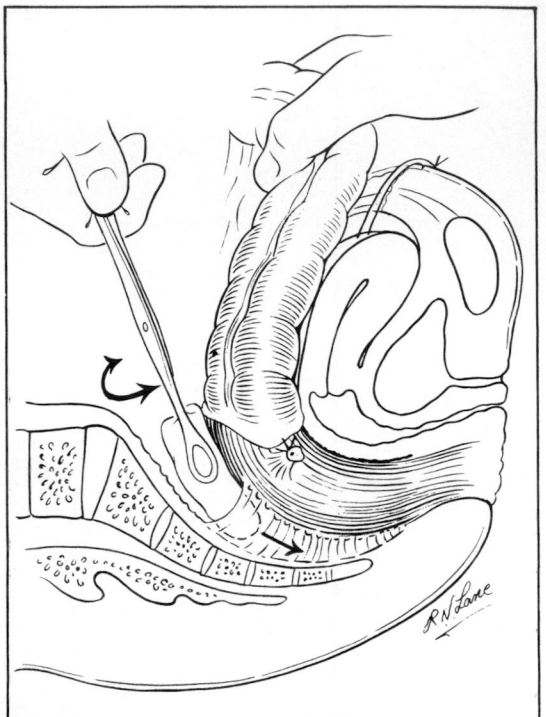

Figure 55–12. To fully mobilise the rectum, the presacral fascial attachments of the posterior and lateral walls of the rectum are separated by gentle blunt dissection with a sponge. (See also Fig. 55–11, top.)

for a low anterior resection (in young males the division of the lateral ligaments is omitted so as to avoid the possibility of impotence).

With the rectum mobilised, a piece of synthetic mesh, approximately 5 to 7 cm by 8 to 10 cm, is prepared. The rectum is then drawn forward and the mesh placed against the mesorectum and sutured in such a fashion that it is stretched and attached to it by fine monofilament synthetic sutures. These sutures are inserted into the edges of the mesh and into the mesorectum and the lateral ligaments using a bunching technique. The upper part of the mesh is then sutured with 0 monofilament nylon to the sacral promontory, having displaced away the iliac vessels with the index finger. A closed suction drain, if needed, is placed in the presacral space. Originally, reperitonealisation was carried out, but this is no longer performed.

Throughout the procedure it is essential not to use silk, cotton, or linen suture materials.

Only synthetic monofilament sutures should be employed for the fixation of the mesh. The ligaturing of vessels is performed with catgut or synthetic sutures. The reason for strict adherence to special synthetic suture materials is that if infection should occur, then the presence of silk, cotton, or linen materials predisposes to sinus formation, and until these suture materials are removed, the sinuses will persist whenever associated with a mesh implant.

This procedure suspends the rectum and promotes adhesions and thickening of the posterior wall, with the result that downward displacement of the rectum is prevented. The author finds it to be an extremely simple and rapidly performed technique and in over 100 cases performed since 1967 has had no operative mortality, minimal morbidity, no need for abdominal reoperation for any reason, and so far no recurrences. Hilsabeck (1981) favours a similar procedure and recently Keighley (1983) reported similar results in 100 cases.

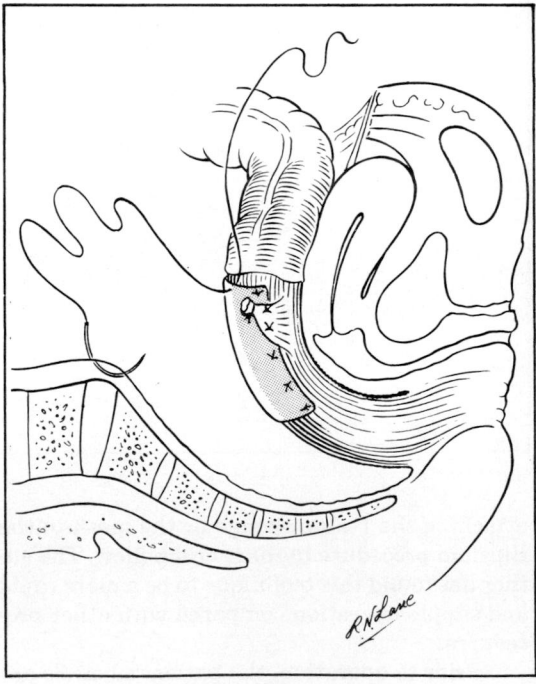

Figure 55–13. After the rectum is fully mobilised, the mesh is attached to posterior wall of rectum and lateral ligaments. The upper portion of the mesh is then sutured to the sacral promontory with two sutures of monofilament nylon. The final result is seen in Figure 55–9.

Rectosacral Suture Fixation

Yet another technique of rectopexy consists of simply suturing the mobilised rectum to the sacrum after the rectum has been mobilised from the sacrum down to the tip of the coccyx. By carefully avoiding the presacral vessels the posterolateral margins of the rectum are fixed on each side of the third and second sacral bodies and the sacral promontory with pairs of stitches.

Carter (1983) reported its success in 32 patients treated in this manner over a period of 12 years, with only 1 recurrence in a demented patient.

Treatment After Rectopexy

Although the newer techniques of rectopexy have succeeded in preventing the rectal prolapse, many of the patients will remain partially incontinent. This is due to the neuromuscular defect in the pelvic floor resulting in inadequate anal sphincters and poor rectal sensation. In most series, approximately 60 percent of the patients with rectal prolapse are classified as being partially incontinent despite a successful repair. Because of the incompetent anal sphincters, the patient is left with the equivalent of an anal colostomy. Management must be continued with regulation of the patient's bowel habit, usually using bulk-producing agents and anal suppositories to stimulate defaecation. Unfortunately pelvic faradism and anal electronic type stimulators (Hopkinson and Lightwood, 1966) have failed to improve the results. In the experience of the author and others, operations aimed at repair of the anal orifice do not seem to benefit in the management of incontinence. Parks (1967) has reported some success with the technique of postanal repair.

Some patients who have had a successful abdominal repair may still have some residual mucosal prolapse. This may be cured by ligature and excision, as previously described.

BIBLIOGRAPHY

Broden B, Snellman B: Procidentia of the rectum studied with cineradiography: A contribution to the discussion of causative mechanism. Dis Colon Rectum 11:330, 1968
Carter AE: Rectosacral suture fixation for complete rectal prolapse in the elderly, the frail and demented. Br J Surg 70:522, 1983
Davidian VA, Thomas CG: Trans-sacral repair of rectal prolapse. Am J Surg 123:231, 1972
Ellis H: The polyvinyl sponge wrap operation for rectal prolapse Br J Surg 53:675, 1966
Goligher JC, Hughes ESR: Sensibility of the rectum and colon: Its role in the mechanism of anal incontinence. Lancet 1:543, 1951
Goligher JC: Surgery of the Anus, Rectum and Colon, 3 edt. Springfield, Illinois: Charles C Thomas, 1975, p 292
Gordon PH, Hoexter B: Complications of Ripstein procedure. Dis Colon Rectum 21:277, 1978
Hawe A, Rastelli GC: Late deterioration of intra-cardiac Ivalon sponge patches. J Thorac Cardiovasc Surg 58:87, 1969
Hilsabeck JR: Transabdominal posterior rectopexy using an inverted T of synthetic material. Arch Surg 116:41, 1981
Hopkinson BR, Hardman J: Silicone rubber perianal suture for rectal prolapse. Proc R Soc Med 66:1095, 1973
Hopkinson BR, Lightwood R: Electrical treatment of anal incontinence. Lancet 1:297, 1966
Keighley B, Alexander-Williams J: Results of Marlex mesh abdominal rectopexy for rectal prolapse in 100 consecutive cases. Br J Surg 70:229, 1983
Launer DD, Fazio VW, et al: The Ripstein procedure. A 16 year experience. Dis Colon Rectum 25:4145, 1982
Miles WE: Rectal prolapse. Proc R Soc Med 26:1445, 1973
Morgan CN, Porter NH, et al: Ivalon (polyvinyl alcohol) sponge in the repair of complete rectal prolapse. Br J Surg 59:841, 1972
Moschcowitz AV: The pathogenesis, anatomy, and cure of prolapse of the rectum. Surg Gynecol Obstet 1:7, 1912
Notaras, MJ: The use of Mersilene mesh in rectal prolapse repair. Proc R Soc Med 27:930, 1973
Parks AG: Post anal perineorrhaphy for rectal prolapse. Proc R Soc Med 60:920, 1967
Penfold JCB, Hawley PR: Experiences of Ivalon sponge implant for complete rectal prolapse at St. Marks Hospital 1960–1970. Br J Surg 59:846, 1972
Porter NH: A physiological study of the pelvic floor in rectal prolapse. Ann R Coll Surg Engl 31:379, 1962
Ripstein CB: Treatment of massive rectal prolapse. Am J Surg 83:68, 1952
Stephens FD: Minor surgical conditions of the anus and perineum (in pediatrics). Med J Aust 1:244, 1958
Thorlakson RH: A modification of the Thiersch procedure for rectal prolapse using polyester tape. Dis Colon Rectum 25:1, 1982
Todd IP: Etiological factors in the production in rectal prolapse. Postgrad Med J 35:97, 1959
Wyatt AP: Perineal rectopexy for rectal prolapse. Br J Surg 68:717, 1981

56. Tumours of the Rectum and Anal Canal

Harold Ellis

CARCINOMA OF THE RECTUM

Nearly half the cancers of the large bowel occur in the rectum, rectosigmoid junction, and anus, and these account for approximately one third of all the deaths from large bowel cancer. The office of Population Censuses and Surveys gives the following figures for registrations of cancers of the large bowel in England and Wales in 1980:

Males:	Colon	6103
	Rectum, rectosigmoid junction, and anus	5044
Females:	Colon	7740
	Rectum, rectosigmoid junction, and anus	4236

In males, cancers of the large bowel were second in incidence of registration only to carcinoma of the lung (26,925 cases) and in females second only to cancer of the breast (21,148 cases). Note that there is a very slight male preponderance for rectal cancers compared with the slight excess of female patients with colonic growths.

In the Registrar General's Statistical Review for England and Wales in 1982 there were 16,009 deaths from cancers of the large bowel, of which 9490 were situated in the colon and 5519 in the rectum, rectosigmoid, and anus.

Aetiology

The aetiologic factors in the development of carcinoma of the rectum are identical with those of carcinomas elsewhere in the large bowel.

Pathology

Carcinoma of the rectum is equally common in the upper, middle, and lower thirds of the rectum but is relatively less common 1 to 2 cm above the dentate line. The lesion may be a malignant polyp, that is, a pedunculated adenoma in which carcinomatous change has occurred to a lesser or greater degree, or it may arise in an obvious villous papilloma. However, most carcinomas are either polypoid or ulcerative growths (Fig. 56–1); a few occur as infiltrating plaque-like lesions. As a general rule, the flatter the growth the more likely it is to be highly malignant. Multiple tumours occur in about 5 percent of patients (Fig. 56–2) and some 10 percent produce excessive mucus and show a colloid appearance on the cut surface of the tumour—the so-called colloid carcinoma.

About 85 percent of carcinomas of the rectum are adenocarcinomas. Between 10 and 15 percent are colloid (mucoid) tumours, which include the pure signet-ring cell type, which is unusual. About 20 percent are well differentiated, 60 percent moderately differentiated, and the remaining 20 percent poorly differentiated adenocarcinomas.

Spread

Carcinoma of the rectum spreads locally, via the lymphatics and by the bloodstream. Late dissemination by the transcoelomic route may occur.

Direct Spread. The tumours of low and average grade of malignancy extend slowly, infiltrating the adjacent mucosa and penetrating into the muscle layers. The ulcerative lesions will extend in a circumferential manner rather than

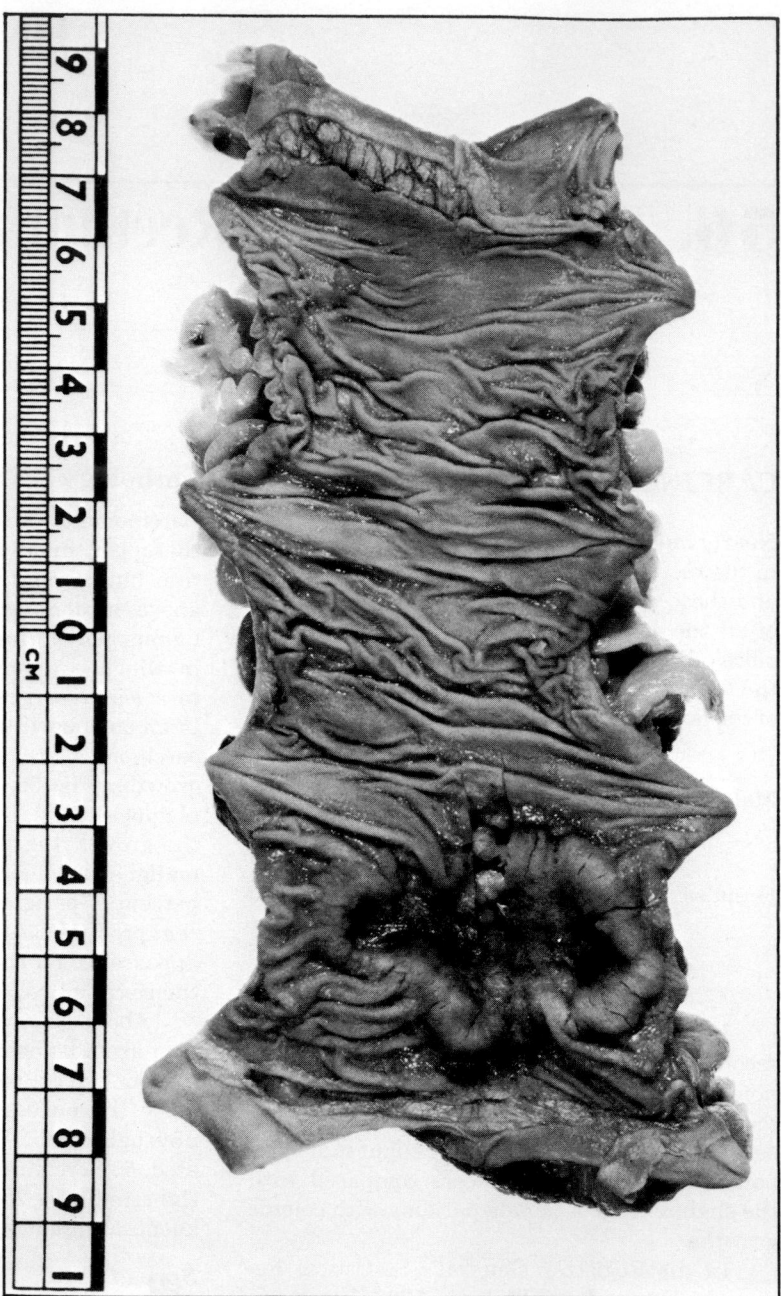

Figure 56–1.

longitudinally until a complete annular growth results, so that when the whole of the ampulla of the rectum has been invaded, the carcinoma may be only 3 to 4 cm in its long axis. In an average case, it is estimated that it will take approximately 6 months for the growth to travel around one quarter of the circumference. Deep penetration through perirectal fat is slow and the tumour is limited by the fascia propria for a considerable time. Indeed, the latter does not seem to be invaded until at least three quarters of the circumference of the bowel has been encompassed, indicating that the disease has existed for about 18 months. Thus a tumour of average grade, situated behind the prostate, very rarely infiltrates through the fascia of De-

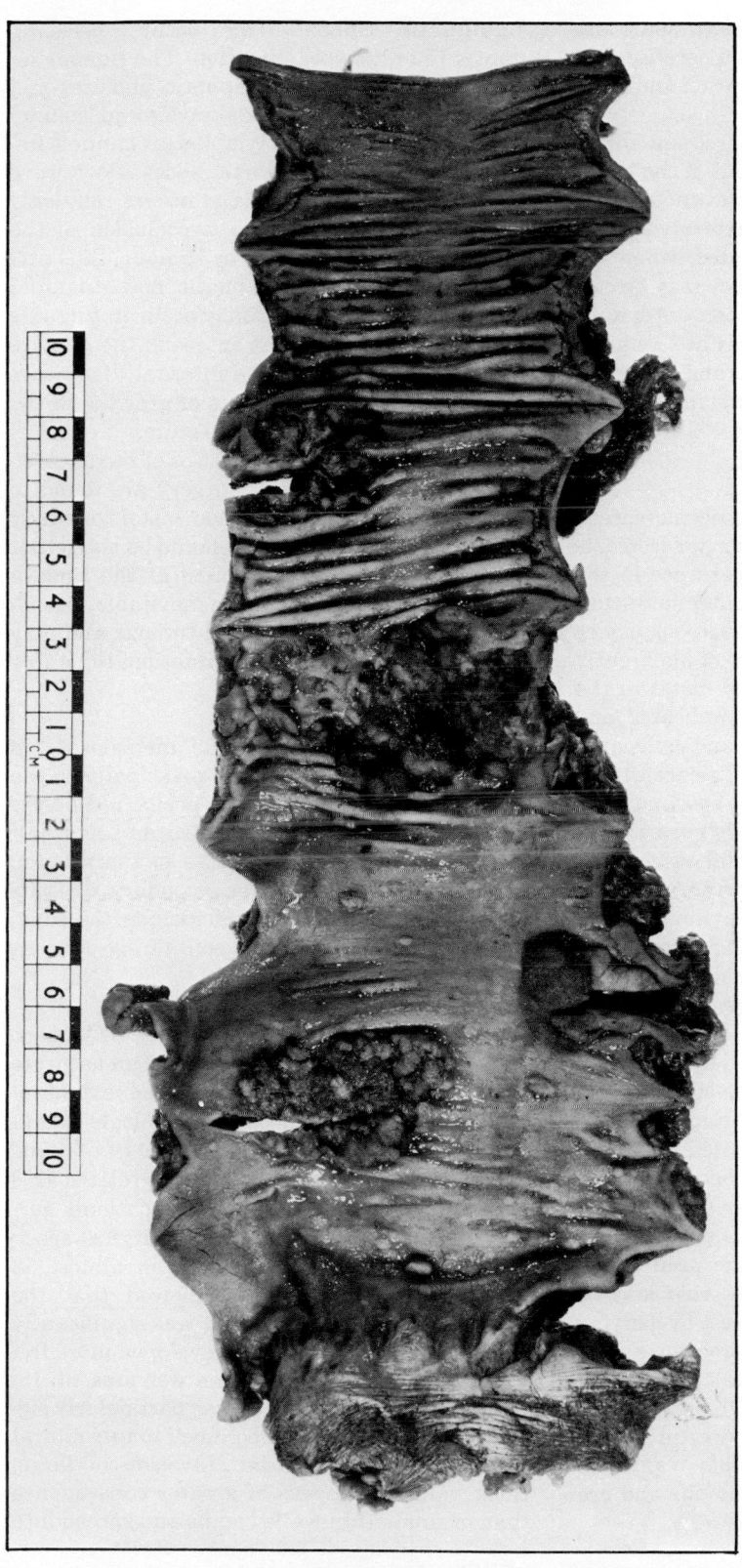

Figure 56–2.

nonvilliers. Poorly differentiated tumours are flat plaques, often with minimal ulceration and with extensive submucous infiltration and rapid growth.

In the upper third of the rectum direct spread will involve the serous coat of the bowel and peritoneal nodules in the rectovesical pouch occur, but they are not usually extensive unless the tumour is poorly differentiated, when the whole of the pelvic peritoneal floor may be covered with almost confluent deposits. Adjacent organs may be invaded—the prostate, seminal vesicles, base of bladder, vagina, and uterus. A loop of sigmoid colon or small bowel may become adherent to a cancer of the upper third of the rectum and a fistula can result.

Distal Spread. The distal microscopic spread of a rectal carcinoma beyond its macroscopic margin is clearly of crucial importance in the development of local recurrence after sphincter-saving resections. The standard textbook advice until recently has been that 5 cm of apparently normal bowel should be resected distal to the tumour if the cancer is to be eradicated and recurrence prevented. Williams and colleagues (1983) in Leeds have carried out a careful and important study of 50 consecutive specimens obtained in the course of potentially curative abdominoperineal resection for rectal carcinomas that were situated 5 to 10 cm from the anal verge and that were examined for the presence of microscopic distal intramural spread. Thirty eight patients (76 percent) were found to have no distal intramural spread. Seven patients (14 percent) had spread for 1 cm or less and only 5 patients (10 percent) had spread of more than 1 cm; these were 1.5, 2, 2.5, 3.5, and 5 cm from the macroscopic distal margin. Each of these patients had a poorly differentiated Dukes' C carcinoma and each was dead or dying from distant metastases within 3 years of the operation. These authors concluded that when the tumour lies 5 to 10 cm from the anal verge, the rigid application of the 5 cm rule may be detrimental to the patient's interest by denying the chance of a sphincter-saving procedure without improving chances of survival. Admittedly a few patients might be left with microscopic deposits of the tumour in the anorectal stump, but such patients would be incurable in any case because of the nature of their tumour and are likely to die of widespread metastases.

Lymphatic Spread. This occurs predominantly in an upward direction. The tumour invades the intramural lymphatic plexuses and passes to the haemorrhoidal nodes and then up the inferior mesenteric lymphatic channels until it reaches the paraaortic nodes. Downward and lateral lymphatic spread occurs relatively late and only when there is occlusion of the normal upward pathways by tumour, thus producing a retrograde lymphatic flow. Inguinal lymph node involvement may occur in tumours of the lower rectum that encroach the dentate line. Lateral spread to the internal iliac nodes may occur in advanced cases of growths in the extraperitoneal part of the rectum.

About 50 percent of all cases of rectal carcinoma undergoing radical surgery are found to have lymphatic metastases on histologic study of the resected specimen. It should be noted that enlarged regional nodes, found at the time of surgery, may result from the inevitable secondary infection of the ulcerated tumour and may be shown, on histologic examination, to be free of tumour deposits.

Venous Spread. Blood-borne metastases via portal tributaries take place principally to the liver, and indeed secondary deposits in the liver are found in between one third and one half of patients dying of carcinoma of the rectum. Other sites of blood-borne secondary deposits are much less common and include the lung, brain, and the red marrow containing portions of the skeletal system.

CLINICAL SIGNIFICANCE OF VENOUS INVASION. Talbot et al (1980) have carried out an accurate appraisal of the the presence and extent of invasion of rectal veins on the histologic examination of surgically excised specimens of carcinoma of the rectum and have correlated this with metastasis to the liver and patients survival rates. Examination of 703 surgical specimens revealed venous invasion in almost 52 percent. Follow-up studies showed that the corrected 5-year survival rate was significantly worse and liver metastases developed more frequently when venous invasion was present. Invasion of extramural veins was particularly significant, whereas spread confined to intramural veins was less important. Invasion of large, thick-walled veins was of greater consequence than of small, thin-walled veins and spread into

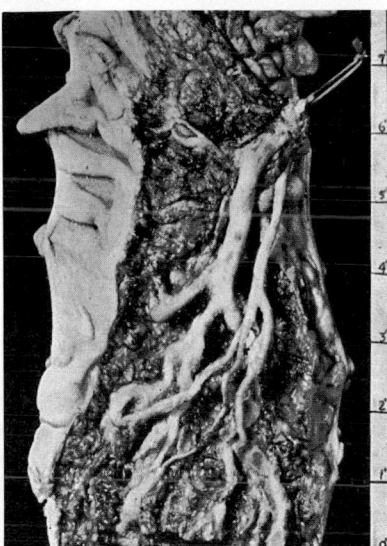

Figure 56–3. Venous spread in rectal cancer. Dissection of haemorrhoidal veins in perirectal fat. Sections showed these vessels to be permeated by carcinoma. (*Source: From Dukes CE, 1957, with permission.*)

thick walled extramural veins had the greatest adverse influence of all (Fig. 56–3). As examples, where venous invasion was not demonstrated, the 5-year survival rate was 73 percent. This fell to 66 percent with intrinsic venous invasion and 33 percent if the extrinsic veins showed involvement. Invasion of extramural thick-walled veins gave a corrected 5-year survival rate of only 19 percent. Hepatic metastases developed in 14.2 percent of patients where venous invasion was not demonstrated, 23.4 percent of those with intramural spread, and 40.4 percent of those with extramural invasion, whereas invasion of thick-walled extramural veins was followed by hepatic metastases in 57 percent of the patients. Observation of venous spread provides a precise assessment of the likely behaviour of rectal carcinoma and supplements, although does not replace, other indices, such as the Dukes' stage (see the following) or the number of lymph node metastases in routine use.

Dukes' Classification

Dr. Cuthbert Dukes (1940), of St. Mark's Hospital London, classified large bowel cancers according to the spread of the tumour in the surgically resected specimen:

- *A cases* are those in which the carcinoma is limited to the wall of the rectum, there being no extension into the extrarectal tissues and no metastases in the lymph nodes.
- *B cases* are those in which the carcinoma has spread by direct continuity to the extrarectal tissues but has not yet invaded the regional lymph nodes.
- *C cases* are those in which metastases are present in the regional nodes.

This method of classification is based on the proved depth of malignant spread; direct spread in or through the rectal wall can usually be judged by naked eye inspection of the freshly cut surface and is confirmed microscopically. The determination of nodal metastases requires microscopic proof, and Dukes found that, on the evidence of their gross characteristics alone, a guess that malignant invasion of lymph nodes had taken place, when subjected to microscopic proof, was incorrect in 60 percent of the total (Fig. 56–4).

The 5-year survival rate following surgery correlates closely with the Dukes' staging of the tumour and typical figures, shown in the form of corrected survival rates, is demonstrated in Table 56–1.

The C cases can be further subdivided into C1 and C2. The C1 group comprises those pa-

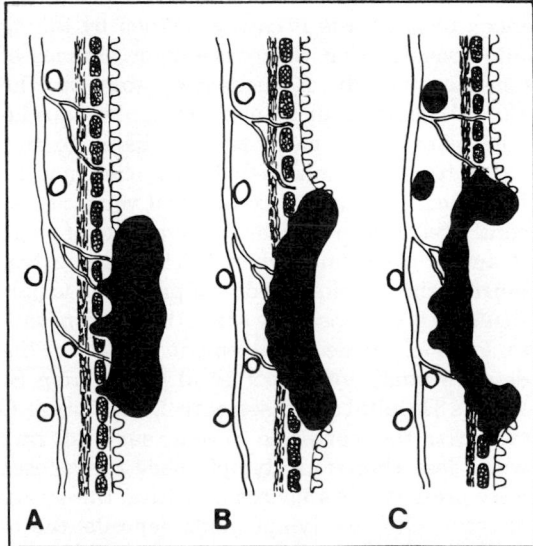

Figure 56–4. Dukes' classification of rectal and colonic tumours.

TABLE 56–1. PROGNOSIS AND DUKES' CLASSIFICATION

Authors	Total No. of Cases		Corrected 5-Year Survival (%)		
			A	B	C
Dukes (1957) (London)	2256 { Male		99.9	76.0	31.3
	Female		93.8	82.0	32.7
Hojo et al (1982) (Tokyo)	423		96.8	78.8	33.3
Pihl et al (1980) (Melbourne)	728		88.0	76.0	41.0
Whittaker & Goligher (1976) (Leeds)	550		91.9	71.3	37.7

tients in which the lymph node involvement is close to the primary, with normal lymph nodes between them and the level of pedicle ligation. The C2 cases are those in which there is involvement of lymph nodes up to the level of pedicle ligation.

Another way in which the C cases can be expressed is to record the number of node metastases. The survival rate falls in an almost arithmetic fashion as the involved nodes increase in number. Dukes summed it up by saying that "Patients with five or more metastases rarely live for 5 years." Hojo and colleagues (1982), in a study of 423 patients following surgery for rectal cancer, found that there was a 70.8 percent 5-year survival in patients with a single node involved, falling to 15 percent when five or more nodes were affected.

Although the Dukes' staging is a consistent index of prognosis it can be refined by taking into consideration the presence or absence of venous invasion. By superimposing on the Dukes' classification an evaluation of venous involvement, those patients most likely to succumb from disseminated disease can now be identified. Invasion of extramural veins significantly reduces the 5-year survival rate of stage B and C cases and, when thick-walled extramural veins are involved, the prognosis is particularly poor, especially when there is concomitant lymph node involvement. Thus in the detailed study by Talbot et al (1980) from St Mark's Hospital for cases with Dukes' stage C tumours, the corrected 5-year survival rate when less than four lymph node metastases were present was 43 percent. Within this group of cases with few lymph node deposits, the 5-year survival rate was considerably higher (59 percent) when venous invasion was demonstrated and the lowest corrected survival rate of 30 percent was related to the presence of

growth in extramural veins. The corrected 5-year survival rate of patients with four or more lymph nodes involved was 17 percent and within this group, when there was extramural venous spread, the survival rate fell to only 8 percent.

Clinical Manifestations

Accurate diagnosis of cancer of the rectum is based on the history and physical examination, which includes, of course, digital examination of the rectum, proctoscopy, and sigmoidoscopy, together with biopsy of the lesion and, if necessary, colonoscopy, and barium enema x-ray examination by the air contrast technique.

Symptoms

The symptoms will vary according to the position of the tumour, its type, and its duration of growth. Lesions of the rectal ampulla are, as a rule, insidious in their progress, whereas tumours of the anal canal quickly declare themselves. If these latter lesions are excluded, the most common early symptoms of rectal cancer include the passage of blood, blood-stained mucus, or blood-stained faecal matter, tenesmus, alteration of bowel function, and lower abdominal cramp-like pains. Local pain is a late and grave manifestation except in connection with malignant lesions of the anal canal itself.

Rectosigmoid Junction. Growths in this situation generally conform to the type encountered in the left colon in that they rapidly involve the circumference of the bowel and produce stenosis. Both the proliferative and the annular types occur in this region and each is attended by a different train of symptoms.

A papillary carcinoma in the rectosigmoid gives rise to excessive mucus secretion and therefore causes diarrhoea, which, although slight at first, tends in time to become more marked. The slimy motions are frequently blood-stained but when a large fragment of growth becomes detached there may be a sharp haemorrhage. After a variable interval, the diarrhoea, which has become excessive, ceases, and an attack of intestinal obstruction supervenes, either from intussusception of the bulky, fleshy mass into the rectum or from impaction of faeces (or barium after radiologic examination) above the strictured area.

In contrast, the annular carcinoma that encircles the bowel is associated in its early stages with alteration of bowel habit, comprising increasing constipation accompanied by colicky abdominal pains, borborygmi, and flatulence. As the constipation becomes more obstinate, the patient may take more and more aperients in order to obtain a bowel action. Eventually the constipation becomes almost complete, with abdominal distension and colicky abdominal pain. In some cases, an attack of acute intestinal obstruction is the first indication of the presence of a stenosing cancer of the rectosigmoid.

Most surgical series show that more than 95 percent of cancers of this segment of the bowel are operable because they come under observation at a comparatively early date on account of the urgency of the symptoms produced.

Ampulla of the Rectum. The ampulla of the rectum is capacious and its mucous membrane is insensitive unless it is stretched. Malignant lesions situated there do not therefore give rise to any symptoms during their early stages of growth until they ulcerate and bleed. The earliest objective sign of the existence of the tumour is streaking of the stools with blood.

As the exuberant mass bulges into the lumen of the rectum, there may be sensation of fullness in the rectum or an impression of incomplete emptying after defaecation. Secretion of mucus from a proliferative growth produces mucous diarrhoea. When the growth penetrates the rectal wall, local suppuration in the pelvirectal fatty tissues may follow and pain, sometimes severe and becoming even more marked during the act of defaecation, is experienced.

At a late stage of the disease, large quantities of pus, mucus, blood, and watery faeces are passed frequently by day and night; tenesmus follows each bowel movement; there is progressive loss of weight and marked pallor. Later still, owing partly to the extent of the circumferential involvement of the ampulla by tumour and partly to the wide fixation of the diseased segment of rectum to neighbouring viscera or to pelvirectal suppuration, there is increasing difficulty in obtaining a bowel action. Eventually the narrowed lumen of the rectum is obstructed by impaction of faecal matter and this is accompanied by abdominal distension with alternating attacks of constipation and diarrhoea heralding the onset of complete obstruction.

During the terminal stages of the disease, pain is of two types. First, abdominal colicky pain due to the large bowel obstruction and second, pelvic pain produced by invasion of the neighbouring structures, including the sacral plexus. There may be a constant gnawing pain over the sacrum radiating down the thigh along the course of the sciatic nerve.

Spread of the tumour to the prostate, bladder, vagina, uterus, and adnexae add symptoms referable to disease of these organs. Pelvirectal suppuration may eventually lead to the formation of ischiorectal abscess and fistula. The cancerous mass may protrude through the anal verge and attack the perianal skin. This may be accompanied by spread to the inguinal lymph nodes. Finally, there is hepatomegaly, jaundice, and ascites, blatantly confirming the presence of generalised carcinomatosis.

Physical Examination

The surgeon performs a general assessment of the patient, checking for clinical signs of loss of weight, anaemia, or jaundice.

Careful abdominal palpation is performed to determine if the liver is enlarged, whether faecal impaction has occurred in the sigmoid colon above the growth and whether ascites is present. The latter is found in advanced tumours with extensive peritoneal involvement. The inguinal regions are carefully palpated for evidence of metastatic spread to the lymph nodes and the supraclavicular area is palpated for late spread along the thoracic duct to Virchow's node.

Rectal examination is, of course, of supreme importance since all malignant growths of the rectum proper should be capable of being felt by the examining finger. Tumours at the rectosigmoid junction may be beyond the reach of the finger, but some of them can be felt through the intervening rectal wall or may be "tipped" if the patient strains. The left lateral position should be adopted for this examination.

A cancer of the ampulla can readily be felt as a protruberant mass or as an ulcer with an indurated edge. If the carcinoma has developed in a preceding adenoma or papilloma, although a part of the mass may be soft, the portion in which malignant change has developed will feel hard and may be ulcerated. The polypoid malignant growths are nodular, protruberant, sessile masses, which are friable and which bleed freely when palpated with the examining finger. At a later stage, they present an ulcerated surface with overhanging indurated edges. The flat plateau-like growth is at first movable in all directions and involves only the mucosa, but later on it presents all the typical characteristics of the malignant rectal ulcer—a crater with raised and indurated everted margins.

As previously stated, some rectosigmoid growths can be felt digitally. In other instances, it may be possible to feel a mass in the lower sigmoid through the rectal wall or, in the case of an intussuscepting growth, to sweep a finger around in the sulcus between the tumour mass and the rectal wall. If the patient strains, a tumour just out of reach of the finger may now become palpable. Difficulties are presented by the very obese or muscular patient, particularly if not relaxed during the examination.

It should be remembered that an ampullary adenocarcinoma may extend downward and invade the anal canal.

As the disease progresses, the rectal tumour becomes more deeply ulcerated and more fixed until a stage is reached when it is adherent to neighbouring structures (bladder, prostate, vagina, or sacrum). As the tumour advances and becomes more deeply ulcerated, there is frequently considerable surrounding inflammation, which may lead the surgeon to believe that the tumour is more advanced than it actually is.

In the female, a vaginal examination must always be performed to ascertain the extent of the tumour. Abdominal examination with bimanual pelvic examination will frequently give helpful information in advanced disease.

Endoscopy

It is, of course, important to obtain visual and histologic confirmation of the presence of a growth in the rectum.

The following points should be noted on sigmoidoscopy:

1. The exact distance of the lower edge of the tumour from the anal verge.
2. The position, extent and character of the growth.
3. The presence of other tumours. The sigmoidoscope is passed beyond the tumour if this can be done easily. A second carcinoma may be present or, more frequently, adenomatous polyps may be visualised.
4. Exclusion of other associated conditions. It is important to make certain that the carcinoma is not associated with familial polyposis or ulcerative colitis, for both of which total colectomy and ileostomy is the appropriate curative treatment.

Two or three generous biopsy specimens should be obtained through the sigmoidoscope, ensuring, as far as possible, that tumour tissue rather than heaped up normal adjacent mucosa is obtained. It goes without saying that the surgeon should not proceed to radical surgery, particularly abdominoperineal excision of the rectum, until histologic confirmation both of the nature of its tumour and of its grade of malignancy has been obtained. Occasionally the pathologist will report that only normal tissue has been obtained. Under these circumstances, repeat endoscopy should be carried out and multiple further biopsies taken.

Special Investigations

Barium Enema. X-ray examination is advised by some authorities but this author certainly does not use this as a routine. If there is an obvious tumour that can be visualised endoscopically and confirmed by histologic examination of a biopsy, a barium enema is avoided. It is uncomfortable to the patient and makes it still more difficult to obtain adequate preoperative emptying of the bowel. There is, of course, the possibility that there are other synchronous tumours elsewhere in the colon and certainly careful examination must be made of the whole of the large bowel at laparotomy. A barium enema is requested where there is any suspicion of polyposis and in any patient with preexisting ulcerative colitis, in both of whom there is a much greater chance of multiple lesions being present. A barium enema also is ordered in the occasional case where it is difficult to identify a suspected lesion at the rectosigmoid through the sigmoidoscope, especially when the field is constantly being flooded with liquid faeces and altered blood.

Search for Liver Secondaries. Liver function tests may be entirely normal even in the presence of hepatic metastases. However, a raised serum alkaline phosphatase is certainly a worrisome finding and patients with clinically undetectable hepatic deposits will be found to have this value raised in about one third of cases. Ultrasound of the liver is a useful, inexpensive, and noninvasive screening of the liver. There may, however, be both false-positive and false-negative findings. Even the preoperative suspicion of hepatic metastases does not, of course, prevent the surgeon from carrying out a laparotomy since, even in the presence of small hepatic deposits, palliative resection of the primary growth may be well worthwhile.

An intravenous pyelogram is carried out in patients with a clinically advanced rectal carcinoma. This will provide useful information as to whether the ureters (particularly the left ureter) have become implicated in the tumour mass.

A chest x-ray, electrocardiogram, and full blood count are performed routinely in the general medical assessment of the patient preoperatively.

Before operation, the surgeon should be in possession, therefore, of the following facts:

1. The exact site of the carcinoma
2. Its fixity or otherwise to surrounding tissues and viscera
3. The grade of malignancy as determined on the preoperative biopsy
4. The presence or absence of metastases, as far as can be ascertained clinically or by laboratory studies
5. The general condition of the patient and an assessment of the patient's chances of withstanding a major operation

Differential Diagnosis

The differential diagnosis of carcinoma of the rectum must be made from:

1. Diverticular disease of the distal sigmoid loop
2. Chronic ulcerative colitis or proctitis
3. Crohn's disease involving the rectum
4. Simple ulcer of the rectum

5. Lymphogranuloma, amoebic granuloma, and bilharzial granuloma
6. Gas cysts of the colon and rectum
7. Endometriosis involving the rectum
8. Benign epithelial or connective tissue tumours
9. Malignant connective tissue tumours (lymphoma, leiomyosarcoma)
10. Malignant tumours arising outside the rectum and invading it from without, e.g., carcinoma of the sigmoid colon, cervix, or prostate
11. Implants in the pelvic shelf from carcinoma of the stomach, ovary, etc.

Prognosis

Most reports on prognosis of carcinoma of the rectum (and indeed of most of the major cancers) stem from surgical series of major specialist centres. It should be admitted, however, that a better idea will be given from studying reports of regional cancer centres, which include records of all the cases of cancer in that particular region. These figures will include those cases admitted to hospitals of all sizes and calibres, often with advanced and hopeless disease, many of whom are not transferred to surgical units, and indeed will include patients who never reach hospital at all (Goligher, 1981).

An excellent study of this type from the Birmingham Regional Cancer Registry in 1950–1961, with a 98 percent registration rate of a total population of nearly five million people, is reported by Slaney (1971), and the results make depressing reading. Of a total of 5800 patients with rectal cancer, the overall crude 5-year survival rate was 21.9 percent (29.2 percent age corrected). This increased to 39.8 percent (48.6 percent age corrected) in the 3005 patients treated by radical surgical resection and plunged dramatically to 3.5 and 1.9 percent respectively, in those patients receiving palliative or purely exploratory surgery. No less than 1282 patients received no treatment whatsoever, with a not unexpected crude 5-year survival rate of 1.8 percent. The majority of patients not undergoing surgery were in a terminal state at first referral and died within a few weeks of first being seen. Slaney concludes "these facts clearly demonstrate the fallacies of attempting to evaluate the validity or effectiveness of the current management of carcinoma of the large bowel by analyses of surgical series alone, since by so doing we are only considering one facet, albeit a most important one, of the problem."

In the individual case, prognosis depends upon the histologic grade of the tumour, its local spread, and the involvement of the lymph nodes and extramural veins. Distant metastases are virtually a death sentence. Other factors include the age, general condition, and sex of the patient, the position of the tumour, and operative mortality.

Although for each stage of the tumour, the histologic grade of malignancy affects prognosis, it should be noted that there is also a close correlation between the histologic grade of malignancy and the extent of spread. For example, some 20 percent of Dukes' A cases are well-differentiated tumours but this drops to the region of 3 to 4 percent in Dukes' C cases.

The correlation between the Dukes' grading and 5-year prognosis (Table 56–1) and how this can be refined still further by taking into consideration the extent of extramural venous spread has already been discussed.

Wide dissemination of the tumour renders the prognosis almost hopeless. As an example, Pihl et al (1980) found that of 211 patients undergoing palliative surgery for rectal cancer in which there was either residual local tumour or distant metastases left behind after resection, no patients survived beyond 4.5 years and the median survival was only 11 months. Slaney's depressing figures for patients beyond even palliative surgery were mentioned earlier.

The relationship of age to prognosis is complex. Young patients withstand radical excision of the rectum better than the elderly but the chances of recurrence are greater in the former because of the higher incidence of poorly differentiated tumours.

Naturally the patient's general condition is important and indeed cases will be encountered from time to time whose cardiovascular and pulmonary function are so poor that radical surgery is precluded.

The 5-year survival rate is better in women than in men and indeed in some series this amounts to as much as a 5 percent difference. Probably this is due to the fact that the wider female pelvis permits a readier dissection and mobilisation of the rectum.

Contrary to what might have been expected, the longer the history of symptoms before the patient presents to the surgeon the better on average the prospects of survival (Slaney,

1971). Possibly this denotes that the longer history is likely to represent the patient with the slower growing, less rapidly disseminating tumour.

The site of the tumour within the rectum is of prognostic importance, survival being greater the higher the lesion. Stearns and Binkley (1953), in a study of 369 patients surviving abdominoperineal excision, noted the crude 5-year survival rate according to the level of the lower margin of the cancer on preoperative sigmoidoscopy as follows: 0 to 6 cm, 52.8 percent; 6 to 11 cm, 61.8 percent; and above 11 cm, 72.5 percent.

Operative mortality of radical excisional surgery will vary from centre to centre depending on such factors as patient selection and the skills of the surgical and anaesthetic teams. The results from centres of excellence are those against which every surgeon must judge personal statistics. Lockhart-Mummery et al (1976) report from St. Mark's Hospital that the operative mortality for rectal cancer resections has fallen overall from 7 percent in the years 1948–52 to 2.1 percent in 1968–72. During those last 5 years of the study there was only 1 death in 229 abdominoperineal excisions of the rectum (0.5 percent) and 7 deaths in 172 anterior resections (4.1 percent). However, of these postoperative deaths only one was due to peritonitis, which might have been a technical fault, the other deaths being due to cardiac or pulmonary complications, which might equally well have occurred following abdominoperineal excision.

RARE MALIGNANT TUMOURS OF THE RECTUM

Carcinoid. Rectal carcinoid tumours are uncommon. Most present as small hard submucous nodules that are seldom larger than 1 cm in diameter. These usually present as incidental findings on rectal or sigmoidoscopic examination and may be treated successfully by local excision. A second group comprises large tumours (above 1 cm in diameter) which are ulcerated and may metastasise. The carcinoid syndrome has been reported in association with rectal carcinoid but is extremely rare.

Malignant Lymphomas. Malignant lymphoid tumours may occur in association with generalised malignant lymphoma or may be found as a primary tumour. The latter may present either as an annular thickening or as a bulky protruberant growth that ulcerates and may be indistinguishable clinically from a carcinoma. The diagnosis can only be made as a result of histologic examination. Lymph nodes are involved in about half the cases.

Leiomyosarcoma. This tumour is much less common in the large bowel than in the small intestine. The growth spreads principally by direct extension into the wall of the bowel and into the perirectal tissues. Lymph node metastases are rare but venous spread results in deposits in the liver.

Secondary Tumours. The most common secondary tumour found in the rectum is in fact a carcinoma of the colon, usually the sigmoid, that prolapses down into the rectovesical pouch. Prostatic carcinoma may rarely infiltrate through the fascia of Denonvilliers and present in the rectum.

Secondaries from carcinomas of the ovary, stomach, and breast can present as extrinsic rectal tumours owing to transcoelomic spread into the pouch of Douglas.

TUMOURS OF THE ANAL CANAL

Malignant tumours of the anal canal are unusual. They need to be differentiated from those of the rectum because of differences in their aetiology, pathology, clinical features, management, and prognosis. The 204 cases reviewed by Beahrs and Wilson (1976) over a 20-year period at the Mayo Clinic accounted for only 2 percent of all their cancers of the large bowel and the 29 patients studied by Lewi and McArdle (1982) at the Royal Infirmary Glasgow made up 3.2 percent of all the malignant tumours of the large bowel at the Glasgow Royal Infirmary.

The malignant tumours can be classified pathologically as follows:

1. Squamous carcinoma, amounting to some 90 percent of all cases
2. Malignant tumours of connective tissue origin—leiomyosarcoma, rhabdomyosarcoma
3. Lymphoid—lymphomas
4. Tumours of cutaneous origin—Bowen's disease, Paget's disease, rodent ulcer (basal cell carcinoma)
5. Malignant melanoma

Careful differentiation must be made from adenocarcinoma of the rectum invading downwards to implicate the anal canal.

Squamous carcinomas in this region need to be subdivided into those of the anal canal proper (Fig. 56–5), astride or above the dentate line, and tumours of the anal margin below the dentate line (Lewi and McArdle, 1982). Anal canal carcinoma is nearly three times more common than cancer of the anal margin, although the age incidence is the same, with most cases presenting between 55 and 70 years of age. Anal canal cancer is more common in women than men although anal margin carcinoma is more common in men. Most carcinomas of the anal canal are of the ordinary squamous type whereas typical prickle cell carcinomas, usually producing much keratin, are rare. The opposite is seen in anal margin tumours, which are mostly prickle cell tumours typical of skin cancer (Morson and Pang, 1968).

Basaloid carcinomas may be found in the anal canal and mostly arise from the junctional zone above the dentate line. They are so called because their histology resembles basal cell carcinoma. They are sometimes termed cloacogenic carcinomas. It should be noted that true basal cell carcinoma (rodent ulcer) of the hair-bearing skin of the anal margin may occur but is very uncommon.

We have reported (Leach and Ellis, 1981) two young male homosexuals who developed carcinomas at this transitional zone. Both had had gonorrhoea but in neither could we demonstrate herpes simplex antibodies. Cooper and colleagues (1979) reported four similar cases.

Anal carcinomas spread locally to involve perianal skin and subcutaneous tissues. In the female the posterior vaginal wall is frequently involved, although in the male the fascia of Denonvilliers forms at least a temporary barrier to the invasion of the urethra, prostate, and seminal vesicles.

Lymphatic spread from carcinomas of the anal canal pass both to the intraabdominal and inguinal nodes, although tumours of the anal verge drain only to the latter.

Blood-borne spread to the liver takes place in advanced cases (about 10 percent of patients) whereas pulmonary metastases are uncommon.

Connective tissue sarcomas are rarely seen, but leiomyosarcoma arising from the internal sphincter and perianal rhabdomyosarcomas have been reported.

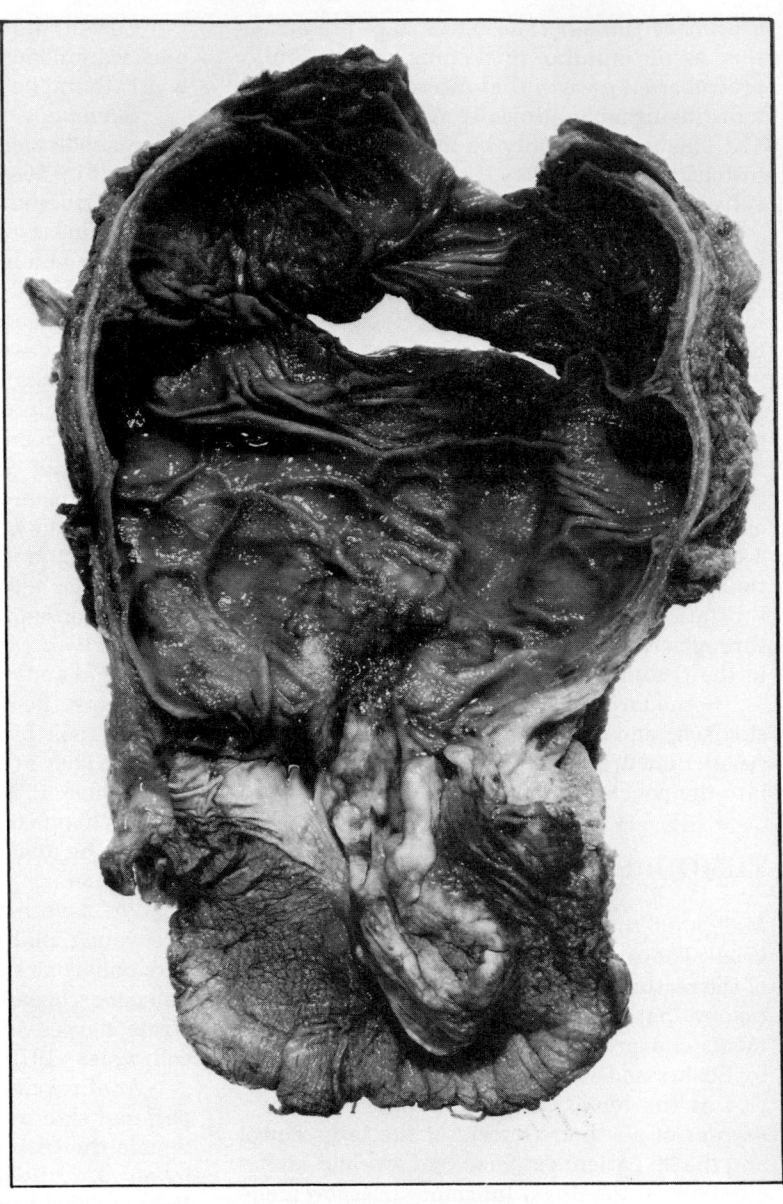

Figure 56–5.

Malignant lymphoma involving the anus is rare, although benign lymphoid polyps may be found in the upper part of the anal canal just above the dentate line.

Bowen's disease, a slow growing intraepidermal squamous carcinoma, is rare in the perianal skin but appears as a red encrusted flat lesion with irregular edges.

Paget's disease, histologically identical to Paget's disease of the breast, is rarely found in elderly subjects of both sexes.

Basal cell carcinoma (rodent ulcer) rarely occurs in the perianal skin. Its naked eye appearance is identical with the common rodent ulcers of the face. Spread to the inguinal lymph nodes does not occur even though these may be enlarged from infection of the ulcerated area.

Malignant melanoma accounts for some 1 percent of all cases of the anal canal. The tumour presents as a large ulcerating pigmented mass, often protruding from the anal verge. Rapid extension locally, to the regional nodes and viscera, particularly liver, is usually very rapid (Fig. 56–6). In the two patients this author

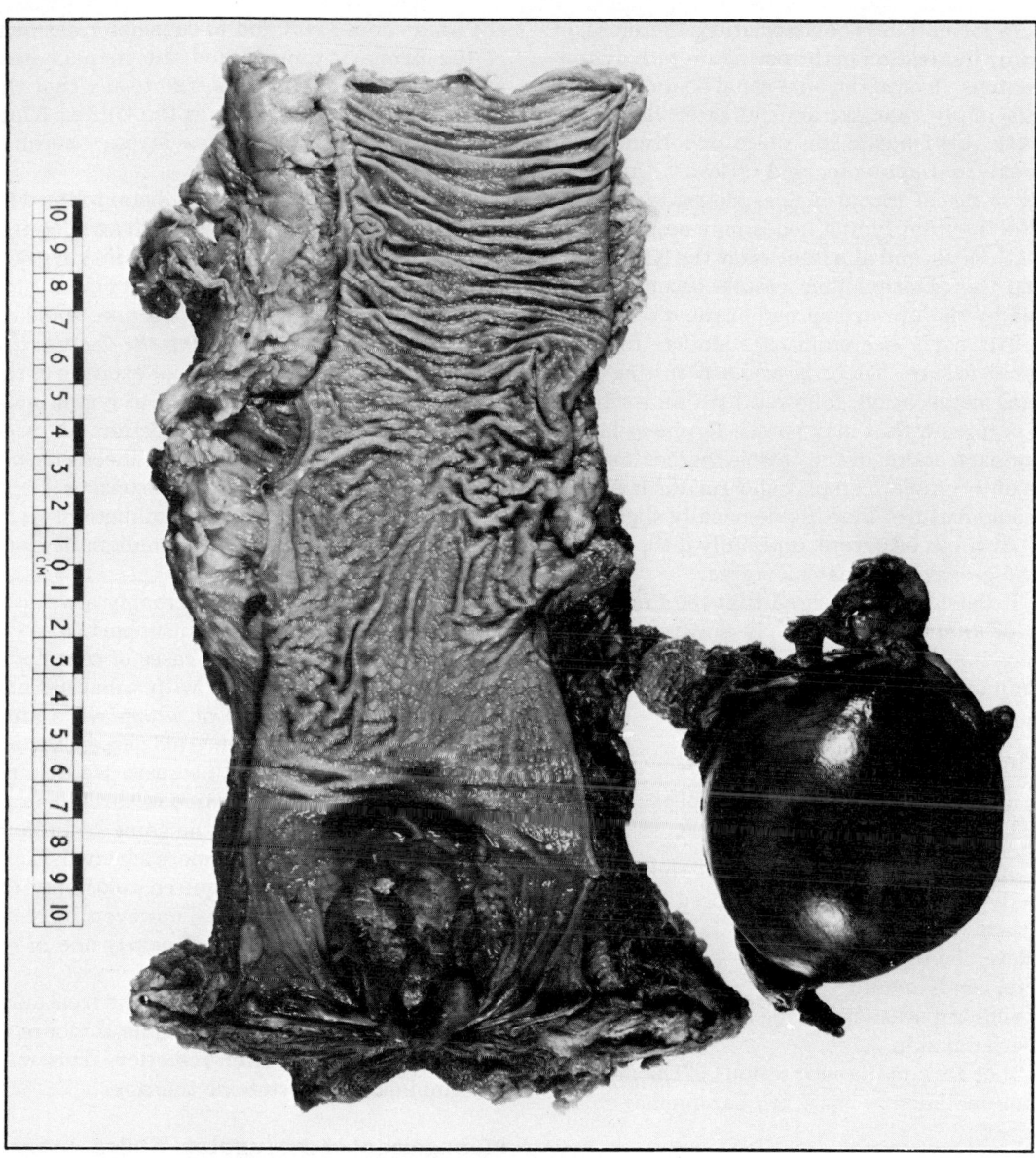

Figure 56–6.

has treated personally this was certainly the case, one dying of haemorrhage from metastases to the stomach. Freedman (1984) records two cases of prolonged survival, where the patients were alive and well and clinically free of recurrent disease 10 years after abdominoperineal excision. His review of previous cases revealed only five further examples who had survived for 10 years.

Clinical Manifestations

Cancers of the anal canal present as a flat infiltrating growth with a raised uneven ulcerating surface and hardened rolled-out edge. The tumour generally grows downward and invades the skin of the perineum rather than extending upward into the rectum. Perforation may occur into the ischiorectal fossa with suppuration and fistula formation. The association, therefore, of brawny induration in the perineum with a carcinomatous ulcer of the anal canal does not necessarily imply that extramural extension of the growth itself has taken place. Involvement of the external sphincter and of levator ani may lead to faecal incontinence. Metastatic spread to the inguinal lymph nodes may occur on one or both sides, and at a later stage the lymphatics along the external iliac vessels become implicated by the upward spread of the disease.

The early symptoms are similar to those of anal fissure. There is a sharp cutting pain during defaecation, followed by a dull ache in the perineum that may persist for many hours. After each action of the bowels there is a sensation of incomplete emptying. Pruritus is a troublesome feature. Bleeding is usually slight, but may at times be severe, especially if the surface of the growth becomes ulcerated.

It must be emphasised that the first symptom of anal cancer is nearly always pain and as this is often severe it generally leads to early examination and consequent early diagnosis.

Differential Diagnosis

The differential diagnosis of an anal canal carcinoma must be made from:

1. Common benign conditions of the anal canal—fissure in ano, thrombosed piles, anal warts
2. Rarer benign anal lesions—syphilitic chancre, condylomata
3. Crohn's disease involving the anal canal and perianal skin
4. Other rare malignant lesions of the anal canal (melanoma, basal cell carcinoma)

Management of Carcinoma of the Anus and Anal Canal

Anal carcinomas are rare and the only large series published come from specialist referral centres such as the Mayo Clinic, where Beahrs and Wilson (1976) were able to review their results in 204 patients. It is not surprising that there are diverging opinions about the treatment of these lesions, particularly in the debate comparing surgery with radiotherapy, which is well reviewed by Goligher (1984). Whatever the treatment modality, it is important to differentiate between tumours of the anal verge and of

the anal canal itself and to consider treatment of the primary tumour and the management of the inguinal nodes. It is true to say that the opinion among authorities in the United Kingdom and the United States favours surgical treatment.

Tumours of the anal verge distal to the dentate line can be locally excised with an adequate (2.5 cm or more) clear margin, even if skin grafting is necessary (Madden et al, 1981).

Tumours of the terminal rectum, anal canal, or anal verge transgressing the dentate line are treated by abdominoperineal excision of the rectum because of the high risk of lymph node involvement along the mesorectum. A wide sweep of perianal skin and subcutaneous tissues is advisable. Abdominoperineal excision is also used in those rare cases of malignant lymphoma, soft tissue tumour, and malignant melanoma of the anal canal.

Radiotherapy has been strongly advocated in the past and receives warm support from Papillon (1982). He reports 19 cases of carcinoma of the anal region treated with cobalt-60 and iridium implantation, 12 of whom were alive at 4 years with no recurrence (63 percent); there was one example of local necrosis. He also records 66 examples of squamous carcinoma of the anal canal treated by the same technique, with a 66 percent 5-year or more survival. Eight of these, however, had required colostomy for radionecrosis. Other centres, however, have reported a radionecrosis rate of nearly one in every four cases.

Radiotherapy may be used in the treatment of locally advanced and inoperable tumours or perineal recurrence after resection. This may be combined with cytotoxic therapy.

Management of the Inguinal Nodes. Involvement of the inguinal lymph nodes occurs in some 40 percent of patients with squamous carcinoma of the anal region, the incidence being rather higher with lesions of the anal margin than of the anal canal. Obviously this is of serious prognostic significance.

If the nodes are not clinically involved, the patient should be kept under close supervision following treatment of the primary lesion and a block dissection advised if the nodes become palpable.

If the nodes are obviously involved (enlarged and hard rather than merely firm) but not fixed so as to be inoperable, a block dissection should be performed on one or both sides, as required, as soon as the patient has recovered from operation on the primary tumour itself. In some instances, soft enlarged nodes will subside once the primary tumour has been removed and in these cases the enlargement can be attributed to septic absorption from the infected and ulcerated anal lesion. Fixed and inoperable inguinal nodes may be controlled, at least temporarily, by palliative radiotherapy.

Prognosis

Carcinoma of the anal margin has a better prognosis than anal canal carcinoma and this is one important reason, apart from other clinical and pathologic differences, for carefully differentiating between these two types of anal tumours. In their important study of carcinoma of the anus at the Mayo Clinic, Beahrs and Wilson (1976) gave the following 5-year survival figures:

Squamous cell carcinoma	57.8 percent in 82 cases
Basaloid squamous carcinoma of anal canal	62.9 percent in 64 cases
Perianal squamous carcinoma	74.2 percent in 31 cases

The squamous cell and basaloid squamous carcinomas of the anal canal had similar overall survival rates, but when lymphatic metastases had occurred, patients with basaloid squamous carcinomas had a rather more favourable prognosis.

BIBLIOGRAPHY

Beahrs OH, Wilson SM: Carcinoma of the anus. Ann Surg 184:422, 1976

Cooper HS, Patchefsky AS, et al: Cloacogenic carcinoma of the anorectum in homosexual men. An observation on 4 cases. Dis Col Rect 22:557, 1979

Dukes CE: Discussion on major surgery in carcinoma of the rectum. Proc R Soc Med 50:1031, 1957

Dukes CE: Cancer of the rectum: An analysis of 1000 cases. J Pathol Bact 50:527, 1940

Freedman LS: Malignant melanoma of the anorectal region, two cases of prolonged survival. Br J Surg 71:164, 1984

Goligher J: Surgery of the Anus, Rectum and Colon, 5 edt. London: Bailliere Tindall, 1984

Goligher J: Results of operations for large bowel cancer, in De Cosse JJ (ed): Large Bowel Cancer. Edinburgh: Churchill Livingstone, 1981

Hojo K, Koyama Y, et al: Lymphatic spread and its prognostic value in patients with rectal cancer. Am J Surg 144:350, 1982

Leach RD, Ellis H: Carcinoma of the rectum in male homosexuals. J R Soc Med 74:490, 1981

Lewi HJE, McArdle CS: Anal carcinoma. J R Coll Surg Edinb 27:282, 1982

Lockhart-Mummery HE, Ritchie JK, et al: The results of surgical treatment for carcinoma of the rectum at St Mark's Hospital from 1948 to 1972. Br J Surg 63:673, 1976

Madden MV, Elliot MS, et al: The management of anal carcinoma. Br J Surg 68:287, 1981

Morson BC, Pang LSC: Pathology of anal cancer. Proc R Soc Med 61:623, 1968

Office of Population Censuses and Surveys. Cancer Statistics Registrations 1980. HMSO, London, 1983

Papillon J: Rectal and Anal Cancers. Conservative Treatment by Irradiation—An Alternative to Radical Surgery. Berlin: Springer-Verlag, 1982

Pihl E, Hughes ESR, et al: Carcinoma of the rectum and rectosigmoid: Cancer specific long term survival. A series of 1061 cases treated by one surgeon. Cancer 45:2902, 1980

Slaney G: Results of treatment of carcinoma of the colon and rectum. Mod Trends Surg 3:69, 1971

Stearns MW, Binkley GE: The influence of location on prognosis in operable rectal cancer. Surg Gynecol Obstet 96:368, 1953

Talbot IC, Ritchie S, et al: The clinical significance of invasion of veins by rectal cancer. Br J Surg 67:439, 1980

Whittaker M, Goligher JC: The prognosis after surgical treatment for carcinoma of the rectum. Br J Surg 63:384, 1976

Williams NSW, Dixon MF, et al: Reappraisal of the 5 centimetre rule of distal excision for carcinoma of the rectum: A study of distal intramural spread and patients survival. Br J Surg 70:150, 1983

57. Anterior Resection and Other Procedures

Harold Ellis

GENERAL CONSIDERATIONS REGARDING OSTENSIBLY CURABLE CARCINOMA

The main objective of a radical operation for carcinoma of the rectum or rectosigmoid is to cure the patient if possible and, if not, to provide good palliation. An important subsidiary aim is to preserve sphincter function whenever this is possible without jeopardising chances of a cure.

There has been a radical change in thought over the last decade. Previously the majority of surgeons thought that abdominoperineal excision should be carried out for any carcinoma that could be palpated digitally. In the United Kingdom as a whole 80 percent of patients were treated by abdominoperineal excision of the rectum and only 20 percent by a restorative procedure. Clearly many patients were having an unnecessary colostomy. With the advent of techniques to enable technically lower anastomoses to be carried out, more patients are having sphincter-saving operations. This is to the advantage of most patients if the swing toward restorative resection is not carried too far, so that preservation of the sphincters becomes the main aim of surgery and the possibility of curing the patient becomes subsidiary. This can occur if the surgeon holds that colostomy is such an unpleasant infliction that it is justifiable to accept some lessening of the chances of complete

eradication of the tumour in order to avoid it. Many patients regularly express dismay and apprehension at the prospect of a colostomy, but the great majority are able to reconcile themselves to it and lead useful active lives with a colostomy.

It is known from the pathologic studies of Westhues (1930, 1934) and Dukes (1940) and even more convincingly from the numerous follow-up studies of the results of clinical practice (Nicholls et al, 1979; Williams et al, 1983) that sphincter preservation can be compatible in suitable cases with a high cure rate. Indeed, if the survival rates of abdominoperineal excision of the rectum and anterior resection are compared, all series show a significantly better survival for anterior resection (Whittaker and Goligher, 1976). This is because more favourable tumours are treated by anterior resection, there being more A cases and less C cases, and more low-grade tumours and less high grade tumours in the group of patients submitted to anterior resection. When a matched group of Dukes' B cases of the middle third of the rectum treated by either anterior resection or synchronous combined excision of the rectum were compared at St. Mark's Hospital there was no statistical difference in the 5-year survival rates. However, this statement begs the question as to which patients are suitable for sphincter-saving resection. The answer to this question must be in those patients in whom the theoretic pathologic requirements of a thoroughly radical sphincter-saving resection can be satisfied by the surgical methods at our disposal with an acceptably low operative morbidity and mortality, and with good sphincter function.

The chapter on choice of operative procedure for rectal cancer in the previous edition was written by Professor John Goligher. This author has merely updated some features of his sage and prudent advice.

Pathologic Requirements of a Radical Sphincter-Saving Resection

It has been well documented that the main lymphatic spread from carcinoma is upward along the inferior mesenteric nodes. Tumours in the lower part of the middle third and the lower third of the rectum will also spread naturally into the lateral ligaments and internal iliac nodes. The ideal scope of a radical sphincter saving resection is depicted in Figure 57–1. No one would dispute that the abdominoperineal excision and anterior resection have an identical excision of tissue in the upward and lateral direction. It was originally pointed out by Dukes that the distal margin of clearance should be 5 cm. This statement was made after studying a large number of specimens and finding that the downward lymphatic and submucosal spread was never greater than 4.5 cm. However, this occurred in very few tumours, all of which were of a high grade of malignancy. In carcinomas of an average or low grade of malignancy, downward permeation rarely exceeds 1 cm— hence the importance of determining the grade of malignancy of the lesion by preoperative biopsy, always realising that there is a sampling error in a small biopsy and parts of the tumour may be of an average grade of malignancy and other parts poorly differentiated or anaplastic. If the tumour is of a high grade of malignancy, every effort should be made to obtain a 5-cm margin below the tumour and, if this proves impossible, to settle for complete removal of the rectum by an abdominoperineal excision. If the tumour is of a low or average grade of malig-

nancy, however, the distal margin can be less if this makes anterior resection possible.

What is the minimum acceptable margin in these tumours? An important recent study by Williams and colleagues (1983) approached this question from two aspects—distal intramural spread and patient survival. In the first part of the study, 50 consecutive specimens, obtained in the course of potentially curative abdominoperineal excisions of rectal cancers situated 5 to 10 cm from the anal verge, were examined for the presence of microscopic distal intramural spread. Thirty eight of the patients (76 percent) were found to have no distal intramural spread whatsoever, a further 7 patients (14 percent) had spread for 1 cm or less, and only 5 patients (10 percent) had spread of more than 1 cm. The measurements were 1.5, 2, 2.5, 3.5, and 5 cm, respectively. Each of these five patients had a poorly differentiated Dukes' C carcinoma and each was dead or dying from distant metastases within 3 years of the operation. Thus, a distal margin of clearance of 2.5 cm would have removed all distal microscopic spread (and all involved lymph nodes) in 94 percent of patients. In those few patients with distal spread, to have taken a small distal margin would, in fact, have made little difference to the outcome because each developed distant metastases and even radical surgery in these patients failed to save their lives. In these authors' experience, the finding of any degree of distal intramural spread in a patient with a Dukes' C tumour meant that the patient was almost certain to die of distant metastases.

In the second part of the study, the results

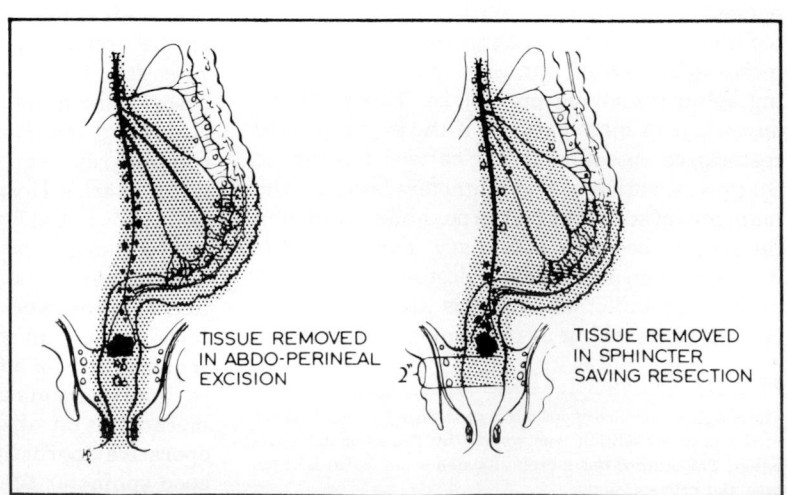

Figure 57–1. *Left:* Tissue removed in abdominoperineal excision. *Right:* Tissue removed in sphincter-saving resection.

TISSUE REMOVED IN ABDO-PERINEAL EXCISION

TISSUE REMOVED IN SPHINCTER SAVING RESECTION

of anterior resection for carcinoma of the rectum were reviewed a minimum of 5 years after operation, to find out whether patients with a wide distal margin of resection had fared better than patients with a small margin. Seventy nine patients had undergone a potentially curative resection, 48 with a distal margin of less than 5 cm (mean 2.8 cm) and 31 with a distal margin greater than 5 cm (mean 6.5 cm). The two groups were well matched for age, sex, degree of differentiation of the tumours, and distance of the lesion from the anal verge. However, 54 percent of patients in the first group had Dukes' C tumours, whereas only 23 percent of the patients in the second group had Dukes' C tumours. Despite the higher proportion of unfavourable tumours in the first group, the outcome, in terms both of survival and of recurrence, were as good in the patients with the small distal margin as in the patients with the wide distal margin of clearance. These authors conclude that the rigid routine application of the "5-cm rule" of distal excision may cause patients with low rectal cancer to lose their anal sphincter unnecessarily.

This study underlines the results of a follow-up of 556 patients who had undergone low anterior resection for rectal carcinoma at the Mayo Clinic reported by Wilson and Beahrs (1976), who found that patients with a 2 to 3 cm distal margin of resection fared just as well in the long term, as did patients with wider margins of resection. The same conclusions were reached in a similar study by Pollett and Nicholls (1981).

Application of Current Methods of Sphincter-Saving Resection

The operations in use in contemporary surgical practise for rectal resection with preservation of the sphincters are anterior resection, either with a sutured anastomosis or one carried out by the automatic circular stapling gun, abdominal–anal resection, either by a pull-through or by a trans-anal technique, and abdominal–sacral resection, either by classical or abdomino-trans-sphincteric technique. Of these methods there is only one that is commonly used as an alternative to an abdominoperineal excision of the rectum and this is the anterior resection (Lockhart-Mummery et al, 1983). Other methods are more complex technically and have been followed by more complications than anterior

resection, although in certain circumstances they will allow a lower anastomosis to be carried out. Furthermore, the quality of functional results afforded by them is sometimes less than perfect. These other procedures are not so much in competition with anterior resection as with abdominoperineal excision, for the care of lesions deemed too low for anterior resection. For most surgeons they will not be used at all, as complete rectal excision with permanent colostomy will be the only alternative considered to anterior resection.

Factors. The factors involved in deciding if a sphincter-saving operation can be undertaken are as follows: the sex and build of the patient, the site of the tumour, the size and histologic grading of the tumour, whether the patient has metastases, and if the colon is well prepared or the patient is obstructed.

Site. The most important factor is the site of the tumour. The level of the tumour is taken to be the distance between the anal verge with the lower margin of the tumour as measured by sigmoidoscopy (Fig. 57–2). It is not the distance between the dentate line and the tumour as recorded in the excised specimen. The rectosigmoid junction is that part of the bowel that lies in front of the sacral promontory and the exact distance will depend upon the build of the patient, but it is usually about 15 cm from the anal verge. Tumours situated between 10 cm and 15 cm will be treated by the majority of surgeons by an anterior resection without too much difficulty. Tumours less than 5 cm from the anal verge will lie in the anal canal or distal centimetre of the rectum and can only be treated by abdominoperineal excision or, in certain cases, by local excision. There remains the group of tumours between 6 and 10 cm, where all options are open to the surgeon. There will be a wide difference of opinion as to the advisability of the sphincter-saving resection and the choice of which particular technique should be used. It is in these difficult resections that the other factors become important, such as the sex and build of the patient. It is obviously much simpler to carry out a low anterior resection in a thin woman than it is in an obese male patient. Indeed, in many women it is possible to divide the rectum, leaving a centimetre cuff above the puborectalis, and to stitch the anastomosis by hand, and in series where surgeons

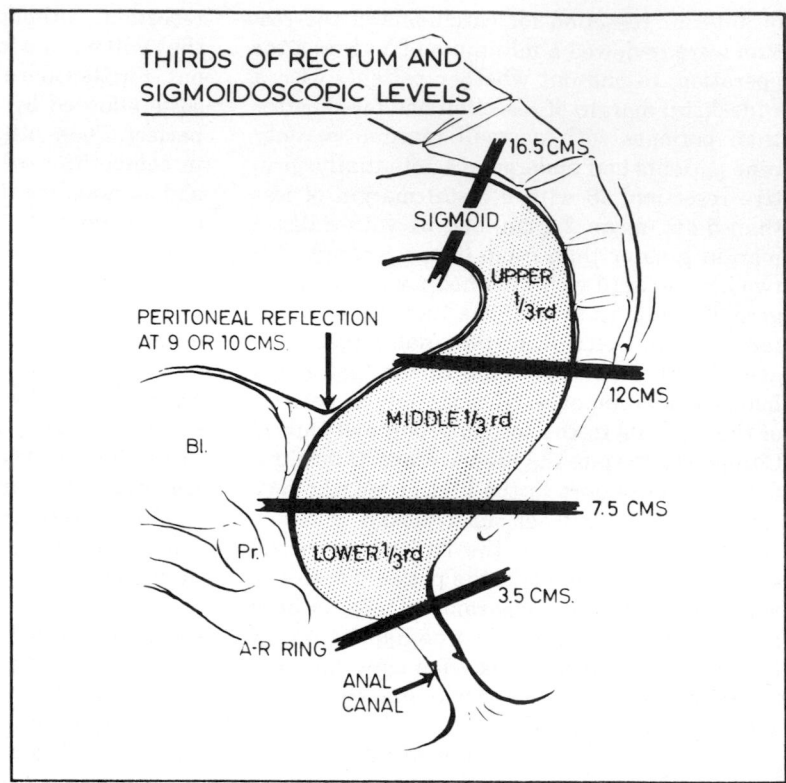

THIRDS OF RECTUM AND SIGMOIDOSCOPIC LEVELS

16.5 CMS.

SIGMOID

UPPER 1/3rd

PERITONEAL REFLECTION AT 9 OR 10 CMS.

12 CMS.

MIDDLE 1/3rd

Bl.

7.5 CMS.

Pr.   LOWER 1/3rd

3.5 CMS.

A-R RING

ANAL CANAL

Figure 57–2. Thirds of rectum and sigmoidoscopic levels.

only use the automatic stapling gun when it is impossible to carry out a hand-sutured anastomosis, most patients in their series will be male. Fortunately, a number of men have a gynaecoid pelvis, which makes working low down relatively easy. A tall, obese man with an android pelvis may make any form of low resection extremely difficult, not only because an anastomosis would be difficult to construct but also because the resection itself may be difficult unless the tumour is approached from the perineum as well as the abdomen.

Size. The size of the tumour may also be important. A small mobile tumour is more amenable to anterior resection than a large partly fixed tumour that fills the pelvis and, again in a male with a small pelvis, it can be virtually impossible to excise the tumour adequately unless an abdominoperineal excision is carried out, preferably by a two-team synchronous combined approach.

Histologic Grade. As has already been mentioned, the histologic grade of the tumour on

rectal biopsy is important, as the distance of clearance below the tumour to the level of transection of the rectum must be 5 cm in the tumour of a high grade of malignancy but can be compromised to 2 or 3 cm in an average- or low-grade tumour. It must be remembered that at operation, when the rectum is completely mobilised from the puborectalis upward, the tumour will become very much higher than appeared on sigmoidoscopy and a sphincter-saving operation may be possible (Fig. 57–3).

Metastases. The presence of metastases will influence the surgeon as to the type of operation to be carried out. If the patient has liver metastases and a short expectation of life, the surgeon may compromise on the distal margin of excision in order to perform an anterior resection. An anterior resection will be carried out if it can be easily performed without a covering colostomy. However, when the choice of procedure is between an abdominoperineal excision with an end colostomy and a difficult low anterior resection or a coloanal anastomosis requiring a defunctioning colostomy to be carried out, it

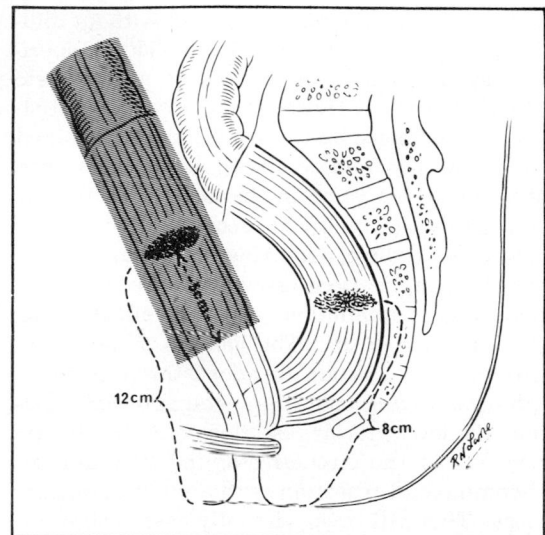

Figure 57–3. Diagram to show that when the rectum is fully mobilised at operation it straightens out and lengthens so that a growth that lay at 8 cm from the anal verge on preoperative sigmoidoscopy rises to perhaps 12 cm from the anus.

is in this author's experience always better to carry out the abdominoperineal excision rather than carry out a more difficult procedure with a higher risk of complications and leave the patient with a transverse colostomy that may never be closed before the patient's death. If the patient has no distant metastases but there is extensive local spread, either directly to the lateral wall of the pelvis or there are positive internal iliac lymph nodes, such a patient will require postoperative radiotherapy and there will be a high incidence of local recurrence. In such circumstances it is unwise to carry out an anterior resection even if this is technically feasible, as the patient is much better served by having an end colostomy constructed. In such cases, after complete mobilisation of the tumour and discovering the extent of local spread confirmed by frozen section, there is no point in carrying out an abdominoperineal excision and in these circumstances this author divides the rectum below the tumour and carries out a low Hartmann's procedure.

Preparation of the Colon. If the tumour is causing obstruction and the proximal colon is loaded with stool and distended, the surgeon must decide whether it is better to carry out

an abdominoperineal excision or a Hartmann's procedure, to perform a preliminary colostomy, or to empty the colon at operation and carry out an anastomosis with a defunctioning colostomy. The decision will depend upon the ease with which the procedure can be carried out and the expectation of life of the patient.

General Condition of the Patient. Finally, the age and general condition of the patient must be taken into account. There is no doubt that an abdominoperineal excision of the rectum, particularly if carried out as a synchronous combined operation by experienced surgeons, is a more straightforward operation with a lower morbidity and mortality, than a difficult low anterior resection. The mortality for abdominoperineal excision at St. Mark's Hospital is 1 percent; it is 2.8 percent for anterior resection generally but for those patients who have difficult low anterior resections, possibly with a peranal anastomosis, the mortality is over 5 percent. This also takes no account of the increased morbidity of the difficult procedures. Mature judgement of the surgeon may indicate that in a particular patient an abdominoperineal excision with permanent colostomy may be a better procedure than the technically feasible difficult low anterior resection. On several occasions this author has carried out a difficult procedure on an elderly patient that has been followed by complications and has made the patient's remaining months a misery when the patient would have been much better served by an abdominoperineal excision and a permanent colostomy.

Alternatives to Anterior Resection

Clearly if anterior resection is the only form of sphincter-saving resection being used by a surgeon a proportion of patients, particularly men with carcinomas of the lower part of the rectum that could on pathologic grounds be regarded as suitable for removal with conservation of the sphincters, will inevitably be treated instead by abdominoperineal excision with colostomy. The proportion of patients falling into this category will vary slightly from surgeon to surgeon and will be approximately 10 to 15 percent of patients. As for the choice between the alternative methods, each surgeon must make a decision on the basis of training, experience, and aptitude.

There is no doubt that the employment of the automatic circular stapling gun has extended anterior resection quite significantly for most surgeons. Although it has made no difference at all to the number of patients avoiding a permanent colostomy in specialised centres, it has undoubtedly influenced general surgical practice as a whole. Every surgeon who treats carcinoma of the rectum must be familiar with the circular stapling gun and be prepared to use it. It must be remembered that when the stapling gun is used a further centimetre of rectum is excised. The lowest level at which the gun can be conveniently used is when there is a cuff of rectum 1 cm to 2 cm above the puborectalis. This will place the anastomosis at the level of the puborectalis or sometimes a little below. It may be impossible to place a purse string suture at this level in a man and this has been inserted through the anal canal with an operating proctoscope in place.

Abdominoanal Resection

What will commend some variant of abdominoanal resection, particularly to surgeons in Britain, is that the patient is placed in the modified lithotomy Trendelenburg position and is thus immediately available for an extended anterior resection or synchronous combined excision of the rectum if either of these procedures becomes necessary during the course of the operation. These anastomoses used to be undertaken as a pull-through procedure, leaving a rectal stump 5 or 6 cm long. However, complications are more common and functional results are inferior to low anterior resection and they have never been popular in Britain. The alternative method of anastomosis is the peranal anastomosis of Parks (1982) when the colon is sutured to the anal canal, either end-to-end or sleeved to the dentate line through an anal retractor. Although there is a high incidence of complications, the final functional results are good and patients are continent much more quickly than after the earlier pull-through procedures.

Abdominosacral Resection

The abdominosacral resection has the advantage of leaving the anal canal and sphincters quite undisturbed by stretching, turning inside out, cutting, or being deprived of their lining. Localio (1978) has been the modern exponent of this method and operates with the patient in the right lateral position, which makes it possible to change the operative plan without difficulty if this proves necessary. An abdominoperineal excision can be carried out as in the classic Miles' technique. However, the average British surgeon, schooled on the synchronous combined operation, has had relatively little experience of perineal dissection in the lateral position. It is unlikely that many surgeons will adopt this type of procedure, requiring a perineal wound and the complications associated with it in addition to an abdominal wound when anastomosis is to be carried out. The general trend today will be for surgeons to adopt three types of sphincter-saving operation—the anterior resection, the low anterior resection occasionally carried out by the circular stapling gun, and an abdominoanal resection with a peranal anastomosis. This will cover virtually every eventuality.

Local Excision or Destruction of the Primary Growth

A controversial issue is the use of a purely local excision or local destruction by diathermy or contact irradiation for ulcerated or protruberant carcinomas of the rectum. This does not include polypoid adenomas that, on snaring, turn out to have carcinomatous foci that usually require no further treatment. Unless the patient is unfit for a radical resection, carcinomas treated by local means should be those that require an abdominoperineal excision if local treatment is not undertaken. They will therefore usually be within 5 or 6 cm of the anal verge, they should be small and rarely more than 3 cm in diameter and should be protruberant lesions rather than deeply ulcerating. On rectal examination they must be freely mobile and confined to the submucosa, with early involvement of the underlying muscle coat. There must be no hard lymph nodes palpable in the mesorectum.

The choice of method of local treatment, whether diathermy fulgaration, endocavity contact irradiation, or local excision, is a personal decision for the individual surgeon, depending on inclination and the available facilities. However, local peranal incision has many advantages and can be carried out readily if the criteria for local excision mentioned above are not extended. The tumour is removed with the full thickness of the rectal wall and a surrounding margin of 1 cm of normal tissue. If the lower edge of the tumour extends to the puborectalis, part of the underlying internal sphincter muscle will be removed with the tumour. The specimen is pinned out on cork and fixed for the pathologist to evaluate histologically.

It must be explained to the patient that the operation undertaken is a total excisional biopsy, which may be adequate treatment or further surgery may be advised when the pathologist has evaluated the tumour. If the pathologist finds that there are any parts of the tumour that are of a high grade of malignancy or there is evidence that local excision is not complete, then an abdominoperineal excision is advocated. With this kind of close pathologic control, approximately 5 percent of all rectal carcinomas can be managed in this way. Local excision should not be undertaken by the transsphincteric or Mason approach, with division of the anal sphincters and the rectal wall, as it is very easy technically to excise much more extensive tumours that are quite inappropriate for this method, resulting in a high incidence of local recurrence. Results of local disc excision are superior to diathermy fulgaration and at St. Mark's Hospital over 90 percent of patients treated with this method are alive at 5 years.

Hartmann's Operation

This operation consists of resecting the upper rectum and lower sigmoid, closing the top of the remaining rectum by suture and bringing out the colon as an iliac colostomy. It can be extended to treat tumours of the middle and lower third of the rectum provided an adequate margin of distal clearance is obtained. Of course the vast majority of patients will have restorative resection and anastomosis carried out. There are occasions, however, when it is more appropriate to avoid an anastomosis. When there is local spread involving the lateral pelvic wall and the internal iliac nodes and there is virtual certainty of local recurrence, the surgeon should alter plans for an anastomosis and construct an end colostomy. If the residual pelvic tumour responds to radiotherapy and after a suitable interval the patient appears cured, reanastomosis can be carried out. When the patient has a recurrence after an anterior resection it is inappropriate to carry out a further anterior resection and if the recurrent tumour can be excised without carrying out an abdominoperineal excision a Hartmann's operation is appropriate. If a low Hartmann's operation is

undertaken it is sometimes difficult to close the rectal stump. In these cases this author leaves it open and drains the pelvis with a catheter placed through the anus.

Multivisceral Resections

Neighbouring organs that have become adherent to a carcinoma of the rectum or to the sigmoid colon can often be excised in total or in part along with the rectum with a reasonable prospect of cure. Fortunately the adhesion is not infrequently due to an inflammatory reaction and not to malignant invasion. Even if it is due to malignant invasion a lasting success is sometimes obtained by a multivisceral resection, as we have already confirmed (Pittam et al, 1984). Of course some adjacent organs are relatively easily removed in conjunction with a rectal excision, for example, a loop of small bowel, the uterus, posterior vaginal wall, seminal vesicles, or a disc of bladder wall.

The 5-year crude survival rate for synchronous combined excision of the rectum with another organ or part of another organ involved is 40 percent. However, excision of the entire urinary bladder with the seminal vesicles and prostate is a much more formidable excision, involving as it does the establishment of a urinary conduit. It is fortunate that total cystectomy is very rarely required in this connection as compared with cases of uterine cancer. It should only be contemplated when the tumour is otherwise highly favourable apart from its close adherence to and strongly presumed infiltration of the bladder, it should be free posteriorly and laterally, there should be no suggestion of distant metastases or gross lymph node involvement, and the biopsy should have shown a well-differentiated tumour.

Adjuvant Radiotherapy or Chemotherapy

Much interest centres at the moment on the possibility of enhancing the curative value of surgical excision of rectal carcinoma by the administration of preoperative low-dose irradiation. A controlled trial at the Memorial Hospital in New York failed to show any benefit from the addition of radiotherapy, but another multicentre trial at U.S. Veterans Hospitals did suggest that irradiation might improve the 5-year survival rate by as much as 10 percent. The divergence of this opinion led the Medical Research Council in Britain to set up a multicentre trial of preoperative irradiation (Smith, 1984). Eight hundred twenty four patients with operable rectal carcinoma were randomly allocated to be treated by surgery alone, 2000 rad in 10 daily fractions, and 500 rad as a single fraction. No difference was demonstrated in the actuarial survival rates to 5 years. The local recurrence-free and metastasis-free rates were similar in all groups. There was also no evidence that the preoperative radiotherapy benefited patients in subgroups by Dukes' staging. The complication rates were also similar in the three treatment groups.

There is no statistical evidence that prophylactic chemotherapy given during or after radical surgery confers any benefit in treatment for curable, dubiously curable, or recurrent carcinomas.

GENERAL CONSIDERATIONS REGARDING PALLIATION

Excision of the Tumour Mass

It is now generally agreed that even if a rectal or rectosigmoid carcinoma is incurable, as from multiple hepatic metastases, and if a rectal excision can be performed without undue difficulty or risk, the patient's period of survival will be much more comfortable than if left to die with the primary lesion in situ. In other words, rectal excision is the best form of palliation. Obviously there are limits to the use of this form of treatment and if the liver is almost totally replaced by tumour or there are multiple peritoneal metastases, or the primary lesion is fixed in a frozen pelvis, attempts at rectal excision will confer little benefit to the patient.

Reference should be made to the report from the Mayo Clinic by Wilson and Adson (1976) on the treatment of hepatic metastases in patients undergoing colorectal resection for carcinoma. There were a number of 5-year survivors after removal of solitary hepatic secondaries, often by local excision rather than formal hepatic lobectomy. Yet patients with multiple metastases did not do well. However, if there are one or two small metastases these should always be removed if easily accessible, as in a few patients this will represent the only spread of the tumour and cure is still possible.

Reoperation for recurrent rectal carcinoma, as strongly urged by Wagensteen, is rarely curable. Only occasionally can recurrence after an anterior resection be successfully removed by subsequent abdominoperineal excision. More often the recurrent tumour is found to be beyond the reach of surgery but a palliative excision of the rectum and colostomy, together with radiotherapy, or chemotherapy, will often give the best form of palliation. More recent follow-up studies by the regular measurement of carcinoembryonic antigen, together with the use of scanning techniques, may reveal metastases or local recurrence at an earlier stage with a possible hope of further radical surgery. This topic is further discussed in Chapter 66.

Colostomy

A loop iliac colostomy proximal to an irremovable carcinoma has little palliative value and should only be carried out if the patient is obstructed.

Radiotherapy or Chemotherapy

Radiotherapy and chemotherapy are the agents to which the surgeon often resorts when faced with an inoperable or recurrent carcinoma. Radiotherapy is especially indicated for pain in the sacral or sciatic region. The trend toward the chemotherapeutic use of two or three agents simultaneously, such as 5-fluorouracil, methyl-CCNU, and mitomycin C, have shown that these rarely confer on the patient any more benefit than can be obtained with 5-fluorouracil alone and the side effects of drug combinations are significantly greater. Although statistically survival is little improved by chemotherapy, an occasional patient will respond dramatically to 5-fluorouracil and have prolonged palliation.

Nerve Block

In patients suffering from severe perineal sacral or sciatic pain that has not been improved by irradiation to the pelvis symptomatic relief may be obtained occasionally from either a subarachnoid injection of phenol or a lateral spinal tractotomy in the hands of a neurosurgeon. It is important to remember, however, that this treatment is not always successful and that it may cause difficulties with micturition and have other side effects.

ANTERIOR RESECTION OF THE RECTUM

The author has drawn very heavily on the excellent description of this operation by Professor John Goligher of Leeds in the previous edition. For descriptive purposes, two varieties of anterior resection are recognised.

The preoperative care of the patient and bowel preparation are as described in Chapter 53.

Low anterior resection is used for tumours of the rectum proper and involves full mobilisation of the rectum from the sacral concavity, the distal line of resection transversing the extraperitoneal rectum and the final anastomosis being made between the colon and a low rectal stump beneath the peritoneal reflection.

High anterior resection is suitable for growths of the rectosigmoid and distal end of the sigmoid colon. It is conducted entirely above the pelvic peritoneum, without disturbing the rectum from its sacral bed.

Sometimes the technique employed, however, is a compromise between these two methods, some some freeing of the rectum from the sacrum, but without division of the lateral ligaments.

Position of the Patient. For both the high and low anterior resection, the patient is placed in the modified lithotomy–Trendelenburg position as for synchronous combined abdominoperineal excision of the rectum. This facilitates access to the anal canal for the purpose of irrigation of the rectum during the operation and it also allows an easy change of operative plan in the light of the findings on exploration of the abdomen to an abdominoanal or synchronous combined excision. It is also important if a stapling anastomosis is to be used after anterior resection.

An indwelling self-retaining urethral catheter is passed and an intravenous drip is set up before the operation commences.

Low Anterior Resection

The initial steps of this operation are identical with those of the abdominal phase of the abdominoperineal excision. The abdomen is explored through a long left lower paramedian or midline incision, extending upward from the pubis. The sigmoid loop is mobilised by division of the con-

genital adhesions on the lateral side of the mesosigmoid. The left ureter is identified. In order to allow the anastomosis to be carried out without tension, adequate mobilisation of the left colon must be performed by dividing its lateral peritoneal attachment, and this may need to be continued as far as the splenic flexure.

The inferior mesenteric vessels are now exposed through incisions in the peritoneum on either side of the base of the mesocolon, extending upward on the right side in front of the abdominal aorta toward the lower border of the third part of the duodenum. The inferior mesenteric pedicle is then doubly ligated with thread and divided, usually at the level flush with the origin of the artery from the front of the aorta, unless the resection is being carried out as a palliative procedure in the presence of hepatic secondaries, in which case a lower site is chosen.

Fashioning the Colon Stump. The sigmoid colon is spread out to display its vessels preparatory to transection of the mesosigmoid from the point of ligation of the inferior mesenteric vessels obliquely to a point on the sigmoid adjudged capable of extending without tension to the top of the future rectal stump (Fig. 57–4). Finally, the bowel is divided between two obliquely applied Parker–Kerr clamps.

Mobilisation of the Rectum. The rectum must now be freed from its surroundings in the pelvis in exactly the same way as in the abdominoperineal excision. The lower ends of the incisions in the peritoneum on either side of the base of the mesosigmoid are extended downward around the brim of the pelvis to meet anteriorly at the deepest part of the peritoneal pouch. The rectum is then lifted forward and the almost avascular presacral plane opened up by inserting the hand in the presacral space. Separation is completed to the tip of the coccyx.

Next, by a mixture of scissor and blunt dissection, the bladder, vasa deferentia, seminal vesicles and prostate (or posterior vaginal wall in the female) are separated from the front of the rectum and its lateral ligaments. Finally, the lateral ligaments are divided with long scissors.

As a result of this mobilisation, the rectum can now be lifted straight out of the pelvis from the anorectal junction without following its usually anteroposterior and lateral curves. As already mentioned (Fig. 57–3) the effect of this

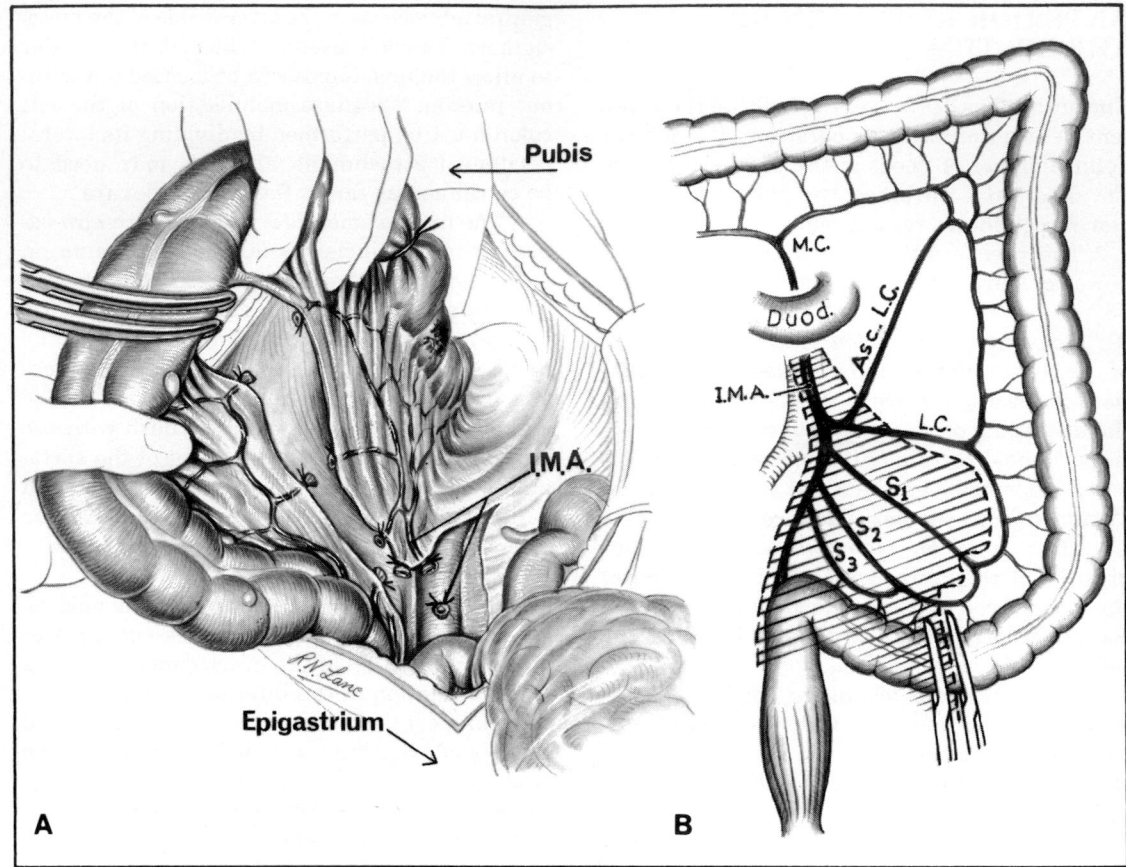

Figure 57–4. Low anterior resection. **A.** The inferior mesenteric artery (IMA) has been tied and divided on the front of the aorta, and the sigmoid mesocolon has been transected obliquely from this point to the sigmoid colon, which is then doubly clamped preparatory to division. **B.** The vascular arrangements of the colon stump.

"lengthening" of the bowel is to elevate the position of the growth, often 2 or 3 inches (5 to 7.5 cm), rendering some lesions that appeared previously too low for anterior resection now quite suitable for it. At this stage, therefore, the surgeon should make a final decision as to the feasibility of a resection with a 2 to 5 cm distal margin of clearance (depending on the factors already discussed) and a rectal stump that will be accessible for a secure colorectal anastomosis.

Preparation of the Rectal Stump. If it is decided to proceed with a low anterior resection, the next step is to separate the mesorectum from the back of the rectum at the level selected for transection of the bowel below the growth

and to divide it between clamps (Fig. 57–5). The higher up on the rectum this distal line of resection, the easier it is to define the mesorectum in this way. Lower down, the mesorectal tissues fan out onto the back of the rectum so that in a really low anterior resection, definition of the mesorectum as described may not be feasible or necessary.

The rectum itself is now clamped across with a crushing clamp at a point corresponding to the top of the intended rectal stump (Fig. 57–6). Different surgeons will have their own favourite angled clamps for this purpose but I find that a nontoothed bronchus clamp is ideal for this purpose.

An assistant now passes a proctoscope per anum and irrigates the rectal stump below the

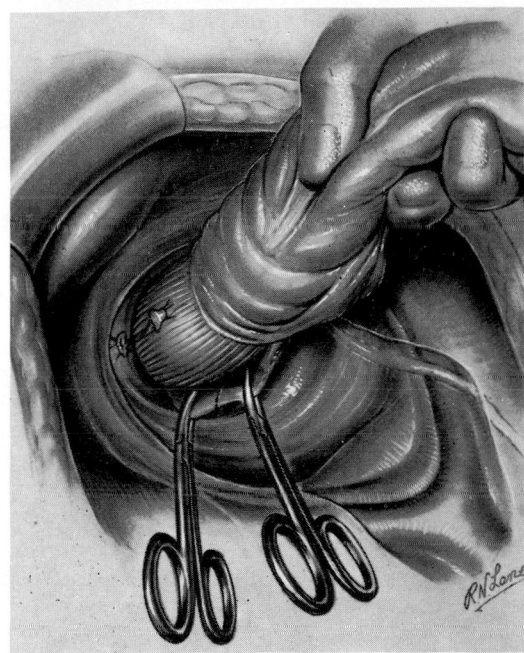

Figure 57–5. Low anterior resection. The rectum has been freed from its surroundings in the pelvis, and the mesorectum is defined and divided. Often in really low anterior resections the mesorectal tissues are so fanned out on the back of the rectum that they are difficult to define in this way.

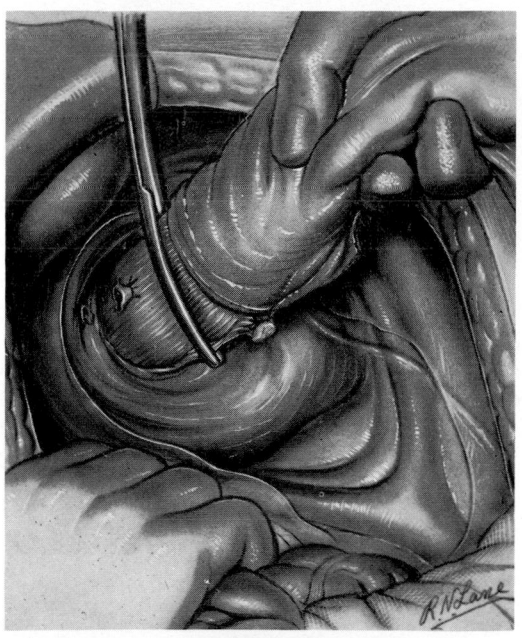

crushing clamp with 1 to 2 pints of a 1 percent solution of cetrimide. This acts not only as a cleansing agent to remove all faecal material, blood, and mucus but it is also cytotoxic to any free-floating cancer cells.

Anastomosis can be performed by either a two-layer or layer suture technique or by using the stapling "gun."

Two-Layer Suture Anastomosis. In preparation for the anastomosis, the sigmoid and upper rectum are pulled vertically upward to lift the lower rectum as far as possible out of the pelvis, since this facilitates the insertion of suture into it (Fig. 57–7). The clamp controlling the end of the colon stump is rested on the left edge of the abdominal wound with its mesenteric border lying posteriorly. In that position it is separated by a few inches from the rectum immediately below where it is clamped (Fig. 57–7). A posterior outer layer of a series of interrupted Lembert-style mattress sutures of 2/0 thread are now inserted and each is held in an artery forceps. If a handle of each forceps is threaded onto long artery forceps held upward by the assistant, this prevents successive sutures from becoming snared with each other. The colon is then slid down on the sutures until the colonic and rectal walls are roughly in apposition. The stitches are then tied and cut except for the first and last, the tails of which are retained long as stay sutures.

The next step is to excise the two crushing clamps from the colon and rectal stumps, respectively, by running a scalpel along the deep aspect of each clamp. In the case of the rectal clamp, this means also, of course, removal of the operative specimen (Fig. 57–8). The result is to leave two open lumina, the cut edges of which are then brought together by a continuous suture of 2/0 thread, as shown in Figure 57–9. A simple over-and-over stitch is used, turning the corner by means of a Connell stitch. The anastomosis is completed by inserting the anterior layer of outer Lembert mattress sutures (Fig. 57–10).

One-Layer Anastomosis. Some surgeons prefer a one-layer technique of anastomosis on the

Figure 57–6. Low anterior resection. Application of the Parker–Kerr clamp across the rectum in the sagittal or anteroposterior plane at the distal limit of resection.

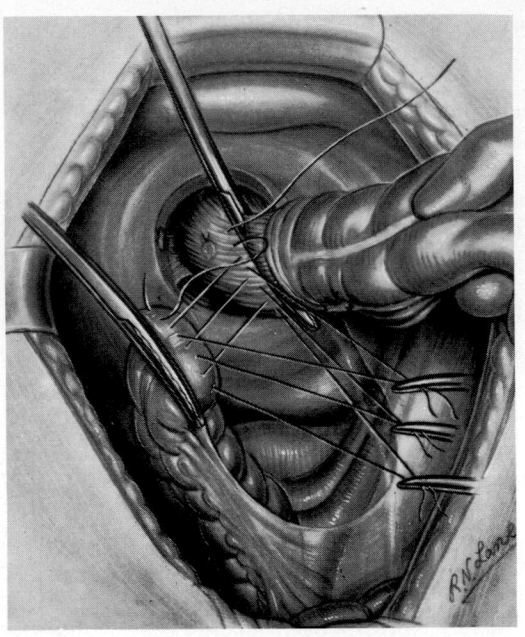

Figure 57–7. Low anterior resection by two-layer technique of anastomosis. Commencement of anastomosis between the colon and rectum by insertion of the first half of the outer row of sutures as a series of mattress stitches left long until all have been placed.

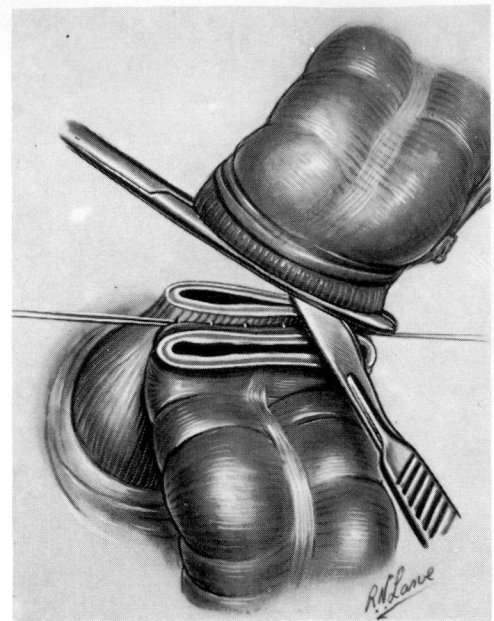

Figure 57–8. Low anterior resection by two-layer technique of anastomosis. The clamp on the colon stump has been "excised," and that on the rectal stump is in the process of being similarly removed, taking with it the growth and specimen.

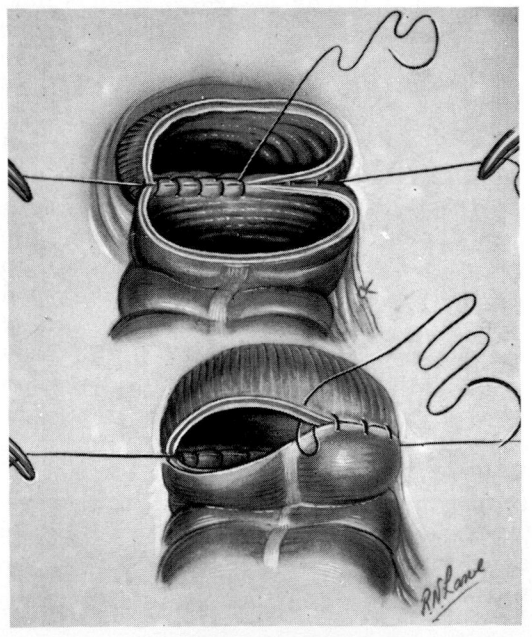

Figure 57–9. Low anterior resection by two-layer technique of anastomosis. The cut edges of the stumps of colon and rectum are being brought together with a continuous through-and-through stitch. Note that at the right posterior corner the suture assumes the Connell or loop-on-the-mucosa pattern for the second half in order to secure good mucosal inversion.

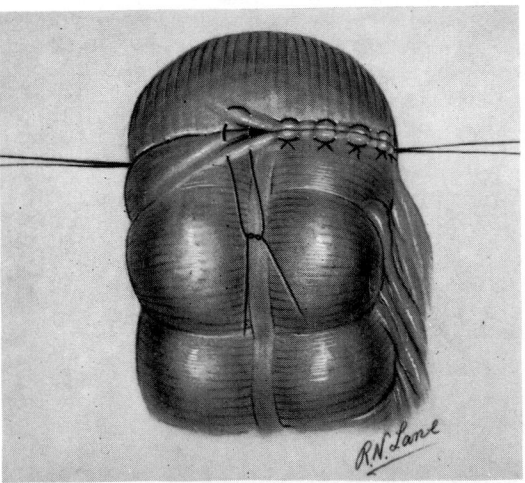

Figure 57–10. Low anterior resection by two-layer technique of anastomosis. The second half of the outer row of mattress sutures is inserted.

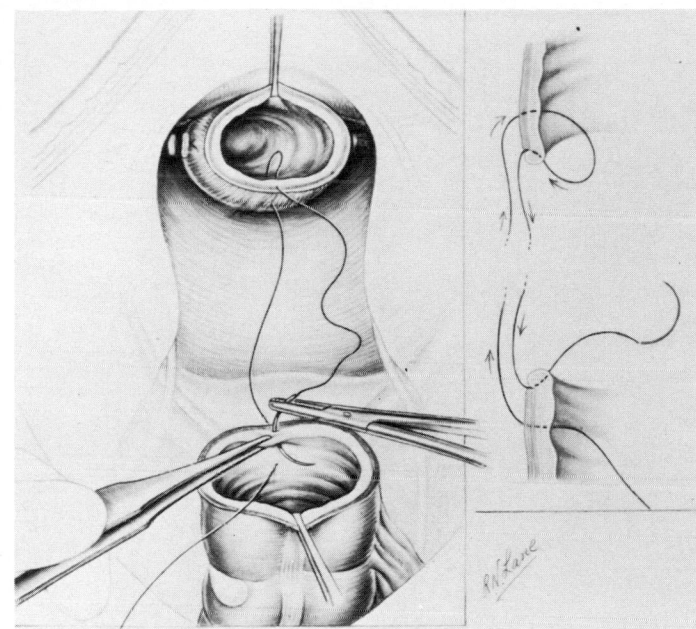

Figure 57–11. Low anterior resection. One-layer technique of anastomosis. Method of inserting vertical mattress sutures in one-layer technique of anastomosis for low anterior resection. (*Source: From Goligher JC, et al, 1977, with permission.*)

grounds that the blood supply to the large bowel may be somewhat tenuous and is less likely to be impaired by one layer of sutures than by two. However, it is controversial whether there is any difference in the likelihood of subsequent anastomotic leakage depending on whether a one- or two-layer technique is used. Everett (1975), in a controlled trial of one- and two-layer techniques of anastomosis, found a significantly smaller incidence of leaks after the one-layer technique for low anterior resection, but no difference could be demonstrated for high resection. Matheson and colleagues (1975, 1981) had remarkably few anastomotic dehiscences in a large uncontrolled experience with a one-layer technique. However, Goligher et al (1977), in a large controlled study of the two techniques, found only a slight difference in the frequency of dehiscence and this was in favour of the two-layer method.

This author's personal preference is for the two-layer technique, but this may be a matter more of habit than of science. However, I have certainly used the one-layer method on many occasions without regret. It really comes down to the surgeon's personal preference; the factors of a good blood supply, absence of tension, and a well-prepared bowel are far more important than the exact suturing method employed.

In performing the one-layer technique, var-

ious suture materials are employed, both absorbable and nonabsorbable. Most surgeons prefer nonabsorbable material and this author personally uses thread. Also the technique of suture may vary slightly, with particular reference as to whether the stitch traverses all coats of the bowel wall and is tied with its knot on the mucosal aspect, or is inserted from the outside, penetrating only the seromuscular and submucous layers and is tied on the serosal aspect. Personally, I use the former technique with 2/0 thread; this is the one to be described.

When the operation has been taken to the stage illustrated in Figure 57–7 (i.e., with the end of the colon stump controlled by a clamp and the second clamp placed across the rectum at the level selected for the distal line of the resection, but without the Lembert sutures shown in that illustration), the clamp on the colon is excised, leaving an open-ended colon stump, and the rectum is similarly divided with a scalpel immediately below the clamp on that piece of bowel, which removes the clamp and the specimen and which leaves an open rectal stump. Bleeding from the cut edges of these two stumps may need to be checked by means of diathermy coagulation. With the stumps separated by a gap of about 15 cm, a series of vertical mattress sutures of 2/0 thread are then inserted as shown in Figures 57–11 and 57–12, corre-

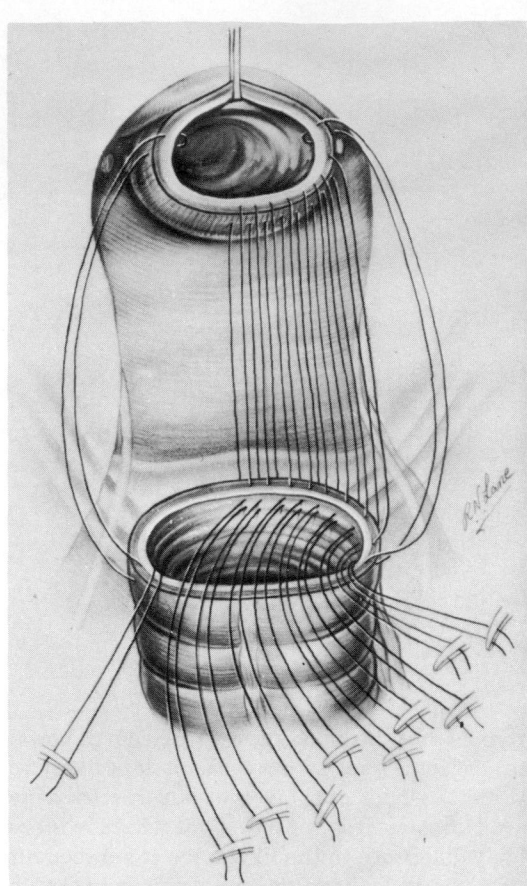

Figure 57-12. Low anterior resection. One-layer technique of anastomosis. Sutures corresponding to the posterior two thirds of the bowel circumference are placed while the colonic and rectal stumps are separated. The stitches have been inserted in the right posterior third but yet to be inserted in the left posterior third. They are left untied until all are in position.

sponding to the posterior two thirds of the bowel circumference. The sutures are held long in artery forceps. Next, the colon is slid down on these sutures, which are tied with the knots on the colonic mucosa (Fig. 57–13). Finally, the gap in the anterior third of the anastomosis is closed by further interrupted sutures, inserted usually as horizontal Lembert sutures because of the greater ease of placement of this type of stitch compared with a vertical stitch in the deep pelvis (Fig. 57–14).

Many surgeons now complete the procedure by suturing the pelvic peritoneum over the anastomosis as shown in Figure 57–15. Some surgeons allege that this leads to accumulation of serosanguineous fluid in the pelvic cavity that may burst through the anastomosis and that in any event anastomoses heal better when exposed to the general peritoneal cavity. Like many others, this author leaves the pelvic peritoneum unsutured but, as far as I am aware, this has never been submitted to any sort of controlled trial.

Drainage of the Pelvic Cavity. The majority of surgeons advise drainage of the pelvic cavity, either transperitoneally or inserted extraperitoneally from the main wound or from stab wounds in the right or left iliac region beneath the parietal peritoneum of the iliac fossa to the region of the anastomosis, as shown in Figure 57–15.

It should be noted that the use of such drains is based more on tradition than science. Indeed, the effectiveness, therapeutic indications and efficiency of drains remain unresolved controversies (Moss, 1981). There is experimental evidence that positive harm may be caused to the anastomosis by the presence of drains. Manz and colleagues (1970) compared nondrained left-sided colonic anastomoses in dogs with those with a Penrose latex drain. In the first group of 14 animals there were no deaths. At sacrifice there were no strictures and only three had filmy adhesions. By contrast, of 20 dogs in the drained group, 9 died from anastomotic breakdown and peritonitis and the rest

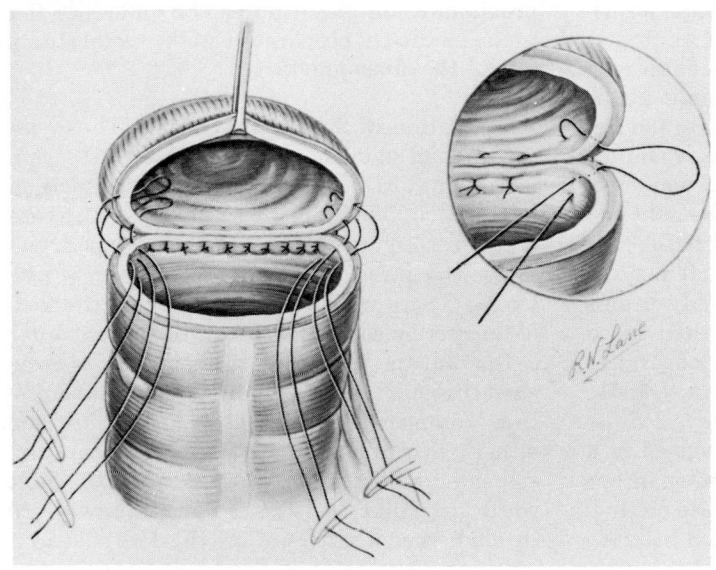

Figure 57–13. Low anterior resection. One-layer technique of anastomosis. Colon stump has been slid down on the sutures until it makes contact with the rectal stump, when the sutures are tied with their knots on the colon mucosa. Note that the two lateral "corners" are well turned in by this technique. (*Source: From Goligher JC, et al, 1977, with permission.*)

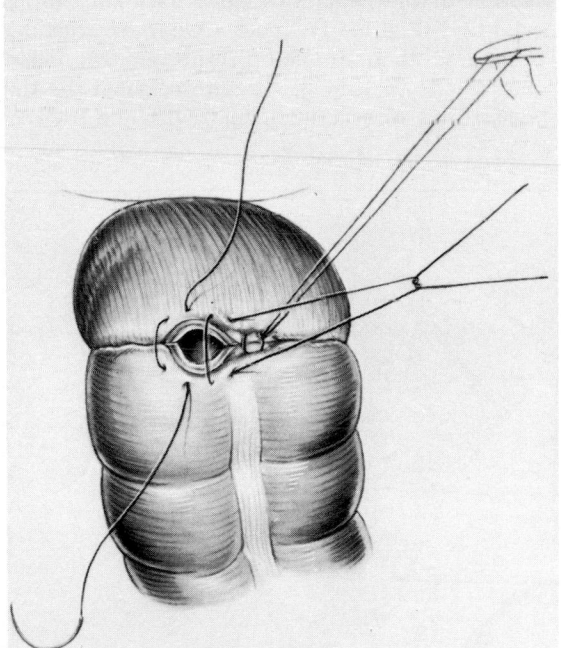

Figure 57–14. Low anterior resection. One-layer technique of anastomosis. The gap corresponding to the anterior third of the anastomosis is closed by horizontal Lembert sutures. (*Source: From Goligher JC, et al, 1977, with permission.*)

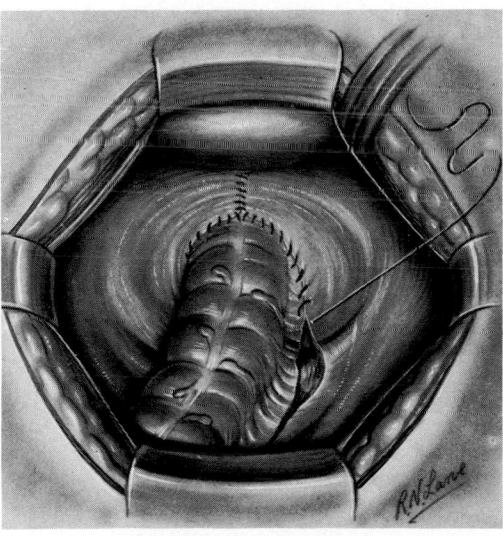

Figure 57–15. Low anterior resection. The pelvic peritoneum can be sutured over the anastomosis and to the colon stump and its mesocolon, but more usually is left unsutured.

had extensive adhesions and stricture formation.

The mechanism of this harmful effect may be as follows. A small area of ischaemia at the anastomosis would normally stimulate the formation of an adhesion to itself. This would act as a vascular graft to sustain the tissue temporarily until it is revascularised. If the adhesion is prevented by foreign material, the tissue may die and the anastomosis may leak. It may be suggested that the surgeon who only drains anastomoses when in doubt about their blood supply, tension, or integrity actually jeopardises those most in need of protection (Lennox, 1984).

On the basis that drains might have definite disadvantages, we are currently involved in a randomised trial to test this hypothesis in our colonic and rectal anastomoses. To date no obvious difference has been demonstrated between our drained and nondrained groups.

High Anterior Resection

The part of this operation leading up to and including ligation of the inferior mesenteric vessels and the construction of the colon stump is exactly the same as in a low anterior resection, except that a slightly shorter length of proximal colon may suffice. The difference lies in the method of preparation of the rectal stump and of the anastomosis.

Preparation of the Rectal Stump. The upper rectum and sigmoid with the related mesocolon is held upward and to the left, while the incision in the peritoneum on the right side of the base of the mesosigmoid, that was used to expose and ligate the inferior mesenteric vessels, is prolonged downward with scissors to reach the back of the rectum some 5 cm below the lower border of the tumour (Fig. 57–16). This incision is deepened through the underlying fat and in the process a number of small vessels are divided and either tied or coagulated. The upper rectum and sigmoid are then drawn upward and to the right while a similar incision is carried downward through the peritoneum on the left side to a corresponding point at the back of the rectum on the left (Fig. 57–17). The posterior part of this incision is also deepened and, in the anterior part, the trunks of the superior haemorrhoidal vessels are identified on the posterior aspect of the rectum, divided between clamps and tied (Fig. 57–17, inset). A curved crushing clamp is then applied in the sagittal plane across the rectum at the site selected for the distal line of resection (Fig. 57–18) and the rec-

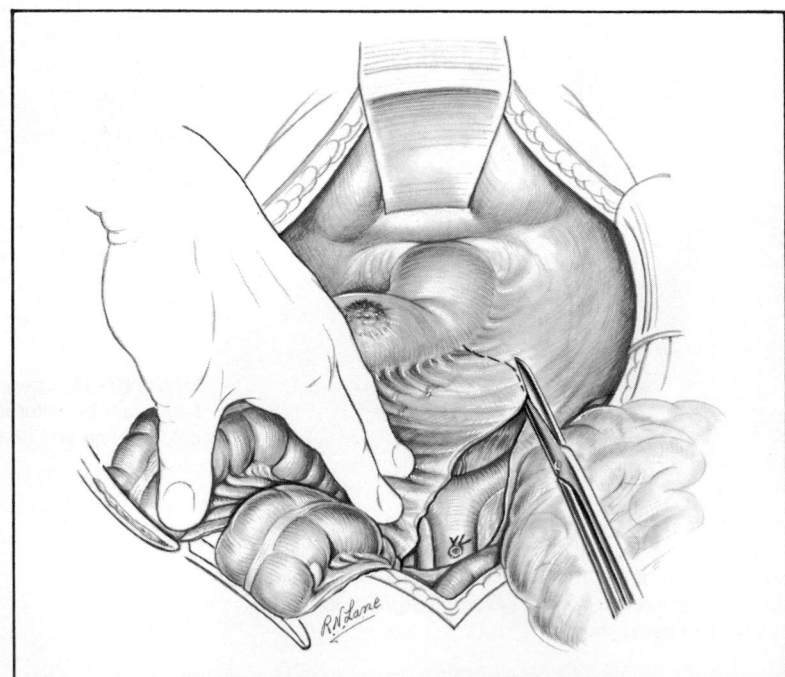

Figure 57–16. High anterior resection. Cutting the peritoneum of the right leaf of the mesorectum down to a point 2 inches below the lower edge of the growth.

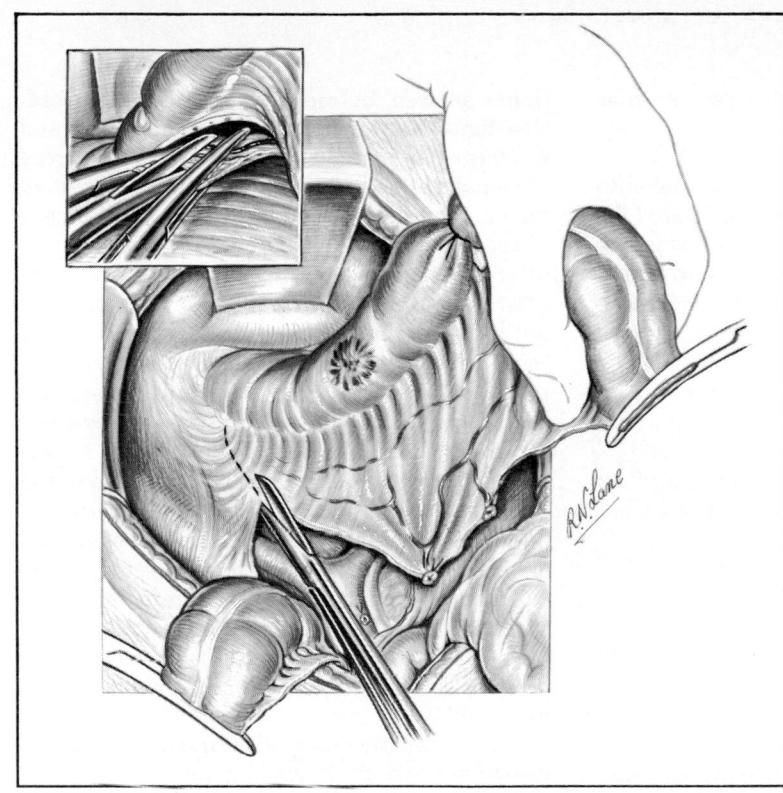

Figure 57–17. *Inset:* High anterior resection. Cutting the peritoneum of the left half of the mesocolon to a similar point on the back of the rectum. Isolation and division of the superior haemorrhoidal vessels on the back of the rectum.

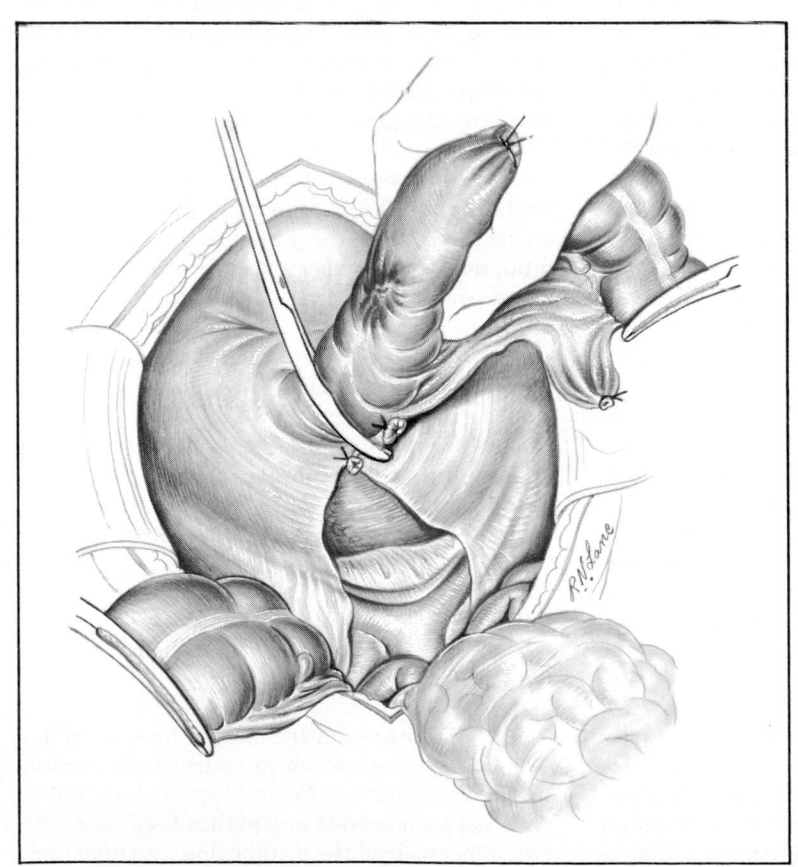

Figure 57–18. High anterior resection. Application of a Parker–Kerr clamp across the intraperitoneal rectum in the sagittal plane, preparatory to irrigating the rectal stump from below and carrying out the anastomosis.

1487

tum below this clamp is irrigated per anum as already described.

Anastomosis. The anastomosis of the colon to the rectal stump follows the lines indicated for low anterior resection and can be performed by either a suture technique in one or two layers or by the stapling method. In the United Kingdom the suture technique is on the whole preferred. The final result is an entirely intraperitoneal union between the colon and a cuff of intraperitoneal rectum.

Anastomosis by Means of the Stapling Gun. This is discussed fully in Chapter 61.

Preliminary or Simultaneous Transverse Colostomy

If at laparotomy the colon is found to be very loaded, it is safer to be content with providing a simple transverse colostomy in the first instance. Such a colostomy should be placed in the extreme right end of the transverse colon through a small transverse wound in the right subcostal region. This will leave the left half of the abdomen unencumbered by a stoma at the subsequent resection and will also not interfere with adequate mobilisation of the left colon. Subsequent anterior resection can be carried out 3 weeks or so later.

A simultaneous transverse colostomy should be carried out with a very low resection, when technical difficulties have been encountered or if the surgeon is at all unhappy about the quality of the anastomosis. A temporary colostomy will not prevent the occurrence of anastomotic breakdown but will less the dangers of this complication and facilitate its management.

When a preliminary or simultaneous colostomy has been provided, it is retained until the anastomosis has been shown on subsequent sigmoidoscopy and/or radiologic examination after a Gastrografin enema to be well healed. In the absence of evidence of leakage this can be carried out 4 to 6 weeks after the resection.

Morbidity and Mortality Rates

Although after anterior resection patients are exposed to all the hazards of a major laparotomy, perhaps the most specific complication that may occur, and certainly the one that is most feared, is anastomotic dehiscence. Go-

ligher showed, by means of regular postoperative digital and sigmoidoscopic examination and Gastrografin enema studies that minor degrees of leakage are common, even in the most skilled hands. Leakage was demonstrated in 37 percent of cases after high resection and in 58 percent after low resection. Many of the breakdowns after high resection are virtually subclinical, but a considerable proportion of those after low resection are gross dehiscences associated with major pelvic sepsis. The causes of leakage are multifactorial and have recently been reviewed by Khoury and Waxman (1983) but the important factors include the general condition of the patient (protein deficiency, vitamin C deficiency, jaundice, uraemia) and local factors, which include blood supply, distraction and tension, faecal loading and bacterial contamination, and surgical technique. Circular intraluminal stapling gives results comparable with those of sutured anastomoses (Beart and Kelly, 1981; Waxman, 1983).

The operative mortality rate after anterior resection has been shown in many series of cases to be of the same order as that after abdominoperineal excision of the rectum. Indeed, because anterior resection is often done in more favourable cases, the figures in some series may favour anterior resection. Whitaker and Goligher (1976) report a 6.8 percent mortality for anterior resection between 1955 and 1968, while Lockhart-Mummery and colleagues (1976) reporting on rather selected cases seen at St. Mark's Hospital, note an operative mortality varying from 2 to 4 percent over the years between 1958 and 1972.

As regards ultimate cure of the carcinoma, many follow-up studies have now been conducted and they suggest that the 5-year survival rate after anterior resection is at least as good as that after abdominoperineal excision (Lockhart-Mummery et al, 1976; Nicholls et al, 1979; Whitaker and Goligher, 1976).

RESECTION AND COLOANAL ANASTOMOSIS FOR RECTAL CARCINOMA

Various pull-through techniques have been described for resections of tumours of the rectum with preservation of the anal sphincters. These have not gained wide acceptance because of the risk of necrosis of the distal colon, the high incidence of pelvic sepsis and variable functional

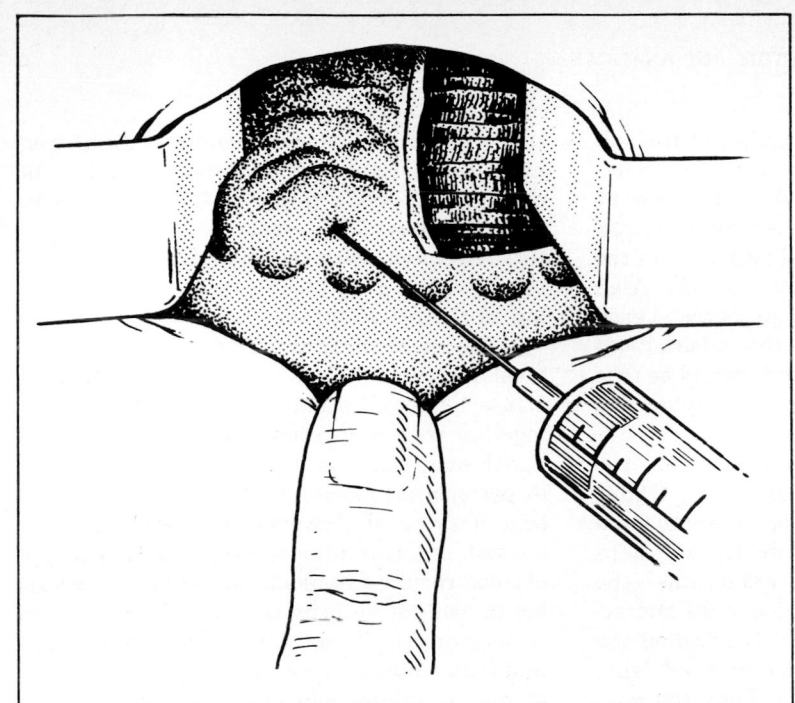

Figure 57–19. Adrenalin 1:300,-000 is infiltrated into the submucosa above the dentate line. On the left, a strip of mucosa has already been excised from the rectal stump. (*Source: Adapted from Parks AG, Percy JP, 1982, with permission.*)

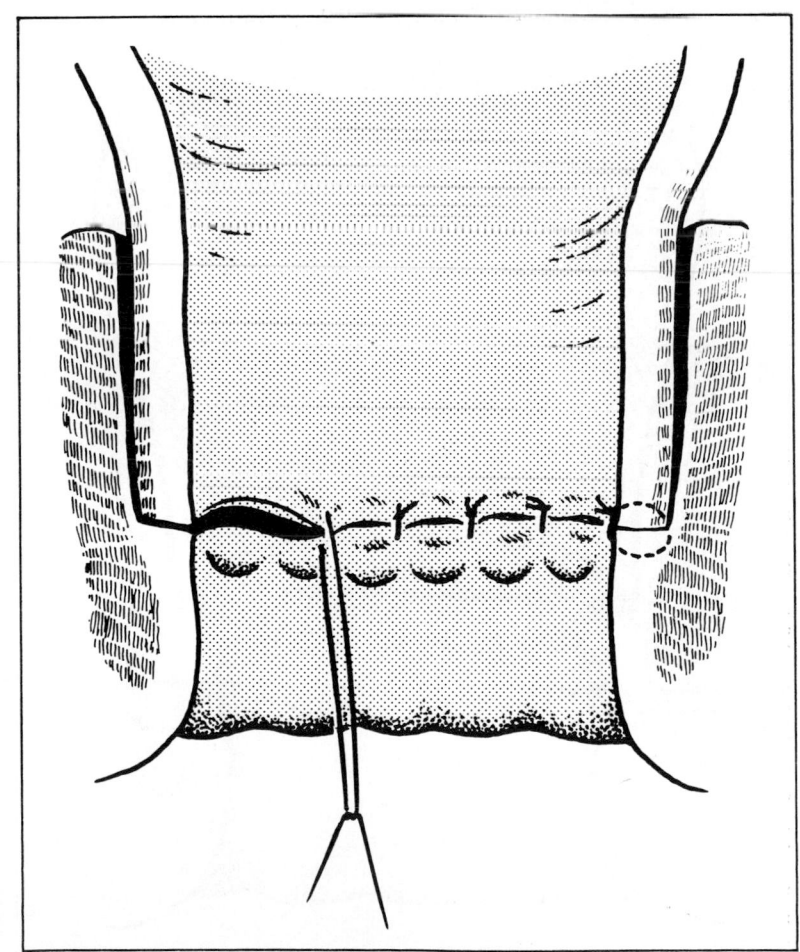

Figure 57–20. Coloanal canal anastomosis with interrupted 3/0 Dexon sutures. (*Source: Adapted from Parks AG, Percy JP, 1982, with permission.*)

results. Moreover, the introduction of the stapling technique for anterior resection of the rectum has enabled sphincter-saving surgery to be performed in most any instance where the surgeon feels that adequate distal clearance of the tumour can be achieved. The late Sir Alan Parks (1972) described a technique of rectal excision with peranal anastomosis that he practiced and taught with great skill, but it would be true to say that few general surgeons employ this procedure.

The following description is based on the excellent account by Parks and Percy (1982).

The patient is positioned as for an abdominoperineal combined excision and the first steps of the operation are essentially the same—the resection of rectum is taken down to the anorectal junction. The pararectal fat is lifted off the levator ani muscles, which are exposed lying beneath their investing fascia. The rectum is cross-clamped below the tumour and the anorectal stump irrigated from below. Usually the midsigmoid colon is employed for the anastomosis, but it may be necessary to mobilise the entire left colon up to the splenic flexure until bowel with a good blood supply can be placed low in the pelvis without tension.

The anastomosis is performed from the perineal approach. A Parks self-retaining retractor is inserted into the anal canal to expose its wall, together with any residual rectum. If only the upper anal canal is left, it may be necessary to perform an anastomosis directly to the cut edge of the canal. However, because of the inherent risk of terminal necrosis in the long length of colon required to reach the canal, it is desirable to achieve an overlapping or "sleeve" type of anastomosis. To do this it is necessary to denude the mucosa from the remaining rectal stump. A dilute solution of adrenalin (1 in

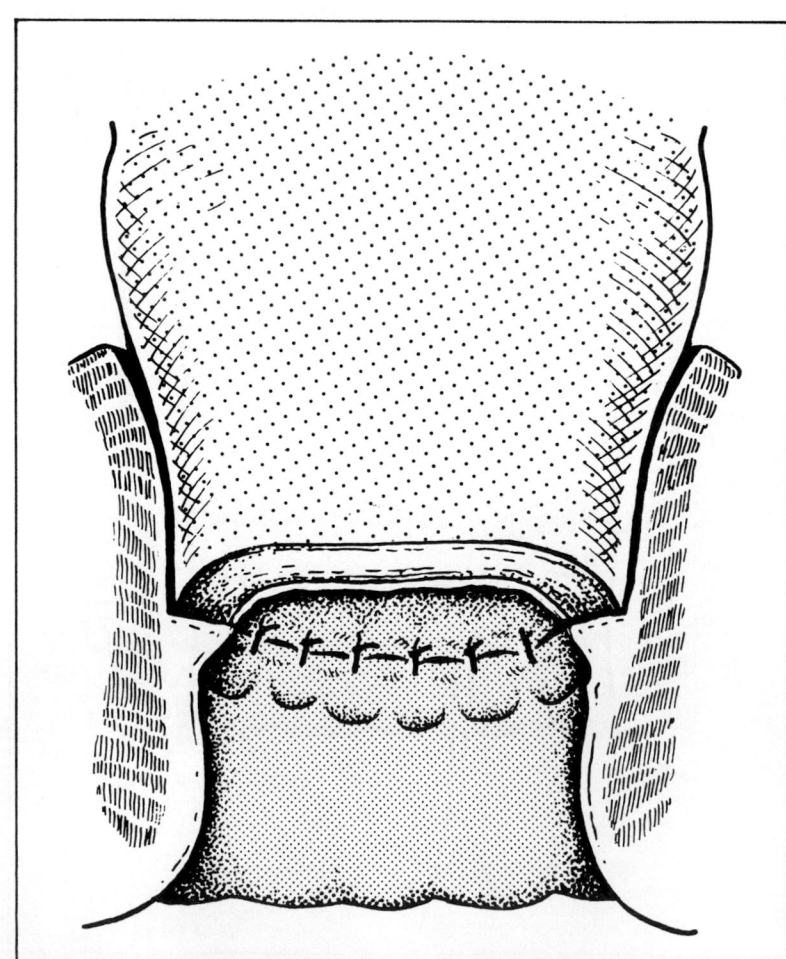

Figure 57–21. The completed anastomosis. The colon lies within the sleeve of the denuded rectal stump. (*Source: Adapted from Parks AG, Percy JP, 1982, with permission.*)

300,000) is injected into the submucosa of the rectal stump to lift the mucosa off the underlying muscle and the submucosal plexus of vessels (Fig. 57–19). The mucosa is removed from just above the dentate line, using scissors dissection. The colon, the end of which has been closed with a purse string suture, is drawn down between the blades of the retractor and through the denuded rectal stump to the lower end of the mucosal excision. The anastomosis is carried out in the anal canal using interrupted sutures of 3/0 polyglycolic acid. Each suture incorporates the mucosa of the anal canal, a portion of the upper internal sphincter and full thickness of the colon in a one-layer anastomosis (Fig. 57–20). The colon lies within a sleeve of denuded upper internal sphincter and rectal muscle (Fig. 57–21). A drain is placed in the hollow of the sacrum and is brought out through a stab incision in the perianal skin. A temporary transverse loop colostomy is performed.

Parks and Percy report on 76 patients undergoing this procedure between 1973 and 1980. There were two anastomotic breakdowns. Sixty nine of the 70 patients who were able to be assessed were either completely normal functionally or had only minor deficiencies of bowel function. The follow-up results of this group of patients are comparable with those seen following abdominoperineal excision of the rectum for similarly sited tumours.

BIBLIOGRAPHY

Beart RW, Kelly KA: Randomized prospective evaluation of the EEA stapler for colorectal anastomoses. Am J Surg 141:143, 1981

Dukes CE: Cancer of the rectum: An analysis of 1000 cases. J Path Bact 50:527, 1940

Everett WG: A comparison of one layer and two layer techniques of colorectal anastomosis. Br J Surg 62:135, 1975

Goligher JC, Lee PWG, et al: A controlled comparison of one- and two-layer techniques of suture for high and low colorectal anastomoses. Br J Surg 64:609, 1977

Khoury GA, Waxman BP: Large bowel anastomoses. The healing process and sutured anastomoses. A review. Br J Surg 70:61, 1983

Lennox MS: Prophylactic drainage of colonic anastomoses. Br J Surg 71:10, 1984

Localio SA, Gouge TH, et al: Abdomino-sacral resection for carcinoma of the midrectum: 10 years experience. Ann Surg 188:745, 1978

Lockhart-Mummery H, Heald RJ, et al: A Colour Atlas of Anterior Resection of the Rectum. London: Wolfe, 1983

Lockhart-Mummery HE, Ritchie JK, et al: The results of surgical treatment for carcinoma of the rectum at St Mark's Hospital from 1948 to 1972. Br J Surg 63:673, 1976

Mason AY: Trans-sphincteric exposure of the rectum. Ann R Coll Surg Engl 51:320, 1972

Matheson NA, Irving AD: Single layer anastomosis after rectosigmoid resection. Br J Surg 62:239, 1975

Matheson NA, Valerio D, et al: Single layer anastomosis in the large bowel: 10 years experience. J R Soc Med 74:44, 1981

Manz DW, La Tendresse C, et al: The detrimental effects of drains on colonic anastomoses. An experimental study. Dis Colon Rectum 13:17, 1970

Moss JP: Historical and current prospectives on surgical drainage. Surg Gynecol Obstet 152:517, 1981

Nicholls RJ, Ritchie JK, et al: Total excision or restorative resection for carcinoma of the middle third of the rectum. Br J Surg 66:625, 1979

Parks AG: Transanal technique in low rectal anastomosis. Proc R Soc Med 65:975, 1972

Parks AG, Percy JP: Resection and sutured coloanal anastomosis for rectal carcinoma. Br J Surg 69:301, 1982

Pittam MR, Thornton H, et al: Survival after extended resection for locally advanced carcinoma of the colon and rectum. Ann R Coll Surg Engl 66:81, 1984

Pollett WJ, Nicholls RJ: Does the extent of distal clearance affect survival after radical anterior resection for carcinoma of the rectum? Gut 22:872, 1981

Smith AN: The evaluation of low dose pre-operative x-ray therapy in the management of operable rectal cancer: Results of a randomly controlled trial. Second report of an MRC working party. Br J Surg 71:21, 1984

Waxman BP: Large bowel anastomoses. The circular stapler. A review. Br J Surg 70:64, 1983

Westhues H: Uber die Entstehung und Vermeidung des lokalen Rektum karzinom-Rezidivs. Arch Klin Chir 161:582, 1930

Westhues H: Die Pathologisch-Anatomischen Grundlagen der Chirurgie des Rektum karzinoms. Leipzig: Thieme, 1934

Whittaker M, Goligher JC: The prognosis after surgical treatment for carcinoma of the rectum. Br J Surg 63:384, 1976

Williams NS, Dixon MF, et al: Reappraisal of the 5 centimetre rule of distal excision for carcinoma of the rectum: A study of distal intramural spread and of patients' survival. Br J Surg 70:150, 1983

Wilson S, Adson MA: Surgical treatment of hepatic metastases from colorectal cancer. Arch Surg 111:330, 1976

Wilson SM, Beahrs OH: The curative treatment of carcinoma of the sigmoid, rectosigmoid and rectum. Ann Surg 183:556, 1976

58. Abdominosacral Resection

S. Arthur Localio
Kenneth Eng

INTRODUCTION

Anterior resection is widely employed for treatment of cancer of the upper third of the rectum. Abdominoperineal resection is generally practiced for lesions of the lower two thirds. Although a number of operations have been advocated for sphincter-saving resection of midrectal cancers, application of these operations has been limited by questions concerning: (1) technical difficulties in achieving a sound anastomosis, (2) functional results, and (3) ultimate cure rate after resection of lesions at this level.

In our experience, the operation that best answers the requirements for resection with adequate margins, safe anastomosis, and excellent sphincter function is abdominosacral resection. The rectum is mobilized completely as in the other radical operations. The superior hemorrhoidal lymphovascular pedicle is divided and the lateral ligaments are taken at the pelvic sidewalls as far down as possible. However, the adequacy of both lateral and distal clearance may be very difficult to determine by the abdominal approach alone, particularly in the male subject, in whom the distal dissection may be blind. The addition of a transsacral incision as described by Kraske in 1885, avoids this uncertainty by providing the necessary exposure. The lower portions of the lateral ligaments, which often remain after the abdominal mobilization, are encircled and divided via the posterior incision to obtain wide lateral clearance down to the distal margin. The distal margin is measured with no tension on the bowel. The rectal wall is cleared of fat at this level and an accurate end-to-end anastomosis is done without disturbing the sphincters and their innervation. Sphincter function is consistently preserved.

Abdominosacral resection has been performed with morbidity and mortality rates and long-term survival rates comparable to anterior resection and abdominoperineal resection.

SELECTION OF PATIENTS

The level of the cancer is determined by sigmoidoscopy in the knee–chest position. The distance is measured from the anal verge to the lowest gross extension of the tumor. Men with lesions 7 to 11 cm from the anal verge and women with lesions at 5.5 to 10 cm are candidates for abdominosacral resection. Lesions above these limits are treated by anterior resection. Lesions below the midrectal level are treated by abdominoperineal resection. This method of selection has been applied to all removable growths whether the operation is palliative or curative.

Measurement of the level of the lesion by sigmoidoscopy has certain limitations. A loose extraperitoneal rectum may yield measurements considerably shorter than actually exist after mobilization of the bowel. Measurement in the knee–chest position allows the rectosigmoid to straighten and provides a more accurate estimate of the ultimate level of the lesion.

The greater ease of operating in a wide female pelvis and a more mobile extraperitoneal rectum account for the lower limits set for sphincter-saving resection in women. Individual variations in the patient's habitus are accounted for at operation. A rough estimate of the feasibility of abdominosacral resection may be determined by digital examination. The lower limit of the operation is at or just below the puborectalis sling. If the tumor lies 2 to 3

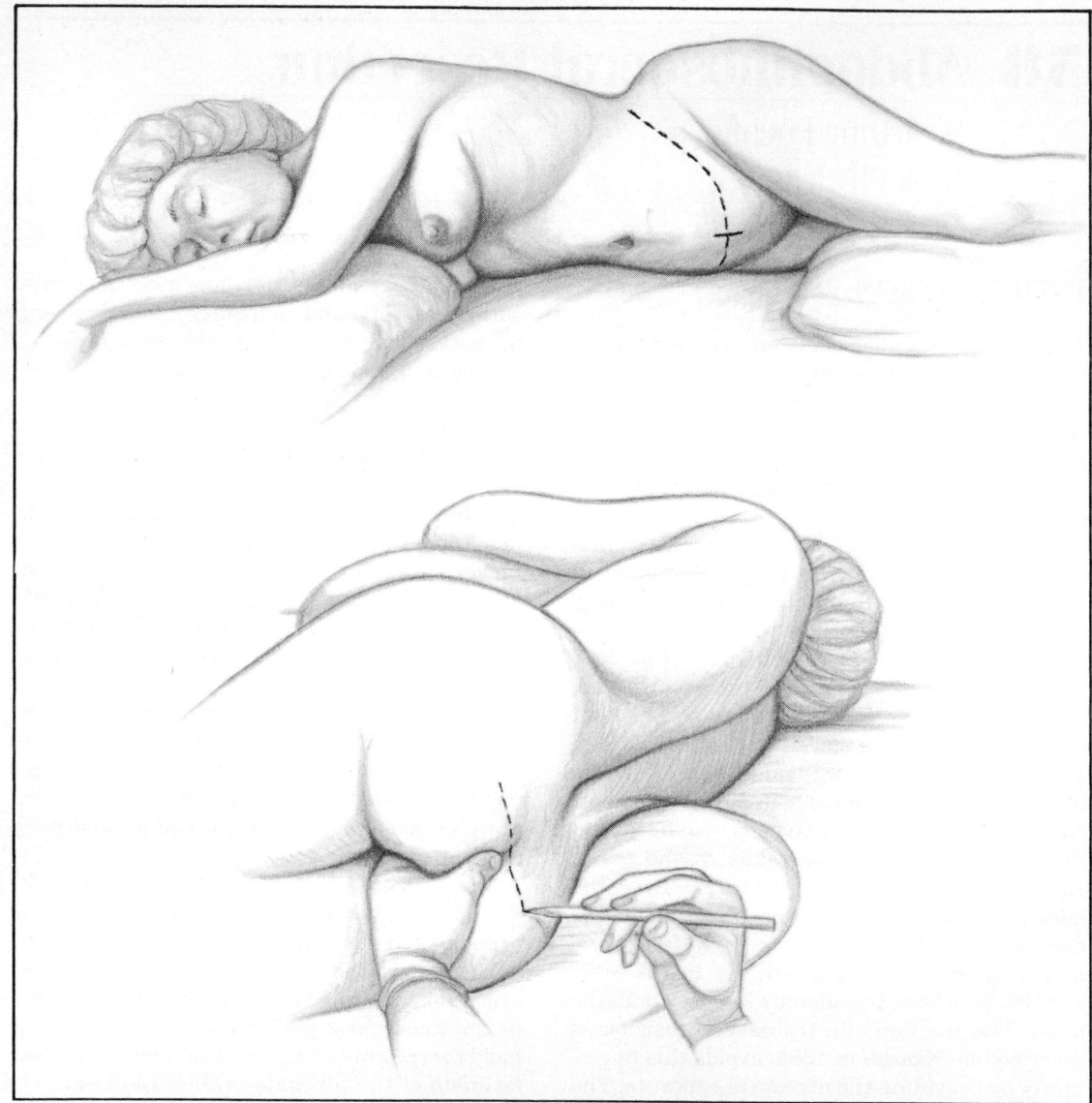

Figure 58–1. The patient is placed in the right lateral position with the buttocks and the right scapula at the edge of the operating table. The abdominal incision is marked as indicated in this figure. The posterior transverse incision is marked at the level of the sacrococcygeal joint.

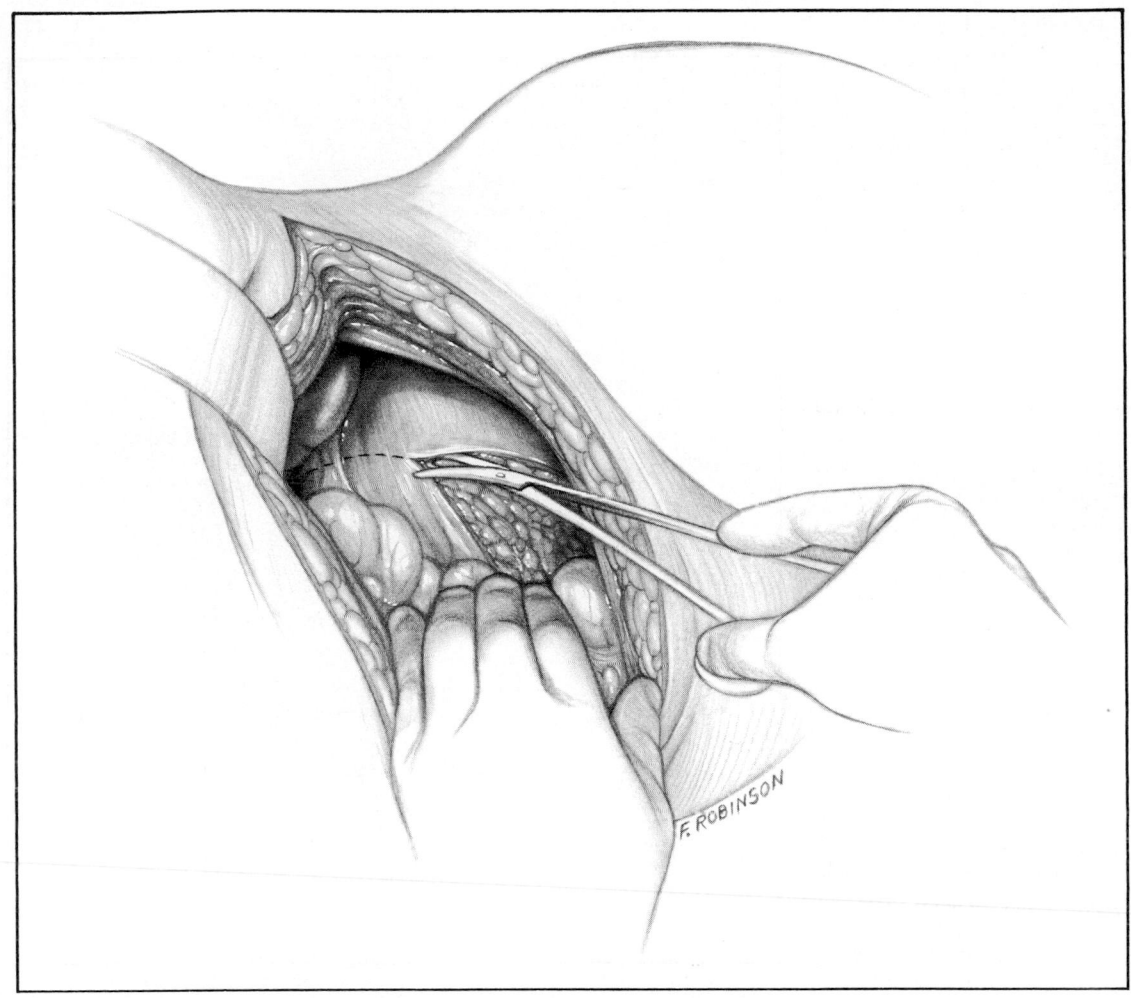

Figure 58–2. The spleen is readily seen at the lateral pole of the wound. Mobilization of the splenic flexure of the colon begins with division of the phrenocolic ligament.

cm above the puborectalis on digital exam, a 3 cm margin or more will probably be obtainable after mobilization.

Candidates for abdominosacral resection are explored in the lateral position. In about 20 percent, after mobilization of the rectum, the exposure is adequate to complete the resection and anastomosis entirely through the abdominal approach. Only rarely has abdominosacral resection been abandoned in favor of abdominoperineal resection because an adequate distal margin could not be obtained. The preoperative measurements therefore predict quite accurately whether sphincter-saving operation will be possible.

OPERATIVE TECHNIQUE

Position. The patient is placed in the right lateral position with the back and buttocks at the edge of the table (Fig. 58–1). An indwelling catheter is placed in the bladder and taped to the thigh. The rectum is irrigated with normal saline until clear returns are obtained and then with water to lyse exfoliated tumor cells. The incisions are marked, the skin prepared, and the patient is draped to provide simultaneous access to the abdominal and posterior wounds.

The abdominal phase of the operation is identical to the other radical operations for rectal cancer, but the surgeon must reorient the

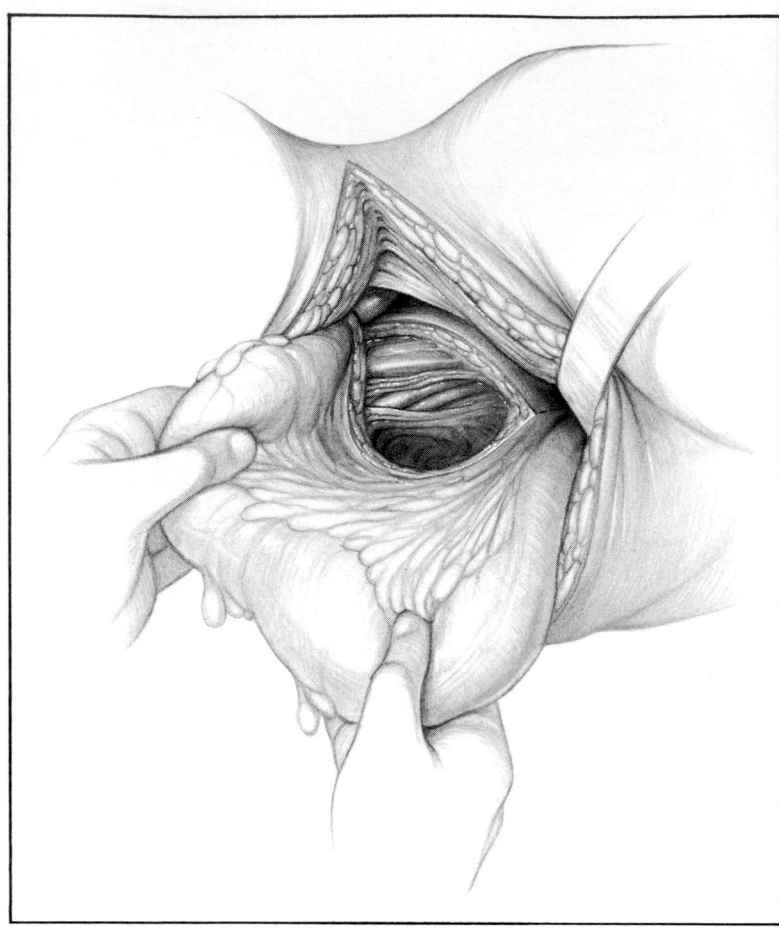

Figure 58–3. The peritoneal incision is carried down the left lumbar gutter. The colon is drawn downward to the patient's right. The left ureter is identified and traced distally. The left ureter and gonadal vessels are displaced laterally (upward).

anatomic view from the horizontal to the vertical plane. This approach facilitates mobilization and delivery of the rectosigmoid stump and proximal colon through the posterior wound and obviates the need for turning and redraping the patient. The surgeon can return to the abdomen to further mobilize the proximal colon to avoid tension on the colorectal anastomosis. If a protective colostomy is deemed necessary, it can be performed at this time. The advantages of abdominosacral resection in the lateral position are analogous to the advantages of synchronous abdominoperineal resection.

Finally, in the event that resection and anastomosis can be achieved through the abdomen alone, or in the event that an adequate distal margin cannot be obtained, anterior resection or abdominoperineal resection may be performed without repositioning and redraping the patient.

Abdominal Incision. The abdomen is opened through an oblique incision starting between the left costal margin and the iliac crest, running parallel to the inguinal ligament and curving across the rectus muscles above the pubis (Fig. 58–1). The incision is carried through all layers of the abdominal wall.

The oblique incision affords excellent exposure of the splenic flexure and the pelvic organs. After thorough exploration of the abdomen, the small bowel is delivered from the abdomen and protected by laparotomy pads. Little retraction is needed to keep the small bowel out of the way in the lateral position since this maneuver is aided by gravity.

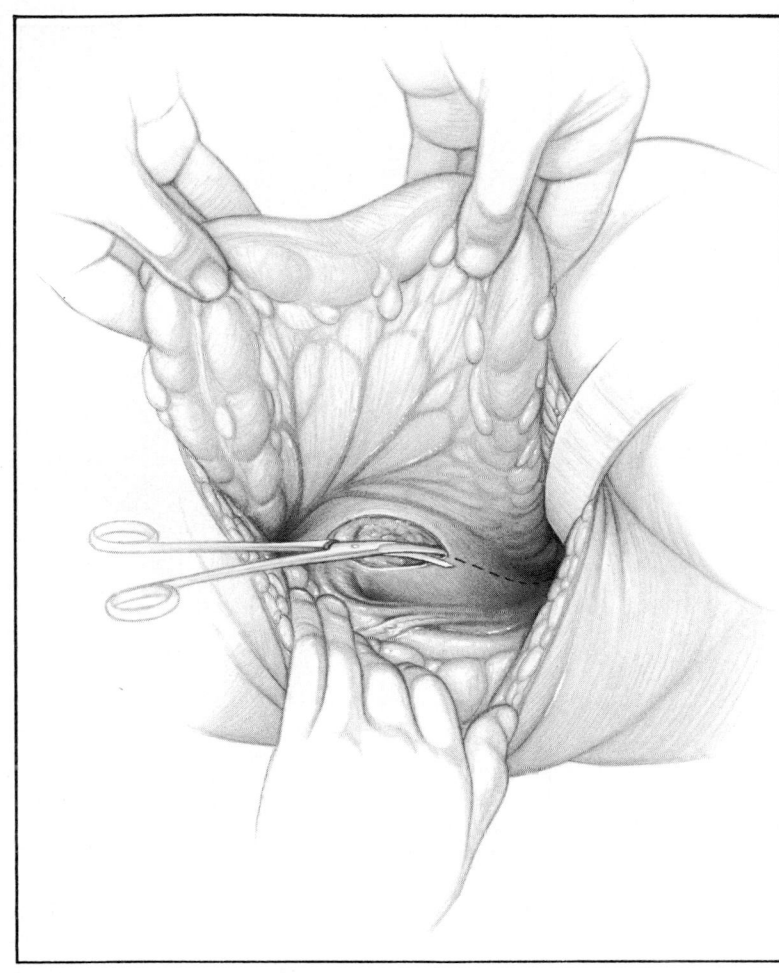

Figure 58–4. The colon is drawn upward by the first assistant. The right ureter can usually be seen through the peritoneum as it crosses the iliac vessels. The peritoneum at the base of the sigmoid mesentery is incised and the right ureter is swept laterally out of harm's way.

Mobilization of the Colon. Mobilization of the splenic flexure begins with division of the phrenocolic ligament (Fig. 58–2). The omentum is separated from the transverse colon by sharp dissection in the embryonic fusion plane. This is carried far enough to the right to allow the transverse colon to rotate on the middle colic artery. The attachments of the omentum to spleen may be divided at this time to allow the omentum to reach the pelvis. The left colon is drawn downward to the patient's right and its lateral peritoneal attachments are divided. The peritoneal incision is carried down the lumbar gutter into the pelvis. The left gonadal vessels and the left ureter are identified and swept laterally (Fig. 58–3)

The colon is then drawn upward to the patient's left and the right leaf of the sigmoid mesentery is incised at its base (Fig. 58–4). The right ureter is identified and swept laterally. The sigmoid mesentery containing the superior hemorrhoidal vessels and lymphatics is now easily swept upward from the aorta. This lymphovascular pedicle is isolated, clamped, divided, and suture ligated, usually at the level of the origin of the left colic artery (Fig. 58–5).

Mobilization of the left colon should be sufficient to allow it to lie loosely in the pelvis conforming to the curve of the sacrum. The left colic artery may be divided at its origin when additional length is necessary because the left colon is often tethered by this vessel. In that case, the marginal artery must be preserved since the blood supply to the colon stump is now based on the middle colic artery. The mesosigmoid is divided to the site selected for the proxi-

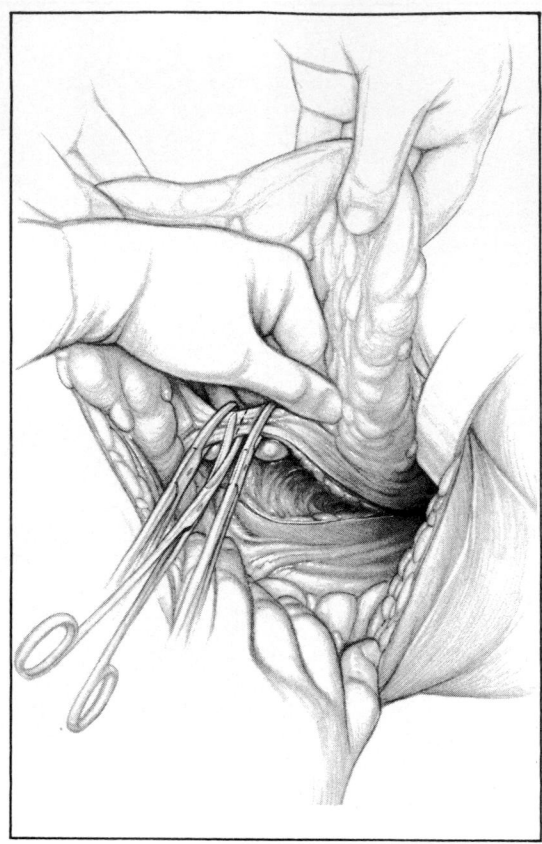

Figure 58–5. The superior hemorrhoidal vessels are divided.

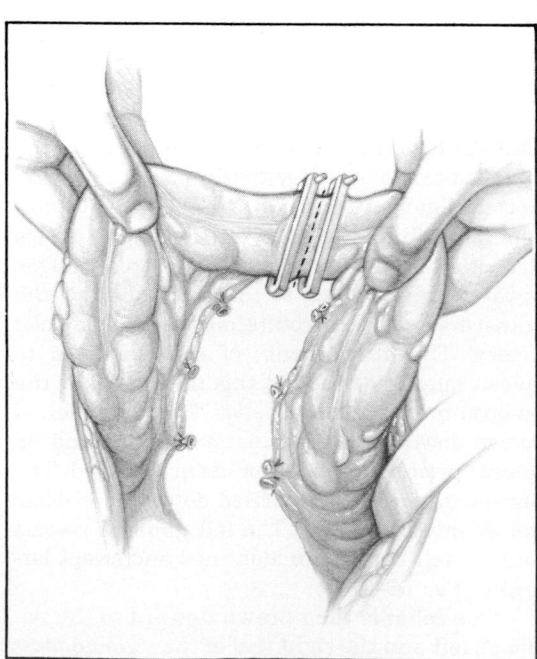

Figure 58–6. Division of the colon at the proximal limit of resection between Cope–deMartel clamps. (The latch of the Cope–deMartel clamp may be used as a marker to prevent axial rotation.)

With the anterior and posterior dissections completed, the lateral ligaments of the rectum containing the middle hemorrhoidal vessels are identified. The left lateral ligament is divided first. The broad band of tissue, which is the lateral ligament, is dissected as far distally as possible, encircled with the finger, clamped near the pelvic sidewall, divided, and ligated (Fig. 58–9). Upward displacement of the rectum now exposes the right lateral ligament which is also encircled, divided, and ligated (Fig. 58–10).

The rectum has now been mobilized as completely as possible. The seminal vesicles or upper vagina are visible. The tip of the coccyx, the levator ani muscle diaphragm, and the puborectalis sling are palpable. If mobilization provides sufficient length to permit anterior resection, the operation is completed through the abdomen. However, with very low lesions, particularly in men, the tumor may be barely in view. Determination of an adequate distal margin will be uncertain, and the anastomosis will be hazardous. Therefore, abdominosacral resec-

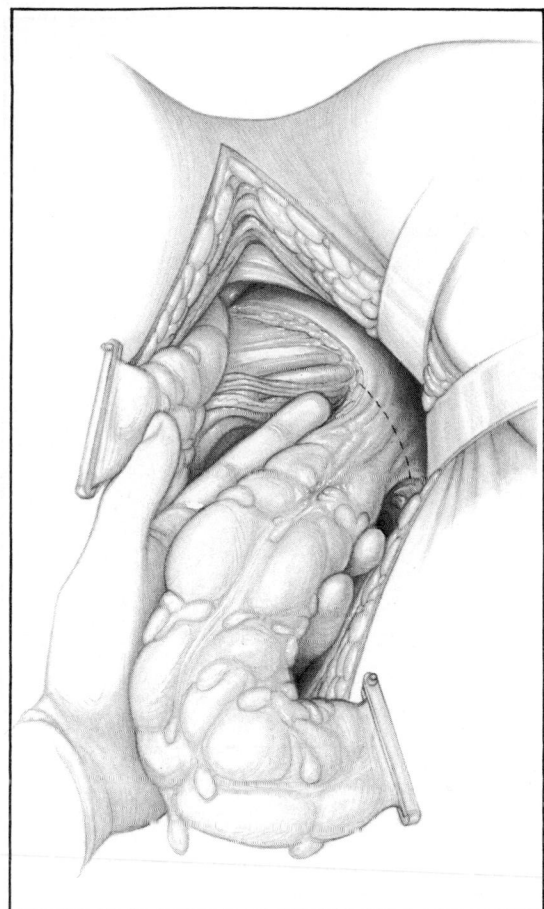

Figure 58–7. The rectum is mobilized from the hollow of the sacrum in the loose areolar plane anterior to the middle sacral vessels and the presacral plexus of veins.

mal margin. Cope–deMartel or other appropriate clamps are applied at this site and the colon is divided (Fig. 58–6). The left border of the colon is marked with a stitch to aid in avoiding axial rotation when the proximal colon is delivered through the posterior wound.

MOBILIZATION OF THE RECTUM. The rectum is mobilized from the hollow of the sacrum by blunt dissection in the loose areolar plane anterior to the middle sacral artery and presacral venous plexus (Fig. 58–7). The peritoneal incisions at the base of the mesosigmoid are continued anteriorly to meet in the cul-de-sac and the anterior wall of the rectum is freed to the level of the seminal vesicles or upper vagina (Fig. 58–8).

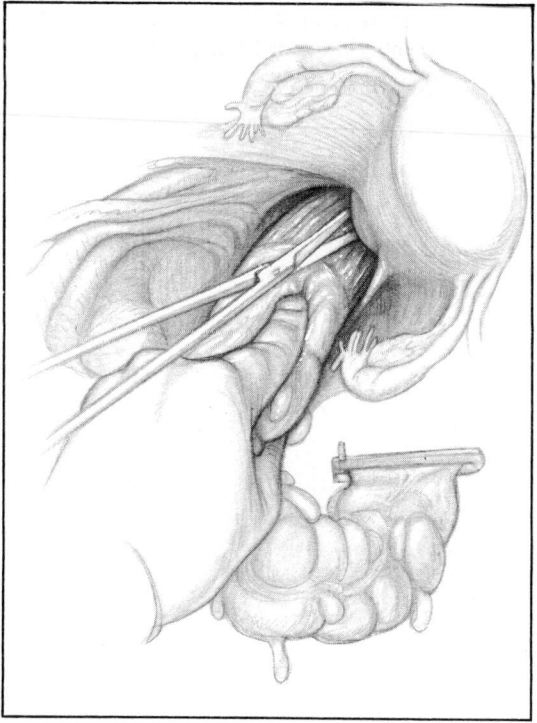

Figure 58–8. The peritoneum of the cul-de-sac is incised and the anterior wall of the rectum is separated from the seminal vesicles or the upper vagina.

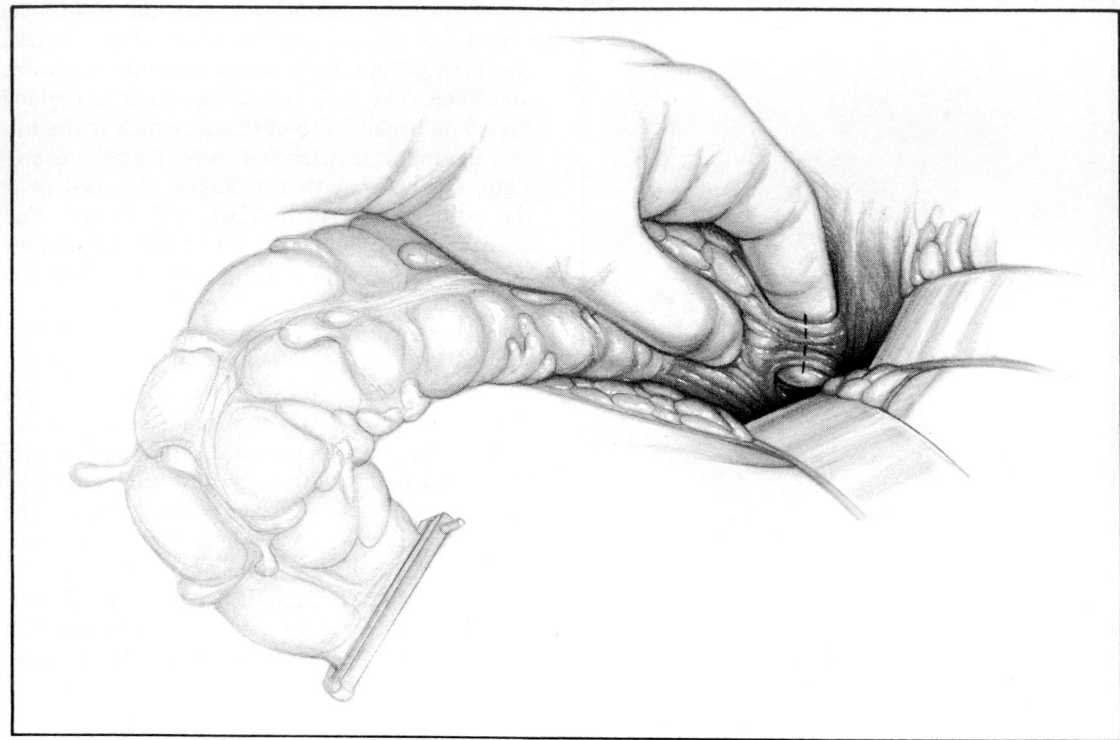

Figure 58–9. The left lateral ligament containing the middle hemorrhoidal vessels is encircled first, then divided and ligated.

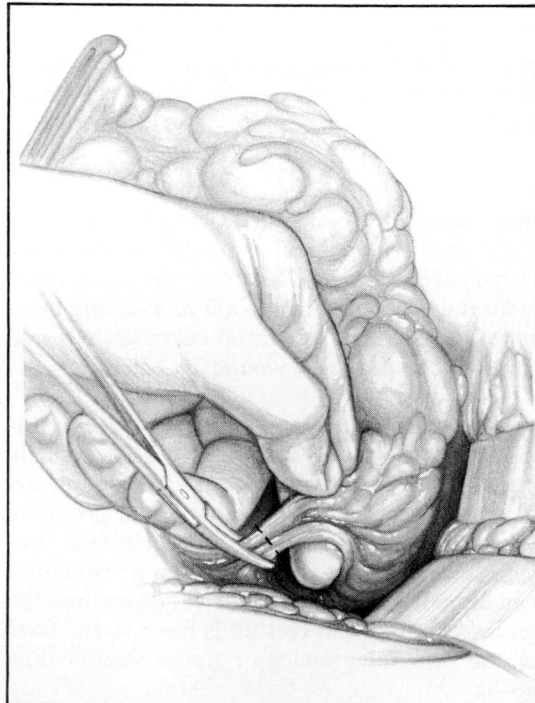

Figure 58–10. Upward displacement of the rectum now readily exposes the right lateral ligament that is also encircled, divided, and ligated.

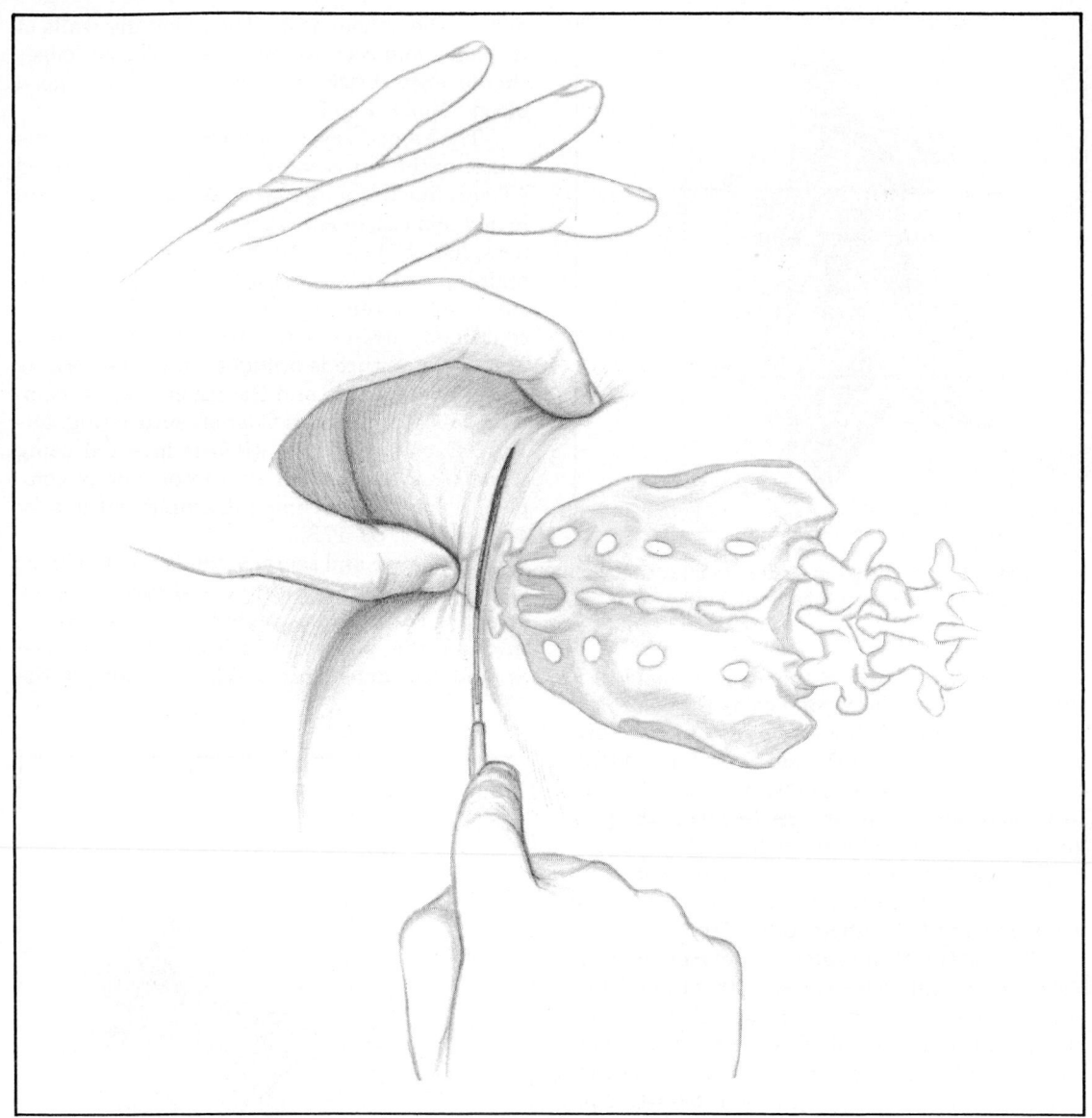

Figure 58–11. Posterior transverse incision is made over the sacrococcygeal joint. Depression of the coccyx defines sacrococcygeal joint and this cartilaginous joint is easily disarticulated with a knife.

tion will be necessary. Before proceeding to the posterior incision, the pelvis is irrigated with saline and meticulous hemostasis is achieved.

Posterior Dissection. A transverse incision is made over the sacrococcygeal joint (Fig. 58–11). Depression of the tip of the coccyx defines this cartilaginous junction. Disarticulation can usually be accomplished with a knife. The coccyx

is excised. The posterior attachments of the levator muscles are separated with scissors to enter the presacral space (Fig. 58–12). The opening is enlarged by blunt dissection, splitting the levators in the direction of their fibers. A transverse incision is suitable because it may be lengthened without limitation by the sacrum or the anus. If necessary, the gluteal muscles may be split for further exposure.

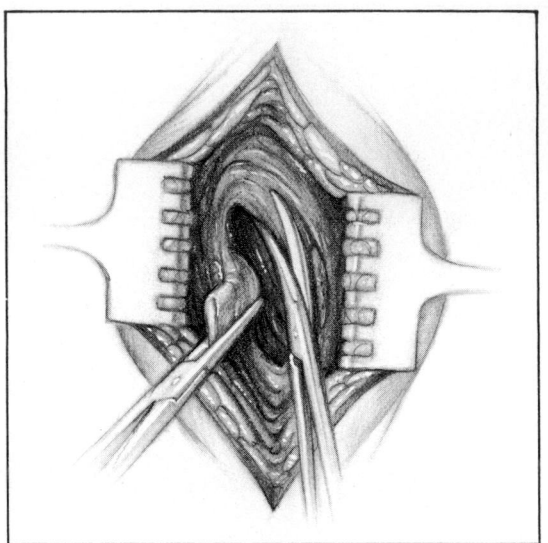

Figure 58–12. The coccyx has been disarticulated and dissected from the fibers of the levator ani.

The rectosigmoid stump is now delivered through the posterior wound using the deMartel clamp as a handle. The lower rectum can now be mobilized further for wide lateral and distal clearance. The lowest portions of the lateral ligaments, which remain, are divided at the pelvic sidewalls. The anterior surface of the rectum can be freed from the prostate or the lower vaginal wall. The posterior surface of the rectum is dissected to the puborectalis sling.

The extent of the tumor is determined and the distal margin is measured with a ruler. This site, at least 3 cm from the lowest extension of the cancer, is cleared of fat down to the bare longitudinal muscle. A right angle renal pedicle clamp is applied at this site (Fig. 58–13). The proximal colonic stump is then delivered, taking care to avoid axial rotation of the bowel. The latch of the deMartel clamp or the marking stitch is a convenient guide for maintaining proper orientation of the colon (Fig. 58–14). An extra 3 to 4 cm of proximal colon is pulled through posteriorly as illustrated. This allows the suturing to be done without hinderance by the deMartel clamp.

Anastomosis. A series of interrupted Cushing stitches of 4-0 silk are placed (Fig. 58–14), taking care that the sutures in the rectum are at right angles to the longitudinal muscle. After all the sutures have been placed, they are tied and cut, retaining the first and the last to mark the cor-

ners of the anastomosis. The adjoining walls of the colon and rectum are incised. The cut edges should show brisk bleeding indicating a good blood supply (Fig. 58–15).

The second row of sutures is started at the center of the anastomosis, using a double armed 4-0 chromic catgut or Dexon suture. This suture is tied and run in both directions as a full thickness, loosely locked stitch (Fig. 58–16). The remaining wall of the rectum is divided and the specimen is removed. Excess proximal colon contained within the deMartel clamp is excised. The catgut suture is brought out at the corners of the anastomosis and the inner layer is completed as a continuous Connell suture (Fig. 58–17A). Each silk corner stitch is inverted using a mattress suture and the outer row is completed using interrupted Cushing sutures of 4-0 silk (Fig. 58–17B).

The pelvic and sacral wounds are now thoroughly irrigated with saline and careful hemostasis secured. The omentum is delivered through the posterior incision and wrapped around the anastomosis. The position of the

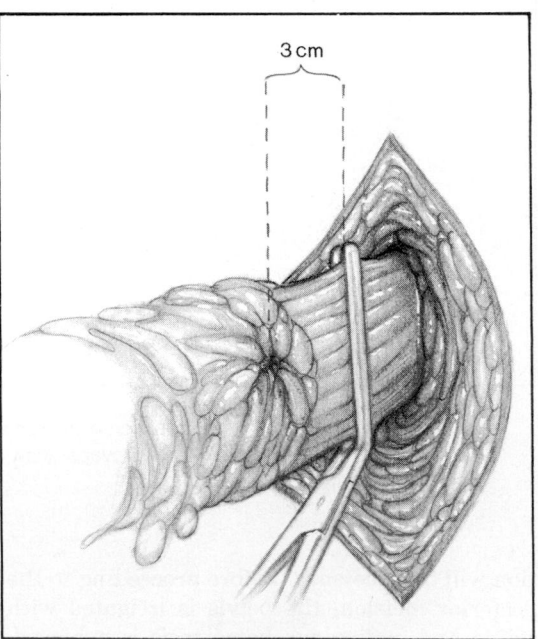

Figure 58–13. The distal (rectosigmoid) colon has been delivered through the posterior incision. Further mobilization is done as necessary to obtain adequate lateral and distal clearance. The distal margin is measured, the rectal wall is cleared of fat, and a right angle clamp is applied at this point, which is at least 3 cm below the palpable limit of the tumor.

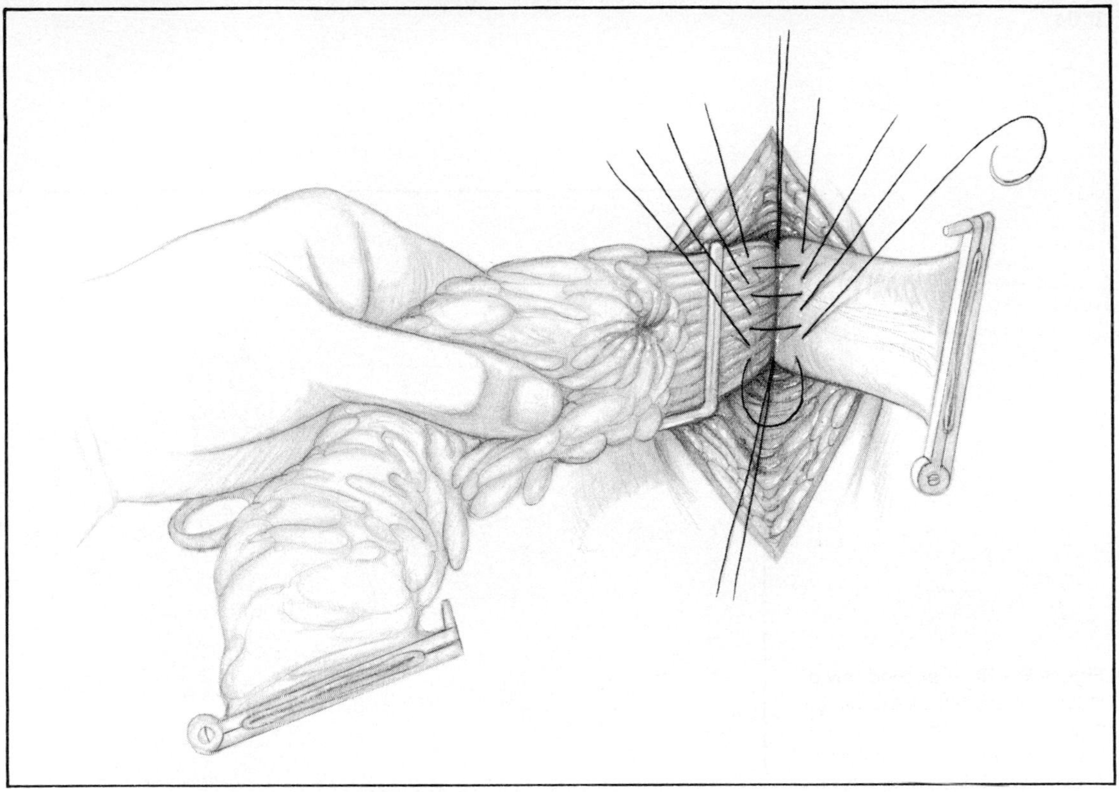

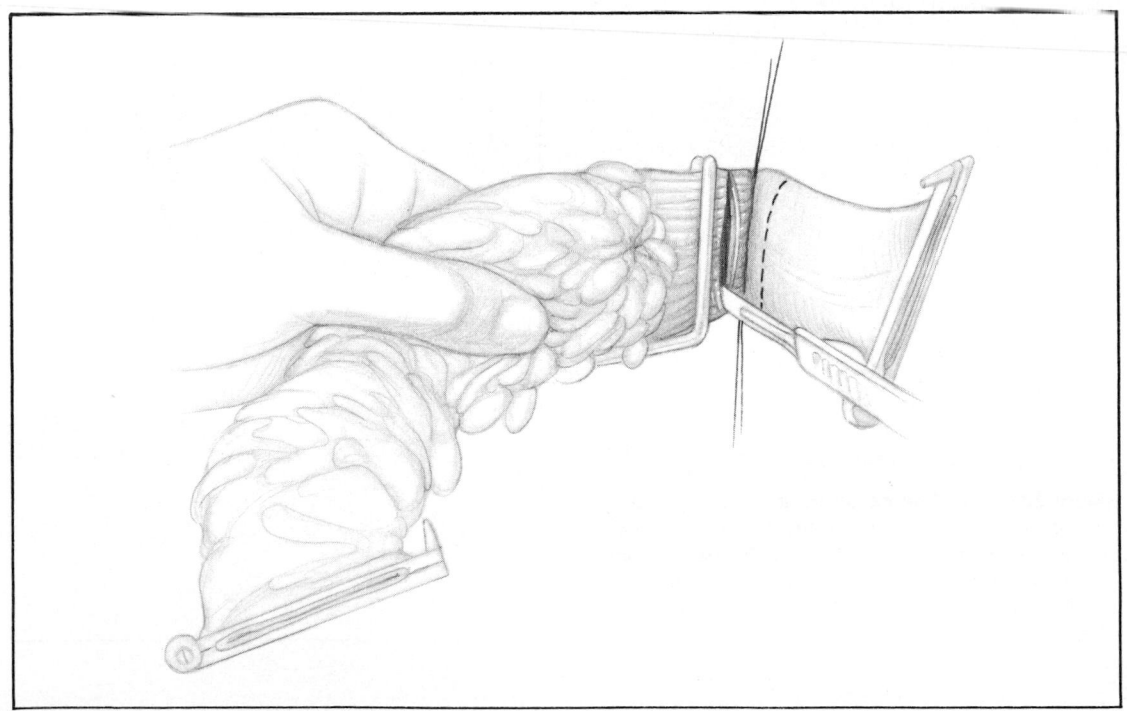

Figure 58–14. Proximal colon has been delivered through the posterior incision. A series of interrupted 4-0 silk Cushing sutures are placed.

Figure 58–15. The rectum and descending colon are incised.

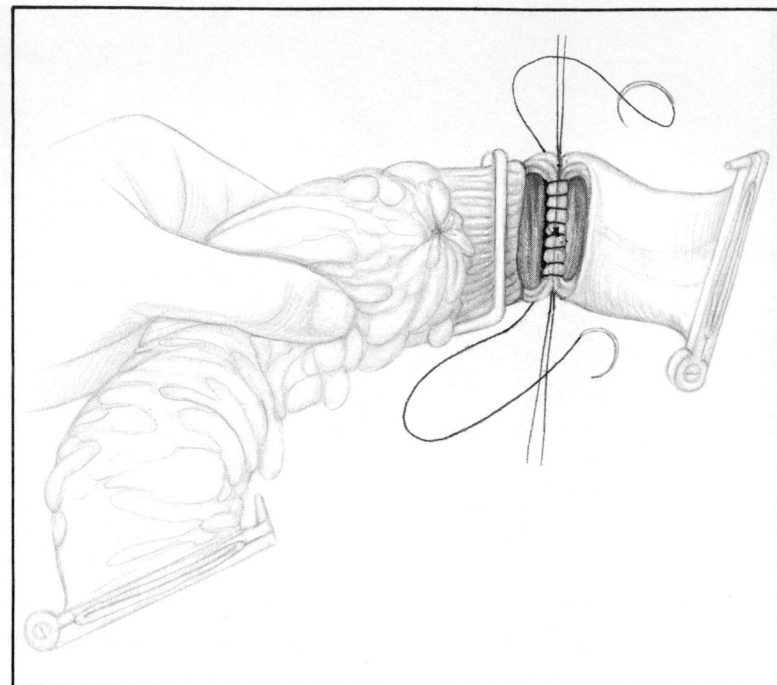

Figure 58–16. A second row of sutures is started at the center of the anastomosis using a double-armed 4-0 chromic catgut or Dexon suture. This suture is tied and run in both directions as a full thickness, loosely locked stitch.

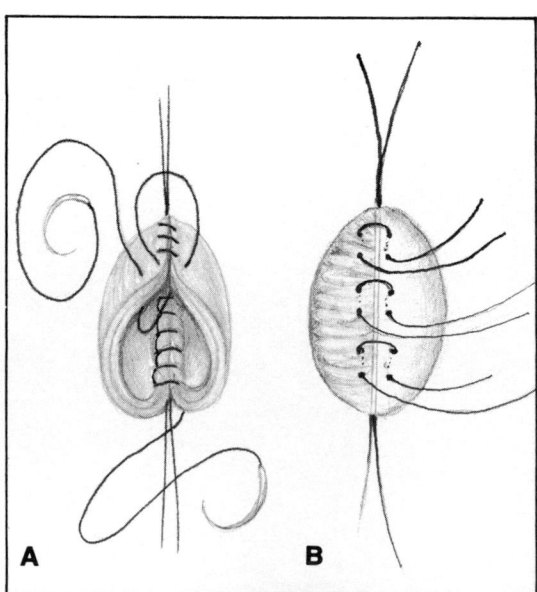

Figure 58–17. A. The catgut suture is brought out at the corners of the anastomosis and the inner layer completed as a continuous Connell suture. **B.** The anastomosis is completed with a series of 4-0 silk interrupted Cushing sutures. A purse string suture is placed at each corner.

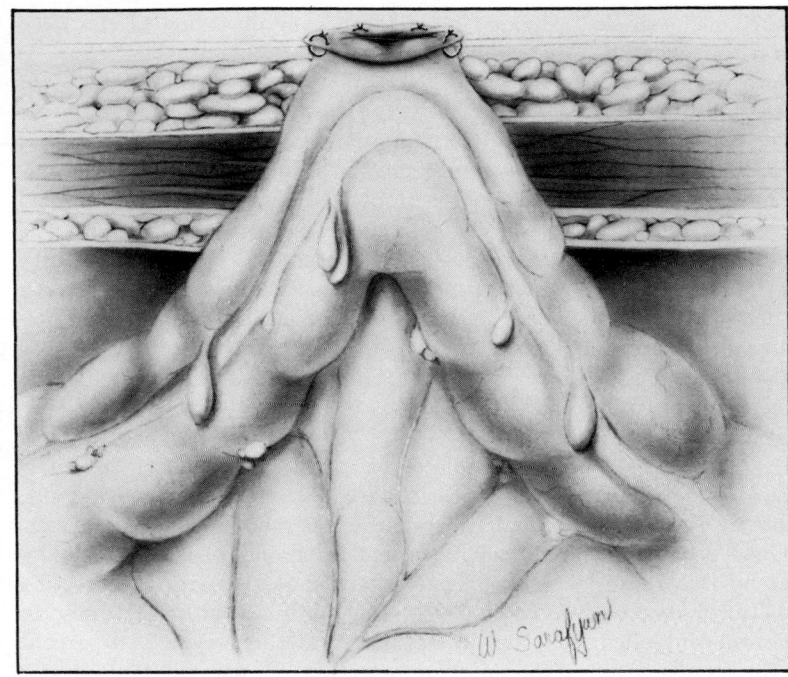

Figure 58–18. Simplified colostomy. A 2 cm skin aperture and a long incision in the peritoneum, muscle, and fascia produce a conical defect in the abdominal wall. A short incision is made in the antimesenteric wall of the colon, and the intestine is sutured to the skin only. (*Source: From Eng K, Localio SA, 1981, with permission of Surgery, Gynecology & Obstetrics.*)

omentum may be maintained by tacking it to the levator ani with several sutures.

No attempt is made to close the defect in the pelvic peritoneum. Loops of small bowel will fill the pelvic dead space and fluid accumulating in the pelvis can drain into the peritoneal cavity. As an added precaution, a soft closed suction drain of silicone rubber may be left in the pelvis. Drainage volumes of 100 to 250 cm³ are not unusual in the first 48 hours. The drain is removed as soon as possible.

Protective Colostomy. Our early experience indicated that anastomotic complications occurred most frequently in young men, presumably due to a narrow pelvis with a heavy muscular pelvic diaphragm. Therefore, colostomy is employed routinely in men 65 years or younger. We do not hesitate to add a colostomy if any doubt exists as to the integrity of the anastomosis. We have employed completely diverting colostomy, loop colostomy, and cecostomy in this setting. More recently, we have constructed a simplified colostomy which consists of a small skin aperture and a large defect in the abdominal wall (Fig. 58–18). This allows the colon to rise to the skin level where a small lateral opening is sutured to the skin only. With adequate mechanical bowel preparation and a satisfac-

tory anastomosis complete diversion is unnecessary. In the first 5 to 9 days intraluminal contents consist of only liquid and gas. A lateral opening, which bleeds off liquid and gas, prevents distention and offers sufficient protection. In fact, when bowel function returns, almost all stool is discharged through this lateral stoma. This colostomy may be closed in several weeks, often under local anesthesia.

RESULTS

In a 15-year period, 646 consecutive patients with primary adenocarcinoma of the rectum were assigned to operation according to the level of the lesion as outlined in the section on selection of patients. The operation was anterior resection in 320, abdominosacral resection in 175, and abdominoperineal resection in 151.

Mortality and Morbidity

The mortality and morbidity risk of abdominosacral resection is comparable to anterior resection and abdominoperineal resection. The mortality rate was 2.2 percent after anterior resection, 2.3 percent after abdominosacral resection, and 2.0 percent after abdominoperineal resection. Morbidity following each of the three operations was also comparable with the exception of anastomotic complications.

Anastomotic leaks were detected in 4 percent of 495 patients after anterior resection and abdominosacral resection. There were three leaks after 320 anterior resections (1 percent) and 17 after 175 abdominosacral resections (9.7 percent). Anastomotic leaks occurred more frequently in men (12.5 percent) than in women (6.3 percent). The leak rate was highest in young men which led to the routine use of protective colostomy in men 65 years or younger. There has been some improvement in the leak rate from 12 percent in the first 100 patients to 6.7 percent in the last 75.

The presence of the posterior wound in abdominosacral resection undoubtedly increased the detection rate for small leaks because of the easy egress of fecal matter by this route. In fact, most of the leaks (13 of 17) after abdominosacral resection resulted in well-controlled posterior fistulas. Nonetheless, the anastomosis after abdominosacral resection is lower than that after anterior resection and is therefore inherently more tenuous. Moreover, the posterior wound in close proximity to the anastomotic suture line may actually predispose to leakage. For this reason, the omentum is interposed between the anastomosis and the posterior wound whenever possible. All fistulas healed after temporary diversion of the fecal stream.

CONTINENCE

Sphincter function following abdominosacral resection is normal in every case. As in all low rectal resections, the loss of the rectosigmoid reservoir results in frequent small stools in the early postoperative period. However, the ultimate functional results following abdominosacral resection are indistinguishable from anterior resection.

Long-Term Survival

The crude 5-year survival rate after 360 curative operations was 60.6 percent. Five-year survival rate was 66.2 percent for anterior resection, 62.9 percent for abdominosacral resection, and 43.4 percent for abdominoperineal resection (Table 58–1). For patients with no tumor in lymph nodes, survival rates were 73.9 percent for anterior resection, 75 percent for anterior resection, and 59.5 percent for abdominoperineal resection. With tumor in regional nodes, survival rate fell to 45.2 percent for anterior resection, 37.9 percent for abdominosacral resection, and 17.2 percent for abdominoperineal resection. Patients fared no worse after abdominosacral resection than after anterior resection and somewhat better than after abdominoperi-

TABLE 58–1. CRUDE 5-YEAR SURVIVAL AFTER 360 CURATIVE RESECTIONS FOR RECTAL CANCER (1966–1976)

Operation	Dukes' Classification	No. of Patients	5-Year Survivors	5-Year Survivors (%)
Anterior resection	A	62	57	91.9
	B	80	48	60.0
	C	53	24	45.3[a]
	All	195	129	66.2[b]
Abdominosacral resection	A	31	27	87.1
	B	29	18	62.1
	C	29	11	37.9
	All	89	56	62.9[b]
Abdominoperineal resection	A	21	17	80.9
	B	26	11	42.3
	C	29	5	17.2[a]
	All	76	33	43.4[b]

[a] Abdominoperineal resection vs anterior resection $p < .001$; abdominoperineal resection vs abdominosacral resection $p < .02$.
[b] Dukes' classification: Abdominoperineal resection vs anterior resection $p < .02$.

neal resection. Survival rate was determined by stage of disease and, to a certain extent, the level of the tumor, but not the operation performed.

Pelvic recurrence rate was 13.3 percent after anterior resection, 14.6 percent after abdominosacral resection, and 13.3 percent after abdominoperineal resection. Pelvic recurrence rate, like survival rate, was determined by the stage of disease and not by the operation performed.

CONCLUSIONS

Abdominosacral resection is the most reliable radical sphincter-saving operation for midrectal cancers, which are too low for anterior resection. The posterior incision provides maximum exposure for wide resection of the tumor, a measured distal margin, and an accurate anastomosis. The procedure can be carried out consistently to the pelvic floor without disrupting the anal sphincters and their innervation. Sphincter function is consistently preserved. Mortality rate is no higher than for other radical rectal resections. Morbidity can be limited by the se-

lective use of protective colostomy. Abdominosacral resection is applicable to a large proportion of patients with rectal cancer. In the treatment of 646 consecutive patients with rectal cancer, fewer than 25 percent (151) required abdominoperineal resection. More than 50 percent of the patients (175) with lesions too low for anterior resection were spared a permanent colostomy by the use of abdominosacral resection. Abdominosacral resection provides the maximum clearance around the tumor and long-term follow-up has revealed no greater risk of local recurrence or death from cancer.

BIBLIOGRAPHY

Eng K, Localio SA: Simplified complementary transverse colostomy for low colorectal anastomosis. Surg Gynecol Obstet 153:734, 1981

Kraske P: Zur extirpation hochsitzender mastdarmkrebs. Verh Dtsch Ges Chir 14:464, 1885

Localio SA, Eng K: Malignant tumors of the rectum, in Ravitch MM (ed): Current Problems in Surgery. Chicago: Yearbook, 1975

Localio SA, Eng K, et al: Abdominosacral resection for midrectal cancer: 15 years experience. Ann Surg 198:81, 1983

59. Abdominoperineal Resection

Harold Ellis

In the management of any given condition, one treatment frequently stands out as the standard against which all others must be measured in terms of safety and effectiveness. The Miles operation or abdominoperineal resection is that treatment for carcinoma of the rectum. It has become a classic surgical procedure, and its details have changed little since it was first described by Miles in 1908. The purpose of the operation is to remove the rectum: the site of the tumour, the anus, and the distal colon (sigmoid), along with the perianal and perirectal tissues and the mesentery of the sigmoid colon. In so doing, the three areas of regional lymphatic spread are excised en bloc with the primary tumour: the area proximally along the superior haemorrhoidal vessels, the area laterally along the lateral attachments of the rectum and the middle hemorrhoidal vessels, and the area of spread distally along the inferior vessels (Fig. 59–1). Unfortunately, cancer of the rectum also spreads by blood vessel invasion, and when this has occurred the operative procedure becomes palliative in that the local operation does not remove the areas of distant spread.

In this operation the entire anus, anal canal, and rectum, together with surrounding levator ani muscles and fatty tissues, are removed. The pelvic mesocolon together with lymphatic vessels and lymph nodes, the peritoneum lining the floor as well as most of the walls of the true pelvis, and a portion of the sigmoid loop are also removed. Since the anus and rectum are removed in the Miles operation, a permanent colostomy is established as a site of evacuation of bowel content. This is essential when regional spread of disease has occurred. However, it is unfortunate when a colostomy is established when unnecessary and when it does not contribute to the future well-being of the patient. This further leads to the use of alternative operations that preserve anal function: low anterior resection, pull-through operations, abdominosacral procedures, and local operations such as local excision, electrocoagulation, cryosurgery, and radiation treatment.

Although Miles deserves the credit for proposing the procedure as a planned operation for cancer of the rectum, it is of interest that in 1884 Czerny, while attempting to excise a high rectal growth by the posterior approach, was forced to open the abdomen to complete the operation. The patient died, but the idea was born. In 1904 Charles Mayo described a technique of combined abdominoperineal excision. In 1903 he mentioned that Quenu and Gaudier of Lille proposed such an operation for complete removal of the growth with its lymphatic fields.

In the classic Miles operation the abdominal and perineal portions of the dissection are performed sequentially and carried out by one surgical team. Generally speaking, the patient will be in the supine position for the abdominal portion; then, after the abdominal incision is closed, the patient will be placed in the lithotomy position, and the perineal portion of the procedure will be carried out. It is interesting that Mayo's description in 1904 recommends doing these procedures in a combined fashion with essentially a two-team approach: "If the surgeon has a good assistant, the perineal operation, with the removal of the rectum, can be performed by him during the same time the abdominal work is advancing above."

In Britain, synchronised or combined excision of the rectum was first performed by Lloyd-Davies and Morgan at St. Mark's Hospital in 1938. This procedure offers the advantage of being performed by two teams simultaneously. Certainly in the United Kingdom this technique

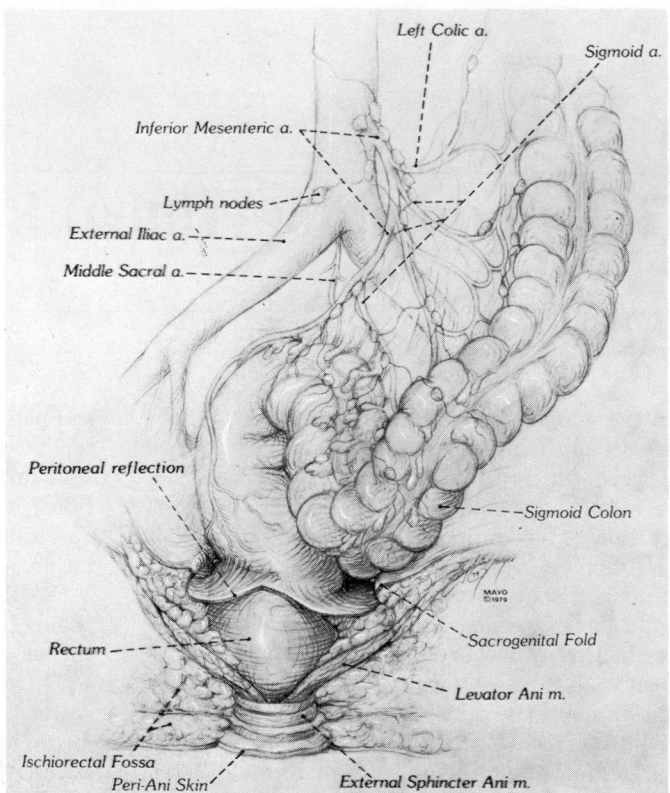

Figure 59–1. Tissues sacrificed in the abdominoperineal resection should include not only the primary cancer in the lower rectum but also the areas of regional spread—proximally, laterally, and distally.

is almost invariably employed, and it is the synchronous combined operation that will be described here. If necessary, however, one surgeon can perform the abdominal and then the perineal dissection.

OPERATIVE TECHNIQUE

Abdominal Dissection

Much of this section is based on the excellent description of this operation by Lloyd-Davies from the previous edition. Preliminary bowel preparation is as described for other major elective large bowel operations.

In synchronous combined excision of the rectum, both the abdominal and perineal fields are exposed at one and the same time. It is a team operation, two surgeons working synchronously, one from the abdominal aspect and the other from the perineum.

The patient is placed in a modified lithotomy position, using special leg rests designed in 1938 by Lloyd-Davies. These extend the thighs away from the abdomen (Fig. 59–2). The sacrum is raised upon a sandbag or sacral rest so that the sacrococcygeal region projects over the end of the table, giving an adequate exposure of the coccyx for the perineal operator. The rest also tilts the pelvis anteriorly and thus lessens the degree of Trendelenburg tilt required by the abdominal operator. A full Trendelenburg is often required, and the Frankis Evans epaulette shoulder rests are highly satisfactory and give full protection to the brachial plexus. The arms should be well protected and placed at the sides.

As soon as the patient is anaesthetised, a self-retaining catheter is passed and connected to a sterile collecting bag that is suspended under the table. The penis and scrotum are strapped to the right thigh.

An intravenous infusion is essential and is set up before the start of the operation, using Hartmann's solution and blood during the operation.

A long left paramedian muscle-sliding inci-

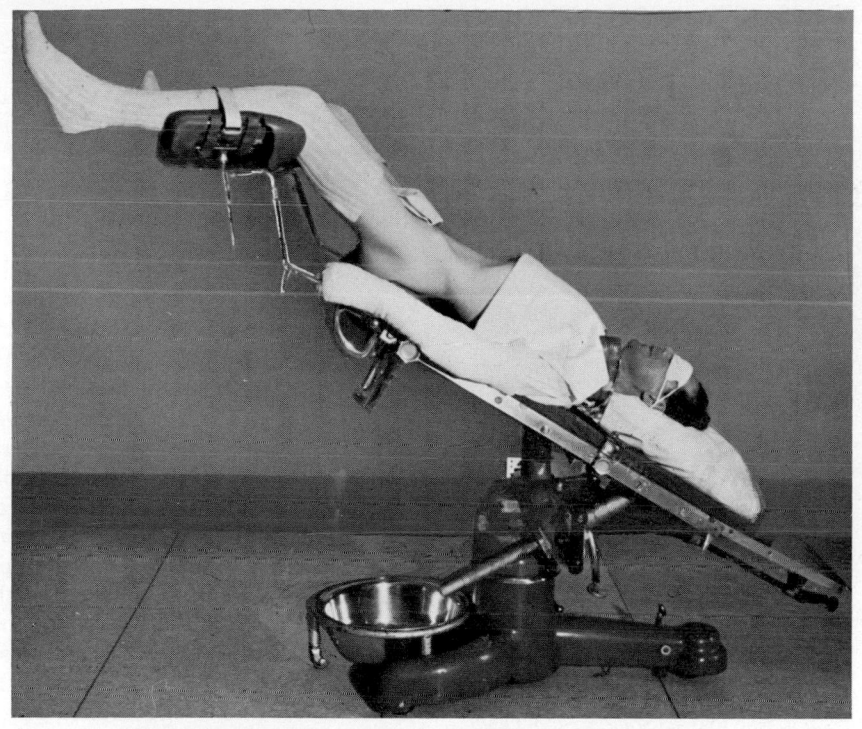

A

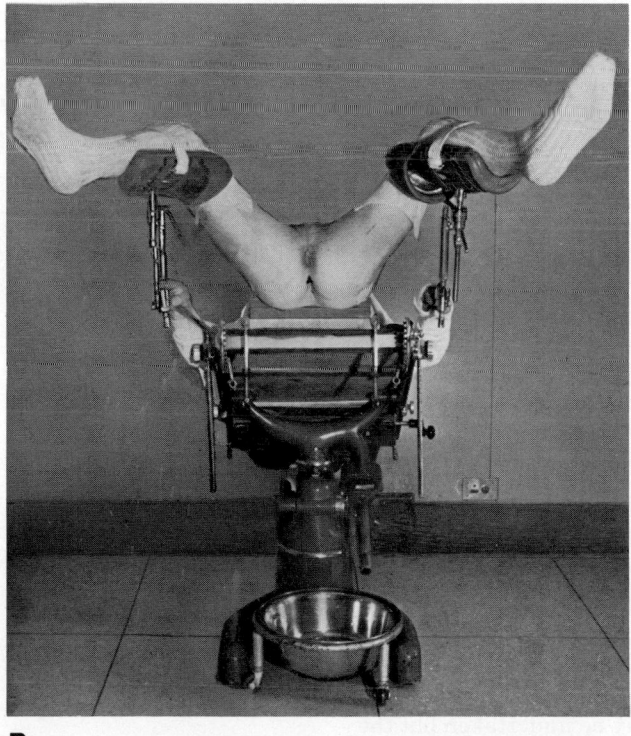

B

Figure 59–2. Lithotomy-Trendelenburg position using special leg supports. (*Source: From Lloyd-Davies OV: Abdomino-perineal excision of the rectum, in Rob C, Smith R (eds): Operative Surgery, 2 edt. London: Butterworths, 1969, with permission.*)

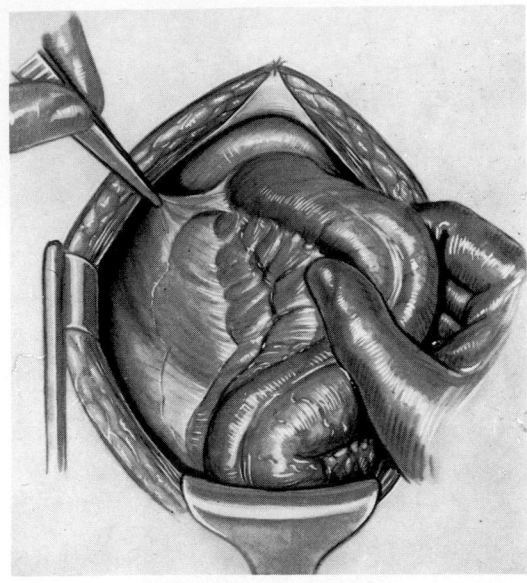

Figure 59–3. Dissection of congenital peritoneal folds attaching iliac colon to iliac fossa. (*Source: From Lloyd-Davies OV: Abdomino-perineal excision of the rectum, in Rob C, Smith R (eds): Operative Surgery, 2 edt. London: Butterworths, 1969, with permission.*)

Regarding fixity, no case should be abandoned until determined trial dissections have been made upon the fixed aspects of the bowel, because fixity is frequently caused by perirectal inflammation.

Following the assessment of the case, both operators commence the dissection, but the abdominal aspect will be described first:

The first step is the careful packing away of the abdominal viscera, apart from the sigmoid loop, into the upper abdomen so that the pelvis is emptied of all but the lower bowel. Next is the careful freeing of the iliac colon from the left iliac fossa (Fig. 59–3). This part of the colon is always found to be partially fixed by a variable number of adventitious peritoneal folds; their attachment to the lateral aspect of the mesocolon is indicated by a whitish serrated line. Division of these folds at the apex of their attachment is carried out with a pair of light curved dissecting scissors until the full length of the mesocolon is exposed. In this way sufficient peritoneum will be preserved to cover the upper part of the pelvic floor at the end of the operation.

sion has been found to give the best exposure. The abdomen is systematically examined, commencing with the liver and concluding in the pelvis. The position, size, fixity of the tumour, and the lymphatic and peritoneal spread are assessed, and a decision is made upon the operability and type of operation required. Growths situated at and above the pelvic peritoneal reflection may frequently be dealt with radically by a restorative resection (e.g., anterior resection). Most growths situated *below* the peritoneal reflection require a combined excision to give the patient the greatest possible chance of cure.

Regarding liver metastases, it has been found to be of definite benefit to proceed with the excision of the primary growth to prevent sacral pain and rectal discharge, provided the liver is not grossly involved and enlarged by the deposits. In favourable cases, where deposits are present in only one lobe of the liver, a right or left hepatectomy may be undertaken but the decision about this is best left for an interval of 3 months after the excision operation, when a more accurate determination can be made as to whether only one lobe is involved.

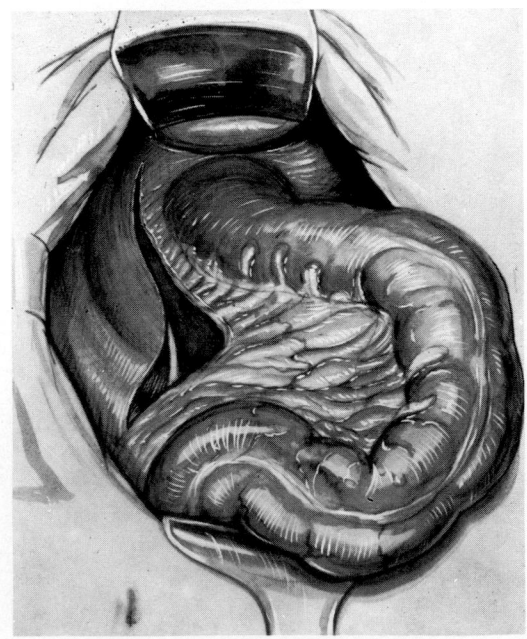

Figure 59–4. Exposure of left ureter. (*Source: From Lloyd-Davies OV: Abdomino-perineal excision of the rectum, in Rob C, Smith R (eds): Operative Surgery, 2 edt. London: Butterworths, 1969, with permission.*)

An incision is then made on the lateral aspect of the base of the mesocolon as it crosses the common iliac vessels, and the left ureter is exposed (Fig. 59–4). A finger placed over the ureter sweeps it away from the posterior aspect of the mesocolon and prevents any possibility of its being included in the main ligature. The vessels to the pelvic mesocolon, which are often quite variable, are then inspected and the site of division of the main pedicle selected (Fig. 59–5).

Some surgeons advocate ligation of the blood supply to the rectum at the origin of the inferior mesenteric artery. However, ligating the vessel at this point does not increase the effectiveness of the operation and it does entail the potential risk of devascularisation of the left colon. Miles himself was always opposed to ligation of the inferior mesenteric artery near its origin and tied the pedicle at the level of the bifurcation of the aorta, a landmark that is easily found, even in the obese patient. At this level, the superior haemorrhoidal artery will be tied at its origin from the inferior mesenteric artery.

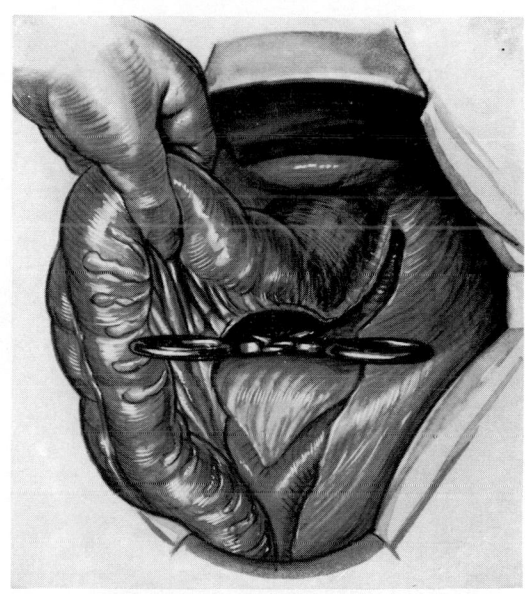

Figure 59–6. Opening of postrectal space. (*Source: From Lloyd-Davies OV: Abdomino-perineal excision of the rectum, in Rob C, Smith R (eds): Operative Surgery, 2 edt. London: Butterworths, 1969, with permission.*)

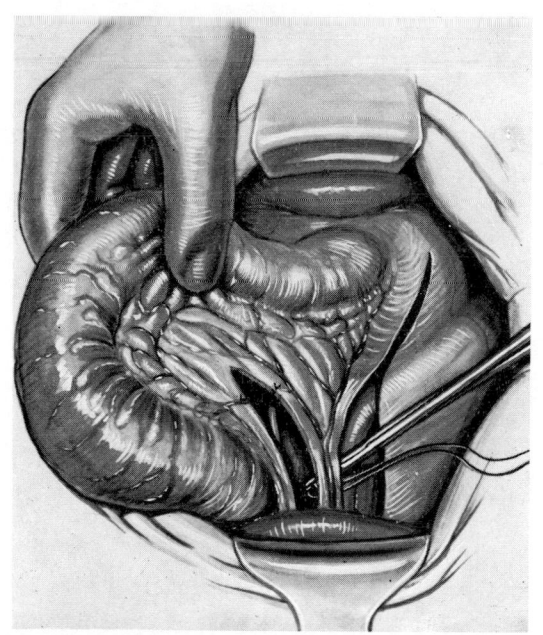

Figure 59–5. Ligation of main pedicle. (*Source: From Lloyd-Davies OV: Abdomino-perineal excision of the rectum, in Rob C, Smith R (eds): Operative Surgery, 2 edt. London: Butterworths, 1969, with permission.*)

The peritoneum on the medial aspect of the mesocolon is then divided from just below the sacral promontory to the site selected for ligature. Then the mesentery is elevated from the anterior surface of the aorta with the finger, and the vascular pedicle is isolated, double tied with stout thread or silk, and divided.

The pelvic dissection is commenced by lifting the rectosigmoid angle forward from the promontory of the sacrum and inserting a pair of blunt-nosed scissors downward and backward immediately in front of the first piece of the sacrum and behind the mesorectum (Fig. 59–6). A presacral plane of cleavage is thus produced. The fingers and finally the whole hand are inserted into this presacral space, and the mesorectum is deliberately pushed forward from the front of the sacrum and lateral pelvic walls as far downward as the coccyx, any tough strands of fascia being divided with scissors. By sweeping the hand from side to side, the posterior aspects of the upper parts of the lateral ligaments are made prominent. At this stage, the abdominal and perineal dissections meet behind the mesorectum, the rectum being completely freed posteriorly.

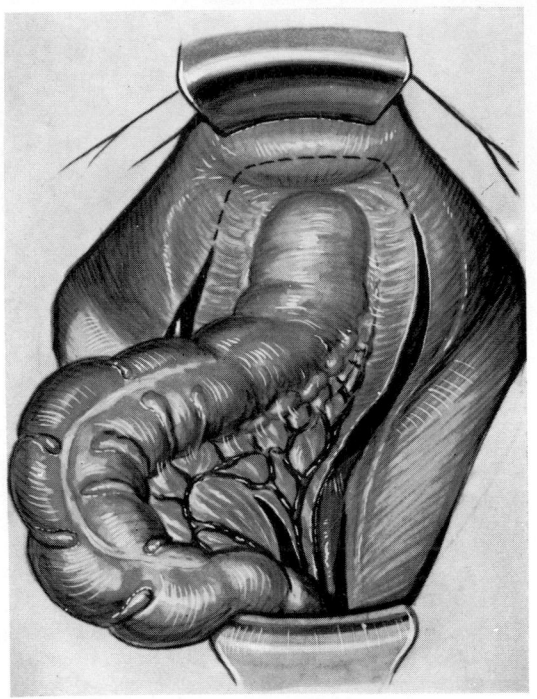

Figure 59–7. Division of pelvic peritoneum and subperitoneal tissue. (*Source: From Lloyd-Davies OV: Abdomino-perineal excision of the rectum, in Rob C, Smith R (eds): Operative Surgery, 2 edt. London: Butterworths, 1969, with permission.*)

laterally to define the anterior borders of the lateral ligaments. Each lateral ligament is in turn made taut by displacing the rectum to the opposite side with the left hand and divided with scissors well out on the pelvic wall and as far downward as possible. Any remaining portions will be divided by the perineal operator. The middle haemorrhoidal vessels will require ligation.

In females, in order to make the operation as radical as possible, it is quite often necessary, especially in low and bulky tumors, to remove the whole of the posterior vaginal wall; thus the division of the vagina through the posterior fornix and into the peritoneal cavity is dealt with by the perineal operator.

These steps result in the lateral ligaments being dealt with at a later stage in the operation and a greater part of them being divided by the perineal operator than in male patients. The uppermost portions, however, should be divided by the abdominal operator who should be fully aware of the exact course of the ureters (Fig. 59–9).

The peritoneum and subperitoneal tissues are then incised widely on either side of the bowel as far down as the peritoneal reflection, and the two incisions are joined anteriorly just in front of the peritoneal pouch (Fig. 59–7). The course of the ureters must be carefully noted at this stage, and in cases of bulky tumours in the midpelvis both ureters should be exposed throughout their course to the bladder.

In males, the apex of the incised peritoneum is drawn upward and the posterior surface of the vesicles exposed by blunt-nosed scissors dissection. At this point in the procedure, the fascia of Denonvillier is frequently found to be incised; alternatively, if the fascia is stout it may be seen lying between the anterior surface of the rectum and the base of the vesicles and is incised transversely (Fig. 59–8). Following this, a distinct plane of cleavage extending down to the apex of the prostate will be found with the fingers.

While in the space, the fingers are swept

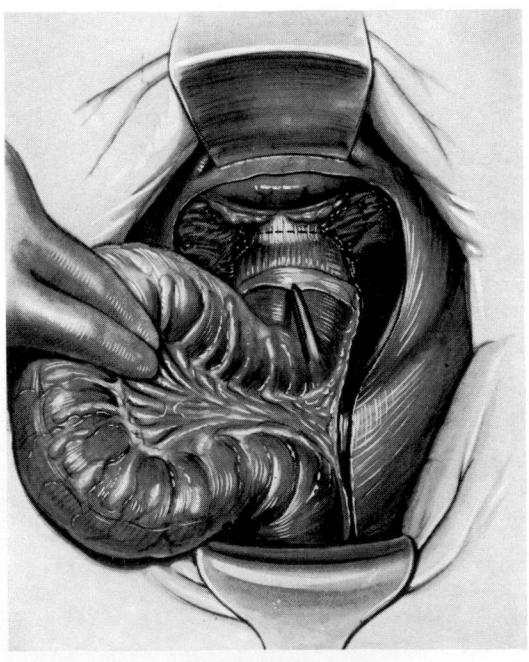

Figure 59–8. Anterior dissection from abdomen showing site of division of Denonvillier's fascia. (*Source: From Lloyd-Davies OV: Abdomino-perineal excision of the rectum, in Rob C, Smith R (eds): Operative Surgery, 2 edt. London: Butterworths, 1969, with permission.*)

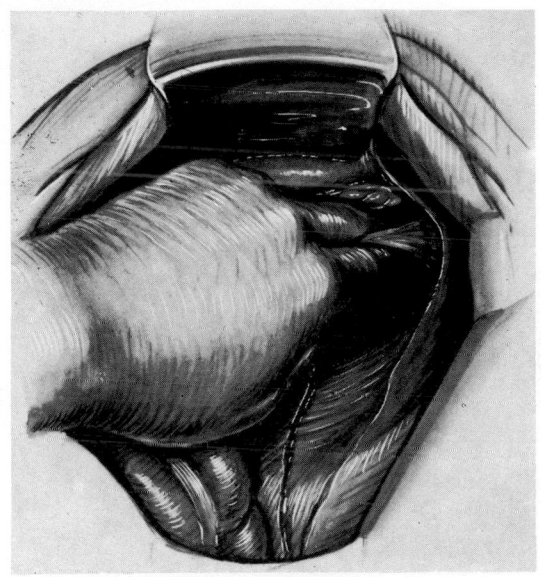

Figure 59–9. Division of upper portions of lateral ligaments. (*Source: From Lloyd-Davies OV: Abdomino-perineal excision of the rectum, in Rob C, Smith R (eds): Operative Surgery, 2 edt. London: Butterworths, 1969, with permission.*)

The colon is then prepared for division by carefully preserving the marginal vessels and dividing them at right angles to the bowel at a site that will allow 5 cm of viable bowel to project through the abdominal wall at the site selected for the colostomy. The bowel is divided between small clamps, such as those of Cope, using proper aseptic care, and the whole specimen is passed through the perineum when the perineal dissection is completed.

Colostomy

A circle of skin is excised at a point about 5 cm along the line from the anterior superior iliac spine to the umbilicus (Figs. 59–10 and 59–11).

Owing to the centrifugal traction of the surrounding skin, the removal of a half-inch circle will usually produce an adequate permanent orifice. A stab incision is made through the muscle layers, the external oblique fibres being divided transversely to avoid constriction of the bowel.

During this procedure, the lateral margin of all layers of the laparotomy wound is drawn toward the midline by holding forceps so that

correct positioning of the colostomy may be made.

In order to obviate the possibility of a loop of small bowel herniating through a narrow foramen between the colostomy and the lateral abdominal wall, this space must be obliterated by one of two techniques. The upper sigmoid colon can be passed through a retroperitoneal tunnel to the site of the stoma, which is the technique this author usually employs, or the defect between the bowel and the lateral abdominal wall may be closed. To carry this out, the lateral margin of the laparotomy wound is elevated by passing a long artery forceps through the colostomy incision, and the paracolic gutter is exposed (Fig. 59–12). A thread suture is inserted from the lateral border of the colostomy incision, including some muscle fibres of the abdominal wall, this is continued under the peritoneum of the paracolic gutter to the mesenteric border of the colon. When this suture is tied, the space to the outer side of the colostomy is

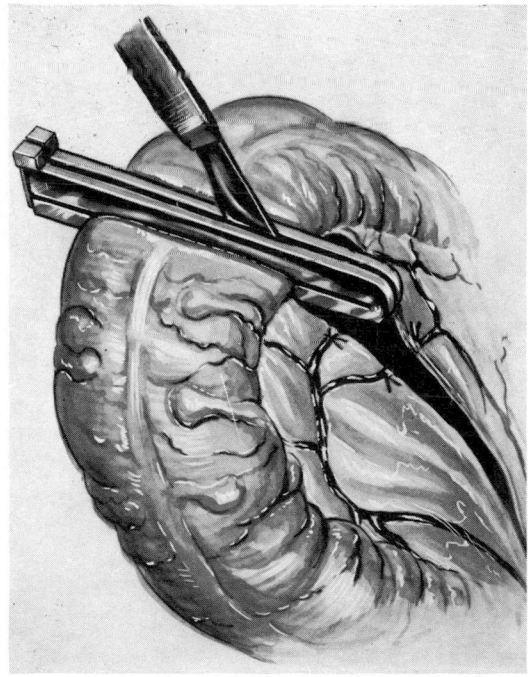

Figure 59–10. Division of the colon between Cope's clamps at site selected for colostomy. (*Source: From Lloyd-Davies OV: Abdomino-perineal excision of the rectum, in Rob C, Smith R (eds): Operative Surgery, 2 edt. London: Butterworths, 1969, with permission.*)

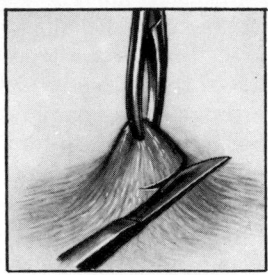 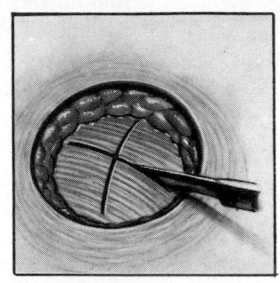 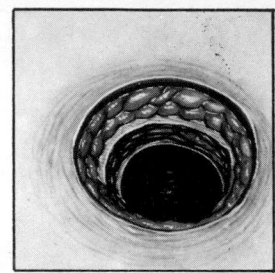

Figure 59–11. Method of formation of colostomy site. (*Source: From Lloyd-Davies OV: Abdomino-perineal excision of the rectum, in Rob C, Smith R (eds): Operative Surgery, 2 edt. London: Butterworths, 1969, with permission.*)

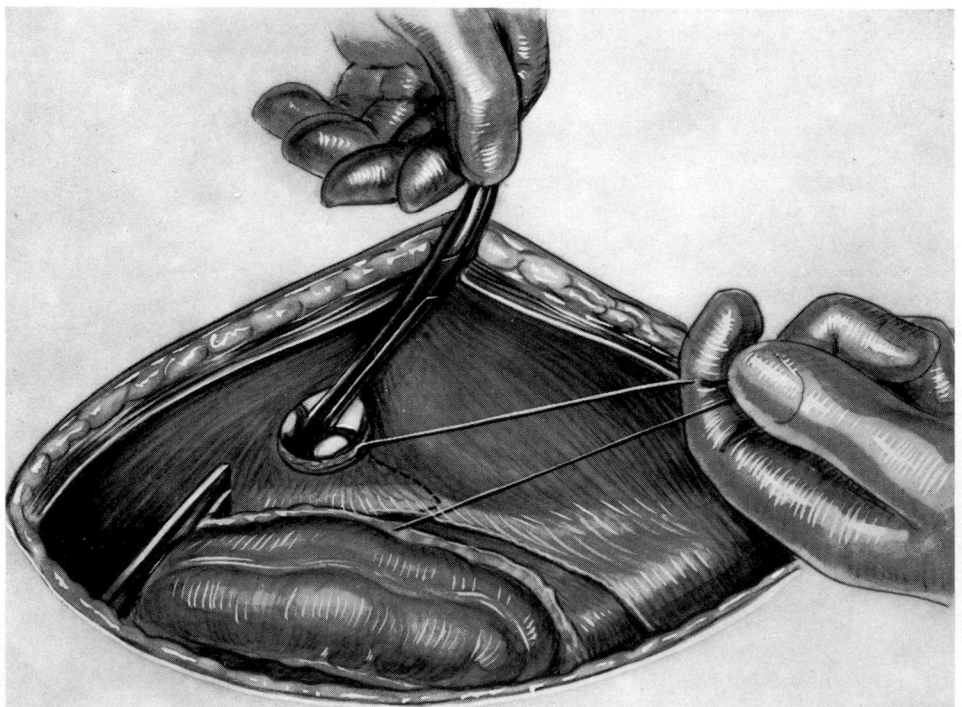

Figure 59–12. Closure of lateral space to outer side of colostomy with purse string sutures. (*Source: From Lloyd-Davies OV: Abdomino-perineal excision of the rectum, in Rob C, Smith R (eds): Operative Surgery, 2 edt. London: Butterworths, 1969, with permission.*)

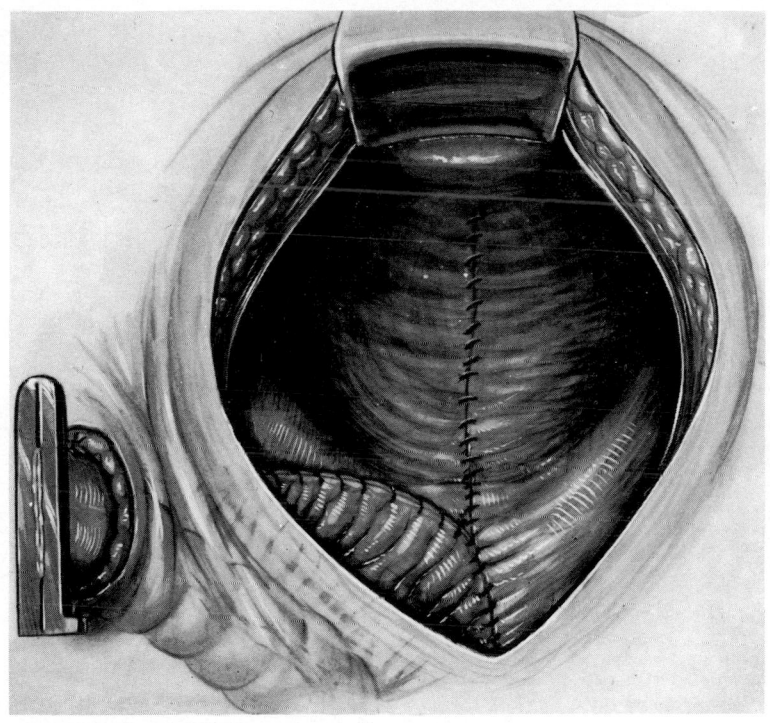

Figure 59–13. Closed pelvic floor. (*Source: From Lloyd-Davies OV: Abdomino-perineal excision of the rectum, in Rob C, Smith R (eds): Operative Surgery, 2 edt. London: Butterworths 1969, with permission.*)

obliterated. The proximal clamped colon is then passed out through the colostomy orifice.

At this stage, pelvic haemostasis is completed, and this is aided by the collaboration of the surgeon working from the perineum.

If there is an adequate amount of remaining peritoneum (this can be further mobilised from the lateral pelvic walls and iliac fossa with the fingers), the peritoneal pelvic floor is closed with a continuous thread suture (Fig. 59–13). If, however, this can only be achieved with a good deal of tension, it is safe practice to leave the pelvic floor widely opened; a small defect in the repaired pelvic floor may lead to strangulation of a knuckle of small intestine.

The abdomen is now closed and covered with a sterile dressing.

Next we turn our attention to the colostomy. The Cope clamp is removed from the protruding stump on the abdominal wall, and the edges of all the coats of the colon orifice are sutured to the surrounding skin using 00 chromic catgut. This produces a very satisfactory stoma with no tendency to skin stenosis (Fig. 59–14). A Stomahesive colostomy bag is applied to the stoma.

Perineal Dissection

The anus is closed with two purse string sutures of strong thread to prevent soiling. The dissection is not commenced until the abdominal surgeon has completed the exploration and decided that a combined excision is the correct procedure.

The principles underlying the perineal dissection are those of an encircling movement. The most difficult and intricate part of the dissection is the anterior portion, and for this reason the posterior and lateral aspects of the rectum are dealt with first, thus giving unhindered access to the anterior attachments.

This author employs an elliptical skin incision around the anus. Others use a transverse incision 5 cm in length made in front of the anus and midway between it and the bulb of the urethra. Lateral incisions are now made from its extremities, and these extend backward to meet over the sacrococcygeal articulation (Fig 59–15). These incisions are deepened through the perianal fascia to expose the lobulated ischiorectal fat, and posteriorly the coccyx is exposed.

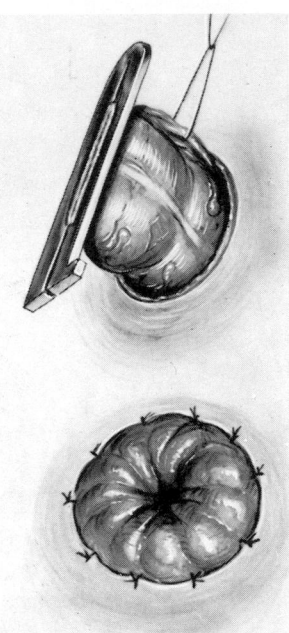

Figure 59–14. Formation of colostomy with direct suture of colon wall to skin. (*Source: From Lloyd-Davies OV: Abdomino-perineal excision of the rectum, in Rob C, Smith R (eds): Operative Surgery, 2 edt. London: Butterworths, 1969, with permission.*)

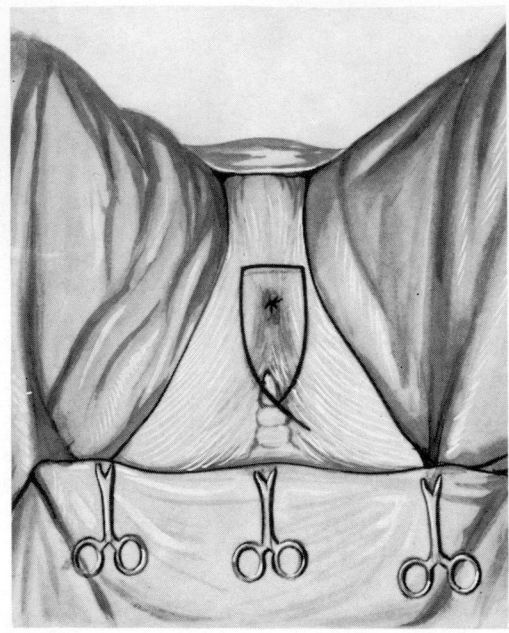

Figure 59–15. Towelled perineum showing skin incision. (*Source: From Lloyd-Davies OV: Abdomino-perineal excision of the rectum, in Rob C, Smith R (eds): Operative Surgery, 2 edt. London: Butterworths, 1969, with permission.*)

This author usually opens the plane in front of the coccyx by means of scissors dissection into the presacral space, but many surgeons remove the coccyx. To perform this, the coccyx is flexed to open up the sacrococcygeal joint, and the point of a scalpel is inserted. The distal portion of the coccyx is removed, care being taken to keep the knife close to the superior surface of the bone to avoid damaging the rectum (Fig. 59–16). The middle sacral vessels may require ligation or fulguration by diathermy at this stage.

Small lateral incisions are next made on either side of the coccyx through the fibrous attachment of the coccygeus muscle, and a finger is inserted on each side in a forward and outward direction to separate the iliococcygeus muscles from the underlying rectal Waldeyer fascia (Figs. 59–17 through 59–19). As the finger passes forward on the superior surface of the iliococcygeus, a gap will be found between the medial border of this muscle and the lateral aspect of the pubococcygeus, which lies in a different plane and covers the rectum. With the finger still in this position to protect the rectum, all the overlying structures (the iliococcygeus muscle, the ischiorectal fossa fat, and the inferior haemorrhoidal vessels and nerves) are divided well out on the lateral pelvic walls. The vessels will require ligation.

A self-retaining perineal retractor (such as the St. Mark's Hospital pattern) is now placed in position, and when the freed posterior portion of the rectum is elevated, Waldeyer's fascia will be seen posteriorly extending from the bony and ligamentous pelvic outlet to the region of the anorectal junction. This fascia is firmly attached to the periosteum of the sacrum and must on no account be stripped up but should be divided with a semicircular incision at the pelvic bony outlet.

The mesorectum—yellow fat enclosed in visceral pelvic fascia—will be seen, and it can then be safely separated (by the hand) from the hollow of the sacrum as far upward as the promontory (Fig. 59–20). The hand is also swept from side to side to free the areolar attachments of the ampulla of the rectum from the

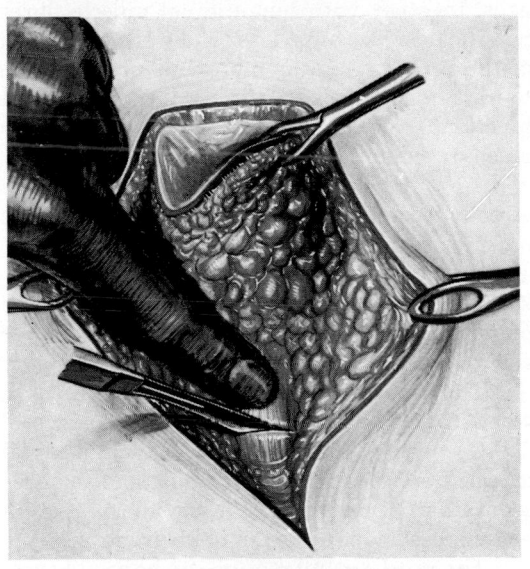

Figure 59–16. Excision of the coccyx. (*Source: From Lloyd-Davies OV: Abdomino-perineal excision of the rectum, in Rob C, Smith R (eds): Operative Surgery, 2 edt. London: Butterworths, 1969, with permission.*)

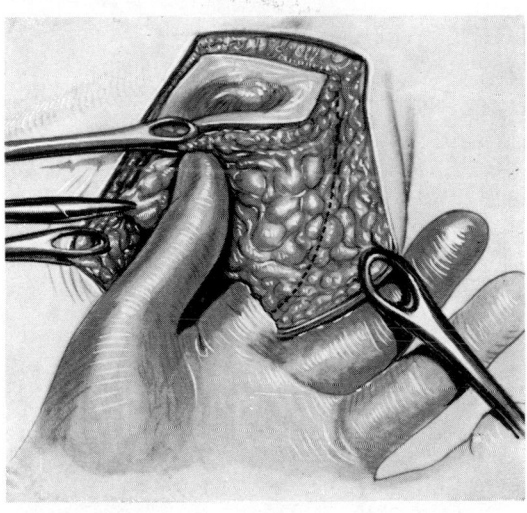

Figure 59–17. Finger inserted above ileococcygeus muscle preparatory to dividing overlying structures. (*Source: From Lloyd-Davies OV: Abdomino-perineal excision of the rectum, in Rob C, Smith R (eds): Operative Surgery, 2 edt. London: Butterworths, 1969, with permission.*)

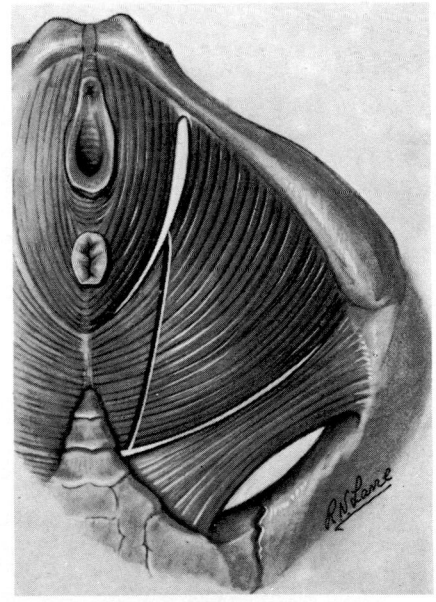

Figure 59–18. Pelvic floor muscles. (*Source: From Lloyd-Davies OV: Abdomino-perineal excision of rectum, in Rob C, Smith R (eds): Operative Surgery, 2 edt. London: Butterworths, 1969, with permission.*)

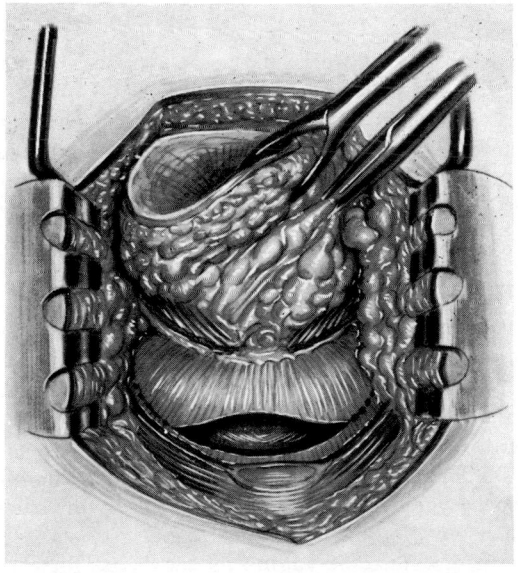

Figure 59–19. Division of Waldeyer's fascia. (*Source: From Lloyd-Davies OV: Abdomino-perineal excision of the rectum, in Rob C, Smith R (eds): Operative Surgery, 2 edt. London: Butterworths, 1969, with permission.*)

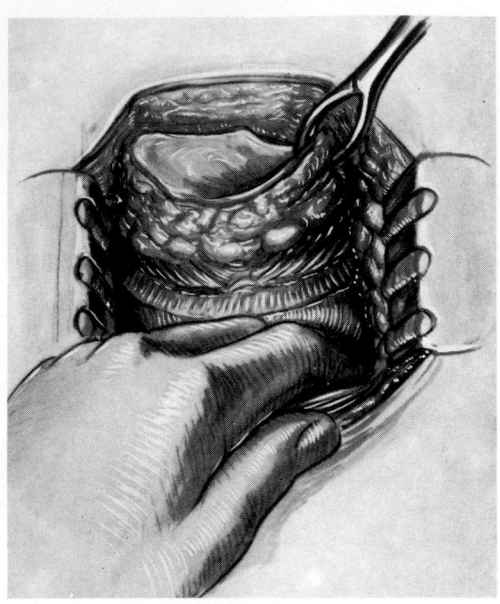

Figure 59–20. Sweeping the mesorectum from the sacral hollow. (*Source: From Lloyd-Davies OV: Abdominoperineal excision of the rectum, in Rob C, Smith R (eds): Operative Surgery, 2 edt. London: Butterworths, 1969, with permission.*)

The thick inferior borders of the pubococcygeus, together with longitudinal muscle fibres passing from the anterior rectal wall to the apex of the prostate and membranous urethra (rectourethralis muscle), still hold the anorectal junction forward in the middle line. This barrier is separated into two bundles by inserting a pair of artery forceps in the middle line toward the already located apex of the prostate; the forceps must be parallel to the posterior plane of the gland to avoid injury to the urethra (Fig. 59–23). When the forceps are gently opened, the puborectalis muscles will be identified on either side and can be separated.

The separated muscle bundles are then divided in turn and the prostatic capsule exposed.

Occasionally a thin layer of longitudinal muscle fibres obscures the capsule and requires separate division to avoid injury to the rectum and expose the true plane of cleavage.

The prostate and rectum can be readily separated by blunt dissection with the fingers, but on either side stout and vascular visceral layers of pelvic fascia still hold the rectum to the sides of the prostate and require division (Fig. 59–24).

posterolateral walls of the pelvis. Both operators meet in this plane.

Traction is now made on the isolated skin in front of the anus, and by transverse incisions on either side the wound is deepened to expose the superficial and then the deep transverse perineal muscles (Fig. 59–21). The plane of dissection must be behind these muscles in order to avoid any injury to the urethra, and when the deep transverse perineal muscles are completely exposed by dividing the decussating fibres of the deep external sphincter in the midline, the whitish longitudinal fibres of the anterior rectal wall will immediately be seen.

The broad fleshy strap-like fibres of the pubococcygeus muscles will now be seen on either side, enveloping the lateral aspects of the rectum, prostate, or vagina as they pass forward to their pubic attachments (Fig. 59–22).

A finger is then inserted above the superior borders of these muscles, separating them from the lateral aspects of the mesorectum whilst they are being divided as far forward as possible on either side. The lateral aspects of the prostate can then be easily felt and the plane of the posterior aspect of the gland determined.

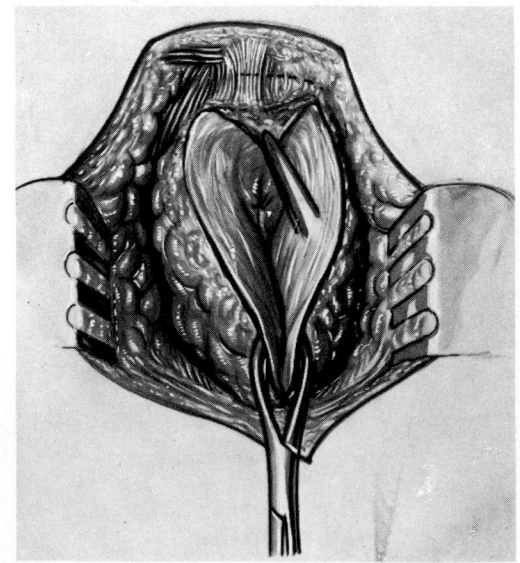

Figure 59–21. Anterior dissection showing central point of perineum with partially exposed transverse perineal muscles—dissection continues behind this muscle plane. (*Source: From Lloyd-Davies OV: Abdomino-perineal excision of the rectum, in Rob C, Smith R (eds): Operative Surgery, 2 edt. London: Butterworths, 1969, with permission.*)

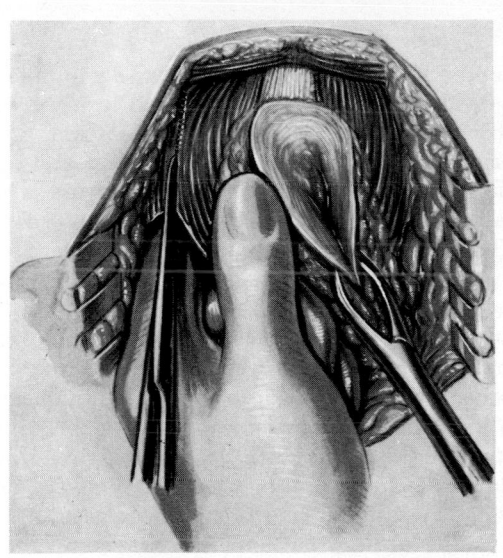

Figure 59–22. Fully exposed transverse perineal muscles; longitudinal muscle coat of the rectum in the centre and the division of the pubococcygeus muscle laterally. (*Source: From Lloyd-Davies OV: Abdomino-perineal excision of the rectum, in Rob C, Smith R (eds): Operative Surgery, 2 edt. London: Butterworths, 1969, with permission.*)

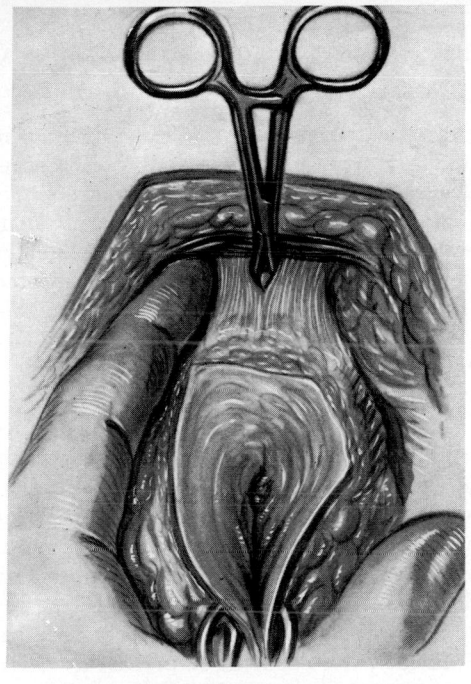

Figure 59–23. Separation of the rectourethralis muscle into two bundles to facilitate its division. (*Source: From Lloyd-Davies OV: Abdomino-perineal excision of the rectum, in Rob C, Smith R (eds): Operative Surgery, 2 edt. London: Butterworths, 1969, with permission.*)

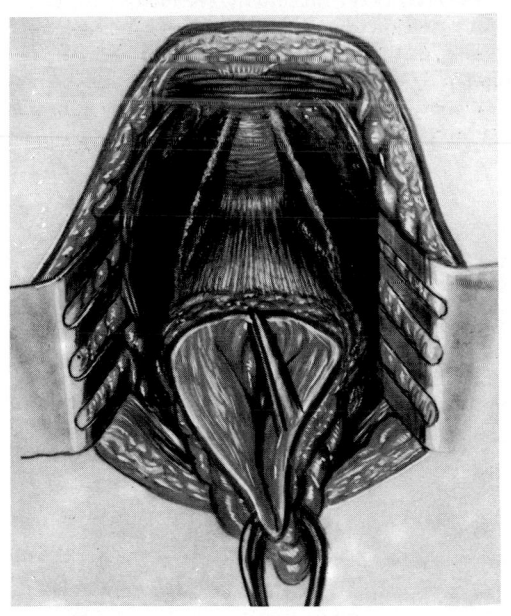

Figure 59–24. Vascular visceral pelvic fascia passing forward from the rectum to the lateral aspect of the prostate before division. (*Source: From Lloyd-Davies OV: Abdomino-perineal excision of the rectum, in Rob C, Smith R (eds): Operative Surgery, 2 edt. London: Butterworths, 1969, with permission.*)

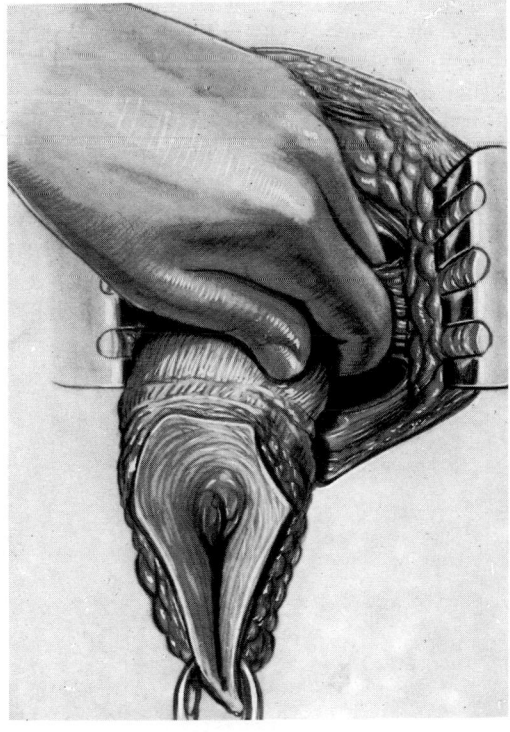

Figure 59–25. Division of the lower portions of the lateral ligaments from the perineum. (*Source: From Lloyd-Davies OV: Abdomino-perineal resection of the rectum, in Rob C, Smith R (eds): Operative Surgery, 2 edt. London: Butterworths, 1969, with permission.*)

The two surgeons will at this time have met anteriorly. The anterior and posterior aspects of the rectum are then completely isolated, and all that remains to be done is the division of the stout lower portions of the lateral ligaments (Fig 59–25). The bowel is alternatively displaced to the opposite side and the stretched ligament divided close to the pelvic wall. The freed bowel is passed down from the abdomen and delivered through the perineum.

Haemostasis is now secured with the cooperation of the surgeon working from the abdominal end. Miles packed the perineal wound open and permitted it to heal by secondary intension, which at times took as long as 3 to 6 months. Very occasionally, unpleasant vascular oozing still leads the surgeon to pack the perineal wound, although this is now rarely necessary.

In fact, the perineal or presacral cavity is only a potential space. After the intraabdominal pressure has returned, it becomes almost obliterated by descent of the pelvic floor (when the pelvic peritoneum has been closed), the uterus in the female and the bladder and prostate in the male, together with other adjacent pelvic structures. Most surgeons now close the perineal wound entirely. It will be found possible easily to produce a satisfactory closure of the divided fatty tissues using interrupted Dexon sutures and then to suture the skin with inter-rupted nylon stitches. A catheter drain is first passed into the pelvic cavity and brought out through one or other ischiorectal fossa. This drain is placed on a low suction pump, and suction is continued until no blood or serum is obtained—usually a period of only 2 or 3 days. The results of this technique are very satisfactory provided careful haemostasis has been obtained before closure. In those cases in the female where the posterior vaginal wall has been excised, the perineal wound is closed and the pelvic cavity drained into the vagina by means of a corrugated drain passed through the vulva and into the defect in the posterior vaginal wall. Rapid regeneration takes place with a very satisfactory cosmetic and functional result.

The urinary catheter is connected into a sterile drainage system and is removed on the fifth postoperative day.

BIBLIOGRAPHY

Lloyd-Davies OV: Lithotomy-Trendelenburg position for resection of rectum and lower pelvic colon. Lancet 2:74, 1939

Miles WE: A method of performing abdomino-perineal excision for carcinoma of the rectum and of the terminal portion of pelvic colon. Lancet 2:1812, 1908

60. Ileostomy and Colostomy

David G. Jagelman

ILEOSTOMY

On occasion, patients with ulcerative colitis, Crohn's disease of the colon, and familial polyposis coli require surgery necessitating an ileostomy. Some patients following various surgical procedures may require a loop diverting ileostomy, often on a temporary basis. Some patients with ulcerative colitis or familial polyposis may be offered or may prefer a continent ileostomy to the standard end ileostomy.

End Ileostomy

The method of colectomy that precedes the fashioning of an ileostomy may facilitate its subsequent establishment. The ileum is transected flush with the ileocecal valve. The mesentery of the right colon is divided and ligated close to the colonic wall up to the hepatic flexure. This will serve two purposes; first, preservation of the blood supply to the terminal ileum and second, it allows enough mesentery to suture to the abdominal wall at the end of the procedure. This final maneuver prevents volvulus occurring around the fixed point of the ileostomy. The exact site for the ileostomy has to be selected preoperatively as it is individualized for each patient. With the patient sitting and lying, a site in the right rectus muscle is chosen to allow for a flat surface for the appropriate ileostomy equipment. The avoidance of scars, dimples, body fat creases and rolls, and the subsequent incision should be taken into consideration. The stomal opening should exit preferentially through the right rectus muscle to reduce the long-term risks of parastomal hernia and prolapse (Fig. 60–1). The exact site can then be marked with a pinprick tattoo of India ink. Following proctocolectomy the stomal opening is made (Fig. 60–2). A circular disc of skin approximately 2 cm in diameter is excised at the previously marked site. The rectus muscle is incised longitudinally followed by separation of the rectus muscle fibers. No tissue is removed to allow for a snug stomal opening. The posterior rectus sheath and peritoneum are also incised longitudinally. The abdominal opening should be a snug two fingers in diameter (Fig. 60–3). The terminal ileum is then brought out through the stomal opening with an excess of intestine above skin level of approximately 5 to 6 cm (Fig. 60–4). The mesentery may need to be trimmed to allow exit of the intestine without tension. If there is any difficulty due to the thickness of the mesentery of the small bowel, lengthening of the peritoneal incision may help easier exiting of the ileum. When adequate ileostomy length is obtained the cut edge of the residual right colon mesentery is then sutured to the peritoneum of the anterior abdominal wall up to the ligamentum teres. Interrupted nonabsorbable sutures are used and on completion will prevent volvulus around the ileostomy. The main abdominal incision can then be closed. Maturation of the ileostomy involves placing 3-0 catgut sutures from the seromuscular layer of the ileum to Scarpa's fascia to stabilize the ileostomy. Four of these sutures are placed, one in each quadrant. Final circumferential 3-0 catgut sutures are placed, suturing the full thickness of the ileum to the subcuticular layer of the stomal opening (Fig. 60–5). Suturing to the subcuticular layer avoids the troublesome implantation of ileal mucosa to the skin around the ileostomy. This technique produces a predictable ileostomy via a snug stomal opening in the rectus muscle which thereby minimizes the chance of short-term or long-term complications.

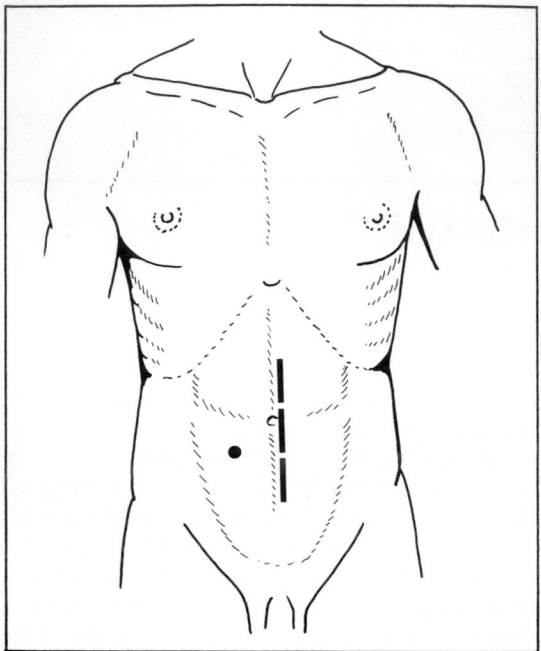

Figure 60–1. Preoperative stomal marking, preferably through the right rectus muscle.

Loop Ileostomy

For patients requiring a diverting loop ileostomy the following techniques will allow the production of a loop ileostomy that projects, functions, and indeed looks like a regular end ileostomy. A loop of ileum is selected that appears to be able to be brought out of the stomal opening without tension. A linen tape is placed through the mesentery at the apex of the loop being careful to avoid damage to the mesenteric vessels. The loop is then gently brought out of the abdominal aperture in such a way that the defunctioned or distal end of the loop is uppermost, i.e., cephalad. Instead of opening the loop at its apex at the time of maturation it should be opened at skin level in its uppermost part in the distal loop (Fig. 60–6). This will allow an excess of ileum that will project like a regular end ileostomy when final maturation is complete. The linen tape previously passed through the mesentery is then replaced with an ileostomy rod. Final maturation of the stoma is then completed with 3-0 chromic catgut suture, taking bites of full thickness of the intestinal wall

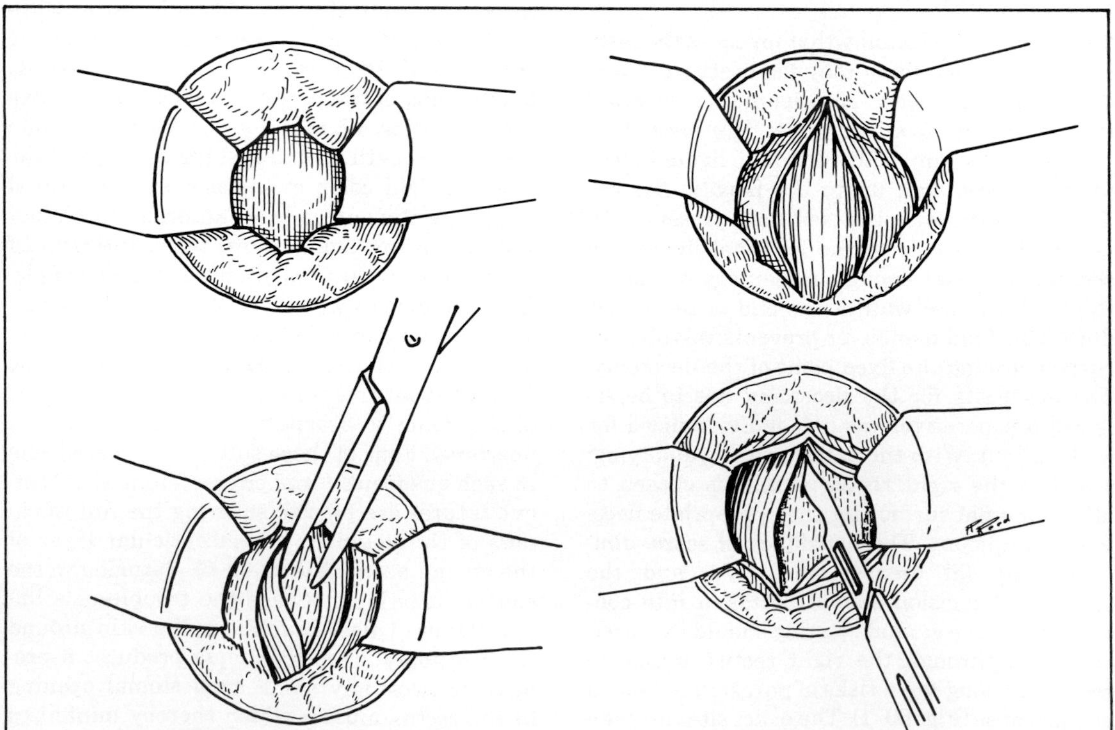

Figure 60–2. Creating the stomal opening in the right rectus muscle.

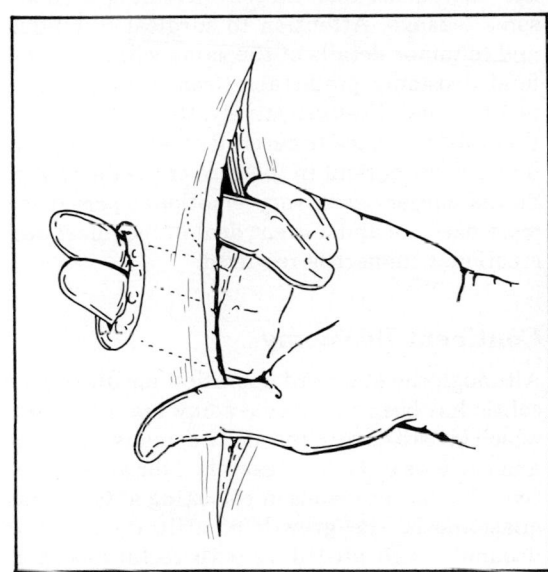

Figure 60–3. The stomal opening should be a snug two fingers in diameter.

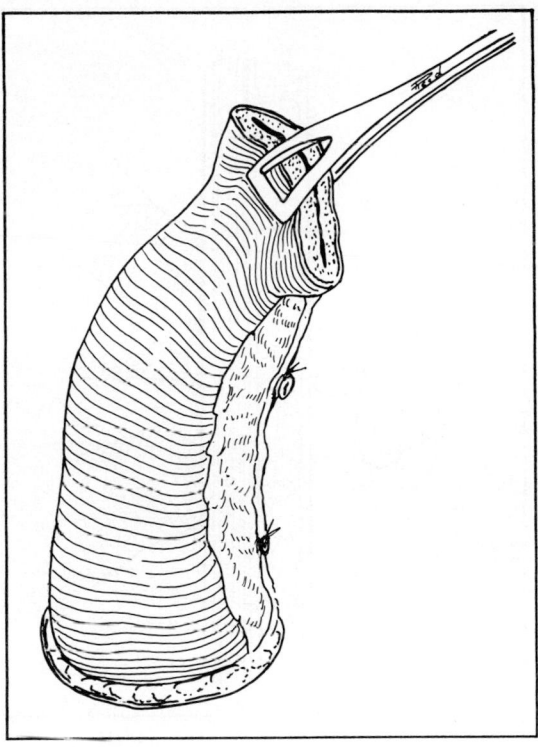

Figure 60–4. Terminal ileum brought out with intact mesentery.

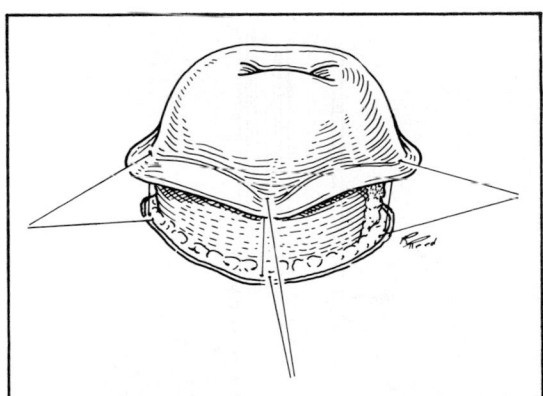

Figure 60–5. Final maturation is achieved by suturing the bowel wall to the subcuticular layer.

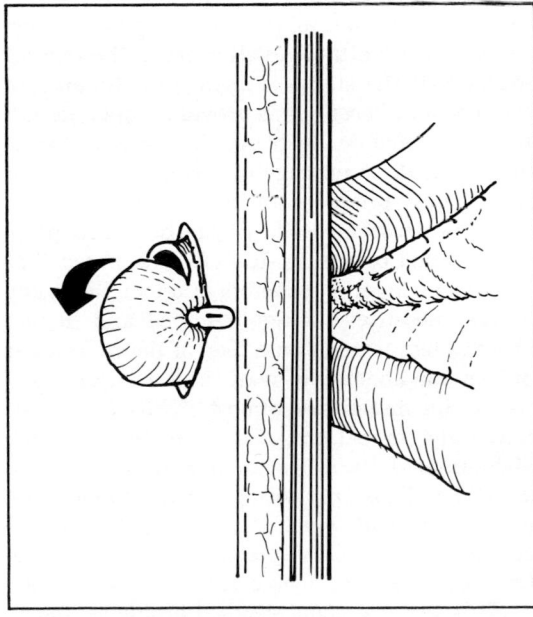

Figure 60–6. Loop ileostomy opened at skin level in the uppermost part rather than at the apex of the loop.

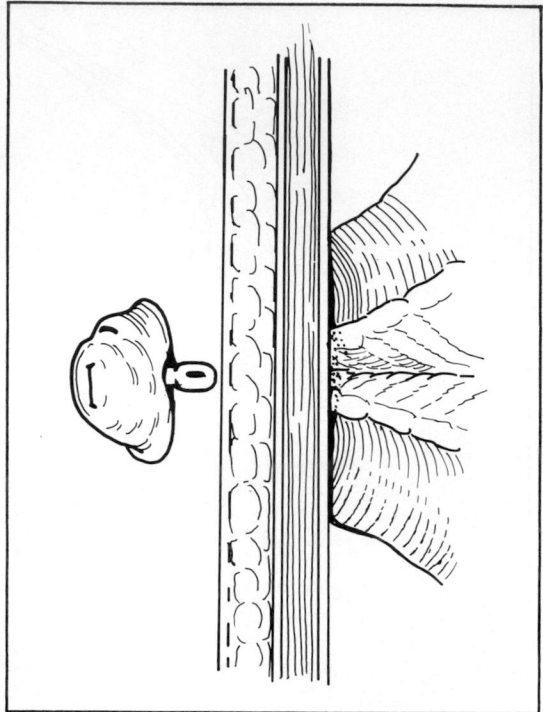

Figure 60–7. Final maturation creates a loop that projects from the skin in a similar fashion to an end ileostomy.

Appropriate stomal surgery to achieve a good result requires close liaison between stoma therapist, surgeon, and patient. Preoperative stomal marking is mandatory in all cases to avoid difficulties for the patient in maintaining the equipment and thereby avoiding troublesome leakage. Attention to surgical technique and to minor details of the same will make the final ileostomy predictable from a mechanical point of view. Postoperatively, the enterostomal therapist will need to carefully measure, fit, and instruct the patient in the care of the ileostomy. Stoma surgery is a very emotional period for most patients and a great deal of technical and emotional support is required.

Continent Ileostomy

Although the standard operation for ulcerative colitis has been proctocolectomy and ileostomy which gives a cure of the disease, many surgeons and patients alike have searched for an alternative. The recent trends in relooking at ileorectal anastomosis, the growth of utilization of the ileoanal pouch procedure with rectal mucosectomy, and the development of the continent ileostomy attests to this search for another option. Although the life of the regular ileosto-

and the subcuticular layer of the skin (Fig. 60–7). The sutures are all placed and by tying them individually the stoma will evert in the regular manner. If the stoma is opened at the apex of the loop and ileostomy is provided that does not project, a double flush opening is left that is very difficult to manage in terms of equipment and usually produces an inadequate result.

The ileostomy rod is usually left in place for a period of 7 days. It should be noted that there is no layer of ischemia in a loop ileostomy as the mesentery is not trimmed and in fact there is less tension on a loop of ileum brought out on the abdominal wall than a regular end when the mesentery almost invariably needs trimming. In patients with obesity and thick abdominal walls, it is even more difficult to create an end ileostomy with predictable blood supply and without tension. In these patients, one can utilize the positive features of the loop ileostomy by creating a loop end ileostomy (Fig. 60–8). This will overcome surgical problems associated with obesity, the stoma being opened and created in just the same way as described for a loop ileostomy in continuity.

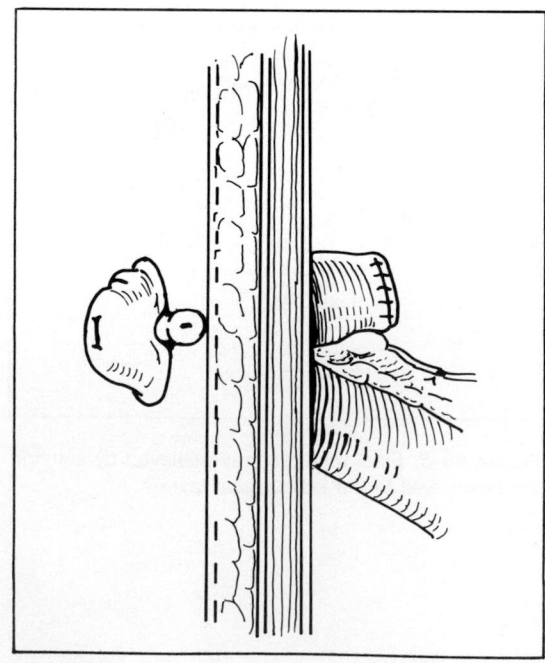

Figure 60–8. A loop end ileostomy may be useful in obese patients.

mate has improved with improvements in surgical technique, the development of enterostomal therapy and better equipment, there are still problems, both physical and emotional—the potential for skin irritation and leakage, awareness of a bulge under the clothes, concerns of younger patients with an ileostomy in dating and sex, to name a few. The continent ileostomy allows a new freedom in that a bag is not required and continence is achieved, both very positive emotional features. Professor Nils Kock in 1969 described the surgical creation of an ileostomy reservoir. The pouch was constructed from 30 cm of terminal ileum. The first patients were not provided with a continence valve, relying only on the rectus muscle to provide this function, but were supplemented with intubation to empty the reservoir. Although this was regarded as a success by the patients, there was still some leakage. Kock later modified the technique to create a so-called nipple valve by intubating the efferent limb of the conduit upon itself. As long as the valve stayed in place, continency of the pouch was assured. Unfortunately there is a tendency for the valve to prolapse allowing partial continence and partial incontinence, the worst of both worlds. The large number of variations in surgical technique have all been aimed at improving the predictability of the valve mechanism. The use of three loops of ileum instead of the originally described two loop pouch, the use of staples on the valve inside the pouch; suturings of various types at the entering pouch of intussusception, fascial slings around the neck of the valve were all tried. Improved methods of attaching the pouch to the anterior abdominal wall help prevent a pulling away action of the pouch and subsequent prolapse of the valve. Overzealous attempts to hold the valve in place surgically have created the danger of fistulas forming around the valve. The development of valve prolapse and incontinence or fistula formation dictates the need for surgical correction. There is a dilemma because surgical intervention is needed to correct incontinence rather than for disease. The problem has been that nearly all patients who have experienced the freedom associated with a continent ileostomy have requested repeat surgery to correct the valve if and when it slipped rather than returning to a regular incontinent ileostomy. Many of the other complications associated with the procedure have been ironed out and even though it is regarded as a major abdominal operative procedure the

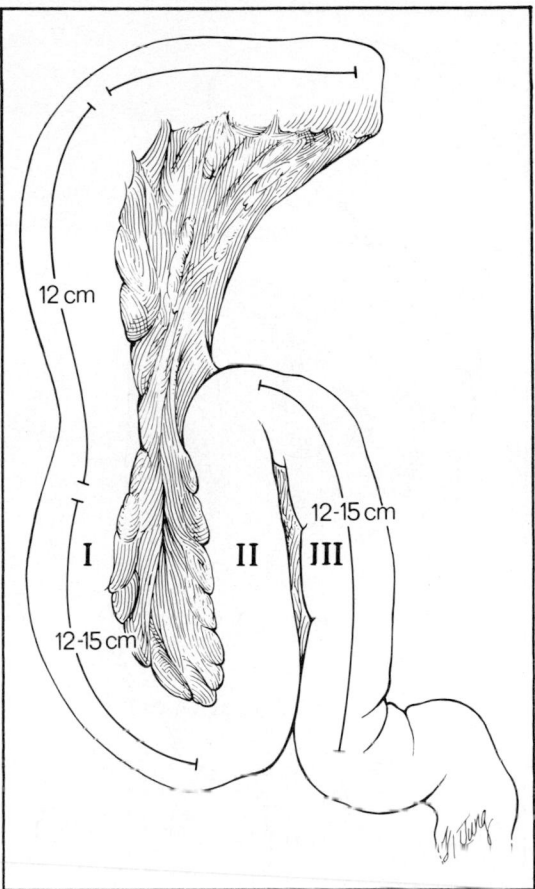

Figure 60–9. Measured segments of ileum to create a continent ileostomy.

mortality has been gratifyingly low. Kock et al reported a mortality of 2.2 percent in the first 299 patients with no mortality in the subsequent 152 patients. The continent ileostomy is not for every patient who requires an ileostomy. It is specifically contraindicated in patients with Crohn's disease and may also be inappropriate in some other patients depending on their age, habits, and life-styles, both working and social. Even though the reoperation rate for valve slippage has been reported between 10 and 20 percent, it should be remembered that similar reoperation rates have been reported for patients with a regular end ileostomy.

Presented here are the surgical techniques that we have developed over the years and our present method of construction of the continent ileostomy. The colonic pathology of all patients is carefully reviewed prior to surgery to exclude patients with Crohn's disease. Preoperatively, the patients are prepared with mechanical

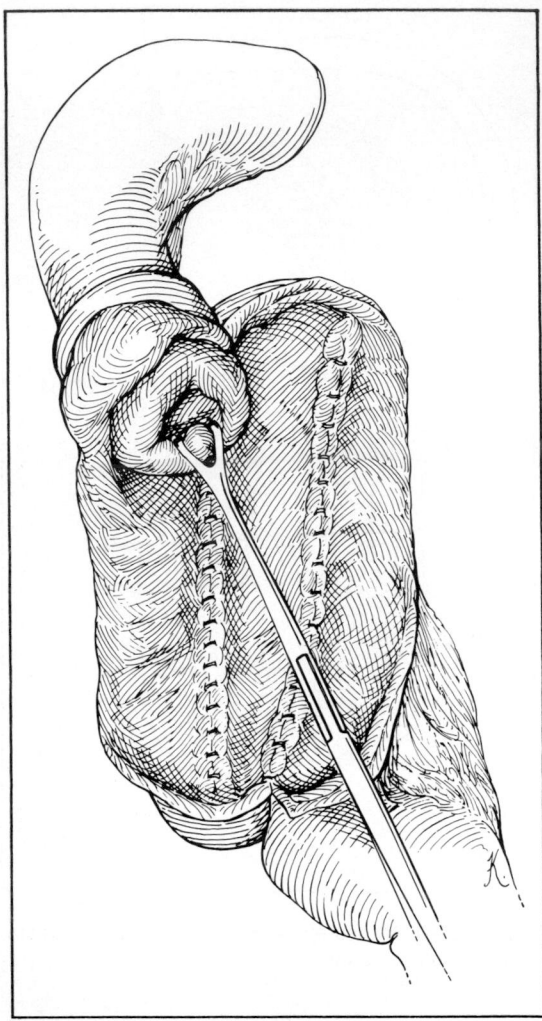

Figure 60–10. The nipple valve is created by intussuscepting the segment into the open pouch.

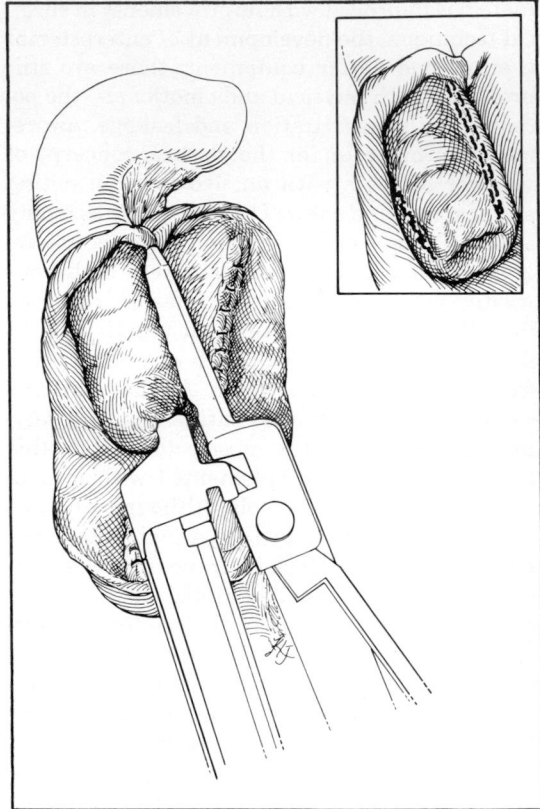

Figure 60–11. Linear stapling of the nipple valve.

bowel preparations of 1000 ml of 10 percent mannitol the day before surgery as an osmotic laxative and perioperative systemic broad spectrum antibiotics. The terminal ileum is transected with a linear row of intestinal staples. Accurate measurements of the ileum are required: 10 cm is left for the efferent limb, 12 cm for the nipple valve, and three 15 cm segments to construct a three loop reservoir (Fig. 60–9). The bowel is clamped proximal to this length of ileum to avoid intestinal spillage. The loop of bowel is then irrigated with 10 percent povidone–iodine to decrease the risk of sepsis. The three 15-cm segments are joined with a running 4-0 Ethibond suture. The pouch is opened

close to the Ethibond suture line and the cut edges cauterized for hemostasis. The side-to-side ileal anastomoses are completed using through-and-through 3-0 chromic catgut sutures.

The valve is created from the 12-cm segment by passing a Babcock forceps from within the pouch catching the midportion of the valve segment and intussuscepting it into the pouch (Fig. 60–10). The nipple valve is completed with two rows of TA-55 or five GIA staples (Fig. 60–11), the valve being maintained at 5 cm in length. The reservoir is then closed in two layers using 3-0 chromic catgut and a superimposed 4-0 Ethibond layer. Finally, a Mersilene mesh strip is placed circumferentially around the fundus of the pouch, suturing it in place with 4-0 Ethibond sutures (Fig. 60–12). Four anchor sutures of 1-0 Ethibond are placed in the Mersilene mesh and these will help to fix the fundus to the anterior abdominal wall (Fig. 60–13). A catheter is then inserted into the pouch through the valve, 150 cc saline is injected into the reser-

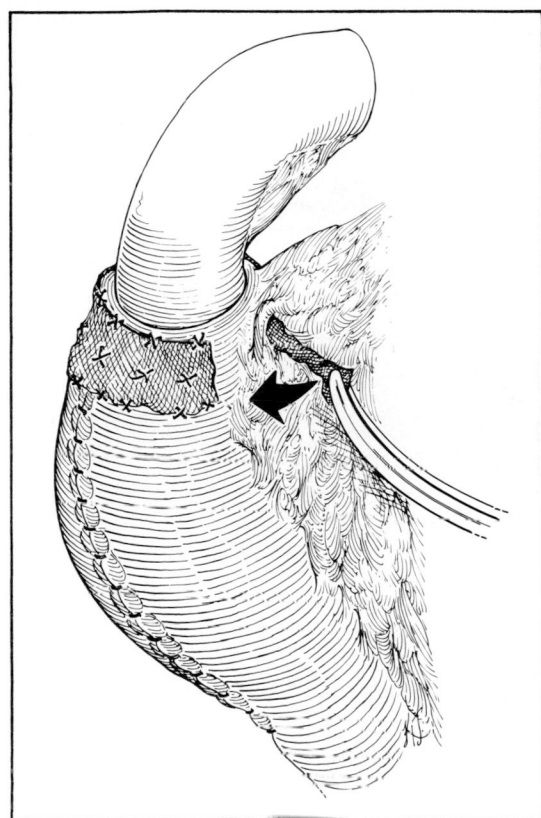

Figure 60–12. Placement of the Mersilene sling around the neck of the pouch.

voir to check for leakage of the reservoir and continence of the valve. The efferent limb of the reservoir is then brought out of the abdominal wall aperture. The 4-0 Ethibond anchor sutures are then sutured to the posterior abdominal wall with deep bites to fix the pouch firmly. The excess extending ileum is then trimmed and the ileostomy matured flush with the abdominal wall skin using 3-0 chromic catgut. A drainage catheter is then placed through the stomal opening for continuous postoperative drainage and decompression and sutured to the skin to prevent it from slipping out. Postoperative care includes regular saline irrigation of the catheter to prevent its obstruction. It seems beneficial to maintain continuous intubation of the stoma and pouch for as long as 3 to 4 weeks. During this period, the catheter should be changed in position slightly to prevent pressure necrosis and possible perforation. Following continuous intubation, the patient empties the pouch every 2 to 3 hours for the next 2 weeks and then as

required. Utilizing this technique, we have achieved eventual continence rates of 86 percent with a reoperation rate of 23 percent. It would seem that if the valve does not slip by 3 months, it is unlikely to do so later. The continent ileostomy has certainly been controversial surgically but sought after and appreciated by many patients. There seems to be a leaning curve in the development of the surgical technique that adds to the predictability of the final result.

COLOSTOMY

End Descending Colostomy

Abdominoperineal excision of the rectum for cancer necessitates an end colostomy. Although the number of patients requiring a permanent colostomy has been reduced with improvement of lower and lower colorectal anastomotic techniques, notably with the various stapling devices, there are still a number of patients in which there is no other alternative than a permanent end descending colostomy. Adequacy of resection for rectal cancer demands total en bloc lymphatic resection. This necessitates a ligation of the inferior mesenteric artery at its origin on the aorta. Following this maneuver the blood supply of the left colon is served from the middle colic artery via the marginal artery (Fig. 60–14). It is this author's belief that the blood supply of the sigmoid colon is unpredictable under these circumstances, it being the most distant point from the middle colic artery. On this basis, this author's practice is to resect the sigmoid colon in all abdominoperineal resections or low colorectal anastomoses. The end colostomy is thus created in the descending colon. This will necessitate some mobilization of the left colon to avoid tension on the subsequent colostomy. The site selected for the colostomy will have been marked before the operation with the patient lying and sitting so as to avoid skin creases, previous incisions, and abdominal fat rolls. This author prefers to create the stomal opening in the left rectus muscle, a more medial position than previously suggested (Fig. 60–15). The classic colostomy opening is situated outside the rectus muscle and is associated with a high incidence of parastomal hernia in almost all patients in the long term. The rectus muscle is a much stronger area for stoma production and

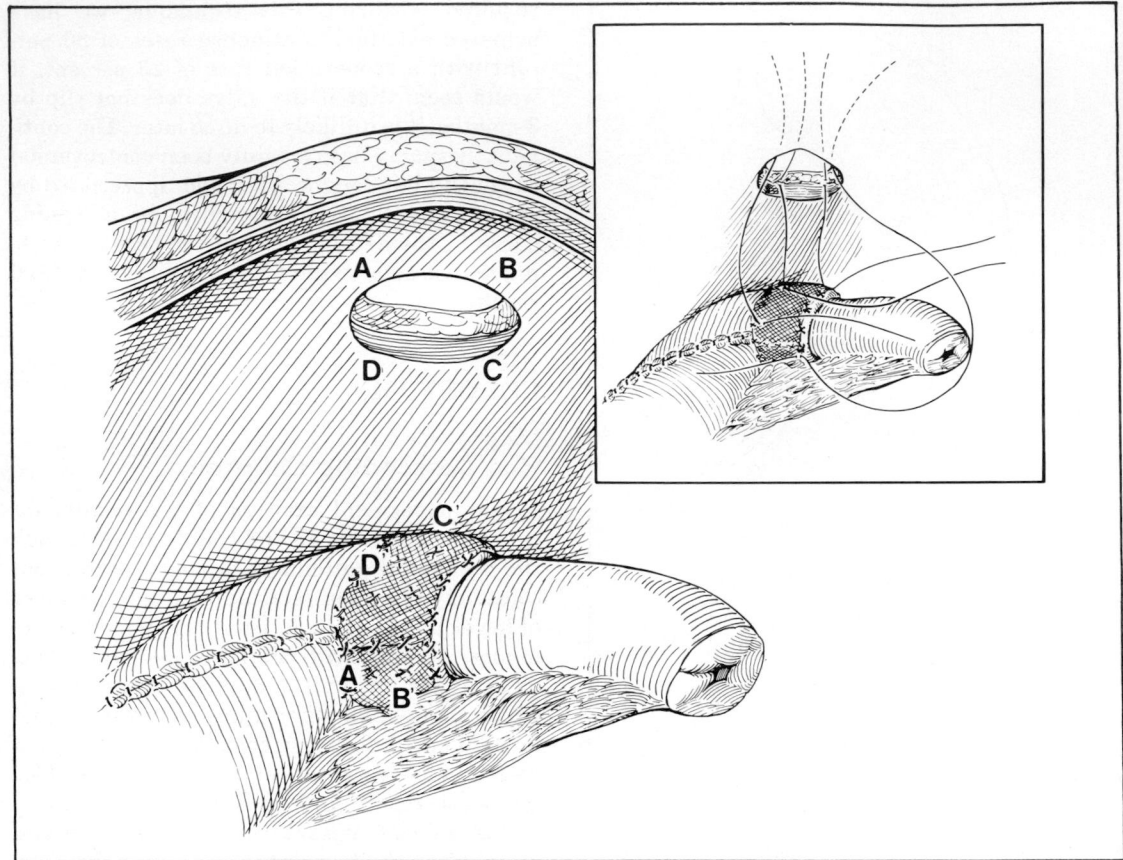

Figure 60–13. Fixation of the pouch to the anterior abdominal wall.

this author believes that it reduces the incidence of parastomal hernia and prolapse. Creation of the stoma through the left rectus muscle also creates a large lateral colostomy space. This negates the need for closing the space as is customary in a more lateral stoma position. It also makes extraperitoneal colostomy production, which has been proposed as an alternative to avoid closing the space, an unnecessary technique. The site of the opening in the abdominal wall having been selected and marked for each individual patient before surgery can now be opened. It is important to make the opening snug and never more than 2.5 cm in diameter. Too large an abdominal opening leads to herniation and maybe prolapse. Therefore the exiting descending colon is snug in the abdominal wall opening and no tissue is removed in creating the abdominal aperture. The rectus sheath is divided longitudinally and the fibers are separated longitudinally. The descending colon is then brought out of the abdominal opening so that approximately 2 cm of excess colon is produced. It is important that there is no tension on the stoma; if there is any doubt, further mobilization is required. Three or four nonabsorbable sutures are placed intraabdominally suturing the semimuscular layer of the colon to the posterior rectus sheath to take the tension off the mucocutaneous layer of sutures. Primary maturation is then achieved using 3-0 catgut mucocutaneous sutures circumferentially, the sutures being placed a few millimeters apart. The stoma does not need to protrude as in an ileostomy and can be made flush with the skin (Fig. 60–16). The final skin level maturation of the stoma is, of course, only performed following closure of the main abdominal incision. The ab-

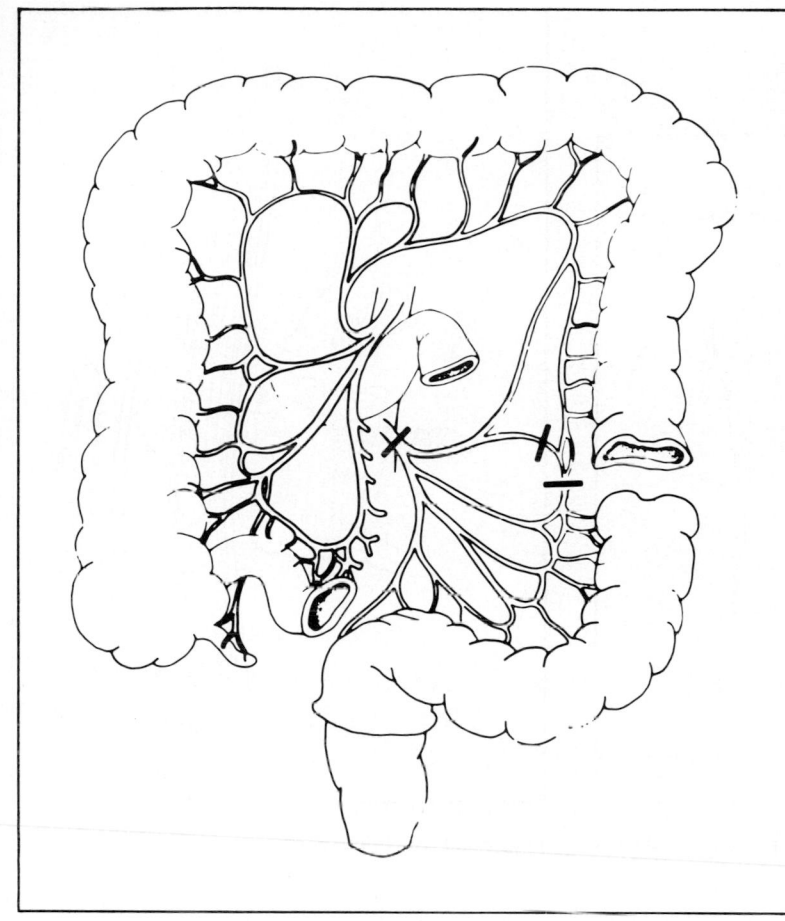

Figure 60–14. Diagrammatic representation of colonic blood supply. Note marginal artery and transection of colon at junction of descending and sigmoid region to avoid ischemia.

dominal incision, due to the site selected through the rectus made for the colostomy, is a midline muscular incision with its cutaneous component made just to the right side of the umbilicus.

Diverting Transverse Colostomy

It is sometimes necessary to divert the fecal stream from the left colon following low colorectal anastomosis, Hirschsprung's disease, rectal trauma, and unresectable disease of the sigmoid colon. It has been debated over the years as to whether a loop transverse colostomy in continuity effectively diverts the fecal stream. Some have suggested dividing the colostomy and bringing it out at two separate ends. Barium and radioisotope swallow studies have demonstrated that a skin level transverse loop colostomy in continuity does totally divert the fecal

stream. Also diverting the transverse colon makes subsequent closure much more of an ordeal for surgeon and patients. In general, it is better to make a transverse colostomy through a separate incision in the right upper abdomen through the rectus muscle. It is possible on occasion, if it is only thought to be required for a short period of time, to fashion the transverse colostomy through the main midline abdominal incision in its upper portion. A 5- to 7-cm continuous transverse incision is made over the right rectus muscle. The skin, subcutaneous fat, deep fascia and rectus sheath are divided transversely. The fibers of the rectus muscle are not divided but rather separated longitudinally. This allows for a smaller abdominal aperture with more support and, as this author believes, it reduces the chance of later colostomy prolapse. The posterior peritoneum is then divided

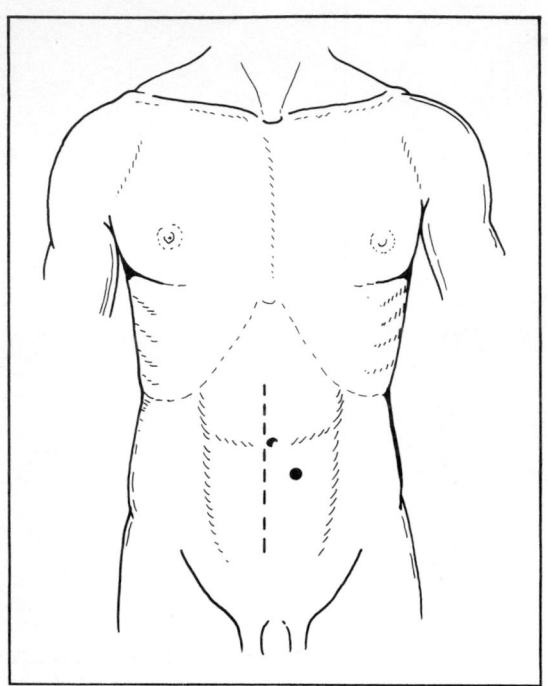

Figure 60–15. Preferred site for end colostomy via the left rectus muscle.

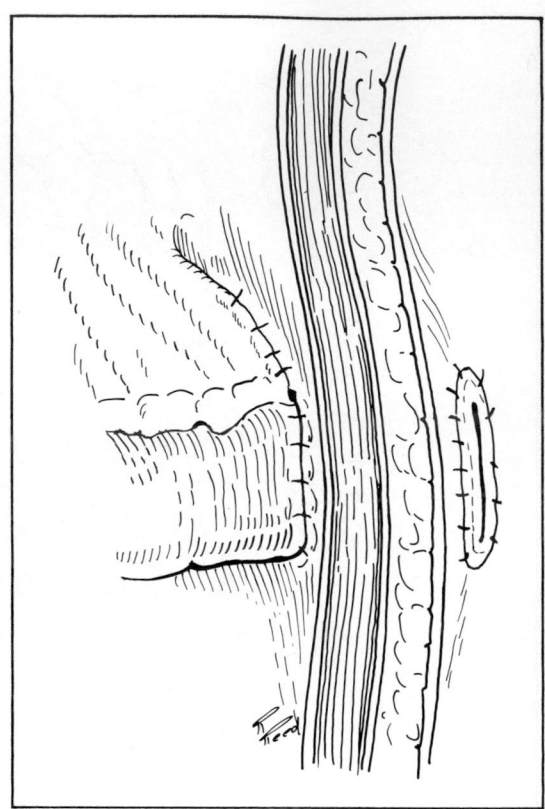

Figure 60–16. Primary maturation of end colostomy flush with skin.

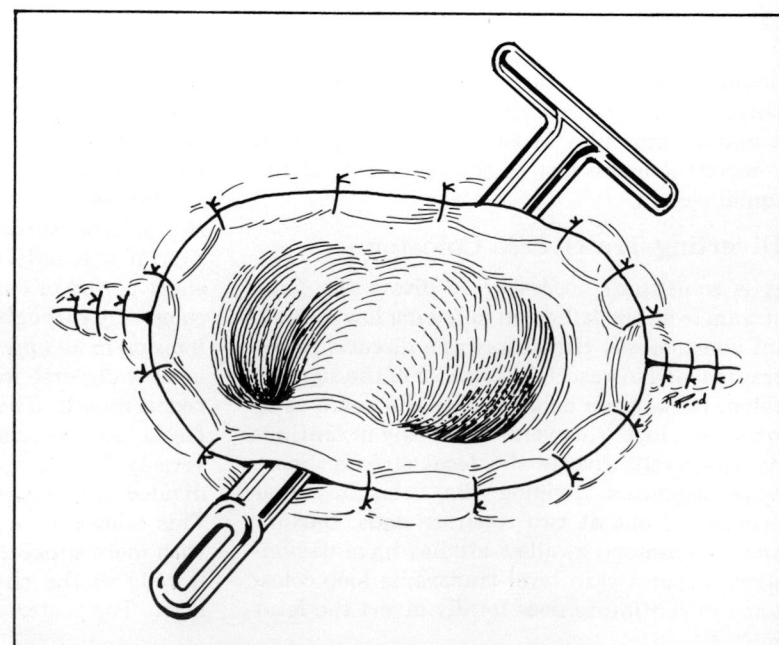

Figure 60–17. Transverse colostomy with rod in place after primary maturation showing central bridge effect for adequate diversion.

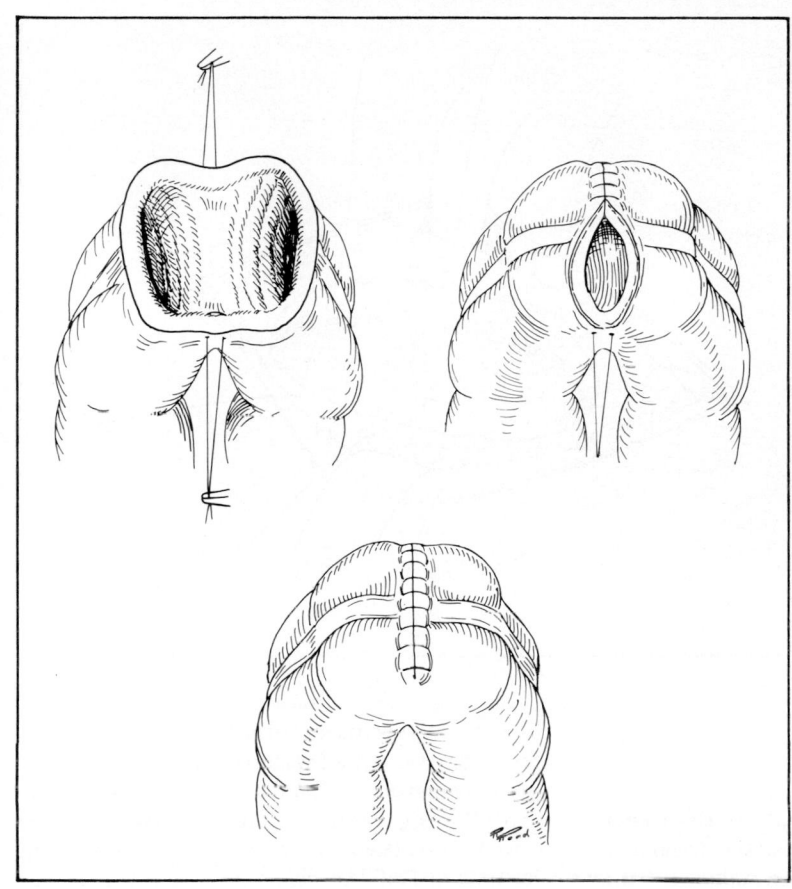

Figure 60-18. Two-layer interrupted suture closure of colostomy in transverse plane.

transversely allowing access to the peritoneal cavity. A loop of transverse colon is then selected and a linen tape is placed through the mesentery at the apex of the loop. Care should be taken to keep the tape close to the bowel wall to avoid damage to the marginal artery. In obese patients, mobilization of the transverse colon, including the hepatic flexure, may be necessary to avoid tension at the colostomy at maturation. Before bringing the loop of colon through the abdominal aperture, interrupted 2-0 chromic catgut sutures are placed in the divided rectus sheath and are not tied on each side. Indeed more sutures than necessary can be placed leaving only a small central opening for the transverse colon. The loop of colon is then brought through the abdominal wall and the rectus sheath sutures tied from outside inward. If there are too many catgut sutures and the closure is too tight around the loop, the last few can be removed; but the closure should be tight and snug. It is not necessary to have a

large amount of extruding colon but just enough to achieve a colostomy at skin level. A plastic or glass rod then is placed through the mesentery to replace the linen tape. It is not necessary to delay maturation of any stoma and, therefore, primary maturation can be achieved immediately on the operating table. The transverse colon is then opened longitudinally at its apex. The longitudinal opening and the effect of the rod maintain the central bridge of the colostomy and effectively control fecal diversion (Fig. 60-17). Primary maturation involves interrupted 3-0 catgut sutures of full thickness of colon to skin placed a few millimeters apart. It is not necessary to suture the colostomy rod to the skin as it can be controlled by placing the colocutaneous sutures close to the rod on both sides. A few skin sutures may be required if the cutaneous incision is larger than the colostomy. The rod is easily removed after 7 days. In this way a small, snug totally diverting transverse colostomy can be achieved.

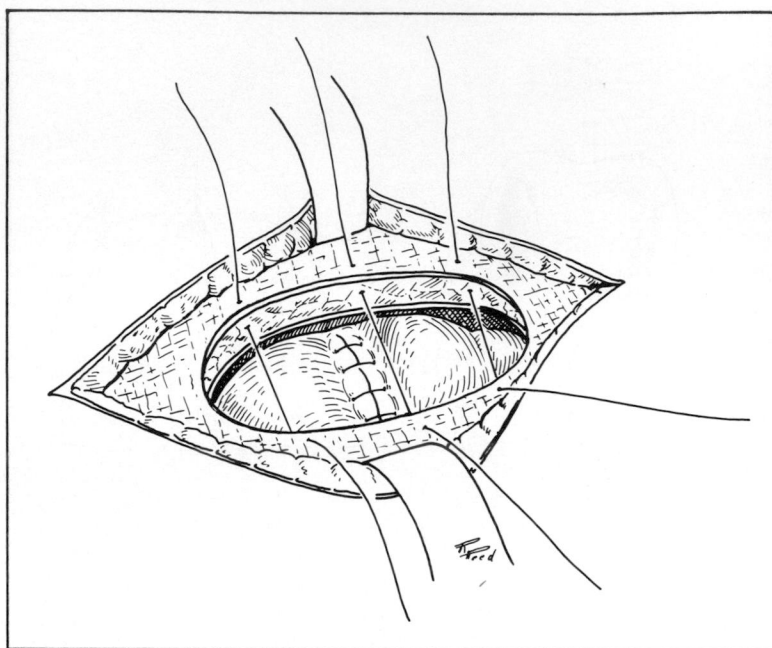

Figure 60–19. All muscular layer closure of abdominal wall. The skin is left open to heal by secondary intention.

Closure of Loop Colostomy

The longer a colostomy is in place, the easier it is closed and in some series, the incidence of postclosure complications are reduced if the stoma is closed after 10 weeks. In most cases it is possible to close the temporary colostomy before 10 weeks and, with careful technique, closure can be achieved without serious complications. Because of the significant complication ratio of fecal fistula reported in some series, some have recommended extraperitoneal closure. This has not been our practice because with appropriate technique a colostomy can be closed in an intraperitoneal manner without significant complication. Following skin preparation with antiseptic solution, a small surgical swab is placed in the afferent limb to prevent inadvertant contamination. The patient will have undergone a simple 1-day mechanical bowel preparation using a fluid diet and 1 L of 10 percent mannitol drunk over a 2-hour period the day before surgery. This type of preparation has been our simple 1-day bowel preparation for all colonic surgical cases for the past 3 years. An incision is made in the skin around the margins of the colostomy a few millimeters from the mucocutaneous junction. The dissection is continued downward keeping close to the colonic wall circumferentially to enter the peritoneal cavity. All adhesions are divided to free up the transverse colon from all the wound margins allowing enough room for closure of the wound. The attached skin is then removed from the margins of the colostomy, the opening in the colon is then closed in a transverse manner (Fig. 60-18). Chromic catgut (3-0) interrupted seromuscular sutures are placed as the first layer closure followed by an outer layer of 3-0 Ethibond interrupted sutures. Closure in the transverse plane minimizes narrowing at the closure site. The colon is then returned to the peritoneal cavity. The abdominal incision is then closed with interrupted figure-eight nonabsorbable mattress sutures. The sutures include all the muscular layers of the abdominal wall (Fig. 60-19). The skin is left open and loosely packed with gauze soaked in antiseptic solution which eliminates postoperative wound infection. The wound heals over during the following 2 weeks in a simple way with minimal scarring. Most patients can resume oral fluid within 24 hours and are able to leave the hospital in 4 to 5 days. If, during mobilization, there is trauma to the colon due to the density of the adhesions, such as seromuscular tears or a generally ragged segment of colon, it is better to resect the transverse colostomy and perform a regular end-to-end anastomosis.

BIBLIOGRAPHY

Ileostomy

Brooke BN: Management of an ileostomy including its complications. Lancet 2:102, 1952

Brooke BN, Walker FC: A method of extensive revision of an ileostomy. Br J Surg 49:401, 1961

Cohen Z: Symposium on the treatment of inflammatory bowel disease in children and adolescents. 4— Evolution of the Kock continent reservoir ileostomy. Can J Surg 25:509, 1982

Dozois RR, Kelly KA, et al: Factors affecting revision rate after continent ileostomy. Arch Surg 116:610, 1981

Kock NH, Darle N, et al: Ileostomy. Curr Prob Surg 14:6, 1977

Kock NG, Myrvold HE, et al: Continent ileostomy: An account of 314 patients. Acta Chir Scand 147:67, 1981

Ritchie JK: Results of surgery for inflammatory bowel disease. A further survey of one hospital region. Br Med J 1:264, 1974

Turnbull RB, Fazio VW: Advances in the surgical technique of ulcerative colitis surgery. Endoanal proctectomy and two-directional myotomy ileostomy. Ann Surg 7:315, 1975

Turnbull RB Jr, Weakley FL: Atlas of Intestinal Stomas. St. Louis: CV Mosby, 1967

Colostomy

Barron J, Fallis LS: Colostomy closure by the intraperitoneal method. Dis Colon Rectum 1:466, 1958

Knox AJS, Birkett FDH, et al: Hazards of colostomy closure. Br J Surg 4:380, 1971

Marino AWM Jr, Mancini HWN, et al: Colostomy simplified. Mod Treat 8:892, 1971

Patey DH: Primary epithelial apposition in colostomy. Proc Roy Soc Med 44:423, 1951

Pemberton LB: Immediate mucocutaneous suture for loop colostomy. Surg Gynecol Obstet 135:793, 1972

Thomson JPS, Hawley PR: Results of closure of loop transverse colostomies. Br Med J 3:459, 1972

SECTION X
Staplers in Surgery

61. Staplers in Gastrointestinal Surgery

Mark M. Ravitch
Felicien M. Steichen

INTRODUCTION

Successful intestinal anastomosis and closure had rarely been accomplished before the beginning of the nineteenth century; the principles of intestinal suturing and healing had not yet been studied and defined and anesthesia and operating rooms equipped with basic amenities were still to be developed. In exploring the healing of intestinal wounds—some sporadic reports of success using a variety of sutures and operative techniques often relying on fistula formation were available by then—surgeons started to use mechanical devices as well as manual sutures employing gross needles and heavy thread, apparently devoting similar interest and effort to both methods. In what became an experimental and clinical study of ever-increasing intensity by surgeons in various clinics, manual and mechanical techniques were continually refined, methods of investigation became more and more sophisticated, and the results obtained provided better understanding of the basic principles involved. Although much of the initial impetus was toward the creation of continually improving mechanical devices, culminating in the presentation by Murphy and Ramaugé of their anastomotic buttons, manual suture techniques emerged progressively as the preferred method by the turn of the century. For immediate practical clinical purposes the anastomotic buttons were added to the surgeon's armamentarium late in the development of intestinal surgery. As a concept, however, for further investigation and possible future clinical application the harmonious initial co-existence of mechanical and manual suture techniques should have been maintained, so as to guarantee the earlier momentum and knowl-edge gained by both methods. However, as surgeons learned from the work of Travers, Lembert, and Halsted to suture the intestines and to trust that healing would take place—with the availability of continuously refined suture materials—they relied increasingly on manual skills acquired through long and hard years of apprenticeship in their craft. The earlier debate between two schools of thought continues unabated to this day and is charmingly illustrated by the words of the French surgeon Jeannel, commenting in 1902 on the ingenious button by Ramaugé, first presented in 1893:

> I believe I know how to sew, yet I side with the "boutonnistes." The ranks of the "suturistes" include only the prestidigitators of our profession. But I beg these skilled men to consider that they are the exception, that they cannot have a monopoly of intestinal surgery. . . . Is it to be denied that for the average surgeon it is easier to apply an anastomotic button than to suture an anastomosis? And friends, when the suturists point to the failures of the buttons, have they forgotten their own failures? Who would dare to say that suturing has not had and will not have more victims than the buttons?

As is so often the case, problem areas are identified and—often similar—solutions are proposed by independent workers during similar time periods. The study of and practical solution to intestinal sutures and healing are no exception. In 1812, Benjamin Travers, Ashley Cooper's distinguished student and colleague, showed very clearly that everting anastomoses in the dog would heal quite safely. To this day the contribution of Travers is misunderstood or misinterpreted inasmuch as it is often stated that Travers described the necessity for inverting sutures. This misconception may even be due to Lembert, who in 1826 suggested that the "lovely experiments" of Travers were in accord with his own beliefs. It was in fact Lembert who established the surgical dogma that the safe healing of intestinal closures depends on inverting, serosa-to-serosa sutures. During that same year two mechanical suture devices were introduced, one for inverting and the other one for everting end-to-end anastomoses. On February 24, 1826, Denans presented before the Société Royale de Médecine de Marseille a simple but elegant anastomotic device that had been used successfully in two dogs. In 1826 also, Henroz of Liège reported in his doctoral thesis the successful experimental use of articulated rings armed with alternating pins and holes. The bowel ends were everted over the rings and caught by the pins; the pins and holes of the two rings engaged, producing a mucosa-to-mucosa everting anastomosis. It remained for Halsted to demonstrate in 1887 that it was the tough submucosa that had to be included in the sutures if the anastomosis was to heal reliably.

The most popular mechanical anastomotic instrument certainly was the button introduced by John B. Murphy in 1892. However, given the simultaneous recognition and practical solution of problems, often when newer materials become available as illustrated by the history of intestinal sutures and the development of many other advances in medicine and surgery, various authors working independently and often without awareness of preceding experiences come to similar conclusions. In this case, Ramaugé of Buenos Aires described an elegant button of his own in 1893, independently of Murphy. However, it was Murphy's design that became most popular and was widely used, imitated, improved, and modified in various clinics here and in Europe, up to the present.

The first stapling instrument was introduced by Humer Hültl of Budapest in 1908 at the Second Congress of the Hungarian Surgical Society. Hültl defined the two principles that all stapling instruments have had in common since then, namely, compression and immobilization of the tissues to be stapled, followed by the introduction of the staples and their closure in B-shape. His instrument placed two double rows of fine steel wire staples, similar to those used today, so that the stomach or duodenum could be transected, leaving the ends closed with a double row of staples. Although Hültl's stapler

was well known at that time, the simpler instrument of Aladar von Petz presented in 1921 at the Eighth Annual Meeting of the Hungarian Surgical Society gained greater popularity. However, this instrument and many that followed used single rows of heavier, flat German silver staples and could only be relied upon to close the viscus, allowing for the placement of reinforcing manual sutures. Although widely known, these instruments were not widely used.

A variety of instruments were then developed in Germany, Hungary, and Japan, of which the most innovative was that of Friedrich of Ulm. One squeeze of the handle approximated the jaws gently compressing the tissues. By switching a release, a second squeeze of the handle drove in the staples, which were like those of von Petz. Friedrich's instrument was the first to provide interchangeable staple magazines, so that the instrument could be used repeatedly during the same operation.

The use of staples in surgical operations received its greatest impetus from the work of the Scientific Research Institute for Experimental Surgical Apparatus and Instruments in Moscow, beginning in 1950 with Gudov's vascular stapler. Three general types of instruments were developed in Russia:

1. A series of linear staplers, of which the American equivalents are the TA 30, TA 55, and TA 90, usually allowing the placement of a double staggered row of staples and, in the case of the American instruments, producing a mucosa-to-mucosa closure of the bowel
2. A linear anastomosing instrument, of which the American equivalent is the GIA. Although the Russian instrument places only one row of staples on each side of a dividing blade, the United States instrument allows for the placement of two staggered rows of staples on each side of the dividing knife
3. A tubular end-to-end or end-to-side, minimally inverting anastomotic stapler, of which the United States equivalents are the EEA and the ILS

In a first step, the American manufacturer* whose instruments are used in the operative techniques to be discussed, created lighter and better balanced instruments capable of accept-

---

* United States Surgical Corporation, Norwalk, Connecticut.

ing disposable, preloaded, sterilized cartridges, comprising all the moving parts that drive the individual staples. In a second step, the instruments have become available in totally disposable form. The TA incorporates a hinged cartridge and anvil unit, including a tissue retaining pin that moves automatically in place when the cartridge closing lever is activated. The disposable GIA contains shorter and finer staples with a closer arrangement so as to ensure better hemostasis. In yet a third refinement, premium instruments have now become available. In these the metal instrument includes all the new modifications and accepts as well the new cartridges. The disposable EEA has been improved by making a curved version available. There has also been devised in this country an instrument—the LDS—for ligature of omental and mesenteric vessels, which simultaneously places two clips and divides the tissue between them. The disposable, powered form of this instrument is preferred by us over the original metal instrument.

Limitations of space preclude a detailed discussion of the history of mechanical and manual intestinal sutures, as well as of the historical stapling instruments, the Russian contribution to surgical stapling, and the specifications and various applications of the United States instruments. These aspects have been dealt with elsewhere and therefore only highlights have been provided.

The use of staples in gastric, intestinal, biliary, and colon surgery in a series of operative drawings and accompanying descriptions is now presented.

OPERATIONS FOR COMPLICATIONS OF GASTROESOPHAGEAL REFLUX

The Combined Collis–Nissen Procedure for Shortened Esophagus (Fig. 61–1)*

A. The operation, performed through a low left posterolateral thoracotomy, is indicated in patients with dilatable strictures and shortening of the esophagus due to reflux esophagitis. The fundus of the stomach is pulled

up through the enlarged hiatus and with the GIA instrument a 5- to 6-cm gastric tube is created in continuity with the esophagus.

B. The caliber of the gastric tube is greater than that of the original esophagus, so as to allow for a reinforcing running suture line, used routinely only when the GIA instrument is applied to both walls of the stomach.

C. With vasa brevia and vessels along the lesser curvature ligated to allow gastric mobilization, a Nissen plication of the remaining fundus is performed. The sutures used to wrap the stomach fundus around the gastric tube are all anchored in the thick wall of this tube.

D. The stomach is then replaced below the diaphragm, positioning the fundoplication intraabdominally and the hiatus is closed around the gastric tube, distal to the stricture.

With the cure of esophageal reflux the stricture will soften and open up, either spontaneously or with a few postoperative dilatations.

Transverse Colon Interposition for Fixed, Fibrous Stricture (Fig. 61–2)

This operation is indicated in patients with fixed, fibrous stricture from reflux esophagitis that cannot be dilated pre- or intraoperatively. The approach is through an upper midline abdominal incision and a separate low left lateral thoracotomy.

A. The segment of transverse colon required is divided proximally and distally with the GIA instrument.

B. The gastric fundus having been stapled and divided, the esophagus is freed proximal to the stricture. The colon is brought up alongside the esophagus in the posterior mediastinum. The GIA arms are inserted through stab wounds in esophagus and colon and the anastomosis made before the specimen is resected.

C. Placing the TA 55 instrument obliquely permits staple closure of the esophagus, excluding the specimen and the now common GIA introduction site. The specimen is then cut away, using the TA jaw edge as a guide for the scalpel.

D. An end-to-end, inverting esophagocolostomy obtained by passing the EEA instrument

---

* Throughout this chapter, the letters in the lists refer to parts of the figures cited in the heading immediately above.

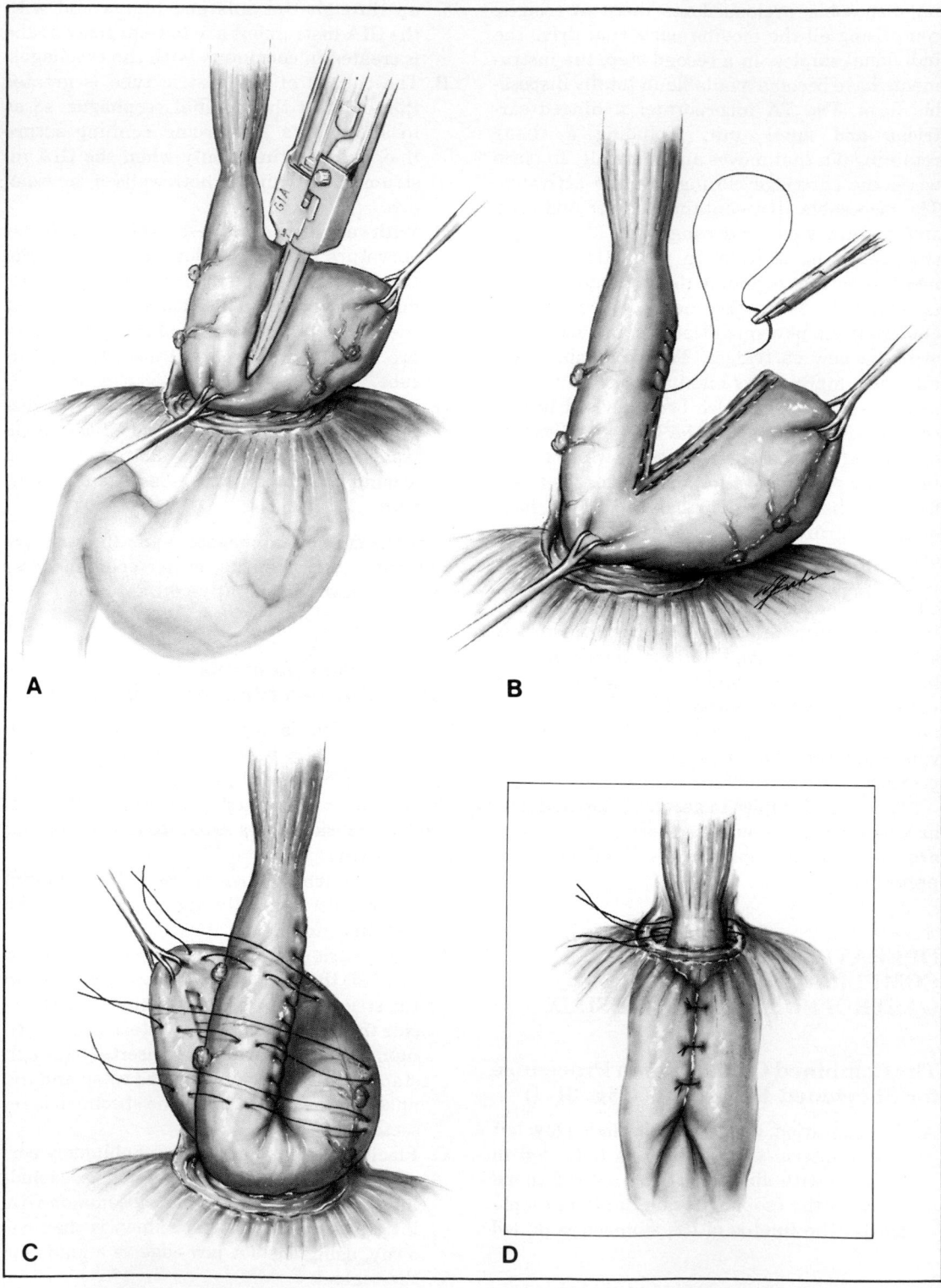

Figure 61–1. The combined Collis–Nissen procedure for shortened esophagus. (*Source: From Steichen FM, Ravitch MM, 1983, with permission.*)

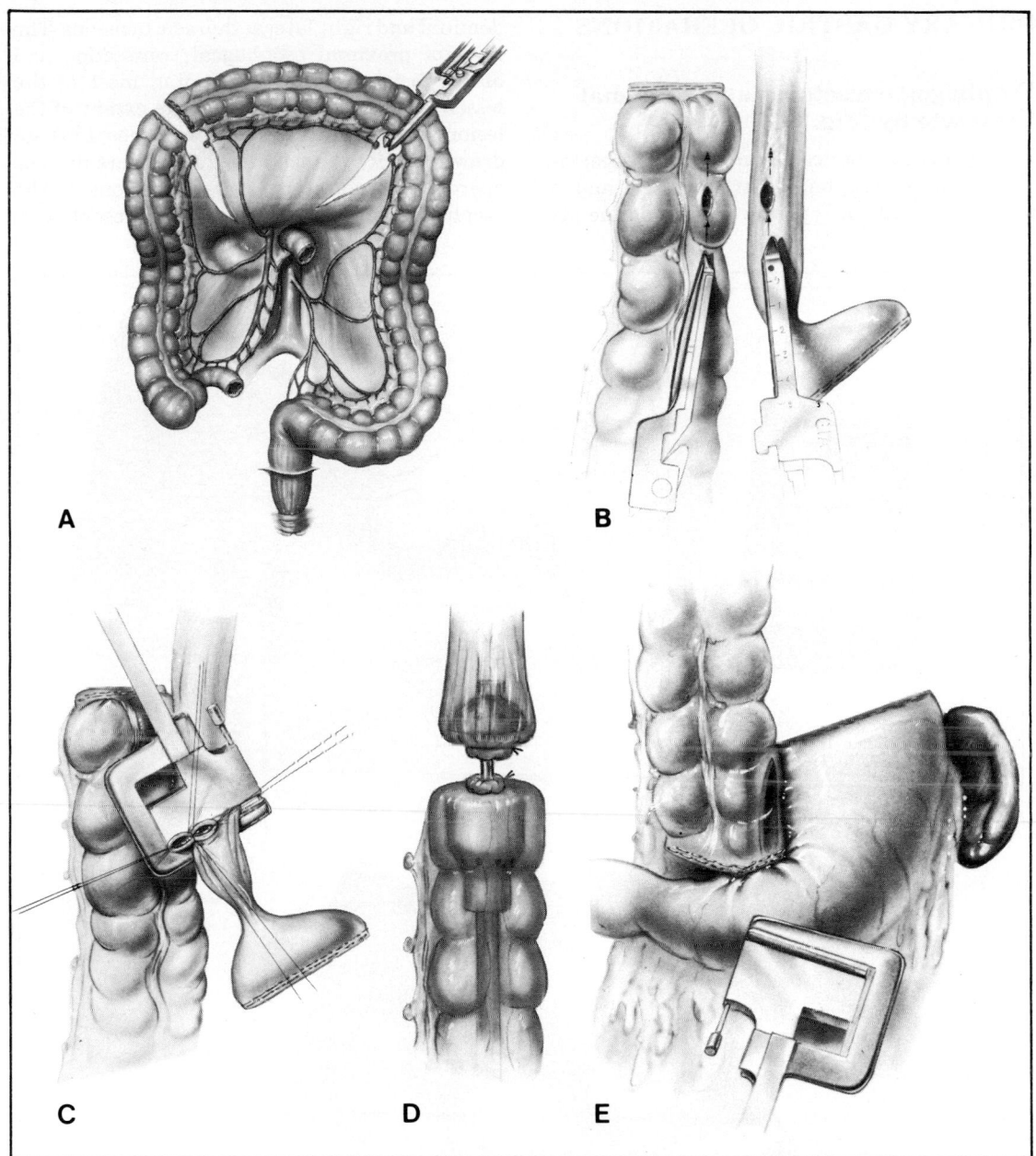

A

B

C   D   E

Figure 61–2. Transverse colon interposition for fixed, fibrous stricture. (*Source: Figs. A,B,C,E from Steichen FM, Ravitch MM, 1983, with permission.*)

through the open lumen of the colon segment from the abdomen represents an alternate solution for the proximal anastomosis.

E. The colonic segment is anastomosed end-to-side to the anterior wall of the stomach, near the lesser curvature, with the GIA instru-

ment prongs inserted through a cutaway corner of the colic staple line (or the entirely open colic lumen, if the EEA was used) and through a stab wound in the stomach. The common GIA opening is closed with the TA 55.

PRIMARY GASTRIC OPERATIONS

Esophagogastrectomy and Proximal Gastrectomy (Fig. 61–3)

This operation is indicated for malignant lesions at or near the esophagogastric junction and is performed through separate upper midline ab-dominal and right lateral thoracic incisions. The level of proximal esophageal transection and distal gastric division—including most of the lesser curvature—depends on the extent of the lesion and the presence of celiac nodes. In these drawings only the basic use of staplers for this operation is demonstrated. For lesions of the esophagus proper we prefer total esophagec-

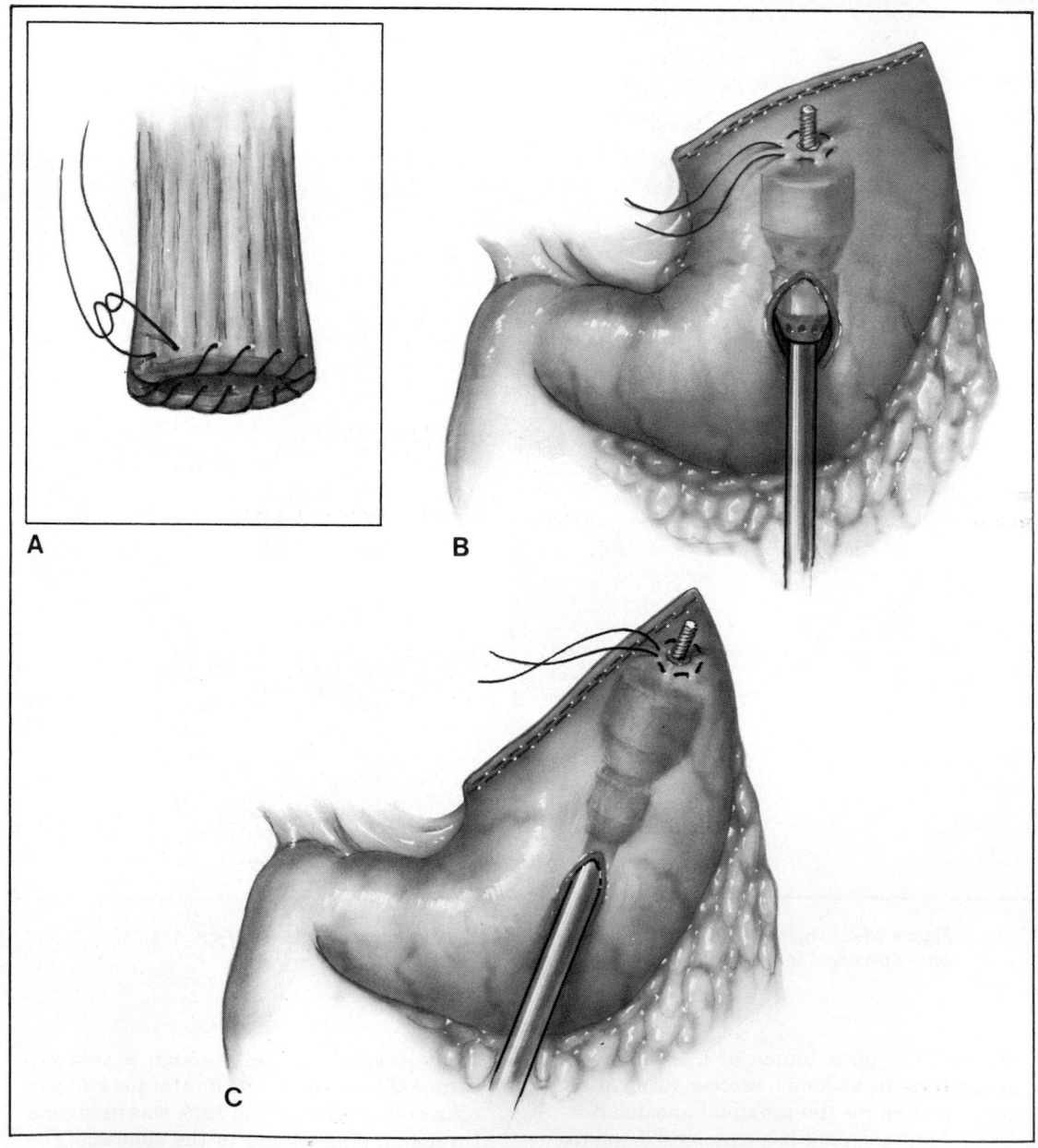

Figure 61–3. A through **G.** Esophagogastrectomy and proximal gastrectomy. (*Source: Figs. B,D,E,F,G from Steichen FM, Ravitch MM, 1980, with permission.*)

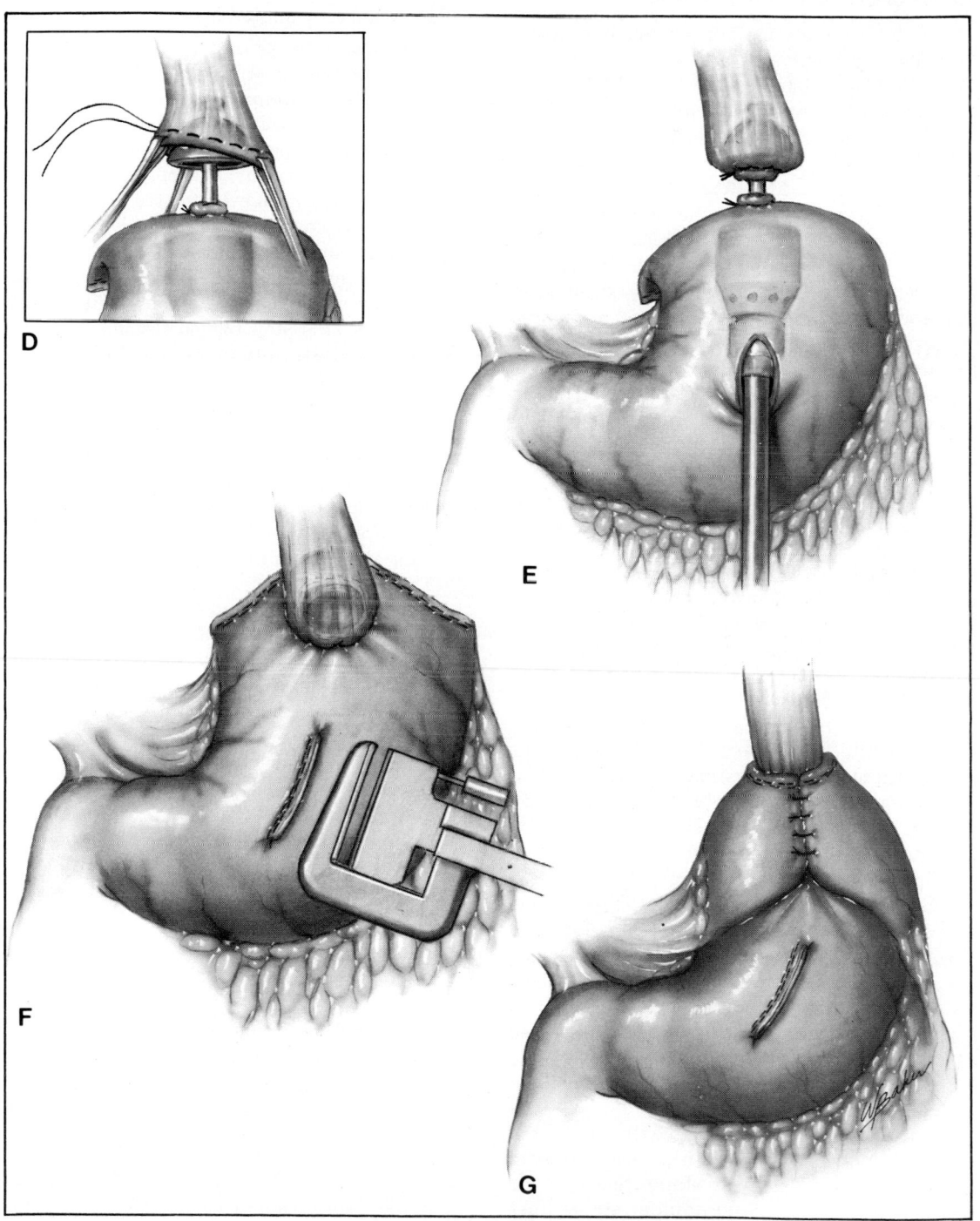

Figure 61–3. *Continued*

tomy and replacement with a gastric tube or colon segment, and in large lesions of the proximal stomach total gastrectomy with jejunal reservoir is the operation of choice.

A. Following resection of the specimen, the remaining esophagus and stomach are prepared for anastomosis with the EEA instrument. As a matter of routine, the division of the body of the stomach will take place along the upper edge of the TA 90 instrument. (Fig. 61–3B) after it has been applied a second time to close the remaining distal stomach. In case of a thick esophageal wall—as illustrated in Figure 61–3A—the esophagus is transected first and an over-and-over purse string suture is placed around the open esophageal end. If the esophageal wall is relatively thin, the modified Furniss clamp purse string instrument is placed across the proximal esophagus at the level chosen for resection and the purse string suture is placed, followed by transection of the esophagus along the lower edge of the purse string instrument (see Fig. 61–14A).

B. The mid-anterior wall of the stomach is incised, the EEA is introduced into the gastric lumen without the anvil, and the center rod is passed through a small puncture in the anterior gastric wall, some 2 to 3 cm distal to the TA 90 closure. A purse string suture may be placed if the central rod does not fit snugly in the gastric opening and if the anastomosis requires manipulation in narrow anatomic spaces where the EEA is used to "carry" the stomach up toward the esophagus.

C. In patients in whom most or all of the lesser curvature has to be removed, the remaining stomach assumes the shape of an elongated tube along the greater curvature. To provide maximum length, the central rod is best brought out in the angle formed by the TA 90 closure and greater curvature or passed through the excised corner of the gastric closure (as illustrated in Fig. 61–4F for distal gastrectomy).

The placement of the center rod of the EEA instrument through a corner or even the center of a linear staple line and the crossing of linear and annular staple lines as the end-to-end inverting anastomosis is performed, had been used by the authors

with great caution initially. Experimental data and a gradually increasing clinical experience have shown the safety of this approach in gastrectomy and low anterior resection. Whenever possible, the areas of overlapping linear and annular staple lines are reinforced by one or two sutures. Should the EEA annular blade not cut clear through the tissues, then the anvil should be separated from the cartridge and the anastomosis inspected through the existing gastrotomy (or a newly created proximal colotomy in case of low anterior resection). Usually small attachments of the purse string doughnuts to the inner aspect of the circular anastomosis are then quite easily severed. This step has so far not been required in a steadily mounting clinical experience, but is reserved to surgeons who have a great experience with stapling in general.

D. The anvil nose cone is attached to the central rod, the gastric purse string tied and the anvil advanced into the esophagus.

E. The esophageal purse string is tied and the two organs approximated by turning the wing nut on the instrument.

F. The end-to-side inverting anastomosis has been accomplished and the EEA instrument removed with the two complete doughnuts of tissue containing the purse strings. The gastrotomy used for the EEA placement is closed mucosa-to-mucosa with the TA 55 instrument.

G. If possible, a gastric wrap is manually sutured about the anastomosis, to reinforce it and prevent reflux. Often there is not enough stomach available for this purpose, especially if the technique shown in Figure 61–3C has been used.

Distal Gastrectomy and Billroth I Reconstruction (Fig. 61–4)

A. The liberation of the lesser and greater curvatures is the same, regardless of the ultimate technique of reconstruction, and is performed with the LDS instrument. Each operation of this instrument fires two staples and divides the tissue between them.

B. For a Billroth I reconstruction, the purse string clamp is applied just distal to the pylorus and the monofilament purse string suture placed. The duodenum is then divided

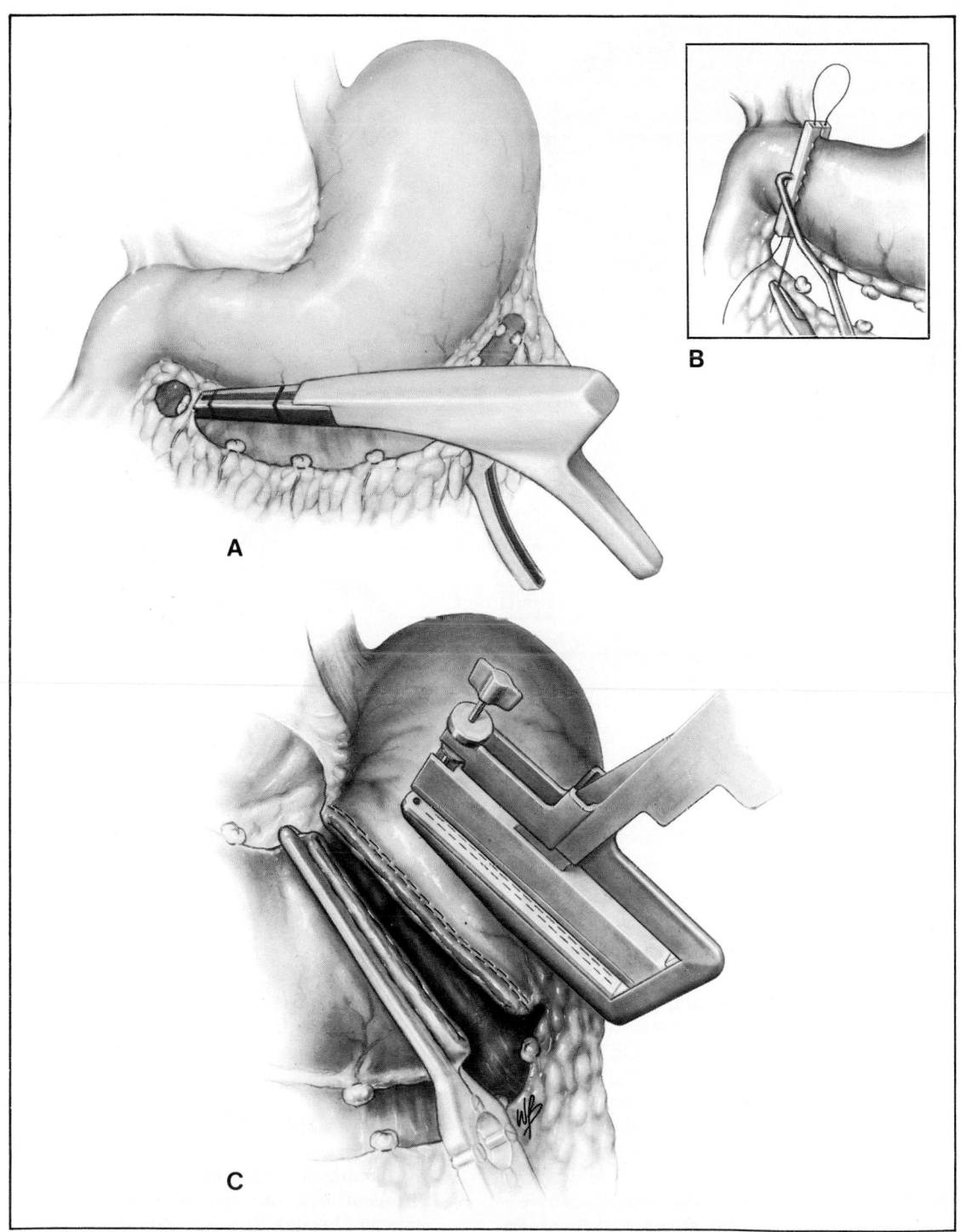

Figure 61–4. A through **G.** Distal gastrectomy and Billroth I reconstruction.

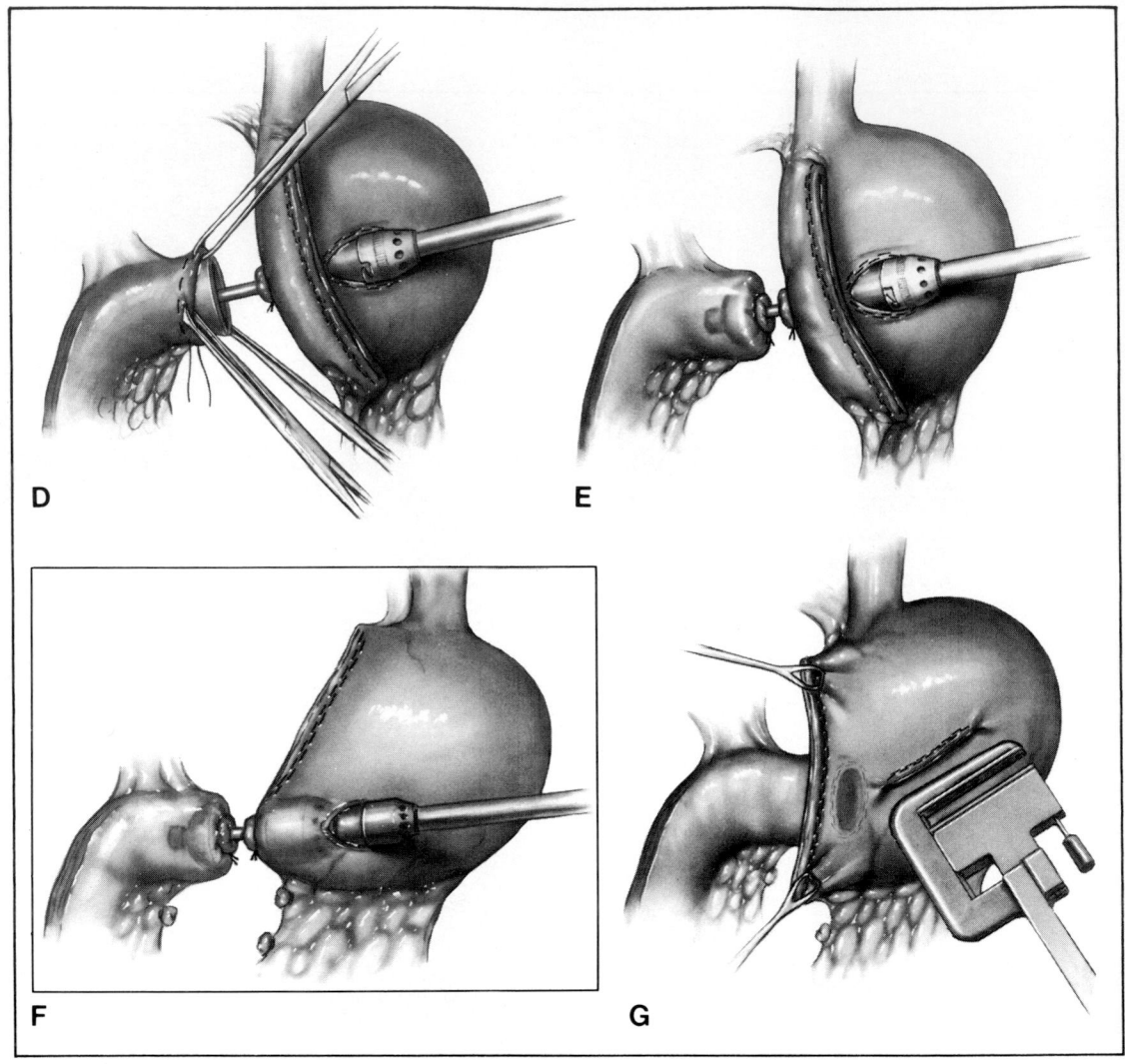

Figure 61–4. *Continued*

on the proximal edge of the purse string clamp.

C. The stomach has been stapled at the elected level of resection and transected between the edge of the TA 90 instrument and a Payr clamp. Usually one will observe a light blush of blood, attesting to the viability of the gastric edge beyond the staple line. An occasional spurting blood vessel will have to be secured with a suture.

D. The EEA instrument—without the anvil—is introduced into the stomach through an anterior gastrotomy and the central rod is advanced through a stab wound in the cen-

ter of a purse string suture, placed in the posterior wall of the stomach, some 3 to 4 cm proximal to the gastric closure. The anvil is attached to the central rod and advanced into the duodenum, held open by three Adson clamps.

E. The duodenal and gastric purse string sutures are tightened around the central rod, and anvil and cartridge are brought together by turning the wing nut of the EEA.

F. Alternatively the central rod can be advanced through the excised corner of the gastric closure, near the greater curvature. A purse string suture is used to secure this opening around the central rod. The passage of the EEA center rod through a linear staple line is described in greater detail in Figure 61–3C.

G. The anastomosis has been accomplished and the EEA instrument removed. The anterior gastrotomy is closed mucosa-to-mucosa with the TA instrument.

Distal Gastrectomy and Billroth II Reconstruction (Fig. 61–5)

A. Liberation of the greater and lesser curvatures is performed with the LDS instrument, which places two staples by one squeeze of the handles and divides the tissues between them.
B. The duodenum, stapled with the TA instrument, is transected between this instrument and a small Payr clamp placed on the stomach.
C. At the site of gastric resection, the proximal stomach is closed with the TA 90 instrument and transected between this instrument and a Payr clamp, using the lower edge of the TA 90 as a guide for the scalpel.
D. Reconstruction of continuity is established by gastroenterostomy on the posterior gastric wall, some 2 to 3 cm proximal to the gastric closure. For this purpose the proximal jejunum and posterior wall of gastric stump are placed side-by-side and stab holes made near the greater curvature in the stomach and in the antimesenteric wall of the jejunum. The GIA limbs are inserted, the instrument halves are locked and the anastomosis is performed (Fig. 61–5E).
E. Alternatively the GIA can be placed through the cut away greater curvature corner of the stomach and the gastroenterostomy performed medial and parallel to the greater curvature.
F. Following removal of the GIA instrument, the anastomosis is inspected. Persistent bleeding points are closed with a figure-eight catgut suture. The common GIA introduction site is then closed with the TA instrument.

Distal Gastrectomy and Billroth II Reconstruction with Roux-Y Loop (Fig. 61–6)

In view of the relatively low, but definite and distressing incidence of alkaline reflux gastritis after Billroth I and II reconstruction following distal gastrectomy, DuPlessis proposed the primary use of a Roux-Y jejunal loop in reestablishing gastrointestinal (GI) continuity. In such operations a vagotomy is always necessary.

A. Stomach and duodenum are closed with staples and transected as in the gastrectomy with Billroth II reconstruction and the jejunum is divided with the GIA instrument, some 10 to 15 cm from the ligament of Treitz.
B. The distal jejunal loop is anastomosed to a convenient point on the posterior wall of the stomach in an end-to-side fashion with the familiar GIA and TA technique.
C. Bowel continuity is reestablished at 40 cm from the gastroenterostomy by Roux-Y anastomosis of the proximal jejunum to the distal, efferent jejunal limb, using the GIA and TA instruments.

Total Gastrectomy and Primary Jejunal Reservoir (Fig. 61–7)

Following total gastrectomy for cure in patients with gastric malignancy, or in case of a Zollinger–Ellison syndrome, whenever possible we prefer to reconstruct intestinal continuity with a Paulino or Hunt–Lawrence pouch to restore reservoir capacity. The various combinations of use of the GIA, TA, and EEA make this an attractive, safe, and functionally sound alternative to simple esophago-duodenostomy or -jejunostomy.

A. The jejunum is divided with the GIA instrument, 20 to 25 cm below the ligament of Treitz. This is our preferred mode of transection of the bowel, for whatever purpose, between the ligament of Treitz and the rectum, simultaneously sealing both ends.
B. The proximal end of the distal jejunal loop is brought up and may be—as shown in Figure 61–7B—anastomosed manually to the esophagus in an end-to-side ("handle of the cane") fashion. The excess jejunum is stapled off with a TA instrument and resected peripheral to the blade of the instrument. The duodenojejunal segment distal to the ligament of Treitz is apposed to the loop that has been anastomosed to the esophagus so as to have an isoperistaltic single limb of jejunum 35 to 40 cm between the esophagus and the 15 to 20 cm jejunojejunostomy.

C. The duodenojejunal segment can be stapled to the long, efferent jejunal limb isoperistaltically as in this case. The GIA instrument inserted through a stab wound in the long jejunal limb and through the cutaway antimesenteric corner of the duodenojejunal limb, is passed upward and activated, creating a 5-cm anastomosis. Five centimeters

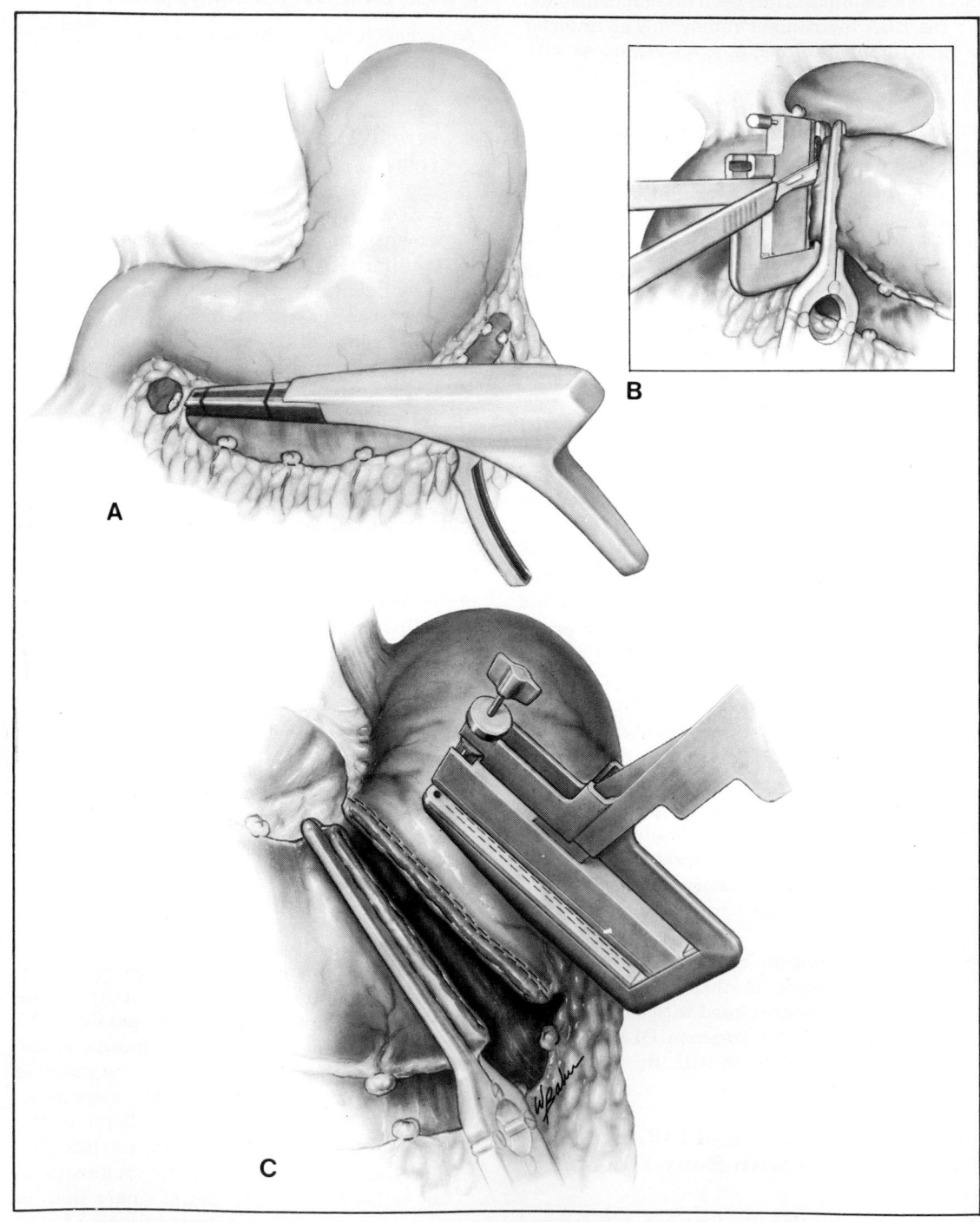

Figure 61–5. A through **F.** Distal gastrectomy and Billroth II reconstruction.

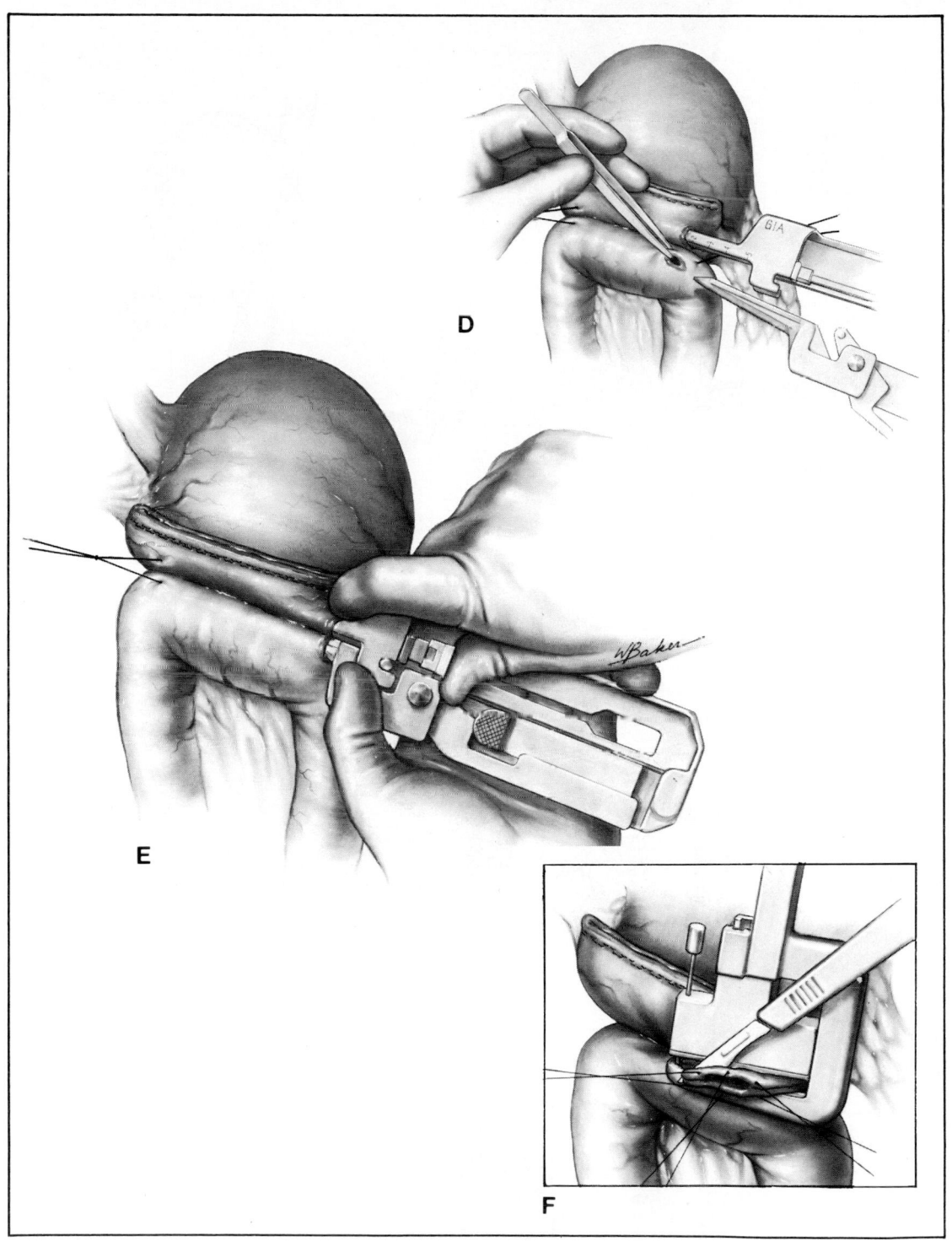

Figure 61–5. *Continued*

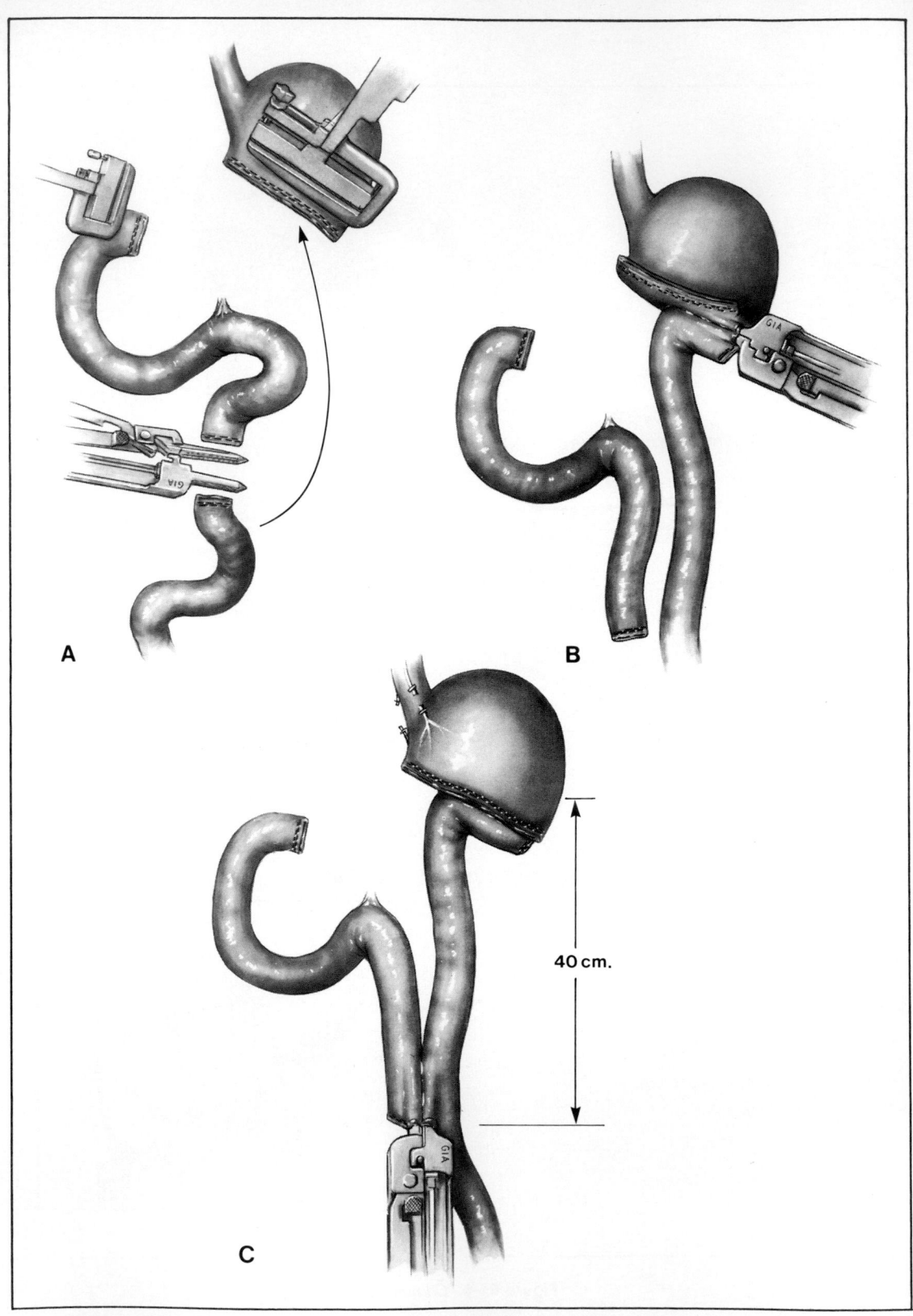

Figure 61–6. Distal gastrectomy and Billroth II reconstruction with Roux-Y loop. (*Source: From Steichen FM, Ravitch MM, 1983, with permission.*)

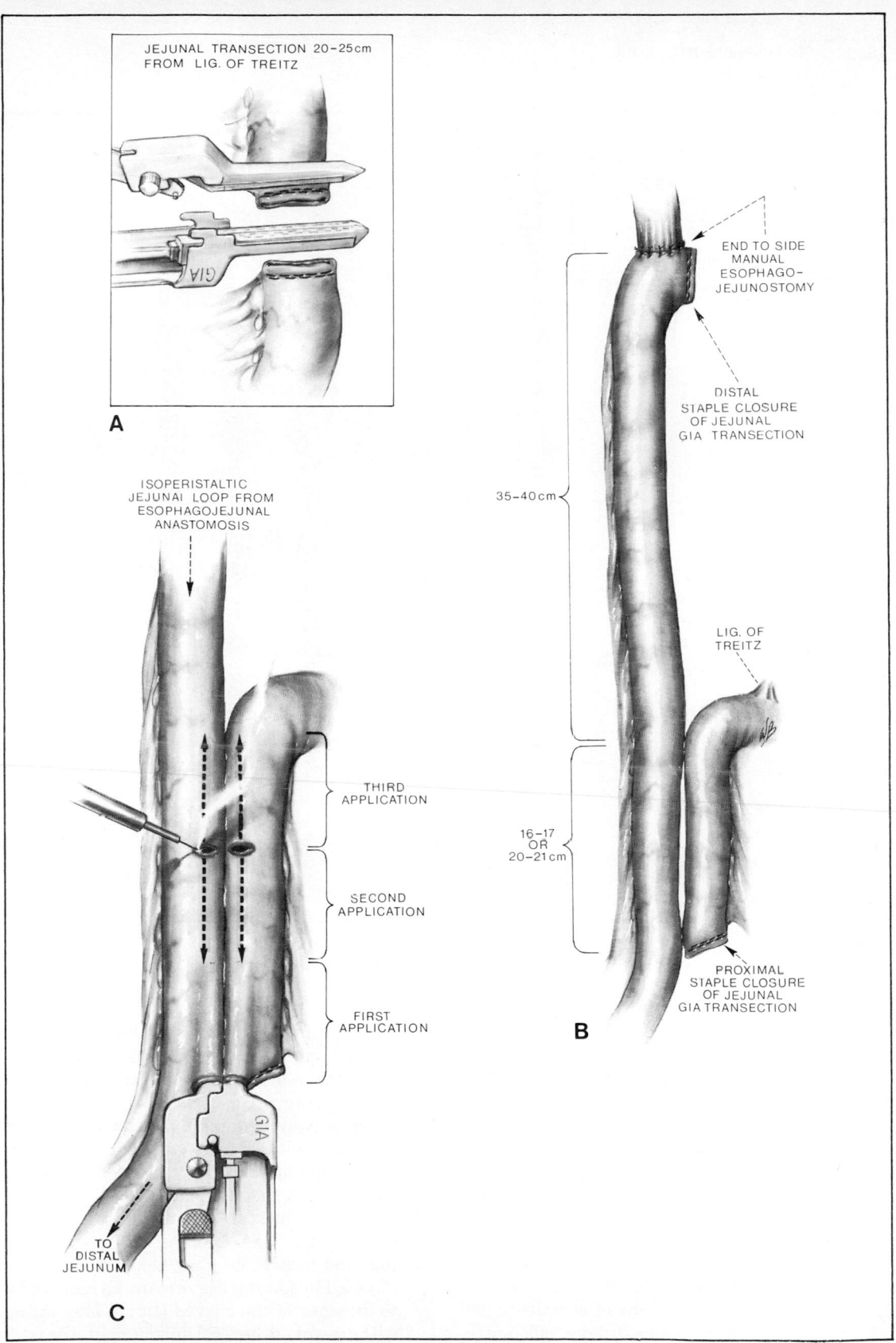

Figure 61–7. A through **G.** Total gastrectomy and primary jejunal reservoir. (*Source: Figs. A through E from Steichen FM, Ravitch MM, Ann Surg, 1972, with permission; Figs. F and G from Steichen FM, Ravitch MM, 1983, with permission.*)

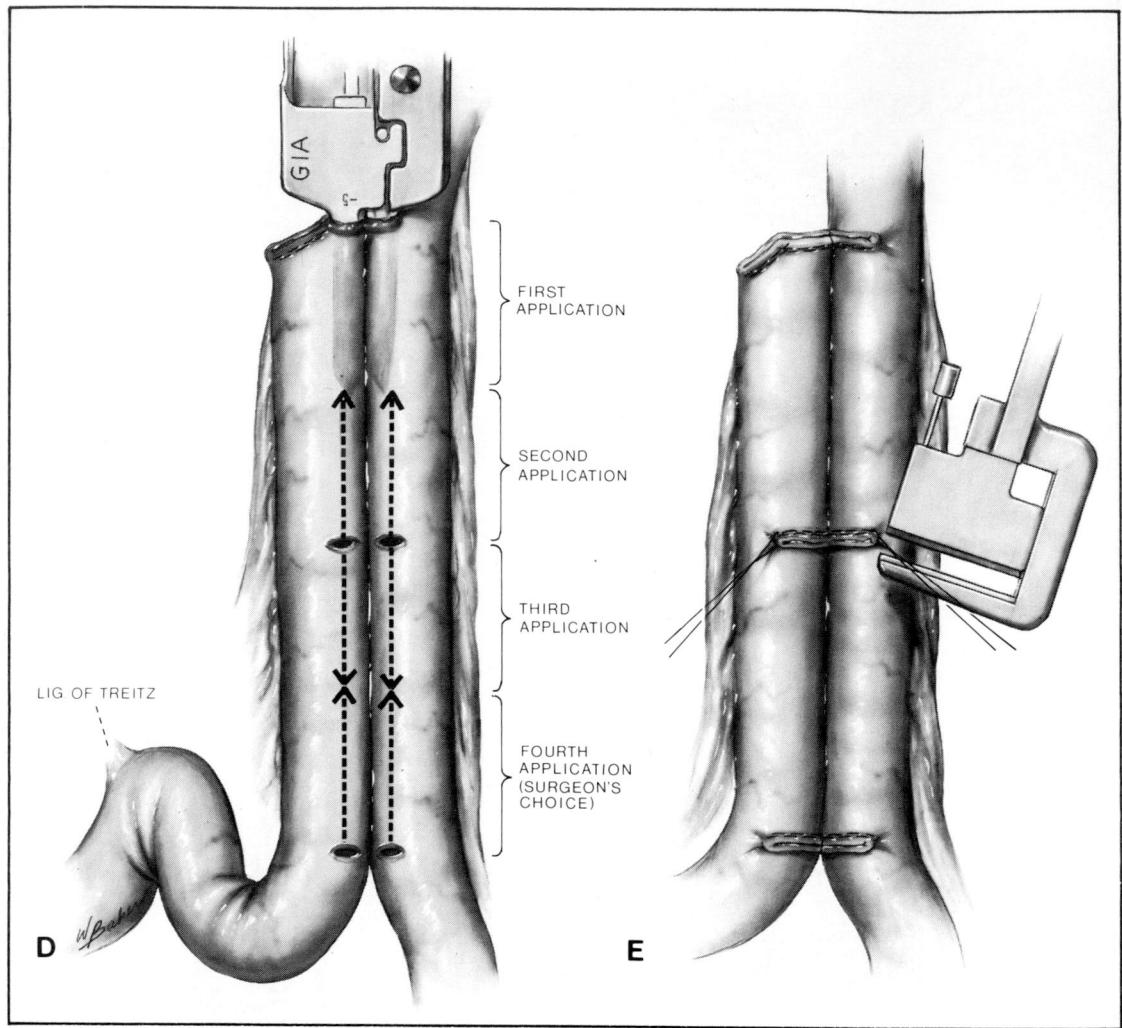

D

E

LIG OF TREITZ

FIRST
APPLICATION

SECOND
APPLICATION

THIRD
APPLICATION

FOURTH
APPLICATION
(SURGEON'S
CHOICE)

Figure 61–7. *Continued*

above the end of this anastomosis, matching stab wounds are created in the two loops and the GIA instrument inserted first distally and then proximally, resulting in three connecting 5-cm anastomoses.

D. The same technique can be employed with the duodenojejunal segment used antiperistaltically. If a larger pouch is desired, the GIA instrument is used four times.

E. The openings left at the withdrawal of the GIA instrument are closed transversely mucosa-to-mucosa with the TA instrument. Complicated constructions of substitute organs are performed much more efficiently with minimal exposure of the open bowel lumen, improved hemostasis, and diminished trauma to the bowel as compared to manual sutures.

F. Alternatively, the jejunum can be doubled back on itself and a 15- or 20-cm Hunt–Lawrence jejunojejunostomy created with the GIA and TA instruments.

G. The EEA instrument is passed upward through the GIA opening and the inverting end-to-side esophagojejunostomy constructed by joining the remaining esophagus to the apex of the curved jejunal loop. After withdrawal of the EEA instrument, the GIA

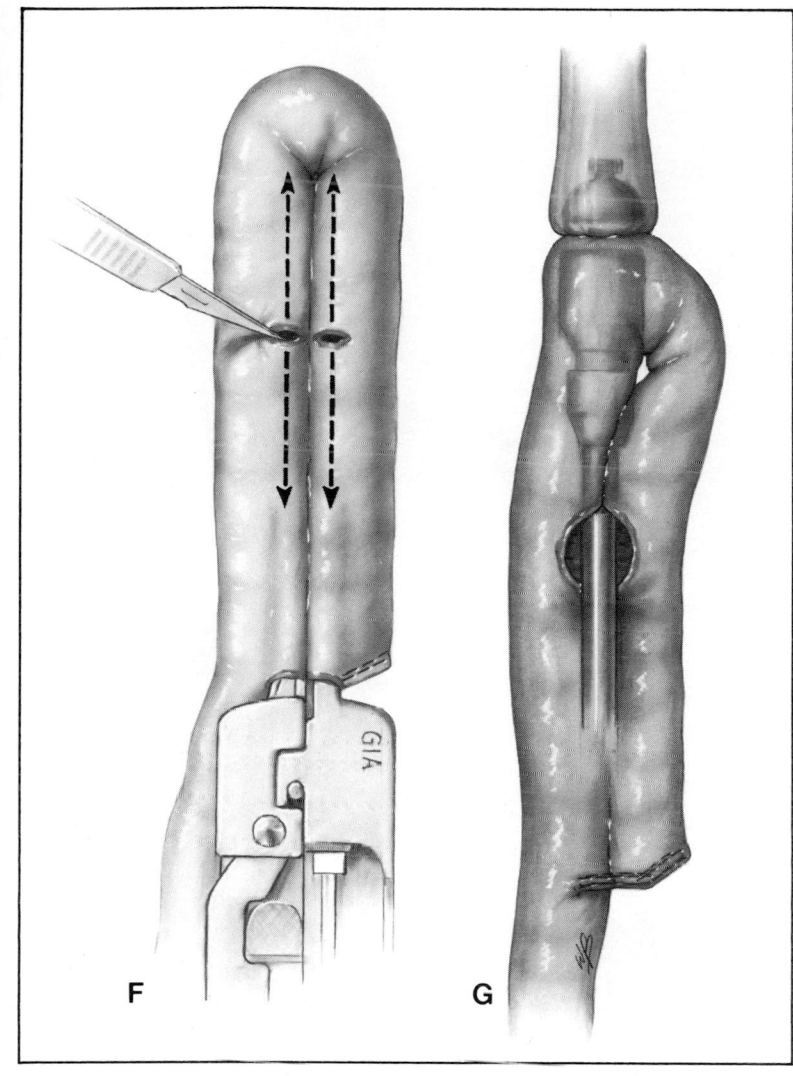

F

G

Figure 61–7. *Continued*

stab wound is closed mucosa-to-mucosa with the TA instrument. The proximal jejunum is then anastomosed some 35 to 40 cm below the jejunal reservoir by a Roux-Y technique as shown in Figures 61–6C and 61–8B.

REMEDIAL GASTRIC OPERATIONS

Roux-Y Conversion of Billroth II Gastroenterostomy (Fig. 61–8)

In a patient with bile gastritis, or with afferent loop obstruction, after gastrectomy and Billroth II reconstruction, it is remarkably simple with the stapling instruments to make the conversion to a Roux-Y. If it had not been part of the original operation, a vagotomy should be added at the time of conversion.

A. The afferent jejunal loop is divided close to the stomach with the GIA.

B. The stapled blind end of the proximal loop is brought down along the efferent loop and anastomosed some 40 cm from the gastroenterostomy with the GIA in end-to-side Roux-Y fashion. The TA clamp is used to close the GIA opening in a mucosa-to-mucosa fashion.

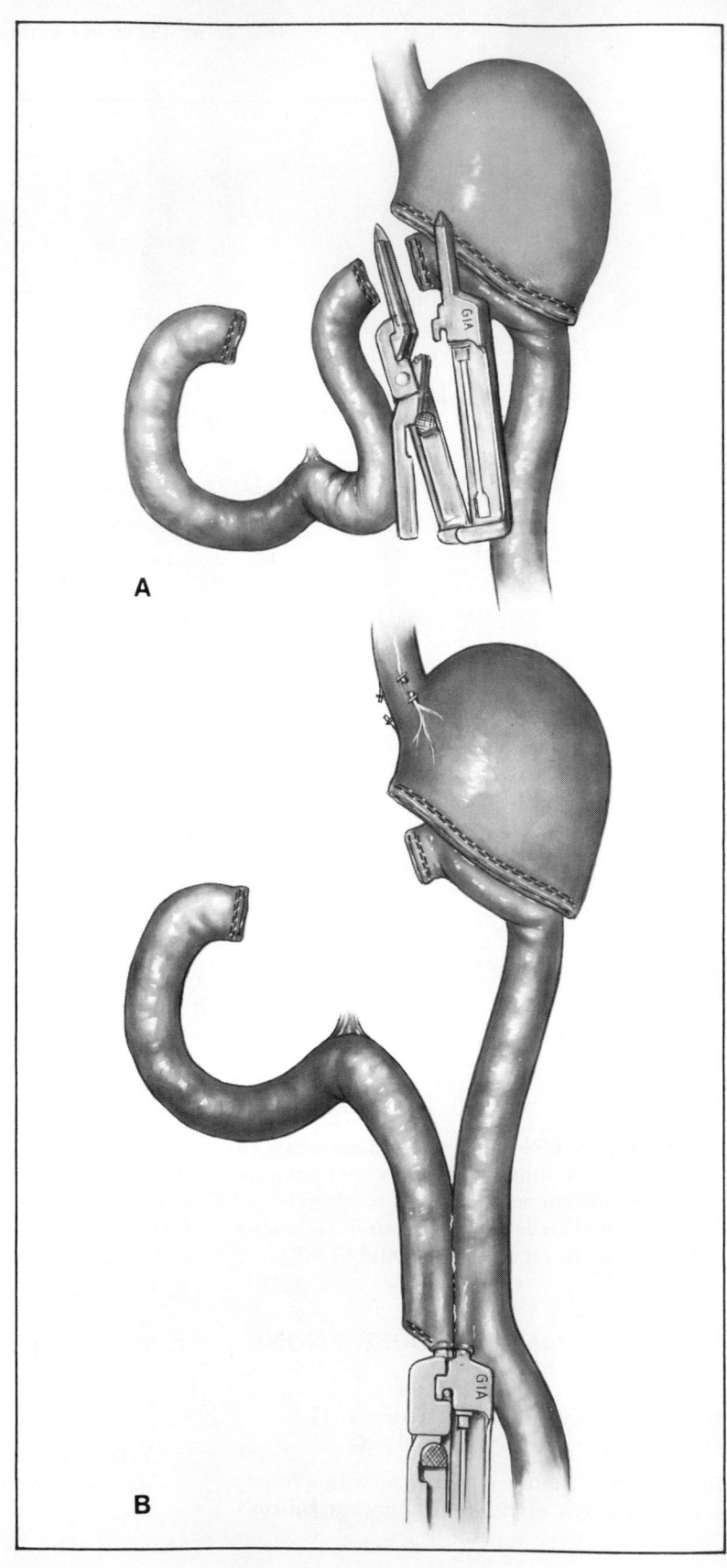

A

B

Figure 61–8. Roux-Y conversion of Billroth II. (*Source: From Steichen FM, Ravitch MM, 1983, with permission.*)

Resection of a Retrocolic Gastroenterostomy and Reconstruction of Normal Anatomy (Fig. 61-9)

A. The dissection of the gastroenterostomy is limited to the creation of a posterior channel to place the index finger behind the anasto-

mosis and guide the lower jaw of the TA 55 instrument through the same channel.

B. The instrument is then passed up on the stomach, just above the anastomosis, and the stomach is closed and transected above the anastomosis, on the TA. The jejunum will be divided with the GIA instrument on either side of the gastroenterostomy.

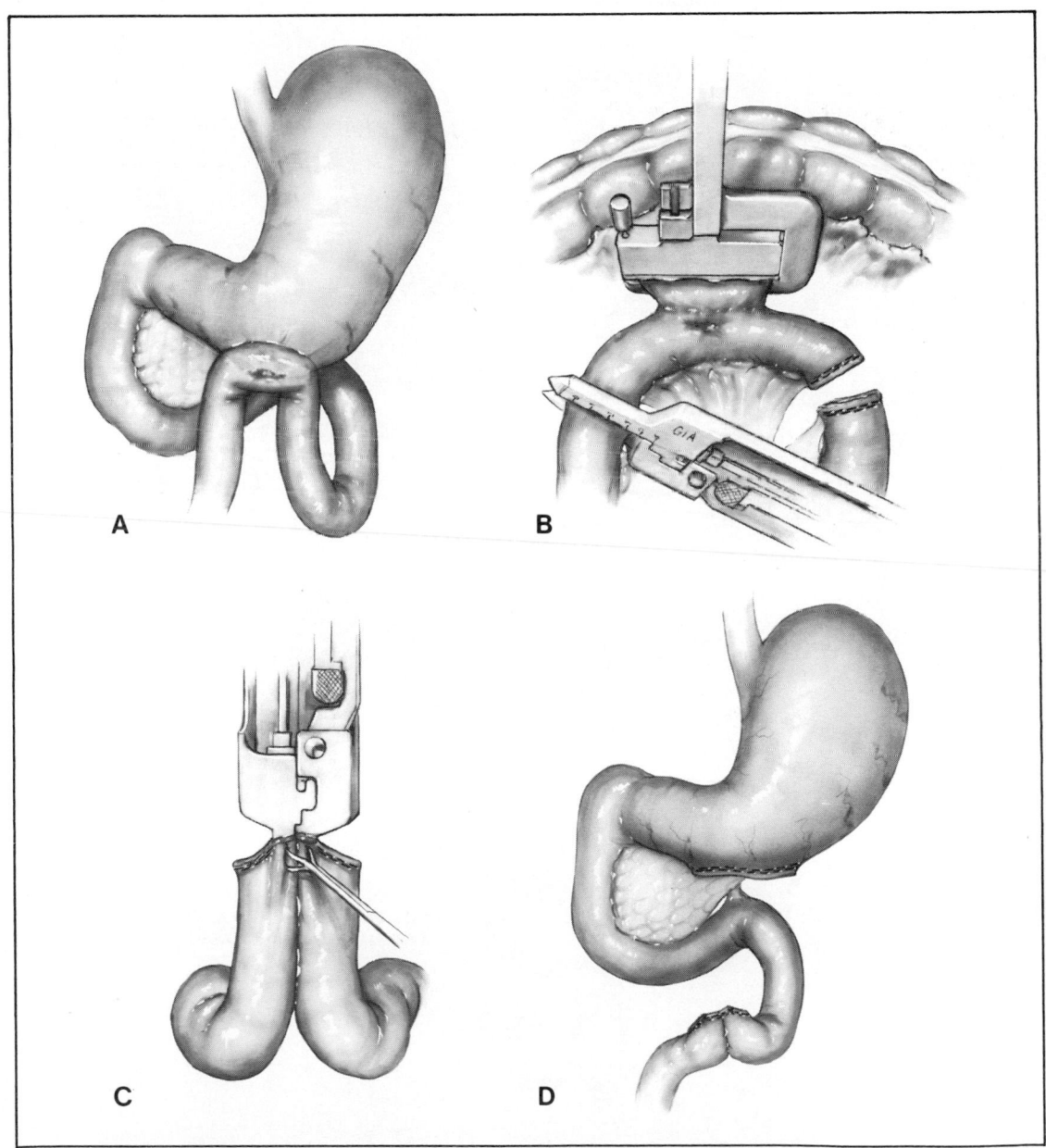

Figure 61-9. Resection of retrocolic gastroenterostomy. (*Source: From Steichen FM, Ravitch MM, 1983, with permission.*)

C. The two jejunal limbs are apposed in gun-barrel fashion and the antimesenteric corners of the jejunal closures are cut away. One blade of the GIA instrument is placed into each bowel lumen and the instrument

operated, achieving an anatomic side-to-side anastomosis.

D. A TA instrument (not shown) is then applied across the GIA introduction site so as to transform the side-to-side anastomosis into

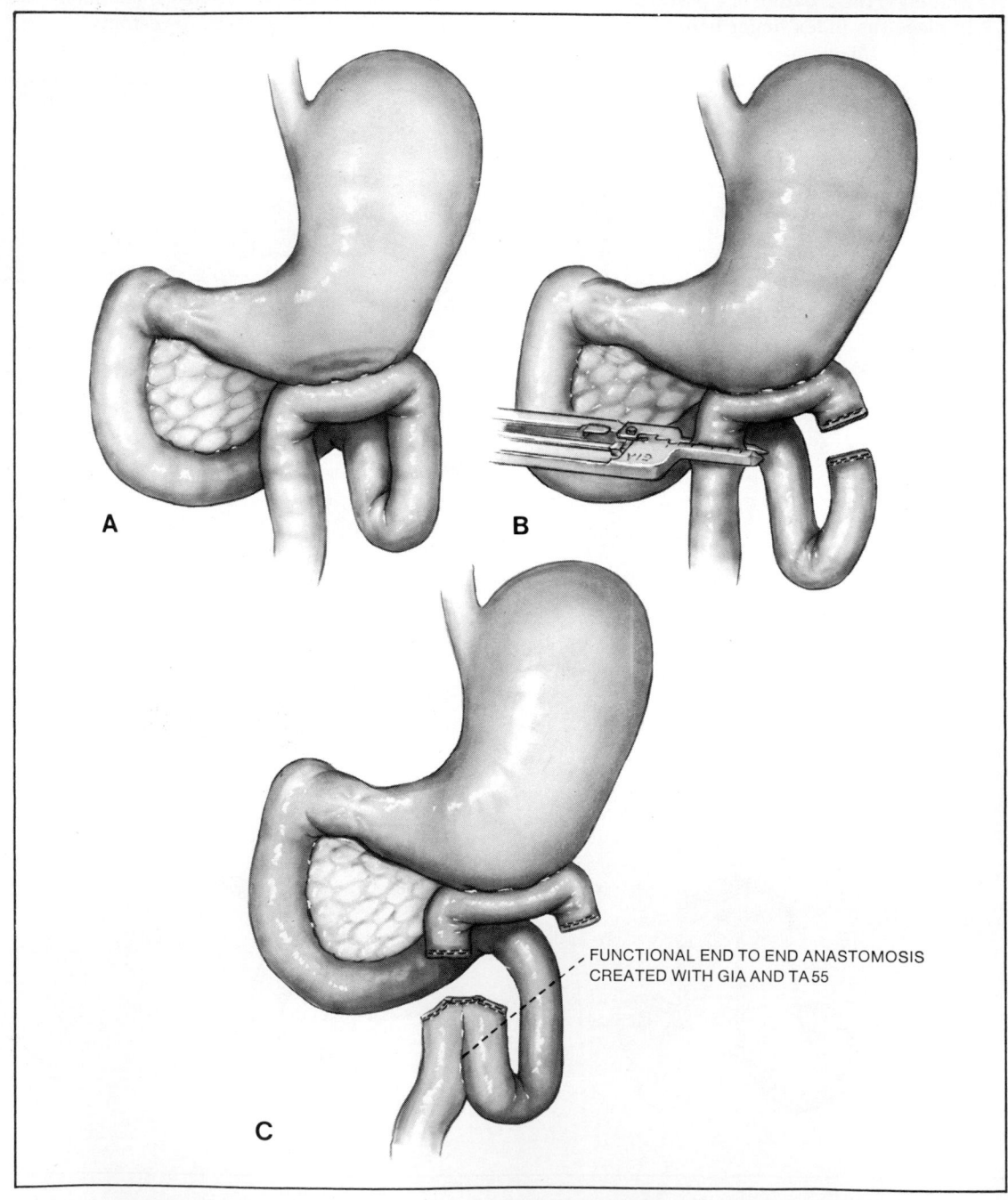

FUNCTIONAL END TO END ANASTOMOSIS
CREATED WITH GIA AND TA 55

Figure 61–10. A through **F.** Resection of gastroenterostomy with distal gastrectomy and Billroth II. (*Source: From Steichen FM, Ravitch MM, 1983, with permission.*)

what is a U-shaped, functional end-to-end anastomosis.

Resection of Gastroenterostomy with Distal Gastrectomy and Billroth II Gastroenterostomy for Persistent Duodenal Ulcer (Fig. 61–10)

A. The gastroenterostomy is close to the pylorus and can therefore not be retained for the Billroth II reconstruction.

B. The afferent and efferent jejunal loops are divided and closed with the GIA instrument.

C. The usual functional end-to-end anastomosis, with the GIA and the TA 55 instruments, restores intestinal continuity.

D. At the elected site for resection, the stomach is stapled and transected on the lower edge of a TA 90 stapling instrument.

E. Through the appropriate stab wound, one arm of the GIA instrument is inserted into the proximal jejunum and the other one into

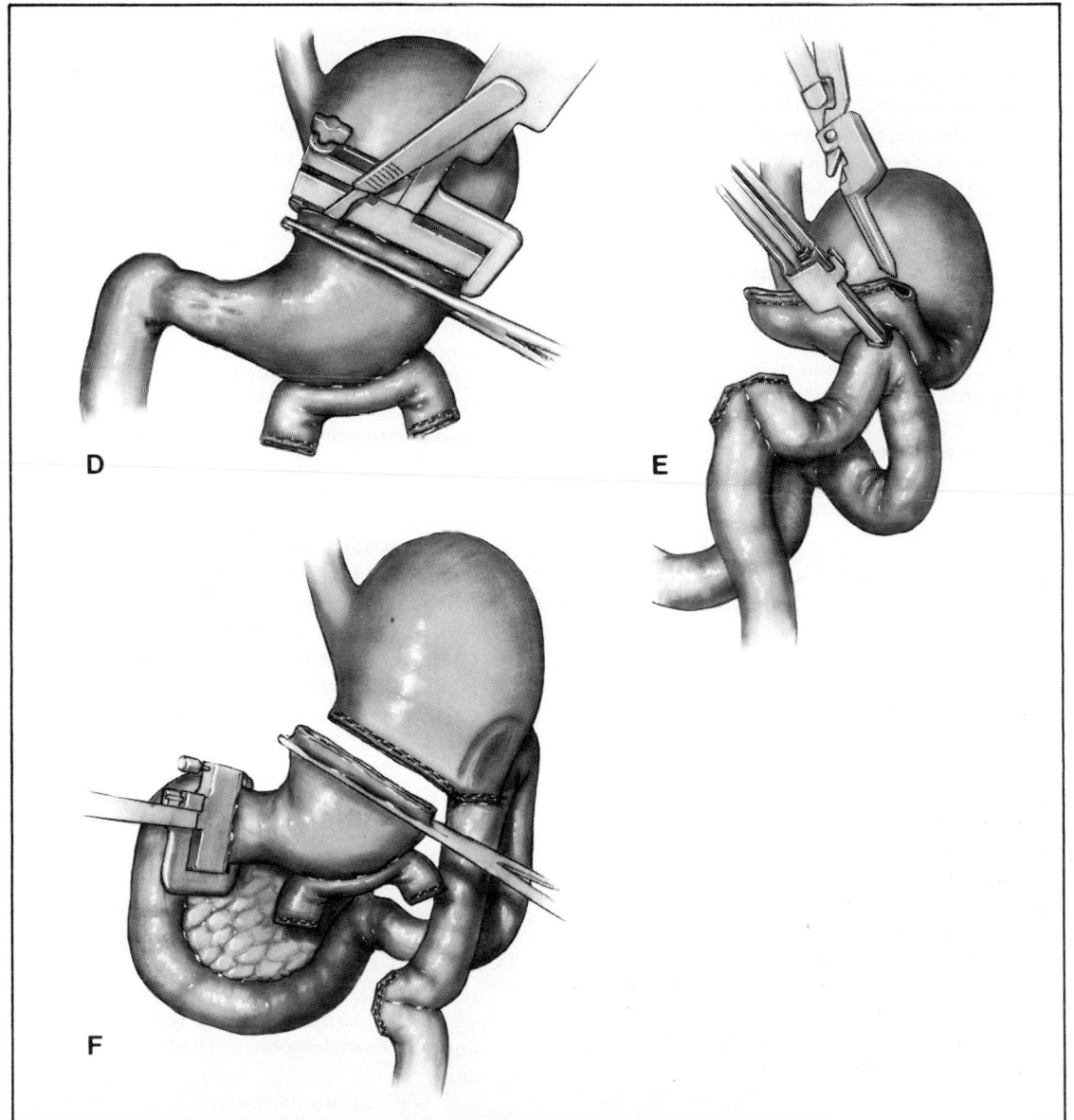

Figure 61–10. *Continued*

the stomach through the excised greater curvature end of the gastric staple closure.

F. The anastomosis thus created has its long axis more or less parallel to the greater curvature. Some surgeons choose to anchor the upper extremity of the jejunal loop to the stomach with a single silk stitch. The mucosa-to-mucosa TA 55 closure of the GIA opening made for construction of the anastomosis crosses the staple line of the stomach and we often place a three-cornered stitch to reinforce this angle. The duodenum is closed with the TA 55 instrument and amputated along the edge of the instrument, preferably distal to the ulcer. If the closure is proximal to the ulcer, one should avoid excessive manipulation of the instrument that may elevate the ulcer away from the pancreas, inviting a leak, which may subsequently be interpreted as a "duodenal stump leak."

Resection of Gastrojejunocolic Fistula with Billroth II Reconstruction (Fig. 61–11)

The efficiency, speed, and freedom from bleeding or contamination afforded by the use of these instruments make them particularly useful in the resection of complicated compound lesions, especially when inflammatory adhesions or invasion with carcinoma add to the difficulty of the procedure.

A. The colon proximal and distal to the lesion has been divided and closed with the GIA instrument. The jejunum immediately proximal and distal is treated in the same fashion. This permits elevation of the stomach and attached viscera. Division of the vessels supplying the segments being resected with the LDS instrument is made safe by the exposure obtained.

B. Continuity of the colon and of the jejunum has been restored by functional end-to-end anastomosis.

C. Because of the gastrojejunocolic fistula and attendant inflammatory mass, the duodenum is divided first. In most patients with duodenal ulcer only, we divide the stomach first to provide better exposure of the duodenum. If the operation is performed for carcinoma of the distal stomach, we usually transect the duodenum first to provide better exposure of the stomach.

D. The proximal stapling and transection of the stomach have been completed and a GIA–TA 55 gastroenterostomy has been performed on the posterior stomach wall.

OPERATIONS UPON THE SMALL AND LARGE BOWEL

Functional Enteroenterostomy (Fig. 61–12)

Shown in Figure 61–12 are two open loops of small bowel. More often this anastomosis is performed with bowel that has been stapled and transected earlier in the procedure.

A. The GIA limbs are inserted into their respective loops, so that the instrument will close along the antimesenteric borders. The depth to which the calibrated instrument is inserted determines the size of the anastomosis. Allowance must be made for the amount to be amputated (see Fig. 61–12D).

B. The instrument is activated, creating an anatomic side-to-side anastomosis.

C. After the instrument has been withdrawn, the ends of the two GIA staple lines are held apart with stay sutures.

D. The TA 55 instrument is applied to close the bowel, with the cut edges of the GIA stapled bowel held widely apart. Since the cut edges of the bowel peripheral to the GIA staples are viable, it is possible, and has happened on rare occasions, that the cut edges will adhere if the TA instrument is applied at right angles to the plane here shown. In point of fact, we have not ourselves had that experience but know that it has happened. Serosa and mucosa must be visible beyond the TA stapler. Scissors are used to cut away the lip of bowel beyond the instrument, since one will be cutting across the two GIA staple lines.

E. The final result: After some months the anastomosis will look like an end-to-end anastomosis, occasionally with a small bulge, if the application of the TA instrument in Figure 61–12D has not been such as to make the length of the anastomosis equal to the diameter of the bowel on either side.

With staple transection and anastomosis of the bowel little or no devascularization

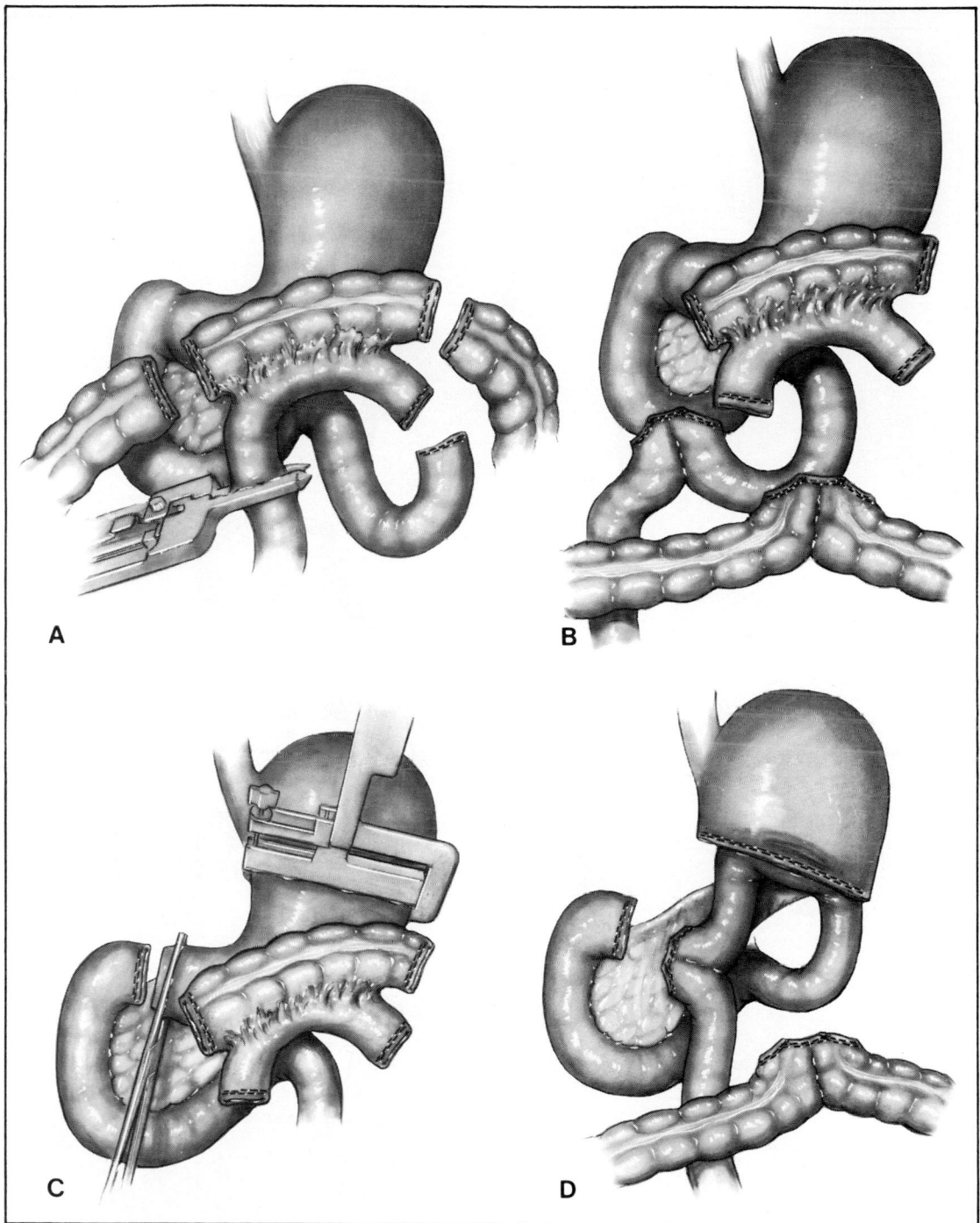

Figure 61–11. Resection of gastrojejunocolic fistula. (*Source: From Steichen FM, Ravitch MM, 1983, with permission.*)

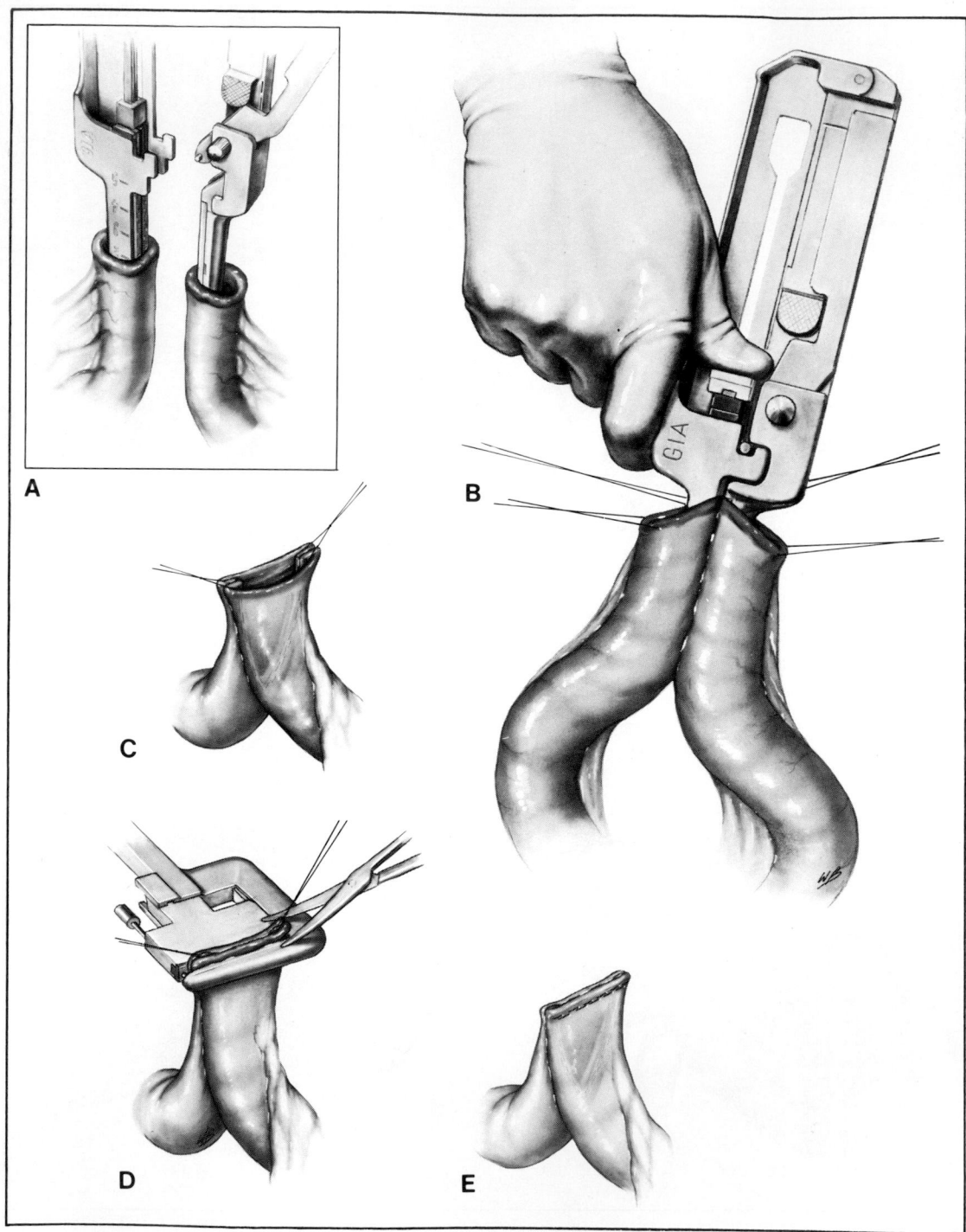

Figure 61–12. Functional enteroenterostomy. (*Source: From Steichen FM, Ravitch MM, 1983, with permission.*)

is necessary for transection, and none for anastomosis. In a manual anastomosis, on the other hand, too little clearing of the mesentery may make anastomotic suturing insecure, too much may jeopardize the viability of the bowel end. In all the variations shown of the functional end-to-end anastomosis, one is careful to insert the GIA instrument on the antimesenteric surfaces, and to be sure no other loop of bowel—or mesentery— is caught between the two loops being anastomosed.

Functional Colocolostomy (Fig. 61–13)

A. The segment of colon is resected between two applications of the GIA instrument. The specimen and the remaining colon are always sealed, and risk of contamination is minimal.
B. The antimesocolic corners of the staple lines in the bowel ends to be anastomosed are excised, and the GIA limbs inserted.
C. A side-to-side anastomosis is created that ideally should be of the same length as the transverse diameter of the bowel. This is determined by the depth of insertion of the GIA limbs and the level at which the TA 55 instrument is placed.
D. The opening, remaining when the GIA instrument is withdrawn, is shown being closed mucosa-to-mucosa with the TA 55 instrument. We usually prefer to apply the TA instrument at right angles to the position shown to hold the anastomosis wide open.
E. The final result. The transparency indicates an anastomosis which is of the same size as the diameter of the bowel on either side.

True End-to-End Colocolostomy (Fig. 61–14)

A. The purse string is shown being placed on the distal colon. The EEA instrument has been inserted through a colotomy in the proximal colon, the purse string already tied about the central rod.
B. The anvil is advanced into the distal lumen, which is held open by three stay sutures.
C. The distal purse string has been tied around the central rod and the anvil is closed against the cartridge.
D. The EEA instrument, having been fired, is

opened and withdrawn. A traction suture, as shown across the anastomosis, may be useful in withdrawal of the opened EEA instrument.
E. The procedure is completed by transverse TA 55 closure of the colotomy made for insertion of the EEA instrument.

The proximal colotomy or enterotomy technique for insertion of the EEA instrument obviously permits end-to-end or end-to-side anastomosis anywhere in the intestinal tract, and this technique has many advocates. In general, we prefer to employ a natural orifice, or an opening necessarily made in the bowel for purposes of the resection, rather than to make a proximal enterotomy with its additional suture line and increased opportunity for intraoperative soiling.

REMEDIAL SMALL AND LARGE BOWEL OPERATIONS

At present, there exists a substantial population of patients with jejunoileal shunts who do require reconstruction of normal intestinal anatomy. The stapling instruments greatly facilitate the multiple disconnections and anatomic restorations needed in such cases. Shown here are examples of what can be achieved with the help of stapling instruments when reconstruction of intestinal anatomy is indicated.

Takedown of Scott Jejunoileal Shunt and Reconstruction of Intestinal Continuity (Fig. 61–15)

A. The region of the old end-to-end jejunoileostomy in which the bowel tends to be dilated and thickened, and is frequently inflamed, is resected with two applications of the GIA instrument.
B. The ileocolostomy draining the terminal end of the bypassed bowel is taken down by a single application of the TA 90 instrument, placed tangentially along the border of the colon. A clamp on the distal end of the bypassed bowel prevents soiling. The bypassed terminal ileum just proximal to this anastomosis will be thickened, requiring excision of several inches by application of the GIA or the TA instrument. The newly stapled distal end of the bypassed bowel is now anas-

1562

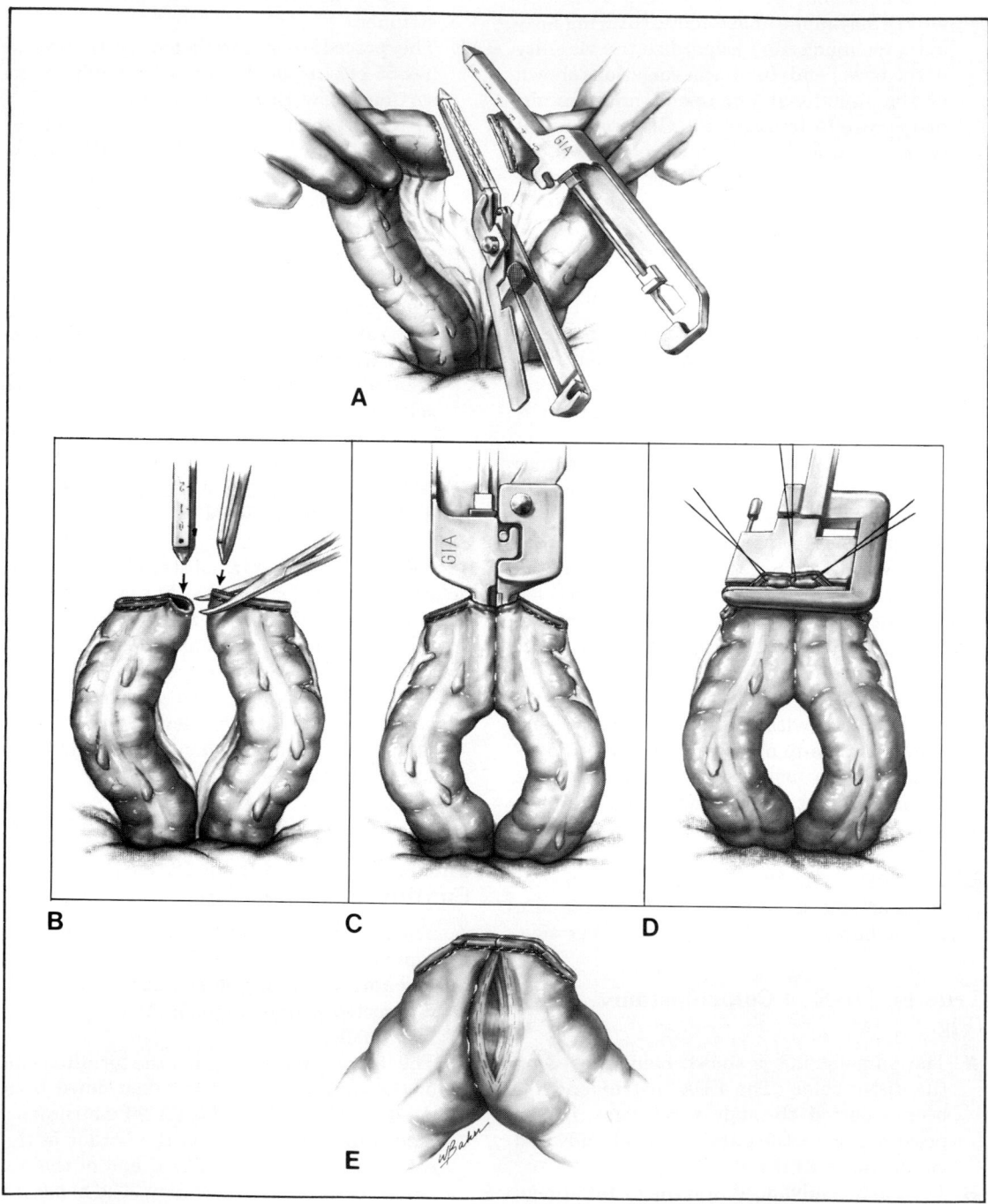

Figure 61–13. Functional colocolostomy. (*Source: From Ravitch MM, Steichen FM, 1972, with permission.*)

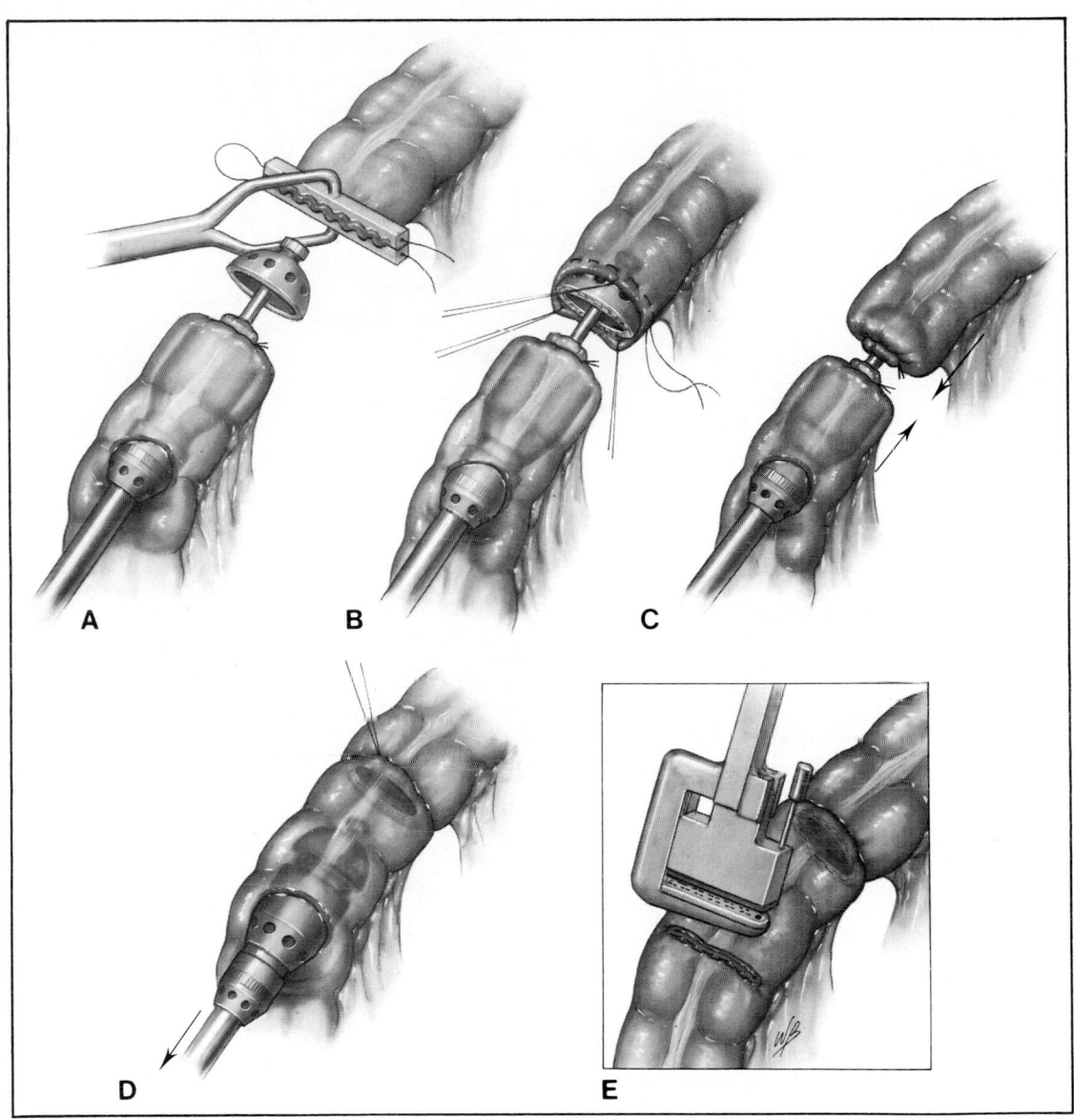

Figure 61–14. True end-to-end colocolostomy. (*Source: From Steichen FM, Ravitch MM, 1983, with permission.*)

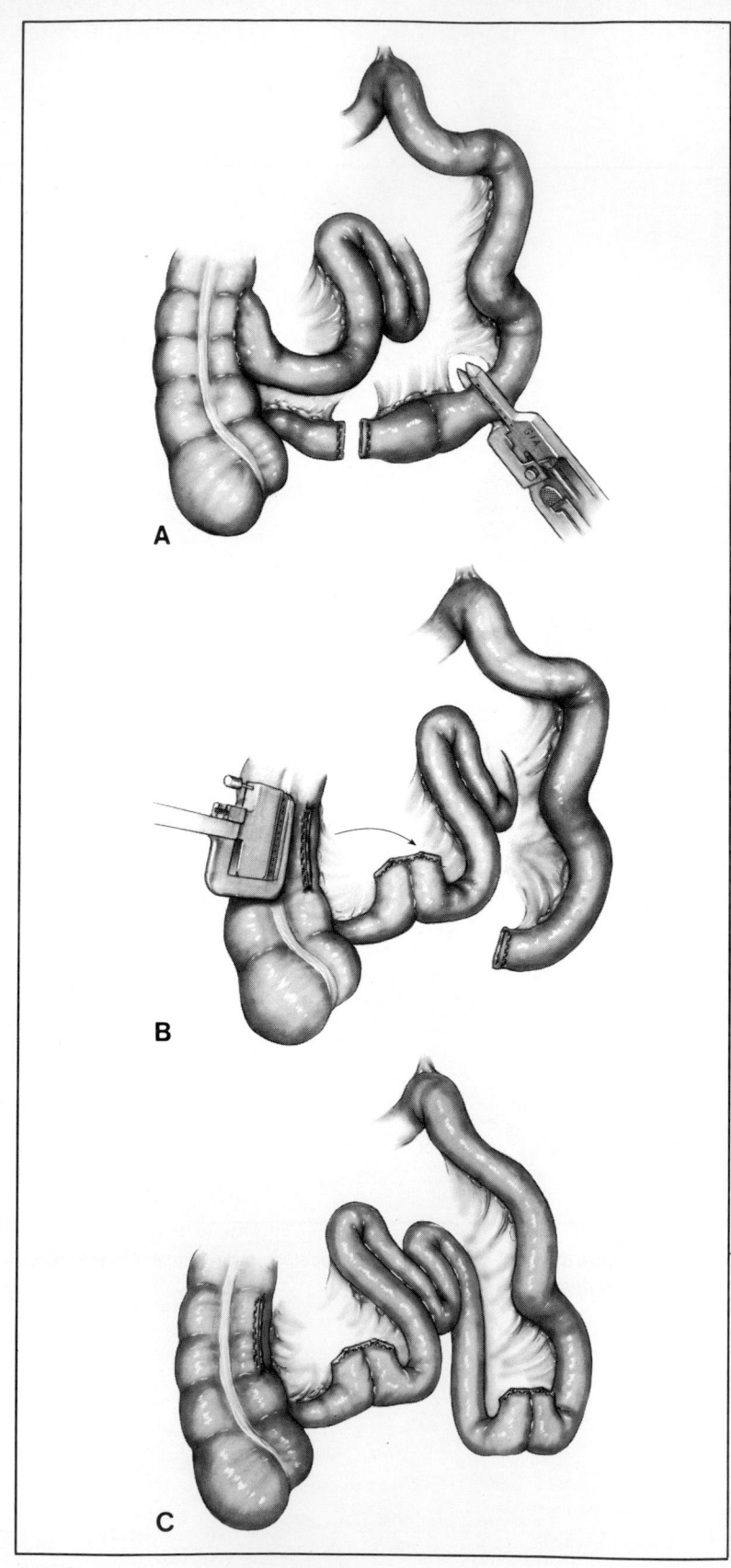

Figure 61–15. Takedown of Scott jejunoileal shunt. (*Source: From Steichen FM, Ravitch MM, 1983, with permission.*)

tomosed to the stump of the terminal ileum by a functional end-to-end anastomosis.

C. The blind, closed, proximal end of the bypassed bowel is anastomosed to the proximal jejunum by a functional end-to-end anastomosis with GIA and TA instruments.

Takedown of Payne Shunt and Reconstruction of Intestinal Continuity (Fig. 61–16)

A. The TA 55 instrument will be applied to close the jejunoileal anastomosis and transect the jejunum on the edge of the instrument, which is placed so that the closure will be transverse on the ileum, thus avoiding the risk of constriction. The proximal jejunum will be divided with the GIA instrument several inches above the anastomosis to resect the short, distended, hypertrophied segment of jejunum (not shown in Fig. 61–16).

B. The proximal end of the bypassed bowel is joined to the proximal jejunum by functional end-to-end anastomosis. Close to the ileocecal valve one can see the transverse stapled closure of the original jejunoileostomy in the terminal ileum.

Takedown of Duodeno- and Gastrocolic Fistulas in the Course of a Pancolectomy (Fig. 61–17)

A. Mobilization of the transverse colon was hampered by an intimate connection between the third portion of the duodenum and the colon and of the stomach and the transverse colon. The extensive inflammation and, for the duodenum, the considerable depth of the lesion, might have posed some problems for conventional excision and closure. In this instance, it was possible to create a tunnel and to pass a finger around the fistulas, facilitating the placement of the lower blade of the TA 55 instrument, first behind the duodenocolic connection. The staples were placed tangentially on the duodenum without significantly narrowing it. A clamp on the colon prevented leakage.

B. The same technique was employed on the stomach. The specimen showed a small fistula in each site, the existence of which had not been demonstrated by the preoperative radiologic studies.

Particularly in hard to reach situations of this sort, and in cases of inflammatory disease, the staplers make it possible to liberate the specimen, securely closing the attached normal portion of the GI tract without risk of bleeding or soiling.

OPERATIONS IN WHICH THE ANASTOMOSIS IS DONE FIRST FOLLOWED BY RESECTION OF THE SPECIMEN

This technique, in which the anastomosis is performed before removing the specimen, can be applied at various levels of the GI tract. In esophageal reconstruction it is shown in the illustrations on the colon interposition (Figs. 61–2B,C) in which the GIA esophagocolonic anastomosis is performed first, followed by excision of the specimen distal to the blades of the TA 55 stapler, simultaneously closing the esophageal lumen and the GIA introduction site. This same approach can be used for distal gastrectomy as first described by Welter, for functional enteroenterostomy and enterocolostomy as first described by Ravitch, and for functional enteroileostomy with appendectomy.

Billroth II Gastrojejunostomy First, Gastrectomy Second (Welter) (Fig. 61–18)

A. The gastrojejunostomy is performed at the elected level of gastric resection on the posterior surface of the stomach near the greater curvature. The duodenum has already been closed.

B. The placement of the GIA limbs may be parallel to the future closure of the gastric remnant as in Figure 61–18A or may be parallel to the greater curvature, making for a safer application of the TA 90.

C. After removal of the GIA instrument, and assurance of hemostasis in the gastroenterostomy, the TA 90 stapler is placed so as to safely surround the now common GIA stab wound consisting anteriorly of the anterior gastric wall and posteriorly of the posterior jejunal lip, near the greater curvature. The TA 90 instrument includes also both walls of the gastric remnant toward the lesser curvature. At the level of the future

1566

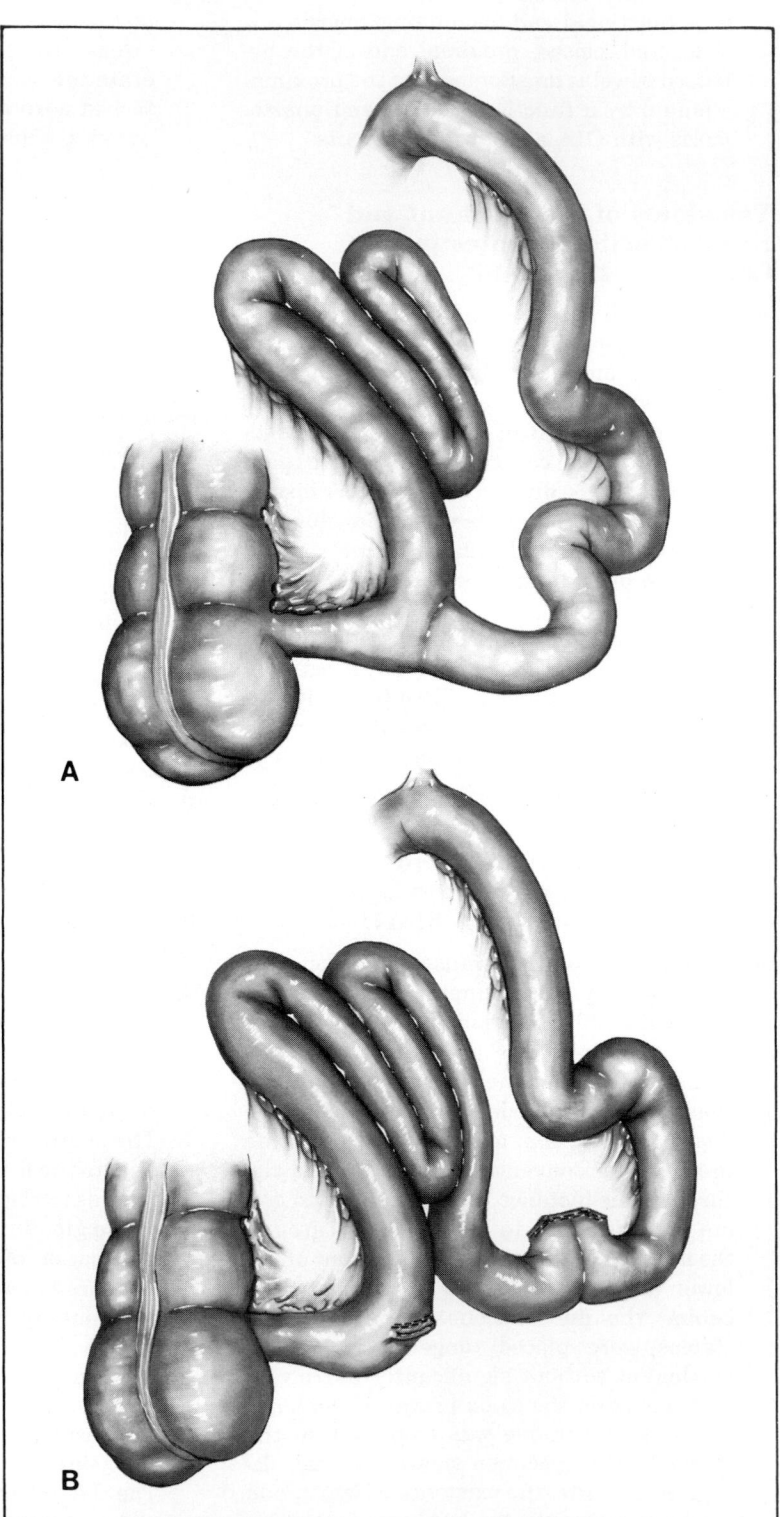

A

B

Figure 61–16. Takedown of Payne shunt. (*Source: From Steichen FM, Ravitch MM, 1983, with permission.*)

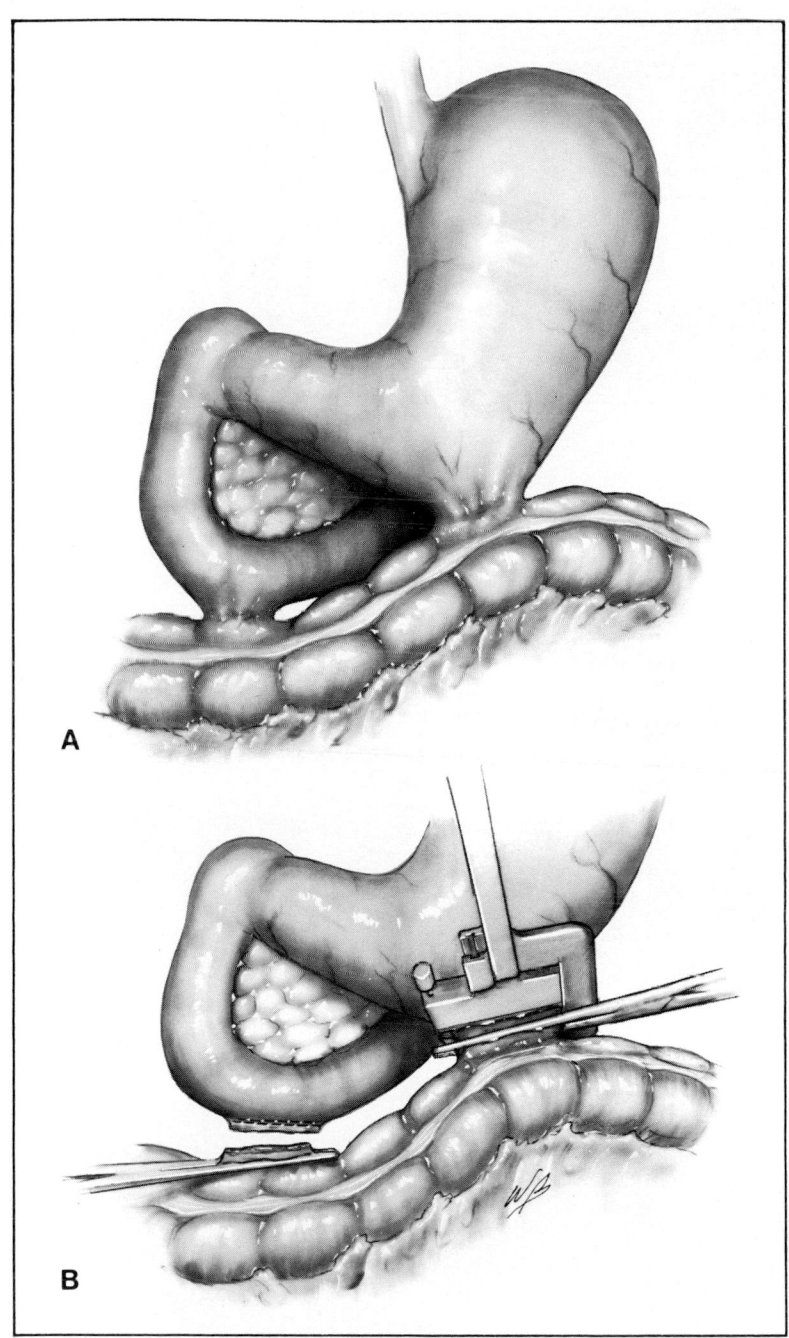

A

B

Figure 61–17. Takedown of duodeno- and gastrocolic fistulas. (*Source: From Steichen FM, Ravitch MM, 1983, with permission.*)

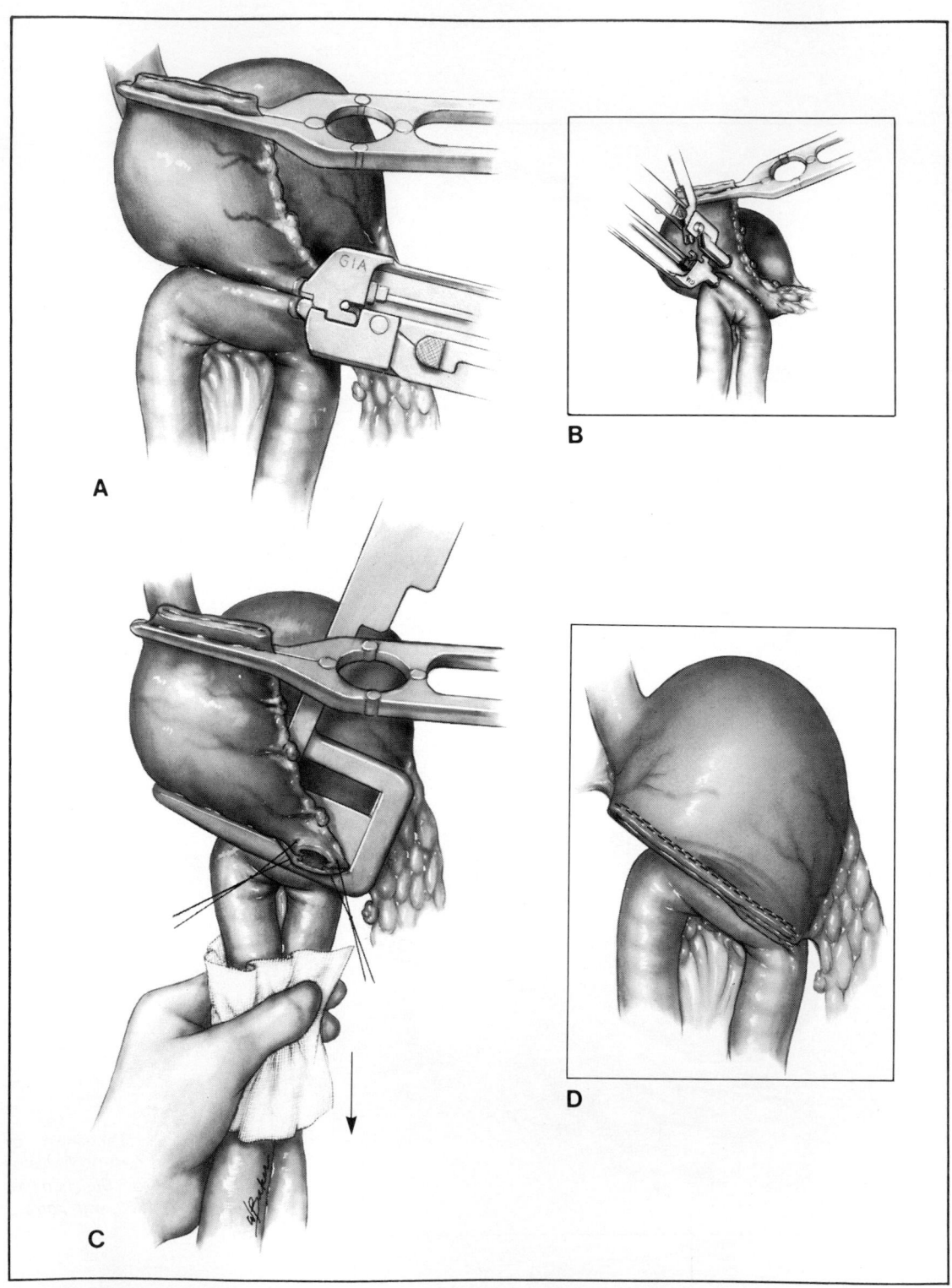

61–18. Billroth II gastrojejunostomy first, gastrectomy second (Welter). (*Source: From Steichen FM, Ravitch MM, 1983, with permission.*)

gastric stump, great care is taken not to include other structures, pads, etc., in the TA 90 closure. Including an excessive amount of the lips of the anastomotic opening would result in a stenosis; therefore, at the time of the TA 90 application and closure, gentle traction is exerted on the afferent and efferent jejunal loops so as to make them conform to the legs of a pair of pants. Following closure with the TA 90 instrument, the excess tissue—e.g., the posterior lip of the jejunal stab wound and the anterior lip of the gastric stab wound along the greater curvature, as well as the distal stomach—is excised, using the TA 90 jaw as a guide, thus delivering the specimen.

D. After completion of the TA 90 suture line and excision of the gastric specimen, the closure is composed of anterior gastric wall to jejunal loop wall toward the greater curvature, and anterior to posterior gastric wall toward the lesser curvature.

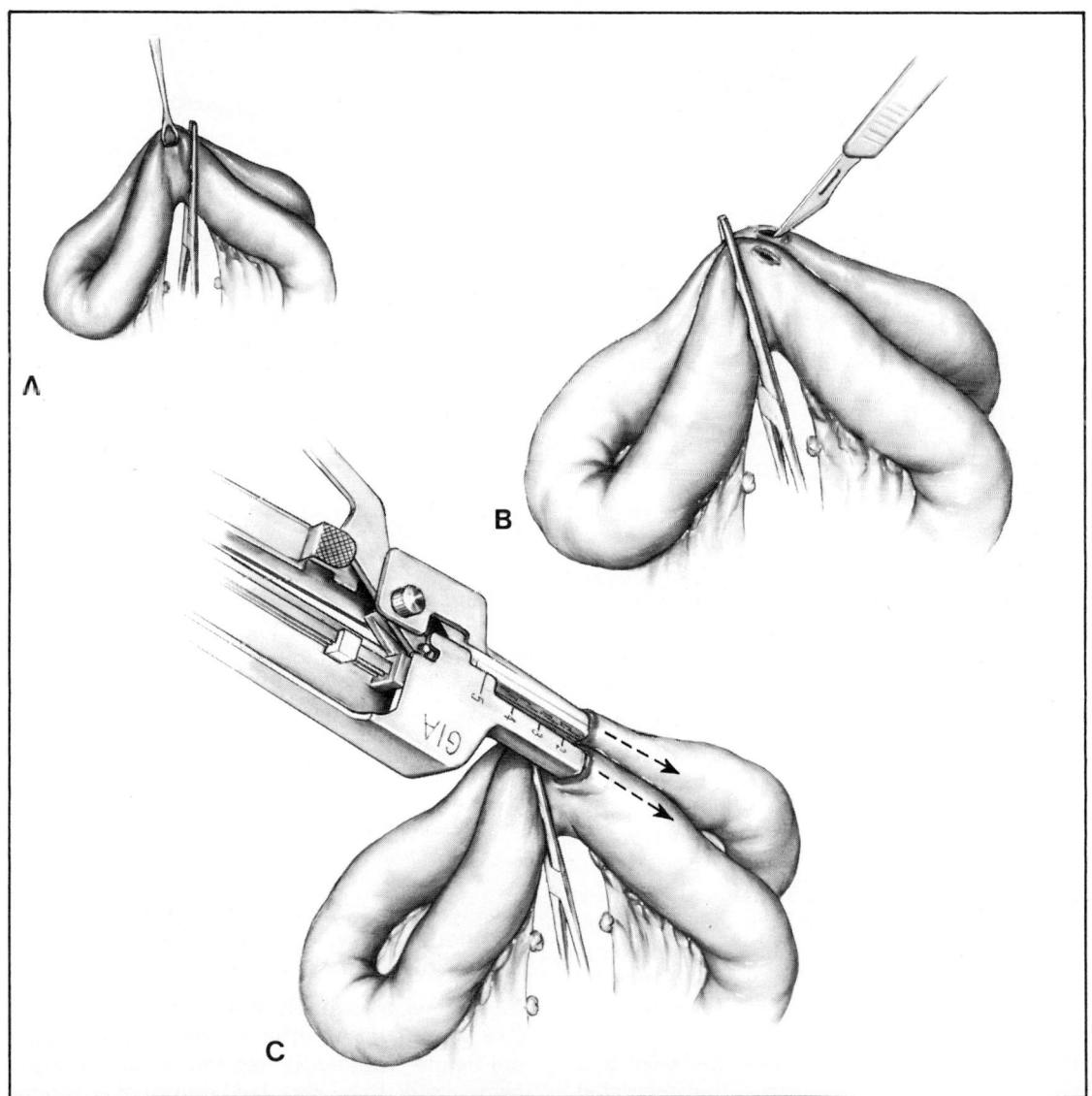

Figure 61–19. A through **F.** Enteroenterostomy first, bowel resection second (Ravitch).

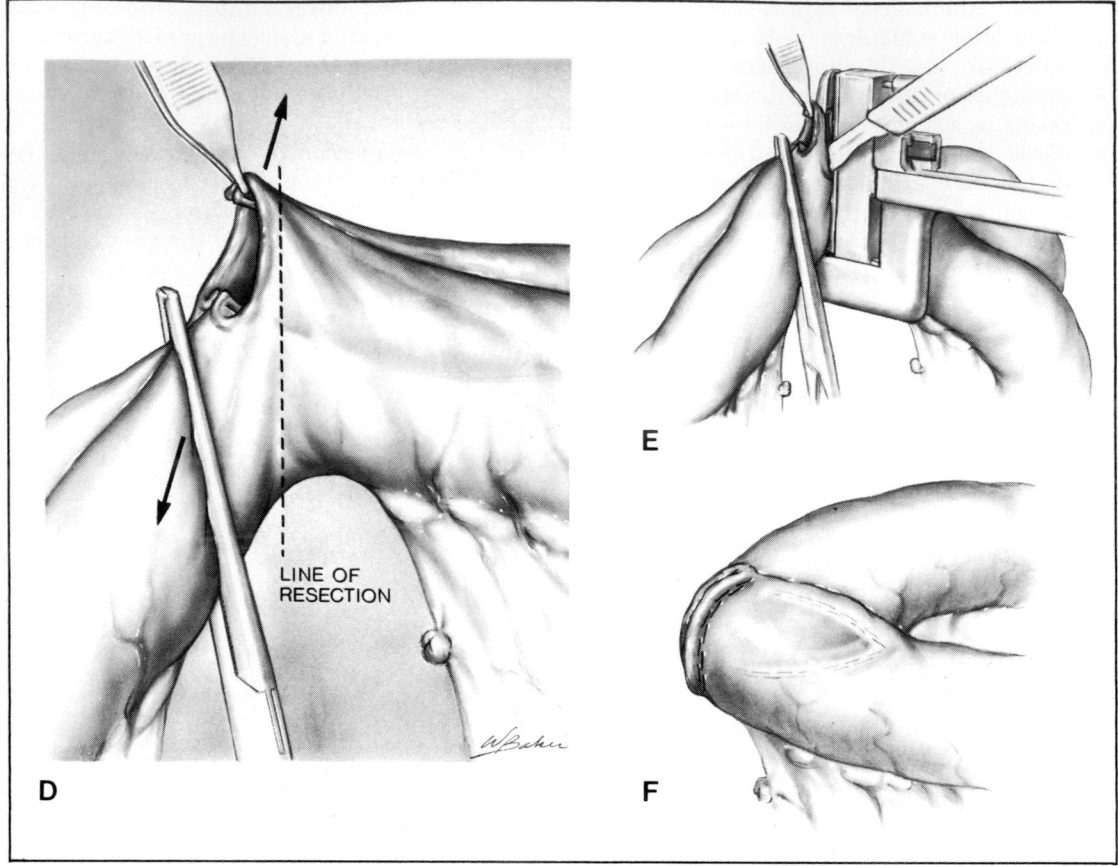

Figure 61–19. *Continued*

Enteroenterostomy First, Bowel Resection Second—Modified Functional End-to-End Anastomosis (Ravitch) (Fig. 61–19)

A. The segment of bowel to be resected has been isolated. The antimesenteric borders are matched at the junction of viable and nonviable bowel and fixed in that position with a Kocher clamp placed just barely on the specimen side.

B. Openings for the GIA instrument are made on the antimesenteric surface of the viable bowel that will be part of the anastomosis.

C. The partially assembled limbs of the GIA instrument can be inserted simultaneously into the two openings.

D. The side-to-side anastomosis has been completed and the GIA suture line inspected.

E. The TA 55 instrument is placed across the two loops so as to exclude the GIA opening

and the specimen is amputated, with the final result seen in Figure 61–19F.

This technique obviates the stapling and division of the bowel at either end of the resection and reduces to a matter of seconds the opportunity for possible contamination. We have used this technique in various resections of the small bowel and in segmental colectomies.

Resection of Terminal Ileum, Ileocecostomy, Followed by Appendectomy (Fig. 61–20)

In patients, most often women, requiring extensive pelvic surgery after irradiation, the terminal ileum—frequently exposed in the radiation field—needs to be resected because of advanced radiation damage. Sigmoid colon and rectum also often require excision because of radiation

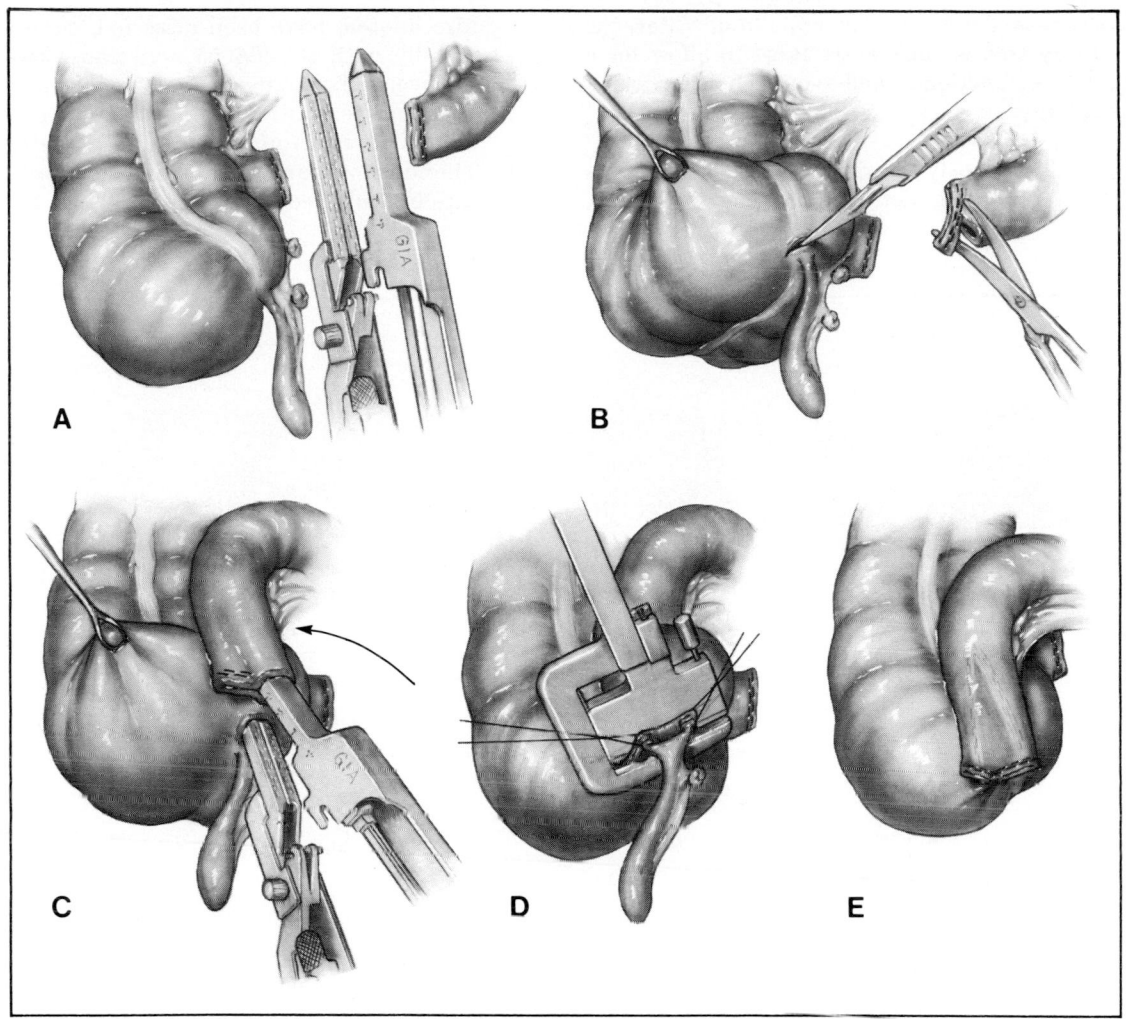

Figure 61–20. Resection of terminal ileum, ileocecostomy, followed by appendectomy.

damage and/or direct involvement with tumor. Operations related to the rectosigmoid are dealt with in another section.

Stapling greatly facilitates the excision and reanastomosis of various bowel segments in complicated, prolonged pelvic operations.

A. The injured terminal ileum is excised between two applications of the GIA instrument.
B. The antimesenteric corner of the closed proximal ileum is excised and the cecum at the base of the appendix is incised.
C. The limbs of the GIA instrument are placed into the ileum and cecum and a side-to-side anastomosis is performed.

D. The TA 30 instrument is applied across the base of the appendix and the GIA stab wound, and the appendix is removed.
E. The GIA introduction site of the ileum closed against the wall of the cecum with the appendix removed.

PALLIATIVE CHOLEDOCHOJEJUNOSTOMY AND GASTROENTEROSTOMY AND ROUX-Y JEJUNOJEJUNOSTOMY (FIG. 61–21)

In many patients with obstructive jaundice due to an inoperable malignancy of the head of the pancreas, duodenum, or ampulla of Vater, the biliary tree is sufficiently large to allow for a stapled functional end-to-end choledochojejunostomy.

A. The greatly enlarged common hepatic duct and a long, densely adherent cystic duct,

also dilated, have been dissected, closely distally with the TA 55 and transected.

B. To avoid cholecystectomy, a side-to-side anastomosis between the cystic and common ducts is accomplished with the GIA.

C. The curve of the distal jejunal loop usually can be adjusted comfortably along the

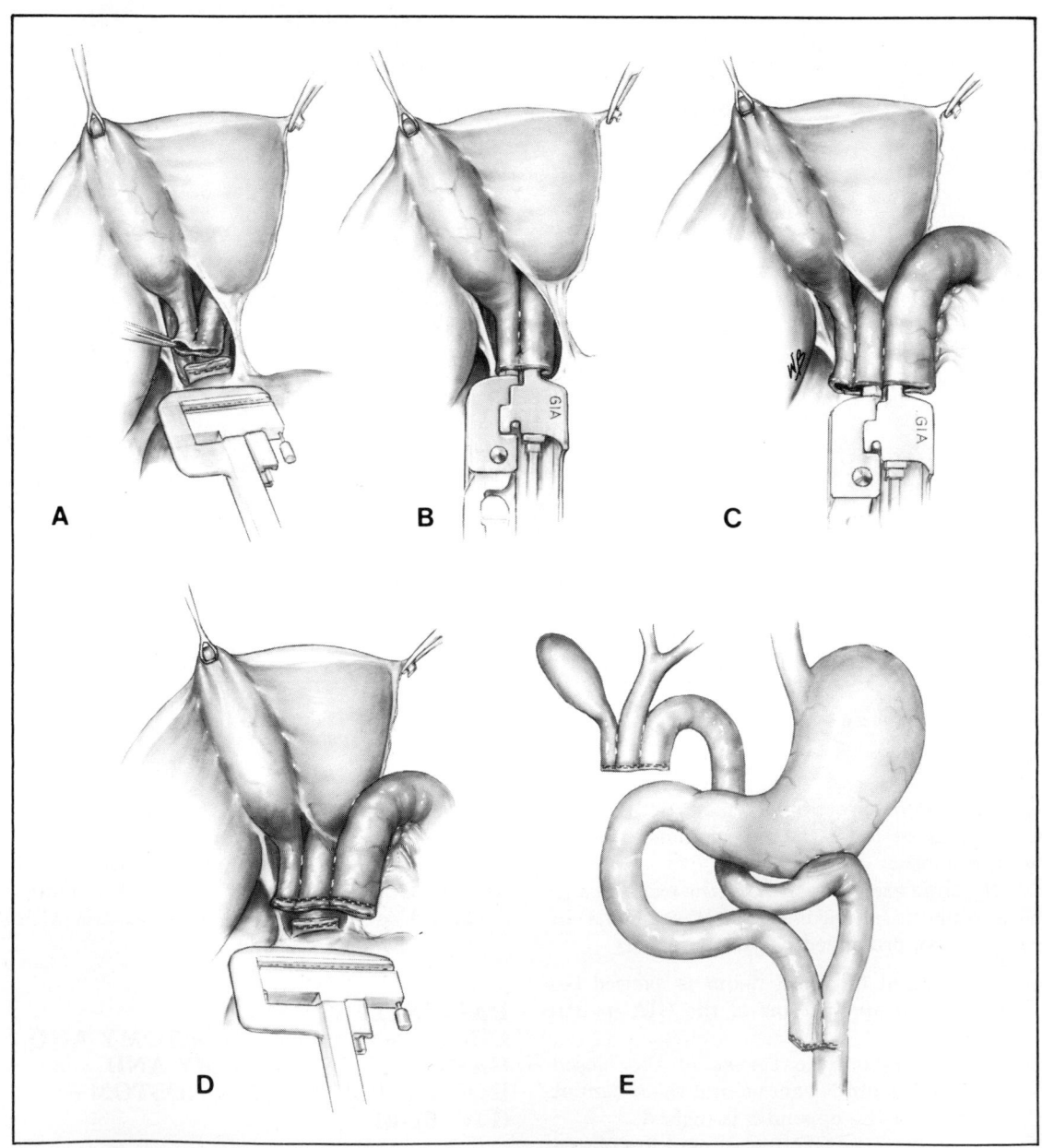

Figure 61–21. A through G. Palliative choledochojejunostomy, gastroenterostomy, and Roux-Y jejunojejunostomy.

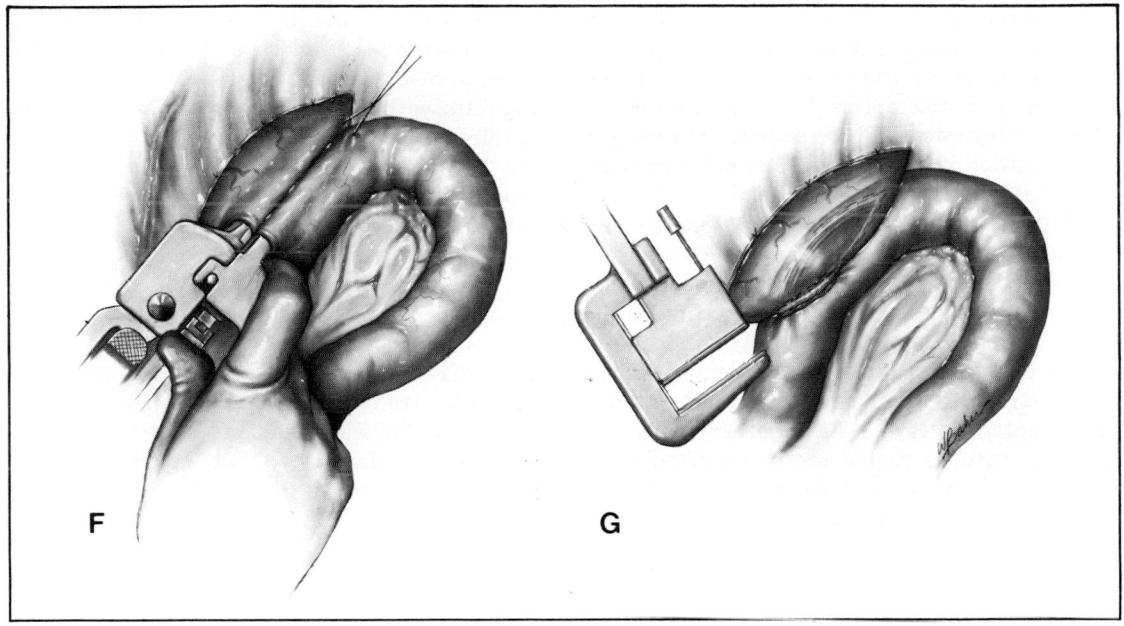

Figure 61–21. *Continued*

PITFALLS AND MISHAPS

All new techniques require a period of learning, which for the surgical resident is best incorporated into the years of training and for the established surgeon is acquired by spending time in the laboratory and watching other, more experienced, surgeons before undertaking—first under supervision—operations with stapling instruments.

With the introduction of the totally disposable TA, GIA, LDS, and EEA instruments or the new cartridges for the TA and GIA premium instruments, many of the previous purely mechanical mishaps have been eliminated. These included improper assembly of the instruments,

common duct and a choledochojejunostomy with the GIA is performed.
D. The open cystic and common ducts, and jejunum are closed transversely with the TA 55 instrument.
E. A retrocolic, posterior gastroenterostomy is performed and bowel continuity is reestablished by Roux-Y jejunojejunostomy as shown.
F,G. Details of the gastroenterostomy are demonstrated.

forgetting the use of the tissue pin in the TA instruments, mismatching anvil and cartridge, and improper placement of the blade-staple pusher assembly of the GIA instrument.

Other pitfalls remain to be watched for by the surgeon and are avoided with increasing and guided experience. They may range from mistakes of lack of attention and poor habit (such as using an empty cartridge, forgetting to fire the staples, cutting the viscus on the patient's side in TA closures and neglecting to close the instrument within the range where staples form properly), to mistakes in judgment (such as relying on staples other than the LDS for hemostasis in mesenteric vessels, closing and transecting the bowel larger than the GIA staple lines, submucosal placement of one or both GIA blades, failure to include full bowel thickness and circumference in TA closures, especially of GIA stab wounds, failure to inspect GIA anastomoses for bleeding, and excessive compression and trauma of edematous tissues).

Potential problems that are more specific to the use of the EEA instrument include splitting the bowel with an oversized cartridge, failure to tie the purse string suture tightly around the central rod, leaving a large tissue rim beyond the purse string suture, resulting in a large mass of tissue in the closed cartridge, devascularizing the bowel end in preparation for the purse string placement, failure to advance the circular knife so that the bowel is not cut through, and attempting to withdraw the instrument before it has been opened or by violent manipulation if the cartridge has not separated clearly from the anastomosis.

Just as for a manual suture that is introduced without undue tension on the tissues, stapled closures and anastomoses should be placed by avoiding leverage and forceful pulling on the tissues, especially since relatively small movements of the instrument handle may result in tissue stress and hidden tears at the cartridge and staple line levels. As a general rule, mechanical sutures should not be expected to be safe and reliable in performing a task that one would not entrust to manual sutures.

PRINCIPLES OF CURRENT CLINICAL USE

The ever-increasing number of publications concerning the clinical use of mechanical sutures brings out the general satisfaction with stapling, which most authors consider to be at least as safe as manual suture techniques, although we are not aware of any satisfactory controlled prospective studies comparing the two techniques. The benefits of stapling techniques to the patient have been sufficiently convincing, so that we have not felt it necessary to undertake a comparative study of our own.

Gross and microscopic comparison in the experimental animal show tissue edema and ecchymoses, with tags of mucosa and loose sutures in manual closures and anastomoses examined at different time intervals, when stapled closures and anastomoses distinguish themselves by minimal edema, hemorrhage and necrosis, when examined at comparable time intervals.

The appropriate and competent use of stapling instruments and techniques results in shortened operating room and anesthesia times, in a significant reduction of soiling from open bowel lumina, in less tissue trauma and therefore a potential for diminishing rates of postoperative infections.

However, stapling instruments do not absolve the surgeon from respecting general principles: Tissues without their proper blood supply do not heal; viscera that are the seat of active

disease such as tuberculosis, cancer, inflammation, postradiation effect, etc., cannot be relied upon to heal. Careful hemostasis, gentle tissue handling with minimal operative trauma, bowel closure and anastomosis in healthy tissue without tension, aspiration and evacuation of all blood and secretions, drainage only when absolutely indicated, no unnecessary dissection of tissue planes and creation of dead spaces and all the other principles acquired and recognized through a surgical lifetime, are just as important with staples as they are with manual sutures. The stapling instruments will not automatically transform a marginal surgeon into a virtuoso. They may, in fact, exacerbate defects in manual dexterity and coordination of thought and motion.

BIBLIOGRAPHY

Barrocas A: The use of stapling devices in the management of postgastrectomy syndromes. Am Surg 45:656, 1979

Denans FN: Nouveau procédé pour la guérison des plaies des intestins. Recueil de la Société Royale dé Medecine de Marseille (Séance du 24 fev. 1826, rédigé par M.P. Roux) Imprimerie d'Archard, Marseille, Tome I:127, 1827

Du Plessis DJ: Gastric mucosal changes after operations on the stomach. S Afr Med J 36:471, 1962

Friedrich H: Ein neuer Magen-Darm-Nähapparat. Zentralbl Chir 61:504, 1934

Gudov VF: A method for the application of vascular sutures by mechanical means. Khirurgila 12:58, 1950

Halsted WS: Circular suture of the intestine—an experimental study. Am J Med Sci 94:436, 1887

Henroz JHF: Dissertatio inauguralis critica medico-chirurgica de methodis ad sananda intestina divisa adhibitis, in Qua Nova Sanationis Methodus Proponitur. Universitate Leondiensi June 1826. PJ Collardin, Typographi Academici, 1826

Hültl H: II Kongress der Ungarischen Gesellschaft für Chirurgie, Budapest, May 1908. Pester Med-Chir Presse 45:108, 121, 1909

Knight CD, Griffen FD: Techniques of low rectal reconstruction. Curr Probl Surg 20:387, 1983

Lembert A: Mémoire sur l'entéroraphie. Rep Gen d'Anat et de Physiol Pathol II:101, 1826

Murphy JB: Choleycsto-intestinal, gastro-intestinal, entero-intestinal anastomosis, and approximation without sutures (original research). Med Rec NY 42:665, 1892

Murphy JB: Cholecysto-intestinal, gastro-intestinal,

entero-intestinal anastomosis, and approximation without sutures (original research). Chicago Med Rec XIII:803, 1892

Ramaugé A: Enteroplexis. Consideraciones preliminares, in Peuser J (ed): Memoria presentada al jurado del concurso de Medicine International Sudamericano. 1893, p 7

Ramaugé A: Enteroplexo. Revista de la Sociedad Medica Argentina 2:667, 1902

Ravitch MM, Steichen FM: Techniques of staple suturing in the gastrointestinal tract. Ann Surg 175:815, 1972

Ravitch MM, Ong TH, et al: A new, precise, and rapid technique of intestinal resection and anastomosis with staples. Surg Gynecol Obstet 139:6, 1974

Steichen FM: The use of staplers in anatomical side-to-side and functional end-to-end enteroanastomoses. Surgery 64:948, 1968

Steichen FM: The creation of autologous substitute organs with stapling instruments. Am J Surg 134:659, 1977

Steichen FM, Ravitch MM: Mechanical sutures in esophageal surgery. Ann Surg 191:373, 1980

Steichen FM, Ravitch MM: History of mechanical devices and instruments for suturing. Curr Probl Surg 19:1, 1982

Steichen FM, Ravitch MM: Stapling in Surgery. Chicago: Year Book, 1983

Travers B: An inquiry into the process of healing in repairing injuries of the intestines. London: Longman, 1812

von Petz A: Zur Technik der Magenresektion. Ein neuer Magen-Darmnähapparat. Zentralbl Chir 5:179, 1924

von Petz A: Aseptic technique of stomach resections. Ann Surg 86:388, 1927

Welter R, Turbelin JM, et al: Gastrectomie avec anastomose gastro-jejunale "premiere." Technique originale d'emploi des procedes de suture mecanique. Nouv Presse Med 10:247, 1981

SECTION XI
Liver

62. Injuries of the Liver

Alexander J. Walt
Jeffrey S. Bender

INTRODUCTION

The approach of the surgeon to liver wounds continues to change as technology advances, relevant data are critically analyzed, and the aura of fear that has surrounded the liver increasingly dissipates. The standard approach to liver trauma will be reviewed and areas of controversy and current uncertainty will be explored in this chapter.

From the time of Hippocrates to Pirogoff, the great Russian military surgeon of the mid-nineteenth century, liver wounds were thought to be uniformly fatal except in rare and bizarre circumstances, such as presented by the young man who spontaneously extruded a sequestrum of liver through his stab wound, as described by Fabricius Hildanus in the early sixteenth century. With the advent of anesthesia and antisepsis, and the American Civil War and the Franco–Prussian War, the last quarter of the nineteenth century saw a rapid increase in experimental work on a wide variety of wounds created in animals. Surgeons soon recognized that hemorrhage from the larger intrahepatic vessels in these specifically designed injuries could be controlled and in 1887 Burkhardt stated that immediate laparotomy and suturing of the bleeding area was the only rational way of treating a liver injury. From 1890, studies were made of the amount of liver that could be resected with the prospect of adequate regeneration. By 1908, when Pringle described temporary occlusion of the portal triad, all the methods used today for the treatment of hepatic injury, except for arterial embolization and the placement of atrial–caval shunts for retrohepatic injuries, had been practiced. The management of hepatic injuries progressed relatively little over the next 60 years.

More recently, the Vietnam conflict established the logical sequence and limitations of extended technical procedures, but battlefield injuries do not accurately reflect the civilian counterparts. A more conservative approach based on experiences in major trauma centers therefore evolved in the 1970s. The past decade has seen a steady refinement of diagnostic methods by newer technology such as arteriography, isotopic imaging, ultrasonography, and computed tomography (CT) scanning. These have altered some of our concepts of the natural history of hepatic injuries, revealing intrahepatic lesions in essentially asymptomatic patients. The frequency of spontaneous resolution of these has been studied and a selective policy of watchful waiting cautiously advocated. A shift towards conservatism at laparotomy is also discernable. Gauze packing, with or without hepatic artery ligation, is now sometimes used in carefully selected patients instead of heroic but predictably doomed resections. Even in the presence of active bleeding, other techniques such as intraarterial embolization by the interventional radiologist to stem intrahepatic bleeding in hemobilia may successfully obviate the need for a hazardous operation. In summary, the trend has been toward relative conservatism.

Today, the mortality rate for hepatic injuries has plateaued between 6 and 20 percent. This wide range reflects the condition of the patient when first seen, the spectrum and severity of injury in different series, and the skill of the surgical team. Each aspect may be separately analyzed. The condition of the patient may be improved by the ready availability of well-trained emergency medical services; the degree of injury may be reduced by public action that reduces drunken driving and the indiscriminate use of firearms; and the surgical mor-

TABLE 62-1. LIVER INJURIES (WAYNE STATE UNIVERSITY)

Injury	1961-1968	1969-1973	1974-1976	1980-1983	Total
Gunshot	151	427	199	90	867 (54.4%)
Stab	235	153	92	81	561 (35.3%)
Blunt	50	57	40	17	164 (10.3%)
Total	436	637	331	188	1592 (100%)

bidity may be lowered by the adoption of a logically tailored approach to each hepatic injury.

The main basis for the conclusions expressed in this chapter, which attempts to provide a modern perspective, is a study of 1592 patients with hepatic injury operated on by members of the Department of Surgery at Wayne State University in the years 1961–1976 and 1980–1983, mainly at Detroit Receiving Hospital (Table 62–1).

ETIOLOGIC FACTORS

As the largest of the intraabdominal organs, the liver is the most frequently injured in both blunt and penetrating abdominal wounds. In the majority of stab wounds, the hepatic injury is isolated. In contrast, with blunt injury, concomitant damage to other intraabdominal organs or to extraabdominal structures, such as the lungs, heart, long bones, or cranial contents, is present in about 90 percent. This difference has a profoundly adverse effect on morbidity and mortality rates.

The type and velocity of the injuring object is obviously critical but in special circumstances, such as pregnancy, peliosis, sickle cell anemia, large primary hepatic carcinoma, and hepatic adenoma, the liver may be unusually fragile and be fractured by a minor blow. Rarely, bleeding appears to occur spontaneously. Whatever the cause of injury, the resulting hemorrhage may be massive and the degree of bleeding encountered cannot always be correlated with the extent of tissue damage. A small but deep stab may sever a large intrahepatic vessel; in contrast, a large crushed segment of parenchyma may cease to bleed spontaneously. Although blood is present in the peritoneal cavity following most liver injuries and may be considerable in about 60 percent of patients with blunt injury, active bleeding has often ceased by the time of laparotomy and is only really difficult to control in about 20 percent.

CLINICAL MANIFESTATIONS

The clinical picture is extremely variable. About 25 percent of patients with hepatic injury are normotensive on admission to the emergency department. Patients with minor injury and minimal bleeding may be virtually asymptomatic. Even with substantial intraparenchymal damage as documented by CT scan and later confirmed at operation, the patient may complain of little more than moderate discomfort in the right upper quadrant or epigastrium. Patients with detached sequestra of liver that have stopped bleeding spontaneously have been known to delay for up to 36 hours before presenting to the hospital. Even then, fever rather than substantial pain may be the dominant symptom. On occasion, the patient may have little more than slight guarding for a few days and the severity of the hepatic injury only becomes apparent when an intrahepatic hematoma ruptures into the peritoneal cavity with consequent hypovolemic shock. When this sequence of events occurs in women, rupture of an hepatic adenoma or an ectopic pregnancy may be simulated.

In extensive hepatic injury by a high-velocity missile or severe crushing injury, pain and rapid blood loss will almost invariably dominate the picture from the start. The patient develops deep shock, severe pain, and an enlarging abdomen to the point of presenting with a tight tamponade. The presence of abdominal tamponade in conjunction with recalcitrant hypotension that does not respond to the rapid infusion of crystalloids and blood should serve as a warning that sudden collapse and death is a potential complication almost immediately after the peritoneum is opened at operation. The dramatic nature of this collapse was at one time attributed to air embolism but it is now recognized to be the result of exsanguination on release of the tamponade. Three alternatives should be considered in this circumstance. The first is a preliminary left thoracotomy and occlusion of the thoracic aorta just above the diaphragm to try to ensure reasonable control of bleeding when the abdomen is opened. A second alternative is the insertion of a large Fogarty catheter through the common femoral artery, with the inflated balloon used to occlude the aorta above the diaphragm. The third and most often used alternative is to have the team prepared to open the lesser omentum to obtain immediate control of the aorta just below the diaphragm manually, by pressure on a sponge stick or by application of a vascular clamp, much as is done for a leaking abdominal aortic aneurysm. If the thoracic approach is used, the potential hazards of acute hypertension with left ventricular strain, spinal cord ischemia, and subsequent renal failure should be recognized and precautions taken to combat these, mainly by moving the clamp on the thoracic aorta down to the abdominal aorta as soon as feasible. A disadvantage of the thoracotomy is that the bleeding is sometimes found to originate from a large vein or from the infrarenal aorta or a branch and not from the liver, in which case an abdominal incision would obviously have been better in the first place. Patients with this degree of tamponade and hypotension do not tolerate indecision or continuing blood loss.

In penetrating wounds, the entrance and exit wounds or the site of lodgment of the missile indicate the overwhelming probability of liver damage. However, such assumptions may be incorrect when the patient has been bent over at the time of injury or when the missile has opened tissue planes just outside the liver. While entering the abdomen from the right chest, the missile may pass immediately adjacent to the bare area of the liver, miss the liver completely, and end in the left upper quadrant, damaging the stomach or the spleen. In addition, one must entertain the possibility that any stab wound below the fourth intercostal space on either side may penetrate the diaphragm and injure the liver, especially when the stab is on the right side.

The diagnosis of hepatic injury may be difficult. History is important, and a blow to the upper abdomen from a boot, the steering wheel of a car, a tire, or an inappropriately worn seat belt is always suggestive. A subcutaneous hematoma or ecchymosis in the abdominal skin should greatly heighten clinical suspicion. A plain roentgenogram of the abdomen is seldom helpful in the diagnosis of a liver injury per

se, although it may reveal concomitant injuries, as evidenced by free or retroperitoneal air, an obscured psoas shadow, a fractured vertebra, or fractured ribs. Peritoneal paracentesis or lavage may confirm the presence of blood but in a few cases where bleeding is contained either within the liver capsule or is walled off by omentum or old adhesions, lavage may be falsely negative. Peritoneal lavage should not be done if a CT scan is contemplated, as the lavage interferes with the subsequent interpretation of the scan.

For a time, isotopic hepatic scanning and arteriography were advanced as helpful diagnostic measures. Unfortunately, the former, although productive of excellent results, is seldom readily available at night or as an emergency while the latter is excessively invasive, too expensive to be used in the relatively minor injury, and too often the cause of delay in the moderately to severely injured patient who needs laparotomy urgently. Arteriography has a place of primacy in the detection of suspected hemobilia, with the catheter serving as a vehicle for embolization when a lesion is shown to be present. Ultrasonography is very useful in the tracking of parenchymal or subcapsular hematomas in a cooperative patient once conservative treatment is instituted, but it is the CT scan that gives the most accurate and reproducible delineation of hepatic damage. The yield of the CT scan as a routine investigation in the stable nonrestless patient with blunt injury of the torso is still being explored. Early data are extremely promising but, as in any injured patient, the patient's general condition must be carefully assessed before moving to the radiologic suite and a physician equipped to deal with any sudden deterioration must always be in attendance.

Hepatic injury should always be suspected in the presence of a right-sided hemothorax or fractured ribs, a fractured pelvis after falls from heights, or an injury of the spinal column in a patient who was wearing a seat belt at the time of injury. Myocardial contusion is suspected in those patients who do not respond appropriately to adequate fluid resuscitation or whose cardiac output remains low in the presence of a stable hematocrit. Paraplegic patients may be particularly deceptive in that they have no local abdominal pain. Furthermore, hypotention in the paraplegic may or may not reflect blood loss as the fall in pressure may be due to interruption of the sympathetic nervous system, with concomitant vasodilatation. Peritoneal lavage is especially helpful in this circumstance.

TREATMENT

Preoperative Preparation

The patient is resuscitated as rapidly as possible by restoration of blood volume and the establishment of adequate ventilation and oxygenation. If any hematuria is noted, an intravenous pyelogram (IVP) is performed preoperatively or, when this is not feasible, performed on the operating room table later. Some surgeons feel that an IVP should be done in all patients with blunt abdominal trauma even in the absence of hematuria so as to exclude the possibility of a renal artery occlusion or a silent ureteric transection.

If the chest x-ray reveals any rib fractures, a No. 36 chest tube is inserted through the fifth intercostal space in the anterior axillary line before general anesthesia is begun to obviate an intraoperative pneumothorax which may develop subtly but lethally. In severe multiple injuries, when massive blood transfusions and a stormy course is predictable, a pulmonary artery catheter should be inserted. The ECG is scanned for arrhythmias in case a cardiac contusion has occurred and the MB fraction of CPK and LDH enzyme levels may be measured as an indication of cardiac injury. Although pericardial tamponade is very rarely a concomitant of liver injury, this should be looked for also. In blunt injuries, special attention is paid to the mediastinum and the contour of the aortic arch to exclude the possibility of an aortic rupture. When, by virtue of any radiologic sign, aortic leakage is suspected, an arch aortogram

preoperatively or postoperatively is essential. The sequence followed is dictated by the assessment of whether the abdominal lesion or the potential aortic lesion is felt to be the most immediately life threatening; in most cases, care of the liver and other associated intraabdominal injuries take priority.

A nasogastric tube is inserted to decompress the stomach, broad-spectrum antibiotics are administered when it is thought that the gastrointestinal (GI) tract has been transgressed, and a Foley catheter is inserted to monitor urinary output. The administration of an H_2 blocker has been advocated as a prophylactic measure in cases where potential aspiration is feared, but this should be avoided in suspected hepatic injury, as these blockers reduce hepatic blood flow by about 25 percent. Blood is sent to be typed and cross-matched and the blood bank is alerted to the probable need for blood, fresh frozen plasma, and possibly platelets in cases of massive injury. The autotransfusor should be prepared and the patient is placed on a heating blanket to combat the deleterious effects of hypothermia (e.g., acidosis, coagulopathy, vasoconstriction) resulting from the infusion of large quantities of cold crystalloids and blood that may be administered intraoperatively. Whenever possible, the blood should be warmed and crystalloids at about 40°C should be used. Allowance for any hypothermia present must be made in the interpretation of arterial pH, which falls about 0.15 for each 10°C drop in body temperature.

Operative Approach (Table 62–2)

A midline incision is made from the xiphoid to the umbilicus. If the incision is not large

TABLE 62–2. METHODS OF TREATMENT OF LIVER INJURIES (WAYNE STATE UNIVERSITY) (1968–1976 and 1980–1983)

Procedure	No. of Patients (1968–1976)	No. of Patients (1980–1983)
Laparotomy alone	492 (50.8%)	123 (67.5%)
Suture	367 (37.9%)	40 (21.3%)
Debridement	46 (4.8%)	5 (2.7%)
Hemihepatectomy	25 (2.6%)	5 (2.7%)
Hepatic artery ligation	14 (1.4%)	3 (1.6%)
IVC cannulation	8 (0.8%)	2 (1.0%)
Packs	3 (0.3%)	6 (3.2%)
Death on table or details unavailable	13 (1.4%)	4 (2.1%)
Total	968 (100%)	188 (100%)

enough to provide the exposure needed for hemostasis or the identification of nonhepatic lesions, the incision should be generously extended without delay. In selected cases, the incision is continued as a median sternotomy to give access to the heart, the inferior vena cava (IVC), and the hepatic veins. Less commonly, the incision may extend across the costal margin into the seventh or eighth interspace to provide exposure of any damaged right lung tissue or diaphragm.

An attempt is made to obtain rapid hemostasis by the application of manual pressure against one or more large laparotomy sponges. Where both posterior and anterior wounds of the liver are present or when injury involves the relatively inaccessible dome of the liver, it may be necessary to cut the coronary ligaments rapidly to permit mobilization of the liver and efficient bimanual compression. Theoretically, transection of these ligaments is undesirable if the hepatic artery is to be ligated as collaterals to the parenchyma on which restoration of blood supply may depend are interrupted. Unfortunately, the surgeon does not often have the desired prescience at this point of the operation.

In the face of major venous bleeding in the region of the hepatic veins, direct pressure packs placed behind the liver may be more effective. Attempts to inspect any posterior hepatic wound should be resisted as long as the patient is unstable, as each attempt at exposure may cost the patient 100 to 250 ml of blood, depending on the source of the bleeding. Furthermore, retraction on a liver that is not fully mobilized may further enlarge the parenchymal wound with disastrous consequences. This is particularly true in cirrhotics in whom the liver is firm.

With bleeding substantially, albeit temporarily, controlled by the assistant's manual pressure, the surgeon conducts a rapid but systematic inspection of the rest of the peritoneal cavity for other injuries. If a perforated intestine is found, a series of Babcock or similar tissue forceps is applied in order to limit further spillage of intestinal content. The degree and sequence of attention to other injuries varies with the individual circumstances but precedence should be accorded to the colon to reduce continuing contamination.

When bleeding continues despite direct manual pressure or recurs when pressure on the liver is released, the portal triad is occluded by a vascular clamp or by a cloth-covered intestinal clamp gently applied (Pringle maneuver). If bleeding still continues unabated, the probability is that either a large hepatic vein (most often, the right hepatic vein) or the IVC is lacerated. Under these conditions, pressure should be relied upon while the incision is enlarged, the sternum is split, blood volume is restored and instruments are made available (such as vascular clamps, a No. 36 chest tube or endotracheal tube for IVC cannulation and a Roumel tourniquet). Attempts at venous repair should be delayed until the patient's vascular volume has been replenished and vital signs are at a reasonable level. The autotransfusor may be invaluable at this point. Most surgeons balk at its use in the presence of frank intestinal content in the peritoneal cavity, but there is no question that many patients have received contaminated autotransfused blood with a successful outcome. Alternatively, and less often, uncontrolled bleeding may be due to an anomalous hepatic artery that has not been included in the clamp on the portal triad. The left hepatic artery originates from the left gastric artery in about 15 percent of patients and the right hepatic artery from the superior mesenteric artery in about 12 percent. Note is made of the color of the blood. When the blood originates from the hepatic veins or inferior vena cava, it will be relatively dark, in contrast to the redness of arterial bleeding in the presence of adequate oxygenation. In most cases, bleeding is substantially reduced by the Pringle maneuver and the clamp is advanced distally to occlude more precisely the specific hepatic arterial or portal venous supply to the area of the damaged tissue while the feasibility of obtaining control of the intrahepatic bleeding points is determined. To succeed in this goal, good exposure of the liver wound is essential. In some cases, it may even be necessary to enlarge the hepatic wound deliberately to gain access to its depths, where the offending vessel may be clearly visualized and suture-ligated with 3-0 silk or hemoclipped. The latter technique is somewhat less dependable. This enlargement of the wound is achieved by a modification of the finger-fracture technique or by use of the knife handle. Any ischemic tissue observed in the area is debrided, as would be done in any other wound.

The maximal period of safety for occlusion of the portal triad has long been debated. Traditionally, 15 minutes has been fixed as the permissible outer limit and although often challenged, this remains a good guide in the shocked, bleeding, acidotic, hypothermic, multiply-transfused patients. Unquestionably, much longer periods of occlusion have been followed by successful outcomes but clamping time should be kept at a minimum. Pachter suggests that protection of a liver deprived of its splanchnic blood supply may be enhanced through cooling of the liver to 27 to 30°C by pouring 1 L of iced Ringer's lactate on the liver surface, with the addition of 0.5 L each 15 minutes. In addition, he has advocated administration of 30 to 40 mg/kg of methylprednisolone succinate before occlusion of the portal triad. With this technique, no cases of liver failure occurred in 30 patients in whom the portal triad was occluded for longer than 20 minutes, in the 17 patients in whom occlusion time exceeded 30 minutes, and in the 3 patients where occlusion time exceeded 1 hour. These two additions have not been widely used by others as yet and the scientific basis for their reported efficacy remains to be explored.

Debridement need not follow segmental lines precisely as long as adequate venous outflow is protected. When extensive hepatic debridement has been performed—and as much as 300 to 400 g may be excised on occasion—the hepatic cavity may be left open after meticulous hemostasis has been obtained or it may be filled with pedicled omentum. Some advocates of the pedicled omentum technqiue use the omentum as a tight tamponading plug, others simply as loose tissue to obliterate dead space, and still others as a tissue purported to have valuable hemostatic properties. It should be noted, however, that the use of the omentum as a plug may be hazardous, as blood trapped beneath the attached omentum may collect under considerable pressure. As an alternative, some surgeons favor the application of microcrystalline collagen to the debrided surface for further hemostasis. As a dry field is required for its efficacy, the value of this substance in this circumstance is questionable. Care must be taken to avoid spillage of the powder in the peritoneal cavity to avoid subsequent adhesions.

Through-and-through wounds of the right lobe of the liver may present difficult problems when deep in the parenchyma. Bleeding superficial wounds lend themselves to easy tractotomy, direct exposure of the track and ligation of the bleeding vessels and leaking bile ducts. In contrast, deep wounds necessitate an incision through many square centimeters of parenchyma, a much more formidable undertaking. The options are limited. Direct manual pressure may stop bleeding spontaneously in some but others require more definitive measures. In this latter difficult but fortunately infrequent group, some surgeons favor the pragmatic application of a series of deep, blindly placed catgut sutures with reliance for hemostasis on firm approximation of the wound edges—and an element of chance. This technique, although crude, is frequently successful. A few surgeons advocate the insertion of a catheter into the track to produce pressure on the walls and to provide objective evidence of any continuing bleeding, but this approach carries considerable risk. If hemostasis is not achieved, however—or occasionally as a primary alternative—ligation of the hepatic artery close to the liver may produce a dramatic result. Whatever technique is selected, the temptation to close both ends of a missile track or the point of entry of a deep stab wound should be resisted in case bleeding continues silently in the depths until a huge intraparenchymal hematoma has been produced with a final sudden and catastrophic rupture. If none of these methods are successful, there is no alternative but to incise through the parenchyma of the liver, identify and ligate the bleeding point, and settle for what may become essentially a partial segmentectomy. The use of a special liver clamp or a Penrose drain employed as a tourniquet across the mobilized lobe may substantially reduce the volume of blood loss as this is done. Before the abdomen is closed, the liver wound should be observed during a period of normotension to be certain that the hemostasis obtained is not primarily a function of a lowered blood pressure.

Formal hepatic lobectomy has a limited place in trauma and should not be equated with a lobectomy performed under elective circumstances. The injured patient who requires resection will amost by definition have been in deep shock subsequent to injury, will have been the recipient of a large volume of banked blood, probably has a grossly disturbed acid–base balance, may well be hypothermic, and will often have a number of other injuries. The operating team is likely to be physically tired if the operation is performed at night, and conditions are usually less than optimal in these nonelective procedures. Balesegeram claims a mortality rate for lobectomy in trauma of only 10.5 percent in Malaysia (the overall mortality rate in his series of 379 liver injuries was 15.8 percent). The mortality rate for lobectomy in trauma in North America, however, ranges from about 35 to 70 percent with an overall mortality rate ranging from 6 to 15 percent. The inclusion of nearly moribund patients temporarily rescued by an excellent EMS presumably plays some part in selection and may paradoxically account for the poor results of lobectomy, which is reserved for the essentially smashed lobe or the lobe that continues to bleed despite the most vigorous attempts at hemostasis after extensive debridement. Although, in a sense, lobectomy is the least desirable of approaches, the decision to pursue this course should not be a last resort only embarked upon in desperation after other failed techniques have rendered the patient virtually moribund. If possible, the situation should be assessed rapidly and a relatively early decision made.

Controversial Areas

Packing

In view of the high mortality of resection, alternative approaches have been explored and the technique of packing has recently acquired tenuous respectability again. The packing of liver wounds was anathema to surgeons between the two world wars because of its failure to produce hemostasis and because of the high incidence of subsequent sepsis in the small group of survivors. These poor results are attributable in large measure to the poor selection of patients for the procedure with concomitant failure to apply local methods of hemostasis or to attend appropriately to associated intraabdominal injuries. In addition, today's supportive measures such as antibiotics and ventilators were not available earlier and there was a tendency to leave the packs in situ for too long a period.

We have successfully used packs to control bleeding in six patients when other methods have failed. Calne and Feliciano have now reported large series and the indications are much clearer: (1) inability to achieve adequate hemostasis due to the nature of the lesion, for example, a transverse crack of the liver across both lobes with less than adequate response to ligation of the hepatic artery; (2) lack of facilities, blood, or experience in an institution in which case temporary packing with transfer of the pa-

tient to a more sophisticated hospital will reduce the mortality of maneuvers that are predestined to failure in an inadequately equipped hospital; (3) the presence of bleeding from a low-pressure retrohepatic lesion when atriocaval shunting is felt not to be feasible or desirable, or when shunting and local repair has failed; (4) continuing bleeding after debridement, segmentectomy, or lobectomy; and (5) an established coagulopathy.

If packs are used, these large abdominal rolls of gauze should be inserted so as to produce direct firm pressure on the bleeding area without occlusion of the venous return to the heart through the IVC. The abdomen should be closed and the packs should not be brought to the outside. Although 5 to 7 days used to be regarded as the optimal time for removal of the packs, most surgeons now agree that 24 to 72 hours is preferable. The packs should be removed in the operating room in the course of a formal laparotomy that amounts to a second-look procedure. In most cases, the field will remain dry after the packs are removed but if bleeding recurs, the chance of clear identification of the bleeding point is enhanced.

Hepatic Artery Ligation (HAL)

Temporary occlusion of the hepatic artery may be very helpful but permanent ligation is only necessary in about 1 to 2 percent of patients. The procedure is not nearly as innocuous as was implied by some of its advocates in the early 1970s. In the light of further experience, however, those institutions that were performing HAL in 14 to 31 percent of patients with hepatic injury have now reduced their use of this procedure considerably. Rebleeding occurs in about 10 to 20 percent of patients even when the appropriate hepatic artery is ligated, as collaterals to the damaged liver tissue are established within 12 hours. Furthermore, ischemia of the subtended liver tissue is inevitable, increasing the incidence of sepsis and death from this cause. Increased mortality from this latter factor is present in series where HAL was frequently performed. Nevertheless, HAL may be invaluable if the following points are recognized:

1. HAL is not a substitute for assiduous attempts to obtain hemostasis locally at the site of the parenchymal injury.
2. As a procedure, HAL is in competition with lobectomy rather than local debridement.

3. The potential efficacy of HAL should first be tested with temporary occlusion of the artery as close to the damaged lobe as possible.
4. Variations in the anatomy of the hepatic artery should be anticipated.
5. When both lobes are injured, the common hepatic artery rather than the hepatic artery proper should be ligated, as occlusion of the latter is more hazardous.
6. Cholecystectomy is necessary when the right hepatic artery is ligated.
7. Antibiotic coverage against biliary tract organisms should be given intra- and postoperatively for 3 to 5 days and, in view of the potential hepatic and intestinal ischemia, coverage of anerobic organisms should also be provided.
8. The splanchnic blood supply and oxygenation should be protected as far as possible, but there is no convincing evidence that Glucagon is helpful in this respect.
9. The bowel should be kept at rest and hepatic function supported by appropriate parenteral hyperalimentation.

Postoperative Drainage

It has been customary over the years to add perihepatic drainage to most hepatic injuries on the premise that collections of blood and necrotic tissue predispose to sepsis and that bile leakage may lead to bile peritonitis. The extent, type, and duration of drainage advocated has varied with the severity of the injury and the prejudice of the surgeon. At one extreme, removal of the right twelfth rib was proposed, with creation of a posterior exit for drainage tubes that was wide enough to admit four fingers. Others advised that sump drains, with or without Penrose drains, be brought lateral to the intact twelfth rib in an attempt to ensure a measure of dependent drainage. Still others have used Penrose drains alone through generous anterior stab wounds. Fischer et al, in a study of 254 patients, however, have cast considerable doubt on the necessity and desirability of the use of drains and have suggested that these may cause sepsis rather than prevent infection. The tendency of trauma surgeons in the past five years, in parallel with the increasingly conservative approach to peritoneal drainage in elective procedures, has been to use drains only in specific circumstances. In liver injuries, these indications at present are limited to: (1) massive bursting injury when lurking doubts exist about the efficiency of the hemostasis and bilostasis obtained, (2) the presence of gross contamination of the peritoneal cavity at the time of laparotomy by feces or small bowel content, and (3) the presence of concomitant pancreatic injury. No prospective randomized study of the advantages of drains, if any, has been published.

When drains are used, no unanimity exists as to the most desirable varieties and in many institutions both sump drains and Penrose drains are carefully placed to provide dependent drainage. Care is taken to obviate damage to intraabdominal organs such as the colon by pressure from the drains. In addition, drains are left in place for much less than the 10 to 14 days previously advocated and are retained only as long as they are producing results. The local extraabdominal care of drains is often neglected and as drains may be responsible for the ingress of organisms, the area of entry of the drains into the abdominal wall should be meticulously cared for.

The routine use of T-tubes between 1963 and the early 1970s has been shown to be unnecessary and highly undesirable. In a prospective randomized study on 189 patients, Lucas and Walt demonstrated that complications, most notably sepsis, were significantly increased. If the intraoperative delineation of ducts is desired, fluid may be injected directly into the common bile duct through a needle inserted above a soft occluding clamp. Sometimes minor hepatic parenchymal extravasation has to be accepted, especially in the severely injured patient where operative time cannot be extended without a price being paid. Perfection is not always attainable at the initial operation. Use of a T-tube is only justified when an extrahepatic biliary radical has been injured.

Management of Hemobilia

Hemobilia is an uncommon occurrence in hepatic trauma. We have encountered only 4 cases in this series of 1592 patients but it must be recognized that hemobilia may only become evident many months after the patient is discharged from hospital. For this reason, all patients who have sustained an hepatic injury should be informed on discharge that any subsequent hematemesis or melena may originate from the liver and should not necessarily be attributed to peptic ulceration or erosive gastritis.

About 50 percent of cases declare themselves by gastrointestinal bleeding more than 1 month after injury. Bleeding may be staccato over days or weeks but may be massive from the start or at least early on. Jaundice is frequently present and colic may be apparent. Fever as a manifestation of sepsis may occur when the hemobilia is due to an intraparenchymal mycotic abscess.

It is surprising that hemobilia is not more common than it is. With increased use of arteriography, it has been conclusively shown that arteriovenous fistulas occur with many hepatic injuries and that most of these occlude spontaneously. Given the intimate anatomic relationship of the intrahepatic bile ducts to the intrahepatic vessels, it is reasonable to anticipate that biliary radicles will frequently be damaged as they lie in immediate juxtaposition to the injured vessels. Fortunately, spontaneous closure would seem to be the rule rather than the exception despite the tendency of bile to dissolve blood clots.

Arteriography should be performed as an emergency when hemobilia is suspected. With the lesion demonstrated, embolization of Gelfoam, muscle, coils, or whatever the interventional radiologist selects should be attempted. This technique has been highly successful, with a reduction in morbidity and mortality when compared with surgical intervention. Despite the fact that postembolization arteriography may show almost total obliteration of the intrahepatic arterial tree, these patients show little clinical disturbance beyond elevation of the liver enzymes.

Operation is reserved for patients in whom embolization is unsuccessful or unavailable. In most of these cases, the source of the intrahepatic bleeding is identified at operation by the external appearance of the hepatic surface or by palpation which reveals a softened area. Needle aspiration confirms the site of bleeding and a Pringle maneuver is performed. The area of injured liver is then opened after adequate exposure has been ensured. Old clot and ischemic tissue is removed and bleeding vessels and leaking ducts are suture-ligated. As extra insurance, the appropriate hepatic artery may also be ligated close to the liver. If an infected cavity remains, the area is drained. Lobectomy is rarely necessary today.

Some patients—mainly children with peripheral bleeding lesions demonstrated arteriographically—have been successfully observed

without the institution of any definitive local treatment, but these constitute the exception. Their lesions are presumably small and the onus for this conservative course of treatment is very much on the surgeon.

Nonoperative Observation of Large Liver Lesions

Modern technology has revealed that in blunt torso injury, the liver may contain a large intraparenchymal or subcapsular hematoma even though the patient is relatively asymptomatic. In a series of 283 patients with severe blunt torso trauma, Geis detected severe liver injury in 65 (23.3 percent). Three quarters of these had explosive damage necessitating immediate and obvious hepatic operation, but 16 patients had their intrahepatic hematoma (IHH) demonstrated on isotopic scans done only 1 to 3 days later. Similar experience is increasingly reported with the spreading use of CT scans, ultrasonography, and early arteriography. Complications of intraparenchymal lesions unrecognized at the time of hospital observation or improperly treated at operation have been appreciated for many years. Olsen described 21 patients with complications of central liver injuries 1 week to several years after the initial injury. In some patients, the complications reflected the unfolding of the natural history of IHH but in 62.5 percent of this series, iatrogenic factors such as the inappropriate suturing of both ends of a track or ligation of the hepatic artery were responsible for the complication.

As far back as 1972, Ritchie et al suggested that subcapsular hematomas may safely be observed, obviating the need for operation and Sugimoto has reported six CT demonstrated posttraumatic intrahepatic "cysts" separated by weeks from the time of injury, 3 of these in the 14 patients with blunt trauma who had routine CT scans as follow-up.

Conservatism is currently the order of the day and the clear demonstration that these intrahepatic lesions have the capacity for spontaneous healing forces new decisions on surgeons. Although it is recognized that some patients may develop delayed complications such as sepsis or hemorrhage, the majority do not. If a nonoperative approach is adopted, the patient should be kept in the hospital for 7 to 10 days at least, warned against any contact sport for at least 6 weeks, given detailed written instructions about potential complications, advised about actions to be taken if complications are suspected, and presented a plan for careful follow-up by ultrasonography or CT scanning. A sudden rise in serum alkaline phosphatase should raise suspicion. Nevertheless, not all such lesions can be safely observed and special attention must be given to patients who have been on anticoagulants at the time of injury. The unquestionable indications for immediate operation are:

1. A deterioration in the clinical condition of the patient, with any suggestion of blood loss, such as a fall in the hemoglobin level
2. An increase in symptoms such as pain in the right upper quadrant or epigastrium
3. An increase in size of the liver demonstrated either clinically or by ultrasonography or other methods, and
4. The occurrence of fever for which no other explanation is obvious

The use of percutaneous aspiration of a hepatic hematoma as a technique for reducing the size of the lesion, while also providing material for Gram smears and cultures, needs to be explored. Hepatostomy by a dePezzer or similar catheter in selected cases of IHH is known to be a successful maneuver and percutaneous hepatic aspiration is merely a simpler form of this.

Atrial–Caval Shunting (ACS)

Atrial–caval shunting was proposed by Shrock in 1968 as a method of providing return of caval blood to the heart while isolating a retrohepatic caval or hepatic venous injury to permit surgical repair. Since then, a number of different approaches have been suggested, including the passage of appropriate large catheters, with or without occluding balloons, inserted through the inferior vena cava below the renal veins or through the common femoral vein.

Injury to the IVC or large hepatic veins carries a high mortality; most patients die before reaching hospital. Those who arrive in the emergency department may have a relatively small injury, as evidenced by a large retroperitoneal hematoma that, arising from a low-pressure system, is contained and tamponaded. This group is best left undisturbed. Most injuries to an hepatic vein in stable patients do not present with a large amount of blood in the peritoneal cavity at operation. The hematoma is usually contained and significant hemorrhage only begins when the liver is mobilized. Almost invariably, a right or left lobectomy becomes neces-

sary in the course of securing control with vascular repair of the injury. When injury is confined to the right hepatic vein, which varies in length but averages about 1.5 cm, successful direct repair without a shunt has been reported, but this technique must be extremely difficult. Ligation of the right hepatic vein without resection of the area that is drained results in venous congestion and necrosis and should be avoided.

The decision to open a large retroperitoneal hematoma in this area is therefore a serious undertaking that should be preceded by the excellent exposure provided by a median sternotomy and the immediate availability of the appropriate cannula. Results have not been good and a move away from this procedure is clearly discernible. Our own experience with ACS at Detroit Receiving Hospital continues to be dismal and we have had no successes in the ten patients who have been treated in this manner. The chief proponents in the past—the group at the Ben Taub Hospital in Houston—have preferred the judicious use of packing in recent years. It seems likely that some of the earlier successes were obtained in relatively minor hemorrhages that are amenable to packing and, conversely, some of the failures may have been avoided by the less aggressive approach of packing.

A review of 18 patients treated at the San Francisco General Hospital (SFGH) between 1968 and 1982 by atrial–caval shunting permits the development of a better perspective on the indications. Thirteen of the 18 patients in this series died rapidly and 1 died after 45 days. The four survivors had in common the following features: (1) all had predominantly hepatic injuries; (2) all had penetrating injuries—no patients with blunt injury survived ACS; (4) all had a systolic blood pressure of greater than 70 mm Hg; and (5) the decision to insert an atrial–caval shunt was made rapidly and before the patient deteriorated to the point of being unstable. In addition, the team involved in this series was experienced and practiced.

Nutrition

Patients with massive hepatic injury inevitably suffer a severe catabolic insult which is likely to be magnified by an inability to eat for days or weeks if associated injuries are present. Some surgeons, allowing for this period of starvation, insert a jejunal catheter at the original operation for purposes of early enteral feeding. Alternatively, total parenteral nutrition via a subclavian or jugular catheter may be used but this carries with it the attendant potential complications of this procedure, such as septicemia, pneumothorax, and thrombosis.

Following resection of a moderate to large amount of liver tissue, a hyperbilirubinemia up to approximately 5 mg/dl is common in addition to elevations of the serum alkaline phosphatase and other liver enzymes for about 1 week. A serum bilirubin level that climbs above 5 mg/dl is usually indicative of sepsis. Transient hypoglycemia may occur and hypoalbuminemia should be expected. It is seldom necessary to infuse albumin to restore reasonable levels in the blood and indeed attempts to do so may be harmful. If the serum albumin should fall below 2.5 g/dl despite TPN, the administration of single donor plasma or fresh frozen plasma should be considered. Patients depleted to this extent, especially if they have a reduced blood volume, are much less able to withstand any fresh insult such as sepsis or further bleeding.

Antibiotics

If spillage of intestinal content is encountered, cefazolin, an aminoglycoside, and clindamycin are given intraoperatively to cover both aerobic and anaerobic microorganisms in the peritoneal cavity, with due consideration given to any history of hypersensitivity and reduced renal function. If it is necessary to continue the aminoglycosides, peak and trough levels are desirable on a daily basis and are mandatory in the presence of oliguria.

The decision to use antibiotics is more difficult in the absence of frank contamination. Many of these patients have marked intestinal ischemia and hepatic hypoxia early on, and an unavoidable suppression of reticuloendothelial function and the threat of the numerous indwelling catheters in an ICU setting later. The surgeon with strong convictions will usually stop any antibiotics soon after operation in this group, but the majority of surgeons tend to administer one or more antibiotics for a few days. In fact, no satisfactory data are available on which to base a rational decision in this complicated setting.

COMPLICATIONS

Bleeding and sepsis, primarily peri- and intrahepatic, are the most common complications of hepatic trauma. These patients are, however, prone to the same wide spectrum of complications that may occur in any abdominal injury. As injury to more than one organ is common, the short- and long-term effects of blood loss and gross bacterial contamination are frequent. In addition, extraabdominal complications associated with injury to other organs such as the brain, lung, heart, diaphragm, kidneys, spleen, and long bones need to be combated in their own right. Pulmonary contusion, fractured ribs and intraperitoneal sepsis may all have profound effects on ventilation and gas exchange. Consequently, patterns of ventilation, changes in blood gas tensions and acid–base alterations are carefully tracked. Ventilatory support may need to be prolonged both to prevent and to treat any evidence of the adult respiratory distress syndrome. The endotracheal tube should not be removed prematurely in serious hepatic injuries and allowances must be made for occult concomitant pulmonary dysfunction.

Coagulopathies are frequent in major hepatic injury. It is essential that distinctions be made between oozing that originates from the platelet deficiency of the "wash-out" syndrome of massive transfusion and that caused by a transfusion mismatch or a frank disseminated intravascular coagulation. The following prophylactic measures can be taken against these hematologic misadventures: the administration of blood less than 24 hours old whenever possible, one unit of fresh frozen plasma after each 4 units of blood, platelet concentrates after every 8 to 10 units of blood (and certainly if the platelet count falls below 20,000/mm^3), and calcium chloride (1 g intravenously) after each 4 to 6 units of blood; careful checking of each unit of blood even in the middle of exsanguinating hemorrhage; and avoidance of excessive acidosis, hypothermia and residual necrotic tissue. It is not necessary to treat laboratory data alone and a low platelet count or a prolonged prothrombin time (up to 5 seconds or so) does not require reversal unless pinpointed as the cause of abnormal bleeding.

Renal failure is prevented by curtailing the length and depth of hypotension and by ensuring urinary flow throughout the operative procedure and beyond. Conversely, polyuria should be recognized as possibly being a reflection of the early hemodynamic changes of sepsis and should not automatically trigger an order to reduce fluid administration precipitously.

Acute erosive gastritis is a frequent concomitant of sepsis and should be guarded against by the administration of carefully controlled hourly antacid designed to keep gastric pH above 5.0, with or without an H_2 blocker, which, on balance, has not been effective in these conditions.

The nonspecific complications referred to above are common and are discussed in detail elsewhere. A few specific complications associated with hepatic injury merit special consideration.

Biliary Fistulas: Cutaneous, Pleural, and Bronchial

Most biliary fistulas which track through a drain site or the main wound will close spontaneously within 1 to 6 weeks if there is no distal obstruction. If drainage persists or is excessive, attempts to delineate the source may be made by direct fistulography, percutaneous hepatic cholangiography, isotopic scanning, or endoscopic retrograde cholangiography (ERCP). Of these, the fistulogram is by far the easiest to do and the most rewarding. Further operation is seldom called for except for marked ductal damage, often unrecognized at the initial operation, or in the presence of continuing local sepsis. Patience should be exercised and vigorous attempts made to ensure that the patient is kept in an optimal metabolic state. Biliary–pleural fistulas are rare, occurring in about 0.1 to 0.3 percent of hepatic injuries. The presence of bile in a pleural effusion mandates the insertion of a thoracostomy tube which is left in place until all drainage has ceased. In some cases, this may be enough but in others where the hepatic leak does not seal spontaneously, diaphragmatic repair, hepatic debridement, subcostal drainage and decortication may be necessary.

Biliary–bronchial fistulas are even less common and more dangerous as bile may flood the bronchial system. Many weeks may elapse between the initial injury and the clinical appearance of the fistula. With the diagnosis made by identification of bile in the sputum, immediate attempts must be instituted to find and eliminate the source. These efforts are likely to be difficult, as the lower lobe of the lung, the diaphragmatic hole, and the hepatic source of the bile are usually buried in a conglomeration of adhesions and necrotic tissue. Through an abdominal incision, the liver is debrided and the diaphragm closed. An omental pedicle brought

to the area may be an invaluable adjunct and a lower lobe lobectomy or segmentectomy through a separate thoracic incision is often essential to cure.

Traumatic Hepatic Arteriovenous Fistula

With the more frequent use of arteriography, the presence of traumatic hepatic arteriovenous (A-V) fistulas is increasingly demonstrated. The vast majority of these acute intraparenchymal lesions close spontaneously within a few days and cause no symptoms. Persistent fistulas, however, are rare and tend to be large. As occurs with similar congenital fistulas over time, a hyperdynamic large fistula may result in portal hypertension and even esophageal varices which may bleed. The presence of this occurrence after a liver injury in a nonalcoholic patient should prompt urgent arteriography. Although smaller A-V fistulas may be occluded by radiographic transcatheter embolization, larger lesions are most effectively treated by a direct surgical attack on the area of the fistula.

Cause of Death in Liver Injury

Of patients with liver injury who die, hemorrhage is the cause in approximately 60 percent, sepsis in 20 percent, and cranial or thoracic injuries in 20 percent. In many, the injuries are so widespread and severe that the surgeon's task is hopeless from the start. Ironically, an improved emergency medical service may deliver to the emergency department a patient who is alive but in extremis and who would, in a less efficient system, have died at the scene of injury or en route to the hospital. Such improvements in prehospital care may affect hospital statistics, and consequently any study of various series should always take this aspect into account. In addition, other factors must be considered, such as the elapsed time between the injury and the commencement of definitive treatment, the presence and degree of shock, and the type and extent of associated injuries. Patients with suspected liver injury should be taken directly to a trauma center, as injuries of the liver, other than stab wounds, are seldom isolated. Furthermore, the bleeding that causes death may originate mainly in perihepatic vessels, e.g., mesen-

TABLE 62–3. MORTALITY OF LIVER INJURIES (1974–1976 and 1980–1983)[a]

Agent	No. of Patients (1974–1976)	Deaths	No. of Patients (1980–1983)	Deaths
Gunshot Wound	186	28 (15.1%)	87	8 (9%)
Stab	91	1 (1.1%)	80	4 (5%)
Blunt	40	8 (20.0%)	17	5 (29%)
Shotgun	13	3 (23.1%)	3	1 (33%)
Iatrogenic	1	0	1	0
Total	331	40 (12.1%)	188	18 (13.8%)

[a] Mortality in 1961–1968 was 10.5% (46/436); in 1969–1973 14.6% (93/637).

teric and portal vessels, rather than in the liver itself.

In the 331 patients we analyzed between 1974 and 1976, 40 (12.1 percent) died. Of the deaths, 25 (62.5 percent) were from bleeding, 6 (15 percent) from sepsis, and 9 (22.5 percent) from other reasons, such as myocardial infarction or head injury. Between 1980 and 1983, 26 of 188 patients (13.8 percent) with liver injury treated in Detriot Receiving Hospital died (Table 62–3). Of the 26, 8 patients (30.8 percent) died in the operating room before definitive treatment could be given and these patients had obvious multiple injuries and severe hemorrhage. Five patients died in the operating room after definitive treatment of the hepatic bleeding had been accomplished; all were so depleted by the effects of deep and extended shock, massive blood transfusions or extrahepatic injury that they could not be salvaged. Five patients died within 24 hours of operation, 4 of adult respiratory disease syndrome (ARDS), and 1 of continued oozing due to disseminated intravascular coagulation (DIC). Eight patients died later, one 36 hours postoperatively of a myocardial infarction, 1 of ARDS 10 days postoperatively, and 6 of sepsis 10 to 79 days later.

It is obvious, then, that to improve the outcome, the surgeon must concentrate on: (1) early diagnosis, (2) rapid restoration of blood volume, (3) immediate operation in those who continue to deteriorate significantly despite vigorous resuscitative measures, (4) control of bleeding at laparotomy, (5) prevention or reduction of sepsis, (6) identification and care of nonhepatic injuries, with priorities assessed at the time of operation in the light of concomitant circumstances, e.g., fecal spill, splenic bleeding, pregnancy, ruptured thoracic aorta, and (7) meticulous postoperative monitoring and the restoration toward normal of the myriad of physiologic changes.

CONCLUSION

About 80 percent of liver injuries pose few if any problems in clinical or technical judgment. In about another 10 percent, major decisions may be made logically on the basis of sequential, standard, widely accepted surgical approaches. In something less than 10 percent, however, judgment becomes paramount and improvization may be necessary. Paradoxically, more than in most trauma, iatrogenic mortality stems as much from the attempt to do too much as from a reluctance to do enough. Over the past decade, surgeons have moved from an attitude of almost universal surgical machismo to a thoughtful, more cautious, selective approach to hepatic trauma. This latter evolution appears to be improving the overall mortality results.

BIBLIOGRAPHY

Balasegaram MB, Joisny S: Hepatic resection: The logical approach to surgical management of major trauma to the liver. Am J Surg 142:580, 1981

Bass EM, Crosier JH: Percutaneous control of post-traumatic hepatic hemorrhage by gelfoam embolization. J Trauma 17:61, 1977

Burkhardt: Beit. z. Behandlund der Leber Verletzungen. Centralbl f Chir S 88, 1887

Calne RY, McMaster P, et al: The treatment of major liver trauma by primary packing with transfer of the patient for definitive treatment. Br J Surg 66:338, 1979

Carmona RH, Lim RC, et al: Morbidity and mortality in hepatic trauma—A 5 year study. Am J Surg 144:88, 1982

Cheatham JE, Smith EI, et al: Nonoperative management of subcapsular hematomas of the liver. Am J Surg 140:852, 1980

Clagett GP, Olsen WR: Coagulopathies causing hemorrhage in severe liver injury. Ann Surg 187:369, 1978

DeFore WW, Mattox KL, et al: Management of 1590 consecutive cases of liver trauma. Arch Surg 111:493, 1976

Feliciano DV, Mattox KL, et al: Intra-abdominal packing for control of hepatic hemorrhage: A reappraisal. J Trauma 21:285, 1981

Fischer RP, O'Farrell KA, et al: The value of peritoneal drains in the treatment of liver injuries. J Trauma 18:393, 1978

Flint LM, Polk HC: Selective hepatic artery ligation: Limitations and failures. J Trauma 19:319, 1979

Franklin DC, Mathai J: Biliary pleural fistula: A complication of hepatic trauma. J Trauma 20:256, 1980

Geis WP, Schulz KA, et al: The fate of unruptured intrahepatic hematomas. Surgery 90:689, 1981

Gewertz BL, Olsen WR: Hepatostomy for central hepatic hematomas. J Trauma 15:271, 1975

Golan A, White RG: Spontaneous rupture of the liver associated with pregnancy: A report of five cases. S Afr Med J 56:133, 1978

Goodnight JE, Blaisdell FW: Hemobilia. Surg Clin North Am 61:973, 1981

Jander HP, Laws HL, et al: Emergency embolization in blunt hepatic trauma. AJR 129:249, 1977

Kudsk KA, Sheldon GF, et al: Atrial-caval shunting (ACS) after trauma. J Trauma 22:81, 1982

Lambeth W, Rubin BE: Nonoperative management of intrahepatic hemorrhage and hematoma following blunt trauma. Surg Gynecol Obstet 148:507, 1979

Lawrence D, Dawson JL: The secondary management of complicated liver injuries. Ann R Coll Surg Engl 64:186, 1982

Lim RC, Giuliano AE, et al: Postoperative treatment of patients after liver resection for trauma. Arch Surg 112:429, 1977

Ledgerwood AM, Kazmers M, et al: The role of thoracic aortic occlusion for massive hemoperitoneum. J Trauma 16:610, 1976

Levin A, Gover P, et al: Surgical restraint in the management of hepatic injury: A review of charity hospital experience. J Trauma 18:399, 1978

Lockwood TE, Schorn L, et al: Nonoperative management of hemobilia. Ann Surg 185:335, 1977

Lucas CE, Walt AJ: Analysis of randomized biliary drainage for liver trauma in 189 patients. J Trauma 12:925, 1972

Mathisen DJ, Athanasoulis CA, et al: Goal in treatment of extrahepatic and post-traumatic intrahepatic aneurysms of the hepatic artery. Ann Surg 196:400, 1982

Missavage AE, Jones AM, et al: Traumatic hepatic arterio-venous fistula. J Trauma 24:355, 1984

Moon KL, Federle MP: Computed tomography in hepatic trauma. AJR 141:309, 1983

Olsen WR: Late complications of central liver injuries. Surgery 92:733, 1982

Pachter HL, Spencer FC, et al: Experience with the finger fracture technique to achieve intra-hepatic hemostasis in 75 patients with severe liver injuries of the liver. Ann Surg 197:771, 1983

Pachter HL, Spencer FC: Recent concepts in the treatment of hepatic trauma. Ann Surg 190:423, 1979

Pilcher DB, Harmon PK, et al: Retrohepatic vena cava balloon shunt introduced via the saphenofemoral junction. J Trauma 17:837, 1977

Popovsky J, Wiener SN, et al: Liver trauma: Conservative management and the liver scan. Arch Surg 108:184, 1974

Pringle JH: Notes on the arrest of hepatic hemorrhage due to trauma. Ann Surg 48:541, 1908

Richie JP, Fonkalsrud EW: Subcapsular hematomas of the liver: Non-operative management. Arch Surg 104:781, 1972

Ryan KG, Lorbor SH: Traumatic fistulae between hepatic artery and portal vein. N Engl J Med 279:1215, 1978

Sandblom P: Hemorrhage into biliary tract following trauma: Traumatic hemobilia. Surgery 24:571, 1948

Sandblom P, Mirkovitch V: Hemobilia: Some silent features and their causes. Surg Clin North Am 57:397, 1977

Schmidt B, Bhatt GM, et al: Management of post-traumatic vascular malformations of the liver by catheter embolization. Am J Surg 140:332, 1980

Schrock T, Blaisdell W, et al: Management of blunt trauma to the liver and hepatic veins. Arch Surg 96:698, 1968

Sclafani SJA, Nayaranaswamy T, et al: Radiologic management of traumatic hepatic artery portal vein arteriovenous fistulae. J Trauma 21:576, 1981

Stone HH, Lamb JM: Use of pedicled omentum as an autogenous pack for control of hemorrhage in major injuries of the liver. Surg Gynecol Obstet 141:92, 1975

Sugimoto T, Yoshioka T, et al: Post-traumatic cyst of the liver found on CT scan—A new concept. J Trauma 22:797, 1982

Svoboda JA, Peter ET, et al: Severe liver trauma in the face of coagulopathy: A case for temporary packing and early re-exploration. Am J Surg 144:717, 1982

Uthoff LB, Wyffels PL, et al: A propsective study comparing nuclear scintigraphy and computerized axial tomography in the initial evaluation of the trauma patient. Ann Surg 198:611, 1983

Walt AJ: The mythology of hepatic trauma or Babel revisited. Am J Surg 135:12, 1978

Yellin AE, Chaffee CB, et al: Vascular isolation in the treatment of juxtahepatic venous injuries. Arch Surg 102:566, 1971

63. Pyogenic and Amebic Abscesses

Seymour I. Schwartz

The diagnosis and treatment of hepatic abscesses was a consideration of Hippocrates, who suggested that the prognosis could be altered by the character of the drainage. Clinical manifestations and pathologic correlations were not described until 1836 by John Bright. In 1922, Sir Leonard Rogers presented the Lettsonian Lectures on amebic liver abscess. The first comprehensive review of hepatic amebic abscesses in the American literature was presented by DeBakey and Ochsner in 1951. A landmark review of pyogenic liver abscess in the preantibiotic era is credited to Ochsner, DeBakey, and Murray in 1938.

Abscess of the liver has become more frequently recognized with refinement in radiographic studies. The formation of a hepatic abscess is related to two distinct groups of pathogens—the pyogenic bacteria, and endomoeba histolytica. The frequency of amebiasis in warmer climates accounts for a difference in geographic incidence. Distinctive features in the clinical manifestations, and also in the therapy of pyogenic and amebic abscesses, necessitate separate consideration.

PYOGENIC ABSCESS

Incidence

Ochsner and associates reported a postmortem incidence of 0.45 percent for patients hospitalized prior to 1938. In the experiences at this author's hospital, hepatic abscesses were demonstrated in 0.63 percent of autopsies performed from 1925 to 1960. A condition prevalence of 0.016 percent was reported for the Massachusetts General Hospital and this was paralleled by a frequency of 0.013 percent reported by the Johns Hopkins Hospital. In 1981, Balasegaram, reporting on a 17-year experience, indicated an incidence of documented pyogenic abscesses of 0.85 percent of total hospital admissions in Malaysia.

No significant predisposition for race or sex has been demonstrated. With a declining association of hepatic abscesses complicating appendicitis, there has been a shift in age prevalence from the third to the later decades of life. Many series report an average age in the sixth and seventh decades. This can be attributed to an aging population, and the incorporation of neoplastic diseases as an etiologic factor.

Etiology

Pyogenic abscesses of the liver result from: (1) ascending biliary infection, (2) hematogenous spread via the portal venous system, (3) generalized septicemia, with involvement of the liver by way of the hepatic arterial circulation, (4) direct extension of an intraperitoneal infection, and (5) other causes, including hepatic trauma. In a recent review by McDonald and Howard, biliary tract disease, principally obstructive, represented the most common cause, accounting for 33 percent of the patients. This included patients with cholecystitis, but the overwhelming majority of patients had biliary tract obstruction, often on a neoplastic basis. Abscesses due to biliary obstruction are generally multiple, involving both lobes of the liver in up to 90 percent of cases.

The portal venous route of infection had been very common prior to the antibiotic era. No segment of the intestinal tract, drained by the portal vein, can be excluded as a cause of pyogenic liver abscess. In the report of Ochsner et al, 22 percent of hepatic infections were attributed to sepsis within the portal venous system. Present series indicate that this route is implicated in about 22 percent of cases. Twenty one percent of liver abscesses are termed "cryptogenic" because their source is unknown. About 13 percent are of hematogenous origin via the hepatic artery and are associated with generalized sepsis in a compromised host. Contiguous liver infection, trauma, and liver metastases each accounts for less than 5 percent of liver abscesses. In the Malaysia experience extrahepatic duct disease accounts for 47 percent of the abscesses. Primary or metastatic tumors of the liver are associated in 16 percent of cases, whereas 12 percent of cases indict a portal venous route. Contiguous infection from perforated viscera account for 5 percent of patients, while cryptogenic abscesses account for approximately 5 percent.

Bacteriology

Positive cultures from the material of pyogenic abscesses have been reported in about 50 percent of cases. Presently, *Escherichia coli* is the most frequent pathogen in pyogenic liver abscesses, reported by McDonald and Howard in 37 percent of cases in which cultures were positive. *Proteus* and *Klebsiella enterobacter* species accounted for 13 and 12 percent, respectively. *Streptococcus* abscesses were present in 23 percent of patients, generally noted in cases of hematogenous spread. Two thirds of the cultures are mixed. More recently, because of improved culturing techniques, the so-called sterile abscesses were encountered in only 7 percent of patients. Pitt and Zuidema have reported a statistically significant increase in the prevalence of anaerobic infections. Improvement in culture techniques for anaerobes has focused attention on these organisms, and as the incidence of anaerobic liver abscesses increases, the incidence of so-called sterile abscesses decreases. Sabbaj and associates reported a prevalence of 45 percent of anaerobic infections in all liver abscesses seen over an 11-year period. In 76 percent of these patients anaerobes were present in pure culture. The anaerobic infections have been implicated in patients with pyogenic abscesses due to infection of hepatic metastatic lesions.

Pathology

Pyogenic abscesses may be solitary, multilocular, or multiple. Ochsner and associates found multiple abscesses in only 45 percent of cases; more recent series have indicated that these occur more frequently than a single abscess. When a single abscess is present, it is usually located in the posterosuperior segment of the right lobe, usually near the dome of the diaphragm. Abscesses that seed via the biliary tract and arterial circulation often involve both lobes. *Pyogenic abscess* was initially described by Waller in 1846 as a disease characterized by suppurative thrombophlebitis of the portal vein and the formation of single or multiple abscesses. Shortly after this description, the occurrence of pylephlebitis was emphasized as a sequela of appendicitis; later it was appreciated that no area of the intestine drained by the portal vein could be excluded as a cause. The fact that multiple abscesses are characteristically located in the right lobe of the liver and associated with pylephlebitis secondary to appendicitis has been ascribed to a streaming effect of two currents of blood in the portal vein. Recent experimental and clinical studies have refuted this theory. Abscesses secondary to diverticulitis of the left colon have been noted in the right lobe of the liver.

In pylephlebitic abscesses of the liver many radicals of the portal vein contain clots and bacteria. Dilatation of these veins is characteristic. Extending from the involved veins are areas of destruction of hepatic parenchyma, and peripherally, inflammation with lymphocytic and polymorphonuclear leukocytic infiltration is present. The pyogenic abscess membrane is initially pinkish grey, while in older lesions an abundance of foam cells is responsible for a yellow color. Ultimately a grey fibrous tissue capsule develops. In the evolution of pylephlebitic abscesses, bile ducts are frequently eroded, making impossible the differentiation between a pylephlebitic abscess and that of a cholangitic origin.

Cholangitic Abscesses. Cholangitic abscesses in general correspond to the anatomy of the biliary radicals. The bile duct involvement is evidenced by a yellowish-green color of the purulent material and of the abscess membrane. In the late stage, involvement of the portal veins is so extensive that these abscesses are indistinguishable from pylephlebitic abscesses.

Embolic Abscesses. These are usually widely disbursed throughout both lobes of the liver and rarely reach significant dimensions individually.

Clinical Manifestations

Since the great majority of pyogenic hepatic abscesses are secondary to other significant infections, it is difficult to ascribe a symptom or symptom complex to the hepatic abscess per se. Clinical manifestations are not specific. Fever is the most common symptom, present in approximately 80 percent of patients. In general, the temperatures are in the range of 40 to 41°C. A "picket fence" configuration of temperature chart has been noted in the presence of multiple abscesses of both cholangitic and pylephlebitic types. Associated rigors have been reported in 40 to 80 percent of patients with fever. Pain is a relatively late symptom and characteristically occurs 1 to 3 weeks after the onset of chills and fever in a patient with a solitary abscess. The pain is located either in the right upper quadrant, or has a pleuritic nature and distribution. Other symptoms that occur in less than one third of patients include nausea, vomiting, weight loss, anorexia, and malaise.

Hepatomegaly and associated tenderness are the most constant physical findings, but these are present in only 50 percent of cases. Jaundice is relatively uncommon, occurring in less than one third of patients. Ascites is an extremely rare finding.

The clinical manifestations are variable. When laparotomy is carried out for fever of unknown origin, hepatic abscesses were noted by Rothman et al in approximately 12 percent of cases.

Leukocytosis with white cell counts averaging between 18,000 and 20,000 is noted in a great majority of patients. Anemias are associated with long-standing infection. Positive blood cultures have been demonstrated in approximately 30 percent of patients.

The liver function tests are not diagnostic. An abnormal serum bilirubin has been reported in about one third of cases. The most significant chemical abnormality is an elevation of the serum alkaline phosphatase. Grossly raised serum levels of vitamin B_{12} (2000 to 4000 pg/ml) have been reported present in pyogenic liver abscesses.

Diagnostic Studies

Radiologic Findings. Characteristically there is elevation and immobility or restriction of motion of the right leaf of the diaphragm. This may be coupled with obliteration of the right cardiophrenic angle on the posterior anterior chest film, and obliteration of the anterocostophrenic angle on the lateral film. Pulmonary consolidation and pleural effusion may be noted. A similar reaction occurs in the left chest in about half the patients in whom a pyogenic abscess of the left lobe is diagnosed. Hepatomegaly may be demonstrated in both supine and erect position films. In about 5 percent of patients an air fluid level in the region of the liver may suggest the diagnosis.

Radionuclide Scanning. Technectium-99m sulfur colloid is injected intravenously and selectively taken up into the Kuppfer cells, where the Tc-99m undergoes isomeric transition to the lower-energy Tc-99 state. The gamma radiation released is detected by a photon-sensitive inorganic crystal. The detection of a space-occupying lesion by this method rests on the difference in the phagocytic activity between adjacent regions of the liver. A decreased uptake of tracer may define the presence of hepatic abscess. Gallium citrate also has been used for diagnosis of hepatic abscesses because of the avidity of the substance for inflammatory lesions. The scan has the disadvantage that it usually requires 2 to 3 days to complete, and the delay may be critical.

Ultrasonography. Grey scale ultrasound study may define the presence of a space-occupying lesion of the liver. The mobility of this technique makes it applicable to bedside diagnosis in critically ill patients. Ultrasonographically controlled drainage of hepatic abscesses may be accomplished.

Computed Tomography (Fig. 63–1). A computed tomographic (CT) scan differentiates areas of density within the liver and can be used to define any intrahepatic lesion, including an abscess. CT scanning is generally regarded as more precise than ultrasonography, and the accurate location that it achieves permits guidance for percutaneous drainage of hepatic abscesses.

Angiography (Fig. 63–2). Angiography is infrequently applied to the diagnosis of hepatic abscess. Characteristically the lesions present as avascular masses with hyperemic rims. Angiography is useful in differentiating hepatic abscesses from hepatocellular carcinomas. The technique employs selective hepatic arteriography by percutaneous catheterization of the femoral artery.

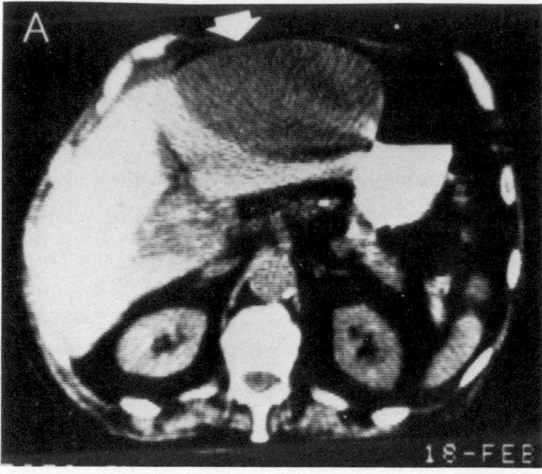
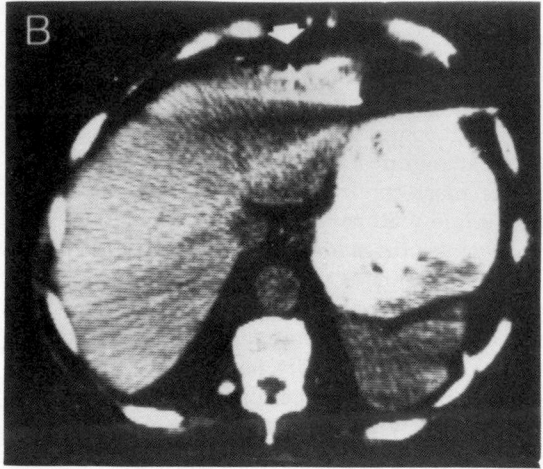

Figure 63–1. CT scan showing percutaneous drainage of the liver abscess. **A.** Before drainage (*arrow*). **B.** After complete drainage of abscess. (*Source: From Mandel SR, Boyd D, et al: Drainage of hepatic, intraabdominal, and mediastinal abscesses guided by computerized axial tomography. Am J Surg 145:120, 1983, with permission.*)

Endoscopic Retrograde Cholangiography. In patients in whom a diagnosis of biliary sepsis and associated hepatic abscess is entertained, this technique has been used to delineate the biliary tree and to provide detail of the intrahepatic biliary radicals. The displacement of major biliary radicals around a space-occupying lesion is suggestive of the diagnosis.

Treatment and Prognosis

Treatment is based on appropriate antibacterial therapy combined with drainage. Since approximately two thirds of infections are due to gramnegative enteric bacteria, broad-spectrum coverage is indicated. An appropriate aminoglycocide or cephalosporin, used in conjunction with an antianaerobic agent, such as clindamycin or metronidazole, generally will provide coverage. Once the abscess itself has been cultured by aspiration or drainage, the appropriate bactericidal agent can be defined.

Drainage is indicated for solitary, large abscesses, or for large, multiple abscesses. If there is no specific need for laparotomy in order to define underlying pathology or to direct efforts at another lesion, drainage can be accomplished by ultrasonographically or computer tomographically controlled insertion of a large percutaneous pigtail catheter. Mandel and associates,

based on a cumulative experience of 252 patients managed by these techniques, reported an 83 percent success rate, with a minimal incidence of complications. Under ultrasonographic or CT control, the liver is punctured with a Chiba needle to confirm the lesion and to localize it better by introducing a small amount of contrast material. Once the lesion has been localized and visualized, it is directly punctured with an 18-gauge sheathed needle. A guidewire is introduced into the abscess cavity, and the sheath is removed. Over this wire a drainage catheter, consisting of a multiple side hole ring catheter, measuring No. 8 or 9 French, or for smaller abscesses, a No. 7 French catheter with six side holes is inserted. The catheter is left to gravity drainage (Fig. 63–3).

If an operative approach is required for drainage, this can be facilitated by localization of the lesion preoperatively. Posterior lesions in the right lobe of the liver are best approached via rib resection. Transpleural drainage is advocated for high-lying posterior lesions. The anterior approach of Clairmont and Meyer is used for more anteriorly situated lesions. It is now felt that there is no increase in morbidity and mortality associated with transperitoneal drainage. Laparotomy provides excellent exposure for suitable drainage. In selected cases (see Fig. 63–4), hepatic lobectomy has been performed.

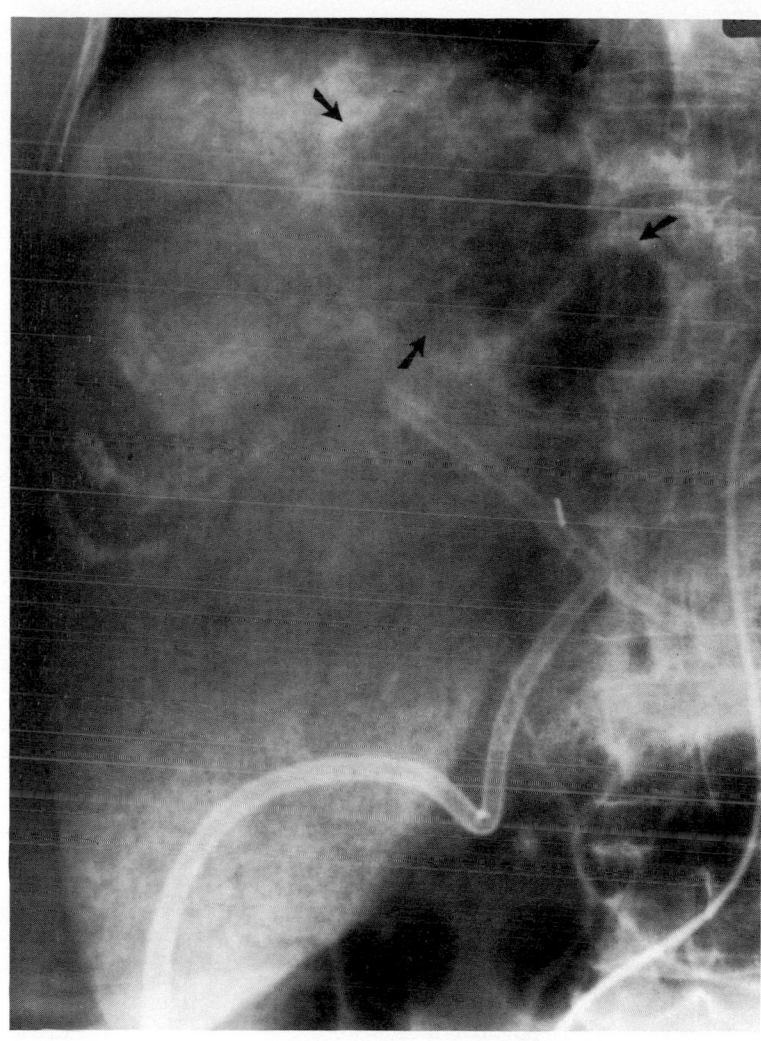

Figure 63–2. Capillary phase of angiogram demonstrating a loculated, lucent lesion with a hyperemic peripheral rim (*arrows*). (*Source: From Gutierrez OH, Schwartz SI: Atlas of Hepatic Tumors and Focal Lesions. New York: McGraw-Hill, 1984, p 122, with permission.*)

Prognosis and Complications

Ochsner and associates reported a fatality rate of 95 percent with multiple abscesses, compared to 37.5 percent for solitary liver abscesses in the preantibiotic state. The mortality rate for multiple hepatic abscesses remains high, ranging from 61 to 100 percent in several series. Higher mortality rates are reported for patients over the age of 50, and in patients with generalized debility and hepatic dysfunction. By contrast, mortality rates of 10 to 20 percent are reported for patients with solitary abscesses.

Complications frequently associated with hepatic abscess include extension of the suppurative process into the pleural space or into the lung itself, rupture of the hepatic abscess into the peritoneal cavity and development of subphrenic abscess.

AMEBIC ABSCESS

Incidence

Endamoeba histolytica, the pathogen responsible for the formation of an amebic abscess, has been found wherever coprologic surveys have been made on the human population—from Saskatchewan, Canada (North 52° 30′) to the Strait of Magellan (South 52°). Amebiasis affects 15 to 30 percent of the population of Mexico. Craig and Faust indicated that at least 10 percent of

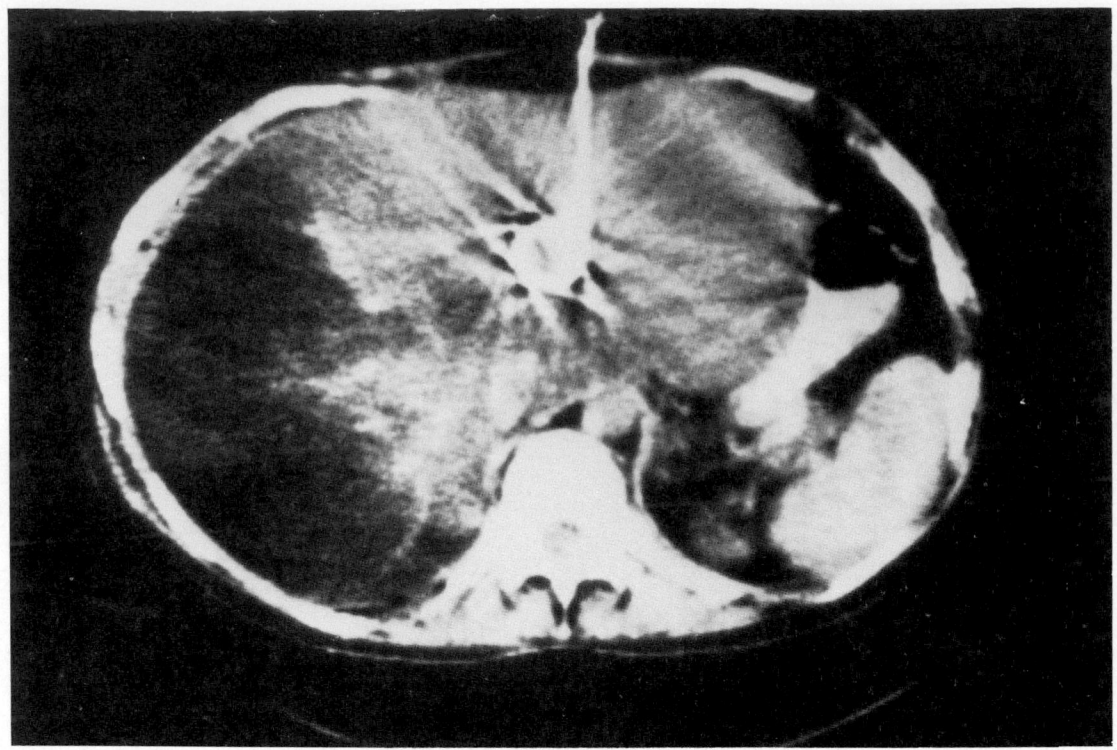

Figure 63–3. Abscess drained extrasonographically with pigtail catheter. (*Source: From Schwartz SI: Liver, in Schwartz SI, et al (eds): Principles of Surgery, 4 edt. New York: McGraw-Hill, 1984, p 1266, with permission.*)

the population of the United States was affected by this parasite.

The incidence of amebic involvement of the liver is more difficult to assess. In autopsy cases, an average of 3.6 percent has been reported for some regions. Amebic abscess of the liver is a disease of the middle-aged adult; the greatest number of cases occurs in the third, fourth, and fifth decades. The disease predominates in the male sex, with a ratio of 9:1 reported.

Pathogenesis and Pathology

In 1883, Koch initially demonstrated amebas in the capillaries and tissues adjoining the wall of the liver abscess. In 1887, *E. histolytica* was first recovered from the wall of an hepatic abscess by Kartulis.

The liver is involved secondarily to a primary disease of the intestine, with the amebas reaching the liver by way of the portal venous system, from a focus of ulceration in the bowel wall. Most amebas become engulfed in a small, interlobular vein of the liver, and undergo de-

generation. Some escape, however, through the walls of the smaller radicals of the portal venous system and invade the connective tissue of the portal triads, where they produce small areas of liquefaction and necrosis. The destructive process extends concentrically by invasion of amebas along open veins, coalescence of small, multiple lesions, and infarction due to thrombosis of contiguous radicals. This results in the typical large, single abscess.

Amebas are the only organisms apart from pyogenic microorganisms capable of producing pus in tissues. The purulent material that has the appearance of anchovy paste contains crenated and noncrenated red blood cells as well as white blood cells. Amebas can be demonstrated in the contents of hepatic abscesses in fewer than one third of cases.

Amebic abscesses are usually spherical lesions with a wall that is only a few millimeters thick and consists of granulation tissue. There is little or no fibrosis and three zones are recognized microscopically: (1) a necrotic center, (2) a middle zone with destruction of parenchymal

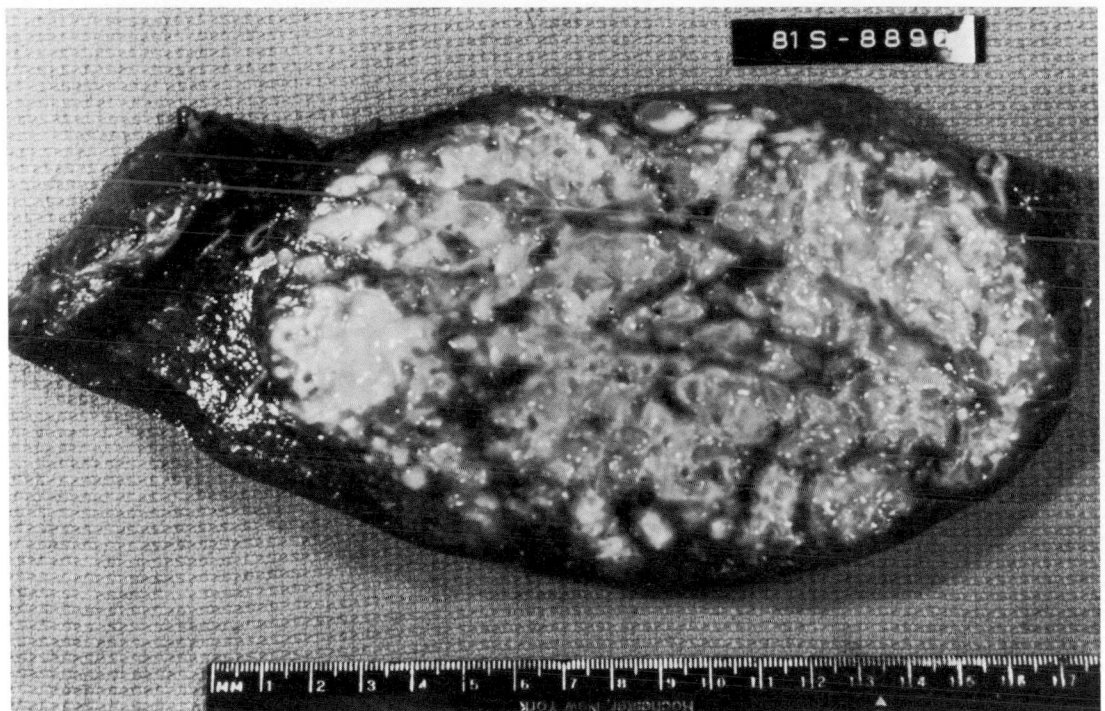

Figure 63–4. The specimen weighed 1950 g; the majority of the specimen was a large, yellow-ish-green tumor that replaced the parenchyma. Within the tumor were multilocular spaces and thick yellowish-green fluid. A normal hepatic parenchyma was present at the edge of the resection. Multiple sections were examined and no evidence of neoplasm was found. There was extensive necrosis and fibrosis associated with the process, and the lesion was diagnosed as a multilocular hepatic abscess. The initial hepatic culture had no aerobic and anaerobic growth. One week later the drainage grew coagulase-negative *Staphylococcus* and diphtheroids. (*Source: From Gutierrez OH, Schwartz SI: Atlas of Hepatic Tumors and Focal Lesions. New York: McGraw-Hill, 1984, p 127, with permission.*)

cells but with some persistence of stroma, and (3) relatively normal tissue in which amoebas may be demonstrated (Fig. 63–5). Amebic abscesses are usually sterile when cultured for bacteria, but they may become secondarily affected, at which time the pyogenic process dominates. The abscess material is then more purulent, and has a dirty yellow appearance. Although the location and number of amebic abscesses vary, they are usually single, and occur in the right lobe of the liver either near the dome or in the inferior surface in juxtaposition to the hepatic flexure of the colon.

Clinical Manifestations

The onset of symptoms of hepatic abscess may be sudden or gradual, and the chief complaints are pain and fever. Pain in the region of the liver is by far the most common symptom in patients with hepatic abscess; it was present in 88 percent of patients in the DeBakey and Ochsner series. It is usually described as a constant ache, or an intermittently sharp pain, and typically is only of moderate severity and is aggravated by motion, inspiration, or coughing. The pain pattern depends on the location of the hepatic abscess. An abscess located in the portion of the liver below the right lower chest wall is accompanied by pain and tenderness over the right lower intercostal spaces. There may be associated bulging of these inner spaces, and pitting edema of the subcutaneous tissue. Right lobe abscesses that are present in the superior surface of the liver, and lie immediately below the diaphragm result in pain referred to the right shoulder. Abscesses presenting in the bare area of the liver have no contact with the serosal surface, and are latent as far as pain is con-

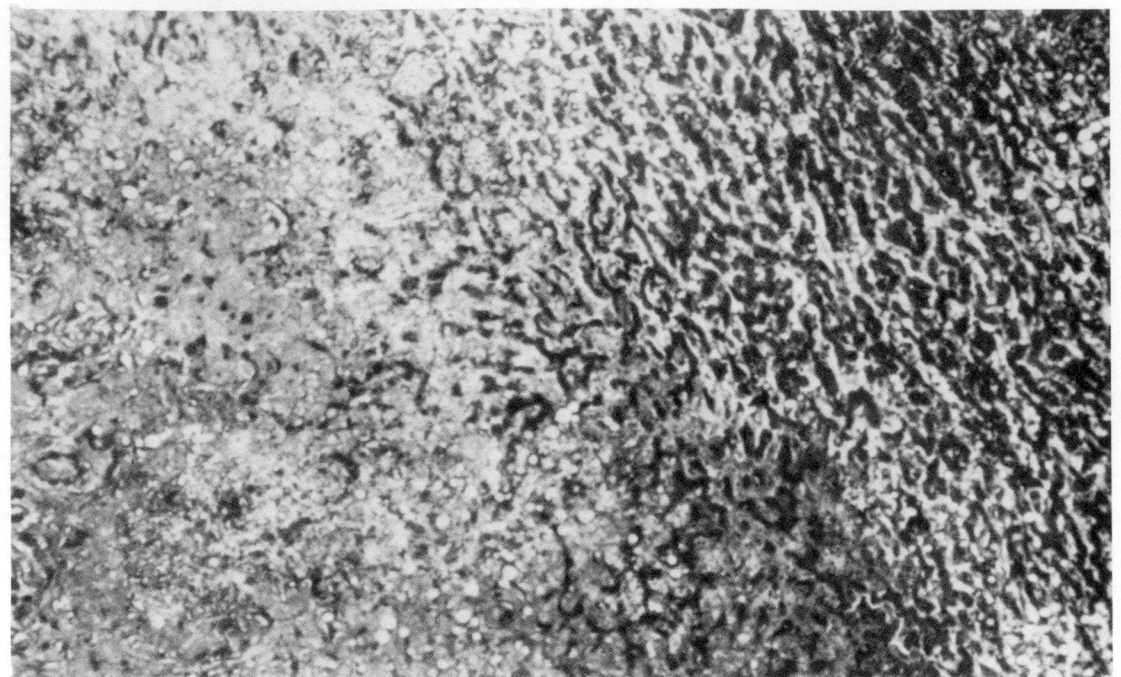

Figure 63–5 Microscopic pathology of amebic abscess of liver. Note central necrosis and inflammatory cells interspaced between liver chords peripherally. (*Source: From Schwartz SI: Hepatic Abscess, in Surgical Diseases of the Liver. New York: McGraw-Hill, 1964, p 153, with permission.*)

cerned. Left lobe abscesses are responsible for painful epigastric swelling.

Fever accompanied by chills and sweating is present in about two thirds of patients, and is frequently of a low-grade, intermittent type, spiking toward nightfall and not returning to normal. Weakness and weight loss occur in over half the patients. Nausea and vomiting are uncommon. One third of the patients give a history of antecedent diarrhea.

The protean manifestations of amebic abscesses often resemble an acute surgical abdomen, mimicking acute cholecystitis and acute appendicitis.

Hepatomegaly is present in one half to three quarters of the patients and is usually accompanied by tenderness in the area. With an abscess of the left lobe of the liver, a tender epigastric swelling, that moves with respiration, may be noted. Right lobe abscesses located on the anterior surface below the chest wall may simulate hydrops or empyema of the gallbladder. Patients with amebic abscesses of the liver may appear acutely or moderately ill. Jaundice

is an uncommon finding, noted in 0 to 14 percent of cases in several series.

Diagnostic Studies

The hematologic findings are related to the duration of the disease. Patients with short histories tend to show no anemia, but appreciable leukocytosis; those with prolonged illness have anemia and less marked leukocytosis. Leukocytosis is typically less pronounced than that associated with a pyogenic abscess. An extremely high white cell count and marked shift to the left is suggestive of a secondary bacterial infection, but differentiation between amebic and pyogenic hepatic abscesses is not possible on the basis of the leukocyte count alone.

In general, examination of the stool does not offer a high diagnostic yield, and trophozoites have been reported in 15 to 30 percent of cases. Liver function tests are not diagnostic, and an elevation of the transaminase level and the alkaline phosphatase levels of a moderate degree occur in over half the patients. Serologic

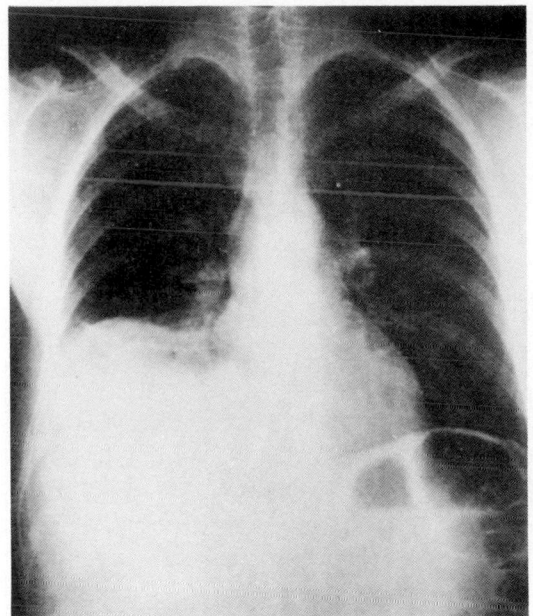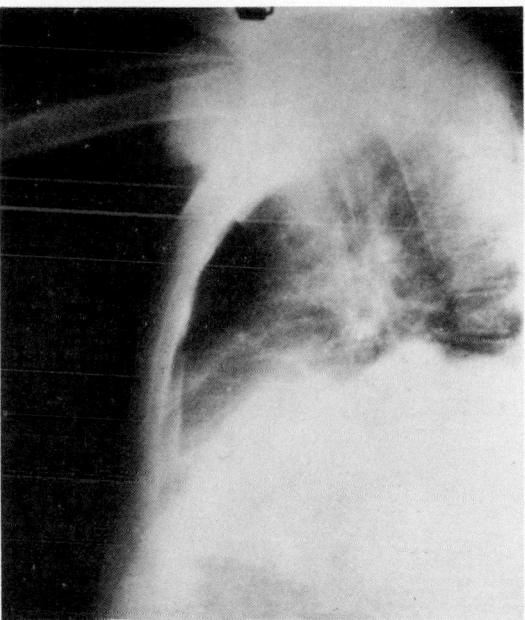

Figure 63–6. X-ray of patient with amebic abscess of right lobe of liver. *Left:* Posteroanterior view; note obliteration of cardiophrenic angle and medial elevation of diaphragm. *Right:* Lateral view; note obliteration of anterior costophrenic angles and anterior elevation of diaphragm. (*Source: From Schwartz SI, in Surgical Diseases of the Liver. New York: McGraw-Hill, 1964, p 156, with permission.*)

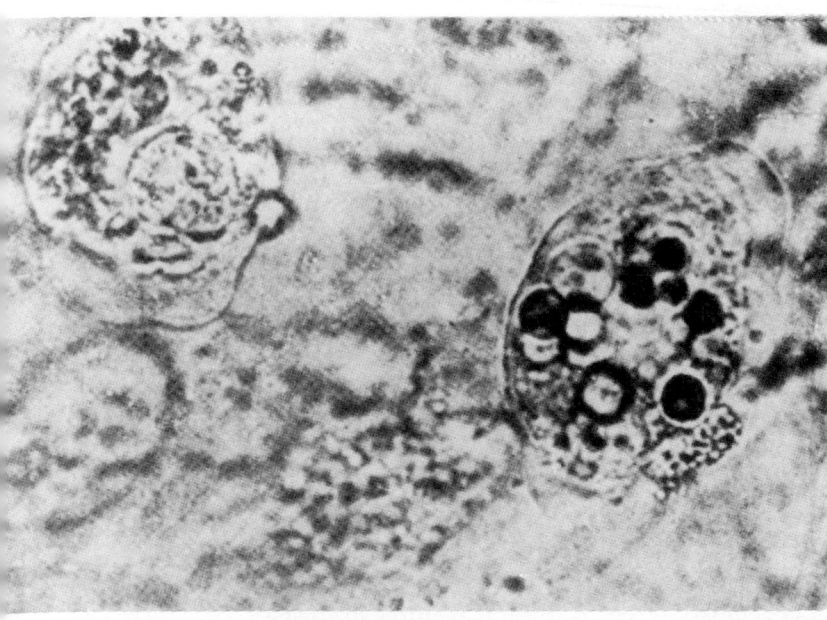

Figure 63–7. *Endamoeba histolytica* trophozoites. Note ingested red blood cells. (*Source: From Schwartz SI, in Surgical Diseases of the Liver. New York: McGraw-Hill, 1964, p 158, with permission.*)

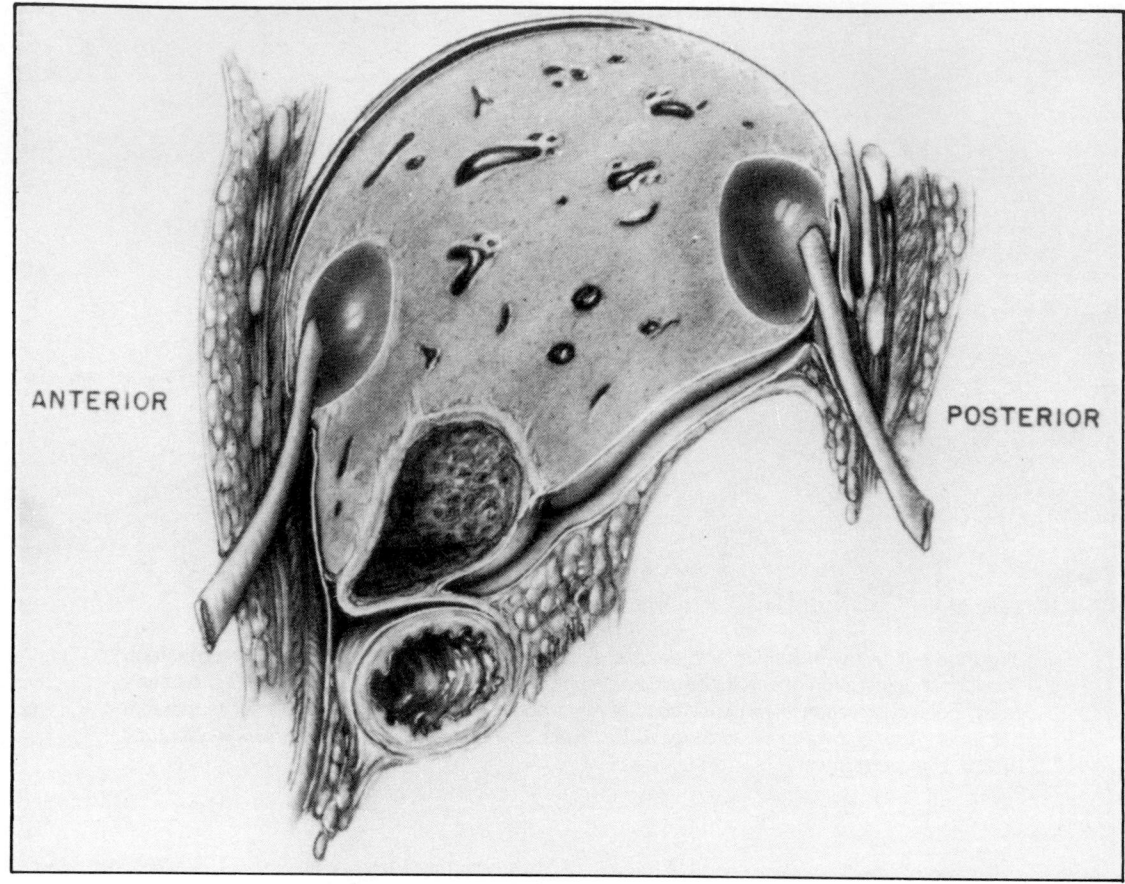

ANTERIOR

POSTERIOR

Figure 63–8. Extraserous drainage. Extraperitoneal drainage of anterior and posterior abscesses is demonstrated. (*Source: From Schwartz SI, in Surgical Diseases of the Liver. New York: McGraw-Hill, 1964, p 161, with permission.*)

testing for amebiasis either by hemagglutination or gel-diffusion precipation was positive in all patients studied by Abuabara and associates.

The radiologic findings are similar to those reported for pyogenic abscess. The classic findings on plane x-ray are: (1) obliteration of the right cardiophrenic angle on the anterior-posterior film, and (2) obliteration of the anterocostal angle on the lateral film (Fig. 63–6). The latter finding is in contrast to the subphrenic abscess in which the posterior cardiophrenic angle is obliterated. Characteristically a single abscess located near the dome of the liver in the posterior superior region or the inferior surface near the hepatic flexure of the colon is defined.

Needle Aspiration. This is infrequently required as a diagnostic test since, if the patient is thought to have an amebic abscess, therapy

is initiated and the size of the lesion is followed by one of the diagnostic studies. If a diagnostic aspiration is performed with proper precaution and a sterile technique, it is a relatively inocuous procedure. The "chocolate sauce," "anchovy paste" aspirate is considered pathognomonic of an amebic abscess. In about one third of cases, however, the abscess content is creamy white even though there is no secondary bacterial infection. Amebic trophozoites are demonstrated in the aspirate of fewer than one third of patients (Fig. 63–7). Direct smears and cultures should be performed to rule out secondary bacterial infection, which influences the therapy because it requires drainage.

Treatment

The majority of patients can be managed with medical treatment alone, using metronidazole,

750 mg orally three times a day for 10 to 14 days. This has replaced emetine as the drug of choice for hepatic amebiasis since emetine is known to have toxic effects and to require a subcutaneous or intramuscular route. Chloroquine phosphate has proved effective in the treatment of hepatic amebiasis, either alone or in combination with emetine. The recommended dose is 0.9 g daily for 10 days, followed by 0.6 g daily for 20 days, resulting in a total dose of 21 g during a 30-day period.

Ultrasonographically directed drainage is required infrequently, and surgical drainage is now reserved for those patients with secondary pyogenic infection who did not improve with the previously described techniques.

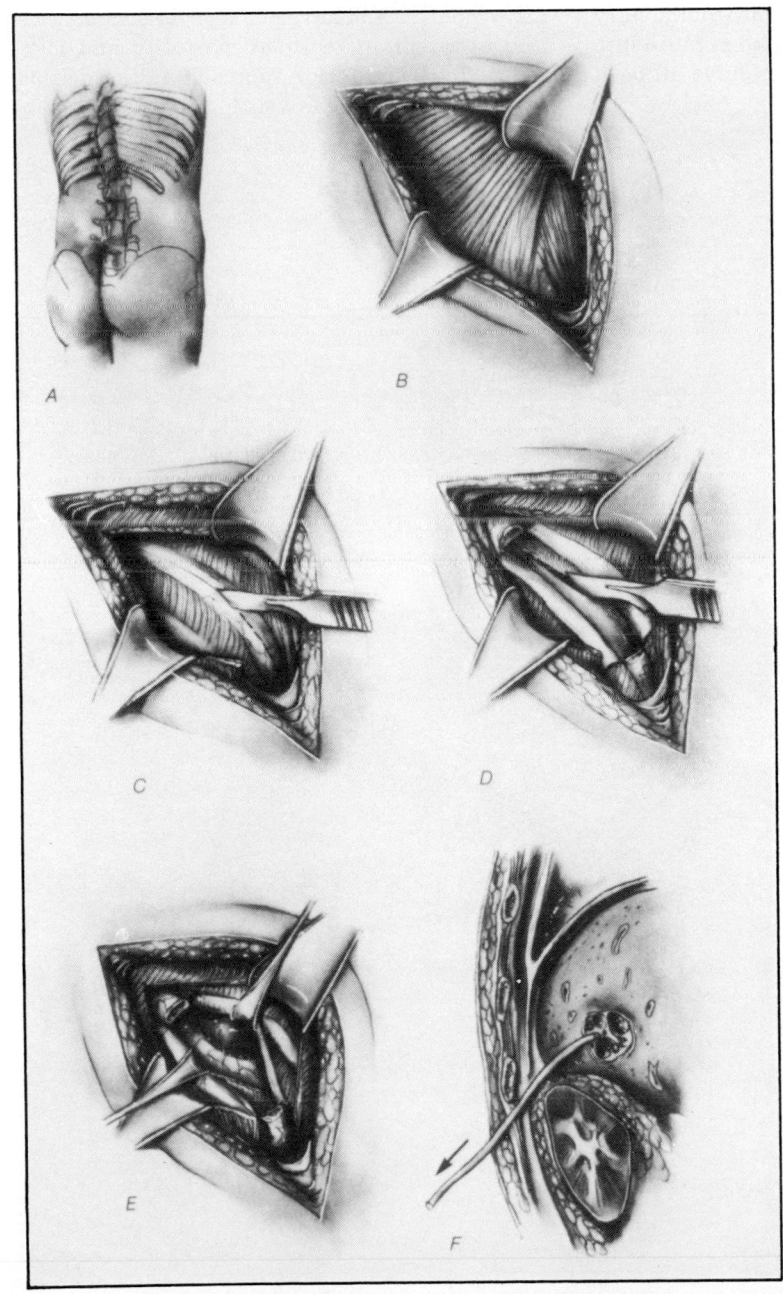

Figure 63–9. Extraserous transthoracic drainage. **A.** Incision is made posteriorly over right twelfth rib. **B.** Latissimus dorsi muscle exposed. **C.** Periosteum of twelfth rib incised. **D.** Twelfth rib removed subperiosteally and bed incised. **E.** Diaphragm is detached and peritoneum is reflected from the inferior surface of diaphragm. **F.** Schematic drawing of position of drain. (*Source: From Schwartz SI: Liver, in Schwartz SI, et al (eds): Principles of Surgery, 4 edt. New York: McGraw-Hill, 1984, p 1267, with permission.*)

Prognosis and Complications

A mortality rate of 5 percent or less is now reported, and a graver prognosis is generally associated with multiple lesions. The presence of complications significantly increases the mortality rate. The most common complication is a secondary infection of the amebic abscess, with pyogenic organisms occurring in approximately 10 percent of patients. Rupture of an amebic abscess accounts for the next most common group of complications. Intrapulmonary rupture, intrapleural rupture, and rupture into the pericardium and peritoneum have all been recorded.

SURGICAL DRAINAGE OF HEPATIC ABSCESSES

In the past drainage through an extraserous approach (Fig. 63–8) was strongly favored. The formation of extensive adhesions frequently permits extraserous drainage of amebic abscesses located anteriorly or posteriorly. With the advent of antibiotics, transperitoneal and transpleural drainage, combined with specific antibiotic therapy, are the techniques usually employed and have not been associated with any apparent increase in mortality and morbidity. In the posterior approach a skin incision is made over the twelfth rib and a sub-

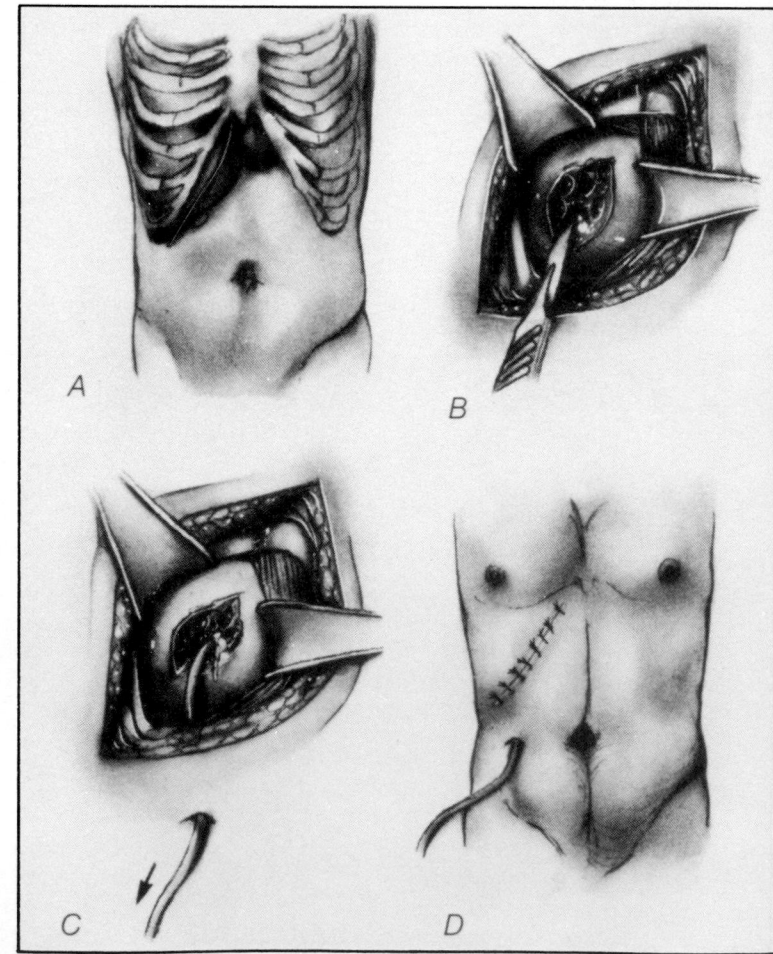

Figure 63–10. Transabdominal drainage. **A.** Subcostal incision. **B.** Peritoneum has been entered and abscess incised. **C.** Drain is positioned in abscess and brought out through the stab wound. **D.** Closure of wound and position of stab wound. (*Source: From Schwartz SI: Liver, in Schwartz SI, et al (eds): Principles of Surgery, 4 edt. New York: McGraw-Hill, 1984, p 1268, with permission.*)

periosteal resection of that rib is carried out. A transverse incision is made through the bed of the twelfth rib at the level of the spinous process of the first lumbar vertebra. Access to the retroperitoneal space, located between the upper pole of the kidney and the inferior surface of the liver is obtained. The parietal peritoneum is mobilized from beneath the diaphragm, and the abscess can then be drained without contamination of the peritoneal cavity (Fig. 63–9).

Transabdominal Approach (*Fig. 63–10*)

Transperitoneal exploration has the advantage of permitting thorough exploration of the abdomen and the liver to rule out multiple abscesses. A right subcostal incision is made through the anterior rectus sheath and the external oblique muscles are divided. The rectus muscle is transected or retracted medially and the posterior rectus sheath and internal oblique muscles are divided. The peritoneal cavity is entered and the abdomen is explored to define the point of fluctuation. Needle aspiration may be required to determine the location of deeply seated lesions. The liver is then incised at an appropriate place. A drain is positioned in the abscess and brought out through a stab wound, following which the major incision is closed.

BIBLIOGRAPHY

Abuabara SF, Barrett JA, et al: Amebic liver abscess. Arch Surg 117:239, 1982

Balasegaram M: Management of hepatic abscess. Curr Probl Surg 18:283, 1981

Basile JA, Klein SR, et al: Amebic liver abscess. Am J Surg 146:67, 1983

Brodine WN, Schwartz SI: Pyogenic hepatic abscesses. NY State J Med 73:1657, 1973

Craig CF, Faust EC: Clinical Parasitology, 3 edt. Philadelphia: Lea & Febiger, 1943, p 43

DeBakey M, Ochsner A: Collective review. Hepatic amebiasis. A 20 year experience and analysis of 263 cases. Int Abstr Surg 92:209, 1951

Mandel SR, Boyd D: Drainage of hepatic, intraabdominal, and mediastinal abscesses guided by computerized axial tomography. Am J Surg 145:120, 1893

McDonald AP, Howard RJ: Pyogenic liver abscess. World J Surg 4:369, 1980

Ochsner A, DeBakey M, et al: Pyogenic abscess of the liver: An analysis of 47 cases with review of the literature. Am J Surg 40:292, 1938

Pitt HA, Zuidema GD: Factors influencing mortality in the treatment of pyogenic hepatic abscesses. Surg Gynecol Obstet 140:228, 1975

Rothman DL, Schwartz SI, et al: Diagnostic laparotomy for fever or abdominal pain of unknown origin. Am J Surg 133:273, 1977

Rubin RH, Swartz MN, et al: Hepatic abscesses: Changes in clinical bacteriologic and therapeutic aspects. Am J Med 57:601, 1974

Sabbaj J, Sutter VL, et al: Anaerobic pyogenic liver abscesses. Ann Intern Med 77:629, 1972

64. Hyatid Disease

Gabriel A. Kune

It is clear that human cystic hydatid disease was already known to Hippocrates and Galen and that the parasitic nature of this disease was strongly suspected in the 17th century. However, it was only during the present century that significant advances were made in accurate diagnosis and in effective treatment of hydatid disease in the human. After World War II, enormous advances were achieved in surgical techniques and organ imaging techniques, as well as in immunologic diagnosis, so that the stage has been reached when both the diagnosis and treatment of human hydatid disease is at a most effective and sophisticated level. During the past 50 years an increasing understanding of the surgical pathology of human hydatid disease and innovative developments in surgical technique have resulted in a very marked decrease in the mortality of human hydatid disease and, even more importantly, a very significant decrease in the morbidity that, in the past, often followed surgery for hydatid disease.

There are two forms of human hydatid disease:

1. *Echinococcus granulosus,* which causes cystic hydatid disease; this form is discussed principally in this chapter.
2. *Echinococcus alveolaris,* or *multilocularis,* a much rarer form in the human; the pathology, diagnosis, and treatment of this rare form are discussed separately at the end of this chapter.

ECHINOCOCCUS GRANULOSUS

Life Cycle of Parasite

Echinococcus granulosus (*Taenia echinococcus*) has a well-established life cycle, which is shown in a diagrammatic form in Figure 64–1. The ova, which are ingested by the human from the faeces of the tapeworm-infected dog, reach the stomach, where they hatch, then penetrate the wall of the intestine and pass to the liver through a portal vein radicle. Some are destroyed in the liver, others develop there into a hydatid cyst, and still others pass on through the hepatic veins into the lungs. Those that reach the lungs may lodge there and develop as hydatid cysts; others pass through the lung and into the systemic circulation to develop as hydatid cysts anywhere else in the body. In any of these sites, the development of these cysts in the human is very slow, but appears to be variable in its rate, possibly related to the immunologic interplay between the human and the hydatid parasite. It is emphasised that in the human, within the abdominal cavity, extrahepatic hydatids can also develop following either extrusion from the liver of a hydatid cyst or rupture of a hydatid cyst through the liver capsule and dissemination within the abdominal cavity either spontaneously or more commonly during hepatic hydatid cyst surgery.

Prevention

Hydatid disease caused by *Echinococcus granulosus* (*Taenia echinococcus*) is still quite prevalent in Greece, Yugoslavia, Australia, and the Middle East, as well as in South American countries, all countries in which sheep breeding is important and where farmers, sheep, and dogs come into close contact.

In order to interrupt the life cycle of the hydatid parasite, the effective disposal of infested sheep offal is the absolute prime target of prevention of this disease in the human. The most important targets of a preventive pro-

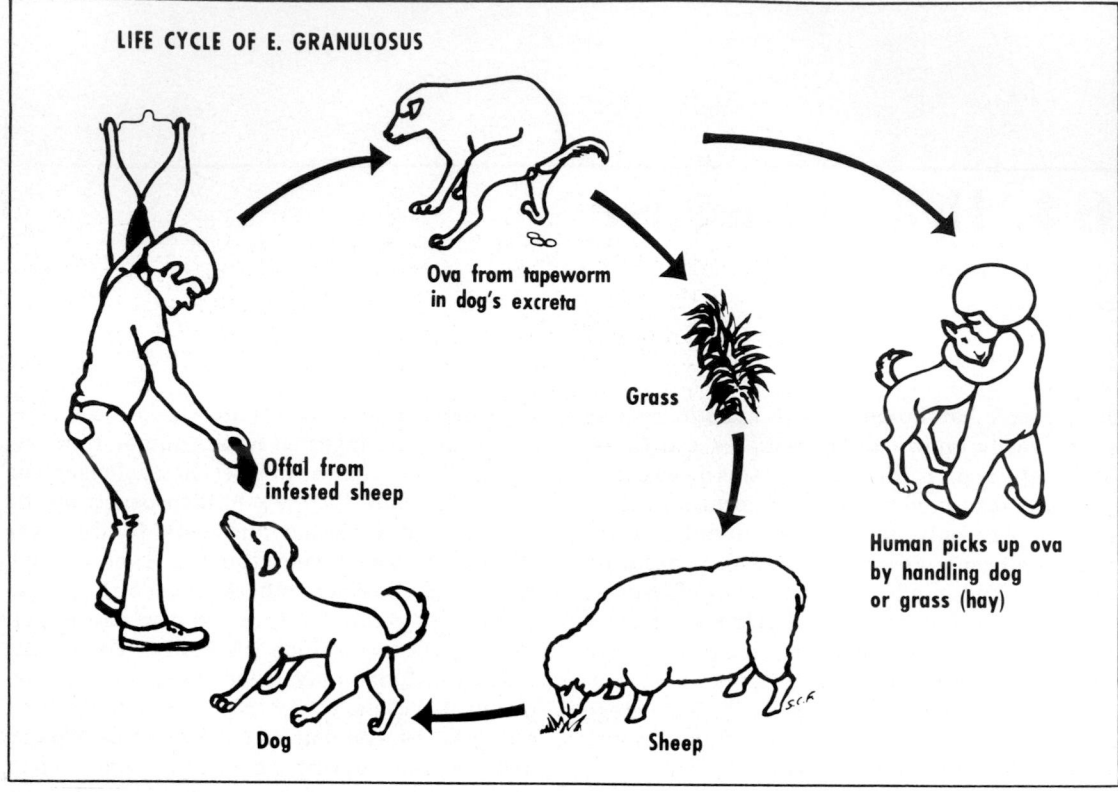

LIFE CYCLE OF E. GRANULOSUS

Ova from tapeworm
in dog's excreta

Grass

Offal from
infested sheep

Human picks up ova
by handling dog
or grass (hay)

Dog

Sheep

Figure 64–1. Life cycle of *Echinococcus granulosus* parasite. (*Source: From Kune GA, Sali A: The Practice of Biliary Surgery, 2 edt. Oxford: Blackwell, 1980, with permission.*)

gramme are the slaughterers of sheep, who feed the offal to the rural dogs, who then in turn transmit the hydatid ova to the human. A secondary and less important measure in prevention is the uniform and regular use of antihelminthic agents, such as praziquantel, administered to rural dogs.

Preventive measures have been extremely effective in the State of Tasmania in Australia, as well as in New Zealand, with a dramatic decrease in the incidence of new cases of human hydatids. Although it may hurt the national pride of those countries in which human hydatid disease is still prevalent, it is clear that relatively simple sanitary measures, combined with public health and educational programmes directed to those dealing with sheep rearing and sheep slaughtering, are the most effective means of dramatically decreasing, if not completely eliminating, human hydatid disease.

Pathology

A review of large collected series of abdominal hydatid cysts indicate that about two thirds of all hydatid cysts in man occur in the liver. In three quarters of cases of liver hydatids, the cyst is solitary and in one quarter there is more than one cyst in the liver.

Hydatid cysts outside the liver but within the peritoneal cavity are uncommon but they have been described in the spleen, in the pancreas, and in the ovaries, as well as disseminated within the abdominal or pelvic cavities: in these latter cases, when found within the abdominal cavity or in the pelvis, they are thought to be derived from a liver hydatid cyst, either by extrusion or by rupture of the liver hydatid.

If hydatid cysts are found outside the liver, it is always a good policy to suspect that hydatids are also present in the liver.

The rate of growth of liver hydatids appears to be dependent not only on the immunologic relationship between parasite and human, as mentioned before, but also on the resistance offered by the enveloping structures, for example, cysts near the surface of the liver, especially in the left lobe, appear to grow more rapidly than centrally located cysts. Similarly, cysts within the peritoneal cavity appear to grow much faster than liver cysts. As a very crude estimate, liver cysts increase their diameter by about 2 or 3 cm each year.

Liver Cysts

Liver cysts are classified as primary cysts, as secondary (also called multivesicular) cysts, or as cysts of secondary implantation.

Primary Cysts. In the liver, these are single cysts within a host capsule consisting of compressed liver tissue as well as scar tissue produced by the human. It is emphasised that this is a reaction to the presence of the parasite and is host tissue: this has an important bearing on the surgical treatment of human hydatids as will be noted later. The actual parasite consists of an outer laminated membrane, lined internally by the growing germinal cells that, with growth and development, give rise to brood capsules, each of which contains a number of protoscolices. Each of these protoscolices resembles a tapeworm's head and can develop in the dog's intestine into a fully grown hydatid tapeworm. Some of these, with growth, round off and drop off into the fluid of the hydatid; should the fluid disseminate elsewhere in the host, such as by rupture, new cysts can develop from these brood capsules.

Multivesicular or Secondary Cysts. Should the primary cyst in the liver rupture, the pieces of the germinal epithelium may also rupture to form daughter cysts, each of which in every respect is similar to the primary cyst, except that it does not have its own host capsule if it remains within the original host capsule of the liver. Similarly, the scolices can develop into cysts within this cavity. Such a collection of daughter cysts is referred to as a multivesicular or secondary cyst. Following rupture, there is an inflammatory reaction resulting in thickening and often in calcification of the host capsule: if there is a biliary communication already pres-

ent, then some of the contents of this secondary cyst becomes bile stained.

Secondary Abdominal Implantation. When a hydatid cyst spills into the adjacent cavities, the pieces of laminated membrane or the protoscolices may become secondarily implanted and may grow to form univesicular cysts that will eventually develop fibrous tissue host capsules that in some cases are also lined by adjacent organs, such as the bowel or the bladder. It is important to know that spillage of living hydatid elements is not invariably followed by secondary implantation and growth, but because spillage is a serious risk during surgery of abdominal hydatids, special techniques have been developed to prevent this type of occurrence.

Natural History of Liver Hydatids

Liver hydatids usually continue to grow. After a number of years, which is variable in different patients, the onset of the complications that will now be described can be seen.

Development of Cyst–Biliary Communications. The surgical pathology of this complication, probably the most common that develops within a liver hydatid, has been well described by Fitzpatrick, whose concept of the development of cyst–biliary connections, a prelude to the cyst rupturing into the biliary ductal system, is shown in Figure 64–2.

As the cyst enlarges, it compresses and stretches bile ducts in its neighbourhood and erosions occur in these overstretched ducts, producing fistulae between the hydatid cyst and the ductal system. These fistulae can be demonstrated during the surgical removal of hydatid cysts, either with an operative cholangiogram or by direct vision after the cyst has been removed (Fig. 64–3). The closure of these biliary communications under vision has become an important part of the modern technique of surgery for liver hydatids.

Intrabiliary Rupture. This is probably the most common type of rupture one sees in long-standing hepatic hydatid cysts. Perhaps because of bile leaking into the primary cyst, rupture occurs and some of the germinal layer or the scolices can enter the ductal system and may cause obstructive jaundice. Almost always, the cause of obstructive jaundice and cholangitis,

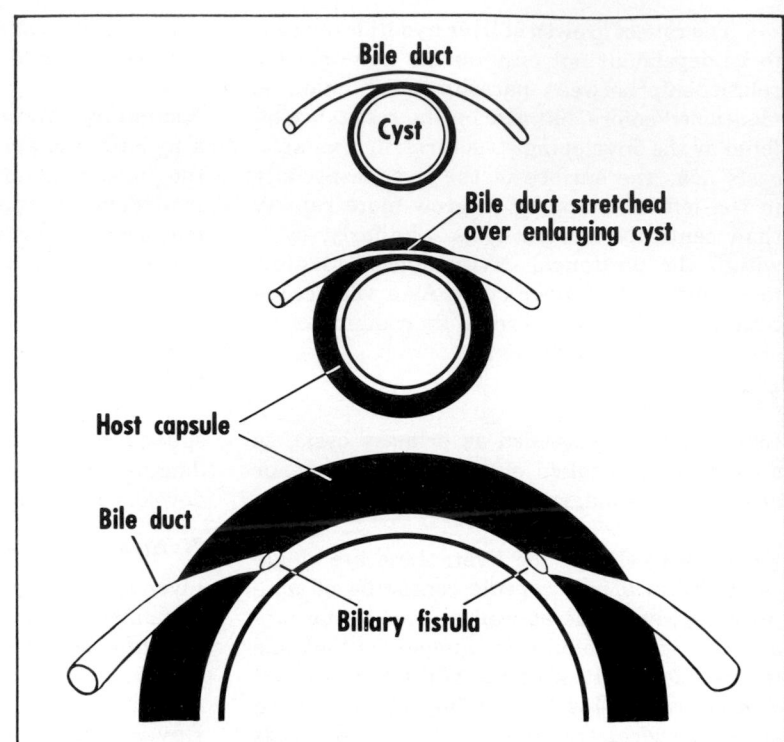

Bile duct

Cyst

Bile duct stretched
over enlarging cyst

Host capsule

Bile duct

Biliary fistula

Figure 64–2. The pathogenesis of cyst–biliary communications. (*Source: From Kune GA, Sali A: The Practice of Biliary Surgery, 2 edt. Oxford: Blackwell, 1980, with permission.*)

in the presence of a hepatic hydatid, is the intrabiliary rupture of hydatid elements. Only rarely is obstructive jaundice caused by extrinsic compression of the main bile ducts in the liver, in the porta hepatis, or in the pancreas (Fig. 64–4).

Intraabdominal Rupture. This usually results in secondary implantation, usually of a multivesicular cyst into the abdominal or pelvic cavity, and only rarely is there an actual extrusion of a univesicular primary cyst from the liver into the peritoneal cavity. Most, but certainly not all, cysts that rupture into the peritoneal cavity survive.

Intrathoracic Rupture. A cyst high under the right hemidiaphragm may erode through the diaphragm and rupture into the right pleural cavity with the development of a hydatid cyst in that area. This may further communicate with radicles of the main bronchi, which eventually may form a bronchial fistula and extrusion of hydatid elements through the bronchial tree (Borrie and Shaw, 1981). These intrathoracic complications will not be discussed any further;

rarely does a liver hydatid, after eroding the diaphragm, rupture into the pericardial space.

Infection of Hepatic Hydatid. Infection of a hepatic hydatid is an uncommon complication if the hydatid elements in themselves have not ruptured into the biliary ductal system. What was once taken to be pus in an infected hydatid cyst is now generally found to be merely very thick, bile-stained material containing white cells. It is sterile on culture, which usually means that bile ruptured into the hydatid, forming what appears to be an abscess within it. As will be noted later, it is important to distinguish between a true bacterial infection of a hydatid cyst and one that merely contains thick, bile-stained material, as the surgical treatment of the two is different.

Cyst Death. The frequency of complete death of a hepatic hydatid cyst is unknown and it is thought to occur when bile through a biliary cyst communication leaks into the cyst and destroys the germinal epithelium. When the cyst dies, the host capsule calcifies, as does the broken-up laminated membrane, so that the cyst

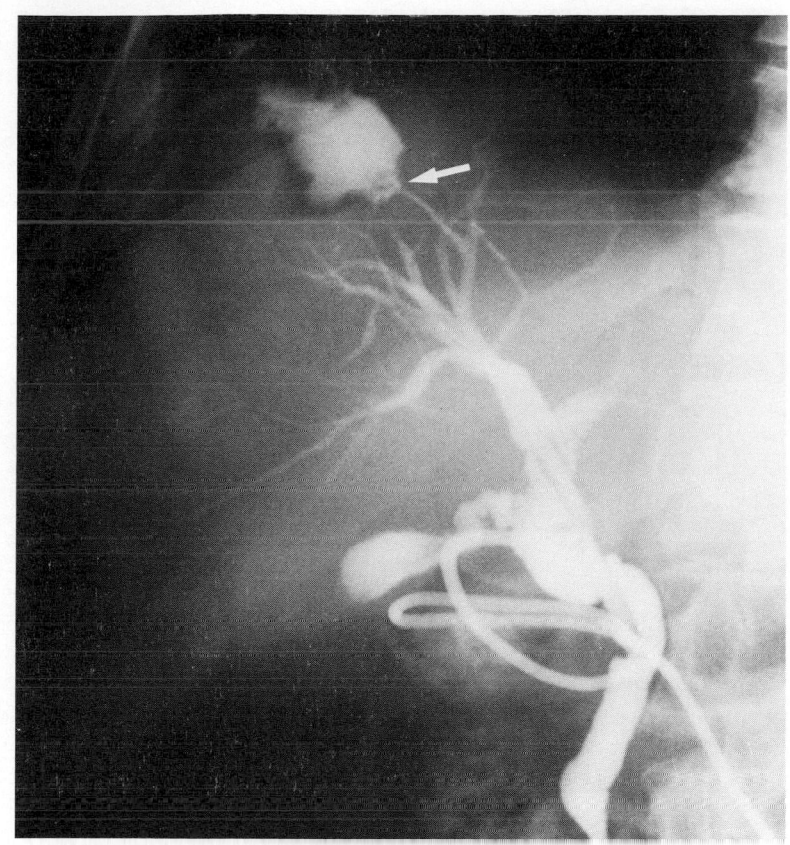

Figure 64–3. An operative T-tube cholangiogram showing a biliary–cyst cavity communication between a radicle of the right hepatic duct and a hydatid cyst cavity in the right lobe of the liver.

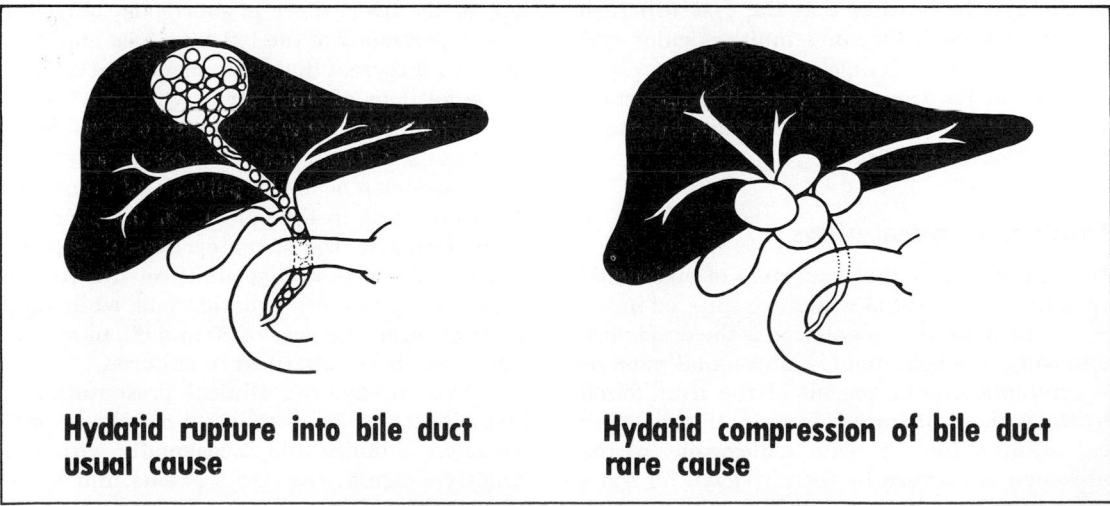

Hydatid rupture into bile duct usual cause

Hydatid compression of bile duct rare cause

Figure 64–4. The ways in which hydatids can cause obstructive jaundice. On the left is the usual cause, hydatid tissue entering the biliary ductal system. (*Source: From Kune GA, Sali A: The Practice of Biliary Surgery, 2 edt. Oxford: Blackwell, 1980, with permission.*)

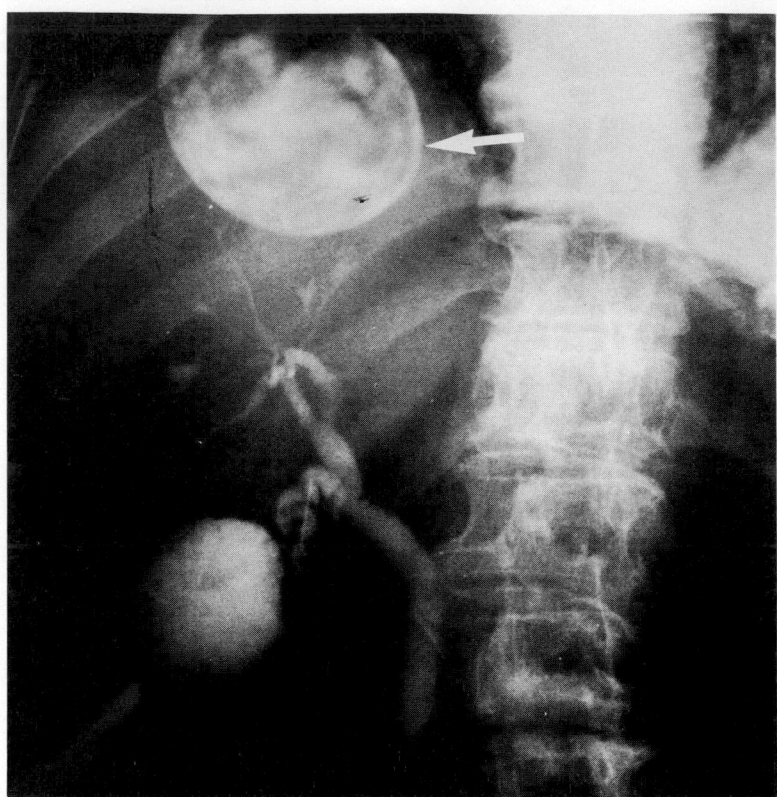

Figure 64–5. Plain radiograph of a dead hepatic hydatid found accidentally during an operative cholangiogram performed during cholecystectomy for gallstones. Note the thick calcified outline of the cyst as well as the crenated irregular calcified contents of the dead cyst.

shrinks and the calcification appears as a thick-walled irregular crenated outline (Fig. 64–5). It is emphasised that minimal peripheral calcification of the host capsule does *not* mean death of the cyst but rather that the cyst will turn out to be a secondary or a multivesicular cyst (Fig. 64–6). If the clinician is in doubt about whether or not the cyst is dead, it is important to go ahead and perform immunologic investigations (described later).

Clinical Manifestations

In approximately three quarters of abdominal hydatid cases, most of which are situated in the liver, the mode of presentation is the accidental discovery of a symptomless abdominal mass or a symtomless enlargement of the liver found by the patient during self-examination, by clinical examination, by plain radiography of the abdomen performed by the physician for some other incidental problem, or during laparotomy performed for some other illness, such as gallstones. A cyst in the left lobe of the liver tends to present in front of the stomach and colon and appears as a mobile mass that moves on respiration into the upper and central abdomen. Sometimes when the hydatid cyst is in the right lobe of the liver, there is enormous compensatory hypertrophy of the left liver lobe and clinically an incorrect diagnosis made of a tumour of the left lobe of the liver.

In the presence of secondary peritoneal hydatid cysts, a lump may be present anywhere in the abdomen or in the pelvis, and eventually turns out to be in the spleen, in the pancreas, in the ovary or free in the peritoneal or pelvic cavities. There is no age limit on the clinical presentation of these hydatid cysts; while most occur between the ages of 20 and 60, numerous cases have been described in children.

Occasionally, the clinical presentation is that of biliary colic, usually but not always with transient jaundice and occasionally with cholangitis as signified by rigors, sweats, and fevers. Intraperitoneal rupture of a hydatid is an uncommon mode of presentation: in these cases, patients have features of an acute abdomen and,

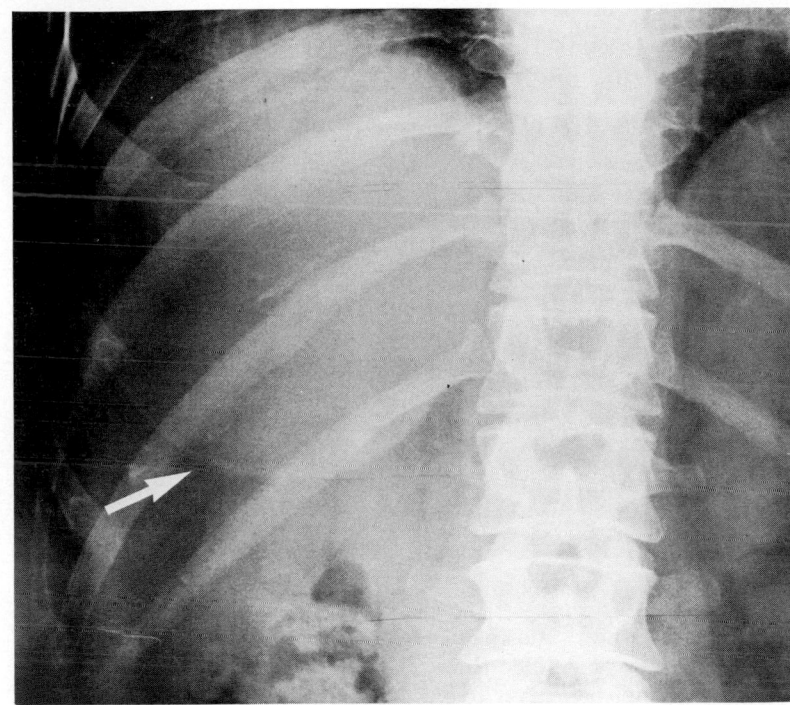

Figure 64–6. Plain radiograph of the abdomen showing a calcified ring in the liver area indicating the presence of a hydatid. Calcification of this kind does *not* indicate a dead cyst.

in some instances, major or minor signs of anaphylactic shock with severe hypovolaemia or minor signs of anaphylaxis with the presence of urticaria. This author has had three patients presenting with an acute abdomen subsequent to an automobile accident while wearing seat belts. At surgery the acute abdominal condition was found to be due to a partial rupture and compression type of seat belt injury to the liver, which was the site of a large hydatid cyst. Rarely, the acute abdominal condition associated with jaundice and high serum amylase is due to a hydatid cyst rupturing into the bile ducts, causing jaundice and cholangitis and also responsible for severe, acute pancreatitis.

Thus, the common mode of presentation of liver hydatids is a palpable mass in the abdomen, which is usually the liver, and less frequently, it is an enlarged liver with a palpable mass within it.

Because of these modes of clinical presentation of abdominal hydatid disease, organ imaging techniques are now used after clinical presentation: only after these have been done does one proceed with immunologic diagnosis. It is therefore rational to describe the diagnostic techniques in that order.

Diagnostic Studies

Imaging Techniques

For many years, it was known that a plain radiograph of the abdominal area showing calcification or a calcified ring in the liver zone was an important signal that a hydatid cyst was likely to be present in the liver (Fig. 64–6). As previously mentioned, a calcified ring of this nature does *not* mean that the hydatid cyst is dead. In the past decade, there have been dramatic advances in organ imaging diagnosis of intraabdominal hydatid disease, principally because of the advent of such effective techniques as radionuclide scanning, ultrasonography, and computed tomography (CT).

Radionuclide Scanning. Hydatid cysts of the liver will show up as filling defects on radionuclide scanning. A "dynamic" radionuclide scan, using agents such as technetium, will distinguish these filling defects from solid vascular masses such as malignant tumours of the liver (Fig. 64–7). A real problem with radionuclide scanning is that small cysts situated peripherally in the liver, especially in its left lobe, can

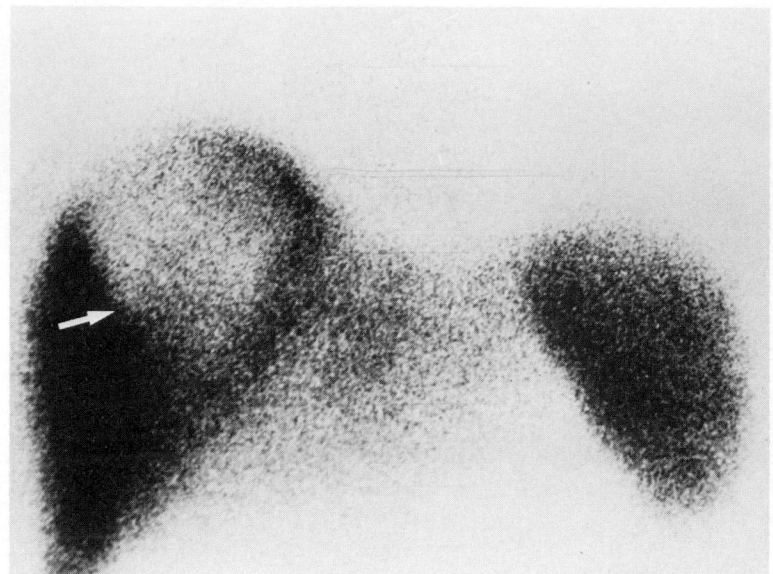

Figure 64-7. Radionuclide scan of the liver showing avascular filling defect caused by a large hydatid in the right lobe. (*Courtesy of Drs. B. Arkles and G. Gill, Melbourne.*)

be missed; also, accurate localisation within the liver, especially in the right lobe, is not always possible. For these reasons, ultrasonography and CT are used more and more frequently in abdominal organ imaging to detect the presence of hydatid disease.

Ultrasonography. Ultrasonography is best in detection of fluid collections, especially when these are situated in otherwise solid organs, and therefore liver hydatids are shown superbly by ultrasonography (Fig. 64-8 and 64-9). The presence of daughter cysts gives a pathognomonic ultrasound appearance, as may be seen in Figure 64-9.

Small cysts of the order of 2 cm in diameter or less, especially if they are peripherally located in the left lobe of the liver, can be missed by ultrasonography. Also, it can be a diagnostic problem to distinguish single univesicular cysts without daughter cysts (such as shown in Fig. 64-8) from simple benign liver cysts. In such cases, immunologic methods of diagnosis are complementary in making a final diagnosis. If a hydatid cyst becomes secondarily infected, the sonographic appearances are those of a nonspecific abscess, and here only the presence of either other cysts or positive immunology in the case of a single cyst is sufficient to make the diagnosis.

Computed Tomography. CT shows up liver hydatids extremely well, but this investigation has been shown to be no more sensitive or specific than ultrasonography. In the presence of liver hydatids, there exist problems of differential diagnosis similar to those described with ultrasonography (Schulze et al, 1980).

The particular value of CT in liver hydatid diagnosis lies in an accurate anatomic localisation of the cyst or cysts (Fig. 64-10). This accurate intrahepatic localisation is of special value to the operating surgeon in making an accurate preoperative decision, whether an abdominothoracic or thoracic surgical approach will or will not be required for a right lobe cyst. As will be seen later, the abdominothoracic approach has been used with increasing frequency in hydatid cysts located high in the right lobe of the liver, and this improvement in exposure has considerably decreased risks of recurrence and other forms of postoperative morbidity. Thoracic or abdominothoracic exposure is rarely needed for a cyst in the left lobe of the liver.

CT, however, is the method of choice when it is necessary to document preoperatively the presence of hydatid involvement in the abdomen but outside the liver itself, it can more accurately diagnose extrahepatic intraabdominal hydatid disease than can ultrasonography.

Immunologic Diagnosis

Immunologic diagnosis using hydatid serology has become extremely sophisticated in the past few years and has assumed an increasing role,

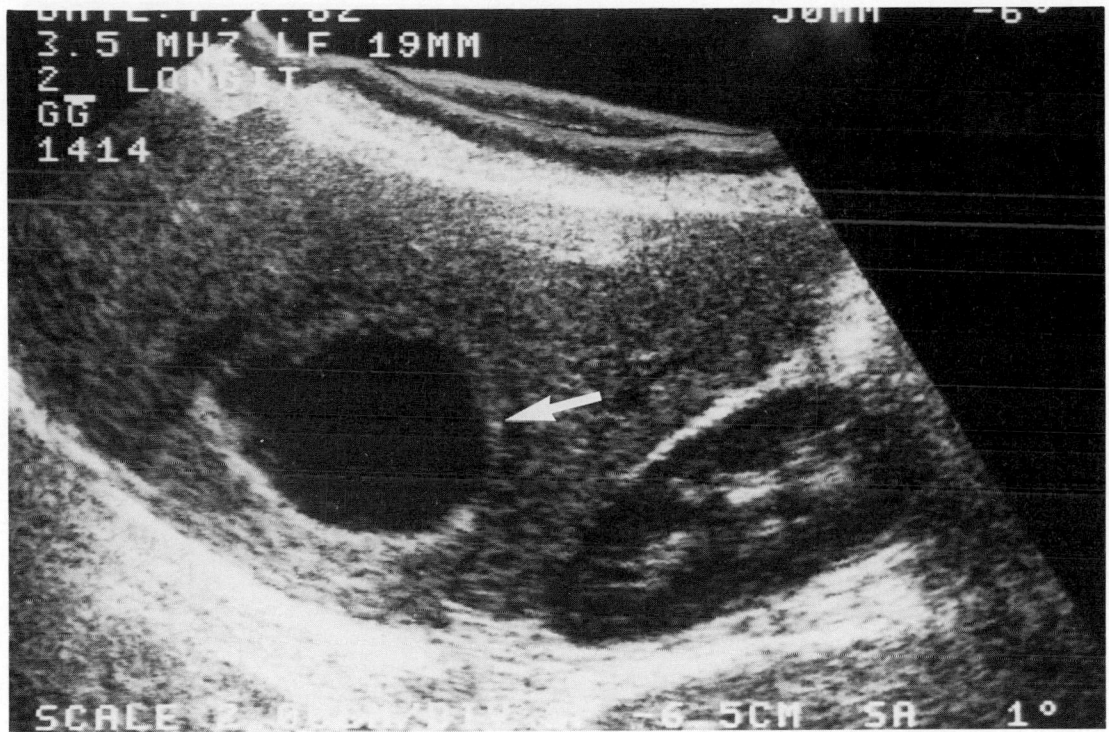

Figure 64–8. Ultrasonographic appearance of a single univesicular cyst in the liver without daughter cysts. This may be difficult to distinguish from that of a simple benign nonparasitic liver cyst. (*Courtesy of Drs. B. Arkles and G. Gill, Melbourne.*)

not only in primary diagnosis of hydatid disease, but also in the screening of susceptible populations as well as in the postsurgical follow-up of hydatid cases for recurrent hydatid disease. The whole subject of immunologic diagnosis of human hydatid disease was well reviewed by Rickard in 1979.

It is emphasised that the *Casoni* or *intradermal test,* though time honoured, now has *no place in diagnosis* because of its high rate of false-positives, its persistence after successful treatment, and the occasional problem of anaphylaxis. A number of laboratory tests have been used in recent years, such as the indirect fluorescent test, counter immunoelectrophoresis, and radioimmunoassay, but these have not been shown to offer advantages over the tests described in the following.

Immunoelectrophoresis. This investigation depends on its positivity, upon the formation of a specific arc of precipitation (called "Arc 5"), produced by the interaction of the serum from the hydatid patient with the antigen, as compared to a control. It is highly specific. Positives have been described only with *Echinococcus granulosus* and *Echinococcus alveolaris* (multilocularis) and therefore this test is most valuable in the diagnosis of human hydatid disease. Positive reactions have been described with *Taenia hydatigena* infestations, but fortunately these do not produce hydatid disease in the human, so that cross-reactions do not present a problem of diagnosis. However, it is important to note that in those countries in which both *Echinococcus granulosus* and *Echinococcus alveolaris* exist, the test cannot differentiate by itself between the two types of human hydatid disease. Fortunately, this does not pose a problem in many countries. Because the positive immunoelectrophoresis test requires high levels of antibody to produce precipitin arcs, the test reverts to negative values after successful surgical cure more quickly than any of the other tests discussed herein. It is therefore useful, not only in primary diagnosis, but also in postsurgi-

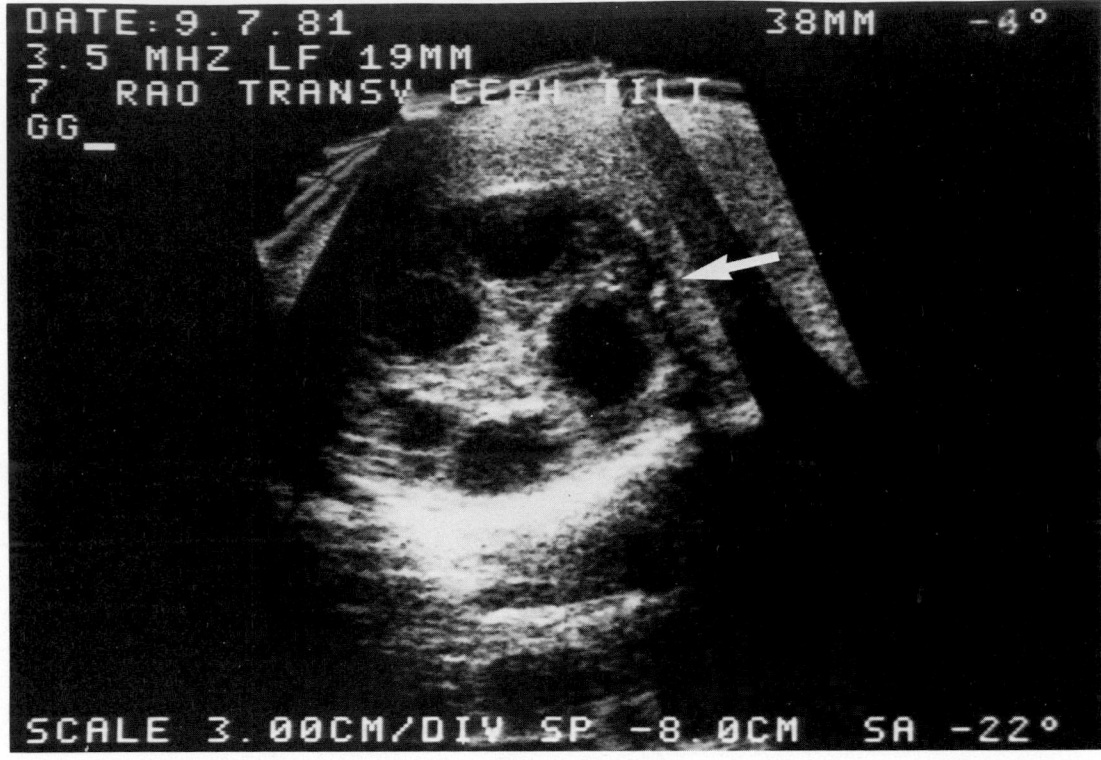

DATE:9.7.81   38MM   -4°
3.5 MHZ LF 19MM
7 RAO TRANSV CEPH TILT
GG_

SCALE 3.00CM/DIV SP -8.0CM SA -22°

Figure 64–9. Ultrasonographic examination of the liver with a large hydatid in the right lobe with internal reflections created by at least five daughter cysts and producing a pathognomonic appearance. (*Courtesy of Drs. B. Arkles and G. Gill, Melbourne.*)

cal follow-up. The test reverts to negative 1 to 2 years after successful surgical treatment, and if it becomes positive again, it almost certainly means that that particular patient has a recurrent hydatid cyst. This investigation is at present the one of choice in primary diagnosis, as well as for postsurgical follow-up.

Indirect Haemagglutination Test. This is a simple and sensitive test. It gives a positive reaction for *Echinococcus granulosus,* but also for other parasitic infestations, such as *Schistosomiasis* and *Nematode* infestations, and this limits its usefulness in primary diagnosis in those countries in which these infestations are common. The test does not revert to negative for long periods after treatment and therefore it is not useful in postsurgical follow-up treatment.

Latex Agglutination Test. This is a reasonably specific, sensitive, and simple test and has

no cross-reactions with other parasitic infestations, so that it is very useful for large scale screening of susceptible populations. Positive titres often persist for long periods after treatment and therefore it is not useful for postsurgical follow-up. However, it is more sensitive than the immunoelectrophoresis test and does produce a number of false-positives.

Complement Fixation Test. This was the first hydatid immunologic investigation and has been used since the beginning of this century. The test is extremely sensitive and therefore has a limited value in the primary diagnosis of human hydatid disease because of an unacceptably high positive reaction in other diseases. However, it rapidly returns to negative and is therefore useful in postoperative follow-up of hydatid patients.

Enzyme-Linked Immunosorbent Assay (ELISA). This investigation has recently been

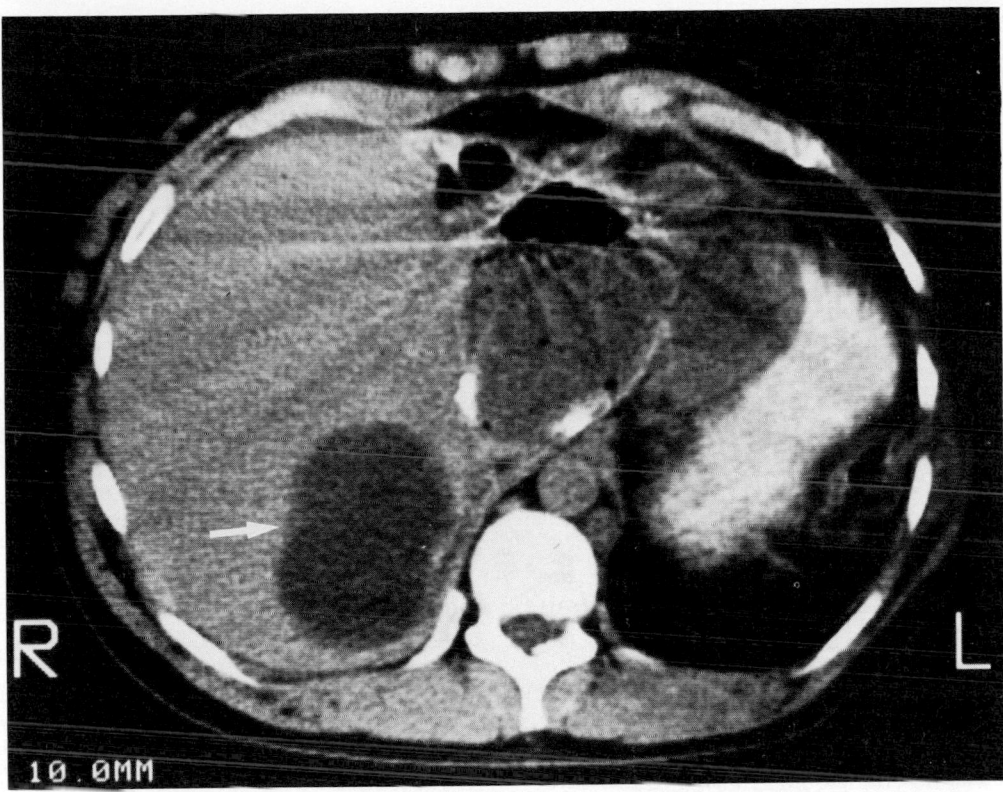

Figure 64–10. CT scan showing the precise localisation of a hydatid cyst, medially in the right lobe of the liver. This can help plan accurate surgical exposure of the cyst through a right thoracic approach.

automated, giving it a great advantage in large-scale screening or in epidemiologic studies of hydatid disease. Only small amounts of hydatid antigen are required, which again makes it most useful for screening of susceptible populations. The value of ELISA in primary diagnosis and in follow-up has not been completely evaluated.

Summary. At present, for primary diagnosis, the hydatid immunoelectrophoresis is the test of choice but, if this is not available, then latex agglutination or indirect haemagglutination tests are useful. ELISA may become the test of choice in the future for primary diagnosis once it has been properly evaluated. The Casoni or intradermal test should now never be used for primary diagnosis.

For postsurgical follow-up of whether there is recurrent hydatid disease, hydatid immuno-electrophoresis is at present the test of choice, but if this test is not available, then the hydatid complement fixation test may be used.

For large-scale screening of susceptible populations, the latex agglutination test or the indirect haemagglutination test may be used, though eventually it seems likely that again ELISA will be the test of choice because of the micro quantities of antigen that are required.

Medical Treatment

In 1977, a preliminary communication by Bekhti et al using the potent oral antihelminthic agent mebendazole demonstrated a marked therapeutic effect on the four patients in whom this was used, and this was most exciting and encouraging. It was already known that praziquantel is a potent antihelminthic, antiparasitic agent in the gastrointestinal (GI) tracts of animals such as dogs, and it was also found to have a marked effect on the cysts of *Echinococcus granulosus* in mice.

Since the initial report in 1977, there has been an evaluation on its effect on human cystic

Echinococcus granulosus in numerous centres around the world. A detailed review of the world literature through the end of 1983 indicates that the drug has been used on several hundred human subjects affected with *Echinococcus granulosus* in the liver. In spite of this very large number treated, thoroughly documented complete disappearance of the liver cysts with reversal of positive immunologic tests has been recorded in only a very few cases. Up to the present, it appears that neither a large collected review of thoroughly documented cases, nor a review by one individual or one centre treating numerous cases (with thorough documentation and thorough follow-up) has appeared in the literature. It thus seems that clinicians are either unprepared, or, more likely, largely unsuccessful in the treatment of human *Echinococcus granulosus* cysts with praziquantel.

For example, in 1982, Braithwaite presented to the Surgical Research Society of Australasia the results of long-term, high-dose praziquantel treatment, which was well controlled and well documented in 12 of 15 cases. In 5 of these 15 cases, there was progression of the hydatid lesions while taking praziquantel, in 6 there was no change, and in only 1 was there a decrease, but not complete disappearance, in the size of the cyst. Only the remaining 3 patients had inadequate control and follow-up. In none of these cases, therefore, was there evidence that long-term, high-dose praziquantel had completely cured the hydatid cyst.

Praziquantel has toxic side effects and abnormal liver function tests are seen not infrequently, while alopecia as well as haematological side effects have also been reported with its use. Praziquantel may be useful to slow progression of disease in patients refusing surgery, or when surgery is contraindicated because of poor general condition, or when there is very extensive widespread and recurrent hydatid disease present after multiple previous operations, but even in these cases, the value of praziquantel is neither clear nor certain. It will be mentioned later that praziquantel may be more useful in the treatment of *Echinococcus alveolaris* (multilocularis). At present, other similar benzimidazole compounds, such as albendazole, are being tested as alternatives to praziquantel in the medical treatment of cystic hydatid disease and the results of these evaluations are being awaited (Morris et al, 1983).

Thus, in the present state of incomplete knowledge of medical treatment of human Echinococcus granulosus cysts, praziquantel is not an alternative to conventional treatment, which at present is surgical excision of the hydatid cysts.

Surgical Treatment

At present, surgery offers the only consistently effective treatment for living abdominal hydatid cysts of the *Echinococcus granulosus* variety, and it is recommended for both symptomatic and asymptomatic cases. It is recommended for asymptomatic cases because, although some cysts die eventually without ever causing symptoms, frequently the natural history is one of growth, onset of complications, and especially rupture of the cyst into adjacent organs and cavities with serious consequences.

In recent years, surgical treatment has become extremely effective with a minimal mortality and, even more importantly, with a very dramatic reduction in morbidity, the latter having been frequent and disabling to the patient in the past. Improved surgical techniques for liver and abdominal hydatids have resulted in simplification of the operation, in almost complete elimination of postoperative biliary fistulae in liver hydatids, in minimisation of postsurgical major sepsis, and in a significant decrease in recurrent cystic hydatid disease, complications that in the past have been common and disabling for the patient, often not only prolonging convalescence, but also necessitating several reoperations.

The problems related to postsurgical morbidity in the past have been due to the inability of the surgeon to prevent spillage of the living hydatid material, which is infectious for the patient or to remove all living cyst elements, as well as problems associated with sterilisation of the residual hydatid cavity because an effective but nontoxic scolicidal agent was not available. In the past, biliary fistulae were frequent, partly because of external drainage of the residual hydatid cavity without closure of the cavity itself but, more importantly, because of a lack of understanding of the surgical pathology, i.e., that these fistulae were due to biliary communications between the bile ducts and the residual hydatid cavity and that such communications require formal surgical closure. An important advance to obtain adequate access and exposure and therefore to decrease the risk of

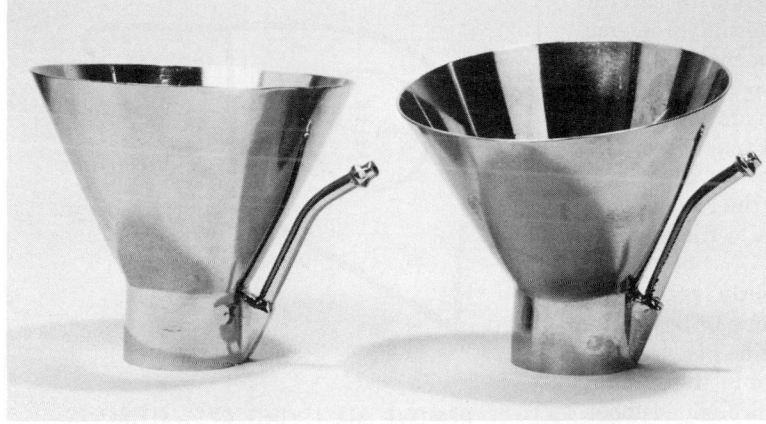

A

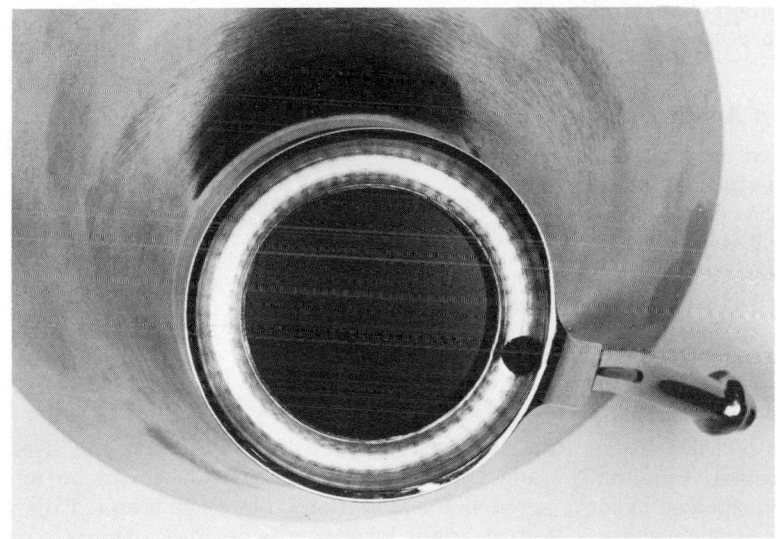

B

Figure 64–11. The hydatid suction cone developed by Aarons in Australia. **A.** Side view of the two cones. **B.** View of the cone base showing the suction mechanisms.

spillage and improve the capacity to completely remove the hydatid cyst when it is large and situated high in the right liver lobe has been the systematic use of a thoracic or a thoracoabdominal exposure. Spillage of hydatid fluid is now very effectively prevented by the use of hydatid cones, through which the operation can be performed, resulting in minimisation of recurrent hydatid disease and also in the prevention of anaphylactic shock during surgery.

In 1971, Saidi and Nazarian described the use of a cryogenic cone, which they adhered to the cyst surface by freezing. They were also the first to advocate the use of freshly prepared 0.5 percent silver nitrate solution as a good scolicidal agent. Since that time it has been found that cetrimide 0.5 or 1 percent is also a suitable alternative as a scolicidal agent. The cryogenic cone developed by Saidi and Nazarian appeared effective but was found to suffer from three potential problems: (1) risk of damage to other structures such as bowel coming into contact inadvertently with the freezing ring, (2) the necessity to excise that portion of the cyst wall damaged by the freezing, and (3) if the cyst fluid at body temperature flowed into the cone the frozen seal may have thawed and therefore the protection may have frequently been lost. Because of these potential problems with the cryogenic cone, a suction cone that adheres to the cyst wall has been developed in Australia by Aarons and Kune (Fig. 64–11). The instrument is simple, safe, and effective and with careful technique has none of the potential problems of the cryogenic cone. It has been used in 42 hydatid cyst cases in Australia without complications and without spillage of hydatid cyst contents. The cones are supplied in sets of two, the first having a conical part vertically above the suction base and the other with the conical part tilted at an angle of 20 degrees to the vertical (Fig. 64–11).

An area of the cyst wall slightly larger than the cone base is exposed, the cone of best fit is placed in position, and suction is applied through the outlet of the groove in the suction base of the cone and connected through a rubber hose to a conventional operating room suction apparatus. When firmly adherent (usually after about 5 to 10 seconds), the operation of removal of the hydatid cyst or cysts can proceed as described below.

Perioperative Management of Anaphylaxis

In all patients who are operated on for cystic hydatid disease, it is desirable to take all possible preventative measures to avoid anaphylaxis during surgery. Patients with a history of allergic rash should have a half- or quarter-dose Casoni test carried performed; if a marked local weal occurs within an hour, desensitisation against hydatid fluid should be considered.

With the premedication, patients should have an antihistamine if general anaesthetic is to be used, and intravenous hydrocortisone should be available to the anaesthetist and administered at the first sign of unexpected hypotensive collapse during surgery. Bronchospasm needs to be treated with conventional intravenous bronchodilators such as aminophylline.

Prevention of spillage of hydatid fluid is of particular importance, especially in sensitive subjects, and methods to avoid this have been described. Unless there has been a considerable blood loss during surgery, the most likely cause of a hypotensive hypovolaemic shock state is anaphylaxis. Should this occur, blood transfusion and the infusion of crystalloid solutions is not indicated, but plasma-expanding solutions should be used in conjunction with the intravenous drug therapy previously described.

Operative Techniques

Surgery of Uncomplicated Liver Hydatids. The surgical approach to uncomplicated liver hydatids depends on the size and position

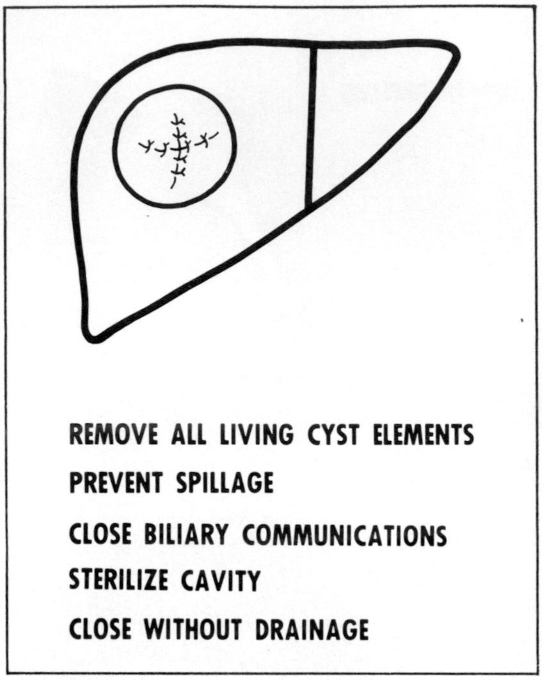

REMOVE ALL LIVING CYST ELEMENTS

PREVENT SPILLAGE

CLOSE BILIARY COMMUNICATIONS

STERILIZE CAVITY

CLOSE WITHOUT DRAINAGE

Figure 64–12. Surgical objectives and the appearance of the liver and residual cyst space at completion of operation for a simple liver cyst. (*Source: From Kune GA, Sali A: The Practice of Biliary Surgery, 2 edt. Oxford: Blackwell, 1980, with permission.*)

of the cyst. Cysts in the left lobe of the liver and those low in the right lobe can be approached abdominally, but cysts situated high in the right lobe usually require a thoracic or a thoracoabdominal approach. The principles of surgical technique and the appearance of the liver at the completion of surgery for a simple hydatid cyst is illustrated in Figure 64–12.

After exposure, the suction cone is applied. Through the cone, two stay sutures are inserted into the wall and brought out over the top edge of the cone to be held by an assistant, who lifts these slightly while also depressing the cone slightly. The cyst wall is then incised between these two sutures and, if the cyst is univesicular, fluid wells up into the cone and is aspirated by a separate sucker, which should be of a wide bore and connected to a suction bottle by a wide-bore tube without any intermediate connectors. The cyst cavity is aspirated until it is empty. The hydatid membrane is then removed, usually in one piece, with the use of plain dissecting forceps and sponge-holding forceps—this entire procedure performed through the operating cone.

Following removal of the fluid and of a univesicular cyst, or of a secondary and multivesicular with numerous daughter cysts, the residual cavity is sterilised using a scolicidal agent. Probably the most effective agent is freshly prepared 0.5 percent silver nitrate solution, but 0.5 or 1 percent cetrimide solution is a suitable alternative. This is instilled into the residual host cavity and left for 5 minutes. Hypertonic saline is no longer used. This author also warns against the use of formalin solutions as scolicidal agents; if this drips into the biliary ductal system through a biliary communication, it will produce irreparable and permanent sclerosis to the biliary ductal system. This was seen by the author in two referral cases of recent years; these had fatal outcomes.

After sucking out the scolicidal agent, the cone and any surrounding packing is removed and the interior of the host capsule is inspected to be sure there is no residual living hydatid tissue that will predispose to recurrence of the cyst. Laminated membrane and daughter cysts are never adherent to the host capsule, but the laminated membrane can fragment and pieces of this material or small daughter cysts may be secreted in folds of an irregularly shaped host capsule. For this inspection, adequate lighting and stretching of the host capsule with sponges is most effective.

Following inspection of the host capsule, an inspection is made for leakage of bile into the residual cyst cavity because this indicates the presence of biliary communications. Again, adequate lighting and careful retraction by an assistant with small retractors within the residual cavity will identify these biliary communications. These can easily be underrun and sutured individually and under vision. This manoeuvre in itself appears to have almost completely eliminated the troublesome postoperative biliary fistula of the past. Finally, the cavity is filled with normal saline and is closed primarily without drainage of either the residual cavity or of the abdomen in the operative area.

In liver hydatidosis of *Echinococcus granulosus* variety, excision of the host capsule or segmental hepatic resection is rarely necessary because the host capsule is part of the liver and is not itself infectious. Also, by leaving the properly treated host capsule, surgery of liver hydatids becomes bloodless and postoperative morbidity is minimised.

The author's experience using this technique taken with the experience of Aarons in Australia now amounts to over 40 consecutive cases in which precisely this technique was used and has resulted in a smooth postoperative convalescence without morbidity and mortality.

Management of Intrabiliary Rupture. This situation can often be predicted before surgery because of the clinical presentation of transient symptoms of cholestasis, such as jaundice, dark urine, pale stools, at times associated with fever and rigors. As has been mentioned, almost always the cause of the jaundice in association with hepatic hydatid cysts is rupture into the biliary ductal system; under these circumstances, an operative cholangiogram is most helpful to diagnose or to exclude the presence of hydatid material in the common bile duct. However, at times the amount of hydatid material in the bile duct is not gross and even then an operative cholangiogram can appear to be completely normal. Hopefully, when the operative cholangiogram is normal, the hydatid elements are so small that they will pass spontaneously if undetected at surgery.

The surgical objectives and the procedures performed in the presence of hydatid material rupturing into the bile ducts is indicated in Figure 64-13. Under these circumstances, the liver cyst is dealt with in exactly the same manner as described for a simple unruptured hydatid cyst with particular care taken to identify and suture the biliary communication or communications responsible for the hydatid elements entering the ductal system. *The cavity should not be drained* but closed after filling with normal saline in the usual way. At some point during the operation, an operative cholangiogram is performed; almost always one needs to open the common bile duct in the usual way, explore it, and extract hydatid elements from the bile ducts. It is probably undesirable in these situations to instill scolicidal agents into the biliary ductal system itself. When the cyst is small and deeply situated so that it does not present to the surface of the liver and is therefore inaccessible, it has been suggested that the bile duct be explored in the usual way, i.e., Fogarty biliary balloon catheters are passed up into the hepatic duct and into the cyst cavity to extract as much as possible of the active hydatid mate-

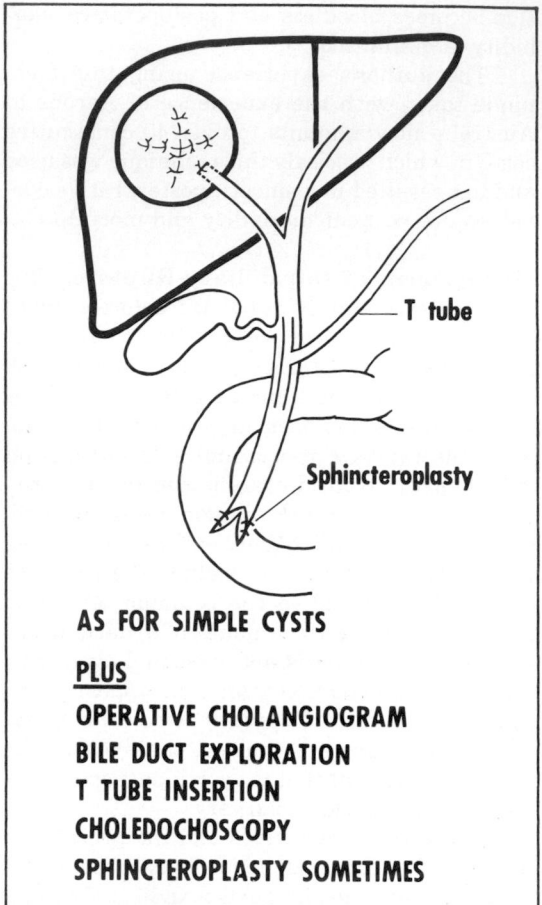

AS FOR SIMPLE CYSTS

PLUS

OPERATIVE CHOLANGIOGRAM

BILE DUCT EXPLORATION

T TUBE INSERTION

CHOLEDOCHOSCOPY

SPHINCTEROPLASTY SOMETIMES

Figure 64–13. Operative procedures performed when a hydatid ruptures into the bile ducts. (*Source: From Kune GA, Sali A: The Practice of Biliary Surgery, 2 edt. Oxford: Blackwell, 1980, with permission.*)

rial. It has been suggested that a transduodenal sphincteroplasty is a wise precaution against future problems related to residual hydatid material within the deeply situated hydatid cyst.

In all cases in which there has been a rupture of the hydatid material into the bile ducts, the author has found it useful, at the completion of bile duct exploration, to perform choledochoscopy to be sure that the bile ducts have been cleared of all hydatid elements, as it is quite easy to see these with the choledochoscope.

These surgical techniques carefully followed have almost eliminated postoperative biliary fistulae. Very occasionally, a large biliary communication resists closure due to calcification of the walls and in such cases, a technique

that is called omentoplasty is useful (described later). In some very persistent cases or cases in which the above techniques have not been followed and, in particular, when the residual cavity had been formally drained, a persistent biliary fistula that does not close within a few months needs reoperation. In the absence of common bile duct obstruction, the most suitable form of secondary surgical intervention is internal drainage of this fistula into a defunctionalised segment of the jejunum.

Management of Infected Cysts. This is an uncommon complication of liver hydatids and usually it is postoperative infection in a hydatid cyst cavity with calcification when the cyst had been removed and the residual cavity had become infected, rather than a spontaneous infection. If a previous operation had not been performed, then the usual cause is an intrabiliary rupture of hydatid elements that were not treated promptly by surgery and that have resulted in infection of the biliary ductal system and spread up through the biliary communication into the hepatic hydatid cyst. Rarely, a late infection can occur in a host cavity that had not become obliterated following surgery and that still has a patent biliary communication. If the clinical picture is compatible with infection and if at surgery infection is confirmed by Gram stain and by the presence of foul-smelling pus, then the cavity should not be closed as described for simple cysts, but rather the hydatid elements removed in the usual way, the biliary communications closed, and a scolicidal injected. The cavity then should be opened widely and an *omentoplasty* performed (Aroney and Souvlis, 1979).

Omentoplasty is a relatively simple operation, in which the greater omentum is mobilised and a piece of its apex is placed into the residual cavity to act as a biologic blotter. The omentum is then loosely sutured with three or four interrupted absorbable sutures to the widely opened mouth of the cavity so that it remains retained in that situation. The actual residual hydatid cavity is not drained directly, but a drainage tube is placed near the cavity in the operative area, as depicted in Figure 64–14. Perioperative antibiotics are also used in the presence of an infected hydatid cyst of the liver.

Postoperative infection of a simple hydatid cyst cavity is most uncommon, but it can result in a liver abscess or the onset of cholangitis. In these cases, the management consists of reop-

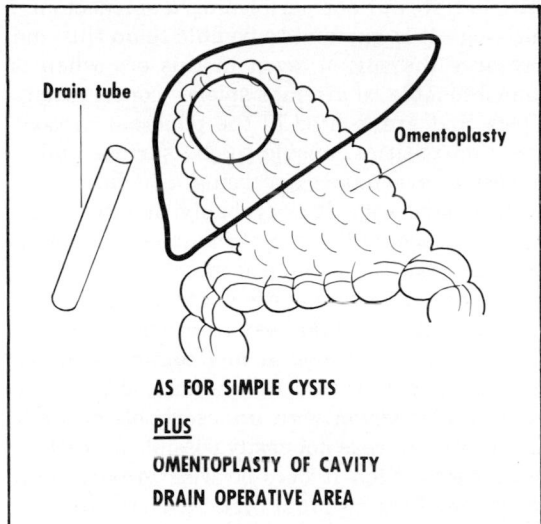

Drain tube

Omentoplasty

AS FOR SIMPLE CYSTS

<u>PLUS</u>

OMENTOPLASTY OF CAVITY

DRAIN OPERATIVE AREA

Figure 64–14. Operative procedures performed in the presence of an infected liver hydatid the "omentoplasty" operation. (*Source: From Kune GA, Sali A: The Practice of Biliary Surgery, 2 edt. Oxford: Blackwell, 1980, with permission.*)

eration with the use of appropriate perioperative antibiotics, the drainage of the residual cavity, with omentoplasty and drainage of the operative area, but drainage tubes are not inserted into the cavity itself.

The operative procedure of omentoplasty has been practiced for some years and many cases have been successfully treated by this method. The advocates of this procedure use omentoplasty, not only with infected liver hydatids, but also as primary treatment for simple cysts (Papadimitriou and Mandrekas, 1970). However, this author prefers the technique described above, rather than omentoplasty, for simple, uninfected cysts and for cysts without infection that have ruptured into the bile ducts, because the former is both easy to perform and effective.

Management of Intraperitoneal Rupture. This is an uncommon complication of hepatic hydatid cysts and usually presents with features of peritonitis with or without features of anaphylactic shock. At operation, the surgeon may find just some clear fluid in the peritoneal cavity. Exploration of the liver shows a partially or fully collapsed hydatid cyst. In other instances, there in fact are pieces of hydatid membrane or daughter cysts found free in the perito-

neal cavity. Almost always, the ruptured cyst is easily found by palpation and exploration of the liver as those that rupture into the peritoneal cavity always present close to the liver surface. It is most important to explore the liver cyst cavity because often there are residual hydatid elements present in it and also it is important to deal with it as for an uncomplicated liver cyst (already described). In addition, the peritoneal cavity, including the pelvis and the perihepatic spaces, is thoroughly searched for hydatid elements. It is probably unwise to instill 0.5 percent silver nitrate into the peritoneal cavity, but 0.5 or 1 percent cetrimide may be used, provided it is followed in 5 minutes by very thorough lavage with large quantities of normal saline.

Management of Intrathoracic Rupture. This is a rare complication and it always implies erosion of the diaphragm, followed by rupture of the liver hydatid cyst into the pleural cavity or a bronchus or into the pericardial cavity (Xanthakis et al, 1981). Occasionally the hydatid cyst ruptures simulta neously into both a bronchus and the pleural cavity. The most common of these rare intrathoracic ruptures is a direct rupture into a bronchus, producing a bronchobiliary fistula; the next most common is rupture into the pleural cavity, followed by rupture into both the pleural cavity and a bronchus, and, finally, rupture into the pericardial cavity.

The surgical management of intrathoracic ruptures essentially involves exposure of both the thorax and the abdomen; therefore an abdominothoracic incision and exposure is almost always obligatory. The liver cyst or cysts are dealt with in the usual way as described previously. Usually the hole in the diaphragm created by the hydatid can also be found and repaired. The fistula into a bronchus, if known to be present from the symptomatology of coughing up bile-stained sputum or occasionally bile-stained sputum mixed with "grape-skins," can usually be located and either the fistula opening repaired or a lobectomy or segmental lung resection carried out. If the rupture is purely into the pleural cavity, then the pleural hydatid components are removed and lavaged safely using 0.5 percent silver nitrate or 0.5 to 1 percent cetrimide in the pleural cavity. The thorax is always drained in the usual way after this type of surgery, whether the surgery be on a bronchus, following a lobectomy, or after removal of pleural cavity hydatid cysts. Occasionally the rupture is a slow one, producing a dumbbell-shaped bilocular hydatid cyst with one component in the liver and another in the pleural cavity communicating through the eroded diaphragm.

The very rare rupture into the pericardial sac is dealt with by further opening the pericardium and removing the hydatid components, but it is unwise to use scolicidal agents of any kind in the pericardial cavity. The pericardial sac is left open to drain into the pleural cavity and it is the pleural cavity that is drained with a drain tube.

Management of Extrahepatic Intraperitoneal Hydatid Cysts. These cysts can be either in a solid organ, such as the spleen or the pancreas, or the ovary, and presumably they are located there because of systemic spread of the original hydatid scolices that have passed through the portal system and through the pulmonary vasculature entering the systemic circulation in that way. The other form of extrahepatic intraperitoneal cystic hydatid disease is called secondary peritoneal hydatidosis, usually the result of spillage of living hydatid material during surgery on a liver hydatid, with implantation and subsequent growth of hydatid elements or daughter cysts following surgery. Rarely, peritoneal hydatids in the peritoneum or in the pelvis are found there because of a slow extrusion of a liver hydatid cyst into the peritoneal or pelvic cavities or because of a relatively silent and asymptomatic rupture of a hydatid cyst into the peritoneal cavity.

Secondary peritoneal hydatidosis may result in the formation of one or up to dozens of hydatid cysts in the peritoneal and pelvic cavity, which may frighten the surgeon when the abdomen is opened. However, they can usually be dealt with individually without significant problems and often each peritoneal hydatid can be removed with its host capsule intact. But when part of the host capsule forms from the bladder, bowel, or some viscus, the cyst should then be treated in a fashion completely identical to simple primary liver cysts.

Cysts in solid abdominal viscera are rare. When they are located in the spleen, the usual surgical treatment is splenectomy, but if there are gross adhesions to the diaphragm, then it may be wiser to evacuate the splenic cyst using a hydatid cone and filling the residual cavity with saline and not performing a splenectomy, although it is unusual to be able to do this and preserve the spleen, even in this era when it is fashionable to attempt splenic conservation. Cysts that are located in the pancreas present their adventitial capsule to the surface and it is best to evacuate these using a hydatid cone in the usual way. It is probably unwise to use scolicidal agents for fear of inducing postoperative pancreatitis, as some of these cysts do erode minor or major pancreatic ducts. Following removal of the hydatid cyst from the pancreas, it is important to look at any communications with the pancreatic ductal system and to suture these under vision with unabsorbable sutures. If this procedure is not easily possible for technical reasons, then it may be wise to perform a drainage of the residual cystic cavity into a defunctionalised segment of jejunum. Otherwise, it is safe to fill the cavity with saline and close it without drainage.

ECHINOCOCCUS ALVEOLARIS OR MULTILOCULARIS

Epidemiology, Pathology, and Natural History

Echinococcus alveolaris is totally different from *Echinococcus granulosus* and is a much rarer form of hydatid disease in the human. It is endemic to parts of the world that are either cold and/or mountainous. The definitive host is the fox, cat, or wild dog and the usual intermediate hosts are rodents, such as field mice and rats, and, occasionally, man. This form of hydatid disease has been reported from Alaska and Canada, the Soviet Union, Bavaria, Switzerland, Japan, and China. It has not been reported in countries where *Echinococcus granulosus* is particularly prevalent.

The adult worm is smaller than the *Echinococcus granulosus*. The infection is acquired by the host through the ingestion of cyst-containing flesh. Man apparently acquires the infection by eating vegetables or berries that are contaminated by the faeces of infected foxes and dogs. The liver is involved in at least 90 percent of cases. The cysts in *Echinococcus alveolaris* infestation are extremely numerous and usually small, varying in size from the microscopic cyst to that of a pea, and contain gelatinous material. Necrosis and the development of an abscess within an area of multiple *Echinococcus alveolaris* cysts is occasionally seen.

Clinical Presentation

Clinically, the condition is characterised by an increase in the liver size and it may be difficult to distinguish this from a liver hepatoma, except by dynamic radionuclide scanning, which will show an irregular and avascular filling defect or defects in the liver. Jaundice frequently develops with involvement of the biliary ductal system. Macroscopically, at operation, the condition can resemble either a mucoid carcinoma that is secondary in the liver or congenital cystic liver disease. Untreated patients progress to a fatal outcome in at least 70 percent of cases. Death is due in part to hepatic replacement, in part to biliary duct obstruction with jaundice and cholangitis, and sometimes from metastatic spread of the parasite (Wilson and Rausch, 1980).

Diagnosis

In a large series of cases reported from Japan (Kasai et al, 1980), immunologic diagnosis had achieved a high rate of detection in the screening of a population of over 140,000 people at risk. Thus, with mass screening, the disease can be recognised at an early stage, with excellent results of treatment. The complement fixation reaction together with indirect haemagglutination and an enzyme immunoassay, achieved a sensitivity of 97 percent in serologic diagnosis.

Organ imaging techniques of diagnosis have shown that radionuclide scanning is useful, particularly with dynamic flow studies using technetium, in demonstrating the presence of an avascular area in the liver, thus differentiating these from vascular lesions such as liver tumours and inflammatory liver disease. It has also been shown that CT is slightly more effective than ultrasonography in the diagnosis of *Echinococcus alveolaris* in the liver.

Treatment

The most effective treatment of alveolar hydatid disease, especially in its early stages, is surgical resection. In the later stages of the disease with gross involvement of the liver, surgical resection is still possible and desirable, but in these cases

it appears that the addition of praziquantel therapy is valuable in arresting the progress of the disease. In advanced alveolar hydatid disease, in which the principal symptom is obstructive jaundice due to involvement of the biliary ductal system, the use of either percutaneous transtubation of the involved bile ducts or peroperative U-tube insertion, has been found to be extremely effective in the control of this symptom, although it may not have affected the long-term survival of the patients. Indeed, it is seriously doubted that in advanced alveolar hydatid disease cure of the condition is ever possible (Mossimann, 1980).

BIBLIOGRAPHY

Aarons BP, Fitzpatrick SC: Hepato-biliary hydatid disease, in Kune GA, Sali A (eds): The Practice of Biliary Surgery, 2 edt. Oxford: Blackwell, 1980, p 399

Aarons BJ, Kune GA: A suction cone to prevent spillage during hydatid surgery. Aust NZ J Surg 53:471, 1983

Aroney M, Souvlis L: Current alternate surgical management of human hepatic hydatid disease with emphasis on omentoplasty. Aust Vet J 55:148, 1979

Bekhti A, Schaaps J-P, et al: Treatment of hepatic hydatid disease with mebendazole: preliminary results in four cases. Br Med J 2:1, 1977

Borrie J, Shaw JH: Hepatobronchial fistula caused by hydatid disease. Thorax 36:25, 1981

Braithwaite PA: Hydatid disease. Med J Aust 1:648, 1981 (letter)

Braithwaite PA: The results of longterm high dose mebendazole for cystic hydatid disease. Proc Surg Res Soc Aust 42, 1982 (abstr)

Grundmann R, Eitenmuller J, et al: Indications for the various surgical procedures in hepatic echinococcosis. Chirurg 52:332, 1981

Kasai Y, Koshino I, et al: Alveolar echinococcus of the liver: Studies on 60 operated cases. Ann Surg 191:145, 1980

Kune GA, Jones T, et al: Hydatid disease in Australia: An update on prevention, clinical presentation and treatment. Med J Aust 1983 (to be published)

Kune GA, Judson R, et al: Solitary liver abscess. Med J Aust 1:151, 1979

Lambert R: Personal communication, 1983

Morl M: Echinococcosis. Rational diagnosis and therapy. Fortschr Med 24:100, 1982

Morris DL, Dykes PW, et al: Albendazole in hydatid disease. Br Med J 1:103, 1983

Mossimann F: Is alveolar hydatid disease of the liver incurable? Ann Surg 192:118, 1980

Papadimitriou J, Mandrekas A: The surgical treatment of hydatid disease of the liver. Br J Surg 57:431, 1970

Rickard MD: The immunological diagnosis of hydatid disease. Aust Vet J 55:99, 1979

Saidi F, Nazarian T: Surgical treatment of hydatid cysts by freezing of cyst wall and instillation of 0.5% silver nitrate solution. N Engl J Med 284:1346, 1971

Schulze K, Aubener KH, et al: Computed tomographic and sonographic diagnosis of echinococcus. ROEFO 132:514, 1980

Wilson JP, Rausch RL: Alveolar hydatid disease. A review of clinical features of 233 indigenous cases of echinococcus multilocularis infection in Alaskan Eskimos. Am J Trop Med Hyg 29:1341, 1980

Xanthakis DS, Katsaras E, et al: Hydatid cyst of the liver with intrathoracic rupture. Thorax 36:497, 1981

65. Cysts and Benign Tumors

Seymour I. Schwartz

Benign tumors of the liver are uncommon, but have been reported with increasing frequency related, in part, to improvements in diagnostic technique and also to the widespread use of contraceptive medication. Edmondson documented the pathologic characteristics of these lesions and formulated the following classification:

1. Focal nodular hyperplasia
2. Adenoma
3. Adrenal rest tumor
4. Cystic mesenchymal hamartoma
5. Nonparasitic cysts
6. Cavernous hemangioma
7. Infantile hemangioendothelioma
8. Teratoma

The adrenal rest tumor and the teratoma are exceedingly rare; the remaining lesions are discussed individually because of unique characteristics.

NONPARASITIC CYSTS

Nonparasitic cysts of the liver may be single or multiple, diffuse or localized, unilocular or multilocular. The rarer varieties include blood and degenerative cysts, dermoid cysts, lymphatic cysts, endothelial cysts (cystadenomas). The more common lesions are retention cysts, which are solitary, simple cysts, or part of polycystic disease.

Incidence

In 1856 Bristowe first reported a case of nonparasitic cystic disease of the liver and emphasized the association with polycystic renal disease. The same year, Michel recorded the first solitary, nonparasitic cyst. Henson et al summarized approximately 500 cases of nonparasitic

cysts from the experience at Mayo Clinic and the world literature up to 1954. Haddad et al brought the total up to almost 900 in their report of 1977. An autopsy incidence of 0.15 to 0.5 percent has been reported. In a retrospective review of 88,000 abdominal operations, Sanfelippo et al found 131 cases of congenital hepatic cysts, only 22 of which were symptomatic.

Cystic disease of the liver has been reported at all ages. The disease most frequently makes its appearance during the fourth, fifth, and sixth decades. The average age of the patients with symptomatic, solitary cysts of the liver is 55 years. Polycystic disease occurs more frequently in the female patient with a 2:1 ratio; solitary nonparasitic cysts occur four times more frequently in the female.

Etiology

Most investigators have regarded the condition as congenital, and it is postulated that aberrant ducts formed during embryonic development enlarge. Cyst formation is attributed to inflammatory hyperplasia of the ducts, or obstruction of the ducts with retention of fluid. Although some investigators believe that solitary cysts and polycystic liver disease are different manifestations of the same process, the opinion is not generally held.

Solitary Nonparasitic Cysts

These cysts are usually located on the anteroinferior surface of the right lobe of the liver. The cysts vary markedly in size from 1 cm to 15 cm. They may be more deeply placed, and some have presented as pedunculated cysts. The external surface is smooth, glistening, and greyish-blue. The cyst wall is usually thin and opalescent or transparent and may be traversed by many dilated blood vessels. The cyst content is a clear, watery, or yellowish-brown material, but may appear bile stained. The cysts characteristically have a low internal pressure, in contrast to the high tension in parasitic cysts. The wall of the solitary cyst is generally composed of three layers: an inner layer of loose, connective tissue that is rich in cellular elements, a circular dense middle layer, poor in cell nuclei, and an outer layer that contains segments of bile ducts and islands of liver cells, and a connective tissue framework that blends into the liver parenchyma. The inner lining may be cuboidal or columnar epithelium, at times ciliated, or there may be no distinct epithelial layer. Communication within the biliary tree may be expected in about one quarter of solitary hepatic cysts.

Polycystic Disease

The affected portion of the liver is enlarged and deformed by numerous cysts of varying size on the surface of the organ (Fig. 65–1). The cysts are surrounded by a capsule of fibrous tissue. On cut section, the appearance is that of a honeycomb with multiple cavities. The cysts contain a clear fluid, usually without bile. They are commonly distributed throughout the liver, but at times one lobe, more frequently the right, is preferentially involved. Hepatic function is seldom appreciably impaired, but polycystic livers have been implicated as a rare cause of portal hypertension. The lesion has been associated with atresia of the bile ducts, cholangitis, and hepatitis. Carcinoma, arising in the cyst wall, has been reported infrequently.

Microscopically the epithelial lining of the cyst varies with the size and stage of development. In the larger cysts, the lining may have degenerated and is absent, or flattened. In medium-sized cysts, the lining is usually cuboidal, whereas columnar cells line the smaller cysts. The lining cells closely resemble those of normal bile ducts. Outside the epithelium, the wall is composed of a thin, collagenous tissue. Numerous nondilated bile ducts are seen in the surrounding tissue, and the islands of hepatic parenchyma between the cysts may be compressed, distorted, or normal.

Unlike the solitary, nonparasitic cyst, which is usually an isolated finding, polycystic disease is frequently associated with cystic involvement of other organs. The kidney is the most commonly involved, usually to a greater extent than the liver. In addition to the kidneys, cystic disease of the liver has been associated with cystic disease of the pancreas, spleen, ovary, and lungs.

Clinical Manifestations

The great majority of patients with hepatic cysts are asymptomatic. Most cysts are incidental findings at operation or autopsy. When symptoms occur, they are usually related to the presence of an enlarging mass in the upper abdomen, coupled with vague, gastrointestinal complaints. The most common presentations of symptomatic cysts are: abdominal mass (55 percent), hepatomegaly (40 percent), abdominal pain (33 percent), and jaundice (9 percent). Complications are rare and may account for symptoms. These include perforation, hemorrhage, and secondary infection. Torsion of a cyst on a pedicle may occur. Jaundice may develop secondary to compression of the common duct, and portal hypertension has been described with polycystic disease.

Diagnostic Studies

Studies of liver function are of little diagnostic aid. Serum bilirubin level and alkaline phosphatase are generally normal. With advanced polycystic disease of the kidneys there are signs of impaired renal function, and excretory urograms are diagnostic. On plain x-ray the diaphragm is frequently elevated, and large cysts displace the colon down and to the left, in contrast to the anterior colonic displacement caused by renal masses. On lateral projection, the anterior location of the extrinsic pressure favors the diagnosis of an hepatic cyst. Isotopic scanning with technetium-99m sulfur colloid may show areas of diminished uptake. Ultrasound examination offers a high yield, and the diagnosis is suggested if an anechoic area is defined. A computed tomography (CT) scan demonstrates a lower attenuation lesion (Fig. 65–2). Ultrasonography may depict cysts as small as 2 cm in diameter. Arteriography, although usually unnecessary, will define an avascular mass.

Differential Diagnosis

Differentiation from primary tumors of the liver and from metastatic lesions is usually not a problem. Generally, differentiation from a hydatid cyst is not difficult; the latter diagnosis is

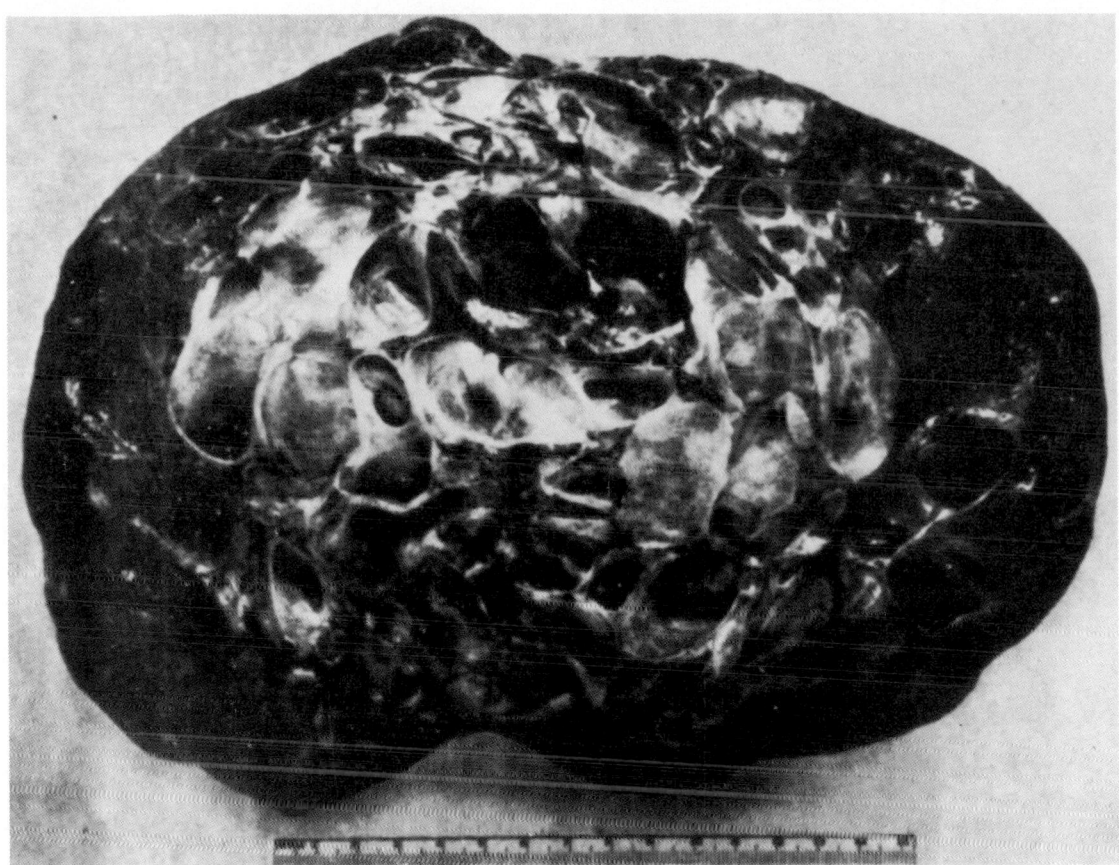

Figure 65–1. Cystic disease of the liver involving the entire left lobe. (*Source: From Schwartz SI: Surgical Diseases of the Liver. New York: McGraw-Hill, 1964, with permission.*)

suggested by eosinophilia, a positive Casoni test, and the deposition of calcium in the walls of the cyst. Calcareous deposits, however, have been noted in benign nonparasitic cysts.

Treatment

Solitary Cysts

With the exceptions of rupture, torsion, and intracystic hemorrhage, the operative treatment is elective, and is based on the size and location of the cyst and the patient's general status. Ideally, excision of the cyst is desirable, but it is hazardous if the cyst is deeply placed within the liver, or if it communicates with the biliary tree. With solitary cysts, a cleavage plane may be developed between the cyst and the liver that permits enucleation of the entire cyst except for the outer wall adjacent to the liver paren-

chyma. Hepatic lobectomy may be necessary for large, complicated cysts.

Most solitary nonparasitic cysts have been treated by partial excision and marsupialization. The cyst is drained to the exterior, and the drainage usually ceases 1 to 2 weeks later. In some instance, however, prolonged drainage has occurred. A variety of sclerosing agents have been used to destroy the cyst lining and to decrease the drainage. External drainage is safer for infected cysts, but internal drainage, into a Roux loop of jejunum is preferable if the cyst contains bile. Aspiration, incision, and drainage into the free peritoneal cavity has been used with success, but recurrence is more frequent with this technique.

Polycystic Disease

If the lesion is located in one lobe, or is preponderant in one lobe, hepatic lobectomy is pre-

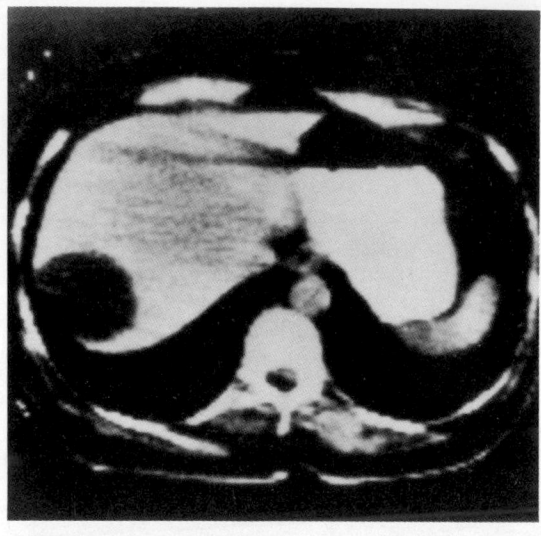

A

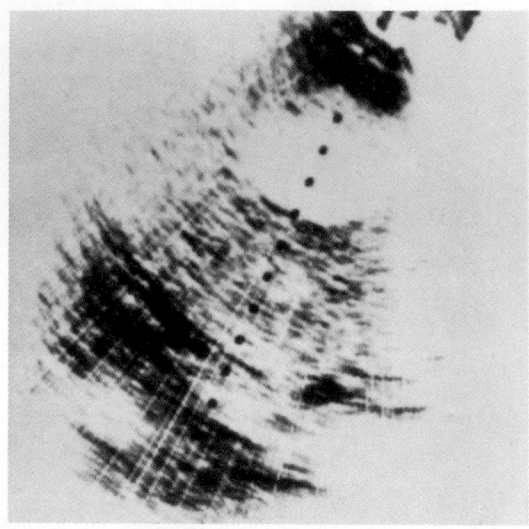

B

Figure 65–2. A. CT scan, 5-cm rounded, low-attenuation cystic lesion in posterosuperior right lobe of liver. Note proximity of cyst to surrounding lung. **B.** Longitudinal sonogram through right lobe. Hypoechoic cyst with well-defined posterior wall. (*Source: From Roemer CE, Ferrucci JT Jr, et al: Hepatic cysts: Diagnosis and therapy by sonographic needle aspiration. AJR 136:1065, 1981, with permission.*)

ferred. If the patient has been relatively asymptomatic, and excision is deemed difficult, definitive therapy is not indicated, and the larger cysts may be unroofed and allowed to drain into the peritoneal cavity. Drainage of large cysts, in this fashion or by puncture, affords only temporary relief.

Prognosis

Although the older literature reports mortality rates in the range of 20 percent for nonparasitic cysts treated by excision, Geist's review reported mortality rates of approximately 5 percent. Limiting the cases to those reported subsequent to 1924, there were only 3 deaths in 122 patients subjected to operation.

Morbidity is usually related to the development of a persistent draining sinus in those patients subjected to marsupialization. Other complications include recurrence, extension of liver damage with hepatic failure, and infection. The prognosis for the polycystic disease of the liver is essentially that of the accompanying polycystic renal disease. When the kidneys are insignificantly involved, the hepatic lesion is compatible with good health and long life. Hepatic

failure, jaundice, esophageal varices, and ascites are extremely rare.

MESENCHYMAL HAMARTOMA

Mesenchymal hamartoma of the liver is a rare, benign tumor of childhood that was first reported by Maresh in 1903. This cystic, hepatic tumor has also been termed "large solitary bile-cell fibroadenoma," "hamartoma," and "large, cavernous lymphangiomatoid lesion."

Incidence

Approximately 50 cases of mesenchymal hamartoma have been reported. The lesion occurs much more frequently in infancy and childhood, but several cases have been reported in adults. The lesion was usually located in the right lobe (37 of 49 reported cases), rarely in the left lobe, and in three cases was present in both lobes. There was approximately an equal number of females and males affected. The diagnosis was made during the first 2 years of life in the great

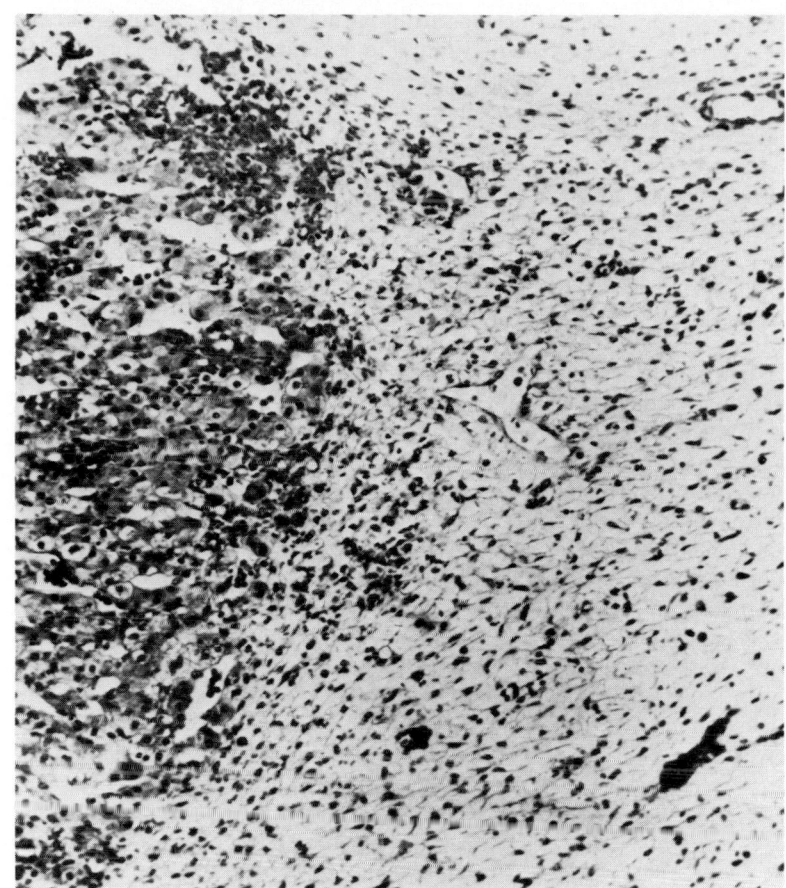

Figure 65–3. This section shows a large island of liver cells with clusters of smaller, darker staining hematopoietic cells on the left and loose mesenchymal tissue on the right. (*Source: From Srouji MN, Chatten J, et al, 1978, with permission.*)

majority of patients; in a few, the diagnosis was made during the first 3 months of life.

Pathology

The lesion usually appears as a single mass bulging from the liver on the inferior surface, and is frequently pedunculated. One case was described as completely intralobar. The tumor is well encapsulated and most frequently cystic. The contained fluid is usually watery; on occasion it has a gelatinous, yellow color but does not contain bile. Histologically, according to Edmondson's criteria, the hamartomas are composed of tissues indigenous to the site. Mesenchymal hamartoma of the liver is characterized by an admixture of ductal structures in a copious, loose connective tissue stroma. The remnants of bile ducts and liver lobules are often associated with recognizable portal triads, all of which are overgrown by mesenchymal elements. These have a tendency to undergo cystic degeneration, and to accumulate fluid in quantities sufficient to create microscopic and macroscopic acellular spaces suggestive of lymphangiomatous channels but without an endothelial lining. Smaller cysts may have one layer of columnar or cuboidal lining cells, probably of bile duct origin (Fig. 65–3).

Clinical Manifestations

Most patients present with symptoms related to accelerated growth rate of the tumor and a rapid accumulation of fluid within the cyst. Symptoms are generally minor. Children present with a right upper quadrant mass that produces a bulge in the abdomen; the general physical condition, however, remains excellent. Occasionally, with large lesions, there is a degree of respiratory distress.

Diagnostic Studies

Tc-99m sulfur colloid scan defines a lack of uptake in the lesion. Angiography, useful in preoperative evaluation by delineating anatomic location, extent, and morphologic features, does not, however, define an abnormal vascularity. Exploration and biopsy are frequently necessary to define the diagnosis.

Treatment

The treatment is surgical excision, which depends on the location of the lesion. Pedunculated lesions are readily removed. If the tumor is well encapsulated, it may be enucleated. When the tumor is localized near the surface of the liver, a partial hepatectomy may be carried out. In rare instances, a formal lobectomy is required. If the lesion is adherent to the inferior vena cava and involves both lobes of the liver, it may be treated by partial excision and marsupialization. Radiotherapy may effect some reduction in size of the lesion, due to hyalinization of the mesenchymal components. Reduction in size should be followed by surgical excision.

HEMANGIOMAS

The most common benign tumor of the liver is the hemangioma, and the liver is the visceral organ most frequently affected by this lesion. Frerich is credited with the first description of hemangiomas of the liver in the medical literature in 1861. Like other benign tumors, the majority are incidental findings, but lesions often reach clinical significance in the adult, where they reach massive proportions and encroach on adjacent viscera or spontaneously rupture. In children, giant cavernous hemangiomas, and infantile hemangioendotheliomas may produce cardiac failure, at times accompanied by a consumptive coagulopathy.

Incidence

Vascular lesions involve the liver with particular frequency. Of 135 reported visceral hemangiomas, 109 occurred in the liver. In a series of 2400 autopsies, cavernous hemangiomas of the liver were demonstrated in 2 percent of the livers. Ten percent of the lesions were multiple.

In the adult hepatic hemangiomas are most frequently found in patients in the third and fourth decades; the average age when the lesion is discovered is 44. Symptomatic hemangiomas in the adult occur in the female five times more frequently. In children most cases present in the first month of life.

Pathology

Hemangiomas are generally classified into two types: capillary and cavernous. The lesions as they appear in the liver are almost always cavernous. They may be single or multiple, and may be limited to the liver or involve other organs. They are occasionally associated with cysts of the liver and pancreas. An association has also been noted between focal nodular hyperplasia and hemangioma of the liver. The size of the hemangioma of the liver varies from 1 g to as much as 40 lb.

The lesions are frequently located immediately beneath the Glisson capsule, and the surface may be depressed, umbilicated, or at times elevated. On cut section, the hemangioma is purplish-red in color, and sponge-like in appearance; there are many cystic spaces filled with blood. The surrounding parenchyma is sharply demarcated, and there is an absence of communication between the tumor and the hepatic parenchyma. With increasing fibrosis, a conditioned termed "sclerosing hemangioma" may be produced.

Histologically, the tumor presents a typical appearance (Fig. 65–4). It is composed of cystic spaces filled with blood and lined with epithelial cells separated by varying amounts of fibrous tissue. The hepatic plates between the blood spaces are absent or markedly compressed, but there is no distortion or compression of the adjacent hepatic parenchyma. Marked fibrosis may be present, contributing to the formation of a sclerosing hemangioma. Malignant degeneration does not occur, and the hemangioma must be distinguished from the hemangioendothelioma. The latter is represented by a widespread area of multicentric lesions, accompanied by vascular involvement of the skin and occurring in children with clinical manifestations in the first week of life.

The other lesion that must be distinguished from the hemangioma is peliosis hepatis, which consists of blood lakes surrounded by tissue without epithelial lining.

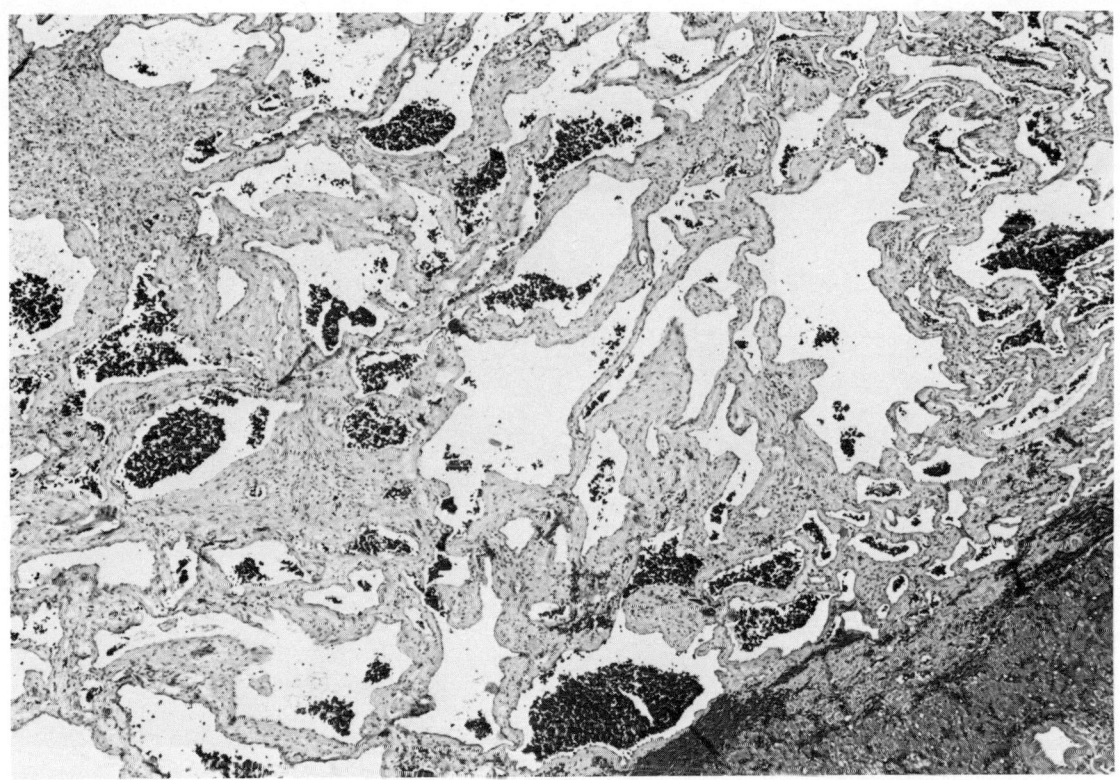

Figure 65–4. Hemangioma histology. Lesion is composed of cystic spaces filled with blood and lined with epithelial cells separated by varying amounts of fibrous tissue. (*Source. From Gutierrez OH, Schwartz SI: Atlas of Hepatic Tumors and Focal Lesions. New York: McGraw-Hill, 1984, p 75, with permission.*)

Clinical Manifestations

Small hemangiomas are usually asymptomatic. Only patients in whom the lesion reaches sizes greater than 4 cm develop symptoms. Larger lesions in adults usually present in one of three ways: as an asymptomatic abdominal mass, with pain or digestive symptoms related to encroachment of the tumor on the abdominal viscera, or as an intraperitoneal rupture. The presentations of giant hemangioma include obstructive jaundice, biliary colic, torsion of a pedunculated lesion, and gastric outlet obstruction. On physical examination, if a mass is palpable, it is most commonly located in the epigastrium or the left upper quadrant. A bruit is heard only rarely. In patients with intraperitoneal hemorrhage, pain precedes shock by a day or more, thus suggesting subcapsular accumulation of blood. Rupture occurs in a greater proportion of children than adults.

Infants frequently present with an abdominal mass, and a high-output frank congestive heart failure. A large liver, out of proportion to the degree of cardiac failure, an abdominal bruit, and cutaneous hemangiomas may be noted. The latter criteria are frequently absent.

Diagnostic Studies

Liver function tests are generally normal. In newborn infants with hepatic hemangiomas, thrombocytopenia is a rare complication, and it is probably due to an increased mechanical destruction of platelets in the hemangioma. In a series of 38 cases reviewed by Linderkamp and associates, thrombocytopenia was present in 6.

Routine x-ray may demonstrate a soft tissue mass, elevation of the diaphragm, displacement of the stomach, or colon. Tc-99m sulfur colloid scan may show single or multiple areas of de-

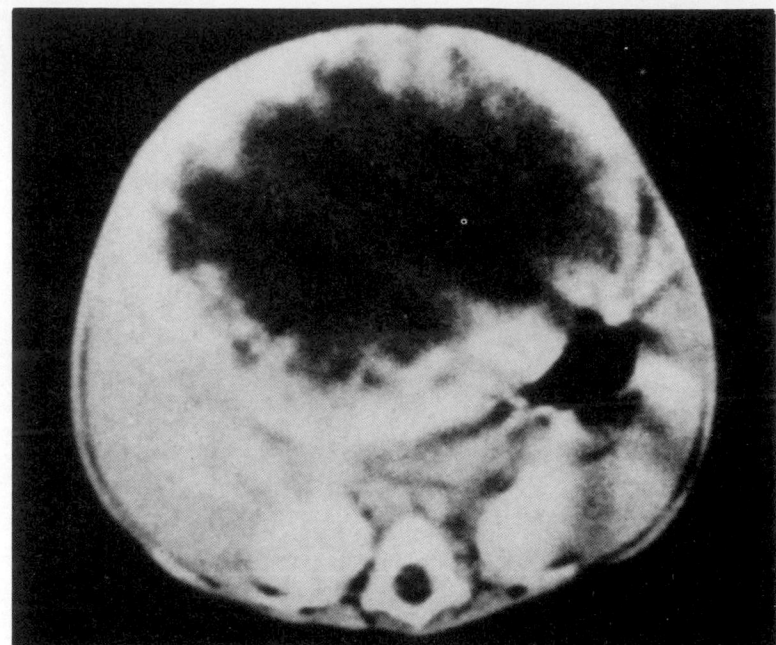

Figure 65–5. CT scan demonstrating early peripheral opacification. (*Source: From Nguyen L, Shandling B, et al, 1982, with permission.*)

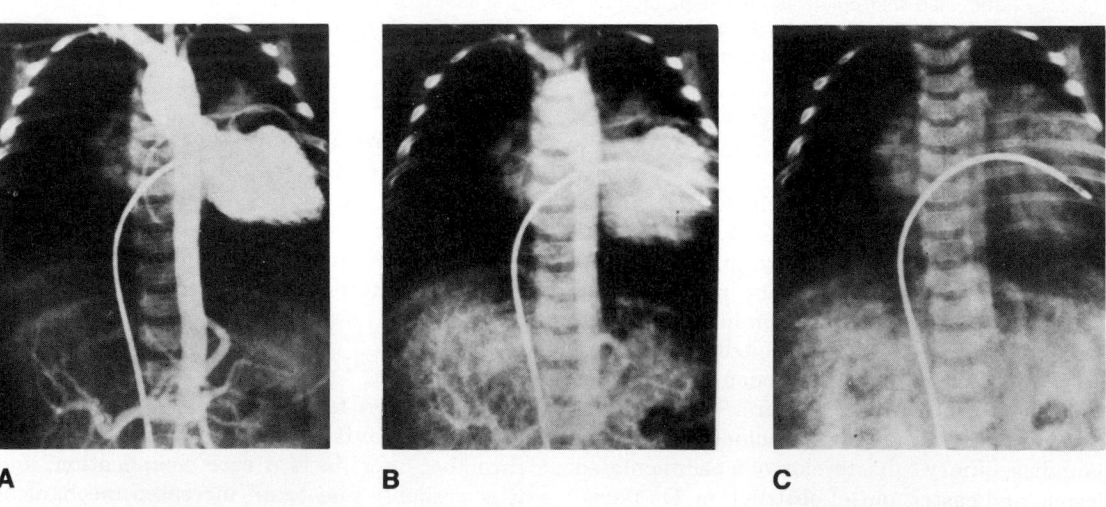

A   B   C

Figure 65–6. A. Large liver and signs of congestive heart failure led to cardiac catheterization. Early roentgenogram of left ventricular injection shows small aorta below hepatic artery. **B.** Late arterial phase shows both hepatic lobes filled with irregular network of abnormal vessels. **C.** Capillary phase shows large draining hepatic veins in both lobes. (*Source: From Slovis TL, Berdon WE, et al, 1975, with permission.*)

creased radioactivity. Although the echogenic pattern is variable, ultrasonography may be helpful in showing the extent of the lesion. A CT scan, when used with contrast material, will show differing degrees of pooling within the tumor (Fig. 65–5). The most valuable examination is the selective angiogram, which demonstrates the vascular character of the tumor, the tortuosity and enlargement of the feeding vessels, and the early venous drainage (Fig. 65–6).

Percutaneous needle biopsy is hazardous because of the danger of hemorrhage.

Treatment

Surgical excision is the preferred treatment of clinically significant hemangiomas of the liver. The extent of resection is dependent upon the size and location of the lesion. Resection of the lesion, plus a rim of normal tissue, is the treatment of choice for selected cavernous hemangiomas of the liver, which can be managed in this fashion. Occasionally large tumors present as predunculated lesions that can be easily excised. The first reported excision of an hemangioma is credited to von Eiselberg in 1893. Larger lesions are best managed by lobectomy along anatomic planes.

Control of bleeding from spontaneous hemorrhage of the cavernous hemangioma has been accomplished with packing and omental tamponade, but resection remains the treatment of choice. Excisional procedures are preferable, since only 1 of 56 patients who underwent excision died postoperatively, while 5 of 11 who did not undergo resection died, as reviewed by Shumacker. Extensive lesions and tumors that are considered nonresectable may benefit from small doses of radiation therapy, which will shrink the size of tumor. Pryles and Heggestad reported the first successful resection of a cavernous hemangioma in an infant. In the review of Linderkamp et al, which considered 38 cases of solitary hepatic hemangioma diagnosed during the first month of life, surgical intervention was performed in 22 patients. Excision of the tumor without lobectomy was possible in 4 cases; there were 14 patients treated by lobectomy, 1 case by partial lobectomy. In three cases an extended lobectomy was performed.

The management of the newborn infant with hemangioma and consequent cardiac failure has proponents of both conservative and aggressive surgical management. Nguyen and associates successfully managed conservatively five children during the first year of life without steroids or radiotherapy. If complications were absent no active treatment was needed, since even large lesions are likely to resolve spontaneously. Goldberg and Fonkalsrud and Touloukian have used steroids successfully in extensive nonresectable tumors. Slovis and associates reported success with a regimen of digitalis and radiation therapy using approximately 350 rads in three treatments. In one patient the size of the tumor regressed within four days. Another patient demonstrated dramatic decrease in liver size and cardiac failure within three days. de Lorimier was the first to report success for hepatic artery ligation as a means of reversing the cardiac failure; it seems the most appropriate method for cardiac failure due to diffuse hepatic hemangiomatosis. Linderkamp's review suggests that in infants with giant solitary hepatic hemangioma, excision of the tumor is the treatment of choice since there was only 1 death among the 22 surgically treated patients with symptoms during the first year of life, whereas 15 of the conservatively treated patients died.

ADENOMA

Both liver cell adenoma and focal nodular hyperplasia occur mostly in females in the menstrual age range. The terms have been used interchangably, and the two lesions have been lumped into a single category of tumors associated with the use of oral contraceptives. Edmondson and Ishak and Rabin consider the two lesions separate entities. Since there are important differences, this chapter presents the two lesions independently and refers to the shared features.

Incidence

In the survey of solid liver tumors conducted in 1974 by Foster and Berman, 37 cases were classified as liver cell adenoma; 34 were in female patients and 27 of the 34 were in the age group between 20 and 40. Nine of the 37 patients, including 4 menstruating females, 2 aged females, and 3 males, had never taken contraceptive medication.

The incidence has increased, as evidenced by the fact that Edmondson found only two hepatic cell adenomas in the review of 418 hepatic tumors in 50,000 autopsies over a 36-year period. Between 1961 and 1980, 23 patients with hepatic adenoma were seen at the Mayo Clinic. A registry for liver tumors associated with oral contraceptives was established early in 1975. This registry collated data on over 90 patients in a 3-year period. Included in the registry are patients with focal nodular hyperplasia, hepatocellular adenoma, hamartoma, and peliosis hepatis, since the terms overlap.

Etiology

Nissen et al, reporting on the role of oral contraceptive agents based on their registry data, indicate that all eight progesterones and both synthetic estrogens have been associated with the appearance of liver tumors. More than 60 percent of the patients were exposed to mestranol only, and 80 percent were exposed to a mestranol product. It is felt that inability to demethylate mestranol in the smooth endoplasmic reticulum of hepatocytes may allow massive accumulative of oncogenic metabolites.

More than half the patients used the pill continuously for over 5 years, and 85 percent of the women were exposed to contraceptive steroids for over 4 years. The shortest duration of use was 6 months, by one patient, and the mean duration of usage was 58.8 months. Peliosis hepatis, i.e., large blood spaces without endothelial linings, which is seen at the periphery of the tumor, has been noted in patients taking oral contraceptives, and also in men on androgenic steroid therapy. Sherlock has reported a hepatic adenoma in a postmenopausal woman receiving hormonal replacement.

An association between oral contraceptive medication and liver cell adenoma is stronger than that for focal nodular hyperplasia. Liver cell adenomas that occur in women on oral contraceptive medication are more likely to undergo necrosis and to rupture than are adenomas occurring in patients who have not taken oral contraceptives. Occurrence of liver cell adenoma has been documented after cessation of oral contraceptives in some patients, but progression has also been reported.

Pathology

On gross examination (Fig. 65–7) the lesions are soft, fleshy tumors with smooth surfaces that occasionally have large vessels coursing over the area. On cross-section there are frequently

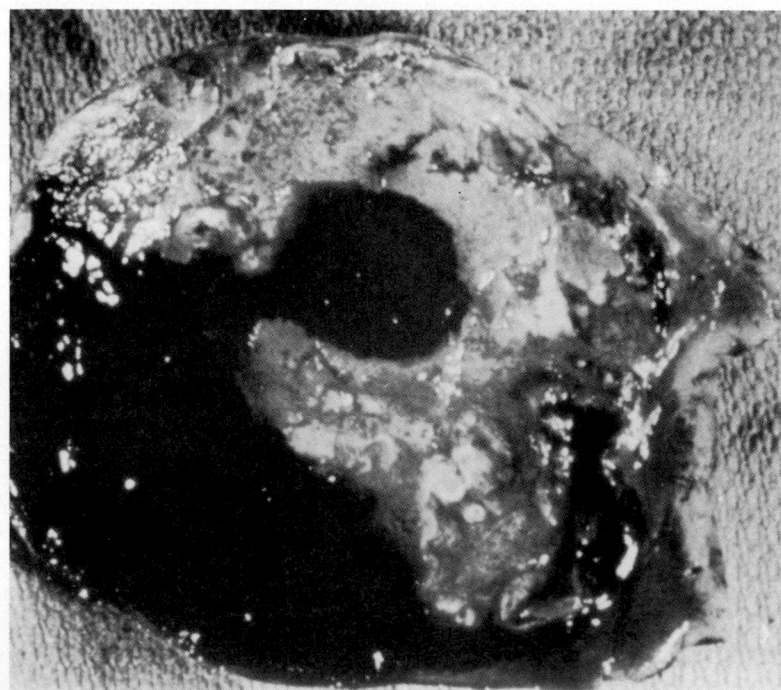

Figure 65–7. Liver cell adenoma resected with a narrow rim of normal liver from a 32-year-old woman with acute abdominal pain and hemoperitoneum. Note light-color tumor, hemorrhage, and necrosis. (*Source; From Foster JH, Berman MM, 1977, with permission.*)

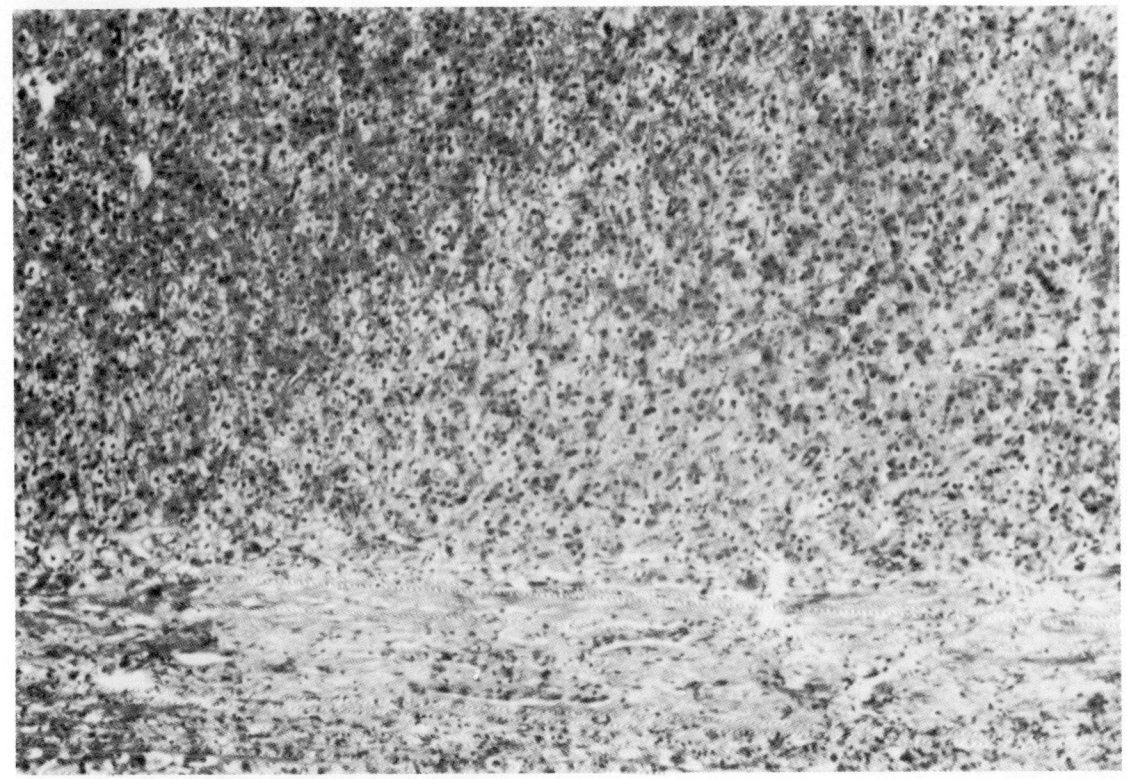

Figure 65–8. Hepatocellular adenoma. Peripheral section of an adenoma with a fibrous capsule component and a homogenous monotonous arrangement of hepatocyte cords without blood vessel or bile duct structures. (*Source: From Foster JH, Berman MM, 1977, with permission.*)

areas of hemorrhage and necrosis. Microscopically, the hepatic adenomas are characterized by monotonous sheets of mature hepatocytes that are often smaller than normal, and may contain glycogen (Fig. 65–8). The lesion is devoid of bile ducts, portal triads, or central veins but may contain areas of peliosis hepatitis. Histologically, large zones of necrotic ghost cells are noted in areas of hemorrhage.

Clinical Manifestations

The lesions present in one of four ways: (1) as asymptomatic tumors noted incidentally during a CT scan, ultrasound, or at operation, (2) as a liver mass, (3) with pain in the upper abdomen, probably indicative of bleeding into the tumor and stretching of the liver capsule, and (4) with shock due to rupture of the lesion and intraperitoneal hemorrhage. Recurrent pallor, diaphoresis, hypotension, and syncope have also been reported. About one third of the reported pa-

tients have presented with intraperitoneal bleeding. The diagnosis should be considered particularly in a woman of childbearing age who has been on oral contraceptive medication and who presents with the triad of right upper quadrant or epigastric pain associated with shock and hemoperitoneum.

Diagnostic Studies

There are no currently available testing methods for identifying a patient at risk. In patients with established hepatic cell adenoma, the liver enzyme values are of limited usefulness. The α-fetoprotein is negative, as is the hepatitis B surface antigen determination. Tc-99m sulfur colloid liver scan will reveal a filling defect in about 85 percent of patients. Ultrasound generally defines a solid, filling defect. CT scan and angiogram are particularly useful (Figs. 65–9 and 65–10). Liver scan demonstrates a filling defect; the angiogram reveals a hypervascular

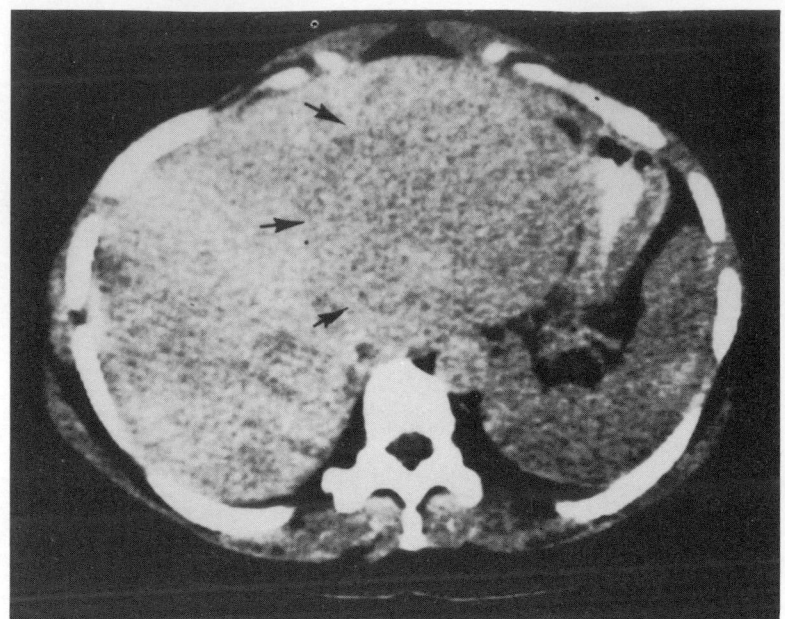

Figure 65–9. CT scan showing a solid, low density mass occupied most of the left lobe of the liver (*arrows*). (*Source: From Gutierrez OH, Schwartz SI: Atlas of Hepatic Tumors and Focal Lesions. New York: McGraw-Hill, 1984, p 83, with permission.*)

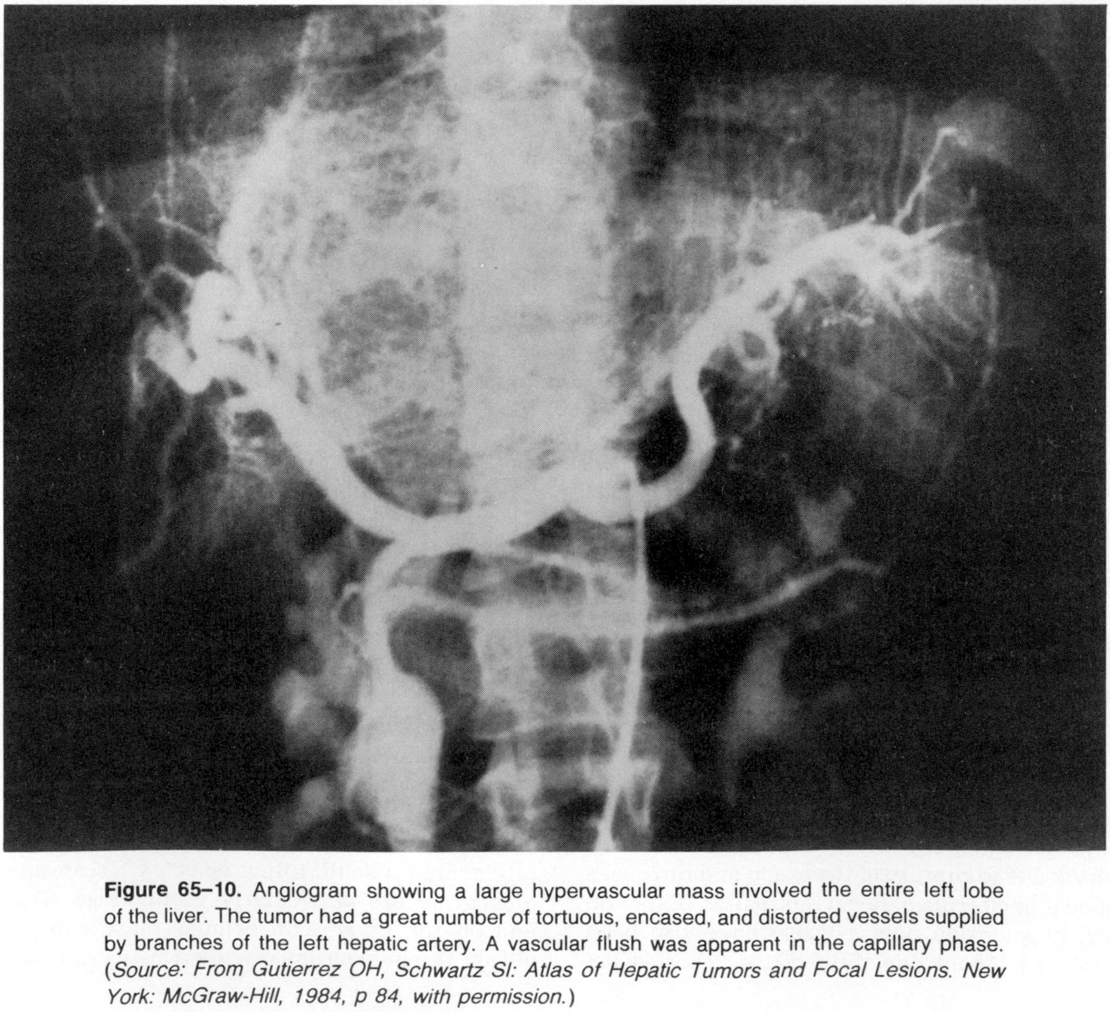

Figure 65–10. Angiogram showing a large hypervascular mass involved the entire left lobe of the liver. The tumor had a great number of tortuous, encased, and distorted vessels supplied by branches of the left hepatic artery. A vascular flush was apparent in the capillary phase. (*Source: From Gutierrez OH, Schwartz SI: Atlas of Hepatic Tumors and Focal Lesions. New York: McGraw-Hill, 1984, p 84, with permission.*)

lesion that may contain hypovascular regions related to tumor bleeding or necrosis. There is frequently distortion and displacement of hepatic vessels, coupled with small, tortuous abnormal vessels in the periphery of the lesion. Needle biopsy of the liver, previously thought to be contraindicated because of the danger of bleeding, is now advocated by some as a method for differentiating benign from malignant lesions. Biopsy of a patient with hepatic cell adenoma frequently demonstrates normal hepatic structure and cellular elements.

Treatment

In general, a conservative approach is reasonable if a malignancy can be ruled out. The asymptomatic patients, presenting with an abdominal mass, require exploratory surgery to define the nature and extent of the lesion. If there is a superficial, solitary, or pedunculated lesion, a wedge resection, including a small portion of normal liver, is preferable. With larger lesions,

incisional biopsy and frozen section will provide the diagnosis. If the tumor displays evidence of hemorrhage, infarction, omental or visceral adhesions, wider excision is indicated.

Regression of liver cell adenoma has been documented after cessation of oral contraceptives by Edmondson and associates. Kent and associates reported enhanced growth of unresected steroid-induced adenomas during pregnancy. This has led to catastrophic consequences, and therefore it is felt that the patient with hormone-dependent tumor should be enjoined from pregnancy and should not receive exogenous steroid hormones. If the patient anticipates a future pregnancy, the lesion should certainly be removed totally. The patient who presents with a suggestive diagnosis of intraperitoneal bleeding due to rupture of such a lesion requires urgent exploration.

It has been the experience of Terblanche that hepatic artery ligation proved adequate to control bleeding. Most cases have required resection, including a narrow margin of liver tis-

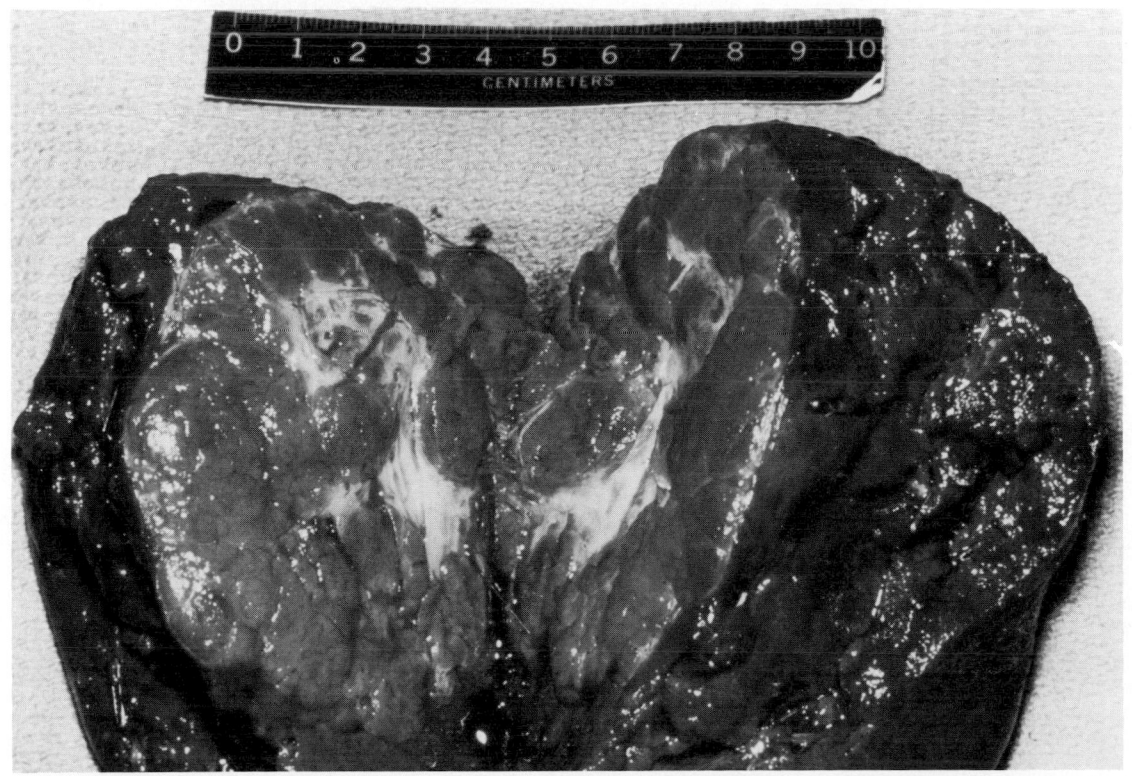

Figure 65–11. Cut section of focal nodular hyperplasia showing lesion with central stellate scar made of fibrous tissue.

sue. If facilities, or the surgeon's experience, preclude resection, packing without ligation of the appropriate hepatic artery may allow time for transfer of the patient to another hospital for definitive therapy.

In the 1974 liver survey, 19 patients had sublobar wedge resection and 3 of these died perioperatively. Nine right lobectomies were done, with one operating room death, and there were three extended right lobectomies, one extended left lobectomy, and two left lobectomies and two left lateral segmentectomies without perioperative deaths. There was no evidence of any recurrent disease in the survivors who were examined from 2 to 101 months after resection.

Total resection was accomplished in 17 of 19 patients in the Mayo Clinic experience; in 2 patients the lesion was deemed unresectable at the time of operation. There was one operative death. The patients discontinued oral contraceptives and remained asymptomatic, and

there was no evidence of recurrence documented with imaging studies.

FOCAL NODULAR HYPERPLASIA

Incidence

In the 1974 liver tumor survey, 63 cases met the criteria for focal nodular hyperplasia, contrasted with the 37 cases categorized as liver cell adenoma. Fifty seven were female, and the majority of cases occurred between age 20 and 50. Eight were seen in patients under the age of 10, the youngest a 10-month-old male infant, and the oldest a 70-year-old female. Focal nodular hyperplasia was also more common in the Mayo Clinic experience, occurring almost twice as frequently as the hepatic cell adenoma. The mean age of the patients with focal nodular hyperplasia was much higher than that in patients with hepatic adenoma, i.e., 41 versus 34 years.

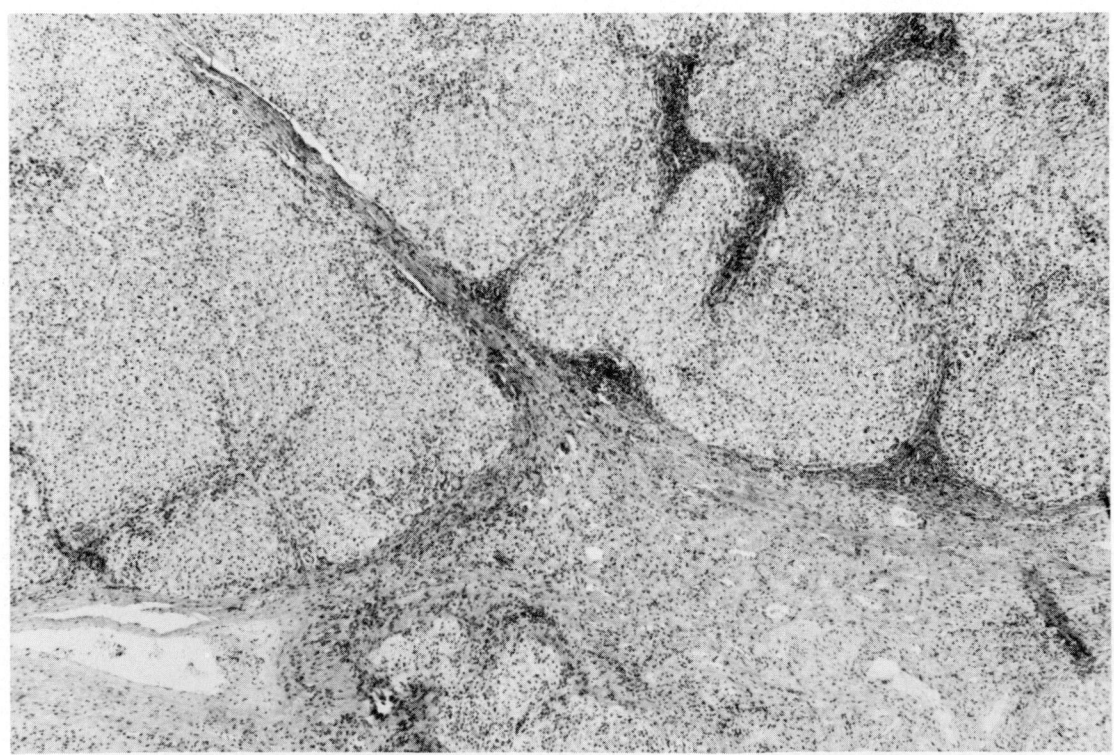

Figure 65–12. Microscopic section of focal nodular hyperplasia showing fibrous band containing bile ducts and surrounding hepatic tissue with nodular appearance. (*Source: From Gutierrez OH, Schwartz SI: Atlas of Hepatic Tumors and Focal Lesions. New York: McGraw-Hill, 1984, p 99, with permission.*)

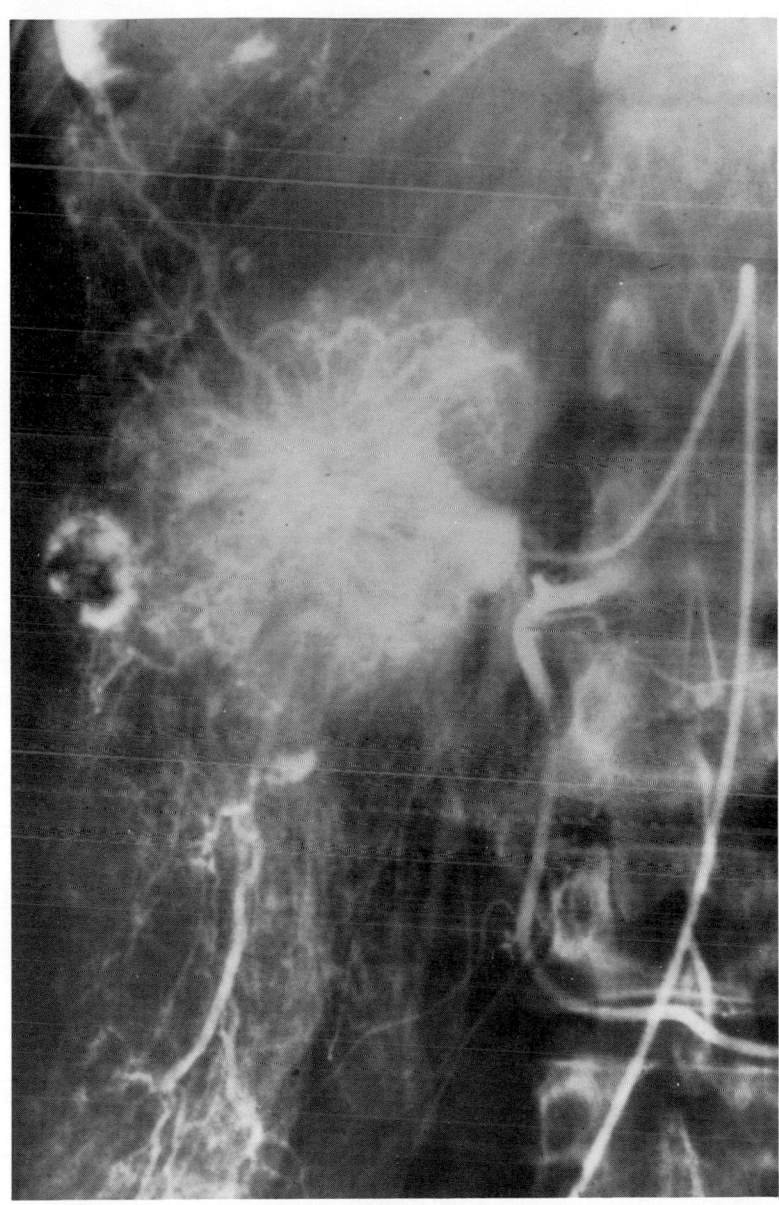

Figure 65–13. Angiogram demonstrating hypervascular tumor and characteristic stellate distribution of blood cells. Note hemangiomas in upper and lower portions of right lobe.

Etiology

Since focal nodular hyperplasias frequently occur in women not on oral contraceptive medication, and in males, many feel that the lesion is neither a neoplasm nor a hamartoma, but rather a reaction to injury. When a reliable history is obtained, only 58 percent of women with focal nodular hyperplasia gave a history of oral contraceptive use, contrasted with almost 90 percent of women with hepatic cell adenoma.

Pathology

The tumors are usually solitary, and less than 5 cm in diameter. They are frequently found near the free edge of the liver; they are grossly nodular with surface scarring and blood vessels. On cut section they are tan in color, and present with a classic central stellate fibrous scar (Fig. 65–11). They may or may not have a capsule. The histologic appearance is characterized by fibrous bands that contain numerous bile ducts.

The hepatocytes are arranged in chords and separated by sinusoids; the cells appear normal. The overall appearance resembles a regenerating nodule with the cirrhotic liver (Fig. 65–12). The nuclei show no evidence of pyknosis or mitosis. Characteristically there is absence of hemorrhage or necrosis.

Clinical Manifestations

The overwhelming majority of cases of focal nodular hyperplasia—90 percent in the Mayo Clinic series—were discovered incidentally. No patient presented with shock or pain due to intraperitoneal rupture of the tumor in that series or in the experience of the 1974 survey by Foster and Berman. A palpable mass was noted in approximately 10 percent of cases; abdominal pain was even a rarer symptom.

Diagnostic Studies

The liver function tests usually reveal no abnormalities. The serum markers for the hepatitis B virus and α-fetoprotein are negative. Tc-99m sulfur colloid scans could detect only half these lesions, and ultrasound and CT examinations also frequently fail to define the lesion, since the major bulk is isodense. The angiogram, however, is diagnostic, demonstrating a hypervascular tumor with large arteries and evidence of arteriovenous shunting. There is a characteristic stellate distribution of the blood vessels (Fig. 65–13).

Treatment

A conservative approach toward this lesion is indicated. When it is found incidentally at laparotomy, a wedge biopsy should be performed to provide diagnosis. Smaller lesions may be removed, but the larger focal nodular hyperplasias should be left. Oral contraceptive medication should be discontinued, and there is no suggestion that pregnancy should be discouraged in these patients because necrosis and rupture of these tumors during pregnancy rarely have been reported. The follow-up of patients subjected to resection for up to 256 months after the operation has failed to reveal a single incidence of persistence, recurrence, or metastasis. There is little to justify the suggestion that hepatic artery ligation be used for unresectable focal nodular hyperplasias.

BIBLIOGRAPHY

de Lorimier AA: Hepatic tumors of infancy and childhood. Surg Clin N Am 57:443, 1977

Edmondson HA: Tumors of the liver and intrahepatic bile ducts, in Atlas of Tumor Pathology. Armed Forces Institute of Pathology, Section VII, Fascicle 25, 1958

Edmondson HA, Reynolds TB, et al: Regression of liver cell adenomas associated with oral contraceptives. Ann Intern Med 86:180, 1977

Foster JH, Berman MM: Solid Liver Tumors. Philadelphia: WB Saunders, 1977

Geist DC: Solitary nonparasitic cyst of the liver. Arch Surg 71:867, 1955

Goldberg SJ, Fonkalsrud E: Successful treatment of hepatic haemangioma with corticosteroids. JAMA 208:2473, 1969

Hadad AR, Westbrook KC, et al: Symptomatic nonparasitic liver cysts. Am J Surg 134:739, 1977

Henson SW, Gray HK, et al: Benign tumors of the liver III. Solitary cysts. Surg Gynecol Obstet 103:607, 1956

Ishak KG, Rabin L: Benign tumors of the liver. Med Clin North Am 59:995, 1975

Kent DR, Nissen ED, et al: Maternal death resulting from rupture of a liver adenoma associated with oral contraceptives. Obstet Gynecol 50:5, 1977

Kerlin P, Davis GL, et al: Hepatic adenoma and focal nodular hyperplasia: Clinical, pathologic, and radiologic features. Gastroenterology 84:994, 1983

Koren E, Lazarovitch I, et al: Cystic hamartoma of the liver. Int Surg 64:21, 1979

Linderkamp O, Hopner F, et al: Solitary hepatic hemangioma in a newborn infant complicated by cardiac failure, consumption coagulopathy, microangiopathic hemolytic anemia, and obstructive jaundice. Eur J Pediat 124:23, 1976

Longmire WR Jr, Mandiola SA, et al: Congenital cystic disease of the liver and biliary system. Ann Surg 174:711, 1971

Moazam F, Rodgers BM, et al: Hepatic artery ligation for hepatic hemangiomatosis of infancy. J Pediatr Surg 18:120, 1983

Nissen ED, Kent DR, et al: Role of oral contraceptive agents in the pathogenesis of liver tumors. Toxicol Environ Health 5:231, 1979

Nguyen L, Shandling B, et al: Hepatic hemangioma in childhood: Medical management or surgical management. J Pediatr Surg 17:576, 1982

Rooks JB, Ory HW, et al: Epidemiology of hepatocellular adenoma. The role of oral contraceptive use. JAMA 242:644, 1979

Sanfelippo RM, Beahrs OH, et al: Cystic disease of the liver. Ann Surg 179:922, 1974

Sherlock S: Progress report. Hepatic adenomas and oral contraceptives. Gut 16:753, 1975

Shumacker HB Jr: Hemangioma of the liver: Discussion of symptomatology and report of patient treated by operation. Surgery 11:209, 1942

Slovis TL, Berdan WE, et al: Hemangiomas of the liver in infants. Am J Roentgen Rad Ther Nucl Med 123:791, 1975

Srouji MN, Chatten J, et al: Mesenchymal hamartoma of the liver in infants. Cancer 42:2483, 1978

Terblanche J: Liver tumours associated with the use of contraceptive pills. S Afr Med J 53:439, 1978

Touloukian RJ: Hepatic hemangioendothelioma during infancy: pathology, diagnosis, and treatment with prednisone. Pediatrics 45:71, 1970

Williamson RCN, Ramus NI, et al: Congenital solitary cysts of the liver and spleen. Br J Surg 65:871, 1978

66. Primary and Metastatic Malignant Tumors

Seymour I. Schwartz

INTRODUCTION

Malignant tumors of the liver include a variety of primary carcinomas originating from epithelial cells and primary tumors deriving from vascular and connective tissue elements, in addition to a broad spectrum of metastatic neoplasms. Although each group possesses a uniqueness, the primary and metastatic lesions are properly considered together because many of the clinical manifestations, diagnostic studies, and therapeutic principles are common to all hepatic tumors. There has been an exponential growth in the reports of liver tumors in the literature; this is related to the increasing surgical concern for hepatic tumors as a consequence of refinements in diagnostic studies and more liberal applicability of resection and isolated perfusion therapy.

HISTORICAL BACKGROUND

Cruveilhier, in 1829, classified cancer as the most serious and frequent disease of the liver. In 1855, Rokitansky distinguished between primary and secondary hepatic malignancies. Virchow's dictum that "organs commonly affected by metastases were rarely the site of primary neoplasia" probably contributed to the delay between the pathologic and clinical recognition of primary carcinoma of the liver. Two cases presented by Kelsch and Kiener in 1876 represent the first distinct clinical report of primary carcinoma of the liver. Major modern additions to our appreciation of solid liver tumors include the contributions regarding pathology by Edmondson and the clinical collations of Foster and Berman.

INCIDENCE

Primary Neoplasms

Primary Epithelial Carcinomas

Liver Cell Carcinoma. The incidence of primary hepatocellular carcinoma varies widely around the world, from less than 1 case per 100,000 in parts of the Western world to over 60 per 100,000 in areas of Africa. The annual incidence of reported cases in the United States is approximately 4 per 100,000 population. Primary epithelial hepatic carcinoma is detected in 0.15 to 0.35 percent of all autopsies. The highest frequency of carcinoma of the liver is observed in Africa, where the postmortem rate averages 1.1 percent, with hepatic carcinoma representing 17 to 53 percent of all cancers. In South African Bantus, the tumor is responsible for over 80 percent of all carcinomas. In Southeast Asia, there has been a reported incidence of 2.4 percent in autopsy series.

Primary epithelial carcinoma of the liver has been reported in all age groups, from the newborn infant to the elderly adult. In children, 53 percent of these tumors occurred under the age of 2, and 68 percent of the patients were male. The majority of the pediatric epithelial carcinomas were of the liver cell type, with a ratio of 60 hepatocellular carcinomas to 3 of bile duct origin. In European adults, the lesion appears mainly in the fifth and sixth decades.

In Africa and Asia, the peak age is between 20 and 40. Cholangiocarcinomas occur at a later age than hepatocellular carcinomas.

Adult primary carcinoma of the liver occurs with greater frequency in the male. The corrected sex ratio for liver cell carcinoma has varied from two to six males for each female patient; this difference also pertains to primary cholangiocarcinoma.

In children, hepatocellular carcinoma accounts for 2 percent of childhood malignancies; males predominate, and the usual age range is about 5 to 15 years. Hepatocellular carcinoma and hepatoblastoma account for two thirds of primary hepatic tumors. Cholangiocarcinoma is virtually nonexistent in childhood.

Hepatoblastoma usually affects children less than 2 years old, with a male to female ratio of 6:1. Fibrolamellar carcinoma, a variant of hepatocellular carcinoma with a propensity for adolescents and young adults, manifests a distinct difference in incidence. The mean age of patients is 26.4 years, and there is equal sex incidence.

Sarcomas

Sarcomas of the liver are rare lesions; the annual incidence is approximately 0.014 cases per 100,000 population. Over the past decade, there has been a significant increase in the number of cases of angiosarcoma.

Secondary Neoplasms

Metastatic neoplasms represent the most common malignant tumors of the liver. The organ is second only to regional lymph nodes as the site for metastasis for intestinal tumors. From 25 to 50 percent of all patients dying of cancer have been found to have hepatic metastases at autopsy. In one large series, the following incidences of liver metastases were established for a variety of primary sites:

Stomach	45 percent
Colon	65 percent
Rectum	47 percent
Pancreas	63 percent
Breast	61 percent
Lung	36 percent
Ovary	52 percent
Kidney	27 percent

In the pediatric age group, metastatic tumors also were significantly more common than primary lesions.

ETIOLOGY AND PATHOGENESIS

Just as almost every type of experimentally induced cirrhosis may be followed by carcinoma of the liver, so a definite association between cirrhosis and primary carcinoma has been noted in the human being. Almost three quarters of the adult cases have been associated with cirrhosis. There is a more pronounced association with hepatocellular type lesions than with the cholangiocarcinomas. In the experience of Edmondson and Steiner, the frequency of cirrhosis was recorded as 89 percent in the liver cell group and 24 percent in the bile duct group.

Laennec's cirrhosis, secondary to malnutrition or to alcoholism, is the type most frequently implicated. Hepatic malignancy was reported to be present in 4.5 percent of approximately 2000 cases of hepatic cirrhosis. Primary hepatic carcinoma is also associated with hemochromatosis, occurring in approximately 10 percent of cases. The question remains unanswered whether hepatitis B virus is a direct etiologic factor or whether it acts through its ability to produce cirrhosis.

A lack of an association with cirrhosis is the principal difference between childhood and adult hepatocellular carcinoma, the incidence of associated cirrhosis in children being only 5 to 6 percent. It has been suggested that birth control pills have a causative relationship with fibrolamellar carcinoma of the liver in young adults. Evidence, however, against oral contraceptive therapy as an etiologic factor is (1) an equal sex incidence in patients and (2) many patients were less than 18 years old and had not been taking contraceptive therapy for 5 years, the time considered necessary for the development of hepatocellular tumors. Another factor associated with hepatocellular carcinoma is aberrant α_1-antitrypsin-pi Z.

A number of specific carcinogens have been associated with angiosarcoma of the liver. A review of 103 cases in the English literature by Locker and associates uncovered 15 patients exposed to thorotrast. There was a mean latency period of 24 years from injection to tumor presentation, with a range of 12 to 35 years. Twenty patients developed angiosarcoma of the liver after vinyl chloride exposure. The mean time from first exposure to development of the tumor was 19 years, with a range of 11 to 37 years. Two patients were exposed to arsenicals with ingestion of Fowler's solution (1 percent arsenic) for 17 and 25 years. One case of hepatic angiosarcoma occurred in a patient who had been treated for breast carcinoma by radium needle implant.

Metastatic neoplasms reach the liver by four routes: (1) through the portal venous circulation, (2) via lymphatic spread, (3) by way of the hepatic arterial system, and (4) by direct extension from adjacent viscera. The venous route of transport is by far the most common. Metastases are found in the liver of approximately half the patients in whom an organ drained by the portal vein is involved. Primary colonic carcinoma heads the list as a consequence of the frequency of the lesion itself. Carcinoid is the most common small intestine lesion that involves the liver with metastatic implantation. Although hepatic involvement from carcinoma of the genitourinary system is less common, malignancies from these organs can invade tributaries of the portal vein in adjacent tissues and reach the liver by this route. Hepatic involvement via the lymph channels also occurs in organs drained by the portal venous system. In addition, the lymphatic route is implicated in the development of liver metastases from primary sites in the breast and lung, draining via the mediastinal nodes. The hepatic arterial system offers another avenue from both primary and secondary neoplasms of the lung and melanoma, either of the cutaneous or ocular type. Local spread by direct extension applies to carcinoma of the biliary tract, stomach, and colon. Direct spread from carcinoma of the gallbladder is reported in 50 to 72 percent of patients.

PATHOLOGY

Malignant tumors of the liver may be classified as primary epithelial carcinomas (including hepatocellular carcinoma, cholangiocarcinoma, and hepatoblastoma), mesenchymomas, mixed tumors, sarcomas, and secondary tumors.

Gross Pathology

Gross patterns of hepatocellular carcinoma include nodular, massive, and diffuse types. The right lobe is more frequently involved than the left, probably because it represents a greater portion of hepatic mass. The nodular type of lesion consists of an aggregate of clusters of similarly sized nodules that are closely packed and surrounded by a thin, fibrous capsule. The massive type consists of a single, large, predominant

mass and may be associated with satellites. The diffuse type, which is the rarest, is characterized by a widespread fine nodular pattern, usually involving the entire liver. Umbilication is rare, but central necrosis of the tumor is common.

On cut section, hepatocellular carcinomas are usually soft and vascular, and the color varies in accordance with the degree of cellular maturity, the presence of bile, necrosis, and hemorrhage. The more mature lesions have a light brown appearance, and the immature ones are grey. Grossly apparent venous thrombosis occurs with relative frequency in hepatocellular carcinomas, and in one series tumor thrombi were macroscopically demonstrated in one third of the patients within the portal veins or the hepatic veins or their major branches.

Cholangiocarcinomas also exhibit massive nodular or diffuse patterns, but they are usually greyish white in color and less vascular. Necrosis of these lesions is uncommon, and venous invasion is rare.

On gross examination, hepatoblastoma is generally a single, lobulated, or nodular mass, with a mean diameter of 10 to 12 cm, occupying the right lobe of the liver in about two thirds of patients. Multinodular or diffuse involvement of both lobes is present in about one third of patients. A thin, compressed rim of fibrous tissue is frequently noted at the periphery of the lesion.

The fibrolamellar carcinoma of the liver may present as a large solitary tumor or in the multinodular fashion. The anatomic distribution of this tumor is unusual in that 75 percent of the recorded cases have been in the left lobe. The tumor may have a prominent depressed fibrous scar in the central area, and many of the lesions have weighed more than 1200 g.

The mesenchymal tumors, including mixed tumor, rhabdomyosarcoma, angiosarcoma, and undifferentiated sarcoma, vary in appearance. The rhabdomyosarcoma has a glistening, greyish-tan, mucoid appearance. The tumor may extend throughout the hepatobiliary tract, and there are frequently areas of hemorrhage and necrosis. The malignant mesenchymal tumor, also known as an undifferentiated sarcoma, may present as a large solitary circumscribed tumor, which, on cut surface, is demarcated from the adjacent parenchyma. The central portion is frequently cystic in nature, and hemorrhagic areas may be noted. Angiosarcoma has a greyish appearance and is very vascular as it extends throughout the hepatic mass.

Metastatic lesions are generally located immediately beneath Glisson's capsule and generally present as multiple nodules that vary in size and color. The individual nodules are usually discrete, and metastases from intestinal primary tumors have a characteristic umbilicated appearance. In the child, the most common tumor metastatic to the liver is neuroblastoma; in this circumstance the liver is enlarged, and there may be different types of involvement. Frequently, large, multiple, greyish tan nodules, 1 to 3 cm in diameter, are noted, but the tumor may present with small miliary lesions. Hepatic metastases from the Wilms' tumor also may be single or multiple and are soft, greyish masses, usually with a diameter greater than 1 cm.

Microscopic Pathology

Hepatocellular Carcinoma. This lesion is characterized by cells that possess an acido-philic cytoplasm and large nuclei containing acidophilic nucleoli (Fig. 66–1). In well-differentiated cases, they are also strikingly similar to normal liver cells, whereas in more anaplastic cases, the similarity becomes decreasingly apparent. The basic structure appears to be trabecular (Fig. 66–2); the trabeculae may be small and thin or plump. The plates contain several bile canaliculi and are surrounded by sinusoids and an argentaffin network. Under low power magnification, a pseudolobular appearance may be noted, particularly when the reticulum becomes collagenized because of pressure of the expanding tumor. Hepatocellular carcinomas frequently invade branches of the veins, causing vascular dilatation, which, in itself, contributes to the nodular appearance of the liver. Hemorrhage and central necrosis may be apparent. The formation of giant cells is a feature of hepatocellular carcinoma, and a predominance of such cells produces a relatively rare "giant cell carcinoma" in which the trabecular structure

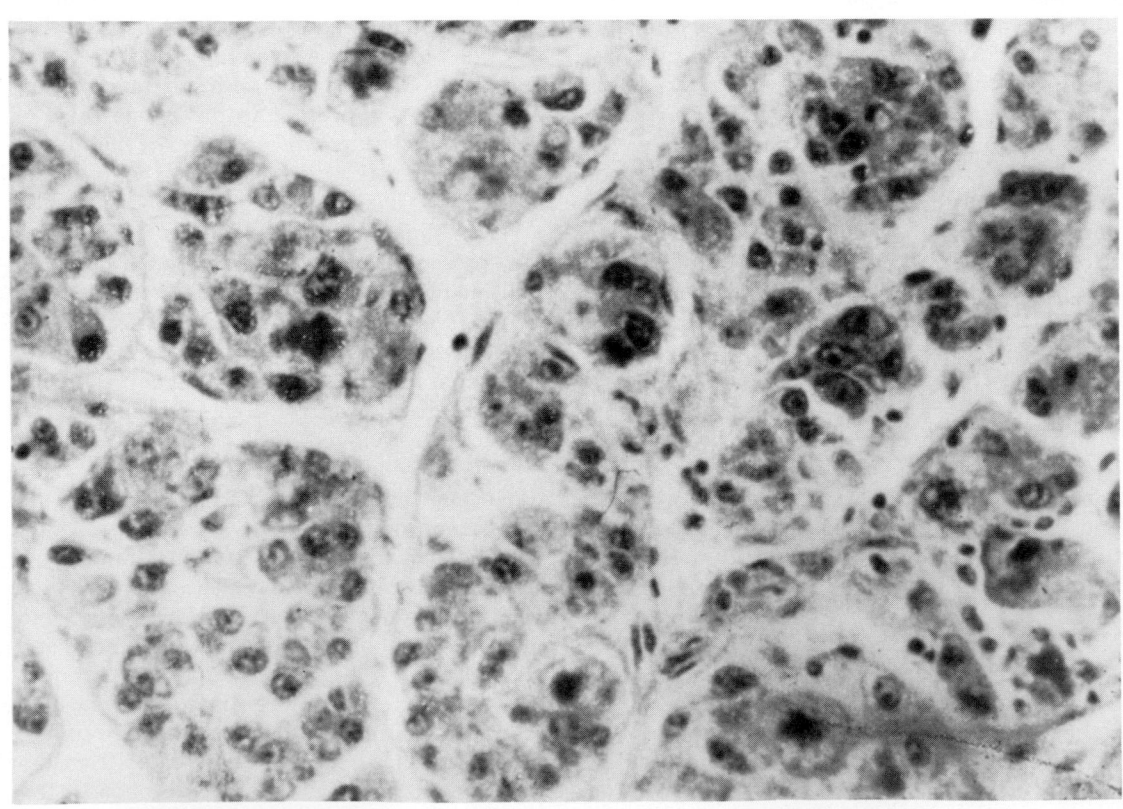

Figure 66–1. Higher magnification of carcinoma cells. (*Source: From Schwartz SI, 1964, with permission.*)

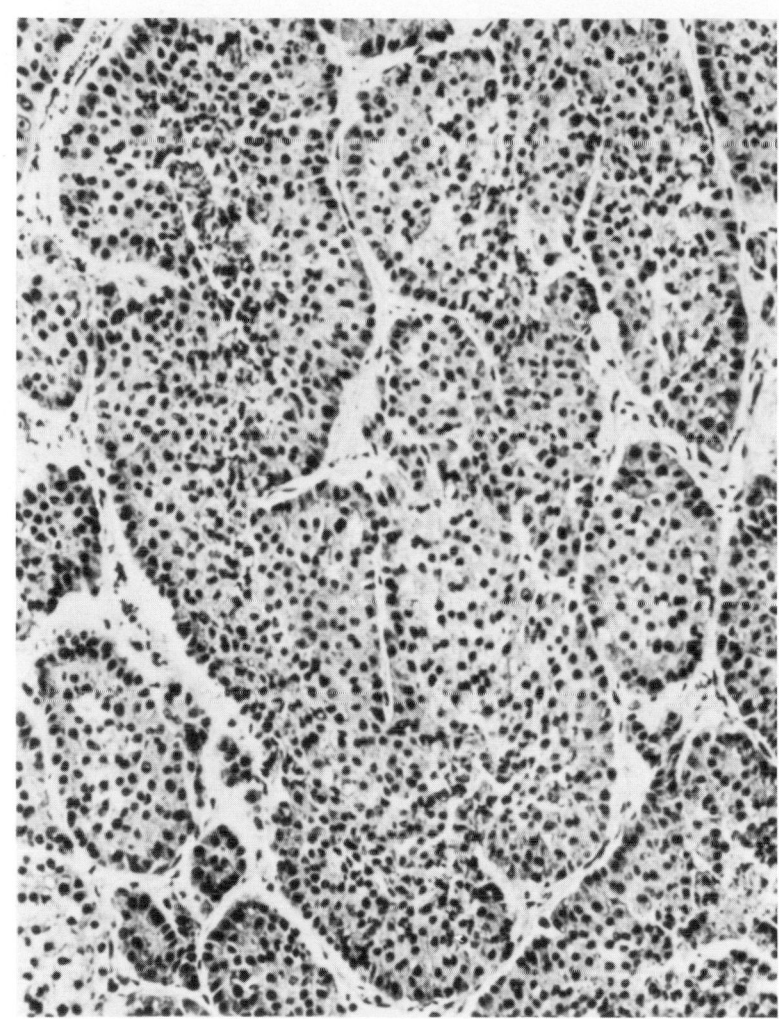

Figure 66–2. Histologic section of a liver cell carcinoma, grade II. Plump cells in closely packed trabecular configuration. (*Source: From Edmonson HA, 1954, with permission.*)

is usually absent. Hepatocellular carcinoma in childhood does not differ from the adult counterpart in its pathologic features.

Fibrolamellar carcinoma of the liver is a variant of hepatocellular carcinoma, with distinctive morphologic features. Two characteristic features of this variant are (1) deeply eosinophilic hepatocytes and (2) abundant fibrous stroma arranged in thin parallel bands around the tumor cells. The malignant hepatocytes have varying shapes, ranging from polygonal to spindle forms, with eosinophilic granular cytoplasm. About half the tumors have isolated tumor cells that contain sharply defined, pale, cytoplasmic bodies, the margins of which are distinct. Mitotic figures are rare, and occasional foci of multinucleated hepatocytes are present. Large areas of necrosis or pelioid patterns may

be noted. The tumors are of medium grade and are never highly anaplastic. The fibrous stroma divides the eosinophilic hepatocytes into thin columns of two to six cells or into larger nodules of hundreds of cells or grows as trabeculae into the tumor (Fig. 66–3). The fibrous stroma comprises many thin, hyalinized bands in layers, suggesting a laminated composition and leading to the term "fibrolamellar." The bands may coalesce and form thick bands and scars, producing a central depression and accounting for the gross similarity to focal nodular hyperplasia.

Cholangiocarcinoma. The histologic appearance of this lesion is that of an adenomatous tumor with a scirrhous background (Fig. 66–4). The cell type is columnar, with a small nucleus and a less prominent nucleolus. Bile is never

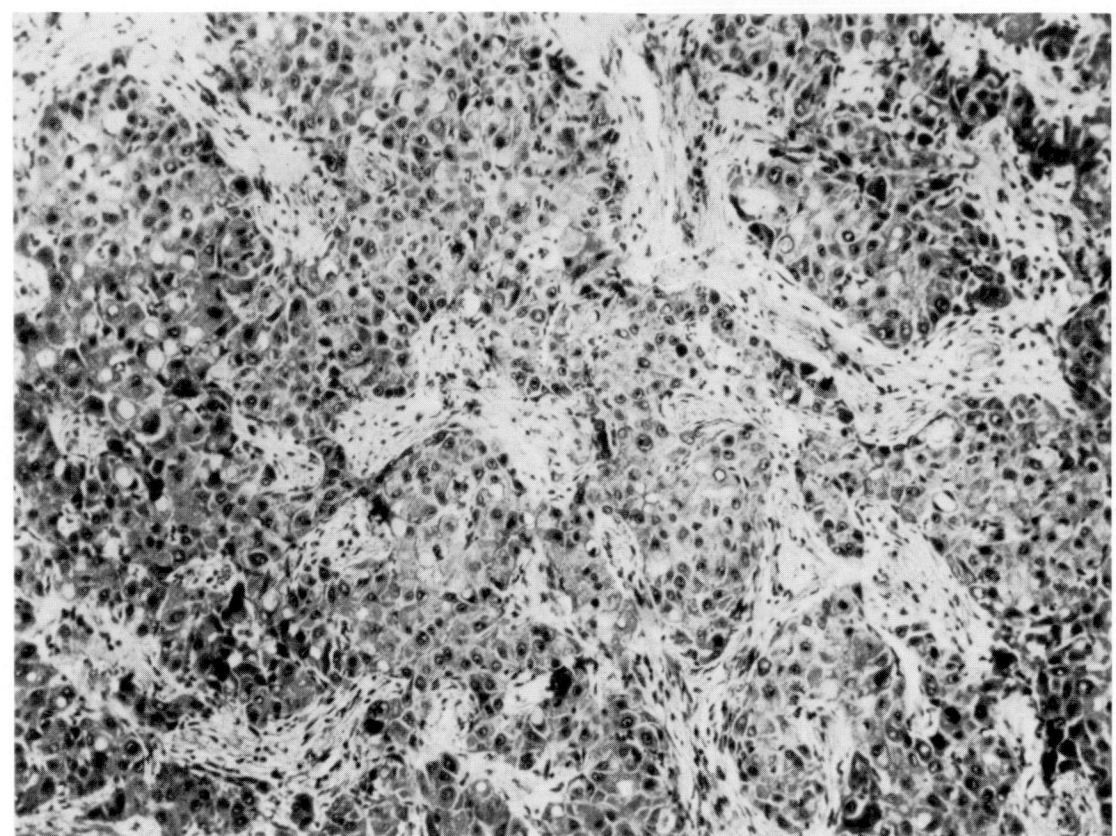

Figure 66–3. Mixture of lamellar fibrosis with moderate sized trabeculae of fibrolamellar carcinoma (×120). (*Source: From Craig JR, Peters RL, et al, 1980, with permission.*)

seen in the acini or cells, whereas mucus formation is quite common. The degree of connective tissue varies from extreme to moderate. The growth is frequently papillary in arrangement, and invasion of blood vessels is less characteristic than it is with hepatic cell carcinomas. The abundance of connective tissues explains the characteristic firm gross appearance. Mixed hepatocellular–cholangiocellular carcinoma shows the distinct histologic features of both types. Three combinations have been noted: (1) separate tumors composed of single cell types, (2) contiguous tumors, each of which has a different cell type, and (3) individual lesions containing both cellular elements.

Hepatoblastoma. Histologically, hepatoblastoma may present as a pure epithelial lesion or a mixture of epithelial and mesenchymal elements. The fetal cells are smaller than adult hepatocytes and are arranged in solid sheets with the substructure of cords and plates of two-cell thickness (Fig. 66–5). There are varying amounts of glycogen and/or lipid in the cytoplasm. Nuclear abnormalities and mitoses are infrequent. Extramedullary erythropoiesis is characteristically present in the fetal cell areas. Misugi and associates distinguished two types of tumors. The first occurred in infants and children up to the age of 3 and was characterized by a combination of embryonal liver parenchyma and mesenchyme, with an ultrastructure that showed a limited number of cytoplasmic organelles. The second type occurred in children older than 6 years and was characterized by increased mitochondria and irregular endoplasmic reticulum.

Malignant mesenchymal tumors have a distinctive microscopic pattern, with a thick fibrous pseudocapsule. The tumor consists of ducts surrounded by poorly differentiated anaplastic cells that are particularly prominent around the

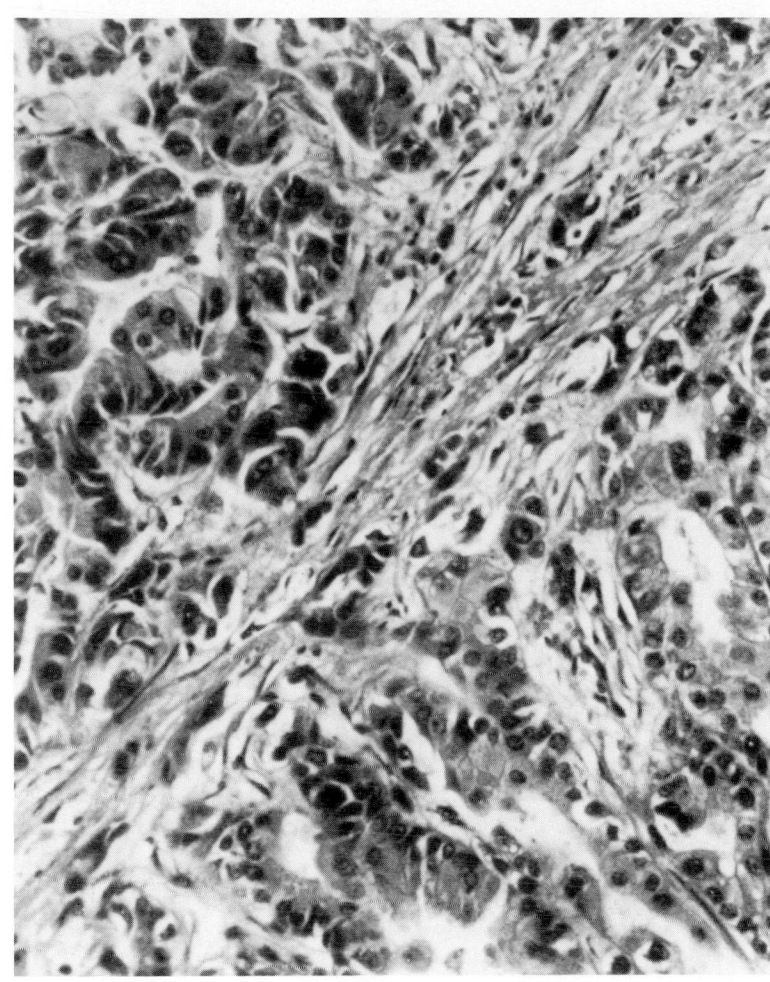

Figure 66–4. Cholangiolar carcinoma (microscopic). (*Source: From Schwartz SI, 1964, with permission.*)

ducts (Fig. 66–6). The background may have an edematous or myxoid quality. Bizarre nuclei are frequently seen within pale acidophilic vacuolated cytoplasm. Mitoses are frequent.

Angiosarcomas are made up of malignant endothelial cells with hyperchromatic nuclei and multiple mytoses. The cells may form a single layer within the blood vessels or may constitute multiple small channels within larger vessels. There is no distortion of the liver cords, but individual groups of liver cells may be surrounded by tumor cells or by a layer of connective tissue containing tumor cells (Fig. 66–7).

CLINICAL MANIFESTATIONS

In the adult, the clinical manifestations of primary carcinoma are varied, and no one manifes-

tation may be considered pathognomonic. None of the symptoms aids in distinguishing primary carcinoma of the liver from metastatic lesions. The most common symptoms are weight loss and weakness, which occur in approximately 85 percent of patients. Abdominal pain is present in about one half to two thirds of patients. The location of pain is variable but is usually situated in the epigastrium and the right upper part of the hypochondrium. It may be referred to the back or chest. Pain is described as dull but persistent; it is rarely severe enough to force the patient to seek immediate medical attention. The sudden onset of acute abdominal pain has been described by patients with intraperitoneal hemorrhage secondary to rupture of a necrotic nodule or erosion of a blood vessel on the surface of the liver. This occurs in 8 to 10 percent of patients.

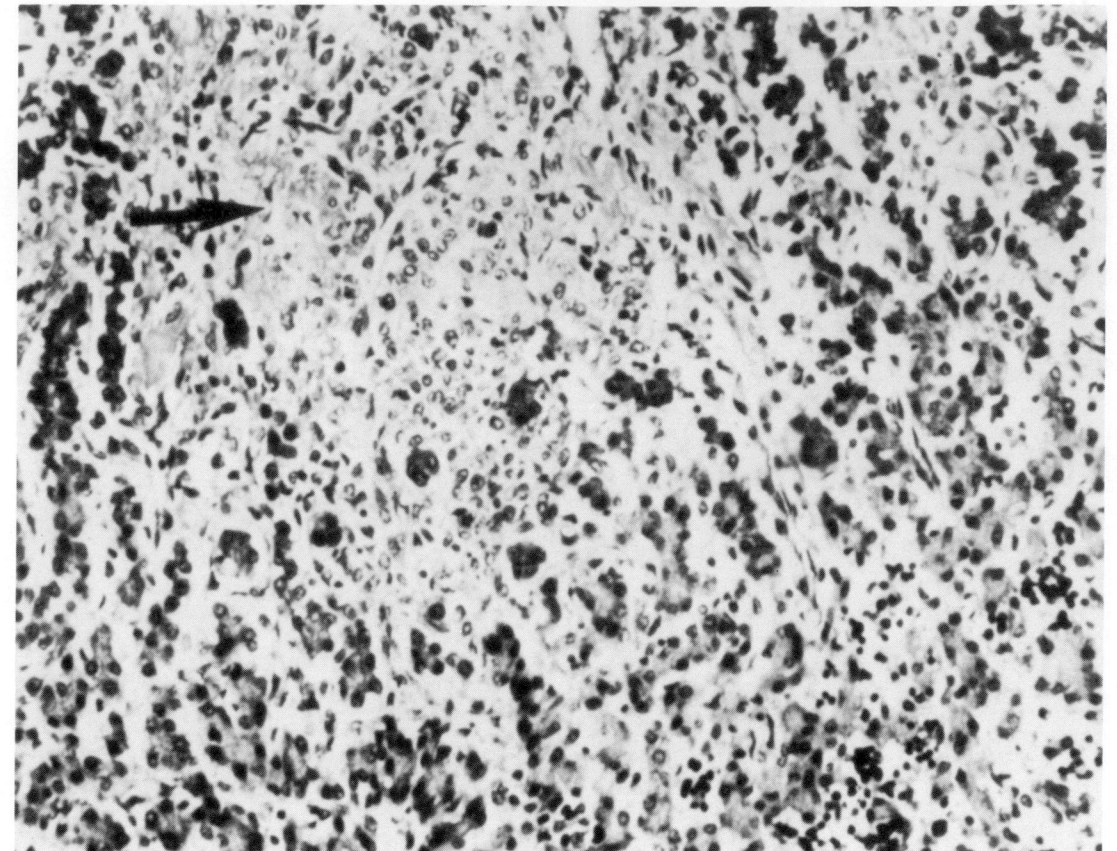

Figure 66–5. Fetal pattern of hepatoblastoma, showing small interrupted cords of differentiated hepatocytes and numerous foci of extramedullary hematopoiesis in the sinusoids. An area of early osteoid formation is present in the upper central field *(arrow)*. (*Source: From Dehner LP, 1978, p 231, with permission.*)

Weight loss varying between 10 and 25 pounds is frequently noted, and anorexia is present in about one third of cases. Fever occurs in one third to one half of patients, and a septic type of fever is suggestive of necrosis or abscess formation within a rapidly growing tumor nodule.

On physical examination, the liver is almost always enlarged, often to a remarkable degree. Significant liver tenderness is noted in fewer than one third of patients. Splenic enlargement and other signs of portal hypertension are present in about one third of cases. Ascites is present in one half to three quarters of patients, and when paracentesis is performed, the fluid is hemorrhagic in one third of these cases. Virilizing and feminizing effects are occasionally apparent.

Among the major problems in diagnosis are the differentiation between primary carcinoma of the liver and cirrhosis and, more particularly, the diagnosis of a hepatic carcinoma in a patient known to have cirrhosis. The clinical picture of a rapid increase in symptoms and signs associated with cirrhosis is suggestive of hepatic carcinoma, particularly when there is an inexplicable acceleration of symptoms in a person with quiescent cirrhosis. The development of abdominal pain in a patient with hemochromatosis should arouse suspicion that a malignant change in the liver has occurred. In addition, the sudden amelioration of diabetes and occasional hypoglycemic intervals should be viewed as indicative of a neoplastic change.

In over half the cases in the pediatric age group, the first evidence of neoplasm is an ab-

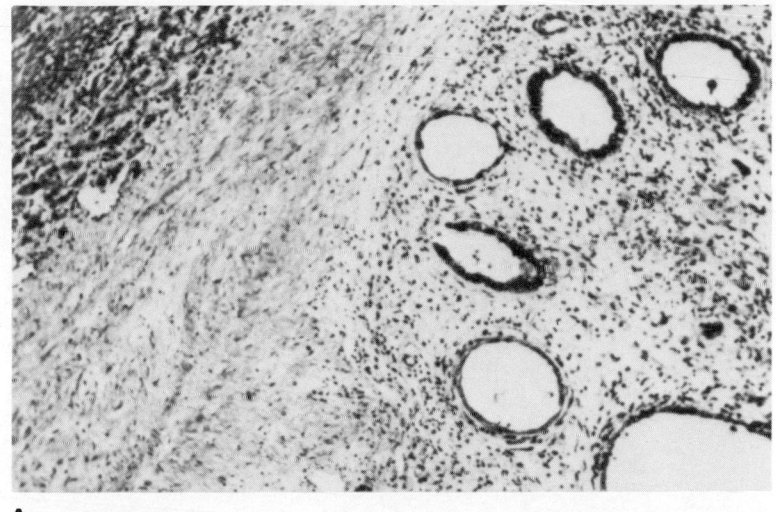

A

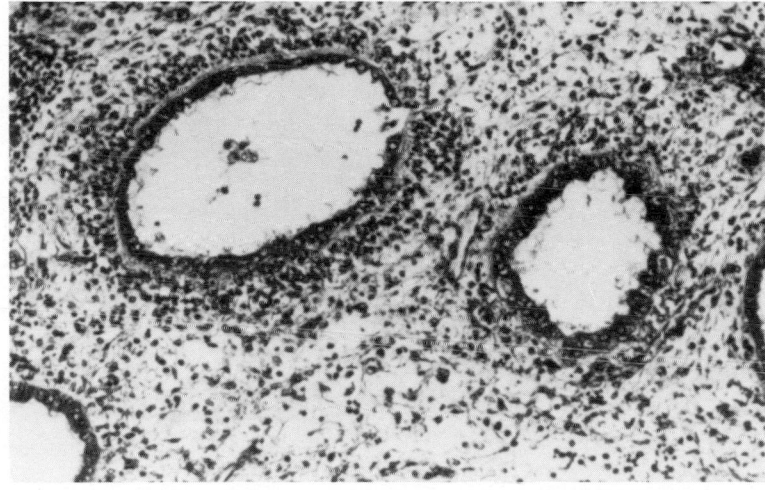

Figure 66–6. Malignant mesenchymal tumor (undifferentiated sarcoma) of the liver. **A.** A pseudocapsule typically separates the tumor from the liver. (H&E, ×75) **B.**The stroma is composed of undifferentiated tumor cells and the ducts are lined by atypical cuboidal epithelium. (H&E, ×125) (*Source: From Dehner LP, 1978, p 256, with permission.*)

B

dominal mass. Fever, abdominal pain, anorexia, and weakness are found in about 25 percent of children. Jaundice and ascites are uncommon. Other associations with hepatoblastoma include hemihypertrophy in 2 to 3 percent of patients and sexual precocity, secondary to ectopic gonadotropin production.

Fibrolamellar carcinomas are distinctive in that the mean age of patients is 26, significantly lower than that for other hepatocellular carcinomas, and there is an equal sex incidence. Ab-

dominal pain occurs in 75 percent of these patients but, more often, hepatomegaly or an abdominal mass leads to hospitalization.

Malignant mesenchymal tumor of the liver also affects males and females equally. Abdominal mass, fever, and pain are the most common clinical manifestations.

Angiosarcoma generally has nonspecific clinical features. Abdominal pain is the most common complaint, followed by weakness and fatigue. Some patients are asymptomatic and

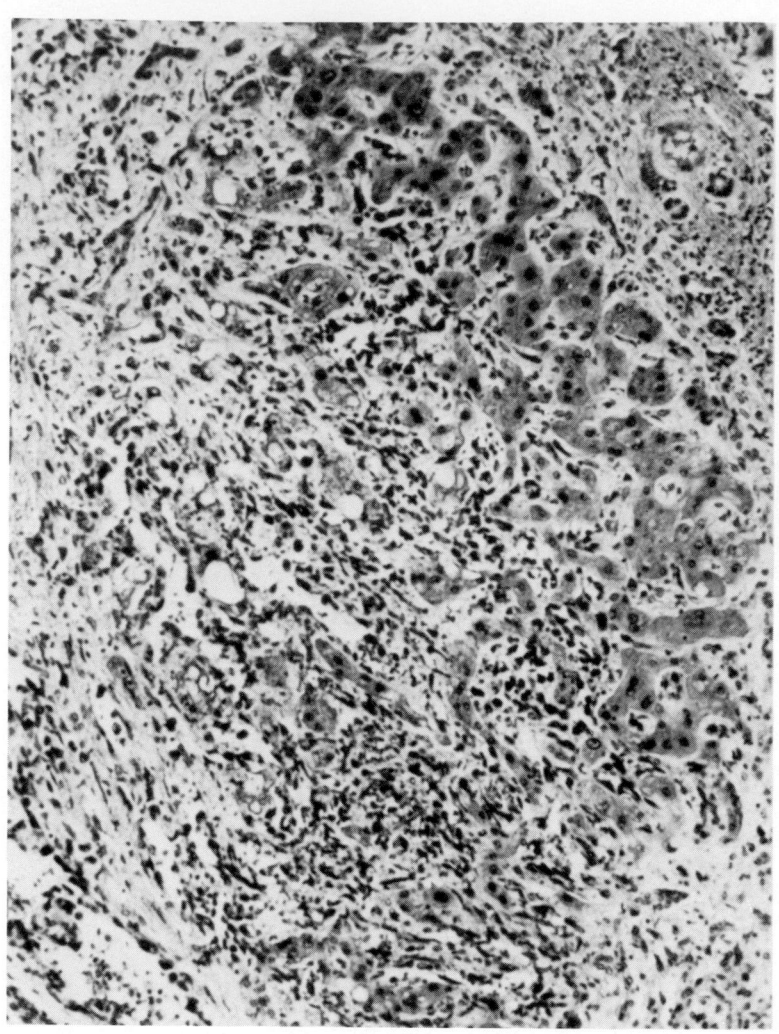

Figure 66–7. Histologic section showing invasion and replacement of the liver lobule by angiosarcoma. The actual process of invasion appears to be via preexisting sinusoids. (*Source: From Edmondson HA, 1954, with permission.*)

have been diagnosed by routine screening. Hepatomegaly, ascites, and jaundice are the three most common presenting physical findings.

Patients with *metastatic involvement of the liver* present with major symptoms referable to the liver in 67 percent of cases. These symptoms include hepatic pain, hepatomegaly, ascites, and jaundice. Anorexia and weight loss are almost constant findings. On physical examination, hepatomegaly and hepatic tenderness are frequently noted, and palpation may reveal a distinct nodularity of the liver in about half the cases. A friction rub is audible over the organ in 10 percent. In patients with carcinoid syndrome, hepatic metastasis is considered causative. These patients present with flushing and profuse, watery diarrhea.

DIAGNOSTIC STUDIES

Laboratory Determinations

The hemogram is of little diagnostic significance, and the anemia is usually indicative of advanced hepatic dysfunction. There are no laboratory tests that consistently define the presence of either a primary or metastatic hepatic carcinoma or aid in the differentiation of the two. The most consistently altered liver function test is the alkaline phosphatase. In various series, 13 to 94 percent of adult patients with primary carcinoma of the liver had elevations, while children showed elevations in 36 percent of hepatoblastoma cases and 45 percent of hepatocellular carcinomas. Adult patients with cholangiocarcinomas were more likely to have increased alkaline phosphatase levels than were patients with hepatocellular carcinoma.

Primary liver cancers were associated with increases in the SGOT in 17 to 87 percent of adult patients and in almost half of the children. In one series, 5'-nucleotidase was elevated in 45 of 51 adult patients with primary cellular carcinoma. α-fetoprotein testing is extremely useful in the diagnosis of hepatocellular carcinoma, particularly if the result is positive. Detection of α-fetoprotein in patients with hepatocellular carcinoma has ranged from 30 to 75 percent; it is not positive in patients with cholangiocarcinoma but has been noted to be present in as many as 38 percent of patients with active hepatitis, most commonly in those with bridging necrosis. Hepatitis-associated antigen is detected in a significant number of patients with primary hepatocellular carcinoma, but it has not been resolved if its presence is related to the underlying liver injury or the tumor itself.

In patients with metastatic neoplasm, the serum alkaline phosphatase level is the most consistently altered determination. The carcinoembryonic antigen (CEA) is often elevated in patients who have colorectal carcinomas with hepatic metastases, but about 20 percent of patients in this category will not show an elevation, and patients with other benign and malignant lesions of the liver may demonstrate elevated levels of CEA.

A prospective study of the ability of laboratory tests to detect hepatic metastases was reported by Kemeny et al. No single laboratory test had greater than 65 percent accuracy in the detection of lesions. The tests evaluated were CEA, GGTP, SGTP, LDH, alkaline phosphatase, SGOT, LAP, and 5'-nucleotidase. No combination of the laboratory tests increased the accuracy. Tartter and associates reported that serum alkaline phosphatase and carcinoembryonic antigen did provide a sensitive and economic way of screening for liver metastases in patients with colorectal cancer. If the alkaline phosphatase was greater than 135 IU and/or carcinoembryonic antigen was greater than 10 ng/ml, the sensitivity was 88 percent. The false-positive rate was 12 percent. The 5-hydroxyindole acetic acid has provided a relatively sensitive method for detecting metastatic carcinoid tumors within the liver, particularly in symptomatic patients.

In children with liver tumors, α-fetoprotein was noted to be a reliable biologic marker in the majority of patients with hepatoblastoma and in about 90 percent of children with hepatocellular carcinoma. Following resection, the levels disappear. The reappearance and growth of these lesions are accompanied by a parallel rise in the level of α-fetoprotein. A similar relationship to B_{12}-binding protein has been demonstrated in the serum of certain children with primary tumors of the liver.

The most striking abnormality in patients with angiosarcoma of the liver is thrombocytopenia, reported in one half to two thirds of patients. The alkaline phosphatase and SGOT are elevated in between 70 and 85 percent of these patients; none has had a positive α-fetoprotein marker. Hypercalcemia may be noted in some of these patients, just as it is present in about 7 percent of patients with hepatocellular carcinoma and is thought to result from the production of an ectopic parathormone-like substance.

Radiologic Studies

The four major radiologic modalities for evaluating focal intrahepatic disease are nuclear imaging, grey-scale ultrasonography, computed tomography (CT), and angiography.

Nuclear Imaging. Radionuclide imaging of the liver is based on the ability of Kupffer cells to phagocytize foreign particles. The most common approach for liver scanning is the administration of sulfur colloid labeled with technetium-99m. Scintigraphy is a relatively nonspecific test, with a 30 percent false-positive rate and a 15 percent false-negative rate for metastatic lesions. On the other hand, 92 percent of primary malignant tumors of the liver have been demonstrated by liver scan.

Ultrasonography. This imaging modality is a low cost, useful method for detecting lesions and assessing the tumor response to therapy. The major disadvantage relates to interference by abdominal gas and the difficulty in performing an adequate examination in patients with marked abdominal tenderness. It is particularly helpful in distinguishing cystic lesions and abscesses from metastatic tumors.

CT. Intrahepatic space-occupying lesions may be detected by CT when the attenuation values

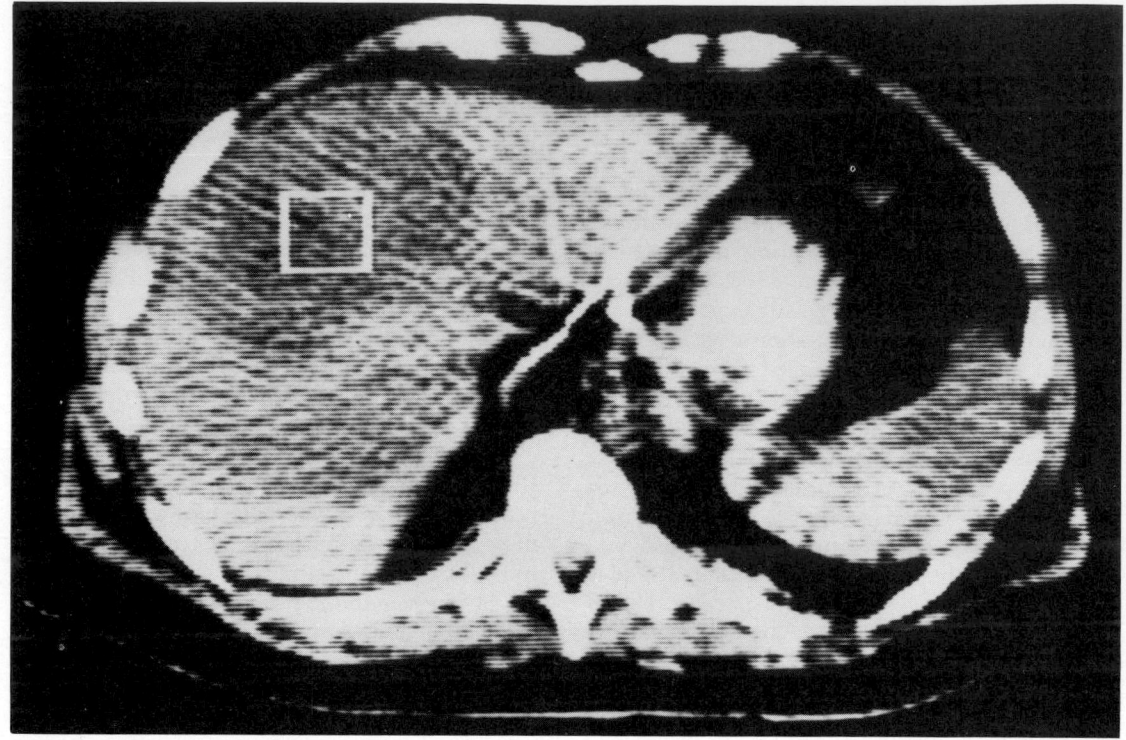

Figure 66–8. A nonenhanced CT scan of the upper portion of the abdomen demonstrated a large, well-demarcated, solid mass located laterally in the right lobe of the liver. (*Source: From Gutierrez OH, Schwartz SI, 1984, with permission.*)

of the x-rays differ significantly from those of the surrounding liver parenchyma. Intravenous urographic contrast medium or the administration of contrast medium directly into a hepatic artery, followed by CT, increases the density of the hepatic tissue and will exaggerate differences between the lesion and the normal liver. The advantages of CT in defining hepatic malignancies are that it is noninvasive, it is the optimal method of detecting left lobar disease, it defines hypovascular and peripheral lesions and hepatic masses associated with diffuse disease, and it distinguishes between solid and cystic lesions. CT is superior to angiography in demonstrating hepatic tumors that are associated with cirrhosis of the liver or tissue undergoing necrosis and secondary infection.

Angiography. Selective angiography is the most useful test supplying information regarding a patient with hepatic malignancy. The advantages of angiography include: (1) definition of the vascular supply and anatomic variations of the major blood vessels, (2) determination of involvement of the portal vein and inferior vena cava, (3) definition of small hypervascular lesions, and (4) determination of the extent of the disease. For appropriate information, celiac angiography, followed by selective hepatic angiography in both the anteroposterior and right posterior oblique views, must be obtained. At times selective catheterization and injection of both the right and left hepatic arteries may be necessary. Superior mesenteric angiography is performed when a replaced hepatic artery originates from that vessel. Angiography is consistently better than CT scanning in determining hypervascular lesions less than 2 cm in diameter. The definition of a hypervascular lesion will serve as a contraindication for needle biopsy. It is also the best method of distinguishing an intrahepatic from an extrahepatic location of a tumor contiguous to the liver.

Figures 66–8 and 66–9 are representative of a CT scan and angiogram of a primary hepatocellular carcinoma. Figures 66–10 and 66–11 are

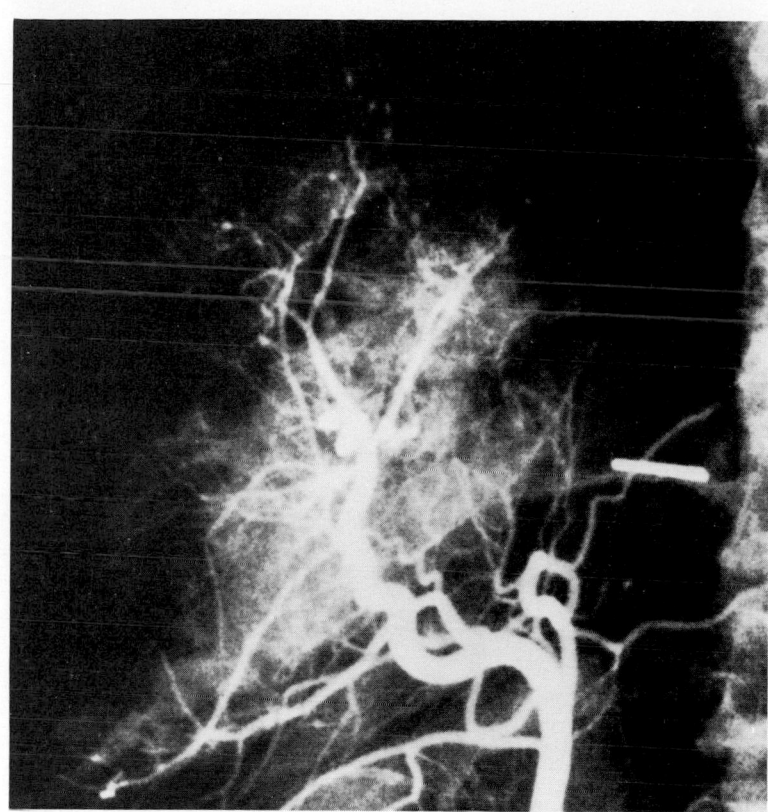

Figure 66–9. An 11 by 16 cm tumor mass occupied the bulk of the right lobe of the liver, mainly posterosuperiorly. The mass consisted of an increased number of irregular, tortuous, and encased vessels with a large, poorly marginated avascular portion laterally. (*Source: From Gutierrez OH, Schwartz SI, 1984, with permission.*)

the CT and angiogram of a patient with a hepatoblastoma. The characteristic findings in a patient with angiosarcoma are shown in Figures 66–12 and 66–13. In contrast to the marked hypervascularity of the previously presented studies, the CT scan (Fig. 66–14) and hepatic angiogram (Fig. 66–15), define a hypovascular metastatic lesion.

Peritoneoscopy

This procedure, which can be performed under local anesthesia, has enjoyed greater popularity in Europe and South America than in the United States. It has helped in establishing the diagnosis and in evaluating the operability of patients with hepatic malignancies. In most patients, the entire left lobe of the liver and the anterior surface of the right lobe can be visualized. Peritoneoscopy may be used to guide the needle for a liver biopsy. The procedure is limited in regard to lesions located in the region of the dome of the liver and deep within the parenchyma.

Needle Biopsy

Percutaneous needle biopsy of the liver should only be performed after normal coagulation studies and platelet count have been defined. Most investigators have been unable to find any evidence to support the view that the presence of hepatic malignancy enhances the hazard of liver biopsy, with the exception of highly vascular angiosarcoma. Sixteen percent of all liver biopsies in patients with angiosarcoma required multiple transfusions. This applied to both open and closed biopsies. Angiographic definition of the vascularity of the tumor should be established prior to performing the liver biopsy.

TREATMENT

The definitive treatment of primary carcinoma of the liver is surgical excision. Certain criteria should be met before resection for primary carcinoma is performed. The carcinoma should be localized to a resectable portion of the liver,

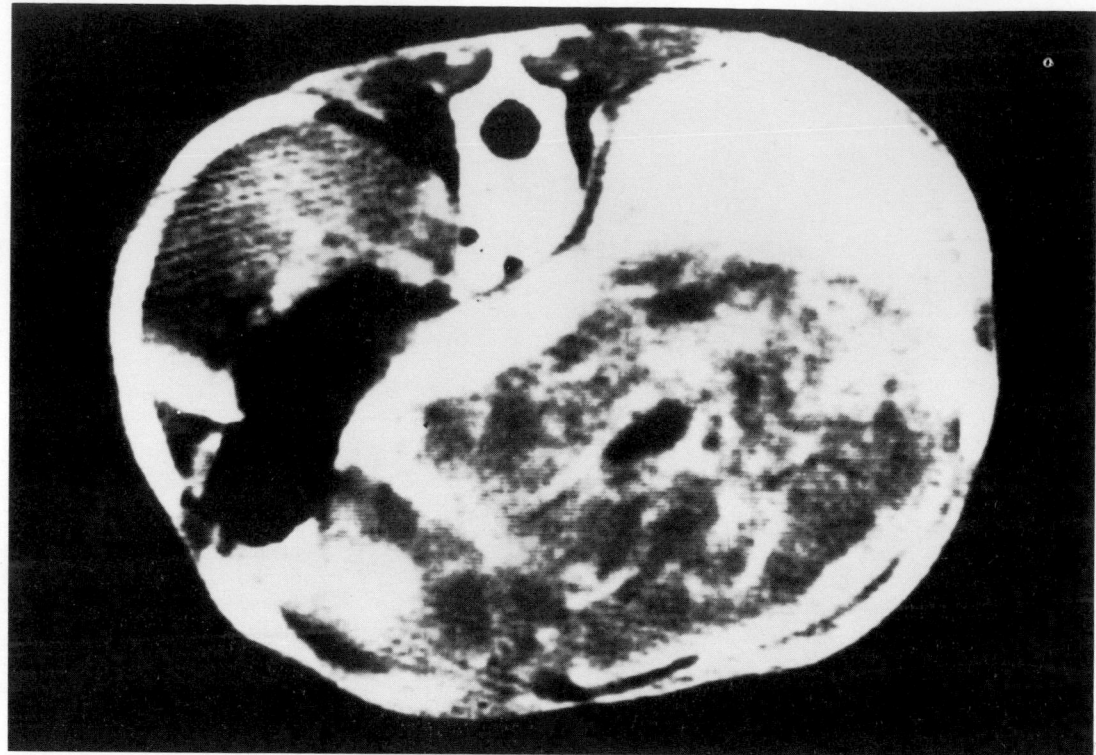

Figure 66–10. CT scan. The midportion of the liver was replaced by a 10 by 12 cm mixed density mass involving both the right and left lobes of the liver. (*Source: From Gutierrez OH, Schwartz SI, 1984, with permission.*)

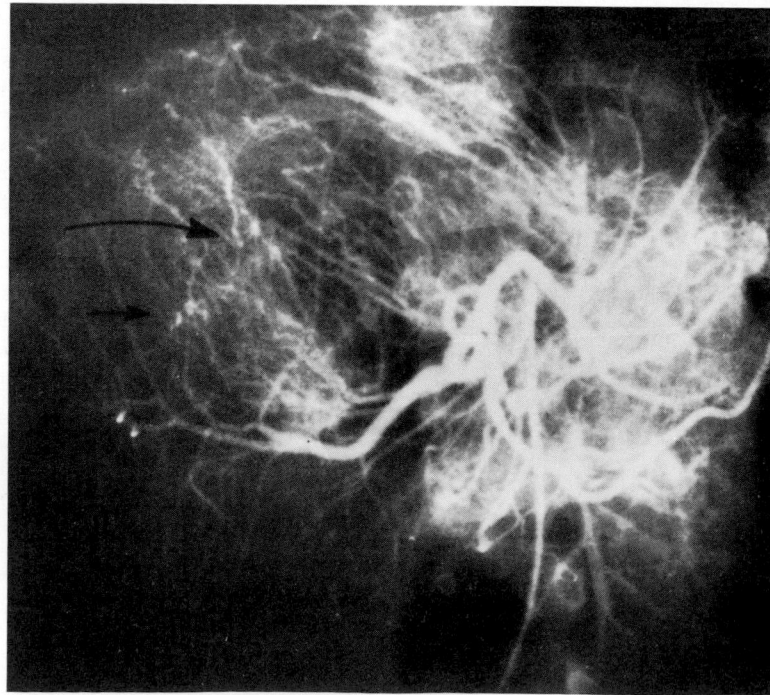

Figure 66–11. Hepatic angiogram. The liver was markedly enlarged, with a 14 by 11 cm hypervascular mass supplied by dilated and tortuous left hepatic arterial branches (*arrows*). There were gross neovascularity and puddling of contrast medium. (*Source: From Gutierrez OH, Schwartz SI, 1984, with permission.*)

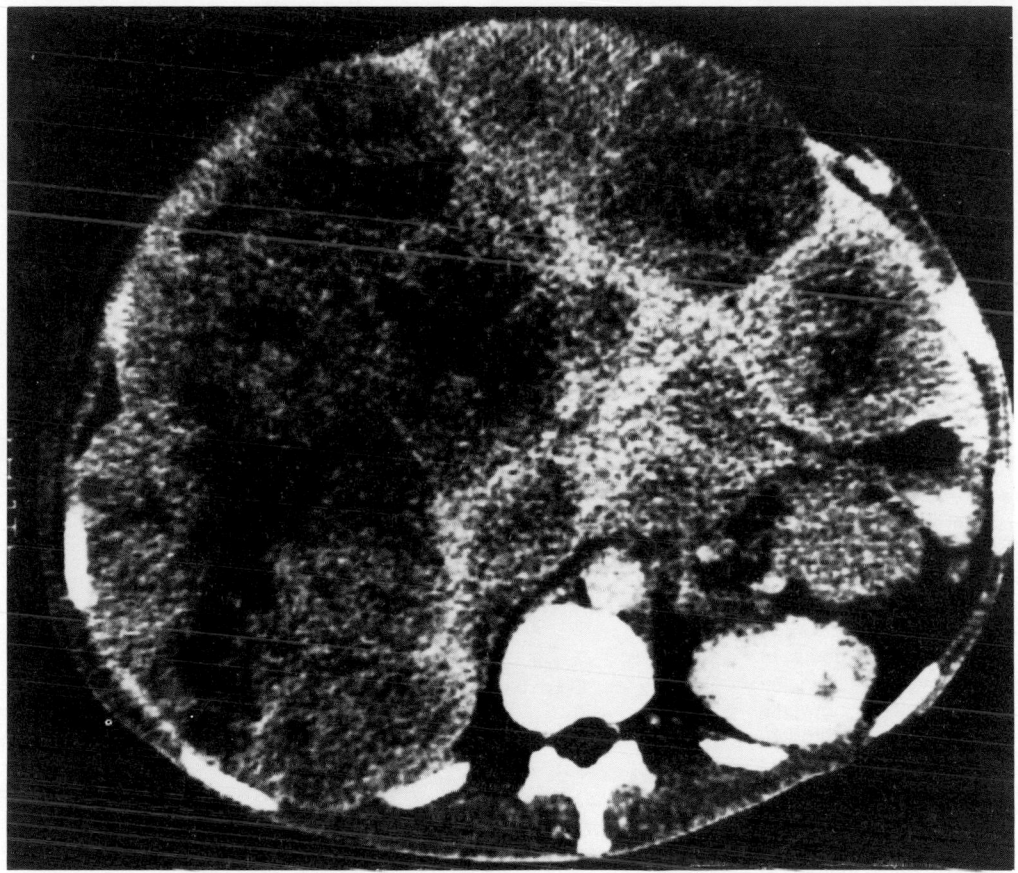

Figure 66–12. CT scan. The liver was enlarged. The entire parenchyma was diffusely infiltrated with rounded, low-density masses. (*Source: From Gutierrez OH, Schwartz SI, 1984, with permission.*)

there must be no evident lymph node, blood vessel, or extrahepatic bile duct involvement, and the presence of distant metastases should be ruled out.

Resection of primary hepatocellular carcinoma superimposed on cirrhosis is compromised by increased vascularity of the liver and attendant increased operative morbidity and an inability for the cirrhotic liver to regenerate. Fibrolamellar carcinomas have an increased resectability. Primary angiosarcoma of the liver is generally nonresectable and might benefit from combined radiation therapy and Adriamycin.

In general, radiation therapy has little to offer in effecting a cure for carcinoma of the liver. Chemotherapy in itself has not been curative, but preoperative chemotherapy in children with hepatoblastoma has converted nonresecta-

ble lesions into resectable ones. Mahour and associates reported seven patients with unresectable tumors treated by chemotherapy alone or in combination with radiation therapy for a mean period of 6 months before a second-look celiotomy was performed. Six of these patients had significant reduction in the size of the tumor and underwent resection; five of these were alive without disease 2.5 to 7 years after diagnosis. Weinblatt and associates also reported on the use of preoperative chemotherapy for unresectable primary hepatic malignancies in children. Adriamycin was used in all drug regimens, usually in combination with cyclophosphamide, vincristine, and 5-fluorouracil. Seven of eight children exhibited a pronounced response, with reduction in the size of the primary tumor, and four were able to have complete, uncomplicated surgical resection of residual disease. Three of

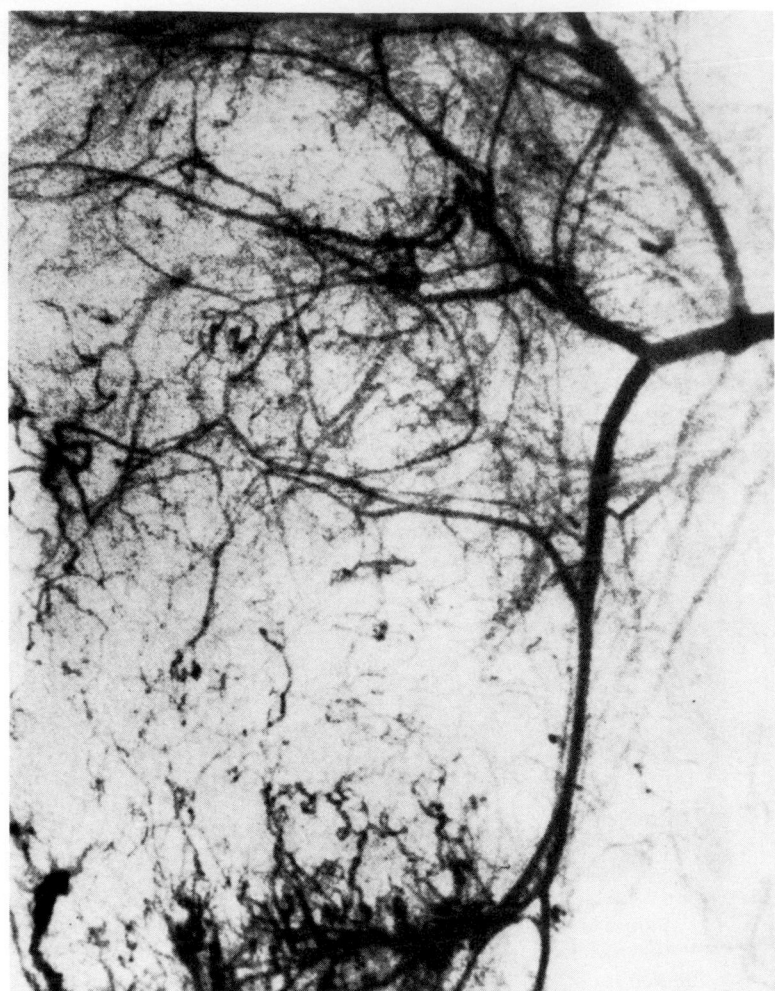

Figure 66–13. Hepatic angiogram. Both the right and left lobes of the liver were grossly enlarged. Most intrahepatic vessels appeared markedly stretched, and some were crowded together toward the dome of the liver. Neovascularity in the form of large vascular networks and lakes was present throughout the liver, particularly in the lower aspect of the right and left lobes. A bizarre appearance was due to persistence of contrast material within parenchymal pools and tumor vessels. (*Source: From Gutierrez OH, Schwartz SI, 1984, with permission.*)

the four are alive and well and off therapy. One patient with hepatocellular carcinoma had complete disappearance of the disease with chemotherapy alone.

In the case of metastatic neoplasms of the liver, only surgical excision can possibly effect a cure. The most encouraging results are associated with patients who have metastases from primary tumors located in the colon and rectum and Wilms' tumors. In patients with metastases secondary to colonic and rectal carcinomas, the microscopic extension of the lesion is rarely more than 1 mm beyond that which is perceived by the naked eye. It is, therefore, appropriate to remove the lesion by wedge resection, if this is feasible. In many instances, hepatic lobectomy or even trisegmentectomy is required to effect total extirpation of the tumor.

Palliation for patients with metastatic colon and rectal carcinoma and for some patients with primary hepatocellular tumors has been achieved by regional hepatic chemotherapy using an implantable drug infusion pump (Fig. 66–16).

A laparotomy is performed, and a catheter is inserted into the hepatic artery, generally via the gastroduodenal artery, in order to provide perfusion of both the right and left hepatic arterial circulations. If these circulations have separate origins, two catheters can be inserted and connected to a newly devised dual pump. A subcutaneous pump pocket is established on the anterior abdominal wall, and the catheter is brought out from the peritoneal cavity to the pump pocket and connected to the pump. FUDR is administered at a rate of 0.3 mg/kg per day

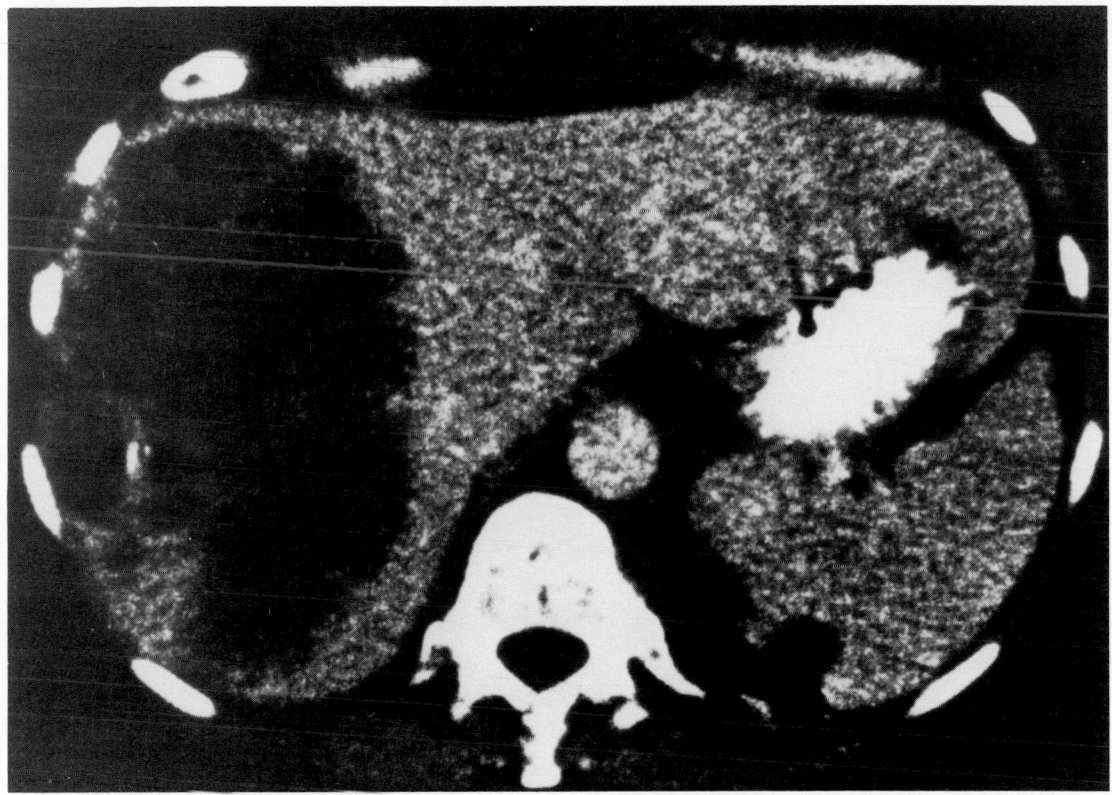

Figure 66–14. Axial CT scan. A large, low-density, solid mass replaced two thirds of the right lobe of the liver. The mass appeared partially calcified in its most lateral aspect; the left lobe was unremarkable. (*Source: From Gutierrez OH, Schwartz SI, 1984, with permission.*)

in 2-week cycles, alternating with saline. The pump is refilled with the chemotherapeutic agent at 15-day intervals as an outpatient procedure.

Balch and associates have reported the results of a prospective evaluation of regional FUDR chemotherapy, using the totally implantable drug infusion pump. An 88 percent response rate occurred, as evidenced by a fall in the serum CEA levels by one third or greater after two cycles of chemotherapy. The regional chemotherapy patients had an improved survival rate, compared to the controlled series. This improved survival rate was not influenced by the extent of tumor involvement or whether the patient had symptomatic disease. As an alternative to a surgical procedure to position the catheter, angiographically controlled percutaneous catheterization of the hepatic artery through the transaxillary route has been employed.

Symptomatic carcinoid disease of the liver has been successfully managed by resection, dearterialization, and radiographically controlled hepatic embolization. Maton and associates reported 13 patients who received a preembolization regimen of cyproheptadine, fenclonine, aprotinin, methylprednisolone, tobramycin, flucloxacillin, and metronidazole and then were subjected to hepatic embolization. Dramatic improvement occurred in the nine patients in whom the embolization was successfully carried out, with abolition of flushing, severe abdominal pain, wheezing, and a reduction in diarrhea. The urinary excretion of 5-hydroxyindole acetic acid fell immediately. Similar results have been achieved by dearterialization or a debulking resection of the majority of the tumor.

The complication of intraperitoneal bleeding, associated with spontaneous rupture of a primary hepatoma, can be managed by hepatic

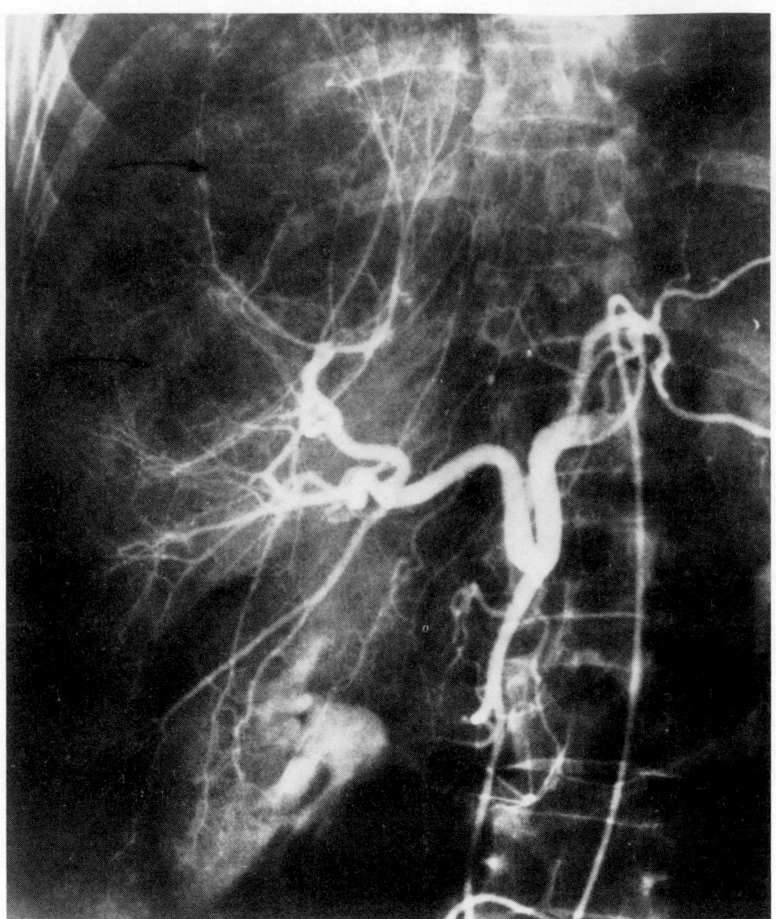

Figure 66–15. Hepatic angiogram. There was a 20 by 14 cm hypovascular mass in the superoposterior aspect of the right lobe of the liver, with stretching of major vessels, arterial encasement, and neovascularity (*arrows*). (*Source: Gutierrez OH, Schwartz SI, 1984, with permission.*)

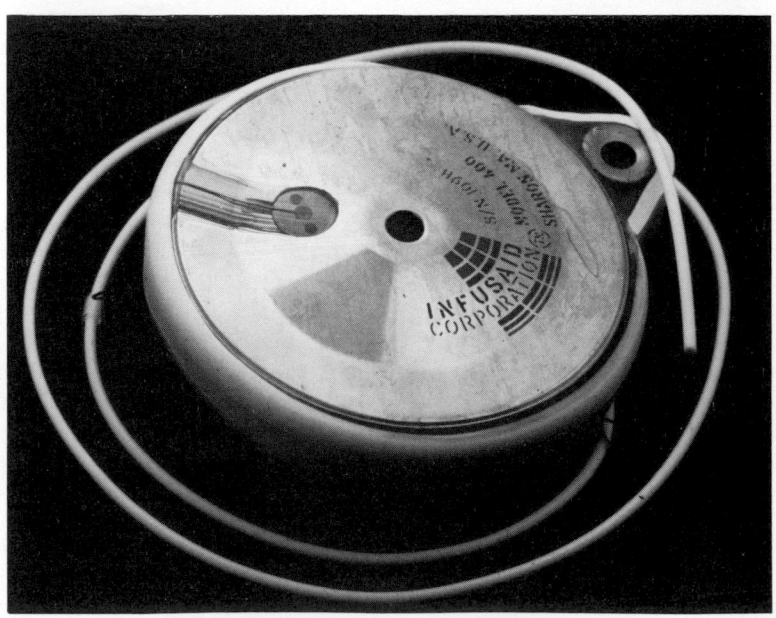

Figure 66–16. Infusaid pump.

artery ligation or embolization. In one series, hepatic artery ligation was employed in 26 patients, with a 54 percent mortality, but bleeding stopped in 92 percent. This should be compared with other conventional surgical measures, such as packing, suture, and cauterization, which are associated with a 90 percent mortality.

PROGNOSIS

The 1974 liver survey of Foster and Berman provides very meaningful data related to prognosis. The survival after resection for cure, excluding operative deaths, in adult patients with primary epithelial carcinoma was 34 percent at 5 years in the noncirrhotic group and 0 of 8 cirrhotic patients. In patients with epithelial cancer in the pediatric age group, 8 of 14 children under the age of 2 with hepatoblastoma survived, while only 1 of 5 over the age of 2 with this tumor survived 5 years. In the pediatric group with hepatocellular carcinoma, none of 3 under the age of 2 survived, while 4 of 11 over the age of 2 survived. Adson and Weiland reported a 5-year survival rate of 36 percent for primary malignant tumors of the liver. A significant improvement in survival rate is associated with resection for fibrolamellar carcinoma of the liver. Survival of patients with primary hepatic angiosarcoma is poor; only 3 percent live longer than 2 years.

In patients with metastatic carcinoid disease and the carcinoid syndrome, the 5-year survival was about 20 percent. Foster has reported a 22 percent 5-year survival for 206 collected patients with metastases from carcinoma of the colon and rectum subjected to hepatic resection, either by wedge excision or by total lobectomy. Adson and van Heerden have reported a 28 percent 5-year survival rate for 60 such patients. Morrow and associates reported 30 patients with synchronous resection of the primary colon carcinoma and hepatic resection with a 26 percent 5-year survival, whereas 34 patients with a metachronous resection had a 5-year survival rate of 30 percent. Patients who underwent resection of multiple metastases had essentially the same survival rate as those with isolated metastases. These data all support an aggressive approach to resection of metastases in the liver that originate from the colon and rectum. An even better yield is achieved for patients with primary Wilms' tumor and hepatic metastases.

BIBLIOGRAPHY

Adson MA: Diagnosis and surgical treatment of primary and secondary solid hepatic tumors in the adult. Surg Clin North Am 61:181, 1981

Adson MA, Van Heerden JA: Major hepatic resections for metastatic colorectal cancer. Ann Surg 191:576, 1980

Adson MA, Weiland LH: Resection of primary solid hepatic tumors. Am J Surg 141:18, 1981

Baggenstoss AH: Pathology of tumors of liver in infancy and childhood, in Pack GT, Islami AH (eds): Tumors of the Liver. New York: Springer-Verlag, 1970

Balch CM, Urist MM, et al: A prospective phase II clinical trial of continuous FUDR regional chemotherapy for colorectal metastases to the liver using a totally implantable drug infusion pump. Ann Surg 198:567, 1983

Bengmark S, Ericsson M, et al: Temporary liver dearterialization in patients with metastatic carcinoid disease. World J Surg 6:46, 1982

Berg NO, Erikkson S: Liver disease in adults with alpha-1-antitrypsin deficiency. N Engl J Med 287:1264, 1972

Chearanai O, Plengvanit U, et al: Spontaneous rupture of primary hepatoma. Cancer 51:1532, 1983

Cohen AM, Kaufman SD, et al: Regional hepatic chemotherapy using an implantable drug infusion pump. Am J Surg 145:529, 1983

Craig JR, Peters RL, et al: Fibrolamellar carcinoma of the liver. Cancer 46:372, 1980

Dehner LP: Hepatic tumors in the pediatric age group: A distinctive clinicopathologic spectrum. Perspect Pediatr Pathol 4:217, 1978

Edmondson HA: Progress in pediatrics: Differential diagnosis of tumors and tumor-like lesions of liver in infancy and childhood. Am J Dis Child 91:168, 1956

Edmondson HA: Tumors of the liver and intrahepatic bile ducts. Section VII, Fascicle 25, Atlas of Tumor Pathology, AFIP, 1958

Edmondson HA, Steiner PE: Primary carcinoma of the liver; a study of 100 cases among 48,000 necropsies. Cancer 7:463, 1954

Farhi DC, Shikes RH, et al: Hepatocellular carcinoma in young people. Cancer 52:1516, 1983

Foster JH: Survival after liver resection for secondary tumors. Am J Surg 135:389, 1978

Foster JH, Berman MM: Solid Liver Tumors. Philadelphia: WB Saunders, 1977

Gutierrez OH, Schwartz SI: Atlas of Hepatic Tumors and Focal Lesions. New York: McGraw-Hill, 1984

Kemeny MM, Sugarbaker PH, et al: A prospective

analysis of laboratory tests and imaging studies to detect hepatic lesions. Ann Surg 195:163, 1982

Lack EE, Neave C, et al: Hepatocellular carcinoma. Cancer 52:1510, 1983

Locker GY, Doroshow JH, et al: The clinical features of hepatic angiosarcoma: A report of four cases and a review of the English literature. Medicine 58:48, 1979

Mahour GH, Wogu GU, et al: Improved survival in infants and children with primary malignant liver tumors. Am J Surg 146:236, 1983

Maton PN, Camilleri M, et al: Role of hepatic arterial embolisation in the carcinoid syndrome. Br Med J 287:932, 1983

Misugi K, Okijima H, et al: Classification of primary malignant tumors of liver in infancy and childhood. Cancer 20:1760, 1967

Morrow CE, Grage TB, et al: Hepatic resection for secondary neoplasms. Surgery 92:610, 1982

Randolph J, Chandra R, et al: Malignant liver tumors in infants and children. World J Surg 4:71, 1980

Schwartz SI: Surgical Diseases of the Liver. New York: McGraw-Hill, 1964

Tartter PI, Slater G, et al: Screening for liver metastases from colorectal cancer with carcinoembryonic antigen and alkaline phosphatase. Ann Surg 193:357, 1981

Weinblatt ME, Siegel SE, et al: Preoperative chemotherapy for unresectable primary hepatic malignancies in children. Cancer 50:1061, 1982

67. Hepatic Resection

Seymour I. Schwartz

INTRODUCTION

The evolution of hepatic resection—from an imprecise removal of portions of the liver, frequently accompanied by extensive hemorrhage, to a controlled, anatomic procedure with acceptable risk—represents a major advance in modern surgery. This accomplishment has been made possible by: (1) an appreciation of the segmental distribution of blood vessels and bile ducts within the liver, (2) recognition of the functional reserve of the liver and the extreme potential for hepatic regeneration, (3) a better understanding of hepatic function and the metabolic needs of the liver, (4) improvements in surgical technique that have reduced the hazard of uncontrollable hemorrhage, and (5) data that have made a strong case for improved survival following resection of primary and metastatic malignancies to the liver.

HISTORICAL BACKGROUND

The first surgical removal of a portion of the liver was recorded in 1716 by Berta, who amputated the protruding portion of the liver in a patient with a self-inflicted knife wound. In 1870 Bruns resected a lacerated portion of the liver in a soldier wounded during the Franco-Prussian war. In 1886, Lius excised a solid tumor of the left lobe of the liver by cutting through a pedicled lesion; death due to hemorrhage from the stump occurred 6 hours later. In 1888 Langenbuch successfully excised a pedicled tumor of the left lobe of the liver; the patient had a long and difficult postoperative course but eventually recovered. Tiffany, in 1890, was the first American surgeon to report a case of hepatic resection for tumor. He excised a walnut-sized mass from the convex surface of the left lobe, using scissors and cauterization. In the United States, the first reported removal of a true neoplasm was accomplished by Keen who, in 1892, resected a cystic lesion from the edge of the right lobe of the liver. Keen resected an angioma in 1897 and a large primary carcinoma of the left lobe in 1899. Wendel has been credited with the first authentic case of near-total right lobectomy performed in 1910 for a primary tumor; the patient survived 9 years. The right hepatic artery and the right hepatic duct were ligated at the hilus of the liver, but Wendel did not attempt ligation of the right portal vein in its extrahepatic position. In 1949, Wangensteen removed the entire right lobe of the liver for metastatic carcinoma of the stomach.

The modern era of anatomic hepatic lobectomy dates from the 1952 report of Lortat-Jacob and Robert, who used a thoracoabdominal approach and a technique designed to control hemorrhage by extrahepatic ligation of the contributing vessels. In 1953, Quattlebaum reported three cases of major hepatic resection, two by guillotine technique. The other represents the first recorded right hepatic lobectomy performed for primary hepatocellular carcinoma. In this patient, the technique of primary hilar ligation of the vessels and ducts was employed.

Digitoclasia, or finger fracture, of the hepatic parenchyma has evolved over the last 30 years. In 1953, Quattlebaum, in his classic article, described breaking the liver with the handle of a knife and clamping the vessels within the plane of transection. In 1956, Fineberg and associates reported on right hepatic lobectomy for primary carcinoma of the liver; they carried out a quick parenchymal dissection with the finger or the back of the scalpel. In 1958, Tien Yu Lin et al introduced a new technique in which the thumb and index finger are inserted into the liver tissue, after which the surgeon "fractures and crushes the tissue between the fingers, and when resistant vessels or ducts are encountered they are tied and divided." In 1963, Ton That Tung modified this technique by occluding the portal pedicle prior to finger fracture.

INDICATIONS

The indications for hepatic resection include: (1) parasitic and nonparasitic cysts, (2) granulomatous processes, (3) benign primary neoplasms, (4) malignant primary tumors, and (5) secondary tumors that involve the liver by direct extension or metastasis. The technique of planned anatomic resection is generally reserved for lesions that are large or located so that resection along an anatomic plane provides the opportunity for the most complete removal, coupled with the best control of vascular supply. Resection along anatomic planes with vascular control is rarely indicated for trauma, where the preferred approach is limited resectional debridement that permits removal of devitalized tissue and control of bleeding.

Advanced cirrhosis generally precludes a major hepatic resection, since intraoperative bleeding from collaterals and parenchymal vessels is significantly increased. The incidence of liver failure with resection is increased because of lack of reserve; hepatic regeneration is impaired, and reported cures for malignant tumors in cirrhotic patients are negligible.

SURGICAL ANATOMY

Ligamentous Attachments

The peritoneal relationships of the liver relate to the embryologic development. Since the liver develops as a forward extension between two layers of ventral mesentery, a prehepatic and posthepatic portion of this original mesentery results. The ventral mesentery extends only to the umbilicus; the dorsal mesentery extends the entire length of the gut. The prehepatic portion of the ventral mesentery persists in the adult as the falciform ligament (Fig. 67–1). The liver is connected with the anterior abdominal wall and the diaphragm by the falciform ligament, the lower free border of which is termed the "ligamentum teres" and contains the obliter-ated left umbilical vein. The posthepatic portion of mesentery becomes the lesser omentum (gastrohepatic ligament) connecting the stomach with the liver. The lowermost portion of the lesser omentum extends beyond the stomach onto the duodenum. The lateral free portion of the lesser omentum is termed the "hepatoduodenal ligament."

The common pleuroperitoneal cavity is divided by the pleuroperitoneal membrane arising from the septum transversum and extending to the dorsal abdominal wall, becoming the diaphragm. This results in an anterior and posterior reflection of the serous lining of the abdominal cavity upon the liver. The reflection of the diaphragmatic peritoneum onto the parietal surface of the liver is termed the "anterior coronary ligament," present on both the right and left sides. Posteriorly, a similar reflection exists, forming the right and left posterior coronary ligaments. The anterior and posterior coronary ligaments remain separate on the posterior surface of the liver; thus, the bare area of the liver maintains an extraperitoneal position. The anterior and posterior coronary ligaments on each side fuse laterally and become the right triangular ligament and the left triangular ligament, which is longer than its counterpart on the right side (Fig. 67–2).

Structures within the Hepatoduodenal Ligament

Bile Ducts. The relational anatomy of structures in the hepatoduodenal ligament is shown in Figure 67–3. The most lateral structure in the hepatoduodenal ligament is the extrahepatic bile duct system. The right and left hepatic ducts form the common hepatic duct in the porta hepatis, where the latter lies anteriorly in relation to other structures in this area. The common hepatic duct then descends a variable distance in the lateral portion of the hepatoduodenal ligament and is joined by the cystic duct coming in from the right side at a variable angle. These two ducts, the common hepatic on the left and the cystic to the right, and the liver above form the cystohepatic triangle of Calot, where the cystic and right hepatic arteries as well as aberrant segmental right hepatic ducts and arteries, are frequently found.

The common hepatic duct averages about 4 cm in length but varies considerably, depend-

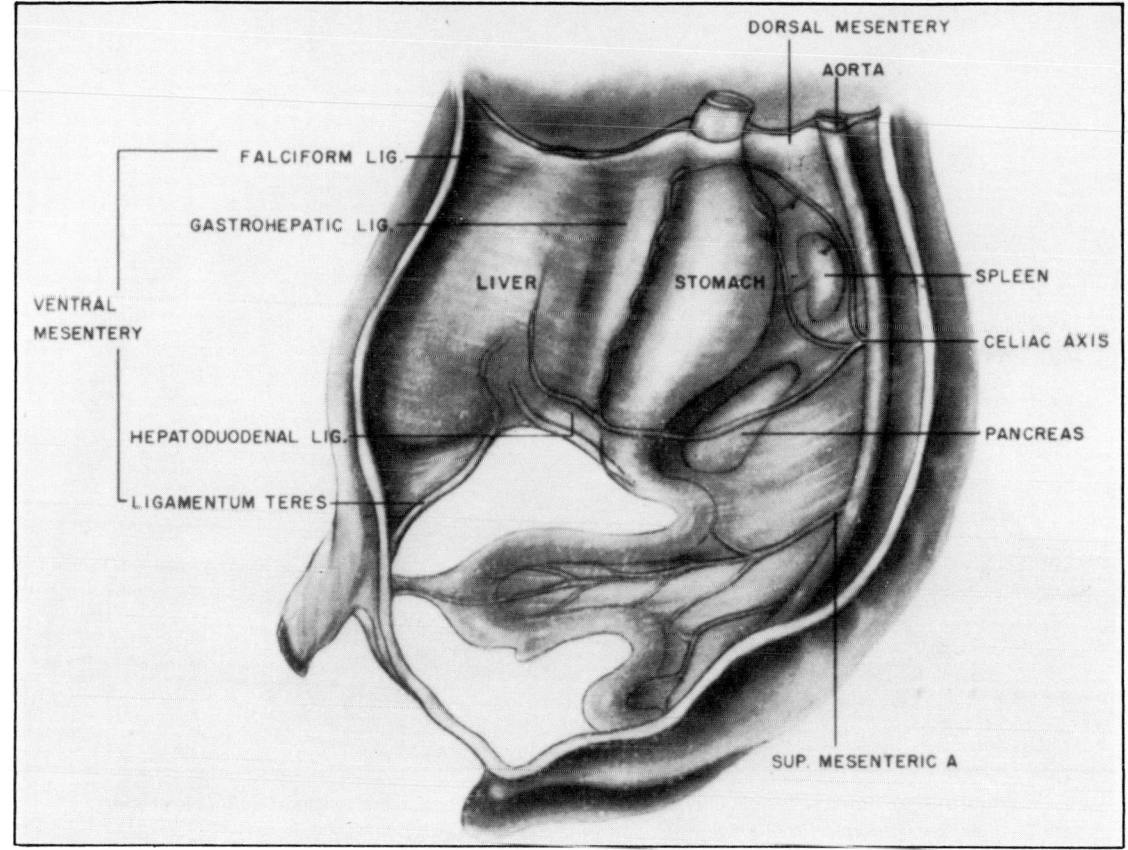

Figure 67–1. Embryonal stage showing relationship of the liver to the ventral mesentery. (*Source: From Healey JE, Schwartz SI, 1964, with permission.*)

ing upon the point of union with the cystic duct, which usually occurs 2.5 cm above the upper border of the duodenum. The common bile duct descends along the right margin of the hepatoduodenal ligament to the right of the hepatic artery and anterior to the portal vein. This supraduodenal portion continues beyond the first portion of the duodenum as a retroperitoneal portion.

Hepatic Arteries. The common hepatic artery derives from the celiac artery and proceeds through the lesser omentum at the upper border of the first portion of the duodenum, where it gives rise to the right gastric artery and the gastroduodenal artery and continues as the hepatic propria, which ascends in the hepatoduodenal ligament to the left of the common bile duct and anterior to the portal vein. In its

ascent, the hepatic propria bifurcates into a right and left branch; the bifurcation occurs at a variable point between the origin of the vessel and the porta hepatis. In the porta hepatis, the bifurcation is always to the left of the main lobar fissure and, as a consequence, the right hepatic artery is the longer of the two terminal branches. The above described origin of the common hepatic artery occurs in over 90 percent of cases. The most frequent aberrant site of origin is directly from the superior mesenteric artery.

After its origin from the hepatic propria, the right hepatic artery courses to the right behind the common hepatic duct in 87 percent of cases; in 11 percent it passes in front of the duct, and in 2 percent there is no true right hepatic artery, and there are separate branches of the anterior and posterior segmental arteries

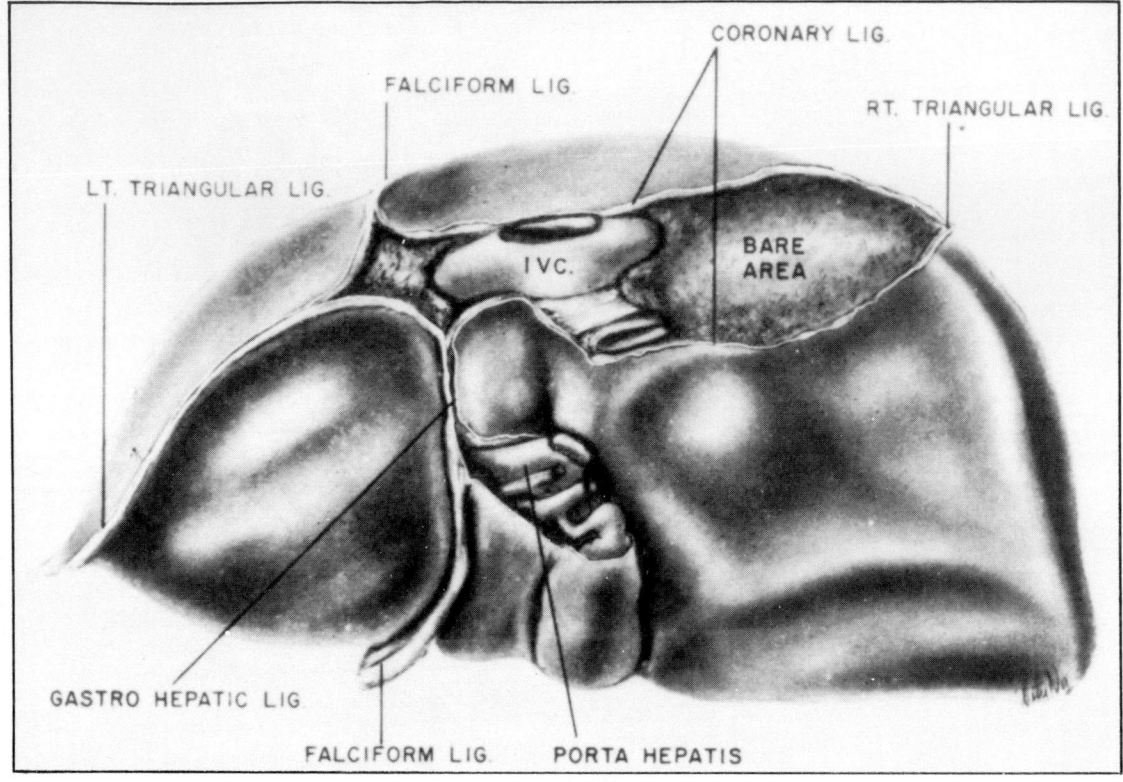

Figure 67–2. Peritoneal reflections: Rear view of the superior and visceral surfaces of the adult liver. (*Source: From Healey JE, Schwartz SI, 1964, with permission.*)

to the right lobe. The termination of the right hepatic artery is its division into an anterior and posterior segmental artery, which may occur within the hepatic parenchyma, extrahepatically in the porta hepatis to the right of the common hepatic duct, in the cystohepatic triangle, or rarely, extrahepatically to the left of the common hepatic duct.

After originating from the hepatic propria in the region of the porta hepatis, the left hepatic artery courses obliquely upward to the left for only a short distance before it divides into its two terminal branches, the medial and lateral segmental arteries. The medial segmental artery arises from the undersurface of the left hepatic artery and descends into the portion of the liver known as the "quadrate lobe" and divides within the liver parenchyma into its superior and inferior branches. The lateral segmental artery ascends in the porta hepatis to gain a variable relationship with the lateral segmental bile duct and is located either on the superior or the inferior border of this duct.

A variety of abnormalities occur in the arte-

rial circulation, and this is a major reason to mandate angiography in a patient who will undergo hepatic resection. In 17 percent of cases the superior mesenteric artery is the site of origin of aberrant arteries to the right lobe of the liver. An aberrant right hepatic artery courses anteriorly and to the right of the portal vein in the hepatoduodenal ligament. The most frequent site of origin of an aberrant left hepatic artery is the left gastric artery (Fig. 67–4).

Portal Venous System. The portal vein is formed behind the pancreas between the head and neck by a confluence of the splenic vein and the superior mesenteric vein and, in about 25 percent of cases, the inferior mesenteric vein. The portal vein passes from its origin behind the first portion of the duodenum and then enters the hepatoduodenal ligament between the two layers of the lesser omentum in front of the foramen of Winslow. In the hepatoduodenal ligament, it ascends in an essentially straight line and resides posteriorly in relation to the hepatic artery and the bile ducts. In the porta hepatis, the portal vein divides into two branches; a short, wide right branch enters the right lobe, and a longer, narrower left branch passes transversely to the left of the porta hepatis and supplies the left lobe and the quadrate lobe. In the porta hepatis, the branches of the hepatic artery maintain their anterior relationship to the branches of the portal vein.

A variety of tributaries may enter the main portal vein; these include the coronary vein, the pyloric vein, the superior pancreaticoduodenal vein, an accessory pancreatic vein, and a cystic vein (Fig. 67–5). The coronary vein (left gastric vein) passes from left to right in the lesser omentum along the lesser curvature of the stomach. It enters the portal vein, or the confluence of the splenic and mesenteric veins in about 75 percent of cases. It enters the portal vein itself in the hepatoduodenal ligament above the pancreas in about 25 percent of cases.

Hepatic Veins. The hepatic venous system begins as a central vein of a liver lobule. The central vein receives sinusoids from all sides and

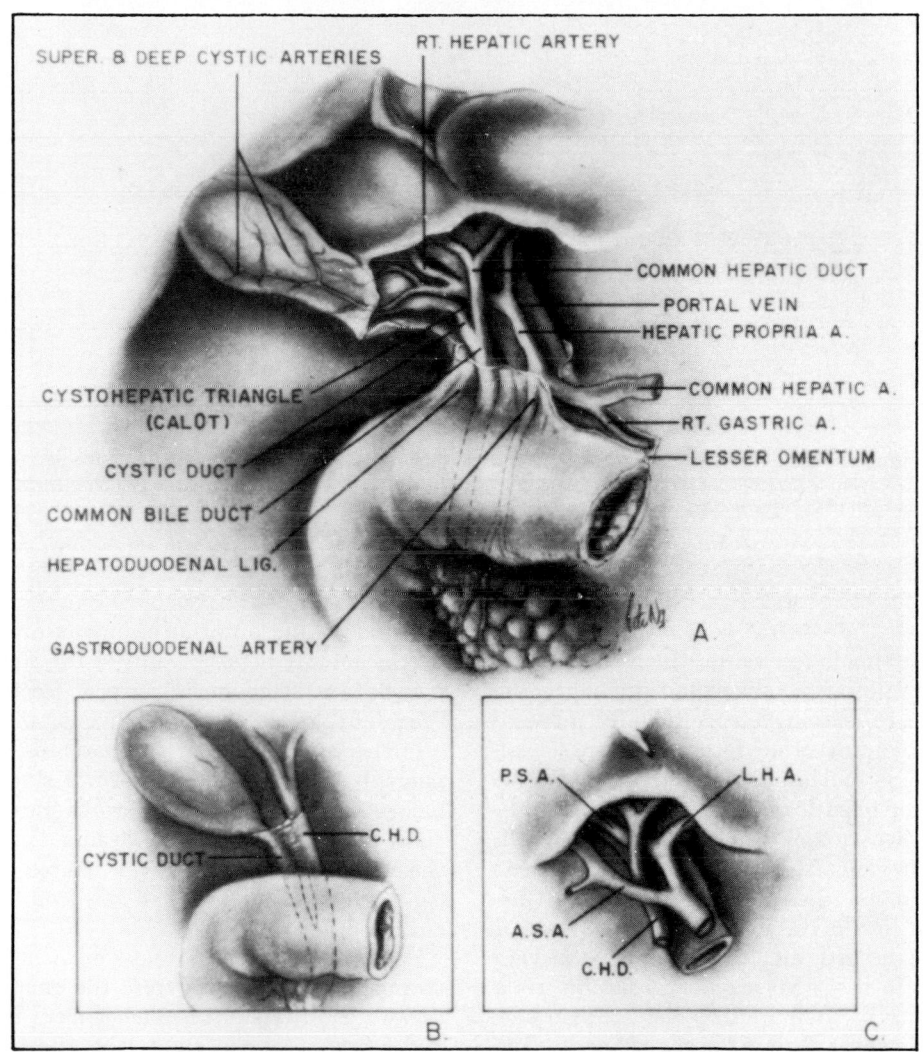

Figure 67–3. Relational anatomy of structures in the hepatoduodenal ligament. **A.** Normal anatomy. **B.** Frequent variation of the union of the cystic and common hepatic ducts (C.H.D.). **C.** Rare variation: Separate origin of the anterior (A.S.A.) and posterior (P.S.A.) segmental arteries. L.H.A. = left hepatic artery. (*Source: From Healey JE, Schwartz SI, 1964, with permission.*)

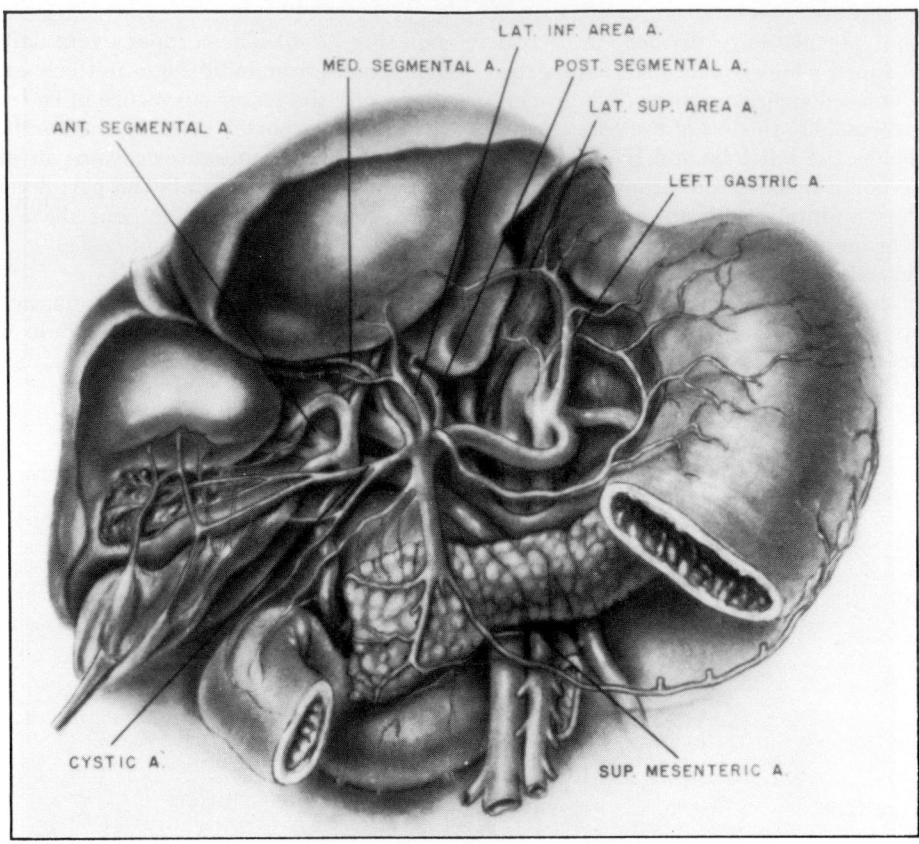

Figure 67–4. Findings in an adult cadaver in which five hepatic arteries were present, each supplying a specific segment or subsegment of the liver. (*Source: From Healey JE, Schwartz SI, 1964, with permission.*)

unites with the central vein of other lobules to form the sublobular veins, which fuse to form collecting veins from various subsegments of the liver. The collecting veins gradually increase in size by joining other large intrahepatic collecting veins and finally coalesce to form the three major hepatic veins.

The three major veins are the right, left, and middle vein (Fig. 67–6). The middle hepatic vein lies in the main lobar fissure, the left hepatic vein lies in the upper portion of the left segmental fissure, and the right hepatic vein is located in the right segmental fissure. As a consequence of their intersegmental positions, the hepatic veins drain adjacent segments. The left hepatic vein drains the entire lateral segment and the superior area of the medial segment. The right hepatic vein drains the entire posterior segment, as well as the superior area of the anterior segment. The inferior areas of the middle and anterior segments are drained by the middle hepatic vein. In the French nomenclature segment is termed "sector," and "segment" represents a subdivision of a sector.

The middle and left hepatic veins, in 60 percent of cases, unite to form a single trunk before emptying into the inferior vena cava. The right hepatic vein usually drains directly into the vena cava. At the caval orifices, both the right and left veins vary in size from 0.8 to 2.0 cm in diameter.

In addition to the main branches, one or two constant branches from the caudate lobe, as well as inconstant branches from the posterior segment of the right lobe, may enter directly into the inferior vena cava caudad in relation to the entrance of the main hepatic veins. There are frequent variations in size and number of the hepatic veins entering the inferior vena cava.

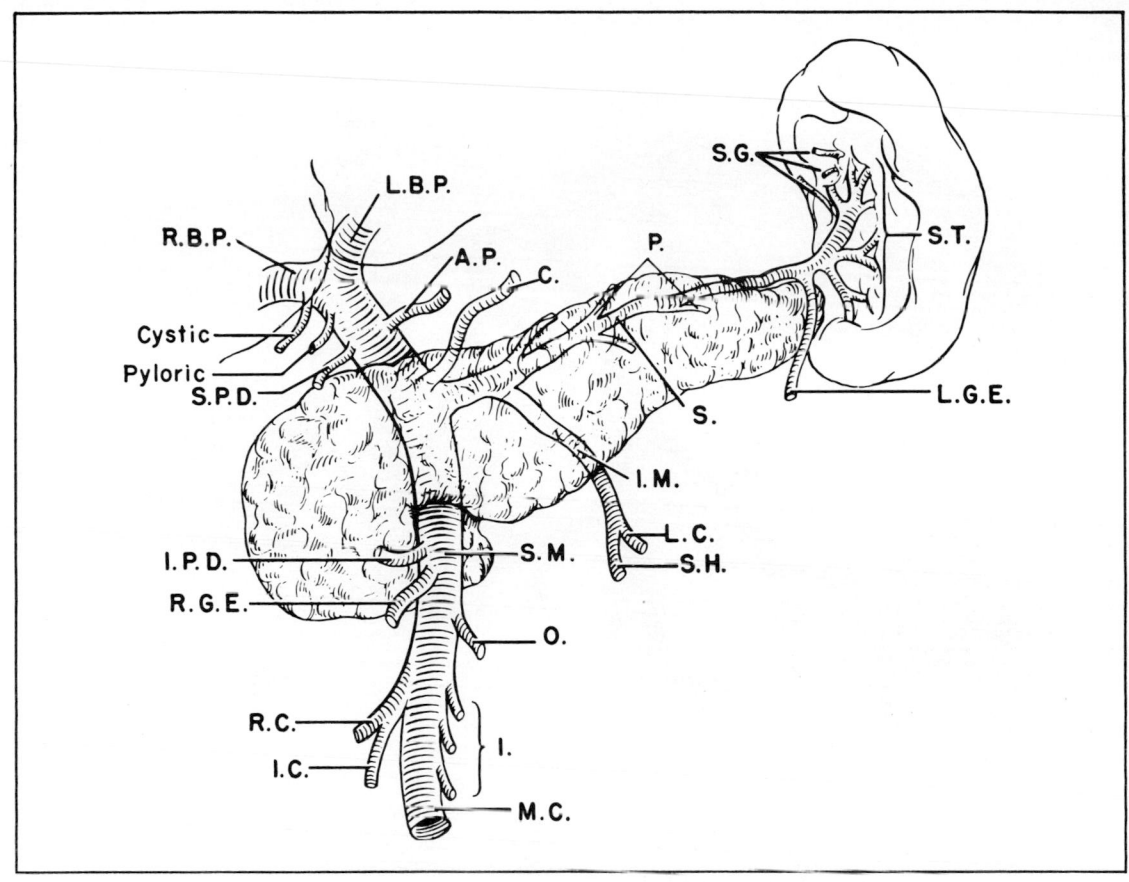

Figure 67–5. Anatomy of the extrahepatic portal venous system, anterior aspect. The termination of each vein is shown as it was encountered most frequently in the 92 dissections. The pancreas is represented by the shaded area. A.P. = accessory pancreatic vein, C. = coronary vein, Cystic = cystic vein, I. = intestinal veins, I.C. = ileocolic vein, I.M. = inferior mesenteric vein, I.P.D. = inferior pancreaticoduodenal vein, L. = liver, L.B.P. = left branch of portal vein, L.C. = left colic vein, L.G.E. = left gastroepiploic vein, M.C. = middle colic vein, O. = omental vein, P. = pancreatic veins, Pyloric = pyloric vein, R.C. = right colic vein, R.G.E. = right gastroepiploic vein, R.B.P. = right branch of portal vein, S. = splenic vein, S.G. = short gastric veins, S.H. = superior hemorrhoidal vein, S.M. = superior mesenteric vein, S.P.D. = superior pancreaticoduodenal vein, S.T. = splenic trunks. (*Source: From Healey JE, Schwartz SI, 1964, with permission.*)

Lobar Anatomy of the Liver

An appreciation of the lobar, or so-called functional, anatomy of the liver was initiated by Cantlie in 1898, and was followed by the works of McIndoe and Counseller, Hjorstjo, Couinaud, and Goldsmith and Woodburne. This concept, which is applicable to hepatic resection, is based on a description of hepatic segmentation related to the distribution of the portal pedicles and the location of the hepatic veins.

The liver is divided into two lobes, or hemi-livers, by the main portal fissure (scissura), which is also called Cantlie's line. The main portal fissure describes a 75 degree angle with a horizontal plane and extends from the antero-inferior gallbladder fossa posterosuperiorly to the left side of the inferior vena cava. The main portal fissure is a constant feature.

On each side of the main portal fissure, the organization of the right and left lobes of the liver is identical. Adjacent to the fissure there

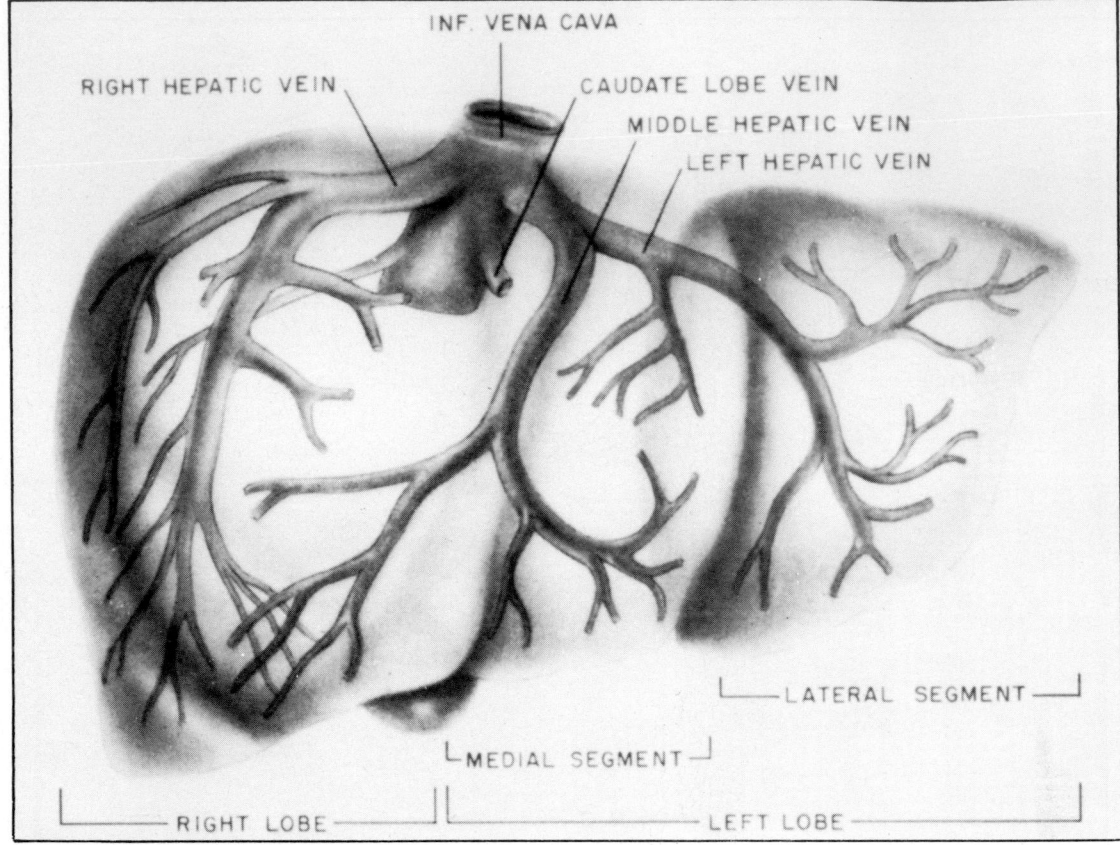

INF. VENA CAVA

RIGHT HEPATIC VEIN

CAUDATE LOBE VEIN

MIDDLE HEPATIC VEIN

LEFT HEPATIC VEIN

LATERAL SEGMENT

MEDIAL SEGMENT

RIGHT LOBE

LEFT LOBE

Figure 67–6. Prevailing pattern of drainage of hepatic veins in the human liver. (*Source: From Healey JE, Schwartz SI, 1964, with permission.*)

is a right or left paramedian sector. Lateral to each of these sectors there is a fissure, which is variable and without anatomic boundaries, separating the paramedian sector from the distal sector known as the right or left lateral sector (Figs. 67–7 and 67–8).

The left lobe of the liver consists of the hepatic tissue to the left of the falciform ligament, plus the quadrate lobe and the caudate lobes of the old anatomic nomenclature. The right hepatic lobe consists of remaining hepatic tissue.

The right portal fissure divides the right lobe into an anteromedial and posterolateral sector. The right hepatic vein courses along this fissure. There is no external landmark to define this fissure. According to Couinaud, it extends from the anterior surface of the liver midway between the right angle of the liver and the right side of the gallbladder to the confluence between the inferior vena cava and the right

hepatic vein posteriorly, describing an angle of 40 degrees with the transverse plane (Fig. 67–9).

The left portal fissure divides the left lobe into an anterior and posterior sector, and it is in this fissure that the left hepatic vein courses. The left portal fissure is located posteriorly in relation to the ligamentum teres.

The liver is further divided into segments that, according to Couinaud, represent the smallest anatomic unit of the organ. In the right lobe, each of the two sectors is divided into two segments: the anteromedial sector is divided into segment V anteriorly and segment VIII posteriorly, while the posterolateral sector is divided into segment VI anteriorly and segment VII posteriorly. In the left lobe, the anterior sector is divided by the umbilical fissure into segment IV, the anterior part of which is the quadrate lobe, and segment III, which is the anterior part of the left lobe. The posterior sec-

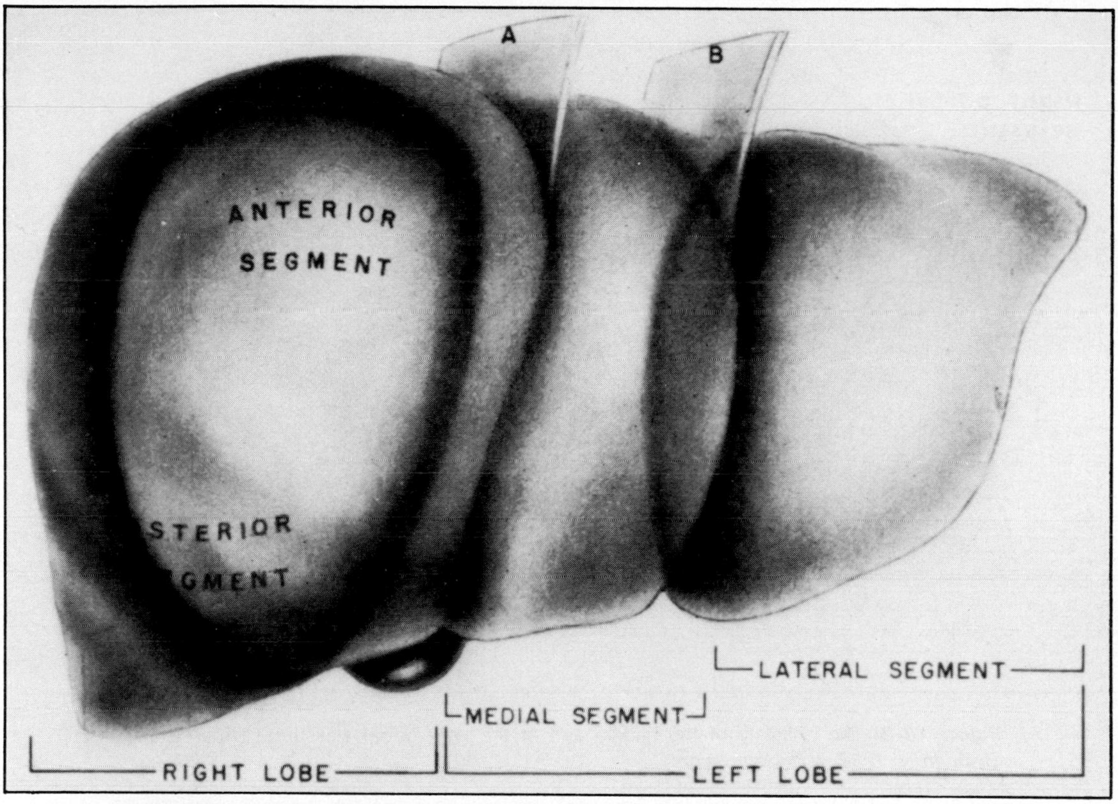

Figure 67–7. Lobar and segmental divisions of the liver. **A.** Lobar fissure. **B.** Left segmental fissure. A right segmental fissure divides the right lobe into its anterior and posterior segments. (*Source: From Healey JE, Schwartz SI, 1964, with permission.*)

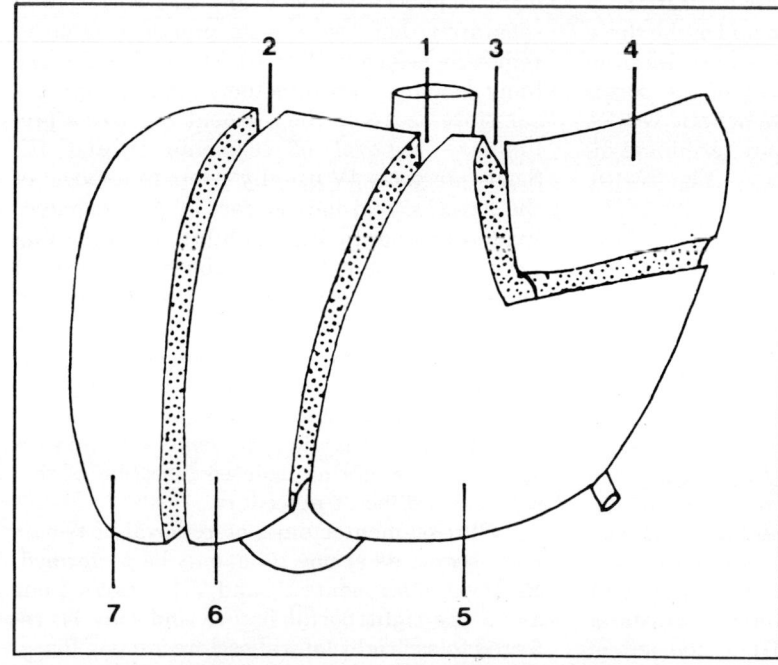

Figure 67–8. Symmetrical organization of the right liver. 1. main portal fissure, 2. right portal fissure, 3. left portal fissure, 4. left lateral sector, 5. left paramedian sector, 6. right paramedian sector, 7. right lateral sector. Human liver is characterized by the atrophy of the left lateral sector. (*Source: From Couinaud C, 1981, with permission.*)

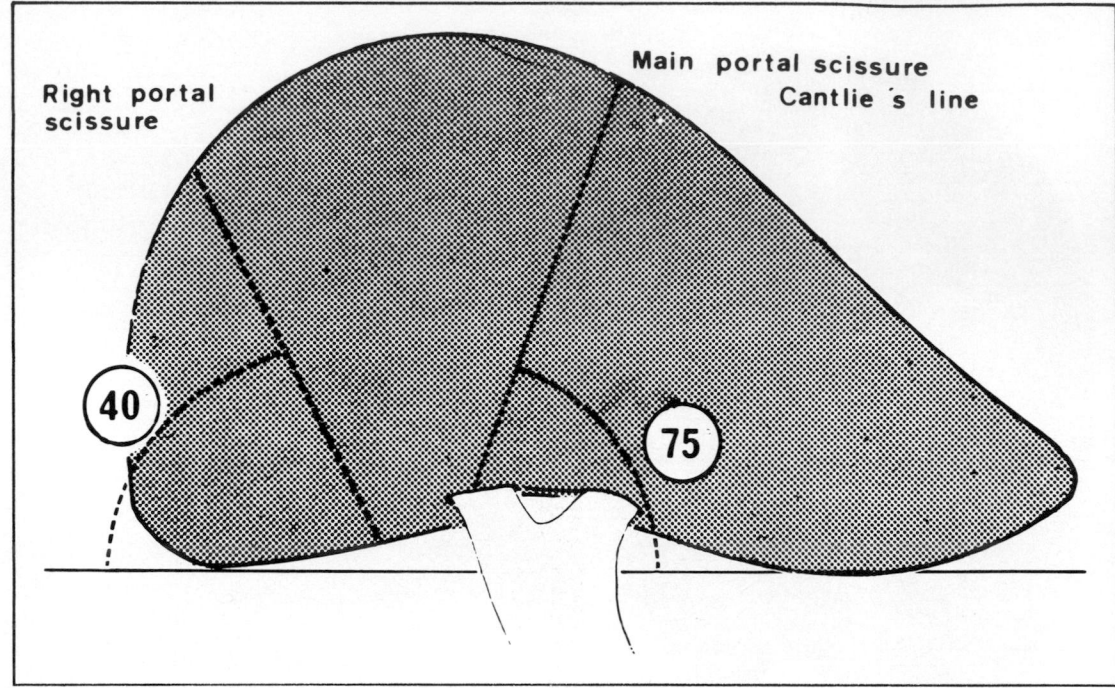

Figure 67–9. The obliquity of the middle and of the right portal scissurae. (*Source: From Bismuth H, 1982, with permission.*)

tor is comprised of only one segment, II, which is the posterior part of the left lobe. The Spigel lobe, or segment I, is considered an autonomous segment, since it receives its vascularization independent of the portal division and of the three main hepatic veins. It receives tributaries from both the right and left branches of the portal vein and hepatic artery, and its hepatic venous drainage is independent and may terminate directly into the inferior vena cava (Fig. 67–10).

NOMENCLATURE OF HEPATIC RESECTION

Resection along the main portal fissure, separating the right and left lobes of the liver, is termed a right or left hepatic lobectomy (right and left hepatectomy in French nomenclature). Resection of the entire right lobe and the medial segment (sector) of the left lobe, i.e., the hepatic parenchyma to the right of the falciform ligament and ligamentum teres, is termed a right extended lobectomy (trisegmentectomy). Left lateral segmentectomy (lobectomy) consists of removal of segments II and III to the left of

the falciform ligament and ligamentum teres.

Unisegmentectomy refers to the removal of a single segment. Theoretically, each of the eight segments of the liver could be removed separately, but there is no practical value to removing segment II or III as a unisegmentectomy. Isolated segmentectomy I is also impractical, since access to the segment requires a preliminary removal of segments II and III. Segmentectomy IV usually refers to removal of the anterior and mobile part of that segment, located anterior to the liver hilus, corresponding to the quadrate lobe. Resection of segment VI alone, i.e., that portion of the liver anterior to the level of the hilus located to the right of the right lateral fissure, is rarely indicated. Segmentectomy VIII consists of resection of the superior part of the right paramedian segment. It is connected with the intrahepatic vena cava and with segment I, rendering isolated resection of this segment a difficult procedure.

Plurisegmentectomy, or removal of two or more segments at one time, may be performed. Removal of segments VI and VII is carried out along the right portal fissure and may be referred to as "right lateral sectorectomy." Biseg-

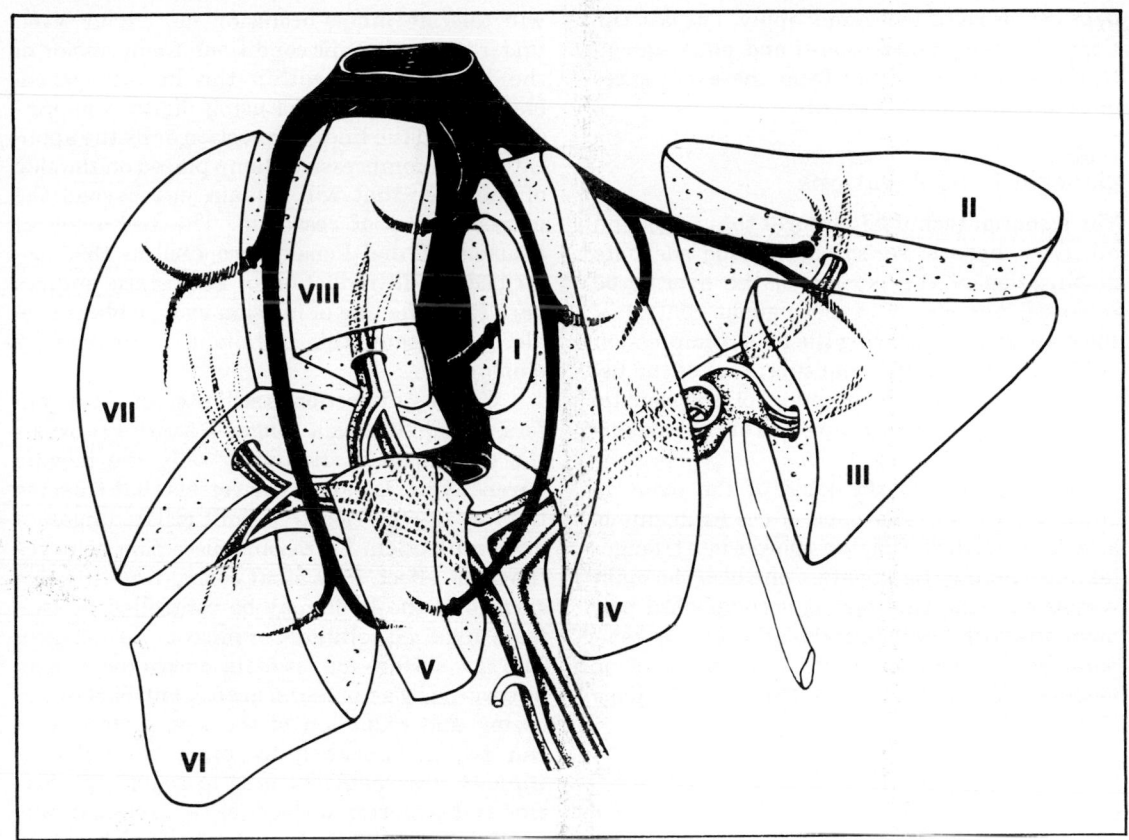

Figure 67–10. The functional division of the liver and the segments according to Couinaud's nomenclature. (*Source: From Bismuth H, 1982, with permission.*)

mentectomy IV and V finds its applicability in patients with carcinoma of the gallbladder extending into the liver. Bisegmentectomy V and VI is rarely performed. Removal of IV, V, and VI may be carried out as treatment for carcinoma of the gallbladder, since the cystic veins may enter in the portal branch of segment VI.

Removal of a small portion of the liver, either within a single segment or traversing segmental planes, constitutes a *wedge resection.*

PREOPERATIVE MANAGEMENT

An essential feature of the preoperative protocol is angiography of both the celiac and the superior mesenteric arteries to define the extent of hepatic involvement and thus the resectability, and also to demonstrate the vascular anatomy and segmental supply. A venous phase to determine involvement of the portal vein should be included. Computed tomography performed while radiopaque medium is infused directly into the hepatic artery provides the best definition of intrahepatic pathology.

The serum albumin, prothrombin time, activated partial thromboplastin time, and platelet count are all to be performed and, if abnormal, corrected. A cephalosporin is instituted on the day of operation. Significant blood loss should be anticipated, and an autotransfusion apparatus is made available for use intraoperatively.

OPERATIVE TECHNIQUE

The more commonly performed major lobectomies and segmentectomies will be considered. Right hepatic lobectomy will be described in detail, and the description of left hepatic lobectomy will be omitted, since all of the principles detailed for right lobectomy apply. The descriptions of unisegmentectomies and plurisegmentectomies derive mainly from the experiences of Couinaud and of Bismuth.

General Considerations

The essential technical features that transcend all major hepatic resections include adequate mobilization of the portion of the liver to be removed, temporary or permanent control of the main vessels entering the liver, compression of blood vessels within the substance of the hepatic parenchyma, transection of the hepatic parenchyma, and efforts directed at the raw surface.

Mobilization of the lobes of the liver requires complete transection of the ligamentous attachments, including the appropriate triangular and coronary ligaments. Control of the main vessels entering the liver is accomplished permanently with ligature and transection or, temporarily, by occlusion using vascular tapes or vascular clamps. It is now known that the liver

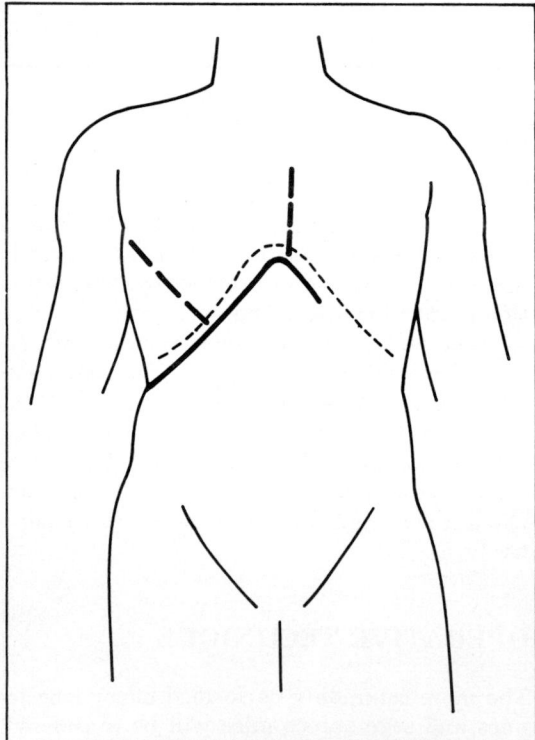

Figure 67–11. Choice of incisions for right hepatic lobectomy.

will tolerate inflow occlusion for 1 hour, even under normothermic conditions. Compression of the blood vessels within the hepatic parenchyma can be achieved using digital compression beyond the lines of resection or by the application of a compressive clamp placed on the side of the liver that will remain just beyond the proposed line of resection. The technique of Kouznetzoff and Pensky, proposed in 1896, described the introduction of hemostatic sutures parallel to the line of incision using a blunt needle. At present, this technique is not usually employed.

Cautery dissection is still used in many centers, but digitoclasia (finger fracture) provides the advantage of disrupting only the hepatic parenchyma, isolating the vessels that traverse the line of resection to permit isolated ligation and transection. Ultrasonic dissection achieves the same effect. Persistent oozing from the raw surface of the liver may be controlled by Gelfoam, oxidized cellulose, or micronized collagen. The raw surface may remain uncovered or may be covered by an omental graft. Control of minor oozing and reduction of the raw surface area can be accomplished by tying through-and-through absorbable sutures to coapt the anterior and posterior surfaces of Glisson's capsule.

Right Hepatic Lobectomy

A right subcostal incision is preferred, either with a left subcostal extension in a chevron fashion (Fig. 67–11) or with an extension craniad over the xiphoid process. The incision should be placed high enough to permit placement of an overhead retractor so that the sternum can be retracted toward the ceiling. The entire right rectus muscle is transected, and the oblique muscles are split laterally almost to the tip of the right tenth rib. Transection of the medial portion of the left rectus muscle usually provides sufficient exposure. A thoracic extension placed perpendicualr to the right subcostal incision and extending through the seventh intercostal space is rarely used and is reserved for large lesions in the dome of the right lobe of the liver, with diaphragmatic involvement or encroachment on the suprahepatic inferior vena cava.

Mobilization

Mobilization should be accomplished so that the right lobe can be delivered into the wound. The ligamentum teres is transected; a clamp can be left on the hepatic end to facilitate traction. The triangular ligament supporting the right lobe is divided, and the dissection is continued by transecting the anterior and posterior leaflets of the right coronary ligament to the inferior vena cava (Fig. 67–2). This permits the entire right lobe of the liver to be mobilized toward the left. At times, complete mobilization is impaired by attachment of two or three small hepatic veins, and these may be ligated at the point where they enter the inferior vena cava. Following mobilization, laparotomy pads may be placed behind the right lobe of the liver to make the hilus more accessible.

Hepatoduodenal Dissection

The cystic artery and duct are ligated and divided prior to dissection of the hepatoduodenal structure. It is generally easier to remove the gallbladder at this time, but it is sufficient to dissect the medial half of the gallbladder from the liver bed, since this will expose the interlobar fissure. The peritoneal reflection overlying the structures within the hepatoduodenal ligament is incised, and the right main hepatic artery is identified as the first step of the dissection, since it is the most anterior structure encountered. A vascular tape is placed around this vessel, and care is taken to insure that the

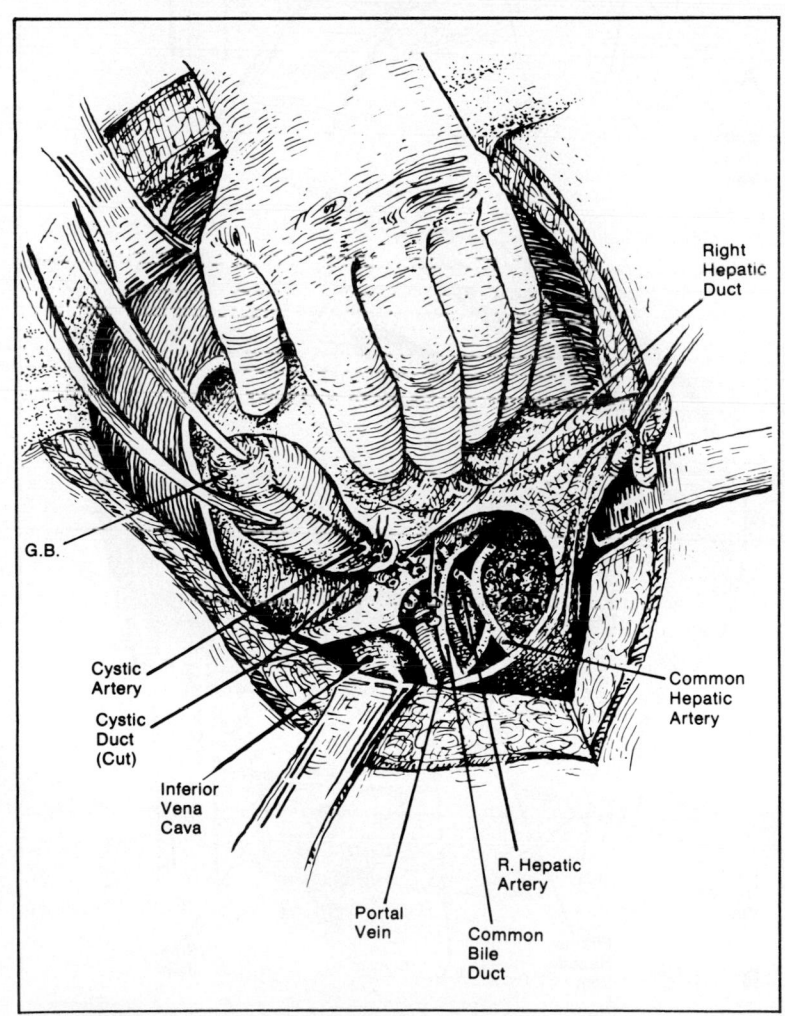

Figure 67–12. Hepatoduodenal dissection. (*Source: From Schwartz SI, 1981, with permission.*)

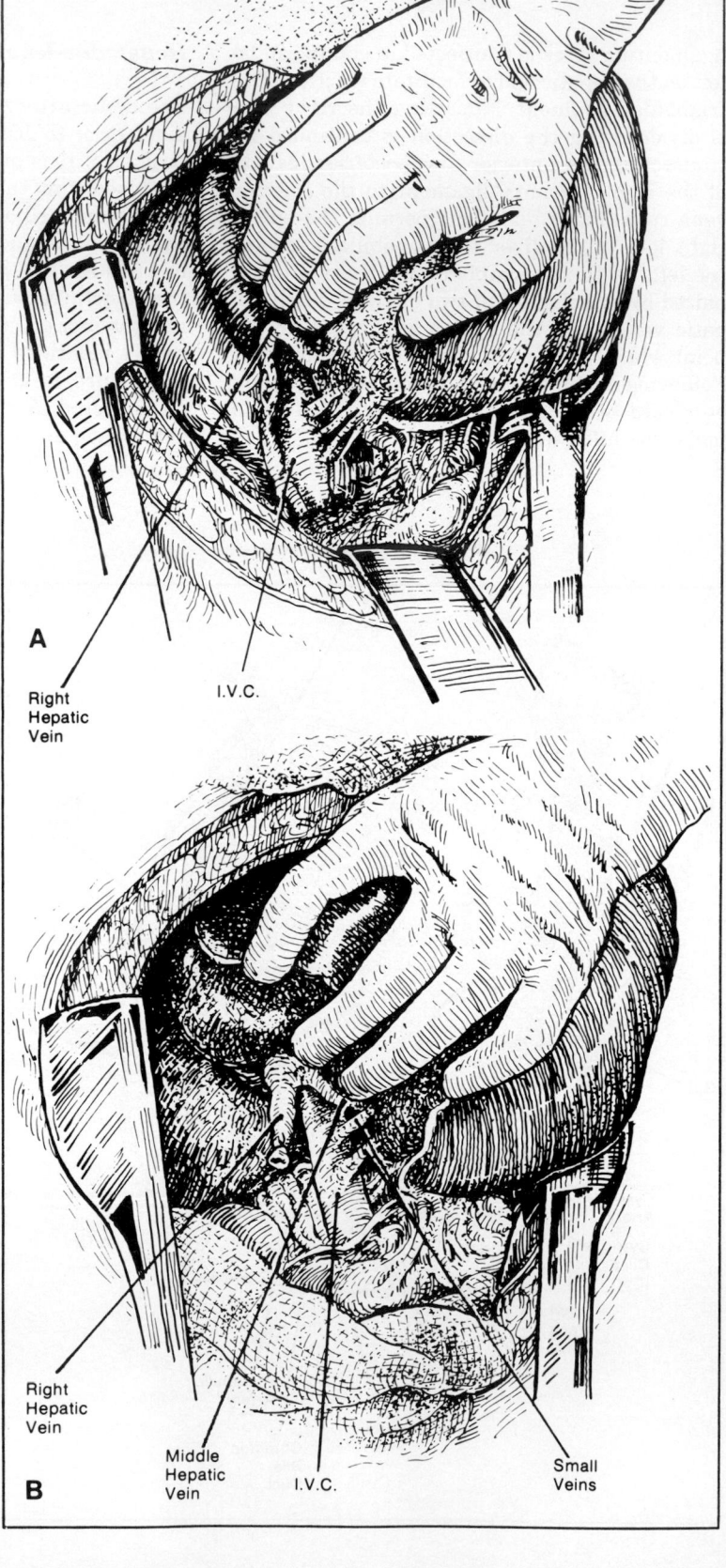

Figure 67–13. A and **B**. Retrohepatic dissection to achieve control of hepatic veins. (*Source: From Schwartz SI, 1981, with permission.*)

A

Right Hepatic Vein

I.V.C.

B

Right Hepatic Vein

Middle Hepatic Vein

I.V.C.

Small Veins

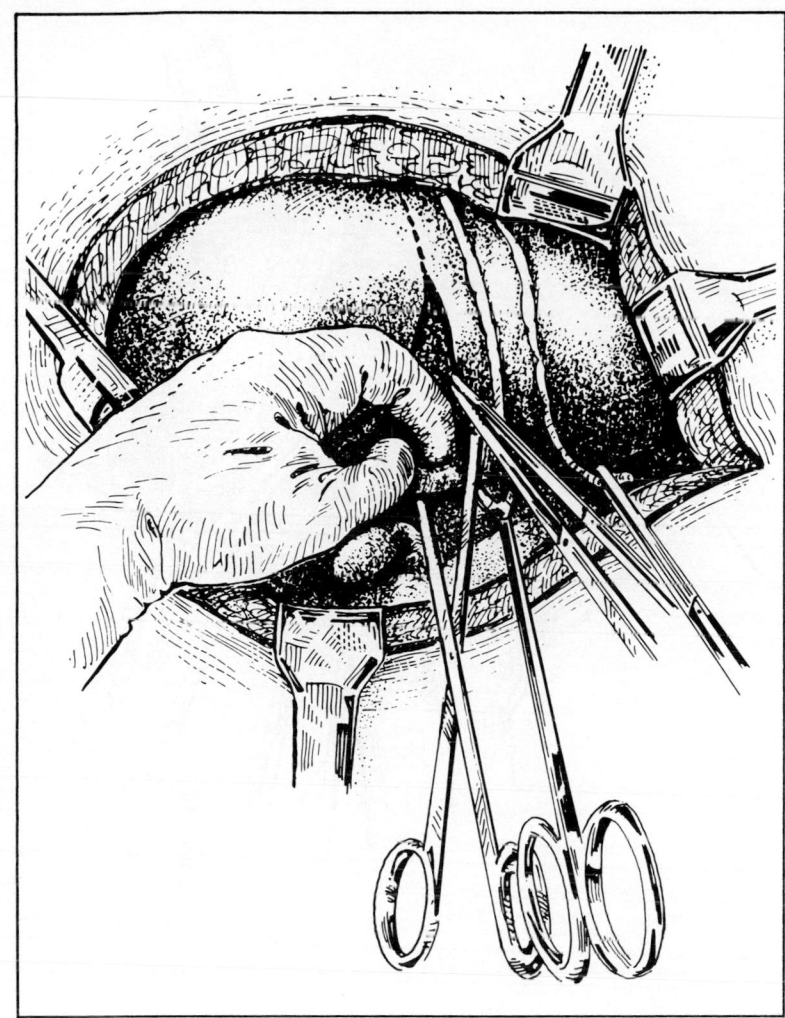

Figure 67-14. Finger fracture technique: Anteroinferior intraparenchymal dissection of portal structures. (*Source: From Schwartz SI, 1981, with permission.*)

left main hepatic artery is protected. The right hepatic artery may be displaced and may arise from the superior mesenteric artery; this is readily defined by preoperative angiogram.

Dissection is continued craniad, and the right branch of the portal vein is identified in the posterior portion of the hepatoduodenal ligament. Exposure is frequently facilitated by rotating the mobilized right lobe of the liver anteriorly. A vascular tape is then passed around the right branch of the portal vein, taking care to protect the left main portal vein. The right main hepatic duct is then dissected free and a tape is passed around it. This maneuver represents the most craniad step in the dissection. The right hepatic artery, the right portal vein, and the right hepatic duct may then

be doubly ligated in continuity, and divided, or the vascular tapes may be snugged up to provide temporary occlusion (Fig. 67-12).

After the structures in the porta hepatis have been ligated and divided or temporarily occluded, there are two potential approaches to the completion of hepatic lobectomy. The first involves securing the hepatic veins outside the liver as they drain into the inferior vena cava. In this circumstance the right lobe is rotated in a clockwise fashion, and the veins are isolated from below upward (Fig. 67-13A,B). The main right hepatic vein is large and is best managed by applying a Satinsky or Derra vascular clamp to the anterior aspect of the inferior vena cava so that it incorporates the right hepatic vein. A curved hemostat is applied to the hepatic side

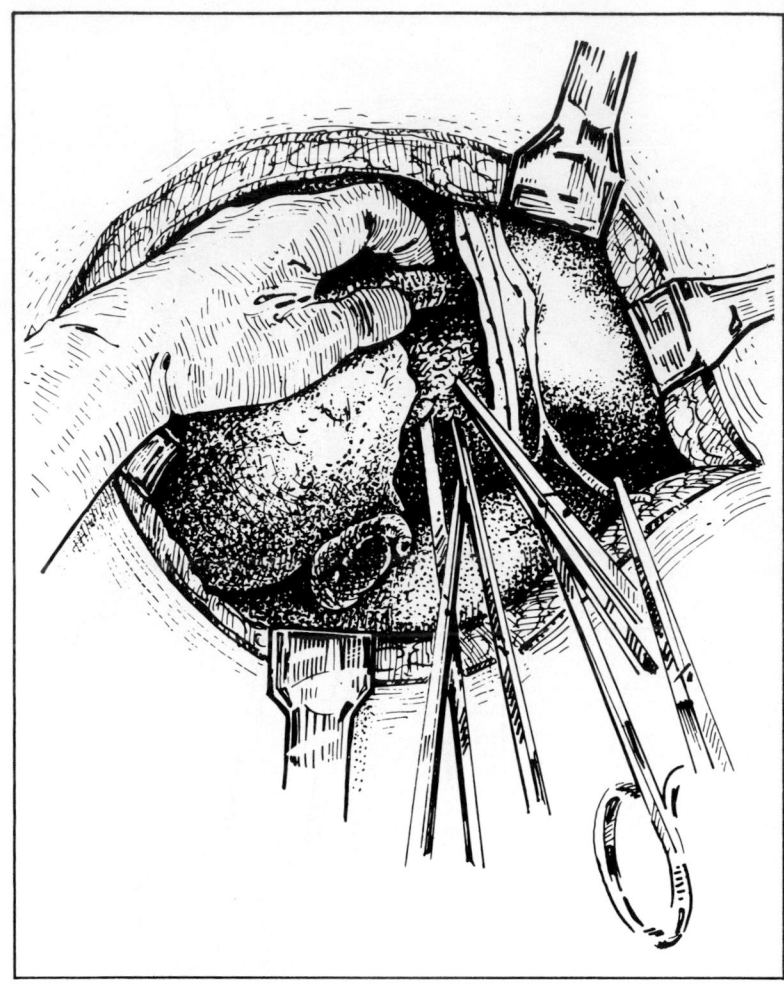

Figure 67–15. Finger fracture technique: Posterosuperior intraparenchymal dissection of right hepatic vein. (*Source: From Schwartz SI, 1981, with permission.*)

of the vein, and the hepatic vein is then transected and the caval side is sewn with continuous Prolene suture. The operation is completed by incising the capsule of the liver and transecting the parenchyma, clamping, dividing, and ligating vessels and ducts as they traverse the interlobar plane.

The second approach, and the one that this author generally uses, involves transection of the hepatic parenchyma in the interlobar plane beginning anteroinferiorly, progressing posterosuperiorly. A compressive liver clamp may be placed to the left of the lobar plane, but this author rarely uses it. Glisson's capsule is incised anteroinferiorly, and the parenchyma is transected by digital dissection, which disrupts the hepatic tissue but does not transect the vessels as they cross the interlobar fissure. These are doubly clamped and transected. The side of the

vessel that will remain is ligated with silk, and the vessels on the specimen side are controlled with hemostatic clips. As the fingers divide the hepatic parenchyma in the anteroinferior portion of the liver, branches of the hepatic artery, portal vein, and duct are defined intrahepatically (Fig. 67–14), doubly ligated, and transected.

The dissection continues posterosuperiorly to the region where the right main hepatic vein is encountered (Fig. 67–15). The hepatic vein is isolated within the substance of the liver and doubly clamped with a vascular clamp applied on the caval side of the vein and a hemostat on the side to be removed. The vessel is then transected, and the caval side of the transected hepatic vein is closed with continuous vascular suture.

This technique has the advantage of avoid-

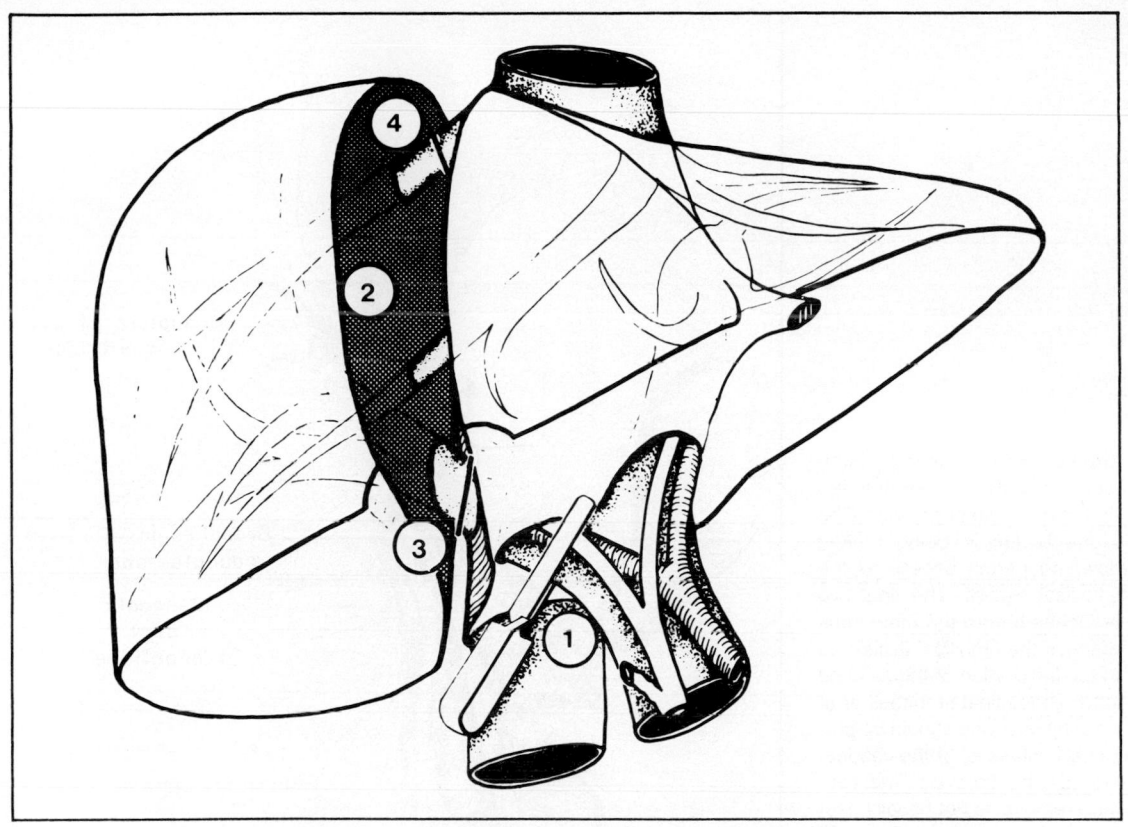

Figure 67–16. Sequence of events: (1) temporary occlusion of structures in hepatoduodenal ligation, (2) anterior parenchymal dissection, (3) parenchymal dissection of portal structures, and (4) parenchymal dissection of hepatic vein. (*Source: From Bismuth H, 1982, with permission.*)

ing inadvertent ligation of a hepatic vein that serves as the efferent conduit from the remaining left lobe of the liver. It is also more rapid.

Transection of the hepatic parenchyma in the interlobar plane may be performed with an ultrasonic scalpel, with a stream of saline irrigating the tip. At 80 to 90 percent of full power the instrument is used in a probing motion, gradually deepening the incision from anterior to posterior. The parenchyma is transected, leaving skeletonized vessels that could readily be controlled by clamps or clips. When the larger vessels are approached posterosuperiorly, the power is reduced to about 70 to 80 percent and the direction of the tip is changed so that it runs parallel to the vessels.

After transection of the parenchyma is complete, the specimen is removed. Following removal of the specimen, the vascular and ductal tapes can be released to determine that the

bleeding and bile leak from the parenchymal surface are completely controlled. If arterial bleeding is encountered, the hepatic artery is ligated in the hepatoduodenal ligament. If portal bleeding is encountered, the portal vein is handled in a similar fashion. If there is evidence of bile leak, the hepatic duct can be ligated within the hepatoduodenal ligament. This is usually not required. The usual sequence that is followed by this author is the same as that endorsed by Bismuth (Fig. 67–16).

The raw surface of the liver may be covered conveniently with pedicled omentum, but this is not necessary. The anterior and posterior portions of the remaining Glisson's capsule can be approximated with interrupted catgut sutures to reduce the raw area and to provide a tamponade effect on the smaller vessels. Soft rubber drains are placed in the subphrenic space that had been occupied by the resected specimen and

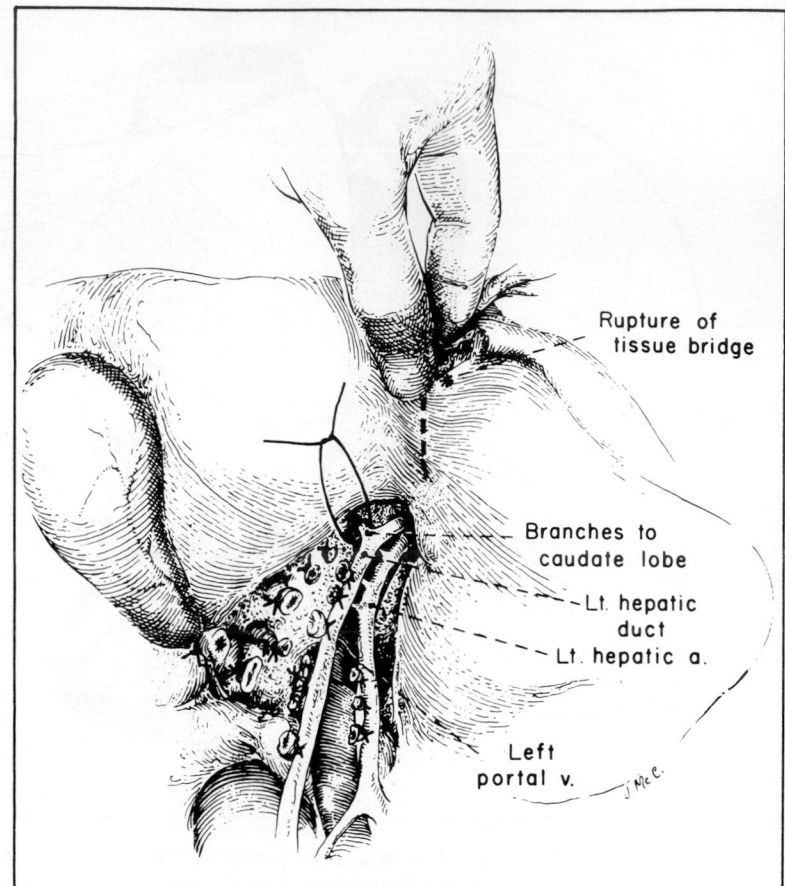

Figure 67–17. Nearly completed mobilization of the left branches of the portal triad. The tissue bridge is being broken down to permit access to the umbilical fissure. The final two branches before the main trunk reaches the umbilical fissure go to the left portion of the caudate lobe. These final branches or at least the last one should be preserved unless all of the caudate lobe is to be removed. Total caudate removal is not usually necessary. (*Source: From Starzl TE, Bell RH, et al, 1975, with permission.*)

Within the figure:
- Rupture of tissue bridge
- Branches to caudate lobe
- Lt. hepatic duct
- Lt. hepatic a.
- Left portal v.

are brought out through one or two large stab wounds, and positioned in a Hollister bag to provide a closed system of drainage. The common bile duct is not drained with a T-tube.

Extended Right Hepatic Lobectomy (Trisegmentectomy)

The initial phases of the operation, including the incision, transection of the ligamentous attachments to the right lobe, and dissection of the hilus proceeds in the same fashion as described for right hepatic lobectomy. The right hepatic artery, right portal vein, and the right hepatic duct are managed similarly.

Dissection in the region of the hilus continues, completing mobilization of the left branches of the portal structures (Fig. 67–17). Two or three branches from the hepatic artery to the caudate lobe are ligated and several branches from the portal vein are also ligated in this region. This dissection is stopped short of the umbilical fissure. The right hepatic vein may be interrupted posteriorly at its junction with the inferior vena cava or might be ligated within the parenchyma itself according to the two options described in the section on right hepatic lobectomy.

An incision is made just to the right of the falciform ligament and the parenchyma is crushed between fingers to permit access to the umbilical fissure. Vessels and ducts passing to the medial segment of the left lobe are divided, preserving the vessels and ducts to the lateral segment of the left lobe. If the right hepatic vein had not been ligated via the posterior approach, it can be managed at this time (Fig. 67–18).

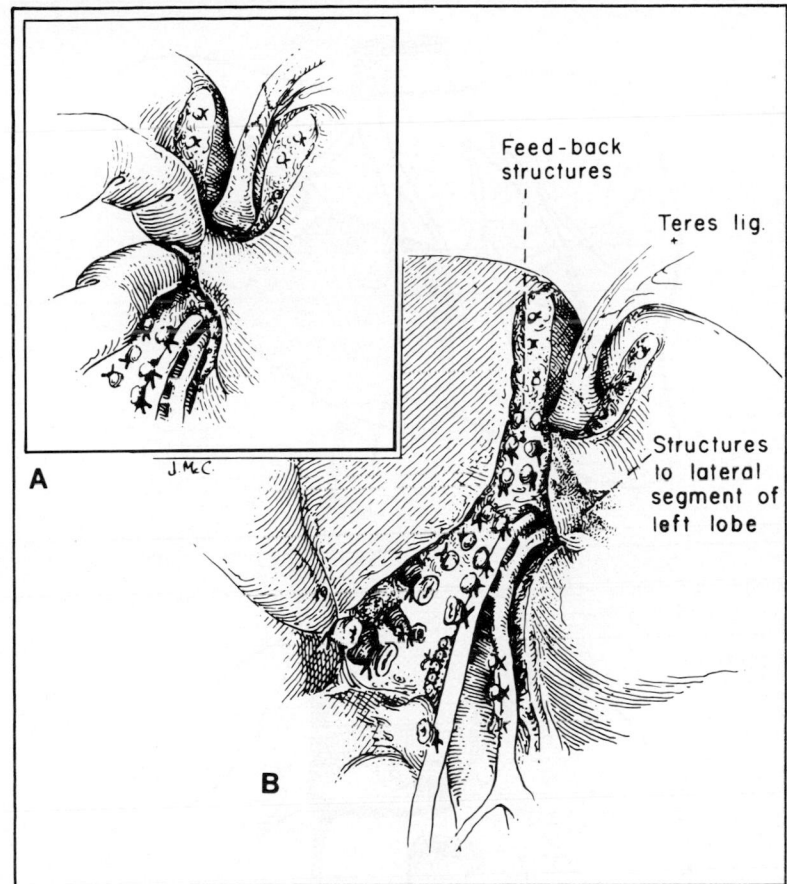

Feed-back
structures

Teres lig.

Structures
to lateral
segment of
left lobe

A

J.McC.

B

Figure 67–18. Structures feeding back from the umbilical fissure to the medial segment of the left lobe. **A.** These are encircled usually by blunt dissection within the liver substances just to the right of the falciform ligament and umbilical fissure without entering the fissure. Note that the hepatic tissue bridge concealing the umbilical fissure has been broken down. **B.** The three segments of the specimen are now devascularized. (*Source: From Starzl TE, Bell RH, et al, 1975, with permission.*)

Left Lateral Segmentectomy (Left Lateral Sectorectomy—Removal of Segments II and III)

This procedure can be performed through the same incision as used for right lobectomy, or through an upper midline incision. The left lateral segment is initially mobilized by dividing its ligamentous attachments, i.e., the left triangular ligament, the left coronary ligaments, and the falciform ligament.

It is then possible to displace the portion to be resected downward and to expose the inferior surface of the porta hepatis. The segmental tributaries of the left branch of the portal vein, the left hepatic duct, and the left branch of the hepatic artery may be dissected within the hepatoduodenal ligament. These may be controlled by vascular tapes, but it may be simpler to temporarily occlude the entire contents of hepato-

duodenal ligament with an atraumatic vascular clamp.

The plane for resection of the lateral segment of the left lobe is located 1 cm to the left of the falciform ligament. In this plane only the terminal branches supplying the lateral segment are encountered. There is no hazard of disturbing the ducts and vessels to the medial segment, since they reside in the umbilical fissure itself. After Glisson's capsule has been incised, the cleavage plane is best established by means of finger fracture to separate the liver parenchyma and to expose the larger ducts and vessels, which may be individually clamped and ligated as they are encountered. The incision is continued posteriorly until the hepatic vein is demonstrated, doubly ligated, and transected. The entire procedure usually can be accomplished with sufficient facility that preliminary vascular inflow occlusion may not be required.

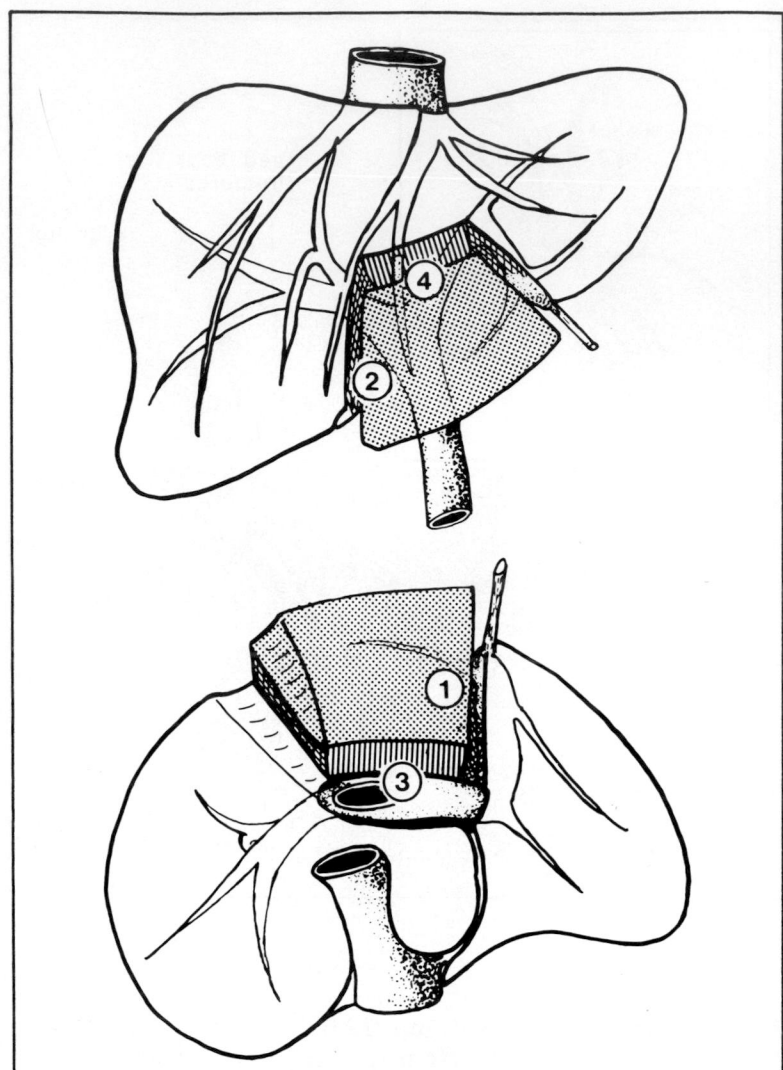

Figure 67–19. Anterior segmentectomy IV or resection of the quadrate lobe. The different steps of the technique: (1) opening of the umbilical fissure, (2) opening of the anterior part of the main scissura, (3) ligation of the portal pedicles entering the posterior part of the quadrate lobe, and (4) transverse transection of the parenchyma. (*Source: From Bismuth H, Houssin D, et al, 1982, with permission.*)

Unisegmentectomy

Anterior Segmentectomy IV (Resection of the Quadrate Lobe)

This was first performed by Caprio and has been used for gaining access to the upper portion of the biliary confluence.

The classic right upper quadrant chevron incision or a midline incision may be used. The anterior portion of the falciform ligament and the ligamentum teres are divided. Resection of the parenchyma begins by dividing the tissue between segments III and IV, by opening the umbilical fissure (Fig. 67–19). The peritoneum at the inferior part of the ligamentum teres is divided, and several arterial and portal pedicles are dissected to the right of the ligamentum teres. The liver is then transected anteriorly along the main fissure, and this dissection is continued up to the hilus. The only vascular elements requiring ligation in this portion of the dissection are the left branches of the middle hepatic vein. Posteriorly, Glisson's capsule is incised in front of the peritoneum overlying the hilus, and arterial and portal branches of the quadrate lobe are ligated and divided. Finally, a transverse incision of Glisson's capsule is

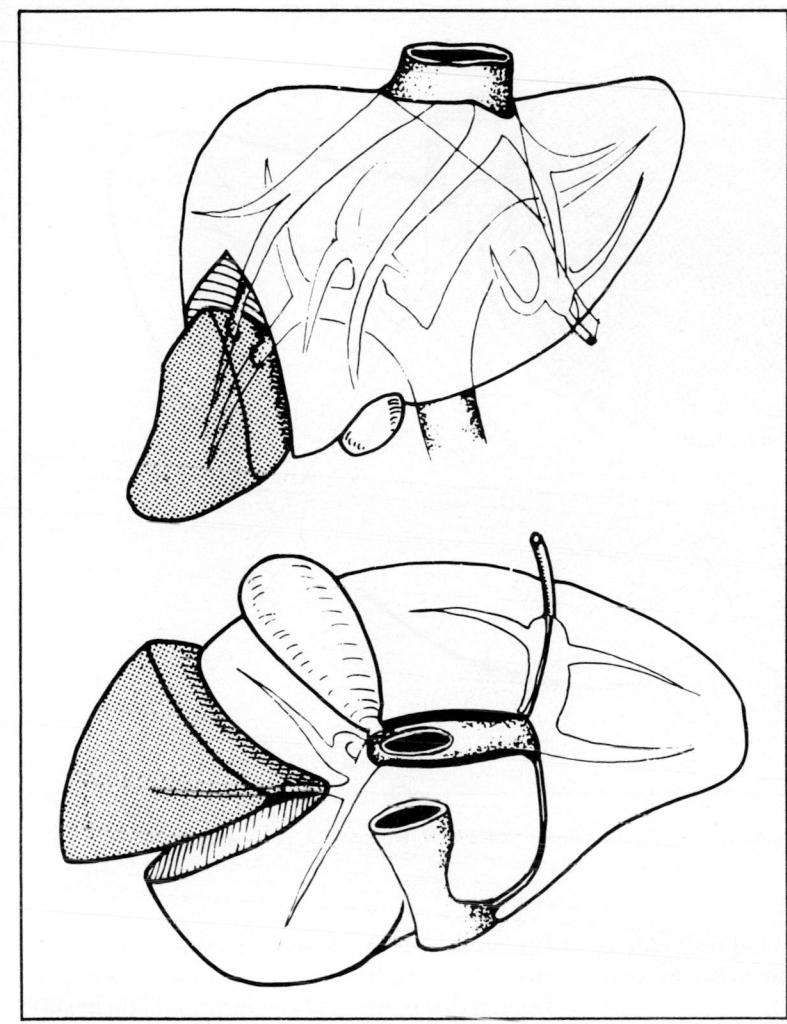

Figure 67–20. Segmentectomy VI. (*Source: From Bismuth H, Houssin D, et al, 1982, with permission.*)

made anteriorly, joining the right and left lines of transection, and the specimen is removed.

Segmentectomy VI

Segmentectomy VI is rarely indicated but is performed with ease after the ligamentous attachments of the right lobe of the liver are divided to permit mobilization. The liver is transected along the right lateral fissure midway between the gallbladder and the right edge of the liver. The transection is continued up to the level of the hilus, where the liver is transected transversely toward its right lateral side. During dissection, the anterior part of the right hepatic vein and the portal pedicle of the segment are ligated (Fig. 67–20).

Segmentectomy VIII

Segmentectomy VIII has been performed on occasions by Ton That Tung for chronic liver abscess situated superiorly in the liver. A right subcostal incision is made, and the falciform and right triangular and coronary ligaments are divided. Temporary hepatic inflow occlusion is effected. The right lateral and the main hepatic fissures are transected from the superior lip at the insertion of the right coronary ligament posteriorly up to the level of the hilus anteriorly. These two lines of transection are joined by two transverse incisions along the insertion of the coronary ligament posteriorly and along the posterior part of the hilus anteriorly. During transection, hepatic veins of segment VIII are

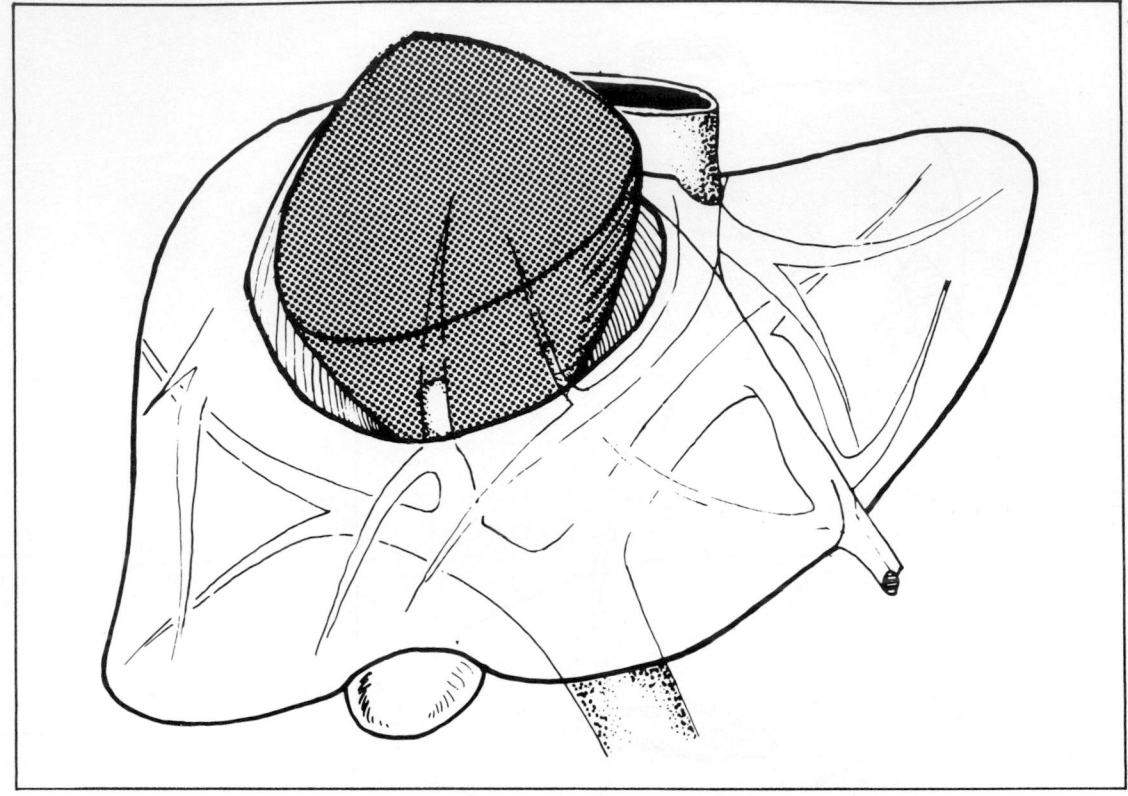

Figure 67–21. Segmentectomy VIII. (*Source: From Bismuth H, Houssin D, et al, with permission.*)

divided; attention must be directed to avoiding injury to the right and middle main hepatic veins (Fig. 67–21).

Plurisegmentectomies

Bisegmentectomy IV, V

This operation is indicated for carcinoma of the gallbladder. Through a subcostal incision the umbilical fissure is opened, and the parenchyma is split to the right of the falciform ligament. The right portal fissure is then opened. The main step in the dissection is ligation of the portal pedicle of segments IV and V, avoiding damage to the main vascular supply to the right and left lobes of the liver. During transection of the hilus, the anterior branch of the large inferior and posterior right paramedian portal pedicle is ligated. The portal branch of the posterior part of the quadrate lobe is then ligated. The final step in the procedure is the posterior

transection of the hepatic parenchyma joining the left and right incisions in front of the hilus. During this maneuver the large, middle hepatic vein is ligated and divided (Fig. 67–22).

Trisegmentectomy IV, V, VI

The initial step is the same as that described for resection of segment IV, with division of the portal pedicles of that segment. The liver is then transected along the umbilical fissure up to the level of the hilus. Anteriorly the Glisson's capsule is incised transversely to the right side of the liver, and the transection is continued deep to provide exposure of the divisions of the portal pedicles of segments V and VI. These are ligated and divided, as are branches of the right and middle hepatic veins (Fig. 67–23).

POSTOPERATIVE MANAGEMENT

Gastric decompression is usually maintained for 1 to 2 days, after which oral intake is begun

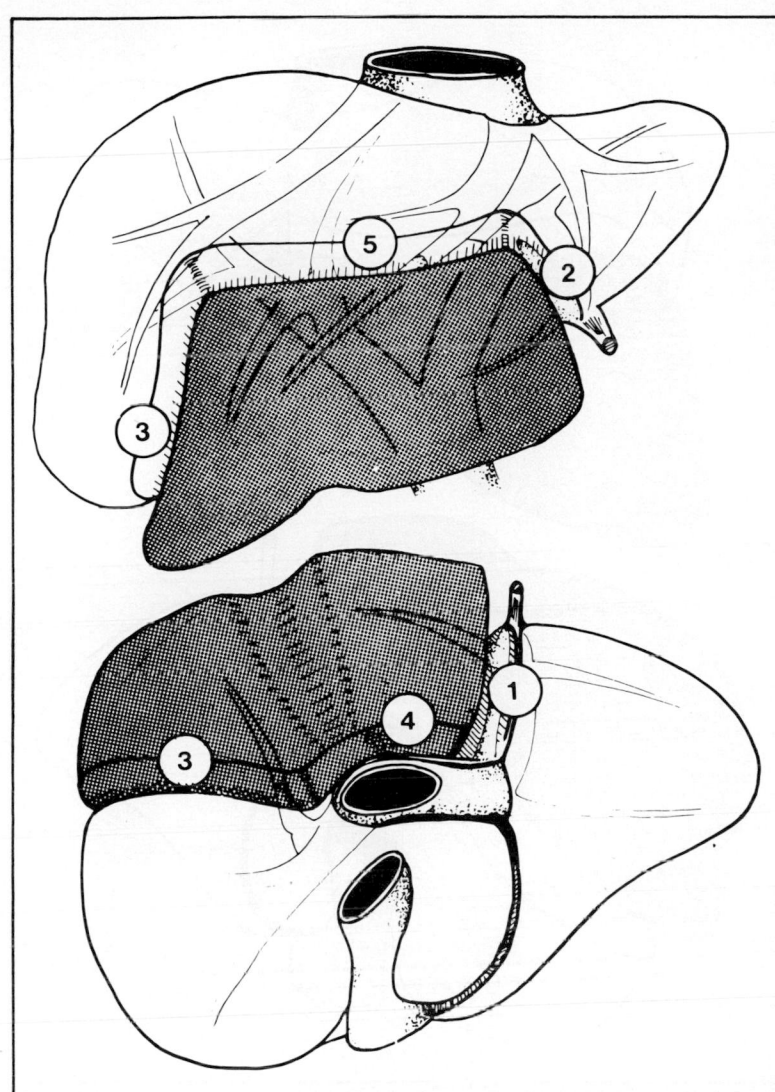

Figure 67–22. Bisegmentectomy IV,V. The different steps of the technique: (1) opening of the umbilical fissure, (2) splitting of the parenchyma to the right of the ligamentum teres, (3) opening of the right portal scissura, and (4) ligation of the portal pedicles of the quadrate lobe and of the anterior portal pedicle of the right paramedian sector. (*Source: From Bismuth H, Houssin D, et al, 1982, with permission.*)

and rapidly advanced. Glucose infusions and albumin are given to maintain normal levels until the oral intake is adequate. Antibiotics are generally continued for 3 days. Following right lobectomy, hyperbilirubinemia and clinical jaundice are anticipated. This usually begins on the second or third day and may continue for as long as 3 weeks. Hypoprothrombinemia also develops but rarely reaches critical levels; if this becomes significant, it is readily corrected with fresh frozen plasma.

Continued bleeding in the immediate pos-toperative period is generally caused by ineffective mechanical hemostasis and not by a coagulopathy; thus, it usually requires early reexploration. Persistent leakage of bile or development of biliary fistula is extremely rare. The most common complication is a subphrenic abscess that usually becomes manifest on the fifth postoperative day. In the past, this required drainage through the lateral aspect of the major incision, but recently it has been managed successfully by ultrasonographically controlled placement of a pigtail catheter.

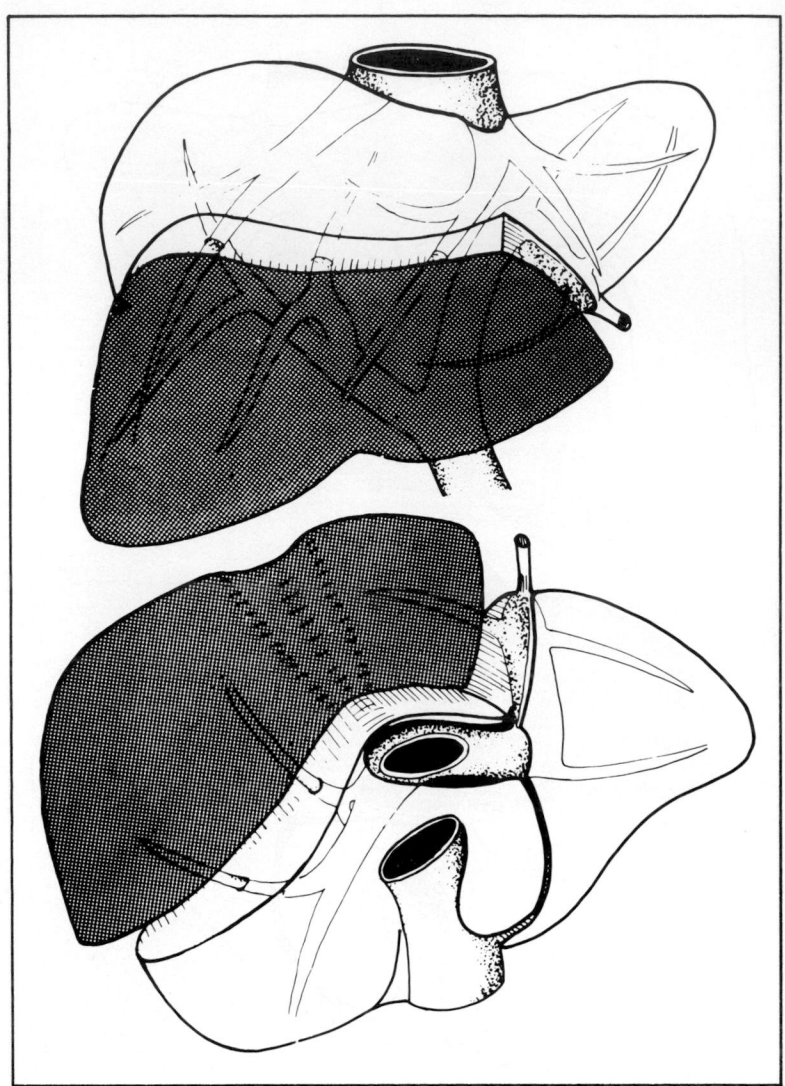

Figure 67–23. Trisegmentectomy IV,V,VI. (*Source: From Bismuth H, Houssin D, et al, 1982, with permission.*)

BIBLIOGRAPHY

Bismuth H: Surgical anatomy and anatomical surgery of the liver. World J Surg 6:3, 1982

Bismuth H, Houssin D, et al: Major and minor segmentectomies "Reglees" in liver surgery. World J Surg 6:10, 1982

Couinaud D: Controlled Hepatectomies and Exposure of the Intrahepatic Bile Ducts. Paris: C Couinaud, 1981

Goldsmith NA, Woodburne RT: Surgical anatomy pertaining to liver resection. Surg Gynecol Obstet 195:310, 1957

Healey JE, Schwartz SI: Surgical anatomy, in Schwartz SI (ed): Surgical Diseases of the Liver. New York: McGraw-Hill, 1964, p 1

Hodgson WJB, DelGuercio LRM: Preliminary experience in liver surgery using the ultrasonic scalpel. Ann Surg 95:320, 1984

Lin TY: A simplified technique for hepatic resection. Ann Surg 180:225, 1974

Schwartz SI: Liver resection, in Modern Technics in Surgery, Abdominal Surgery 10:1, Mt. Kisco, New York: Futura Publishing, 1981

Schwartz SI: Hepatic resection, in Schwartz SI (ed): Surgical Diseases of the Liver. New York: McGraw-Hill, 1964, p 237

Starzl T, Bell RH, et al: Hepatic trisegmentectomy and other liver resections. Surg Gynecol Obstet 141:429, 1975

Tung TT: Les resection majeures et mineures du foie. Paris: Masson, 1979

68. Transplantation of the Human Liver

Thomas E. Starzl
Shunzaburo Iwatsuki
Byers W. Shaw, Jr.

INTRODUCTION

In this chapter, the usual section on historical background has been omitted. The reason is that the first report by C.S. Welch of whole-organ hepatic transplantation in dogs was only 28 years ago. Furthermore, the first clinical attempts at liver transplantation were not described until 1963. Consequently, these, as well as most of the other early articles on liver transplantation, are still of current interest.

Until recently, liver transplantation was considered an experimental operation. At a Consensus Development Conference held in Bethesda, Maryland on June 20–23, 1983, under the sponsorship of several federal agencies, the adjudication was made that the operation had become therapeutic. With this change in classification, it is certain that a number of new liver transplantation centers will spring up in the United States in the next year or two. Thus, for the first time, liver transplantation will become an acknowledged part of the surgical armamentarium available for the treatment of end stage hepatic disease.

AUXILIARY TRANSPLANTATION

There are two general approaches to transplantation of the liver. With one method, an extra liver is inserted at an ectopic site, without removal of the diseased native organ. This was a procedure that Welch envisioned with the ultimate objective of treating patients who were dying of cirrhosis or other nonneoplastic hepatic diseases.

One technique used for auxiliary hepatic transplantation as adapted to human subjects is depicted in Figure 68–1. Here, the extra liver is placed in the right paravertebral gutter or right pelvis. Its hepatic arterial supply is derived from the aorta or an iliac artery. Venous inflow is reconstituted by anastomosing the host superior mesenteric vein to the homograft portal vein. Outflow is into the inferior vena cava.

In theory, the use of auxiliary homografts for the treatment of benign hepatic disease has a special appeal. First, sacrifice of the remaining, albeit limited, function of the ailing recipient liver can be avoided. Thus, in the event of poor initial performance by the homograft due to ischemia or to a severe but reversible rejection, it might be hoped that some assistance would be provided by the diseased host liver during a transition recovery period. This would be predicted to be a particularly significant advantage in patients with biliary atresia, since the synthesizing functions of the liver are often retained until the terminal stages of this disease. Second, it was assumed initially that the placement of an extra liver would be safer and technically less demanding than the orthotopic procedure.

In actual practice, auxiliary transplantation has lost much favor. The results in animals have been inferior to those with liver replacement, partly because co-existing livers have the capacity to damage each other to a variable degree, according to which organ is the "dominant" one. Factors favoring dominance include a splanchnic source of the blood for portal venous inflow, perfect biliary drainage, optimal total hepatic blood flow, and unimpeded venous

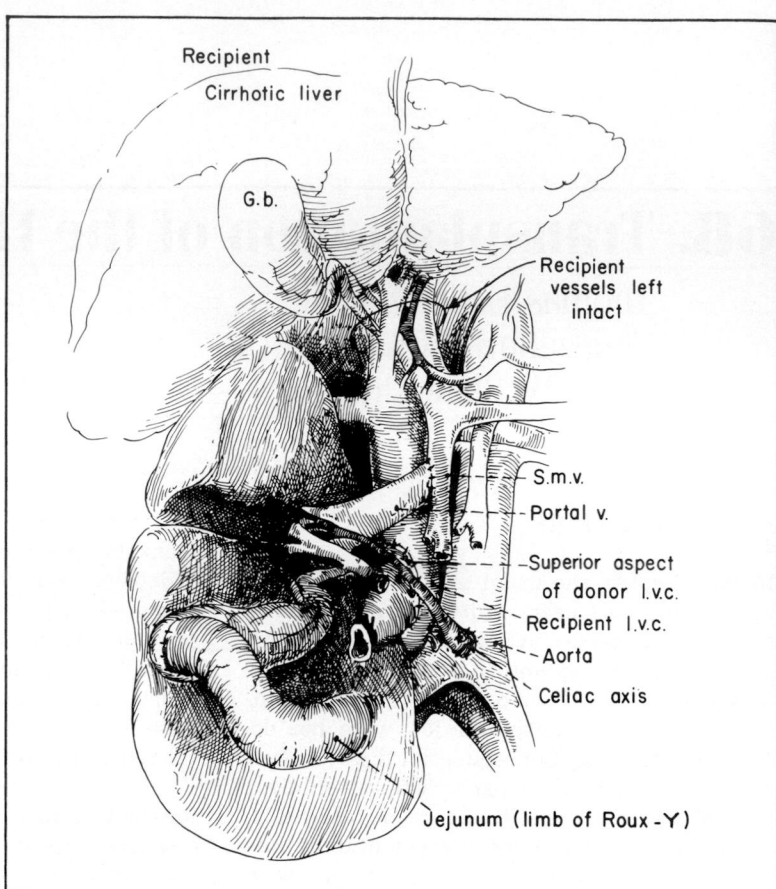

Figure 68–1. Technique of auxiliary liver transplantation that provides splanchnic venous flow for the homograft. Because of portal hypertension caused by the diseased native liver, splanchnic flow will pass preferentially through the homograft. (*Source: From Starzl TE* (*with the assistance of CW Putnam*), *1969, with permission.*)

outflow. An auxiliary canine liver graft, which does not enjoy these advantages relative to the host liver, undergoes rapid atrophy by mechanisms that have been ascribed to "interliver competition." (A detailed discussion of this fascinating topic, often referred to as hepatotrophic physiology, can be found elsewhere.)

Most patients who would be candidates for liver transplantation do not have adequately functioning livers, so that the concept of competition may not be a critical one in clinical practice. Nevertheless, auxiliary liver transplantation for the indication of hepatic failure has resulted in the significant prolongation of life for only two patients. One was a child with biliary atresia who is still well as of August, 1983, more than 10½ years after auxiliary transplantation by Fortner of New York, using a technique similar to that shown in Figure 68–1. The second patient, an adult, treated in Paris had lived for more than 2 years at the time of his reporting in May, 1980.

Failure in the vast majority of patients has been due to a variety of reasons. In many cases good inital homograft function was not obtained due to an ischemic injury during and/or after donor death. In others, the presence of an extra organ within the abdomen was not well tolerated with restriction of diaphragmatic movement and consequent lethal pulmonary complications. Finally, the expectation that the placement of an extra organ would be technically simpler than with liver replacement has not been borne out by actual experience, as evidenced by an extremely high incidence of mechanical complications. Because of the poor clinical results, the number of attempts at human auxiliary transplantation has declined to such a point that this kind of operation will not be considered further herein.

ORTHOTOPIC TRANSPLANTATION

In contrast, there is mounting evidence that the operation or orthotopic hepatic transplantation (liver replacement) will play an increasing role in the future treatment of liver disorders. With this procedure, the diseased host liver is removed, creating a space into which a graft is transplanted with as normal an anatomic reconstruction as possible. Survival in dogs and human subjects has been achieved exceeding 12 and 13⅔ years, respectively. The remarks in succeeding sections will pertain to orthotopic transplantation.

Preoperative Preparation

Virtually all prospective liver recipients are poor risks for a major operation, and many of those with hepatic failure from nonneoplastic diseases appear at first evaluation to be hopeless. Symptomatic relief may be obtained by the performance of procedures such as paracentesis or thoracocentesis. Yet, unfortunately, there is probably little of real value that can be done

TABLE 68-1. INDICATIONS FOR TRANSPLANTATION IN PEDIATRIC PATIENTS (<18 YEARS) FROM MARCH 1963 THROUGH APRIL 1982

Biliary atresia	62[a]
Inborn metabolic errors	21[b]
Nonalcoholic cirrhosis	15
Hepatoma	3[c]
Neonatal hepatitis	3
Secondary biliary cirrhosis	3[d]
Byler's disease	2
Congenital hepatic fibrosis	2
Budd–Chiari's syndrome	1
Total	112

[a] Two had Allagilles' syndrome.
[b] Inborn errors:

α-1-antitrypsin deficiency	13
Wilson's disease	3
Tyrosinemia	2
Type I glycogen storage disease	1
Type IV glycogen storage disease	1
Sea blue histiocyte syndrome	1
Total	21

[c] Seven other patients had incidental malignancies (6 hepatomas and 1 hepatoblastoma) in their excised livers. The principal diagnoses in these 7 cases were biliary atresia (3 examples), congenital tyrosinemia (2 examples), α-1-antitrypsin deficiency (1 example), and sea blue histiocyte syndrome (1 example). The diagnosis of the neoplastic change was known in advance in 4 of the 7 cases.
[d] Secondary to choledochal cyst (2) or trauma (1).

TABLE 68-2. INDICATIONS FOR TRANSPLANTATION IN ADULT PATIENTS (>18 YEARS) FROM MARCH 1963 THROUGH APRIL 1982

Nonalcoholic cirrhosis	47
Primary malignancy	24[a,b]
Alcoholic cirrhosis	15
Primary biliary cirrhosis	12
Sclerosing cholangitis	10
Secondary biliary cirrhosis	6[c]
α-1-antitrypsin deficiency	4
Budd–Chiari's syndrome	3
Acute hepatitis B	1
Adenomatosis	1[a]
Hemochromatosis	1
Protoporphyria	1
Total	125

[a] One patient in each group had previous (1 and 4½ years earlier) right hepatic trisegmentectomy. At transplantation, the regenerated left lateral segment was replaced with a whole liver.
[b] Thirteen hepatomas, 7 duct cell carcinomas (Klatskin), 2 cholangiocarcinomas, 1 hemangioendothelial sarcoma, 1 unclassified sarcoma.
[c] Two examples each of choledochal cyst and trauma; one example each of duct hypoplasia and Caroli's syndrome. All 6 patients had had multiple previous operations.

to reduce the consequent operative hazards short of providing liver tissue. Nevertheless, even patients near death from complications of hepatic disease can be brought through the transplantation procedure with almost immediate improvement providing the homograft functions properly and promptly.

Although little can be done for the preexisting liver failure, secondary abnormalities of other organs can sometimes be effectively ameliorated. For example, the effects of renal failure secondary to the hepatorenal syndrome can be treated with the artificial kidney. Pulmonary manifestations may be improved by simple tracheobronchial toilet, particularly if aspiration has occurred. Transfusions of blood or albumin may be useful for the correction of blood volume or other fluid space abnormalities. If fresh whole blood, fresh frozen plasma, or platelets are judiciously given, some improvement in coagulation may be possible.

Case Selection

Of the 237 patients treated from March 1963 through April 1982, 112 were classed as pediatric recipients (Table 68–1); their ages ranged from 5 months to 18 years. The 125 adults (Table 68–2) were 19 to 68 years old.

It is now clear that none of the disorders for which transplantation has been attempted can be categorically excluded from future trials. At the same time, a fairly complete understanding has evolved with many specific diseases about what advice to give to prospective recipients and their families, when and if the operation should be decided upon, how much risk there is of deterioration and death during the search for a donor organ, and what are the technical difficulties to be anticipated during the transplantation.

At present, candidacy is restricted to patients who are less than 55 years old, who are free of extrahepatic infection, and who do not have an extrahepatic malignancy. Within this group, the two main principles in case selection concern: first, the *propriety* of a decision to proceed and, second, the *feasibility* of an attempt. In the early days of transplantation, the propriety issue was the dominant theme because of anxiety that meaningful life might be foreshortened by a dangerous and unpredictable surgical undertaking. Our general guideline was that transplantation for nonneoplastic liver disease became justifiable with the advent of social and vocational invalidism. This condition usually was reflected in repeated hospitalizations for encephalopathy, variceal hemorrhage, hepatorenal syndrome, uncontrolled coagulation disorders, intractible ascites and other complications of hepatic disease.

According to Underlying Diseases

Hepatic Malignancy. When orthotopic liver transplantation was first attempted in humans, primary liver malignancy was considered to be an outstanding indication for proceeding. Liver replacement was conceived of as a means of extending the limits of resectability in patients who did not have extrahepatic spread of their tumors.

In actual experience our results in our early cases were discouraging. About 80 percent of our patients who had liver replacement for hepatomas, intrahepatic duct cell carcinomas, cholangiocarcinomas, and sarcomas and who lived through the early postoperative interval developed tumor recurrence. Most commonly, the posttransplantation metastases involved the new liver (Fig. 68–2). Deaths from recurrence have occurred as early as 143 days (Fig. 68–2) and longer than 4 years after transplantation.

It is too early to conclude once and for all that liver replacement in the face of hepatic malignancy is a futile undertaking. One of our patients, for whom the primary reason for liver transplantation was biliary atresia, had an incidental hepatoma in the total hepatectomy specimen. Her preoperative serum contained almost 4 mg/dl of α-fetoprotein. After operation in January 1970, the fetoprotein disappeared from the serum (Fig. 68–3) and has not recurred in the

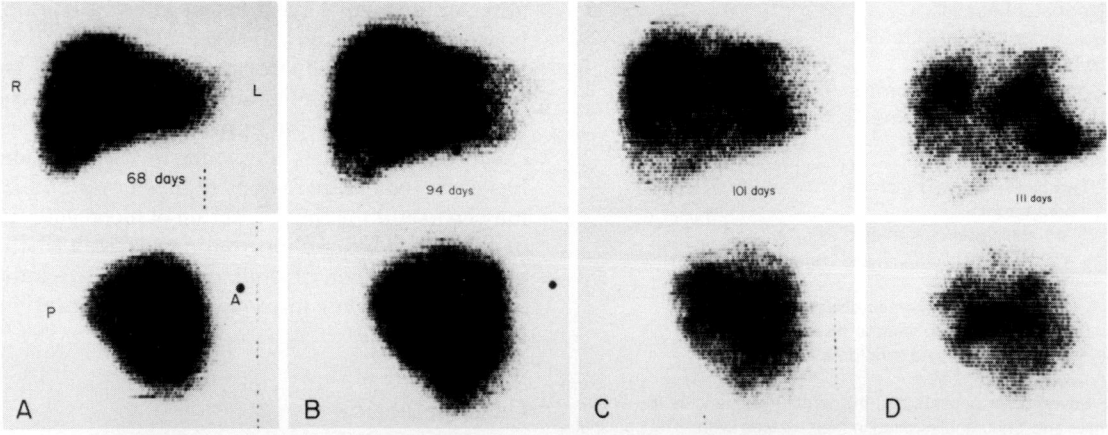

Figure 68–2. Technetium-99m liver scans in a patient whose indication for transplantation was hepatoma. Note progressive invasion of liver homograft by tumor beginning at 94 days. The patient died of carcinomatosis 143 days posttransplantation. At autopsy, the homograft was almost completely replaced with carcinoma. (*Source: From Starzl TE (with the assistance of CW Putnam), 1969, with permission.*)

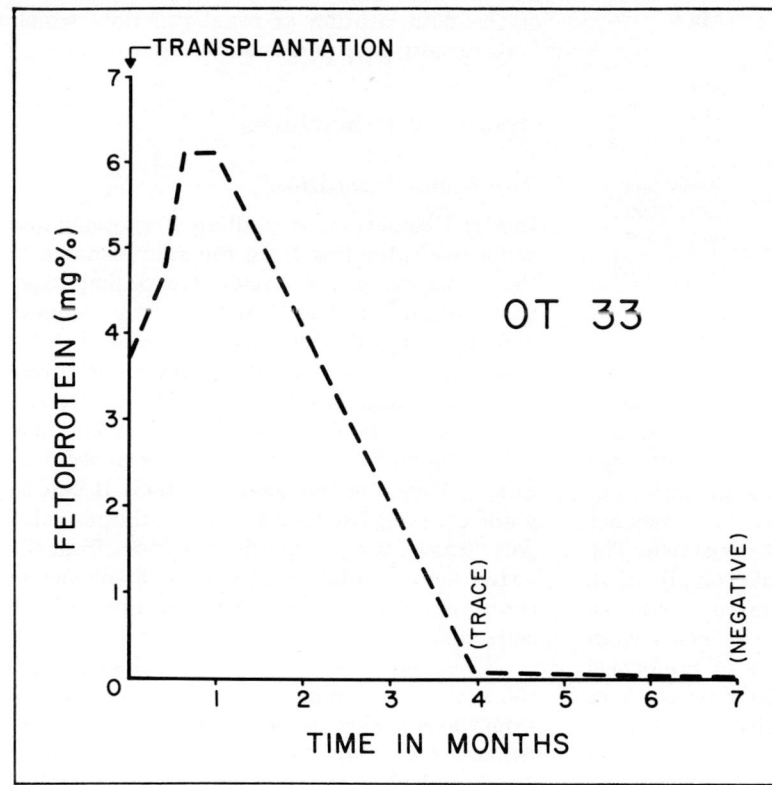

Figure 68–3. α-Fetoprotein determinations in a 3-year-old child who underwent transplantation for biliary atresia. A small hepatoma was discovered within the operative specimen. The child is now 13⅔ years after transplantation. α-Fetoprotein determinations continue to be negative and she remains free of tumor.

13⅔ years of posttransplantation life. Apparently, this child has achieved a cure of her hepatoma. Another of our patients, a 28-year-old woman, is well 6¾ years after transplantation for sclerosing cholangiocarcinoma. Palliation or even cure of primary hepatic malignancies has also been reported by Calne.

Since immunosuppression with cyclosporine and steroids has been used, the incidence of recurrence has been much less. This may only reflect better case selection. However, it cannot be assumed out of hand that cyclosporine does not have some anticancer qualities.

Biliary Atresia. The prime indications for orthotopic liver transplantation have come to be terminal liver diseases of nonneoplastic origin. Of these, extrahepatic biliary atresia is perhaps the least questionable, since death is inevitable after a relatively predictable interval and without any hope in the remaining life for rehabilitation. With intrahepatic biliary atresia, more conservatism is exercised, since some of these children can survive for many years.

Other Benign Diseases. The problem of the proper time for liver transplantation may be a difficult one if alcoholism is a significant etiologic factor that could be eliminated by abstinence. Other common diseases in our series (Tables 68–1 and 68–2) have been chronic aggressive hepatitis, inborn errors of metabolism (Wilson's disease, α-1-antitrypsin deficiency, Types 1 and 4 glycogen storage disease, tyrosinemia, sea blue histiocyte syndrome), sclerosing cholangitis, and primary biliary cirrhosis. Patients with acute liver disease usually are not considered since they may have the capacity to recover spontaneously. Contraindications would include advanced age, a history of sociopathic behavior that would prevent postoperative management, preexisting and untreatable systemic or local infections, or serious disease of organs other than the liver, as, for example, co-existing severe heart disease.

According to Immunologic Criteria

ABO Matching and Cytotoxic Antibodies. When possible, the rules of tissue transfer are

TABLE 68–3. DIRECTION OF ACCEPTABLE MISMATCHED TISSUE TRANSFER

O to non-O[a]	Safe
Rh− to Rh+	Safe
Rh+ to Rh−	Relatively safe
A to non-A	Dangerous
B to non-B	Dangerous
AB to non-AB[b]	Dangerous

[a] O is universal donor.
[b] AB is universal recipient.

followed (Table 68–3). These are designed to avoid the transplantation of an organ into a recipient who possesses performed antidonor isoagglutinins. Violation of these guidelines in kidney transplantation can lead to immediate graft destruction by hyperacute rejection. The liver has proved resistant to this complication, meaning that blood group barriers can be breached in the case of desperate need. Even more surprisingly, the presence of preformed cytotoxic antibodies against donor tissues does not usually cause hyperacute liver rejection.

HLA Matching. The poor correlation in renal, cardiac, and liver transplantation between matching at the A, B, and Dr histocompatibility loci and clinical outcome has led us to ignore the question of tissue matching for liver transplantation. Nor do we even use the most favorable matching as an instrument of selection among a given group of candidates for transplantation. At the present, our major criterion concerns who has the most pressing need.

Donor Procurement

The most common explanation for transplantation of an inadequately preserved liver is preexisting hepatic injury, rather than poor harvesting or preservation technique. Thus, removal of a satisfactory liver for transplantation begins with wise screening of donors and elimination of those whose physiologic situation could jeopardize vital organ function in advance of procurement. Aside from abnormalities in the hepatic function profile, signals that it may be dangerous to the recipient to proceed with the donor hepatectomy are donor cardiovascular instability, a need for excessive vasopressor support, an excessive period (several days) between injury and the pronouncement of brain death,

or the deterioration of renal function, which may suggest poor perfusion of other organs.

Operative Procedures

The Donor Operation

Initial Dissection. A midline sternotomy and celiotomy extending from the sternal notch to the pubic symphysis provides excellent exposure not only of the liver but of the kidneys and other organs which might be needed. After assessing the liver and other organs for gross suitability, anomalies of the hepatic arterial supply are looked for (Fig. 68–4). A common variant is an artery to the left lateral segment arising from the left gastric artery. It can be found coursing from left to right in the gastrohepatic ligament accompanied by fibers from the vagus nerve. This vessel can be preserved in continuity with its left gastric origin and the celiac axis.

The right lobe of the liver (and sometimes the entire liver) may be supplied by a branch from the superior mesenteric artery (Fig. 68–4). Almost invariably this branch lies posterior to the portal vein and can be felt there with a finger placed through the foreamen of Winslow (Fig. 68–5A). On rare occasions, in which the left gastric or superior mesenteric artery branches supply the entire liver, a true common hepatic artery arising from the celiac axis may not be found.

After the anomalies have been identified, the structures of the portal triad are dissected; it is important to stay as far from the liver as possible. Usually, the hepatic artery is dissected retrograde, starting with ligation and division of the gastroduodenal and right gastric arteries (Fig. 68–5). The splenic and left gastric (and sometimes phrenic) branches of the celiac axis are ligated and divided. The proximal dissection is facilitated by cutting the diaphragmatic crura, exposing the origin of the celiac axis and a short segment of the subdiaphragmatic aorta. If a good view of the common hepatic artery, the celiac axis and the aorta cannot be obtained easily with this anterior approach, the spleen and stomach can be mobilized and reflected to the right, and the aorta is approached from the left side (Fig. 68–6). At some time during the dissection, the origin of the superior mesenteric artery is also exposed to that it can be ligated later.

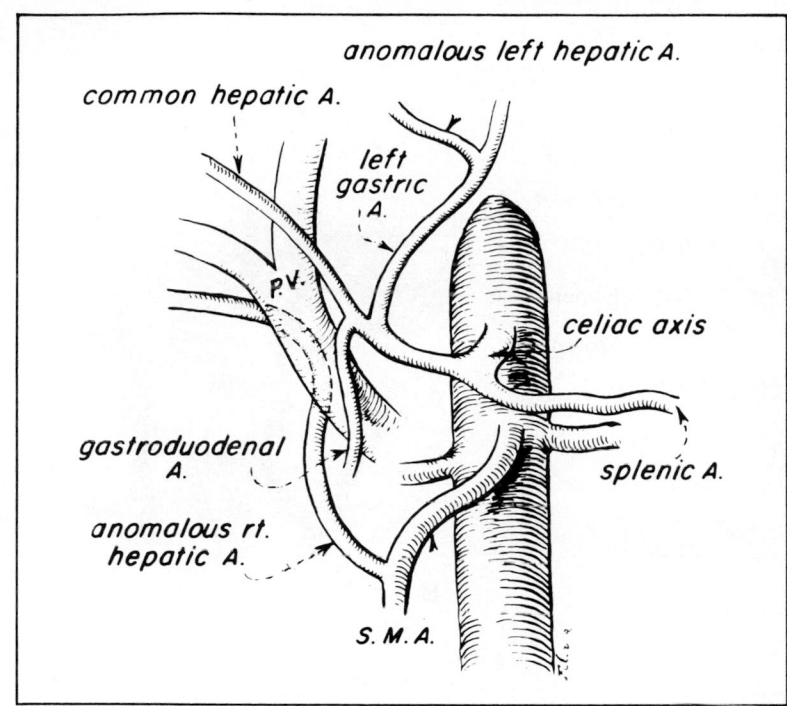

Figure 68–4. Anomalies of hepatic arterial supply. (*Source: From Shaw BW Jr, Hakala T, et al: Combination donor hepatectomy and nephrectomy and early functional results of allografts. Surg Gynecol Obstet 155:321, 1982, with permission.*)

An anomalous superior mesenteric artery branch to the right hepatic lobe (occasionally it is the sole arterial supply of the liver) is best approached by performing a Kocher maneuver and reflecting the duodenum and head of the pancreas to the left. The hepatic artery (Fig. 68–4) can be seen posterior to the portal vein, duodenum, and pancreas and traced back to its takeoff, which is at a right angle from the superior mesenteric artery. Small branches to the pancreas are ligated and divided. The superior mesenteric artery distal to its hepatic branch is dissected so that later ligation is possible. The superior mesenteric artery proximal to this point is cleaned back to its origin from the aorta. This may be most easily done from the left side (Fig. 68–6) or from an inferior approach.

Having completed the dissection of the arterial supply, the portal vein is isolated at the superior border of the pancreas. The pancreas can be divided at this level between two mass ligatures and exposure of adequate lengths of splenic and superior mesenteric veins obtained. All other branches to the portal vein are ligated or divided, the most constant being coronary veins (Fig. 68–5).

The common bile duct is encircled as close to the superior margin of the duodenum as possible. A transverse incision is made high on the fundus of the gallbladder and the extrahepatic biliary tract flushed out with saline to prevent later autolysis of the mucosa by bile.

It remains to dissect the inferior vena cava. The falciform, left and right triangular, and coronary ligaments are divided and the suprahepatic vena cava is encircled (Figs. 68–7 through 68–9). Care is taken to identify, ligate, and divide the right, left, and posterior phrenic veins. The right lobe is retracted anteromedially and the retrohepatic vena cava is dissected free to the level of the renal vein inferiorly (Fig. 68–9). This step requires ligation and division of a large right adrenal vein and occasionally smaller tributaries.

In some cases, retraction of the liver from the liver fossa causes color changes in the organ, reflecting either inflow or outflow obstruction. If the donor mean arterial pressure falls, the cause usually is outflow obstruction with compromised cardiac filling from loss of venous return. In such an event, retrohepatic vena caval dissection is deferred until the final steps.

Our present policy is to carry out in situ infusion of the kidneys and liver, although

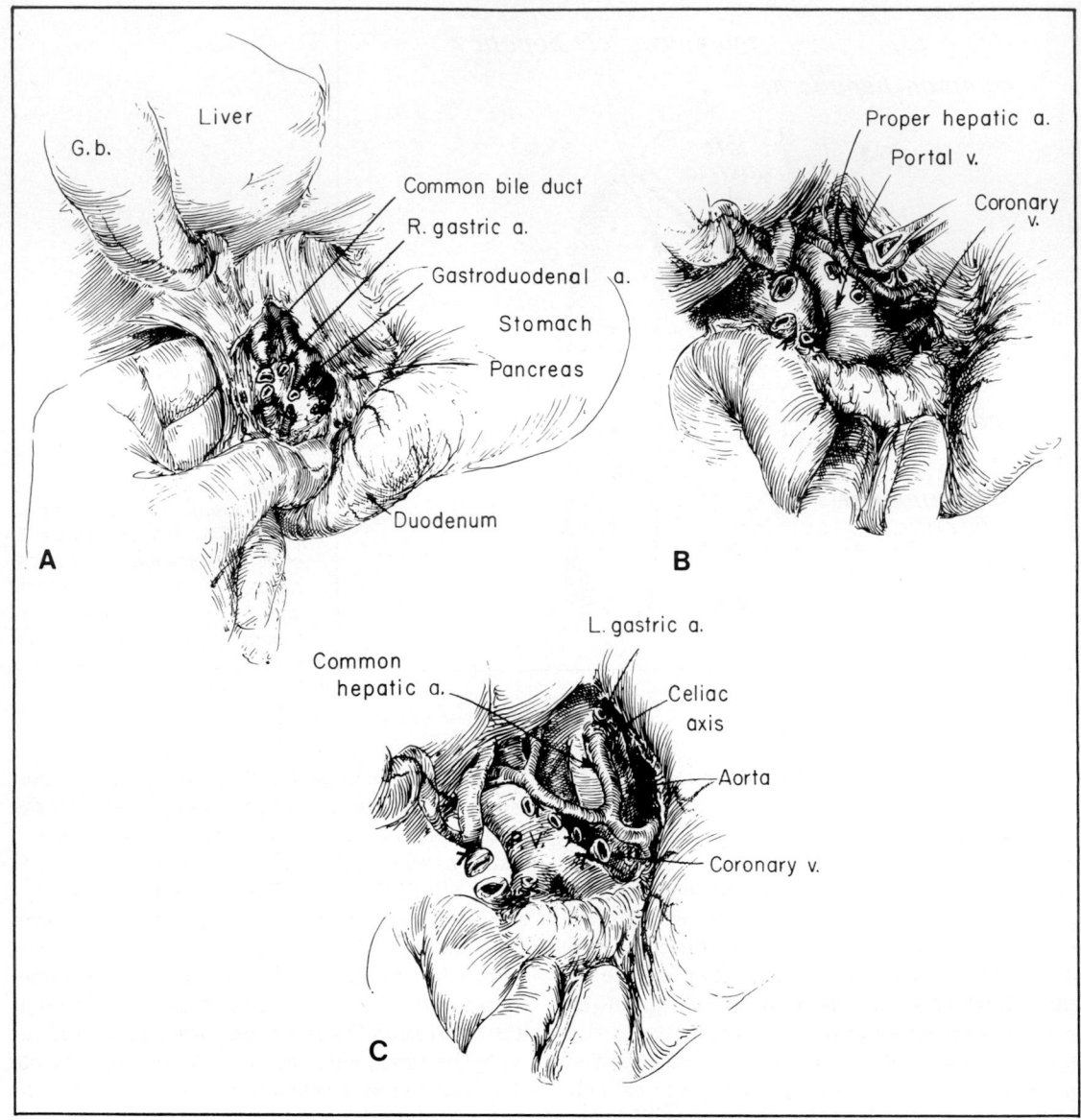

Figure 68–5. Dissection of the portal triad during donor hepatectomy. **A.** The common duct and the gastroduodenal and right gastric arteries are tied and divided. **B.** The hepatic artery has been mobilized far enough so that the anterior surface of the portal vein is uncovered. The coronary vein entering the left side of the portal trunk, or into the splenic vein as shown, is almost always found; this tributary is ligated and divided. **C.** The portal vein has been freed and the celiac axis mobilized. The splenic artery has not yet been ligated and divided. When the liver is removed, all of the celiac axis is usually retained with the specimen, and it may be advisable to include a segment of aorta as well. (*Source: From Starzl TE (with the assistance of CW Putnam), 1969, with permission.*)

many surgeons with whom we collaborate prefer to excise the kidneys at this time and to flush them ex vivo. With either method for the kidney removal, the principles of the hepatectomy are the same. The donor is anticoagu-lated with heparin (300 USP units/kg) and a large cannula is inserted into the distal aorta near the bifurcation to provide for in situ infusion of cold (4°C) preservation solution (Fig. 68–10). A second cannula is placed into the distal

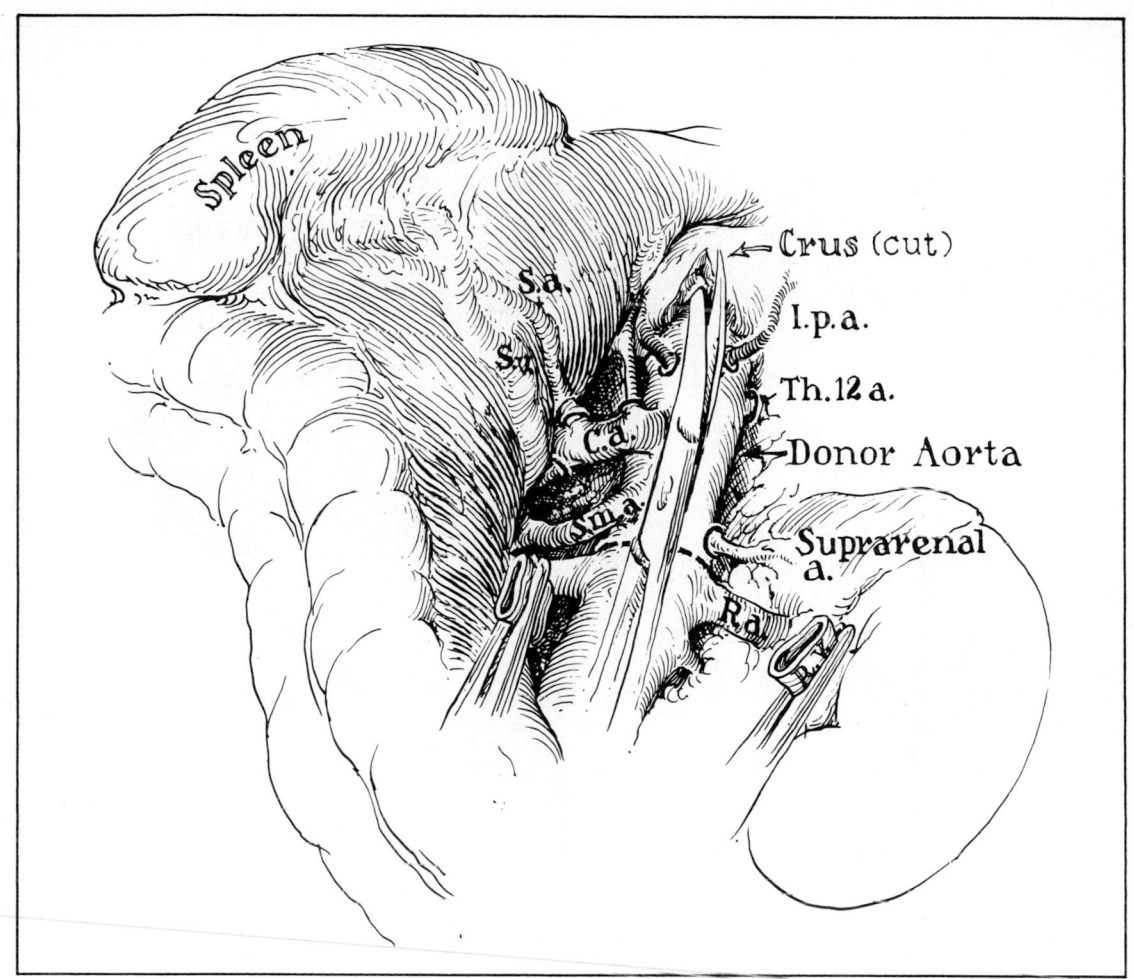

Figure 68–6. Alternative approach to arterial supply of liver. During the initial dissection, all the aortic branches except the celiac axis and superior mesenteric artery are ligated and divided; the latter vessel is cut only after it has been shown not to give rise to an anomalous hepatic arterial branch. A segment of aorta is usually removed in continuity with the celiac axis. (*Source: From Starzl TE (with the assistance of CW Putnam), 1969, with permission.*)

vena cava to allow bleeding off of central venous volume during the subsequent infusion of cold solutions (Fig. 68–10).

Precooling of the Liver. A critical principle in the procurement of satisfactory livers is to bring the infusion of cold solution into the portal vein while there is still an effective donor circulation. This step of hepatic precooling eliminates warm ischemia by reducing the temperature of the liver tissue while an adequate flow of oxygenated arterial blood is still present. At the same time, added protection to the kidney and other organs is provided since donor core temperatures during this precooling phase drift quickly to 28 to 32°C at the same time as the liver temperature drops several degrees below this.

The precooling solution is introduced into the portal vein via a cannula inserted into the previously dissected splenic vein (Fig. 68–10). Cold (4°C) lactated Ringer's solution is rapidly infused and during the infusion the superior mesenteric artery and vein are ligated in that order. Perfusion pressures of 80 to 100 cm of water are maintained by elevation of the infusion reservoir. Central venous hypertension is avoided by intermittently bleeding off blood vol-

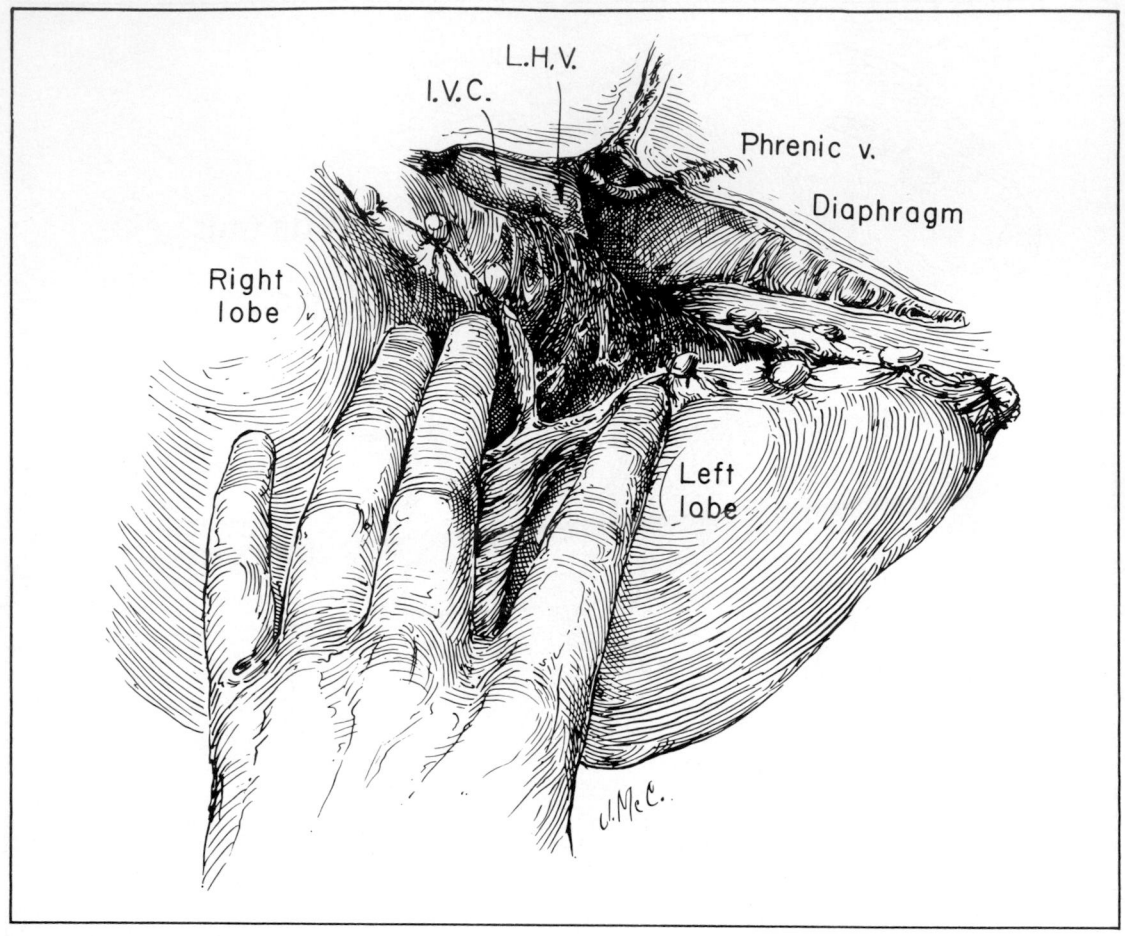

Figure 68–7. Exposure and initial dissection of the suprahepatic vena cava and its tributaries. This is done by entering the raw area formed by divergence of the leaves of the falciform and triangular ligaments. A short segment of the left hepatic vein (L.H.V.) is usually seen first. (*Source: From Starzl TE (with the assistance of CW Putnam), 1969, with permission.*)

ume via the previously placed inferior vena cava cannula. After approximately 1 L of lactated Ringer's solution has been infused, the liver becomes noticeably cool to palpation. Any increased firmness of the organ suggests hepatic venous hypertension and demands immediate lowering of central venous pressures by bleeding off from the caval cannula and slowing of the portal infusion. The infusion is continued until a total of approximately 2000 ml of lactated Ringer's have been given, until donor core temperature reaches 28 to 30°C, or until there is difficulty maintaining the donor blood pressure. During the precooling, a vasolytic agent (e.g., chlorpromazine, phentolamine, tolazoline) is given as an intravenous bolus injection.

Final Stages. As portal precooling is terminated, in situ aortic flushing of the liver, kidneys, or other organs is begun (Fig. 68–10). The abdominal aorta is clamped at the diaphragm and rapid infusion of cold (4°C) modified Collin's solution (Travenol) is begun via the distal aortic cannula at the same time as the vena cava cannula is opened to allow free drainage of blood to a collection bag placed on the floor. The portal vein infusion of lactated Ringer's solution is changed to a modified Collin's solution for a final flush in adult donors of about 500 ml or of a proportionately smaller amount in pediatric donors.

All of the abdominal organs are now cold. The liver is removed first. The suprahepatic

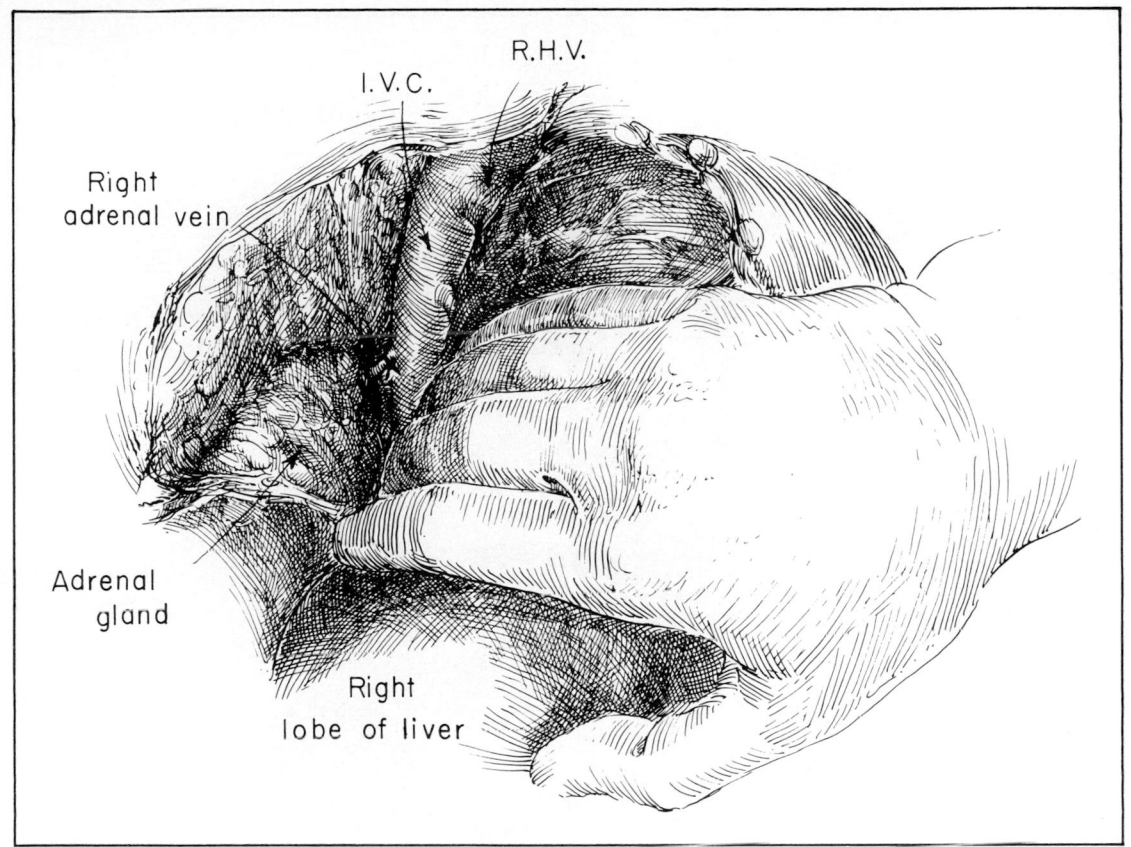

Figure 68–8. Retraction of the liver to the left. The bare area of the right hepatic lobe has been opened, exposing the adrenal gland. The right adrenal vein is ligated and divided. This is usually the only posterior tributary to the retrohepatic vena cava. At this stage of the dissection the right hepatic vein (R.H.V.) can be identified. (*Source: From Starzl TE (with the assistance of CW Putnam), 1969, with permission.*)

vena cava is transected as high as possible (Fig. 68–11). A piece of the right atrium sometimes is included. The liver is peeled out from the retroperitoneum from a superior to inferior direction by gentle anterior traction on the liver, care being taken to ligate all posterior tributaries to the retrohepatic vena cava. The vena cava is transected just superior to the entrance of the renal veins. The aorta is reclamped just distal to the celiac axis so that further infusion of the kidneys may be continued if desired. The liver is removed.

The nephrectomy team proceeds with removal of the kidneys. The most common practice is to remove the organs en bloc with a long segment of aorta and vena cava. The early function of cadaveric kidneys obtained during heart

and liver procurement, or both heart and liver, has been better than that achieved in our center and elsewhere with renal procurement alone. This advantage for the eventual renal recipients probably is due to the more discriminating donor selection and the greater intensity of surgical technical care that are features of the multiple organ harvesting operations. It should be specifically noted that heart and liver grafts can be obtained from the same donor with minor modifications of the described technique.

The chilled liver is placed in a plastic bag that contains Collin's solution. The bag is sealed and packed in ice in a standard picnic refrigerator. Canine livers so processed can support the life of a recipient after storage for 12 to 24 hours, but in humans, an effort is made to keep the

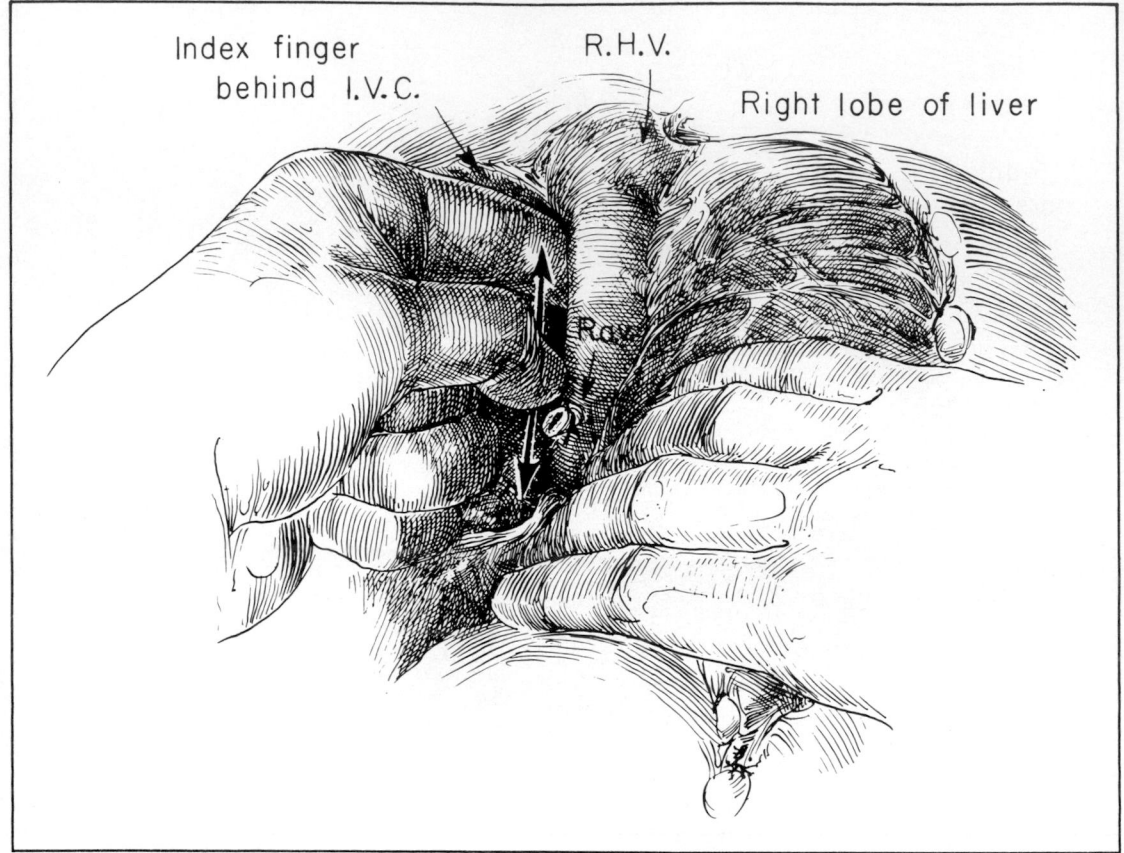

Figure 68–9. Sweeping behind the retrohepatic vena cava with a dissecting finger. This should be possible from the diaphragm to the renal veins. If resistance is encountered, it usually indicates the presence of extra branches which must be ligated and divided. R.A.V. = ligated right adrenal vein. (*Source: From Starzl TE* (*with the assistance of CW Putnam*), *1969, with permission.*)

cold preservation time to less than 6 or 8 hours. Using a different infusion solution, the Cambridge workers have described similar time limitations.

Contingency Vascular Grafts. After the organs are out, the distal aorta and vena cava, the iliac veins, and the iliac arteries are removed and stored separately in balanced electrolyte solution. It is surprising how often these vascular segments have been desperately needed for the subsequent performance of a renal or hepatic transplantation (Fig. 68–12).

The Recipient Operation

A bilateral subcostal incision is used with an upper midline extension through which the xiphoid process is excised (Fig. 68–13). The midline extension with xiphoid removal provides badly needed exposure for dissection of the hepatic ligaments and the suprahepatic inferior vena cava. If it is obvious that there will be a struggle to remove the liver, another extension should be made immediately into the right seventh intercostal space (Fig. 68–13). This is most commonly needed if the liver is unusually shrunken.

The preexisting pathologic changes often necessitate deviations from a standard plan. However, the usual first step is to find the hilum to encircle it (Fig. 68–14), and to dissect the proper and common hepatic artery in the same way as described for the donor (Fig. 68–5). If the artery is of inadequate size, it should be

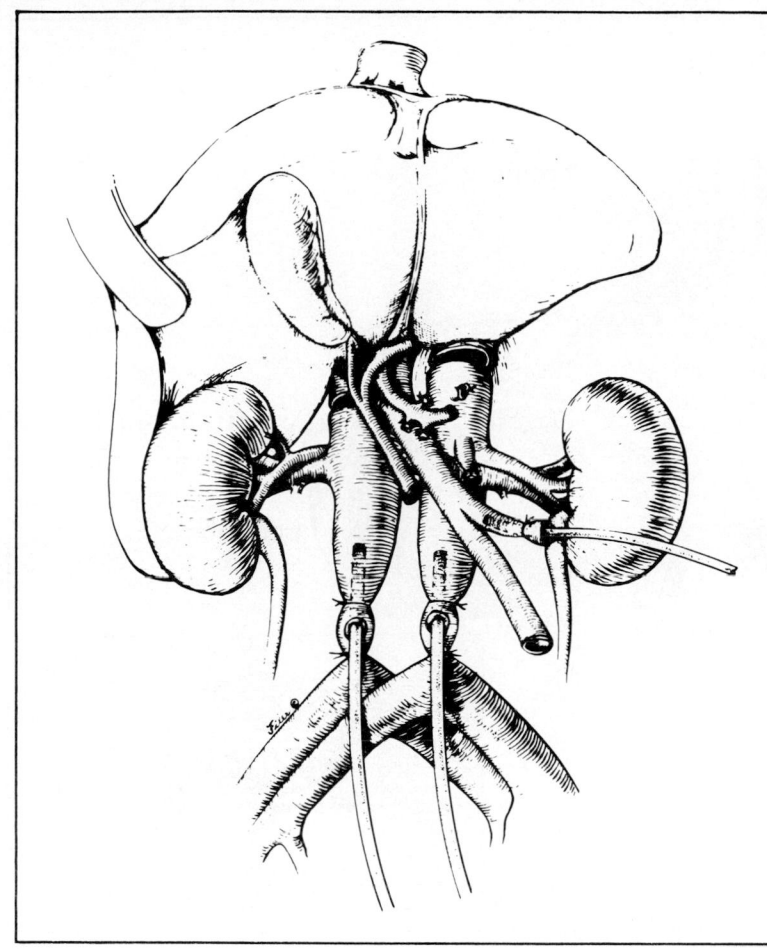

Figure 68–10. En bloc infusion of liver and kidneys. Note the infusion cannulas in the aorta and splenic veins, and the bleed-off cannula in the inferior vena cava. (*Source: From Shaw BW Jr, Hakala T, et al: Combination donor hepatectomy and nephrectomy and early functional results of allografts. Surg Gynecol Obstet 155:321, 1982, with permission.*)

mobilized proximal to the gastroduodenal and right gastric artery. In difficult cases, the proper hepatic artery can be ligated at this time. This can expedite dissection of the other hilar structures and slow hemorrhage from the liver surface later in the procedure. During the hilar dissection, the bile duct (if one is present) is transected as high as possible so that the option of duct-to-duct anastomosis is retained. The portal vein is left intact until later in order not to aggravate the portal hypertension.

The inferior vena cava below the liver is encircled with as little dissection as possible. The left triangular and falciform ligaments are incised until the suprahepatic vena cava can be identified. The suprahepatic vena cava is encircled, usually from the left side with enough dissection to allow the placement of a cross-clamp. In some cases, the encirclement may be easier from the right side. If these maneuvers can be successfully executed, the safety of subsequent steps is increased since, in the event of an accident, such as a laceration of the vena cava, the liver can be removed from the circulation by emergency cross-clamping of the encircled but intact vessels.

In straightforward cases, the right triangular and coronary ligaments are incised and the bare area is entered. With retraction of the liver toward the left, it becomes safer to dissect lengths of the inferior vena cava above and below the liver (Fig. 68–9). If the native disease is an "easy" one (primary biliary cirrhosis for example), adequate cuffs may be obtained with the liver in place and the mobilization of the entire specimen including ligation of the right adrenal vein can be completed now in the same way as with donor hepatectomy (Figs. 68–7

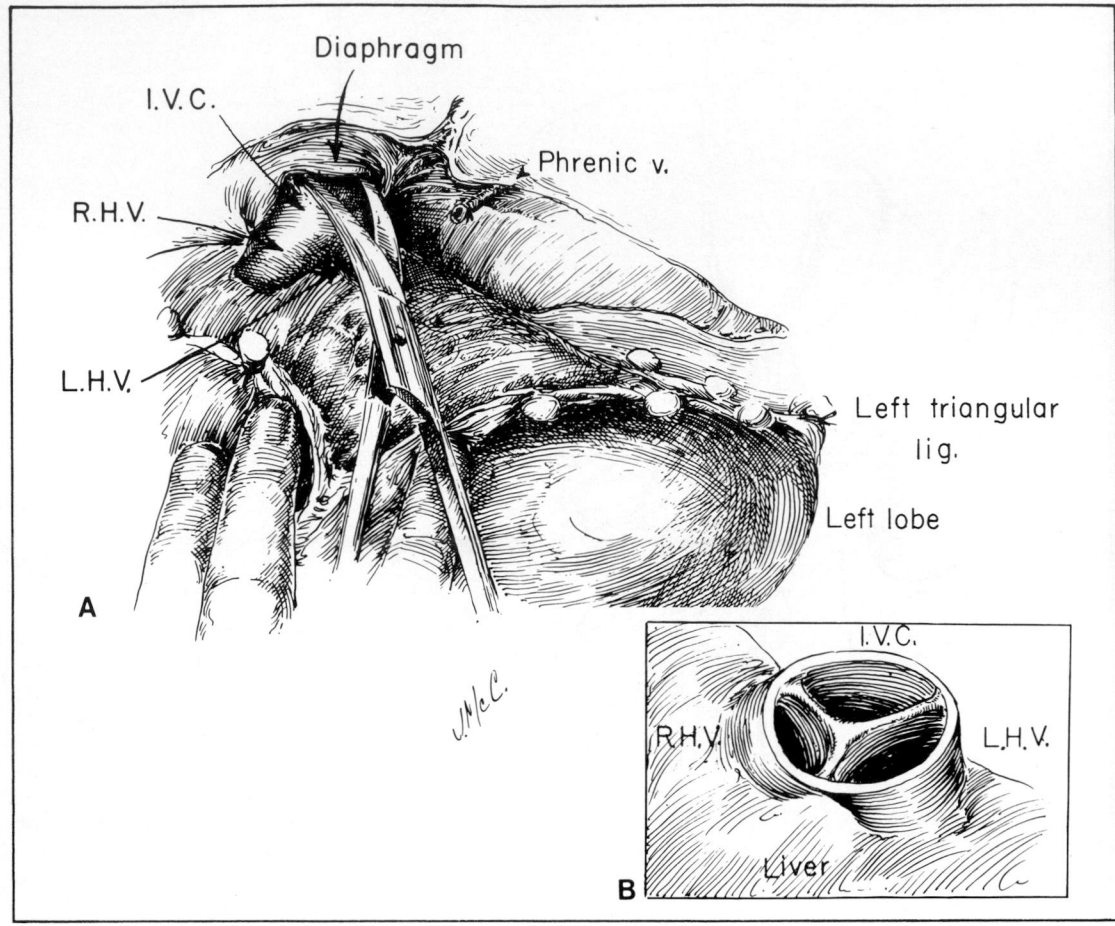

Figure 68–11. Dissection above the liver. **A.** Development of suprahepatic vena caval cuff. At this stage it is desirable to ligate and divide one or more phrenic veins on each side. Extra length can also be obtained by dissecting off the diaphragmatic reflection, as is shown. **B.** Cross-sectional appearance of the venous confluence above the liver as it is seen from above. The cloaca is formed by the junction of the right and left hepatic veins with the inferior vena cava. (*Source: From Starzl TE* (*with the assistance of CW Putnam*), *1969, with permission.*)

through 68–9). If this is feasible the time of later portal and vena caval cross-clamping is only that necessary to transect the vessels and suture in the new liver. The upper vena caval cuff can be fashioned at the entry of the main hepatic veins (Fig. 68–15). If the clamp is placed too superiorly, it is possible to crush the right phrenic nerve (Fig. 68–16).

This phase of the operation often is not easy because of scarring and anatomic distortion above and below the liver and in the retrohepatic area. In patients with cirrhosis, it may be impossible to enter the bare area without causing a lethal hemorrhage. Then the step of liver isolation described earlier may be necessary, with the clamping of the residual hilar structures and the previous encircled vena cava above and below the liver. When this has been accomplished, the liver, including the retrohepatic vena cava, can be peeled out of the hepatic fossa from below (Fig. 68–17) or from above (Fig. 68–18). Cuffs of the suprahepatic and infrahepatic vena cava can be fashioned as the liver is removed. Sufficient infrahepatic vena cava is not difficult to obtain, but the development of an adequate suprahepatic cuff may require

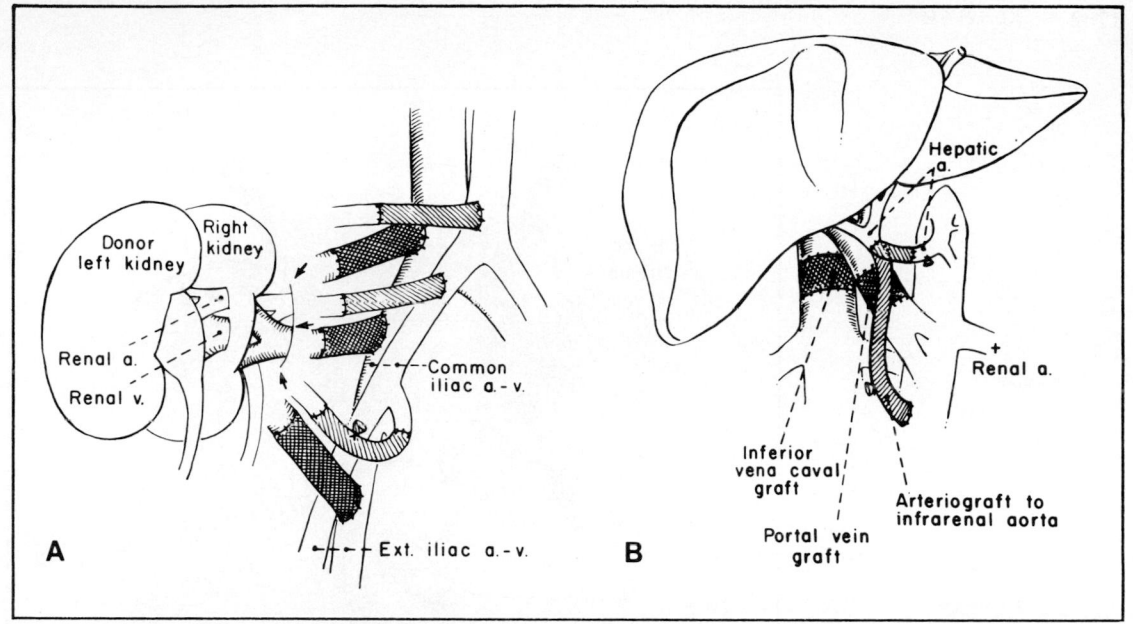

Figure 68–12. The uses to which aortic, vena caval, and iliac vascular grafts have been put in renal **(A)** and hepatic **(B)** transplantation. (*Source: From Starzl TE, Halgrimson CG, et al: Vascular homografts from cadaveric organ donors. (The Surgeon At Work) Surg Gynecol Obstet 149:737, 1979, with permission.*)

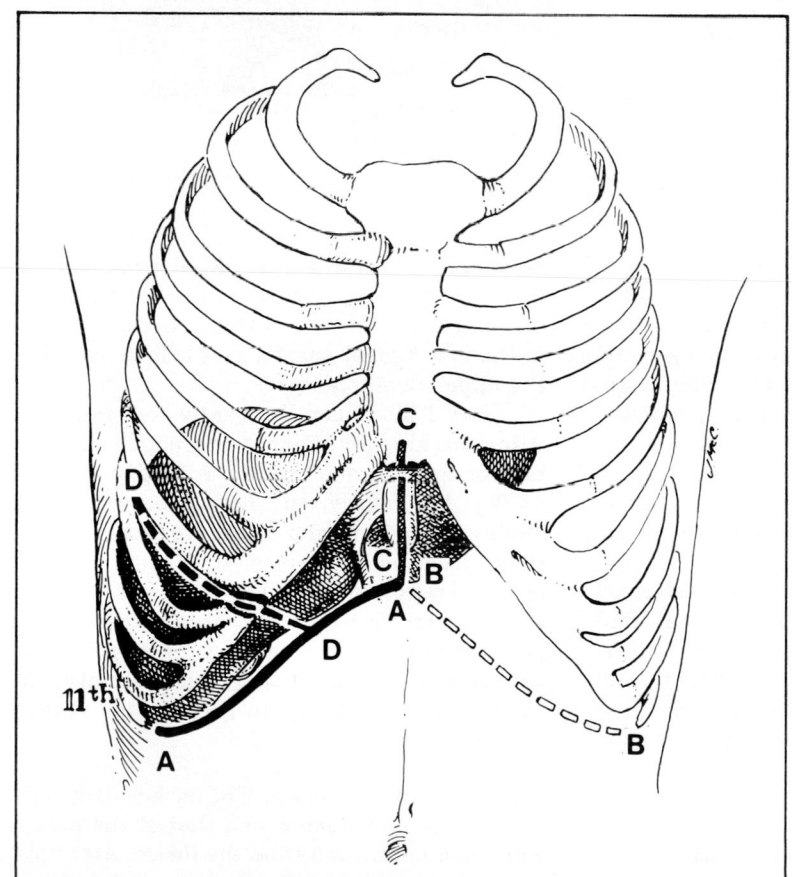

Figure 68–13. Incisions for orthotopic liver transplantations and for hepatic resections, right or left. Note that several extensions may be made from the basic right subcostal incision, A to A, that is almost always used. More than one of the depicted extensions may be required in a given patient. (*Source: From Starzl TE, Bell RH, et al: Hepatic trisegementectomy and other liver resections. Surg Gynecol Obstet 141:429, 1975, with permission.*)

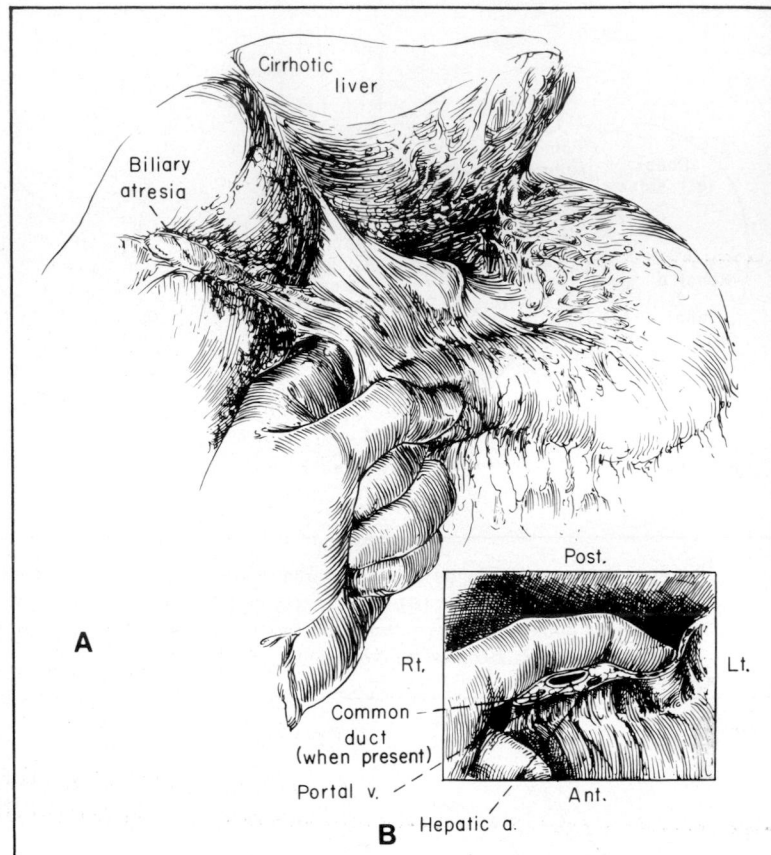

Figure 68–14. A. Encirclement of the portal structures preparatory to their individual dissection. This can be done either from the right side as indicated or from the left through the lesser omental sac. **B.** Spatial relationships of the components of the portal triad. (*Source: From Starzl TE* (*with the assistance of CW Putnam*), *1969, with permission.*)

considerable tailoring of the vena cava, which is mobilized from within the liver (Fig. 68–18). The technique of isolating the liver in this way and peeling it out in the bloodless state permits all residual tissue connections of the right triangular ligament and the bare area, including the right adrenal vein, to be ligated under perfect vision. The penalty is an increased time of portal and vena caval occlusion which, if excessive, can set into motion an irreversible spiral of physiologic deterioration (discussed later).

With the liver out, the wound is checked for major sites of bleeding, realizing that total hemostasis of the bare area and elsewhere is not possible at this time. The suprahepatic and infrahepatic vena caval anastomoses are performed first, followed usually by reconstruction of the portal vein. At a convenient time, air and the potassium-rich preservation fluid in the graft should be washed out (Fig. 68–19) to prevent air embolism or hyperkalemia with revascularization. An alternative to the infusion

technique shown in Figure 68–19 is to flush the liver with the first surge of restored portal blood, allowing the outflow to escape through a vent in the lower caval anastomosis before releasing the upper caval clamp.

Portal blood flow is usually restored first. After checking for major anastomotic leaks, the hepatic arterial anastomosis is performed (Fig. 68–20). Frequently, the new liver is at first swollen and hard, and there is diffuse hemorrhage from all raw areas. With time and the administration of platelets and fresh frozen plasma, the problems are usually reversible, providing a major bleeder has not been missed. Efforts at mechanical hemostasis are continued until it is thought safe to perform the biliary tract reconstruction.

Vascular Anastomoses. The back wall of both vena caval anastomoses and that of the portal vein must be sutured from the inside. Attempts to develop long enough cuffs for external sutur-

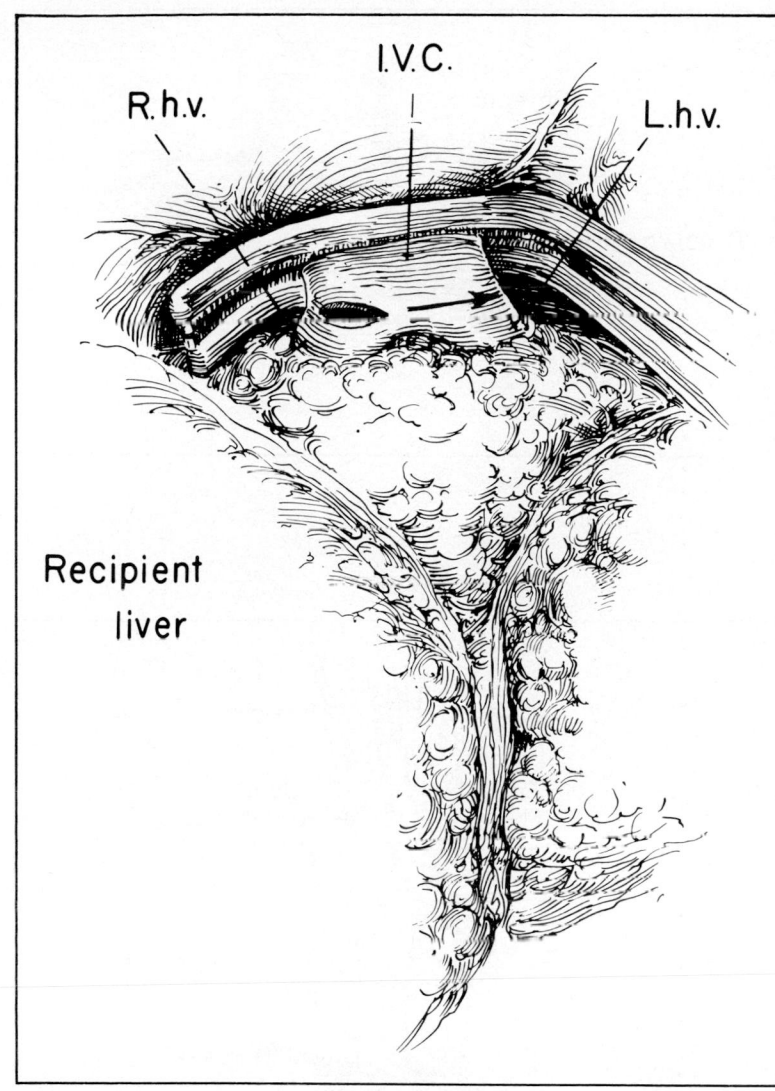

I.V.C.

R.h.v.

L.h.v.

Recipient
liver

Figure 68–15. Transection of the suprahepatic inferior vena cava. Note that the line of incision is kept as close to the liver as possible in order to retain the maximum vessel length for subsequent anastomosis. R.h.v. = right hepatic vein; L.h.v. = left hepatic vein; I.V.C. = inferior vena cava. (*Source: From Starzl TE (with the assistance of CW Putnam), 1969, with permission.*)

ing may be fruitless; if successful, the reconstructed vessels may kink from the excessive length. We have used a continuous intraluminal suturing technique.

The principle of the method, as demonstrated in Figure 68–21, is the immediate formation of intraluminal shoulders in both vessels to be joined. First, sutures are placed in the extremities of the anastomosis. The swaged needle is passed into the posterior part of the lumen of one of the vessels 1 mm from the line of incision (Fig. 68–21A2). A firm bite of the other vessel is then taken, making sure that the entry and exit sites of the needle pass through the intima at some distance from the cut edge (Fig.

68–21A3). The full thickness of the wall is included. The same kind of bite is taken in the back wall of the other vessel. A mound of protruding tissue presents, which makes the similar placement of subsequent sutures easy (Fig. 68–21A4). The back wall is automatically everted. When the opposite end of the posterior anastomotic line is reached, the needle is passed outside (Fig. 68–21A4) and the anterior row is completed with an everting over-and-over suture (Fig. 68–21A5). The steps are almost exactly the same for an end-to-end (Fig. 68–21B) or end-to-side anastomosis (Fig. 68–21C).

The degree of eversion obtained in the back wall is the same as if the sewing were done

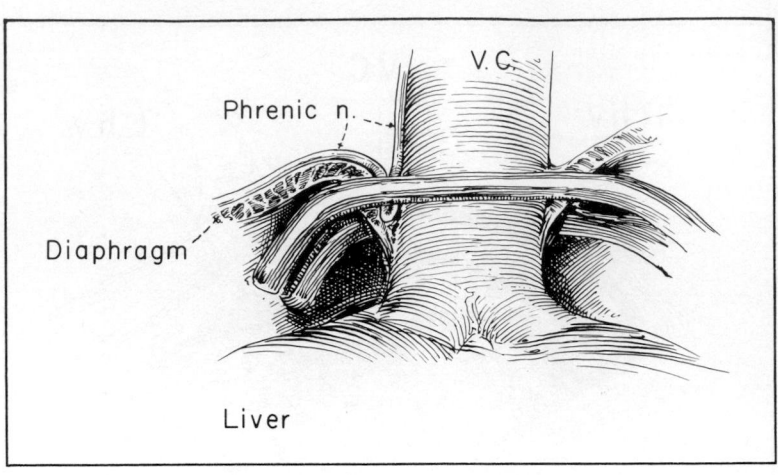

Figure 68–16. Probable mechanism of operative injury of the right phrenic nerve in several pediatric patients. Note the inclusion of the nerve in the bite of the vascular clamp, which has been placed across the suprahepatic vena cava and which has also included a piece of diaphragm. (*Source: From Starzl TE* (*with the assistance of CW Putnam*), *1969, with permission.*)

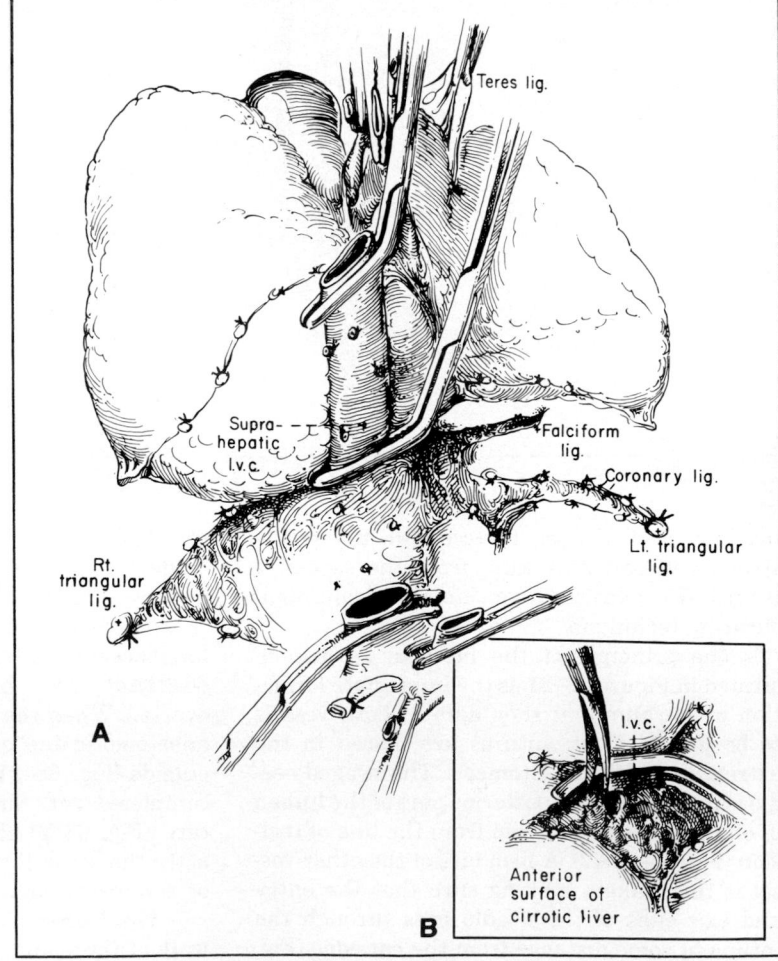

Figure 68–17. A. Operative field after retrograde liver mobilization. The last remaining structure, the suprahepatic inferior vena cava, has been clamped above the liver. **B.** Technique for mobilizing a suitable length of suprahepatic vena cava after placement of clamp. In adults, this usually involves cutting away cirrhotic liver tissue over the frequently distorted and foreshortened right and left hepatic veins. (*Source: From Starzl TE, Porter KA, et al: Orthotopic liver transplantation in 93 patients. Surg Gynecol Obstet 142:487, 1976, with permission.*)

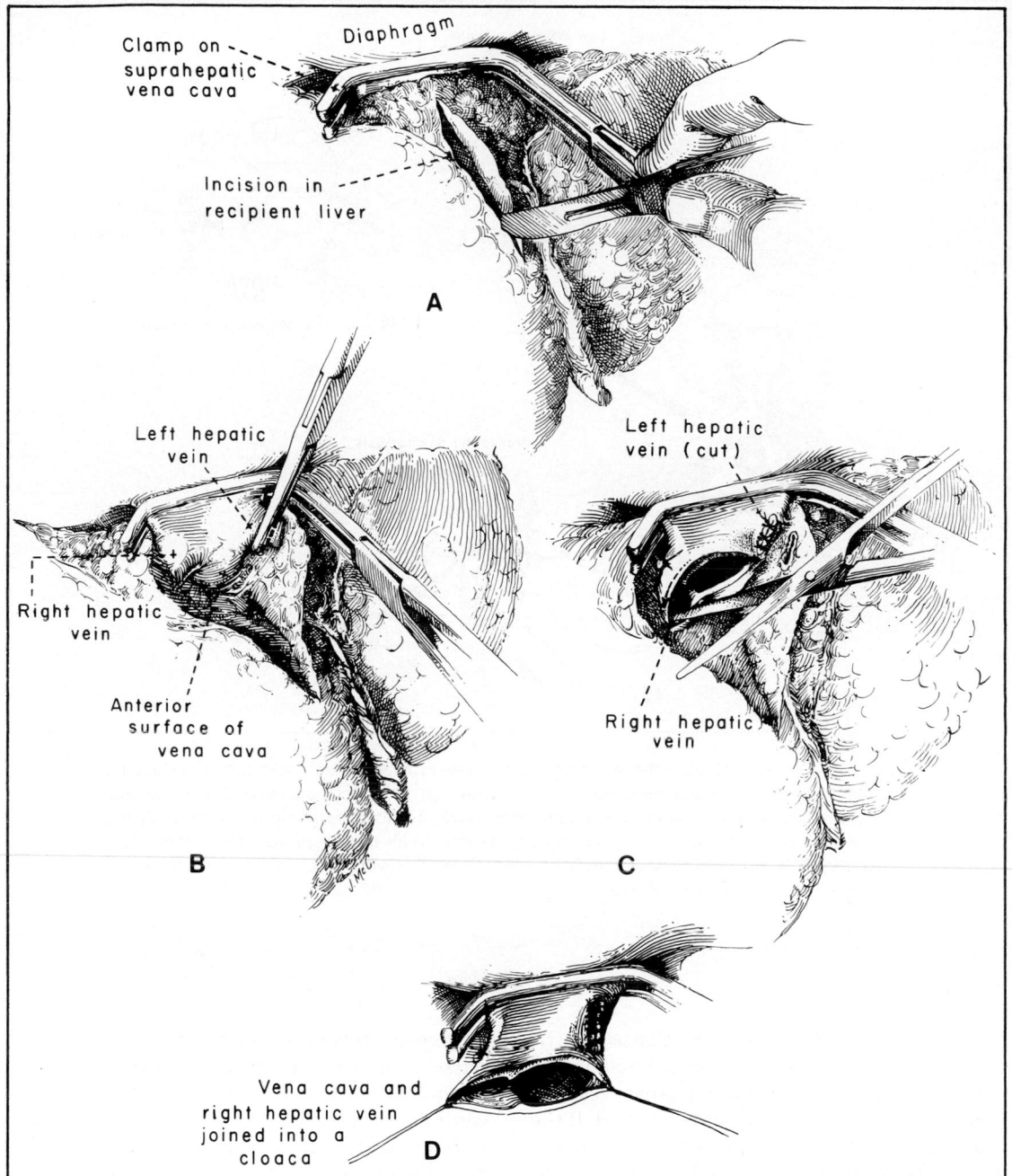

Figure 68–18. Development of a suprahepatic cuff of inferior vena cava. This technique is required most commonly if the native disease is nonalcoholic or alcoholic cirrhosis. Note that the suprahepatic vena cava is encircled and clamped **(A)** and that length is developed by cutting and peeling away the diseased liver tissue and scar **(B).** The eventual cuff usually has a lateral closure of either the left **(C,D)** or right hepatic vein. (*Source: From Starzl TE, Keop LJ, et al: Development of a suprahepatic recipient vena cava cuff for liver transplantation. Surg Gynecol Obstet 149:76, 1979, with permission.*)

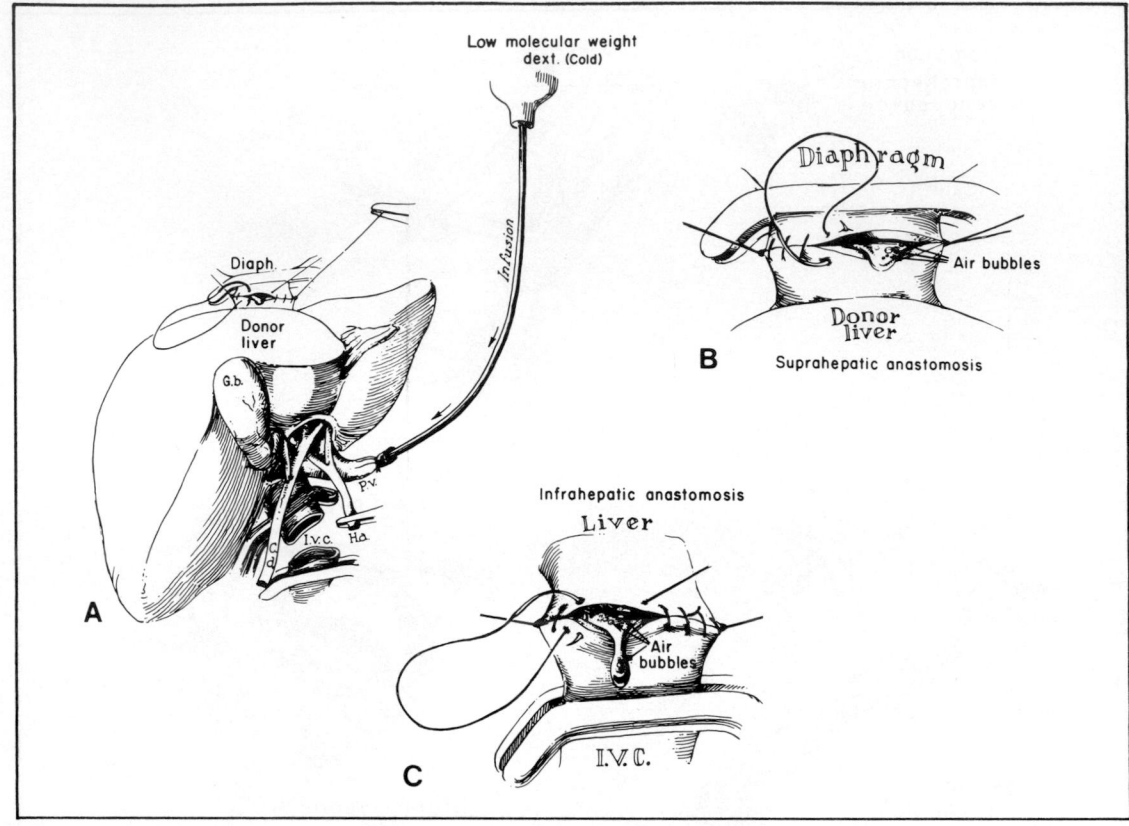

Figure 68–19. Initial steps in the implantation of a new liver. **A.** Infusion with lactated Ringer's solution in order to wash out the potassium rich Collin's solution. **B.** Completion of suprahepatic anastomosis. **C.** Completion of infrahepatic vena cava anastomosis. Note in **(B)** and **(C)** the escape of air bubbles which, if not expelled, could lead to air embolism. (*Source: From Starzl TE, Schneck SA, et al: Acute neurological complications after liver transplantation with particular reference to intraoperative cerebral air embolus. Ann Surg 187:236, 1978, with permission.*)

from the outside (Fig. 68–21A6). Consequently, the amount of intraluminal suture material is not increased. There are other advantages. A perfect intimal coaptation can be assured. If the orifices of tributaries to the anastomosed vessels are identified near the suture line, they can be incorporated into the shoulder, thereby circumventing potential paraanastomotic leaks. Gentle traction on the suture facilitates placement of the next bite, making it unnecessary to grasp or manipulate the vessel wall with forceps.

In the early years of our experience, silk was used for the vascular suturing. More recently we have preferred Prolene, a material that causes little advential pull, but that can purse string an anastomosis because of its easy movement through sutured tissues. A minor purse string effect at the large vena caval anastomosis has not been a concern but special precautions in addition to avoidance of excessive tension on the suture are taken to protect the portal vein and hepatic artery. Half of the continuous anastomosis is performed with one suture (Fig. 68–22A), and its mate is used for the other half of the circumference (Fig. 68–22B). The two are tied where they meet, but the knots are set at a distance from the vessel of about a third of the circumference (Fig. 68–22C). When blood flow is restored, the slippery Prolene pulls back into the suture line and the slack gradually is distributed back toward the opposite end (Fig. 68–22D). The process can be encouraged by gen-

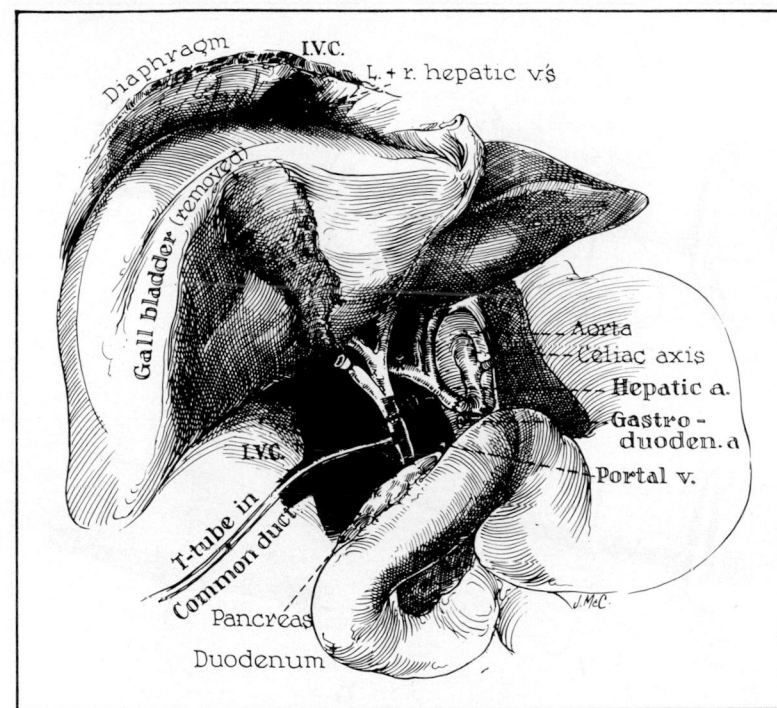

Figure 68–20. Completion of vascular reconstructions at hilum, and duct-to-duct biliary anastomosis over a T-tube stent. (*Source: From Starzl TE, Marchioro TL, et al: Experimental and clinical homotransplantation of the liver. Ann NY Acad Sci 120:739, 1964, with permission.*)

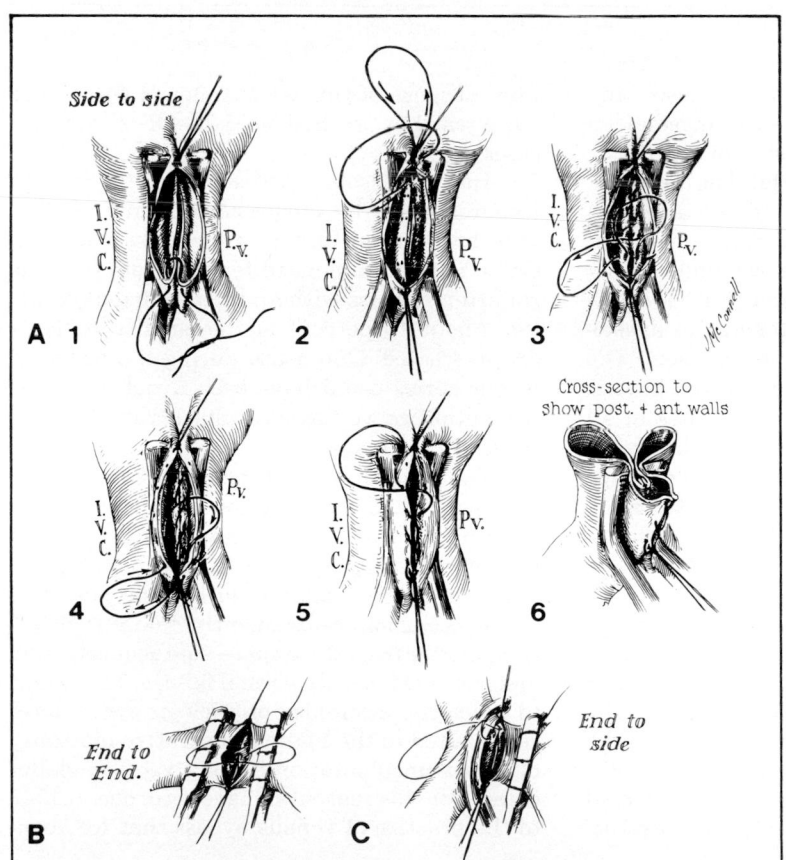

Figure 68–21. Techniques of intraluminal everting vascular suture: **A.** Side-to-side. **B.** End-to-end. **C.** End-to-side. (*Source: From Starzl TE, Groth CG, et al: An everting technique for intraluminal vascular suturing. Surg Gynecol Obstet 127:125, 1968, with permission.*)

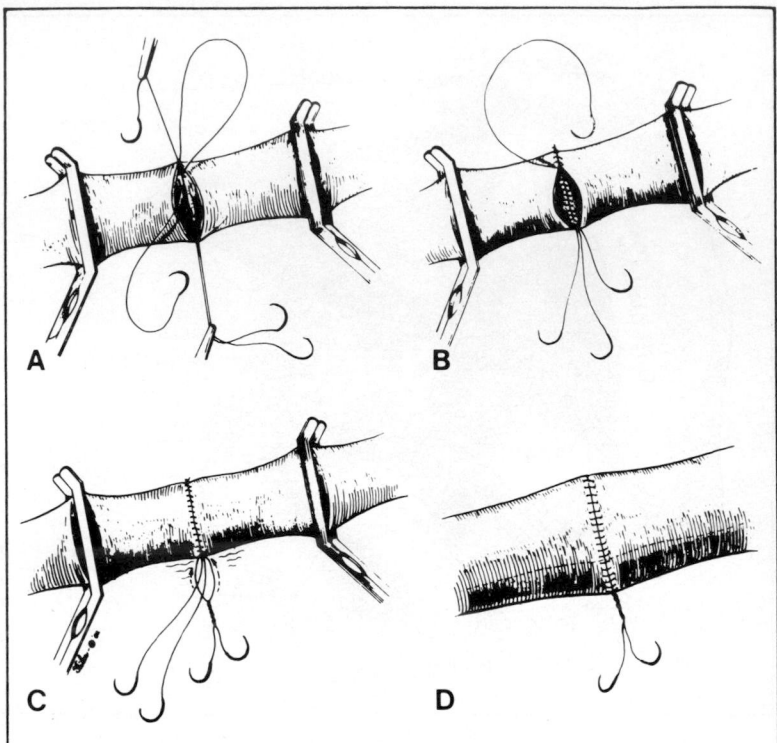

Figure 68–22. Method of avoiding strictures of small vascular anastomoses. (*Source: From Starzl TE, Iwatsuki S, et al: A "growth factor" in fine vascular anastomoses. Surg Gynecol Obstet* (*in press*), *with permission.*)

tle circular kneading of the anastomosis. Any bleeding from resulting gaps in the anastomosis is controlled with additional simple sutures.

The extra suture material has been referred to as a "growth factor." Some observers have been aghast at this seemingly heretical technique until they see the astounding way that small anastomoses expand (Fig. 68–22D), and with little bleeding. Postoperative anastomotic hemorrhage has not been seen. The growth factor technique is used for the hepatic arteries and portal venous anastomoses in all patients. In pediatric recipients, we believe it to be at least as important as the use of loupe magnification in the routine ability to reconstruct these tiny structures at the hepatic hilus.

Venous Bypasses. Portal and vena caval occlusion during the anhepatic phase often is reasonably well tolerated during a 45- to 90-minute anhepatic phase in spite of major declines in cardiac output and variable hypotension. The relative safety of the occlusions depends on the collaterals that develop with human liver disease. The same thing has been demonstrated in dogs subjected to chronic bile duct obstruc-

tion. Because of this we abandoned the venous bypasses that we had used in all of our first cases.

However, some patients can be gravely jeopardized by the venous cross-clamping. If severe hypotension occurs after cross-clamping, Calne has recommended femoral vein to femoral artery bypass with an intervening oxygenator. About 10 percent of the English patients are so treated. One death during the last year in our series could have been avoided by this precaution as well as a cardiac arrest that was successfully treated.

The fact that most patients can recover from portal and vena inferior caval cross-clamping may have created a false impression about the safety of this practice. Usually there is gross swelling of the intestine during the period of portal occlusion. Subsequently, many such patients suffer from third space fluid sequestration and from postoperative renal failure. The extent to which these complex physiologic events have contributed to the high perioperative mortality of liver transplantation has not yet been delineated. For this reason we have returned in 1982 to the practice of venous bypass that we abandoned long ago. Cannulae were placed into the inferior vena caval (through an iliac or femoral vein) and into the portal system through the open end of the transected portal vein. During the anhepatic phase the blood was returned to a reservoir and pumped to one of the large veins in the neck or arm. This kind of bypass required total body heparinization and the amount of bleeding was so excessive and nonresponsive to later protamine reversal that two of the patients died on the operating table.

Eventually, the feasibility of using pump-driven venous bypasses with no heparin was proved in dogs, using heparin-coated tubing and nontraumatic closed-system pumps without a reservoir. Clinical application was promptly undertaken and now this technique is used for all adult recipients. With this change, liver transplantation has become possible with maintenance of better patient physiology and without so much stress on the anesthesiologists and surgeons. Removal of the devascularized liver in a meticulous and deliberate way as well as more

leisurely performance of the vascular anastomoses for the first time has made transplantation a pleasant operation instead of a desperate race against the clock.

Variant Technical Problems and Solutions

THE "FROZEN" LIVER HILUS. Patients with previous operations may have such severe right upper quadrant adhesions that it is virtually impossible to enter the abdomen. In such recipients, it is essential with sharp dissection to develop an exact plane on the undersurface of the liver, and eventually to encircle the portal triad (Fig. 68–14). If the lesser omental sac can be found and entered, through the avascular gastrohepatic ligament, the encirclement usually is easiest from the left side. If it is then impossible to dissect the individual structures of the portal triad, the triad mass can be transected after placement of a vascular clamp (Fig. 68–23). The individual structures can be identified

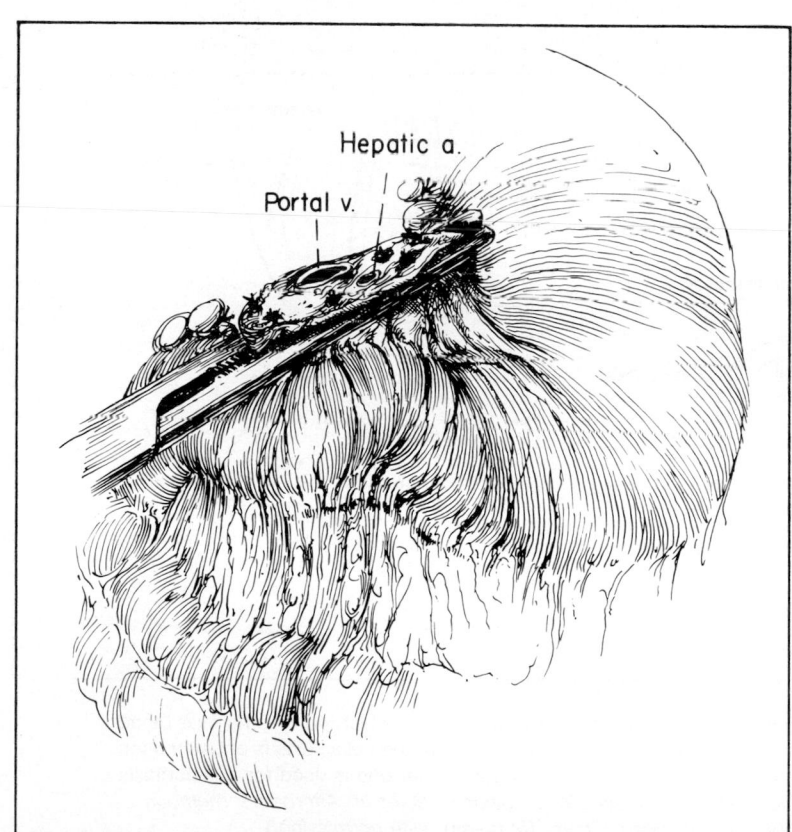

Hepatic a.

Portal v.

Figure 68–23. Incision en masse of the portal triad. This maneuver has been necessary on several occasions when the individual structures could not be dissected free. After the transection, the portal vein and hepatic artery can be liberated enough to permit the vascular anastomoses to be performed. (*Source: From Starzl TE (with the assistance of CW Putnam), 1969, with permission.*)

at the cut surface and traced back for the development of cuffs.

ARTERIALIZATION OF GRAFT ANOMALIES. Problems posed by homograft arterial anomalies (Fig. 68–4) have been described with various technical solutions. A double arterial supply originating from the celiac axis and superior mesenteric artery once was thought to be too troublesome to warrant an effort at reconstruction. In several recent cases, the celiac axis and superior mesenteric artery have been connected (Fig. 68–24), and one or the other end of the superior mesenteric artery has been anastomosed to the recipient hepatic artery.

INADEQUATE RECIPIENT ARTERY. Contingency plans should be made in the event that a recipient hepatic artery is too small or too inconveniently located to permit an effective anastomosis. The most common cause for this circumstance is an anomolous recipient arterial supply such as that described in previous sections.

In our earliest experience in such recipi-

ents, attempts were made to perform an anastomosis of the graft aorta or celiac axis to the aorta of the recipient above the recipient celiac axis. The dissection required to clean off the recipient aorta in this inaccessible area was difficult, and aortic cross-clamping, which was usually required during the anastomosis, had devastating physiologic effects. Consequently this approach has been abandoned.

The easiest solution is to attach the homograft blood supply to the recipient abdominal aorta, inferior to the origin of the renal arteries (Fig. 68–25). The exposure of the distal aorta is relatively easy, even in patients with severe portal hypertension. The ascending colon is retracted to the left. The most convenient site for anastomosis is near the origin of the inferior mesenteric artery. The extra length of graft vessel necessary to reach this location can be provided by retaining the thoracic aorta of the donor in continuity with the celiac axis and by turning the aorta 180 degrees (Fig. 68–25). The occasional need for this technical deviation has prompted the donor team to retain the thoracic aorta with the specimen whenever possible.

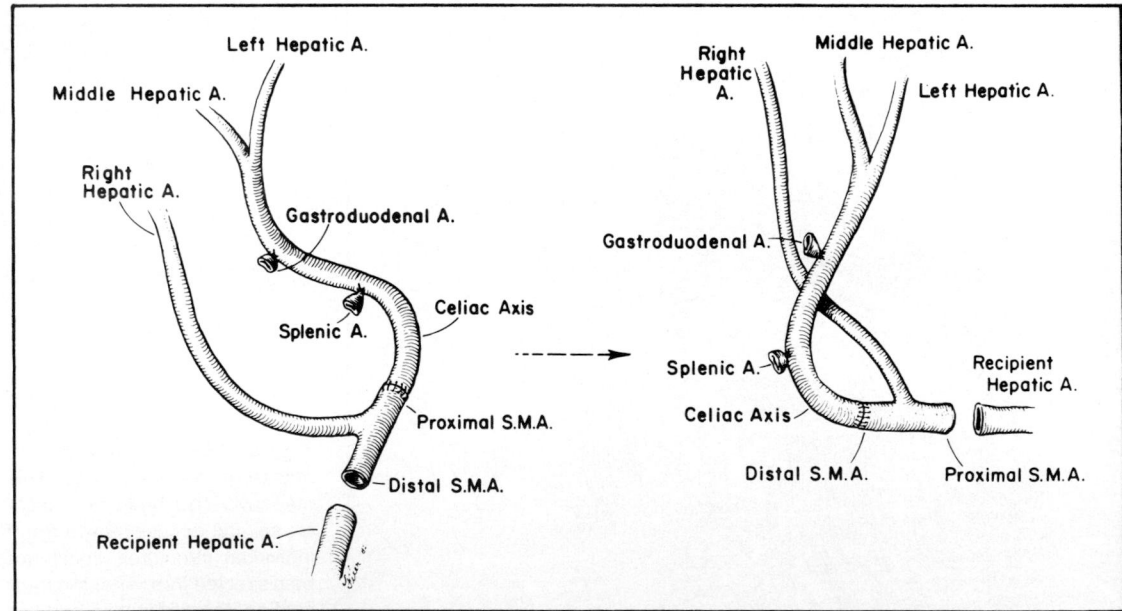

Figure 68–24. The management of a common graft anomaly in which part of the liver blood supply is derived from the superior mesenteric artery. Note that the celiac axis is anastomosed to one end of the main superior mesenteric artery and the other end is used for anastomosis to a recipient vessel. (*Source: From Shaw BW Jr, Iwatsuki S, et al: Alternative methods of hepatic graft arterialization. Surg Gynecol Obstet (in press), with permission.*)

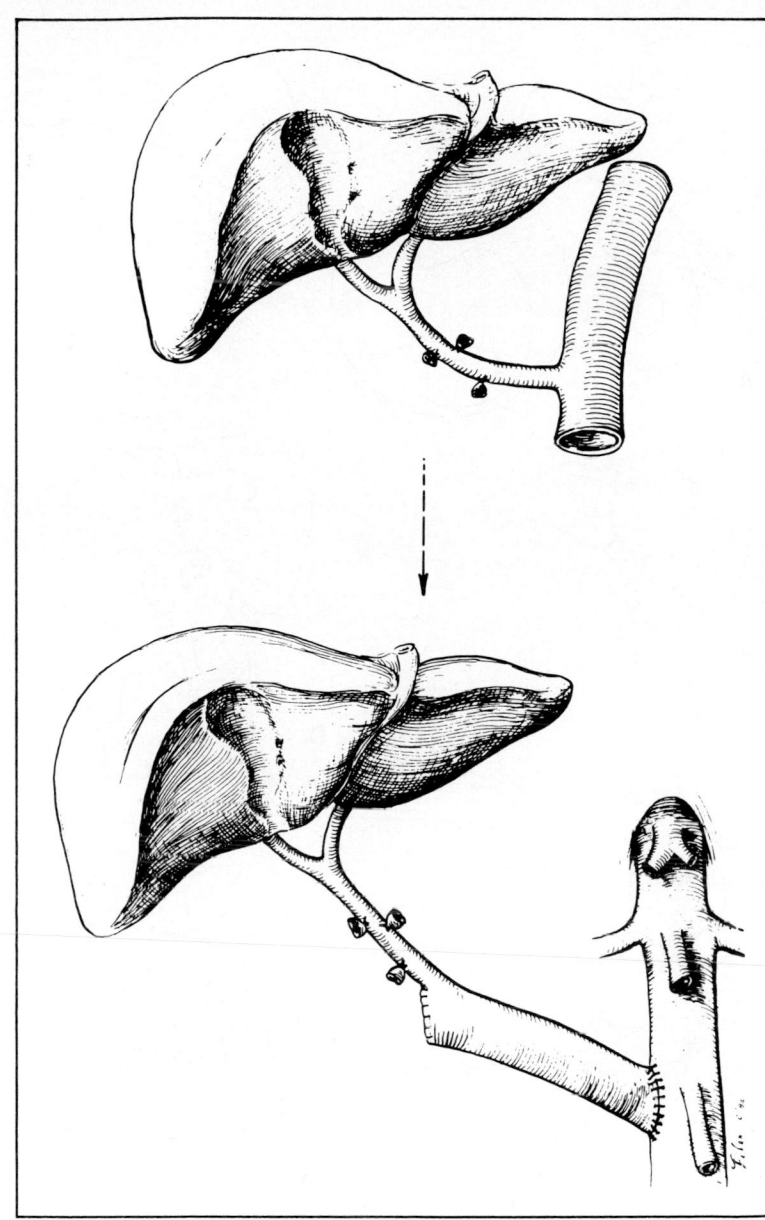

Figure 68–25. Technical solution if an adequate recipient artery cannot be found in the area of the portal triad. A piece of graft aorta in continuity with the graft celiac axis can be anastomosed to the abdominal aorta of the recipient. Alternatively an iliac artery graft can be attached to the recipient aorta with a distal anastomosis to the celiac axis. The latter technique depends upon the availability of contingency grafts procured at the time of the liver harvest (Fig. 68–12). (*Source: From Shaw BW Jr, Iwatsuki S, et al: Alternative methods of hepatic graft arterialization. Surg Gynecol Obstet (in press), with permission.*)

Another option to obtain the needed length is to anastomose the free common iliac artery graft to the same location in the recipient aorta with ligation of the hypogastric artery. The external iliac artery is almost a perfect match for anastomosis to the graft celiac axis.

THROMBOSED OR HYPOPLASTIC PORTAL VEIN. One of the great tragedies of liver transplantation has been the discovery at operation of an unsus-

pected thrombosis or hypoplasia of the portal vein. If effective revascularization of the homograft portal vein has not been accomplished, survival has never been obtained. In two patients, the suprarenal inferior vena cava has been anastomosed to the graft portal vein, providing the liver with systemic venous inflow as with a portacaval transposition. This anastomosis thrombosed in one patient, who died of massive hemorrhage from esophogeal varices a

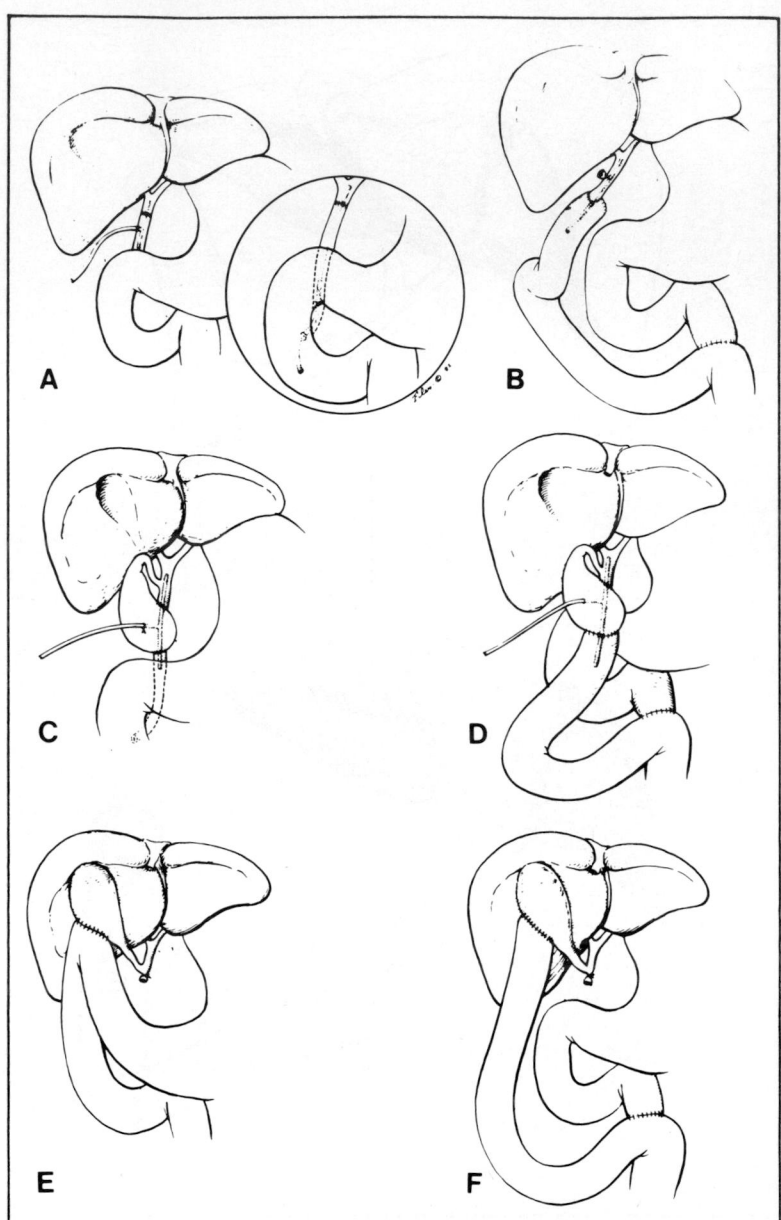

Figure 68–26. Methods of biliary tract reconstruction that have been used with liver transplantation. The techniques shown in (**E** and **F**) are so defective that they have been abandoned. Depending upon the anatomic and clinical circumstances, each of the other methods may be useful in individual cases.

month later; the other patient died of massive graft necrosis.

If the thrombosis (or hypoplasia) has not involved the splenic and superior mesenteric veins, the confluence of these portal tributaries can be dissected free from beneath the pancreas. We have then developed a cloaca at this junction to which an iliac vein graft has been anastomosed to provide added length. The use of an interposition host graft under these circumstances (Fig. 68–12) has been lifesaving.

If thrombosis of the portal vein has been recent, thrombophlebectomy has been accomplished on several occasions. Although a rough intimal surface has been left, the portal venous system has remained open.

BILIARY TRACT RECONSTRUCTION. In the early days of liver transplantation, the now abandoned procedure of cholecystoduodemostomy was frequently used (Fig. 68–26E). Obstruction at the homograft cystic duct occurred in almost half of the cases. Even without obstruction the biliary tract became the site of entry of bacteria (Fig. 68–27). Organisms that could be cultured from the bloodstream were those indigenous to the gastrointestinal (GI) tract. It was envisioned that the liver was being frequently contaminated with enteric contents, followed by systemic dissemination of the bacteria (Fig. 68–27).

The systematic use of a defunctionalized jejunal limb (Roux-Y) to which the gallbladder was anastomosed (Fig. 68–26F) was an improvement. However the problem of cystic duct obstruction in more than one third of the recipients remained (Fig. 68–28), necessitating frequent secondary revisions with conversion to choledochojejunostomy (Fig. 68–26B).

If biliary enteric anastomosis is necessary, we now perform a choledochojejunostomy (Roux-Y) at the first operation (Fig. 68–26B). This is done with a single layer of continuous

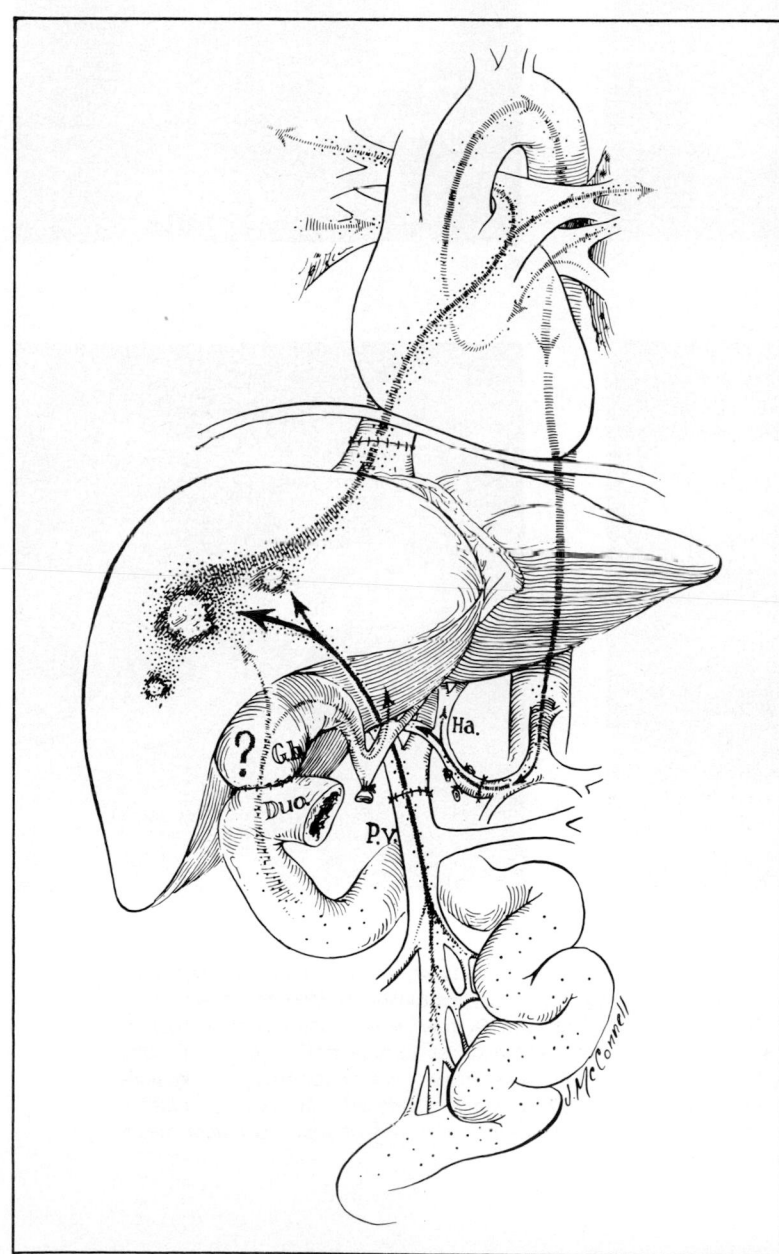

Figure 68–27. Development of regional and systemic infectious complications secondary to contamination and/or partial obstruction of the biliary tract. (*Source: From Starzl TE, Groth CG, et al: Orthotopic homotransplantation of the human liver. Ann Surg 168:392, 1968, with permission.*)

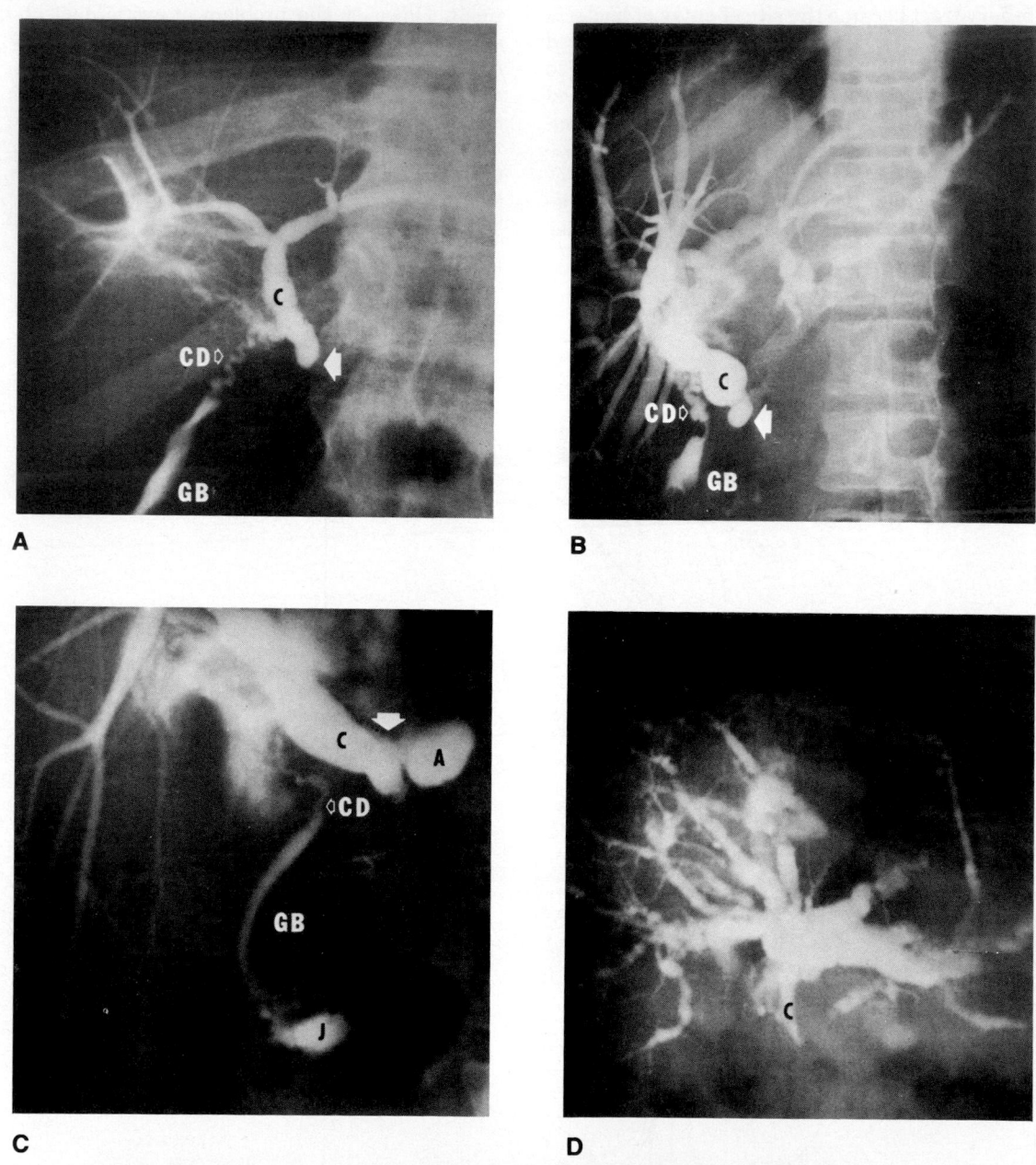

Figure 68–28. Transhepatic cholangiograms in four patients whose original biliary reconstructions were with Roux-Y cholecystojejunostomy. **A.** Minimal obstruction. **B.** Moderate obstruction. **C.** Severe obstruction with leak and abscess formation. **D.** Very severe obstruction; at reoperation the common duct was necrotic. A = leak and abscess formation; C = common duct; CD = cystic duct; GB = gallbladder; J = jejunum; large arrow = site of common duct ligation. (*Source: From Starzl TE, Putnam CW, et al: Biliary complications after liver transplantation: With special reference to the biliary cast syndrome and techniques of secondary duct repair. Surgery 81:212, 1977, with permission.*)

absorbable suture (Fig. 68–29). A few tacking sutures can be used for reinforcement (Fig. 68–29). An internal stent is used (Fig. 68–26B). When choledochojejunostomy is performed, the gallbladder is removed.

Biliary tract reconstruction by duct-to-duct anastomosis was the first one used by the authors and then temporarily abandoned because of a high incidence of biliary leaks, which were lethal in the patients treated 15 to 20 years ago. The duct-to-duct anastomosis (Fig. 68–26A) is performed with interrupted absorbable sutures. A T-tube stent is used whenever possible (Fig. 68–26A), and the T-limb is brought out through a choledochotomy in the recipient portion of the

composite duct. In small children, and occasionally adults, the available T-tubes are too large and an internal stent is used, with the distal tip passed into the duodenum (Fig. 68–26A′).

In 1973, Waddell and Grover recommended that the homograft duct be anastomosed to the graft gallbladder as part of the biliary reconstruction in liver transplantation. Calne has used this technique extensively in the Cambridge program and for him it is the method of choice. The distal anastomosis with the fundus of the homograft gallbladder is made either to the recipient common duct (Fig. 68–26C) or to a Roux limb of jejunum (Fig. 68–26D). In either case, both of the anastomoses are stented

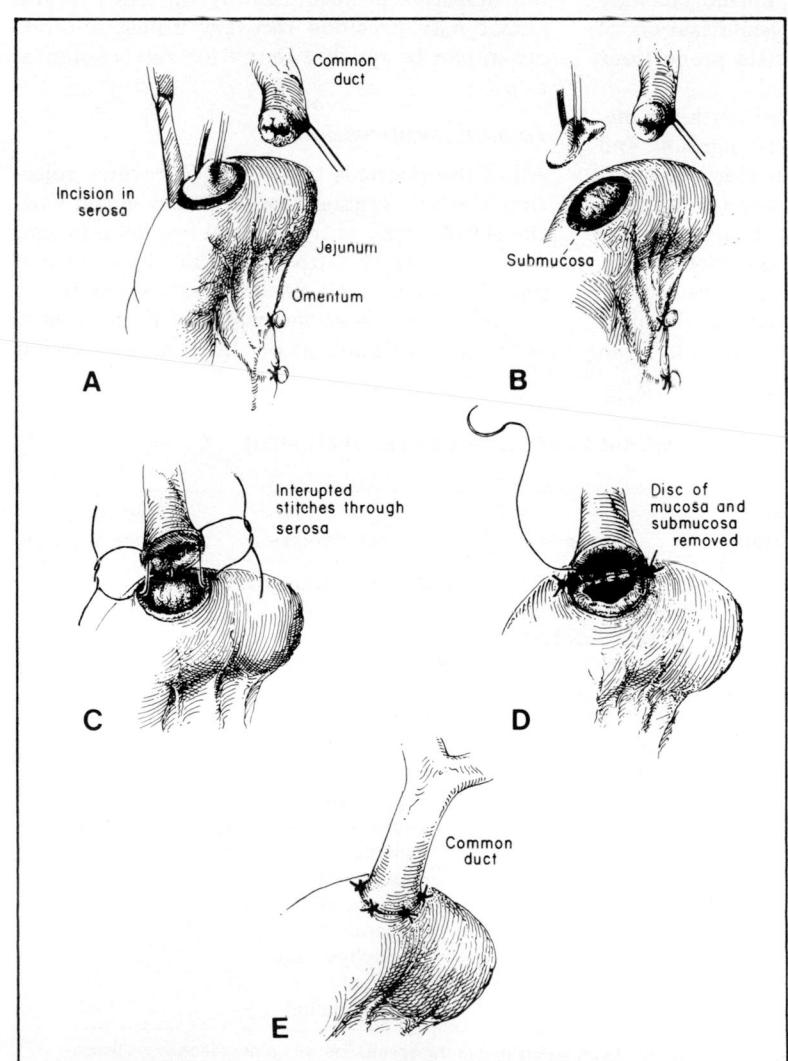

Figure 68–29. Technique of choledochojejunostomy. (*Source: From Starzl TE, Putnam CW, et al: Biliary complications after liver transplantation: With special reference to the biliary cast syndrome and techniques of secondary duct repair. Surgery 81:212, 1977, with permission.*)

with a T-tube which can be used for irrigation. We have used the Waddell–Calne procedure only when the extra length provided by the gallbladder was necessary to bridge a gap between the graft and the distal anastomosis.

In our hands, choledochocholedochostomy and choledochojejunostomy have both provided excellent results. Our experience with the Waddell–Calne procedure has been too limited to warrant comment, but the Cambridge team has been pleased with the results.

CONTROL OF HEMORRHAGE. The most important factor in hemorrhage is portal hypertension with extensive venous collaterals. In addition, coagulation defects must be anticipated routinely with depletion of clotting factors produced by the liver. In addition, fibrinolysis may begin shortly before the revascularization of the homograft and assume crisis proportions shortly afterward.

Control of bleeding must start with the mechanical means of ligation, suture ligation, and cautery. With the new liver in place, there is decompression of the portal system through the new organ, with elimination of the adverse mechanical factor of portal hypertension. If the liver functions well, the perturbations in clotting can be expected to self-correct but this may require hours. In the meanwhile platelets, fresh frozen plasma, and blood constituents may be used as temporary expedients.

Postoperative Care

The most common, early difficulties have been with pulmonary insufficiency requiring prolonged mechanical ventilation, renal failure at the same time that massive fluid shifts are occurring, and persistent clotting abnormalities. These problems are managed with conventional methods of intensive care with great emphasis on biochemical and hemodynamic monitoring. Recovery can be expected from preexisting encephalopathy and the hepatorenal syndrome. Patients who have received well-functioning livers can have an almost miraculous recovery, but defective performance by the graft at the outset may preclude recovery unless another organ can be quickly found for retransplantation.

Immunosuppression

All of the methods to prevent or reverse rejection of whole organs have been developed with the simpler procedure of renal transplantation. These are summarized in Table 68–4, with a notation about their use in liver recipients.

Although there was widespread discontent with all techniques of immunosuppression

TABLE 68–4. CLINICAL IMMUNOSUPPRESSIVE DRUG REGIMENS DEVELOPED WITH KIDNEY TRANSPLANTATION

Agents	Year Reported	Place	Deficiencies	Used for Liver Transplantation
Azathioprine	1962	Boston	Ineffective, dangerous	No
Azathioprine–steroids	1963	Denver; Richmond; Boston; Edinborough	Suboptimal	Yes
Thoracic duct drainage as adjunct	1963[a]	Stockholm	Nuisance; requires 20–30 days pretreatment	Yes
Thymectomy as adjunct	1963	Denver	Unproven value	No
Splenectomy as adjunct	1963	Denver	No longer necessary	Yes
ALG as adjunct	1966	Denver	Still suboptimal	Yes
Cyclophosphamide substitute for azathioprine	1970	Denver	No advantage except for patients with azathioprine toxicity	Yes
Total lymphoid irradiation	1979	Palo Alto; Minneapolis	Dangerous; extensive preparation; not quickly reversible	No
Cyclosporine alone	1978–1979	Cambridge	Suboptimal	Yes
Cyclosporine–steroids	1980	Denver	Under evaluation	Yes

[a] It was not realized until much later that pretreatment for 3 to 4 weeks before transplantation was a necessary condition.

available from 1963 to 1978, improved drug therapy was not possible until the advent of cyclosporine. Cyclosporine is an extract from the fungi *Cylindrocarpon lucidum* and *Trichoderma polysporum*. It was discovered and characterized biochemically by scientists at the Sandoz Corporation, Basel, Switzerland, who showed it to be immunosuppressive in mice, rats, and guinea pigs. The drug depressed humoral and cellular immunity with a quickly reversible action. These effects were not accompanied by the bone marrow depression that had frequently limited the doses of azathioprine and cyclophosphamide.

When cyclosporine A was first used in patients by Calne at Cambridge it was hoped that no other drug would be routinely required. Our experience has been that cyclosporine should be combined with steroid therapy from the outset, although the steroid component with this version of double drug therapy has been smaller than in the past.

Nephrotoxicity is the most serious side effect of cyclosporine (Fig. 68–30). Fortunately the renal complications are promptly reversed by reducing the cyclosporine doses. Most of the other side effects of cyclosporine have not been serious, including hirsutism, gum hyperplasia, tremor, regional flushing or vague abdominal discomfort just after drug ingestion, and the development of breast fibroadenomas in women. Although hepatotoxicity has been seen in about one fifth of cases, this has rarely been serious and it can be controlled by dose reduction.

For liver transplantation, cyclosporine is started a few hours preoperatively with an oral dose of 17.5 mg/kg (Fig. 68–30). Cyclosporine is continued daily, but with reduced intramuscular or intravenous (Fig. 68–31) quantities until diet is resumed. Subsequently an oral dose of 17.5 mg/kg/day is given, usually with half every 12 hours. The doses are reduced subsequently if nephrotoxicity develops. Steroids also are started on the day of operation. For adult patients who leave the operating room in relatively good condition a 5-day burst of prednisolone is given, starting at 200 mg and stopping with a maintenance dose of 20 mg/day. Further reductions of cyclosporine and steroid doses are made on an individualized basis in the ensuing months. Initial maintenance therapy with steroids is scaled down in infants and children (Fig. 68–30).

If rejection occurs in spite of this beginning

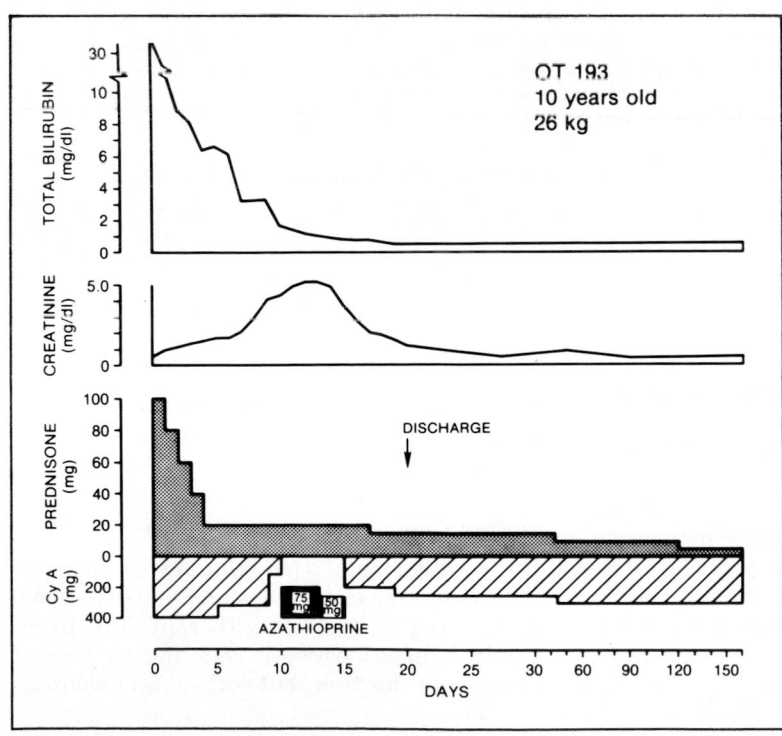

Figure 68–30. Immunosuppression with cyclosporine and steroids (plus temporary azathioprine) in a 10-year-old girl (OT 193). Note that the 5-day opening burst of prednisone therapy was scaled down because of her small size. The temporary discontinuance of cyclosporine and replacement with azathioprine between postoperative days 10 and 15 was because of probable cyclosporine nephrotoxicity. The patient who was of B blood type was given the liver of an A donor. (*Source: From Starzl TE, Iwatsuki S, et al: Evolution of liver transplantation. Hepatology 2:614, 1982, with permission.*)

OT 193
10 years old
26 kg

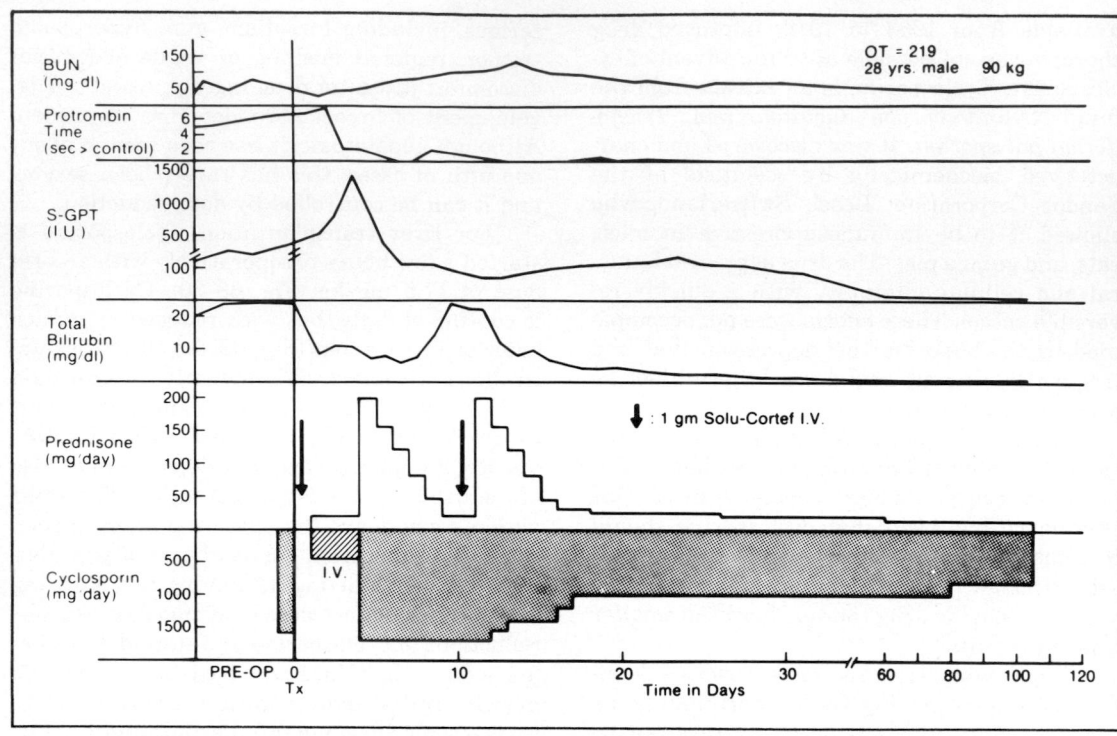

Figure 68–31. Deviation from standard steroid therapy in a patient (OT 219) whose perioperative condition was frail. The 5-day burst of postoperative steroids was begun several days postoperatively but had to be repeated when rejection supervened. Before operation, the patient had hepatorenal syndrome and encephalopathy and he had been on a ventilator for more than 1 week. Because of defective clotting, efforts to place central venous lines before starting transplantation resulted in uncontrolled hemorrhage, with the loss of 20 L of blood. The subclavian and innominate vessels were explored through cervical and thoracotomy incisions, and the bleeding was mechanically controlled before transplantation was started. The blood loss from placement of the vascular lines exceeded that incurred during transplantation. The patient survived because of prompt correction of the coagulation abnormalities. (*Source: From Starzl TE, Iwatsuki S, et al: Evolution of liver transplantation. Hepatology 2:614, 1982, with permission.*)

therapy, the principal responses have been to administer intermittent large doses of hydrocortisone (or prednisolone) intravenously (Fig. 68–31), to repeat the original 5-day burst of steroids (Fig. 68–31), and to settle at a higher maintenance level of steroids. Although cyclosporine is not a drug that permits much dose maneuverability, it has sometimes been possible to increase the amounts given, the limiting factor being nephrotoxicity. Dose adjustments of cyclosporine can be aided by pharmacologic monitoring of plasma or blood levels.

Results After Liver Replacement

The introduction of cyclosporine–steroid therapy has had a major influence upon the results after orthotopic liver transplantation.

Before Cyclosporine (1963–1979)

During this time, 170 patients underwent orthotopic liver transplantation under conventional double-drug or triple-drug therapy. The 1-year survival ranged between 28.8 and 50 percent throughout this time, but without an indentifia-

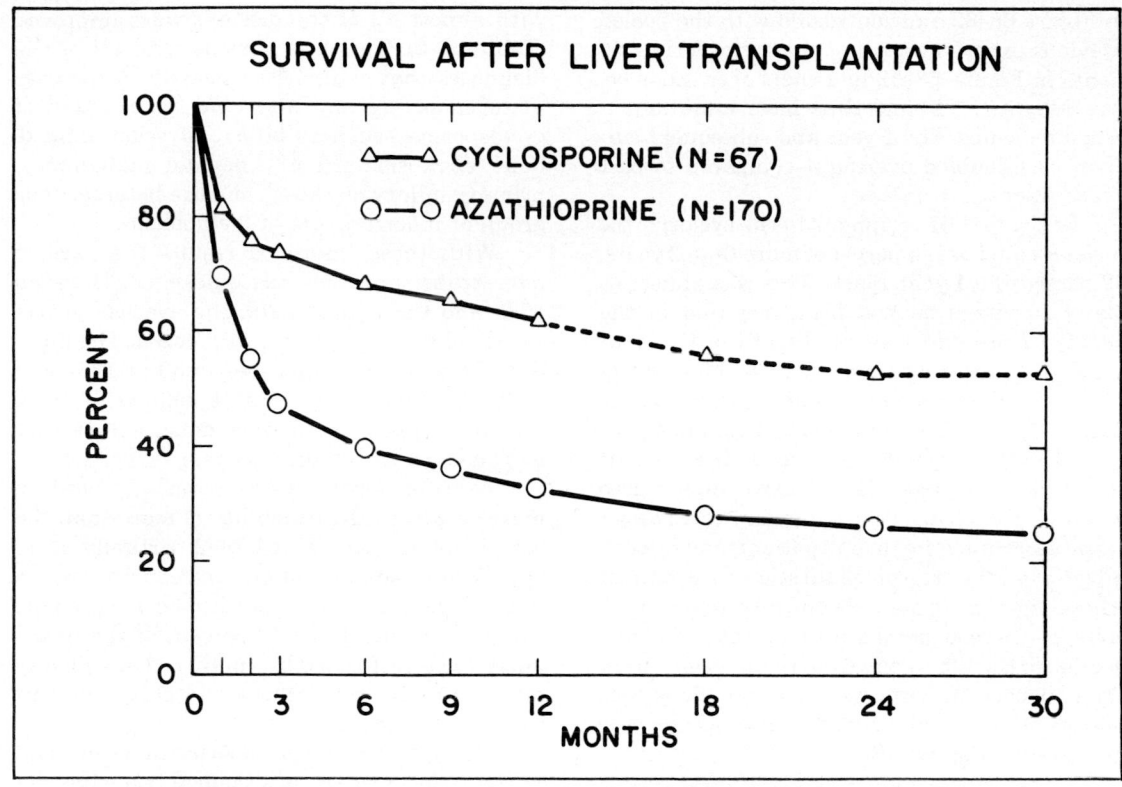

Figure 68–32. The survival of 67 patients treated with cyclosporine and low-dose steroids (minimum follow-up 16 months) compared to the survival obtained under conventional immuno-suppression (azathioprine). (*Source: From Starzl TE, Iwatsuki S, et al: Report of Colorado-Pittsburgh liver transplantation studies. Transplant Proceedings 15:2582, 1983, with permission.*)

ble trend of improvement. The results during this 16-year period are summarized in Figure 68–32.

Of the 170 patients entered into this series, 56 lived out the first postoperative year. Twenty three subsequently died. Although 13 of the 23 late deaths were in the second postoperative year, losses occurred as late as 6 years. Of the original 170 patients, 33 (19.4 percent) are still alive after follow-ups of 3½ to 13⅓ years. Between 1963 and 1979, there was an almost equal division between adult and pediatric recipients (Tables 68–1 and 68–2). From the sixth month onward the younger patients had about a 10 percent survival advantage.

A similar experience of occasional spectacular successes interspersed with a larger number of failures was also heard in the Cambridge–King's College trials from the beginning of that

program in 1968 through early 1980. In the English series, 22 (23.7 percent) of the first 93 recipients lived for at least 1 year, with 11 subsequent deaths during the second to sixth years; at the time of last reporting the 11 survivors had been followed for 1 to 6 years.

The Cyclosporine Era (1980–1982)

The predictability and reliability with which liver transplantation could be carried out improved abruptly with the first trials of cyclosporine–steroid therapy, and this promise has been sustained with subsequent experience. Since 1980, the majority of liver recipients have been brought through the early postoperative convalescence and have been able to leave the hospital for outpatient care (Fig. 68–32).

The survival in the first 67 consecutive recipients in the cyclosporine era is summarized in Figure 68–32 and contrasted with the pooled previous experience. All of the cyclosporine patients in Figure 68–32 had their operations before May 1, 1982, and thus have minimum 1-year follow-ups. The 1-year and subsequent survival was doubled overnight compared to past expectations.

Of the first 67 recipients in the cyclosporine series treated over a period of more than 2 years, 42 passed the 1-year mark. This was almost as many survivors as had been acquired in the nearly 17 preceding years. Six of the 42 1-year survivors subsequently died. In 4 the cause of the late failure was recurrence of the original disease (2 hepatic malignancies, 1 example each of Budd–Chiari's syndrome and B-virus chronic hepatitis). The other late deaths were caused by an airway obstruction secondary to an upper respiratory infection in one patient, and by complications after retransplantation in a patient whose first graft was chronically rejected. In spite of these 6 deaths after 1 year, the late decline of the life survival curve has been slower than in past patients who entered the second postoperative year under azathioprine and prednisone (Fig. 68–32).

A natural question would be if these results could be explained by a sudden change in candidacy criteria or by a difference in the diseases for which transplantation was performed. Analysis according to the recipient diseases showed that this was not the case. Instead, the results

with almost all of the diseases were improved (Table 68–5). This was obvious with all of the diagnoses that contributed heavily to the case material before and after the introduction of cyclosporine—such as biliary atresia, nonalcoholic cirrhosis, primary hepatic malignancy, primary biliary cirrhosis, and the heterogenous group of inborn errors of metabolism.

With these improved results the pace of liver transplantation has quickened. Between 1963 and the end of 1979, the average yearly case load was not much over a dozen. The number of transplantations rose to 30 in 1981 and to 80 in 1982. In the first 4 months of 1983, 34 liver replacements were done, a rate that extrapolates to 100 for this year.

To be of service, a new surgical procedure must be within the capability of more than the occasional surgeon. Until 1982, virtually all of our liver transplantation procedures over a span of 19 years were performed by a single surgeon. During 1982, 40 percent of the procedures were performed by another young faculty member or by the fellows and this year this figure has been 70 percent.

The influence of cyclosporine upon survival in the Cambridge–King's College trials has not yet been clearly defined, in part because the drug has not been used regularly and in part because it has been started late in most cases after an initial course of azathioprine and steroid. Nevertheless, improved results have been

TABLE 68–5. INFLUENCE OF DISEASE UPON 1-YEAR SURVIVAL IN 237 PATIENTS[a]

	Conventional Therapy		Cyclosporine–Steroids	
	No.	1 Year (%)[b]	No.	1 Year (%)[c]
Biliary atresia	51	14 (27)	11	6 (54.5)
Nonalcoholic cirrhosis	46	16 (34.8)	16	9 (56.3)
Primary liver malignancy	18	5 (27.8)	9	6 (66.7)
Inborn errors[d]	15	8 (53.3)	10	7 (70)
Alcoholic cirrhosis	15	4 (26.7)	0	—
Primary biliary cirrhosis	6	1 (16.7)	6	5 (83.3)
Sclerosing cholangitis	7	2 (28.6)	3	2 (66.7)
Secondary biliary cirrhosis	4	3 (75)	5	1 (20)
Budd–Chiari's syndrome	1	1 (100)	3	3 (100)
Miscellaneous[e]	7	2 (28.6)	4	3 (75)

[a] The same case material was analyzed in detail elsewhere but with shorter follow-ups.
[b] Thirty two of these 52 patients are still alive with follow-ups 3½ to 13½ years.
[c] Thirty six of these 42 patients are still alive with follow-ups 1 to 3¼ years.
[d] α-1-Antitrypsin deficiency (17 examples), Wilson's disease (3 examples), Tyrosinemia (2 examples), glycogen storage disease (2 examples), sea blue histiocyte syndrome (1 example).
[e] Neonatal hepatitis (3 examples), congenital hepatic fibrosis (2 examples), Byler's disease (2 examples), adenomatosis, hemachromatosis, protoporphyria, acute hepatitis B (1 example each).

attributed by Calne to the better immunosuppression that they can now provide.

Steps to Reduce Mortality

A glance at the life survival curves from the earlier days of our experience or even in recent times (Fig. 68–32) shows that the highest priority for improved management is reduction of the perioperative mortality. However, the fact that the survival curves continue to decline even after 3 or 4 months means that strategies to circumvent late mortality will also be important. Policy adjustments may have an impact in both periods.

The way in which the original disease dictates the technical difficulty of transplantation and thus the early mortality was not clearly perceived until relatively recently. The consequent hidden risk factor could be improved by trying to treat patients with technically "dangerous" diseases like postnecrotic cirrhosis, alcoholic cirrhosis, and secondary biliary cirrhosis at an earlier time. When such patients have had previous operations at or near the hepatic hilum (such as repeated biliary tract reconstructions or especially portacaval shunts) it may be reasonable to conclude in some cases that liver transplantation is no longer a reasonable option, especially if the patient's physical and metabolic decay is extreme. Almost all of our deaths on the operating table and many not long afterward have been of such patients. We now believe that all adult patients are candidates for veno–venous bypasses. None of the candidates need this advantage more than the patients with previous portacaval shunt.

Incomplete knowledge of the recipient anatomy cannot be accepted in future cases. Of all the adverse possibilities, an inadequate recipient portal vein is the worst and the only one for which there usually is not a technical remedy. Means to detect a defective portal vein with ultrasound are now available.

Liver transplantation for postnecrotic cirrhosis in B-virus carriers and for patients with hepatic malignancies has resulted in disease recurrence in the grafts. There is not yet enough evidence to foreclose this avenue of treatment but it will be important for workers in the field to pool data in order to arrive at a consensus. Too many late deaths from recurrence of these diseases have occurred, a problem that has not been so overwhelming with any of the other disorders that have recurrence potential.

When a transplanted liver fails either early or late from rejection or other causes, aggressive attempts at retransplantation usually offer the only chance for survival. One of the most common judgment errors we have made is to hope vainly for improvement in hepatic function until the hope of reintervention was lost. Despite this, more than 40 patients have undergone retransplantation since 1968. Only recently have these efforts been encouraging. More than 30 patients treated during 1980–1983 had retransplantation a few days to 20 months after primary grafting and the majority are surviving, with subsequent follow-ups of up to 1½ years.

The performance of retransplantation has usually been surprisingly easy. The procedure has been greatly simplified by retaining cuffs from the suprahepatic and infrahepatic vena cava and from the portal vein of the first graft. Usually it has been necessary to perform the arterial anastomosis proximal to the previous site of anastomosis. Failure to do this in a recent case resulted in thrombosis of the arterial segment retained from the failed first graft for anastomosis to the celiac axis of the second liver.

SUMMARY

During the 20 years since transplantation was first attempted in humans, the procedure has gone from an experimental to a difficult but therapeutic procedure. As the manifold problems associated with this complex form of care have been resolved, the survival after liver replacement has improved to the point where two thirds of recipients can now be expected to live through the first postoperative year. Within the next two or three years a national network of cooperating centers providing this form of advanced service can be expected to be well established in the United States.

BIBLIOGRAPHY

Birch AG, Moore FD: Experiences in liver transplantation. Transplant Rev 2:90, 1969

Calne RY, Williams R: Liver transplantation. Curr Probl Surg 16:3, 1979

Calne RY, Williams R, et al: Improved survival after orthotopic liver grafting. Br Med J 283:115, 1981

Schmid R, Berwick DM, et al: National Institutes of Health Consensus Development Conference Statement: Liver transplantation. Hepatology 4:1075, 1984

Starzl TE (with the assistance of Putnam CW): Experience in hepatic transplantation. Philadelphia: WB Saunders, 1969

Starzl TE, Iwatsuki S, et al: Evolution of liver transplantation. Hepatology 2:614, 1982

Starzl TE, Marchioro TL, et al: Homotransplantation of the liver in humans. Surg Gynecol Obstet 117:659, 1963

Welch CS: A note on transplantation of the whole liver in dogs. Transplant Bull 2:54, 1955

69. Portal Hypertension

Seymour I. Schwartz

HISTORICAL BACKGROUND

In his classic monograph, Child presents a historic review emphasizing that although the co-existence of hepatic disease and the manifestations of portal hypertension have long been recognized, the specific role of elevated pressure within the splanchnic venous system has been appreciated only recently. The Ebers Papyrus provides evidence that the Egyptians were aware of the relationship between ascites and diseases of the liver. It was not until the turn of the twentieth century that Gilbert and associates and Pichancourt reasoned that pressure within the portal system was elevated in patients with ascites; they introduced the term "portal hypertension." At the same time, Banti, in the description of a syndrome that bears his name, underscored the association between splenomegaly, anemia, leukopenia, intestinal hemorrhages, ascites, and liver disease; he considered the splenic lesion to be primary.

Also at the turn of the century, several pathologists related the formation of esophagogastric varices to portal venous obstruction. In 1928, McIndoe concluded that portal pressure is elevated with cirrhosis. In 1937, Thompson, Caughy, Whipple, and Rousselot defined the presence of the pathophysiologic state of portal hypertension by manometric studies in which they demonstrated that the splenic venous pressure was consistently higher than the systemic venous pressure in patients with Banti's syndrome.

In 1877, based on animal experiments, Eck suggested application of a portacaval shunt for ascites. In 1894, Banti advised splenectomy for the manifestations of portal hypertension. The early operations for ascites consisted of a variety of omentopexies. These superseded the first Eck fistula in man in 1903, performed by Vidal. The first peritoneovenous shunt for ascites, consisting of an anastomosis between the saphenous vein and the peritoneal cavity, was conducted by Ruotte in 1907. Lenoir, in 1912, performed the first end-to-side portacaval shunt, and the same year Rosenstein performed the first successful Eck fistula in man for the relief of ascites.

The modern era of portal decompressive surgery was initiated by Blakemore and Lord, and Whipple, who performed nonsuture anastomoses of the portal vein to the inferior vena cava and an end-to-end splenorenal shunt for bleeding varices. Two years later Blalock advised suture anastomosis and an end-to-side splenorenal shunt, and Linton championed splenectomy and end-to-side splenorenal shunt with preservation of the kidney. Transesophageal ligation of varices was introduced by Boerema and Crile, in 1949 and 1950, respectively. The superior mesenteric inferior venacaval shunt that had been first performed in 1913 by Bogoras was reintroduced in 1953 by Marion and, independently, in 1955 by Clatworthy, Wall, and Watman.

The use of interposition grafts for effecting a mesocaval shunt was initially reported by deResende-Alves in 1963. Gliedman first inserted a Dacron interposition graft in 1967, but the first English report of this technique is credited to Lord et al.

In 1967, Warren, Zeppa, and Foman introduced selective transsplenic decompression of gastroesophageal varices by a distal splenorenal shunt; three years later, Maillard, Benhamou, and Rueff reported the technique of arterialization of the liver concomitant with a portacaval shunt.

Endoscopic injection of bleeding varices with a sclerosing solution was first described by Craaford in 1939, and more recently popularized by Terblanche et al. The devascularization procedures, studied for years by Womack and associates only to be discarded because of their poor results, are now enjoying recurrent popularity as a consequence of modifications introduced by Sugiura and Futagawa in 1977.

ETIOLOGY

The etiologic factors implicated in portal hypertension can be categorized into four major groups: (1) increased hepatopetal flow, (2) extrahepatic outflow obstruction, (3) obstruction of the extrahepatic portal venous system, and (4) intrahepatic obstruction.

Increased hepatopetal flow is an uncommon cause of portal hypertension; it may be related to a hepatic arterial–portal venous fistula, a circumstance that has been reported fewer than a dozen times. The diagnosis is readily established by angiography and effectively treated by ligation of the hepatic artery and disconnection between the hepatic artery and portal vein. Splenic arteriovenous fistula is also an uncommon lesion with a predilection for females between the ages of 20 and 50. Resection of the fistula itself is therapeutic. The spleen is implicated in this category in patients with massive enlargement as a consequence of tropical splenomegaly or myeloproliferative disorders. Portal hypertension and esophagogastric varices in these patients are corrected by splenectomy alone.

Obstruction of the suprahepatic inferior vena cava or an increased pressure within hepatic veins results in increased sinusoidal pressure and portal hypertension. A web in the suprahepatic vena cava has been reported, particularly in the Japanese population. The more common obstruction is associated with an endophlebitis of the hepatic veins that results in the Budd–Chiari's syndrome. Both an inflammatory process and an accompanying intravascular thrombosis contribute to the obstruction. The hepatic involvement may be isolated, or it may be part of a generalized migrating thrombophlebitis. Involvement of the hepatic veins may represent extension of a process originating in the hepatic segment of the inferior vena cava.

Portal hypertension secondary to obstruction and impairment of flow in the extrahepatic portal venous system is usually not complicated by hepatocellular dysfunction. Congenital atresia of the portal vein, related to changes in the circulation that occur at birth, is rare. More commonly, there is a cavernomatous transformation of the portal vein that may represent a congenital malformation, or may be the result of neonatal omphalitis obstructing the main portal vein, leading to the consequent enlargement of the veins of Sappey, which permit splanchnic venous flow to enter the liver. Isolated splenic vein thrombosis, usually a consequence of alcoholic pancreatitis, may cause esophagogastric varices and "left-sided" portal hypertension that responds only to splenectomy.

Over 90 percent of patients with portal hypertension have intrahepatic obstruction as the etiologic factor. The pathogenic factors include: (1) hepatic fibrosis with compression of portal venules, (2) compression by regenerative nodules, (3) increased arterial blood flow, (4) fatty infiltration and acute inflammation, and (5) intrahepatic vascular obstruction. The most common causative factor of intrahepatic obstruction is nutritional cirrhosis, which in Western countries is most frequently associated with alcoholism.

Both postnecrotic cirrhosis that develops as a progression of hepatitis and primary or secondary biliary cirrhosis may also result in portal hypertension. Hemachromatosis and Wilson's disease are often characterized by the clinical manifestations of portal hypertension. Congenital hepatic fibrosis, which is related to dilatation of the intrahepatic bile ducts, and is usually an autosomal recessive disease, is relatively unique because the manifestations of portal hypertension and cholangitis generally are not accompanied by hepatic dysfunction.

On a world-wide basis, hepatic infestation with *Schistosoma mansoni* is a very important factor. This results in presinusoidal occlusion of the portal venous radicals by the ova of the parasite. In the early phase of the architecture of the liver it is not disturbed and hepatic function may be only minimally impaired.

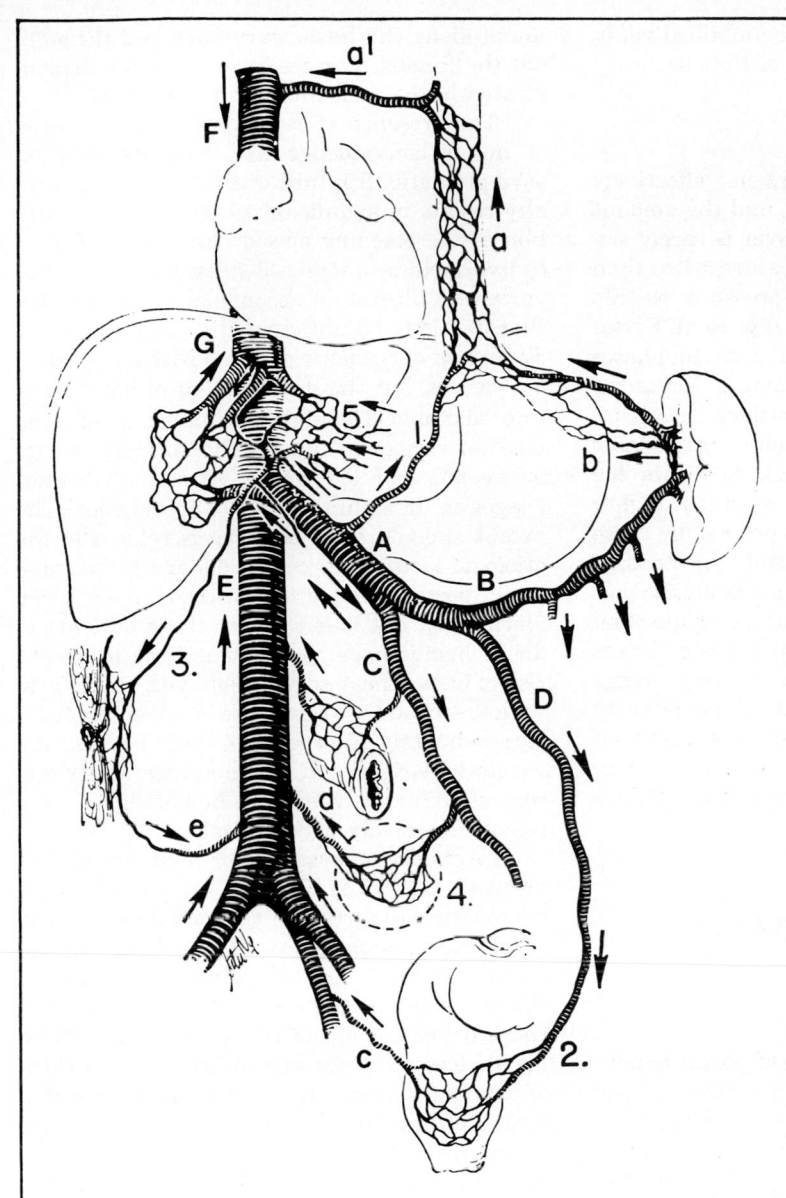

Figure 69–1. Collateral circulation. 1, coronary vein, 2, superior hemorrhoidal veins, 3, paraumbilical veins, 4, veins of Retzius, 5, veins of Sappey, A, portal vein, B, splenic vein, C, superior-mesenteric vein, D, inferior mesenteric vein, E, inferior vena cava, F, superior vena cava, G, hepatic veins, a, esophageal veins, a', azygos system, b, vasa vrevia, c, middle and inferior hemorrhoidal veins, d, intestinal veins, e, epigastric veins. (*Source: From Schwartz SI, 1964, p 292, with permission.*)

PATHOLOGY

Pathologic Anatomy

The collateral vessels that become functional in cases of portal hypertension are classified into two groups: hepatopetal veins that develop when the intrahepatic vasculature is normal and hepatofugal vessels that develop when

there is intrahepatic portal obstruction. The collateral circulation and the course of flow in each of the venous systems is shown in Figure 69–1.

The hepatopetal circulation includes the accessory veins of Sappey, the deep cystic veins, the epiploic veins, the hepatocolic and hepatorenal veins, the diaphragmatic veins, and the veins of the suspensory ligaments. The hepatofugal vessels include the coronary vein, the superior hemorrhoidal veins, the umbilical veins, and the retroperitoneal veins of Retzius.

Pathophysiology

The collateral circulation does not effectively decompress the portal system, and the amount of blood shunted around the liver is rarely significant. The normal portal pressure is less than 200 mm of saline. When the pressure exceeds this level, portal hypertension is present. Portal pressure varies with changes in position, phases of respiration, and intraabdominal pressure. There are also diurnal fluctuations. In all instances of portal hypertension, intrasplenic pressure is elevated. The pressure within the spleen is usually 27 to 81 cm of saline, higher than that of the portal vein per se. In those circumstances in which the portal hypertension is caused by obstruction of the extrahepatic portal venous system, or intrahepatic presinusoidal obstruction, such as congenital hepatic fibrosis and schistosomiasis, the hepatic vein wedge pressure is normal. By contrast, in the majority of cases of portal hypertension, including all those associated with cirrhosis, hepatic vein wedge pressure is elevated, reflecting a postsinusoidal obstruction.

CLINICAL MANIFESTATIONS

Esophagogastric Varices

The four major manifestations of portal hypertension are: (1) esophagogastric varices, (2) ascites, (3) hypersplenism, and (4) encephalopathy.

The submucosa of the esophagus is richly supplied with veins situated both above and below the muscularis interna. Fine anastomoses between the caval and portal circulations exist at the lower end of the esophagus. As the veins become engorged, vessels in the submucosal plexus of the esophagus increase in size and become dilated. To a lesser extent, the submucosal veins in the fundal and subfundal regions of the stomach also become varicose. In the later stages, the submucosa disappears over the large venous dilatations, and the walls of the veins themselves form the lining of the esophagus. Gastric varices occur predominantly in the cardiac end of the stomach, but they also may be found along the lesser curvature and throughout the fundus. Varices have also been demonstrated in the duodenum and the ileum.

The presence of esophagogastric varices is of minor consequence and patients may be asymptomatic. Rupture of these vessels generally results in significant blood loss. Precipitation of the bleeding episode has been ascribed to two factors—increased pressure within the varix and ulceration secondary to esophagitis. Bleeding is to be anticipated in approximately 30 percent of cirrhotic patients with demonstrable varices, but the development of bleeding is unpredictable. The elapsed time from the diagnosis of varices to the first hemorrhage varies between 1 and 187 weeks. Almost all hemorrhages occur within 2 years of observation. The extent and course of bleeding is related to the etiologic factor. Varices secondary to extrahepatic portal venous obstruction may bleed alarmingly, but it is rare for these patients to die of hemorrhage. By contrast, the mortality risk of hemorrhage in a patient with esophageal varices secondary to cirrhosis is extremely high. Approximately 70 percent of these patients die within 1 year of the first hemorrhage. Sixty percent of cirrhotics who have hemorrhaged once rebleed massively within 1 year.

In children, massive hematemesis almost always is caused by bleeding varices. When extrahepatic obstruction of the portal venous system is the etiologic factor, 70 percent of patients experience their first bleeding episode before the age of seven, and almost 90 percent hemorrhage before the age of ten. In the adult, bleeding varices comprise one quarter to one third of cases of massive upper gastrointestinal (GI) tract bleeding. In cirrhotic patients, varices are the source of upper GI bleeding in about 50 percent of patients, whereas gastritis is implicated in 30 percent, and duodenal ulcer in 10 percent. The bleeding from varices and peptic ulceration is characteristically severe; bleeding from gastritis is usually mild to moderate.

Ascites

Impairment of hepatic venous outflow (Budd–Chiari's syndrome) results in the sudden onset of ascites, frequently accompanied by abdominal pain, nausea, and vomiting. By contrast, ascites is not a usual accompaniment of extrahepatic portal venous obstruction. Intrahepatic postsinusoidal obstruction, as is present in patients with cirrhosis, frequently results in ascites.

The factors implicated in the formation of ascites include reduced serum osmotic pressure related to hypoalbuminemia, retention of sodium and water related to increased secretion of adrenal cortical hormones, and natural antidiuretic substances. Ascites may be complicated by the development of an umbilical hernia, necrosis of abdominal wall, or primary peritonitis. The presence of increased intraperitoneal pressure as a consequence of tense ascites results in a parallel increase in pressure within the esophagogastric veins and represents an etiologic factor in acute bleeding episodes.

Hypersplenism

Splenomegaly with engorgement of the vascular spaces frequently accompanies portal hypertension. There is little correlation, however, between the size of the spleen and the degree of hypertension. The hypersplenism associated with portal hypertension has been related to sequestration and destruction of circulating cells by immune mechanisms mediated by the enlarged spleen. A patient may demonstrate reduction of any or all of the cellular elements of blood. The usual criteria for making the diagnosis of hypersplenism are a white blood count below 4000/ml and a platelet count below 100,000/ml. It is unusual for the degree of neutropenia or thrombocytopenia to reach sufficiently low levels that they become symptomatic. Spontaneous ecchymosis and purpura as a consequence of portal hypertension alone are rare. Hypersplenism is a frequent manifestation of schistosomal infestation, and may represent the salient feature. The presence of hypersplenism has been correlated with the size of the spleen, but no correlation has been noted between the degree of anemia or leukopenia and the 5-year survival rates in patients with portal hypertension due to cirrhosis.

Encephalopathy

The development of neuropsychiatric symptoms related to natural and surgically created shunts is a debilitating feature of portal hypertension. This rarely occurs in patients with obstruction of the extrahepatic portal venous system without hepatocellular dysfunction. Nor does it occur in children who have been shunted for hypercholesterolemia and glycogen storage disease in the absence of portal hypertension. The neuropsychiatric syndrome is most commonly associated with cirrhosis and is present to a greater extent in patients with marked hepatocellular dysfunction. The syndrome has been related to hyperammonemia; both exogenous and endogenous causes contribute to the blood ammonia level, accounting for the fact that encephalopathy is a prominent feature in patients with bleeding varices.

The two factors implicated in the disturbed ammonia metabolism are impairment of hepatocellular function and portal systemic collateralization. The neuropsychiatric manifestations include changes in the state of consciousness, altered motor activity, and abnormal findings on psychometric testing. The encephalopathic syndrome has been divided into three stages: delirium, stupor, and coma. In the early stages there is mental confusion and exaggerated reflexes. The characteristic liver flap may be elicited. In the second stage there is an accentuation of muscular hypertonicity to the extent of rigidity; in the final stage there is complete flaccidity.

DIAGNOSTIC STUDIES

The presence of portal hypertension is generally established by occlusive catheterization of a hepatic venule (OHVP) demonstrating a pressure 40 mm saline greater than the free hepatic venous pressure. This pertains in all circumstances of postsinusoidal obstruction. The occluded hepatic vein pressure is characteristically normal in patients with presinusoidal obstruction and when the portal hypertension is due to extrahepatic portal venous obstruction. In this situation, percutaneous splenic pulp manometry can be used to define portal hypertension. This procedure, which is carried out under local anesthesia, is contraindicated in patients with a bleeding tendency, marked ascites, or severe hyperbilirubinemia.

The venous phase of celiac and superior mesenteric angiography defines the pathologic features of the portal circulation. The study provides a demonstration of the collateral veins, particularly esophagogastric varices, and also

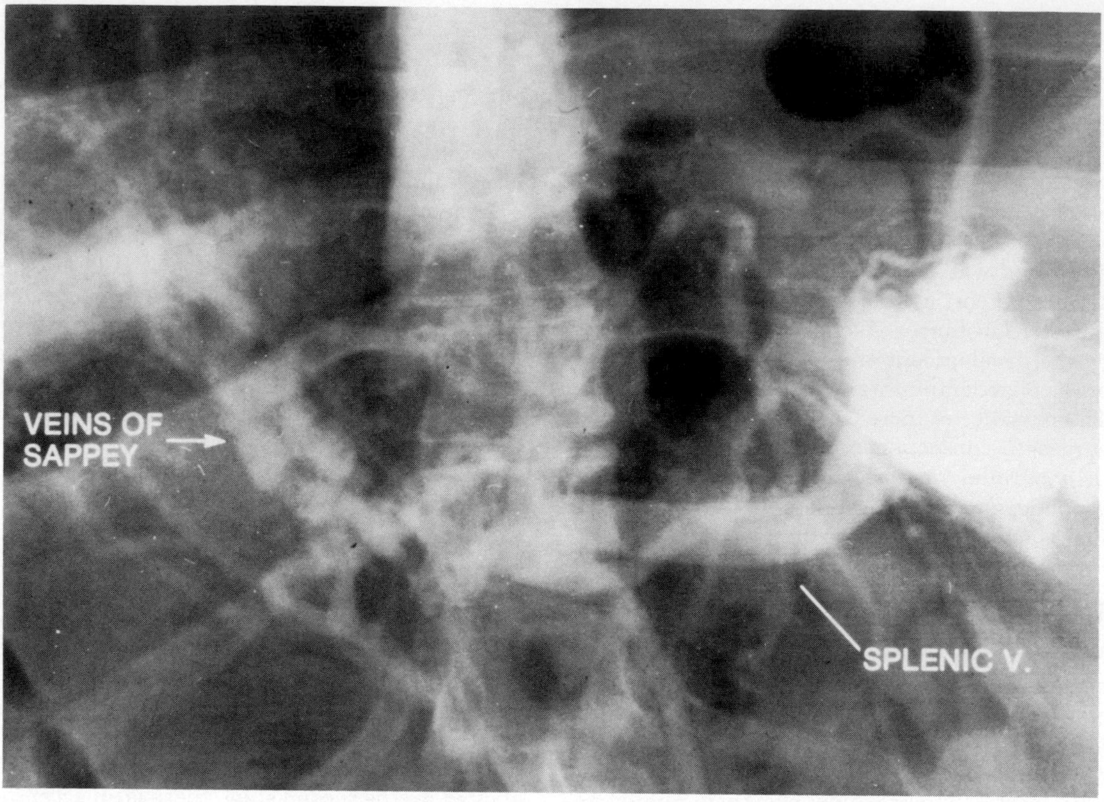

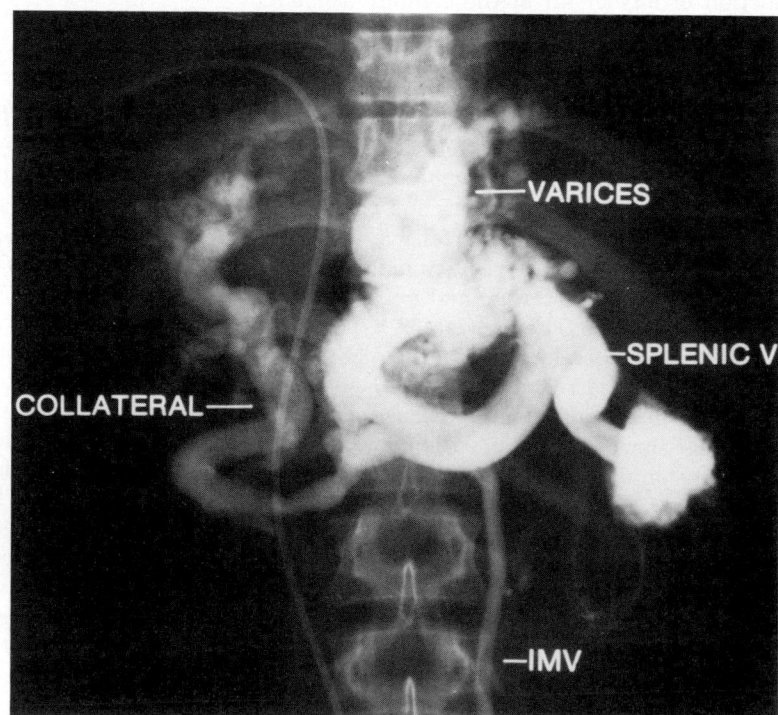

Figure 69–2. Splenoportogram demonstrating veins of Sappey indicative of portal vein thrombosis.

Figure 69–3. Splenoportogram showing varices and other collaterals.

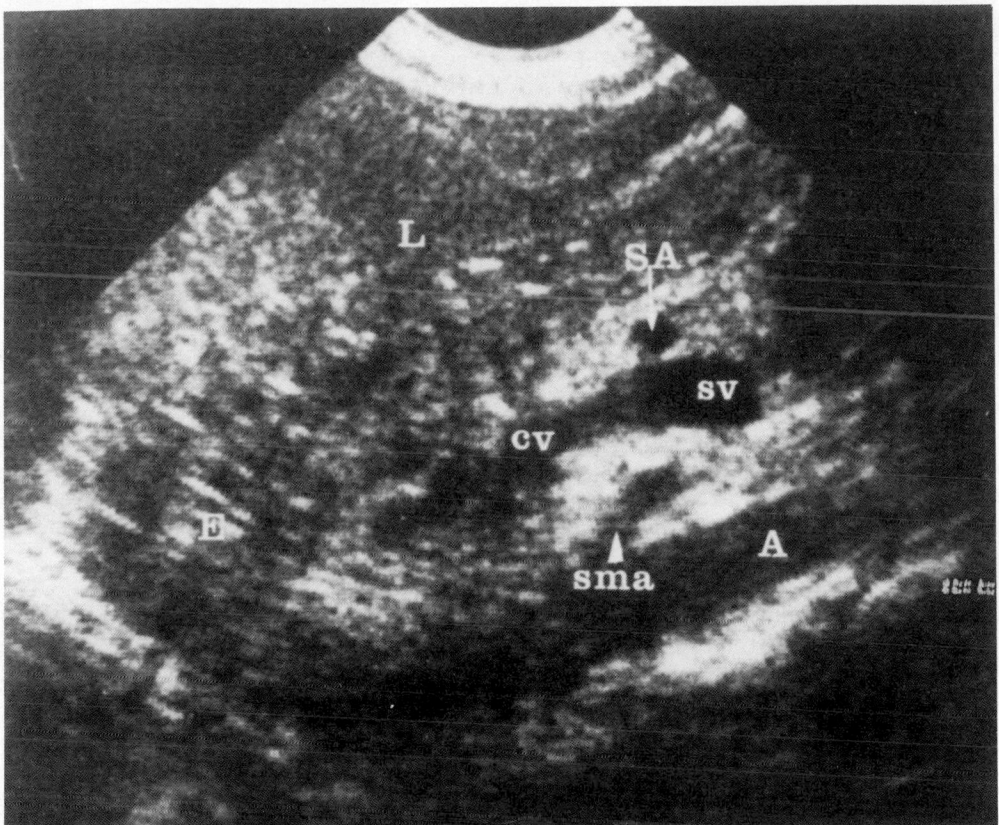

Figure 69–4. Sagittal scan through the liver (L) reveals superior mesenteric artery (sma) origin from aorta (A). A dilated coronary vein (cv) extends from splenic vein (sv) to the esophagus (E). SA, splenic artery. (*Source: From Subramanyam BR, Balthazar EJ, et al, 1983, p 370, with permission.*)

defines the site of obstruction, i.e., intra- or extrahepatic. The absence of a portal vein on angiography is not diagnostic of portal vein obstruction, but the presence of afferent collaterals in the region of the hepatoduodenal ligament should suggest that the etiology of portal hypertension is extrahepatic portal venous obstruction (Fig. 69–2). Isolated thrombosis of the splenic vein is readily diagnosed by celiac angiography. Transhepatic portography and splenoportography (Fig. 69–3) also provide definition of the portal venous system. Real-time ultrasonography has been applied to the assessment of patients suspected of portal hypertension. A portal vein diameter greater than 13 mm is indicative of portal hypertension, with a sensitivity

of 50 percent. The presence of venous collaterals can be demonstrated in about 90 percent of patients suitable for sonography. With this technique (Fig. 69–4), coronary gastroesophageal varices can be seen in about 90 percent of patients when they are large, and in 65 percent when they are small.

The presence of esophagogastric varices is best defined by endoscopy. Nonbleeding varices are readily demonstrated, but massive bleeding may obscure the varices themselves. Upper GI radiologic evaluation of the esophagus by barium swallow has a significantly high percentage of false-negative results related to the diagnosis of esophagogastric varices, and this is increased during the acute bleeding episodes.

TREATMENT

General Considerations

Esophagogastric Varices

Prophylactic Shunt. A prophylactic shunt is not advised for a patient with esophagogastric varices that have not bled, because one cannot predict which patients will bleed, the survival is not improved, and encephalopathy may be induced in a previously asymptomatic patient.

Management of the Acutely Bleeding Varices. The treatment of acutely bleeding esophagogastric varices is somewhat dependent upon the etiology. In the case of extrahepatic portal venous obstruction, although the bleeding may be severe, it frequently stops without any specific measures. This is generally not true in patients with hepatocellular dysfunction. In these patients, rapid control of the bleeding is necessary to avoid the injurious effects of shock on hepatic function, and also to avoid the toxic effects of the absorption of blood from the GI tract. The drug most frequently used to control bleeding by reducing portal hypertension is vasopressin, which acts by constricting the splanchnic arterial circulation and consequently reducing the portal pressure by approximately 40 percent. Effective control has accompanied the intravenous infusion of 0.2 to 0.4 units/ml/min. This method is as effective as infusion into the superior mesenteric artery. Isoproterenol may be given at the same time to reduce the hemodynamic hazards of vasopressin related to its potential effect on cardiac output. Propranolol also reduces portal pressure in cirrhotic patients, and may contribute to the control of acute bleeding. There is preliminary evidence to suggest that it can reduce the rate of rebleeding in patients maintained on the drug. Drug therapy, with either drug, characteristically results in a temporary cessation of bleeding and is associated with a high incidence of rebleeding.

The same characteristics pertain to the use of balloon tamponade, generally employing a Sengstaken–Blakemore tube. After this tube is inserted into the stomach, the gastric balloon should be inflated with 200 ml of air and the lumen to this balloon clamped. The tube is then withdrawn until the gastric balloon is engaged and a minimal amount of tension is maintained by taping the tube to a helmet used for traction

(Fig. 69–5). This maneuver in itself frequently controls the bleeding. If bleeding continues, the esophageal balloon should be inflated to a pressure of 40 mm Hg, monitoring the pressure with an aneroid manometer. The stomach is irrigated and aspirated through the other lumen. If a quadruple lumen tube is used, the fourth lumen provides suction in the upper esophagus. If the four-lumen tube is not available, a small nasogastric tube should be inserted in the upper esophagus to prevent aspiration.

Balloon tamponade has reduced the mortality and morbidity from bleeding varices in good risk patients, but little change has been noted in poor-risk patients. Failure to control hemorrhage has been reported in 25 to 50 percent of patients, and it is important to release the pres-

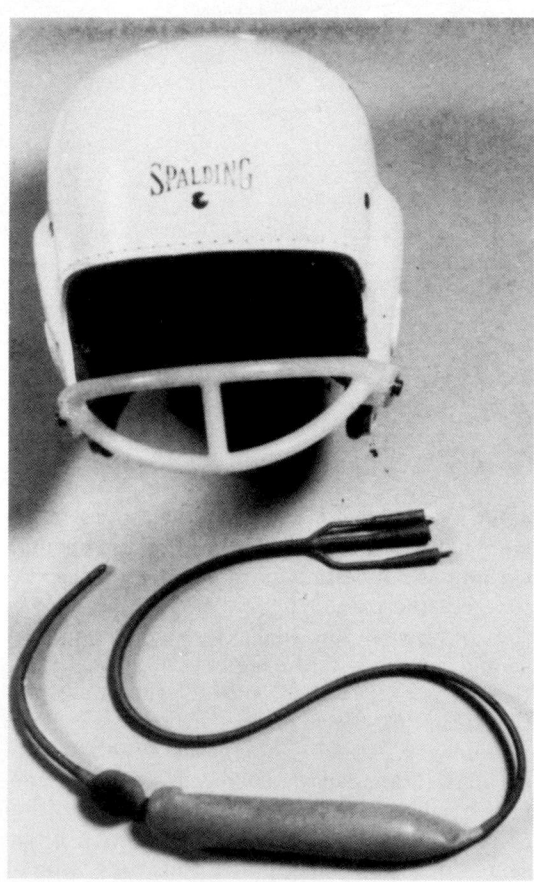

Figure 69–5. Sengstaken–Blakemore tube and helmet to permit the tube to be taped after traction is applied. (*Source: From Schwartz SI, 1964, p 301, with permission.*)

sure within the esophageal balloon every 12 hours to avoid significant esophageal erosion.

Recently there has been enthusiasm for the use of transendoscopic sclerotherapy, based on the favorable results reported by Terblanche and others. Acute bleeding episodes have been controlled and repeat injections of the sclerosing solution has avoided subsequent bleeding episodes. Cello, Crass, and Trunkey have noted that endoscopic sclerotherapy in Child's class III patients did not improve survival. Others have reported a dampening of enthusiasm for this method of primary treatment of bleeding varices.

The introduction of the end-to-end stapler has rekindled interest in direct attack on the varices, originally proposed by Boerema and Crile. In a report of 30 patients in whom esophageal transection and paraesophagogastric devascularization was performed as an emergency measure for uncontrolled variceal bleeding, immediate success was achieved in all patients, but death occurred within 1 month in 17 patients, and two later died of bleeding varices, leaving an overall survival incidence of 30 percent. Hoffmann's review of the role of stapler transection for bleeding esophageal varices led to the conclusion that it is not unequivocally better than medical treatment, endoscopic sclerotherapy, or the performance of an emergency portacaval shunt.

Orloff and associates have advised a more liberal use of emergency portacaval shunts for the cirrhotic patient whose bleeding cannot be controlled by tamponade or vasopressin. They reported an operative survival of 48 percent, and an actuarial 7-year survival of 42 percent in consecutive, unselected patients with alcoholic cirrhosis and bleeding varices operated on within 8 hours of admission. There was no correlation between survival and the patient's Child's classification, and no significance could be attributed to the presence of jaundice; ascites, when present, was associated with a marked reduction in survival rate.

In general, however, most surgeons would prefer to temporize, using conservative approaches in order to avoid operating on an acutely bleeding patient. The supportive measures that pertain to patients with massively bleeding varices include fresh blood or frozen red cells, and fresh frozen plasma to correct the coagulopathy. Therapy directed at preventing hyperammonemia and encephalopathy consists primarily of removing the blood from the GI tract, catharsis, gastric lavage, and enemas. A reduction in bacterial flora with nonabsorbable antibiotics also contributes to the prevention of coma.

Elective Management of Varices That Have Bled. There is no unanimity of opinion regarding the role of elective surgery for the prevention of recurrent variceal hemorrhage. In children with extrahepatic portal venous obstruction, although there is a voice of conservatism suggesting that patients can be treated satisfactorily and safely without operation despite repeated episodes of variceal bleeding, the results of major shunting procedures are encouraging. The central splenorenal shunt, the cavamesenteric shunt, and the selective splenorenal shunt have all been applied. The incidence of postoperative encephalopathy with any of these procedures has been negligible.

Alvarez and associates reported on 76 children with portal vein obstruction who underwent a portasystemic shunt for severe GI bleeding. Although significant regression of varices, as viewed endoscopically, was often delayed postoperatively for up to 6 months, the children with a proved, patent shunt had no further episode of GI bleeding, displayed no signs of encephalopathy, and often exhibited a significant increase in growth velocity.

The prevention of recurrent bleeding from varices in adult patients with presinusoidal intrahepatic obstruction relates to the etiologic factor. In patients with hepatic fibrosis, the results of a decompressive procedure are gratifying and provide the patient with an essentially normal life expectancy. In patients with schistosomiasis, because of their great propensity to postshunt encephalopathy, only a distal splenorenal shunt or a devascularization procedure with esophageal transection should be performed.

Patients whose bleeding varices are associated with sinusoidal portal hypertension, particularly cirrhotic patients, invariably have a complicated, impaired hepatic function. The presence of an active intrahepatic process such as hyalin necrosis, active hepatitis, or acute fatty infiltration usually precludes intervention. Ascites that fails to respond to medical therapy, a prolonged prothrombin time that does not respond to administration of vitamin K, and a bilirubin above 3 mg/dl, plus a serum albumin less than 2.5 g/dl, are all associated with poor postoperative prognosis according to Child's studies. These assessments of hepatic function are not completely predictive, however. The case for surgical intervention is based on the precept that a patient who has bled from varices is likely to rebleed, and that subsequent bleeding episodes are associated with a higher mortality than an elective operation. Recently, Zeppa and associates have shown that when both nonalcoholics and alcoholics were subjected to distal splenorenal shunts, the improved survival occurred in the nonalcoholics.

Ascites

The medical treatment of ascites consists of bedrest to reduce the functional demand on the liver, a diet high in calories with an excess of carbohydrates and protein, and a daily intake that is low in sodium (10 to 20 mEq). Fluid is usually not restricted, but potassium supplements are provided to treat the potassium depletion that accompanies the formation of ascites. A variety of diuretics, including chlorothiazide, furosemide, and aldosterone antagonists, are employed. Abdominal paracentesis should not be performed as a repeated procedure; it merely depletes the protein and contributes to the development of systemic hyponatremia. Several attempts have been made to construct a permanent peritoneovenous shunt with flow-activated valves. These were unsuccessful due to technical problems related to shunt patency. LeVeen developed a new device with a competent valve activated by pressure greater than 2 to 4 cm of water; this resulted in consistent patency. Subsequently, the Denver shunt that incorporates a pumping mechanism has been applied to clear the valve mechanism and to minimize the chance of occlusion.

The peritoneovenous shunt is indicated in patients with ascites secondary to cirrhosis, who are truly intractable to medical therapy. The presence of severe active liver disease with encephalopathy, infected ascitic fluid, or coagulation abnormalities all represent relative contraindications for peritoneal venous shunting. Severe cardiac failure, unrelated to the effects of ascites also is a contraindication due to the risk of initiating or aggravating pulmonary edema. Greig and associates used the peritoneovenous shunt to treat 23 patients with intractable ascites due to portal hypertension. Favorable results were obtained in 20 of the 23,

including 3 of 5 with acute hepatorenal failure, but 74 percent had significant complications in the first postoperative month, including technical complications, infections, and thrombocytopenia. Four patients developed spontaneous bleeding due to disseminating intravascular coagulation requiring platelet and factor replacement. One patient died of massive vericeal bleeding.

Technique (Fig. 69–6). Local anesthesia is preferred, particularly in advanced cirrhotics. A urinary catheter is placed before the operation begins. With the patient's neck slightly extended, an incision is made, usually on the right side, at the insertion of the sternocleidomastoid muscle. The space anterior to the internal jugular vein is opened, permitting lateral and medial retraction of the clavicular and sternal heads of the sternocleidomastoid muscle. The internal jugular vein is encircled and freed of surrounding tissue. The vagus nerve is protected during the dissection. The cephalad portion of the internal jugular vein is ligated with a nonabsorbable suture and the caudad portion of the vein is looped with a ligature.

The abdominal incision is then made on the same side of the body as the cervical incision to minimize the length of the subcutaneous tunnel. A transverse incision is made over the rectus muscle about five finger breadths below the costal margin and below the liver edge. The anterior sheath of the rectus is incised transversely, and the muscle is split. A purse string suture is placed in the posterior rectus sheath, and an incision is made in the center of the circle. The peritoneal tube is inserted and directed toward the pelvis. The valve is placed in the extraperitoneal pocket, and the purse string suture is tied tightly around the nipple on the extraperitoneal surface of the valve.

The proposed subcutaneous tunnel is anesthetized with local anesthesia and a tunnel is passed up to the neck just beneath the skin anterior to the pectoral fascia and the clavicle. The tubing is then passed into the neck and inserted into the interior jugular vein with a gentle curve. Approximately 9 to 11 cm are directed into the jugular vein and the suture that was previously placed to encircle the caudad portion of the jugular vein is then tied to secure this tube in place. An x-ray is taken to confirm the position of the proper placement of the tube.

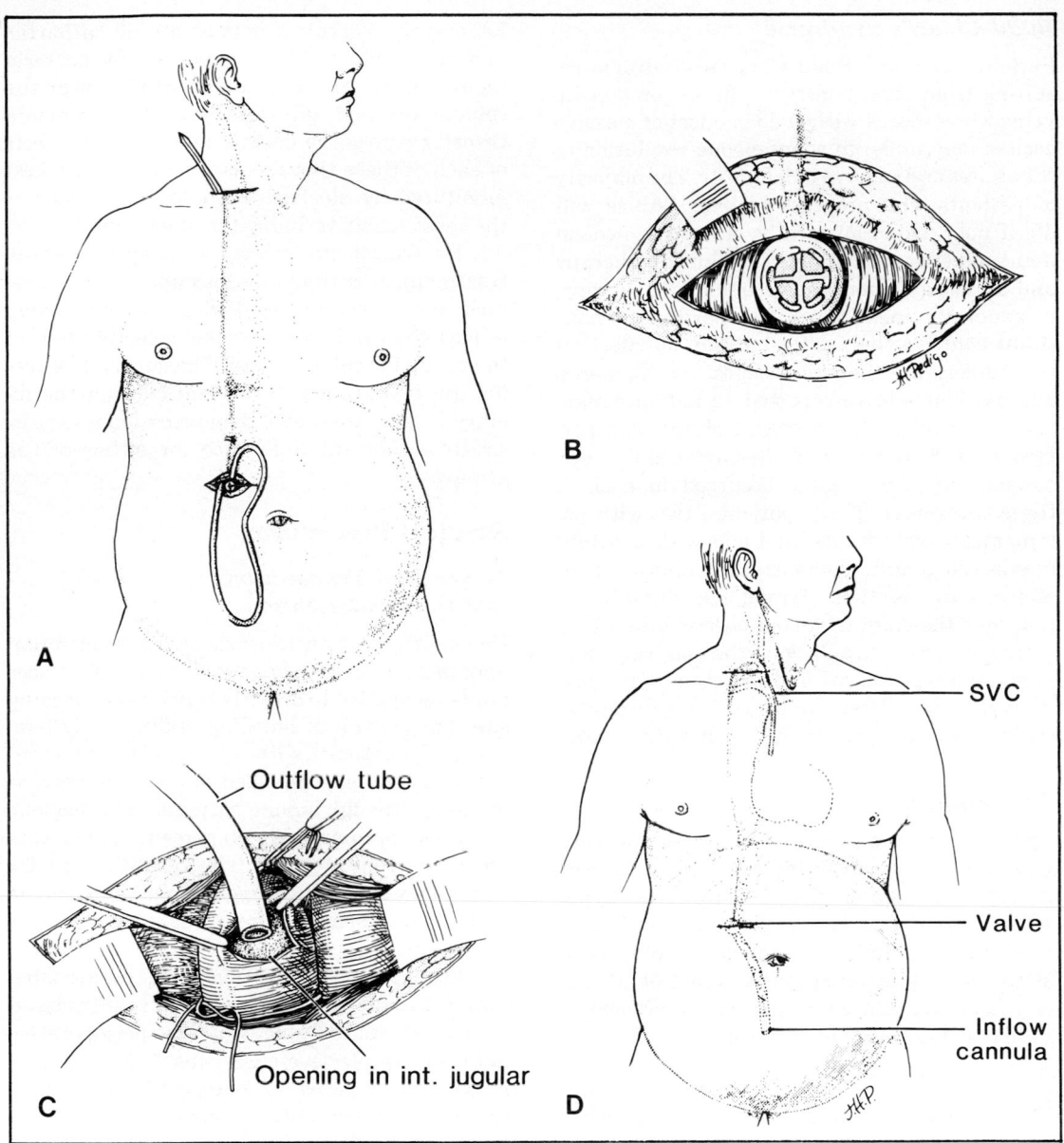

Figure 69–6. Insertion of peritoneovenous shunt. **A.** Position of catheter insertion into peritoneal cavity and cervical incision and tunnel. **B.** One-way valve is positioned superficial to posterior rectus sheath. **C.** Insertion of outflow tube into interior jugular vein. **D.** Position of venous and peritoneal cannulae. (*Source: From Greenlee HB, Stanley MM, 1982, with permission.*)

The wounds are then closed without drainage.

Postoperatively 20 mg of furosemide is given intravenously and for the next 2 or 3 days 60 mg of furosemide, four to six times per day, is administered intravenously to effect a marked diuresis. The application of an elastic binder to increase abdominal pressure is postponed for about 5 or 6 days. Sodium restriction and diuretic therapy is continued in accordance with the patient's monitored weight loss.

Budd–Chiari's Syndrome

Patients with the Budd–Chiari's syndrome resulting from occlusion from the major hepatic veins who present with sudden onset of massive ascites may undergo spontaneous resolution of the ascites and survive indefinitely. The majority of patients who progress to liver failure will die if not treated surgically, since the medical management, consisting of a diuretic therapy and anticoagulation and thrombolytic therapy, is generally ineffective. The peritoneovenous shunt controls the ascites but has no effect on the underlying hepatic congestion. Cameron and associates have reported 12 patients managed surgically: A mesocaval shunt was performed in 5 and in 7 a mesoatrial shunt was carried out. Two deaths occurred in each of these categories. Three patients, two with patent mesocaval shunts, and one with a patent mesoatrial shunt, demonstrated improvement of liver architecture. Sennig has directly approached the point of venous obstruction. Using extracorporeal circulation the suprahepatic caval vein was incised and resection of the juxtacaval hepatic tissue that had been thrombotically involved resulted in free hepatic venous flow.

Hypersplenism

Splenectomy or decompression of the portal venous system is rarely indicated for treatment of hypersplenism associated with portal hypertension. Each of the major portal decompressive procedures, including the selective splenorenal shunt, is accompanied by reduction of the size of the spleen and correction of hypersplenism in about two thirds of the cases.

Encephalopathy

The treatment of encephalopathy is supportive, and directed at reducing nitrogenous material within the intestinal tract, reducing the production of ammonia from this nitrogenous material, and increasing ammonia metabolism. Protein is reduced to 400 g daily or less and glucose is added to the diet since it inhibits ammonia production by bacteria. Prompt control of GI bleeding is indicated to reduce the addition of an ammonia load from the blood. The protein substrate on which bacteria acts within the gut may be reduced by cathartics and enemas to purge the intestinal tract. Bacteria within the bowel are reduced in numbers by administering nonabsorbable antibiotics such as neomycin or kanomycin. Lactulose acts as a mild cathartic, and the products of its oxidation by bacteria include lactic and acetic acid which lower the colonic pH and interfere with the ammonia transfer across the colonic mucosa. The effects of each of these therapeutic modalities are best monitored by electroencephalogram, which is the most sensitive indicator of changes.

Partial colectomy has been suggested as the treatment of intractable encephalopathy. Resnick and associates studied a matched group of patients randomly selected, selecting half of the group for colon bypass. The survival figures for the two groups were identical and the dietary protein tolerance demonstrated no statistically significant difference for either of the groups.

Surgical Procedures

Esophageal Transection and Devascularization

Using either a transthoracic or transabdominal approach, transesophageal ligation of varices has been applied to directly control the bleeding site. The control of bleeding is frequently temporary. In patients without cirrhosis, recurrent bleeding has been reported in about 28 percent of cases, although among patients with alcoholic cirrhosis approximately 50 percent of survivors have recurrent bleeding. The mortality rate for emergency procedures performed in patients with acutely bleeding varices is approximately 50 percent.

Esophageal transection with paraesophageal devascularization was initially introduced by Sugiura and Futagawa. The perioperative mortality in elective cases was 2 percent and, in emergency cases, 12 percent. Hepatic function was not disturbed; postoperative encephalopathy did not occur. In a recent report, radiographic and endoscopic examination of 101 patients subjected to transabdominal esophageal transection and devascularization demonstrated improvement in essentially all patients who survived the procedure. Posttransection bleeding was observed in 14 of 89 survivors followed from 1 to 13 years.

A variety of modifications has occurred over the years. Transection of the esophagus is now generally accomplished by the EEA stapler, using the largest size cartridge possible. The procedure usually incorporates a highly selective vagotomy rather than the originally proposed selective vagotomy, because this obviates the need for pyloroplasty. Because of a significant incidence of esophageal reflex, a Nissen fundoplication has been added as part of the protocol by many.

Technique. Esophageal transection is generally performed transabdominally through an upper midline incision, exposing the esophagogastric junction. The lower 3 to 5 cm of the esophagus is mobilized, and care is taken to avoid the vagus nerves. The paraesophageal veins are ligated. A high vertical incision is made in the anterior wall of the stomach and the EEA stapler is inserted. The esophagus is tied over the center rod, 2 cm above the gastric junction. The instrument is fired, resulting in simultaneous transection and reanastomosis of the esophagus (Fig. 69–7). The original Sugiura procedure (Fig. 69–8) is performed through two incisions; one is an upper abdominal incision through which a splenectomy, paraesophageal

and gastric devascularization, and pyloroplasty and selective vagotomy are performed. The other incision, a left lateral thoracotomy, is then performed to devascularize the esophagus up to the arch of the aorta, dividing all connections between the azygous and hemiazygous system and the esophagus. The esophagus is then transected, the varices ligated, and the esophagus reanastomosed.

The procedure is now more commonly performed either through an abdominal approach or a thoracoabdominal incision (Figs. 69–9 and 69–10). The spleen is removed and devascularization begins with the lesser curvature, ligating the left gastric artery and vein. The abdominal esophagus and cardia are devascularized from the lesser curvature and the posterior part of the stomach up to the esophagus, and then the greater curvature is devascularized and the spleen is removed. The main vagus trunks are preserved and a highly selective vagotomy is carried out at the time of dissection of the lesser

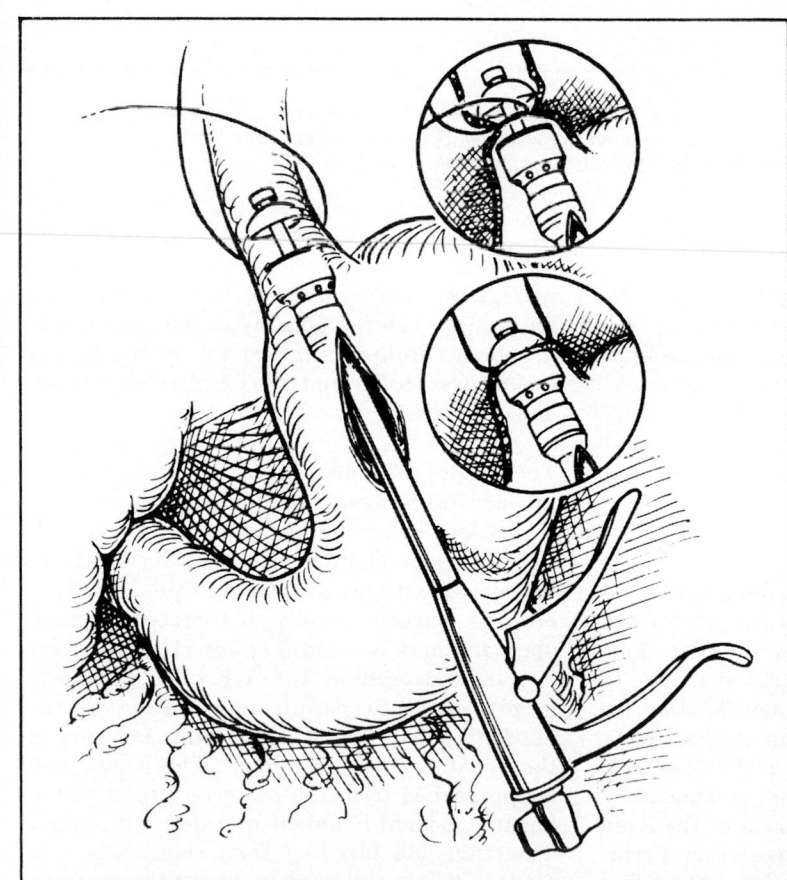

Figure 69–7. The EEA stapler is introduced and the esophagus securely tied over the center rod 2 cm above the gastric junction. The instrument gap is closed and the trigger fired, completing the simultaneous transection and reanastomosis. (*Source: From Schwartz SI: Liver, in Schwartz SI, Shires GT, et al (eds): Principles of Surgery, 4 edt. New York: McGraw-Hill, 1984, p 1290, with permission.*)

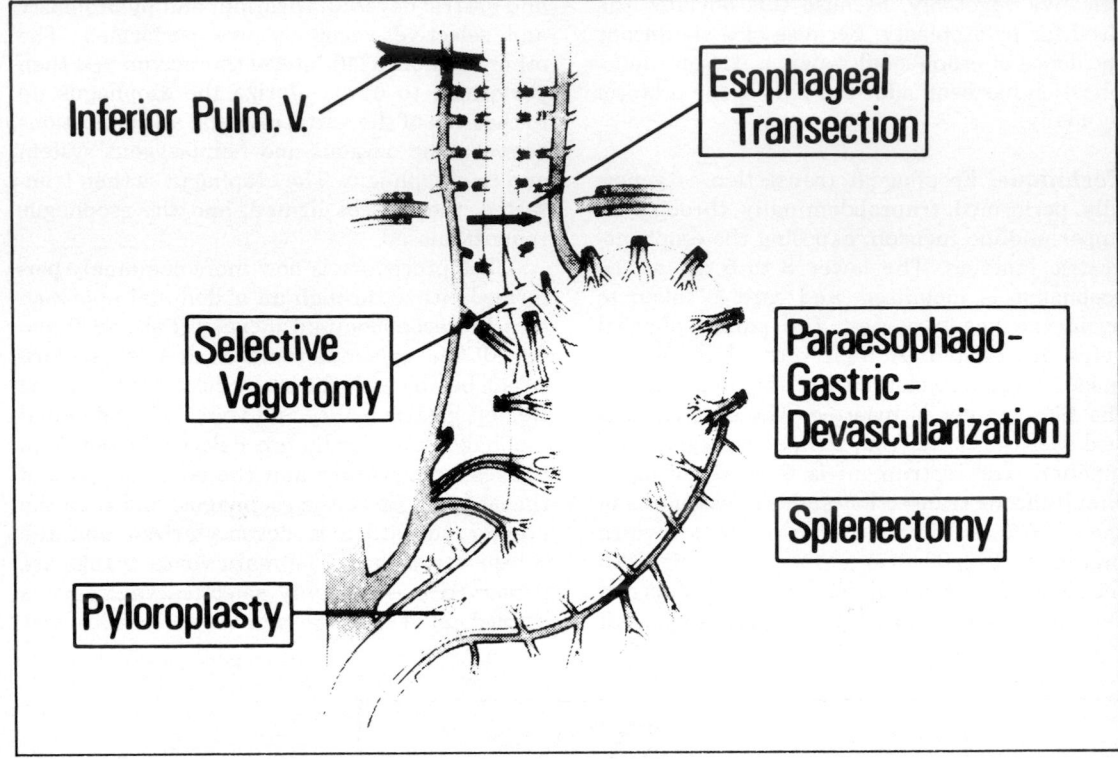

Figure 69–8. Esophageal transection with paraesophagogastric devascularization (Sugiura procedure). (*Source: From Schwartz SI: Liver, in Schwartz SI, Shires GT, et al (eds): Principles of Surgery, 4 edt. New York: McGraw-Hill, 1984, p 1290, with permission.*)

curvature of the stomach. Multiple veins directly entering the esophagus and draining into the azygous and hemiazygous system are individually ligated and the esophagus is transected with the EEA stapler. The operation is completed by a loose Nissen fundoplication around the lower end of the esophagus covering the esophageal anastomosis.

Portacaval Shunt

The major indication for establishing a portacaval shunt is esophageal varices that are rather actively bleeding or have bled in the past. Both end-to-side and side-to-side portacaval shunts have been applied to this situation. Another indication for a portacaval shunt is the Budd–Chiari's syndrome with rapidly evolving ascites, in which case a side-to-side shunt is mandatory in order to provide decompression of the liver in addition to the splanchnic circulation. Portacaval anastomosis has been carried out in a few

patients without portal hypertension as therapy for familial heterozygous hypercholesterolemia in whom cardiovascular complications pose a major threat to life and also for glycogen storage abnormalities.

Technique (Fig. 69–11). A long, right, subcostal incision is most commonly employed with the patient either in the supine position or with the right side slightly elevated (Fig. 69–11A). In unusual patients with markedly enlarged livers and extreme obesity, a thoracoabdominal approach may be used (Fig. 69–11B). The liver is retracted craniad and a Kocher maneuver is performed to permit mobilization of the duodenum (Fig. 69–11C). Dissection is begun in the hepatoduodenal ligament. The portal vein is approached from the posterior aspect of the hepatoduodenal ligament in order to minimize dissection and bleeding from collaterals, and also to obviate the need to dissect the common

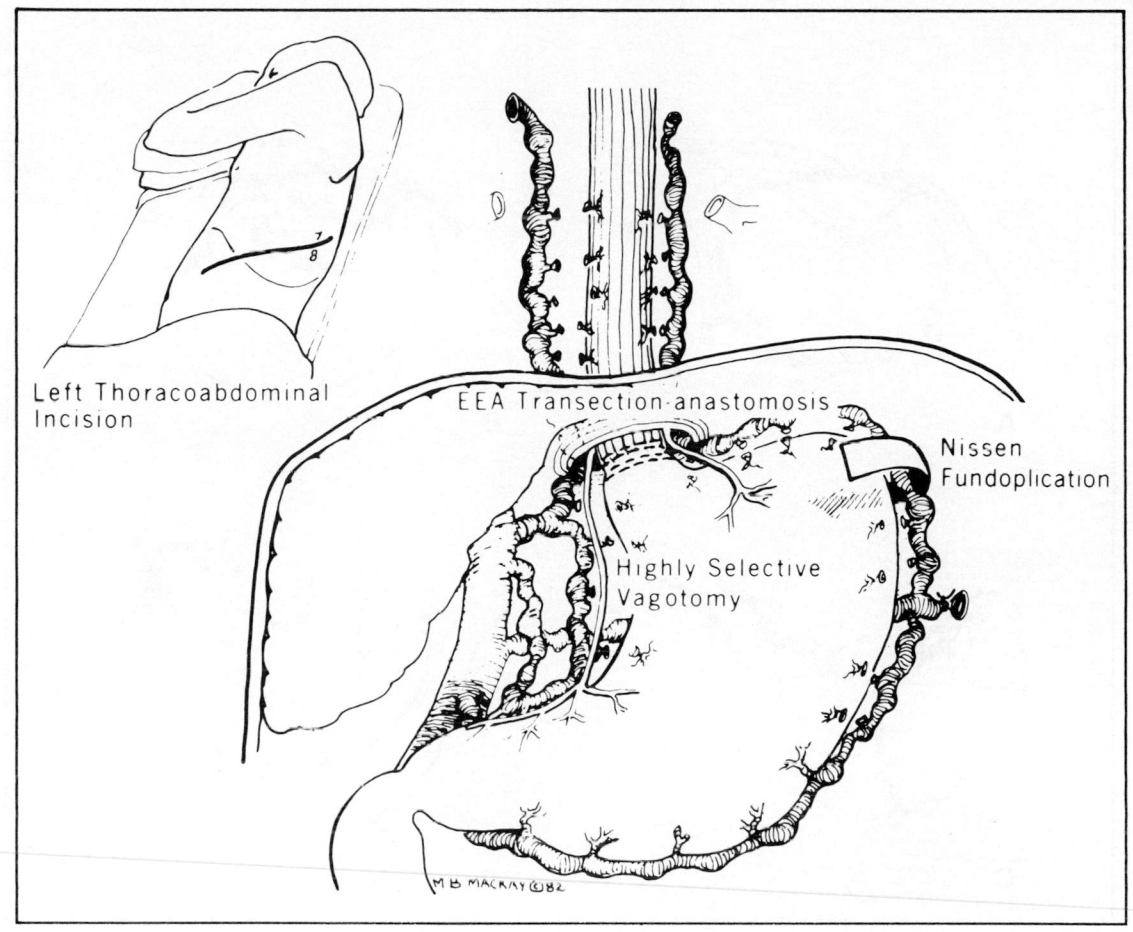

Left Thoracoabdominal
Incision

EEA Transection-anastomosis

Nissen
Fundoplication

Highly Selective
Vagotomy

M B MACKAY©82

Figure 69–9. Thoracoabdominal approach, highly selective vagotomy with no gastric drainage, transection and anastomosis with the EEA stapler, and Nissen fundoplication. (*From Ginsberg RJ, Waters PF, et al, 1982, p 259, with permission.*)

bile duct (Fig. 69–11D). Usually no branches are encountered during this dissection, but at times there are several small branches including the cystic vein and small pyloric veins located on the medial aspect. An umbilical tape can be passed around the portal vein, and the tissue in the hepatoduodenal ligament posterior to the portal vein should be removed to avoid angulation of the vein when it is anastomosed to the inferior vena cava.

Attention is then directed to the inferior vena cava. The retroperitoneum is incised and the anterior and medial and lateral aspect of the inferior vena cava are dissected free from surrounding tissue. The length of cava exposed usually extends from the right renal vein to

the point where the vessel passes retrohepatically. Vascular clamps are applied to the portal vein proximally where it is in juxtaposition to the pancreas and distally where it bifurcates (Fig. 69–11E). The portal vein is transected (Fig. 69–11F) as far distally as possible and the hepatic stump is oversewn with continuous 5-0 vascular suture. Two stay sutures are placed in the proximal transected end of the vein in order to assure proper orientation. A partially occlusive Satinsky clamp is applied to the anterior aspect of the inferior vena cava, which is incised between the jaws of the clamp. A small ellipse may be excised from the inferior vena cava, but this is not necessary if the caval incision is at least one and one half times the diame-

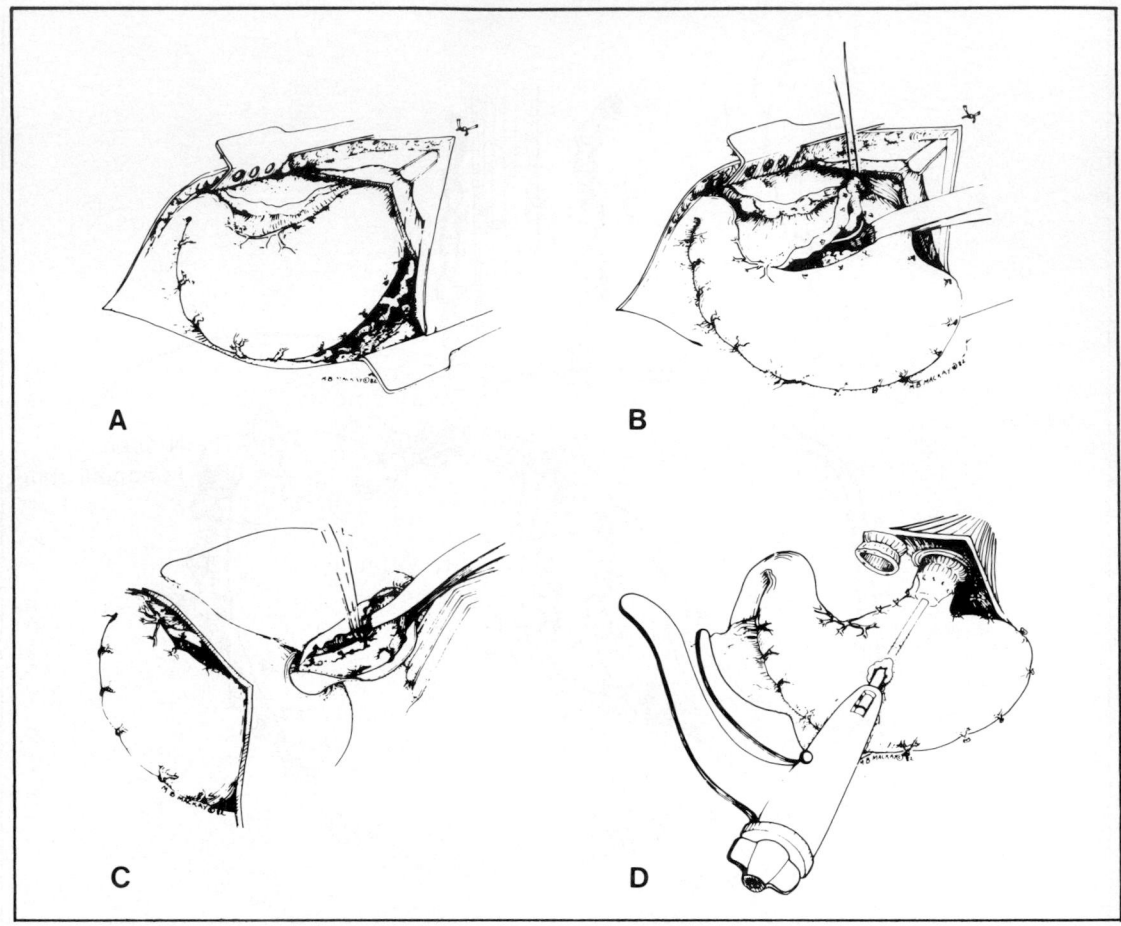

A

B

C

D

Figure 69–10. A. Splenectomy and gastric devascularization. **B.** Lower esophageal devascularization and highly selective vagotomy. **C.** The esophageal devascularization extends up to the inferior pulmonary vein and preserves all longitudinal veins. **D.** Transection and anastomosis with the EEA stapler. (*From Ginsberg RJ, Waters PF, et al, 1982, pp 260–261, with permission.*)

ter of the transected portal vein. A continuous vascular suture of 5-0 Prolene (Fig. 69–11G) is used to suture the posterior aspect of the portal vein to the medial aspect of the inferior vena cava. It is appropriate to place several of these sutures prior to approximating the portal vein to the medial aspect of the inferior vena cava and then sliding the two structures together as tension is applied to the suture (Fig. 69–11H). The anterior row of the anastomosis is performed with either interrupted horizontal mattress sutures (Fig. 69–11I) or with a continuous suture that begins at the upper pole and continues to the lower pole of the caval stoma.

After completing the anastomosis (Fig. 69–11J), the clamp is removed from the inferior

vena cava and distention is demonstrated. This is followed by removal of the clamp from the portal vein. A thrill should be palpable in the inferior vena cava. Pressure is then directly recorded from the portal vein to define the efficacy of the shunt. There should be minimal gradient between the portal venous and the inferior venacaval pressure.

The side-to-side portacaval shunt is performed following a similar dissection. Bulldog clamps are applied (Fig. 69–11K) to occlude the portal vein proximally and distally. A longitudinal incision is made both in the portal vein and in the inferior vena cava. This should be one and one half times the width of the portal vein. A side-to-side anastomosis is effected with Prolene sutures, using a continuous technique interrupted at the upper and lower poles (Fig. 69–11K).

Mesocaval Shunt

The original mesocaval shunt was applied in children with cavernomatous transformation of the portal vein and employed only native tissue, anastomosing the end of the inferior vena cava to the side of the superior mesenteric vein. This was modified for adults with cirrhosis by interposing a prosthetic conduit between the superior mesenteric vein and the inferior vena cava in order to minimize dissection and intraoperative blood loss.

Technique: End-to-Side Cavamesenteric Shunt (Fig. 69–12). The peritoneal cavity is entered through a midline or a right paramedian incision, extending from the xiphoid to well below the umbilicus. Upper traction on the trans-

verse colon exposes the superior mesenteric vessels (Fig. 69–12A). The superior mesenteric vein is identified and dissected free. The lateral reflection of the ascending colon is then incised along its entire length to permit medial displacement of the transverse and ascending colon, and medial reflection of the ascending mesocolon. This exposes the inferior vena cava and the third portion of the duodenum. The inferior vena cava is mobilized from its origin up to the entrance of the right renal vein (Fig. 69–12B). The paired lumbar veins are ligated and transected. Vascular clamps are then applied immediately below the renal veins and at the confluence of the iliac veins. The inferior vena cava is transected as far distad as possible, and the caudal stump is ligated (Fig. 69–12C). The right iliac vein may be left attached to the vena cava to achieve greater length. A window is created in the mesentery of the small intestine between the iliocolic and the origin of the main ileal

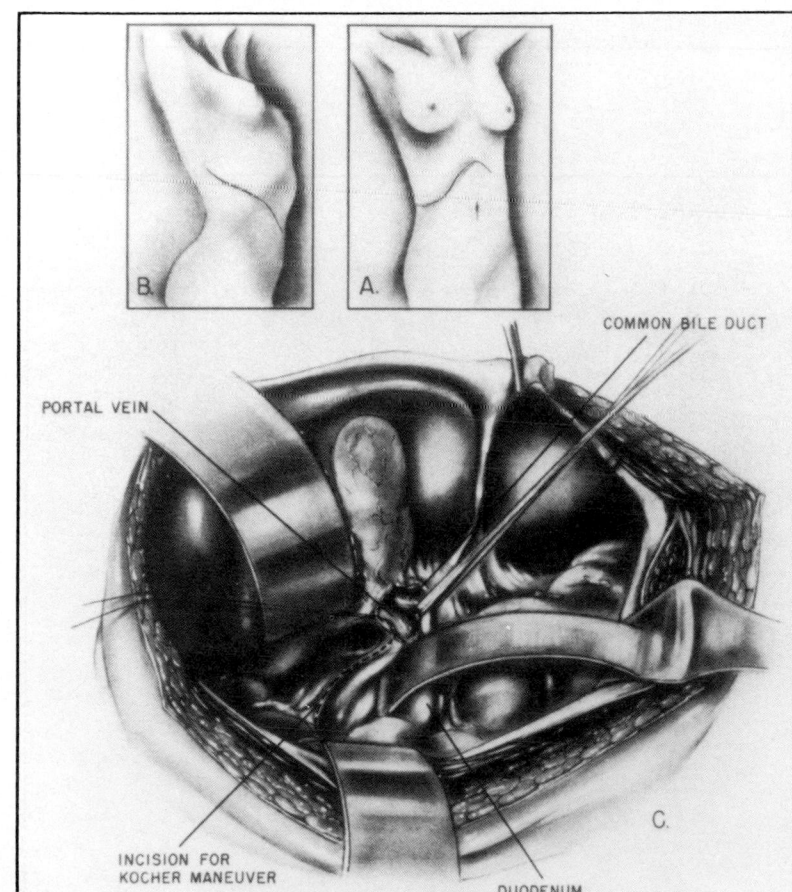

Figure 69–11. 1 and **2.** Two kinds of portacaval shunt. **1.** End-to-side portacaval shunt. **A.** Subcostal transabdominal incision. **B.** Thoracoabdominal incision over ninth intercostal space. **C.** Line of incision for Kocher maneuver. Initial dissection of hepatoduodenal ligament, with isolation and retraction of the common bile duct and exposure of the portal vein.

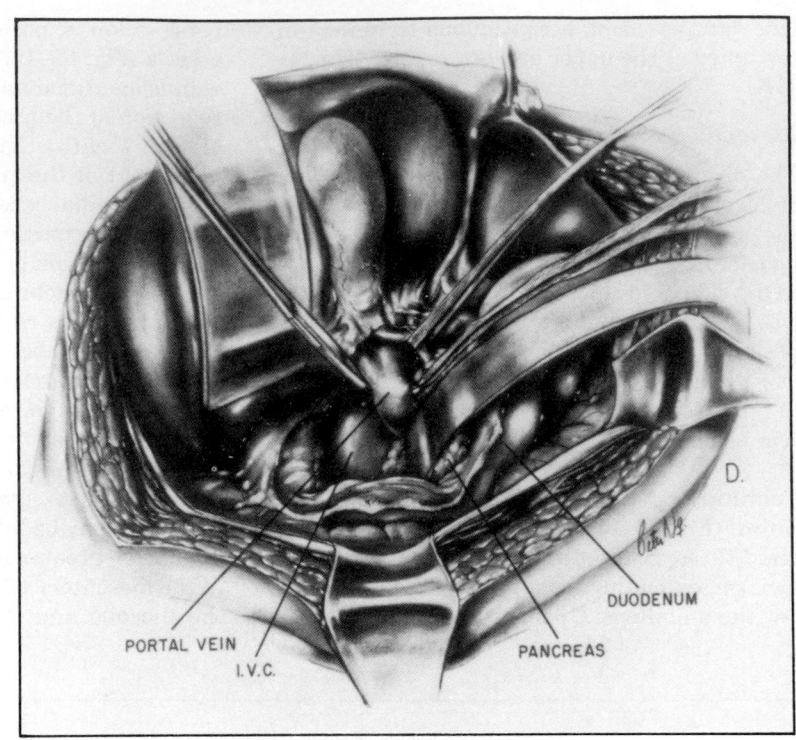

Figure 69–11. 1. *Continued* **D.** Completion of dissection of portal vein, with demonstration of bifurcation in porta hepatis. Dissection of retroperitoneum to clear inferior vena cava.

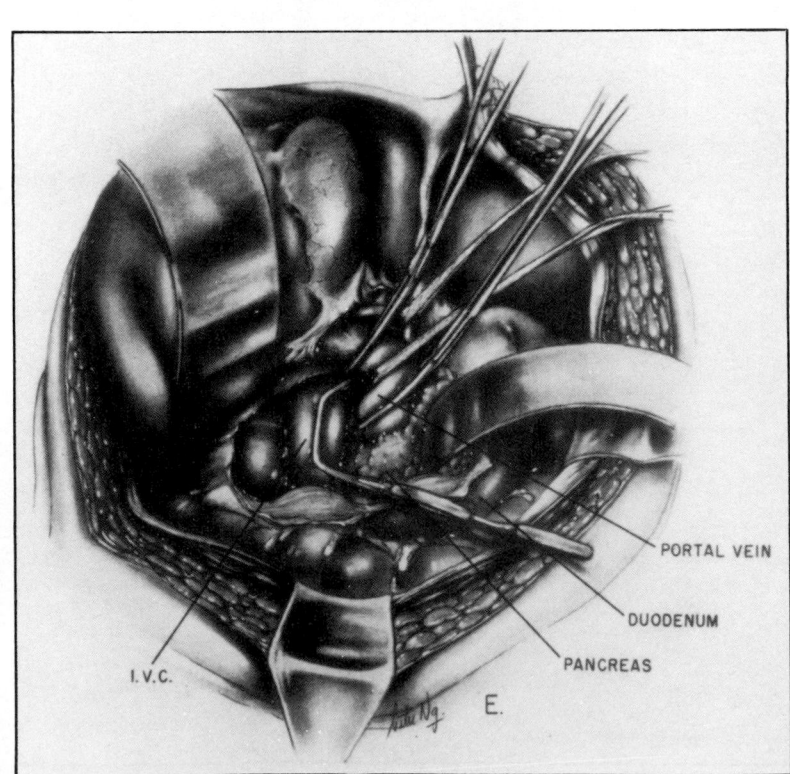

Figure 69–11. 1. *Continued* **E.** Technique for end-to-side anastomosis. Note partially occluding clamp on the anteromedial aspect of the inferior vena cava. Atraumatic clamps are applied to the proximal and distal portions of the portal vein.

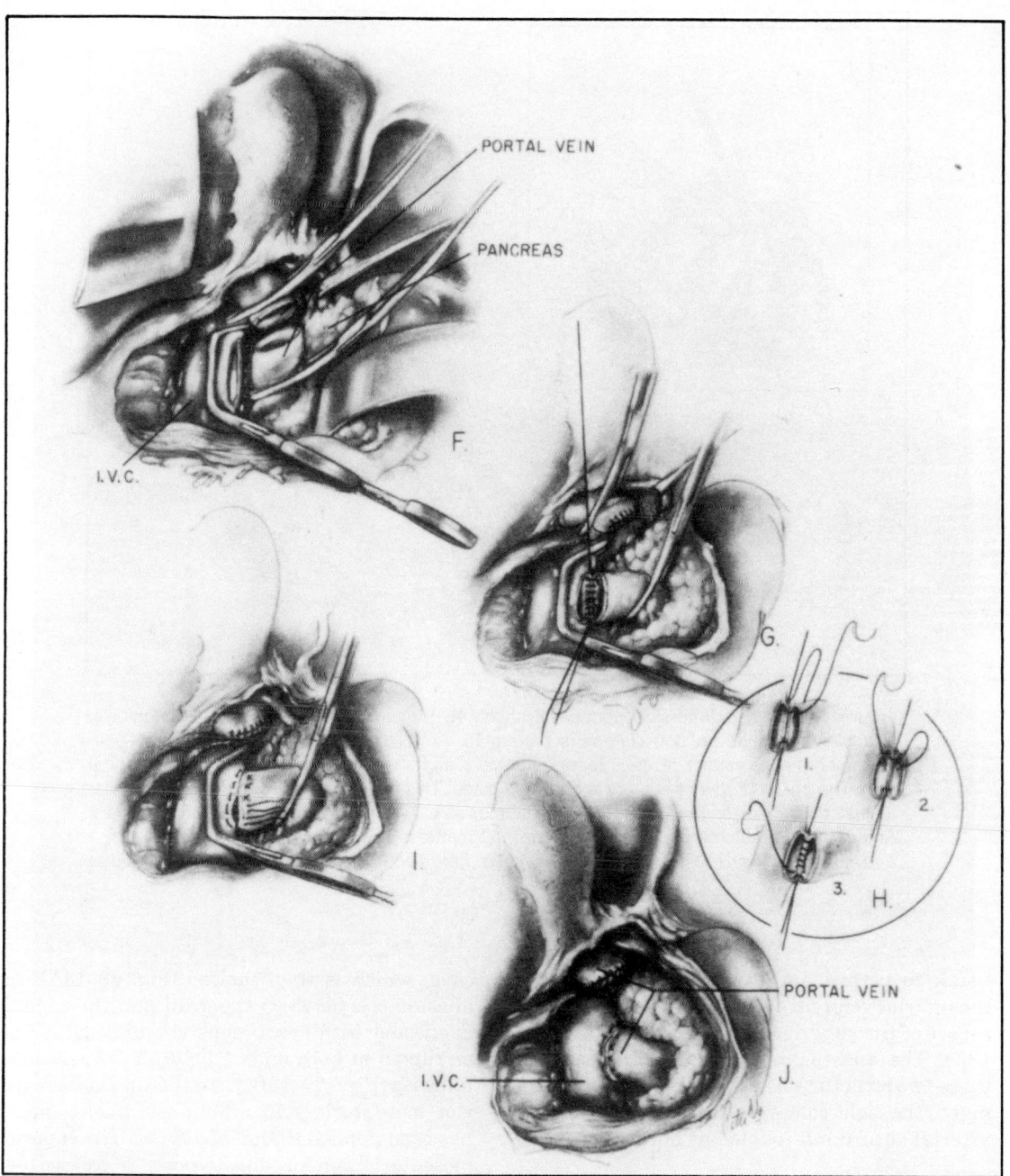

Figure 69–11. 1. *Continued* **F.** An ellipse has been removed from the inferior vena cava. This should measure one and one half times the diameter of the portal vein. The portal vein has been transected. **G.** The distal end of the portal vein has been oversewn with continuous silk sutures. (This may be handled by ligature and transfixion ligature.) The portal vein has been approximated to the stoma of the inferior vena cava. Two stay sutures are initially tied, and the posterior layer is in place. **H.** Placement of the posterior layer of sutures is facilitated by passing the cranial suture into the lumen of the portal vein and continuing this suture to the caudal limb of the portal vein where it is then passed to the outside and tied. **I.** Closure of the anterior row is accomplished with interrupted horizontal mattress sutures. (A continuous suture may also be used.) **J.** Completed anastomosis.

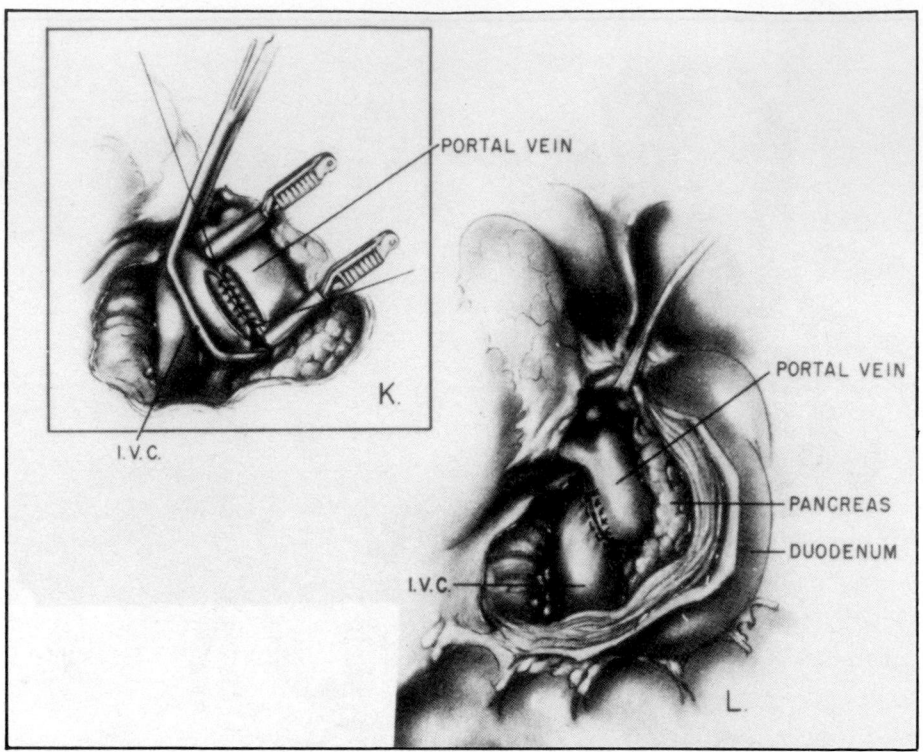

Figure 69–11. 2. Side-to-side portacaval shunt: **K.** Beginning of side-to-side anastomosis. Use of rubber-shod bulldog clamps is preferable. An ellipse has been removed from both the anteromedial aspect of the inferior vena cava and the anterolateral aspect of the portal vein. The posterior row of sutures is shown in place. This is accomplished in a manner similar to that described for the end-to-side anastomosis. **L.** Completed side-to-side anastomosis. Anterior row of sutures is placed in a horizontal mattress fashion. (*Source: Figures 69–11, 1 and 2, from Schwartz SI: Portacaval anastomosis. Mod Tech Surg 12:1, 1982, with permission.*)

trunk to permit approximation of the end of the inferior vena cava to the right posterolateral aspect of the superior mesenteric vein (Fig. 69–12D). The anastomosis (Fig. 69–12E) between these two structures is usually performed proximal to the right colic vein utilizing a continuous arterial suture interrupted at both ends.

Technique: Mesocaval Interposition Graft (Fig. 69–13). A woven Dacron or Goretex graft is interposed between the inferior vena cava and the superior mesenteric vein. The dissection of the superior mesenteric vein is similar to that described above. The anterior, medial, and lateral surfaces of the inferior vena cava are then dissected as in the case of an intended portacaval anastomosis. A Satinsky clamp is applied to the anterior surface of the inferior vena

cava, which is then incised (Fig. 69–13A). An anastomosis between the graft and the conduit is effected with continuous vascular suture interrupted at both ends. The graft is then anastomosed (Figs. 69–13B, C) to the side of the superior mesenteric vein after an occlusive clamp has been applied to that structure. The superior mesenteric venous anastomosis is carried out with a continuous suture from within after two stay sutures have been secured (Fig. 69–13D). The anterior row of sutures is performed from without (Fig. 69–13E). The completed anastomosis usually requires a conduit of 4 to 6 cm in length, 10 to 20 mm in diameter (Fig. 69–13F).

Central Splenorenal Shunt (Fig. 69–14)

This procedure is usually performed electively for patients with varices that have previously

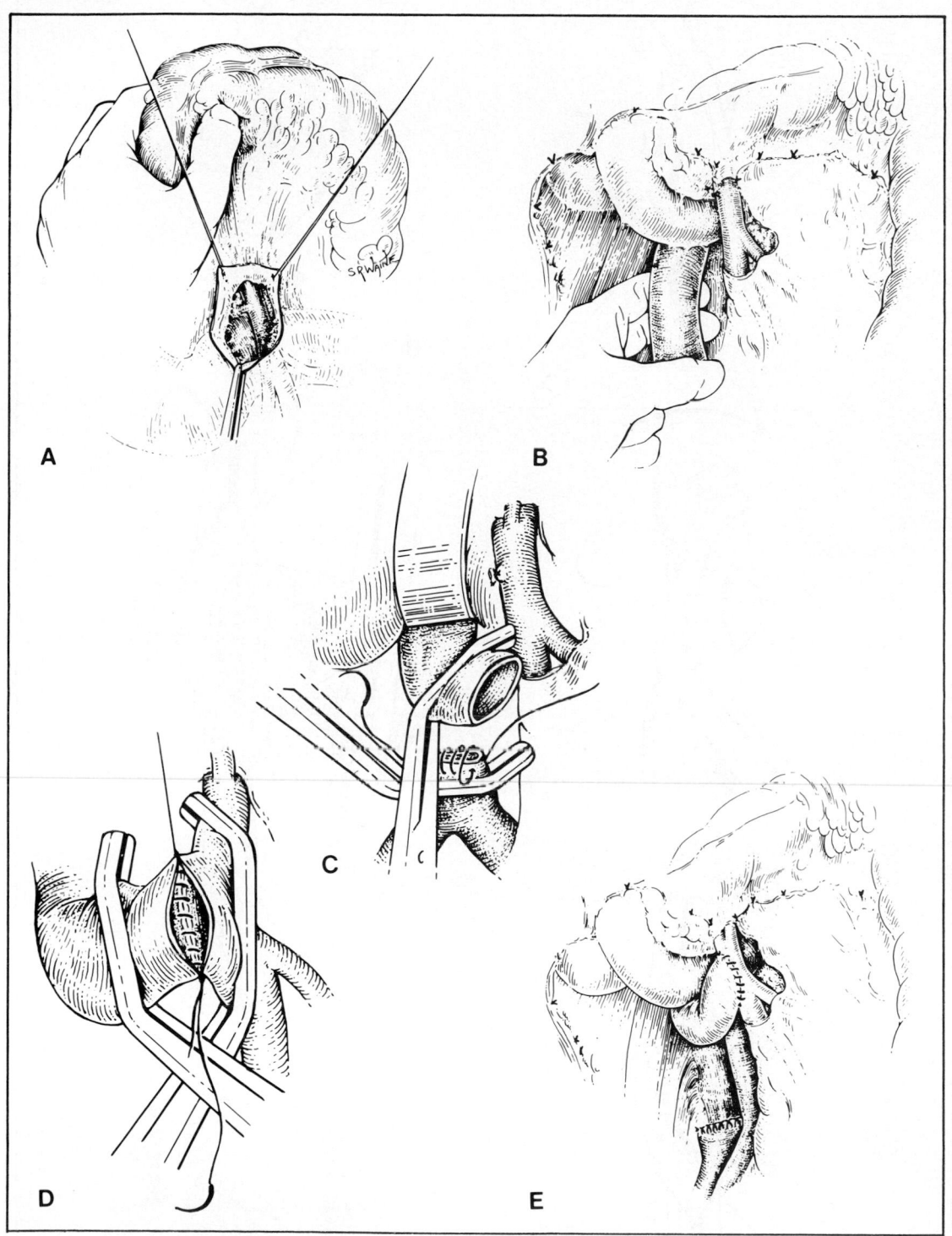

Figure 69–12. A through **E.** End-to-side cavamesenteric shunt. **A.** Exposure of superior mesenteric vein. **B.** Mobilization of inferior vena cava. **C.** Distal end of cava oversewn. **D.** Posterior row of cavamesenteric anastomosis. **E.** Completed anastomosis. (*Source: From Gliedman ML, 1982, with permission.*)

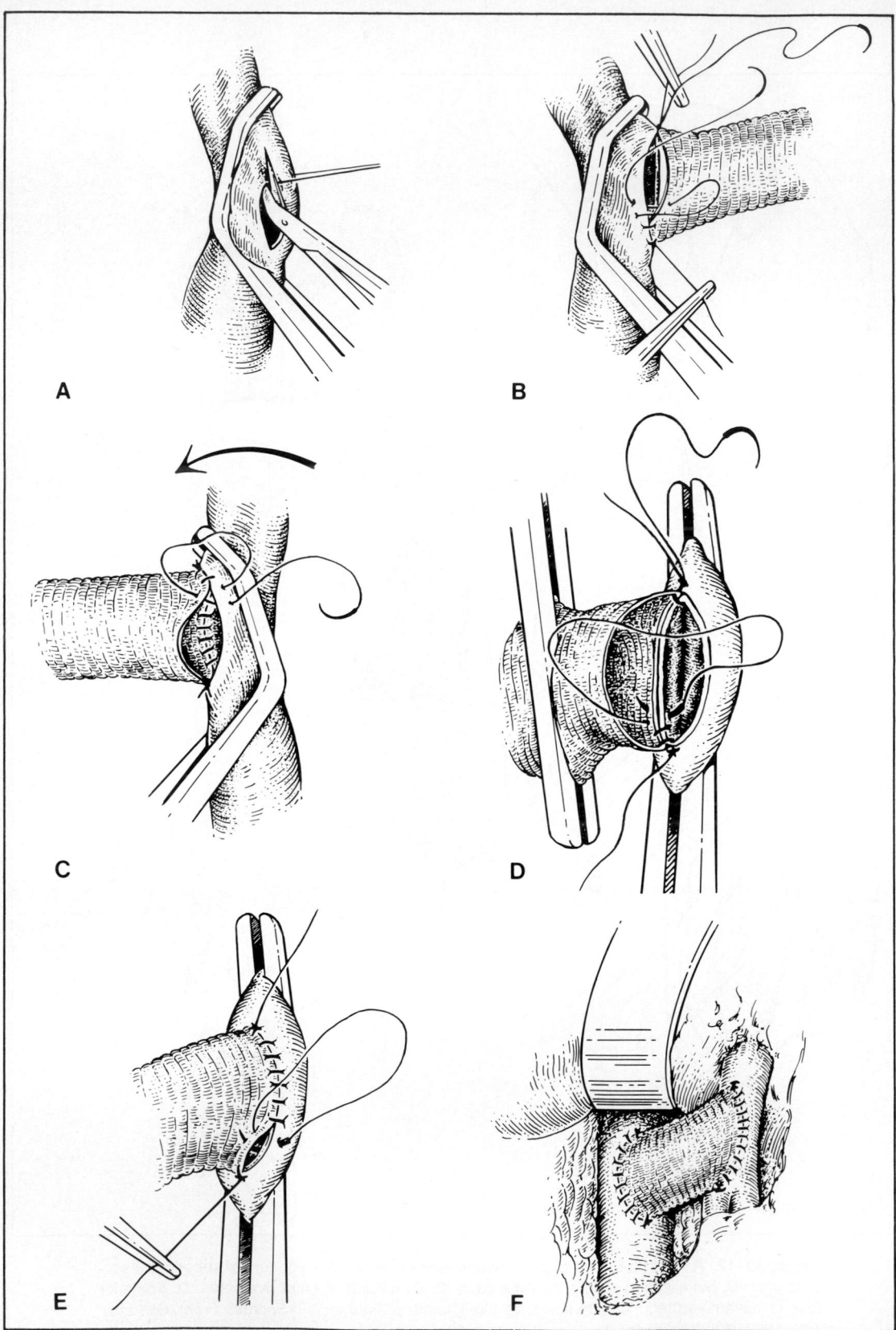

A

B

C

D

E

F

bled. The advocates of the procedure suggest that it may allow blood to course to the liver, providing the liver with positive trophic effects. Others feel that it, like the mesocaval shunt, does not provide the liver with splanchnic flow because blood will preferentially course from the high-pressure portal system directly to the low-pressure systemic venous system, in this case via the renal vein.

Technique. An oblique subcostal incision or a thoracoabdominal approach may be used. The transverse colon and splenic flexure are mobilized and retracted caudad and the short gastric vessels are doubly ligated and transected (Fig. 69–14A). The splenophrenic and splenorenal ligaments are transected and an ultimate pedicle is established in the hilus of the spleen. The splenic artery is ligated (Fig. 69–14B) and the splenic vein is dissected free as it courses along the pancreas (Fig. 69–14C). It is frequently preferable to remove a large spleen prior to carrying out the dissection of the splenic vein, in order to clear the operative field. The retroperitoneum is then incised and the renal vein is identified (Fig. 69–14D). Ligation of the adrenal vein facilitates dissection of the renal vein and permits better mobilization of that vein. The splenic vein is dissected toward its junction with the superior mesenteric vein until adequate length is achieved. During the course of mobilizing the splenic vein multiple small branches draining the pancreas must be ligated. A vascular clamp is then applied to the splenic vein centrally, and a Satinsky clamp is applied to partially occlude the renal vein. Alternatively, tapes may be used to isolate a segment of renal vein (Fig. 69–14E). An ellipse is removed from the top of the renal vein and an end-to-side anastomosis is effected between the splenic vein and the renal vein, using 5-0 Prolene interrupted at either end. Anteriorly the sutures may be placed in an interrupted fashion to avoid compromise of the lumen (Fig. 69–14F).

Selective (Distal) Splenorenal Shunt (Fig. 69–15)

This procedure is carried out specifically to decompress esophagogastric varices for control of hemorrhage while maintaining a high pressure in the splanchnic venous system and preserving flow to the liver. It is well established that it does accomplish this effect, but in some patients, over the course of time, a reduction in adhepatic flow has occurred. The operation is associated with a reduced incidence of postoperative encephalopathy compared with other shunting procedures. It has also been associated with an increased incidence or augmentation of ascites.

Technique. The procedure is carried out through a left upper quadrant oblique chevron incision, beginning in the left anterior axillary line and crossing to the lateral border of the right rectus abdominal muscle (Fig. 69–15A). The round ligament is traced to the liver, and the umbilical vein is ligated at this point. The lesser sac is entered by dividing the gastrocolic ligament from the lowest short gastric vein on the greater curvature of the pylorus (Fig. 69–15B). It is preferable to divide the vessels inside the gastroepiploic arcade to reduce collateralization.

Attention is now directed to mobilizing the splenic vein. The peritoneum overlying the groove between the duodenum and the inferior border of the pancreas is incised and the lower border of the pancreas is mobilized along its entire length (Fig. 69–15C). The gland can then be reflected cephalad and dissection is begun on the splenic vein. The adventitia along the splenic vein is incised and the branches coursing from the pancreas to the splenic vein are ligated and divided (Fig. 69–15D). The inferior mesenteric vein enters the splenic vein and is doubly ligated and transected. A significant length of splenic vein is dissected free from surrounding tissue, up to its point of junction with the superior mesenteric vein to form the portal vein.

Figure 69–13. A through **F.** Mesocaval interposition graft. **A.** Incision into partially occluded inferior vena cava. **B.** Anastomosis between graft and inferior vena cava. **C.** Clamp rotated in order to facilitate anastomosis between clamp and inferior vena cava. **D.** Posterior row of anastomosis between graft and mesenteric vein. **E.** Anterior row of anastomosis between graft and mesenteric vein. **F.** Complete shunt. (*Source: From Gliedman ML, 1982, with permission.*)

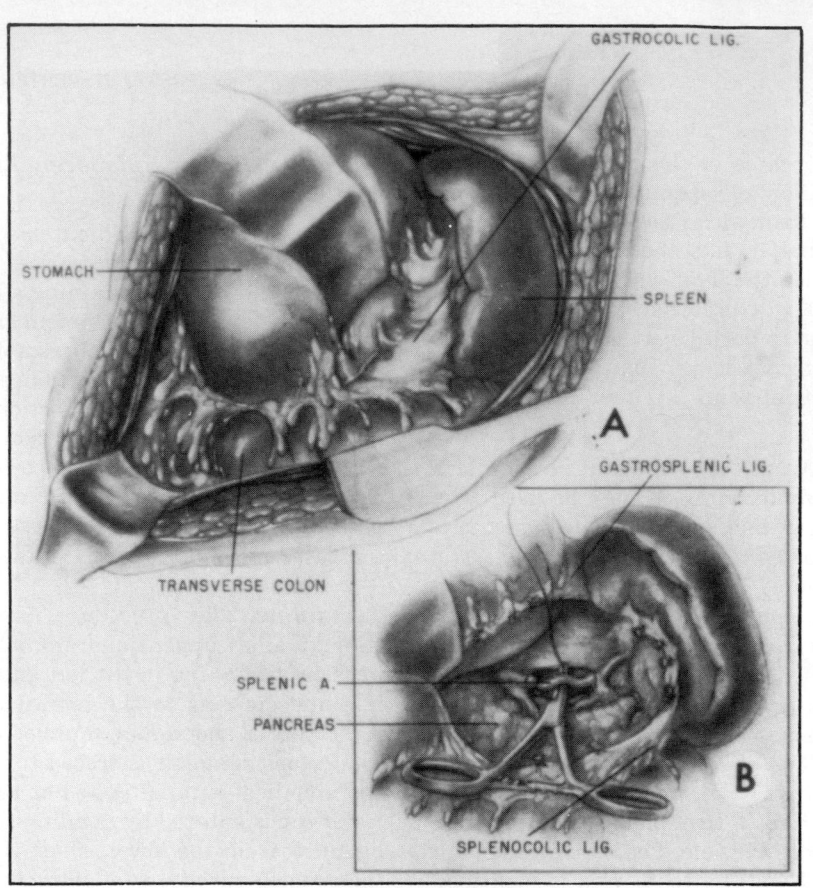

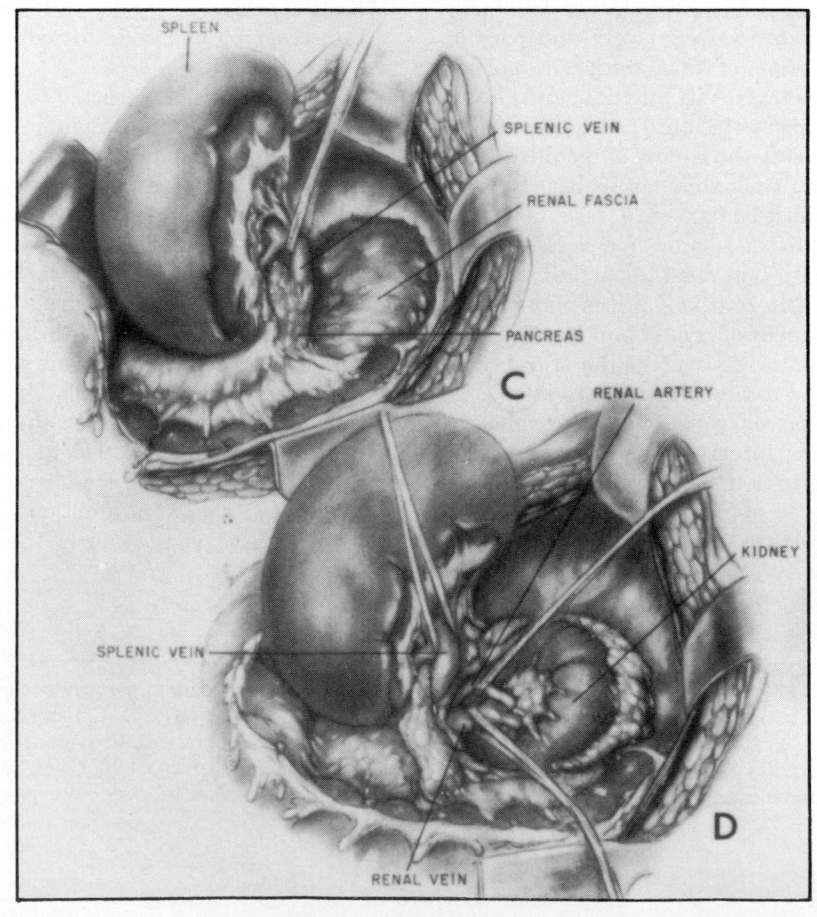

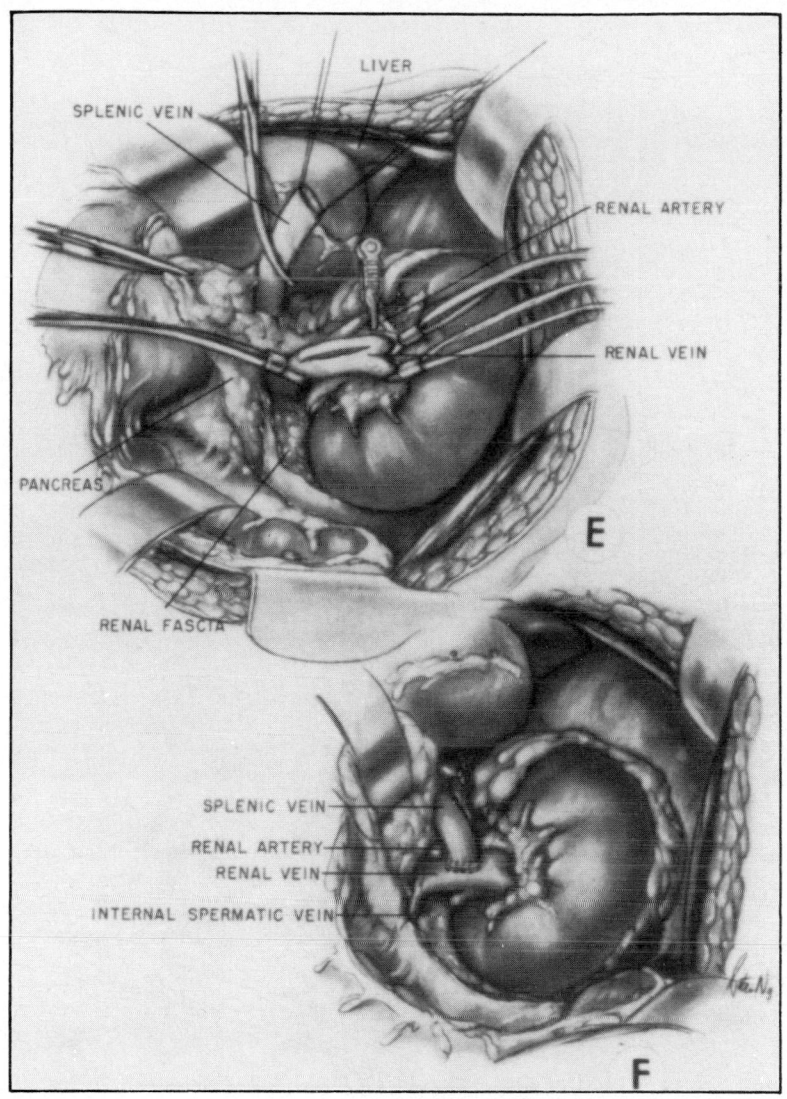

Figure 69-14. A through **F**. Central splenorenal shunt. **A.** Retraction of stomach medially. **B.** Vasa brevia have been transected. Splenic artery is ligated. Gastrosplenic and splenocolic ligament are to be transected. **C.** Spleen is mobilized so that an ultimate pedicle of splenic vein remains. **D.** Retroperitoneum has been incised, and tapes are placed around the renal artery and renal vein. **E.** Tapes are placed around the major tributaries of the renal vein within the hilus of the kidney and around the main renal vein. The renal artery is occluded with a bulldog clamp, and traction is applied to the tapes around the renal vein to secure control. An ellipse is then removed from the anterosuperior aspect of the renal vein. This should be one and one half times the diameter of the splenic vein. A vascular clamp has been applied to the splenic vein, and the spleen is removed; as long a segment of splenic vein as possible is retained. **F.** The splenic vein is brought down and anastomosed to the stoma which has been created in the main renal vein. The occlusive tapes have been removed from the splenic vein and the renal artery. (*Source: From Schwartz SI, 1964, p 334–336, with permission.*)

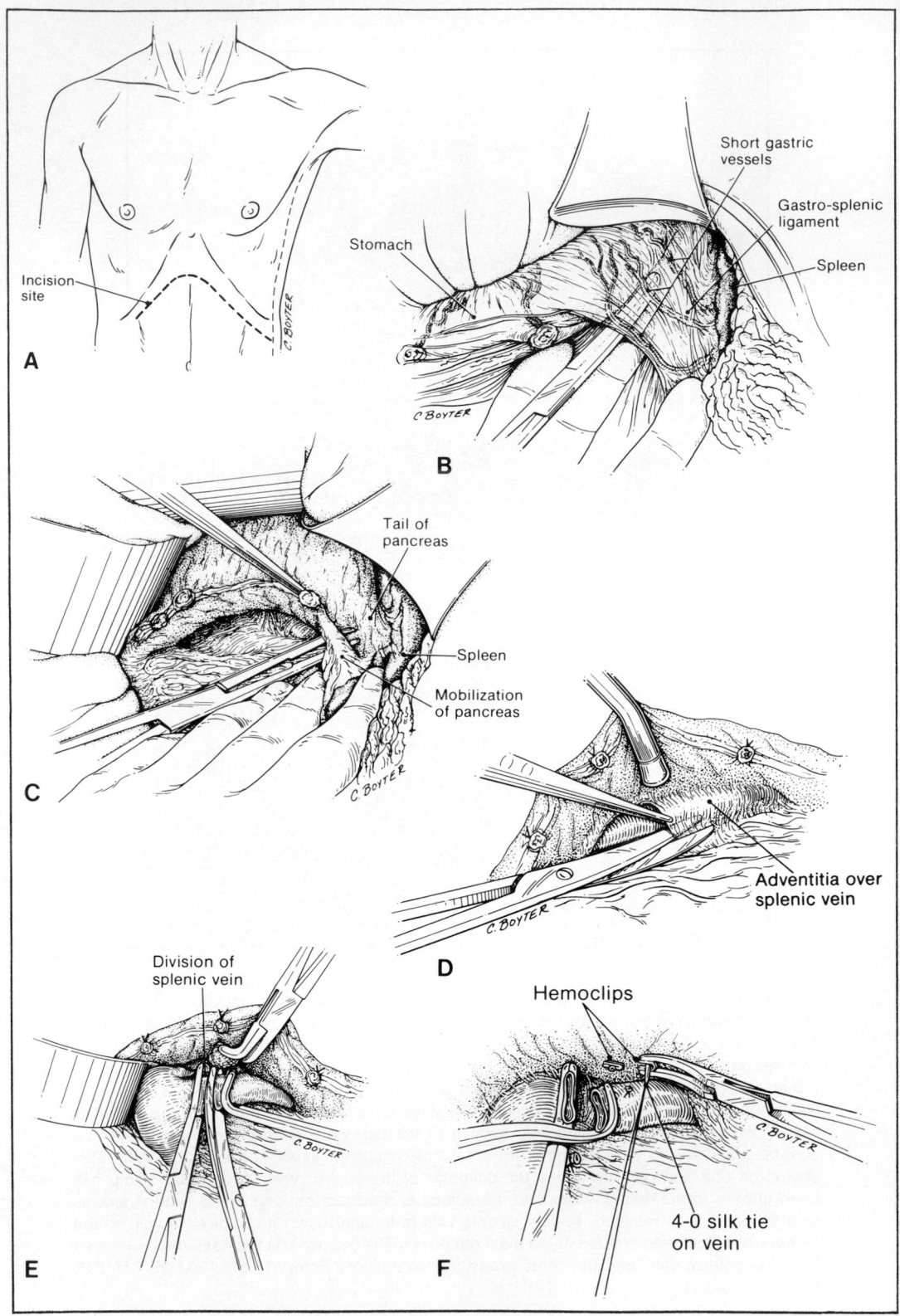

A

Incision site

B

Stomach

Short gastric vessels

Gastro-splenic ligament

Spleen

C. Boyter

C

Tail of pancreas

Spleen

Mobilization of pancreas

C. Boyter

D

Adventitia over splenic vein

C. Boyter

E

Division of splenic vein

C. Boyter

F

Hemoclips

4-0 silk tie on vein

C. Boyter

1748

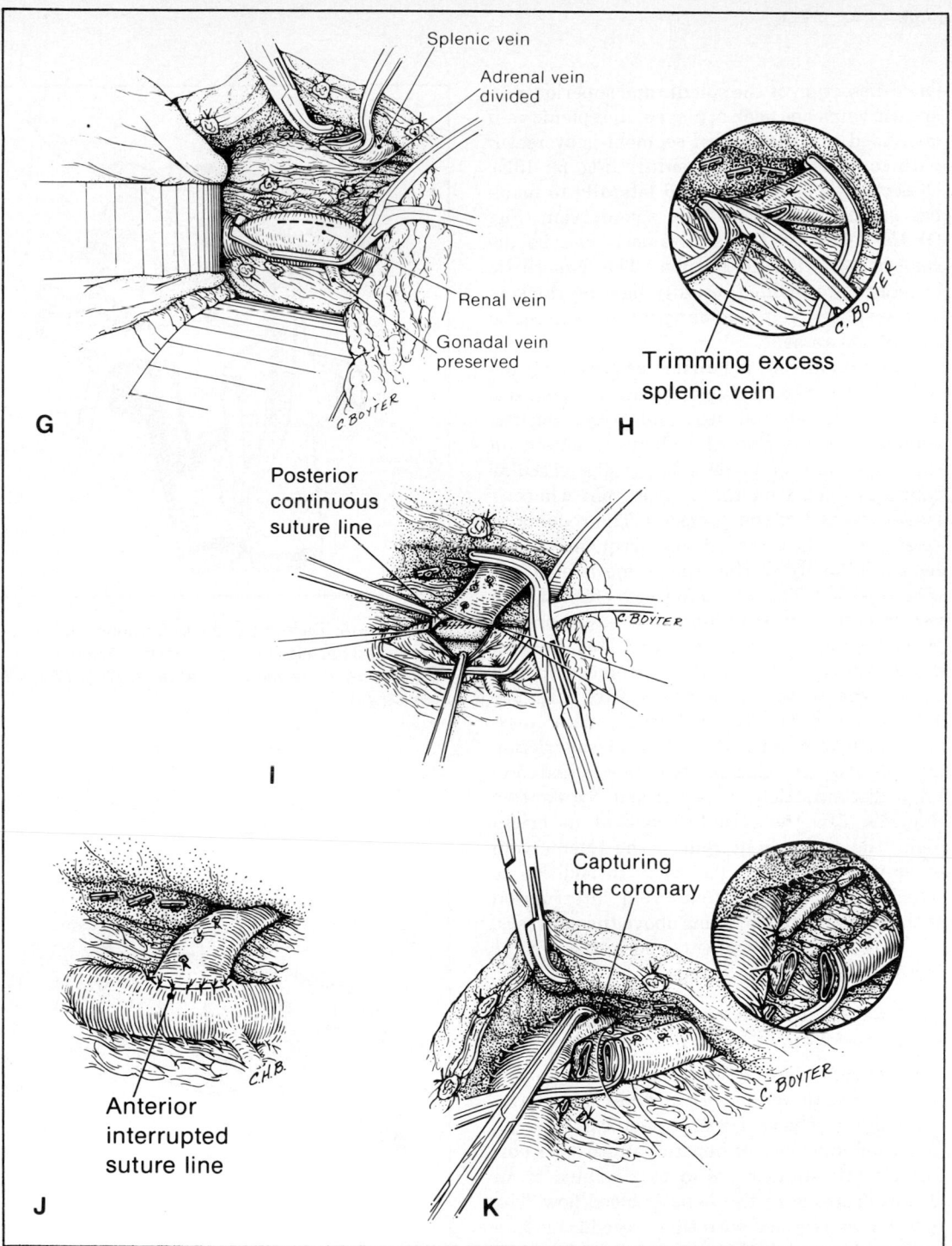

Figure 69–15. A through **K.** Selective (distal) splenorenal shunt. **A.** Incision. **B.** Entrance into the lesser sac. **C.** Mobilization of lower border of pancreas. **D.** Dissection of splenic vein. **E.** Division of splenic vein at its junction with the superior mesenteric vein. **F.** Lateral dissection of splenic vein. **G.** Occlusion of renal vein showing line of incision. **H.** Oblique transection of splenic vein to enlarge stoma. **I.** Posterior row of anastomosis. **J.** Completed anastomosis. **K.** Ligation of coronary vein. (*Source: From Warren WD, Millikan WJ Jr, 1982, with permission.*)

Once dissection of the splenic and superior mesenteric veins has been achieved, the splenic vein is divided and the central segment is oversewn with continuous vascular suture (Fig. 69–15E). Dissection is then continued laterally to mobilize sufficient length of the splenic vein (Fig. 69–15F) so that the anastomosis can be accomplished without tension. The pancreatic branches are divided, usually ligating the side on the splenic vein and clipping the pancreatic side of the vessel.

The renal vein is handled as previously described for the central splenorenal anastomosis, dividing the adrenal vein and preserving the gonadal vein. A Satinsky clamp is placed on the renal vein (Fig. 69–15G), and a vascular clamp is placed on the splenic vein where it leaves the bed of the pancreas. The redundant splenic vein is removed and frequently transected obliquely so that the stoma is enlarged (Fig. 69–15H). The anastomosis is effected with 5-0 vascular sutures. After the posterior row of the anastomosis has been completed, the needle is passed out through the renal vein and tied to the corner anchoring suture (Fig. 69–15I). The anterior row is sutured with interrupted 5-0 vascular suture to avoid constriction (Fig. 69–15J). The clamps are removed, and coronary disconnection is performed by ligating (Fig. 69–15K) the coronary vein at its origin along the superior margin of the splenic vein or as it enters the portal vein. In addition to interruption of the coronary vein, interruption of the retroperitoneal veins above the pancreas, in the splenocolic ligament, and in the greater and lesser omentums is required.

Portacaval Shunt with Arterialization of the Portal Vein

Arterialization of the hepatic stump of the portal vein in conjunction with an end-to-side portacaval shunt is based on the hypothesis that the increased incidence of hepatic failure after portal systemic shunting is in part related to an abrupt decrease in the hepatic blood flow. The reported experience with this procedure is limited to a few hundred cases. Recently, based on 75 cirrhotic patients who underwent the procedure, Otte and associates have concluded that it could be beneficial in respect to operative mortality, late survival, and tolerance.

Technique (Figs. 69–16 and 69–17). The operation is performed through a right subcostal in-

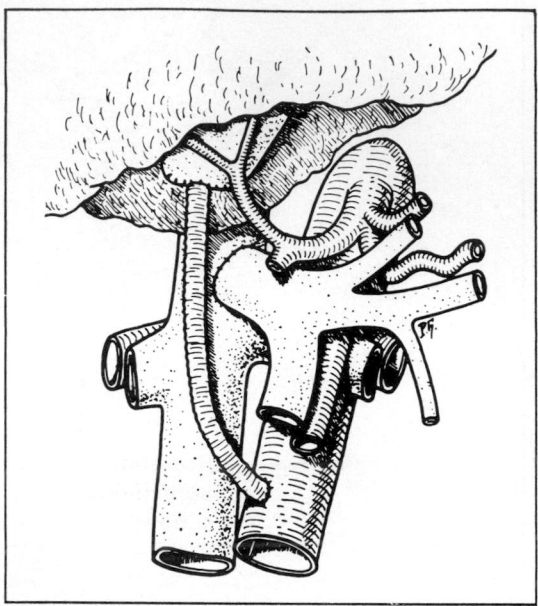

Figure 69–16. Dacron prosthesis between inferior part of aorta and hepatic stump of portal vein. (*Source: From Maillard J-N, Benahmou J-P, et al, 1970, p 884, with permission.*)

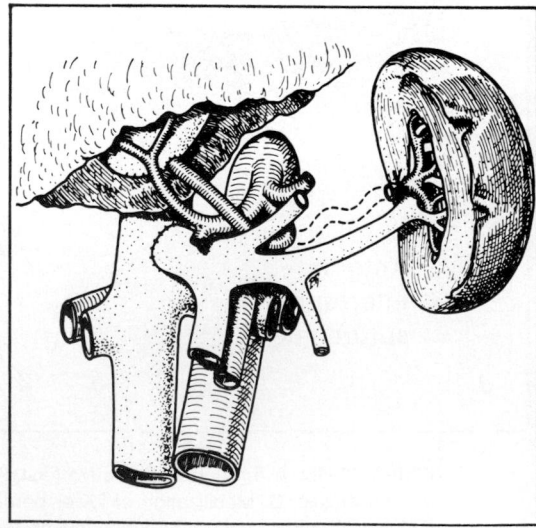

Figure 69–17. End-to-end anastomosis between splenic artery and hepatic stump of portal vein. (*Source: From Maillard J-N, Benahmou J-P, et al, 1970, p 885, with permission.*)

cision and a standard portacaval anastomosis is carried out. Arterialization of the portal circulation is achieved by interposing a saphenous vein graft between the infrarenal aorta and the hepatic stump of the portal vein. It has also been accomplished with an 8-mm prosthetic conduit (Fig. 69–16), or by turning up the splenic artery and anastomosing it in a side-to-end fashion to the portal vein stump (Fig. 69–17).

Selection of Procedure

To date there are no statistically significant data that permit confident selection of an operative procedure for patients with actively bleeding varices or for a patient whose varices have bled. The devascularization procedures and the selective distal splenorenal shunt have the advantage of reduced encephalopathy and, therefore, are theoretically more applicable in patients with Schistosomal cirrhosis and in Child's A cirrhotic patients in whom postoperative cerebral function is a vital element. The distal splenorenal shunt has been shown to provide an improved survival in nonalcoholic cirrhotics when compared to other shunting procedures, but this does not apply to alcoholic cirrhotics.

Large series have shown that pressure and flow determinations can be offered to substantiate an argument for each of the shunting procedures. The end-to-side portacaval shunt is the procedure that has been most commonly performed because it is technically easiest and has been associated with lowest incidence of thrombosis. The presence of a large caudad lobe is less compromising to this procedure than a side-to-side shunt. The Budd–Chiari's syndrome dictates a side-to-side shunt and there is evidence to suggest that a side-to-side shunt is preferable in a patient with significant ascites. To date, a prospective randomized series of alcoholic patients subjected to the various surgical procedures to prevent bleeding varices has failed to reveal any difference in survival.

BIBLIOGRAPHY

Alvarez F, Bernard O, et al: Portal obstruction in children. II. Results of surgical portosystemic shunts. J Pediatr 103:703, 1983

Belghiti J, Grenier P, et al: Long-term loss of Warren's shunt selectivity: Angiographic demonstration. Arch Surg 116:1121, 1981

Bismuth H, Franco D, et al: Portal diversion for portal hypertension in children: First 90 patients. Ann Surg 192:18, 1980

Cameron JL, Herlong HF, et al: The Budd–Chiari Syndrome. Treatment of mesenteric–systemic venous shunts. Ann Surg 198:335, 1983

Cello JP, Crass R, et al: Endoscopic sclerotherapy versus esophageal transection in Child's class C patients with variceal hemorrhage: Comparison with results of portacaval shunt—Preliminary report. Surgery 91:333, 1982

Chojkier M, Groszmann RJ, et al: Controlled comparison of continuous intra-arterial and intravenous infusions of vasopressin in hemorrhage from esophageal varices. Gastroenterology 77:540, 1979

Fischer JE: The technic for central splenorenal shunt. Mod Tech Surg 13:1, 1982

Ginsberg RJ, Waters PF, et al: Modified Sugiura procedure. Ann Thorac Surg 34:258, 1982

Gliedman ML: Mesocaval shunts. Mod Tech Surg 14:1, 1982

Greenlee HB, Stanley HM: Peritoneovenous shunt for ascites. Mod Tech Surg 16:1, 1982

Greig PD, Langer B, et al: Complications after peritoneovenous shunting for ascites. Am J Surg 139:125, 1980

Hoffman J: Stapler transection of the oesophagus for bleeding oesophageal varices. Scand J Gastroenterol 18:707, 1983

Lebrec D, Poynard T, et al: Propranolol for prevention of recurrent gastrointestinal bleeding in patients with cirrhosis: Controlled study. N Engl J Med 305:1317, 1981

Little AG, Moossa AH: Gastrointestinal hemorrhage from left-sided portal hypertension: An unappreciated complication of pancreatitis. Am J Surg 141:153, 1981

Maillard J-N, Benhamou J-P, et al: Arterialization of the liver with portacaval shunt in the treatment of portal hypertension due to intrahepatic block. Surgery 67:883, 1970

Mir J, Ponce J, et al: Esophageal transection and paraesophagogastric devascularization performed as an emergency measure for uncontrolled variceal bleeding. Surg Gynecol Obstet 155:868, 1982

Orloff MJ, Bell RH, et al: Long-term results of emergency portacaval shunt for bleeding esophageal varices in unselected patients with alcoholic cirrhosis. Ann Surg 192:325, 1980

Otte J-B, Reynaert M, et al: Arterialization of the portal vein in conjunction with a therapeutic portacaval shunt. Ann Surg 196:656, 1982

Schwartz SI: Portal hypertension, in Surgical Diseases of the Liver. New York: McGraw-Hill, 1964, p 282

Sennig A: Transcaval posterocranial resection of the liver as treatment of the Budd–Chiari syndrome. World J Surg 7:632, 1982

Smith RB III, Warren WD, et al: Dacron interposition shunts for portal hypertension: Analysis of morbidity correlates. Ann Surg 192:9, 1980

Subramanyam BR, Balthazar EJ, et al: Sonographic evaluation of patients with portal hypertension. Am J Gastroenterol 78:369, 1983

Sugiura M, Futagawa S: A new technique for treating esophageal varices. J Thorac Cardiovasc Surg 66:677, 1973

Terblanche J, Northover JMA, et al: A prospective controlled trial of sclerotherapy in the long-term management of patients after esophageal variceal bleeding. Surg Gynecol Obstet 148:323, 1979

Umeyama K, Yoshikawa K, et al: Transabdominal oesophageal transection for oesophageal varices: Experience in 101 patients. Br J Surg 70:419, 1983

Warren WD, Millikan WJ Jr: Selective transsplenic decompression procedure: Changes in technique after 300 cases. Contemp Surg 18:11, 1981

Warren WD, Millikan WJ Jr: Selective (distal) splenorenal shunt. Mod Tech Surg 15:1, 1982

Wexler MJ: Treatment of bleeding esophageal varices by transabdominal esophageal transection with the EEA stapling instrument. Surgery 88:406, 1980

Zeppa R, Hensley GT, et al: Comparative survivals of alcoholics versus nonalcoholics after distal splenorenal shunt. Ann Surg 187:510, 1978

SECTION XII
Gallbladder and Bile Ducts

70. Anatomy of the Extrahepatic Biliary Tract

Seymour I. Schwartz

NORMAL ANATOMY

Duct System

Hepatic Ducts

The intrahepatic segmental bile ducts unite to form lobar ducts, which, in turn coalesce to form the right and left hepatic ducts that represent the beginning of the extrahepatic biliary system. The right hepatic duct is formed by the intrahepatic confluence of dorsocaudal and ventrocranial branches. It enters with a sharp curve, which accounts for the fact that extrahepatic biliary calculi are less commonly found in this segment. The left hepatic duct is longer than the right and has a greater propensity for dilatation as a consequence of distal obstruction. The junction of the right and left hepatic ducts occurs extrahepatically in almost all instances, but incision and dissection of the fibrous tissue in the "hepatic plate" may be necessary to expose this junction (Fig. 70–1). The common hepatic duct, which begins at the confluence of the right and left hepatic ducts is 3 to 4 cm in length; it is joined by the cystic duct to form the common bile duct.

The Gallbladder

The gallbladder is located in the bed of the liver, in line with the anatomic division of that organ into right and left lobes. It is pear-shaped, has an average capacity of 50 ml, and is divided into four anatomic portions: fundus, corpus or body, infundibulum, and neck. The fundus represents the rounded, blind end that normally extends beyond the liver margin and is covered with peritoneum. It contains most of the smooth muscle of the organ, in contrast to the corpus or body, which is the major storage area and contains most of the elastic tissue. The body is covered extrahepatically by peritoneum and tapers into a neck, which is funnel shaped, and lies in the free border of the hepatoduodenal ligament (lesser omentum). The convexity of the neck may be distended into a dilatation known as the infundibulum, or Hartmann's pouch.

The wall of the gallbladder is made up of smooth muscle and fibrous tissue, and the lumen is lined with high columnar epithelium that contains cholesterol and fat globules. The mucus secreted into the gallbladder originates in the tubular alveolar glands and the globular cells of the mucosa lining the infundibulum and neck.

The gallbladder enters the common duct system by means of the cystic duct that has a variable length, averaging 4 cm. It joins the common hepatic duct at an acute angle, and the right branch of the hepatic artery resides immediately behind it. Variations in reference to the point of union between the cystic duct and the common hepatic duct are surgically important (Fig. 70–2). The cystic duct may lie parallel to the common hepatic duct and actually be adherent to it for a variable length. It may be extremely long, and unite with the hepatic duct in the duodenum. On the other hand, the cystic duct may be absent or very short, and there may be an extremely high union with the hepatic duct; at times the cystic duct enters the right hepatic duct. In some instances, the cystic duct may spiral either anteriorly or posteriorly

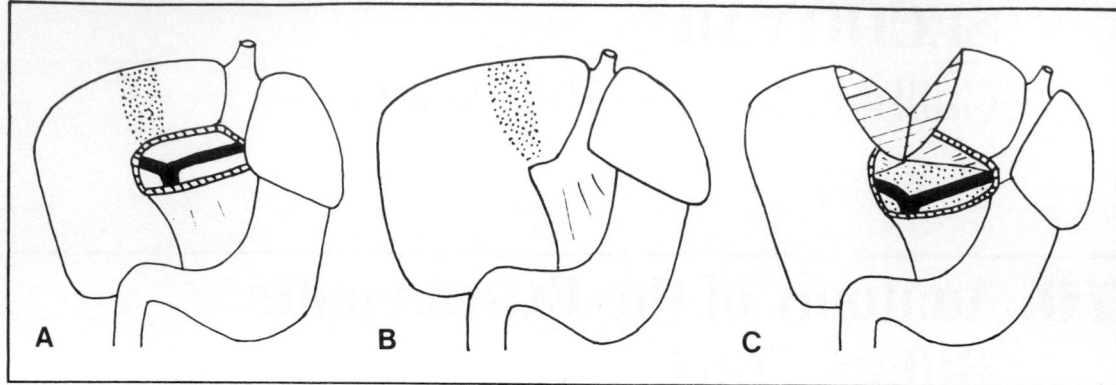

Figure 70–1. Approach to the upper bile confluent within the hilus. **A.** Detachment of the hilar plate; the bile ducts are the most superior structure in the hilus. The left duct is widely exposed throughout its length, and the upper confluent. The approach to the right duct is more limited. **B.** The length of the left duct depends on the width of the quadrate lobe. Here the lobe is triangular with a posterior apex; the exposure is limited. **C.** When opening the anterior portion of the main fissure and detaching the hilar plate, a very large exposure is obtained. (*Source: Adapted from Couinaud C, 1981, with permission.*)

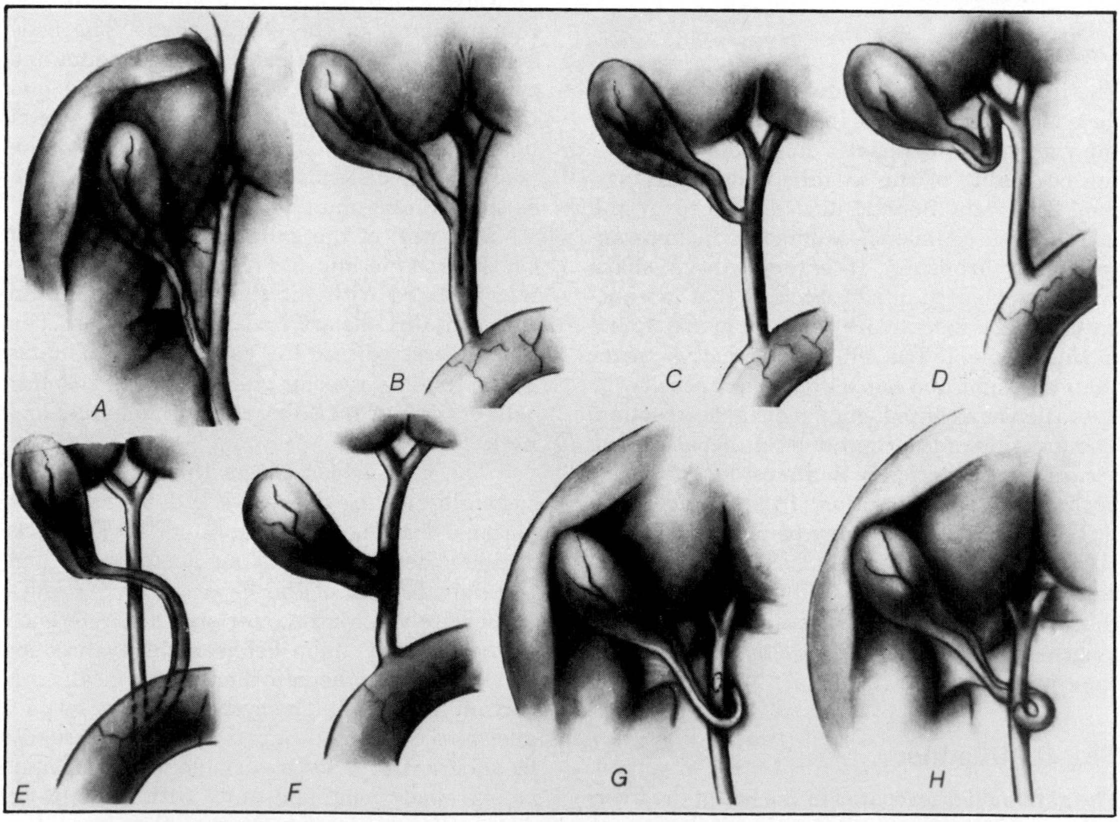

Figure 70–2. Variations of the cystic duct. **A.** Low junction between the cystic duct and the common hepatic duct. **B.** Cystic duct adherent to common hepatic duct. **C.** High junction between cystic and common hepatic duct. **D.** Cystic duct drains into right hepatic duct. **E.** Long cystic duct which joins common hepatic duct behind duodenum. **F.** Absence of cystic duct. **G.** Cystic duct crosses anterior to common hepatic duct and joins it posteriorly. **H.** Cystic duct courses posteriorly to common hepatic duct and joins it anteriorly. (*Source: From Schwartz SI: Gallbladder and extrahepatic biliary system, in Schwartz SI, Shires GT, et al (eds): Principles of Surgery, 4 edt. New York: McGraw-Hill, 1984, p 1307, with permission.*)

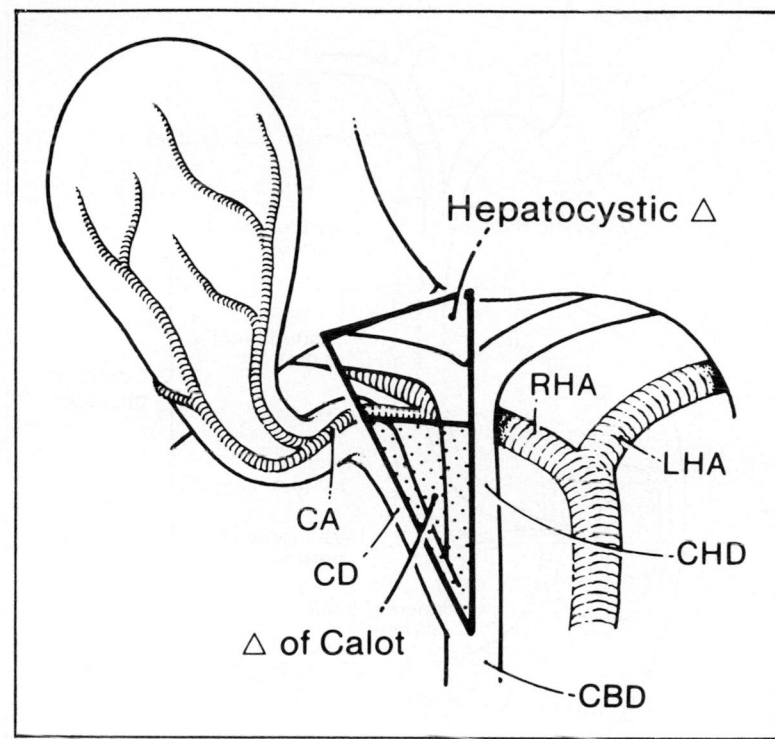

Figure 70–3. The hepatocystic triangle and the triangle of Calot. The upper boundary of the former is the margin of the liver; that of the latter is the cystic artery. The triangle of Calot is stippled. (*Source: From Skandalakis JE, Gray SW, et al, 1983, with permission.*)

in relation to the common hepatic duct and join the common hepatic duct from the left side. The segment of the cystic duct adjacent to the gallbladder bears a variable number of mucosal folds that have been referred to as "valves of Heister" but do not have valvular function.

The Cholecystohepatic Triangle

This anatomic region of surgical importance was originally described by Calot in 1891; it is formed by the cystic duct and the gallbladder below, the right lobe of the liver above, and the common hepatic duct medially (Fig. 70–3). The contents of the triangle include the right hepatic artery that enters posteriorly to the common hepatic duct in 87 percent of cases, and anterior to that duct in the remaining 13 percent. It parallels the cystic duct for a short distance before turning craniad to reach the liver. In about one quarter of cases there is an aberrant right hepatic artery originating from the superior mesenteric artery and coursing through the triangle. The cystic artery arises from a normal or aberrant right hepatic artery within the cholecystohepatic triangle. It usually

divides into a superficial branch that goes to the serosal surface and a deep branch that reaches to the hepatic surface of the gallbladder. Duplication of the cystic artery is found in about 25 percent of patients, and these vessels may arise either from adjacent or separate sites. The cholecystohepatic triangle may contain aberrant or accessory hepatic ducts that enter the cystic or common hepatic duct separately in about 15 percent of cases.

Common Bile Duct

The common bile duct is approximately 8.5 cm in length. The normal external diameter ranges between 4 and 10 mm. Leslie has shown that at diameters of 10.2 mm or above, the probability of obstructive pathology is 50 percent. The upper portion is situated in the free edge of the lesser omentum, to the right of the hepatic artery and anterior to the portal vein. The middle third of the common duct curves to the right behind the first portion of the duodenum, where it diverges from the portal vein and hepatic arteries. The lower third of the common bile duct

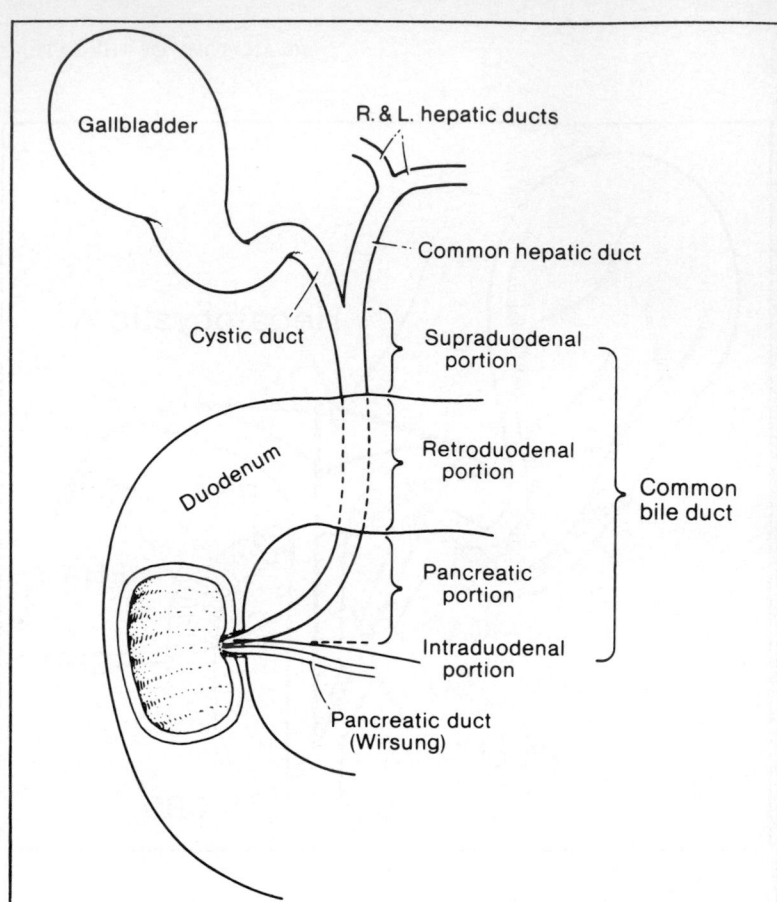

Figure 70–4. The extrahepatic biliary tract and the four portions of the common bile duct. (*Source: From Skandalakis JE, Gray SW, et al, 1983, with permission.*)

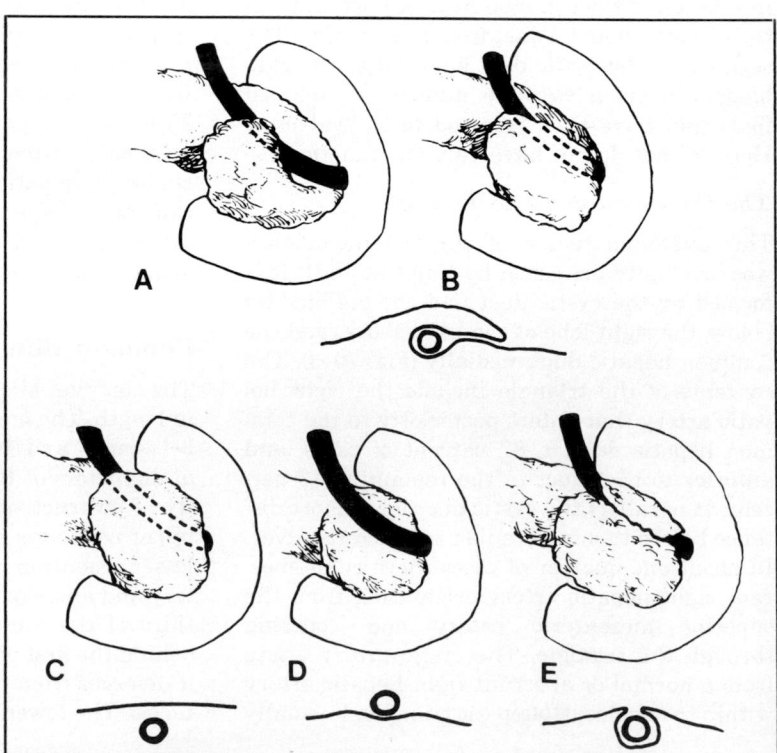

Figure 70–5. Relation of the pancreas and the common bile duct. **A** and **B.** The duct is partially covered by a tongue of pancreas (44 percent). **C.** The duct is completely covered by the pancreas (30 percent). **D.** The duct lies free on the surface of the pancreas (16.5 percent). **E.** The duct is covered by two tongues of pancreas with a cleavage plane between. (*Source: From Skandalakis JE, Gray SW, et al, 1983, with permission.*)

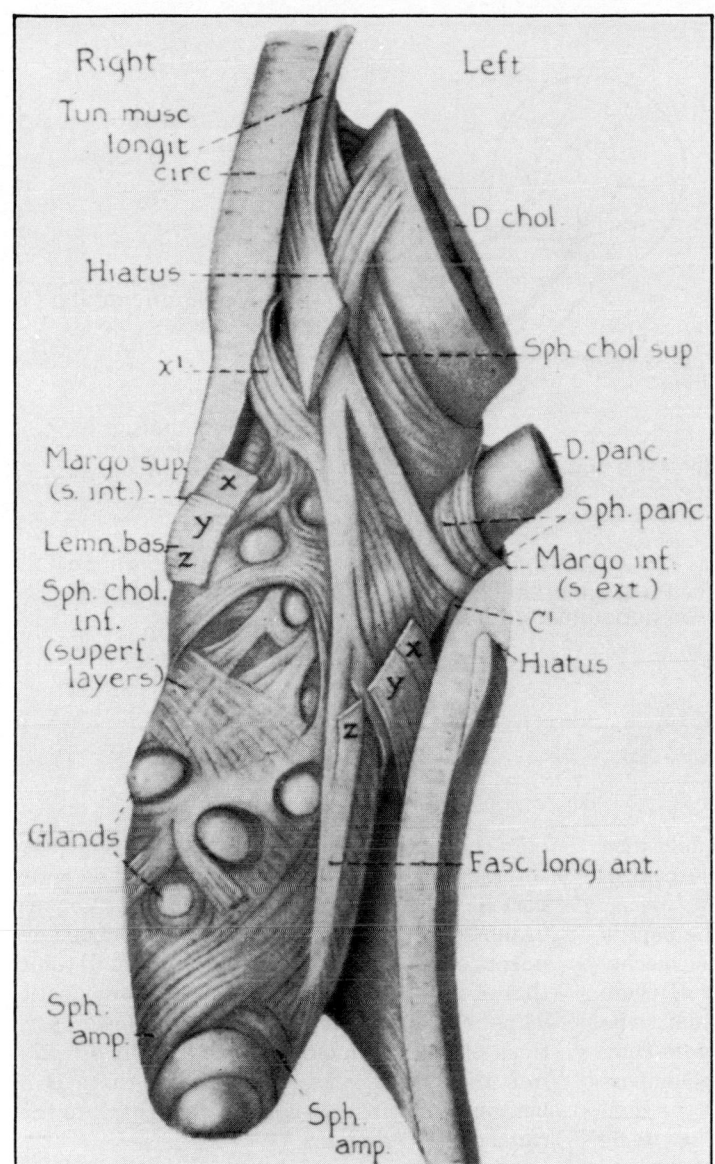

Figure 70–6. Assembly drawing of the human choledochoduodenal junction with major papilla as seen from the anterior side with the tunica mucosa removed. This is a composite drawing designed to illustrate the auxiliary musculature, i.e., the strands passing from the tunica muscularis to the musculus proprius of the ducts and papilla. The anterior longitudinal fascicle has been narrowed somewhat, in order to display relations of underlying layers. Obviously the strongest layer of the sphincter choledochus inferior cannot be seen in this view since it lines the bile duct. (*Source: From Boyden EA, 1957, with permission.*)

curves more to the right beyond the head of the pancreas, which it grooves, and enters the ampulla of Vater, where it is frequently joined by the pancreatic duct. The portions of the duct have been named according to their relationship to the intestinal viscera: supraduodenal, retroduodenal, intrapancreatic, and intraduodenal. The average length of each of these segments is 2, 1.5, 3, and 1 cm, respectively (Fig. 70–4). The pancreatic portion of the common duct is partially covered by pancreatic tissue in about 45 percent of cases and completely covered in

another 30 percent of cases (Fig. 70–5).

The final, intraduodenal or intramural portion of the common bile duct passes obliquely through the duodenal wall with the main pancreatic duct and follows one of three patterns. The structures may unite outside the duodenum and traverse the duodenal wall and papilla; they may join within the duodenal wall and have a common short, terminal portion; they may exit independently into the duodenum. Separate orifices have been demonstrated in 29 percent of autopsy specimens, while injection into cadav-

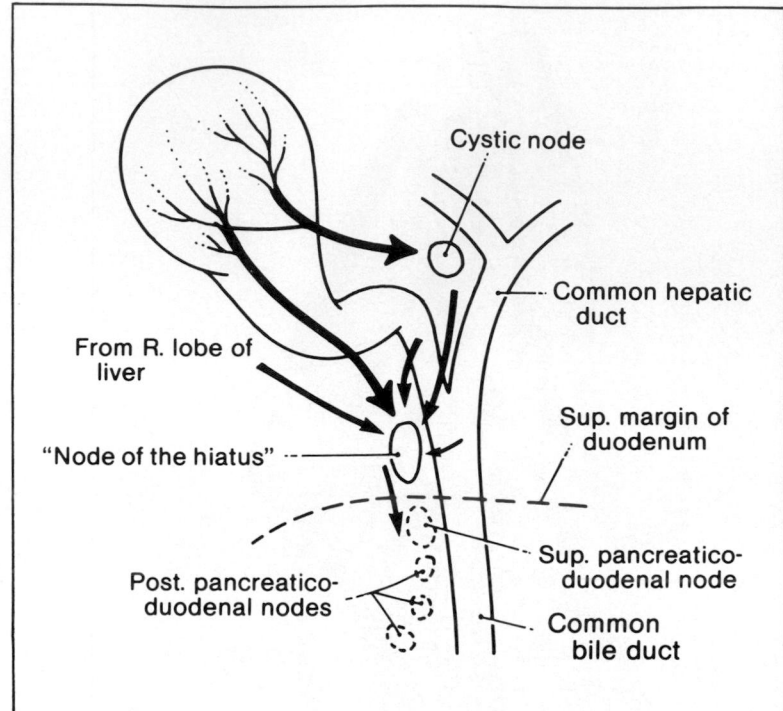

Figure 70–7. Lymphatic drainage of the biliary tract. The cystic node and the node of the hiatus are relatively constant. Drainage from the gallbladder, the cystic duct, and the right lobe of the liver reaches the posterior pancreaticoduodenal nodes. (*Source: From Skandalakis JE, Gray SW, et al, 1983, with permission.*)

ers reveals reflux from the common bile duct into the pancreatic duct in over 50 percent of cases.

The distal common bile duct at the papilla of Vater is regulated by a sphincteric mechanism, originally named the sphincter of Oddi, but more accurately described by Boyden, who has defined a complex of four sphincters composed of circular or spiral smooth muscle fibers surrounding the intramural portion of the common bile duct and pancreatic ducts (Fig. 70–6). The common duct exits into the duodenum at the papilla of Vater. This point can be defined by the junction of a longitudinal mucosal fold meeting a transverse fold to form a T.

Vascular Supply

The gallbladder, hepatic ducts, and upper portion of the common bile duct are supplied by the cystic artery; the lower portion of the common bile duct is supplied by branches of the pancreaticoduodenal and retroduodenal arteries. Northover and Terblanche have emphasized that two arteries run parallel to the common duct at 9 o'clock and at 3 o'clock, and this

may represent a significant supply to the duct. Interruption of these two arteries has been reported to result in ductal stricture. Venous drainage of the gallbladder, hepatic ducts, and upper common duct courses through small veins that enter directly into branches of the hepatic veins within the liver. Veins from lower portions of the common duct may drain directly into the portal vein. Occasionally there is a large cystic vein that carries blood back to the right portal vein.

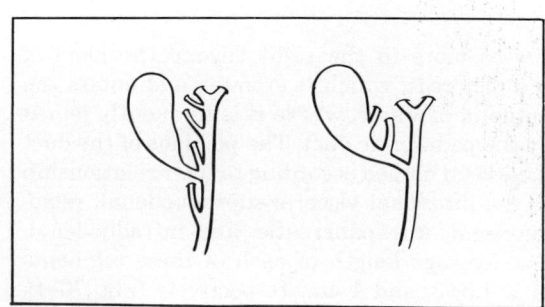

Figure 70–8. Abnormalities of the bile ducts. Accessory hepatic ducts.

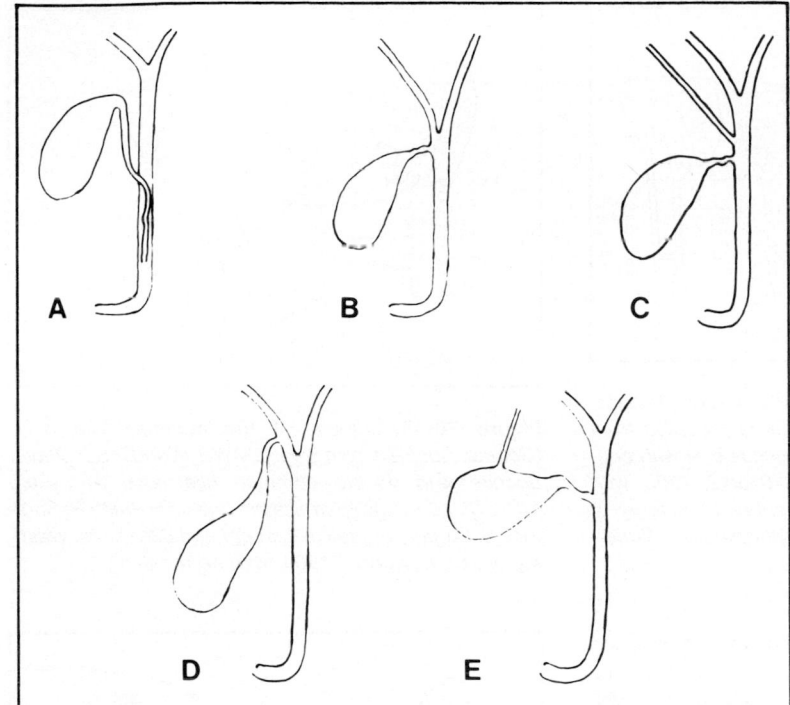

Figure 70–9. Duct anomalies. **A.** A long cystic duct with low fusion with common hepatic duct. **B.** Abnormally high fusion of cystic duct with common hepatic duct (trifurcation). **C.** Accessory hepatic duct. **D.** Cystic duct entering right hepatic duct. **E.** Cholecystohepatic duct. (*Source: From Benson EA, Page RE, 1976, with permission.*)

Lymphatic Drainage and Neural Supply

Lymph flows directly from the gallbladder to the liver and also drains into several nodes along the surface of the portal vein and common bile duct. The collecting lymphatic trunks from the left side of the gallbladder drain into a cystic node, located at the junction of the cystic and common hepatic ducts (Fig. 70–7).

The nerves of the gallbladder arise from the celiac plexus and are located along the hepatic artery. Motor nerves are made up of vagus fibers mixed with postganglionic fibers from the celiac ganglion. The preganglionic sympathetic level is at T8 and T9. Sensory supplies are provided by fibers in the sympathetic nerves coursing to the celiac plexus through the posterior root ganglion at T8 and T9 on the right side.

ANOMALIES

Anomalies of the Extrahepatic Ducts

The atresias are discussed elsewhere, and the variations in the cystic duct have been outlined previously.

Anomalous (accessory) hepatic ducts may open into the cystic duct or into the neck of the gallbladder, enter the right hepatic duct, enter the right side of the common hepatic duct at a point at, or very close to, the site where the cystic and common hepatic ducts join, enter the common duct below the insertion of the cystic duct, or the gallbladder itself (Fig. 70–8). Accessory hepatic ducts are present in about 10 percent of human subjects. An accessory duct is usually the size of a normal cystic duct, but in some cases it may be minute. An undetected injury to one of these ducts may result in no change in the patient's postoperative course, or may produce a biliary fistula. When an accessory duct passes through the cholecystohepatic triangle, it is subject to inadvertent transection and bile leakage. Cystohepatic ducts, which drain bile from the liver directly into the gallbladder are rare. Michels was unable to find an example of such a duct in dissection of 500 cadavers. Cases have been reported, however, in which the right, left, or even both, hepatic ducts enter the gallbladder and ligation of these ducts could result in a surgical catastrophe.

Benson and Page, based on dissection of the

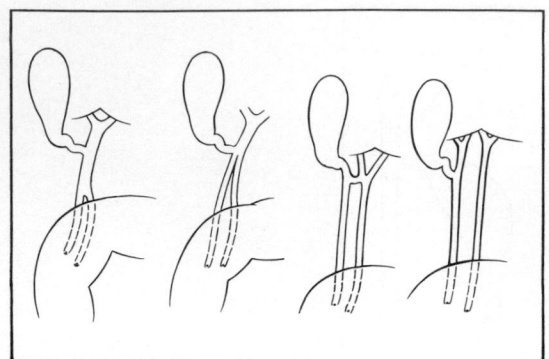

Figure 70–10. Malpositions and partial or complete duplications of the choledochus. (*Source: Adapted from Swartley WB, Weeden SD: Choledochus cyst with double common bile duct. Ann Surg 101:912, 1935, with permission; and from Smith R, Sherlock S: Surgery of the Gallbladder and Bile Ducts. Washington: Butterworths, 1964, with permission.*)

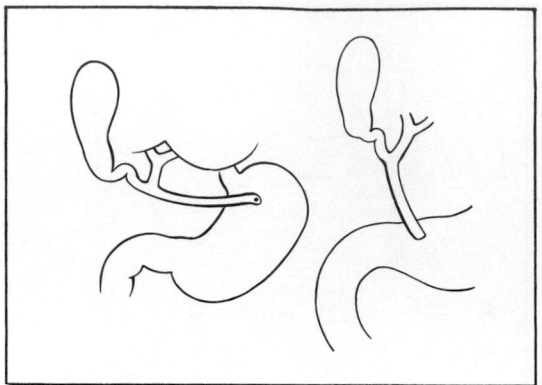

Figure 70–11. Ectopia of the common bile duct. (*Source: Adapted from Swartley WB, Weeder SD: Choledochus with double common bile duct. Ann Surg 101:912, 1935, with permission; and from Smith R, Sherlock S: Surgery of the Gallbladder and Bile Ducts. Washington: Butterworths, 1964, with permission.*)

extrahepatic biliary tree of 65 cadavers, defined five ductal anomalies of surgical consequence (Fig. 70–9). Vigorous traction on a long cystic duct with a low fusion with the common hepatic duct may produce marked angulation of the common hepatic and lobar bile ducts, which may then be caught in a clamp. If there is an abnormal fusion of the right and left hepatic ducts with the cystic ducts, a hepatic duct may be damaged during cystic duct ligation. If there is an accessory hepatic duct from the right lobe that enters the common hepatic duct, it may be inadvertently damaged at operation with consequent prolonged bile leakage. When the cystic duct enters the right hepatic duct, the right hepatic duct may be mistaken for the cystic duct and ligated. Failure to recognize a cholecystohepatic duct of significant size will result in prolonged leakage.

Malpositions and Duplications of the Common Bile Duct (Figs. 70–10 and 70–11)

Malposition and duplication of the main ducts are rare and usually are found at postmortem examination. Five different variations have been reported: (1) the common bile duct empties into the pylorus or into the cardiac end of the stomach (Fig. 70–11), (2) the common bile duct joins the duodenum independent of the pancreatic duct, (3) bifurcation of the common bile duct with separate openings into the duodenum,

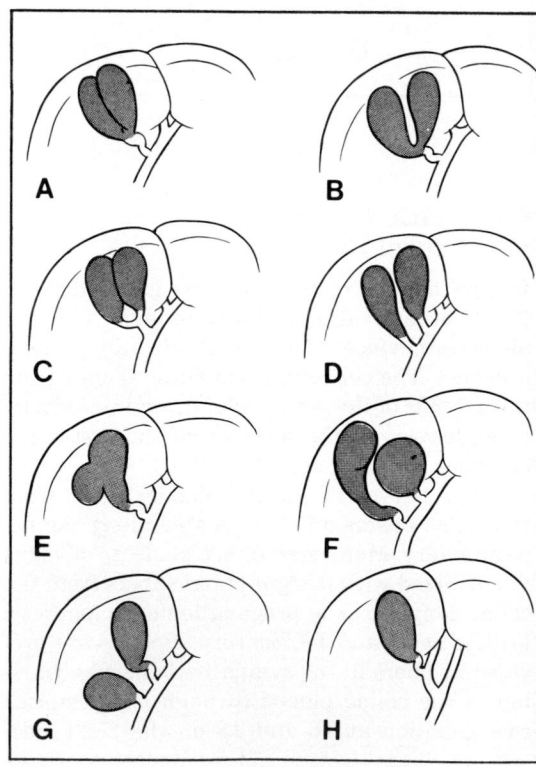

Figure 70–12. Anomalies of the gallbladder. **A, B,** and **C.** The three types of bilobed gallbladder: septal, T-, and Y-shaped. **D, F,** and **G.** The small rounded "gallbladders" are rudimentary in origin. **E.** Diverticulum of the gallbladder. **H.** High position of the gallbladder with its cystic duct draining into the right hepatic duct. (*Source: From Gross RE: Congenital anomalies of the gallbladder. Arch Surg 32:131, 1936, with permission.*)

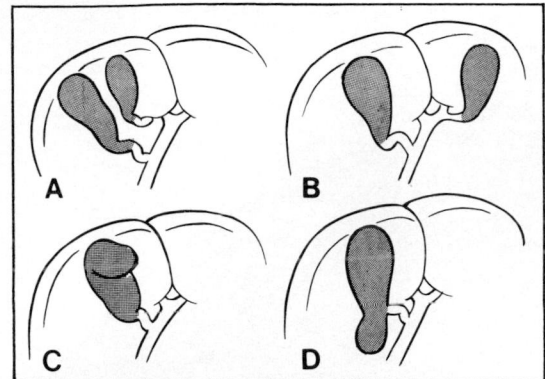

Figure 70–13. Anomalies of the gallbladder. **A.** Double gallbladder. **B.** One gallbladder in its normal position and another on the left side. **C.** Phrygian cap. **D.** Enlarged Hartmann's pouch. (*Source: From Gross RE: Congenital anomalies of the gallbladder. Arch Surg 32:131, 1936, with permission.*)

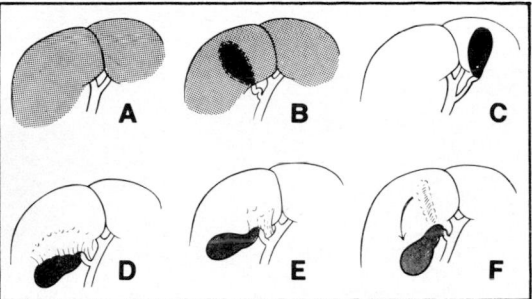

Figure 70–14. Anomalies of the gallbladder. **A.** Absence or agenesis. **B.** Intrahepatic gallbladder. **C.** Gallbladder on the left side. When the gallbladder is situated on the left side, the cystic duct may drain into the left hepatic duct or the common hepatic duct. **D, E,** and **F.** Gallbladder with and without a mesentery. Ptosis or "floating" gallbladder. (*Source: From Gross RE: Congenital anomalies of the gallbladder. Arch Surg 32:131, 1936, with permission.*)

(4) duplication of the main bile ducts (Fig. 70–10), and (5) a bifurcating duct with one branch entering the duodenum and the other entering the stomach.

Anomalies of the Gallbladder

Congenital anomalies of the gallbladder (Figs. 70–12 through 70–14) may be classified as follows: (1) anomalies of number—absence (agenesis) of gallbladder, double or triple gallbladder, replacement by a fibrous nodule, (2) anomalies of form—partitioned, bilobed, septate, hourglass, diverticulum of the gallbladder, kinking of the gallbladder, and Phyrgian cap, and (3) anomalies of position—intrahepatic, transverse, left-sided gallbladder, double gallbladder, one on each side, ptosis of the gallbladder.

Anomalies of Number

Absence of the Gallbladder. Congenital absence or agenesis of the gallbladder is a rare anomaly, with an autopsy incidence of 0.3 percent. Before the diagnosis is made, the presence of an intrahepatic vesicle, or left-sided organ, must be ruled out. Prior to 1978, fewer than 200 recorded cases appeared in the literature. Many of the patients died in the first 6 months of life and there were accompanying malformations and agenesis of the extrahepatic ducts. Most adult cases are associated with choledocholithiasis, part of a general correlation between biliary tract anomalies and cholelithiasis.

Double Gallbladder (Fig. 70–15). In this situation there are two separate organs and two separate cystic ducts. Full duplication of the gallbladder occurs in about 1 in 4000 patients. In the previous edition of this text, Maingot was able to trace 136 cases of double gallbladder in the literature. On occasion one gallbladder was situated on the right side and the other on the left side beneath the lobe of the liver. At times there were small, circular or ovoid accessory, anomalous, or rudimentary gallbladders that arose from the common duct by a narrow neck and lay along the free margin of the hepatoduodenal ligament. These frequently had an intrahepatic component. The rudimentary gallbladders had no remaining function, and measured from 1 to 2 cm in length. In 1958 the first case of a triple gallbladder in man was reported. Two additional cases subsequently have been authenticated.

Anomalies of Form

Bilobed gallbladder represents an anomaly in which the gallbladder has two cavities that drain a common cystic duct. Fewer than two dozen cases have been reported. Three varieties of bilobed gallbladder have been noted: (1) the cavities may be divided by a septum, and the septum may be partial or complete, (2) there may be two cavities that coalesce at their necks to join the cystic duct, and (3) there may be two vesicles of equal size that have their own cystic ducts that unite to form a single duct before this drains into the main bile duct.

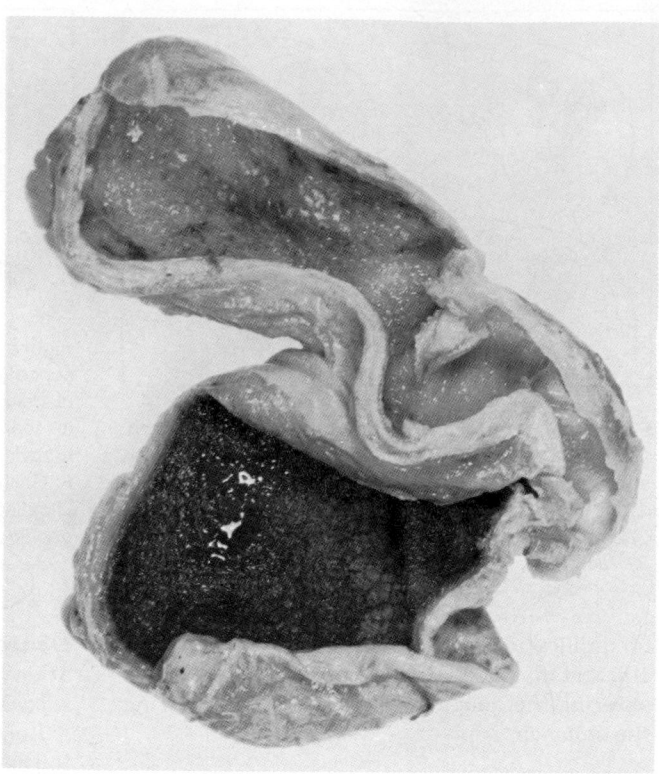

Figure 70–15. Double gallbladder, one cavity showing acute cholecystitis, the other normal. (*Courtesy of Lord Smith and Butterworths, with permission.*)

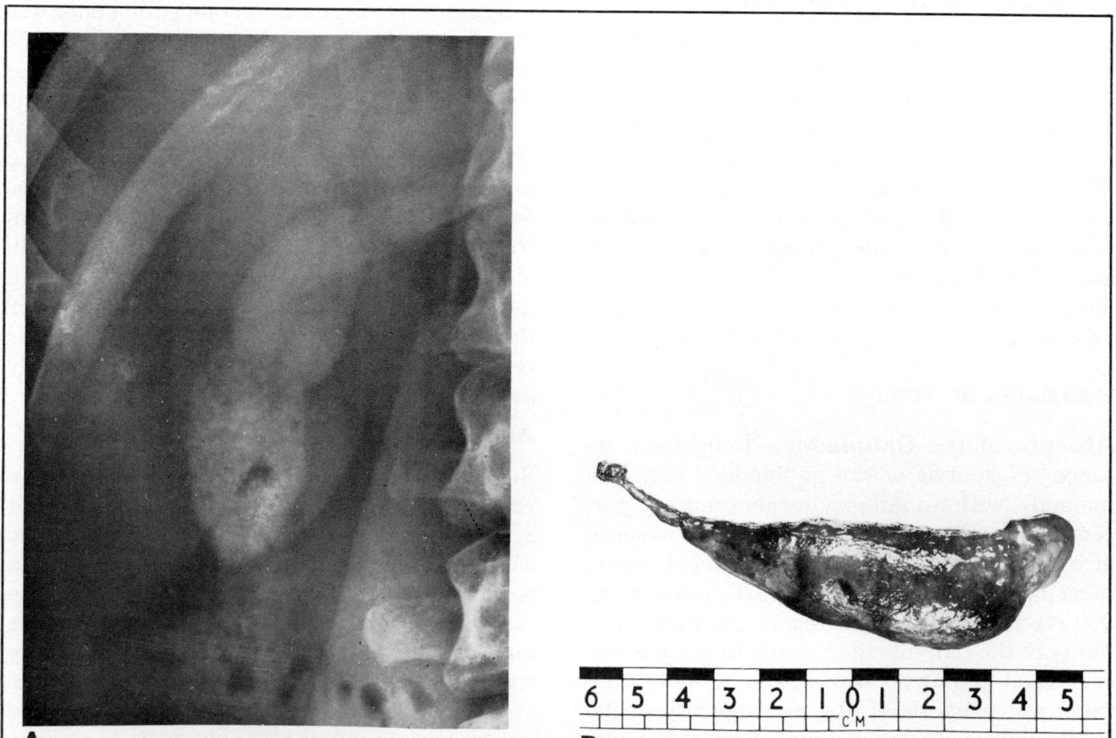

A

B

6 5 4 3 2 1 0 1 2 3 4 5
C M

Another anomaly is the diverticulum of the gallbladder, the most common site of which is in Hartmann's pouch. These diverticula vary in diameter from 0.6 to 9.0 cm. Blalock found diverticula to be present in 0.2 percent of 727 surgically removed gallbladders. Cholecystectomy is indicated when this abnormality produces symptoms or harbors calculi. Multiple diverticula do occur, but they are exceedingly rare. Other malformations of form and contour include dumbbell, or hourglass, gallbladders (Fig. 70–16A), which may be congenital or acquired. Marked kinking between the body and fundus may also occur.

The Phyrgian cap (Fig. 70–16B) has been described as a congenital malformation, the incidence of which is between 3 and 8 percent. It occurs more commonly in women. The septum may vary from one quarter of the diameter to the entire diameter separating the fundus from the body. The gallbladder functions normally and in itself the anomaly has no clinical implication.

Anomalies of Position

Normally formed gallbladders have been found in a number of locations: (1) within the hepatic substance, (2) under the left lobe of the liver (left-sided gallbladder), (3) posteriorly under the inferior aspect of the right lobe of the liver, and (4) horizontally, in the transverse fissure of the liver. Other positional anomalies are retrodisplacement, lumbar, iliac (Fig. 70–17), or pelvic location, and ptosis, or floating gallbladder. There are three types of floating gallbladder: (1) the organ is completely invested by peritoneum and possesses no mesentery, in which case the only attachment between the gallbladder and the liver is the cystic duct and the cystic artery, (2) the gallbladder is suspended from the liver by a complete mesentery (Fig. 70–18), and (3) the cystic duct and neck of the gallbladder have a mesentery in which the cystic artery lies, but the fundus and body are free and ptosed. The condition of ptosis is seen in approximately 5 percent of all gallbladders.

The maximal incidence for symptomatic torsion of the gallbladder is between the ages

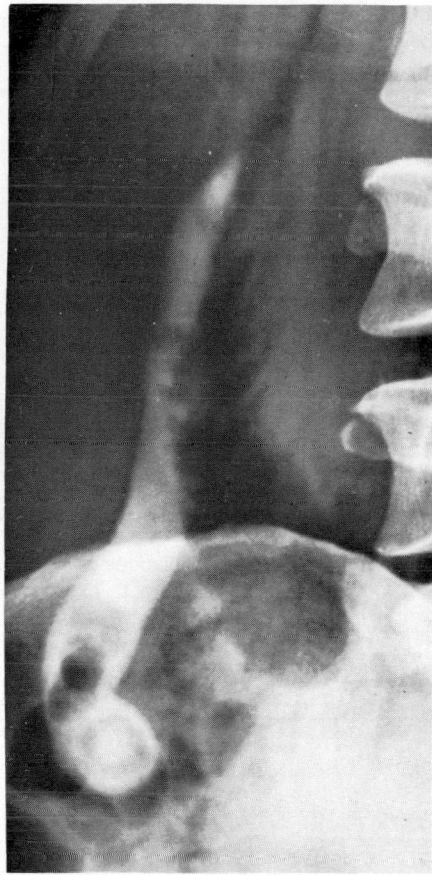

Figure 70–17. Iliac gallbladder. Note the large gallbladder (containing a circular gallstone at the fundus) lying in the right iliac fossa. In such cases the gallbladder usually has a complete mesentery. (*Source: From May RE: An unusual case of torsion of the gallbladder. Br J Clin Pract 21:191, 1967, with permission.*)

of 60 and 80, but cases have been reported in the pediatric age group. The number of reported cases for torsion of the gallbladder is now approximately 300. The onset of acute pain and vomiting without jaundice in an elderly patient and the appearance within a few hours of the onset of a greatly enlarged and palpable gallbladder is suggestive of the diagnosis of acute torsion. Nearly all patients who suffer from torsion are thin, asthenic individuals. The onset of pain is abrupt and occurs below the right

Figure 70–16. A. Hourglass gallbladder. Note that the proximal pouch appears normal on the cholecystogram, but the distal pouch of the hourglass gallbladder contains many small and closely packed gallstones (R. Maingot's patient). **B.** Phyrgian cap.

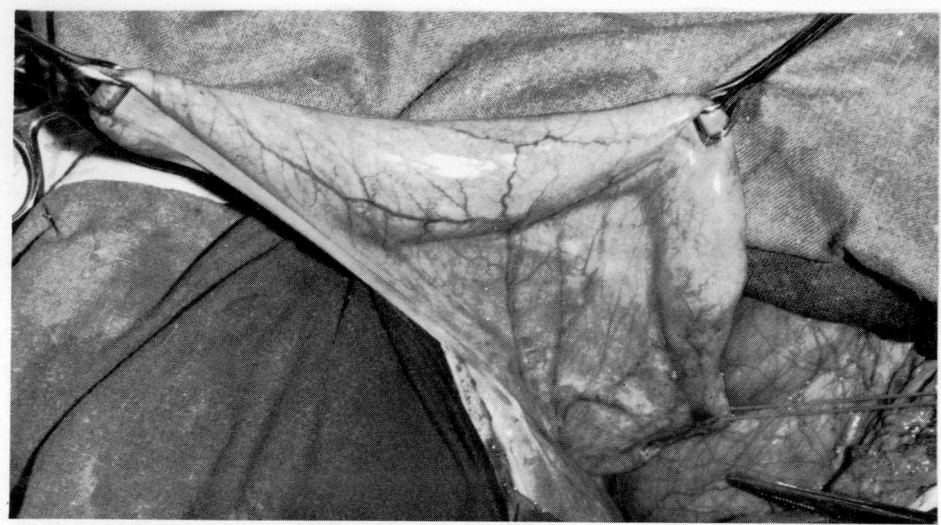

Figure 70–18. Gallbladder with complete mesentery. The cystic artery and the cystic duct have been ligated prior to excision of the gallbladder. (*Source: From May RE: An unusual case of torsion of the gallbladder. Br J Clin Pract 21:191, 1967, with permission.*)

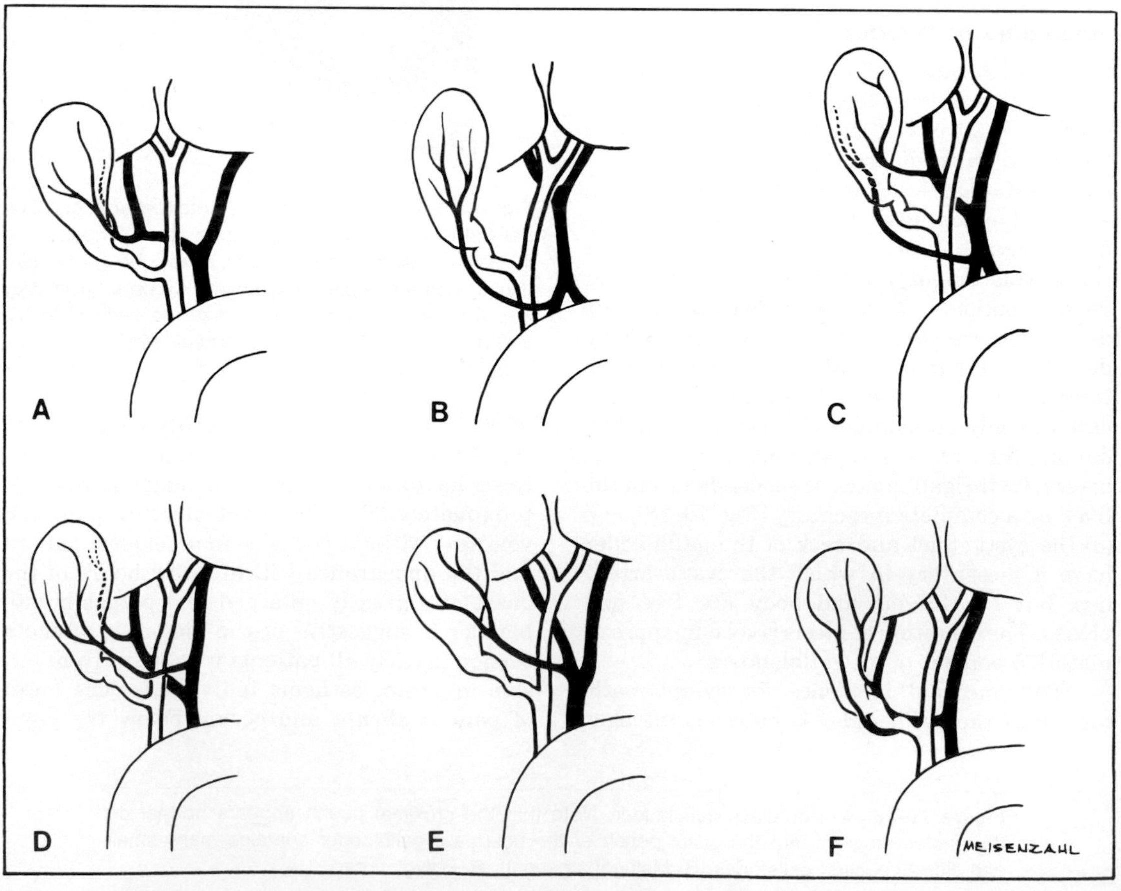

A

B

C

D

E

F

MEISENZAHL

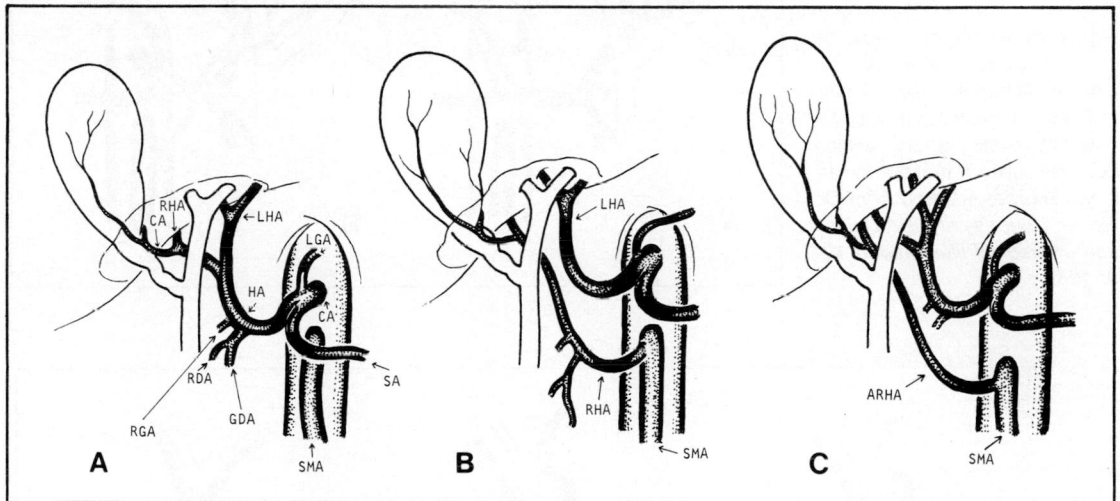

Figure 70–20. Some anomalies of the hepatic arteries. CA = coeliac axis, SA = splenic artery; LGA = left gastric artery, HA = hepatic artery, CHA = common hepatic artery; RHA = right hepatic artery, LHA = left hepatic artery, CA = cystic artery; GDA = gastroduodenal artery; RGA = right gastric artery, SMA = superior mesenteric artery, ARHA = accessory right hepatic artery. **A.** So-called normal anatomic arrangements of the feeding vessels of the liver and gallbladder. RDA = retroduodenal artery. Note the replacing right hepatic artery **(B)** and aberrant or accessory right hepatic artery **(C)**. (*Source: Adapted from Holinshead WH: Textbook of Anatomy, 2 edt. New York: Harper & Row, 1967, with permission.*)

Figure 70–19. Anomalies of the arteries to the gallbladder. **A.** Cystic artery arises from right hepatic artery in 95 percent of cases. **B.** Cystic artery arises from gastroduodenal artery. **C.** Two cystic arteries, one arising from right hepatic artery and the other from common hepatic artery. **D.** Two cystic arteries. Abnormal one arises from left hepatic artery and crosses common hepatic duct anteriorly. **E.** Cystic artery arises from right hepatic artery but courses anterior to common hepatic duct. **F.** Two cystic arteries arising from right hepatic artery. Right hepatic artery is adherent to cystic duct and neck of gallbladder. Posterior cystic artery is very short (a common finding).

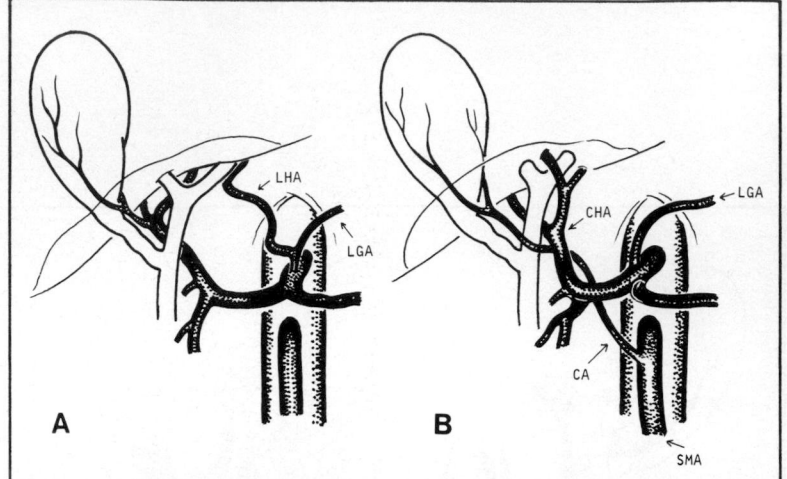

Figure 70–21. Some anomalies of the hepatic arteries. **A.** Replacing left hepatic artery arising from the left gastric artery. **B.** An aberrant cystic artery arising from the superior mesenteric artery. (*Source: Adapted from Dr. Netter. Courtesy of CIBA Collection of Medical Illustrations, Vol 3, 1957.*)

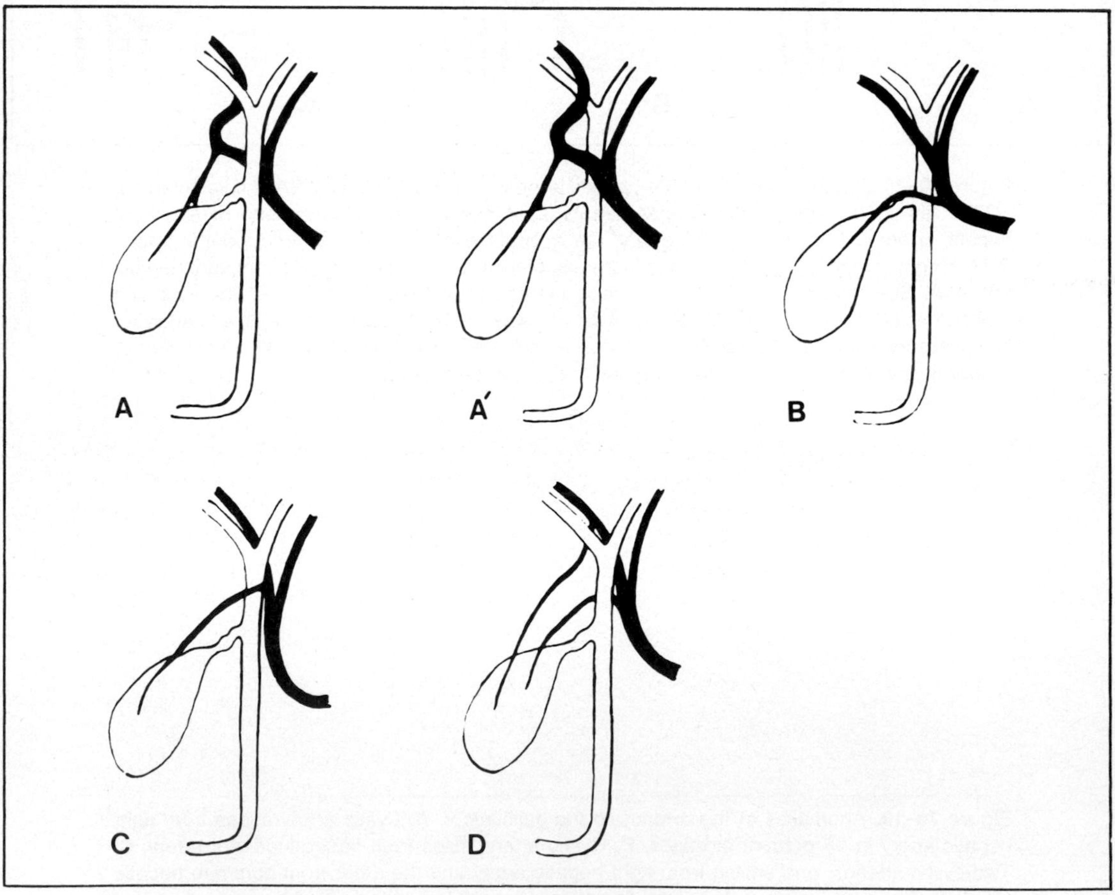

Figure 70–22. Vascular anomalies. **A, A'.** ''Caterpillar hump'' right hepatic artery. **B.** Right hepatic artery anterior to common hepatic (or common bile) duct. **C.** Cystic artery anterior to common hepatic (or common bile) duct. **D.** Accessory cystic artery. (*Source: From Benson EA, Page RE, 1976, with permission.*)

costal margin; the treatment consists of detorsion and cholecystectomy.

Anomalies of the Hepatic and Cystic Arteries

Anomalies of the hepatic and cystic artery are present in about 50 percent of cases (Fig. 70–19). A large accessory left hepatic artery originating from the left gastric artery occurs in about 5 percent of patients, in 10 to 20 percent of cases the right hepatic artery originates from the superior mesenteric artery, and in about 5 percent of cases there are two hepatic arteries, one originating from the common hepatic artery and the other from the superior mesenteric artery. In 3 to 6 percent of cases the left hepatic artery derives its origin from the left gastric, splenic, or superior mesenteric artery, or the aorta. In these situations the artery is in danger during the performance of subtotal gastrectomy. Figures 70–20 and 70–21 depict a variety of anomalies of the arterial system.

The significant arterial anomalies defined in the dissections of Benson and Page are shown in Fig. 70–22. A "caterpillar hump" right hepatic artery can pass in front of, or behind, the common hepatic duct or common bile duct, and may be mistaken for the cystic artery and therefore ligated. Because the cystic artery that arises from the "caterpillar hump" is short, it is easily avulsed from a parent trunk. With the right hepatic artery lying anterior to the common bile duct or common hepatic ducts, or with the cystic artery coursing anterior to these structures, there is risk of injury to either the common hepatic or common bile duct when the cystic artery is being ligated. An accessory cystic artery may be torn if it is not identified. The most common arterial anomaly is the accessory cystic artery.

BIBLIOGRAPHY

Adam Y, Metcalf W: Absence of the cystic duct: A case report, the embryology and a review of the literature. Ann Surg 164:1056, 1966

Benson EA, Page RE: A practical reappraisal of the anatomy of the extrahepatic bile ducts and arteries. Br J Surg 63:853, 1976

Boyden EA: The anatomy of the choledochoduodenal junction in man. Surg Gynecol Obstet 104:641, 1957

Burnett W, Gairns FW, et al: Some observations on the innervation of the extrahepatic biliary system in man. Ann Surg 159:8, 1964

Couinaud C: Controlled hepatectomies and exposure of the intrahepatic bile ducts. Paris: C Couinaud, 1981

Fahim RB, McDonald JR, et al: Carcinoma of the gallbladder: A study of its modes of spread. Ann Surg 156:114, 1962

Ferris DO, Vibert JC: The common bile duct: Significance of its diameter. Ann Surg 149:249, 1959

Flannery MG, Caster MP: Congenital abnormalities of the gallbladder: 101 cases. Int Abstr Surg 103:439, 1956

Frey C, Bizer L, et al: Agenesis of the gallbladder. Am J Surg 114:917, 1967

Harlaftis NS, Gray W, et al: Three cases of unsuspected double gallbladder. Am Surg 42:178, 1976

Langley JR, Hull DC: Congenital absence of the gallbladder: Review of the literature and report of a new case. Am Surg 40:548, 1974

Leslie D: The width of the common bile duct. Surg Gynecol Obstet 126:761, 1968

Michels NA: Blood Supply and Anatomy of the Upper Abdominal Organs. Philadelphia: JB Lippincott, 1955

Northover JMA, Terblanche J: A new look at the arterial supply of the bile duct in man and its surgical implications. Br J Surg 66:379, 1979

Skandalakis JE, Gray SW, et al: Biliary tract, in Skandalakis JE, Gray SW, et al (eds): Anatomical Complications in General Surgery. New York: McGraw-Hill, 1983

71. Evaluation of Jaundice

Seymour I. Schwartz

"Jaundice" is derived from the French word for "yellow" and refers to the presence of an excess of bile pigments in the tissue and the serum. The differential diagnosis and management are dependent upon an appreciation of the normal and abnormal variants of bile pigment metabolism. "Surgical" jaundice may be distinguished from other etiologic factors by relatively simple means in approximately 80 percent of cases, but the remaining 20 percent demand a sophisticated knowledge of metabolism and excretion of bile pigments.

NORMAL BILE PIGMENT METABOLISM

The bile pigment bilirubin is a tetrapyrrole that is transported, conjugated, stored, and excreted by the liver cells. It is derived from several sources, the majority of which are red cells destroyed by the reticuloendothelial (RE) system, either at the end of their natural life-span, or prematurely. To a lesser extent, bilirubin derives from myoglobin breakdown, the turnover of nonhemoglobin heme-containing proteins in the liver, the degradation of hemoglobin during erythrocyte maturation in the bone marrow, and the intramedullary destruction of newly formed erythrocytes. When the red blood cell is destroyed, the heme ring is opened and transformed into biliverdin, which is reduced to become bilirubin. The bilirubin combines with albumin to form a relatively stable complex that is transported to the hepatic parenchymal cell. This complex is a lipoid soluble pigment that gives an indirect van den Bergh diazo reaction only after treatment with alcohol and other substances that split the protein bond. The bilirubin albumin complex is poorly soluble in water and is not excreted in urine.

The complex is transported via the portal vein or hepatic artery into the sinusoidal circulation of the liver, where it is acted upon by the hepatocyte. The albumin is removed and the bilirubin is conjugated with glucuronic acid to form diglucuronide, which is water soluble and excreted into the bile canaliculi. This substance gives an immediate diazo reaction, and is, therefore, termed "direct reacting" in the van den Bergh test. It is readily excreted into the urine. When liver function is impaired, conjugation may take place from the kidney, small intestine, and other tissues. Other hydrophilic groups such as sulfates may be used as conjugates. Normally there is less than 0.3 mg of indirect-reacting serum bilirubin and less than 1.2 mg of direct-reacting serum bilirubin per liter of serum.

The conjugated bilirubin that is excreted via the bile into the intestine is acted upon by bacteria and undergoes a series of reductive reactions leading to the formation of two compounds—the colorless urobilinogen, which is further converted to stercobilin that provides the characteristic brown color of feces, and urobilin. The normal daily fecal excretion varies between 40 and 300 mg. In children, the values are lower, and in newborns, because of the absence of bacterial flora, urobilinogen may be absent. A reduction in enteric bacteria is also responsible for the reduced pigment excretion that accompanies the use of intestinal antibiotics. Some urobilinogen is reabsorbed by the portal system and reexcreted by the liver and kidney.

HYPERBILIRUBINEMIA

Before focusing on the conditions responsible for jaundice, conditions that may simulate jaundice must be ruled out. Hypercarotinemia

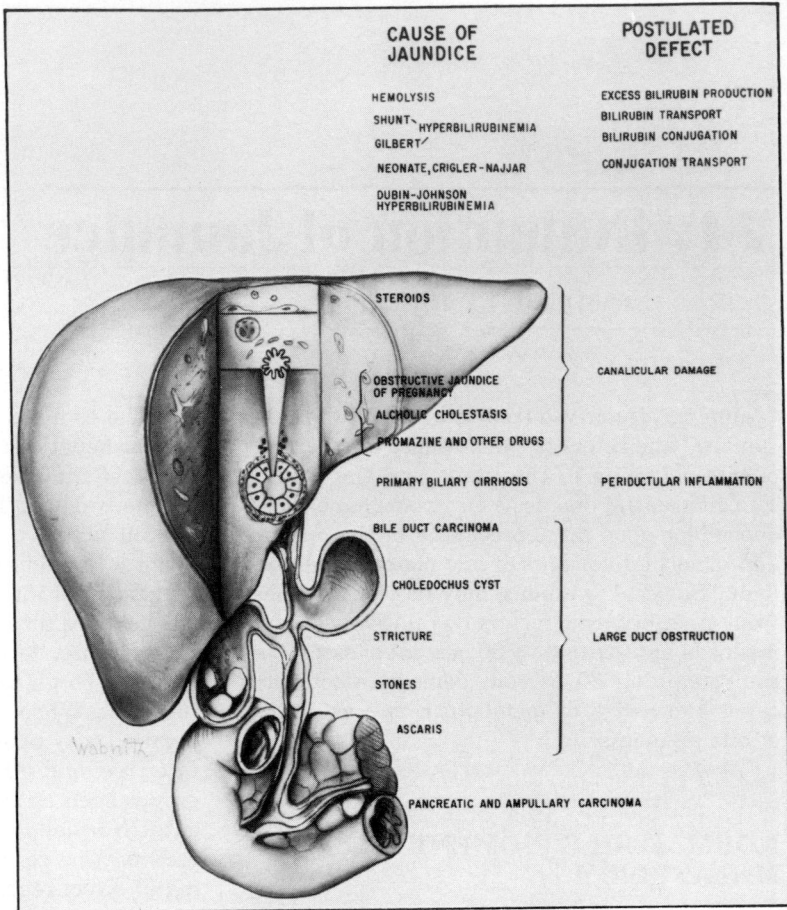

CAUSE OF JAUNDICE

HEMOLYSIS
SHUNT — HYPERBILIRUBINEMIA
GILBERT
NEONATE, CRIGLER-NAJJAR
DUBIN-JOHNSON HYPERBILIRUBINEMIA

STEROIDS

OBSTRUCTIVE JAUNDICE OF PREGNANCY
ALCHOLIC CHOLESTASIS
PROMAZINE AND OTHER DRUGS

PRIMARY BILIARY CIRRHOSIS

BILE DUCT CARCINOMA

CHOLEDOCHUS CYST

STRICTURE

STONES

ASCARIS

PANCREATIC AND AMPULLARY CARCINOMA

POSTULATED DEFECT

EXCESS BILIRUBIN PRODUCTION
BILIRUBIN TRANSPORT
BILIRUBIN CONJUGATION
CONJUGATION TRANSPORT

CANALICULAR DAMAGE

PERIDUCTULAR INFLAMMATION

LARGE DUCT OBSTRUCTION

Figure 71–1. Abnormal bile pigment metabolism. (*Source: From Schwartz SI, Storer EH: Manifestations of gastrointestinal disease, in Schwartz SI, Shires GT, et al (eds): Principles of Surgery, 4 edt. New York: McGraw-Hill, 1984, with permission.*)

is the most common condition in this category. The pigment has an affinity for the palms of the hands, the soles of the feet, the areas of the face covered by sebaceous glands, and the hair; in contrast, jaundice has an affinity for elastic tissue, particularly in the mucous membranes and bulbar conjunctiva. The diagnosis of hypercarotinemia can be established by demonstration of an elevated serum carotene (normal of 40 to 300 μg/dl). Other uncommon forms of yellow pigmentation may come from drugs such as atabrine.

No classification of jaundice is entirely satisfactory. The classification most widely used distinguishes between hemolytic, hepatocellular, and obstructive jaundice and focuses on a distinction between those states in which the bile flow is unimpeded and those types that are associated with impairment of bile flow (Fig. 71–1).

Unconjugated Hyperbilirubinemia

The overproduction of bile pigment from excessive hemolysis creates a situation in which the normal liver is confronted with more pigment than it is able to remove. This occurs in physiologic jaundice of infancy and in all pathologic hemolytic states. The reserve capacity of the liver is great, however, and even when the bilirubin production is increased six-fold, there is a rise in the serum bilirubin of only 2 to 3 mg/dl. Since the material is unconjugated it does not appear in the urine, but there is an increase in fecal and urinary urobilinogen.

Unconjugated hyperbilirubinemia is generally the result of an increased production associated with a variety of the hereditary or congenital anemias such as spherocytosis, nonspherocytic anemia, thalassemia, and sickle cell anemia. An increased production of bilirubin is also a consequence of acquired hemolytic anemia, paroxysmal nocturnal hemoglobinuria, and shunt hyperbilirubinemia. In this circumstance, indirect-reacting bilirubin accumulates in the absence of any reduction of the red cell life-span. Hemolytic states also may be associated with ingestion of a variety of chemical agents, poisons, severe burns, and sepsis.

Increased levels of unconjugated bilirubin also occur with several transport and storage diseases. In Gilbert's disease, where there is hyperbilirubinemia without impairment of the bile flow, there is a defect in the bilirubin transport into the liver cells. This is the most common form of unconjugated hyperbilirubinemia not associated with hemolysis. The serum bilirubin values are usually less than 5 mg/dl and, although the jaundice is present in early childhood, at times it may not be recognized until later in life. The Crigler–Najjar's syndrome has been divided into two types. In Type I, the bilirubin concentration may rise to 30 mg/dl, and kernicterus is frequent. The conjugation defect in these patients is transmitted as an autosomal recessive. In Type II, the bilirubin values are less than 20 mg/dl, and kernicterus does not occur. The conjugation defect in this type is transmitted as an autosomal dominant. In this category, a striking improvement in jaundice occurs within weeks following treatment with phenobarbital. Another familial disorder is the Lucey–Driscoll's syndrome, where there is an unconjugated neonatal hyperbilirubinemia and an accompanying kernicterus. This disorder is caused by a steroid that inhibits glucuronyl transferase activity and is found in the mother's serum. It disappears rapidly in both maternal and infant serum after delivery. The jaundice of neonates can also be caused by abnormal steroids in breast milk.

Conjugated Hyperbilirubinemia

An accumulation of conjugated bilirubin in the blood may be due to impaired hepatic excretion or extrahepatic obstruction. This bilirubin pigment is water soluble and is readily excreted into the urine, which becomes brown.

The intrahepatic impaired excretion may be related to a congenital secretory failure. The excretion of conjugated bilirubin is impaired in the Dubin–Johnson's syndrome, which is associated with normal liver function and the appearance of iron-free pigment in the hepatic cells.

A variant of the Dubin–Johnson's syndrome is the Rotor's syndrome, in which no pigment is found in the liver. Intrahepatic obstruction and impaired excretion occur in cirrhosis and hepatitis, and also in diffuse carcinomatosis, amyloidosis, and granulomatous disease involving the liver.

Jaundice from hepatocellular degeneration is associated with morphologic changes in the parenchymal cells and abnormal liver function. It has been suggested that in these disorders there is regurgitation of bilirubin from the bile canaliculi into tissue spaces. Although there is a reduction in the ability of the liver cell to convert the bilirubin protein to bilirubin glucuronide, this defect causes a rise in both bilirubin and its conjugates. Intrahepatic cholestasis has also been related to a variety of drugs and hepatocellular diseases. Methyltestosterone and norethandrolone damage the microvilli of the bile canaliculi and cause jaundice. Phenothiazine drugs, such as chlorpromazine, may evoke a hypersensitivity reaction in a small percentage of patients and result in a cholangiolitic hepatitis and intrahepatic cholestasis with conjugated hyperbilirubinemia.

Extrahepatic cholestasis is caused by an anatomic obstacle to the flow of bile from the liver to the intestine. The obstacle may be situated anywhere from the junction of the right and left hepatic ducts to the termination of the common bile duct in the duodenum. Atresia, stricture, choledocholithiasis, tumors of the bile duct and pancreas, choledochal cysts, and parasites all have been implicated. Obstruction of the extrahepatic ducts results in an increase of serum bilirubin, particularly of the direct-reacting type, the appearance of bile in the urine, and the passage of clay-colored stools. When the total bilirubin level is above 3 mg/L the increases in both direct and indirect reacting fractions parallel each other. With complete and persistent obstruction, the serum bilirubin levels may plateau. If the obstruction is fluctuating, the levels will change (Fig. 71–1).

PATIENT EVALUATION

History. Congenital and inflammatory diseases occur more commonly in children and young adults. A detailed family history and a history of drug ingestion should be taken. Loss of appetite, fever, and change in smoking habits are particularly suggestive of hepatitis and hepatocellular dysfunction. Inquiry into chronic alcohol ingestion is important. Jaundice secondary to obstruction of the extrahepatic ducts usually starts insidiously and becomes progressively more pronounced. Gastrointestinal (GI) symptoms are uncommon, with the exception of those related to biliary calculi. Although, classically, carcinoma of the head of the pancreas is painless, some 20 to 30 percent of these patients complain of deep epigastric distress or backache. Extrahepatic obstruction is associated with ascending cholangitis and may be accompanied by spiking fevers and abdominal pain. Pruritus occurs more often in obstructive jaundice but can occur with primary cholangitis or with primary biliary cirrhosis; it is almost never associated with hemolytic jaundice.

Physical Examination. Jaundice is apparent when the serum bilirubin level exceeds 2 mg/L. Tissues rich in elastic fibers have a particular affinity for bilirubin, and this accounts for the earlier appearance and greater intensity in the sclerae and in the skin of the face and upper trunk. Jaundice is not a mere reflection of the yellow pigment through the skin from underlying interstitial fluid but, rather, a deposition of pigment in the tissue fibers and cells. Tissues stain more readily with direct bilirubin than with the indirect reacting fraction. There is a failure to stain areas of marked edema and vitiligo.

Inspection of the skin may reveal a rash typical of drug reaction, the spider angiomas of cirrhosis, or excoriations suggestive of pruritus. Splenomegaly may be present with hemolytic jaundice. Hepatomegaly and hepatic tenderness are predominant findings in viral hepatitis. An enlarged, hard, nodular liver is almost certainly indicative of carcinoma. A palpable gallbladder in a patient with extrahepatic obstruction occurs more frequently when the obstruction is related to malignancy distal to the cystic duct entrance into the common duct, and less commonly when the obstruction is due to biliary calculi. This axiom, known as Courvoisier's law, however, is not universal.

An acholic stool is usually a consequence of obstructive jaundice and is characterized by its grey appearance. The fact that bile pigments are contributing to a darkened urine is readily demonstrated by the foam test; this is positive when there is a yellow tint to the foam after the urine is vigorously shaken. A positive reaction occurs in patients with hepatocellular and obstructive jaundice but is not present in patients with hemolytic disease.

Laboratory Studies. Hemolytic jaundice is accompanied by anemia and increased reticulocyte count. Smears for spherocytes, target cells, and sickle cells should be made. These and other tests related to hemolysis are specifically discussed in the section on splenectomy for hematologic disorders. Stools should be assessed for pigment and the presence or absence of guaiac reaction indicative of bleeding. With carcinoma of the pancreas, approximately one third of the patients have guaiac positive stool; this occurs more frequently in patients with obstructive jaundice secondary to carcinoma of the ampulla of Vater.

Serum determinations of the bilirubin including assessment of the 1-minute direct (conjugated soluble) fraction test should be carried out. In patients with jaundice secondary to extrahepatic obstruction or hepatocellular degeneration, the determination of the direct fraction is a more sensitive index of impairment than the total serum bilirubin. In hepatocellular dysfunction there is impaired production of albumin, fibrinogen, and prothrombin, which are formed solely in the liver. With hepatocellular disease, the cholesterol level falls and the esterfied fraction almost disappears; in patients with obstruction the cholesterol level rises. The alkaline phosphatase is a sensitive indicator of obstruction either from extrahepatic causes or a cholangitic process. The transaminases, including the SGOT and the SGPT, are regarded the most valuable of the enzyme determinations, and an elevation generally is indicative of hepatocellular disease. Lower levels of elevation are found in obstructive jaundice while higher levels, especially those in the range of 400 to 500 units or above, are highly suggestive of hepatocellular involvement.

Removal of foreign dye from the liver is dependent upon hepatic blood flow, hepatocellular function, and biliary excretion. Bromsulphalein (BSP), rose bengal, and indocyanine have all been used but the bromsulphalein test is of little value in the icteric patient. The response of prothrombin time to the injection of parenteral vitamin K may be used to differentiate between hepatocellular and obstructive jaundice. An increase in prothrombin time within 48 hours of parenteral administration suggests a diagnosis of obstructive jaundice; a lack of response is more compatible with hepatocellular disease.

Radiologic Studies. An x-ray of the abdomen will reveal gallstones in 20 percent of patients in whom they are present. The oral cholecystogram rarely visualizes the gallbladder or ducts if serum bilirubin is above 1.8 mg/L. Intravenous cholangiography has been replaced by radionuclide scans. The technetium-99m-pyridoxylideneglutamate biliary scan is a safe,

noninvasive means of distinguishing between jaundice due to hepatobiliary disease and that due to partial or complete extrahepatic bile duct obstruction. It is applicable even if the bilirubin is elevated to a 20 mg/L level. Ultrasonography has provided means of detecting biliary calculi and also for identifying dilated intrahepatic and extrahepatic ducts. Computed tomography (CT) will also demonstrate dilatation of intrahepatic and/or extrahepatic portions of the biliary tract. Both percutaneous transhepatic cholangi-

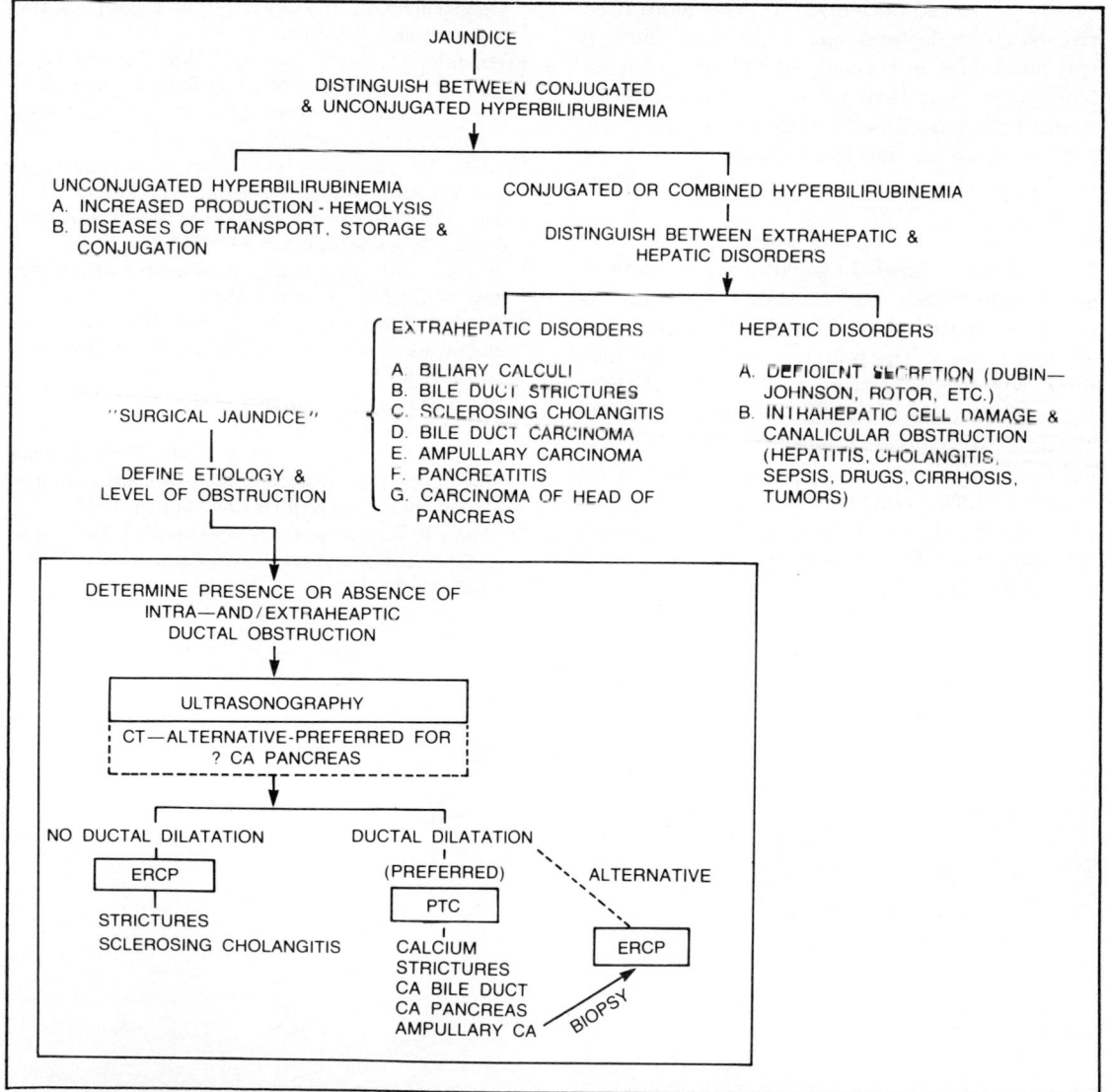

Figure 71–2. Algorithm for differential diagnosis of jaundice; within the box are diagnostic procedures related to "surgical jaundice."

ography (PTC) and endoscopic retrograde cholangiopancreatography (ERCP) may contribute to the diagnosis, providing direct visualization of the duct system. In experienced hands, 90 to 95 percent success rates for ERCP definition of the extrahepatic biliary system have been reported, but in most institutions the yield is less than 65 percent. Cholangitis or pancreatitis are uncommon complications. The technique is uniquely suited for the evaluation of sclerosing cholangitis and carcinoma of the ampulla of Vater; in the latter case a biopsy will establish the diagnosis. In a randomized trial comparing PTC with ERCP for bile duct visualization in deeply jaundiced patients, PTC was more effective when cholestasis had a surgical cause. It was successful in 95 percent of cases with extrahepatic cholestasis and in 25 percent of patients with intrahepatic cholestasis; ERCP was successful in 62 percent of patients with extrahepatic and 76 percent with intrahepatic cholestasis.

Liver Biopsy and Laparotomy. Percutaneous needle biopsy may establish the diagnosis in patients with hepatocellular disease and obviate laparotomy. The patient should be screened for deficiency in clotting mechanism. If there is marked ascites or significant alteration in the clotting mechanism, it may be safer to carry out the liver biopsy as an open procedure under local anesthesia. Laparotomy may be required to establish a diagnosis in an occasional patient. An algorithm for patient evaluation is presented in Figure 71–2.

BIBLIOGRAPHY

Arias IM: The pathogenesis of "physiologic" jaundice of the newborn: A reevaluation. Birth Defects 6:55, 1970

Blumgart LH, Salmon PR, et al: Endoscopy and retrograde cholecochopancreatography in diagnosis of patient with jaundice. Surg Gynecol Obstet 138:565, 1974

Chalmers TC, Alter HJ: Management of the asymptomatic carrier of the hepatitis-associated (Australia) antigen. N Engl J Med 285:613, 1971

Elias E, Hamlyn AN, et al: A randomized trial of percutaneous transhepatic cholangiography with the Chiba needle versus endoscopic retrograde cholangiography for bile visualization in jaundice. Gastroenterology 71:439, 1976

Freimanis AT: Intraabdominal fluid collections, in Gottlieb S, Viamonte M Jr (eds): Diagnostic Ultrasound. Chicago: The American College of Radiology, Committee on New Technology, 1976

Havrilla TR, Hagga JR, et al: Computed tomography and obstructive biliary disease. AJR 128:765, 1977

Jander HP, Galbraith J, et al: Percutaneous transhepatic cholangiography using the Chiba needle: Comparison with retrograde pancreatocholecystography. South Med J 73:415, 1980

Levitt RG, Sagel SS, et al: Accuracy of computed tomography of the liver and biliary tract. Radiology 124:123, 1977

Smith R, Sherlock S: Surgery of the Gall Bladder and Bile Ducts. London: Butterworths, 1964

Williams JAR, Baker RJ, et al: Role of biliary scanning in the investigation of the surgically jaundiced patient. Surg Gynecol Obstet 144:525, 1977

Williams R: Recent advances in jaundice: Medical aspects of investigation and treatment. Br Med J 1:225, 1970

72. Extrahepatic Biliary Atresia

Edward R. Howard

Atresia means "without a lumen," and in extrahepatic biliary atresia bile flow is obstructed by occlusion or even complete destruction of part or all of the extrahepatic bile duct. The incidence in Great Britain is approximately 1 in 14,000 live births. Traditionally, cases were divided into "correctable" and "noncorrectable" types depending on the presence or absence of patent proximal segments of bile ducts. "Correctable" biliary atresia therefore implied the patency of hepatic or proximal bile ducts that could be treated by conventional techniques of biliary–enteric anastomosis. "Noncorrectable" suggested that all attempts at surgical treatment would fail.

Recent surgical results have shown this classification to be inappropriate. Many cases treated as correctable types have failed to drain bile and a number of noncorrectable cases treated by radical excision of the extrahepatic duct system (portoenterostomy) have been cured. The 4-year survival rate in untreated cases is 2 percent but surgical treatment can improve the outlook; a review of recent results suggests that a 5-year survival rate of approximately 35 percent may be achieved when the portoenterostomy operation is performed before 10 weeks of age.

HISTORICAL NOTE

The first major review of 49 cases published by Thomson in 1891 and 1892 concluded that, whatever the aetiology of biliary atresia, it was characterised by a progressive, destructive inflammatory lesion of the bile ducts.

The first suggestion that surgical treatment might be effective in biliary atresia was made in 1916 by Holmes, who collected 120 cases from the literature. He estimated that 16 percent might be correctable by surgery. Ladd (1928) described a further 20 cases in detail; 11 of these underwent operation and 8 were considered correctable (40 percent). Six recovered from the operation, but analysis of these case reports suggests that two were examples of choledochal cysts, two were cases of hepatitis with hypoplastic ducts, and two were rare examples of atresia of the distal common bile duct. In general, the surgical results remained extremely poor; Hays and Snyder reported in 1963 that in most American series less than 5 percent of the patients survived beyond early childhood. These poor results led to trials of partial hepatic resection, insertion of tubes into the hepatic parenchyma, thoracic duct lymph drainage to the oesophagus, and hepatic lymph drainage to the jejunum. These techniques failed to prolong the survival of children. In 1959, Kasai and Suzuki described a new radical operation for "noncorrectable" atresia that was based on the histologic observation that remnants of the extrahepatic ducts in the region of the porta hepatis frequently showed bile-containing ductules up to 300 μm in diameter. It was suggested that anastomosis of this tissue to bowel could lead to effective bile drainage. Approximately 85 percent of cases of extrahepatic biliary atresia are of the "noncorrectable" type and the Kasai (1974) procedure presently is regarded as the only possible treatment. The only alternative appears to be liver transplantation, details of which are beyond the scope of this chapter and are discussed elsewhere.

AETIOLOGY

Although many theories have been suggested, the aetiology of biliary atresia remains unknown. Associated developmental defects such

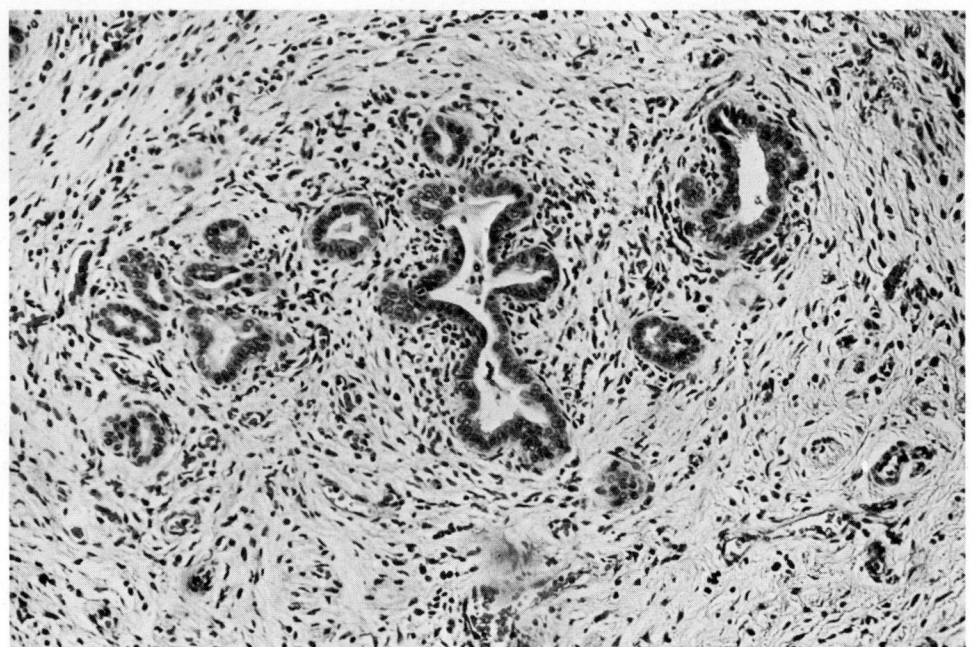

Figure 72–1. The microscopic appearance of residual bile duct tissue excised from the porta hepatis of a 3-month-old infant with "noncorrectable" biliary atresia. Small ductules lined by cuboidal epithelium are visible within the fibrous tissue. (H&E)

as malrotation of the gut, situs inversus, and polysplenia are present in less than 15 percent of cases and experimental occlusion of fetal bile ducts produces choledochal cysts rather than biliary atresia. No relationship has been found with either teratogenic drugs or ionizing radiation and there is no obvious link with ischaemic injury. A viral aetiology has been suggested on several occasions but viral studies in patients have remained inconclusive and electron microscopic examination of tissue resected at surgery has failed to show any infective agent. Abnormalities in the metabolism of L-proline affecting growth of the biliary tract (Vacanti and Folkman, 1979) and monohydroxy bile acids causing bile duct inflammation have also been investigated (Jenner and Howard, 1975). Anatomic studies have suggested the presence, in some cases, of an abnormally long common channel distal to the junction of the bile and pancreatic ducts, but the significance of this observation remains unclear at the moment.

PATHOLOGY (FIG. 72–1)

Histology of the extrahepatic ducts shows a destructive inflammatory process with inflammatory cells of all types and a variable degree of fibrosis (Bill et al, 1977; Haas, 1978). The inflammatory process is not confined to the bile ducts and gallbladder but also affects the periductal tissues and increased vascularity is a prominent feature during surgery. Hyperplastic lymph nodes and enlarged extrahepatic lymphatics are also found in the region of the porta hepatis. Studies of the extrahepatic ducts excised at surgery have been published by Gautier et al (1981), who classified the abnormalities into three types. Type 1 cases showed no residual ductal tissue and few inflammatory cells. Type 2 contained small residual lumina lined with cuboidal epithelium but with a diameter less than 50 μm. Polymorphonuclear leucocytes were seen in this tissue. Type 3 tissues retained obvious central structures resembling residual bile ducts with evidence of columnar epithelium. Bile staining was reported in 68 percent of Type 3 cases, mostly within macrophages.

Intrahepatic bile ducts remain patent during the first 2 to 3 months after birth and studies of the bile ducts in the region of the porta hepatis have revealed that the major ducts divide into many small branches, which terminate in the residual extrahepatic inflammatory ductal tissue. The intrahepatic ducts undergo progressive destruction in the newborn period so that surgery is most effective before 10 weeks of age. *Early and rapid investigation, diagnosis and treatment is therefore mandatory.*

The histologic features of the hepatic parenchyma in biliary atresia include giant cell transformation, focal hepatocellular degeneration, necrosis, pseudoacinous formation, and extramedullary haemopoiesis. The portal tracts are affected by fibrosis, oedema, and inflammatory change, which is accompanied by proliferation of bile ductules that contain bile plugs. Progression of the disease leads rapidly to biliary cirrhosis with increasing periportal fibrosis.

Correlations of postoperative bile flow with numbers and size of luminal structures observed in the tissue of the porta hepatis have shown conflicting results (Gautier et al, 1976). Bile flow seems more successful when the diameter of residual ducts exceeds 150 μm. However, bile flow can occur in the presence of very small ductules and has even been observed in cases in which *no* duct remnants were identified. It is likely that intrahepatic inflammation and fibrosis are probably as important in determining the effectiveness of bile flow as are the histologic features of the extrahepatic tissue in the porta hepatis.

Although the morphology of the extrahepatic bile duct tissue varies widely in atresia, the Japanese Society of Pediatric Surgeons (1980) identified three principal types, which form the basis of their classification now in general use (Fig. 72–2):

Type 1—atresia of the common bile duct
Type 2—atresia of the common hepatic duct
Type 3—atresia of right and left hepatic ducts

Subdivisions of this classification depend on details of the morphology of the gallbladder and distal common bile duct as well as the histologic features of the tissue at the porta hepatis. Non-communicating cystic dilatations of the extrahepatic bile duct tissue may accompany any of these types and may make the macroscopic diagnosis at laparotomy difficult. Confusion with choledochal cyst has sometimes occurred.

CLINICAL MANIFESTATIONS

Infants with biliary atresia commonly have normal birth weights. Jaundice and acholic stools are noted within the first 2 weeks of life in 80 percent of the patients, and enlargement of the liver and spleen are common findings. Conjugated hyperbilirubinaemia in infancy is also a presenting feature of the infective, metabolic, and other medical causes of neonatal hepatitis syndrome as well as inspissated bile syndrome, intrahepatic hypoplasia, choledochal cyst, and spontaneous perforation of the common bile duct (Howard et al, 1976).

Infants with biliary atresia usually appear well nourished during the first few months of life and have no clinical features of chronic liver disease. Failure to thrive occurs only in the later stages of the disease.

DIAGNOSTIC STUDIES

Examination of the stools in a jaundiced infant is most important, for when they are white, or acholic, biliary atresia must be high on the list of differential diagnoses.

Techniques used for the investigation of conjugated hyperbilirubinaemia in infants include:

- Screening tests (infection, metabolic disorders, genetic disorders—especially 1-antitrypsin deficiency, etc.)
- Liver biopsy
- Duodenal intubation for bile (Greene et al, 1979)
- Ultrasonography
- I-131-rose bengal faecal excretion
- Radionuclide hepatobiliary imaging (Jenner et al, 1978)
- Percutaneous cholangiography (Howard and Nunnerley, 1979)
- Laparoscopy
- Operative cholangiography (Leape and Ramenofsky, 1977)

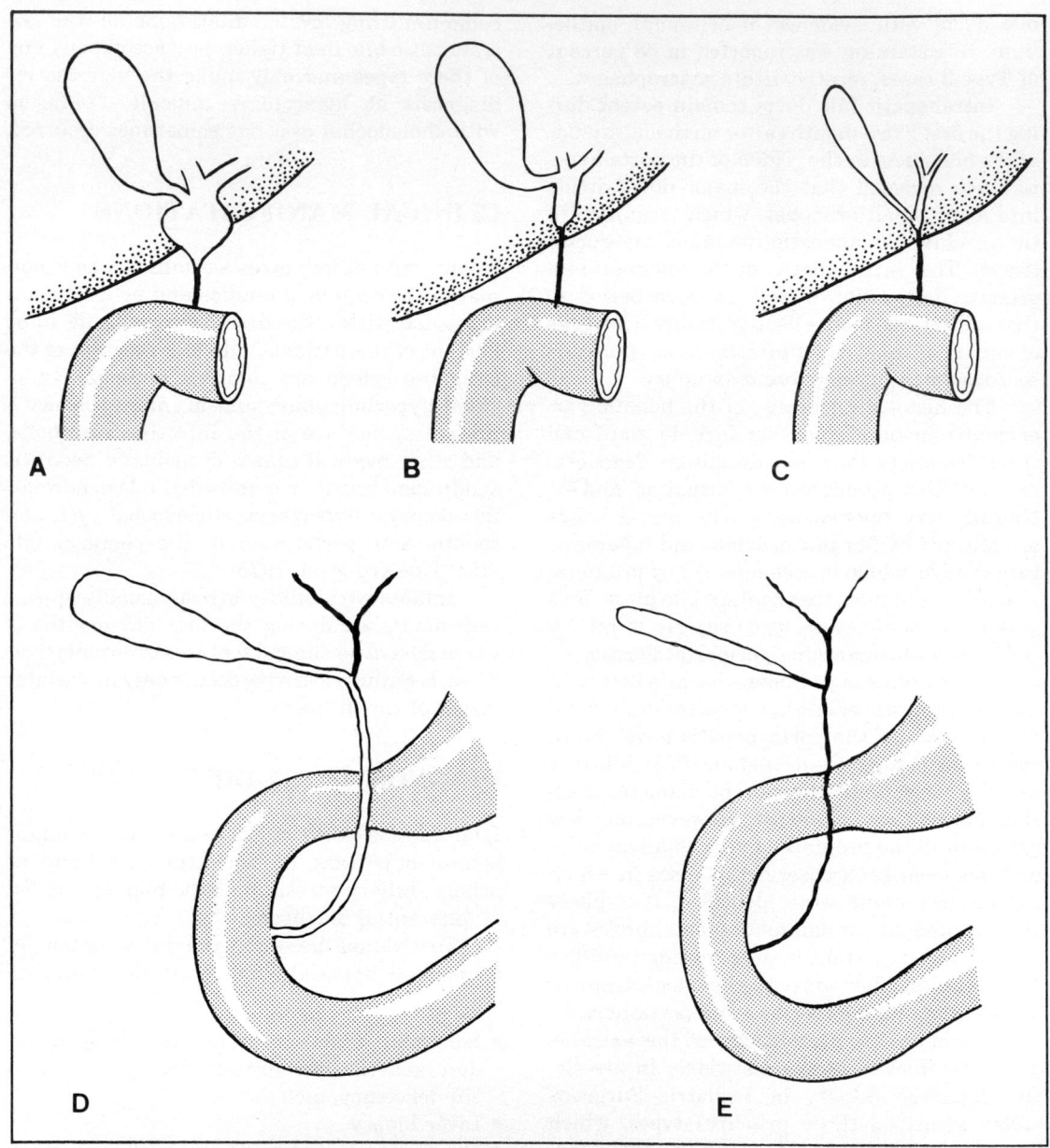

Figure 72–2. Some examples of extrahepatic biliary atresia. **A, B,** and **C** are types of "correctable" atresia in which there is occlusion of the distal common bile duct. **D** and **E** represent the more common varieties of "noncorrectable" atresia with occlusion of the proximal bile ducts.

Standard liver function tests do not differentiate clearly between medical and surgical causes of conjugated hyperbilirubinaemia in early infancy although a low gamma glutamyl transpeptidase value suggests a hepatocellular rather than a bile duct disorder. The specific screening tests for infection, metabolic, or genetic disease identify approximately 30 percent of the causes of hepatitis syndrome, the remainder being termed idiopathic.

An unequivocal diagnosis of atresia on liver biopsy may be made by an experienced pathologist in 80 to 90 percent of cases, but difficulty is encountered when there is marked hepatocellular necrosis, cholestasis, and giant cell transformation, all features of hepatitis. Choledochal cyst in early infancy may cause intrahepatic changes consistent with extrahepatic biliary atresia, but diagnosis of the cyst is usually suspected from displacement of the duodenal loop on barium meal and confirmed by ultrasound examination of the right hypochondrium.

The faecal excretion of an injected dose of I-131-rose bengal gives a measure of bile excretion into the gut (Sharp et al, 1967), and 75 percent may be recovered from a 3-day collection of faeces in a normal infant. An excretion value below 8 percent is very suggestive of biliary atresia. Recently ultrasonography and percutaneous cholangiography have been added to the investigations and patent bile ducts have been demonstrated in infants with hepatitis (Fig. 72–3).

Intrahepatic hypoplasia, which is found in association with patent extrahepatic ducts, must be considered in the differential diagnosis. Liver biopsy may show less fibrous tissue than cases of extrahepatic atresia but bile ducts are either reduced in number or absent from the portal triads. This syndrome, described by Porter et al (1968) and Alagille et al (1975) is often associated with characteristic facial features, vertebral and cardiac anomalies, and is compatible with survival for a number of years.

SURGICAL TREATMENT

Traditionally the surgical treatment of biliary atresia consisted of two stages. At the first operation a minilaparotomy was performed through a small transverse incision in the right hypochondrium and operative cholangiography followed inspection of the liver and biliary tract. A liver biopsy completed this procedure. Definitive surgery was attempted as a second stage a few days later. However, in many cases the two-stage management is unnecessary for atresia can often be diagnosed from the characteristic appearances of the gallbladder and the extent of the atretic process rules out satisfactory cholangiography in nearly 75 percent of cases. Open liver biopsy is now being superseded by preoperative percutaneous biopsy and this is fol-

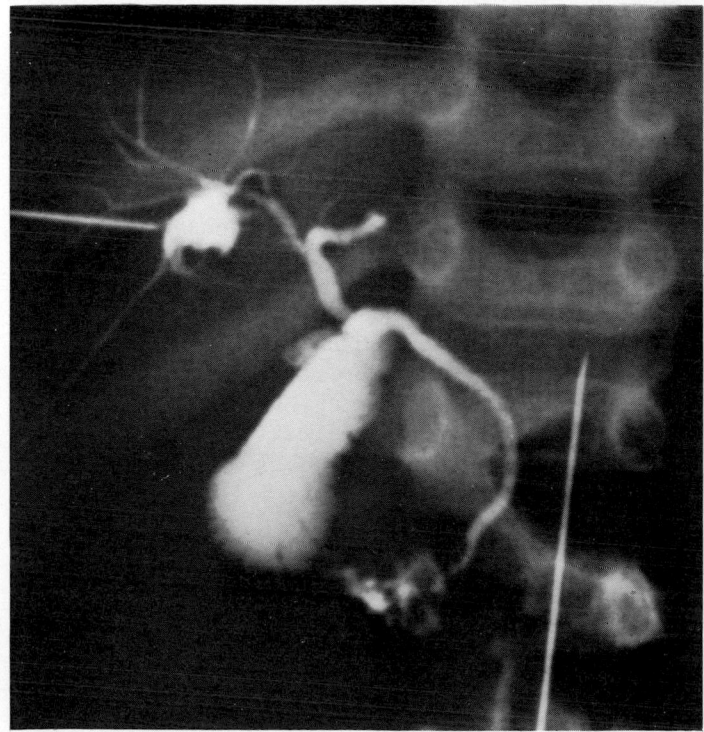

Figure 72–3. Percutaneous cholangiogram in a 5-month-old infant with hepatitis syndrome. Contrast material flows freely into the duodenum. Bile duct size is compared with the 19-gauge needle lying over the spine.

lowed by definitive surgery consisting of a radical resection of the occluded biliary tract and reconstruction with a Roux loop of jejunum.

All of the current radical operations (Bill, 1978; Howard, 1983; Jenner, 1978; Lilly, 1979) are based on the original procedure developed by Kasai (1974, 1978) in Japan following his original observation of residual microscopic bile channels in the fibrous tissue of the porta hepatis. The technique is now applied to the majority of cases, including the 15 to 20 percent who are found at laparotomy to have cystic bile-containing structures in the porta hepatis and in whom conventional bile-duct to bowel anastomoses have been applied in the past ("correctable" atresia). The surgical results for this latter group have been disappointing and the more radical "Kasai" approach is now recommended in most instances.

Preoperative Preparation. Vitamin K (phytomenadione), 1.0 mg/day, is administered intramuscularly for 4 days and oral neomycin (50 mg/kg/day in 6 divided doses) for 24 hours before the operation. One unit of blood is crossmatched and oral fluids are withheld from 4 hours before induction of anaesthesia. An adequate intravenous line is inserted and a nasogastric tube passed. The infant is placed supine on a thermostatically controlled warming pad and an x-ray cassette box must be in position for cholangiography. Intravenous antibiotics (a cephalosporin) are started with the induction of anaesthesia and continued for 5 days. An oral cephalosporin is then substituted for a further 3 weeks as prophylaxis against possible attacks of ascending cholangitis (see the following).

Operation (Original Kasai Portoenterostomy) (Fig. 72–4)

A transverse abdominal incision across the right rectus muscle is sited over the palpable liver edge, and the inferior surface of the right lobe of the liver is exposed. The gallbladder in cases of atresia is usually thick-walled, contracted, and hidden within a cleft of liver. The fundus of the gallbladder is exposed and incised within a purse string suture and a small polythene catheter is inserted. *Operative cholangiography is mandatory whenever bile is found in the gallbladder.* Two or three millilitres of contrast material (25 percent Hypaque*) is injected into the gallbladder and x-rays are taken. The demonstration of patent hepatic and common bile ducts terminates this procedure (Fig. 72–5). In some cases of atresia, the atretic process does not involve the cystic duct or distal common bile duct. Contrast may therefore flow into the duodenum but fails to fill the upper ducts (Fig. 72–6) even after occlusion of the supraduodenal portion of the common bile duct with a soft clamp. The confirmation of atresia is followed by an extension of the abdominal incision across the left rectus muscle.

Exposure of the porta hepatis and hepatoduodenal ligament is increased if the liver is depressed by the positioning of a small pack between the superior surface of the liver and the diaphragm.

Large lymph nodes frequently obscure the extrahepatic ducts, which are most easily identified by an initial mobilisation of the gallbladder from its liver bed. The vascularity of the gallbladder bed is usually increased and bleeding is controlled by the judicious use of diathermy and ligatures.

The cystic artery is ligated and the cystic duct traced to its junction with the fibrotic common bile duct. The distal portion of the common bile duct is divided between ligatures at the level of the upper border of the duodenum (Fig. 72–4D).

Dissection of the extrahepatic bile duct remnants is now performed toward the porta hepatis and meticulous tying with fine ligatures close to the ducts helps to prevent postoperative ascites from lymphatic leaks. The hepatic artery and portal vein are identified during this dissection, and the ductal system is traced above the bifurcation of the latter.

---

* Winthrop Laboratories.

Figure 72–4. The Kasai portoenterostomy operation. **A.** Abdominal incision. **B.** Insertion of cholangiogram catheter into gallbladder. **C.** Mobilisation of gallbladder and occluded bile ducts. **D.** Excision of occluded extrahepatic duct system. **E.** Transection of ductal tissue above bifurcation of portal vein flush with liver capsule. **F.** Anastomosis of Roux-Y loop (30 cm) of jejunum to porta hepatis–posterior layer. **G.** Anterior sutures begun to complete the anastomosis.

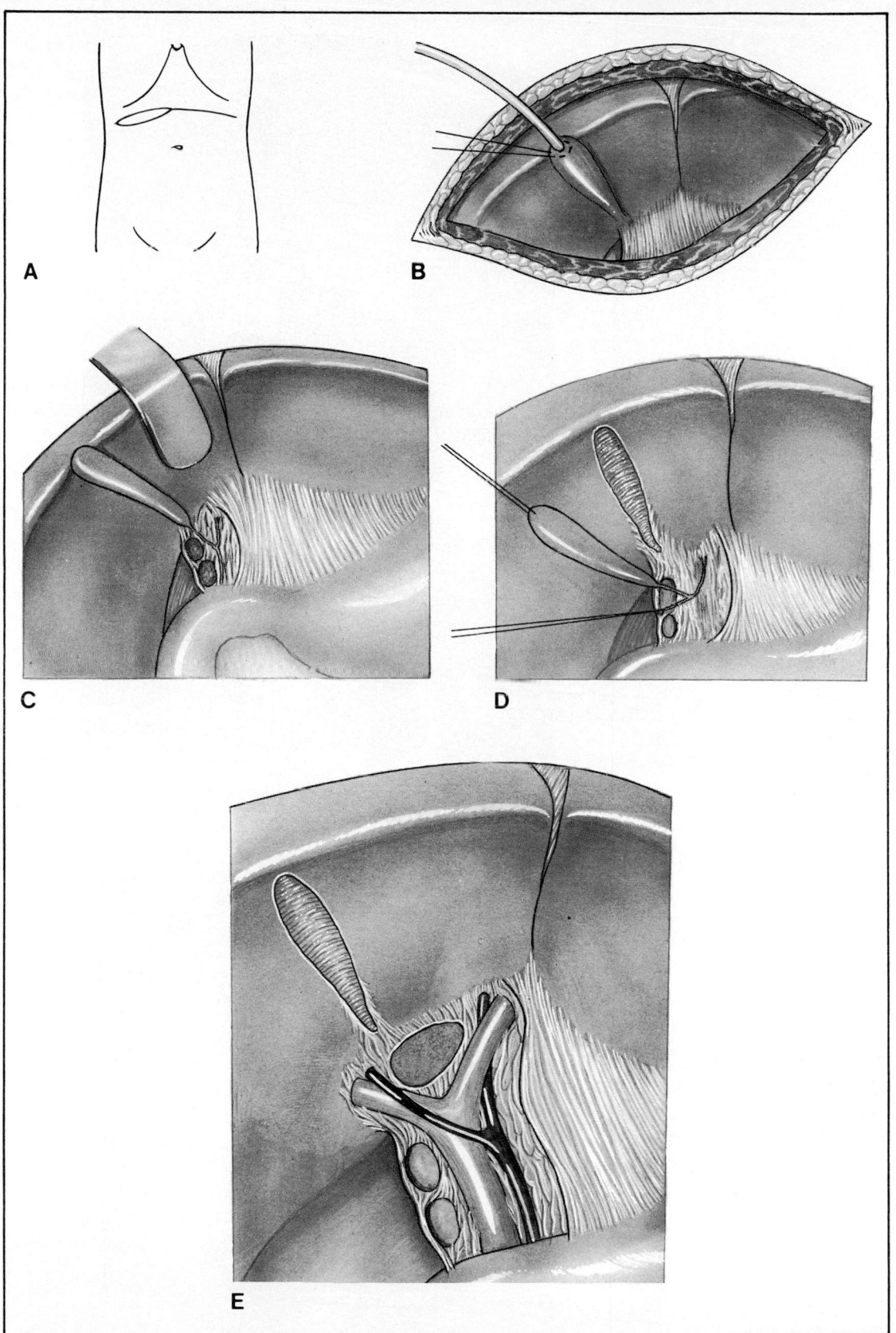

A

B

C

D

E

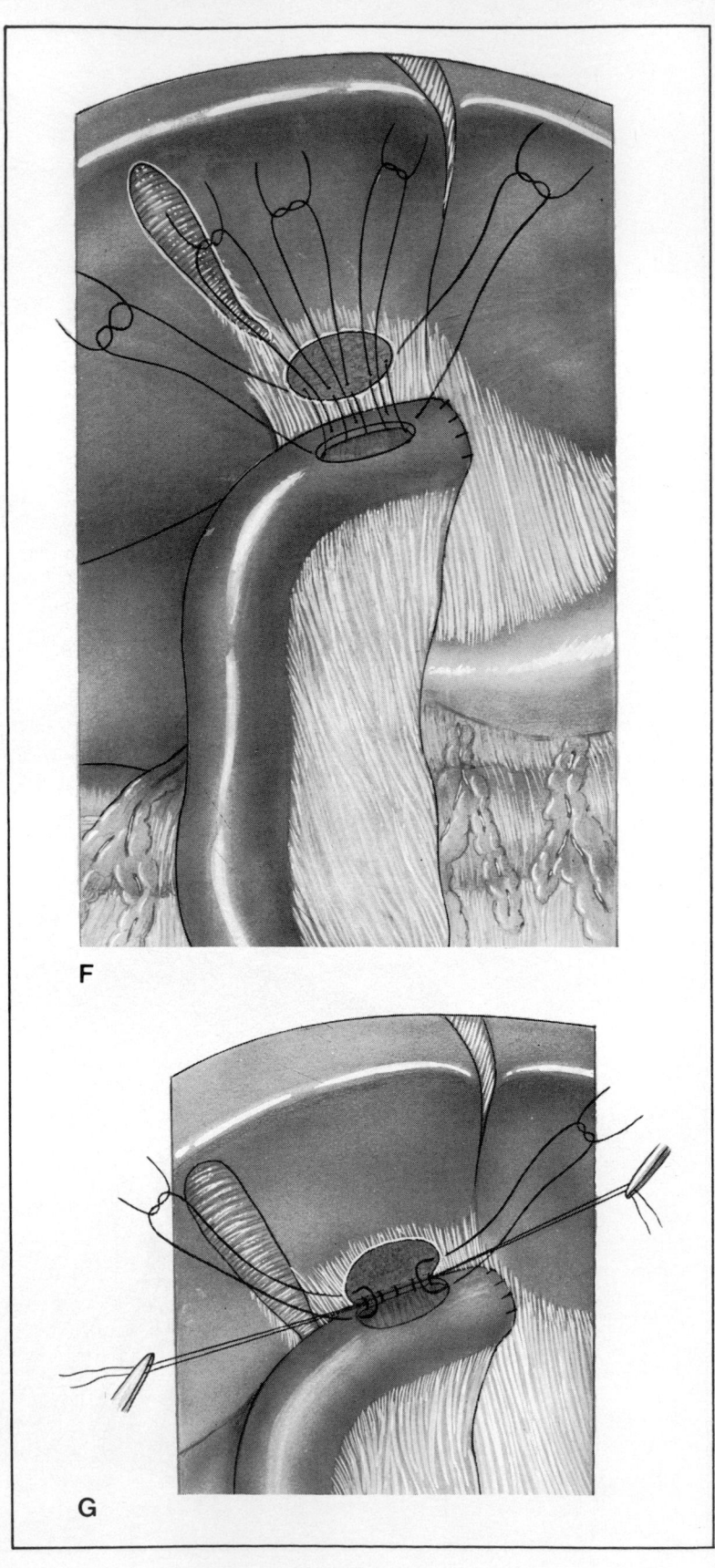

F

G

Figure 72–4. *Continued*

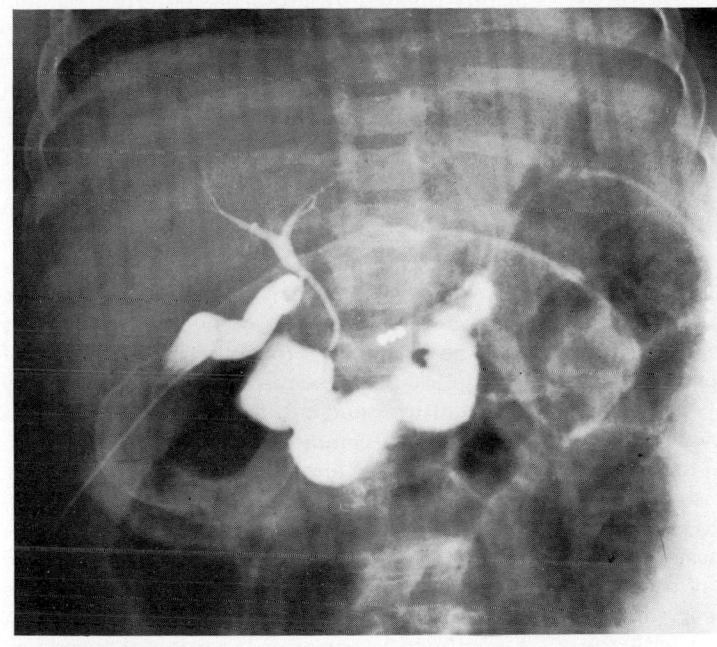

Figure 72–5. Operative cholangiogram in a 3-month-old infant with hypoplastic but patent extrahepatic bile ducts.

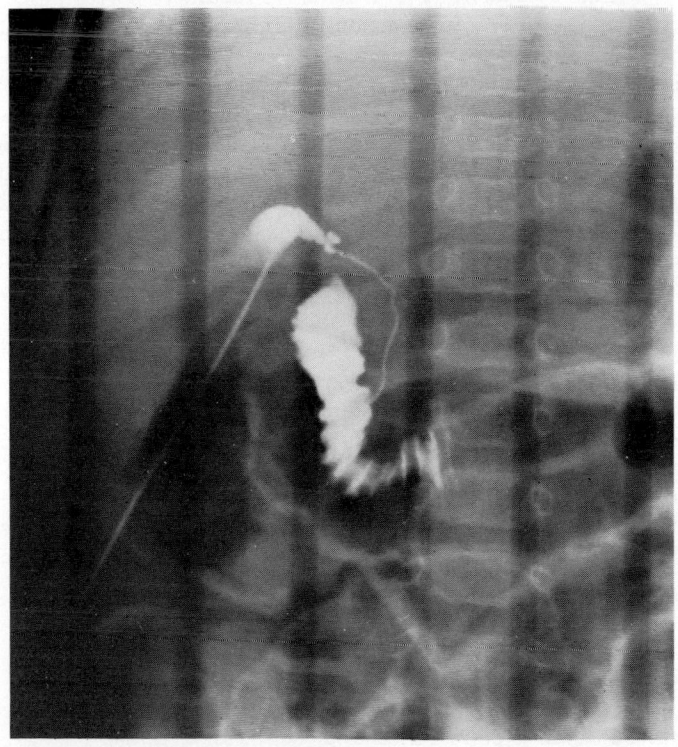

Figure 72–6. Operative cholangiogram in a 3-month-old infant with atresia of the common hepatic duct. The cystic and common bile ducts are patent.

Occasionally a patent segment of hepatic duct ("correctable" atresia) will be discovered that can be used for a choledochojejunostomy. In the majority of cases, however, the dissection proceeds above and behind the bifurcation of the portal vein and hepatic artery, and the tissue is transected at its junction with the capsule of the liver (Fig. 72–4E).

The aim is to expose remnants of the hepatic bile ducts, or to transect bile ductules that may be seen on histologic examination of the transected tissue. If ductules are absent on frozen section examination of the tissue, then deeper dissection into the liver has been advocated. Bleeding from the porta hepatis is controlled by direct pressure.

A Roux-Y loop of jejunum is now prepared. The jejunum is transected just distal to the duodenojejunal flexure. The distal end is oversewn and passed in an antecolic manner to the hilum of the liver. An end-to-side anastomosis is fashioned accurately between the edges of the transected liver tissue and the jejunal loop with interrupted sutures of 4/0 catgut, tied with the knots on the outside. The accessibility of the anastomosis is improved by positioning all of the posterior sutures before they are tied (Fig. 72–4F). The jejunum can then be "railroaded" into position and the sutures tied seriatim. Some improvement in results has been claimed by Suruga et al (1976) when this anastomosis is performed with the aid of an operating microscope.

In the original Kasai procedure intestinal continuity is reestablished by anastomosing the proximal jejunum to the distal loop at approximately 30 cm from the porta hepatis. A small drain is placed in the supraduodenal area before closure of the abdomen.

The frequent occurrence of ascending cholangitis after operation has been thought to be due to ascending infection from the intestine. Many rearrangements of the biliary—enteric anastomoses have been devised to overcome this problem and these have been illustrated diagrammatically (Fig. 72–7). Recent reports, however, suggest that the incidence of cholangitis is un-

affected even when the drainage loop is completely isolated by cutaneous enterostomy, and it has been suggested that the infection may be primarily blood-borne.

Postoperative Management. Histologic analysis of the tissue excised from the porta hepatis may help to predict prognosis. If bile ductules with diameters greater than 150 μm are seen there is a good chance of bile drainage. This, however, may not be effective for several days or weeks (Fig. 72–8). Any sign of cholangitis with pyrexia and worsening of liver function tests must be treated vigorously with large doses of antibiotics. Bacteraemia should be identified by blood cultures and culture of liver biopsy material, and the common organisms detected include *Proteus, Klebsiella,* and *Escherichia coli.*

Bile drainage from a cutaneous enterostomy may be replaced either through a more distal enterostomy if this has been fashioned or into the stomach via a nasogastric tube. The bile fistulae have been closed surgically from 3 months to 1 year after the original operation.

Results of Surgery

The early postoperative results of portoenterostomy have gradually improved during the last 25 years (Adelman, 1978; Carcassonne and Bensoussan, 1977; Kasai et al, 1975; Odiévre, 1978) from 10 to 86 percent satisfactory bile drainage. Operative results are closely related to the age of the patient at operation and we have reported bile drainage in 55 percent of children treated between 8 and 11 weeks of age, compared with 27 percent of older infants.

The oldest survivor after portoenterostomy is now 25 years of age, but most of the long-term patients do show obvious abnormalities of hepatic histology and function. Howard et al (1982), for example, described abnormal liver function tests in most of their survivors, who now range up to 10 years of age.

The postoperative progress of these patients may be complicated by recurrent cholangitis (Kobayashi et al, 1973), increasing intrahepatic

---

Figure 72–7. Diagrams of some of the suggested modifications to the original portoenterostomy operation. The recommended lengths of bowel segments (cm) are indicated. **A.** Original Kasai portoenterostomy. **B.** Kasai (1974) modification to prevent ascending cholangitis. **C, D,** and **E.** Operations suggested by Sawaguchi et al (1980), Suruga et al (1976), and Lilly and Altman (1975). **F.** Portocholecystostomy utilising a patent gallbladder and distal common bile duct.

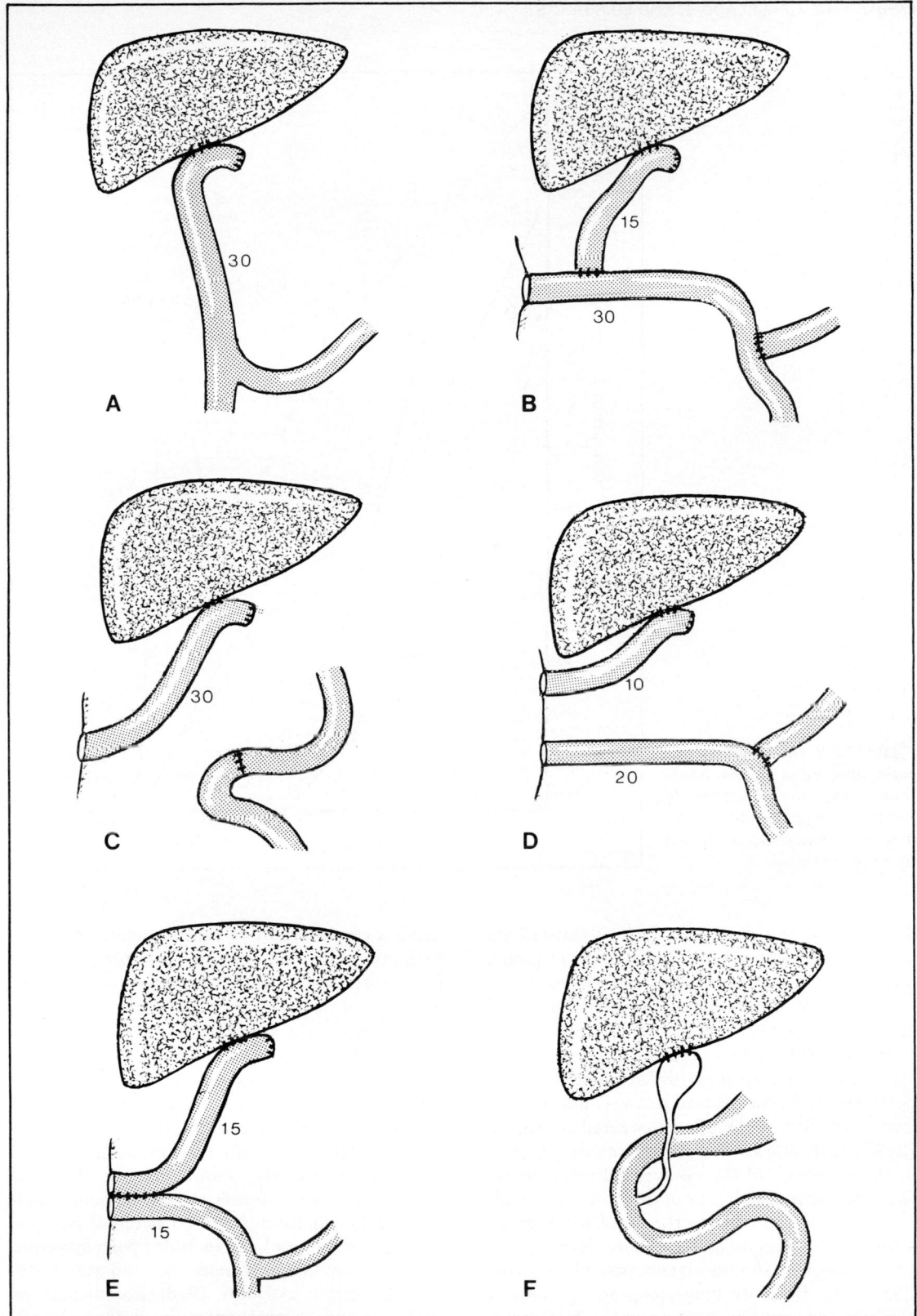

A

B

C

D

E

F

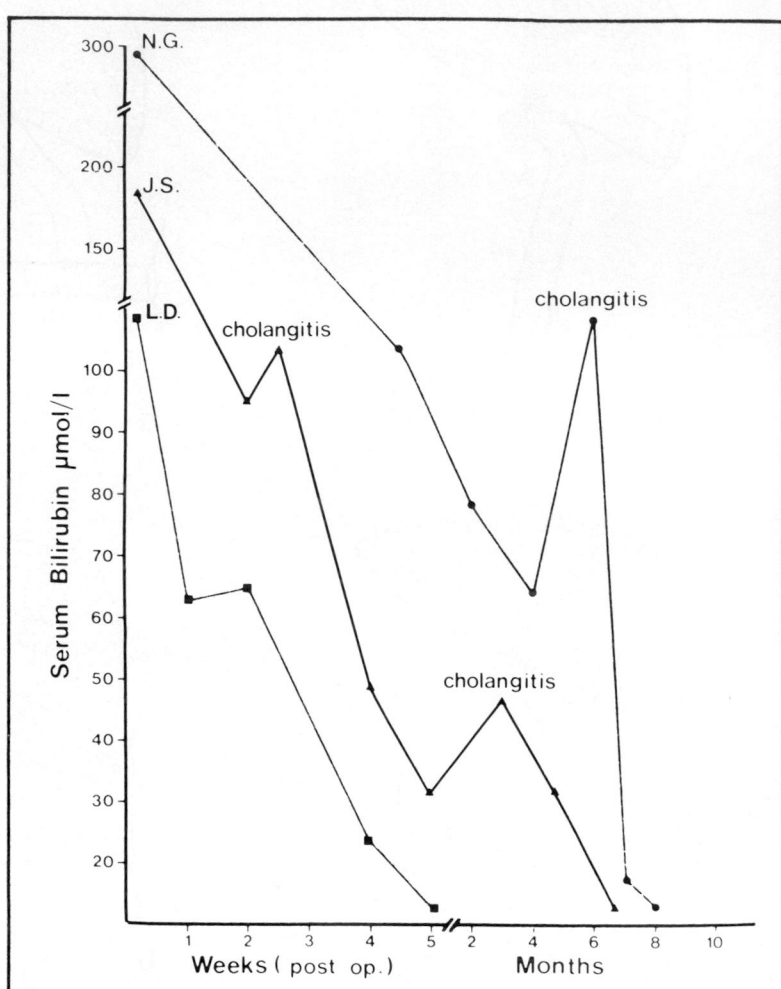

Figure 72–8. Fall in serum bilirubin after three portoenterostomy operations. Episodes of ascending bacterial cholangitis in two cases were accompanied by rises in bilirubin.

fibrosis, and the manifestations of consequent portal hypertension, and liver cell carcinoma has also been recorded in late survivors.

Bacterial infection is diagnosed from a triad of pyrexia, rising serum bilirubin, and a recurrence of acholic stools. Prompt treatment with intravenous broad-spectrum antibiotics is imperative as a deterioration in liver function follows each attack. This is illustrated in Figure 72–8, which shows the postoperative progress in three cases and the rises in bilirubin levels that accompanied attacks of infection. These attacks are maximal during the first 6 to 9 months after surgery and an episode more than 2 years after treatment should suggest possible obstruction in the Roux drainage loop and perhaps a need for reoperation. Assessment of bile drainage in postoperative patients is very satisfactory

using a combination of percutaneous cholangiography and radionuclide scanning and is recommended if there is any possibility of mechanical obstruction to bile flow.

Prophylactic antibiotics have not been shown to have any significant effect on the long-term prevention of ascending cholangitis and cutaneous diversion of bile also remains disappointing in reducing the number of attacks.

Over 50 percent of survivors after portoenterostomy eventually show evidence of portal hypertension and significant oesophageal varices develop in more than 30 percent. Suggestions for treatment have included portasystemic shunts, oesophageal transaction, and gastric devascularisation (Altman, 1976). Recent success with injection sclerotherapy in children bleeding from oesophageal varices indicates, however, that this may be the treatment of choice (Stamatakis et al, 1982).

It is now clear that advances in the surgery and postoperative care of children with biliary atresia have increased the 4-year survival rate from 2 to over 40 percent. Factors that influence operative results include operation before 10 weeks of age, the histology of resected tissue from the porta hepatis, the rapid onset of postoperative bile drainage, and complications from cholangitis or portal hypertension.

BIBLIOGRAPHY

Adelman S: Prognosis of uncorrected biliary atresia: An update. J Pediatr Surg 13:389, 1978

Alagille D, Odiévre H, et al: Hepatic ductular hypoplasia associated with characteristic facies, vertebral malformation, retarded physical, mental and sexual development and cardiac murmur. J Pediatr 86:63, 1975

Altman RP: Portal decompression by interposition mesocaval shunt in patients with biliary atresia. J Pediatr Surg 11:809, 1976

Altman RP: The portoenterostomy procedure for biliary atresia. Ann Surg 188:351, 1978

Bill AH: Biliary atresia. World J Surg 2:557, 1978

Bill AH, Haas JE, et al: Biliary atresia: Histopathologic observations and reflections upon its natural history. J Pediatr Surg 12:977, 1977

Carcassonne M, Bensoussan A: Long term results in treatment of biliary atresia. Prog Pediatr Surg 10:151, 1977

Chandra RS: Biliary atresia and other structural anomalies in the congenital polysplenia syndrome. J Pediatr 85:649, 1974

Clatworthy HW, MacDonald VG: The diagnostic laparotomy in obstructive jaundice in infants. Surg Clin North Am 36:1545, 1956

Gautier M, Eliot N: Extrahepatic biliary atresia: morphological study of 98 biliary remnants. Arch Pathol Lab Med 105:397, 1981

Gautier M, Jehan P, et al: Histologic study of biliary fibrous remnants in 48 cases of extrahepatic biliary atresia. Correlation with post-operative bile flow restoration. J Pediatr 85:704, 1976

Greene HL, Helinek GL, et al: A diagnostic approach to prolonged obstructive jaundice by 24-hour collection of duodenal fluid. J Pediatr 95:412, 1979

Haas JE: Bile duct and liver pathology in biliary atresia. World J Surg 2:561, 1978

Hays DM, Kimura K: Biliary atresia: New concepts of management. Curr Probl Surg 18:546, 1981

Hays DM, Snyder WH: Life-span in untreated biliary atresia. Surgery 54:373, 1963

Hirsig J, Kara O, et al: Experimental investigations into the etiology of cholangitis following operation for biliary atresia. J Pediatr Surg 13:55, 1978

Holmes JB: Congenital obliteration of the bile duct: Diagnosis and suggestions for treatment. Am J Dis Child 11:405, 1916

Howard ER: Extrahepatic biliary atresia: A review of current management. Br J Surg 70:193, 1983

Howard ER, Driver M, et al: Results of surgery in 88 consecutive cases of extrahepatic biliary atresia. J R Soc Med 75:408, 1982

Howard ER, Johnston DI, et al: Spontaneous perforation of the common bile duct in infants. Arch Dis Child 51:883, 1976

Howard ER, Nunnerley HB: Percutaneous cholangiography in prolonged jaundice of childhood. J R Soc Med 72:495, 1979

Jenner RE: New perspectives on biliary atresia. Ann R Coll Surg Engl 60:367, 1978

Jenner RE, Howard ER: Unsaturated monohydroxy bile acids as a cause of idiopathic obstructive cholangiopathy. Lancet 2:1073, 1975

Jenner RE, Howard ER, et al: Hepatobiliary imaging: The use of ^{99m}Tc-pyridoxylidene glutamate scanning in jaundiced adults and infants. Br J Radiol 51:862, 1978

Kasai M: Treatment of biliary atresia with special reference to hepatic porto-enterostomy and its modifications. Prog Pediatr Surg 6:5, 1974

Kasai M, Okamoto A, et al: Changes of portal vein pressure and intrahepatic blood vessels after surgery for biliary atresia. J Pediatr Surg 16:152, 1981

Kasai M, Suzuki S: A new operation for "non-correctable" biliary atresia; hepatic portoenterostomy. Shujitsu 13:733, 1959

Kasai M, Suzuki H, et al: Technique and results of operative management of biliary atresia. World J Surg 2:571, 1978

Kasai M, Watanabe I, et al: Follow-up studies of long-term survivors after hepatic portoenterostomy for "non-correctable" biliary atresia. J Pediatr Surg 10:173, 1975

Kobayashi A, Utsunomiya T, et al: Ascending cholangitis after successful surgical repair of biliary atresia. Arch Dis Child 48:697, 1973

Ladd WE: Congenital atresia and stenosis of the bile duct. JAMA 91:1082, 1928

Lawrence D, Howard ER, et al: Hepatic portoenterostomy for biliary atresia. Arch Dis Child 56:460, 1981

Leape LL, Ramenofsky ML: Laparoscopy in infants and children. J Pediatr Surg 12:929, 1977

Lilly JR: Hepatic porto-cholecystostomy for biliary atresia. J Pediatr Surg 14:301, 1979

Lilly JR, Altman RP: Hepatic portoenterostomy (the Kasai operation) for biliary atresia. Surgery 78:76, 1975

Lilly JR, Chandra RS: Surgical hazards of coexisting anomalies in biliary atresia. Surg Gynecol Obstet 139:49, 1974

Lilly JR, Hitch DC: Postoperative ascending cholangitis following portoenterostomy for biliary atresia: Measures for control. World J Surg 2:581, 1978

Mowat AP, Psacharopoulos HL, et al: Extrahepatic biliary atresia versus neonatal hepatitis. Review of 137 prospectively investigated infants. Arch Dis Child 51:763, 1976

Odiévre M: Long-term results of surgical treatment of biliary atresia. World J Surg 2:589, 1978

Porter SD, Soper RT, et al: Biliary hypoplasia. Ann Surg 167:602, 1968

Sawaguchi S, Akiyama H, et al: Longterm follow-up after radical operation for biliary atresia, in Kasai M, Shiraki K (eds): Cholestasis in Infancy. Tokyo: University of Tokyo Press, 1980, p 371

Sharp HL, Krivit W, et al: The diagnosis of complete extrahepatic obstruction by rose bengal [131]I. J Pediatr 70:46, 1967

Silverberg M, Craig J, et al: Problems in the diagnosis of biliary atresia. Am J Dis Child 99:574, 1960

Sondheimer JM, Shandling B, et al: Hepatic function following portoenterostomy for extrahepatic biliary atresia. Can Med Assoc J 118:255, 1978

Stamatakis JD, Howard ER, et al: Injection sclerotherapy for oesophageal varices in children. Br J Surg 69:74, 1982

Suruga K, Kono S, et al: Treatment of biliary atresia: Microsurgery for hepatic portoenterostomy. Surgery 80:558, 1976

Thomson J: On congenital obliteration of the bile ducts. Edinburgh Med J 37:523, 1891

Thomson J: On congenital obliteration of the bile ducts. Edinburgh Med J 37:604, 1892

Vacanti JP, Folkman J: Bile duct enlargement by infusion of L-proline: Potential significance in biliary atresia. J Pediatr Surg 14:814, 1979

73. Choledochal Cysts

Edward R. Howard

Choledochal cyst may be defined as a rare congenital dilatation of the common bile duct that is associated not infrequently with a congenital or acquired dilatation of the intrahepatic ducts. The condition is most frequently observed in females and is more common in Oriental races. It predisposes to cholangitis, gallstones and carcinoma, as well as to jaundice and portal hypertension. Unremitting jaundice in young children may lead to prompt diagnosis but the presentation in older patients may not be so specific and diagnosis therefore may be delayed. Long-term follow-up studies have shown least complications after cyst excision and this is now the treatment of choice.

HISTORICAL NOTE

The original description of a choledochal cyst is usually accredited to the anatomist Vater in 1748 but the first detailed case was published by Douglas in 1852; this clinical report included details of cyst structure and thoughts on aetiology. The case concerned a 17-year-old girl who presented with jaundice and fever. There was a 3-year history of intermittent abdominal pain and examination showed a large painful swelling in the right hypochondrium. The symptoms lessened after percutaneous drainage of the cyst, but the patient died one month later. Postmortem examination revealed a large choledochal cyst, an undilated gallbladder, and fibrotic changes in the cyst wall.

Early reviews of the subject are listed by Saito and Ishida (1974) and include the paper of Alonso-Lej et al (1959), which contains the most generally used classification of choledochal cysts. The combination of dilatations of both intra- and extrahepatic ducts was first described in detail by Arthur and Stewart in 1964.

Recommended reviews of the subject include those of Tsardakas and Robnett (1956), Alonso-Lej et al (1959), Flanigan (1975), and Yamaguchi et al (1980).

INCIDENCE

The incidence of choledochal cyst in Western countries is between 1 in 100,000 and 1 in 150,000 live births, but it is more common in Japan, where the hospital admission rate (1 per 1000 admissions) is higher than in either the United States (1 per 13,000) or Australia (1 per 15,000). However, the female-to-male-ratio in both Western and Japanese series varies between 3 to 1 and 4 to 1. Approximately 60 percent of cases are diagnosed before the tenth year of life and details of more than 1000 have been published.

AETIOLOGY

It is usually accepted that choledochal cysts are congenital in origin but the mechanism of their formation remains in doubt. Shocket (1955) reported observations on cysts detected in an unborn foetus, a stillborn infant, and a 4-day old infant.

The classic embryologic theory proposed that cystic abnormalities are a result of irregular canalisation of the bile ducts. The biliary passages develop in the foetus from an outgrowth on the ventral aspect of the foregut and during the early stages of development cellular hyperplasia is so marked that the lumen of the ducts becomes obstructed. Recanalisation is not completed until the fifth month. In 1974, Saito and Ishida (1974) proposed that an abnormality of this process could result in a weakness of the bile duct wall and an obstruction of the distal lumen. In support of this hypothesis they pointed out that cysts are found in the newborn and that, although they may be accompanied by biliary tract anomalies such as double common bile duct, double gallbladder, and intrahepatic cysts, they are not usually associated with any other obvious abnormality.

Babbitt (1969) suggested that a congenital malformation of the junction of pancreatic and bile ducts could allow a reflux of pancreatic juice that might cause recurrent cholangitis and eventual fibrosis of the wall of the common bile duct. A small distal common bile duct was shown to enter the pancreatic duct at a right angle 2.0 to 3.5 cm proximal to the ampulla of Vater, allowing pancreatic secretions into the biliary ducts in 19 cases of choledochal cyst.

A cholangiographic study of 22 cases reported by Ono in 1982 showed abnormal pancreaticobiliary junctions on 15 occasions and several studies have revealed common pancreaticobiliary channels greater than 0.5 cm in length. It has been suggested that the anatomic anomaly is the result of faulty budding of the primitive main pancreatic duct from high on the primitive common bile duct. The terminal portion of the pancreatic duct therefore lies proximal to the sphincteric muscles of the ampulla of Vater, allowing free reflux of pancreatic juice. A recent study of human foetuses by Wong and Lister (1981) has shown that the choledochopancreatic junction lies outside of the duodenal wall before 8 weeks of gestation and gradually moves toward the duodenal lumen. Premature arrest of this process could give rise to an anomalous pancreaticobiliary junction.

Experimental studies have shown that simple destruction of bile duct epithelium alone does not cause choledochal cysts. An increase of intraluminal pressure does seem important, however, and ligation of the distal common bile duct in foetal lambs (Spitz, 1977) has produced cystic dilatation. Cysts have also followed anastomosis of the pancreatic duct to the gallbladder in dogs with proliferation of collagen in the bile duct wall and patchy loss of epithelium.

The abnormally long "common-channels" that have been demonstrated on cholangiography distal to the terminal portions of pancreatic and common bile ducts may therefore be important in the aetiology of choledochal cysts (Miyano et al, 1981) and the high amylase content of some cysts, the well-documented complication of pancreatitis, and the experimental evidence support the concept. However, not all cysts contain high levels of pancreatic enzymes, and in two recent cases treated by cyst excision, Standfield (1983) showed that the first contained 140,000 units per litre of amylase and 120,750 units per litre of lipase while the second case, which was associated with intrahepatic duct dilatation of the Caroli type, contained bile with only 80 units per litre of amylase and 25 units per litre of lipase (i.e., less than normal serum enzyme levels). Although the "common-channel" theory remains attractive, developmental factors may still be important; Lilly (1979) has pointed out that abnormal distal anatomy may be only one manifestation of a disordered embryology that may have affected the whole of the extrahepatic duct system.

PATHOLOGY

The widespread use of cholangiography has revealed that cystic dilatation can affect any part of the biliary duct system, and the term "bile-duct cyst" may now be preferable to "choledochal cyst." The size of cysts varies enormously, the smallest measuring 1.0 to 2.0 cm and the largest filling almost the entire abdomen. Characteristially the dilatation of the common bile duct starts 1.0 to 2.0 cm above the duodenum and ends abruptly just below the bifurcation in the common hepatic duct. The cystic duct enters the cystic area but the gallbladder is usually of normal size. The cuboidal biliary epithelium may be intact but in many cases it is ulcerated to such a degree that only small patches of viable cells remain. Flanigan (1975) pointed out that there is no correlation between the state of the epithelium and the type of cystic dilatation. The wall of the cyst, which may vary from 2.0 to 7.5 mm in thickness, is composed mainly of fibrous tissue with occasional fibres of elastic tissue and smooth muscle (Figs. 73–1 through 73–3).

Liver histology in a case of uncomplicated cyst may show little change apart from some inflammatory-cell infiltration of portal tracts and some periportal fibrosis. Proliferation of bile ductules is a feature in infancy and may be associated with interlobular cholestasis in the neonatal period when the biopsy may be confused with the more common biliary atresia.

Several classifications have been proposed for bile-duct cysts but the scheme prepared by Alonso-Lej et al (1959) is used most commonly. Cysts of the common bile duct are divided as follows: Type I—cystic; Type II—diverticulum; and Type III—choledochocele (dilatation of intraduodenal common bile duct). Type IV includes cases with both extra- and intrahepatic cysts (Fig. 73–4).

Extrahepatic cysts may be cystic or fusiform in appearance; with the latter type an abdominal mass is less common and the usual presentation is jaundice with or without abdominal pain.

The classification of Todani et al (1977) divided Type I cysts further into cystic (Fig. 73–5), fusiform (Fig. 73–6), or segmental types and added a Type V for cases in which the dilatation was confined to the intrahepatic ducts (Fig. 73–4).

A recent survey by the Japanese Society of Pediatric Surgeons (Yamaguchi, 1980) showed that 51 percent of cases were of the Type I–cystic variety whereas 10.6 percent were Type I–fusiform. Dilatation of both intra- and extrahepatic ducts occurred in 28.5 percent and intrahepatic ducts alone were affected in 4.6 percent.

This author's series of 11 cases undergoing primary surgical treatment included 5 of Type I–cystic, 3 of Type I–fusiform, and 3 in which there was combined intra- and extrahepatic disease.

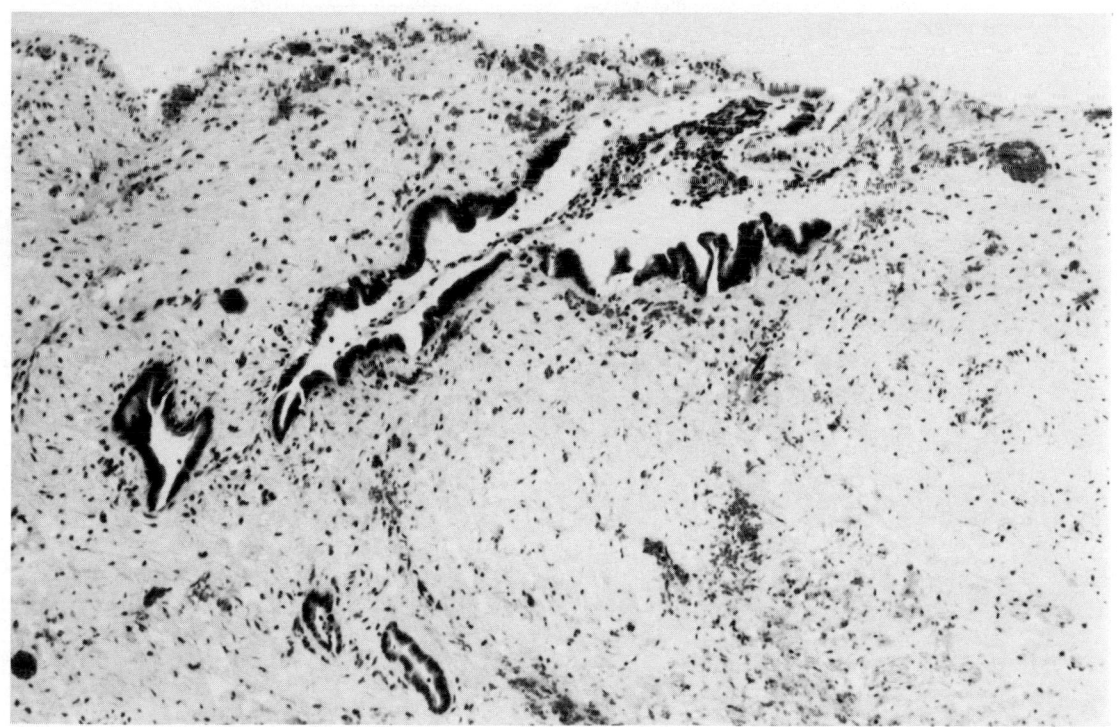

Figure 73–1. Sections showing the wall of a choledochal cyst composed of fibrovascular connective tissue in which there is a moderately heavy chronic inflammatory cell infiltrate. The mucosal surface is mainly granulation tissue with surviving islands of hyperplastic columnar epithelium. (H&E, ×16) (*Courtesy of Dr. Marie Driver.*)

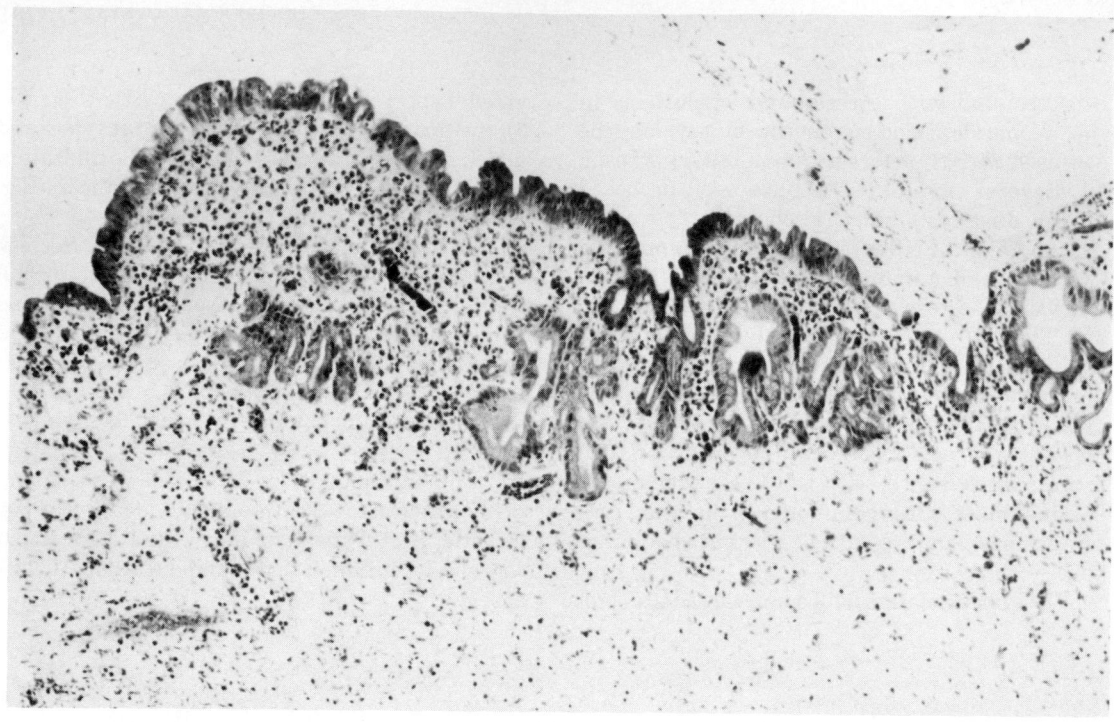

Figure 73–2. The mucosal surface of a choledochal cyst lined by hyperplastic columnar epithelium producing a complex glandular pattern. There is associated chronic inflammation. (H&E, ×10) (*Courtesy of Dr. Marie Driver.*)

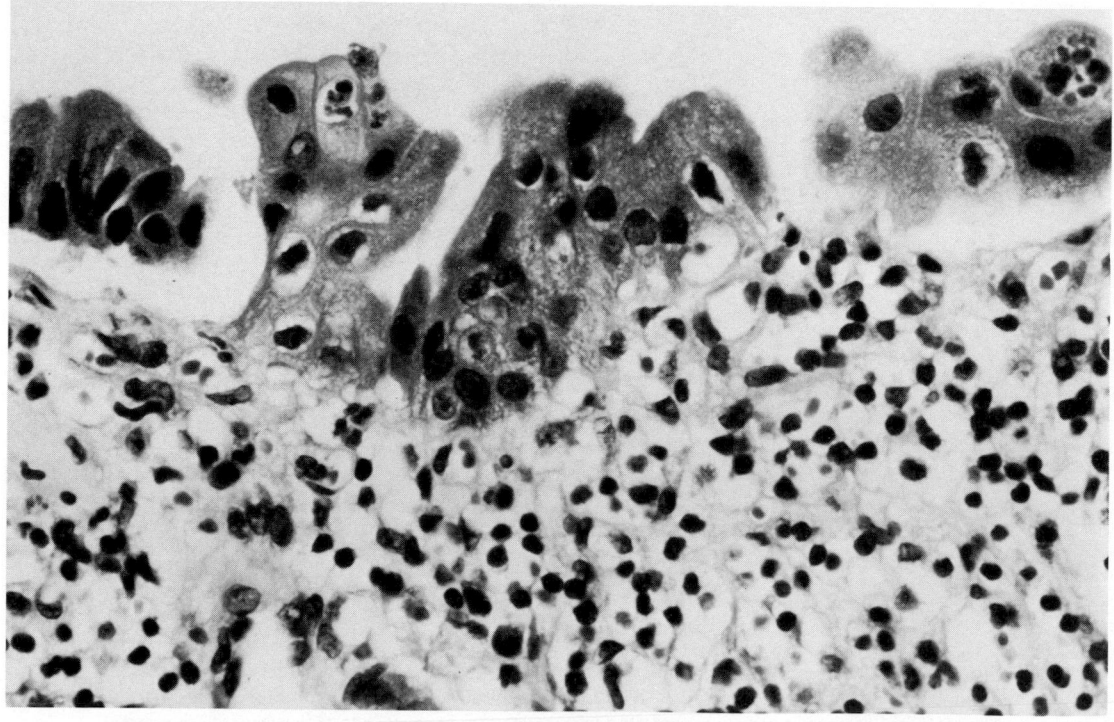

Figure 73–3. Section of acutely inflamed mucosa lined by hyperplastic, regenerating columnar epithelium. (H&E, ×63) (*Courtesy of Dr. Marie Driver.*)

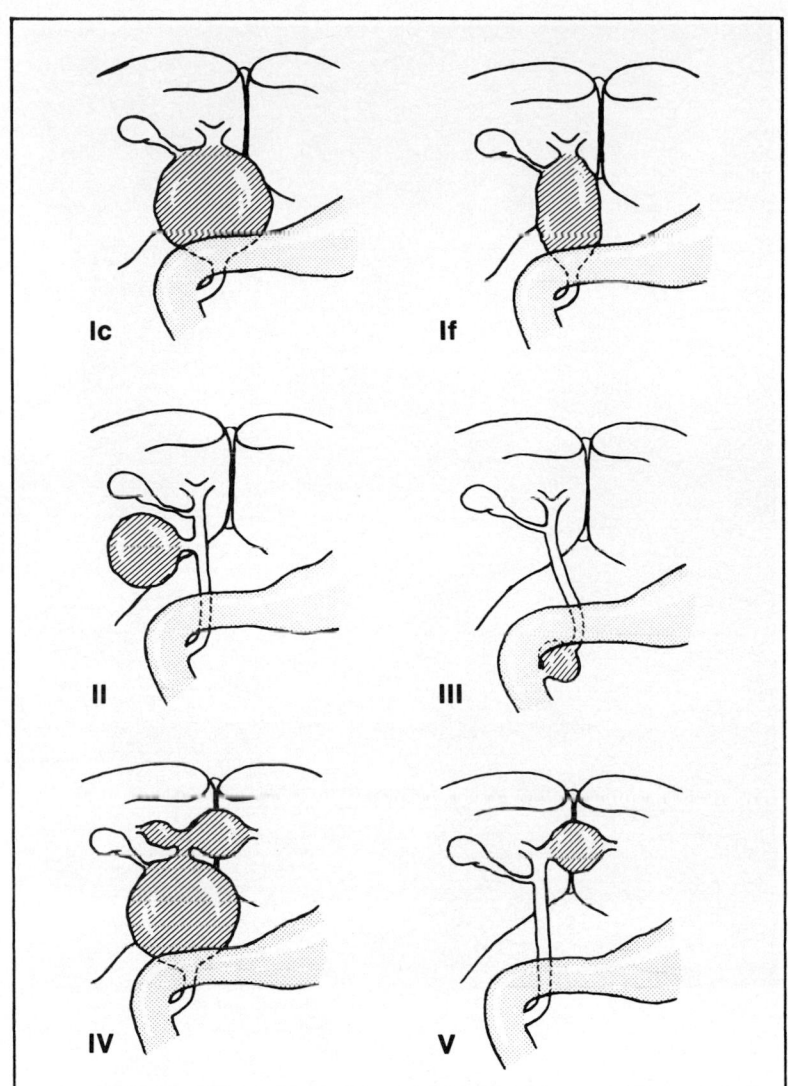

Figure 73–4. Classification of bile duct cysts. Ic = cystic dilatation of common bile duct, If = fusiform dilatation, II = diverticulum, III = choledochocele, IV = combination of extra- and intrahepatic cysts, V = dilatation confined to intrahepatic ducts.

CLINICAL MANIFESTATIONS AND DIFFERENTIAL DIAGNOSIS

Choledochal cyst may present in early infancy; the youngest case in this author's series underwent operation at 7 months of age. The majority of cases—up to 60 percent—are diagnosed in childhood before 10 years of age, but diagnosis may be made at any age and 25 percent of patients are older than 20 years at presentation. Occasional cases have been reported as late as the eighth decade.

The order of frequency of the classic signs of jaundice, pain, and right hypochondrial mass varies from series to series. The occurrence of all three symptoms and signs in the same patient ("classic triad") also varies from 13 to 63 percent of reported series, and fever or vomiting are features in approximately 30 percent of patients.

Obstructive jaundice is typically intermittent and is the main feature in infancy, while a mass is a more common finding in later childhood (Fig. 73–7). Jaundice accompanied by fever

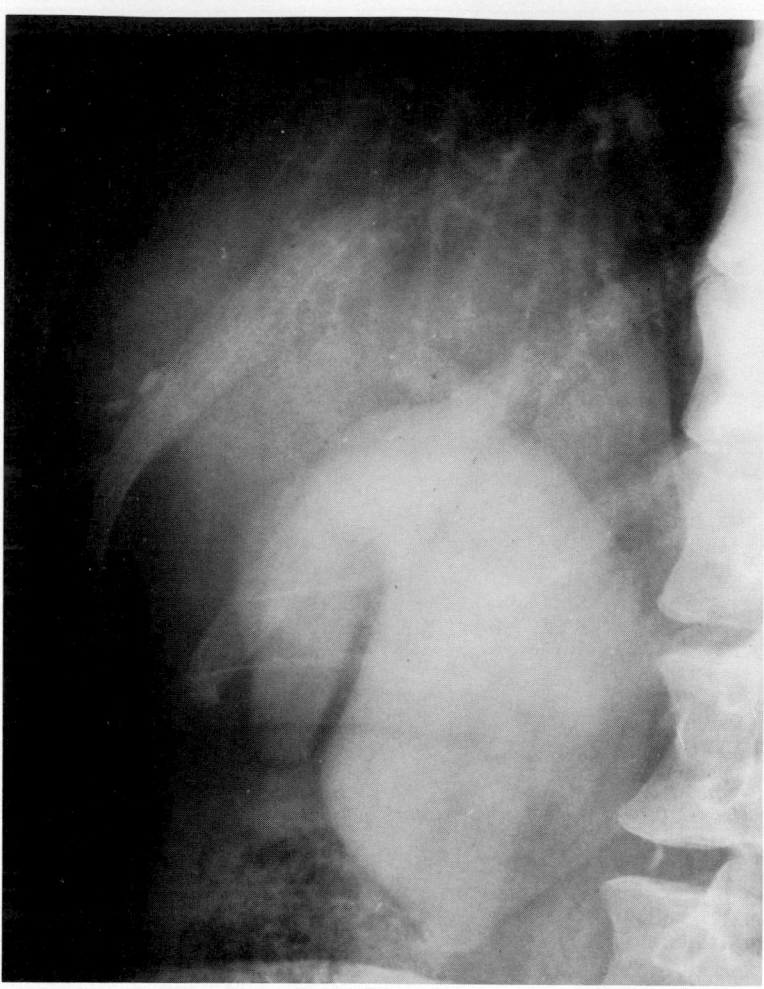

Figure 73–5. Gallbladder and Type I cystic dilatation of the common bile duct imaged by oral cholecystography in a 50-year-old woman who presented with pain in the right hypochondrium.

(cholangitis) is reported more often in adults.

Occasionally patients may present with one of the complications such as cholecystitis, pancreatitis, or haematemesis from portal hypertension. Bile duct cysts must be remembered in the differential diagnosis of all of these conditions.

The differential diagnosis of a cyst presenting with a mass in the right hypochondrium includes mucocele of the gallbladder, hepatic cysts, and tumours, neoplasms and cysts of the pancreas and suprarenal gland, kidney lesions, and the rare spontaneous perforation of the bile ducts in infancy.

Author's Series. Of 15 patients treated during the last 10 years, primary surgical procedures were performed in 11 while 4 were referred af-

ter complications of previous surgery. Ages ranged from 7 months to 50 years, but 13 were under 15 years at presentation. The presenting symptoms and signs are listed in Table 73–1, but of the 11 presenting as "new" cases only 3 (27 percent) had the "classic triad" of symptoms and signs.

Intrahepatic Cystic Dilatation

The aetiologic relationship of classical choledochal cysts to intrahepatic cysts and Caroli's disease is unclear. Recent cholangiographic observations have revealed at least three types of intrahepatic dilatation:

1. Dilatation secondary to long-standing extrahepatic obstruction, which rapidly returns

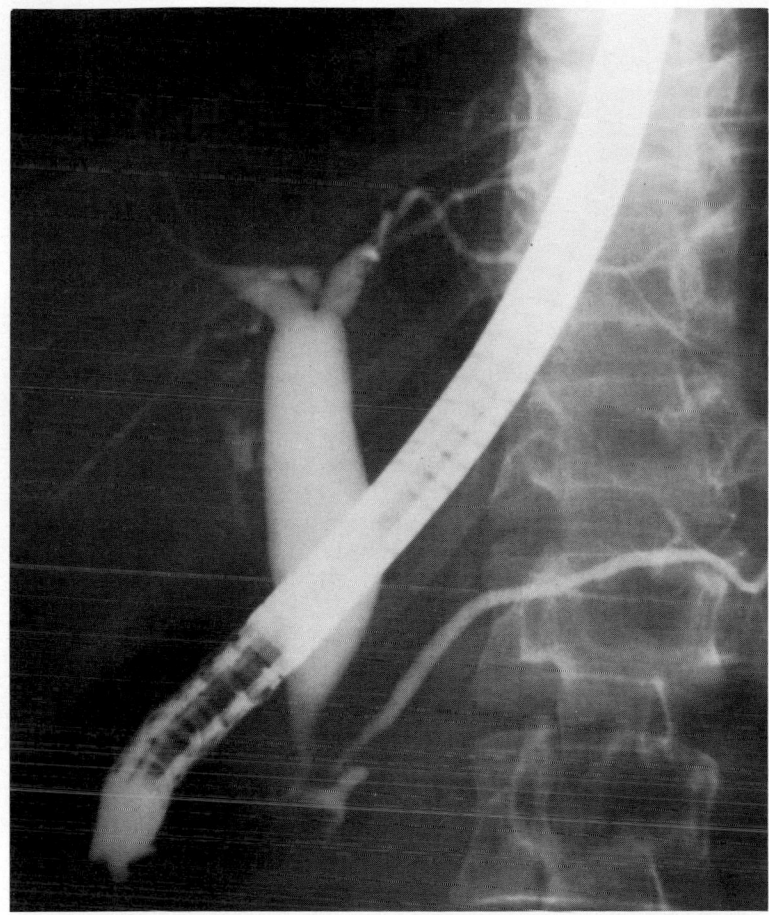

Figure 73–6. Fusiform dilatation of the common bile duct shown by ERCP examination in a 31-year-old man who presented with intermittent abdominal pain. Note the absence of intrahepatic duct dilatation. (*Courtesy of Mr. J.L. Dawson.*)

to normal after excision of the extrahepatic cyst (Fig. 73–8).

2. Cystic dilatation of one or more segments of the primary branches of the intrahepatic ducts with normal peripheral ducts. It may be possible to decompress these at the time of extrahepatic cyst excision (Fig. 73–9).
3. Multiple cysts, either saccular or cylindrical, throughout the biliary tree. These may be restricted to one segment and may therefore be amenable to segmental hepatic resection.

Caroli (1968) was the first to classify intrahepatic cysts into two types, to emphasize their association with extrahepatic cysts, and to point out the complications of recurrent cholangitis and intrahepatic stone formation. Of the two main types of multiple cysts Type I is the rarer and presents with recurrent cholangitis, usually without jaundice. Abdominal pain is associated with the formation of intrahepatic calculi. Type II cysts are associated with hepatic fibrosis, portal hypertension, and renal disease. Recurrent cholangitis may also be a feature of Type II disease and early death is usual. Murray Lyon et al (1972) reported a typical series of five cases, with congenital hepatic fibrosis in four and renal anomalies ("medullary sponge") in three.

Surgery is useful for the management of associated extrahepatic cysts and for calculus formation but has been disappointing for the control of recurrent cholangitis.

DIAGNOSTIC STUDIES (TABLE 73–2)

The diagnosis of choledochal cyst is frequently delayed, as it may not be considered in either the differential diagnosis of rather nonspecific symptoms such as recurrent abdominal pain or

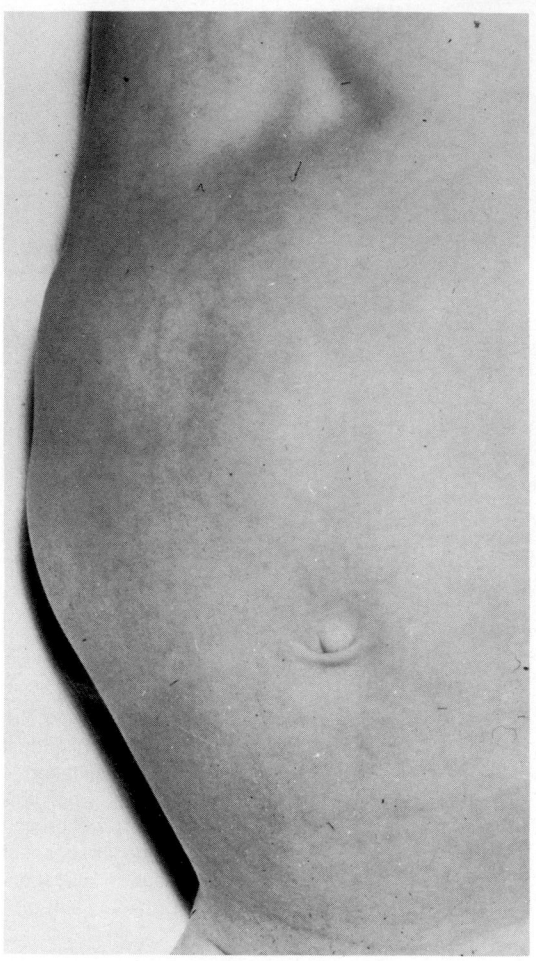

Figure 73–7. Right-sided abdominal mass caused by a Type I dilatation in a 3-year-old female child who was pyrexial but not jaundiced.

TABLE 73–1. SYMPTOMS AND SIGNS AT PRESENTATION IN 15 CASES OF CHOLEDOCHAL CYST (AUTHOR'S SERIES)

Recurrent jaundice	6
Jaundice + pain + mass	3
Recurrent pancreatitis	1
Intraabdominal haemorrhage	1
Complications following previous drainage procedures	4
Total	15

to the left, and may also show oesophageal varices from biliary cirrhosis or from extrahepatic portal vein compression.

Oral and intravenous cholangiography may reveal a cyst (Fig. 73–5), but in most cases contrast concentration is very poor and the diagnosis may be missed. Endoscopic retrograde cholangiography (Marshall and Halpin, 1982), however, gives good visualisation of both extrahepatic cysts and of the intrahepatic ductal anatomy and the technique is now commonly used for preoperative diagnosis and assessment (Fig. 73–10). Recorded complications from retrograde cholangiography include a rise in serum amylase, occasional fatal pancreatitis, and gram-negative septicaemia. Percutaneous transhepatic cholangiography also gives good visualisation, but the author has seen significant bile leaks on two occasions.

Ultrasonography is particularly valuable in the diagnosis of choledochal cyst and is discussed by Dewbury et al (1980), Frank et al (1981), Kangarloo et al (1980), and Yamaguchi et al (1980). Size, contour, and position can all be determined and high-resolution, real-time scanning is very accurate in determining the anatomy of the intrahepatic ducts and the confluence of the extrahepatic ducts. Rare hepatic artery aneurysms have been misdiagnosed as cysts but real-time scanning should allow demonstration of any arterial pulsation and make the diagnosis clear.

The recent widespread introduction of antenatal ultrasonography has allowed the observation of choledochal cysts in two foetuses of 25 and 36 weeks of gestation although the differential diagnosis of liver cyst, mesenteric cyst, and bowel duplication may be difficult. The author was referred a case of possible choledochal cyst diagnosed before birth, but at laparotomy a large ovarian cyst was found in the upper abdomen.

in the investigation of a jaundiced patient in whom the classic triad of jaundice, pain and mass is absent. However, several diagnostic techniques are now available that can accurately define the anatomy of the biliary tree and a preoperative assessment can be made in nearly all cases once the diagnosis has been considered.

A large cyst may be suspected on a plain x-ray from displacement of the gas-filled stomach, duodenum, and colon. Opaque calculi or gas within a cyst have been reported occasionally but these are rare signs. The cyst wall is rarely calcified. A barium meal will confirm the gut displacement, with the first and second parts of the duodenum moved anteriorly and

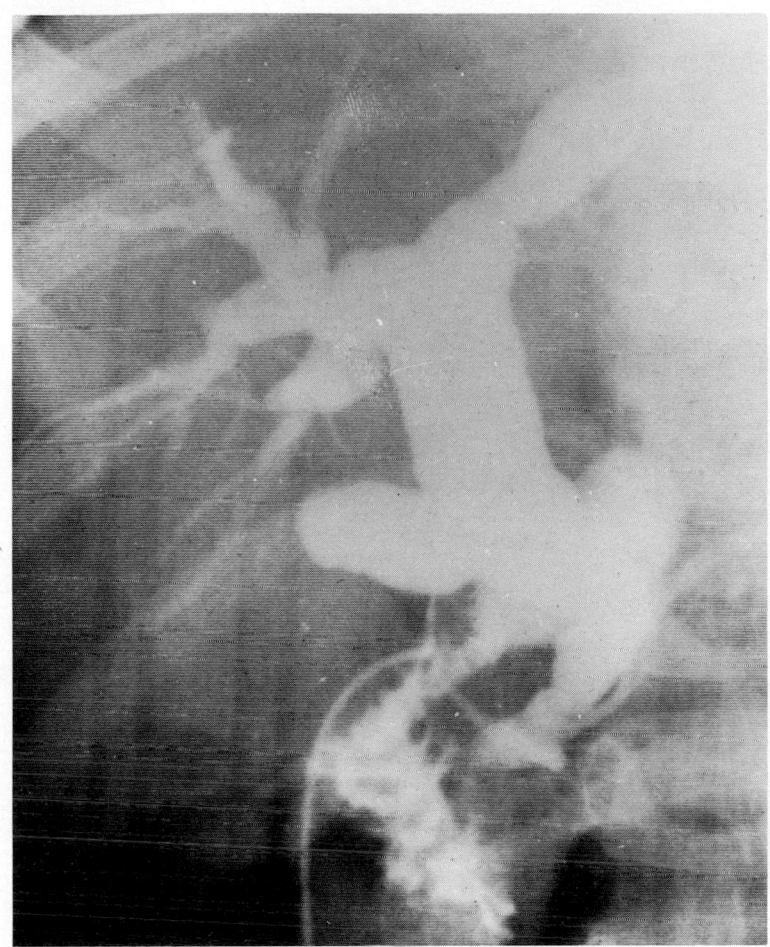

Figure 73–8. Operative cholangiogram showing a fusiform dilatation of the common bile duct, with secondary dilatation of the intrahepatic ducts, in a 3-year-old female child who had suffered several attacks of painless jaundice. Note free flow of contrast to duodenum.

Hepatobiliary scintigraphy with technetium-99m, which is readily available and provides good images, is considered by some to be the investigation of choice (Han et al, 1981; Huang and Liaw, 1982; Parasothy and Somasundram, 1981). Many complexes of Tc-99m are in use, but diethyl IDA (EHIDA) is currently recommended because of fast blood clearance and low renal excretion. An initial filling defect in the liver followed by a gradual increase in the concentration of radioactivity in the cyst on serial scans is pathognomonic and may be seen within 2 hours in a nonjaundiced patient. Diagnosis in a jaundiced patient may take up to 24 hours. Radionuclide scanning is particularly useful for demonstrating the patency of bile duct–bowel anastomoses after surgery.

Computed tomography (CT) also gives a clear demonstration of the size, extent, and cystic nature of the lesion (Araki et al, 1980; Chol-ankeril et al, 1982; Nakata et al, 1981). It is reported as a useful technique in differentiating between congenital and acquired dilatation of the intrahepatic ducts. In choledochal cyst significant intrahepatic duct dilatation is limited to the central parts of the duct system, whereas in acquired disease the dilatation tapers gradually toward the periphery. Difficulties in diagnosis have arisen when the gallbladder has been compressed by a cyst and consequently lost its separate identity or when a large mucocele has been mistaken for a cyst.

Laparoscopy and angiography complete the list of possible methods of diagnosis, but are not generally used as primary methods of investigation.

In summary, most cases of choledochal cyst may be assessed very adequately before operation with a combination of ultrasonography and radionuclide scanning, thus avoiding the possi-

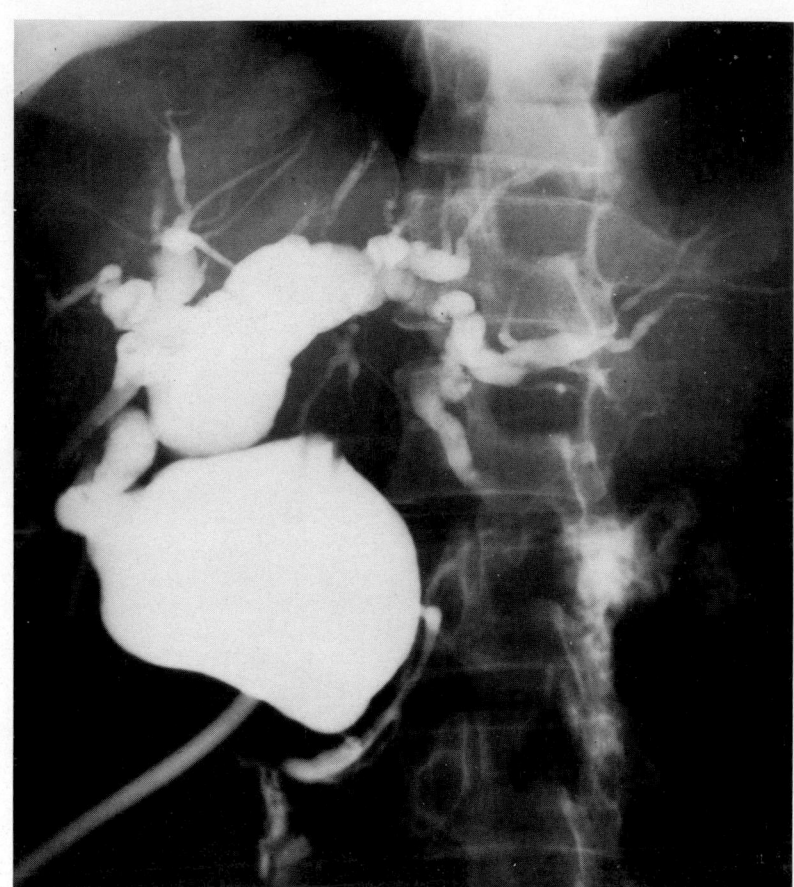

Figure 73–9. Type I cyst associated with segmental dilatation of the left hepatic duct in a 40-year-old woman with a short history of painless jaundice (operative cholangiogram).

ble complications of more invasive techniques. The detailed anatomy of the intrahepatic ducts and pancreaticobiliary communications can be visualised with intraoperative cholangiography, which must be performed directly through the common hepatic duct and lower end of the common bile duct rather than through the cyst it-

self. Injection of contrast medium into the cyst frequently fails to outline the intrahepatic bile ducts and obscures filling of the distal duct.

COMPLICATIONS

Jaundice, recurrent cholangitis, pancreatitis, gallstones, cholecystitis, carcinoma, cyst rupture, hepatic fibrosis, cirrhosis, and portal hypertension have all been recorded as complications of bile duct dilatation. The condition may also complicate pregnancy through a worsening of the symptoms, and 0.7 percent of recorded cases were diagnosed from such an exacerbation. Chesterman (1944) gave details of 14 cases diagnosed or managed during pregnancy, 8 of which had an onset or an exacerbation of symptoms during pregnancy and 4 during the puerperium. Cyst rupture has also been described during pregnancy and after trauma (Blocker et al, 1937; Friend, 1958), but it occurs mostly as

TABLE 73–2. INVESTIGATIONS AVAILABLE FOR THE DIAGNOSIS OF CHOLEDOCHAL CYST

Plain abdominal x-ray
Barium meal
Oral and intravenous cholangiography
Endoscopic retrograde cholangiography
Percutaneous cholangiography
Ultrasonography
Hepatobiliary scintigraphy
Computed tomography
Laparoscopy
Angiography
Intraoperative cholangiography

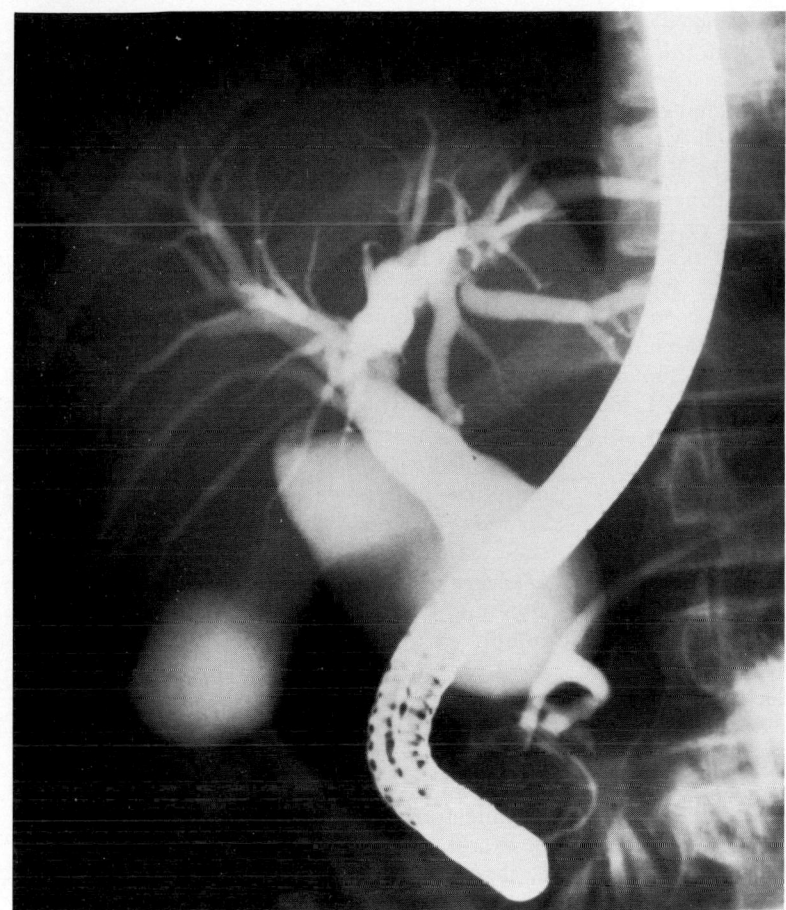

Figure 73–10. Common bile duct–pancreatic channel associated with a choledochal cyst in a 12-year-old girl who presented with recurrent pancreatitis. Note possible calculus in duct of Santorini. (*ERCP examination courtesy of Dr. D. Carr-Locke.*)

a spontaneous event (Tagart, 1956; Yamashero et al, 1982). Review of 16 recorded cases reveals no relationship between cyst size and rupture, and the rupture may affect either the anterior or posterior walls.

Choledochal cyst may be diagnosed in patients with a history of recurrent abdominal pain and elevated serum amylase levels suggesting pancreatitis. The pancreas may or may not appear inflamed at laparotomy and Stringel and Filler (1982) suggested that a high concentration of amylase within a cyst may have ready access to the bloodstream through a duct wall denuded of epithelium. Certainly the presence of a raised serum amylase should not delay cyst excision; the author has excised a cyst without complication at a time when the serum amylase measured 11,000 units per litre. The serum amylase falls rapidly after surgery and there has been no recurrence of hyperamylasaemia in patients treated with cyst excision.

Goldberg et al (1980) reviewed four cases of pancreatitis associated with choledochocele and pointed out that there is often a long history of pain, either with jaundice or pancreatitis, and that the condition may be misdiagnosed as gallbladder disease. Transhepatic cholangiography has shown contrast medium refluxing into the pancreatic duct with peristalsis. Excision of the intraduodenal portion of the cyst wall is effective treatment.

Gallstones are usually considered to be rare in bile duct cysts, but Yamaguchi (1980) reported an 8.0 percent incidence in 1433 cases in Japan. Most of these were within the cysts but pancreatic calculi were found in three cases. Gallstones may also occur as a complication of an inadequate cystoenterostomy operation and the author has reoperated on a 12-year-old girl in whom such an anastomosis had stenosed, allowing the formation of stones in the cyst and causing episodes of recurrent abdominal pain and cholangitis. The possibility of cholecystitis is dealt with by cholecystectomy at the time of cyst excision.

Malignant change within a choledochal cyst was first described by Irwin and Morison in 1944 and 48 cases were reviewed by Kagawa et al (1978) who estimated the incidence to be approximately 3.0 percent. Lesions of the extrahepatic ducts accounted for 32 of the cases, thus emphasising the value of cyst excision whenever feasible. Later reports have been published by Ackerholm et al (1981), Bedikian et al (1980), and Todani et al (1979). The female-to-male ratio of malignant change is 3 to 1 and the average age 34 years, which is much younger than the age of occurrence of primary carcinoma of noncystic bile ducts. Carcinoma of dilated intrahepatic ducts has been reported in nine patients, even after extrahepatic cyst excision, but no case has occurred in undilated ducts. Histology usually shows adenocarcinoma but squamous and undifferentiated lesions have been reported, and rarely may occur in sites other than the bile ducts, such as liver, gallbladder, pancreas, or duodenum.

Portal hypertension may arise from either portal vein compression or biliary cirrhosis and intestinal bleeding may be the presenting sign of the choledochal cyst (Martin and Rowe, 1979; Orenstein and Whitington, 1982). Complete and rapid relief of portal hypertension after cyst surgery is well documented, presumably by decompression of the portal vein.

Abnormalities of liver histology discussed by Kim (1981) in a review of 188 cases included cirrhosis in 32 percent and congenital hepatic fibrosis in 3.7 percent, but Yeong et al (1982) have shown that even biliary cirrhosis may regress after effective surgery, with recovery of normal liver histology and disappearance of portal hypertension.

SURGICAL MANAGEMENT

The operative treatment of choledochal cysts is best summarised according to the type of lesion. The following is based on the classification of Todani et al in 1977.

Type I Cystic Dilatation. Total excision with Roux loop reconstruction is now the procedure of choice, although Schärli and Bettex (1968) and Cahlin (1974) have described two cases in which it was possible to resect the cyst and to anastomose the common hepatic duct to the distal common bile duct. However, if pancreatic reflux is an aetiologic factor then primary reconstruction is perhaps not the optimal treatment. The details of radical excision are described in the following section.

Choledochocystojejunostomy with a Roux loop of jejunum is still a popular form of cyst drainage (Fig. 73–11). Essential points in the technique include a 30- to 40-cm length of jejunum placed in a retrocolic position and a long anastomosis, which is placed at the most dependent part of the cyst. The stoma should be at least 5.0 cm in the older child or adult and is performed with catgut sutures after excision of an ellipse of cyst wall. The technique is useful for cases in which there is severe adherence of the cyst to surrounding structures, or in cases of severe portal hypertension. Radical cyst excision might also be hazardous in the very young infant.

Choledochocystenterostomy may fail to provide completely dependent drainage and might therefore predispose to recurrent cholangitis. Furthermore, as the wall of the cyst is mostly composed of fibrous tissue and deficient mucosa the anastomosis tends to contract, obstruct bile flow and also precipitate recurrent infection. Gallstone formation and malignancy are well-documented complications of this type of drainage.

Type I Fusiform Dilatation. Todani et al (1977) have suggested that transduodenal sphincteroplasty may be effective for this type of cyst and they reported a satisfactory result in one case.

Type II Diverticulum. Excision of the diverticulum and reconstruction of the common bile duct was described in the collective review of Alonso-Lej et al (1959); however, this is the rarest type of choledochal cyst and very few other cases have been recorded.

Type III Choledochocele. Transduodenal sphincteroplasty is effective and has been recommended as the treatment of choice by several authors including Klotz et al (1973) and Todani et al (1977).

Type IV Combined Cysts of Extra- and Intrahepatic Ducts. The intrahepatic cysts

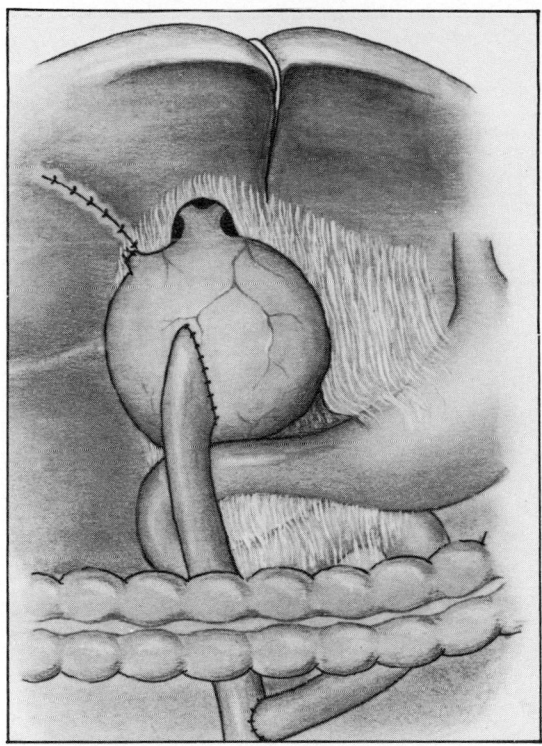

Figure 73–11. Choledochocystojejunostomy with Roux-Y loop anastomosed to the most dependent portion of the cyst. Note that the gallbladder is removed.

are usually inaccessible but biliary tract drainage is improved after excision of the extrahepatic dilatations and Roux loop anastomosis. It is sometimes possible to include dilated segments of hepatic ducts in the length of the anastomosis (see the following).

Type V Intrahepatic Cysts. Surgery is rarely of benefit for cysts confined to the liver unless recurrent cholangitis is associated with calculus formation. Watts et al (1974), in a review of 84 cases, reported recurrent cholangitis after all types of drainage procedures and three patients developed biliary tract carcinoma. Occasionally the dilatation is restricted to one segment and Watts described three such patients who did well after hepatic lobectomy.

EXTERNAL DRAINAGE OF CYSTS. Drainage to the exterior via a T-tube should rarely be necessary except in complicated cases of perforation, uncontrolled cholangitis, or a combination of severe infection and cholelithiasis.

RADICAL EXCISION OF CHOLEDOCHAL CYSTS

This is the recommended treatment for a majority of the more usual types of biliary tract cysts (Filler and Stringel, 1973; Jones et al, 1971).

Preoperative Preparation. Anaemia and coagulation abnormalities are corrected with blood transfusion and vitamin K. Bowel preparation includes colonic evacuation, oral neomycin, and metronidazole. A systemic antibiotic, usually a cephalosporin, is started with the induction of anaesthesia and continued for 5 days postoperatively. Blood is cross-matched. Facilities must be available for intraoperative cholangiography.

Operative Techniques (Figs. 73–12 through 73–14)

A high transverse incision, dividing right and left rectus muscles, gives excellent exposure. The size of the cyst and the presence or absence of ascites are recorded. The gallbladder may or may not be distended and the duodenum is displaced forward over the lower portion of the cyst (Fig. 73–13). Macroscopic appearances of the liver do not give an accurate idea of histologic change unless advanced cirrhosis is present. Evidence of portal hypertension, including splenic size, are noted and the pancreas palpated and inspected for changes of pancreatitis.

Operative cholangiography via the gallbladder is useful for defining the anatomy of small cysts and for fusiform dilatations of the biliary tract but often fails to give adequate visualisation of intrahepatic or pancreatic ducts in patients with the more common, large Type I cystic lesions. Cholangiography in these cases is best deferred until a later stage in the operation, when contrast may be injected into the upper and lower ends of the common bile duct. A sample of bile is removed from the cyst for culture and analysis of pancreatic enzymes before any injection of contrast medium.

Dissection is started between the peritoneum and anterior wall of the cyst. The place is usually found without difficulty and is developed downwards between duodenum and cyst until most of the retroduodenal portion is freed. Sharp dissection may be needed to complete this phase. The lateral walls are now exposed after partial decompression of larger cysts and curved

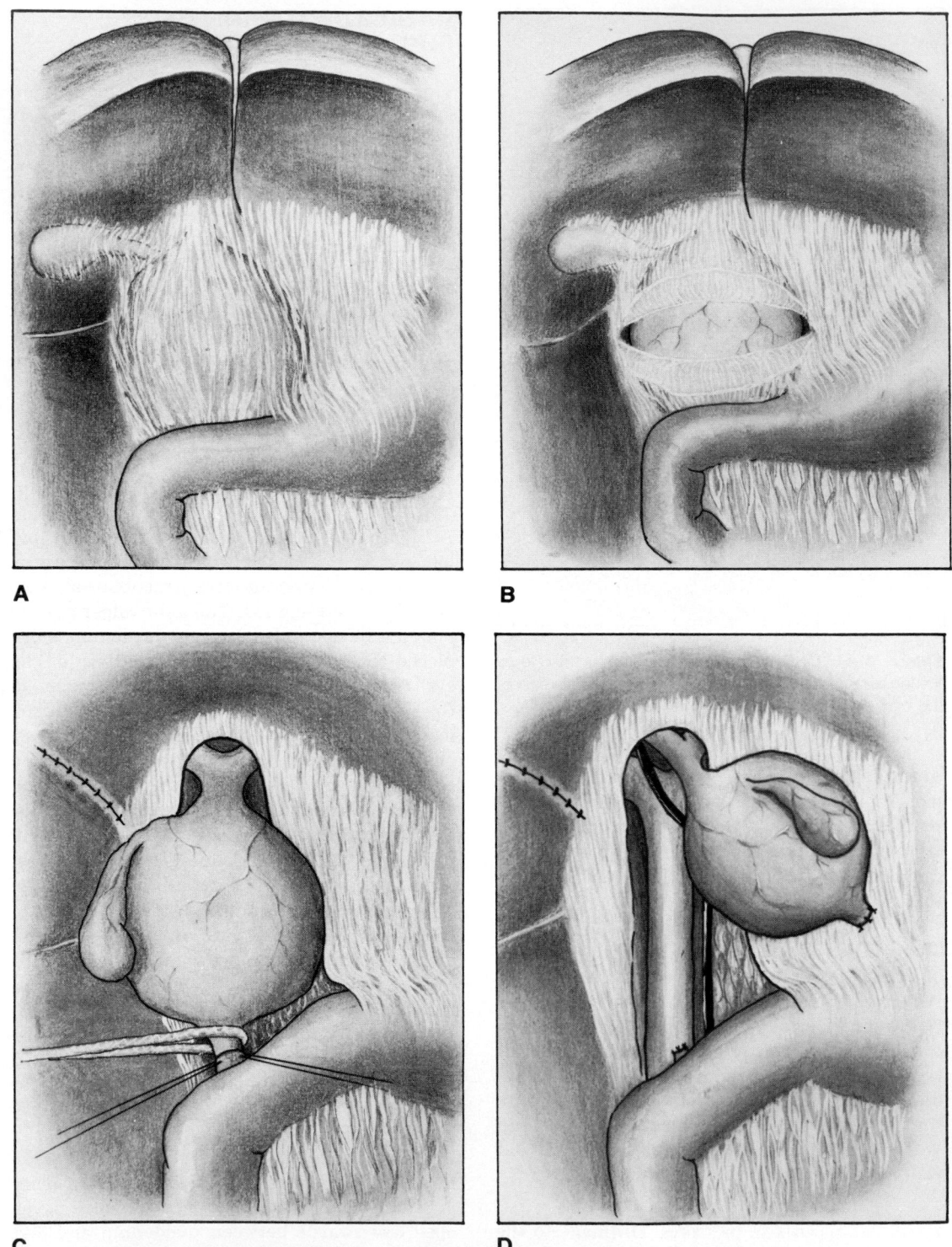

Figure 73–12. A through **G.** Radical excision of a Type I choledochal cyst. **A.** Exposure of cyst and gallbladder. **B.** Division of peritoneum over cyst. **C.** Dissection of gallbladder and narrow segment of distal common bile duct. **D.** Cyst and gallbladder dissected free of portal vein and hepatic artery. Distal common bile duct divided and oversewn.

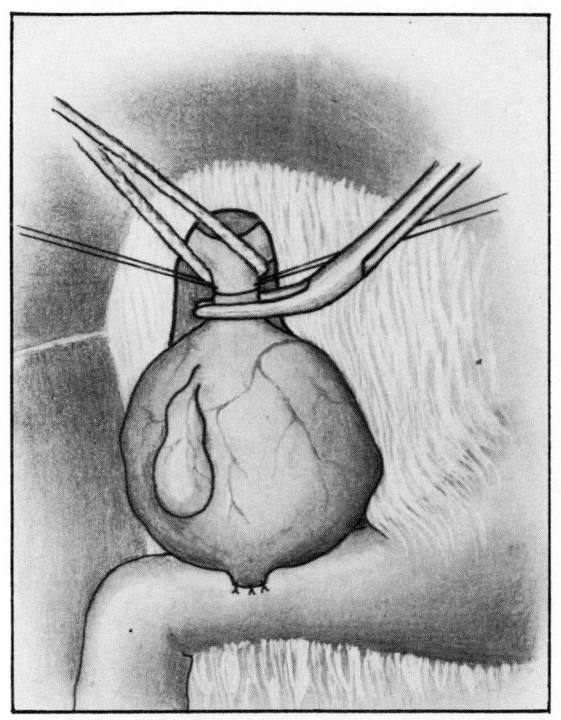

E

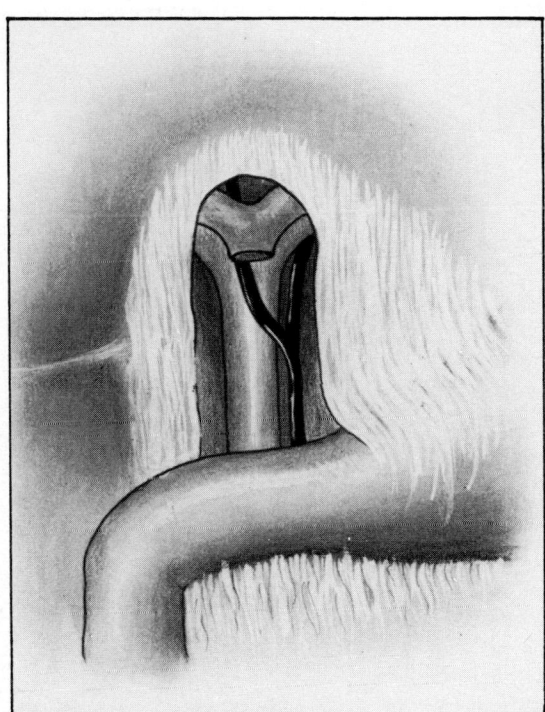

F

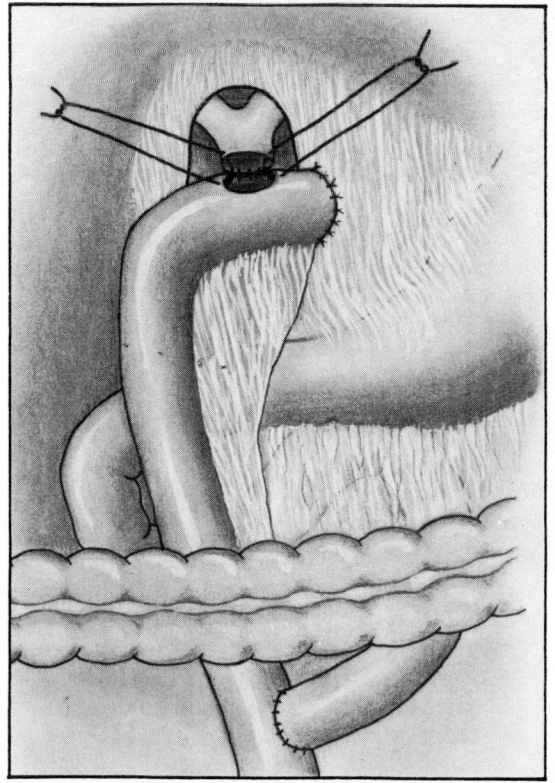

G

Figure 73–12. E,F. Dissection and division of common hepatic duct. **G.** Anastomosis of Roux-Y loop of jejunum (retrocolic) to common hepatic duct.

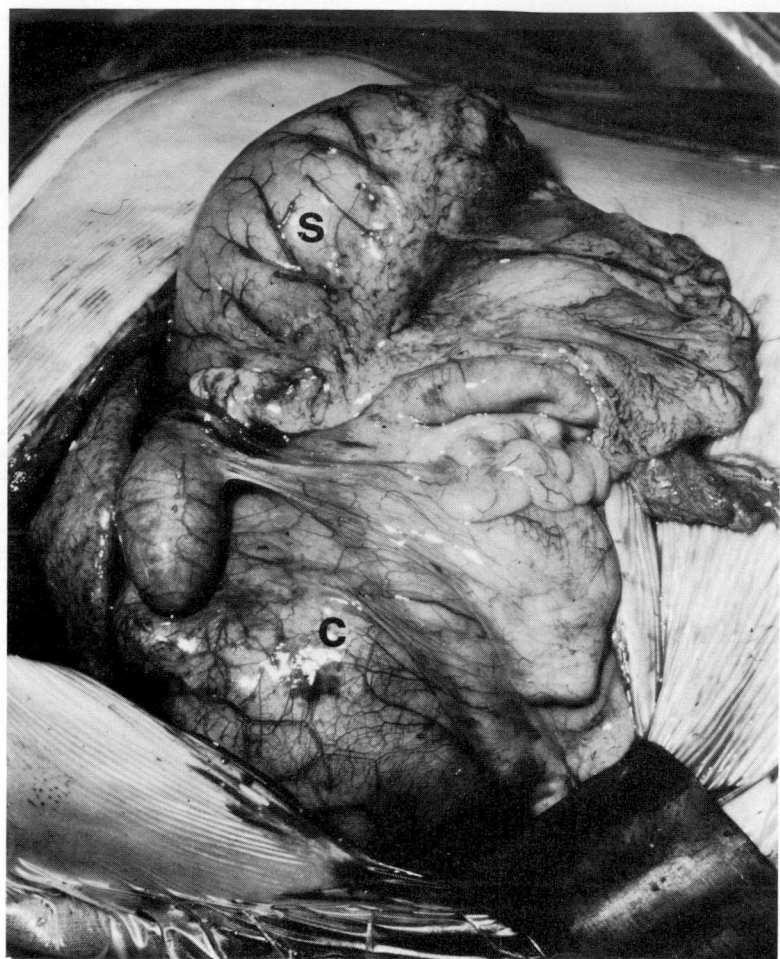

Figure 73–13. Operative photograph of Type I cystic dilatation of common bile duct in a 3-year-old girl showing displacement of the stomach (s) by the huge cyst (c).

forceps are passed around the lower narrow segment of duct behind the duodenum. Division is carried out proximal to the segment, which is densely adherent to the pancreas, thereby avoiding the pancreatic ducts. The anatomy of the latter may be identified by distal cholangiography at this stage of the operation and the distal common bile duct is then oversewn.

The gallbladder and cystic duct are mobilised, with care taken to define the position of the right hepatic artery, which may be adherent to the front wall of the cyst. The cyst is dissected forward from the portal vein and freed completely to the junction with the narrower common hepatic duct. Injection of saline to define tisue planes may help in cases of increased adherence.

The common hepatic duct is divided between stay sutures just below the bifurcation

and the cyst and gallbladder are removed. Intrahepatic cholangiography is now performed.

The operation is completed with a two-layer, end-to-side anastomosis between the common hepatic duct and a 40-cm retrocolic Roux loop of jejunum. Internal splinting of this anastomosis is not necessary.

Modifications of Operative Technique

1. Lilly in 1979 suggested a modification of the resection technique to avoid possible damage to the portal vein and hepatic artery, which may be difficult to identify in cases of severe pericyst fibrosis, or when a previous cyst anastomosis has been performed.

    An initial transverse opening of the cyst, between stay sutures, divides the anterior, lateral, and medial walls but leaves the poste-

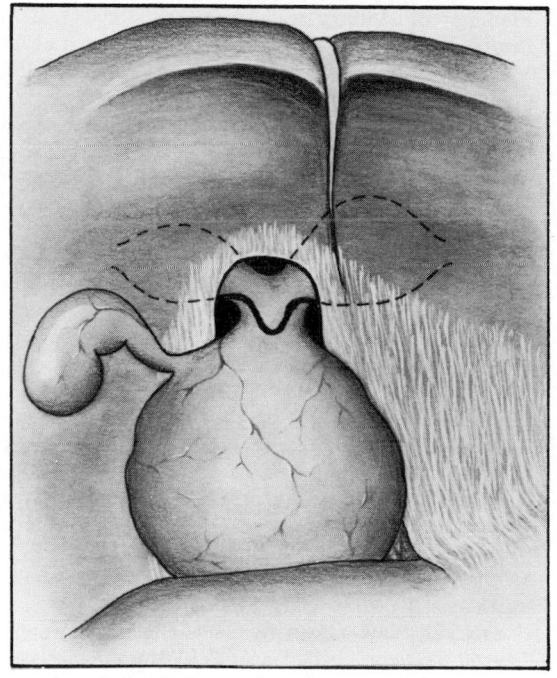
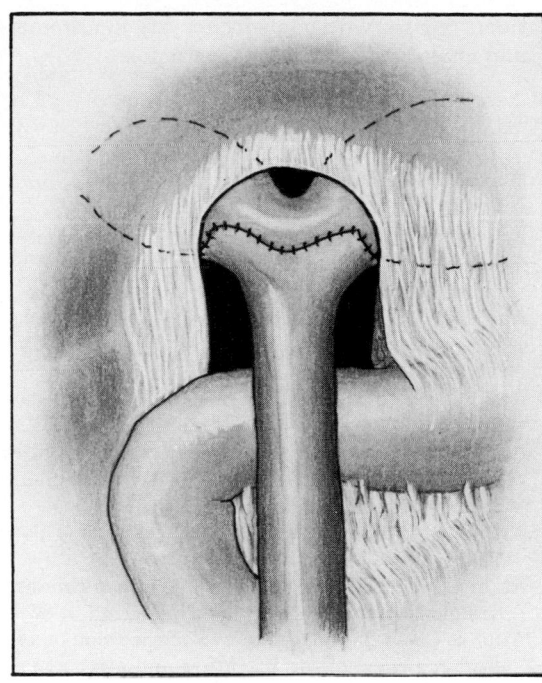

A   **B**

Figure 73–14. Method of incorporating dilated intrahepatic segments in the hepaticojejunostomy anastomosis. **A.** Incision of right and left hepatic ducts (*continuous line*). **B.** Anastomosis completed.

rior wall attached to the vessels. The fibrous posterior wall is then split into thick inner and thin outer layers and the former is stripped out by blunt dissection. Distally the common bile duct is ligated or oversewn in the usual manner and proximally a place of dissection around the common hepatic duct is easily found and transected. The whole of the cyst is then removed except for the thin back wall.

2. Congenital dilatation of the larger intrahepatic ducts is probably more common in cases of choledochal cyst than previously appreciated. They are frequently asymmetric and inaccessible for definitive drainage procedures but occasionally dilatations of the main hepatic ducts can be treated by making lateral incisions into the cysts from the transected bifurcation of the common hepatic duct. The common opening fashioned in this way allows a wide anastomosis with a Roux loop of jejunum (Fig. 73–14).

3. Severe pericyst fibrosis or portal hypertension may occasionally prevent total cyst exci-

sion. Choledochocystojejunostomy with a 40-cm Roux-Y loop of jejunum is the alternative operation of choice (Fig. 73–11).

Summary. The advantages of total cyst excision include removal of a fibrous-walled dilated duct, conservation of which may lead to gallstone formation, infection, or malignancy. The technique can be performed in all age groups and is the definitive treatment for complications occurring in cysts previously anastomosed to the gastrointestinal tract. A review of recent publications suggests that cyst excision is at least as safe as an internal drainage procedure and that late complications of cholangitis and gallstones are reduced to a minimum. Miyano et al (1980), for example, reported a 1- to 13-year follow-up of 22 patients in whom there were no operative deaths and no postoperative complications. The present author has had a smaller but similar experience with eight cases treated by radical excision in the last 9 years. In contrast, Trout and Longmire (1971) reported reoperation rates of 33 and 40.5 percent in patients treated with choledochocystjejunostomies and choledochocystoduodenostomies.

BIBLIOGRAPHY

Ackerholm P, Benediktsdottir K, et al: Cholangiocarcinoma in a patient with biliary cysts. Acta Chir Scand 147:605, 1981

Alonso-Lej F, Rever WB, et al: Congenital choledochal cyst, with a report of 2, and an analysis of 94, cases. Int Abstr Surg 108:1, 1959

Araki T, Itai Y, et al: CT of choledochal cyst. Am J Radiol 135:729, 1980

Arima E, Akita H: Congenital biliary tract dilatation and anomalous junction of the pancreatico-biliary ductal system. J Pediatr Surg 14:9, 1979

Arthur GW, Stewart JOR: Biliary cysts. Br J Surg 51:671, 1964

Atkinson GO, Gay BB: Choledochal cysts in children: Radiologic features. South Med J 75:1215, 1982

Attar S, Obeid S: Congenital cyst of the common bile duct: A review of the literature and a report of 2 cases. Ann Surg 142:289, 1955

Babbitt DP: Congenital choledochal cysts: New etiological concept based on anomalous relationships of common bile duct and pancreatic bulb. Ann Radiol 12:231, 1969

Babbitt DP, Starshak RJ, et al: Choledochal cyst: A concept of etiology. AJR 119:57, 1973

Bedikian AY, Valdivieso M, et al: Cancer of the extrahepatic bile ducts. Med Pediatr Oncol 8:53, 1980

Blocker TG, Williams H, et al: Traumatic rupture of a congenital cyst of the choledochus. Arch Surg 34:695, 1937

Cahlin E: Choledochal cyst: A case operated with excision and anatomical reconstruction. Acta Chir Scand 140:161, 1974

Caroli J: Diseases of intrahepatic bile ducts. Israel J Med Sci 4:21, 1968

Chen W, Chang C, et al: Congenital choledochal cyst: With observations on rupture of the cyst and intrahepatic ductal dilatation. J Pediatr Surg 8:529, 1973

Chesterman JT: Choledochus cyst complicating pregnancy and the puerperium. J Obstet Gynaecol Br Emp 51:512, 1944

Cholankeril JV, Ketyer S, et al: Demonstration of choledochal cyst by computed tomography. Comput Radiol 6:109, 1982

Dewbury KC, Aluwihare M, et al: Prenatal ultrasound demonstration of a choledochal cyst. Br J Radiol 53:906, 1980

Douglas AH: Case of dilatation of the common bile duct. Monthly J Med Sci 14:97, 1982

Filler RM, Stringel G: Treatment of choledochal cyst by excision. J Pediatr Surg 8:529, 1973

Flanigan DP: Biliary cysts. Ann Surg 182:635, 1975

Frank JL, Hill MC, et al: Antenatal observation of a choledochal cyst by sonography. Am J Radiol 137:166, 1981

Friend WD: Rupture of choledochal cyst during confinement. Br J Surg 46:155, 1958

Gallagher PJ, Millis RR, et al: Congenital dilatation of the intrahepatic bile ducts with cholangiocarcinoma. J Clin Pathol 25:804, 1972

Gatrad AR, Gatrad AH: The association of choledochus cyst with congenital hepatic fibrosis. Br J Clin Pract 33:182, 1979

Ghahremani GG, Lu CT, et al: Choledochal cyst in adults. A clinical and radiological study in ten cases. Gastrointest Radiol 1:305, 1977

Goldberg PB, Long WB, et al: Choledochocele as a cause of recurrent pancreatitis. Gastroenterology 78:1041, 1980

Han BK, Babcock DS, et al: Choledochal cyst with bile duct dilatation: Sonography and ^{99m}Tc IDA cholescintigraphy. Am J Radiol 136:1075, 1981

Harris V, Ramilo J, et al: Choledochal cyst with cholelithiasis. J Pediatr Surg 14:191, 1979

Huang MJ, Liaw YF: Intravenous cholescintigraphy using Tc 99m-labelled agents in the diagnosis of choledochal cyst. J Nucl Med 23:113, 1982

Irwin ST, Morison JE: Congenital cyst of the common bile-duct containing stones and undergoing cancerous change. Br J Surg 32:319, 1944

Jaubert de Beaujeu M, Bonjean JA, et al: Congenital cystic dilatation of the common bile duct and acute pancreatitis in children. Chir Pediatr 20:325, 1979

Jensen SR, Nielsen OV, et al: Fat malabsorption in patients with Roux-en-Y hepaticojejunostomy. Surg Gynecol Obstet 147:561, 1978

Jona JZ, Babbitt DP, et al: Anatomic observations and etiologic and surgical considerations in choledochal cyst. J Pediatr Surg 14:315, 1979

Jones PG, Smith ED, et al: Choledochal cysts: Experience with radical excision. J Pediatr Surg 6:112, 1971

Kagawa Y, Kashihara S, et al: Carcinoma arising in a congenitally dilated biliary tract. Gastroenterology 74:1286, 1978

Kangarloo H, Sarti DA, et al: Ultrasonographic spectrum of choledochal cysts in children. Pediatr Radiol 9:15, 1980

Karjoo M, Bishop HC, et al: Choledochal cyst presenting as recurrent pancreatitis. Pediatrics 51:289, 1973

Kasai M, Asakura Y, et al: Surgical treatment of choledochal cyst. Ann Surg 172:844, 1970

Kato T: The etiology of congenital choledochal cyst, in Kasai M, Shiraki K (eds): Cholestasis in Infancy. Tokyo: University of Tokyo Press, 1980, p 241

Kato T, Hebiguchi T, et al: Action of pancreatic juice on the bile duct: pathogenesis of congenital choledochal cyst. J Pediatr Surg 16:146, 1981

Kim SH: Choledochal cyst: Survey by the surgical section of the American Academy of Pediatrics. J Pediatr Surg 16:402, 1981

Kimura K, Tsugawa C, et al: Choledochal cyst. Etiological considerations and surgical management in 22 cases. Arch Surg 113:159, 1978

Kirwan WO: Choledochal cyst. Br J Surg 61:147, 1974

Klotz D, Cohn BD, et al: Choledochal cysts: Diagnosis and therapeutic problems. J Pediatr Surg 8:271, 1973

Lake DNW, Smith PM, et al: Congenital hepatic fibrosis and choledochus cyst. Br Med J 2:1259, 1977

Lilly JR: Common bile duct calculi in infants and children. J Pediatr Surg 15:577, 1980

Lilly JR: Surgery of coexisting biliary malformations in choledochal cyst. J Pediatr Surg 14:643, 1979

Lilly JR: The surgical treatment of choledochal cyst. Surg Gynecol Obstet 149:36, 1979

Lilly JR: Surgical jaundice in infancy. Ann Surg 186:549, 1977

Marshall JB, Halpin TC: Choledochocele as the cause of recurrent obstructive jaundice in childhood: Diagnosis by ERCP. Gastrointest Endosc 28:88, 1982

Martin LW, Rowe GA: Portal hypertension secondary to choledochal cyst. Ann Surg 190:638, 1979

McLoughlin MJ: Congenital cystic disease of the liver. J Can Assoc Radiol 28:243, 1977

Mettler FA, Wicks JD, et al: Diagnostic imaging of choledochal cysts. Clin Nucl Med 6:513, 1981

Miyano T, Suruga K, et al: "The choledocho-pancreatic long common channel disorders" in relation to the etiology of congenital biliary dilatation and other biliary tract disease. Ann Acad Med Singapore 10:419, 1981

Miyano T, Suruga K, et al: A clinicopathologic study of choledochal cyst. World J Surg 4:231, 1980

Miyano T, Suruga K, et al: Abnormal choledocho-pancreatico ductal junction related to the etiology of infantile obstructive jaundice diseases. J Pediatr Surg 14:16, 1979

Muakkasah K, Obeid S, et al: Congenital choledochal cysts. Arch Surg 111:1112, 1976

Murray-Lyon IM, Shilkin KB, et al: Nonobstructive dilatation of the intrahepatic biliary tree with cholangitis. Q J Med XLI:477, 1972

Nakata H, Nobe T, et al: Choledochal cyst. J Comput Assist Tomogr 5:99, 1981

Ohkawa H, Sawaguchi S, et al: Experimental analysis of the ill effect of anomalous pancreaticobiliary ductal union. J Pediatr Surg 17:7, 1982

Oldham KT, Hart MJ, et al: Choledochal cysts presenting in late childhood and adulthood. Am J Surg 141:568, 1981

Ono J, Sakoda K, et al: Surgical aspect of cystic dilatation of the bile duct: An anomalous junction of the pancreatico-biliary tract in adults. Ann Surg 195:203, 1982

Orenstien SR, Whitington PF: Choledochal cyst resulting in congenital cirrhosis. Am J Dis Child 136:1025, 1982

Parasothy M, Somasundram K: Technetium 99m-diethyl-IDA hepatobiliary scintigraphy in the preoperative diagnosis of choledochal cyst. Br J Radiol 54:1104, 1981

Rabinowitz JG, Kinkhawala MN, et al: Rim sign in choledochal cyst. Additional diagnostic feature. J Can Radiol 24:226, 1973

Redo SF: Biliary tract problems in pediatric patients. Major Probl Clin Surg 16:105, 1982

Rento JJ, Bailly G, et al: Congenital choledochal cyst. The value of systematic ultrasound screening starting in the second trimester of pregnancy. J Gynecol Obstet Biol Reprod (Paris) 10:61, 1981

Saito S, Ishida M: Congenital choledochal cyst. (Cystic dilatation of the common bile duct.) Progr Pediatr Surg 6:63, 1974

Saito S, Yura J, et al: A proposal of new classification of congenital biliary dilatation. J Jpn Soc Ped Surg 16:319, 1980

Scharli A, Bettex M: Congenital cyst: Reconstruction of the normal anatomy. J Pediatr Surg 3:604, 1968

Shallow TA, Eger SA, et al: Congenital cystic dilatation of the common bile duct. Case report and review of literature. Ann Surg 117:355, 1943

Shocket E, Hallenbeck GA, et al: Choledochal cyst. Report of cases. Proc Mayo Clin 30:83, 1955

Spitz L: Experimental production of cystic dilatation of the common bile duct in lambs. J Pediatr Surg 12:39, 1977

Standfield N: Personal communication, 1983

Stringel G, Filler RM: Fictitious pancreatitis in choledochal cyst. J Pediatr Surg 17:359, 1982

Tagart REB: Perforation of a congenital cyst of the common bile duct. Br J Surg 44:18, 1956

Tanaka M, Ikeda S, et al: The presence of a positive pressure gradient from pancreatic duct to choledochal cyst demonstrated by duodenoscopic microtransducer manometry: Clue to pancreaticobiliary reflux. Endoscopy 14:45, 1982

Todani T, Tabuchi K, et al: Carcinoma arising in the wall of congenital bile duct cysts. Cancer 44:1134, 1979

Todani T, Watanabe Y, et al: Hepaticoduodenostomy at the hepatic hilum after excision of choledochal cyst. Am J Surg 142:584, 1981

Todani T, Watanabe Y, et al: Congenital bile duct cysts. Classification, operative procedures and review of thirty-seven cases including cancer arising from choledochal cyst. Am J Surg 134:263, 1977

Trout HH, Longmire WP: Long-term follow-up study of patients with congenital cystic dilatation of the common bile duct. Am J Surg 121:68, 1981

Tsardakas E, Robnett A: Congenital cystic dilatation of the common bile duct: Report of 3 cases, analysis of 57 cases and review of the literature. Arch Surg 72:311, 1956

Tsuchida Y, Ishida M: Dilatation of the intrahepatic bile ducts in congenital cystic dilatation of the common bile duct. Surgery 69:776, 1971

Valayer J, Alagille D: Experience with choledochal cyst. J Pediatr Surg 10:65, 1975

Vater A (Dr Abrahamo Vatero): Dissertatio anatomica qua novum bilis diverticulum circa orificum ductus cholidochi. Disputationum Anatomicarum Selectarum 3:259, 1748

Watts DR, Lorenzo GA, et al: Congenital dilatation of the intrahepatic biliary ducts. Arch Surg 108:592, 1974

Wellwood JM, Madara JL, et al: Large intrahepatic cysts and pseudocysts. Pitfalls in diagnosis and treatment. Am J Surg 135:57, 1978

Witlin LT, Gadacz TR, et al: Transhepatic decompression of the biliary tree in Caroli's disease. Surgery 91:205, 1982

Wong KC, Lister J: Human fetal development of the hepatopancreatic duct junction—A possible explanation of congenital dilatation of the biliary tract. J Pediatr Surg 16:139, 1981

Yamaguchi M: Congenital choledochal cyst. Analysis of 1433 patients in the Japanese literature. Am J Surg 140:653, 1980

Yamaguchi M, Sakurai M, et al: Observation of cystic dilatation of the common bile duct by ultrasonography. J Pediatr Surg 15:207, 1980

Yamashiro Y, Sato M, et al: Spontaneous perforation of a choledochal cyst. Eur J Pediatr 138:193, 1982

Yeong ML, Nicholson GI, et al: Regression of biliary cirrhosis following choledochal cyst drainage. Gastroenterology 82:332, 1982

Yotuyanagi S: Contributions to the aetiology and pathogeny of idiopathic cystic dilatation of the common bile duct. With report of three cases: New aetiologic theory. Gan (Tokyo) 30:601, 1936

74. Gallstones—Aetiology and Dissolution

Avni Sali

Gallstone disease is very common in most developed countries; for example, in the United States, it is estimated that 20 million people have gallstones with 500,000 cholecystectomies being performed and approximately 10,000 deaths per year related to this disease. During the last 15 years, our understanding of gallstone formation has been greatly enhanced and stone dissolution has become possible, but more information is needed on the prevention of this disease before it can be adequately controlled.

HISTORICAL BACKGROUND

Cholesterol gallstones have been described in Chilean mummies since the second and third centuries AD. There are also descriptions of stones in the biliary system in Greeks in the fifth century AD, as well as in Persians in the tenth century AD. Vesalius (1514–1564) established the teaching that gallstones were evidence of disease and he associated them with jaundice.

The existence of bile acids has been known for some time. Berzelius (1809) was the first to recognise an acid fraction in bile. Gmelin (1826) studied ox bile and identified both sodium cholate and taurine, whereas Demarcay (1838) showed that cholic acid was the major solid component of bile. The term "bile acid" was coined by Lieberg in 1843. Lehman (1855) recognised glycocholic and taurocholic acids as separate entities.

Substances secreted by the liver, absorbed by the intestine, and resecreted by the liver, have an enterohepatic circulation. Borelius, an Italian mathematician of the seventeenth century, calculated the amount of bile entering the duodenum and postulated that there is a particular circulation of the bile through the abdomen. Credit must be given to Hoffmann (1844) for wondering about some kind of circulation, but it was left to Hoppe-Seyler (1863) to postulate a continuous circulation of bile acids. The existence of the enterohepatic circulation was confirmed when "foreign" bile acid was fed to an animal and subsequently identified in bile by Weiss in 1844.

The idea of dissolving gallstones attracted early interest with Durande in 1782 describing the use of turpentine for in vitro dissolution. In 1892, Naunyn placed human gallstones in dog gallbladders and found that they had disappeared 1 to 2 months later when the dogs were reoperated. Similar dissolution of human cholesterol gallstones has been observed in the gallbladder of pig, goat, monkey, and sheep. The bile of all these animals is less saturated with cholesterol than human bile.

Hawker, in 1897, described the dissolution of bile duct stones by infusing ether and glycerine through a biliary fistula. Best and others, in 1953, tested the gallstone-dissolving powers of a number of substances including bile acids and found chloroform to be the most effective. However, Probstein and Eckert had already found in 1937 that chloroform and ether T-tube infusion caused death in all dogs that were infused, but little notice was taken of their finding although many patients were developing complications from chloroform and ether bile duct infusions. Consequently, the technique was abandoned after many years.

PHYSIOLOGY

Bile Secretion

Bile, which is predominantly water, is produced by the hepatocytes and the cells of ducts continuously at a rate of 500 to 1500 ml/day. The chief constituents of bile, apart from water, are bile acids, cholesterol, phospholipids, and bilirubin (Table 74–1).

Bile is produced as a result of mechanisms in the canaliculi, ductules, and ducts. Osmotically active bile acids are responsible for fluctuations in bile flow and also approximately half of the bile volume. The composition of hepatic bile fluctuates during the 24-hour period, primarily due to the fluctuation of bile acid through the enterohepatic circulation.

The biliary system conveys the bile to the duodenum after a proportion of it is stored and concentrated in the gallbladder. The gallbladder concentrates bile from six- to ten-fold. The pH of hepatic bile varies, but it is generally alkaline and the gallbladder lowers pH. Changes in bile pH may be responsible for inflammation of gallbladder mucosa.

Three quarters of the bile production is canalicular. Also, a constant volume of water is added at the canalicular level independent of bile acid secretion. In the ductules, secretion and absorption of electrolytes plus water occurs unrelated to the canalicular mechanisms. Water and permeable ions flow into the bile ductules to establish isoosmolality and electrical neutrality. Bile duct epithelium has adaptive responses and bile concentration in the common bile duct increases following cholecystectomy in the dog.

The mechanisms by which bile acids influence the biliary secretion of lipids are poorly understood. Bile acid secretion influences the

amount of lecithin and to a lesser extent cholesterol in bile. It is possible that bile-acid-independent cholesterol secretion may contribute to the cholesterol supersaturation of bile during fasting.

Bile Acids

Bile acids are steroid molecules formed from cholesterol by hepatocytes and are a major pathway of cholesterol excretion by the body. To enhance their solubility in bile, bile acids are conjugated to lysine or taurine before excretion as a sodium salt. There are three types of bile acids in bile: primary, secondary, and tertiary (Fig. 74–1). Cholic and chenodeoxycholic acids are primary bile acids, comprising 75 percent of bile acids produced by the hepatocytes. Each day, one third to one quarter of the primary bile acid pool is lost or converted by anaerobic bacteria to secondary bile acids, with cholic acid being converted to deoxycholic acid, and chenodeoxycholic acid to lithocholic and 7-keto lithocholic acid. The 7-keto lithocholic acid which is reabsorbed can be converted, probably in the liver, to ursodeoxycholic acid—a "tertiary" bile acid normally found in man and which comprises about 15 percent of the bile acids.

Functions of Bile Acids. Bile acids, cholesterol, and phospholipids are the principal lipids in bile. Bile acids have a dual function. They are primarily responsible for the transport of

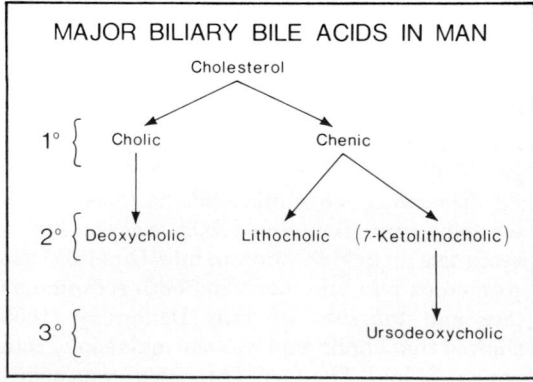

Figure 74–1. Major primary, secondary, and tertiary biliary bile acids in man. Since 7-ketolichocholic acid is reduced to chenodeoxycholic acid and ursodeoxycholic acid during hepatic passage, it is usually not detected in bile. Chenic = chenodeoxycholic acid. (*Source: From Hoffmann AF, 1977, with permission.*)

TABLE 74–1. COMPOSITION OF BILE

	Hepatic Bile (g%)	Gallbladder Bile (g%)
Water	97.0	92.0
Bile acids	1.0	6.0
Bilirubin	0.04	0.03
Cholesterol	0.06	0.35
Lecithin	0.1	0.7

(*Source: From Kune GA, Sali A, 1980, with permission.*)

cholesterol in bile and are also involved in the digestion of fats. Cholesterol is virtually insoluble in water and is carried in bile by the combined detergent action of conjugated bile acids and phospholipids. The cholesterol is mainly transported in water soluble aggregates known as micelles (Fig. 74–2). Above a certain level, bile acids coalesce to form micelles that have a hydrophilic (water soluble) external surface and hydrophobic (fat soluble) internal surface. The water insoluble cholesterol is incorporated into the hydrophobic interior of the micelle. Phospholipids are inserted into the walls of micelles so that they are enlarged. These mixed micelles are then able to hold more cholesterol. Bile acids also act as a solvent for dietary lipids in the intestine and, in addition, aid their intestinal absorption.

Cholesterol

The major site of cholesterol synthesis and excretion is the hepatobiliary tract in the form of cholesterol and its metabolites, the bile acids, and neutral steroids. Cholesterol is derived from dietary ingestion, hepatic and small intestinal synthesis, and, to a lesser degree, synthesis in almost all other body tissues. The relative contributions of each are not known and therefore the influence of each on cholesterol metabolism remains unclear. At each major step in cholesterol metabolism there is a complex feedback relationship, involving both bile salt synthesis and secretion. This complex mechanism explains the difficulty in elucidating changes in cholesterol metabolism.

Hepatic synthesis of cholesterol is from acetyl-CoA and is facilitated by the rate-limiting enzyme hydroxymethyl (HMGCoA) reductase. High calorie diets increase the activity of HMGCoA reductase and hence increase the synthesis and secretion of cholesterol. The effects of cholesterol ingestion are less clear. Fasting appears to decrease cholesterol synthesis and secretion in bile, but even with fasting, there appears to be a diurnal variation in cholesterol secretion.

Phospholipid

The majority of phospholipid in bile is lecithin. Lecithin is synthesised in the liver and secreted into bile. Both the synthesis and secretion are influenced by bile salt secretion in a direct but not linear relationship. With interruption of the enterohepatic circulation and depletion of bile acids, there is a concomitant decrease in bile-salt-stimulated lecithin synthesis. Unlike bile salts, lecithin is not conserved and very little is reabsorbed in the intestine; its hepatic synthesis accounts for the majority of its pool.

Bilirubin Secretion

Bilirubin is produced from the breakdown of red blood cells in the reticuloendothelial (RE) system. Of the 250 to 300 mg of bilirubin secreted each day, the majority is conjugated to form diglucuronide which is water soluble. Most of the bilirubin is excreted as the glucuronide conjugate with unconjugated bilirubin, which is insoluble in water, accounting for approximately 1 percent of bilirubin in bile. Appreciable quantities of monoglucuronide and smaller amounts conjugated to sulphate and other substances are present. Bilirubin is actively transported into the biliary canaliculus by a mechanism shared by several organic anions, such as sulfobromophthalein, but this transport mechanism is separate from that responsible for excretion of bile acids. Complex interferences between bile acid and bilirubin excretion exist, but these are not clearly understood.

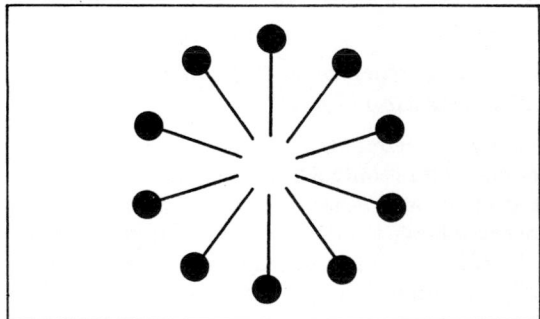

Figure 74–2. A spherical micelle formed by the aggregation of bile acid molecules. The rounded end of each molecule is water-loving (hydrophilic) while the stick end is the hydrophobic part to which the water-insoluble cholesterol is absorbed. (*Source: From Bailey, Love: Short Practice of Surgery, 15 edt. London: HK Lewis, 1964; and courtesy of Prof. A.H. Rains, with permission.*)

Control of Bile Flow

To enable the understanding of gallstone formation and dissolution, it is important to be familiar with the mechanisms controlling bile flow and composition.

Bile flow within the biliary system is regulated by three factors: hepatic secretion, gallbladder contraction, and bile duct sphincteric resistance. Bile secretion is influenced by neural and hormonal stimuli, but it is the enterohepatic circulation of bile acids that primarily influences bile secretion.

Enterohepatic Circulation of Bile Acids

Most people who form gallstones have abnormal bile that is supersaturated or overloaded with cholesterol. This supersaturated bile appears to result from alterations in the enterohepatic cycling of bile salts. The liver secretes 20 to 30 g of bile acid per day, but the total body pool of bile acids at any one time is between 3 and 5 g. The bile salt pool is defined as the total mass of bile salt circulating in the enterohepatic circulation. This pool usually circulates twice each meal; therefore, 6 to 8 times per day. After a meal, about 98 percent of the bile salts entering the intestine are absorbed and returned through the portal vein to the liver, where they are cleared and resecreted into canaliculi (Fig. 74–3). Bile acids, returning to the liver via the portal vein, control hepatic bile acid synthesis

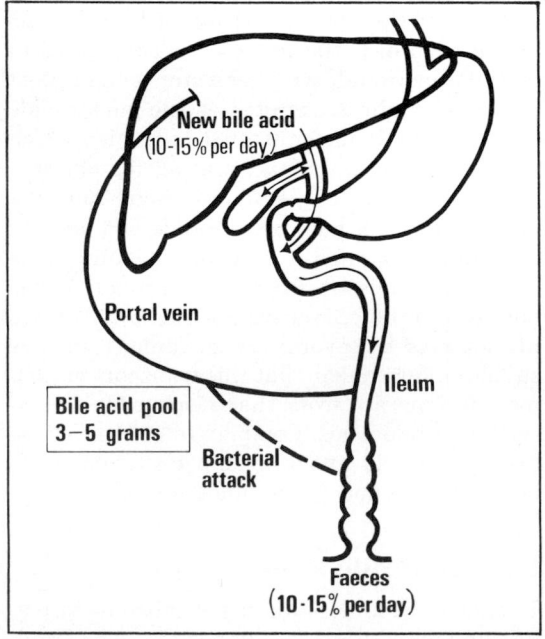

Figure 74–3. Enterohepatic circulation of bile acids. (*Source: From Kune GA, Sali A, 1980, with permission.*)

from cholesterol through a negative feedback mechanism. The details of this feedback mechanism are unclear, but the amount of bile acid produced equals the small amount lost in the faeces. The rate limiting enzyme, cholesterol $7-\alpha$ hydroxylase, mediates bile acid synthesis in the liver. The activity of this enzyme appears to be inversely proportional to the enterohepatic circulation of bile acid. The liver clears bile acids returning via the portal vein efficiently, therefore less than 5 percent of the total bile acids entering the liver enter the systemic circulation. This explains the extremely low serum bile acid level. The liver conjugates deconjugated primary bile acids and secondary bile acids to glycine and taurine before they are resecreted. Only small amounts of new bile acid are added to bile.

The bile acids are primarily actively absorbed in the ileum in the conjugated form. Passive absorption of 15 to 20 percent of unconjugated bile acids does occur in the intestine. Deconjugation of bile acids results from anaerobic bacteria, especially *Bacteroides,* mainly in the colon. About one quarter of the conjugated primary bile acids are deconjugated by bacterial enzymes in the ileum. The bacteria also convert primary bile acids to secondary bile acids. Only one fifth of the lithocholate is reabsorbed whereas one third to one half of the deoxycholic acid is reabsorbed. Each day, one third to one quarter of the primary bile acid pool is lost or converted by anaerobic bacteria to secondary bile acids and there is 500 to 700 mg of bile acid lost in the faeces. This loss is replaced by new bile acid synthesised from cholesterol in the liver.

Vagal and Hormonal Control of Bile Secretion

Animal experiments have shown that neurohormonal factors control bile secretion. Vagus stimulation, as well as secretin and cholecystokinin, increase hepatic bile secretion. The stimulus to bile secretion following ingestion of food is probably neurohormonal.

Bile Canaliculi Ductules and Ducts

Bile flow, down the canaliculi towards the ductules, may be facilitated by contractions of the canalicula. This has been recently demonstrated. Gastrointestinal (GI) hormones, such as vasoactive intestinal peptide (VIP), caerulein, cholecystokinin, and gastrin act on the ductules and influence the volume and composition of bile primarily by diluting canalicular and gallbladder bile.

Gallbladder

The gallbladder, which has a capacity of the order of 20 ml, has two important roles: concentration of bile and delivery of bile into the duodenum after food ingestion. Hepatic bile entering the gallbladder can be concentrated by 90 percent in 4 to 5 hours. Water is absorbed by the gallbladder passively as a result of electrolyte transport. Approximately half of the hepatic bile bypasses the gallbladder during the interprandial state and also overnight, and therefore bile enters into the duodenum directly. The gallbladder can store almost all of the total bile acid pool.

Gallbladder Motility. Gallbladder filling occurs when the common bile duct pressure increases adequately to divert bile into the gallbladder. The regulation of gallbladder relaxation is not fully understood, but pancreatic polypeptide, VIP, and also somatostatin cause relaxation. Sarles' group from France has demonstrated the presence of a hormone which is capable of relaxing the gallbladder. They have called this hormone "anticholecystokinin." The degree of gallbladder relaxation, and also the bile duct pressure regulated by the sphincter of Oddi, determine gallbladder filling. Fasting gallbladder volume is increased with pregnancy and after total vagotomy.

Ivy et al demonstrated in 1928 that the release of cholecystokinin controls gallbladder emptying after meals, probably by acting directly on the musculature of the gallbladder. It is possible that motilin may play some part in the interdigestive gallbladder emptying.

Choledochal Sphincter Motility

The volume of bile entering the gallbladder is mainly influenced by the choledochal sphincter and, to a lesser extent, by duodenal musculature. The choledochal sphincter has a constant rhythmic peristaltic activity, with phases of contraction and relaxation. Contractions of the sphincter of Oddi occur about four times per minute. It is likely that the duration of each phase determines the amount of bile entering the duodenum and also gallbladder filling. However, animal studies have shown that gallbladder filling occurs even after sphincterotomy.

The function of the choledochal sphincter is independent of duodenal musculature. Narcotic drugs, especially morphine and pethidine, increase sphincteric tone whereas anticholinergic drugs and glyceryl trinitrate decrease tone. Meal-induced endogenous cholecystokinin leads to simultaneous gallbladder contraction, sphincter of Oddi relaxation, and hepatic bile secretion.

NATURE OF GALLSTONES

Gallstones are crystalline or amorphous bodies formed from the constituents of bile. The type of gallstone depends on the predominance of one or more constituents. Much is known about those circumstances that predispose bile to precipitate cholesterol, but little is known about the precipitation of bile pigments. Scant information is available about the factors governing crystal formation and growth of stones in bile. Crystallisation takes place almost always in the gallbladder. Primary bile duct stones occur rarely and these are less crystalline than gallbladder stones.

Classification of Gallstones

Human gallstones occur in two main types, classified according to their predominant components. There are predominantly cholesterol gallstones, and also stones with appreciable amounts of calcium bilirubinate and related pigments and very little cholesterol, referred to as pigment stones. "Mixed" stones have appreciable amounts of both pigment and cholesterol, but usually contain over 50 percent cholesterol and are considered as a variant of cholesterol stones.

Gallstones can also be classified by their gross morphology as being either cholesterol or pigment stones. Cholesterol stones are smooth or faceted in shape, 2 to 40 mm in diameter, light tan in colour, and laminated and/or crystalline on cross-section with a distinct dark nucleus, whereas pigment stones are usually multiple, 2 to 5 mm in diameter, irregular to smooth in shape, black to brown in colour, and amorphous or crystalline in cross-section (Fig. 74–4).

Chemical analysis has confirmed the accuracy of visual classification for the major constituents of stones, such as cholesterol, bilirubin,

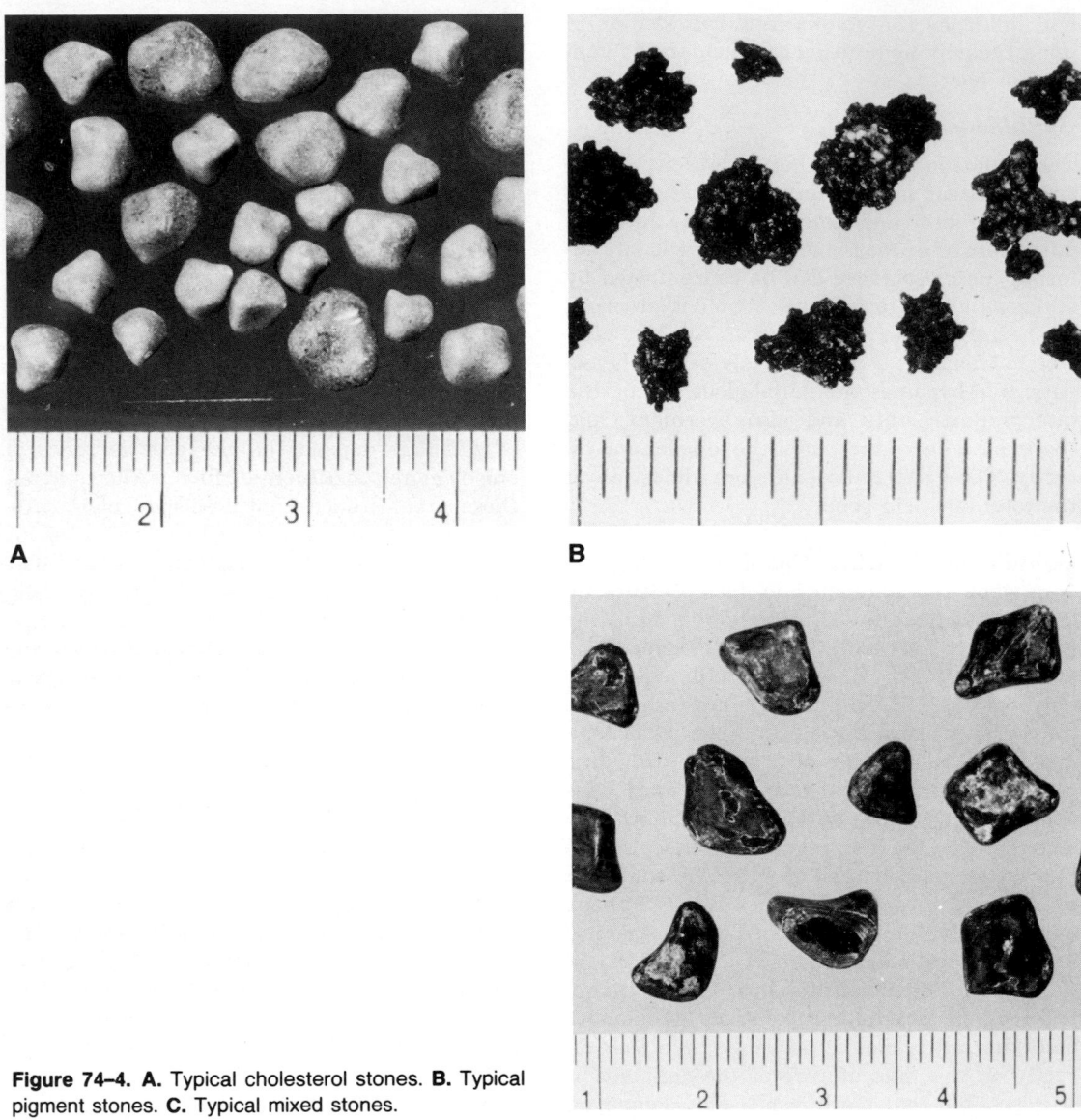

Figure 74–4. A. Typical cholesterol stones. **B.** Typical pigment stones. **C.** Typical mixed stones.

and calcium. Analysis of gallstones shows a continuous spectrum of stone composition, rather than the two distinct types. Pure cholesterol and pigment stones are rare and make up 20 percent of gallstones. Mixed stones composed mainly of cholesterol, pigment, and calcium are the most common type of stone accounting for approximately 70 percent of all stones. Of the mixed stones, the majority (70 to 80 percent) are radiolucent and cholesterol-rich (70 to 75 percent). The radiopaque stones account for 20 percent

of all gallstones and it is estimated that pigment stones account for 60 percent of radiopaque stones.

CHEMICAL COMPOSITION OF GALLSTONES

Cholesterol. Cholesterol is the major component of most gallstones in Western countries and occurs in crystalline form.

Bile Pigment. Bile pigment is the second most common component of gallstones, the majority of which is bilirubin. The pigment in gallstones can be in either the conjugated or unconjugated form. Different types of pigment have been found using complex assays, but only bilirubin can be analysed with ease.

Calcium. Calcium is the third major chemical present in gallstones in Western countries. Its content usually varies from 0.02 to 5 percent and stones with up to 55 percent calcium salts have been described. Calcium in gallstones occurs as the bilirubinate, carbonate, phosphate, and palmitate.

Other Substances. Many other substances can be found in gallstones and these include sodium, potassium, phosphorus, copper, iron, manganese, and fatty acids. Organic compounds, such as triglycerides, polysaccharides, and phospholipids are also found in addition to considerable amounts of bile acid, especially in pigment stones. Gallstones in patients taking oral contraceptive drugs for long periods of time have been shown to have very high levels of copper.

Gallstone Structure

An essential constituent of all gallstones is the matrix, a gel-like substance found to consist of large amounts of glycoproteins. An amorphous mass of calcium, bilirubinate, and protein, with or without copper ions, occurs at the centre of most cholesterol gallstones (Fig. 74–5). Surrounding this core, there may be cholesterol crystals either with or without calcium salts. Highly calcified stones also have a central pigment. Pigment stones are amorphous conglomerates and consist primarily of bile pigments with variable amounts of calcium.

Primary Common Bile Duct Stones

In 1923, Aschoff described in detail the features of a "primary biliary stasis stone" based on morphologic characteristics. He described these stones as being brownish yellow, "earthy," soft, frequently laminated, and easily crushed (Fig. 74–6). Madden et al in 1968 used these macroscopic features to differentiate primary from secondary common bile duct stones. There have been variable reports on the incidence of primary common duct stones, ranging from 2.5 to 56 percent of bile duct stones. Saharia and others, in 1977, included the following criteria before stones could be classified as primary common bile duct stones: preexploration for choledocholithiasis, previous cholecystectomy, 2-year asymptomatic period after cholecystectomy, characteristic morphologic features, and no evidence of a long cystic duct stump or stricture from the previous operation. This group confirmed the presence of abnormal functional

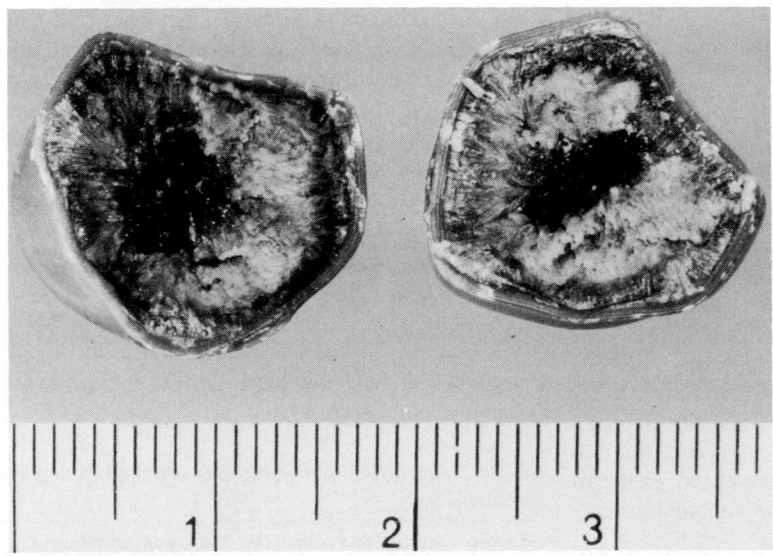

Figure 74–5. Cross-section of cholesterol stone with distinct dark nucleus.

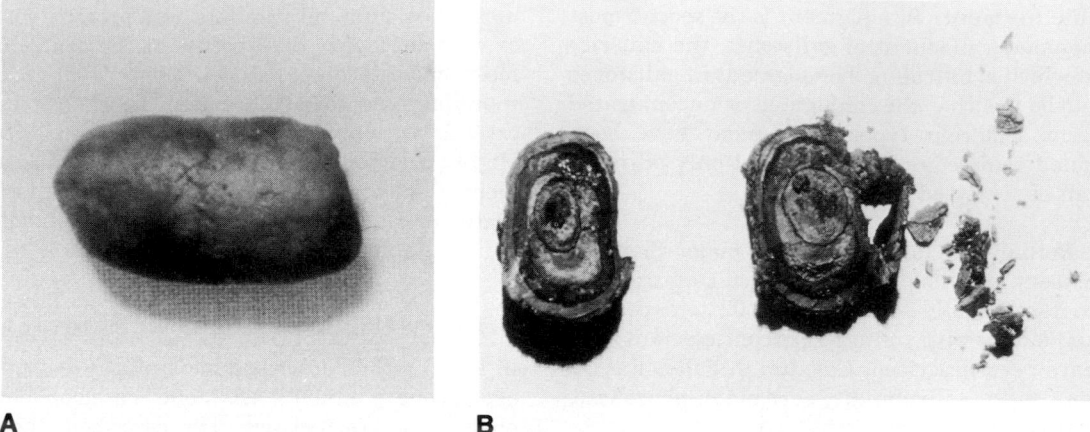

A   **B**

Figure 74–6. A. Primary common bile duct stone with typical shape. **B.** Transverse section showing laminated appearance and fragmentation.

dilation of the bile duct observed by others. It is suggested that primary common bile duct stones may result from stasis, changes in bile composition, and also infection.

Until recently, there was no information on the chemical composition of these stones. In an extensive analysis of primary common bile duct stones, the author's group has shown that these stones have a similar chemical composition to pigment stones but are clearly very different morphologically. Another Australian group has also analysed bile duct stones and found that stones with morphologic characteristics typical of primary duct stones have less than 25 percent cholesterol.

Gallbladder Stones

The pathogenesis of gallstones and the mechanisms thought to underline the various risk factors for the development of cholelithiasis will be discussed. The causes of cholesterol gallstone formation are understood in greater depth and detail than those for pigment stone formation and are therefore discussed in more detail. Gallstone composition is different in the Western countries where stones are predominantly of cholesterol, compared to most Oriental countries where they are usually pigment. An emphasis on human findings is presented, as it can be difficult to extrapolate from the variable results of animal experiments.

PATHOGENESIS OF CHOLESTEROL GALLSTONES

For almost 150 years, stasis, obstruction, and inflammation were known as aetiologic mechanisms in cholelithiasis. Although these concepts were important and could contribute to a particular mechanism of stone formation, such as the formation of primary bile duct stones, general theories based on any one of these phenomena could not explain the overall process of gallstone formation. Much of the early information relating to the various theories of gallstone formation has been reviewed extensively by Rains in his comprehensive monograph.

Small, in 1980, postulated that gallstone formation occurs in four stages (Table 74–2). Current concepts have been aimed at understanding the pathogenesis of gallstones by focusing heavily on the physicochemical properties of bile and the formation of saturated bile. Initiation of stone formation and stone growth mech-

TABLE 74–2. STAGES OF GALLSTONE FORMATION

- Formation of saturated bile
- Formation of microcrystals
- Nucleation
- Stone growth to detectable size without passing into duodenum

(*Source: Adapted from Small DM, 1980, with permission.*)

anisms are equally important, but less information is available regarding these factors.

It is known that bile supersaturated with cholesterol is frequently found in hepatic gallbladder bile of healthy people. Gallstones may not form in this latter group because supersaturation is not present long enough to initiate precipitation and there may be inhibitors of nucleation. They may also have more optimum biliary tract motility.

Solubility of Cholesterol in Bile

The three major biliary lipids—cholesterol, lecithin, and bile salts—form soluble mixed micelles in bile. Cholesterol can precipitate from the mixed micelle depending on the relative proportions of the three biliary lipids. Admirand and Small in 1968 were first to propose a graphic analysis on the ability of bile acid micelles to solubilise cholesterol. Their in vitro model system consisted of three major bile lipids: bile salts, lecithin, and cholesterol. The relative molar percentages of the three biliary lipids were graphically illustrated by a triangle (Fig. 74–7). The presence or absence of insoluble cholesterol or bile supersaturated with cholesterol was determined by the relative concentration of bile salt, lecithin, and cholesterol.

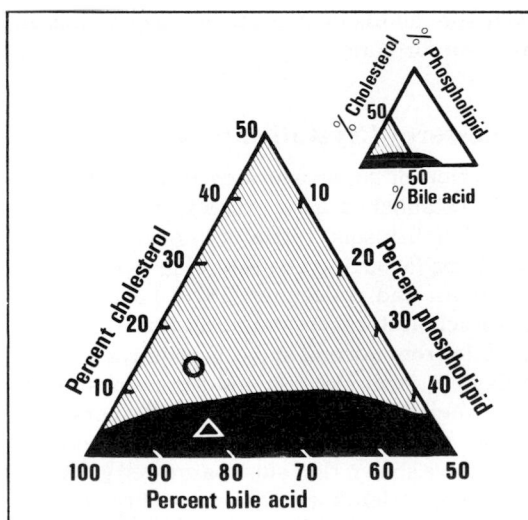

Figure 74–7. Triangular coordinates illustrating gallbladder bile composition. The larger triangle is an expanded section of the phase diagram. △ = bile in the micellar zone, ○ = bile in the supersaturated zone. (*Source: From Kune GA, Sali A, 1980, with permission.*)

Since this report, it has become apparent that the physical chemistry of cholesterol solubility in bile is more complex. Other techniques for preparation and identification of cholesterol crystals have found that maximum cholesterol solubility is less than originally proposed. It is possible for bile to be supersaturated with cholesterol without cholesterol precipitating. This is called the metastable state. In contrast, bile in a labile state enables cholesterol to precipitate rapidly. In vitro experiments have shown that in a metastable state, bile is supersaturated but crystal growth does not occur or is slow, whereas in the labile state with supersaturated bile, the quantity of cholesterol is sufficient for rapid crystallisation.

Carey and Small (1970) have also reported that factors other than relative concentration of cholesterol, bile acids, and phospholipids can influence the capacity to hold cholesterol in micelle solution. These factors include ionic strength and water content; of these considerations, the water content of bile appears to be most important. As bile acids become more concentrated, their aggregation into micelles with additional cholesterol solubilising capacity is enhanced. Thus, dilute bile is less capable of cholesterol solubilisation than concentrated bile of the same relative lipid composition and, although hepatic bile may become progressively more saturated during an overnight fast because of low secretion rates of bile acids, gallbladder bile simultaneously may become more capable of cholesterol solubilisation because of the concentrating action of the gallbladder mucosa. The major causes of supersaturated bile are high water content, high cholesterol content, and a low bile acid and phospholipid content.

Bile supersaturated with cholesterol can occur in one of three ways: by a decreased synthesis and secretion of either bile acids or phospholipids, or by an increased synthesis and excretion of cholesterol. The available evidence implicates altered hepatic metabolism of bile acids and cholesterol in the pathogenesis of saturated bile. The following mechanisms are involved.

Bile Salt Pool

The bile salt pool is reduced in most patients with gallstones to about half that of normal. This can result from either impaired bile acid reabsorption or reduced hepatic bile acid synthesis. Malabsorption is almost certainly the cause of supersaturated bile in diseased states, such as regional enteritis, ileal resection or bypass, cirrhosis, and probably during the use of oestrogens and progestins. A small bile acid pool can also result from rapid bile salt circulation within the enterohepatic circulation, as with multiple small meals. Apart from these disorders, impaired hepatic bile acid synthesis seems to be the main cause of diminished pool size.

Because hepatic bile acid synthesis is subject to feedback regulation, the normal response to faecal bile acid loss is a compensatory increase in bile acid synthesis to prevent reduction in the pool size. In vitro studies comparing gallstone patients with those without gallstones have demonstrated diminished activity of 7-α hydroxylase, the limiting enzyme of hepatic bile acid synthesis, and this could explain the impaired bile acid synthesis. However, in vitro assays of the enzyme are difficult to interpret and other studies have not confirmed this finding. It may be that the feedback regulation of bile acid synthesis is abnormally sensitive in such persons, so that despite reduced bile acid pools, the synthesis of bile acids does not increase as it would in a normal person whose bile acid pool was reduced to a similar degree.

There is a poor correlation between the total bile salt pool size and cholesterol saturation. Pool size may influence biliary saturation but it possibly is not the major determinant, although it has been postulated that there may be a subgroup of individuals in whom pool size is a significant determinant.

Hepatic Cholesterol Synthesis and Secretion

Cholesterol saturation in bile and the potential for precipitation occurs when cholesterol constitutes more than 10 percent of the total lipids in bile. Defects in the hepatic synthesis and secretion of cholesterol play a major role in the formation of supersaturated bile. Biliary cholesterol supersaturation could reflect excessive cholesterol secretion in the presence of normal bile salt production. It is possible that a combined defect of decreased bile salt and excessive cholesterol secretion exists in many non-obese gallstone subjects. There is controversy whether the rate-limiting enzyme for cholesterol HMGCoA reductase activity is increased in gallstone disease. Therefore, it cannot be concluded that there is a specific defect in cho-

lesterol synthesis in non-obese subjects with cholelithiasis.

Obesity, lipid lowering drugs and diets, age, and female sex hormones can all cause excessive secretion of cholesterol in bile and predispose to saturation or gallstone formation.

Enterohepatic Circulation

A review by LaMorte and others in 1981 states that most people who form gallstones have bile supersaturation which appears to result from alterations in the enterohepatic cycling of bile salts. These alterations in bile salt circulation result in changes in the synthesis of biliary lipids and their secretion in the liver. The various factors that influence the enterohepatic circulation and their importance in gallstone formation are dealt with in other sections.

Phospholipid

Lecithin in gallbladder bile has been demonstrated to be reduced in absolute amount and concentration in gallstone patients. The relative percentage of phospholipids to the other lipids is also reduced. There is lower secretion of phospholipid in association with the reduced biliary bile salt secretion in non-obese patients with cholelithiasis, compared to normals, but there is no difference in phospholipids from normal in obese subjects. Overall, little is known about the details of the role of phospholipid in gallstone formation.

Cholesterol Crystallisation

Production of supersaturated bile has become firmly established as a prerequisite of cholesterol cholelithiasis. Little is known about the conditions favouring cholesterol growth in bile.

Holan and colleagues (1979) have studied in vitro cholesterol crystal formation and found that bile from normal subjects requires at least 15 days to form crystals and sometimes never does, whereas bile from gallstone formers took a mean of 3 days to develop crystals. Another group have shown that supersaturated gallbladder bile of patients with gallstones has crystals but supersaturated bile in subjects without gallstones does not have crystals.

The role of gallbladder mucus and other substances in forming a nucleus will be discussed later. It is known that the majority of cholesterol gallstones have a central region of bile pigment. There is some evidence indicating that there is an increase in the poorly soluble bilirubin monoglucuronide in the bile of cholesterol gallstone patients, which could explain the presence of the pigment nucleus in cholesterol stones. However, the majority of patients do not have this bilirubin abnormality. Unabsorbable sutures have been found in bile duct stones and are almost certainly a major factor in their aetiology.

Calcium and Bilirubin

Calcium precipitation in bile is a requisite in the pathogenesis of pigment gallstones and may also serve as a nucleus for precipitation of cholesterol to form cholesterol gallstones. Gallbladder bile has a calcium concentration of about three times that of hepatic bile. As part of a detailed study into the solubility of bile, Williamson and Percy-Robb (1980) have determined that micellar binding can account for 80 percent of the calcium binding in hepatic bile but only 50 percent in gallbladder bile. It was suggested that such binding of calcium in this soluble micellar form would lower the activity of calcium in gallbladder bile and therefore its liability to precipitation as gallstone nuclei.

More recently it has been shown that bile acid anions, both in free and micellar form, constitute an important potential buffer for intraluminal calcium in the biliary tree and intestine. Thus, by limiting the ambient ionised calcium concentrations, bile acid anions may protect against calcium precipitation.

The majority of bilirubin in bile is conjugated to glucuronide, the calcium salt that is water soluble. Unconjugated bilirubin (1 percent of total bilirubin) in bile is kept soluble by association with bile salt micelles. Increase in the concentration of calcium does not necessarily cause bilirubinate to precipitate from solution. However, during concentration of bile in the gallbladder, a decrease in the pH of gallbladder bile has been observed. This drop in pH can subsequently alter the solubility properties of both unconjugated bilirubin and calcium bilirubinate. This may then be an important physicochemical factor in the formation of a precipitate and nidus for gallstone formation. The amount of citrate in bile, which has recently been discovered by the author's group, may also determine the availability of free calcium for precipitation as it is a strong calcium binder.

Sulphated glycoproteins have also been implicated in the seeding of gallstones, they have been found to be present in increased amounts in the bile of patients with gallstones, and they are known to bind calcium salts tightly.

Gallstone Growth

Like the process of nucleation, the process of gallstone growth is poorly understood and is probably complex. Scanning electron microscopic studies of gallstones and bile sediments from gallstone patients have been used to investigate gallstone growth. It has been concluded that the basic units of both microscopic and macroscopic stones were laminated cholesterol crystals. These laminated crystals were aggregated randomly, radially, or concentrally and showed evidence of dissolution, suggesting that gallstones result when conditions favouring precipitation predominate over dissolution.

The role of other constituents of mixed cholesterol gallstones in the growth of the cholesterol crystals, such as protein, bile pigments, and calcium salts, remains to be elucidated.

Cholesterol Gallstones

Epidemiology. The epidemiology of cholelithiasis is complex but it holds the key to aetiology. The incidence of gallstones in developed Westernised countries is high. The world incidence of gallstones, based on postmortem studies, is seen in Table 74–3. A postmortem study recently concluded by Vitetta and Sali with predominantly male patients at a Veterans Administration Hospital has shown a gallstone incidence of approximately 50 percent. This study suggests that the incidence of gallstones in Australia is increasing. Unlike malignant diseases,

TABLE 74–3. WORLD INCIDENCE OF GALLSTONES

	Female (%)	Male (%)	Mean (%)
Sweden	57	32	45
Czechoslovakia	50	30	40
England	35	15	25
USA	30	16	23
Australia	26	25	21
Japan	—	—	8
China	—	—	3

cholelithiasis remains undetected during life in approximately 60 to 80 percent of people, as most gallstones are asymptomatic.

In Japan and China, gallstones are much less common. However, if Japanese or Chinese migrate to mainland United States or Hawaii, they have an incidence of gallstones equal to the original inhabitants of that country. It has also been shown that not only is the incidence of gallstones increasing in Japan, but also the cholesterol type of gallstone has become more common over the last 30 years. This information strongly indicates an environmental factor, in particular a dietary factor, as an important cause of gallstones.

Gallstones are much more frequently seen in the white population than in the black population of the United States and South Africa. An extremely low incidence of gallstones in a nomadic East African tribe, despite their higher consumption of cholesterol and fat than the average American, supports a racial factor in cholelithiasis. There are also racial differences in gallstone incidence in Asian countries and also among the eight races in Hawaii.

Apart from racial variations, the frequency of cholelithiasis has a familial relationship. In a study of 100 consecutive patients with gallstones, 72 percent of the primary relatives had gallstones. The incidence of gallstones in parents and siblings of patients with the disease was significantly higher than in matched controls, but there was no increased incidence in spouses. It was also found that the familial incidence of gallstones was greater in those presenting in childhood and adolescence with the disease. In the Pima North American Indians, the incidence of gallstones may be as high as 75 percent. A prospective study on twins has not supported a simple genetic factor. It is possible that some people are genetically susceptible to gallstone formation but require the participation of other factors, such as diet, before the disease manifests.

Age and Sex. Gallstone disease has been shown to occur earlier and with a higher frequency in women than in men for all age groups above 20 years of age. A female-to-male ratio of between 2:1 to 4:1 has been reported. The susceptibility of women to the disease has also been reported from Thailand and India. However, in Japan and Singapore the frequency in men and women is approximately equal. The strong relationship between femininity and parity to cholesterol gallstones does not exist for pigment stones where a similar incidence in both sexes has been found in Western and Oriental countries.

Gallstones are extremely rare before the age of 10 years. Their frequency increases with age. Bile becomes more saturated in older people and this occurs in the absence of any change in bile salt metabolism suggesting that biliary

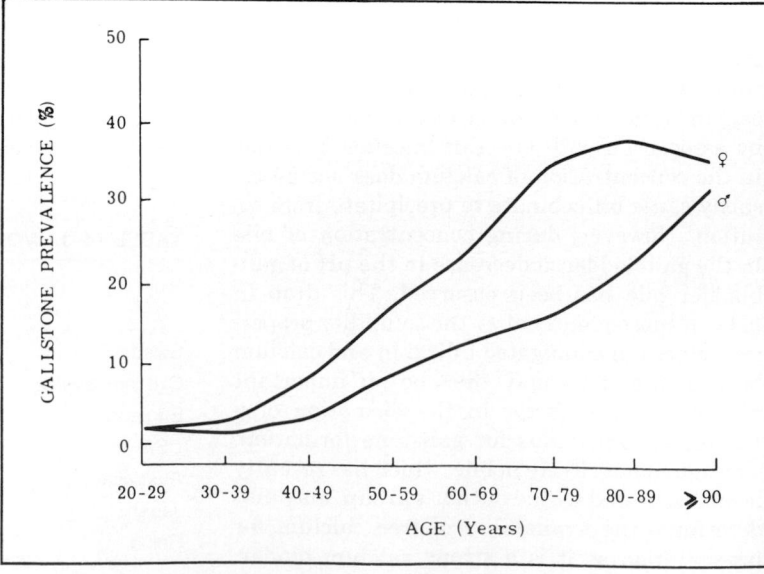

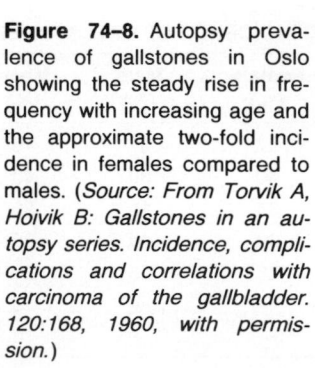

Figure 74–8. Autopsy prevalence of gallstones in Oslo showing the steady rise in frequency with increasing age and the approximate two-fold incidence in females compared to males. (*Source: From Torvik A, Hoivik B: Gallstones in an autopsy series. Incidence, complications and correlations with carcinoma of the gallbladder. 120:168, 1960, with permission.*)

secretion of cholesterol increases with advancing age.

A definite increase in gallstone disease in women is seen from the time of puberty (Fig. 74–8). Autopsy studies have shown that the incidence of white women with gallstones tends to rise sharply up to the 50 to 60 years of age group and from there on rises slowly. White men show a steady rise in incidence, but do not reach the levels associated with white women, except before puberty and after the age of 60 (Fig. 74–9). Therefore, hormonal differences appear to account for the sex-related incidence of gallstones. A number of studies have suggested that endogenous oestrogens and progestins (or both) mediate this phenomenon through an effect on bile saturation and smooth muscle function of the gallbladder and intestine during the phases of menstrual cycle and pregnancy. In contrast, others have found that hormonal changes during the normal menstrual cycle do not alter biliary cholesterol saturation significantly and no male-to-female differences in bile composition have been demonstrated.

The onset of ovarian function in Pima Indian girls has been found to be accompanied by a decrease in the total bile acid and chenodeoxycholic acid pools and a simultaneous increase in bile cholesterol saturation, increasing the possibility of gallstone formation. Similar

changes do not occur in the male Pima Indian. Cessation of ovarian function as a result of surgical castration is accompanied by expansion of the bile acid pool and a decrease in bile cholesterol saturation, suggesting that endogenous oestrogens or progestins, or both, are responsible. Progesterone appears to cause relaxation and impaired emptying of the gallbladder. Sluggish gallbladder contraction has been observed during the midluteal phase of the menstrual cycle and women empty their gallbladders more slowly than men.

Data relating pregnancy with an increased incidence of cholelithiasis has remained highly controversial. A recent study showed that late pregnancy caused incomplete emptying of the gallbladder leaving a large residual volume which could cause retention of cholesterol crystals, a prerequisite for cholesterol gallstone formation. To determine if pregnancy does cause gallstones, the author's group is doing gallbladder ultrasonography at the beginning and soon after the end of pregnancy.

Diet. Epidemiologic and dietary manipulation studies both suggest that diet is emerging as a major determinant of bile composition and, ultimately, the potential to develop gallstones. Striking differences exist among countries and racial populations having a very high or very low incidence of cholelithiasis and atherosclerosis. Moreover, the type and incidence of gallstones, or both, within a population have been well correlated with changes in diet in that country or migration to another country. Dietary factors have also been implicated in Japan to explain the increasing incidence of gallstones and also the change from pigment to cholesterol stones. The unrefined carbohydrate in the Japanese diet has decreased and their protein and fat intake has increased.

Epidemiologic studies suggest that overconsumption of calories and highly refined carbohydrates can be major factors in cholesterol gallstone formation. Moreover, Sarles and others (1971) have found that patients with gallstones have a significantly higher intake of calories irrespective of their dietary composition. Their results suggest that apart from its effect on causing obesity, the ingestion of high calorie diets promotes gallstone formation through an increase in hepatic cholesterol secretion. The rise in biliary cholesterol results from an increase in the activity of HMGCoA reductase,

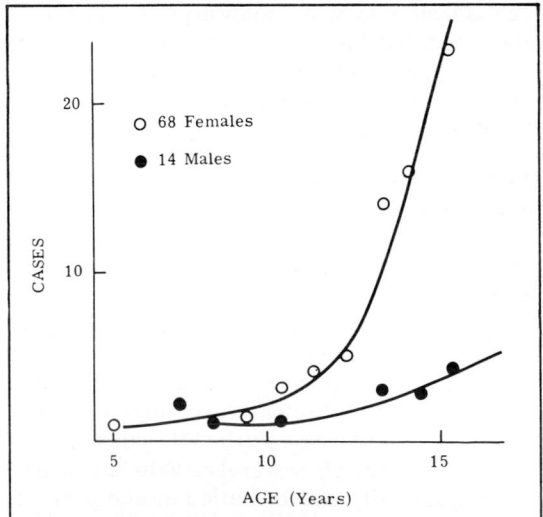

Figure 74–9. Cholelithiasis in children in a Swedish community hospital. Note the increase in females at puberty. (*Source: From Nilsson S, 1966, with permission.*)

the rate-limiting enzyme in cholesterol synthesis. This group has also found that a diet high in protein and calories increases lithogenicity. Wheeler and others (1970) have shown that southern European women who migrated to Australia had a higher prevalence of gallstone disease, probably related to the increased consumption of refined carbohydrates as well as meat.

Increased dietary fibre has been shown to increase the solubility of bile in patients with gallstones. It was found that the synthesis and pool size of chenodeoxycholic acid increased when bran was given. Gallstones have been shown to form in several species fed with fibre depleted carbohydrate. In addition, this phenomenon may account for the low incidence of cholesterol gallstones in populations in which the diet is rich in fibre.

The effects of excessive ingestion of cholesterol are less clear. Gallstones can be produced in a number of animal models by supplementing dietary cholesterol. Human studies have found that an increase in dietary cholesterol causes bile to become more saturated, but other studies have disagreed.

Obesity and Dieting. Epidemiologic, autopsy, and clinical studies closely relate obesity to gallstone prevalence. Gallstone incidence in obese people has been estimated to be about three times that of the general population. A number of studies have shown that a very high percentage of obese patients have bile supersaturated with cholesterol from an absolute and relative increase in cholesterol in bile, without changes in bile acid secretion. The supersaturated state of the bile in these patients may increase even further, in approximately half of them during a weight reduction period. However, after establishing a stable lower weight, bile is consistently less saturated with cholesterol than in the previous obese state. Patients with morbid obesity without gallstones who undergo gastric bypass surgery have been shown to form stones, frequently following rapid weight loss or as a result of operation. The changes in the regulation of biliary lipid metabolism during fasting are complex and not fully understood.

The effect of fasting for periods up to 16 hours on gallbladder bile is to increase transiently its cholesterol saturation. Prolonged fasting from 20 hours to 6 days results in a decrease in cholesterol secretion with a consistent

fall in hepatic and gallbladder bile lithogenicity.

A French group has recently shown that young women aged between 20 and 35 years who do not have breakfast may increase the risk of gallstone formation. This result agreed with previous reports of bile being lithogenic after short-term fasting.

Gastrointestinal Disease

ILEAL DISORDERS. It has been known for some time that ileal disease, resection, or bypass increases the incidence of gallstones. The majority of bile acids are absorbed from the ileum and therefore malabsorption of bile acids at this site interrupts the enterohepatic circulation. This interruption causes bile acid synthesis to increase from the normal range of 500 to 700 mg/day to compensate for faecal loss. When faecal losses exceed the synthetic capacity of the liver, the bile acid pool shrinks until a new steady state is reached in which faecal losses equal hepatic synthesis. With bile acid pools depleted, bile saturation increases and the prevalence of gallstones increases in these conditions. As a result of ileal disease, excessive bile acids enter the large bowel causing diarrhoea.

CYSTIC FIBROSIS AND PANCREATIC INSUFFICIENCY. Gallstones are more common among children with cystic fibrosis. Children with untreated cystic fibrosis have supersaturated bile, and treatment with pancreatic enzyme supplements normalises bile saturation. The supersaturated bile results from bile acid malabsorption and subsequent reduced bile acid pool. There may also be abnormal biliary mucus which could increase nucleation for stone formation or interfere with bile flow, causing stasis and gallstone growth.

TRUNCAL VAGOTOMY. The gallbladder generally dilates to approximately double its size following truncal vagotomy, but its response to cholecystokinin, and therefore emptying, is unaltered. Progressive dilatation of the gallbladder has also been observed after gastrectomy, presumably because in some cases the hepatic branches of the anterior vagus are divided during gastrectomy. Truncal vagotomy is usually followed by an increase in the bile salt pool and a reduction in the cholesterol ratio in bile, which would make gallstone formation unlikely. Moreover, vagotomy does not alter bile composition from the normal micellar zone to the abnormal lithogenic zone.

However, Sali and others have demonstrated that some patients have excess faecal bile salt loss following truncal vagotomy, probably as a result of "intestinal rush" following their drainage procedure. This increased faecal loss could then lead to depletion of bile salt pool, bile cholesterol saturation, and subsequent gallstone formation in this group of patients. A small increased incidence of gallstones following truncal vagotomy and gastrectomy has been noted.

Diabetes. Gallstones occur more frequently in diabetics and gallbladder bile from these patients is supersaturated with cholesterol. The metabolic defect leading to supersaturated bile in maturity onset diabetics is unknown. It is possible that the enterohepatic circulation, and hence bile acid pool size, may be disturbed in diabetics because of autonomic neuropathy, causing defects of intestinal motor activity and small intestinal bacterial overgrowth with interference in bile acids.

Drugs. A number of drugs have a marked influence on hepatic bile secretion or on biliary tract motility, increasing gallstone disease.

ORAL CONTRACEPTIVES. These increase the incidence of gallstones, as do other oestrogenic and also progesterone medications. Contraceptive steroids do not affect gallbladder resting volume or contraction whereas progesterone impairs the gallbladder response to exogenously administered cholecystokinin in animals but has not been tested in man. Apart from the direct action of progesterone as a smooth muscle relaxant, it may also influence the release of cholecystokinin from the intestinal mucosa. Oestrogen given to normal women increases biliary cholesterol saturation and reduces the pool of chenodeoxycholic acid.

HYPOLIPIDEMIC AGENTS. These drugs are used to reduce serum lipids in order to prevent premature vascular disease. Both cholestyramine and thyroxine can produce gallstones in animals experimentally. However, an increased prevalence of gallstones in humans using these drugs has not been documented. Clofibrate mobilises body cholesterol and increases hepatic cholesterol output in bile, and a marked increase in gallstone incidence accompanies its use. This specific mode of action of clofibrate in altering hepatic liver secretion is unknown. Nicotinic acid also increases biliary cholesterol.

Pigment Gallstones

Pigment stones account for 27 percent of gallstones in the United States, rather than the 10 percent which is often quoted. The incidence of pigment stones in the Orient varies from 28 to 70 percent. Almost every gallstone has a pigment centre and both intrahepatic gallstones and stones caused by bile stasis or cirrhosis are composed mainly of pigment.

Pigment stones can be characterised by their typical morphologic features already described. Soloway and others (1977), in their extensive review of pigment gallstones, have defined these stones as containing less than 25 percent cholesterol, whether or not pigment is its major component and irrespective of the nature and proportions of its other constituents.

Although there have been recent advances in analysing pigment gallstone composition, there are still difficulties in detecting and measuring the various pigments and other components present. Only 50 percent of the components can be measured, with pigment being the major one. Bilirubin can be measured quite accurately in these stones and the majority of the pigment is calcium bilirubinate, but other pigments are also present as well as heavy metals, magnesium phosphates, carbonates and sulphates, and calcium salts of fatty acids. Approximately 50 percent of pigment stones are radiopaque and in the United States they constitute two thirds of all radiopaque stones. This information has been very relevant to medical dissolution of gallstones as it decreases the chances of a radiolucent stone being of the pigment type, which does not respond to conventional medical therapy. A retrospective study has shown that 14 percent of radiolucent stones are pigment.

A study from Japan has shown that the incidence of pigment stones is decreasing, especially in the urban areas, and at the same time, there has been an increase in cholesterol cholelithiasis. The incidence of pigment stones in Japan varies from 28 percent in urban areas to 70 percent in rural regions.

Epidemiology. There is a clear difference in the incidence of pigment gallstones when people from rural regions of Oriental countries are compared with those from Westernised countries. Pigment stones are notably rare among American Indians who frequently have cholesterol gallstones. No difference in the incidence of pigment stones has been shown among the blacks and whites in the United States. The shift from pigment to cholesterol gallstones in Japan has been ascribed to the decrease in frequency of parasitic infestation and biliary infection, as well as Westernisation of the Japanese diet. Whereas most pigment stones in Westernised countries are in the gallbladder, in the Orient they are more likely to be intraductal.

Age and Sex. Pigment gallstones are more prevalent with advancing age, as with cholesterol cholelithiasis. In cholecystectomised adolescents, pigment stones account for less than 10 percent of stones, whereas by the seventh decade, pigment stones predominate. It is unknown whether pigment stones form later in life or remain asymptomatic for longer periods of time than cholesterol stones. Autopsy data from patients with cirrhosis and with haemolytic anaemias have shown an increased incidence of pigment stones.

Although there is a strong relationship between femininity and parity in cholesterol gallstones, this has not been found to be true for pigment lithiasis. Men and women with pigment stones are affected equally both in Western countries like the United States and in the Orient, suggesting that the factors affecting pigment lithiasis are independent of the levels of female hormones and their possible effect on bile composition and gallbladder emptying. Therefore, unlike cholesterol stones, sex, obesity, and parity are not associated with pigment stones.

Diet. The role of dietary factors in pigment stone formation is still not defined, although Soloway and co-workers (1977) feel that dietary factors leading to pigment stone formation may inhibit cholesterol stone formation and vice versa. Japanese, on a low protein, low fat diet, produce calcium bilirubinate gallstones more frequently than those on a high protein, high fat diet. Matsushiro and others (1977) have proposed that a low protein, low fat diet lowered the biliary concentrations of glucuro-1,4-lactone, which is an inhibitor of β-glucuronidase that is normally found in bile. It has also been postulated that either tissue or bacterial (*Escherichia coli*) β-glucuronidase activity in the bile may lead to the formation of free bilirubin and subsequent precipitation of calcium bilirubin.

Infection. Bile is normally sterile, but bacterial and parasitic infection is not uncommon. The bile of Japanese patients with calcium bilirubinate stones has been found to be almost invariably infected with some strain of *Escherichia coli*. Moreover, eggs or fragments of cuticles of *Ascaris lumbricoides* have been found in over 50 percent of calcium bilirubinate stones collected in Japan directly after World War II. The eggs are probably effective nucleating agents for precipitation of calcium bilirubinate in vitro and they play a similar part in vivo. By 1970, there had been a dramatic decline in pigment stones in Japan and the incidence of infection had fallen to 1 percent of the population.

The mechanism for stone formation, which has been postulated by Maki, (1966), implicates *Escherichia coli* as a producer of β-glucuronidase, an enzyme that hydrolyses the water soluble bilirubin glucuronide into free water, insoluble bilirubin, and glucuronic acid. He also proposed that the bilirubin would be available to precipitate with ionised calcium to form calcium bilirubin in bile. The activity of the β-glucuronidase is usually inhibited by glucuro-1,4-lactone in bile and Maki demonstrated that the addition of this latter enzyme to bile in vitro can prevent precipitation of calcium bilirubinate.

Infection, however, does not appear to be the major cause of calcium bilirubate stones in the United States and the mechanisms involved are unknown. However, because calcium bilirubinate forms the nidus of most gallstones, including cholesterol gallstones, it seems that precipitation of free bilirubin may be a very important factor in the formation of all gallstones.

Haemolytic Anaemia. Classically, pigment stones are said to occur more frequently in patients with haemolysis but this disease is rare in the general population and, therefore, this is a rare cause of pigment stones. Any condition that shortens the life-span of red blood cells, such as prosthetic heart valves and hereditary spherocytosis, is associated with pigment stones. It has been suggested that these patients have an excess of unconjugated bilirubin as a result of increased secretion by the liver. Another mechanism involves increased total bilirubin content of bile in excess of the ability of bile acids to hold them in solution.

A mouse model of haemolytic anaemia has provided useful information on the pathogenesis of pigment stones and has highlighted the importance of an increased bile content of free unconjugated bilirubin and the role of the gallbladder in providing the conditions suitable for the precipitation of calcium bilirubinate.

Hepatic Cirrhosis. Hepatic cirrhotic patients have been shown to have an increased incidence of gallstones overall, but pigment stones are found more frequently. Little data are available relating to the cause of pigment cholelithiasis in patients with cirrhosis. It is unlikely that the hypersplenism and the mild haemolytic anemia that often accompany cirrhosis influence stone formation as bilirubin has not been shown to be increased in cirrhosis. With cirrhosis, there may be a decrease in bile acid secretion that subsequently increases the chance of bilirubin precipitation because of fewer bile acid micelles to incorporate any unconjugated bilirubin and therefore maintain its solubility.

Bilirubin Saturation. In comparison with cholesterol saturation of bile, very little is known about why and how pigment precipitates from bile. The extremely insoluble unconjugated bilirubin in bile appears to be the major defect in these patients.

An increased concentration of unconjugated bilirubin in the gallbladder bile of patients with pigment stones has been demonstrated. The unconjugated bilirubin originates either from increased hepatic secretion or from excessive hydrolysis of conjugated bilirubin. The hydrogen ion concentration of bile is a critical factor in maintaining unconjugated bilirubin in solution. In Japanese patients, it is likely that the hydrolysis results from infection with *Escherichia coli* producing β-glucuronidase which subsequently hydrolyses bilirubin diglucuronide to the free form. However, not all pigment stones occur in the presence of increased unconjugated bilirubin and therefore other factors, such as calcium availability, must play a role.

Role of Gallbladder Function in Gallstone Formation

The gallbladder is essential for the formation of all gallstones apart from intrahepatic stones of the Orient and primary bile duct stones. It provides the environment for nucleation crystal formation and stone growth. LaMorte and co-workers (1981) have extensively reviewed the literature on the role of the gallbladder and biliary tract motility on cholesterol gallstone formation.

Gallbladder function is considered crucial in cholesterol stone formation, but its role in the formation of pigment gallbladder stones is much less well defined. In the formation of intrahepatic pigment stones, the gallbladder may have no role at all, though it is usually anatomically abnormal in this condition. A number of disturbances of gallbladder function that may lead to cholelithiasis have already been mentioned.

Rate of Gallbladder Emptying. Maudgal and others (1980) have demonstrated that the percentage of gallbladder emptying at 15 and 60 minutes after eating was significantly higher among stone-formers than controls. Increased rates of gallbladder emptying in gallstone patients after cholecystokinin stimulation has also been found by another group. Gallbladder function may influence the composition of biliary lipids. Moreover, rapid bowel transit has been found to decrease the total bile salt pool and also decrease the synthesis of primary bile acids resulting in increased cholesterol saturation of bile. Therefore, an increased rate of gallbladder emptying and intestinal transit increases bile cholesterol as in gallstone forming patients.

In a recent experiment, spincterotomy in dogs decreased cholesterol cholelithiasis. It was speculated that gallstones did not form because gallbladder stasis was prevented. However, pressures can be measured in the common bile duct and the sphincter of Oddi using transendoscopic manometry and no difference in the sphincter of Oddi pressure in controls and gallstone patients has been found. Therefore, it is unlikely that alteration in extrahepatic biliary tract motility is a significant factor in the pathogenesis of gallstones.

Impaired gallbladder contraction occurs with diabetes mellitus, coeliac disease, vagotomy, and pregnancy. Gallstone incidence appears to be increased in each of these conditions. However, some of the effects of a sluggish gallbladder are counteracted by the associated increase in bile salt pool that occurs at the same time as a result of the decreased gallbladder contraction. Therefore, the lithogenic tendency of a poorly contracting gallbladder is somewhat offset by the decreased cholesterol saturation of bile that is produced.

Stratification and Stasis of Bile. Stratification of bile occurs in the gallbladder as a result of the varying cholesterol saturation of bile with time and appears to be resistant to mixing. It would be possible for areas of supersaturation to provide localised zones of crystallisation which could predispose to stone formation. It is suspected that cholesterol crystal precipitation occurs in the region of the gallbladder wall.

Stasis of bile in the gallbladder may also play a role in the formation of gallstones. The impaired evacuation of the gallbladder might contribute to the growth of stones from crystals. It has been observed in certain instances that the gallbladder empties partially in response to a meal. Failure to empty bile from the gallbladder completely has in turn been linked to an accumulation of excess calcium secreted by the gallbladder mucosa and to an inadequate time allowance for calcium salts to precipitate from bile. Recently, bile stasis has been closely related to biliary sludge by Allen and others (1981). Biliary sludge was defined as a suspension of particulate matter consisting of pigment precipitates in bile, part of which was considered to be calcium bilirubinate. Biliary sludge may favour the formation of cholesterol microcrystals. In addition, it was noted also that biliary sludge disappeared after the return of gallbladder contractility.

Mucosal Secretion. The mucosa of the gallbladder secretes substances into its lumen but the mechanisms are poorly understood. A number of factors, such as variations in bile pH at the mucosal surface and some products of diet or drug metabolism found in bile, may produce membrane irritation or inflammation. Calcium ions are known to be secreted with damage to the mucosa.

Lysolecithin may influence gallstone formation. It can be produced by the gallbladder mucosa and is known to have a damaging effect on the mucosa. Lysolecithin could also enhance absorption of fatty acids in bile which are important for maintaining cholesterol in solution in the presence of lysolecithin. Experiments have shown that inflammation of the mucosa could permit absorption of bile salts with consequent cholesterol saturation.

Mucus (glycoproteins) is also secreted by the gallbladder and this may coalesce by itself or after binding with calcium to form a nucleus promoting precipitation of cholesterol crystals and subsequently gallstones. The mucus may also influence gallstone formation by binding bile acids and therefore increase cholesterol saturation. In addition, mucus has been shown to form the matrix for gallstones.

Patients with gallstone disease have an excess of glycoproteins in both gallbladder and hepatic bile and this probably accounts for the increased viscosity exhibited by bile from diseased gallbladders. Studies in experimental animals support the importance of biliary glycoproteins in stone formation.

Besides mucus, substances that can promote heterogenous precipitation in bile include calcium salts such as calcium bilirubinate, bacteria, and desquamated cells from the gallbladder mucosa.

Cholecystectomy. Removing the gallbladder markedly reduces the possibility of gallstone formation in the extrahepatic biliary tree. There are conflicting reports of the effect of cholecystectomy on hepatic bile composition. The enterohepatic cycling of bile acids increases at least two-fold following cholecystectomy and subsequently leads to a decrease in bile acid pool. The turnover of primary bile acids increases and, as a result of longer exposure to intestinal bacteria, this causes a rise in the percentage of secondary bile acids in bile. The decreased bile acid pool size following cholecystectomy does not generally increase the cholesterol saturation of bile. Redinger (1976) observed that with the gallbladder becoming nonfunctioning in patients with cholesterol stones, there was a tendency to desaturation of previously saturated bile. Unfortunately, other groups have not confirmed this finding. Therefore, in some patients, but not in others, cholecystectomy influences bile composition. Factors such as changes in intestinal transit, diet, and weight following cholecystectomy may also be responsible for the variable findings. Sphincterotomy, with an intact gallbladder, decreases the bile acid pool enormously. When cholecystectomy has also been performed, sphincterotomy does not significantly reduce the already diminished pool size.

Summary of Gallstone Formation

It is clear that the development of the majority of gallstones cannot be explained by stasis, obstruction, and inflammation. Physicochemical properties of bile, in particular those relating to the solubility of cholesterol in bile, are important. However, the details involved in the control of synthesis and secretion of cholesterol and bile acid have yet to be clearly elucidated.

Decreased cholesterol solubility in bile is present in people without gallstones as well as in those with gallstones, and therefore this factor in itself is not enough to explain the formation of cholesterol gallstones. There now is increasing evidence that cholesterol crystals can go on to form gallstones once there is a nidus. This nidus consists mainly of calcium bilirubinate and there is no conclusive information regarding the cause of the nidus that is found in most cholesterol gallstones.

A number of risk factors in gallstone patients have been identified. There appears to be a genetic factor responsible for gallstones in the Pima North American Indians. However, the role of genes and gallstones in other populations remains controversial. With cholesterol gallstones, sex, obesity, and parity are important factors in the development; this is not the case for pigment stones. Both cholesterol and pigment stones are more common with increasing age. Diet appears to play an important part in the cause of both types of gallstones. It is clear that populations with a Western diet form cholesterol gallstones predominantly, whereas those with an Oriental diet form primarily intrahepatic pigment gallstones.

Very little is known about the initiation of pigment stones in the absence of biliary infection, but it would seem that this aspect is also important in the development of cholesterol gallstones as most of these, as mentioned previously, have a central pigment nidus.

It is now apparent that gallbladder function, and perhaps the motility of the biliary system in general, is also involved in the cause of gallstones. However, the details of this involvement remain unclear.

GALLSTONE DISSOLUTION

The relevance of cholesterol saturation to cholesterol gallstone disease was clearly documented for the first time in 1968 when Admirand and Small demonstrated that gallbladder bile from gallstone patients, but not from normal controls, is supersaturated with cholesterol. In 1971, Thistle and Schoenfield reported that oral administration of chenodeoxycholic acid in gallstone patients reduces the cholesterol satu-

ration of gallbladder bile. In 1972, gallstone dissolution was reported with chenodeoxycholic acid in two different centres; one in the United States and one in the United Kingdom. Since then many further studies have been carried out that confirm this finding.

Treatment of Gallbladder Stones with Chenodeoxycholic Acid

As mentioned previously, chenodeoxycholic acid is one of the two primary bile acids synthesised by the normal human liver, the other being cholic acid. Thus, chenodeoxycholate therapy involves administration of a naturally occurring substance in a pharmacologic rather than a physiologic dose. Oral administration of chenodeoxycholic acid renders fasting gallbladder bile unsaturated with cholesterol. The bile thus acquires the capacity to dissolve further cholesterol, leading to gallstone dissolution.

Chenodeoxycholate expands the reduced total bile acid pool size in gallstone patients. Initially it was assumed that this effect was the cause of the decreased cholesterol saturation. It now is known that cholic acid administration also expands the total bile acid pool but it does not improve cholesterol solubility, nor does it cause gallstone dissolution. Current evidence suggests that the underlying mechanism of action of chenodeoxycholic acid is a reduction in biliary cholesterol secretion probably due to inability to synthesise endogenous cholesterol in the liver. Cholic acid does not reduce biliary cholesterol secretion.

As mentioned earlier, there is some evidence that patients with gallstones have increased levels of HMGCoA reductase activity which is inhibited by chenodeoxycholate feeding. However, it is still doubtful whether the secretion of cholesterol into bile is linked to hepatic synthesis. It has also been postulated that chenodeoxycholic acid may alter cholesterol intestinal absorption.

Patient Selection. A large number of clinical trials with chenodeoxycholate have now been completed with thousands of patients being treated, including the results of the 5-year national co-operative gallstone study in the United States and Canada. Chenodeoxycholic acid has now been released for general use in many countries.

Sali and Iser (1978) have reviewed the criteria of selection for chenodeoxycholate treat-

TABLE 74-4. CHENODEOXYCHOLATE TREATMENT: CRITERIA FOR SELECTION

Indications:
- Functioning gallbladder
- Radiolucent gallstones
- Stones < 2 cm diameter
- Patients unfit for surgery

Contraindications:
- Chronic liver disease
- Severe symptoms
- Nonfunctioning gallbladder
- Radiopaque gallstones
- Stones > 2 cm diameter

ment (Table 74-4). Radiologic investigation must show radiolucent stones, preferably of 15 mm in diameter and definitely not greater than 20 mm, and a functioning gallbladder. Chenodeoxycholic acid therapy only dissolves cholesterol stones, and for dissolution to occur, unsaturated bile would have to enter the gallbladder.

In one unselected series of patients coming to cholecystectomy, only 20 percent had radiolucent gallstones in a functioning gallbladder and were therefore potential candidates for successful treatment. Another report from Australia by Watts (1980) has shown that approximately 50 percent of the gallstone patients presented acutely and therefore were not suitable for treatment. Of the remaining patients, approximately 60 percent had a functioning gallbladder. Finally, only 70 percent of these had radiolucent stones, but some of these would also be excluded because of stone size and therefore less than 20 percent of all patients with gallstones could be offered medical therapy.

Ideally the patient should not be obese. There is clear evidence that floating stones, which form a horizontal layer in the erect position during cholecystography, are the most suitable for therapy as they are almost invariably cholesterol rich. However, in the author's experience, only 5 percent of patients suitable for medical treatment have this type of stone. Of the radiolucent stones, 10 to 15 percent will be pigment stones and it is fortunate that over 50 percent of the pigment stones are radiopaque. Furthermore, pigment stones are usually irregular in shape and cholesterol gallstones usually have a rounded contour. Gallbladder bile obtained by stimulation of the gallbladder with cholecystokinin after duodenal intubation usually has cholesterol supersaturation when gallstones are of the cholesterol type, whereas with pigment stones, bile is more frequently not saturated with cholesterol.

Radiopaque gallstones have been shown not to dissolve with oral bile acid therapy whether calcification is present in the periphery, centre, or diffusely throughout the stone. A few gallstones with a tiny calcified nucleus of less than 3 mm in diameter have been reported as dissolved with bile acid therapy, but none with diffuse calcification. However, it is possible that these stones have passed into the duodenum at a stage when the gallstone remnant consisted of a tiny calcified centre without being dissolved.

Since use of the Hida scan for testing cystic duct patency, the author and co-workers have shown that a small number of patients have nonfunctioning gallbladders on cholecystography but a patent cystic duct. Some of these patients may be suitable for dissolution therapy.

As discussed previously, obese patients are more likely to develop gallstones. There is some evidence that these patients may respond better to an increased dose of chenodeoxycholic acid as described by Iser and others (1978). Most women of child-bearing age are in good health and should be treated surgically if they prefer a quick and definitive cure. However, it is important that these patients are also given the choice of treatment. Adequate contraception is important if medical treatment is given to these women as the teratogenic potential of these drugs is unknown.

Currently, medical treatment of gallstones could be recommended to those who are judged to be at increased risk at operation, those who fear operation, or those who wish to delay gallbladder surgery. Another group who may benefit from this treatment are those with silent gallstones. To date, no deaths have been attributed to treatment with oral bile acids for gallstone dissolution.

Efficacy, Dose, and Duration. The therapeutic use and the pharmacologic properties of chenodeoxycholic acid have been extensively reviewed by Iser and Sali (1981). There are a number of reasons why the efficacy of bile acid treatment can never reach 100 percent and these include radiolucent noncholesterol stones, nondissolvable residue, the development of a cystic duct obstruction and a nonfunctioning gallbladder during treatment, and the lack of patient compliance in taking a prescribed dose of medication. Correct patient selection is a key factor in the efficacy of medical treatment.

There have been variable reports on the efficacy of medical treatment of gallstones, with one group of enthusiastic physicians claiming a 93 percent success rate compared to a statement by a sceptical surgeon that the drug's efficacy was only 5 to 10 percent. The largest study has been the National Co-operative Gallstone Study which involved the treatment of 916 patients with chenodeoxycholate. After up to 2 years of treatment, there was confirmed complete gallstone dissolution in only 19 percent of patients. Unfortunately, patients in this study received doses of chenodeoxycholate that are generally regarded as too low for successful treatment.

It can be predicted on a physicochemical basis that gallstone dissolution can occur only during chenodeoxycholate therapy if a dose sufficient to render fasting gallbladder bile unsaturated with cholesterol is given. Clinical studies have confirmed this prediction and have also shown that the effects of chenodeoxycholate on cholesterol saturation is dose related. In general, a dose of 15 mg/kg body weight is adequate to make gallbladder bile unsaturated with cholesterol. There is still controversy about timing of the bile acid dose. Most groups favour a conventional divided dose (meal time regimen); Northfield's group (1975) have recommended that the total daily dose of bile acids should be taken at bedtime but this concept is not yet proven.

The National Co-operative Gallstone Study has confirmed the findings of other investigators as to which patients do best on chenodeoxycholate. Also, it has confirmed the value of the first on-treatment oral cholecystogram in predicting subsequent gallstone dissolution. Thus, if the stones are not appreciably smaller after 6 months, it is advisable for drug treatment to be stopped. Most groups have shown that roughly 30 percent of the patients have complete dissolution of stones and approximately 10 percent have partial dissolution (Fig. 74–10).

The duration of treatment is principally governed by stone size, with small stones of less than 5 mm dissolving in 6 months in 78 to 80 percent of patients, but larger stones up to 20 mm in diameter may require more than 2 years of treatment. Cholecystography is performed ev-

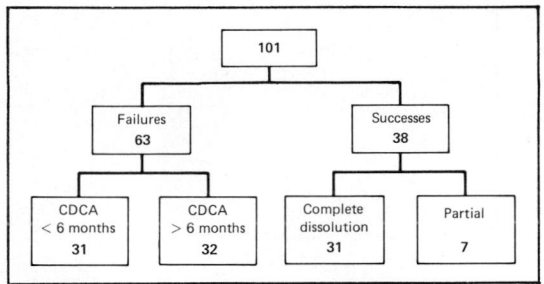

Figure 74–10. Flow chart showing results of treatment in a series of patients accepted for medical dissolution of gallstones.

ery 3 to 6 months to ensure that stones are decreasing in size (Fig. 74–11). Time required for dissolution varies because the rate of dissolution is proportional to the surface area exposed to the solution. Thus, the duration of treatment required with chenodeoxycholate does pose a problem, especially as the drug is expensive. It is therefore important to find a method of enhancing the effect of chenodeoxycholate therapy to reduce the duration and cost of treatment. The role of diet and other agents in trying to achieve this are discussed later.

Side Effects. Diarrhoea is the most common side effect occurring in about 50 percent of patients taking 15 mg/kg of body weight per day. It is dose related and almost certainly due to the cathartic effect of unabsorbed bile acids entering the colon. It is not of any serious medical significance. It almost always responds to a temporary reduction in the dose of chenodeoxycholate and in the majority of patients, tolerance can be achieved by gradually increasing the number of capsules until the full dose of chenodeoxycholate is reached. In very few patients does resistant diarrhoea prevent the patient taking the full therapeutic dose of 15 mg/kg of body weight per day.

Of more serious importance, has been the possibility that chenodeoxycholate might cause liver damage. Hypertransaminasaemia has been reported but, on the basis of hundreds of liver biopsies throughout the world, there has been no evidence of structural liver damage. Hepatotoxicity occurs in experimental animals given either chenodeoxycholate or its bacterial metabolite, lithocholic acid. Hepatotoxicity in animals is most probably due to an accumulation of hepatic lithocholic acid, whereas in man

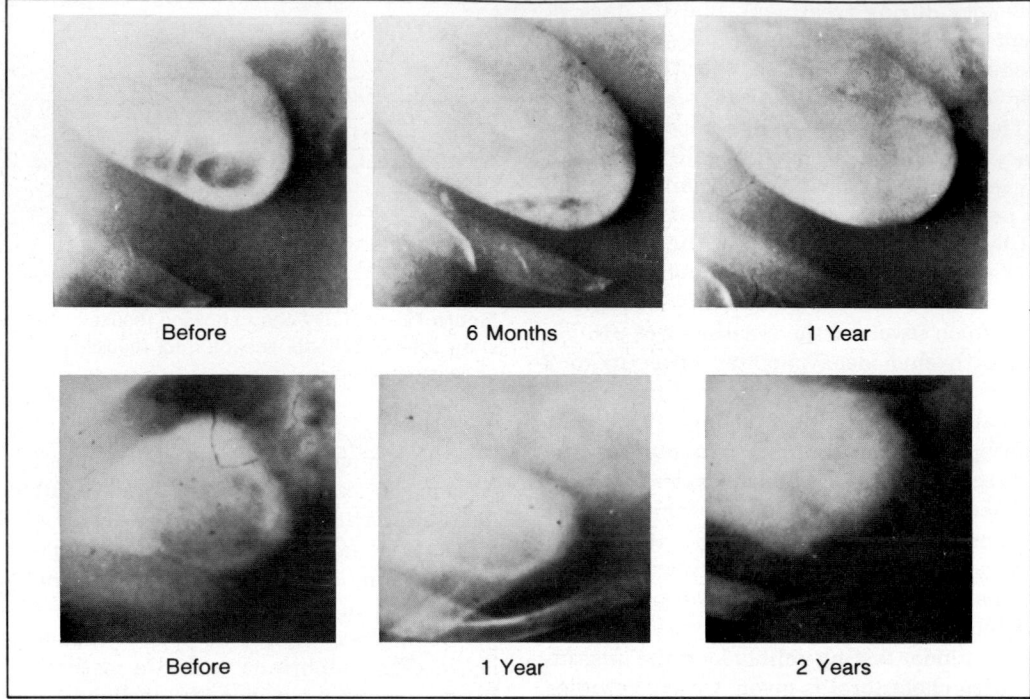

Before   6 Months   1 Year

Before   1 Year   2 Years

Figure 74–11. Gallstone size before and during chenodeoxycholate therapy. *Upper Panel:* Several medium-sized stones were smaller at 6 months and had completely dissolved in 1 year. *Lower Panel:* One large stone (2 cm diameter) was smaller at 1 year but had not yet completely dissolved at 2 years.

it has been shown that this bile acid is rapidly eliminated through an efficient sulfating mechanism.

A major catabolic and excretory pathway of cholesterol is its conversion to bile acids. It was feared that, theoretically, chenodeoxycholate might block endogenous bile acid synthesis from cholesterol and expand the cholesterol pool, which in turn could have the undesirable effect of promoting atherosclerosis. Extensive studies, however, have not revealed any evidence of an increase in either the serum cholesterol level or the size of the cholesterol pool. The possibility of an underlying carcinoma of the gallbladder in association with gallstones exists, but gallbladder cancer is a rare condition and, until now, there have been few reports of this condition being present in patients receiving chenodeoxycholate therapy.

There is a mass of conflicting information concerning the possible links between bile acids and colon cancer. To date, there is no evidence that bile acid therapy for gallstone dissolution increases the risk of developing colon cancer.

There is also no evidence that patients with ileal disease and bile acid malabsorption develop colon cancer more frequently.

Treatment of Gallbladder Stones with Ursodeoxycholic Acid

The only other agent that has been shown definitely to cause dissolution of gallbladder gallstones is ursodeoxycholic acid. This is very closely related chemically to chenodeoxycholic acid and is synthesised from it. A major problem with ursodeoxycholate has been its expense and unavailability, and its long-term usefulness may be governed by these factors.

Ursodeoxycholate has been extracted from the bile of bears by the Japanese and Chinese since ancient times and used for a number of GI problems in Japanese folk medicine. Although it had been credited with making gallstones disappear, the first report was in 1967 by Sugata and Shimizu who reported gallstone dissolution with this agent and the first therapeutic trial of ursodeoxycholate was done in

Japan by Makino in 1978. The efficacy of urso-deoxycholate in producing complete gallstone dissolution is similar to chenodeoxycholate. There, however, has been much less experience with ursodeoxycholate.

The mechanism of gallstone dissolution by ursodeoxycholate may be different from that of chenodeoxycholate, but its effect on bile choles-terol appears similar. The dissolution rate of cholesterol stones in vitro is significantly slower in ursodeoxycholate solution than in chenodeox-ycholate solution, despite its comparable effi-cacy in vivo. Ursodeoxycholate reduces biliary cholesterol secretion, cholesterol saturation, and hepatic HMGCoA reductase at a lower dose than that of chenodeoxycholate. The usual dos-age of ursodeoxycholate is 8 to 10 mg/kg of body weight per day. This advantage, however, is neg-ated by the fact that it is more expensive.

Another advantage of ursodeoxycholate is that it causes fewer side effects: it causes diar-rhoea only if high doses are used, as it does not exert a secretory effect on the colon; no ap-preciable changes occur in biochemical tests of liver function; and histology is unaltered. In contrast to chenodeoxycholate, there is only a slight increase in the hepatotoxic secondary bile acid, lithocholic acid, as only a small portion of ursodeoxycholate is metabolised to this hepa-totoxic substance.

A possible disadvantage may be a tendency to induce calcification of gallstones during treat-ment. Gallstone calcification has also been re-ported in chenodeoxycholate treated patients. It is unknown if the incidence of calcification during treatment is any greater than that occur-ring spontaneously in untreated gallstone pa-tients. Further information is required about biliary calcium, in particular the degree of available calcium for incorporation in gall-stones.

Diet and Gallstone Dissolution

To improve the gallstone dissolution rate, pa-tients have been placed on a low cholesterol diet but this group also was given all of the chenode-oxycholate as a single bedtime dose. Therefore, it is difficult to interpret the effect of the low cholesterol diet. Changes in diet are frequently made by patients for symptom relief. It is advis-able to encourage obese patients to lose weight. Increased dietary fibre in combination with bile acid therapy may have a role in increasing gall-stone dissolution rates, and currently we are testing this hypothesis.

There is still inadequate data to suggest any other changes in diet that may be useful in im-proving gallstone dissolution during bile acid therapy. Gerolami and Sarles (1975) have used β-sitosterol, a plant sterol which modifies cho-lesterol intestinal absorption, to supplement bile acid treatment but its usefulness is still con-troversial. Vitamin C may also improve gall-stone dissolution with chenodeoxycholate.

Alternative Treatment for Gallstones

Citrate. Sali and co-workers first showed in 1980 that citrate is normally present in bile and also that citrate concentration of bile can be increased by an oral citrate load. Subsequently, in vitro studies by this group have shown that calcified pigment stones can be dissolved using citrate solutions alone and calcified cholesterol gallstones can be dissolved using solutions con-taining both citrate and bile acid. More recently, patients with diffusely calcified gallstones have been treated successfully for the first time (Fig. 74–12). Citrate is known to form soluble com-plexes with calcium and therefore calcified stones are probably decalcified because of this characteristic. The cholesterol component of the gallstone would be dissolved by the concomitant use of chenodeoxycholate as shown in our in vitro experiments.

The majority of radiolucent stones that do not respond to chenodeoxycholate treatment have significant amounts of calcium on the stone surface which would prevent cholesterol dissolution. Preliminary studies by Sali have shown a decrease in gallstone size in patients with radiolucent stones resistant to chenodeoxy-cholate therapy.

Most cholesterol gallstones have a central calcium bilirubinate pigment that may act as a nucleus for cholesterol precipitation; calcium bilirubinate precipitation is also important in the cause of pigment stones. Therefore, the con-centration of citrate, which is normally present in bile, may be an important factor in maintain-ing calcium solubility and enhancing preven-tion of gallstone formation.

Mono-terpenes (Rowachol). There have been several reports of radiolucent gallstones disap-pearing after prolonged treatment with Rowa-chol. It may also be effective in dissolving the

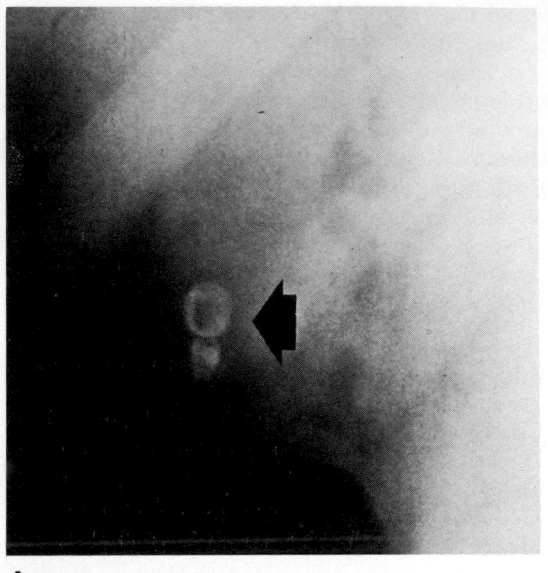

A

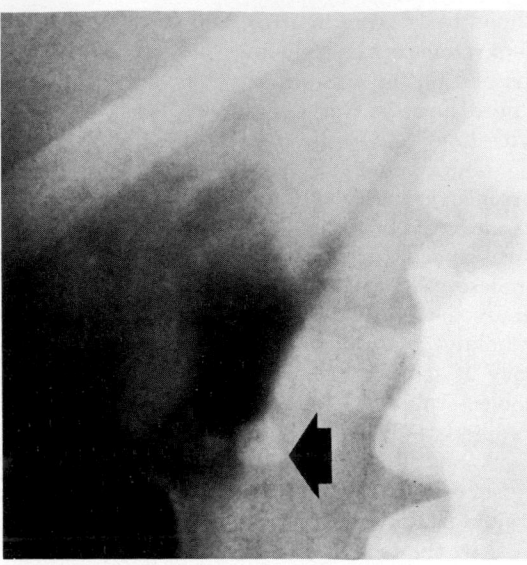

B

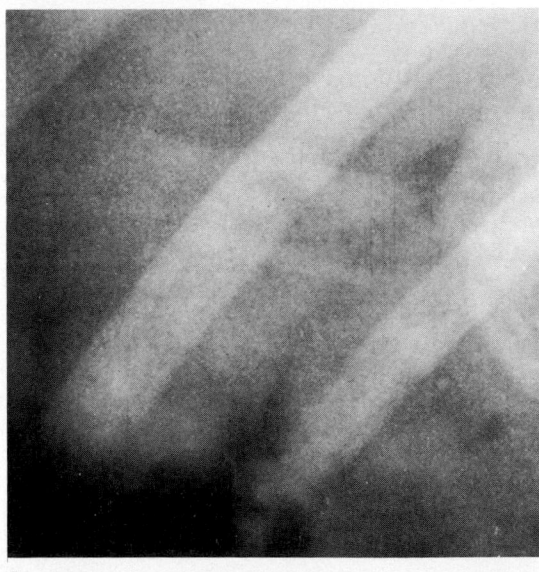

C

Figure 74–12. Plain x-ray of calcified gallstones before treatment with chenodeoxycholate and citrate **(A)**, 1 year after treatment where decreased calcification is noted **(B)**, and at 18 months after treatment, gallstones are decalcified **(C)**.

calcified rim of gallstones. More recently it has been used in combination with chenodeoxycholate to dissolve radiolucent stones and an increased efficacy over bile acid alone is claimed. Rowachol has a slight effect in desaturating bile, but its mode of action is unknown.

Phenobarbitone. Phenobarbitone is a microsomal enzyme inducer and can affect bile acid synthesis, but in its long-term treatment of epileptics it has failed to protect them from gall-

stone formation. In addition, chenodeoxycholate and phenobarbitone has been used without any increased benefit on biliary cholesterol desaturation.

Metronidazole. Recently metronidazole has been shown to decrease bile cholesterol saturation and also bile deoxycholate. This response has been explained by its effect on colonic microflora and the subsequent effect of the new microflora on colonic bile acid metabolism and eventually bile composition. The study suggests that this may be another way of treating gallstones or improving the efficacy of bile acid therapy.

Shock Wave Treatment for Gallstones. Surprisingly, Brendel and Enders (1983) and others from Germany have used shock wave treatments to treat kidney stones in humans by placing the patient in a heated water bath. Recently, this same group has used similar shock waves for successful treatment of gallstones in dogs. It is quite possible that with further development this treatment may be an alternative treatment for gallstones or it may be used in combination with gallstone dissolution therapy.

Recurrence of Gallstones

Bile reverts to its supersaturated state in 1 to 3 weeks when treatment is withdrawn following complete gallstone dissolution. Therefore, chenodeoxycholate only temporarily suppresses the basic metabolic defect or defects that led to the formation of gallstones in the first place. These patients may be at risk of again forming gallstones. Recurrence is maximal in the first 2 years after stopping treatment and increases with time. A follow-up by Dowling and Ruppin (1982) of 60 patients with gallstone dissolution at 3 to 60 months after stopping treatment showed a 50 percent recurrence.

One of the reasons for recurrence may be failure to achieve complete gallstone dissolution. Oral cholecystography may not be sufficiently sensitive to detect the end point of complete stone dissolution, resulting in a falsely high success rate and an increased chance of stone fragments acting as a nidus for stone regrowth once treatment is stopped. The author's group has shown that ultrasound provides a more accurate assessment of treatment end point and a more complete dissolution may result in lower recurrence rates.

Intermittent treatment with chenodeoxycholate is of no value and studies are in progress to determine the lowest dose of continuous treatment that prevents stone recurrence. As mentioned previously, a high fibre diet can decrease cholesterol saturation in gallstone patients. Because of this, Sali and co-workers in 1977 decided to divide patients with complete dissolution into two groups: one group continued with their normal diet and the other began

a high fibre diet. There are not sufficient numbers as yet to analyse the results statistically, but there is less stone recurrence in the high fibre group.

It is not proven if pregnancy causes gallstones, but if this is the case, these patients would be best treated soon after pregnancy as the gallstones would be small and it would be improbable that significant gallbladder damage would have occurred at this early stage. It is very likely that the degree of gallbladder damage, as a result of chronic inflammation, is an important factor in stone recurrence after bile acid therapy.

Role of Gallstone-Dissolving Agents and Their Future

Although initially there were high hopes for chenodeoxycholate and ursodeoxycholate treatment for gallstone dissolution, it has become clear that only a small percentage of patients, ranging from 3 to 25 percent, would benefit from bile acid therapy. However, gallstone disease is very common and if 15 to 20 percent of all patients with gallstones are suitable for treatment, this would still be an enormous number of patients. It is quite obvious that currently the majority of patients are more suitable for cholecystectomy, but when patients are suitable for medical treatment, they should be able to choose between the two. Medical treatment complements surgery rather than competes with it, and it offers an effective alternative treatment to cholecystectomy in selected patients. The cost of cholecystectomy and medical treatment is similar, but operative treatment is a cure in almost all patients, whereas with medical treatment recurrence is possible. A decision will have to be made with each patient with gallstone recurrence as to whether to retreat with dissolution or to recommend cholecystectomy. More patients with gallstones would be suitable for medical treatment if gallstones were diagnosed earlier, with the possibility that recurrence after dissolution may be less in this group because of minimal gallbladder changes resulting from cholelithiasis. The development of treatments such as citrate and the use of shock waves may also improve efficacy of treatment.

A factor of great importance relating to the medical treatment of gallstones has been the vast increase in our understanding of gallstone formation and, hopefully, this information will eventually lead to the prevention of gallstone disease.

Dissolution and Flushing of Bile Duct Stones

In the United States, a half million cholecystectomies are performed each year and 4000 patients are found to have retained bile duct stones. The findings of Glenn in 1974 also reflect the incidence of retained stones (Table 74–5). Circumstances in which stones are likely to be overlooked are comprehensively discussed by Kune and Sali (1980). During the last decade, several alternative treatments have become available (Table 74–6).

Flushing

The flushing technique should be tried initially in patients with a T-tube. Retained stones ideally should be less than 7 mm in diameter for flushing. Bile must be cultured and prophylactic antibiotics given to the patient. The procedure must be explained to the patient to avoid anxiety; in addition, premedication should be given including an anticholinergic agent for sphincter relaxation. Xylocaine is infused into the T-tube and intravenous Glucagon also can be given for further sphincter relaxation. The stone is either flushed under radiologic control or by continuous T-tube infusion of normal saline over 24 hours. Stones may be found in the patient's stool to confirm successful flushing.

Bile Acid Infusion for Dissolution of Cholesterol Bile Duct Stones

Chemical solutions can be infused into bile ducts for the treatment of retained bile duct stones if a T-tube is in situ. Recently a small group of patients with retained or recurrent bile duct stones, but no T-tubes, have had chemical infusion via a long nasobiliary tube inserted endoscopically into the bile duct. A number of solu-

TABLE 74–5. RETAINED BILE DUCT STONES

Incidence	
16,700	Cholecystectomies
24.0%	Duct exploration
46.0%	Duct stones found
1.1%	Retained stones without duct exploration
4.3%	Retained stones after duct exploration

(*Source: Adapted from Glenn F, 1974, with permission.*)

TABLE 74–6. MANAGEMENT OF RETAINED BILE DUCT STONES

- Flushing
- Chemical dissolution
- Instrumental extraction
- Endoscopic papillotomy
- Reoperation
- Leave

tions have been tried in attempts to dissolve bile duct stones, but only two have achieved an acceptable degree of success—cholic acid and mono-octanoin.

In Vitro Gallstone Dissolution

CHOLESTEROL GALLSTONES. A number of solutions have been tested in vitro to determine the best solvent. The bile acid, deoxycholate, is very effective in dissolving gallstones in vitro, but unfortunately it is toxic to the jejunum. Chenodeoxycholate is also effective but difficult to obtain and expensive. Ursodeoxycholate is surprisingly a poor solvent for in vitro gallstone dissolution. Cholate is not as effective as deoxycholate and chenodeoxycholate but has been used extensively as it is safer than deoxycholate and is more freely available and less expensive than chenodeoxycholate.

Mono-octanoin, a monodiglyceride of medium chain length fatty acids, has been found to be superior to bile acids in dissolving cholesterol gallstones.

CALCIFIED GALLSTONES. Calcified gallstones are resistant to bile acid and mono-octanoin in vitro. However, citrate will dissolve noncalcified and calcified pigment gallstones and also, when used in combination with chenodeoxycholate, calcified cholesterol gallstones. Ethylenediamine tetra acetic acid (EDTA) is a calcium-binding agent which will dissolve both noncalcified and calcified pigment stones in vitro.

Cholate T-Tube Infusion. Rewbridge in 1937 used massive doses of oral bile acid, about four times the currently used dose, for partial success in the treatment of bile duct stones. It was not until 1972 that Way and others showed that cholate T-tube infusion dissolved retained cholesterol bile duct stones.

Cholate infusion can be used only if choledochograms show that the retained bile duct stone is not causing complete obstruction. Ideally the stone should be distal to a limb of the T-tube in the bile duct, although it may be possible to move the stone distally by removing the T-tube and replacing it with a catheter for cholate infusion. Patients with multiple bile duct stones are usually not suitable for cholate therapy. Infusion through a cholecystostomy is also rarely effective.

For the treatment of intrahepatic stones, it has been suggested that a catheter can be passed through the T-tube or its track and into the intrahepatic bile ducts, but a recent study has shown that infusion of cholate to this site may be fatal, possibly due to hepatic bile duct mucosal damage and subsequent infection.

Available gallbladder gallstones from the patient should be analysed to ensure that their composition is mainly cholesterol. Bile must be cultured and prophylactic antibiotic given whenever necessary. Flushing should be tried first under radiologic control, then a 24-hour trial of half normal saline infusion at the rate normally used for cholate is given to test patient tolerance. During cholate treatment, patients should have regular liver function tests and amylase estimations.

Treatment takes from 1 to 2 weeks during which time the complications of diarrhoea, impaction of the stone in the region of the ampulla of Vater, pancreatitis, and cholangitis have been reported. At times, pain during infusion can also be a problem. Diarrhoea, which occurs because of the action of bile salts on the large bowel, can usually be controlled with simultaneous oral cholestyramine or, as described by Sali in 1980, with the use of aluminium hydroxide which is free of the problems usually associated with cholestyramine treatment.

T-tube choledochograms are usually carried out at weekly intervals to check for dissolution. A review of the results of cholate infusion shows that there is a 70 percent success rate in most series. However, a flushing technique had not been used in most of these studies initially, and it is possible that a number of these stones may have been flushed out rather than dissolved. The response to cholate infusion is probably due to flushing, partial dissolution, or stone disintegration.

Mono-octanoin T-Tube Infusion. The use of mono-octanoin infusion for retained cholesterol gallstones has confirmed, in in vitro results, that it dissolves cholesterol gallstones more rapidly than cholate. Mono-octanoin is safe for use in humans as it is a monodiglyceride, which is a normal digestion product of medium chain triglycerides.

Initially, mono-octanoin was given in high doses which caused frequent side effects, but Jarrett and others (1981) have proven that good results can be achieved with a low infusion dose which also reduces side effects. The main side effects consist of nausea, biliary pain, and diarrhoea. All of the side effects respond to temporary cessation of the infusion. Jarrett's group also has shown that patients can be mobilised if a portable syringe pump rather than a main driven pump is used. Mono-octanoin has to be kept warm to avoid solidification; this is achieved by body warmth. It is possible to supervise the treatment of some patients with this infusion technique as outpatients. Mono-octanoin is successful in the treatment of retained stones in approximately 70 percent of patients and, if stones are proven to be radiolucent and of the cholesterol type, then a 90 percent success rate is achieved.

Treatment of Retained Bile Duct Pigment and Calcified Stones

EDTA infusion has been used to treat retained radiolucent bile duct pigment stones with success. Citrate should also be successful in treating radiolucent and radiopaque pigment stones because of its in vitro action on these stones. Based on in vitro findings, retained calcified cholesterol gallstones should respond to a combination of citrate and bile acid infusion.

Future of Dissolution Therapy for Choledocholithiasis

Retained bile duct stones can be rapidly removed by either percutaneous T-tube techniques or by using endoscopic sphincterotomy. However, these procedures require specialised equipment and, in particular, expert personnel. Therefore, in situations where these facilities are not available, dissolution therapy for bile duct stones is a suitable alternative. The main disadvantage to dissolution therapy is the increased hospitalisation, but this can be avoided in some patients with portable infusion pumps using mono-octanoin. The useful aspect of this treatment is that one may be able to dissolve stones early after surgery; as with mechanical extraction, a waiting period of 3 to 6 weeks after operation is required.

Dissolution therapy can also be useful in patients who have stones that are too large to be removed by the other two procedures. These stones can be reduced in size by infusing solvents initially and then attempting T-tube instrumental extraction or endoscopic removal.

BIBLIOGRAPHY

Admirand WH, Small DM: The physico-chemical basis of cholesterol gallstone formation in man. J Clin Invest 47:1043, 1968

Allen B, Bernhoft R, et al: Sludge is calcium bilirubinate associated with bile stasis. Am J Surg 141:51, 1981

Anderson F, Bouchier IAD: Phospholipids in human lithogenic gallbladder bile. Nature 221:372, 1969

Anderson JR, McLean Ross AH, et al: Cholelithiasis following peptic ulcer surgery: A prospective controlled study. Br J Surg 67:618, 1980

Bateson MC, Bouchier IAD, et al: Calcification of radiolucent gallstones during treatment with ursodeoxycholic acid. Br Med J 283:654, 1981

Been JM, Bills PM, et al: Microstructure of gallstones. Gastroenterol 76:548, 1979

Bennion LJ, Grundy SM: Risk factors for the development of cholelithiasis in man (first of two parts). N Engl J Med 299:1161, 1978

Bennion LJ, Grundy SM: Risk factors for the development of cholelithiasis in man (second of two parts). N Engl J Med 299:1221, 1978

Blitzer BL, Boyer JL: Cellular mechanisms of bile formation. Gastroenterol 82:346, 1982

Bloom SR, Polak JM (eds): Gut Hormones, 2 edt. Edinburgh: Churchill-Livingstone, 1981

Bogren H: The composition and structure of human gallstones. Acta Radiologica (suppl):226, 1964

Boston Collaborative Drug Surveillance Programme: Oral contraceptives and venous thromboembolic disease, surgically confirmed gallbladder disease and breast tumours. Lancet 1:1399, 1973

Bouchier IAD: Gallstone dissolving agents. Br Med J 286:778, 1983

Bouchier IAD: Biochemistry of gallstone formation. Clin Gastroenterol 12:25, 1983

Braverman DZ, Johnson M, et al: Effects of pregnancy and contraceptive steroids on gallbladder function. N Engl J Med 302:362, 1980

Brendel W, Enders G: Shock waves for gallstones: Animal studies. Lancet 1:1054, 1983

Capron JP, Delamarre J, et al: Meal frequency and duration of overnight fast: A role in gallstone formation? Br Med J 283:1435, 1981

Carey MC, Small DM: The characteristics of mixed

micellar solution with particular reference to bile. Am J Med 49:590, 1970

Coyne MJ, Marks J, et al: Mechanism of cholesterol gallstone formation. Clin Gastroenterol 6:129, 1977

Dam H: Determinants of cholesterol cholelithiasis in man and animals. Am J Med 51:596, 1971

Danzinger RG, Hoffman AF, et al: Dissolution of cholesterol gallstones by chenodeoxycholic acid. N Engl J Med 286:1, 1972

Domschke W, Domschke S: Bilirubin metabolism and bile secretion: Hormonal regulation in liver and bile. Bianchi L, Gerok W, Sickinger K (eds): Liver and Bile. Lancaster: MTP Press, 1977, p 45

Dowling RH: Cholelithiasis: Medical treatment. Clin Gastroenterol 12:125, 1982

Dowling RH, Ruppin DC: Gallstone dissolution and recurrence: Are we being misled? Br Med J 285:132, 1982

Dutt MK, Murray B, et al: Bilirubin solubilisation by mixed micelles and interaction with cholesterol and calcium. Gut 21:A919, 1980

Editorial: Dissolving gallstones. Br Med J 284:1, 1982

Editorial: Dissolving hopes for gallstone dissolution? Lancet 2:905, 1981

Ellis WR, Bell GD, et al: Mechanisms for adjuvant cholelithiolytic properties of the mono-terpene mixture Rowachol. Gastroenterol 80:1141, 1981

Gerolami A, Sarles H: β-sitosterol and chenodeoxycholic acid in the treatment of cholesterol gallstones. Lancet 2:721, 1975

Gerolami A, Sarles H, et al: Controlled trial of chenodeoxychol therapy for radiolucent gallstones, a multicentre study. Digestion 16:299, 1977

Glenn F: Retained calculi within the biliary ductal system. Ann Surg 179:528, 1974

Hand BH: Anatomy and function of the extrahepatic biliary system. Clin Gastroenterol 2:3, 1973

Heaton KW: Bile Salts in Health and Disease. Edinburgh: Churchill-Livingstone, 1972

Heaton KW: The epidemiology of gallstones and suggested etiology. Clin Gastroenterol 2:67, 1973

Heaton KW: Disturbances of bile acid metabolism in intestinal disease. Clin Gastroenterol 6:69, 1977

Hoffmann AF: The enterohepatic circulation of bile acids in man. Clin Gastroenterol 6:3, 1977

Holan KR, Holzbach RT, et al: Nucleation time: A key factor in the pathogenesis of cholesterol gallstone disease. Gastroenterol 77:611, 1979

Holzbach RT, Marsh M, et al: Cholesterol solubility in bile: Evidence that supersaturated bile is frequent in healthy man. J Clin Invest 52:1467, 1973

Iser JH, Maton PN, et al: Resistance to chenodeoxycholic acid (CDCA) treatment in obese patients with gallstones. Br Med J 1:1509, 1978

Iser JH, Sali A: Chenodeoxycholic acid: A review of its pharmacological properties and therapeutic use. Drugs 21:90, 1981

Iser JH, Sali A, et al: Gallstone dissolution: Illustration with oral cholecystography. Aust N Z J Med 13:438, 1983

Ivy AC, Oldberg E, et al: A hormone mechanism for gallbladder contraction and evacuation. Am J Physiology 85:381, 1928

Jarrett LN, Balfour TW, et al: Intraductal infusion of mono-octanoin. Experience in 24 patients with retained common ductal stones. Lancet 1:68, 1981

Kaminski DL, Nahrwold DL: Neurohormonal control of biliary secretion and gallbladder function. World J Surg 3:449, 1979

Kune GA, Sali A: The Practice of Biliary Surgery, 2 edt. Oxford: Blackwell Scientific Publications, 1980

LaMorte WW, Matolo NM, et al: Pathogenesis of cholesterol gallstones. Surg Clin North Am 16:765, 1981

Large AM, Johnston CG, et al: Gallstones and pregnancy: The composition of gallbladder bile in the pregnant woman at term. Am J Med Sci 239:713, 1960

Leuschner U, Wurbs D, et al: Alternating treatment of common bile duct stones with a modified glyceryl-1-mono-octanoate preparation and a bile acid-EDTA solution by naso-biliary tube. Scand J Gastroenterol 16:497, 1981

Low-Beer TS: Diet and bile acid metabolism. Clin Gastroenterol 6:165, 1977

Low-Beer TS, Nutters S: Colonic bacterial activity, biliary cholesterol saturation, pathogenesis of gallstones. Lancet 2:1063, 1978

Mabee TM, Meyer P, et al: The mechanism of increased gallstone formation in obese human subjects. Surgery 79:460, 1976

MacKay C: Bile acids and gallstone disease. Br J Surg 62:505, 1975

MacKay C, Sali A, et al: Phenobarbitone and gallstone disease. Br J Surg 65:362, 1978

Madden JL, van der Heyden L, et al: The nature and surgical significance of common duct stones. Surg Gynecol Obstet 126:3, 1968

Maki T: Pathogenesis of calcium bilirubinate gallstone: Role of E. coli, beta-glucuronidase and coagulation by inorganic ions, polyelectrolytes and agitation. Ann Surg 164:90, 1966

Maki T, Matsushiro T, et al: The role of sulphated glycoprotein in gallstone formation. Surg Gynecol Obstet 132:846, 1971

Makino I, Nakagawa S: Changes in biliary lipid and biliary bile acid composition in patients after administration of ursodeoxycholic acid. J Lipid Res 19:945, 1978

Malt RA, Williamson RCN: Carcinogenesis. Lancaster: MTP Press, 1982

Matsushiro T, Suzuki N, et al: Effects of diet on glucaric acid concentration in bile and the formation of calcium bilirubinate stones. Gastroenterol 72:630, 1977

Maudgal DP, Kupfer RM, et al: Postprandial gallbladder emptying in patients with gallstones. Br Med J 280:141, 1980

Maudgal DP, Kupfer RM, et al: Minimum effective dose of chenic acid for gallstone patients: Reduction with bedtime administration and a low cholesterol diet. Gut 23:280, 1982

Miyake H, Johnston CG: Gallstones: Ethnological studies. Digestion 1:219, 1968

Nakayama F, Miyake H: Changing state of gallstone disease in Japan, composition of the stones and treatment of the condition. Am J Surg 120:794, 1970

Nayman J: Bile duct stasis stones, in Kune GA, Sali A, Jones T (eds): Proc Bil Dis 1980, Melbourne University, 1980, p 100

Nilsson S: Gallbladder disease and sex hormones. A statistical study. Acta Chir Scand 132:275, 1966

Northfield TC, Hoffmann AF: Biliary lipid output during three meals and an overnight fast. I. Relationship to bile acid pool size and cholesterol saturation of bile in gallstone and control subjects. Gut 16:1, 1975

Northfield TC, Kupfer RM, et al: Gallbladder sensitivity to cholecystokinin in patients with gallstones. Br Med J 280:143, 1980

Northfield TC, LaRusso NF, et al: Biliary lipid output during three meals and an overnight fast. II. Effective chenodeoxycholic acid treatment in gallstone subjects. Gut 16:12, 1975

Paumgartner G, Sauerbruch T: Secretion, composition and flow of bile. Clin Gastroenterol 12:3, 1983

Paumgartner G, Stiehl A, et al (eds): Bile Acids and Lipids. Lancaster: MTP Press, 1981

Pomare EW, Heaton KW, et al: The effect of wheatbran upon bile salt metabolism and upon lipid composition of bile in gallstone patients. Dig Dis 21:521, 1976

Ponz de Leon M, Ferenderes R, et al: Bile lipid composition and bile acid pool size in diabetes. Dig Dis 23:710, 1978

Ponz de Leon M, Loria P, et al: Intestinal solubilisation, absorption, pharmico-kynetics and bioavailability of chenodeoxycholic acid. Eur J Clin Invest 10:262, 1980

Rains AJH: Gallstones. London: Heinemann, 1964

Redinger RN: The effect of loss of gallbladder function on biliary lipid composition in subjects with cholesterol gallstones. Gastroenterol 71:470, 1976

Rewbridge AG: Disappearance of gallstone shadows following prolonged administration of bile salts. Surgery 1:395, 1937

Royal College of General Practitioners Oral Contraception Study (Principal Authors: Wingrave SJ, Kay CR; Manchester Research Unit, Manchester, England). Oral contraceptives and gallbladder disease. Lancet 2:957, 1982

Rudick J, Hutchinson JS: Evaluation of vagotomy and biliary function by combined oral cholecystography and intravenous cholangiography. Ann Surg 162:234, 1965

Saharia PC, Zuidema GD, et al: Primary common duct stones. Ann Surg 185:598, 1977

Sali A: Neurohumerol control of hepatic bile secretion. PhD Thesis, Monash University, 1977

Sali A: Bile duct gallstones. The overlooked stone, flushing and dissolving, in Kune GA, Sali A, Jones T (eds): Proc Bil Dis 1980, Melbourne University, 1980, p 110

Sali A, Crowe C, et al: Biliary citrate secretion. Aust N Z J Med 10:114, 1980

Sali A, Iser JH: The non-operative management of gallstones. Aust N Z J Surg 48:484, 1978

Sali A, Murray WR, et al: Bile acid binding properties of antacids. Lancet 2:1851, 1976

Sali A, Vitetta L, et al: Calcified cholesterol gallstones and citrate. Proc 7th World Congress, Collegium Internationale de Chirurgiae Digestivae, 1982, p 52

Sali A, Vitetta L, et al: Composition of primary bile duct stones. Proc 7th World Congress Collegium Internationale de Chirurgiae Digestivae, 1982, p 18

Sali A, Watts JM: Regulation of hepatic bile flow and its composition. Aust N Z J Surg 41:94, 1971

Sarles H: Research and the pancreas, in Kune GA, Sali A, Jones T (eds): Proc First Aust Pancreas Congress, Melbourne, 1978, p 21

Sarles H, Cruite C, et al: Influences of cholestyramine, bile salt and cholesterol feeding on the lipid composition of hepatic bile in man. Scand J Gastroenterol 5:603, 1970

Sarles H, Crotte C, et al: The influence of caloric intake and of dietary protein on the bile lipids. Scand J Gastroenterol 6:189, 1971

Schoenfield LJ, Lachin JM: The NCGS Steering Committee and the NCGS Group: National Co-operative Gallstone Study, a controlled trial of the efficacy and safety of chenodeoxycholic acid for dissolution of Gallstones. Ann Int Med 95:257, 1981

Shaffer EA, Small DM: Biliary lipid secretion in cholesterol gallstone disease. The effect of cholecystectomy and obesity. J Clin Invest 59:828, 1977

Shaffer EA: The effect of vagotomy on gallbladder function and bile composition in man. Ann Surg 195:413, 1982

Sharp KW, Gadacz TR: Selection of patients for dissolution of retained common duct stones with monooctanoin. Ann Surg 196:137, 1982

Small DM: Cholesterol nucleation and growth in gallstone formation. N Engl J Med 302:1305, 1980

Smallwood RA, Jablonski P, et al: Intermittent secretion of abnormal bile in patients with cholesterol gallstones. Br Med J 4:263, 1972

Soloway RD, Trotman BW, et al: Pigment gallstones. Gastroenterol 72:167, 1977

Sugata F, Shimizu M: Re-evaluation of cases with disappearing gallstone shadows. Jap J Gastroenterol 71:75, 1974 (in Japanese)

Sutor DJ, Percival JM: The effect of bile on the crystallisation of calcium carbonate, a constituent of gallstones. Clin Chimica Acta 89: 479, 1978

Sutor DJ, Woolley SE: The nature and incidence of gallstones containing calcium. Gut 14:215, 1973

The Coronary Drug Project Research Group: Gallbladder disease as a side effect of drugs influencing lipid metabolism: Experience in the coronary drug project. N Engl J Med 296:1185, 1977

Thistle JL, Carlson GL, et al: Mono-octanoin—a dissolution agent for retained cholesterol bile duct stones: Physical properties and clinical application. Gastroenterol 78:1016, 1980

Thistle JL, Schoenfield LJ: Induced alterations in composition of bile in persons having cholelithiasis. Gastroenterol 61:488, 1971

Trotman BW, Ostrow JD, et al: Pigment vs cholesterol cholelithiasis: Comparison of stone and bile composition. Am J Dig Dis 19:585, 1974

Thureborn E: On the stratification of human bile and its importance for the solubility of cholesterol. Gastroenterol 50:775, 1966

van der Linden W: Genetic factors in gallstone disease. Clin Gastroenterol 2:603, 1973

Vitetta L, Sali A: The autopsy incidence of gallstones in Australia. Unpublished data.

Vlahcevic ZR, Bell C Jr, et al: Diminished bile acid pool size in patients with gallstones. Gastroenterol 59:165, 1970

Wattchow DA, Hall JC, et al: Prevalence and treatment of gallstones after gastric bypass surgery for morbid obesity. Br Med J 286:763, 1983

Watts JM: Gallstone dissolution, in Kune GA, Sali A, Jones T (eds): Proc Bil Dis 1980, Melbourne University, 1980, p 19

Watts JM, Jablonski P, et al: The effect of added bran to the diet on the saturation of bile in people without gallstones. Am J Surg 135:321, 1978

Watts JM, Toouli J, et al: Gallstone dissolution present and future, in Blumgart LH (ed): The Biliary Tract. Edinburgh: Churchill-Livingstone, 1982, p 17

Way L, Admirand WH, et al: Management of choledocholithiasis. Ann Surg 176:347, 1972

Wheeler HO: Water and electrolytes in bile, in Handbook of Physiology, The Alimentary Canal. American Physiological Society, 1968 p 2401

Wheeler M, Hills LL, et al: Cholelithiasis: A clinical and dietary survey. Gut 11:430, 1970

Williamson BWA, Percy-Robb IW: Contribution of biliary lipids to calcium binding in bile. Gastroenterol 78:696, 1980

Wood M: Eponyms in biliary tract surgery. Am J Surg 138:746, 1979

Wood JR, Svanvik J: Gallbladder water and electrolyte transport and its regulation. Gut 24:579, 1983

75. Cholecystitis

Gabriel A. Kune
Gary D. Gill

Acute cholecystitis is a distinct clinicopathologic entity, irrespective of its cause. In this description, acute cholecystitis is defined as an acute upper abdominal condition that is always associated with macroscopic and microscopic features of acute inflammatory change in the gallbladder. Excluded are other acute changes, such as oedema of the gallbladder, not infrequently seen in association with acute pancreatitis.

The usual precipitating factor in acute cholecystitis is the occlusion of the Hartmann pouch or of the cystic duct by a gallstone and, much less frequently, the obstructive cause is a cancer of the bile duct or of the gallbladder outlet that occludes the cystic duct. Occasionally there is no obstructive cause present, a situation usually referred to as acute acalculous cholecystitis. As an example, in a study of 240 consecutive operative cases of acute cholecystitis, Kune and Birks in 1970 found gallstones the cause in 98 percent, a malignant obstruction in 1 percent and acute acalculous cholecystitis also in 1 percent.

ACUTE CALCULOUS CHOLECYSTITIS

Pathophysiology

The first event is occlusion of the gallbladder outlet by a gallstone; this is followed by an acute inflammatory change in the gallbladder wall that, in the first instance, is chemical rather than bacterial. Numerous bacteriologic studies have consistently shown that bacterial infection is a secondary event and probably the rate of this rises if the obstructive cause remains unrelieved. In 1974, Kune and Schutz found positive cultures in the bile of half of the patients operated on for acute cholecystitis. The organisms are similar to those found in gallstone disease, namely aerobic enterobacteria, such as *Escherichia coli* and only occasionally are anaerobic organisms isolated.

The gallbladder itself is swollen, vascular, and tense, and after 24 to 48 hours the inflammatory process usually spreads to the gastrohepatic omentum to involve the common bile duct, the common hepatic duct, and all the tissues in the porta hepatis.

A transient jaundice is commonly seen during an attack of cholecystitis in the absence of bile duct gallstones; although the pathologic basis of this is unclear, it is likely to be caused by pericholecystic oedema involving the bile duct and creating a functional disturbance of bile transport in the common bile duct.

The acute inflammation settles down spontaneously in the majority of cases, but in approximately 10 percent it progresses to the local complications of empyema formation, with or without gangrene, or perforation, with the formation of a pericholecystic abscess; acute free perforation of the gallbladder, however, with general biliary peritonitis, is a most uncommon sequel.

Diagnosis

Clinical diagnosis of acute cholecystitis can be made with reasonable certainty in most cases. The clinical diagnosis can be strengthened in doubtful cases with the use of ultrasonography, intravenous cholangiography, and radionuclide scanning, so that now almost all cases of acute cholecystitis are diagnosed preoperatively.

1839

The condition commences with an attack of biliary type pain, but in contradistinction to so-called biliary colic, the pain does not settle down and remains unabated for one or several days. There is guarding and tenderness in the right upper quadrant of the abdomen, and with progress of the inflammatory process, a pyrexia develops. In approximately 40 percent, the gallbladder becomes palpable and tender and a mild transient jaundice is noted in 10 to 15 percent of cases, whereas a leucocytosis is present in two thirds of cases.

A plain radiograph of the liver area is useful in the rare acute pneumocholecystitis, which is a fulminating type of acute cholecystitis, with gas-forming organisms being present in the gallbladder. Patients with acute pneumocholecystitis are often male diabetics, have the clinical features of acute cholecystitis, but their general condition shows rapid deterioration and early progression to hypovolaemic shock. A plain radiograph of the abdomen may also show a calcified gallstone, though this finding is not usually of particular value in the diagnosis of calculous acute cholecystitis, as the gallstone may be an incidental finding.

The development of local complications of empyema formation, gangrene of the gallbladder, as well as a pericholecystic abscess, is diagnosed first in a similar way to acute cholecystitis, but the complication can usually be discerned from the clinical course of the patient because both the general condition of the patient, as well as the local abdominal signs, persist and deteriorate progressively. Thus, in these cases, the pyrexia and tachycardia persist and also the local signs show a progression of the area of abdominal guarding, rigidity, and tenderness. Also, the abdominal mass may increase in size during a short period of observation. Unfortunately, in some elderly patients, a local complication of this kind may be discovered unexpectedly at operation unpredicted by the clinical course, hence some advocate early surgery in the elderly patient. Free perforation with general biliary peritonitis is not usually diagnosed before surgery, as these patients present with the features of general peritonitis, the cause of which is uncertain.

Special diagnostic investigations in acute calculous cholecystitis include ultrasonography, intravenous cholangiography, and radionuclide cholescintigraphy. At present, almost all patients would have ultrasonography performed and this, with the clinical findings, can establish a firm diagnosis of acute calculous cholecystitis in about 90 percent of cases. Radionuclide cholescintigraphy is useful in certain selected cases, whereas intravenous cholangiography is being used less and less frequently in diagnosis of acute calculous cholecystitis since the advent of ultrasonography and cholescintigraphy.

Ultrasonography. Ultrasound examination is performed with grey scale B-mode equipment that may be either static or a real-time machine. Real time generally allows a more rapid assessment, and with modern equipment there is no disadvantage in terms of image quality. Transducers with frequencies between 2.25 and 5.0 MHz may be used, depending on the body build of the patient, with 3.5 MHz proving optimum for most patients. In order to obtain ideal images, it is highly desirable that the patient is fasting for at least 6 hours prior to the examination. This is usually not difficult as most patients are fasting anyway because of their illness. The demonstration of gallbladder calculi supports the diagnosis of acute calculous cholecystitis, but because of the prevalence of cholelithiasis, it is not regarded as diagnostic, and other ultrasound evidence is sought to strengthen the clinical diagnosis.

Other evidence, apart from a gallstone, is when a stone is seen to be impacted in the neck of the gallbladder, when there is tenderness over the gallbladder, a sign that has been termed the "ultrasonic Murphy sign," thickening of the gallbladder wall and the presence of a sonolucent layer in the gallbladder wall, dilatation of the gallbladder itself, the presence of echogenic material in the gallbladder, and the presence of pericholecystic collection. Tenderness, specifically over the gallbladder, which has been accurately localised by ultrasound—the so-called ultrasonic Murphy sign—although quite specific is not particularly sensitive and has been found in only two thirds of cases. Thickening of the gallbladder wall and the presence of a sonolucent layer within the wall, thought to be due to inflammatory oedema, are strongly suggestive of acute inflammation, but these findings need to be taken into consideration with the clinical findings, because similar changes may also occur in other conditions such as hypoalbuminaemia, hepatitis, and alcoholic cirrhosis. The presence of medium to coarse nonlayering and nonshadowing echoes within the lumen of the gallbladder, especially if associated with wall changes is a reliable sign of empyaema, as demonstrated by Kane in 1980. Typical examples of ultrasonography findings in acute calculous cholecystitis are shown in Figures 75–1 through 75–3.

Pneumocholecystitis, although uncommon, can be diagnosed ultrasonographically by the presence of highly reflective gas echoes within the lumen of the gallbladder with poorly defined distal acoustic shadows. Gallstones may be missed on ultrasonography in as many as 10 to 15 percent of patients with acute calculous cholecystitis; in this situation, the associated features become more important, particularly gallbladder tenderness, wall changes, and evi-

dence of empyaema or of a pericholecystic abscess. The specificity of ultrasonography is of the order of 90 percent and the sensitivity is of the order of 85 percent. Ultrasound examination also provides assessment of the bile ducts, the liver, and the pancreas. However, there is a small group of patients in whom the gallbladder cannot be seen because of obesity, the patient's inability to cooperate, or an inaccessible gallbladder situation high under the right costal margin.

Intravenous Cholangiography. This investigation is regarded as positive for acute cholecystitis if the gallbladder fails to fill, indicating obstruction of the cystic duct by a gallstone. Al-

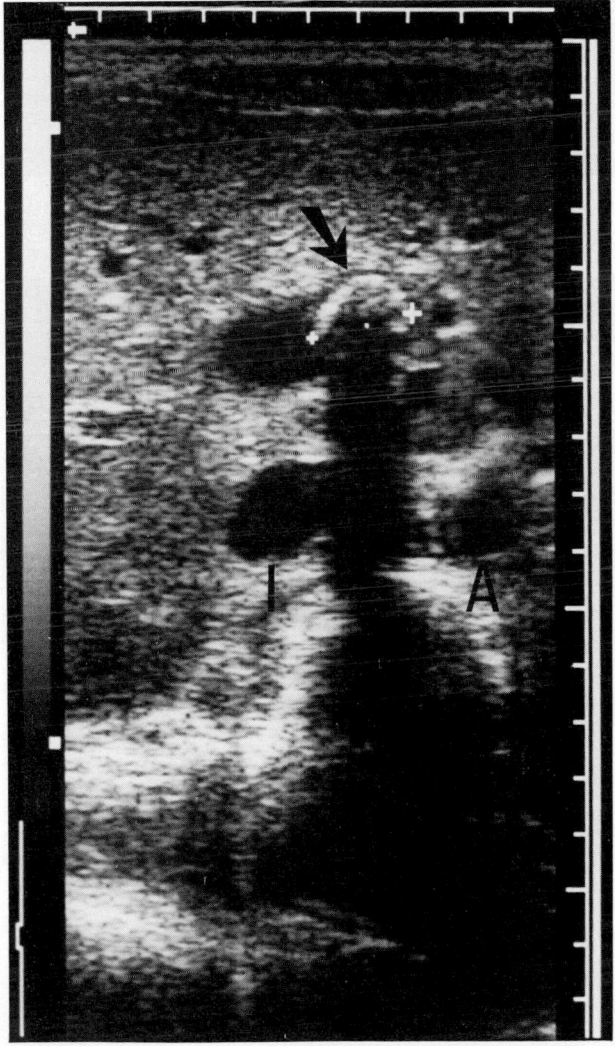

Figure 75–1. Ultrasonogram showing a stone in the neck of the gallbladder. Transverse view of the upper abdomen showing the inferior vena cava (I), aorta (A), and a 19-mm calculus (*arrow*) impacted in the neck of the gallbladder. Note the dense sonic shadow distal to the calculus.

1842

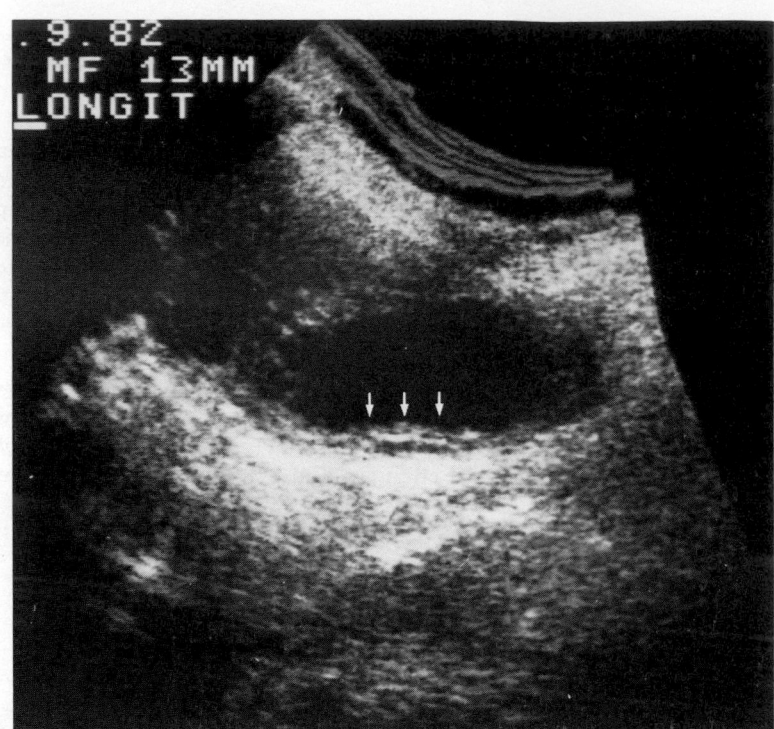

Figure 75–2. Ultrasonogram showing the gallbladder wall (*arrows*) to be thickened and less distinct than normal in a case of acute cholecystitis.

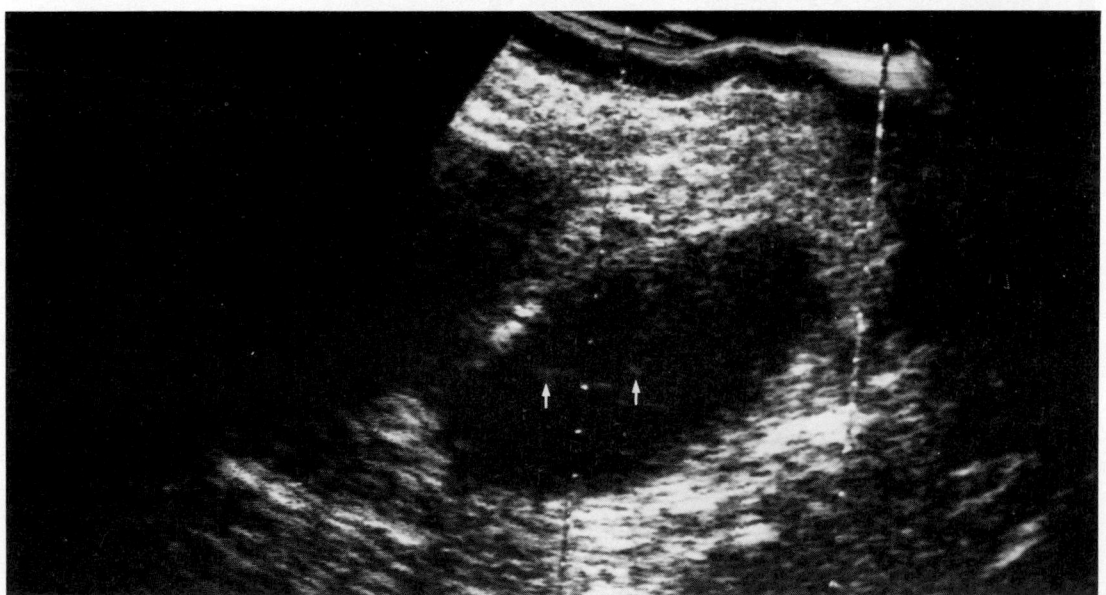

Figure 75–3. Ultrasonogram showing the presence of nonlayering echogenic material (*arrows*), representing pus in the gallbladder lumen in a case of empyaema of the gallbladder.

though high sensitivity and specificity rates have been reported for this investigation, it is now used less and less frequently for the diagnosis of acute calculous cholecystitis because of the risk of hypersensitivity to the contrast medium and also because 24-hour views are required to confirm an abnormal result, as late filling of the gallbladder may occur. The study is also of very limited use in the presence of jaundice. Tomography demonstrating opacification of the inflamed gallbladder wall following infusion of the excretory agent used in intravenous pyelography has been reported to have a sensitivity between 77 and 96 percent but a low specificity of 50 percent due to the high incidence of false-positives.

Radionuclide Cholescintigraphy. The availability of technetium-99m-labelled biliary tract agents has resulted in high-quality visualisation of the hepatobiliary system, enabling study of its morphology, function, and the dynamics of bile flow. Approximately 85 percent of the administered dose is metabolised by the hepatocytes and excreted unconjugated into the biliary system, with the remaining 15 percent rapidly excreted by the kidneys. Amino acid Schiff base complexes such as pyridoxylidine glutamate (PG) have now been almost universally replaced in clinical use by iminodiacetic acid (IDA) compounds. The latter have greater hepatobiliary specificity and more rapid hepatic transit times. IDA compounds in use include dimethyl-IDA (HIDA), p-isopropyl-IDA (PIPIDA), diethyl-IDA (DIDA), and di-isopropyl-IDA (DISIDA). DIDA and DISIDA are more resistant to displacement by bilirubin, attributed to their greater protein binding capacity, and this enhances hepatic excretion. Good-quality biliary tract studies can therefore be performed in the presence of hyperbilirubinaemia up to 10 mg/dl (170 μmol/L). Above this level, the liver and excreted isotope in the gut is visualised but ducts and gallbladder may not be discerned.

The patient must be fasting for at least 2 hours and preferably greater than 4 hours to avoid false-positive results. Following intravenous injection of 5 mCi (185 MBq) of a Tc-99m IDA derivative, anterior gamma camera images are obtained at 2 minutes, 5 minutes, and then serially at 10- to 15-minute intervals for 1 hour, including a right lateral view that may be necessary to separate gallbladder from duodenum if they overlap. The features of a normal study are a good uptake by the liver within 5 minutes, an initial renal activity cleared by 30 minutes, well-seen biliary ducts with the gallbladder seen by 45 minutes, and duodenal activity by 60 minutes (Fig. 75–4). Bile duct visualisation and gut activity in the absence of gallbladder filling is taken to indicate cystic duct obstruction, and in conjunction with the clinical findings, a diagnosis of acute cholecystitis, as shown in Figure 75–5. As there may be delayed filling of the gallbladder, this conclusion should not be drawn unless 4-hour scintiphotos show no gallbladder activity.

Using the criteria mentioned, both the sensitivity and the specificity of cholescintigraphy in the diagnosis of acute cholecystitis has been reported by numerous investigators to lie between 94 and 100 percent. The gallbladder may not be visualised in the absence of acute cholecystitis in patients who have had no oral intake for longer than 48 hours or who have been receiving total parenteral nutrition. A higher incidence of false-positive results has also been reported in alcoholics. However, the presence of acute pancreatitis does not significantly affect the usefulness of cholescintigraphy in the diagnosis of cute cholecystitis. Acute calculous cholecystitis but with a patent cystic duct at the time of the radionuclide scan is most uncommon, but it has been reported as a cause of false-negative studies by Echevarria and Gleason in 1980.

Using radionuclide cholescintigraphy a negative result for acute cholecystitis can be established within 30 minutes and a positive diagnosis of acute cholecystitis can be made within 4 hours. The rapidity with which either a positive or negative diagnosis of acute cholecystitis can be made is a significant advantage over intravenous cholangiography.

Summary of Diagnostic Process in Acute Calculous Cholecystitis. At present a firm diagnosis of acute calculous cholecystitis can be made in approximately 90 percent of cases by the clinical findings taken in conjunction with the results of ultrasonography of the gallbladder. In doubtful cases the addition of radionuclide cholescintigraphy can, in almost every case, confirm or deny the presence or absence of acute calculous cholecystitis. Intravenous cholangiography now has a very limited role in the diagnosis of acute calculous cholecystitis.

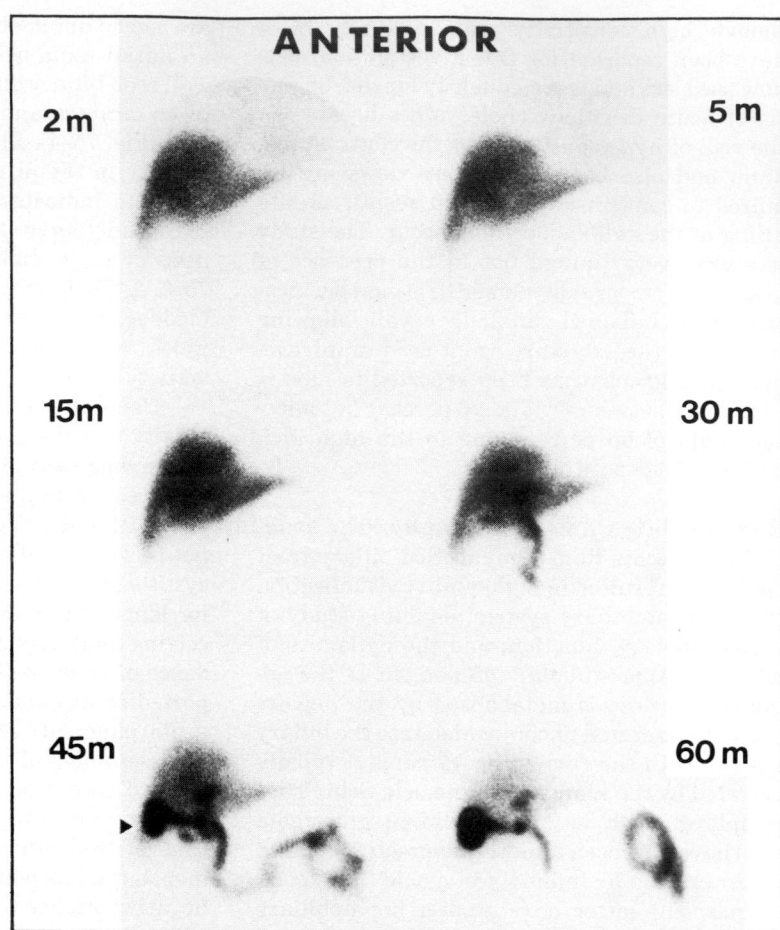

Figure 75–4. Normal cholescintigram. A normal Tc-99m-HIDA biliary tract study. The gallbladder is well visualised by 45 minutes (*arrow*), indicating patency.

Treatment

The management of acute calculous cholecystitis consists of an initial period of medical treatment and resuscitation, according to the needs of the particular patient, followed by surgery. Medical dissolution of the calculi using oral agents such as chenodeoxycholic acid are contraindicated because these agents will not penetrate into the gallbladder bile due to the blocked gallbladder outlet.

Medical Treatment

Medical measures bring the patient into an optimal condition for surgery. Adequate analgesia is given. Cardiorespiratory disease commonly co-exists in elderly patients with acute cholecystitis and this is corrected. Fluid and electrolyte disturbances are uncommon in acute cholecystitis though minimal dehydration is frequent and is corrected before surgery. It has been shown in a number of studies that antibiotics are valueless in decreasing the eventual incidence of local septic complications, such as the formation of an empyema or of a pericholecystic abscess, but can be of value in decreasing the rate of septicaemia of patients who are at risk. Patients at risk are aged over 60 or have a debilitating disease such as diabetes that lowers their resistance to infection, or they already have a septic complication such as a pericholecystic abscess. However, numerous studies have shown that the use of appropriate antibiotics given in the perioperative period will decrease the rate of postoperative septic complications, especially that of wound infections. As the bacteria present in the gallbladder during acute cholecystitis are enterobacteria, broad-spectrum antibiotics such as cephalosporins or cotrimoxizole are usually used.

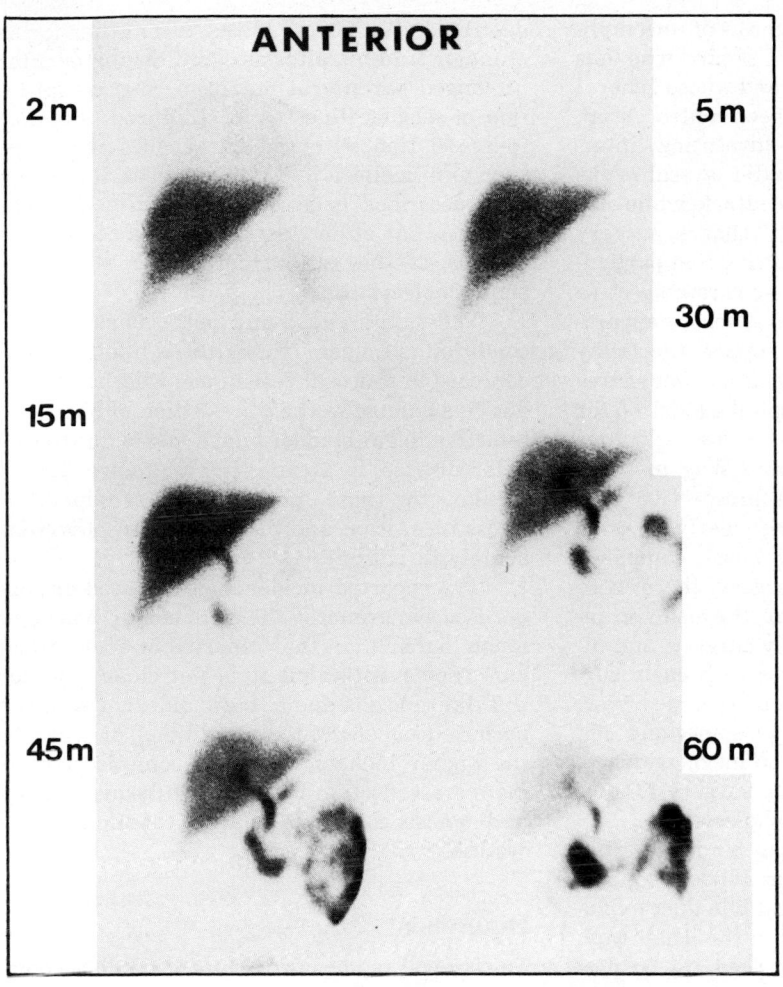

ANTERIOR

2 m

5 m

30 m

15 m

45 m

60 m

Figure 75–5. Abnormal chole-scintigram. Despite normal transit of Tc-99m-HIDA through the liver and bile ducts into the gut, the gallbladder is not seen. There was no gallbladder activity present in the 4-hour scinti-photos, consistent with cystic duct obstruction and therefore acute cholecystitis.

During the period of medical treatment, both the general and local abdominal condition of the patient is frequently observed in order to detect evidence that a local complication, such as a pericholecystic abscess, has not occurred. If the patient continues to be treated medically for some reason, the observations are continued during the whole of the patient's stay in hospital. Medical treatment alone is nowadays used only in the very old or very poor risk patient in whom it is judged that the risks of surgery are greater than the risks of conservative management, and also in the patient who refuses or wishes to delay surgery.

Surgical Treatment

Emergency or semiemergency surgery is advocated for all patients in whom a local complication such as empyaema, gangrene, or perichole-cystic abscess formation is present, or suspected, and also in the rare case of acute pneumocholecystitis, as gangrene and perforation of the gallbladder is common in this group. Patients with acute pneumocholecystitis need to be protected, not only with the usual perioperative use of a broad-spectrum antibiotic, but also with an anti-anaerobic antibiotic, such as the injectable form of metronidazole. Emergency surgery is also necessary when the diagnosis of acute cholecystitis is uncertain and when another acute abdominal condition, which requires urgent surgery, such as a perforated peptic ulcer, cannot be excluded with certainty. In recent years the number of patients in which a diagnosis is a problem has diminished because of the advent of ultrasonography and radionuclide cholescintigraphy, as described earlier.

In the past, the timing of surgery in a typical patient in whom the diagnosis of uncomplicated acute cholecystitis is certain, who has been optimally resuscitated, and whose general condition is satisfactory, has been controversial. Thus, some authorities were advocating "interval surgery," that is, surgery after several weeks or months following the acute attack, while others advocated "early surgery," that is, surgery as a semielective procedure during that particular hospital admission. Numerous retrospective uncontrolled trials, as well as at least four prospective controlled trials, all support the safety and efficacy of early surgery as a semielective operation during a single hospital admission for patients with uncomplicated acute calculous cholecystitis. Thus Motson and Way in 1982, from a collective review of prospective controlled trials, found that with early surgery there were no deaths in 214 cases, compared to 5 deaths with interval surgery, there were no duct injuries in either group, the mean hospital stay was halved with early surgery, and although there were no failures with early surgery, 19 percent failures were recorded with interval surgery. Because of its safety and efficacy, on the basis of a large volume of evidence, the authors recommend early surgery for uncomplicated acute calculous cholecystitis.

Thus, cholecystectomy can be done in the usual way for this condition, and if desired, peroperative cholangiography and bile duct exploration can also be performed in the usual way. Cholecystostomy only rarely needs to be performed in these cases.

ACUTE ACALCULOUS CHOLECYSTITIS

This is an uncommon form of acute cholecystitis and may be defined as acute cholecystitis in the absence of gallstones or of any other form of obstructive pathology at the gallbladder outlet. It accounts for 1 percent or less of all cases of acute cholecystitis.

Aetiology and Pathogenesis

The cause of acute acalculous cholecystitis is unclear, but it may be multifactorial. A number of clinical antecedents have been described, but it is uncertain whether these are aetiologic associations or merely risk factors indicating some other unknown underlying cause or causes. Thus, acute acalculous cholecystitis has been

described after severe burns, after other forms of major trauma, after surgery, during or after prolonged parenteral nutrition, as a complication of serious illnesses in childhood, and also in association with certain specific infections, such as brucellosis and typhoid fever. It has also been described in association with acute pancreatitis, but often this is merely a contiguous oedema of the gallbladder rather than true acute cholecystitis.

The actual cause and pathogenesis of the condition is unclear, though it is likely to be a decrease in mucosal resistance, whether this is due to a change in the composition of bile salts, infection in gallbladder bile, hypoxia due to vascular disease, or some other unknown factors similar to those producing gastroduodenal stress ulceration and bleeding in an otherwise acutely ill patient.

The reported incidence of localised or generalised gangrene of the gallbladder has been much higher than that reported in acute calculous cholecystitis, but it is not clear whether this difference is due to basic differences in the pathogenesis of the two conditions, or whether the higher incidence of local complications is merely a reflection of the more frequent delay in diagnosis compared to acute calculous cholecystitis.

Diagnosis

The clinical syndrome of acute acalculous cholecystitis is similar to the calculous variety, but diagnosis is more frequently delayed or more frequently made only at surgery compared to acute calculous cholecystitis. The reasons for this difference are partly that the clinician does not entertain the possibility of acute cholecystitis in the absence of gallstones and partly because the disease often presents as an intercurrent event in association with another dominant clinical illness such severe trauma, burns, or recent major surgery. The clinical features are similar to calculous acute cholecystitis with upper abdominal pain and tenderness, often with a palpable distended and tender gallbladder.

If the condition is suspected, a firm preoperative diagnosis can be made with ultrasonography and radionuclide cholescintigraphy. With ultrasonography, gallstones are absent but other features previously described for calculous acute cholecystitis are present. A positive cholescintigram, as for calculous cholecystitis, is present in the absence of an anatomic obstruction, presumably due to a "functional" obstruction as a result of marked gallbladder and cystic duct wall oedema. The reported sensitivity and specificity of ultrasonography has been reported to lie between 50 and 100 percent and for cholescintigraphy between 78 and 100 percent, but the data in general support the latter investigation as the more sensitive and the diagnostic procedure of first choice.

Treatment

Semiemergency or emergency surgical treatment is advocated for all cases of acute acalculous cholecystitis after prompt correction of any fluid, electrolyte, and cardiorespiratory deficits. The surgery is best performed under perioperative broad-spectrum antibiotic cover and this should probably also include an antianaerobe.

The surgical treatment consists of laparotomy, establishment of diagnosis, and cholecystectomy. Peroperative cholangiography is useful in order to exclude biliary ductal stones. In children, it has been found that in the absence of perforation or gangrene of the gallbladder, cholecystostomy alone also produces very satisfactory results.

A collected review of the literature indicates that acute acalculous cholecystitis has a much higher mortality than calculous acute cholecystitis, probably because of the frequent delay in diagnosis, the high rate of serious local complications, such as gangrene or perforation of the gallbladder, and the presence of another serious intercurrent illness, trauma, or major surgery.

CHRONIC CHOLECYSTITIS

The diagnosis of chronic cholecystitis is, and should remain, a pathologic and *not* a clinical diagnosis. Thus, a diagnosis of chronic cholecystitis at present can only be made following surgery or postmortem examination and there are no specific tests available to diagnose this entity at a clinical level. Also, it is doubtful whether chronic inflammatory change in the gallbladder wall ever produces clinical symptoms in the absence of other pathology, such as gallstones. The management of patients who have gallbladder gallstones in association with suspected, so-called chronic cholcystitis is straightforward, namely, it is the conventional treatment of the gallstones rather than the treatment of the

suspected chronic inflammatory change in the gallbladder wall. In fact, after surgical excision of gallbladders that contain gallstones, it is quite the usual finding that varying degrees of chronic inflammatory change are present in the gallbladder on histologic examination. These chronic inflammatory changes are regarded as secondary to the gallstones and are not believed to be responsible for any additional symptoms apart from those produced by the gallstones themselves.

For many years claims have been made intermittently that acalculous chronic cholecystitis exists and that this is a clinically diagnosable entity. However, up to the present time, there is no solid evidence for such claims. There is nevertheless a group of patients with typical gallstone symptoms who, upon initial cholecystography or ultrasonography, reveal no gallstones. In a proportion of these, repeat investigations or the addition of other techniques, such as endoscopic retrograde cholangiography, will in fact demonstrate gallstones that have been missed initially.

There remains a residual group of patients who appear to have symptoms emanating from the biliary tract without gallstones or without any other demonstrable biliary pathology, and it is this group that at times has been labelled as "patients with chronic acalculous cholecystitis." Cholecystectomy has been advocated by a number of surgeons over many years with variable success rates, but it is the belief of the present writers, as well as that of other authorities, that the indiscriminate advocacy of cholecystectomy in this group of patients will result in a fairly low postsurgical success rate, as well as a high rate of disabling postcholecystectomy pain. The present writers are in full accord with other authorities, such as Siffert and Ham, who believe that this subgroup of patients should be grouped with other so-called functional disorders of the biliary tract and, for their diagnosis, similar diagnostic criteria to functional biliary tract disorders should be applied before any surgical treatment is undertaken. This implies careful pretreatment evaluation of the patient by the use of discriminative investigations, including cholecystokinin cholecystography, analysis of duodenal bile for cholesterol crystals and bacteria, morphine provocation test with or without a study of emptying of the gallbladder and bile ducts on cholecystography and cholangiography, as well as endoscopic biliary manometry as well as liver biopsy. Only in the pres-

ence of strict criteria of abnormality of one or
several of these investigations is surgical treatment such as cholecystectomy, sphincterotomy
or sphincteroplasty likely to be effective in either the short- or long-term in this group of
patients, who are notoriously difficult to diagnose and difficult to treat effectively.

BIBLIOGRAPHY

Blaquiere RM, Dewbury KC: The ultrasound diagnosis of emphysematous cholecystitis. Br J Radiol 55:114, 1982

Burnett W, Robinson P: The management of acute cholecystitis. Med J Aust 1:770, 1966

Chervu LR, Nunn AD, et al: Radiopharmaceuticals for hepatobiliary imaging. Semin Nucl Med 12:5, 1982

Cheung LY, Chang FC: Intravenous cholangiography in the diagnosis of acute cholecystitis. Arch Surg 113:568, 1978

Croce F, Montali G, et al: Ultrasonography in acute cholecystitis. Br J Radiol 54:927, 1981

Deitch CA, Engel JM: Acute acalculous cholecystitis— Ultrasonic diagnosis. Am J Surg 142:290, 1981

Echavarria RA, Gleason JL: False negative gallbladder scintigram in acute cholecystitis. J Nucl Med 21:841, 1980

Freitas JE, Coleman RE, et al: Influence of scan and pathologic criteria on the specificity of cholescintigraphy. J Nucl Med 24:876, 1983

Gilchrist NL, Boniface GR, et al: Acute cholecystitis: a diagnostic approach using Tc-99m-Diethyl-IDA scintigraphy. Aust NZ J Surg 52:461, 1982

Glenn F, Becker CG: Acute acalculous cholecystitis— An increasing entity: Ann Surg 195:131, 1982

Gupta SM, Owshalimpur D, et al: Radionuclide scanning for rapid diagnosis of cute cholecystitis. Aust NZ J Med 12:265, 1982

Hall AW, Wisbey ML, et al: The place of hepatobiliary isotope scanning in the diagnosis of gallbladder disease. Br J Surg 68:85, 1981

Ham JM: Acalculous benign biliary disease, in Kune GA, Sali A (eds): The Practice of Biliary Surgery, 2 edt. Oxford: Blackwell, 1980, p. 344

Herlin P, Ericsson M, et al: Acute acalculous cholecystitis following trauma. Br J Surg 69:475, 1982

Howard RJ: Acute acalculous cholecystitis. Am J Surg 142:194, 1981

Kane RA: Ultrasonographic diagnosis of gangrenous cholecystitis and empyaema of the gallbladder. Radiology 134:191, 1980

Keighley MRB: Infection in biliary tract surgery, in Watts JMcK, McDonald PJ, et al (eds): Infection in Surgery. Edinburgh: Churchill Livingstone, 1981, p 194

Klingensmith WC, Spitzer VM, et al: The normal fasting and post prandial Tc-99m DISIDA hepatobiliary study. J Nucl Med 22:7, 1981

Kune GA, Birks D: Acute cholecystitis. An appraisal of current methods of treatment. Med J Aust 2:218, 1970

Kune GA, Burdon JGW: Are antibiotics necessary in acute cholecystitis? Med J Aust 2:627, 1975

Kune GA, Sali A: The Practice of Biliary Surgery, 2 edt. Oxford: Blackwell, 1980, p 136

Kune GA, Schutz E: Bacteria in the biliary tract. A study of their frequency and type. Med J Aust 1:255, 1974

Loberg MD, Ryan JW, et al: Hepatic clearance mechanisms of Tc-99m-IDA. J Nucl Med 21:1111, 1980

Matolo N, Stadalnik R, et al: Comparison of ultrasonography, computerized tomography and radionuclide imaging in the diagnosis of acute and chronic cholecystitis. Am J Surg 144:676, 1982

Mauro MA, McCartney WH, et al: Hepatobiliary scanning with Tc-99m-PIPIDA in acute cholecystitis. Radiology 142:193, 1982

Moncada R, Cardosa M, et al: Acute cholecystitis: One hundred and thirty seven patients studied with infusion tomography of the gallbladder. AJR 129:583, 1977

Morrow DJ, Thompson J, et al: Acute cholecystitis in the elderly. Arch Surg 113:1149, 1978

Motsom RW, Way LW: Cholecystitis, in Blumgart LH (ed): Clinical Surgery International. 5. The Biliary Tract. Edinburgh: Churchill Livingstone, 1982, p. 121

Nicholson RW, Herman KJ, et al: The plasma protein binding of HIDA. Eur J Nucl Med 5:311, 1980

Pedersen JH, Nancke S, et al: Ultrasonography 99mTc-DDA cholescintigraphy diagnosis of acute cholecystitis. Scand J Gastroenterol 17:77, 1982

Petersen SR, Sheldon GF: Acute acalculous cholecystitis: A complication of hyperalimentation. Am J Surg 138:814, 1979

Ralls PW, Colletti PM, et al: Prospective evaluation of 99mTc-IDA cholescintigraphy and gray scale ultrasound in the diagnosis of acute cholecystitis. Radiology 144:369, 1982

Shunan WP, Gibbs P, et al: PIPIDA scintigraphy for cholecystitis: false positives in alcoholism and total parenteral nutrition. AJR 138:1, 1982

Siffert G: Chronic non calculus cholecystitis, in Bockus HL (ed): Gastroenterology, 3 edt. Philadelphia: WB Saunders, 1976, vol. 3, p 811

Ternberg JL, Keating JP: Acute acalculous cholecystitis. Complication of other illnesses in childhood. Arch Surg 110:543, 1975

Weissman HS, Badia J, et al: Spectrum of Tc-99m-IDA cholescintigraphic patterns in acute cholecystitis. Radiology 138:167, 1981

Weissman HS, Berkowitz D, et al: The role of Tc-99m-IDA cholescintigraphy in acute acalculous cholecystitis. Radiology 146:177, 1983

76. Cholecystostomy and Cholecystectomy
Harold Ellis

INTRODUCTION

Sir Zachary Cope (1965) has left us a fascinating account of the evolution of the diagnosis and treatment of acute cholecystitis. Gallstones have been found in ancient mummies and we must assume that their malign effects date back to the earliest times. Gallstones were recorded in the autopsy reports of Benevieni, published in 1507; Morgagni, in 1761, related 20 postmortem examinations in which gallstones were found. The surgeon who first fully discussed inflammatory conditions due to gallstones was Petit (1674–1750), who taught that in cases of inflammation of the gallbladder, if the organ were not adherent to the abdominal wall there should be no operative intervention, but if there were signs of an abscess or of adhesion of the gallbladder to the parietes, drainage could be effected, either by puncture with a trocar or by lithotomy.

Formal laparotomy with removal of the gallstones by cholecystotomy was first performed in the United States by Bobbs in 1866 in a female aged 30 in whom a preoperative diagnosis of ovarian cyst had been made. The gallbladder was opened, gallstones were evacuated, and the edges of the gallbladder incision were sewn to the margins of the abdominal wound so that any further stone that appeared might be seized. The patient recovered.

The account by Bobbs was published in the *Transactions of the Indiana State Medical Society* in 1867 but was overlooked by surgeons on both sides of the Atlantic so that, 10 years later, when other surgeons performed similar operations, no reference was made to Bobbs. Three surgeons performed cholecystotomy in 1878—Sims, Kocher (who performed a two stage operation), and Keen. The following year, Tait of Birmingham performed a successful cholecystotomy and did much to pioneer the operation.

By 1892 he listed 71 cholecystotomies with only 4 postoperative deaths.

The first cholecystectomy was performed by Langenbuch of Berlin in 1882; the patient, a male aged 43, recovered. Langenbuch suggested that the common bile duct might be opened for removal of stones contained therein. This was first carried out by Kummell in 1884 and first performed successfully by Thornton in 1889.

CHOLECYSTOSTOMY

Cholecystostomy is nearly always a procedure of compromise, but it is frequently a life-saving one. It is a measure that meets the immediate demand to save the patient's life, and it also paves the way for safety at a later date for the performance of a definitive operative procedure.

Indications

Acute Cholecystitis with Gallstones. Cholecystostomy is indicated in these circumstances; (1) when the patient is aged and infirm, perhaps with serious renal, cardiovascular, or pulmonary complications, (2) when cholecystectomy presents unusual technical difficulties, for example anatomic obscuration or extreme obesity, so that the surgeon has serious fears for the possibility of injury to the bile ducts, and (3) when there is some anaesthetic problem during the early stages of the exploratory laparotomy and there is the need for rapid termination of the operation.

Chronic Calculous Cholecystitis. When the surgeon lacks experience in operating on the biliary tract, and when the risk involved in excising the gallbladder appears to be unusually great in the particular case, cholecystostomy represents a safer procedure.

Acute Pancreatitis with Obstructive Jaundice. When committed to operation for such a grave event, the surgeon would be well advised to adopt the simplest procedure—cholecystostomy or, possibly, T-tube choledochostomy.

In Some Instances of Carcinoma of the Pancreas. It is only very occasionally these days that the surgeon encounters a patient with a carcinoma of the head of the pancreas or of the periampullary region with very severe jaundice and in poor general condition and yet in whom the tumour itself is eminently resectable. In such instances, percutaneous or endoscopic drainage of the distended gallbladder can often be carried out as a preliminary while the patient's general condition improves. The situation may be encountered at laparotomy where the surgeon decides to perform preliminary drainage of the gallbladder by means of a fine polyethylene tube with the intent of carrying out a formal resection as soon as the patient's general condition has improved, usually within 1 or 2 weeks.

Operative Technique

An upper right paramedian or a right subcostal (Kocher) incision gives excellent approach to the region. In the usual situation, where cholecystostomy is being performed for acute calculous cholecystitis, a full laparotomy is not indicated, but gentle exploration of the gallbladder region is carefully performed. Having decided that preliminary drainage, rather than emergency cholecystectomy, is the wiser course, the edges of the wound and the region around the gallbladder are carefully packed off with saline-soaked abdominal pads. Inflammatory adhesions, and in particular inflamed oedematous omentum that is walling off the gallbladder, should be disturbed as little as possible.

The tense gallbladder must now be decompressed before any further procedure can take place. Its contents are aspirated with a wide-bore needle or, if this proves unsatisfactory, the isolated fundus is punctured with a Mayo–Ochsner trocar and cannula, and the infected bile removed by suction (Fig. 76–1). A specimen of the bile is immediately despatched in transport medium for bacteriologic culture.

The fundus is seized with Allis or Babcock tissue forceps on either side of the puncture spot

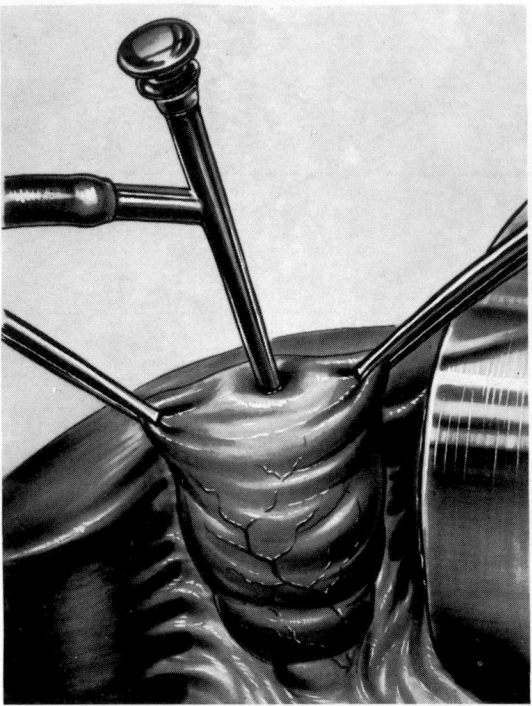

Figure 76–1. Cholecystostomy. The contents of the gallbladder are withdrawn by suction through a Mayo–Ochsner trocar and cannula. (*Source: From Maingot R: Cholecystostomy, in Rob C, Smith R (eds): Operative Surgery, 2 edt. Philadelphia: JB Lippincott, 1969, p 392, with permission.*)

to prevent the gallbladder from retracting when it is empty and also to prevent any leakage when the needle or cannula is withdrawn. An incision of sufficient length to admit the finger is then made through the fundus, a suction tube is introduced into the gallbladder, and the septic bile and inflammatory debris and gravel are withdrawn (Fig. 76–2). The gallbladder should by then be collapsed, unless its walls are thickened and rigid with inflammatory exudate or unless stones occupy its interior. The index finger is passed under the cystic duct and the neck of the gallbladder, and the stones are worked upward with the fingers towards the opening in the fundus. The calculi may be expressed through this opening or may be extracted from the gallbladder with special scoops or forceps (Fig. 76–2). When no further stones can be palpated, either in the cystic duct or in the gall bladder, the forefinger of the right hand is once again introduced into the gallbladder to feel for

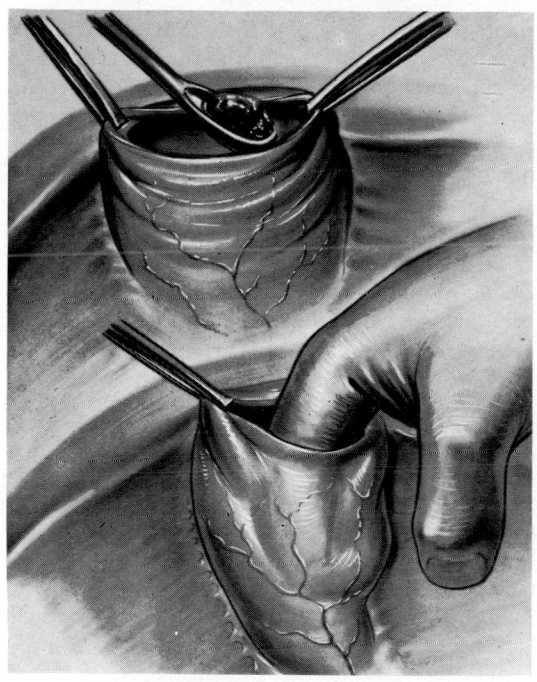

Figure 76–2. Cholecystostomy. Removal of gallstones by scoops and exploration of the interior of the gallbladder with the index finger.

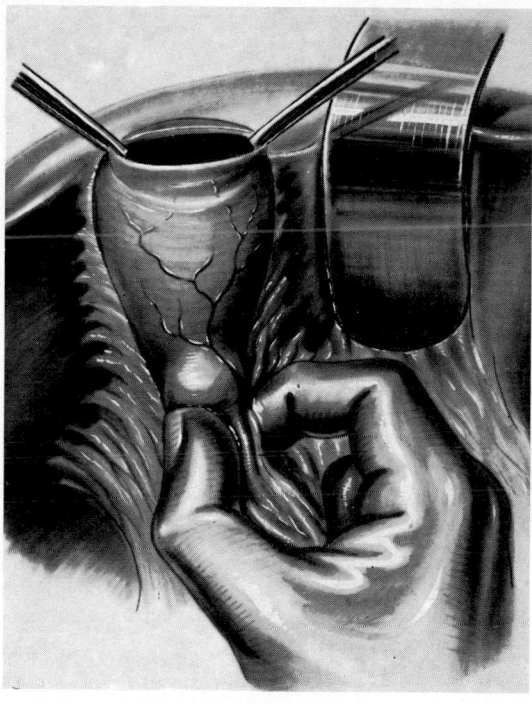

Figure 76–3. Cholecystostomy. Dislodging a stone impacted in the neck of the gallbladder.

any remaining fragments or grit; these may be removed by passing strips of gauze into the gallbladder with dissecting forceps, packing the gauze strips firmly in, and then withdrawing them. Small particles will become entangled in the gauze mesh and can then be extracted. If there is much inflammatory debris or putty-like pigment substance, the gallbladder should be gently irrigated with warm normal saline solution by means of a catheter attached to a syringe. The returning fluid should be aspirated at once with a suction tube.

When calculi are felt to be firmly impacted in the neck of the gallbladder or in the cystic duct, it is usually possible to milk them back into the gallbladder (Fig. 76–3). This is done by passing the finger and thumb down and along the outer side of the neck of the gallbladder until the finger tip enters the foramen of Winslow. In this way the lowest part of the cystic duct is reached. From this point the fingers are worked gently upward, pushing any stones that may be encountered back into the gallbladder. If a stone is firmly lodged in the cystic duct,

firm pressure is applied with the finger and thumb to the duct's lower end, thus coaxing the stone back into the gallbladder. If the stone cannot be dislodged or if the cystic duct or neck of the gallbladder is inadvertently torn during this manoeuvre, cholecystectomy should be carried out if this is technically possible.

When the surgeon has made quite sure that no more stones or debris remain in the gallbladder and that the cystic duct is patent, a Foley or Malecot self-retaining catheter with an outside diameter of 10 mm is passed through the fundal incision so that its tip lies comfortably within the body of the gallbladder. The incision in the gallbladder is then closed around the tube, either by a series of interrupted sutures or by means of one or two purse string sutures of either Dexon or catgut (Figs. 76–4 through 76–6). When the walls of the gallbladder are very thick or friable, interrupted sutures will have to be used but when the walls are sufficiently flexible and firm, a purse string is preferred.

Adjacent omentum is next brought up and

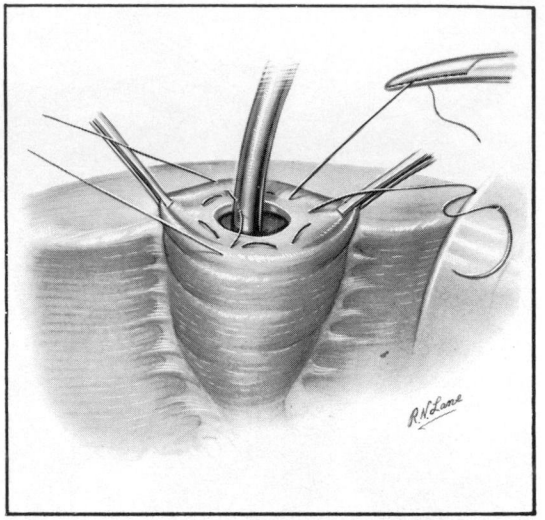

Figure 76–4. Cholecystostomy. The purse string method of closure of the opening in the fundus of the gallbladder. Note how the tube is stitched to the adjacent walls of the gallbladder.

the tube either brought through it or the omentum tacked around the fundus of the gallbladder to afford assurance against leakage (Fig. 76–7). Some surgeons advocate suturing the fundus of the gallbladder to the parietal peritoneum but this step is unnecessary and indeed these stitches may tear out. It is much safer to use the omentum as protection.

The cholecystostomy tube is brought out through a separate small stab incision and either a corrugated or a Penrose drain is placed below the gallbladder and brought out through a separate stab. The cholecystostomy tube is attached to a sterile plastic bag (Fig. 76–8) and the laparotomy wound closed.

In some instances in which the fundus of the gallbladder is, or appears to be, gangrenous and yet cholecystectomy is contraindicated owing to the poor condition of the patient or technical difficulties, it may be advisable to excise the major portion of the distal end of the gallbladder (subtotal cholecystectomy) and then to drain the

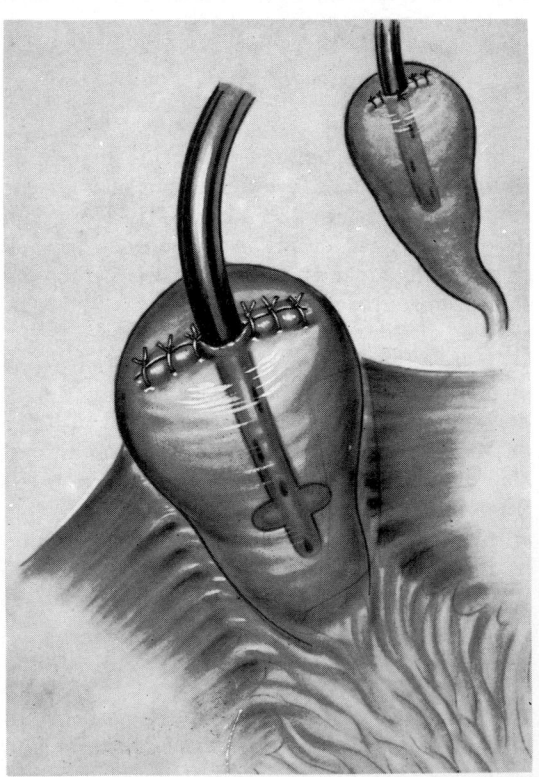

Figure 76–5. Cholecystostomy. A Malecot catheter is used to drain the gallbladder.

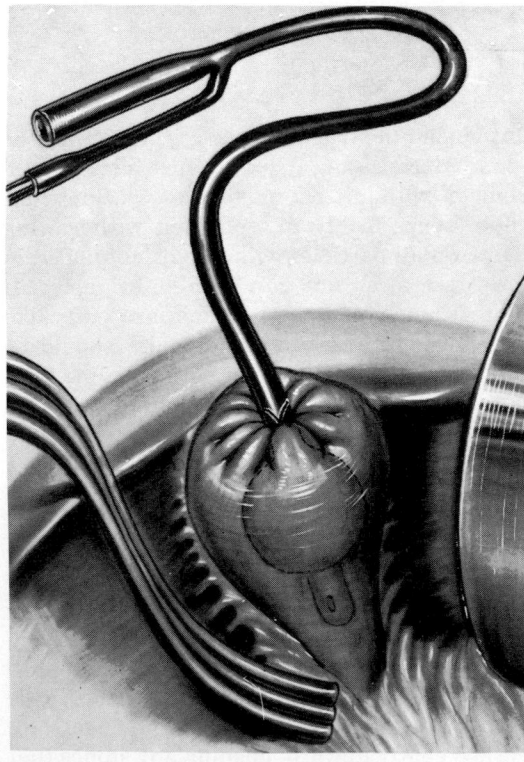

Figure 76–6. Cholecystostomy. The Foley catheter method. (*Courtesy of Butterworths, London.*)

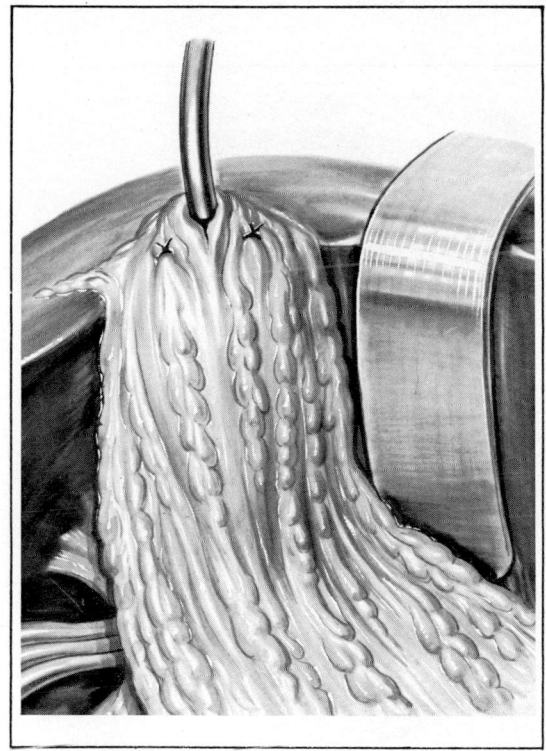

Figure 76–7. Cholecystostomy. Completion of the operation. Note the position of the tubes and also the method of cloaking the gallbladder with the greater omentum.

taken after injection of radiopaque contrast material down the cholecystostomy tube. This will enable the biliary tree to be outlined and the presence or absence of residual stones can be determined.

The cholecystostomy tube should not be removed until it works loose. This usually takes place between the twelfth and fifteenth postoperative days.

Prognosis

The majority of cholecystotomies are performed as emergencies and constitute the preliminary to a second-stage elective cholecystectomy. If the cholangiogram reveals residual stones in the gallbladder or in the common bile duct, the fistulous track leading from the gallbladder fundus to the skin surface is unlikely to heal and, provided the patient's general condition is satisfactory, cholecystectomy will need to be carried out within a few weeks.

What if the cholangiogram shows that the biliary system is entirely clear? Is cholecystectomy still indicated? The long-term results of cholecystotomy as an elective procedure are well documented and are not at all encouraging.

Long and Webster (1957) traced 22 patients

remnant of the gallbladder with an indwelling Foley catheter (Fig. 76–9).

Antibiotic Prophylaxis. These cases are nearly always infected. Intravenous gentamicin or one of the newer cephalosporins (this author prefers cefuroxime) is commenced immediately preoperatively and continued for the three postoperative days, changing the therapy only if necessary in the light of subsequent bacteriologic studies of the bile.

Management of the Cholecystostomy Tube. The tube should be secured firmly to the abdominal wall with adhesive tape and free drainage instituted into a sterile plastic bag. The amount of discharge should be measured daily. The drain to the gallbladder region is shortened on the second day, and removed on the third postoperative day.

Within a few days of operation, when the patient's condition is satisfactory, x-rays are

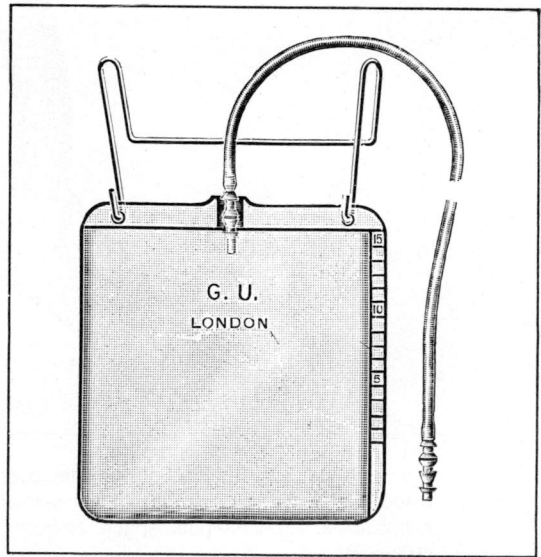

Figure 76–8. Uri-Bag. (*Courtesy of Genitourinary Manufacturing Co.*)

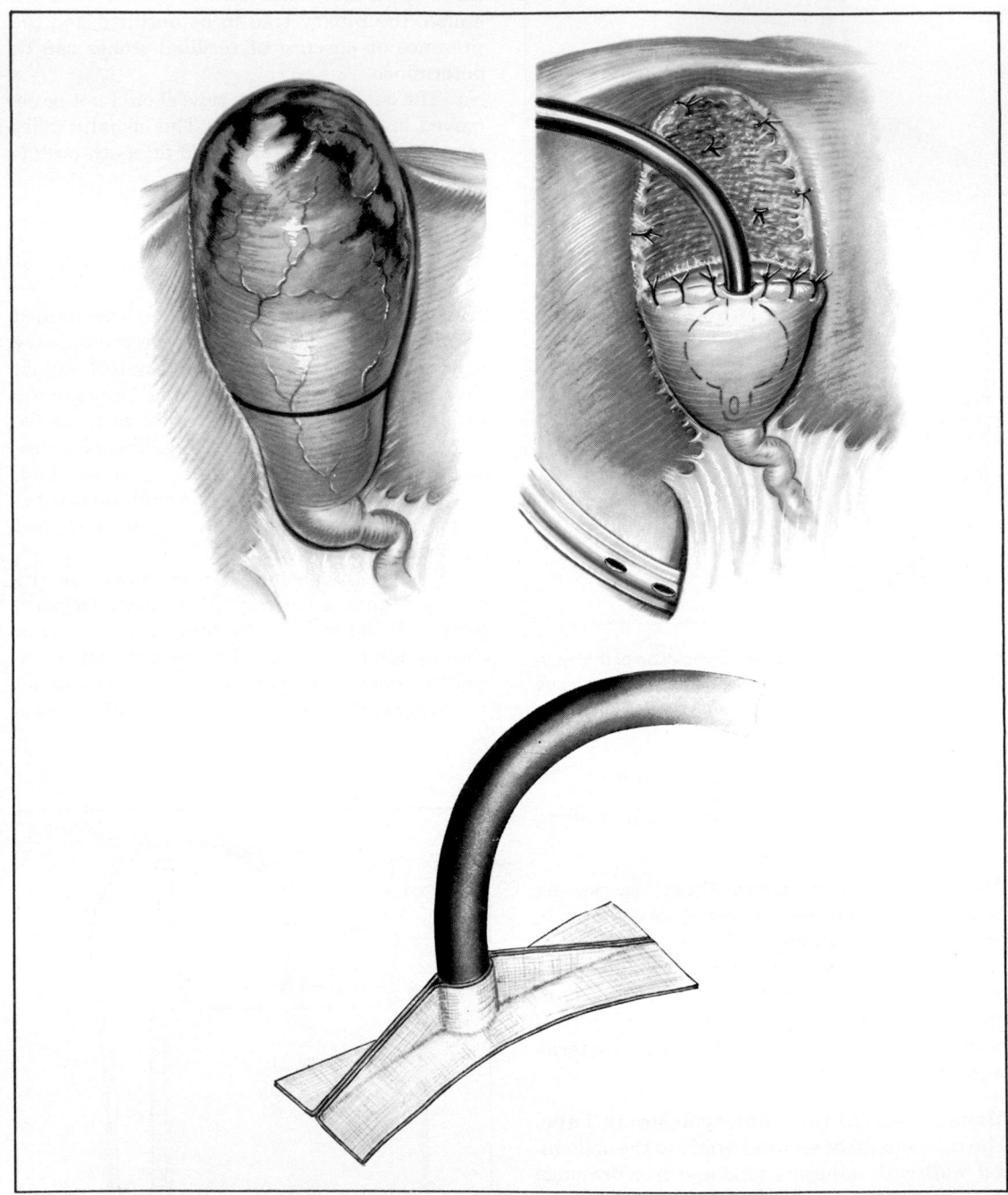

Figure 76–9. *Top:* Subtotal cholecystectomy for gangrene localised to the fundus of the gall-bladder. The remaining portion of the gallbladder is drained with a Foley catheter and a drain is passed to the subhepatic space. *Bottom:* The drainage tube is securely held in place with strapping.

operated upon between 19 and 21 years previously who had stones removed from functioning gallbladders. Two of the patients were still free from symptoms. Nine had required subsequent cholecystectomy between 3 and 10 years from the initial cholecystotomy, all by now having developed stones. The remaining 11 patients all had moderate or severe symptoms and cholecystograms performed on 9 of these revealed calculi in 6 cases. Norrby and Schonebeck (1970) carried out a similar study on 53 patients who had had stones removed from macroscopically normal gallbladders that were functional on the original cholecystogram. Forty eight of these patients were available for reexamination 15 years later. Thirty three had already been operated upon (32 for stone recurrence and 1 for noncalculous cholecystitis); the remaining 15 patients were all submitted to cholecystography and 7 of these had developed further stones. Fifty percent of the recurrences had taken place within 3 years of the original cholecystolithotomy. Welch and Malt (1972) studied 77 patients in whom cholecystostomy had been performed for acute cholecystitis, either because of the poor condition of the patient or because of distorted anatomy. The severity of the disease was shown by the fact that 12 of the patients had a gangrenous gallbladder, in 8 the gallbladder had perforated, and in a further 8 there was an empyema of the gallbladder. The poor condition of these patients is demonstrated by the high mortality; no less than 18 died during their hospital admission (23 percent). Of the 59 survivors, 11 were lost to follow-up and, of the remaining 48, followed up from 2 to 10 years later, 25 had required cholecystectomy and 20 were free from symptoms. In those patients in whom cholangiography shows residual stones, the majority develop recurrent symptoms within a few months.

Castle et al in 1982 have reported 7 cases of carcinoma of the gallbladder in patients previously undergoing cholecystotomy, collected over a period of 50 years. They represent 6.7 percent of their 105 cases of tumours of the gallbladder.

In summary, it is good practice to advise cholecystectomy if the postoperative cholangiogram shows residual stones, and this should be carried out as soon as the patient's condition is satisfactory. If the patient is elderly and in poor general condition with a normal cholangiogram, it is reasonable to leave well alone, but in younger fit patients under these circumstances, an elective cholecystectomy is advisable.

CHOLECYSTECTOMY

Today cholecystectomy is the most common elective operation performed by general surgeons throughout the Western world. It is estimated that some 40,000 cholecystectomies are performed annually in England and Wales, and a quarter of a million each year in the United States. In most cases, when carefully performed, it is one of the simplest and safest of all abdominal procedures and is associated with a low operative mortality rate, certainly less than 1 percent, and gratifying immediate and late results. However, it may be a most difficult and hazardous procedure, demanding the greatest technical skill, experience, and endurance. Inadequate knowledge of the anatomy of the biliary system and its vascular supply, inadequate visualisation of the operative field, undue haste, and continuing to operate in a difficult case where preliminary cholecystostomy would be safer are factors that are responsible for most major postoperative complications such as ductal stricture or fistula and bile peritonitis.

Indications

The indications include:

1. The presence of a gallstone, or gallstones—with or without symptoms.
2. Acute or chronic cholecystitis, with or without gallstones.
3. Torsion of the gallbladder.
4. As a second stage after a preliminary cholecystostomy or where there is persistent biliary or mucus discharge following cholecystostomy for calculous cholecystitis or in patients who have recurrent symptoms due to overlooked or reformed gallstones following a previous cholecystostomy.
5. Traumatic rupture of the gallbladder or cystic duct, an unusual complication of abdominal trauma.
6. Cases of biliary peritonitis, with or without demonstrable perforation.
7. Carcinoma of the gallbladder. Usually the

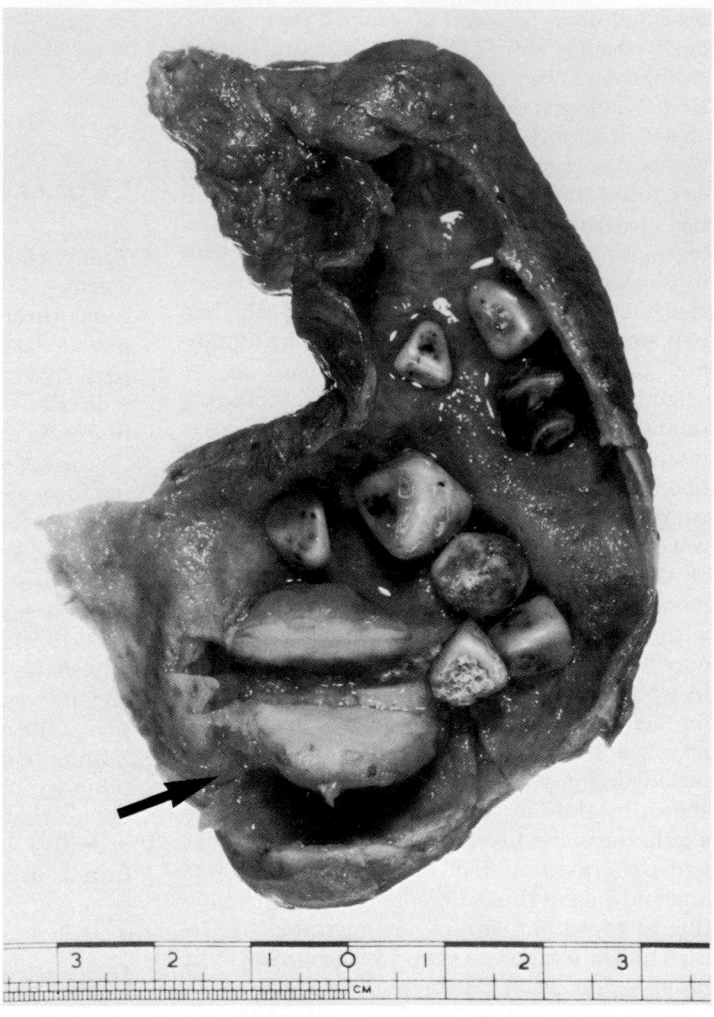

Figure 76–10. Carcinoma of the gall-bladder found incidentally at cholecystectomy for calculous disease. (The tumour is arrowed.)

situation is only operable when the tumour is a chance finding at laparotomy for calculous disease (Fig. 76–10).

Contraindications

Gallstones that are asymptomatic or producing little in the way of trouble in poor-risk, aged, and feeble patients are better left alone. The same consideration applies to patients with other grave complicating medical disorders. If patients in these categories are subjected to recurrent or intractable attacks of colic, perhaps associated with bouts of pyrexia, rigors, and/or jaundice, the gratifying results of judicious, expeditious, and skillful surgical intervention, assisted by preliminary medical treatment to get the patient into the best possible condition, should be carefully weighed against the calcu-

lated risks that are entailed by performing cholecystectomy on this type of patient.

The mortality and morbidity of cholecystectomy are increased in old age, in the presence of jaundice, and in cases of liver damage caused by recurrent attacks of cholangitis or obstruction of the bile duct. Cholecystectomy in a patient with cirrhosis is particularly hazardous. Schwartz was the first to focus on this problem (1981). An important study by Aranha et al (1982) demonstrated this most clearly. Of 429 patients undergoing cholecystectomy at the Hines Veterans Administration Hospital in Illinois, the mortality was 1.1 percent in 374 patients with normal livers. This rose to 9.3 percent in the 43 patients with mild cirrhosis. However, of 12 patients with severe cirrhosis and with a prothrombin time more than 2.5 sec-

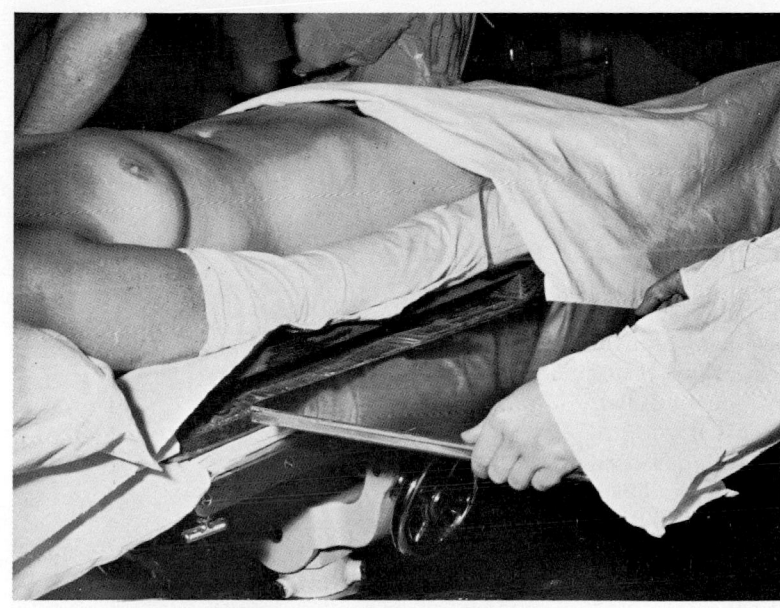

Figure 76–11. Preexploratory cholangiography. The patient is shown in position on the operating table, lying on a box into which the x-ray cassettes can be inserted. For clarity, the towels are not in position but the cassettes can easily be inserted beneath the towels without contaminating the operative field.

onds above the control, there were no less than 10 deaths (83 percent). Lethal complications included hepatic encephalopathy, ascites, sepsis, and haemorrhage. Obviously biliary surgery in such patients should only be performed in the presence of the life-threatening complications of empyema, perforation, or ascending cholangitis.

Operative Technique

Since operative cholangiography is to be carried out, the patient is placed on an operating table fitted with a compartment in which the x-ray cassettes can be placed (Fig. 76–11). In order to avoid obscuring the films, towels should be fixed to the patient with sutures or adhesive film and not with clips.

An upper right paramedian or a right subcostal (Kocher) incision gives excellent approach to the region.

The gallbladder may be removed by starting the dissection from the fundus (retrograde dissection) or from the cystic duct end. When the dissection commences from the fundal end, the blood oozes from the raw surface of the liver and tends to obscure the field of operation, thus rendering isolation of the cystic artery and duct difficult. Nevertheless, when the gallbladder is encompassed by dense adhesions, when a very large ovoid or barrel-shaped stone occupies Hartmann's pouch and by its bulk distorts and obscures the ducts, or when in some cases of

acute cholecystitis these vital structures are hidden by oedematous peritoneal bands and membranes rendering dissection precarious, the plan of excising the gallbladder by starting the dissection at the fundus end may be recommended. Warren (1960) disagrees with this view:

> Many surgeons prefer to remove the gallbladder from above downward, waiting to identify the precise anatomical structures, including the cystic artery, the cystic duct and the common bile duct, until the gallbladder has been mobilised to the general level of these structures. This procedure has been employed for a sufficient number of years by so many surgeons that it can be performed with relative safety. Our concern with the protection of the common bile duct is so acute, however, that we never mobilise the gallbladder until the vital structures around the common duct have been identified. Once these structures have been identified, clamped and divided and the stump of the cystic artery and cystic duct secured, it makes very little difference whether the gallbladder is removed from below upward or from above downward. We are reluctant to accept the premise that it is safe to remove the gallbladder from above downward, leaving the identification of the vital structures until the region of the common duct has been approached.

Cholecystectomy Starting at the Cystic Duct

It should be emphasised that this is the procedure of choice of the great majority of surgeons, including this author. The cystic artery and duct are displayed early in the operation, cholangiography performed, and only then is the gallbladder freed from its liver bed and removed. The operation is greatly assisted by ensuring the maximum degree of exposure of the gallbladder and bile ducts. This is obtained by the following means:

1. The use of an adequate right upper paramedian or Kocher's incision.
2. Excellent illumination of the operative field.
3. The right hand is passed between the liver and the diaphragm and the liver retracted downward to facilitate the introduction of air into the subphrenic space. This downward displacement of the liver brings what often seems to be an almost inaccessible gallbladder adequately into the operative field.
4. Adhesions between the gallbladder and adjacent viscera are carefully freed before any further procedure is carried out.
5. In some cases, a particularly tense gallbladder may require aspiration by means of a needle passed through the fundus.
6. The fundus of the gallbladder is grasped with sponge-holding or tissue forceps and drawn firmly downward and outward into the wound.
7. The operative field is packed as follows:

A gauze pack is placed over the hepatic flexure of the colon and another over the first part of the duodenum and the stomach. The assistant's hand, or a Deaver's retractor, judiciously placed over the packs, effectively exposes the region of the gallbladder neck and the duct system. The third gauze pack is folded and applied to the right lobe of the liver medial to the gallbladder to draw the undersurface of the liver upward and this is held in place by means of a retractor (Fig. 76–12). If the packs, retractor and assistant's hand have been correctly placed, the stomach, duodenum, hepatic flexure of the colon, and the omentum are not seen throughout the next essential steps of the operation.

Hartmann's pouch is now picked up with a second sponge-holding or tissue forceps and is drawn downward and to the right while the forceps on the fundus are pulled upward, thereby putting the cystic duct on the stretch so that this structure and Calot's triangular space above it, in which the cystic artery lurks, may be readily recognised.

A small incision is made in the peritoneum

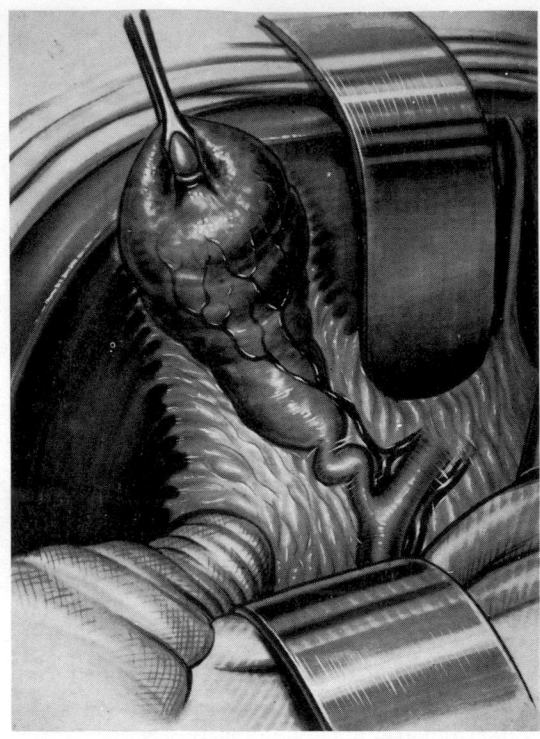

Figure 76–12. Cholecystectomy. Note the positioning of the Deaver retractors.

over the neck of the gallbladder and the serofatty tissues in this region are cautiously dissected away until the supraduodenal portion of the common bile duct and the cystic duct can be clearly defined (Fig. 76–13). The dissection then proceeds a little further inward and upward in order to display the cystic artery and the common bile duct, the right margin of the hepatic duct and point where the cystic duct joins the common ducts (Fig. 76–14).

In the chapter on anatomy the various anatomic points in connection with the cystic artery, and how the right hepatic artery may be mistaken for it and be inadvertently ligatured, have already been discussed. As a rule, the cystic artery lies in a more posterior plane than the cystic duct, slightly above it and in close proximity to the liver. A little dissection in this obscure area will reveal the artery as it travels toward the gallbladder. It should, when possible, be traced from its point of origin from its parent vessel to the point where it enters the wall of the gallbladder, usually near the neck. When it has been isolated, an aneurysm needle armed

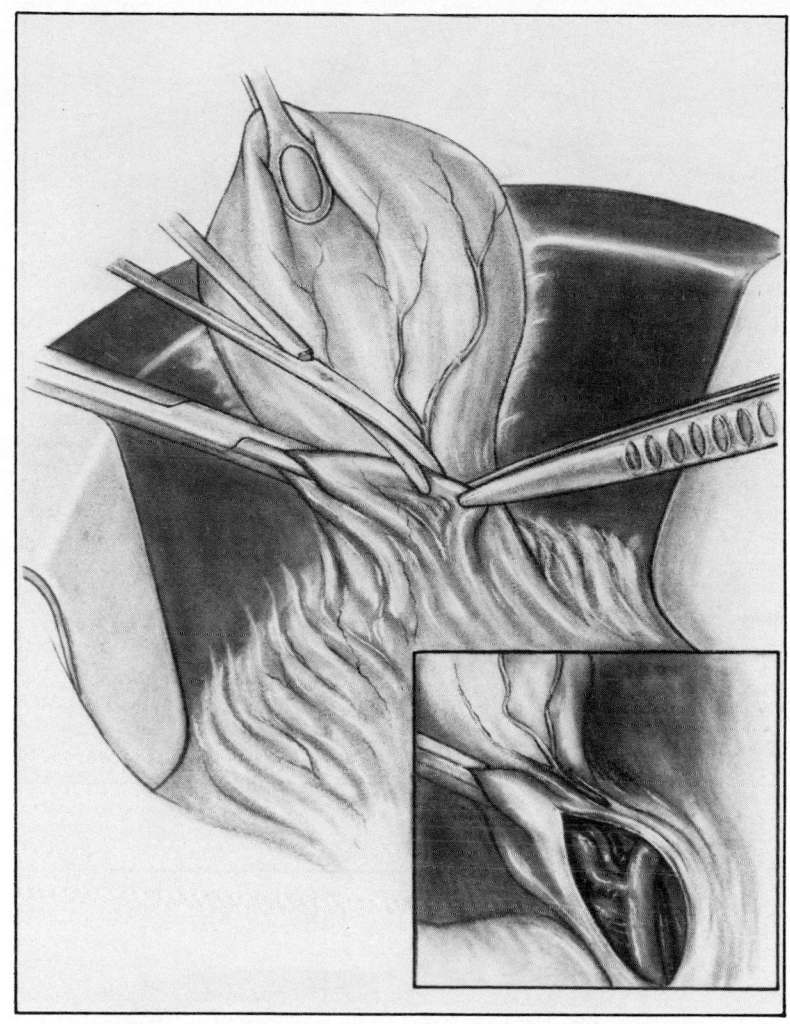

Figure 76–13. Cholecystectomy. The three ducts are exposed.

with thread, or a thread held on a fine curved artery forceps, should be passed behind the artery and the vessel tied three times—twice proximally and once distally, well away from the right hepatic artery or its parent trunk and close to the gallbladder itself. The artery is then divided close to the distal ligature (Fig. 76–15).

The cystic artery is usually a small vessel; it should be handled gently and with the greatest care. Large artery forceps are often clumsy instruments and it is advisable not to use them to catch this delicate structure. The passage of a ligature around the vessel by means of an aneurysm needle or fine artery forceps is the method that ensures a neat and precise ligation of the vessel.

The surgeon must always be on guard when an *unduly large cystic artery* is seen. Here,

again, the dissection cannot be too meticulous, and the vessel must be cautiously freed to demonstrate its true anatomic relationships. Too often what the surgeon considers to be a large cystic artery is, in fact, the right hepatic artery. The surgeon should also proceed with circumspection when the right hepatic artery has a caterpillar-like hump or when it jostles the cystic duct on its way to the right lobe of the liver, as the cystic artery in these cases is often stumpy and hidden behind the neck of the gallbladder. The surgeon should constantly bear in mind that the right hepatic artery frequently runs parallel to, and in close company with, the cystic duct and the neck of the gallbladder. The surgeon should proceed cautiously with the dissection of the cystic artery when the gallbladder possesses a mesentery, as in such instances the

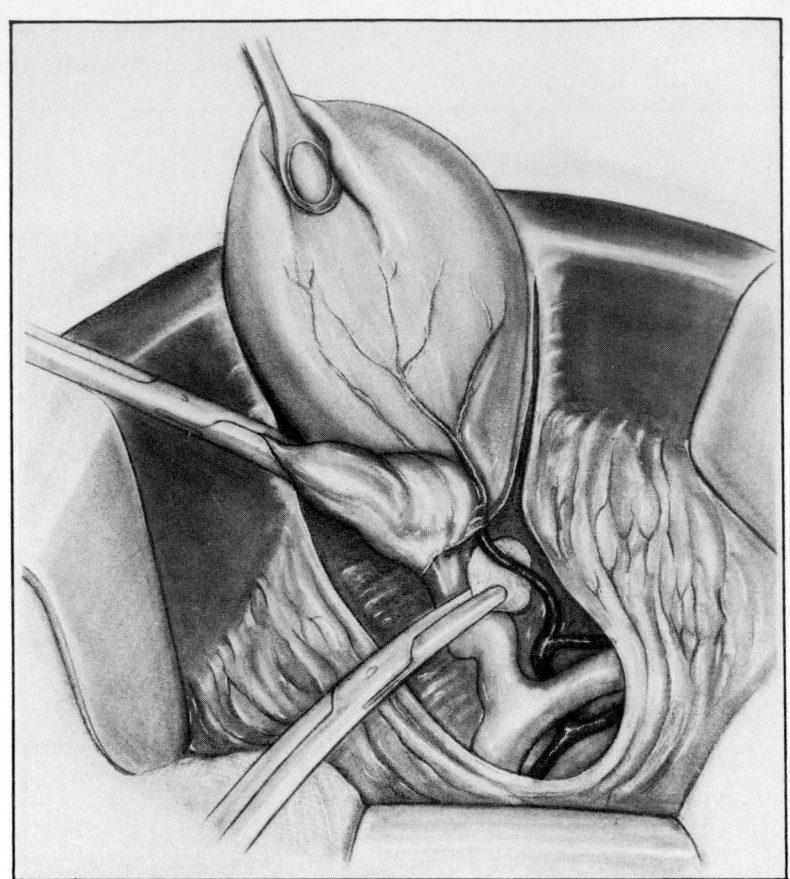

Figure 76–14. Cholecystectomy. Dissection of the cystic artery. (*Source: Adapted from Maingot R: Cholecystectomy, in Rob C, Smith R (eds): Operative Surgery, 2 edt. Philadelphia: JB Lippincott, 1969, p 402, with permission.*)

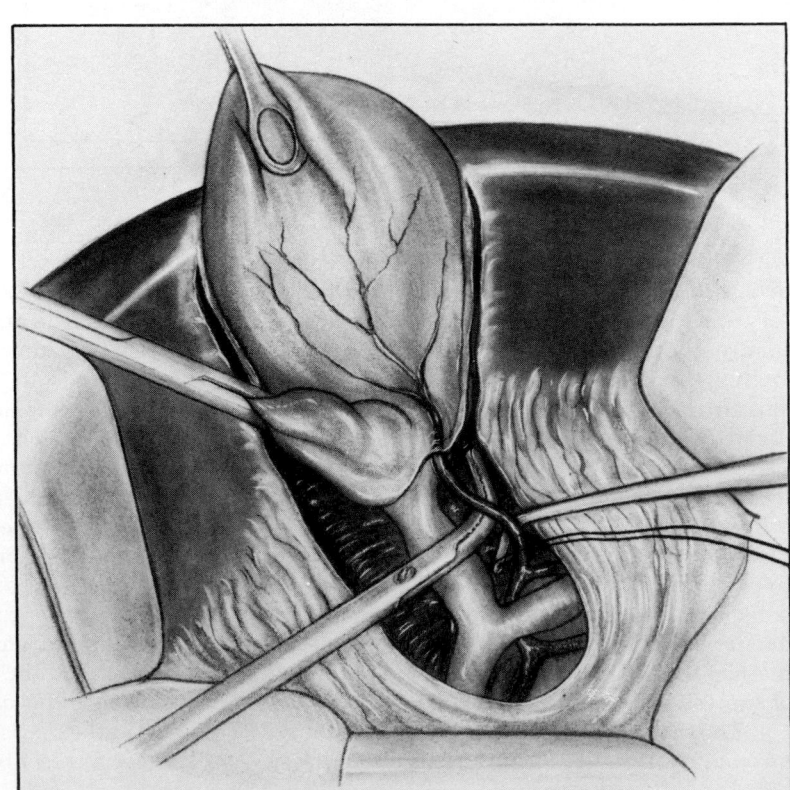

Figure 76–15. Cholecystectomy. Isolation of the cystic artery. This artery must be dissected free and displayed where it gives off its anterior and posterior branches to the gallbladder. Its site of origin should, in most instances, be identified. Here the cystic artery is arising from the right hepatic artery.

right hepatic artery (or the common hepatic artery itself) may course through this structure on its way to the porta hepatis. Again, a meticulous search should always be made for two or more cystic arteries and for the slender trunk of an accessory hepatic bile duct. The cystic duct lymph node nearly always lies on top of the cystic artery and is a good guide to this vessel.

By securing the cystic artery first, three things are accomplished:

1. The subsequent dissection is carried out in a relatively dry field.
2. When the cystic artery is divided and released from the gallbladder, the convolutions of the cystic duct can be straightened out and the junction of this duct with the common duct more clearly and accurately defined (Fig. 76–16).
3. It eliminates the danger of serious bleeding from tearing the cystic artery through traction on the gallbladder.

It should be remembered that an accessory cystic artery is found in about 12 percent of cases and that in 8 percent of cases two cystic arteries arise from the right hepatic artery.

The cystic duct is never ligatured until it has been followed upward into the neck of the gallbladder and inward to the point where it unmistakably joins the common ducts, and it is a good rule at this stage to demonstrate to an assistant the three ducts as they are clearly displayed.

Cholangiography is now carried out (see the following), followed by ligation and division of the cystic duct with Dexon.

Dissection of the gallbladder from its liver fossa is now performed. The stump of the cystic duct is seized with curved artery forceps and rotated outward. The peritoneum at the gallbladder margin is incised and the plane between the gallbladder and the liver developed, using gauze pledgets held in artery forceps (Fig. 76–17). Vessels in the gallbladder bed should be

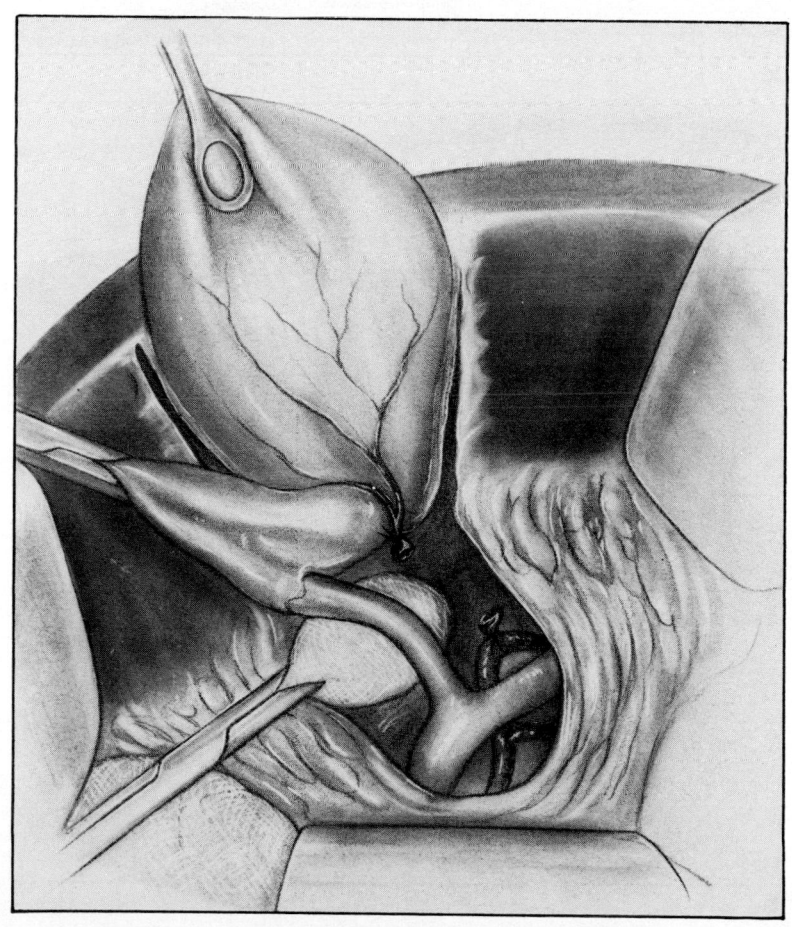

Figure 76–16. Cholecystectomy. Ligation and division of the cystic artery. Note how the cystic duct straightens out after division of the cystic artery.

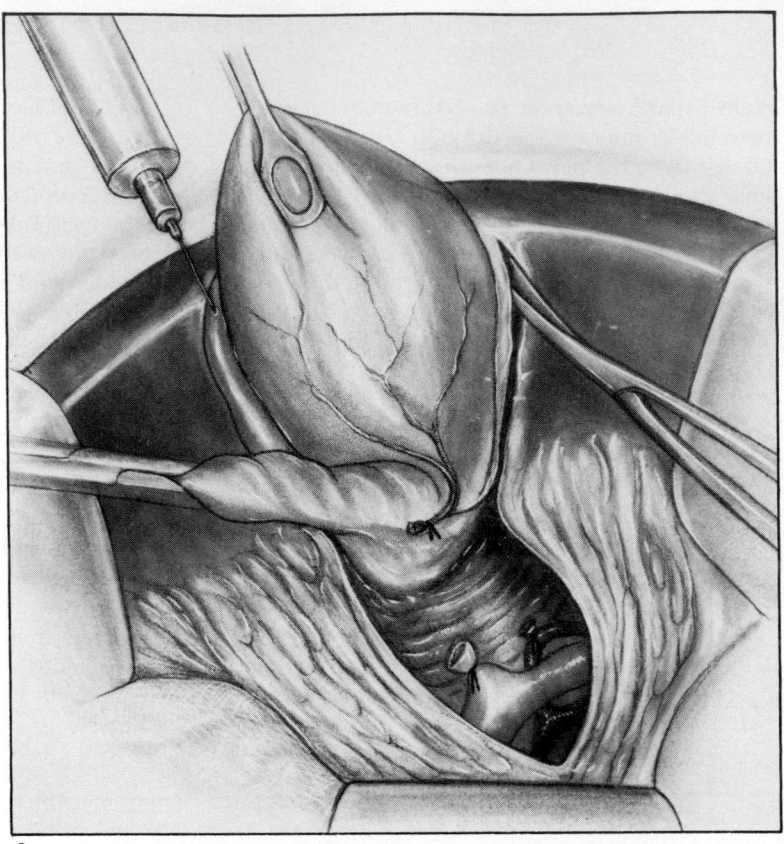

A

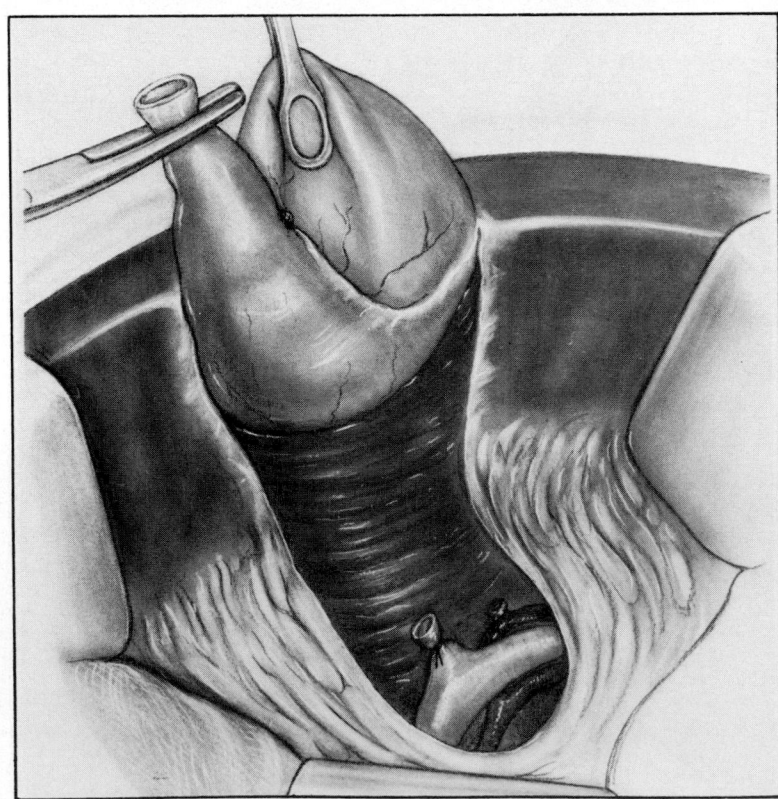

Figure 76–17. Cholecystectomy. In order to facilitate division of the peritoneal reflections of the gallbladder, saline solution may be injected underneath the peritoneum, where it is reflected from the gallbladder onto the liver. **A.** Injection of saline. **B.** Completion of the dissection.

1862

B

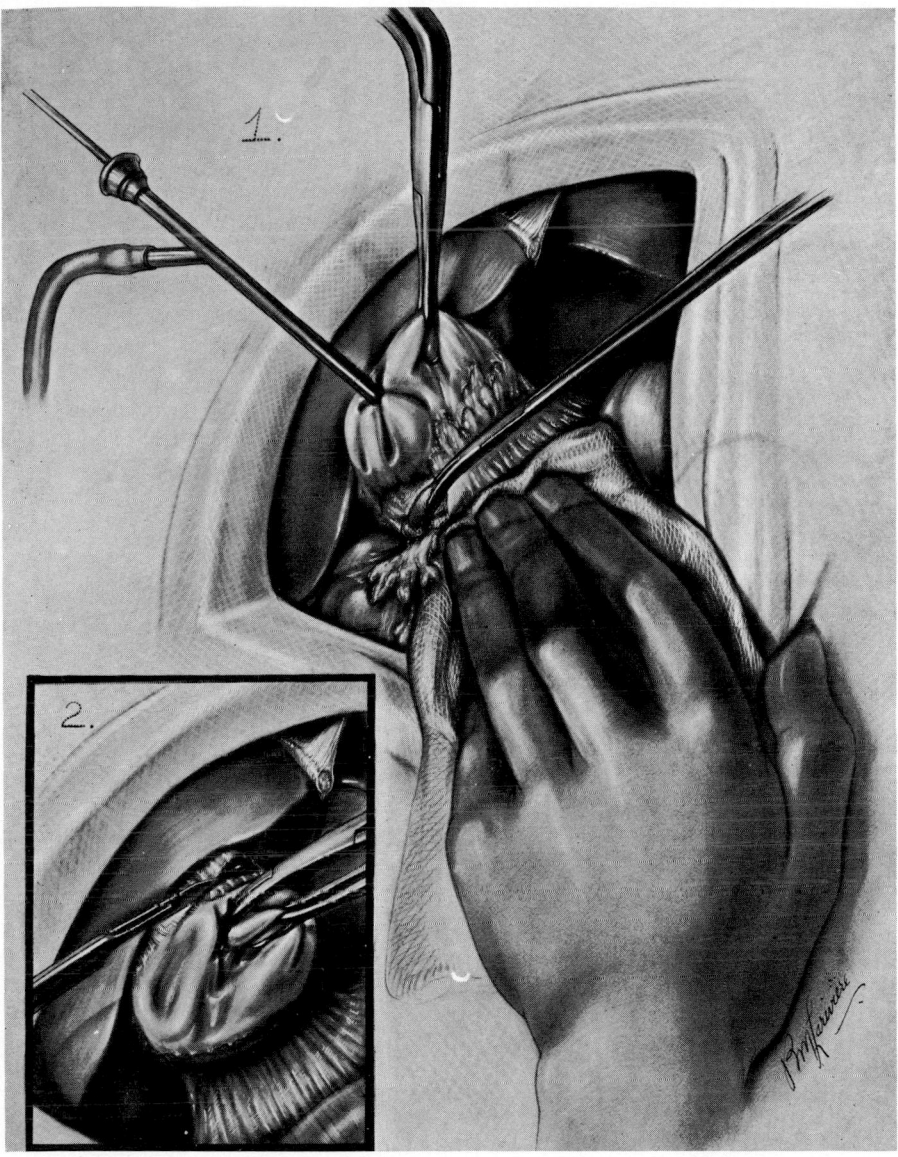

Figure 76–18. Retrograde cholecystectomy, starting the dissection from the fundus end. The gallbladder contents should be emptied with a trocar and cannula before proceeding with the dissection.

seen before dividing them and controlled by diathermy coagulation.

A swab soaked in warm saline is applied to the gallbladder fossa to control oozing, but if any bleeding points remain after this, they are dealt with by diathermy coagulation. It is not this author's practice to reperitonealise the gallbladder bed since it is known from both clini-cal and experimental studies that denuded serosa undergoes rapid regeneration.

Cholecystectomy Starting at the Fundus

First Method. A trocar and cannula are plunged into the cavity of the gallbladder (Fig. 76–18). The cannula is attached to a suction apparatus and the gallbladder is emptied of its

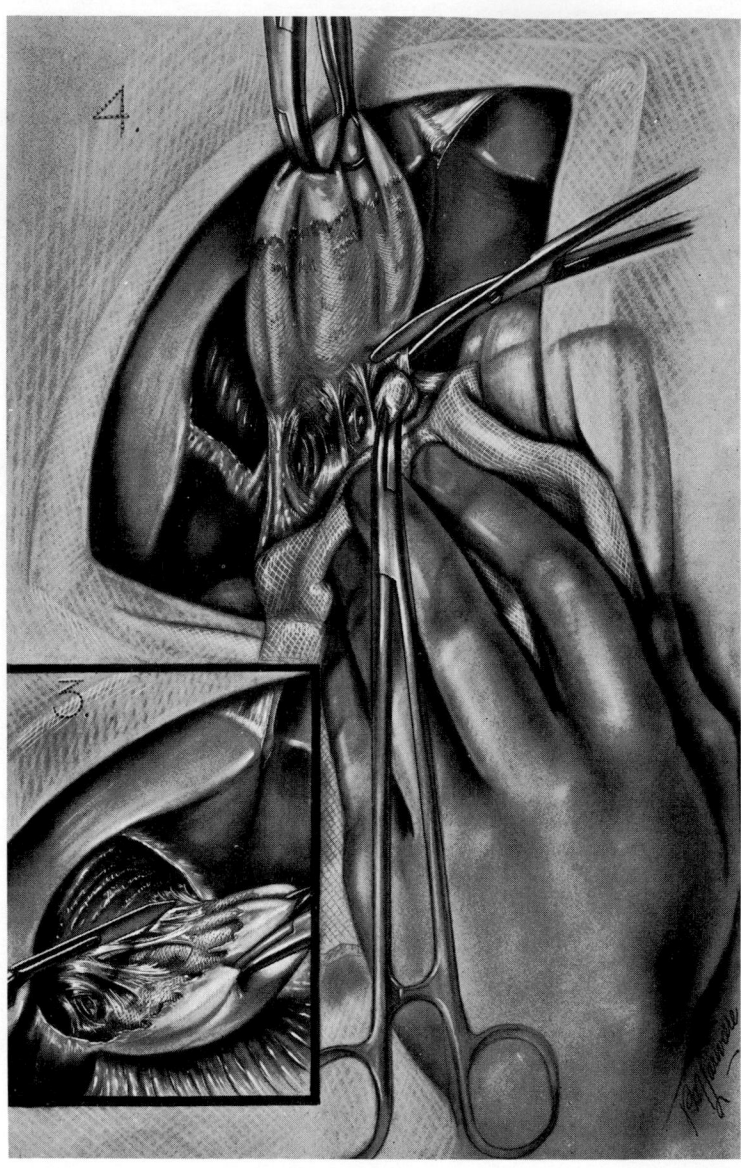

Figure 76–19. Retrograde cholecystectomy, starting the dissection from the fundus. Adhesions
are being separated cautiously.

contents. When this instrument is withdrawn,
the puncture hole in the fundus is immediately
grasped in the jaws of a sponge-holding or tissue
forceps to prevent any leakage of bile during
subsequent manipulations. The adhesions between the gallbladder and adjacent viscera are
cautiously separated, as shown in Figure 76–
19, and the organ is gradually detached from
its vascular bed by dissection with the point of
a knife. When the neck of the gallbladder is
reached, great care must be taken to isolate the
cystic artery and to tie it in continuity close
to the gallbladder, using an aneurysm needle

or long curved (Moynihan) artery forceps. It is
advisable to tie the cystic artery proximally
twice with thread.

After the artery has been double tied and
divided, the fatty envelope around the cystic
duct is dissected clear and the duct itself is
traced to its junction with the common hepatic
duct and the common bile duct.

Second Method. By this method, which was
advocated by Lahey, no clamp or haemostat is
applied to the friable wall of the gallbladder.

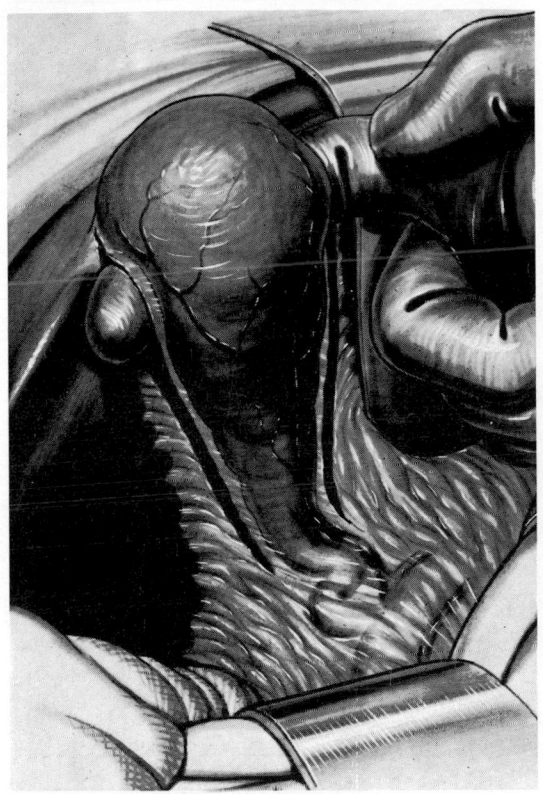

Figure 76–20. Cholecystectomy by the so-called retro-grade method. Mobilisation of the gallbladder. (*Source: From Lahey FH, Pyrtek LJ: Experience with the operative management of 280 strictures of the bile ducts. Surg Gynecol Obstet 91:25, 1950, with permission.*)

The gallbladder and its contents are removed intact.

The operation is performed by incising the medial peritoneal reflection of the gallbladder close to the liver and well above the neck of the viscus, so as to avoid the cystic artery, and by passing a finger behind the gallbladder into the loose layer of tissue that lies between the gallbladder wall and the layer of fascia over the liver. The finger is swept upward and readily detaches the body and fundus of the gallbladder from its fossa, after which the cystic duct is cleared and the cystic artery is displayed (Figs. 76–20 and 76–21).

The cystic artery and the three ducts are clearly brought into view by drawing the gallbladder downward and cautiously clearing the fibrofatty tissues that obscure these vital structures. The cystic artery is ligated twice and di-

vided to permit the cystic duct to be straightened out by traction and gauze dissection.

Operative Cholangiography

Regardless of the technique used to mobilise the gallbladder and to expose the cystic duct and artery, once the stage is reached at which the cystic duct has been clearly dissected, a routine operative cholangiography is performed.

Using a curved cholecystectomy forceps, a thread ligature is tied at the junction of the cystic duct and the gallbladder; this is to prevent fragments of stone being inadvertently manipulated down the duct during the subsequent procedures. A loop of Dexon is threaded more distally around the cystic duct and a small incision made in the duct (sucking away any bile that escapes). A malleable probe is passed along the duct into the common bile duct and then the duct is cannulated by means of an umbilical catheter, which is threaded about 2 cm into the common bile duct. To avoid introducing bubbles of air into the ductal system, it is essential, before insertion of the catheter, to attach it to a syringe filled with normal saline and to maintain a steady flow of saline through the catheter during insertion (Fig. 76–22). Unless the duct has been straightened and gently dilated by means of a probe beforehand, the catheter will often impact in the spiral valve of Heister in the cystic duct. After insertion of the catheter, a few millilitres of saline are injected to test that flow is perfectly free.

Before taking x-ray films, all instruments and packs that contain radiopaque markers are removed. A towel is placed over the operation area and the x-ray apparatus wheeled into position. The syringe containing saline is replaced with one filled with 20 ml of 25 percent sodium diatrizoate (Hypaque) or 60 percent meglumine Iothalamate (Conray 280). Care is taken to clamp the proximal end of the catheter when the syringes are exchanged in order to prevent the introduction of air bubbles. Films are exposed after the injection of 3 and then 7 ml of contrast material, the anaesthetist being asked to arrest all respiratory movement at the time of each exposure.

It is essential that the first film be taken after a small volume of medium has been injected. If this is not done, the image of the lower part of the common duct may easily be obscured by contrast medium in the duodenum, with the result that small stones and other abnormalities

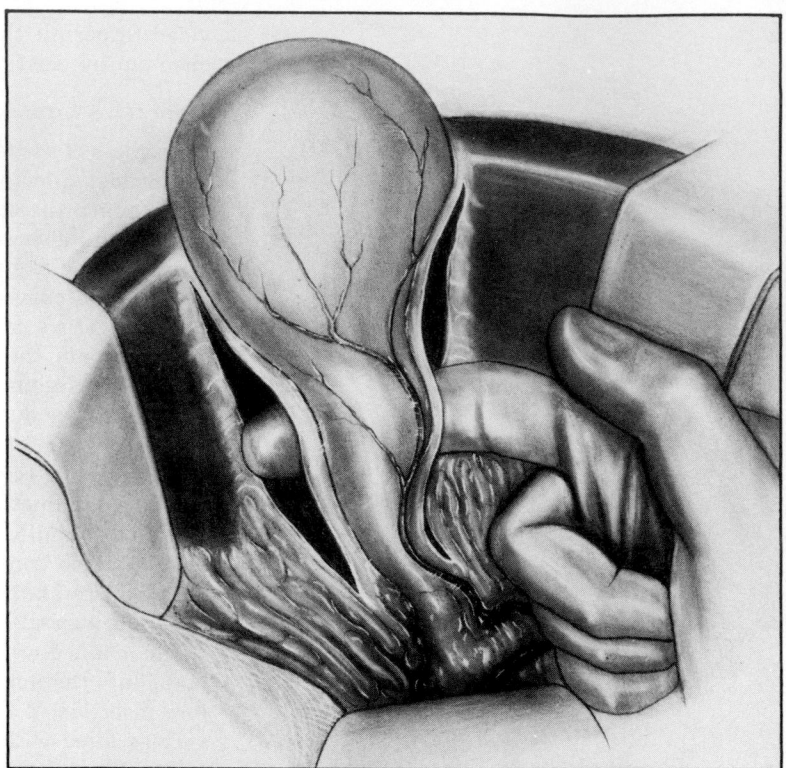

A

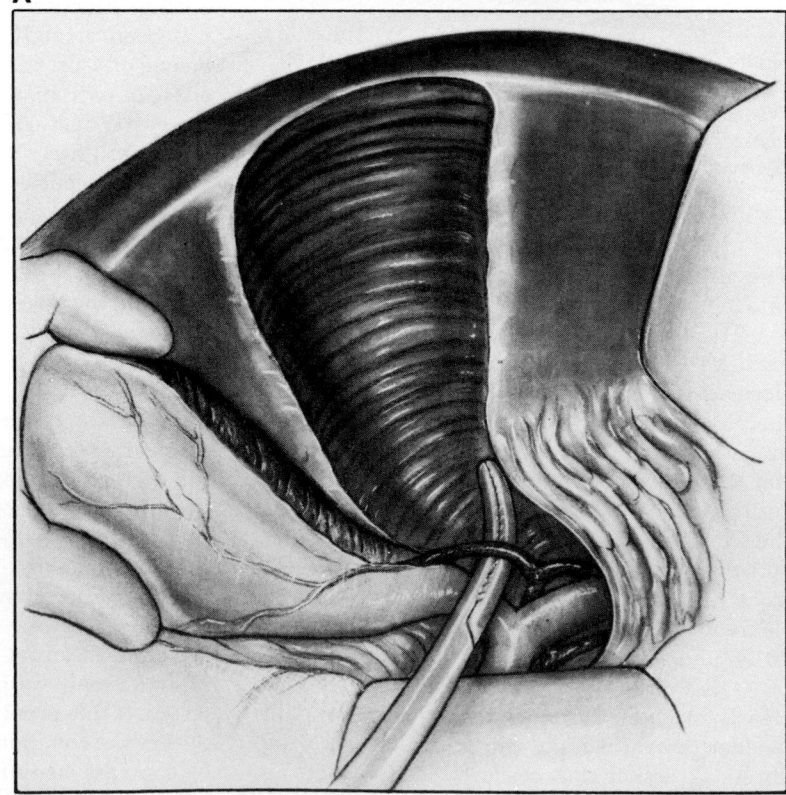

Figure 76–21. Cholecystectomy by the retrograde method. **A.** Dissection of gallbladder from hepatic bed. **B.** Dissection completed. Clamp passed under cystic artery, which will be ligated. Following this, the cystic duct is ligated. (*Source: From Maingot R: Cholecystectomy, in Rob C, Smith R (eds): Operative Surgery, 2 edt. Philadelphia: JB Lippincott, 1969, p 406, with permission.*)

B

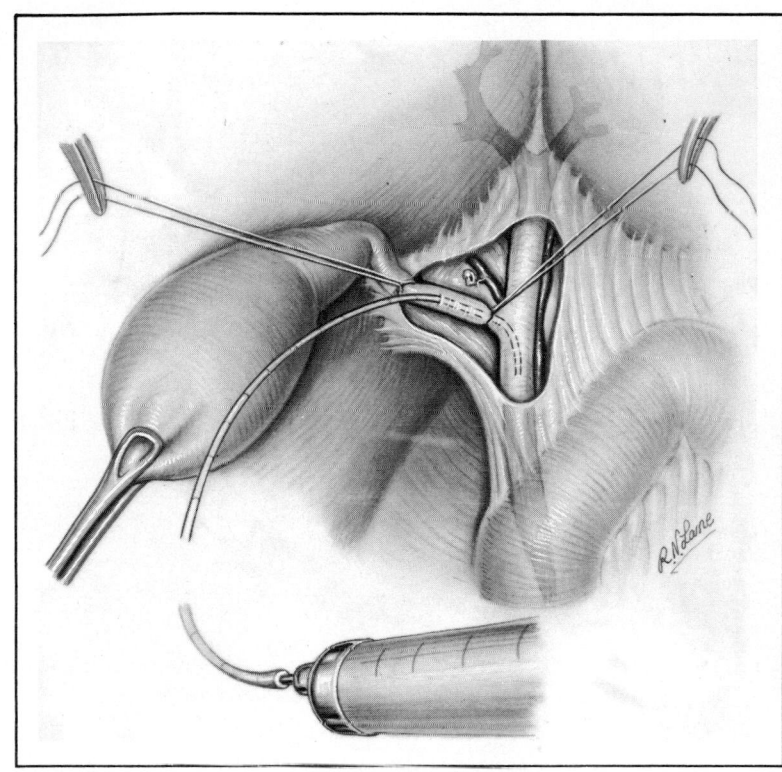

Figure 76–22. Operative cystic duct cholangiography (*Courtesy of Butterworths, London.*)

can be missed. Failure to appreciate this point may be the cause of misleading results (Fig. 76–23).

If stones are revealed on the operative cholangiogram, exploration of the duct must be carried out, as will be described in Chapter 77. If the ducts are clear radiologically, the catheter is removed and the cystic stump double tied with catgut or Dexon (Fig. 76–24). Nonabsorbable suture materials such as silk should not be used, as they may give rise to common duct calculi. Newman and Hamer (1975) review this topic and report a patient in whom, following cholecystectomy and ligation of the stump of the cystic duct with black silk, a round calculus 1 cm in diameter was found in the common bile duct 1 year later at operation. The stone contained the knot and the two tails of the black silk ligature.

Drainage

It would be accurate to say that the great majority of surgeons routinely place a drain down to the gallbladder bed following cholecystec-

tomy. The rationale is that this will allow the escape of any collection of blood from an oozing gallbladder bed or collection of bile from an overlooked biliary leakage from the same source or from a slipped cystic duct ligature. However, reports of cholecystectomy without drainage have been appearing for the last 70 years with claims of an actual improvement in postoperative results. Recently a number of carefully controlled trials of cholecystectomy with and without drainage have been reported in elective and uncomplicated cholecystectomies (Gordon et al, 1967; Edlund et al, 1979; Man et al, 1977). The first two groups found no difference between their drained and undrained patients with regard to postoperative fever or wound infection whereas the third group actually found diminution in their sepsis rate in the undrained cases. Budd et al (1982), in a prospective trial of 300 cholecystectomies randomised to no drainage, Penrose drainage, and sump drainage, found a higher incidence of pyrexia and wound infection in the drainage groups. An increased incidence of pulmonary complications was attributed to

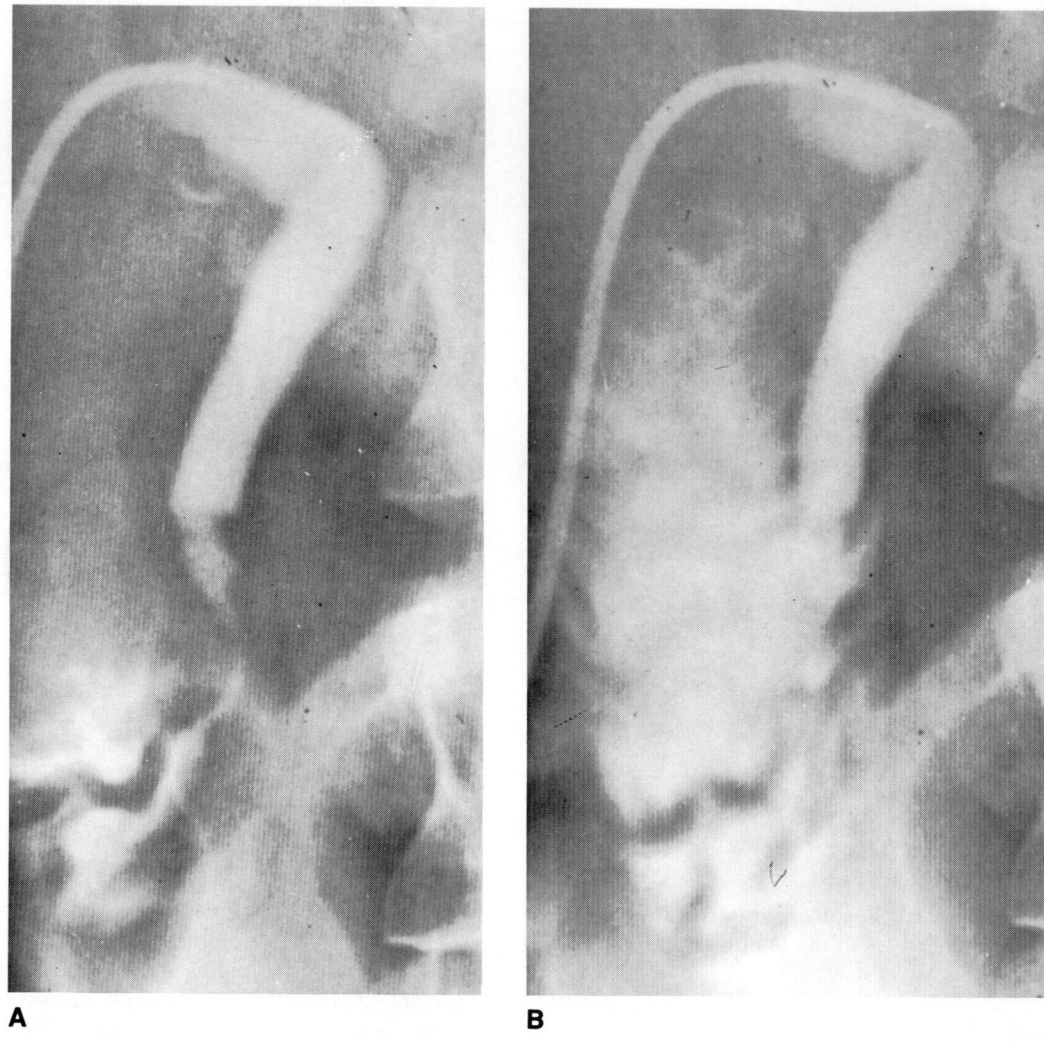

A   **B**

Figure 76–23. The first **(A)** and second **(B)** films from a preexploratory cholangiogram, illustrating how the flow of contrast material into the duodenum can easily obscure the detail of the terminal segment, thus emphasising the importance of the first film taken after the injection of only 2 to 3 ml of contrast medium.

the increased discomfort of the drain and the increased sepsis rate to the two-way conduit effect of the drain passing between the skin and the peritoneal cavity. The argument that a drain is a safety precaution against the occasional accumulation of bile was refuted in their study. The only two examples of bile peritonitis in the series both had drains (one a Penrose the other a sump drain), yet neither failed to prevent this complication.

Although once a firm believer in drainage following cholecystectomy, this author has forsaken this practice in the last few years. A corrugated drain led out through a stab wound is still employed in complicated biliary procedures, including exploration of the common bile duct, choledochoenterostomy, and transduodenal removal of common duct stones. Whether there is any real justification or not for this practice must be the subject for future trials.

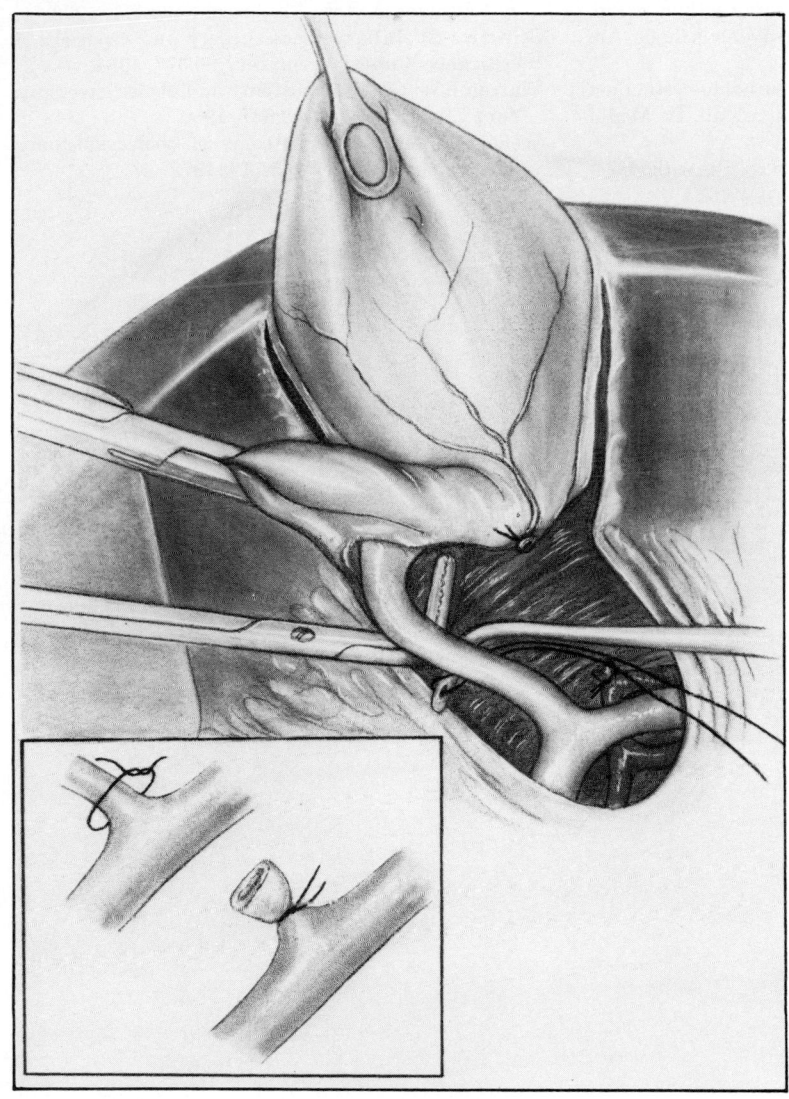

Figure 76–24. Cholecystectomy. Ligation and division of the cystic duct.

BIBLIOGRAPHY

Aranha GV, Sontag SJ, et al: Cholecystectomy in cirrhotic patients: A formidable operation. Am J Surg 143:55, 1982

Budd DC, Cochran RC, et al: Cholecystectomy with and without drainage. A randomized, prospective study of 300 patients. Am J Surg 143:307, 1982

Castle WN, Wanebo HJ, et al: Carcinoma of the gallbladder and cholecystostomy. Arch Surg 117:946, 1982

Cope Z: A History of the Acute Abdomen. London: Oxford University Press, 1965

Edlund G, Gedda S, et al: Intraperitoneal drains and nasogastric tubes in elective cholecystectomy. A controlled clinical trial. Am J Surg 137:775, 1979

Ellis H: The aetiology of post-operative adhesions. An experimental study. Br J Surg 50:10, 1962

Gordon AB, Bates T, et al: A controlled trial of drainage after cholecystectomy. Br J Surg 63:278, 1976

Langenbuch C: Ein Fall von exstirpation der Gallenblase wegen chronischer Cholelithiasis. Heilung. Berliner Klinische Wochenschrift 48:725, 1882

Lang RC, Webster DR: Cholecystolithotomy in functioning gallbladders. Surgery 42:837, 1957

Man B, Kraus L, et al: Cholecystectomy without drainage, nasogastric suction and intravenous fluids. Am J Surg 133:312, 1977

Newman CE, Hamer JD: Non-absorbable cystic duct ligatures and common bile duct calculi. Br Med J 4:504, 1975

Norrby S, Schonebeck J: Long-term results with chole-cystolithotomy. Acta Chir Scand 136:711, 1970

Schwartz SI: Biliary tract surgery and cirrhosis: A critical combination. Surgery 90:577, 1981

Warren KW: Choledochostomy and cholecystectomy. Surg Clin North Am 40:681, 1960

Welch JP, Malt RA: Outcome of cholecystostomy. Surg Gynecol Obstet 135:717, 1972

77. Symptoms After Cholecystectomy

Ward O. Griffen, Jr.

INTRODUCTION

The title of this chapter was chosen carefully in order to avoid confusion with the so-called "postcholecystectomy syndrome." Most patients with upper abdominal discomfort, excessive flatulence, "indigestion," and other nonspecific symptoms eventually undergo oral cholecystography. If there is nonvisualization of the gallbladder or it contains stones, they are convinced that removal of the gallbladder will relieve their symptoms. Unfortunately, many surgeons tend to make a cause-and-effect relationship with this finding and too often fall into the trap of assuring the patient that their symptoms will disappear when the obviously diseased gallbladder is removed. Nevertheless, in large series of patients followed for an extended period after the cholecystectomy, a significant number of patients continued to have problems. Unlike appendectomy for appendicitis, where the relief of symptoms is almost 100 percent, the removal of the gallbladder is followed by relief of symptoms in only about 75 to 80 percent of the patients.

When investigations are carried out in symptomatic patients, however, three distinct groups can be identified. There is a group of patients who either had extrabiliary disorders in association with their gallbladder disease and at least some, if not all, of the symptoms were the result of that disease. It is possible that these disorders may have developed after their cholecystectomy. Investigation into the continuing symptoms of these patients will often disclose hiatal hernia, peptic ulcer disease, pancreatitis, or even pancreatic carcinoma. The second group of patients are those who have an abnormality of the biliary tract that was unrecognized or was created at the time of the cholecystectomy.

The conditions present in this group include retained common duct stones, cystic duct remnant, and problems associated with the duodenal papilla or sphincter of Oddi.

In a very small percentage of patients symptoms continue despite the fact that there are no gross abnormalities of the extra- or intrahepatic biliary ductal system. Even this group is being decreased in size by more modern diagnostic techniques (see the following), so that only a small number of patients have what is apparently a perfectly normal anatomic and physiologic biliary tree and who still have symptoms after cholecystectomy—the true postcholecystectomy syndrome patient. In fact, some surgeons feel that there is no such entity as postcholecystectomy syndrome; others believe it does exist and may be related to abnormalities of bile acid metabolism rather than some form of mechanical or other postoperative changes. As more accurate diagnostic methods have been developed, the number of patients who fit into the category of postcholecystectomy syndrome has become exceedingly small, although it probably is a true entity.

DIAGNOSTIC MODALITIES

A physician, when confronted with a patient who has had a cholecystectomy, and who now has postprandial upper gastrointestinal (GI) distress, excess flatulence, "heartburn," perhaps some radiation of pain around or through to the back, and some food intolerances, should not immediately leap to the conclusion that the patient is suffering from the postcholecystectomy syndrome. There are two valid reasons for not reaching that conclusion. First is the fact that it is much more likely that appropriate diagnostic studies will uncover a cause for the symptoms that can then be treated. Second, the therapy for true postcholecystectomy syndrome is nonspecific and often unrewarding.

Today there are a variety of diagnostic maneuvers available that carry very little morbidity, yield a great deal of information, and are generally cost effective. In contrast, there are some diagnostic techniques that should be used sparingly, and even some that should be abandoned altogether. In the latter category is the intravenous cholangiogram. First of all, it can only be used in the nonjaundiced patients, and often the patient who comes for medical aid following a cholecystectomy is jaundiced. More importantly, however, is the fact that the intravenous cholangiogram carries about a 15 percent morbidity, which includes everything from nausea and mild reaction to the contrast agent to anaphylactic reaction and renal failure. It has a significant mortality of 1 in 5000 and therefore really is a diagnostic test of historical interest only. Upper GI barium studies in evaluating patients following cholecystectomy are probably only occasionally necessary. Often the patient has an upper GI x-ray taken prior to the cholecystectomy. This is particularly true if the patient is over the age of 45 or 50 since many physicians (without a great deal of scientific justification) feel that such an x-ray in a patient with gallstones is routine. If the symptoms the patient describes do not fit totally with the diagnosis of cholelithiasis even though gallstones exist, then a preoperative evaluation of the GI tract is in order. Nevertheless, if the symptoms occurring in the postcholecystectomy patient suggest esophageal disease or a peptic ulcer disorder, an upper GI tract x-ray may be the first test to be performed.

However, a variety of other diagnostic tests can be performed to evaluate the postcholecystectomy patient. Some are not invasive; some are moderately or significantly invasive; but all are done in sufficient frequency in most medical facilities so as to carry a very low morbidity and practically no mortality. In addition, the yield from these diagnostic tests is great. For example, the radionuclide scans now available for evaluating both the morphology as well as the physiology of the extrahepatic biliary tract can be used despite jaundice. The specific diagnostic modalities with their advantages and disadvantages are as follows:

1. *Grey Scale Ultrasonography*—this is a totally noninvasive test that is effective in detecting biliary tract calculi and is about 85 percent accurate in identifying dilatation of intra- and extrahepatic biliary ducts. There is no radiation risk. However, gas in the GI tract interferes with ultrasonographic detection, particularly of ductal dilatation.

2. *Computed Tomography (CT)*—this technique of producing sagittal section tomograms of the abdomen is extremely useful in detecting mass lesions, particularly intrahepatic lesions or a mass in the head of the pancreas or enlargement thereof. It is occasionally valuable in detecting dilatation of the extrahepatic biliary tract but only when it is grossly enlarged; it is of no value for biliary tract calculi. It has the distinct disadvantage of exposing the patient to some radiation.

3. *Cholescintigraphy with Technetium-99m Labeled Analogue of Imminodiacetic (IDA)*—this is an excellent technique for identifying both the morphologic and physiologic situation with regard to the biliary tract. Using serial scintigrams over a specified time frame, one can determine whether the anatomic structure in question fills as well as empties in a normal fashion. It can be used in a patient who is jaundiced. It does give the patients a slight amount of irradiation. A distinct disadvantage of the technique is that should ductal obstruction be present, the obstructing mechanism cannot be identified.

4. *Morphine–Prostigmine Test*—the so-called Nardi test was originally designed to detect obstruction to bile flow at the sphincter of Oddi. It gained some popularity and then fell into disrepute, but has recently been resurrected. It may be useful in detecting stenosis of the papilla, an entity that is being recognized with increasing frequency as a cause of upper abdominal complaints both de novo as well as following cholecystectomy.

5. *Esophagogastroduodenoscopy*—with the advent of fiberoptic flexible endoscopic equipment, both the ease and the safety with which the mucosal surface of the esophagus, stomach, and duodenum could be viewed increased enormously. Already upper GI endoscopy has displaced various studies in the patient with acute GI bleeding. It may well be that endoscopic evaluation of the esophagus, stomach, and duodenum will displace upper

GI x-ray in the evaluation of the patient with pain and other problems following cholecystectomy. The great disadvantage of this technique is its invasive quality and expense. Nevertheless, the esophagus can be viewed for both the presence of reflux as well as esophagitis. Ulcers or other lesions of the stomach or duodenum can be identified with the endoscope. When the duodenal papilla has been identified, the papilla can be cannulated so that contrast media may be injected into both the common bile duct as well as the pancreatic duct to provide for further diagnostic yield. If endoscopic retrograde cholangiopancreatography (ERCP) is used, an additional disadvantage of the procedure is exposure to irradiation.

6. *Percutaneous Transhepatic Cholangiography (PTC)*—With the use of a thin needle, this technique is becoming extremely safe, although it still has a disadvantage of being an invasive diagnostic maneuver. When successful (the success rate is now close to 95 percent), it does provide an excellent means of evaluating the intra- and extrahepatic biliary ductal system. In addition to the disadvantage of being invasive, it exposes the patient to some irradiation.

7. *Angiography*—this very invasive test with selective catheterization of the celiac axis and superior mesenteric artery provides excellent information about normal and abnormal arterial vessels to the stomach, duodenum, pancreas, and liver. It is only occasionally necessary in evaluating patients for pain following cholecystectomy, but carries the usual risk of arterial invasion as well as exposure to irradiation.

CLINICAL MANIFESTATIONS

Approximately 75 percent of patients undergoing cholecystectomy will be rendered asymptomatic. Of the remaining patients, the occasional abdominal pain or nausea they experience may be so mild as to be inconsequential. However, 5 to 10 percent of patients will have persisting recurrent or new symptoms of such severity that investigation is required. The interval between the cholecystectomy and the onset of problems may be as short as 2 days after the operation or as long as 40 years later.

However, about two thirds of this group of patients will have developed their problem within 1 year of the operation. Very few patients will be asymptomatic for years only to develop symptoms 25 to 40 years after the cholecystectomy.

Extrabiliary Disorders

The first group of patients who develop symptoms after cholecystectomy are those who have some disorder outside of the biliary tract such as hiatal hernia with gastroesophageal reflux, peptic ulceration, acute or chronic pancreatitis, and, rarely, pancreatic or bile duct carcinoma. In evaluating the patient with upper abdominal complaints and known gallstones, it is important to take a careful history with regard not only to the location of the abdominal pain, but precipitating factors and its relationship to meals. If there is any suspicion that the patient may have hiatal hernia with reflux or peptic ulceration, preoperative endoscopy to make the diagnosis and some form of nonoperative therapy prior to the cholecystectomy may be indicated. If the patient's symptoms disappear with this approach, then whether the gallbladder should be removed becomes a question of the management of "silent" gallstones. Particularly in the case of hiatal hernia, if the symptoms of which the patient complains appear to be a combination of hiatal hernia and gallstone etiology, the appropriate approach may well be cholecystectomy in combination with some form of antireflux procedure.

In general, the patient with mild symptoms of peptic ulceration in association with gallstone disease can be treated for ulcer disease with nonoperative means. In this author's and others' experience, the most unhappy postoperative patients have been those who have had a cholecystectomy for truly symptomatic gallstones and also an "incidental vagotomy and pyloroplasty" because the surgeon was not absolutely certain that some of the patients' complaints were not due to peptic ulcer disease. The justification for the peptic ulcer operation has often been duodenal deformity on upper GI series. The point to be made is that if an extrabiliary disorder is felt to be present, it should be completely evaluated and perhaps treated nonoperatively before the gallbladder is removed.

Another extrabiliary problem that may not come to the forefront until after the cholecystectomy is pancreatitis. The acute form of the disease may occur early in the postoperative period because of retained common duct stones (see the following) and rarely it may be a major immediate complication of cholecystectomy. On the other hand, the patient may have chronic pancreatitis because of sufficient episodes of acute pancreatitis during the course of the gallstone disease that there are now fibrotic changes within the pancreas, or the patient may be an alcohol abuser, which was not fully appreciated prior to the cholecystectomy. In either instance, the chronic pancreatitis may gradually increase in severity until it becomes the cause of recurrent or upper abdominal pain following cholecystectomy. Again, a careful history and thorough physical examination preoperatively is essential. Following this, appropriate diagnostic steps should be taken to evaluate the pancreas if it is suspected that pancreatitis is the underlying cause for some or all of the patient's symptoms.

Nevertheless, some patients will undergo cholecystectomy for symptomatic gallstones only to develop new or recurrent upper abdominal complaints that do not appear to have their basis in biliary tract disease. In these patients it is essential to try to detect the offending organ on clinical grounds and then confirm the diagnosis with appropriate diagnostic evaluation. If the patient is suspected of having hiatal hernia with reflux or peptic ulceration, fiberoptic endoscopy is essential in this evaluation. If the patient is suspected of having acute or chronic pancreatitis or chronic pancreatitis with acute exacerbations, a careful alcohol and drug history must be obtained. Following this, a CT scan of the abdomen may reveal pancreatic enlargement or an ERCP may show ductal changes consistent with pancreatitis.

Regardless of what extrabiliary problems are uncovered, the first form of therapy is nonoperative. If the patient has hiatal hernia with reflux and is overweight, as is often the case, then antacids, an H_2 blocker, diet, changing the eating pattern to the big meal in the middle of the day, and elevation of the head of the bed should be undertaken. If symptoms persist and are of sufficient severity, an antireflux procedure may be recommended. If the patient is found to have peptic ulcer disease, antacids, H_2 blockers, avoidance of certain foods, cessation of smoking, and other measures may be instituted. Only if the patient developed severe and

significant peptic ulcer disease should an operation for the condition be considered. If pancreatitis is the problem, the etiology should be sought and eliminated. There are a number of drugs currently on the market that are associated with development of pancreatitis and these should be avoided. If the patient has a history of alcohol abuse, alcohol is contraindicated. The use of pancreatic enzymes may help in decreasing the symptoms, and, again only if the patient has significant complications of the pancreatitis should operative intervention be considered.

Biliary Tract Problems

The second group of patients developing symptoms after cholecystectomy are those who have continued biliary tract problems. In most series describing problems following the removal of the gallbladder, continuing biliary tract disorders are the major reason for such continuance of symptoms. The conditions comprising this group are (1) residual common duct stones, (2) cystic duct remnant, (3) stenosis at the sphincter of Oddi, and rarely (4) bile duct stricture.

Residual Common Duct Stones

Today, removal of the gallbladder is almost always accompanied by operative cholangiography. When performed and evaluated properly, this addition to cholecystectomy does not prolong the procedure, is associated with no greater morbidity, and in most instances will prevent the problem of a retained stone in the common duct following cholecystectomy. Additional means of evaluating the common duct for the presence of calculi include operative ultrasonography and, if the common duct is being explored, choledochoscopy. All of these maneuvers should reduce the incidence of retained common duct stones to a minimum and virtually eliminate this disorder as a cause of postcholecystectomy symptoms. Unfortunately, there are still some surgeons who do not practice routine or almost-routine operative cholangiography, and one can expect about a 5 percent incidence of retained common duct stones in these patients since that is about the incidence of unsuspected choledocholithiasis in the hands of those who use operative cholangiography routinely.

The patient with a retained common duct stone may present simply as a recurrence of the symptoms prior to the cholecystectomy or may develop obvious obstructive jaundice or even ascending cholangitis as a complication of the impaction of a common duct calculus. Acute pancreatitis occurring 2 months or longer after a cholecystectomy should raise suspicions of a common duct stone.

Whenever a retained common duct stone is suspected, ultrasonography can be used to confirm the presence of the stone and radionuclide studies with IDA analogues will demonstrate the ductal obstruction. The latter can be used in the jaundiced patient and will show dilatation of the common duct and perhaps delayed emptying as manifested by retained radioactivity in the common duct at 2 hours or even increased radioactivity at 2 hours as compared to 1 hour. The etiology of the obstruction can then be accurately elucidated either by ERCP or transhepatic cholangiography if appropriate.

The definitive management of this condition is currently undergoing significant changes. The patient can be subjected to a second operation with exploration of the common duct and extraction of the stone or stones, but that carries with it some morbidity and mortality. Endoscopic papillotomy in association with ERCP is now becoming popular; based on the

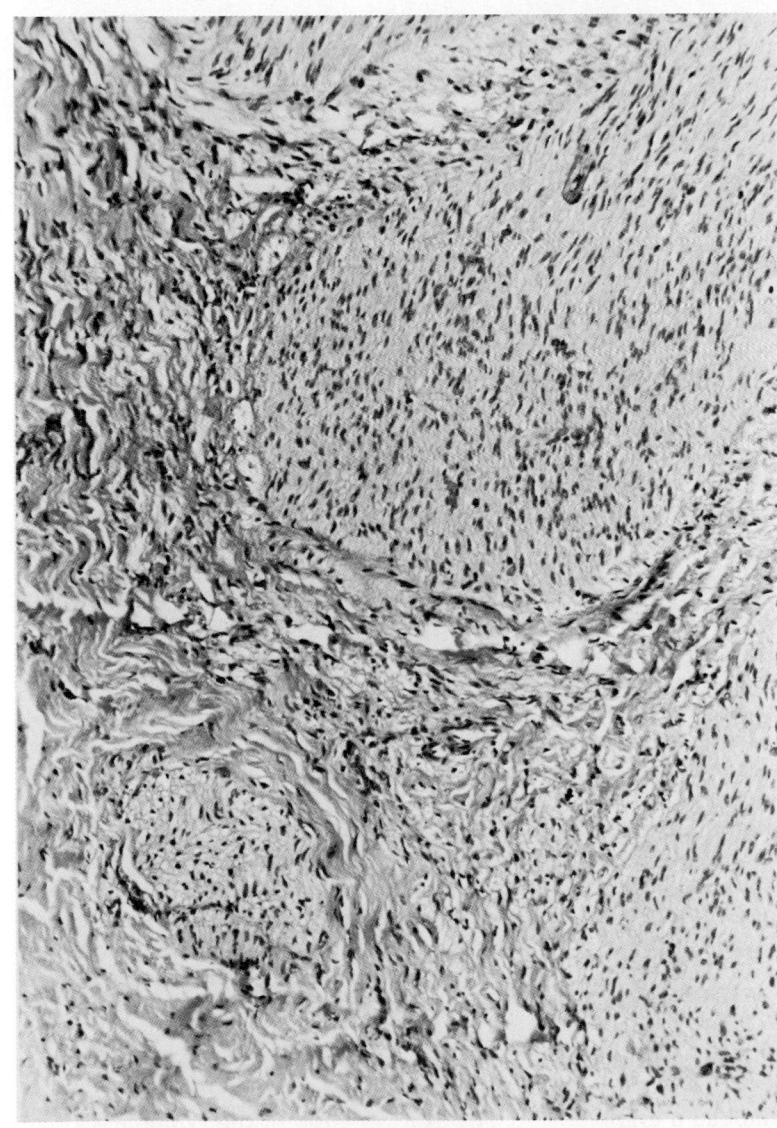

Figure 77–1. Neuroma of cystic duct in patient with persistent pain postcholecystectomy.

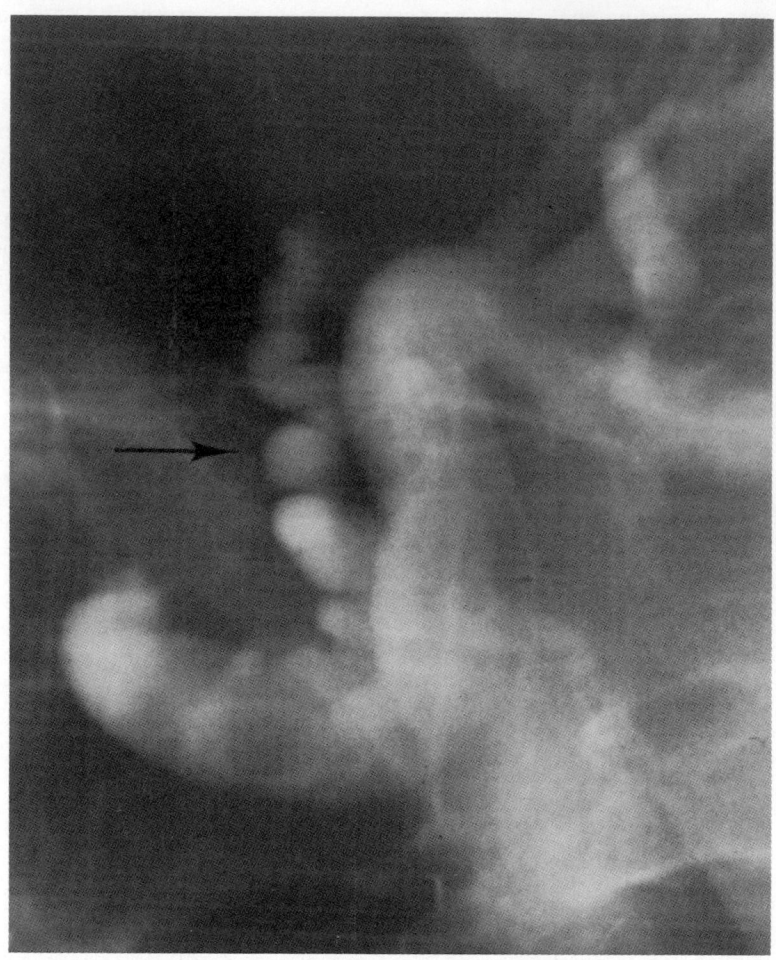

Figure 77–2. Cystic duct remnant in patient after cholecystectomy.

results to date, it must be viewed as a relatively safe technique and it does avoid an operative procedure. Finally, on the horizon is percutaneous transhepatic extraction of the stone, which at this time is in its infancy but also may prove to be a technique that is safe and also avoids an operative procedure. Although the goal of treating a patient with a residual stone in the common duct after cholecystectomy is to remove the stone, the first objective for any surgeon is to avoid the problem of retained common duct stone by evaluating the biliary tract by some means during the performance of the cholecystectomy.

Cystic Duct Remnant

In 1912, Florcken reported on a "reformed gallbladder which contained stones." In 1936, Beye described a series of patients who had a cystic duct remnant and recurrent symptoms of nausea, upper abdominal pain, and occasional biliary colic, ascribing all of it to the cystic duct remnant. Since that time a major cause of recurrent, continuing, or new symptoms following cholecystectomy has been ascribed to the presence of a cystic duct remnant, which is defined as a residual cystic duct greater than 1 cm in length. In fact, several decades ago it was axiomatic that in a patient who developed symptoms following cholecystectomy and was shown to have a cystic duct remnant, operative excision of the cystic duct remnant was mandatory. Subsequent to that time, several series were reported where cholangiography was performed routinely after cholecystectomy and a cystic duct remnant was found in many patients who were totally asymptomatic.

The exact etiology of the symptoms associated with cystic duct remnant was then questionable. There is no doubt that some cystic duct remnants are long enough so that the most distal end of the cystic duct contains gallbladder mucosa capable of concentrating bile, thus possibly leading to new stone formation. In fact, cystic duct remnants with stones within their lumen have been described radiographically as well as at the operation. The possibility of a neuroma forming on the cystic duct stump and producing pain was emphasized by Womack almost 40 years ago and does appear to be a rare cause of symptoms associated with a cystic duct remnant (Fig. 77–1). More than half of the patients with a demonstrable cystic duct remnant, however, have been found to have unsuspected common duct stones, a likely cause of the symptoms.

The diagnosis of cystic duct remnant and problems associated with it can be made by a variety of techniques. Occasionally, ultrasonographic evaluation of the biliary tract may clearly demonstrate a cystic duct remnant. It may also show a stone within the remnant. The PIPIDA scan is a very good way of demonstrating the cystic duct remnant and also may show common duct dilatation and delay of emptying, which would raise the suspicion of a retained or new common duct stone. With good filling of the common bile duct during ERCP, a cystic duct remnant can often be identified, and the technique also will allow one to evaluate the common duct for unsuspected calculi (Figs. 77–2 and 77–3). When a cystic duct remnant is identified even though stones may be present in the common duct, the cystic duct remnant should be excised at the same time that the common duct is explored for stones. The cystic duct remnant may be the source of stone formation. This will continue to be the case even should endoscopic papillotomy or transhepatic extraction of the stone be performed. In addition, the rare instance of a neuroma of the cystic duct may be the cause of the pain, and that symptom will

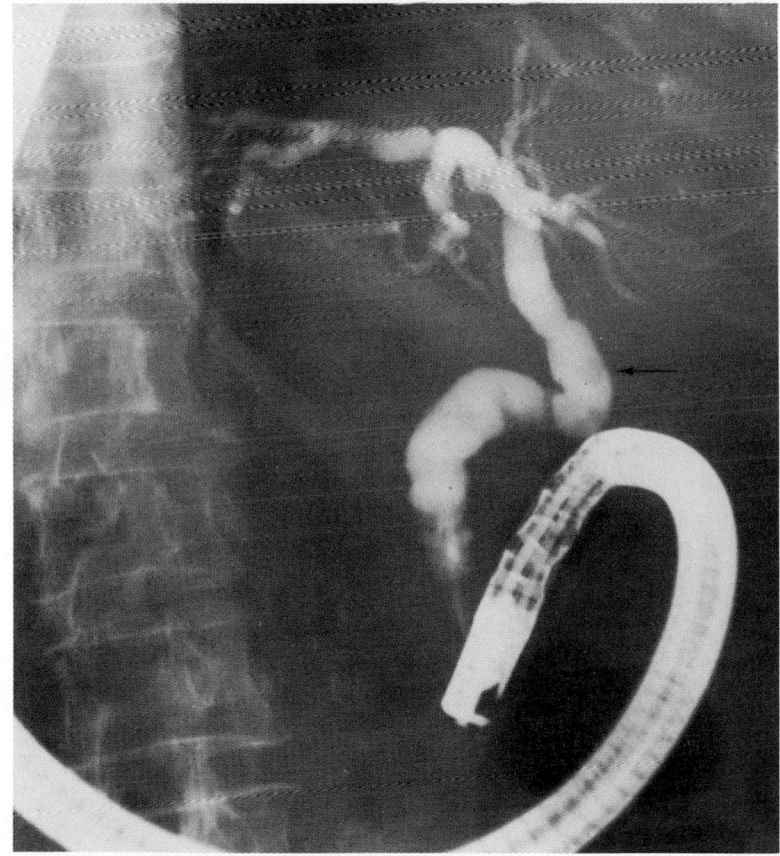

Figure 77–3. Retained common duct stone diagnosed by ERCP.

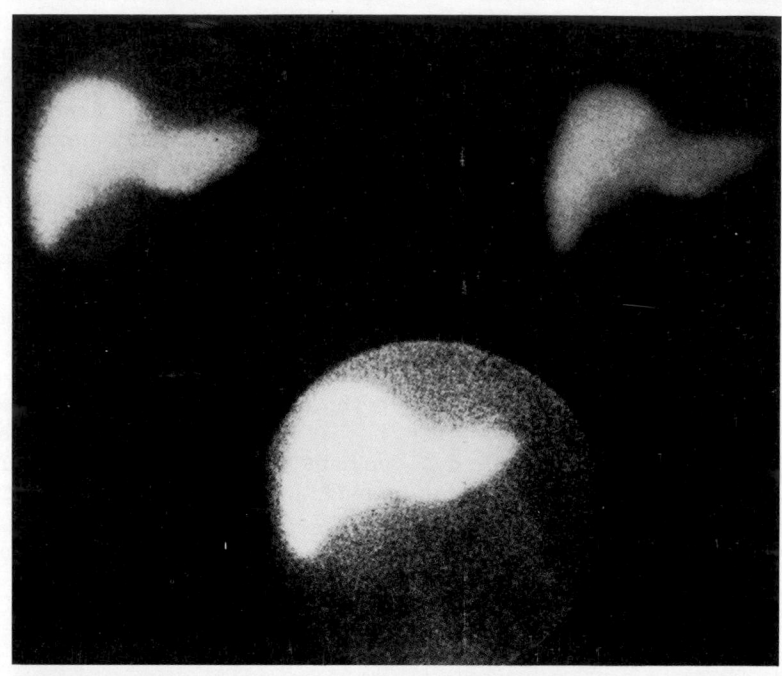

A

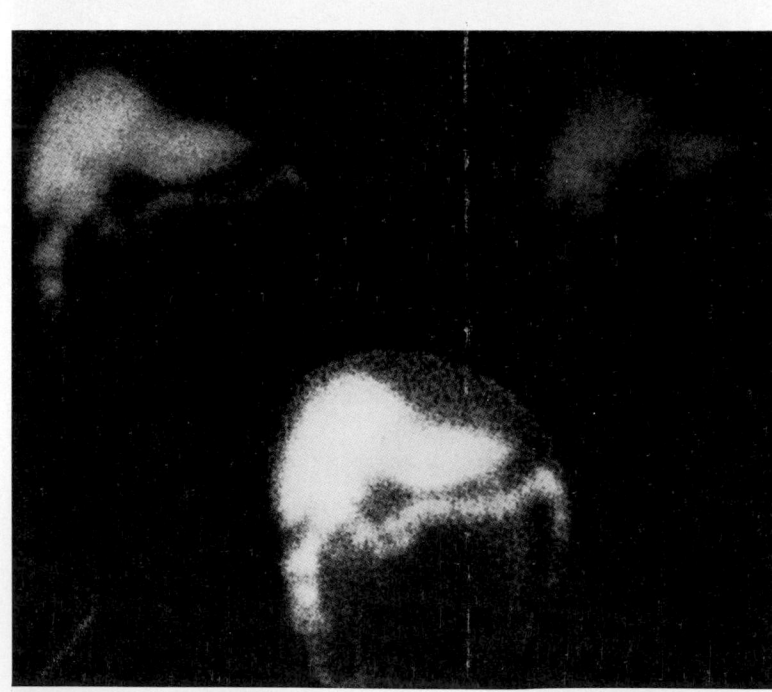

Figure 77–4. Cholescintigram at 1 hour **(A)** and at 24 hours **(B)** showing marked delay in emptying. Patient had papillary stenosis relieved by sphinctero-plasty.

B

only be relieved if the cystic duct remnant is excised. However, one should be forewarned that the mere presence of a cystic duct remnant without evidence of abnormalities of the remainder of the biliary tract is not an indication for excision of the cystic duct remnant for relief of symptoms.

Papillary Stenosis

Anatomically the extrahepatic biliary tree has two areas of narrowing, namely the cystic duct and the sphincter of Oddi. From the standpoint of the gallbladder two potential sites of obstruction occur in sequence. It is likely that partial obstruction plays a role in the development of gallstones. Inflammation or fibrosis of either the cystic duct or the papilla may result in bile stasis and stone formation. The gallbladder will be more likely to develop calculi because of increased concentration of cholesterol, lecithin, and bile acids. Generally, it is cystic duct obstruction that leads to cholelithiasis. Under that circumstance cholecystectomy will be followed by symptomatic relief. However, if papillary fibrosis co-exists with cystic duct dysfunction, it may be the primary cause for symptoms, and cholecystectomy will not relieve the pain.

Unfortunately neither oral cholecystography nor biliary tract ultrasonography, the two most utilized modalities for diagnosing cholelithiasis, can evaluate whether papillary stenosis, and hence mild common bile duct obstruction, exists. During cholecystectomy, operative cholangiography may not demonstrate papillary stenosis, so the operation is terminated. It is the patient with unrecognized papillary disease who is likely to develop symptoms early in the postoperative course as the bile flow in the common duct increases subsequent to the loss of the storage and concentration function of the gallbladder.

When a patient who has had a cholecystectomy presents with symptoms similar to the preoperative ones or new symptoms suggesting further difficulties with the biliary tract, ultrasonography is unlikely to delineate the problem. An elevated serum bilirubin may be confirmatory of CBD obstruction, but since papillary stenosis produces partial obstruction, serum bilirubin is often normal. Alkaline phosphatase, on the other hand, will often show persistent elevation when partial obstruction exists. Cholescintigraphy using one of the IDA analogues is the ideal diagnostic maneuver (Fig.

77–4). It is capable of showing morphologic dilatation and also can identify obstruction to bile flow by making serial examinations over several hours. Unlike the dog, the human common bile duct does *not* dilate after cholecystectomy except when obstruction occurs. Demonstrable enlargement of the CBD on scintigram is evidence of obstruction. If there is delay in transit of the radionuclide from the CBD to the bowel or if the concentration of radionuclide is greater on the 2-hour study than on the 1-hour study, partial obstruction to bile flow is present. The mechanisms of obstruction, e.g., stone, fibrosis, or tumor, cannot be elucidated by radionuclide imaging. However, as a screening test, it is invaluable.

Once CBD obstruction is suspected and then confirmed by cholescintigraphy, other diagnostic tests can be conducted to elucidate the etiology of the obstruction. ERCP may be attempted, but if the stenosis is sufficiently tight, ERCP may be unsuccessful. Of course, this can be construed to indicate an obstructive problem at the papilla. Thin needle percutaneous transhepatic cholangiography, on the other hand, is very likely to be successful and will usually demonstrate the offending lesion (Fig. 72–5). If papil-

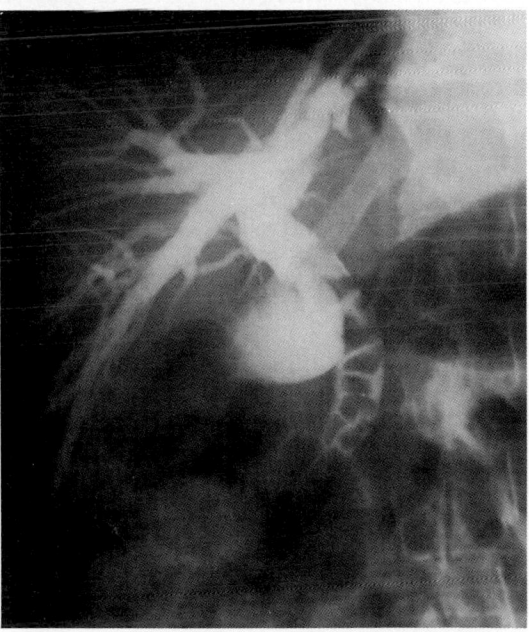

Figure 77–5. Percutaneous transhepatic cholangiogram showing retained common duct stones.

lary stenosis exists, sphincteroplasty, septectomy, or choledochoenteric anastomosis to bypass the lesion are the choices of operative procedures. The role of endoscopic papillotomy as therapy remains to be evaluated for long-term benefit. If it proves to be worthwhile, it will make ERCP for diagnosis an attractive technique.

POSTCHOLECYSTECTOMY SYNDROME

After all of the diagnostic modalities have been completed on a patient who has new, recurrent, or persistent symptoms following cholecystectomy, there remains a very small group of patients who have no demonstrable abnormality. These patients can be said to be suffering from the postcholecystectomy syndrome. Interestingly enough, they often are patients who had symptoms for a long period of time and whose history and workup is not typical of biliary colic or gallbladder disorder. In retrospect, it is often contended that these patients did not have typical symptoms before the operation and continued to have the same or similar symptoms after the operation. A high percentage of these patients are women, have functioning gallbladders on oral cholecystogram, have stones as opposed to cholecystitis, or have acalculous cholecystitis. Stanley Hoerr of the Cleveland Clinic once stated a corollary to his original surgical axiom as: "If you remove an organ which is not causing the problem, the symptoms will persist." This is the situation in the very few patients who have true postcholecystectomy syndrome. Their abdominal discomfort is being used for some other purpose and can be construed as a functional disorder. Under this circumstance the appropriate maneuver is to work with the patient and a psychiatrist, if the patient will permit it, in order to unravel the difficult situation that has led to the patient's psychosomatic illness.

"SUMP SYNDROME" AFTER CHOLEDOCHOENTEROSTOMY

It is almost 100 years since Riedel performed the first choledochoduodenostomy. During the past decade this operation has been used with increasing frequency on patients with benign obstruction at the distal end of the common bile duct. It has been seen following both choledochoduodenostomy as well as choledochojejunostomy and produces symptoms secondary to partial obstruction of the new anastomosis. The patient develops chills, fever, obstruction of the common duct as evidenced by jaundice, increased serum bilirubin, and increased alkaline phosphatase. The latter may be increased in the absence of jaundice. The etiology of the syndrome is thought to be due to a combination of some narrowing of the stoma between the common bile duct and the bowel, along with stagnation of debris and other material in the distal common duct that with bacterial action on the bile produces lithogenic bile that leads to frank stone formation or stone-like material in the "sump" portion of the common bile duct.

The treatment of the "sump syndrome" is prevention; it can be accomplished by placing the choledochoenterostomy as far distal on the common duct as possible or by doing an end-to-side choledochoenterostomy if feasible. Once the syndrome has occurred, it can be diagnosed by ERCP, which should be done under covering intravenous antibiotics and then relieved by endoscopic papillotomy. Transduodenal sphincteroplasty or conversion of the side-to-side choledochoenterostomy to an end-to-side one will also relieve the condition.

BIBLIOGRAPHY

Beye HL: Conditions necessitating surgery following cholecystectomy: An analysis of 66 cases and a discussion of certain technical problems concerned in removal of the gallbladder and in operations upon the common bile duct. Surg Gynecol Obstet 62:191, 1936

Blumgart LH, Carachi R, et al: Diagnosis and management of post-cholecystectomy symptoms: The place of endoscopy and retrograde choledochopancreatography. Br J Surg 64:809, 1977

Bodvall B, Overgaard B: Computer analysis of postcholecystectomy biliary tract symptoms. Surg Gynecol Obstet 124:723, 1967

Christiansen J, Schmidt A: The postcholecystectomy syndrome. Acta Chir Scand 137:789, 1971

Classen MM, Safrany L: Endoscopic papillotomy and removal of gallstones. Br Med J 4:371, 1975

Florcken H: Gallenblasenregeneration mit steinrecidive nach cholecystectomie. Dtsch Z Chir 113:604, 1912

Garlock JH, Hurwitt ES: The cystic duct stump syndrome. Surgery 29:833, 1951

Glenn F, Johnson G Jr: Cystic duct remnant, a sequela of incomplete cholecystectomy. Surg Gynecol Obstet 101:331, 1955

Glenn F, McSherry C: Secondary abdominal operations for symptoms following biliary tract surgery. Surg Gynecol Obstet 121:979, 1965

Gregg JA, Clark G, et al: Postcholecystectomy syndrome and its association with ampullary stenosis. Am J Surg 139:374,1980

Hopkins SF, Bivins BA, et al: The problem of cystic duct remnant. Surg Gynecol Obstet 148:531, 1979

Hunt DR: Investigation of post-cholecystectomy problems. Med J Aust 1:214, 1982

Iwamura K: Pathogenetic significance of bile acid metabolism in the post-cholecystectomy syndrome. Tokai J Exp Clin Med 5:217, 1980

Larmi TKI, Modda R, et al: A critical analysis of the cystic duct remnant. Surg Gynecol Obstet 141:48, 1975

LeQuesne LP, Whiteside CG, et al: The common bile ducts after cholecystectomy. Br Med J 1:329, 1959

Moody FG, Berenson MM, et al: Transampullary systectomy for post-cholecystectomy pain. Ann Surg 186:415, 1977

Nardi GL, Acosta JM: Papillitis as a cause of pancreatitis and abdominal pain: Role of evocative test, operative pancreatography and histologic evaluation. Ann Surg 164:611, 1966

Nardi GL, Michelassi F, et al: Transduodenal sphincteroplasty: 5–25 year follow-up 89 patients. Ann Surg 198:453, 1983

Pribram BOC: Postcholecystectomy syndromes. JAMA 142:1262, 1950

Siegel JHP: Biliary bezoar: The sump syndrome and choledochoenterostomy. Endoscopy 14:238, 1982

Stefanini P, Carboni M, et al: Factors influencing the long term results of cholecystectomy. Surg Gynecol Obstet 139:734, 1974

Taylor TV: Postvagotomy and cholecystectomy syndrome. Ann Surg 194:625, 1981

Weed TE, Blalock JB: "Sump syndrome" after choledochoduodenostomy. South Med J 75:370, 1982

Weissmann HS, Gliedman ML, et al: Evaluation of the postoperative patient with ^{99m}Tc-IDA cholescintigraphy. Semin Nucl Med XII:27, 1982

Womack NA, Crider RL: Persistence of symptoms following cholecystectomy. Ann Surg 126:31, 1947

78. Choledocholithiasis

Harold Ellis

A stone in the common bile duct is one of the most common and most serious of the complications of gallstones. The great majority are associated with calculi in the gallbladder, although there is debate regarding the proportion of stones in the common bile duct that originate in the gallbladder and pass down the cystic duct and those that form in situ. Stones can undoubtedly form per primam in the common bile duct; this is shown by the fact that calculi may develop therein in patients who have previously undergone cholecystectomy and in whom, at that time, cholangiography proved without doubt that the duct system was free from stones. An origin in the gallbladder is suggested by the presence of multiple faceted stones in the gallbladder, a dilated cystic duct, and the presence of similar multiple faceted stones in the bile ducts. In the absence of fistula formation, only relatively small stones can pass into the common duct but, once in this duct, they may enlarge as the result of the deposition of soft pigment and debris on their surface. When this occurs, the stones may become barrel-shaped and mutually congruent (Fig. 78–1). On section, such stones will usually be found to contain in their centre a small, hard, and often faceted calculus, betraying their origin from the gallbladder. Soft concretions of biliary mud, however, suggest primary origin in the bile duct and Madden (1978) argues that, contrary to generally accepted beliefs, such primary duct stones are found almost twice as frequently as secondary stones originating from the gallbladder.

Stones may form in the bile ducts in the type of suppurative cholangitis seen in the Far East.

INCIDENCE

Stones in the common duct may be single or multiple, one hundred or more sometimes present in a dilated duct (Fig. 78–2).

The incidence of stone in the common duct is difficult to determine with accuracy, partly because some such stones may not give rise to symptoms, because stones in the common duct may be overlooked, and because comparison of reported series of patients may be misleading owing to the differing composition of the various series. The latter is particularly important in relation to the age of the patients in any series, for the incidence of stones in the common bile duct increases with age. Havard (1970) observed that the incidence of this complication was 6.5 percent in patients under the age of 40 undergoing cholecystectomy, rose to 42 percent in patients between 70 and 80, and reached 50 percent in those over the age of 80.

In 1981 Bolton and Le Quesne reviewed a dozen reports from leading surgical centres published over the last 30 years where the incidence of stones found in the common bile duct at the time of cholecystectomy ranged from 6 to 19.5 percent. Glenn (1967), in a meticulous study of 4677 patients operated upon for nonacute cholecystitis, usually associated with gallstones, reported an 8.8 percent incidence of choledocholithiasis.

FATE OF COMMON DUCT STONES

There is no doubt that some stones that enter the common duct pass on into the duodenum. Evidence in support of this outcome is provided

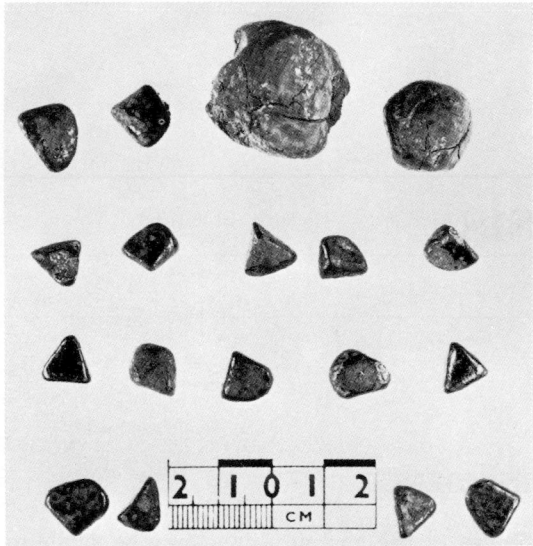

Figure 78–1. Multiple stones removed from a dilated common bile duct. Many of the stones are faceted, revealing their origin in the gallbladder. The two large, barrel-shaped stones were impacted in the intrapancreatic portion of the duct: They are covered with a layer of soft pigment and debris laid down in the duct, and are mutually congruent where they have been in contact.

by patients who pass gallstones per rectum and who, at subsequent operation, are shown to have no fistula between the gallbladder and the bowel. Occasionally, radiographic examination may provide similar evidence (Fig. 78–3). Gardner et al (1966) described seven patients with "disappearing gallstones" in whom the stones were clearly visualised on cholecystography and then, after attacks of biliary colic, they either disappeared or were reduced in number at further cholecystography or surgical exploration. How often this occurs is not known and it may well be that small stones are passed more often than is realised. It is believed that the majority of stones within the common bile duct remain there until removed surgically, but there is no real evidence in support of this belief, particularly with regard to small calculi.

Rarely, stones in the common bile duct are symptomless—a chance finding at x-ray, laparotomy, or autopsy. Much more commonly, the stone either impacts at the narrow lower end of the duct to produce an acute obstruction or

moves up and down to produce chronic intermittent obstruction.

Acute obstruction is caused partly by the presence of the stone itself, which usually impacts in the intrapancreatic portion of the duct at the junction of its main portion with the terminal segment, and partly by oedema of the duct wall, perhaps enhanced by sphincteric spasm. The obstruction to the flow of bile is rarely complete, so that although the stools are pale they contain some bile pigment and, accordingly, some urobilinogen is usually present in the urine. Furthermore, the degree of obstruction tends to vary from day to day, with the result that the jaundice is characteristically fluctuant. In the majority of cases, the stone either passes on into the duodenum, or, when the oedema and spasm subside, free flow of bile recommences; in either case, the jaundice clears.

Chronic intermittent obstruction may produce repeated and transient episodes of jaundice. Chronic obstruction results in progressive dilatation of the ducts, which may become twice their normal calibre. Infection in the duct is a common complication.

Chronic obstruction also gives rise to changes in the liver, which eventually result in biliary cirrhosis. However, this is usually marked only in patients with long-standing obstruction of a severe degree, as in patients with a stricture of the duct. The essential change in the liver is the deposition of fibrous tissue in the portal tracts, which spreads out to surround the liver lobules. Together with this, there is proliferation of the bile canaliculi and the formation of bile thrombi in the smaller ducts. These changes, when mild, are reversible following relief of the obstruction (Fig. 78–4).

CLINICAL MANIFESTATIONS

Stones may be present in the common duct for months or years without causing symptoms, but sooner or later the great majority give rise to the typical picture of severe upper abdominal pain, accompanied or followed by jaundice, with pale stools and dark urine. Often these attacks are precipitated by the ingestion of a fatty meal and characteristically they occur in women who have previously experienced symptoms suggestive of stones in the gallbladder.

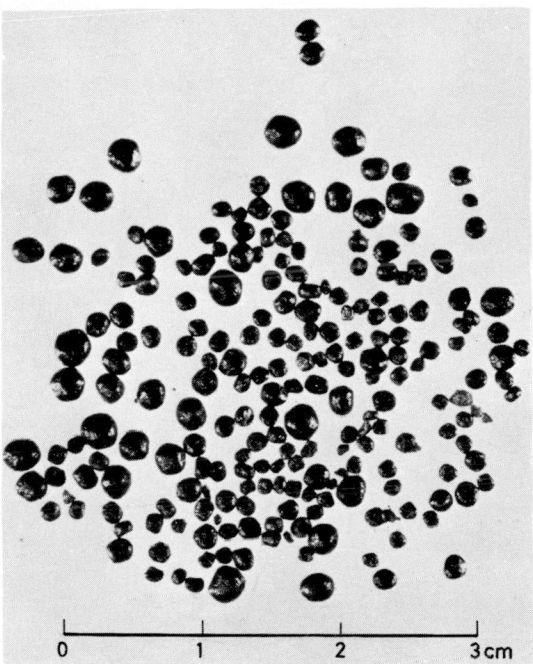

Figure 78–2. Multiple small stones removed from the common bile duct.

The pain is usually sudden in its onset, rapidly reaches its maximum intensity, and then may last continuously for several hours or until relieved by an opiate injection. Surprisingly, many textbooks describe the pain as intermittent, but a carefully taken history from any group of patients will reveal that this is not so (an interesting account of this simple piece of clinical investigation was described by French and Robb in 1963). The pain is commonly epigastric and right subcostal but not uncommonly it radiates across to below the left costal margin. Referred pain to the lower pole of the right scapula is also common. During the attack, the patient is usually restless, doubled-up in agony, often sweats, and commonly feels sick or actually vomits. There is usually tenderness in the upper right quadrant of the abdomen.

In a typical attack, the pain usually subsides within 12 to 24 hours; toward the end of which time, or shortly afterward, the patient may become jaundiced and excrete pale stools and dark urine. The jaundice is rarely intense, so that pruritus is uncommon. Often within a few days or weeks there is recurrence of the pain with reappearance of the icterus.

Examination reveals a patient obviously in pain. Jaundice should be sought in natural light; a tinge of jaundice may not be apparent when viewed in yellow artificial illumination. There is frequently pyrexia and tachycardia. There is usually tenderness in the right upper abdomen with a positive Murphy's sign but a palpable distended gallbladder is rarely found in obstructive jaundice caused by a stone, in contrast to the jaundice in association with carcinoma of the head of the pancreas (Courvoisier's law). The reason for this difference between the two common causes of obstructive jaundice is two-fold: First, in patients with calculous obstruction, the gallbladder is affected almost invariably by chronic cholecystitis with fibrosis, and so cannot readily dilate; in patients with carcinoma of the pancreas, the gallbladder is usually normal and therefore distensible. Secondly, in patients with stone in the duct, the obstruction is usually incomplete so that the pressure in the ductal system does not rise as high as in malignant obstruction when, once established, the obstruction is usually complete and continuous.

If there is an associated cholangitis, in general the illness is altogether more severe. In addition to the pain and jaundice, there is a high fever, often with severe sweating and rigors. The fever tends to be intermittent (Charcot's intermittent hepatic fever). The blood culture is often positive. The problems of infection in relation to stone in the common duct are discussed more fully later in this chapter.

Patients with obstructive jaundice are at significant risk of developing renal failure following surgery. This is associated with the presence of bacterial endotoxin in the peripheral blood. Cahill (1983) has shown that the administration of the bile salt sodium deoxycholate preoperatively prevents endotoxin absorption from the gut by direct action on the endotoxin molecule and is an effective prophylactic against renal damage in obstructive jaundice.

By no means do all patients with stones in the common duct present with a typical picture. As already mentioned, patients can harbour stones in their common duct with no symptoms or only insignificant ones. They may present with jaundice that is not accompanied by pain and then there is very real difficulty in differentiating from a carcinoma of the head

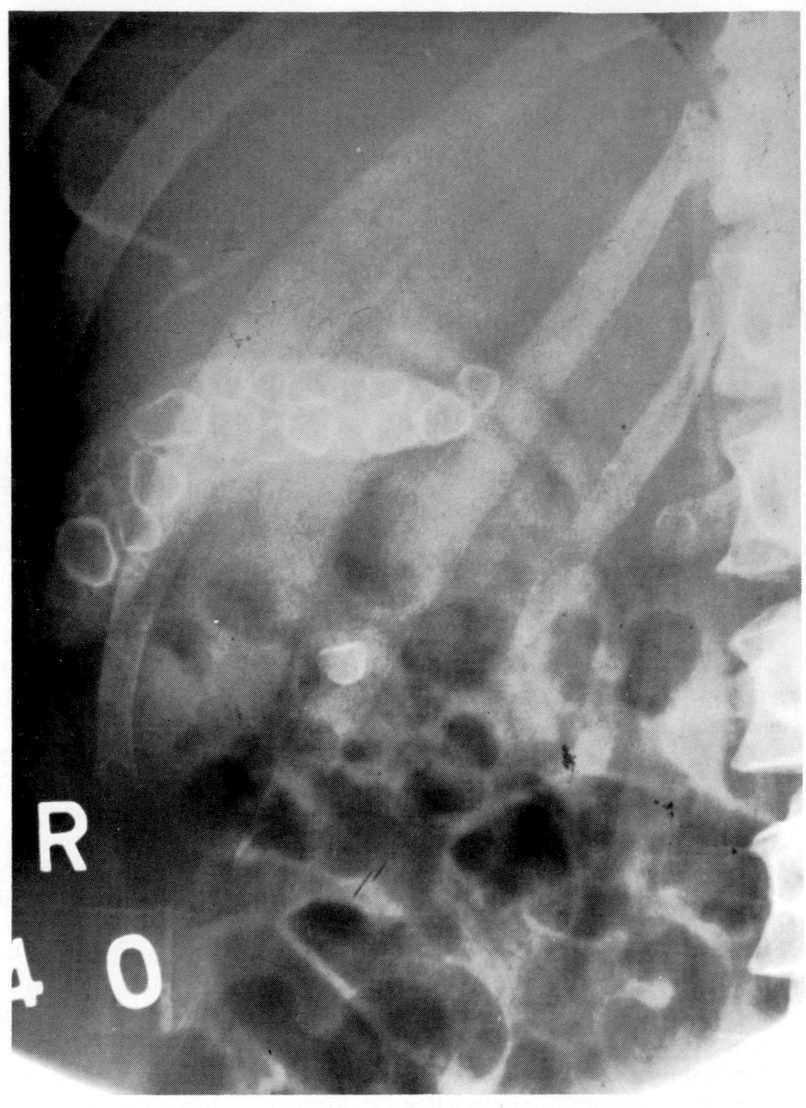

Figure 78–3. Intravenous cholangiogram showing multiple stones in the gallbladder, with a single faceted calculus lying separate from the gallbladder, probably in the colon. Subsequent x-rays showed this separate stone to have disappeared, and operation showed no fistula between the gallbladder and intestines.

of the pancreas; alternatively they may complain of pain without jaundice. A recent interesting review by Rubin and Beal (1983) of 60 patients with common duct calculi showed that 53 described classic biliary pain while 7 were free from this symptom. Fifty percent of the patients had jaundice and 22 were febrile. Of the 60 patients, 21 had one symptom, 22 had two, 15 had all three symptoms, and 2 were asymptomatic.

Although an attack of severe biliary pain with jaundice commonly indicates the presence of a stone in the common bile duct, this is certainly not always the case. Watkin and Thomas

(1971) conclude that the incidence of choledocholithiasis in patients with acute cholecystitis and jaundice is about 70 percent. The cause of the jaundice in the remaining cases has been the subject of a good deal of speculation. Among the mechanisms suggested have been associated pancreatitis, cholangitis, compression of the common bile duct by an acutely enlarged cystic lymph node, and oedema around a stone impacted in the cystic duct. None of these explanations are particularly convincing. However, Nolan and Espiner (1972) studied three patients with acute cholecystitis in whom displacement and narrowing of the common bile duct was

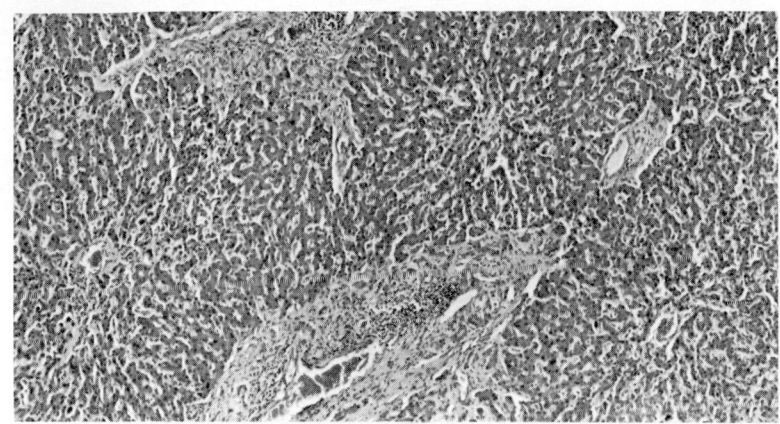

Figure 78–4. Section cut from a liver biopsy obtained at operation from a patient with multiple stones in a dilated common duct, showing the changes of biliary cirrhosis. Note the periportal fibrosis, with bile-duct proliferation and bile thrombi. (X50)

demonstrated by intravenous cholangiography. At emergency surgery, the acutely inflamed and enlarged gallbladder was found to be compressing the porta hepatis. These authors suggest that compression of the duct system by the acutely distended gallbladder readily accounts for the jaundice in those patients in whom stones are not found within the common duct.

Differential Diagnosis

The differential diagnosis of stones in the common duct involves a large number of conditions and, to a considerable extent, depends upon whether jaundice or pain is the predominant symptom. If jaundice is prominent and pain unobtrusive or absent, it must be distinguished not only from other causes of obstructive jaundice (notably carcinoma involving the lower end of the common duct) but also from viral hepatitis, drug-induced jaundice, and secondary deposits in the liver. Classically the jaundice caused by malignant obstruction to the common duct is accompanied by a palpably distended gallbladder (Courvoisier's law), although in practice this is only found in about 50 percent of cases.

Depending upon its exact location and accompanying features, the pain produced by stones in the bile duct may have to be distinguished from a wide range of diseases, including not only other abdominal lesions but also various intrathoracic diseases. Thus, the pain of a myocardial infarction may closely resemble that of a stone in the common duct. Of the various abdominal lesions that may give rise to pain similar to that of a duct stone, the most common are peptic ulcer, chronic pancreatitis, and pancreatic carcinoma.

DIAGNOSTIC STUDIES

In most instances, the diagnosis of a stone in the common bile duct is fairly clear on clinical grounds; biochemical, radiologic, and imaging studies are required mainly to confirm the diagnosis. In some instances, however, the diagnosis may be difficult even with the help of all possible aids. Among the difficulties are:

1. Failure to visualise very small calculi.
2. A stone firmly impacted in the lower end of the common bile duct that may closely mimic an ampullary carcinoma.
3. Liver disease concomitant with calculous obstruction.
4. The occasional association of stones in the biliary system with a pancreatic cancer.

With regard to the last, this author has performed two Whipple operations in which stones in the gallbladder and the common bile duct were present in addition to the pancreatic neoplasm; in both cases the preoperative diagnosis of the exact cause of the obstructive jaundice was not clear, and the operative diagnosis was only established after careful dissection.

Laboratory Studies. The jaundice of calculous obstruction is characterised by a moderately raised serum bilirubin concentration that wanes over several days. A firmly impacted stone, however, may result in a persistently elevated bilirubin level and, to complicate matters, jaundice due to an ampullary carcinoma may also disappear completely. The jaundice of calculous obstruction is accompanied by a raised serum acid phosphatase. The serum glutamic pyruvic transaminase (SGPT) and serum glutamic oxaloacetic transaminase (SGOT) may show a slight rise if there is an associated cholangitis (Gitnick, 1981).

Plain Abdominal Radiography. A plain film of the upper abdomen may show radiopaque calculi. Such stones are usually in the gallbladder and it is uncommon to demonstrate a stone in the duct by this technique (Fig. 78–5). Failure to demonstrate the presence of gallstones in no way invalidates the diagnosis, since only some 10 to 15 percent of gallstones are radiopaque. At the same time, the demonstration of gallstones does not necessarily prove the diagnosis, as symptomless gallstones are quite common, especially in women over the age of 40, and may be an incidental finding in a patient jaundiced for some other reason.

Ultrasonography. Grey scale and real-time ultrasonography have been used with increasing frequency in the investigation of the jaundiced patient because they are expedient, noninva-

sive, relatively simple in application and may be used in pregnant patients, in those who cannot ingest drugs orally, and in those who have an elevated serum bilirubin level. It is valuable in the differentiation between hepatic and obstructive jaundice, the latter being correlated with dilatation of the biliary radicles and dilatation of the common bile duct. Taylor and Rosenfield (1977), for example, in 150 consecutive patients with cholestatic jaundice, could differentiate between intrahepatic and extrahepatic obstruction in no less than 145 of the cases (97 percent). The 5 errors occurred in the 22 patients with calculous obstruction where transient occlusion was not associated with duct dilatation.

Stones within the gallbladder itself can be diagnosed with a high degree of accuracy; thus Cooperberg and Burhenne (1980) missed only 5 out of 261 cases proved to have gallstones at operation. The technique is much less accurate in determining the presence of common bile duct stones; only about 55 percent of these can be positively identified. (Dewsburg et al, 1979; Graham and Lees, 1980).

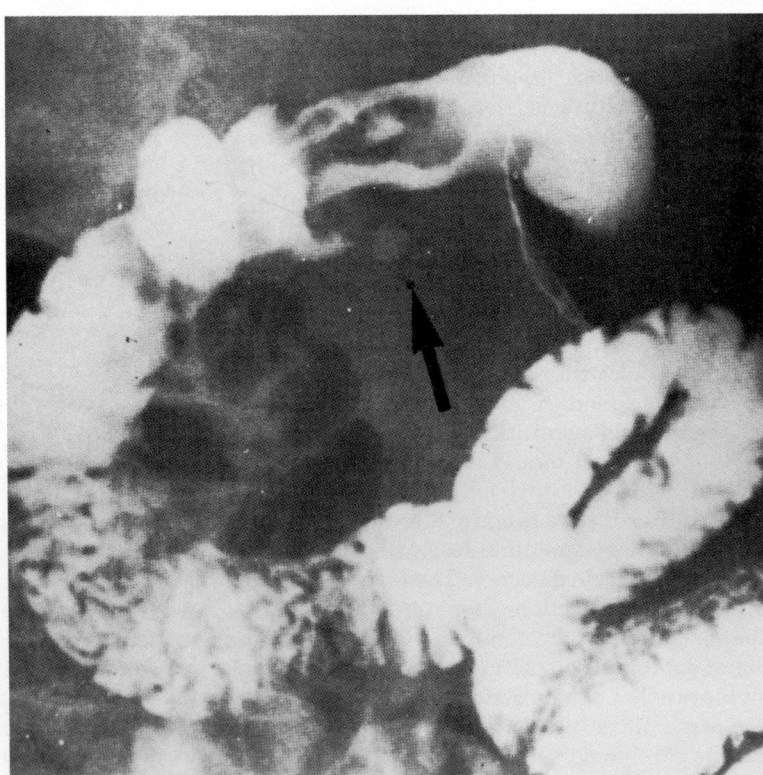

Figure 78–5. Barium meal film from a patient with obstructive jaundice. A rounded shadow is seen below the pylorus (*arrow*); operation confirmed a stone in the common duct. The pyloric mucosa is deformed by oedema in the pylorus and pancreas resulting from impaction of the stone.

A full discussion of abdominal ultrasound is given in Chapter 2.

Computed Tomography. This is much more expensive, more time consuming, and less widely available than ultrasound. It is useful in patients in whom ultrasonography is difficult—the obese and those with a good deal of gas in the bowel. It will give good evidence in the jaundiced patient of the level and cause of the obstruction (Levitt et al, 1977). Thus Pedrosa and colleagues (1981) report a 97 percent overall accuracy in determining the site of the obstruction and a correct cause in 94 percent in a series of 67 cases of obstructive jaundice. Seventeen of these were due to common duct stones and in 14 the calculi were visualised.

Computed tomography (CT) is not particularly helpful in the specific diagnosis of gallstone disease. Although it will demonstrate the dilated gallbladder, it may fail to show stones within it (Cooperman et al, 1977). Stones in the common duct may be dense and readily visualised but in many cases the stones may be only slightly denser than surrounding structures and relatively pure cholesterol stones may even have a lower density than bile.

Cholecystography. Neither oral nor intravenous cholangiography are of any assistance in the diagnosis of common bile duct stones in the presence of jaundice, since no opacification of the biliary tree will be seen. Following the clearance of jaundice, it is wise to wait at least 2 weeks after the serum bilirubin level has returned to normal before ordering cholecystography so that liver function has recovered sufficiently to allow good opacification. In a patient who has been recently jaundiced, the demonstration on intravenous cholangiography of a stone or stones in the common duct (Fig. 78–6) is clearly of diagnostic significance, but a failure to demonstrate such stones does not exclude their presence. Indeed, calculi can only be demonstrated in about 60 percent of cases. A dilated common duct, of a calibre over 13 mm, almost invariably indicates an obstruction, but it is important to note that stones may be present even in ducts of a normal diameter and with no stones demonstrated radiologically.

Invasive Diagnostic Techniques. The differential diagnosis and investigation of obstructive jaundice may involve the use of the invasive

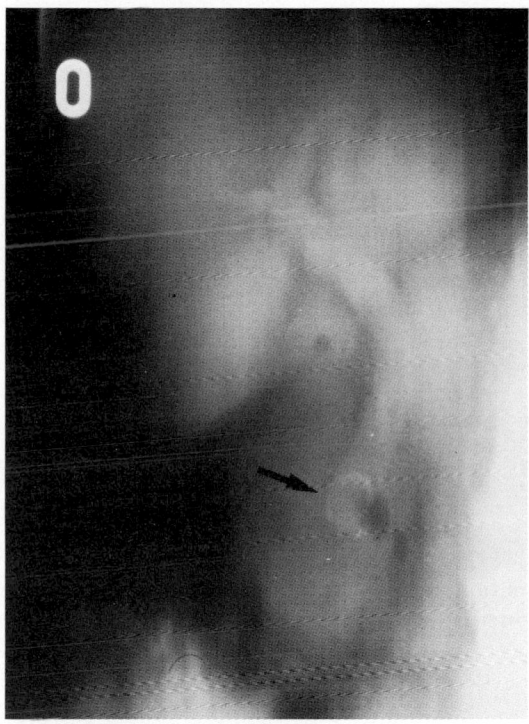

Figure 78–6. Intravenous cholangiogram of a stone in the common bile duct (*arrow*).

techniques of percutaneous transhepatic cholangiography, in cases where duct dilatation is seen on scanning but more information is still required, or endoscopic retrograde cholangiography, particularly if the ducts are not dilated (Wild et al, 1980).

In the great majority of cases, however, the clinical features of pain and recurrent jaundice, together with the findings on oral cholecystography and ultrasound, give the surgeon quite enough information to warrant laparotomy with a firm preoperative diagnosis of calculous biliary disease. The final diagnosis of stones in the common bile duct will be made at laparotomy as a result of careful palpation of the duct system, combined with operative cholangiography and/or choledochoscopy.

Operative Cholangiography

Modern imaging techniques have greatly improved the accuracy of preoperative diagnosis of common duct stones, but there still exists a proportion of false-positive and false-negative findings. The surgeon needs to know, with a high degree of accuracy, whether or not the common duct contains stones at the time of laparotomy, and operative cholangiography makes a major contribution to accurate diagnosis. Introduced by Mirizzi in 1932 by injection of contrast medium into the opened common bile duct, the technique was at first unsatisfactory owing to the use of oil contrast material, but with the development of water-soluble media, its value was soon appreciated.

Two types of operative cholangiogram can be performed:

1. Before the duct is explored (preexploratory cholangiography)
2. After the duct has been explored (postexploratory cholangiography)

The purpose of the preexploratory examination is to determine whether the common duct contains a stone or stones and hence whether it requires exploration. The postexploratory examination is to determine whether exploration has succeeded in removing all the stones from the duct.

To produce reliable films capable of critical interpretation, preexploratory cholangiography demands scrupulous attention to details in technique (see Chapter 76). A normal preexploratory cholangiogram shows the following features:

1. There is a free flow of contrast medium into the duodenum on the first film.
2. The narrow terminal portion of the duct is clearly seen.
3. The main portion of the duct is of normal calibre; as measured on the x-ray film, the diameter of the duct is usually 10 mm or less, and a diameter in excess of 12 mm should be considered abnormal.
4. There are no filling defects in the ducts.
5. There is no excess retrograde filling of the intrahepatic radicles (Fig. 78–7).

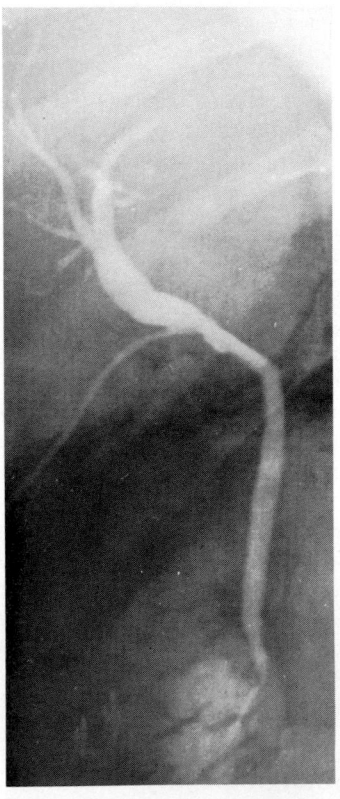
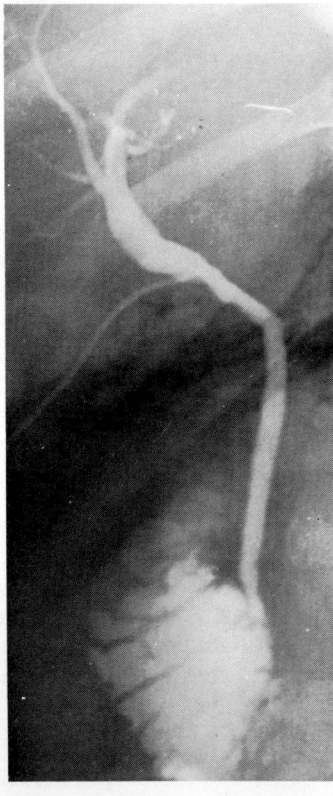
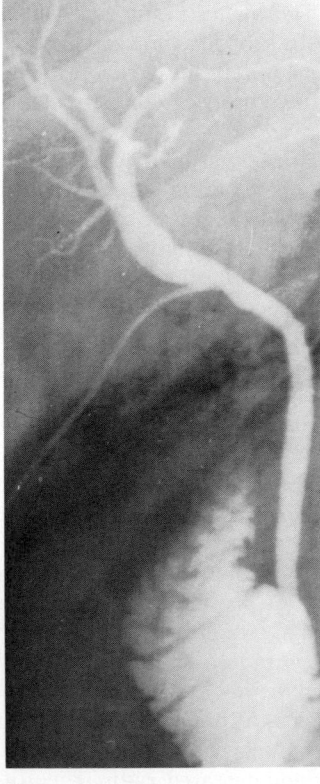

A **B** **C**

Figure 78–7. Three films from a normal, preexploratory cholangiogram. Note the free flow of contrast material into the duodenum, the clear delineation of the narrow terminal segment in **(A)**, the normal calibre of the duct, and the absence of filling defects.

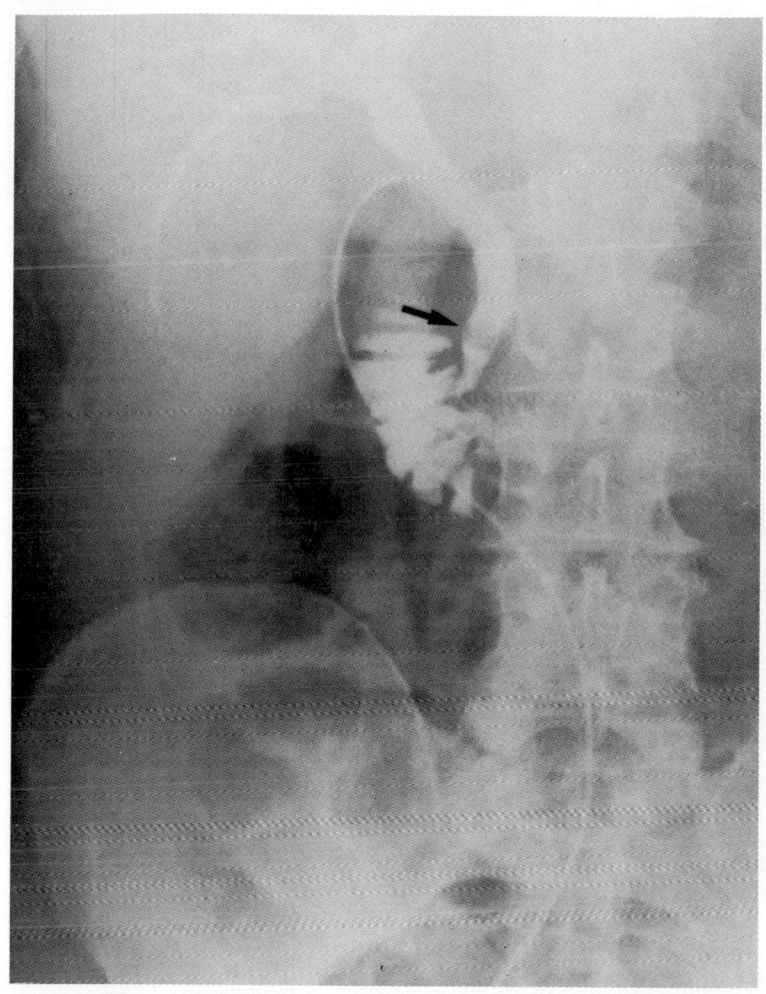

Figure 78–8. A single stone in the common bile duct at operative cholangiography (*arrow*).

If all these criteria are strictly fulfilled, the cholangiogram can be relied upon as evidence of a normal duct that does not require exploration. If, however, the films show any abnormality, this should be taken as evidence of an abnormal duct that probably requires exploration. The only exception to this rule is failure to demonstrate flow into the duodenum in the first film; if the examination is in all other respects normal, particularly if the narrow segment is seen in the first film, it can be taken as indicating a normal duct.

The most obvious indication of a stone in the common duct is a filling defect, which may be single or multiple (Figs. 78–8 and 78–9). Often the defect is accompanied by dilatation of the duct, lack of flow of contrast medium into the duodenum, failure to demonstrate the terminal narrow segment, and excess retrograde filling of the intrahepatic ducts (Fig. 78–10).

In some cases a filling defect is not seen and the only evidence of stone is failure of flow of contrast medium into the duodenum with failure to visualise the narrow segment. If this also is associated with dilatation of the duct and excess retrograde filling, these findings strongly suggest the presence of a stone or sludge at the lower end of the duct (Fig. 78–11).

It must be emphasised that the examination should be accepted as indicating a normal duct that does not require exploration *only* if it fulfills the criteria set out previously.

The presence of bubbles in the duct occasionally can give rise to difficulties in interpretation, although these should be eliminated by attention to details in technique. The fact that

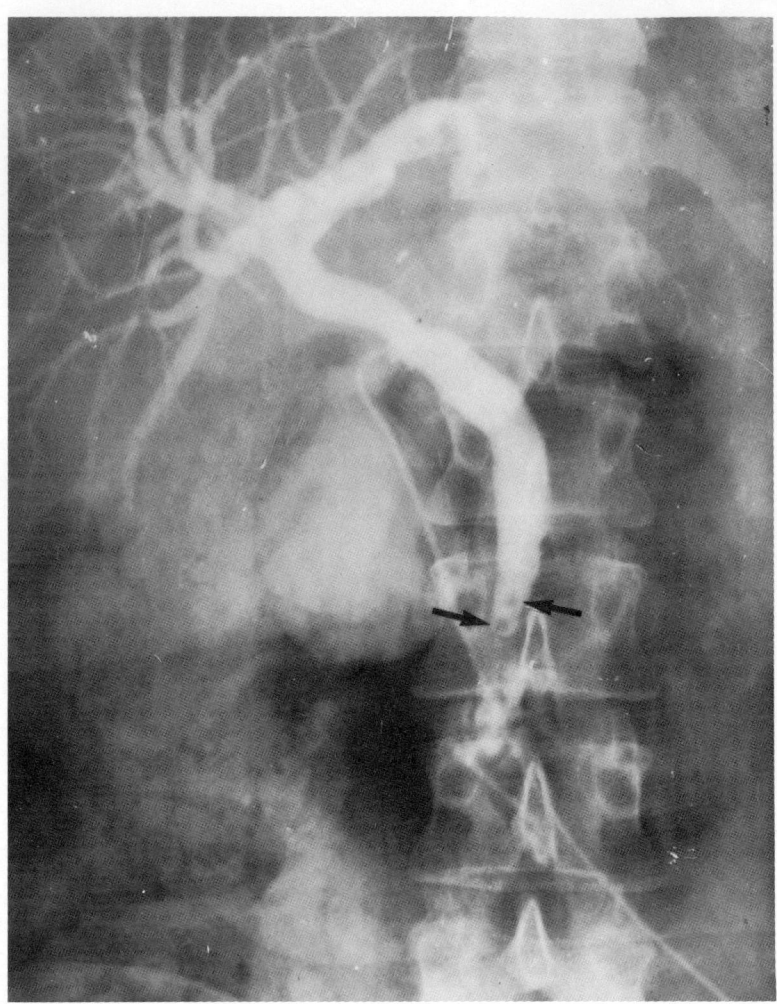

Figure 78–9. Multiple stones in the common bile duct at operative cholangiography (*arrows*).

a filling defect is caused by an air bubble is usually suggested by the circular outline and a cholangiogram that is in all other respects normal. If the presence of a bubble or bubbles is suspected, the difficulty can usually be resolved by repetition of the examination after thoroughly flushing the duct with normal saline (Fig. 78–12).

Occasionally, difficulties also can arise as the result of spasm of the sphincteric mechanism surrounding the terminal portion of the duct for reasons other than the presence of a stone in the duct. Spasm will prevent flow of the contrast medium into the duodenum and also visualisation of the terminal segment of the duct. Usually these abnormalities are caused by the presence of a stone in the duct

or by pancreatitis, but occasionally they may be due to extraneous causes, such as the preanaesthetic agents. If this is thought to be the case, the examination may be repeated after asking the anaesthetist to give the patient amyl nitrite by inhalation. In the absence of a stone in the duct, this will usually relax the spasm, resulting in a normal cholangiogram. If the appearances are still abnormal, then exploration is indicated.

Value of Cholangiography. In assessing the value of preexploratory cholangiography, the critical question to be faced is not whether this form of examination can demonstrate stones in the common duct (for this is manifestly the case), but whether the information it gives is more accurate in the diagnosis of stone in the

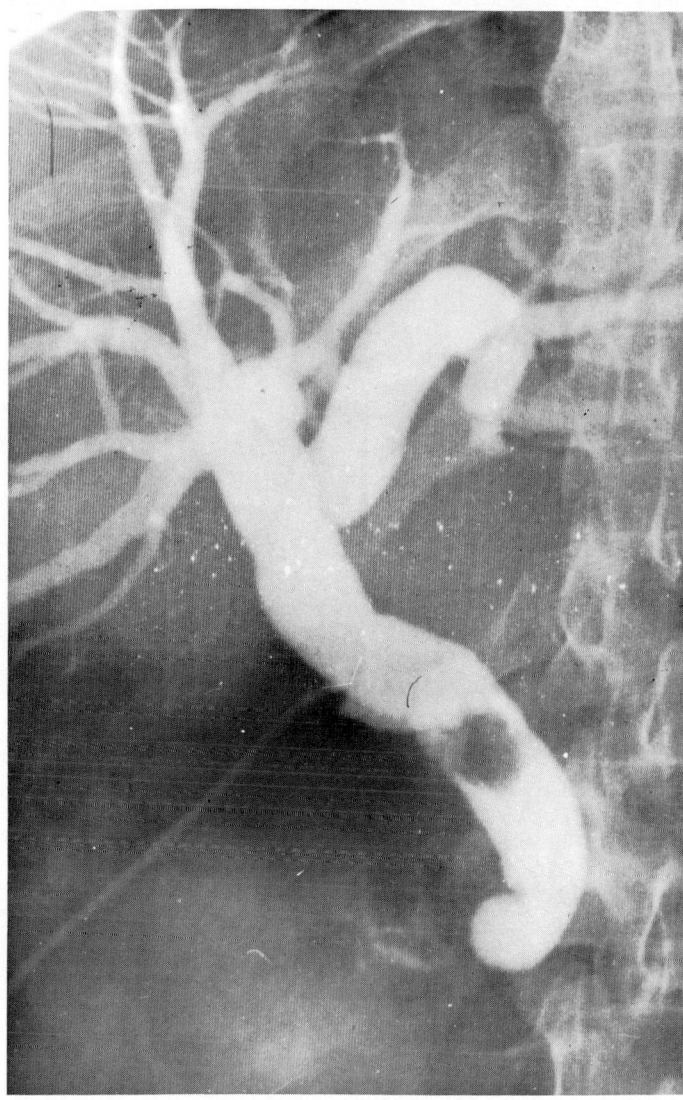

Figure 78-10. Preexploratory cholangiogram showing a large stone in a dilated duct. Note also the absence of flow of contrast material into the duodenum and failure to delineate the terminal segment.

duct than is provided by a combination of the clinical assessment of the patient and operative palpation of the ducts. To pose the problem in a different way:

Does the use of preexploratory cholangiography reveal stones that might otherwise have been overlooked and does it cut down the incidence of negative, and hence unnecessary, explorations of the duct? Numerous studies over the past three decades quite clearly indicate that the answer to both these questions is unequivocally yes.

The use of preexploratory cholangiography will identify stones in the common bile duct in up to 5 percent of patients undergoing cholecys-

tectomy that would have been missed without this investigation, and in addition it will lead to reduction in the numbers of ducts explored and in the incidence of negative exploration by about 50 percent.

A very large number of publications have now appeared on the value of preexploratory cholangiography. Indeed, there now is documented evidence on many thousands of cases. Schulenburg (1969) details his experience in 1000 consecutive operative cholangiograms with only seven technical failures. In 286 common bile ducts explored, only 12 had false-positive cholangiographic findings. In 4 percent of cases, stones that were not palpable were dem-

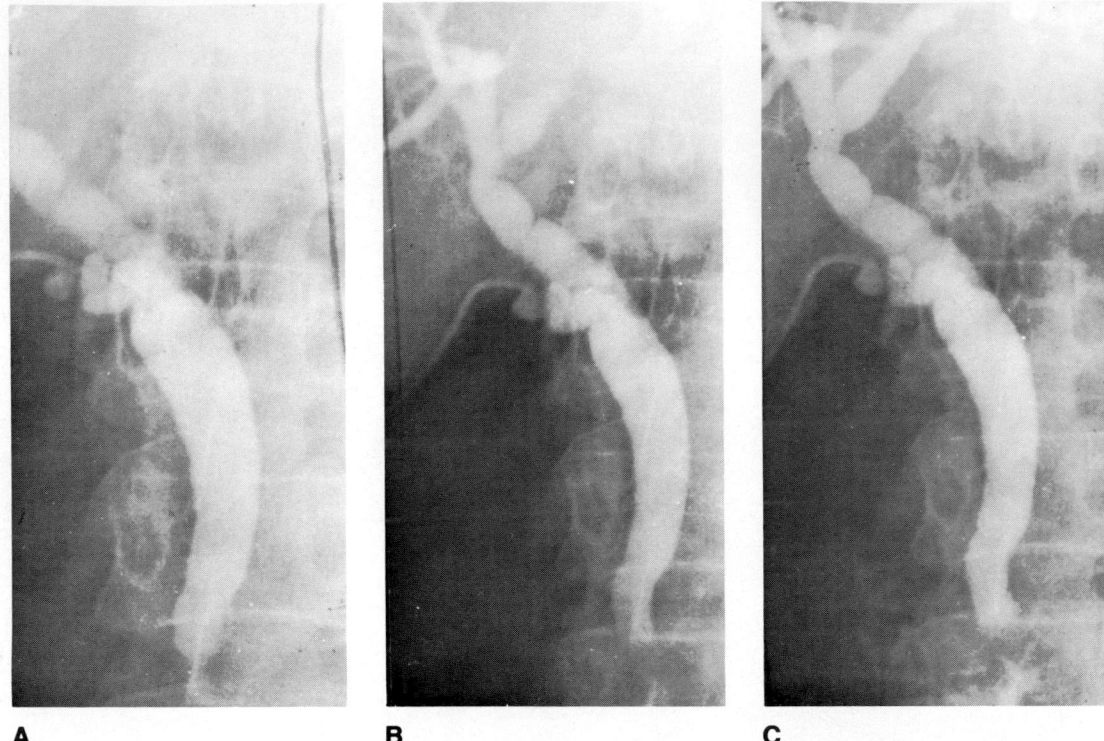

A   B   C

Figure 78–11. Three films from a preexploratory cholangiogram showing a duct of normal calibre with no filling defect, but with no flow of contrast material into the duodenum, and failure to demonstrate the terminal segment. Repetition of the examination after the inhalation of amyl nitrite showed no change in these appearances, and on exploration a stone was found in the lower portion of the duct. Note the superimposition of the duct image on that of the spine, owing to failure to tilt the table sufficiently.

onstrated radiologically and in 5.6 percent of cases stones were shown on x-ray although there had been no jaundice. In contrast, exploration of the common ducts was avoided in 50 cases despite a history of jaundice or the actual presence of jaundice. Saltzstein and colleagues (1973) carried out cystic duct cholangiography in 423 patients undergoing cholecystectomy. Seventy nine of these had clinical evidence that would have led to exploration of the common duct but 39 had normal cholangiograms, thus obviating duct exploration in 50 percent of these cases. Eight patients with no clinical evidence to suggest exploration were found to have stones on cholangiography (1.8 percent).

A study by Kakos and colleagues (1972) provides an interesting demonstration of the value of cholangiography. They review 3012 cholecystectomies in the 20-year period from 1951 to 1970. The use of preexploratory cholangiogra-

phy rose from 2.9 percent in the first 5-year period to 93 percent in the last. Comparison of these two 5-year periods showed that the increased use of the technique was associated with a decrease in the incidence of exploration of the bile ducts from 41 to 25 percent, and by a striking increase in the incidence of positive explorations from 28 to 62 percent. In addition, 4 percent of patients were found to have common duct calculi that had been unsuspected on clinical criteria.

Faris and colleagues (1975) demonstrated a positive benefit from preexploratory cholangiography for 19 percent of their 400 consecutive patients. If clinical and operative criteria alone had been used, 16 patients (4 percent) would have had common duct stones overlooked and 48 patients would have had unnecessary common duct explorations (15 percent). On the basis of cholangiographic evidence, 27 percent of the

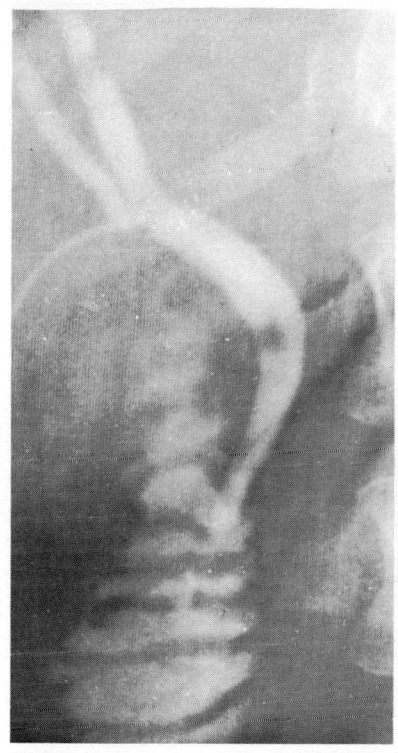 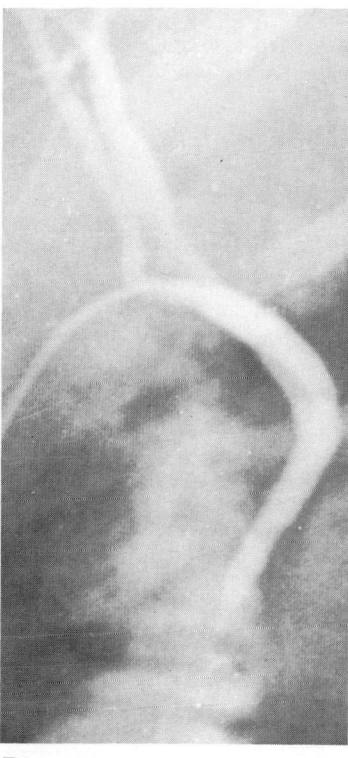

A **B**

Figure 78–12. Preexploratory cholangiogram. **A.** A defect due to an air bubble in the duct. Note that the defect is circular and that the cholangiogram is normal in all other respects. After flushing the duct with saline, a repeat cholangiogram **(B)** showed a normal duct with no defect. Note that in this patient the cystic duct joins the right hepatic duct.

patients had the common duct explored and stones were found in 71 percent of these. The limitations of the sole use of noncholangiographic criteria for exploration are further emphasised by two other findings from this study. Patients with a history of jaundice were as likely to have stones solely in the gallbladder as they were to have a stone in the common bile duct, and the incidence of multiple stones in the gallbladder was the same in those with and those without common duct stones. The only noncholangiographic criteria of value are the finding of a palpable stone or stones in the common bile duct and frank jaundice at the time of laparotomy.

One further question concerning the accuracy of preexploratory cholangiography remains to be answered. What is the incidence of residual stones in those whose duct was not explored on the basis of a normal preexploratory cholangiogram? A follow-up study of 19 patients with this criterion was carried out by Chapman et al (1964). All patients were reviewed 1 year or more after operation (12 to 50 months, average 31 months), and in all an intravenous cholangiogram was performed at the time of this review; in no patient was there any clinical or radiographic evidence of a residual duct stone. Burnett and Bolton (1972) reported that in 247 patients followed up for 2 to 8 years after a normal preexploratory cholangiogram, not one developed clinical evidence of a residual stone.

The examination has an additional advantage in that it may demonstrate abnormalities in the bile duct system. Indeed, Schulenburg (1969) reported significant variations from the normal in no less than 22 percent of his series. The most important abnormalities that the examination may reveal are drainage of the cystic duct into the right hepatic duct and a low insertion of the cystic duct into the common bile duct.

Attempts to identify a select group of patients in whom cholangiography is indicated on clinical and operative criteria is not recommended. At least 4 percent of patients will have common bile duct stones overlooked if this policy is adopted. The widely held view that a large solitary stone in the gallbladder is not associated with ductal stones is not supported by the

1972 study of Mullen and colleagues, who concluded that 4 percent of patients with a large solitary stone in the gallbladder had associated stones in the common duct.

Preexploratory cholangiography is often omitted in patients who are jaundiced at the time of surgery or who have a palpable stone in the common bile duct. Although these findings are certainly absolute indications for duct exploration, a cholangiogram can provide valuable information concerning the number and site of the stones as well as the local ductal anatomy before choledochotomy is performed.

TECHNIQUE OF COMMON DUCT EXPLORATION

Exploration of the common duct usually is performed after the cholangiogram has confirmed the presence of common duct stones and before removal of the gallbladder. Before exploration of the common duct, the cystic duct is ligated. This obviates the risk that manipulation of the gallbladder will force small stones down the cystic duct and into the common duct after the latter has been explored.

Exploration of the common duct through the stump of the cystic duct does not give adequate access and is not recommended.

The decision to explore the common duct having been taken, the area of the free edge of the lesser omentum is exposed by the suitable positioning of packs, retractors, and the assistant's hand. The essential steps are retraction of the right lobe of the liver upward, displacement of the duodenum downward, and the retraction of the stomach to the left. The peritoneum over the anterolateral surface of the common duct is divided and the duct exposed by clearing away any overlying fatty tissue. A small swab held in a long artery forceps is invaluable for this.

Before opening the common duct, a sample of bile is taken by needle aspiration and is sent for bacteriologic examination. Two stay sutures of 2/0 chromic catgut are inserted on the anterior surface of the duct about 2 cm above the superior border of the duodenum (Fig. 78–13) and the duct opened longitudinally between them with a scalpel (Fig. 78–14). The incision is enlarged to a length of about 2 cm and should terminate immediately above the duodenum. Any escaping bile is removed by a sucker. If

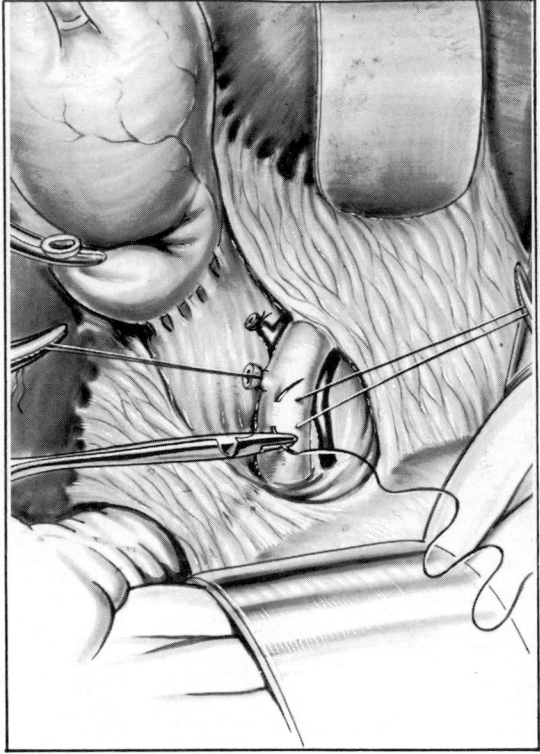

Figure 78–13. Exploration of the common duct: Insertion of the stay sutures.

this initial incision exposes calculi, they should be removed immediately.

With the margins of the incision held open by the stay sutures, the ducts are explored by means of Desjardin's forceps. These are passed first upward into the common hepatic and right and left hepatic ducts, any calculi encountered being extracted. Removal of stones from the region of the junction of the two ducts is often difficult, and sometimes they are more easily removed by the insertion of a fine sucker up the duct. A small modified Fogarty catheter is another useful instrument for removal of small stones.

On completion of exploration of the proximal ducts, if it is suspected that the lower reaches of the common duct contain many stones, it is wise to insert a small swab into the common hepatic duct to prevent stones passing up toward the liver during subsequent manipulation; a marker length of suitable ligature material must be attached to this swab and care

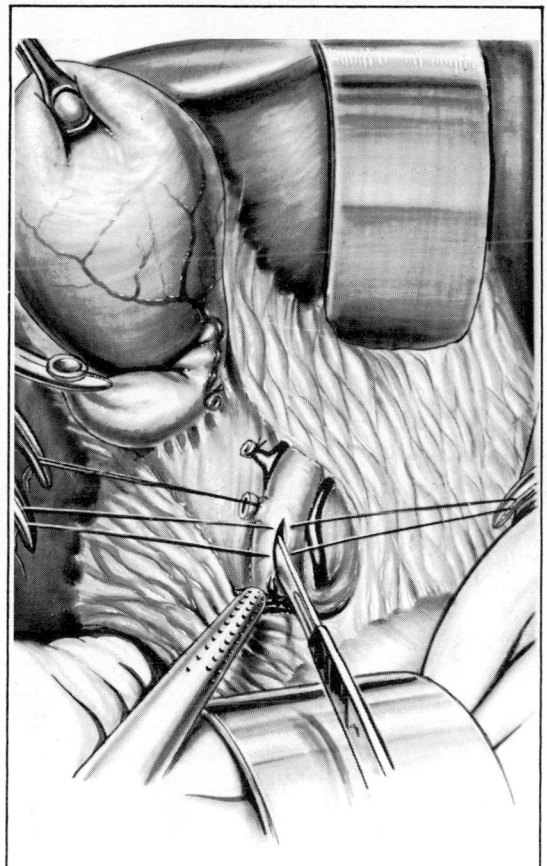

Figure 78–14. Exploration of the common duct: The duct is incised between the stay sutures. Note the sucker, to remove escaping bile.

taken to see that it is removed at the end of the operation (Fig. 78–15).

Any stones in the lower part of the duct are now removed by passing Desjardin's forceps down toward the duodenum. If there is a large stone in the intrapancreatic portion of the duct, it may only be removed by mobilising the duodenum and head of the pancreas by Kocher's manoeuvre and manipulating the stone with the fingers inserted behind the head of the pancreas at the same time as attempts are made to grasp it with the forceps passed down the duct through the choledochotomy incision. If the duct contains many small stones, sludge, or grit, it is necessary to irrigate the duct with normal saline via a catheter.

It is in just these circumstances, especially if the common duct is grossly dilated and there

are many small stones in the hepatic ducts, that it is often advisable to perform either a sphincterotomy or choledochoduodenostomy, as will be described. Failure to be able to remove a stone impacted at the lower end of the duct is also an indication for duodenotomy and transsphincteric removal.

To complete exploration of the duct, the Desjardin forceps or a Bakes' dilator is passed down the duct into the duodenum (Fig. 78–16). In doing this it is very easy to push the duodenal papilla forward against the anteromedial wall of the duodenum and on palpation it may appear that the instrument has entered the duodenal lumen when, in fact, it is still within the duct. To be sure that the instrument has entered the duodenum, it is essential either to feel the cuff of the papilla around the instrument where it is entering the duodenum (Fig. 78–17) or to feel the instrument several inches down the duodenum, well beyond the opening of the duct.

Some surgeons complete the exploration by dilating the terminal portion of the duct by the passage of increasingly large bougies. There is no concrete evidence that this is of any value and this author believes that traumatising the sphincter in this way may lead to later stricture formation.

Having cleared the ducts as carefully as possible of stones, many surgeons at this stage perform *choledochoscopy*, using either the flexible fibre-optic instrument or the rigid choledochoscope. If the duct is of small diameter this technique is not possible and may actually produce trauma to the duct. The instrument is particularly useful in searching the widely dilated duct system in which multiple stones have been discovered. Any residual stones or debris discovered at this examination are removed either by a balloon catheter or wire basket (Ashby, 1978).

Whether or not choledochoscopy is performed, a T-tube is now placed in the choledochotomy incision and the duct closed around the tube with 2/0 Dexon or chromic catgut as a continuous suture. There are a number of important points in the technique of T-tube drainage. The limbs of the T should be cut short, each limb being about 1 cm in length. A long length of tube that may project down through the sphincter may occasionally precipitate pancreatitis and in any case a long T may traumatise the duct on removal. The T-tube should be brought out at the lower extremity of the bile duct incision to avoid pulling on the suture line

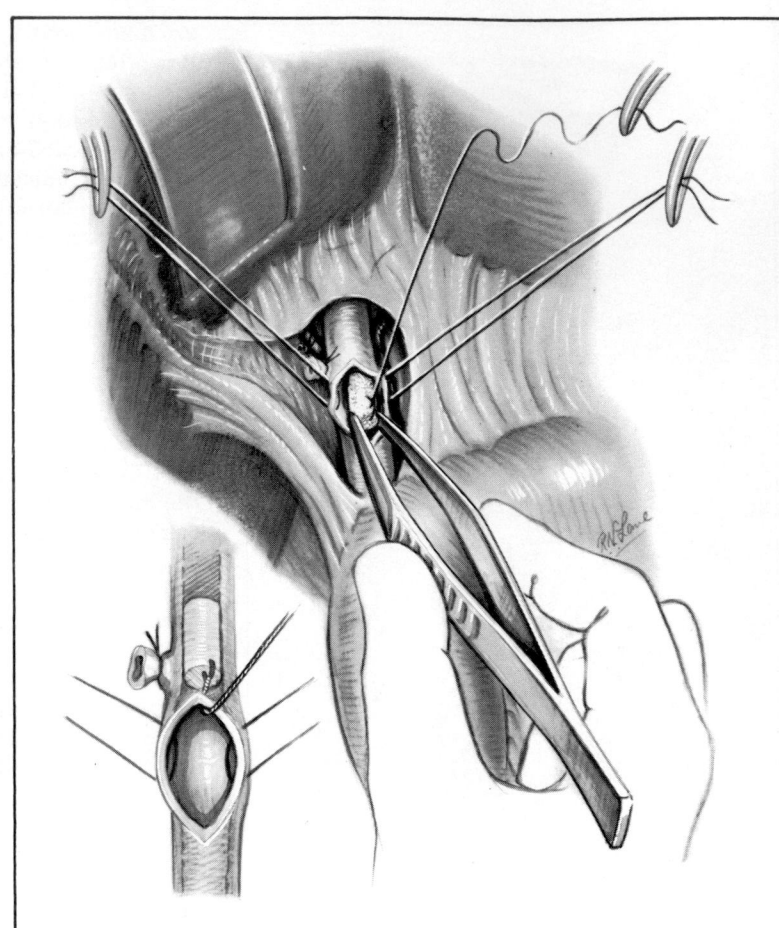

Figure 78–15. Exploration of the common duct: Insertion of a small swab into the common hepatic duct. When the lower duct is thought to contain small stones and debris this manoeuvre is useful in preventing the passage of small stones up into the proximal duct. Note the stay suture attached to the swab.

when the tube is removed (Figs. 78–18 and 78–19). It is important that the T-tube be made of latex rubber and not of polyvinylchloride or other plastic materials, as such materials are so inert in the tissues that they cause no adhesive reaction, with the result that on removal of the tube a biliary leak or bile peritonitis may develop. Winstone and colleagues (1965) have described four such cases.

Postexploratory Cholangiography. Cholangiography should now be carried out once again via the T-tube in order to determine whether exploration of the duct has succeeded in removing all stones or whether some still remain. As with the preexploratory examination, all instruments and other radiopaque objects must be removed from the operation site. A difficulty in this examination is to rid the common duct of air bubbles. To effect this, the T-tube is flushed with normal saline, first to check that a water-

tight closure has been obtained (Fig. 78–20) and then to wash all the bubbles from the duct. Once this is achieved, a syringe containing a water-soluble radiopaque solution (Conray 280) is substituted for the saline, care being taken that air is not introduced into the T-tube while changing syringes. Owing to the dead space within the T-tube, larger quantities of contrast medium have to be injected than in the preexploratory examination. Two films should be exposed, the first after injection of 5 ml and the second after the injection of 10 ml of the medium. If the duct is markedly dilated, even larger quantities may be required.

Apart from the problem of the presence of air bubbles, the interpretation of the films of a postexploratory cholangiogram is further complicated by the fact that failure to demonstrate flow of contrast medium into the duodenum and to visualise the terminal segment of the duct is common, presumably as a result of

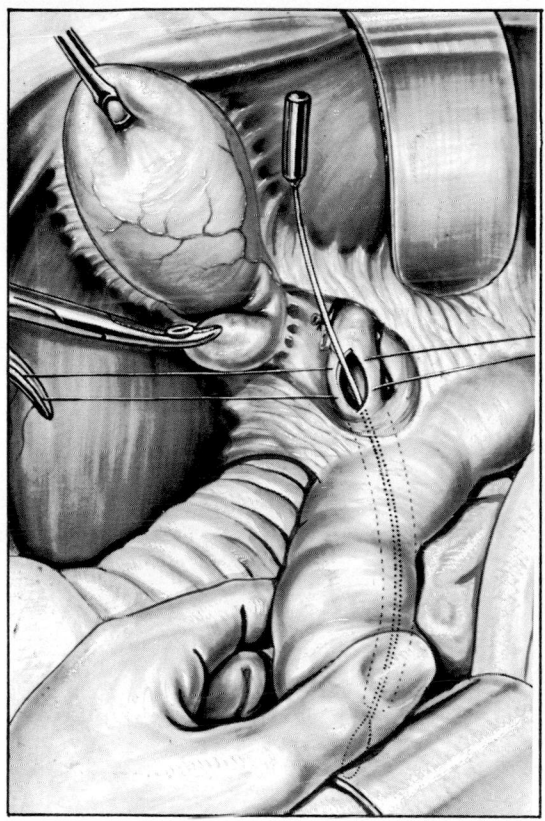

Figure 78–16. Exploration of the common duct: Passage of a sound down the duct into the duodenum.

attached to a sterile plastic bag. In addition, a corrugated drain is passed down to the region of the common duct before closing the abdominal wound and this is brought out through the abdominal wall through a second stab incision. Although this author now rarely drains a routine cholecystectomy, common duct explorations are always drained because of the risk of some bile leakage around the side of the T-tube.

Controversial Points. There are surgeons who practice primary closure of the common bile duct after exploration and others who decry the use of postexploration of T-tube cholangiography. In this author's opinion, neither group has proved its case to satisfaction.

It is perfectly true that the common bile duct can be closed safely by primary suture with little risk of leakage. Sawyers et al (1965) reported the results in 250 patients undergoing exploration of the common duct with T-tube drainage compared with 250 patients undergoing the same operation with primary closure of the duct; they encountered no untoward results in the first group on the grounds of postoperative morbidity or mortality and there was certainly a shorter stay in hospital compared with the conventional technique of T-tube drainage. Collins (1967) performed primary closure of the common duct in 57 out of 70 common

spasm. Ginzburg et al (1967) found that 30 out of 56 postexploratory cholangiograms showed obstruction to the contrast at the level of the sphincter but only one of these had a stone on reexploration. All demonstrated flow into the duodenum at a subsequent postoperative cholangiogram. Accordingly, the only reliable indication of a residual stone in the duct is a filling defect (Fig. 78–21) and to this extent postexploratory cholangiography is not so sensitive a method of investigation as the preexploratory examination. Should the T-tube cholangiogram demonstrate one or more stones then, of course, the duct must be reopened, the stones removed, the T-tube replaced, and a further check cholangiogram performed. This whole procedure may be quite a tedious affair, but it fades into insignificance against the very real morbidity to the patient if a stone is left within the duct.

Before proceeding to the completion of cholecystectomy, the T-tube should be brought out through the lateral abdominal wall via a small stab wound; at the end of the operation it is

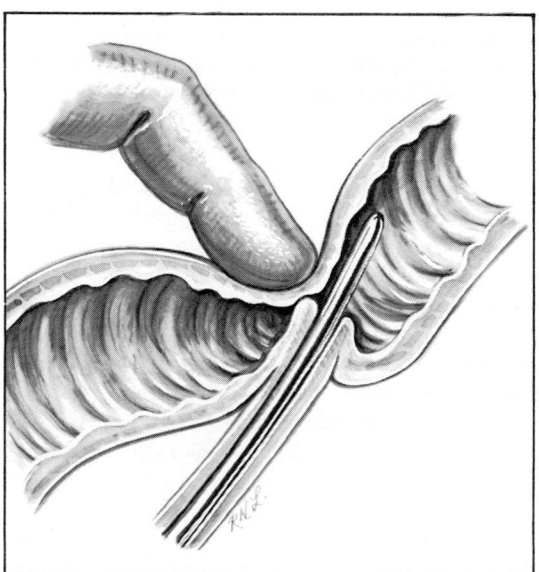

Figure 78–17. Exploration of the common duct: Palpation of the papilla as a cuff surrounding the bougie, to make certain that the bougie has entered the duodenum.

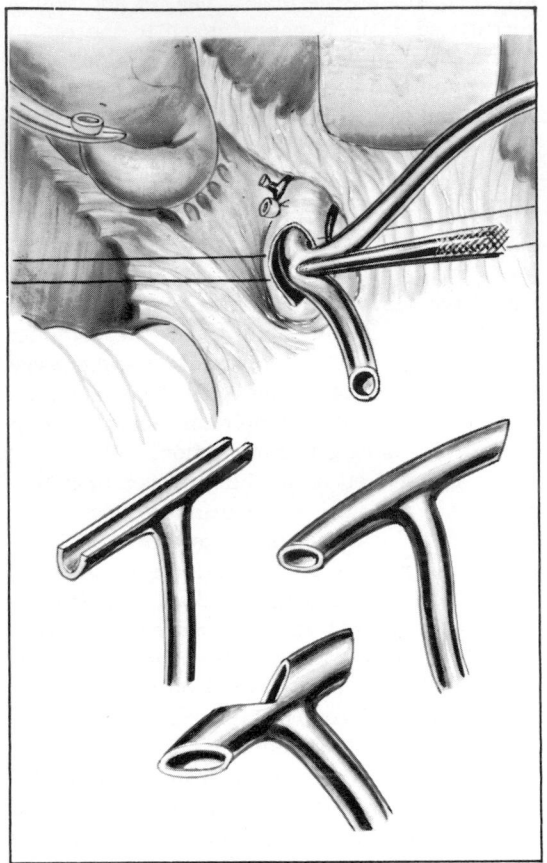

Figure 78–18. Exploration of the common duct: Insertion of the T-tube. Insert shows the various types of T-tubes available: Maingot's split tube (*top left*) is that most commonly used, and is the easiest to insert. Before inserting the tube, its patency should be tested by flushing it with saline.

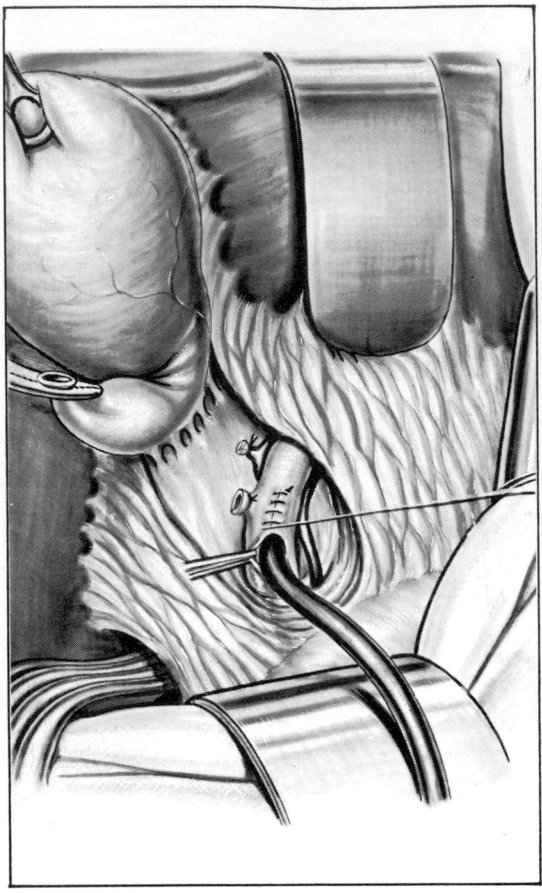

Figure 78–19. Exploration of the common duct: Closure of the duct, with fine Dexon on an atraumatic needle, around the emergent T-tube. Note that the tube protrudes from the lower end of the incision. The corrugated drain to the subhepatic space is shown in position.

duct explorations without complications. His contraindications to this procedure were undue trauma to the duct (for example removal of an impacted stone), suppurative cholangitis, and associated pancreatitis, where transduodenal procedures on the ampulla had been carried out and when the common bile duct was of narrow calibre and thin walled and where stenosis might follow primary suture. Similar recommendations were made by Sawyers and colleagues.

The importance of T-tube drainage is not the prevention of biliary leakage but the fact that, even after the most meticulous precautions, a proportion of patients will demonstrate residual stones on the postoperative T-tube cholangiogram and only this technique will give a completely reliable answer as to whether or not the duct has been completely cleared. Moreover, the T-tube track in such cases provides access to the duct for percutaneous removal of such residual stones.

Although postexploratory cholangiography has its limitations, it is still of great value in picking up overlooked stones—for example, Nienhuis (1961) reported the demonstration of residual calculi in 3 out of 36 patients and others have reported similar figures. It is true that stones can be missed. Millward (1982) has recently reported 37 patients studied by postexploratory operative cholangiography in which one stone was found which would otherwise have been missed. A further six were overlooked and only demonstrated on subsequent postoperative cholangiography. However, even the demonstration of this single stone, with the prevention

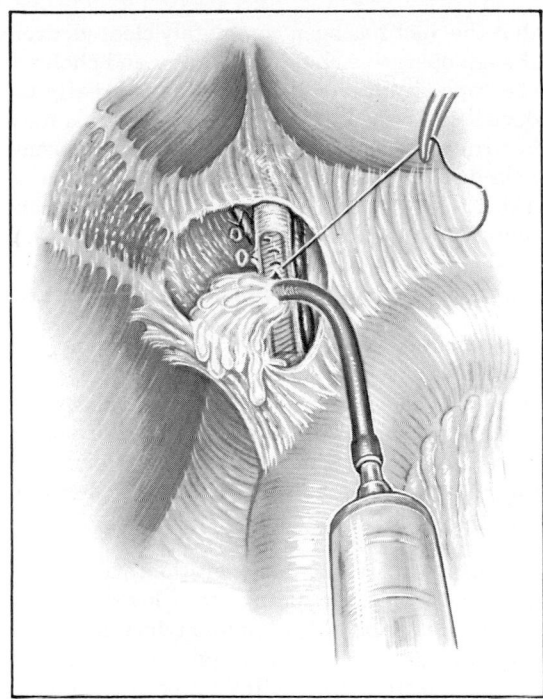

Figure 78–20. Postexploratory cholangiography: To remove bubbles from the duct, the T-tube is flushed with saline at intervals during closure of the duct.

of all the problems of its subsequent removal, made a few extra minutes in the operating theatre well worthwhile.

There seems little doubt that the most certain way of ensuring clear common duct is to carry out choledochoscopy (provided that the duct is dilated) followed by an immediate T-tube cholangiography. Choledochoscopy alone cannot be guaranteed to reveal every stone. Keighley and Kappas (1980), for example, report 73 patients where operative choledochoscopy was performed after exploration of the bile ducts. In 13 instances, further stones were seen and removed and in the remaining 60 the ducts appeared clear; however, 9 of these patients were found to have further stones, 4 on subsequent T-tube cholangiography and 5 because of the development of later problems.

To conclude, the surgeon must take every precaution after exploring the common bile duct to ensure the duct is clear. The choledochoscope should be used if available, if the surgeon is skilled in its use, and if the duct is dilated. This should be supplemented by a T-tube cholangiogram on the operating table, even with the im-

perfections of this technique. Because there is still a risk of retained stones, a T-tube drainage is obligatory to allow postoperative cholangiography, which will either confirm that the ducts are clear or allow access for percutaneous or endoscopic transphincteric manipulation should there still be, in spite of every care, retained calculi within the common duct.

Antibiotic Prophylaxis. Stones in the common bile duct, especially in the presence of jaundice, are associated with a high incidence of infected bile (Keighley and Burdon, 1979). The aerobic organisms usually present are *Escherichia coli, Klebsiella aerogenes,* and *Strepto-*

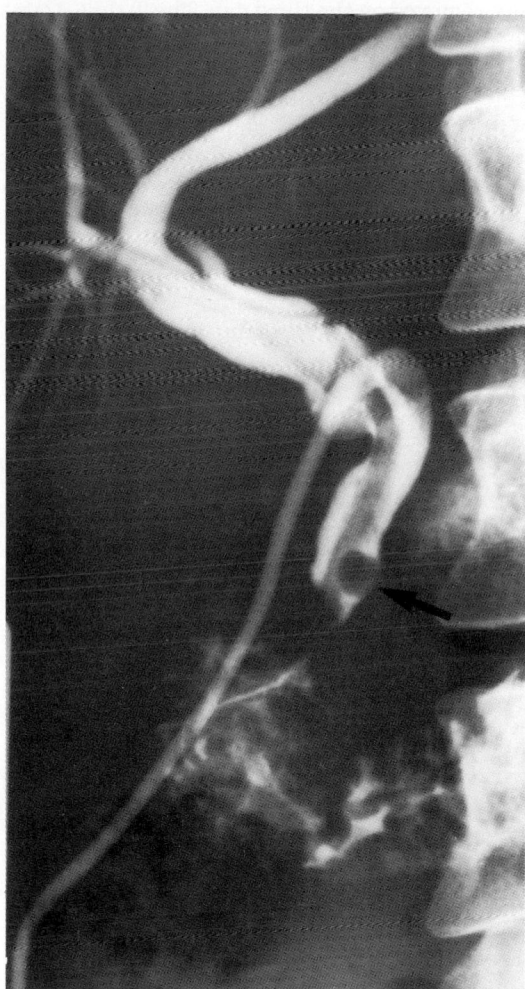

Figure 78–21. Residual stone in common bile duct (*arrow*) demonstrated on T-tube cholangiography.

coccus faecalis. The common anaerobes are *Clostridium perfringens* and *Anaerobic streptococci.* The genus *Bacteroides* is extremely uncommon in bile.

Exploration of the common bile duct should be covered with antibiotic prophylaxis, using an aminoglycoside (e.g., gentamicin) or a cephalosporin. My current practice is to use cefuroxime. The particular antibiotic regime may need to be modified as a result of the bacteriologic study of the bile.

The subject of infection in biliary tract surgery is considered in detail later in this chapter.

Postoperative Care. The T-tube is allowed to drain freely postoperatively into a sterile plastic bag. A separate corrugated drain is covered by a sterile bag, shortened after 48 hours, and usually removed on the third day. The T-tube drainage is recorded daily. Preparatory to its removal, the T-tube is clamped for an increasing time each day, starting with a period of 2 to 4 hours on the fourth day and ending with continuous occlusion on the eighth or ninth day after operation. Alternatively, the sterile bag is raised by attaching it to the patient's hospital gown so that the hydrostatic pressure in the drainage system enables the bile to flow down the duct into the duodenum.

Postoperative cholangiography is performed in the x-ray department on the seventh day by the injection of water-soluble contrast medium down the T-tube. Very careful precautions are taken to ensure that gas bubbles are not introduced into the system. Provided that the cholangiographic findings are normal, the T-tube is removed on the tenth day. This is done by gentle firm traction and causes little pain. Usually there is only a slight discharge from the tract for a few hours, after which time it dries up completely.

ADDITIONAL DRAINAGE PROCEDURES: CHOLEDOCHODUODENOSTOMY, SPHINCTEROTOMY, AND SPHINCTEROPLASTY

Indications. The removal of multiple stones from the lower end of the common bile duct through a supraduodenal choledochotomy incision may be a difficult procedure and, particularly if there are small stones and debris in a dilated duct, it may be impossible to be certain that the duct has been completely cleared, even though operative cholangiography and choledochoscopy, as already discussed, have greatly reduced this risk. In other cases, a calculus may be firmly impacted at the lower end of the common duct. Under these circumstances, there is a risk that the patient may have further symptoms from residual or recurrent stones. For this reason, an additional operative procedure is often thought wise. The available procedures are:

CHOLEDOCHODUODENOSTOMY. The purpose of this operation is to construct a wide, new stoma between the common duct and the duodenum, providing free drainage of bile, even if stones have been overlooked or new calculi form at a later date (Capper, 1961; Hosford, 1957; Johnson and Rains, 1972; Madden et al, 1970).

SPHINCTEROTOMY. In this operation, part of the musculature surrounding the lower, intraduodenal portion of the common duct is divided (Fig. 78–22) to allow thorough exploration of the duct from below. After its performance, a postoperative T-tube cholangiogram is indistinguishable from normal. The sole purpose of this procedure, in relation to the operative treatment of choledocholithiasis, is to provide access to the lower reaches of the common bile duct (Carter, 1983).

SPHINCTEROPLASTY. In this operation, the entire length of the musculature surrounding the lower end of the common duct is divided (Fig. 78–22). Not only does this procedure allow thorough exploration of the duct from below, but it is also designed to give free drainage of the bile through a wide opening. It is, in effect, an internal choledochoduodenostomy and is described fully in Chapter 81.

Choice of Drainage Procedure

From the reported results of experienced surgeons, there is no evidence that there is a significant difference in the mortality of the three surgical drainage procedures of choledochoduodenostomy, sphincterotomy, and sphincteroplasty. All three give excellent long-term results. The important questions in relation to these operations are:

1. Under what cirumstances should an additional procedure be added to supraduodenal exploration of the common bile duct?
2. What procedure should be used?

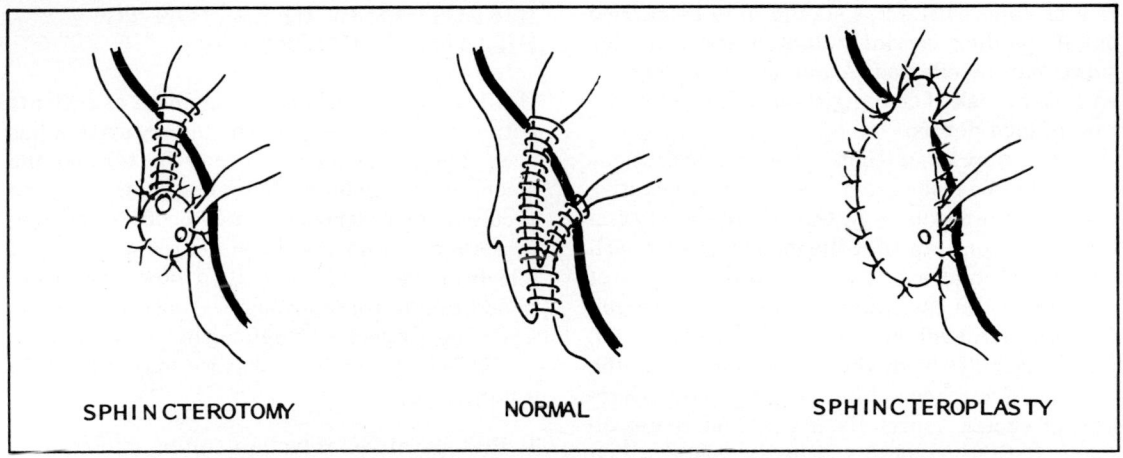

SPHINCTEROTOMY   NORMAL   SPHINCTEROPLASTY

Figure 78–22. Diagrammatic representation of the difference between the operations of sphinc-terotomy and sphincteroplasty. In the operation of spincterotomy, the greater part of the intra-duodenal portion of the sphincteric musculature surrounding the lower end of the common duct is divided, but a major portion remains undisturbed. Spincteroplasty involves division of the whole length of the sphincter, and of necessity involves an incision through the full thickness of the posteromedial wall of the duodenum.

With regard to the first, clearly if as a result of an impacted stone, or the presence of quantities of grit and sludge, it is impossible to clear the lower reaches of the duct by supraduodenal exploration, then a further procedure is indicated. Even if there is no impaction of stone at the lower end of the duct but this is widely dilated and there has been obvious infection, particularly if the surgeon is now operating on recurrence of common duct stone after previous exploration, it can be argued that to prevent subsequent stone formation a procedure is required to provide free drainage from the duct. Under these circumstances many surgeons, including myself, would perform a choledochoduo-denostomy.

With respect to the choice of procedure, there are few comparative studies but Thomas et al (1971) report that both sphincterotomy and choledochoduodenostomy were effective in over-coming obstruction and preventing recurrent symptoms.

In their own series of 53 sphincterotomies there were 4 deaths (2 from pancreatitis) compared with 2 deaths in 57 choledochoduodenos-tomies. The morbidity and follow-up results (at an average of 3 years later) were comparable. The same authors collected a large series of pub-lished reports of the two operations, again with very similar results (Table 78–1).

Sphincterotomy carries with it a slight risk of postoperative pancreatitis and should proba-bly be avoided if there have been previous epi-sodes of pancreatitis. It has the advantage of leaving the patient with a duct draining through an apparently competent sphincter, and the long-term results are satisfactory. *Cho-ledochoduodenostomy* does not carry the same

TABLE 78–1. COLLECTED RESULTS OF SPHINCTEROTOMY AND CHOLEDOCHODUODENOSTOMY

Operation	Sphincterotomy	Choledochoduodenostomy
Number of papers reviewed	10	10
Dates of publication	From 1956	From 1946
Number of cases	1061	733
Hospital mortality	4.6%	3.0%
Postoperative pancreatitis	1.1%	1.0%
Postoperative cholangitis	0.8%	0.8%

(Source: From Thomas CG, Nicholson CP, et al, 1971, with permission.)

risk of pancreatitis but should only be carried out if the duct is widely dilated and if a wide stoma can be effected. A narrow stoma carries with it the risk of cholangitis and the accumulation of food debris.

It is now clear that these two operations should not be looked upon as simple alternative additional procedures in the treatment of common duct stone but that the indications for each are rather different, although with an area of overlap. If the essential problem is the search for, and removal of, stones (particularly impacted calculi) from the lower portion of the common duct, then sphincterotomy is the operation of choice, especially if the duct is not dilated. If this procedure is to be performed, it is wise to make the decision as soon as possible in the course of the operation, rather than after prolonged fruitless attempts to remove an impacted stone. If, however, the essential problem is the provision of drainage of a widely dilated and infected duct, then choledochoduodenostomy is the preferred procedure, particularly if there has already been a previous exploration of the duct and one is dealing with recurrent stone. Again it must be emphasised that this operation should not be performed unless the common duct is dilated.

With regard to *sphincteroplasty,* the evidence of Jones (1973) suggests that it is a safe and effective procedure, but it does involve an incision through the full thickness of the posteromedial wall of the duodenum; the majority of surgeons would advocate a simple sphincterotomy under the circumstances delineated previously.

The situation is further complicated by the fact that more and more common duct stones are being removed nowadays by endoscopic sphincterotomy. This is particularly true for recurrent or residual calculi following common duct exploration. It may be that in the future, the majority of cases of stones in the common duct will be dealt with by the endoscopic route if long-term studies confirm the efficacy of this technique. This will apply particularly to elderly and infirm patients (Dowling, 1983). A recent report by Salvioli and colleagues (1983), from Modena, Italy, on the dissolution of radiolucent biliary duct stones in 7 out of 14 patients treated with ursodeoxycholic acid gives rise to hope for medical treatment, at least in a proportion of such cases.

INFECTION IN RELATION TO BILIARY SURGERY

Until recent years, the management of patients with calculous disease of the biliary system has been dominated by what may be termed the mechanical problems they present, that is, the problems of diagnosis, removal of stones, and preservation and provision of free drainage of bile into the duodenum. It is now clear that, in addition to these problems, those of infection are more important than hitherto recognised.

Infection in biliary disease may present in a number of ways:

1. Postoperative infection after cholecystectomy is still common. In many cases this amounts to nothing more than minor wound infection, but there may be the serious complications of septicaemia, liver abscess, hepatic failure, disseminated intravascular coagulation, renal failure, and endotoxaemia, with, inevitably, an associated mortality.
2. Sepsis may be a presenting feature of calculous biliary disease. There may be local pain, pyrexia, and rigors or even the classic features of Charcot's intermittent hepatic fever, with pyrexia, pain, and jaundice. Occasionally patients may present in shock because of an extreme septicaemia.
3. Septicaemia may also occur after such manipulations as transhepatic cholangiography and endoscopic retrograde catheterisation of the bile duct, when there is introduction of contrast material under pressure into the infected biliary tract.

Bacteriology. Normal bile is sterile, but there is a wide range of incidence of bacteria in the bile in patients with calculous disease, positive cultures being obtained in about 10 percent of patients with a normally functioning gallbladder containing stones, rising to 80 percent in patients undergoing emergency surgery for acute cholecystitis or in cases of stones or stricture in the common duct. Gunn (1976) found positive bile culture in 19 percent of the elective cholecystectomies and 35 percent of emergency operations. It was found that infected bile is likely to be associated with elderly patients, recent acute cholecystitis, and an obstructed and dilated common bile duct.

Keighley et al (1976) studied 181 patients undergoing biliary tract surgery. They were able to define eight variables that were more common in patients with infected than with noninfected bile: jaundice at the time of operation, recent rigors, emergency operation or one within 4 weeks of an emergency admission, age over 70 years, previous biliary operation, common bile duct obstruction, and stones in the common duct. In patients where one or more of these high-risk factors was present, the bile contained organisms in 53 percent. When four high-risk factors occurred in the same patient, organisms were isolated in 87 percent compared with the low-risk group in which the incidence of infected bile was 19 percent.

The predominant organisms in bile are *Escherichia coli, Klebsiella,* and *Streptococcus faecalis. Bacteroides fragilis* is extremely uncommon in patients with stones although it is frequently recovered after a previous anastomosis between the biliary tract and the intestine, especially if there is a recurrent stricture. *Clostridium welchii* can be recovered in about 10 percent of bile specimens in gallbladder disease and is frequently found in acute acalculous cholecystitis. Keighley (1982) has shown that the bile is usually colonized by more than one organism. He isolated a single bacterial species in 38 percent of patients with a positive bile culture, two species in 29 percent, three in 20 percent, four in 12 percent, and more than four different isolates in 1 percent.

In the majority of instances, these organisms cause no overt changes in the bile, bile ducts, or liver, but in the presence of significant obstruction they give rise to cholangitis with acute inflammatory changes in the wall of the bile duct, spreading up into the portal tracts, and in severe cases the bile ducts become full of purulent bile and liver abscesses may develop.

Clinical Manifestations. Just as in the majority of instances the infection gives rise to no overt changes in the duct, so also the majority of patients show no clinical evidence of this infection, save for an increased incidence of septic postoperative complications. Keighley (1982) reviewed a series of 181 biliary tract operations where no antibiotic cover was employed. The overall incidence of wound sepsis was 20 percent and there was a significantly higher incidence after emergency surgery (41 percent) than after elective operations (18 percent). In the elective operations, the incidence of wound sepsis was three times greater when the common duct was explored than after cholecystectomy alone.

In some patients, however, the biliary tract infection may produce obvious clinical effects, the most common being the occurrence of fever in a patient with so-called biliary colic, which is sometimes accompanied by a rigor. In such patients, a blood culture may well confirm the presence of a transient septicaemia. Usually the fever settles, but in some patients it recurs, producing a picture of *Charcot intermittent hepatic fever.*

In some patients the infection dominates the clinical picture. Occasionally a patient with a stone in the common duct may present with fever and rigors, but little or no pain and no history suggesting the presence of gallstones. In these circumstances the diagnosis may be elusive. By far the most serious condition in which the infective element dominates the picture is that of acute, obstructive suppurative cholangitis, well reviewed by Faber and colleagues (1978). This condition is caused by calculus obstruction of the common duct, leading to accumulation of infected bile under pressure within the biliary system and leading in turn to septicaemia with shock and liver damage. Clinically the condition is characterised by a diagnostic pentad of abdominal pain, fever, jaundice, mental confusion, and shock. If untreated, it often causes acute renal failure. Unless diagnosed promptly and treated correctly there is a significant mortality.

If pain is a prominent feature of the acute illness, and if there is a previous history indicative of gallstones, the diagnosis may be relatively easy. However, in many instances there is no such previous history, and if pain is absent or only mild and the patient admitted to hospital with such a degree of mental confusion that a clear story cannot be given, then the overall clinical picture can be confused with a number of other medical conditions not requiring prompt operative treatment for their relief. The introduction of the new investigative techniques of ultrasound and endoscopic retrograde cholangiography provides important assistance in achieving a correct diagnosis.

Treatment. Many studies have demonstrated that the incidence of wound infection following cholecystectomy can undoubtedly be reduced by means of prophylactic systemic antibiotic therapy. For example, Stubbs (1983) noted an incidence of wound infection of 15 percent for cholecystectomy alone and 30 percent when the common duct was explored before routine prophylaxis was introduced, which fell to 3.6 and 3.4 percent, respectively, when antibiotic cover was given. It has been suggested that immediate Gram staining of bile at the time of operation can define those patients at risk and give an indication of the specific antibiotic regime. McLeish and colleagues (1977) gave gentamicin if gram-negative organisms were seen and ampicillin for gram-positive organisms. Using this technique in a controlled trial, they reduced their wound sepsis rate from 22 percent in the control group receiving no antibiotics to 7 percent in the treated group.

Our own regimen is to use cefuroxime as a routine in two doses, one at the time of premedication and the second 12 hours later.

If the patient's presenting symptoms of pain, jaundice, and so on are accompanied by a fever and/or rigors, a blood culture should be performed and antibiotic therapy commenced. A cephalosporin or gentamicin is the drug of choice. In the majority of instances, the fever will subside, but despite this, operation should be undertaken without undue delay, as the condition may well recur. If the fever does not subside promptly, continued conservative treatment is unlikely to be beneficial and operation to remove the stones should be performed before the more serious complications of cholangitis develop. Usually it is safe to perform a cholecystectomy with formal exploration of the common duct, but in a seriously ill patient whose condition is deteriorating, simple drainage of the common duct may be all that is possible at first operation. It is probable that in these instances endoscopic sphincterotomy will prove to be the emergency treatment of choice.

By far the most serious manifestation of infection complicating biliary calculi is acute, obstructive, suppurative cholangitis. The essential steps in the management of this condition are:

1. To administer appropriate antibiotics
2. To give adequate appropriate intravenous fluids
3. To establish promptly free drainage from the common duct

A very serious complication is the development of acute renal failure. Patients with this condition should be treated on the same lines as outlined above but in severe cases dialysis may be required.

Cahill (1983) has demonstrated that prophylactic administration of the bile salt sodium deoxycholate in patients with obstructive jaundice prevents postoperative endotoxaemia by a direct effect on the endotoxin and greatly reduces the risk of renal failure.

BIBLIOGRAPHY

Ashby BS: Fibreoptic choledochoscopy in common bile duct surgery. Ann R Coll Surg Engl 60:399, 1978

Bolton JP, Le Quesne LP: Choledocholithiasis, in Smith, Lord, SS (ed): Surgery of the Gall Bladder and Bile Ducts, 2 edt. London: Butterworths, 1981, p 257

Burnett W, Bolton PM: Operative cholangiography in the surgery of gallstones: Implementation of a policy decision in a consecutive series of 327 patients. Aust NZ J Surg 42:14, 1972

Cahill CJ: Prevention of postoperative renal failure in patients with obstructive jaundice—the role of bile salts. Br J Surg 70:590, 1983

Capper WM: External choledochoduodenostomy. An evaluation of 125 cases. Br J Surg 49:292, 1961

Carter AE: The transduodenal per-ampullary approach to common bile duct calculi. Ann R Coll Surg Engl 65:183, 1983

Chapman M, Curry RC, et al: Operative cholangiography. An assessment of its reliability in the diagnosis of a normal, stone-free common bile duct. Br J Surg 51:600, 1964

Collins PG: Further experience with common bile-duct suture without intraductal drainage following choledochotomy. Br J Surg 54:854, 1967

Cooperberg PL, Burhenne HJ: Real-time ultrasonography. Diagnostic technique of choice in calculous gallbladder disease. N Engl J Med 302:1277, 1980

Cooperman AM, Haaga J, et al: Computed tomography: A valuable aid to the abdominal surgeon. Am J Surg 133:121, 1977

Dewbury KC, Joseph AEA, et al: Ultrasound in the evaluation and diagnosis of jaundice. Br J Radiol 52:276, 1979

Dowling RH: Management of stones in the biliary tree. Gut 24:599, 1983

Faber RG, Ibrahim SZ, et al: Gallstone disease presenting as septicaemic shock. Br J Surg 65:101, 1978

Faris I, Thomson JP, et al: Operative cholangiography. A reappraisal based on a review of 400 cholangiograms. Br J Surg 62:966, 1975

French EB, Robb WAT: Biliary and renal colic. Br Med J 2:135, 1963

Gardner AM, Holden WS, et al: Disappearing gall-stones. Br J Surg 53:114, 1966

Ginzburg L, Geffer A, et al: Pseudo-obstruction following post-choledochotomy cholangiography. Ann Surg 166:83, 1967

Gitnick G: Assessment of liver function. Surg Clin North Am 61:197, 1981

Glenn F: Choledochotomy in non-malignant disease of the biliary tract. Surg Gynecol Obstet 124:974, 1967

Graham N, Lees WR: The problem of gallstones in the ultrasonographic diagnosis of jaundice. Br J Radiol 53:619, 1980

Gunn AA: Antibiotics in biliary surgery. Br J Surg 63:627, 1976

Havard C: Operative cholangiography. Br J Surg 57:797, 1970

Hosford J: Treatment of stone in the common bile duct. Br Med J 1:1202, 1957

Johnson AG, Harding Rains AJ: Choledochoduodenostomy. A reappraisal of its indications based on a study of 64 patients. Br J Surg 59:277, 1972

Jones SA: Sphincteroplasty (not sphincterotomy) in the treatment of biliary tract disease. Surg Clin North Am 53:1123, 1973

Kakos GS, Tompkins RK, et al: Operative cholangiography during routine cholecystectomy. A review of 3012 cases. Arch Surg 104:484, 1972

Keighley MRB: Infection and the biliary tree, in Blumgart LH (ed): The Biliary Tract. Edinburgh: Churchill-Livingstone, 1982, p 219

Keighley MRB, Burdon DW: Antimicrobial Prophylaxis in Surgery. Tunbridge Wells: Pitman Medical, 1979, p 70

Keighley MRB, Flinn R, et al: Multivariate analysis of clinical and operative findings associated with biliary sepsis. Br J Surg 63:528, 1976

Keighley MRB, Kappas A: Evaluation of operative choledochoscopy. Surg Gynecol Obstet 150:357, 1980

Kocher T: Ein Fall von Choledochoduodenostomie intern wegen Gallenstein. Corresp Bl Schweiz Ärz 25:193, 1895

Letton AH, Wilson JP: Routine cholangiography during biliary tract operations: Technic and utility in 200 consecutive cases. Ann Surg 163:937, 1966

Levitt RG, Sagel SS, et al: Accuracy of computer tomography of the liver and biliary tract. Radiology 124:123, 1977

McBurney C: Removal of biliary calculi from the common duct by the duodenal route. Ann Surg 28:481, 1898

McLeish AR, Keighley MRB, et al: Selecting patients requiring antibiotics in biliary surgery by immediate Gram stains of bile at operation. Surgery 81:473, 1977

Madden JL: Primary common bile duct stones. World J Surg 2:465, 1978

Madden JL, Chun JY, et al: Choledochoduodenostomy. An unjustly maligned surgical procedure? Am J Surg 119:45, 1970

Millward SF: Post-exploratory operative cholangiography: Is it a useful technique to check clearance of the common bile duct? Clin Radiol 33:535, 1982

Mirizzi PL: La colangiografia durante las operaciones de las vias biliares. Bol Soc Cirug B Aires 16:1133, 1932

Mullen JL, Rosato EF, et al: Gallstone characteristics in the diagnosis of choledocholithiasis. Ann Surg 176:718, 1972

Nienhuis LI: Routine operative cholangiography. Ann Surg 154 (suppl):192, 1961

Nolan DJ, Espiner HJ: Compression of the common bile duct in acute cholecystitis. Br J Radiol 45:821, 1972

Pedrosa CS, Casanova R, et al: Computed tomography in obstructive jaundice. The cause of obstruction. Radiology 139:635, 1981

Peel ALG, Bourke JB, et al: How should the common bile duct be explored? Ann R Coll Surg Engl 56:124, 1975

Rubin JR, Beal JM: Diagnosis of choledocholithiasis. Surg Gynecol Obstet 156:16, 1983

Saltzstein EC, Evani SV, et al: Routine operative cholangiography. Arch Surg 107:289, 1973

Salvioli G, Salati R, et al: Medical treatment of biliary duct stones: Effect of ursodeoxycholic acid administration. Gut 24:609, 1983

Sawyers JL, Herrington JL, et al: Primary closure of the common bile duct. Am J Surg 109:107, 1965

Schulenburg CAR: Operative cholangiography: 1,000 cases. Surgery 65:723, 1969

Sprengel OGK: Über einen Fall von Exstirpation der Gallenblase mit Anlegung einer Communication zwischen Ductus choledochus und Duodenum. Arch Klin Chir 42:550, 1891

Stubbs RS: Wound infection after cholecystectomy: A case for routine prophylaxis. Ann R Coll Surg Engl 65:30, 1983

Taylor KJW, Rosenfield AT: Grey-scale ultrasonography in the differential diagnosis of jaundice. Arch Surg 112:820, 1977

Thomas CG, Nicholson CP, et al: Effectiveness of choledochoduodenostomy and transduodenal sphincterotomy in the treatment of benign obstruction of the common duct. Ann Surg 173:845, 1971

Watkin DFL, Thomas GG: Jaundice in acute cholecystitis. Br J Surg 58:570, 1971

Wild SR, Cruikshank JG, et al: Grey-scale ultrasonography and percutaneous transhepatic cholangiography in biliary tract disease. Br Med J 281:1524, 1980

Winstone NE, Golby MGS, et al: Biliary peritonitis: A hazard of polyvinyl chloride T-tubes. Lancet 1:843, 1965

79. Choledochoduodenostomy

Marvin L. Gliedman
Michael S. Gold

INTRODUCTION

Choledochoduodenostomy is now the accepted operative procedure for primary or secondary choledocholithiasis in the presence of a dilated common bile duct. Numerous studies involving large numbers of cases, many with long-term follow-up, confirm the technical ease, low mortality rate, and excellent results of this procedure. Providing that the essential criteria are met, choledochoduodenostomy is clearly superior to choledochotomy with T-tube or transduodenal sphincteroplasty.

In 1888, Riedel was the first to perform choledochoduodenostomy for common duct stones. The patient died 9 hours postoperatively and at autopsy was found to have a disrupted anastomosis. Sprengel, in 1890, performed the first successful choledochoduodenostomy and gave the procedure its name. In 1913, Sasse reported 10 successful cases and recommended its use routinely in patients with common duct stones to avoid problems with retained calculi. Allen in 1945, reported the occurrence of cholangitis following choledochoduodenostomy when the length of the stoma was less than 2.5 cm. The first United States study was published by Sanders in 1944, reporting 26 cases with 2 deaths postoperatively. Madden reviewed 1255 cases reported in published series from 1946 to 1968 with an overall incidence of cholangitis of 0.4 percent and mortality rates from 0 to 8 percent. Contributions by Degenschein, Schein, and Gliedman continue to attest to the procedure's safety and technical ease.

Choledochoduodenostomy provides a needed solution to a complex problem. Thirty percent of patients undergoing cholecystectomy will have common duct exploration. The overall incidence of common duct stones is approximately 15 percent, ranging from 6.4 percent in patients under age 30 to 33 percent in patients over age 80. Retained stone rates following cholecystectomy, either with or without common duct exploration, range from 1 to 10 percent, averaging 5 percent in many series. As many as 5 to 7 percent of patients require reoperation after cholecystectomy for retained or residual stones. Secondary common bile duct exploration is reported to carry a mortality rate twice that of primary choledochotomy and four times that of simple cholecystectomy. The overall mortality rate for reoperation on the biliary tree is at least 2 percent, with higher rates in elderly patients.

Two basic technical criteria are essential for a successful choledochoduodenostomy. We agree with the majority of authors who consider a dilated common bile duct to be essential. Although the definition of dilatation varies, we now consider a common duct of 1.4 cm diameter to be the usually smallest accepted size. A stoma size of 2.5 cm is essential.

Of the first 100 choledochoduodenostomies performed at the Montefiore Hospital and Medical Center reported by Schein et al in 1978, the majority were done as a secondary procedure, most patients having had cholecystectomy and/or common duct exploration in the past. In their publications in 1980 and 1981, Gliedman and Schein reported an additional 100 choledochoduodenostomies, the majority of which were done as an initial biliary operation in an increasingly elderly population. In the earlier series 17 percent of patients were 80 or over. By the 1981 report 33.3 percent were above 80 years old. The percentage done as a secondary operation decreased from 54 to 33.3 percent. Gaining increasing confidence, more surgeons are relying on choledochoduodenostomy as the primary biliary tract operation. In 1980, Engleberg reported a large series in which 70 percent had choledochoduodenostomies performed as the primary biliary procedure. More recent series of choledochoduodenostomies contain at least 50 percent that were done at the initial biliary tract surgery. This represents a significant increase over the older literature.

INDICATIONS

Multiple Common Bile Duct Calculi (Fig. 79–1)

The technical difficulty of removing all calculi, or sludge, is well known to all who operate on the biliary tree. Even when combining operative cholangiography and choledochoscopy, a significant number of common duct stones will remain. The best available statistics, combining all operative modalities, still result in a retained stone rate of at least 1 percent, with numerous reports continuing to suggest a significantly higher rate. It has been well shown that hepatic bile after cholecystectomy remains lithogenic. The combination of biliary stasis, a dilated common bile duct, and lithogenic bile will inevitably result in a significant number of late primary common duct stones in these patients. Even with negative operating room cholangiography, the number of patients requiring reoperation after T-tube drainage is as high as 10 percent when followed over 10 years. As well, the time

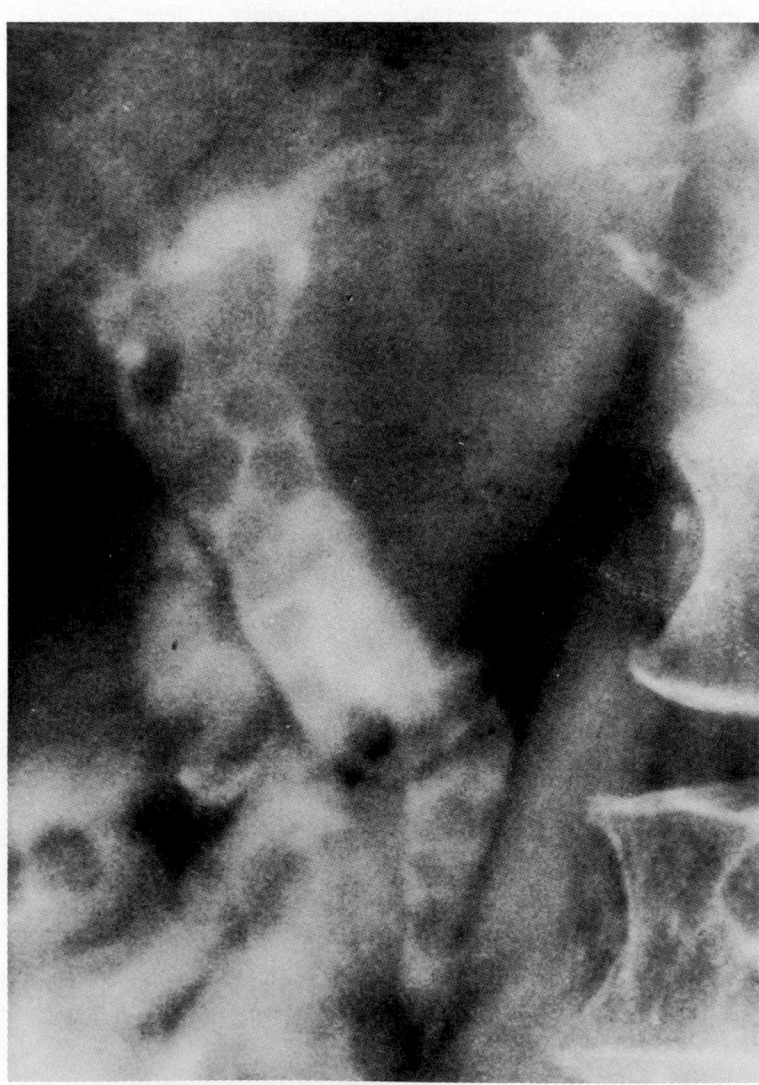

Figure 79–1. Intravenous cholangiogram showing a "cast of stones" in a dilated common bile duct.

involved in cholangiography, choledochoscopy, T-tube placement, repeat cholangiography, and the potential necessity for T-tube removal and reoperation in a missed stone far exceed the time needed to do the choledochoduodenostomy.

Papillary Stenosis (Fig. 79–2)

Diagnosis of this condition is made preoperatively by failure of radionucleatide (IDA scan) to enter the intestinal tract or by the continued and increasing concentration of intravenous contrast in the common bile duct. At operation, the diagnosis is made on cholangiography with the failure of contrast to enter the duodenum in the presence of a dilated common duct without evidence of an impacted distal stone. Failure of a 3-mm dilator to pass into the duodenum is also considered suggestive evidence. A charac-

teristic pattern of the loss of normal tapering of the distal bile duct on cholangiography is often seen. Careful palpation of the ampulla via the duodenotomy prior to choledochoduodenostomy must be done to avoid overlooking an ampullary neoplasm.

Impacted Distal Stone (Fig. 79–3)

Concern with performing choledochoduodenostomy above an impacted distal stone has been put to rest by a large volume of data. In numerous reports no postoperative pancreatitis has been reported although theoretical objections have been raised. Vigorous attempts at manual distal stone removal in a dilated duct are hazardous and should not be done. Direct surgical approach to the sphincter, i.e., sphincterotomy or sphincteroplasty, must be reserved for an im-

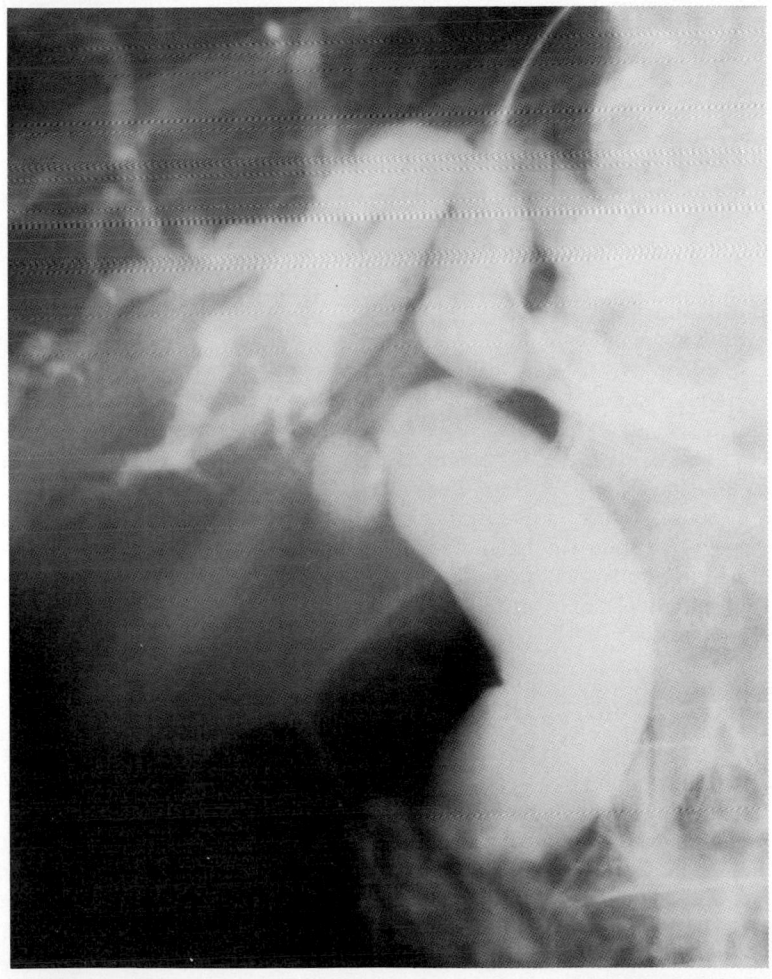

Figure 79–2. Massively dilated duct with lack of tapering and no stones.

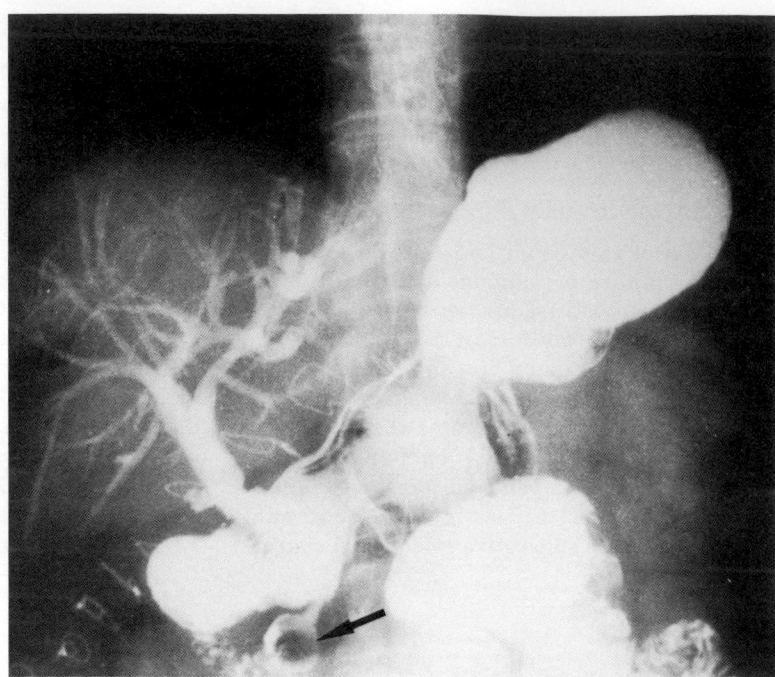

Figure 79–3. Ten-year postoperative upper GI series showing good reflux into biliary tree. Arrow indicates impacted distal stone. The distal bile duct is constructed around the stone.

pacted obstructing stone in a duct considered too small for safe choledochoduodenostomy or when acute pancreatitis is present at surgery.

Intrahepatic Calculi

Any stone lodged in the intrahepatic biliary tree will easily pass through an adequate sized choledochoduodenostomy. Simi et al reported an incidence of 1.3 percent of intrahepatic stones in 2700 biliary procedures. As many as one third of all retained common bile duct stones are felt to be intrahepatic. An adequate choledochoduodenostomy allows easy passage of these stones into the duodenum. Rarely, postoperative endoscopic retrieval through the choledochoduodenostomy will be required if the intrahepatic stone does not descend to the stoma.

Narrow Distal Common Duct Segment (Fig. 79–4)

Benign distal narrowing with proximal common duct dilatation, whether due to inflammatory changes secondary to stones or pancreatitis, represents an ideal indication for choledochoduodenostomy. The length of the narrowed segment together with the risk of pancreatitis make sphincteroplasty contraindicated. The possibility of a distal common bile duct neoplasm must be carefully excluded by biopsies if any suspicion exists.

Perivaterian Duodenal Diverticuli (Fig. 79–5)

A dilated common bile duct with recurrent bouts of cholangitis may be seen in conjunction with a perivaterian diverticulum with or without common duct calculi. This represents an obvious indication for choledochoduodenostomy. Recurring symptoms following bypass have not been seen in our series or reported in the literature. Direct resection of the diverticulum is hazardous, and sphincterotomy and endoscopic papillotomy are contraindicated.

Dilated Common Duct Without Stones

Massive ductal dilatation, often large enough to be categorized as adult choledochal cyst, may be seen in elderly patients without evidence of calculi. A dilated duct without obvious cause accounts for 5 percent of the indications for choledochoduodenostomy in many series, and this should be considered the therapy of choice.

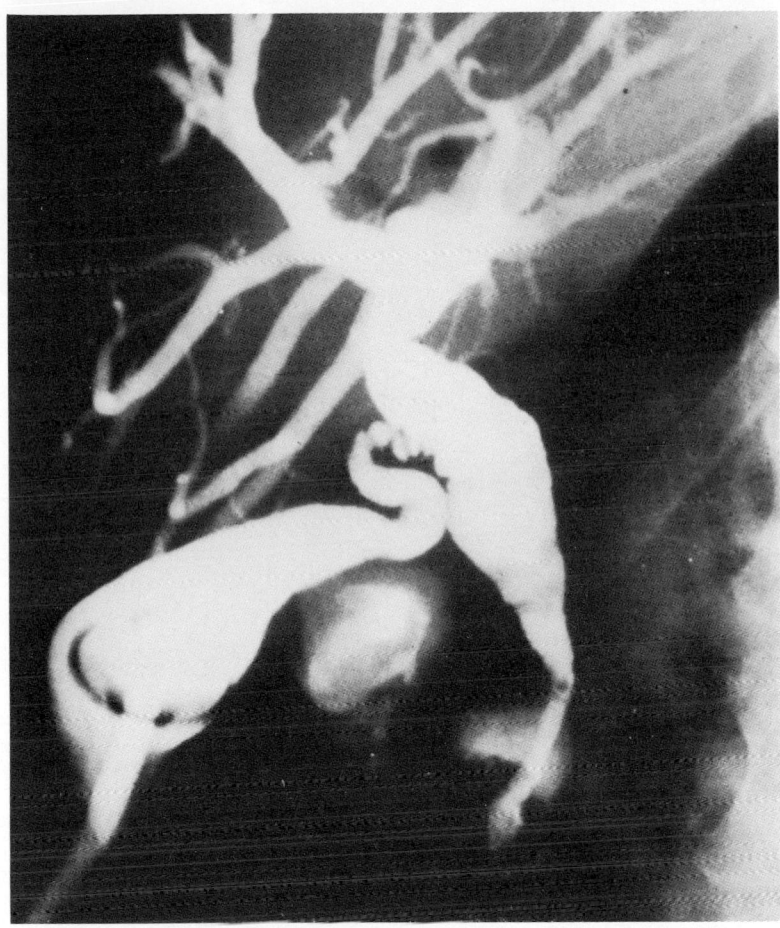

Figure 79–4. Cholecystostomy study in patient with stenosis secondary to pancreatitis. A small stone can be seen in the narrow segment.

Primary Common Duct Stones

The incidence of primary stone formation in the common duct varies in the literature according to the criteria of the author. Saharia, utilizing the strict criteria of a previous cholecystectomy, a minimum of 2 years since any biliary surgery, sludge, or soft easily crushable stones, found 30 primary stones in 785 common duct explorations (4 percent). Madden et al, using only the criteria of soft easily crushable stones, found 54.5 percent of common duct stones to be considered primary stones. Most authors agree that primary common duct stones represent an indication for choledochoduodenostomy even with an intact gallbladder.

Residual Stones

Secondary common duct exploration in the presence of a dilated duct must be considered safer with a choledochoduodenostomy even if the surgeon feels that all stones have been removed.

Low Iatrogenic Stricture

Previous surgical damage to the common duct that occurred low enough to allow a 2.5-cm choledochoduodenostomy proximal to the stricture is well treated by this procedure. Herman reported favorable results in 90 percent of a large series of ductal injuries corrected with choledochoduodenostomy. He recommended this as the preferred procedure when technically feasible.

To conclude, in reviewing indications for choledochoduodenostomy it is important to keep in mind that the majority of patients will have more than one indication. We now feel that choledochoduodenostomy is indicated in any benign biliary tract obstruction in a patient having a common bile duct over 1.4 cm in diameter. Cho-

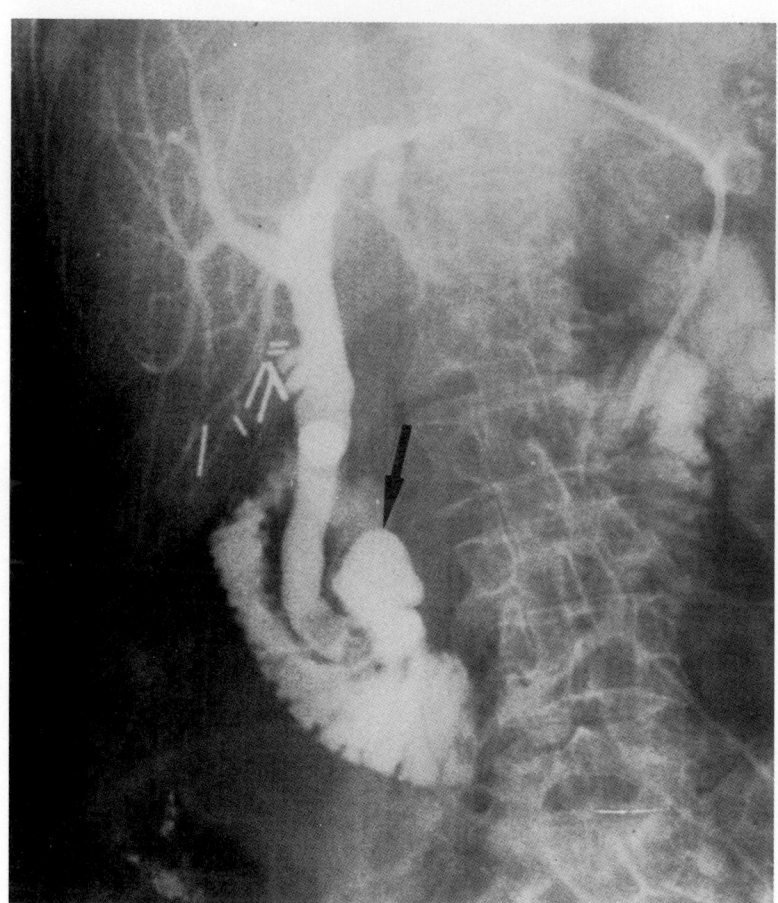

Figure 79–5. Transhepatic cholangiogram in a patient postcholecystectomy with a perivaterian diverticulum (*arrow*) and stones in the distal duct

ledochoduodenostomy is indicated in any patient with an equivocal intraoperative cholangiogram in contrast to attempting additional efforts at vigorous common duct exploration or repeated cholangiography.

CONTRAINDICATIONS

Nondilated Common Duct

Nearly all authors agree that choledochoduodenostomy should not be done in a nondilated duct, though we have successfully used the technique in patients with repeated episodes of cholangitis with an undilated common duct and an ampullary diverticulum.

Sclerosing Cholangitis

Choledochoduodenostomy is generally not effective for this entity. There may be rare occasions where sufficient proximal ductal dilatation exists to allow a 2.5-cm stoma to be made. We have not been fortunate enough in encountering sclerosing cholangitis of this variety. Most authors, however, feel that sclerosing cholangitis is not amenable to simple surgical bypass in the majority of cases.

Decompression of the Pancreatic Duct for Pancreatitis

Generally, choledochoduodenostomy does not provide effective pancreatic duct decompression. We have treated one patient with repeated episodes of pancreatitis with a periampullary diverticulum successfully with a choledochoduodenostomy. When chronic pancreatitis gives rise to a distal stricture this is quite amenable to bypass with choledochoduodenostomy. One cannot leave an impacted distal stone with pancreatitis and do a choledochoduodenostomy expecting the pancreatitis to subside.

Malignant Obstruction

Although many authors have included malignant obstruction in their indications for choledochoduodenostomy, the incidence of recurrent obstruction with cholangitis is unacceptably high and other methods of biliary bypass should be used. In reviewing choledochoduodenostomy for benign and malignant conditions, Fry et al found that 4 of 19 choledochoduodenostomies done for malignancy required reoperation for recurrent obstruction. They concluded that Roux-Y choledochojejunostomy was the preferred method.

Significant Duodenal Edema or Inflammation

The presence of an acute inflammatory process involving the postbulbar portion of the duodenum, whether due to acute cholecystitis with secondary duodenal inflammation or active peptic ulcer disease, should contradict choledochoduodenostomy. The edematous, inflamed duodenum holds sutures poorly. An inflamed choledochus does not present a problem, a significant percentage of our patients having had acute suppurative cholangitis at operation. The inflamed duodenum may be at risk for anastamotic disruption. A previous Billroth II gastrectomy is not a contraindication, as we have seen no difficulties in our series with patients having undergone previous gastric or duodenal surgery.

CHOLEDOCHODUODENOSTOMY VERSUS T-TUBE

The data comparing choledochoduodenostomy to T-tube insertion emphasize the numerous advantages of biliary bypass. The reported mortality for common duct exploration with or without cholecystectomy varies from 2.1 to 4.7 percent. The occurrence of retained stones after positive common duct exploration is between 7 and 10 percent; after negative exploration it is between 2 and 3 percent. The great majority of these patients require reoperation or endoscopic manipulative stone retrieval. Reporting on 341 patients undergoing common duct exploration as a secondary procedure for retained stones, McSherry and Glenn report a 2.1 percent mortality rate. In 1973, Saharia et al found an 18 percent incidence of stone recurrence in patients undergoing choledochotomy and T-tube insertion for primary common duct stones. Seventy five percent of these patients required a third operation. With appropriate indications and technique no patient who undergoes a choledochoduodenostomy performed in a dilated common duct should require reoperation. The complication rate is no different than T-tube placement and the mortality rate for choledochoduodenostomy is significantly lower.

CHOLEDOCHODUODENOSTOMY VERSUS SPHINCTEROPLASTY

Although not strictly comparable, many authors consider both choledochoduodenostomy and sphincteroplasty to be interchangeable in many instances. In several collected series the mortality rate for sphincteroplasty is 5 to 10 percent. Comparing the two procedures in equivalent patients, Thomas et al in 1971 found a mortality rate of 3.5 percent for choledochoduodenostomy and 7 percent for sphincteroplasty with two deaths from pancreatitis in the latter group. They concluded that choledochoduodenostomy should always be done where technically possible. In Vogt and Hermann's series of 91 choledochoduodenostomies, 2 were performed for failed sphincteroplasties. Transduodenal sphincteroplasty should be reserved for benign distal obstruction or an impacted stone in a small duct. The procedures are not competitive, but should be viewed as complimentary. It is important for the surgeon to decide between choledochoduodenostomy and sphincteroplasty before performing a duodenotomy, as the incision must be placed differently for the two procedures.

TECHNIQUE

Our method of performing choledochoduodenostomy has been refined in more than 300 operative procedures. All patients receive perioperative antibiotics; generally one or two doses of cephalosporin are given preoperatively and continued for 24 hours postoperatively. We have found this to significantly reduce the incidence of wound sepsis.

The entire second and third portions of the duodenum and head of the pancreas must be mobilized so that the postbulbar dudodenum may be brought to the hilus of the liver (Fig.

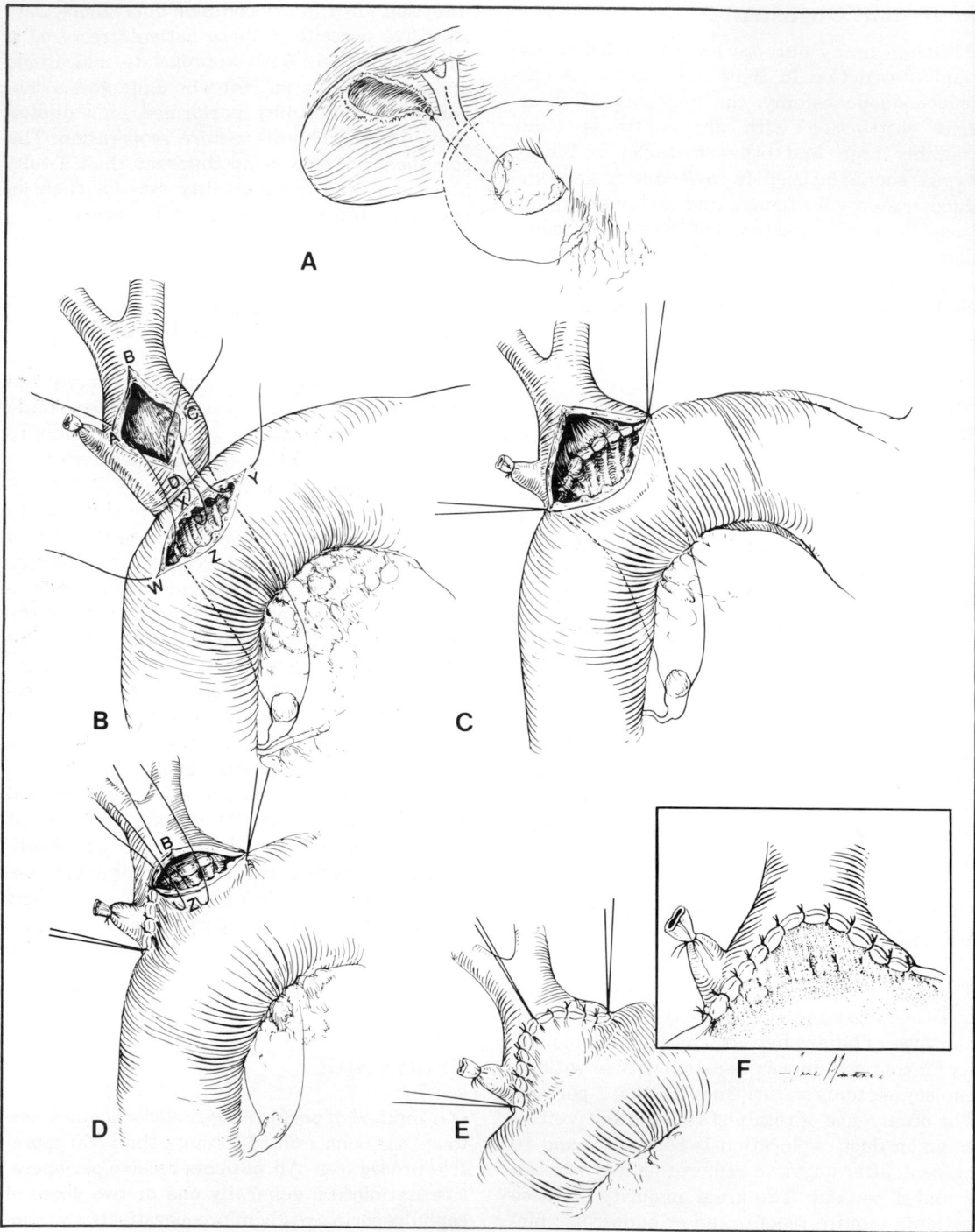

Figure 79–6. A. Dotted lines indicate placement of choledochal and duodenal incisions. **B.** Incisions have been made. Corner sutures have been placed. **C.** Posterior row completed. Knots seen on inside. **D.** One half of anterior row completed with knots on outside. **E.** Anterior row completed. **F.** Shaded area with posterior row visible behind. Funnel effect can be seen.

79–6A). This will assure the lack of anastomotic tension.

A longitudinal choledochotomy is made to the point where the common duct becomes retroduodenal (Fig. 79–6B). Several small arteries cross the common duct at this point, and extending the incision too far inferiorly may cause troublesome bleeding. Careful measurement of the choledochotomy must be made to ensure that it is at least 2.5 cm in length. In the vast majority of patients a choledochotomy of adequate length will extend above the cystic duct entrance onto the common hepatic duct. The duodenum is incised toward its lateral edge in a peristaltic direction. This incision may be 2 or 3 mm shorter than the length of the choledochotomy, as the duodenal incision will stretch slightly. At this point the ampulla should be carefully palpated to ensure that a tumor is not overlooked.

A single interrupted layer of absorbable sutures is used for the anastomoses. This may be 2 or 3-0 chromic cat-gut, Dexon (polyglycolic acid) or Vicryl (Polyglactin 910). Our experience has convinced us of the advantages of the single-layer anastomosis. A two-layered anastomosis will produce too large a ridge and may result in a narrowed opening. Silk sutures, either as an outer layer of a two-layered anastomosis or as a single layer, have been shown to result in recurrent stone formation or inflammation. Although Madden recommends a single layer of 4-0 silk, in 1981 Lewis reported two cases with endoscopic evidence of recurrent stone formation on choledochoduodenostomies using a single layer of 4-0 silk sutures. Akiyama et al performed annual endoscopies on 15 patients for up to 5 years following choledochoduodenostomies that utilized a two-layered interrupted technique of 3-0 silk and 3-0 chromic. There was evidence of residual intraluminal silk sutures with inflammation of the stoma in 4 of the 15

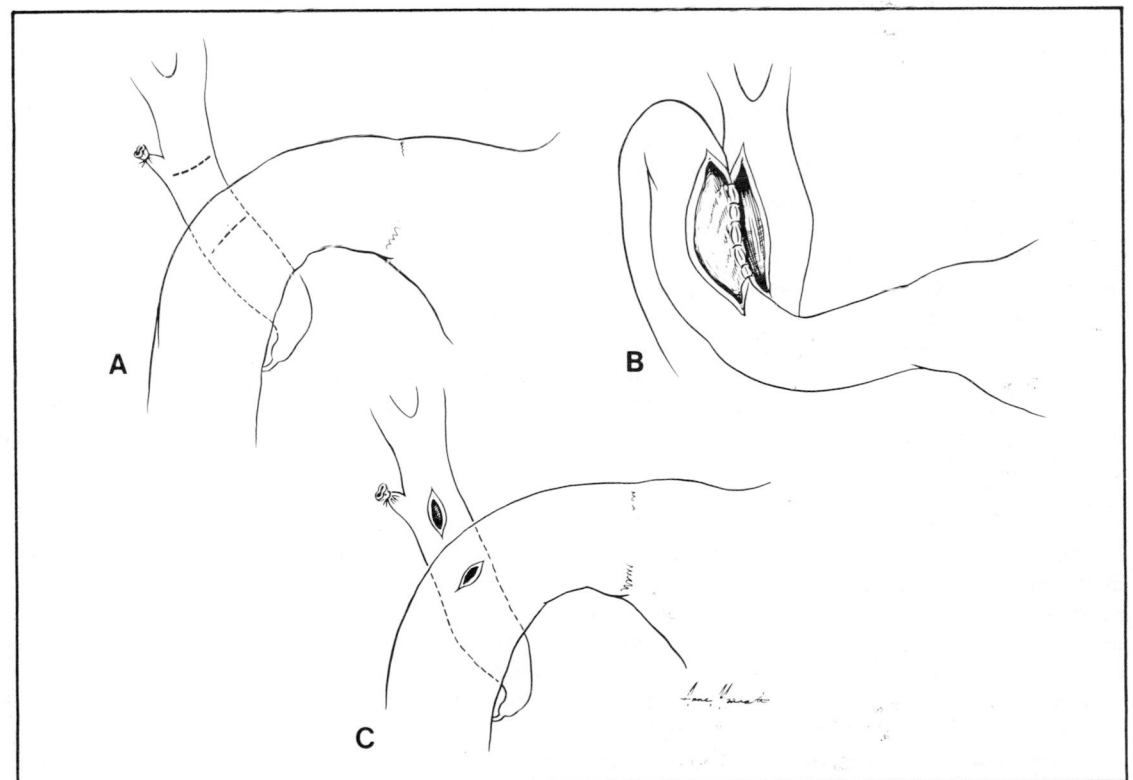

Figure 79–7. A. Choledochotomy and duodenotomy are transverse and cannot be of adequate length. **B.** Side-to-side anastomosis fails to provide the funnel effect. **C.** Stoma too small. May result in cholangitis.

patients. They concluded that silk sutures were contraindicated and recommended a single layer of absorbable sutures.

A triangulated anastomosis is performed (Figs. 79–6B through 79–6E). The corner sutures (A-W and C-Y) are placed initially and are used for traction to properly align the anastomosis. These are passed from outside-in, then inside-out, resulting in the knots tied on the outside. The posterior row of sutures is next placed with interrupted stitches 2 to 3 mm apart, with the knots tied on the inside of the lumen (Fig. 79–6C). As an option, the middle suture (D-X) may be placed initially to aid in alignment. Figure 79–6C shows the completed posterior row. The corner sutures are kept long and are used for traction when performing the anterior row.

The anterior row of sutures is done with the knots tied outside. No attempt at inversion is made. When beginning the anterior row, it is sometimes helpful to place the middle suture (B-Z) first. This is not tied, but with gentle anterior traction helps protect the posterior row and further align the anastomosis. Figure 79–6D shows one half of the anterior row completed. Generally, 10 to 12 sutures will be needed to complete each row. In Figure 79–6E the completed anterior row is illustrated. Utilizing our triangulated technique, a tongue of duodenum will overlie the common duct. Figure 79–6F shows a portion of the anterior duodenal wall shaded. The inner portion of the stoma can be seen to have a funnel-like appearance, which maintains separation of the edges and promotes prompt emptying.

Figures 79–7A through 79–7C show several common errors. A transverse choledochotomy will not allow the formation of a 2.5-cm stoma in the vast majority of cases. Performing the anastomosis side-to-side without triangulation may allow the edges to co-apt and will not produce the desired funnel effect. Too small a choledochotomy or duodenotomy prevents adequate drainage, produces stasis, and impedes passage of residual calculi or debris, resulting in the possibility of cholangitis or sump syndrome. Anastomotic stents are not used. If the choledochotomy is properly long (2.5 cm), it will be technically difficult to insert a T-tube; there is no real reason for a T-tube. Drains are optional, but generally we do not drain secondary procedures having had a previous cholecystectomy.

RESULTS

The postoperative course has been remarkably benign, and is significantly simpler than with a T-tube in the common bile duct. The risks of postoperative T-tube cholangiography are not present. The majority of our patients were eating by the third postoperative day, and many were ready for discharge by 1 week. The average hospital stay in several collected series was 15.23 days with an average age in this group of patients of 65 years.

The mortality rate of choledochoduodenostomy varies from 0 to 8 percent. Madden, reviewing 1255 choledochoduodenostomies from 1946 to 1968, found an overall mortality rate of 2.7 percent. The incidence of cholangitis in this series was 0.4 percent. A review of 1466 choledochoduodenostomies reported in the literature from 1969 to 1982 shows a mortality rate now reduced to an overall 1.8 percent. The incidence of cholangitis is 0.9 percent (Table 79–1). This must be considered the minimum mortality of operating on an elderly group of patients often under emergency conditions.

One criticism of choledochoduodenostomy has been ascending cholangitis from either retained calculi and debris or food particles entering via the newly created anastomosis. In our personal series we have no cases of cholangitis in over 300 choledochoduodenostomies done as described due to distal stones or ampullary problems. We have had one patient with a stenosis of a secondary right hepatic duct who had cholangitis years later due to obstruction behind the stenosis. Review of the first postcholedochoduodenostomy upper gastrointestinal (GI) series shows a previously unappreciated stenosis to be present at the original position. The patient has been controlled by antibiotics. Indeed, when performing a biliary colic anastomosis in dogs there is no evidence of cholangitis if a stoma of 2.5 cm is created. McSherry et al, in 1981, reported five cases of recurrent stones and cholangitis following biliary enteric anastomosis. In none of their cases is the initial duct size, stoma length or operative technique described. The representative x-rays in this report demonstrate significant anastomotic narrowing in all cases. Cholangitis will not occur unless the anastomosis is too small.

Another criticism of choledochoduodenostomy has been the creation of a "blind" segment

TABLE 79–1.

Author	Year	Total No. Cases	Total No. Cholangitis	Cholangitis Rate (%)	Total No. Mortality	Mortality Rate (%)
Farrar	1969	36	1	2.7	0	0
Thomas	1971	57	0	0	2	3.5
Johnson	1972	64	0	0	0	0
Stuart	1972	44	1	2.2	0	0
White	1973	24	0	0	2	8.3
Degenschein	1974	175	2	1.1	5	2.8
Rutlege	1976	13	0	0	0	0
Freund	1977	27	1	3.7	0	0
Engin	1978	60	0	0	3	5
Hagan	1978	36	0	0	0	0
Engleberg	1979	55	2	5.6	1	1.8
Kaminsky	1979	79	0	0	0	0
Berlatzky	1980	60	1	1.6	0	0
Krauss	1980	51	2	3.9	4	7.8
Gliedman & Schien	1981	200	0	0	6	3.0
Lygidakis	1981	342	0	0	0	0
Vogt & Hermann	1981	50	2	4.0	0	0
Fry	1982	24	0	0	1	4.1
Moesgard	1982	49	0	0	2	4.1
Total		1446	13	0.9	26	1.8

or pouch between the anastomosis and the papilla of Vater, the "sump syndrome." It is postulated that this blind segment serves as a sump and promotes stasis and cholangitis by permitting food particles, infected bile, and residual calculi to remain in the distal portion of the common bile duct. Although often alluded to, no clearly documented cases of sump syndrome have been reported, and there is a total lack of agreement as to the importance of this concept. Akiyama noted residual food debris distally in 4 of 15 patients with choledochoduodenostomies who were endoscoped annually. In three of the four, the material was floating free and easily washed out. In the fourth patient the material was adherent to residual silk sutures. There were no symptoms of cholangitis in any of these patients. It is important to note that all of these patients had a stoma size of at least 2.5 cm. A number of our patients with retained distal stones have been without sequelae for 10 years.

Johnson et al reported a slight bile leak in 5 percent of patients. This was generally benign and usually subsided within a few days. Gliedman et al noted 4 transient leaks in 175 cases without any constitutional symptoms, and 3 closed spontaneously. In 75 consecutive cases receiving perioperative antibiotics Gliedman also noted no wound infections. Other authors have reported wound infection rates of 2 to 5 percent.

The overall complication rate is acceptably low, although difficult to compare due to a lack of agreement as to what constitutes a reportable complication. The rate is certainly no higher than in simple cholecystectomy in the aged and relates primarily to the problems of a laparotomy in an elderly, ill population with purulence in the common bile duct.

Comparison of choledochoduodenostomy with endoscopic papillotomy is inevitable. Safrany, tabulating the experience of multiple centers with 3618 endoscopic papillotomies, found an overall success rate of 93.9 percent, a complication rate of 7 percent, and a 1.4 percent mortality. Three percent of patients in the series required emergency surgery. The failure rate with stones greater than 1 cm in diameter increases to 30 percent, and as many as 75 percent of patients require multiple endoscopic procedures. There are no long-term follow-up results yet available for endoscopic papillotomy. Its role in that group of overlapping patients suitable for choledochoduodenostomy still remains to be clearly defined.

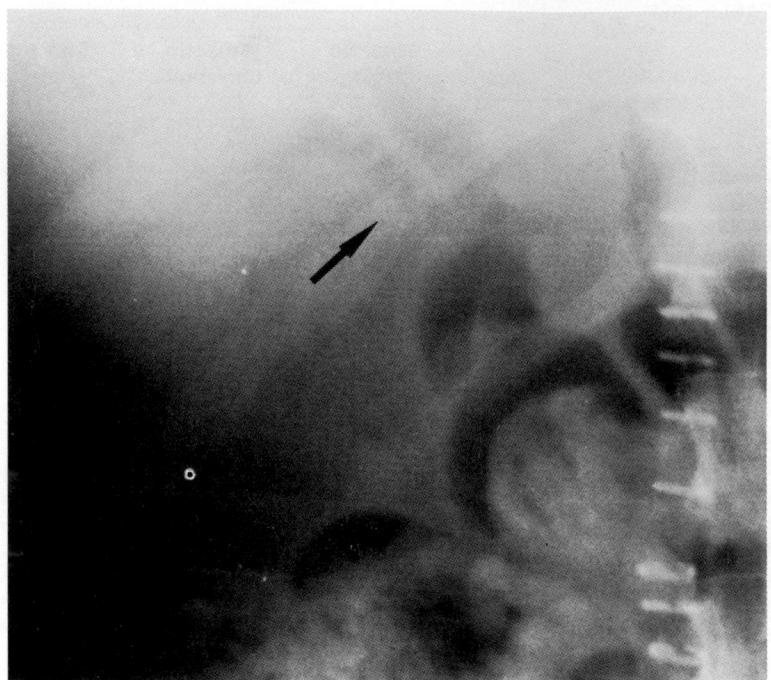

Figure 79–8. Plain film of abdomen. Arrow denotes air in biliary tree.

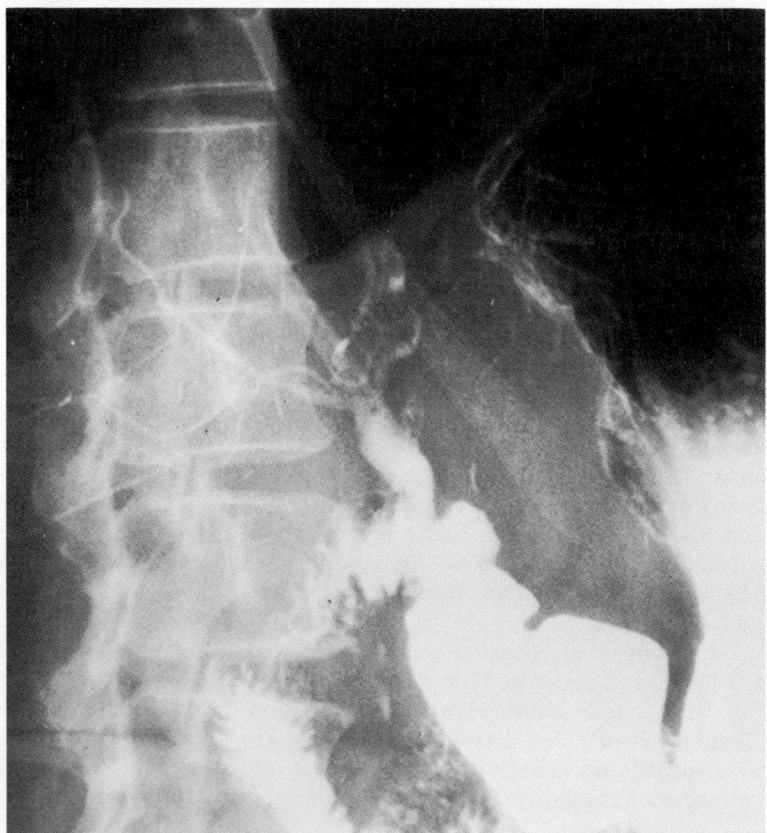

Figure 79–9. Postoperative upper gastrointestinal series showing prompt filling and emptying of the biliary tree.

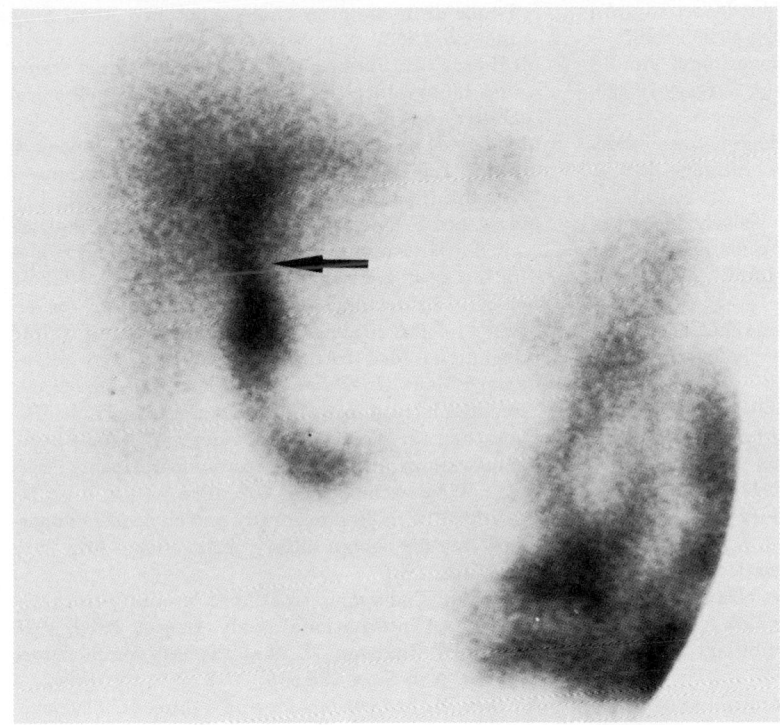

Figure 79–10. IDA scan with contrast promptly entering duodenum.

POSTOPERATIVE EVALUATION

The evaluation of a choledochoduodenostomy postoperatively is important. All patients should have air in the biliary tree on a plain x-ray of the abdomen (Fig. 79–8). When evaluation of a choledochoduodenostomy is needed, two options exist. An upper GI series should show prompt filling of the biliary tree, and complete emptying should occur by 12 hours and certainly no later than 24 hours (Fig. 79–9). Currently we evaluate choledochoduodenostomy function with the IDA scan. With a properly functioning stoma the biliary tree will empty in 45 minutes (Fig. 79–10).

CONCLUSIONS

Providing that the basic requirements of a stoma size of at least 2.5 cm in length and a common duct diameter of at least 1.4 cm are adhered to, the overall results of choledochoduodenostomy are excellent. Numerous authors with large numbers of cases followed for as long as 20 years have shown a remarkably low long-term incidence of problems. Evidence to support the clinical significance of retained food matter causing cholangitis or sump syndrome are not documented. Retention of debris within the defunctionalized segment does not represent a problem if an adequate stoma is constructed. The operation is strongly recommended as a safe, definitive procedure. Every surgeon operating on the biliary tree should be familiar with the techniques and indications.

BIBLIOGRAPHY

Akiyama H, Ikezawa H, et al: Unexpected problems of external choledochoduodenostomy. Fiberscopic examination in 15 patients. Am J Surg 140:660, 1980

Allen AW: A method of re-establishing continuity between the bile duct and the gastrointestinal tract. Ann Surg 121:412, 1945

Barkin JS, Silvis S, et al: Endoscopic therapy of the "sump" syndrome. Dig Dis Sci 25:597, 1980

Berlatzky Y, Freund H: Choledochoduodenostomy in the treatment of benign biliary tract disease. Am J Surg 141:90, 1981

Capper WM: External choledochoduodenostomy. An evaluation of 125 cases. Br J Surg 49:292, 1961

Degenshein GA: Choledochoduodenostomy: An 18 year study of 175 consecutive cases. Surgery 76:319, 1974

Degenshein GA, Hurwitz A: The techniques of side-to-side choledochoduodenostomy. Surgery 61:972, 1967

Engelberg M, Avrahami I, et al: Choledochoduodenostomy—a useful procedure in the management of benign disorders of the biliary tract: A review of 53 cases. Am Surg 46:344, 1980

Engin A, Haberal M, et al: Side-to-side choledochoduodenostomy in the management of choledocholithiasis. Br J Surg 65:99, 1978

Farrar T, Painter MW, et al: Choledochoduodenostomy in the treatment of stenosis in the distal common duct. Arch Surg 98:442, 1969

Freund H, Charuzi I, et al: Choledochoduodenostomy in the treatment of benign biliary tract disease. Arch Surg. 112:1032, 1977

Fry DE, Buchignani E, et al: Applications of choledochoduodenostomy in biliary tract obstruction. Am Surg 48:149, 1982

Glenn F, McSherry CK: Calculous biliary tract disease. Curr Probl Surg, June, 1975

Gliedman ML, Schein CJ: The use and abuse of choledochoduodenostomy, in Najarian JS, Delaney JP (eds): Hepatic, Biliary, and Pancreatic Surgery, Miami: Symposia Specialists, 1980, p 91

Herman RE: Diagnosis and management of bile duct strictures. Am J Surg 130:519, 1975

Johnson AG, Rains AJ: Choledochoduodenostomy. A reappraisal of its indications based on a study of 64 patients. Br J Surg 59:277, 1972

Johnson AG, Rains AJ: Prevention and treatment of recurrent bile duct stones by choledochoduodenostomy. World J Surg 2:487, 1978

Johnson AG, Stevens AE: Importance of the size of the stoma in choledochoduodenostomy. Gut 10:68, 1969

Jordan GL: Choledocholithiasis. Curr Probl Surg, Dec, 1982

Kaminski DL, Barner HB, et al: Evaluation of the results of external choledochoduodenostomy for retained, recurrent, or primary common duct stones. Am J Surg 137:162, 1979

Kraus MA, Wilson SD: Choledochoduodenostomy. Importance of common duct size and occurrence of cholangitis. Arch Surg 115:1212, 1980

Lewis JW, Urdaneta LF: Stone formation on silk suture after choledochoduodenostomy. South Med J 74:1280, 1981

Lygidakis NJ: Choledochoduodenostomy in calculous biliary tract disease. Br J Surg 68:762, 1981

Lygidakis NJ: Surgical approaches to postcholecystectomy choledocholithiasis. Arch Surg 117:481, 1982

Lygidakis NJ: Surgical approaches to recurrent choledocholithiasis. Choledochoduodenostomy versus T-tube drainage after choledochotomy. Am J Surg 145:636, 1983

McSherry CK, Fischer MG: Common bile duct stones and biliary–intestinal anastomosis. Surg Gynecol Obstet 153:669, 1981

Madden JL, Chun JY, et al: Choledochoduodenostomy. An unjustly maligned surgical procedure? Am J Surg 119:45, 1970

Moesgaard F, Nielsen ML, et al: Protective choledochoduodenostomy in multiple common duct stones in the aged. Surg Gynecol Obstet 154:232, 1982

Orr KB: External choledochoduodenostomy for retained common duct stone: Reappraisal of an old technique. Med J Aust 2:1027, 1966

Reidel BMCL: Uber den zungenformigen forsatz der rechten leberlappens und seine pathognotische. Beduntung für die erkrankung der gallenglase nebst bemerkungen uber gallensteinoperationen. Berl Klin Wchneschr 25:577, 602, 1888

Rutledge RH: Sphincteroplasty and choledochoduodenostomy for benign biliary obstructions. Ann Surg 183, 476, 1976

Safrany L: Endoscopic treatment of biliary-tract diseases. An international study. Lancet 2:983, 1978

Saharia PC, Zuidema GD, et al: Primary common duct stones. Ann Surg 185:598, 1977

Sanders RL: Indications for and value of choledochoduodenostomy. Ann Surg 123:847, 1944

Sasse F: Uber choledocho-duodenostomie. Arch Klin Chir 100:969, 1913

Schein CJ, Beneventano TC, et al: Choledochoduodenostomy—roentgen considerations. Surgery 60:958, 1966

Schein CJ, Shapiro NL, et al: Choledochoduodenostomy as an adjunct to choledocholithotomy. Surg Gynecol Obstet 146:25, 1978

Schein CJ, Gliedman ML: Choledochoduodenostomy as an adjunct to choledocholithotomy. Surg Gynecol Obstet 152:797, 1981

Schwartz F, Benshimol A, et al: Choledochoduodenostomy. Surgery 46:1020, 1959

Sprenger O: Uber einen fall von Exstirpation der Gallenblase mit anlegung einen Communication Znischen Ductus Choledochus and Duodenun. Arch Klin Cir 42:550, 1891

Stuart M, Hoerr SO: Late results of side-to-side choledochoduodenostomy and of transduodenal sphincterotomy for benign disorders. Am J Surg 123:67, 1972

Szanto I, Bozalyi I, et al: Purulent cholangitis and hepatic abscess after choledochoduodenostomy diagnosed by ERCP. Endoscopy 1:70, 1979

Thomas CG, Nicholson CP, et al: Effectiveness of choledochoduodenostomy and transduodenal sphincterotomy in the treatment of benign obstruction of the common duct. Ann Surg 173:845, 1971

Tompkins RK, Pitt HA: Surgical management of benign lesions of the bile ducts. Curr Prob Surg 19, 1982

Vogt DP, Hermann RE: Choledochoduodenostomy, choledochojejunostomy or sphincteroplasty for biliary and pancreatic disease. Ann Surg 193:161, 1981

Way LW: Retained common duct stones. Surg Clin North Am 53:1139, 1973

Way LW, Admirand WH, et al: Management of chole-docholithiasis. Ann Surg 176:347, 1972

White TT: Indications for sphincteroplasty as opposed to choledochoduodenostomy. Am J Surg 126:165, 1973

Wright NL: Evaluation of the results of choledocho-duodenostomy. Br J Surg 55:33, 1968

80. Stenosis of the Sphincter of Oddi

George L. Nardi

INTRODUCTION

Stenosis of the sphincter of Oddi is a clinical entity that is not well recognized by the clinician. It is responsible for intermittent or continuous pain in the epigastrium, with radiation to the back rarely associated with jaundice or dilatation of the biliary passages. It may occur at any age and routine clinical studies are negative precipitating the physician into a premature psychosomatic diagnosis. Symptoms may persist after cholecystectomy and this condition has been termed postcholecystectomy syndrome but perhaps should be more aptly called precholecystectomy syndrome.

Langenbuch first suggested in 1884 that stenosis of the sphincter of Oddi might cause biliary symptoms and first proposed transduodenal division of the sphincter. Kocher, in 1894, advised suturing the cut edges of the papillotomy describing the operation as an internal choledochostomy. It was Archibald in 1913, however, who defined the classic operation of sphincterotomy.

In 1926 Del Valle achieved excellent results with "papillosphincterotomy" in a large number of patients suffering from the pain of what he described as "sclerosing choledocho-Odditis." In 1956, Doubilet and Mulholland claimed excellent results from sphincterotomy but felt that spasm rather than fibrosis produced reflux of bile into the pancreatic duct to cause symptoms. Cattell, however, felt that fibrosis was a distinct entity and that any exploration of the common bile duct should be considered incomplete unless the surgeon has ruled out obstruction of the ampulla of Vater.

Acosta et al found that, in 38 sphincter biopsies, 22 (57 percent) showed histologic abnormalities consisting of fibrosis of the papilla in 10

instances, acute or chronic inflammatory infiltration in 9, and pseudopolyps composed of granulation tissue in 3. Muscular hypertrophy and cystic glandular dilatation accompanied the fibrosis or chronic inflammation. Fibrosis was the predominant pathologic change in 10 instances (16 percent).

Stenosis of the sphincter of Oddi is three times more common in women than men. The condition may occur at any age but is most common between the ages of 30 and 50.

DIAGNOSIS

Clinical Manifestations. The condition is basically an obstructive biliopancreatopathy and symptoms and signs vary depending on the effect on each system. Obstructive jaundice, duct dilatation, and cholangitis may occur, but much more frequently epigastric pain radiating to the back, presumably secondary to pancreatitis, is the predominant symptom.

There is a frequent history of previous surgery, most commonly cholecystectomy. Not uncommonly a history of duodenal ulcer can be obtained. Whether or not the latter could have any etiologic significance is unclear at present.

Frequent bouts of loose stools may occur and is suggestive of pancreatic exocrine insufficiency.

Papillitis and stenosis may be associated with alcoholism and in this situation papillitis may only be a part of a pathologic complex involving the liver and pancreas.

Laboratory Studies. Occasionally elevation of serum alkaline phosphatase may provide a clue to diagnosis. Serum bilirubin and pancreatic enzymes are rarely elevated.

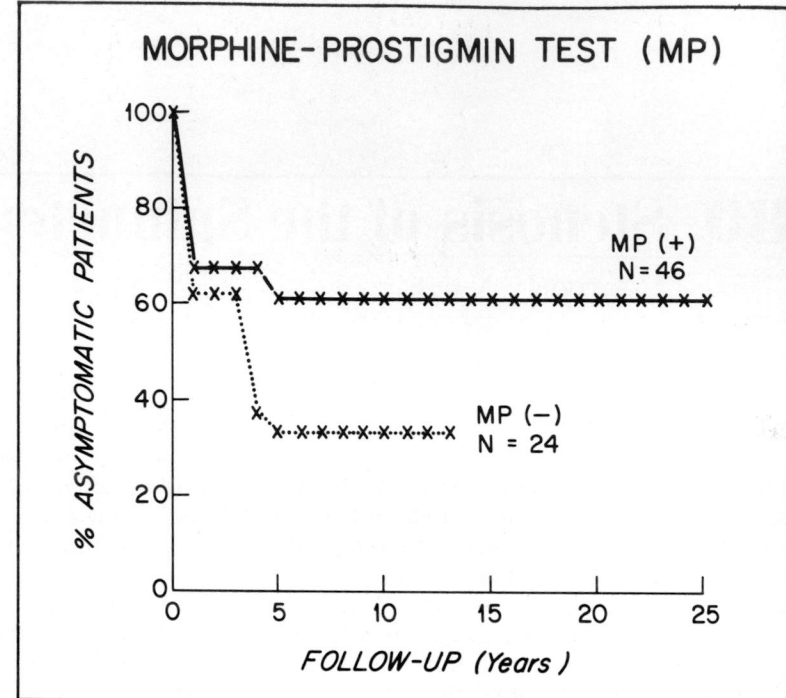

Figure 80–1. Comparison of successful surgical outcome in patients who had positive or negative morphine–prostigmin tests.

The morphine–prostigmin evocative test has been shown to be a reasonable screening test. This consists of an intramuscular injection of 10 mg of morphine and 1 mg of prostigmin methylsulfate. Serum amylase and lipase are measured before and 1, 2, and 4 hours after injection. A test is considered positive when enzyme levels rise to a value greater than three times normal. Patients with a positive evocative test have a significantly better chance of a good result from surgery (Fig. 80–1). When combined with the patient's history this test becomes an even more reliable diagnostic aid and predictor of response to surgery (Fig. 80–2).

Figure 80–2. Successful surgical outcome when result of morphine–prostigmin test combined history of previous surgery, diarrhea, alcoholism, or drug abuse.

CLINICAL RESULTS OF SPHINCTEROPLASTY		
	M – P TEST	
	(+)	(–)
● GOOD RESULT	60%	35%
● HISTORY OF		
DRUG ABUSE	65%	30%
DIARRHEA	65%	15%
ABD. SURGERY	75%	15%
EtOH	65%	0

Radiologic Studies. The only worthwhile radiologic examination is endoscopic retrograde cholangiopancreatography (ERCP). In one single examination hiatus hernia, peptic ulcer disease, residual biliary calculi, and other pathology can be ruled out and the status of biliary and pancreatic ducts can be defined. The size of the orifice of the papilla can be estimated and the rate of emptying of injected contrast substance can be assessed to verify a diagnosis of papillary stenosis.

In approximately 5 percent of examinations pancreas divisum or failure of fusion of the pancreatic ductal anlage is found. This condition in the symptomatic patient is believed to be related to stenosis of the minor papilla. When combined with a proper history and a positive morphine–prostigmin test, findings of papillary narrowing justify surgical correction.

OPERATIVE TREATMENT

The operation of ampullary sphincteroplasty is best performed through a right paramedian or midline incision.

The hepatic flexure is mobilized downward and the duodenum extensively mobilized through its third portion to the superior mesenteric vessels.

A choledochotomy may be performed to pass a probe through the papilla for easier identification, but after some experience this step may be omitted and the major papilla exposed directly through a longitudinal duodenotomy.

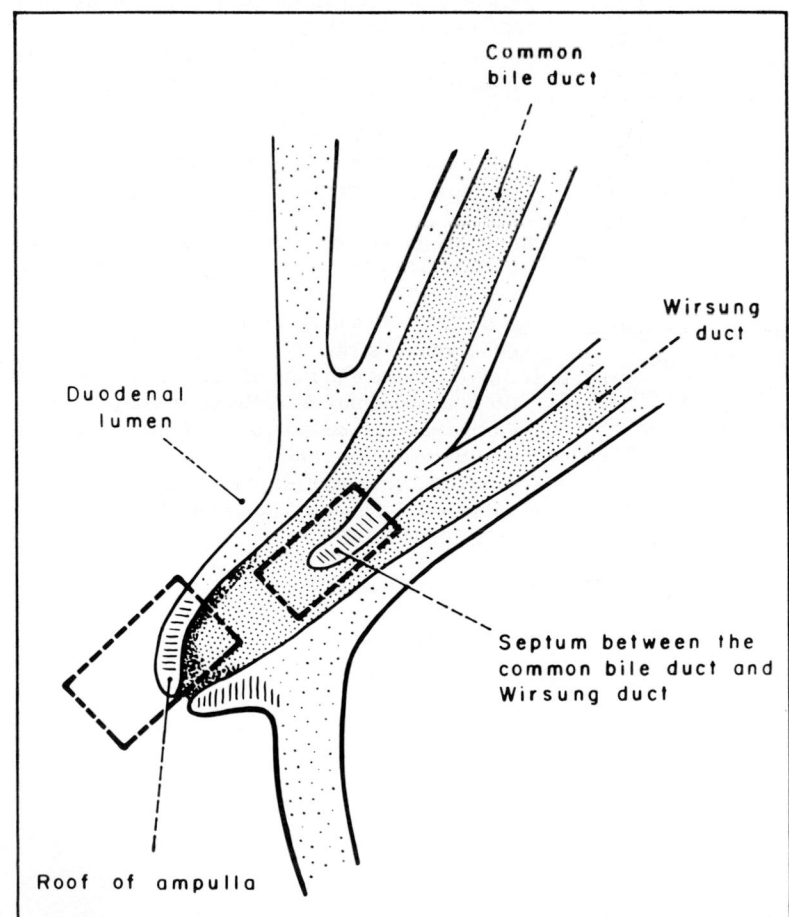

Figure 80–3. Longitudinal section of the ampulla of Vater, common duct, Wirsung's duct, and duodenum. Dotted blocks represent sites of biopsies. Operative unroofing was carried further. (*Source: From Acosta JM, Nardi GL, 1966, with permission.*)

The papilla is dilated with lacrimal probe dilators and a Doubilet sphincterotome is inserted to perform a 1-cm sphincterotomy (papillotomy) and obtain a simultaneous tissue biopsy. The roof of the common duct is further divided for 1 cm with scissors, thus completely dividing all the musculature and achieving a sphincteroplasty. The cut edges are then carefully sutured.

The orifice of the pancreatic duct is then identified in the floor of the common duct and the roof of Wirsung's duct, i.e., the septum between the common and pancreatic ducts is divided for a distance of approximately 1 cm. This will usually allow passage of a number 3 Bakes' dilator. This septectomy is a most important step since the inflammatory reaction involving the sphincter of Oddi may extend to the musculature surrounding the termination of the duct of Wirsung. The extent of the procedure is shown in Figure 80–3.

The duodenotomy is carefully closed longitudinally with two layers of sutures and the retroduodenum drained with a suction catheter.

A complementary gastrostomy is performed and left on drainage for 4 days. Then it is gradually occluded until its removal on the tenth postoperative day. This procedure is most desirable since delayed gastric emptying secondary to the duodenotomy is not unusual. The gastrostomy eliminates the distressing nasogastric tube and provides a simple means for assaying and controlling gastric residuals.

Antibiotics are administered perioperatively and for the first 3 postoperative days.

Mortality of the procedure is approximately 3 percent and usually results from the complications of postoperative pancreatitis. Postoperative elevations of serum amylase and lipase are usually present but are rarely of clinical significance.

BIBLIOGRAPHY

Acosta JM, Civantos F, et al: Fibrosis of the papilla of Vater. Surg Gynecol Obstet 124:787, 1967.

Acosta JM, Nardi GL: Papillitis: Inflammatory disease of the papilla of Vater. Arch Surg 92:354, 1966

Archibald E: Ideas concerning the causation of some cases of pancreatitis. J Med Surg 33:263, 1913

Bartlett MK, Nardi GL: Treatment of recurrent pancreatitis by transduodenal sphincterotomy and exploration of the pancreatic duct. N Engl J Med 262:643, 1960

Del Valle D, Donovan R: Coledoco-Odditis esclero-retractil cronica. Concepto clinico y quirurgica. Arch Argentinos enf ap Digestiv y Nutricion 1:4, 1926

Doubilet M, Mulholland JH: Eight years study of pancreatitis and sphincterotomy. JAMA 160:521, 1956

Gregg, JA, Taddeo AE, et al.: Duodenoscopy and endoscopic pancreatography in patients with positive morphine prostigmin tests. Am J Surg 134:318, 1977

Kocher T: Ein fall von Choledochoduodenostomia interna wegen Gallensteines. Korrespondinz—blatt für aerzte 7:193, 1895

Langenbuch, cited in Grage TB, Laher PH, et al: Stenosis of the sphincter of Oddi. A clinicopathologic review of 50 cases. Surgery 48:304, 1960

Madura, JA, McCammon, RL, et al: The Nardi test and biliary monometry in the diagnosis of pancreatobiliary sphincter dysfunction. Surgery 90:588, 1981

Moody FG, Berenson MM, et al: Transampullary septectomy for postcholecystectomy pain. Ann Surg 186:415, 1977

Nardi GL: Acute suppurative cholangitis due to ampullary fibrosis. Surg Clin North Am 50:1137, 1970

Nardi GL, Acosta JM: Papillitis as a cause of pancreatitis and abdominal pain: Role of evocative test, operative pancreatography, and histologic evaluation. Ann Surg 164:611, 1966

Nardi GL, Michelassi F, et al: Transduodenal sphincteroplasty: 5–25 year followup of 89 patients. Ann Surg 198:453, 1983

81. Transduodenal Sphincteroplasty in the Prophylaxis and Treatment of Residual Common Duct Stones

S. Austin Jones

INTRODUCTION

The finding of residual bile duct calculi following biliary surgery is one of the most distressing complications confronting the abdominal surgeon. The overall incidence of residual stones in the United States following initial choledocholithotomy is 10 percent, and 5 percent in patients who have had a negative duct exploration. It is especially important to realize that when a patient is operated upon for residual stones, the occurrence of further residual calculi averages 25 percent. Morbidity and mortality increase with repeated operations.

Residual ductal calculi are divisible into two types. First there are stones that originated in the gallbladder, passed into the common duct, and were overlooked at the time of the initial ductal exploration. At reoperation, there may be only one or a few faceted cholesterol calculi remaining. The bile is clear and thin, and no evidence of distal duct obstruction is present, either by ductal dilatation, operative cholangiography, or papillary narrowing checked by gentle calibration using a red rubber catheter. Under these circumstances, removal of the stones should solve the problem. The second type of residual stone is the stasis stone that is truly reformed. The bile is viscous and filled with mud and sludge, and the calculi may form a rough cast of the duct. When stones of this type are encountered, the surgeon can be certain that a distal ductal obstruction exists, that bile stasis has resulted in stone formation, and that the distal obstruction must be eliminated

if one is to expect permanent clearing of the ducts. It is possible that both types of residual calculi can occur in the same individual, in which case the distal ductal obstruction must be corrected in addition to mechanically clearing the ducts. Stones in the hepatic ducts may be unrecognized or irremovable and eventually pass into the common duct, producing distal obstruction. The management of irremovable hepatic duct stones will be discussed under indications for sphincteroplasty.

Table 81-1 outlines the results of various operative techniques designed to insure complete clearing of the ducts at surgery. These are the figures obtained by experts in the field and are not representative of those of the general surgical population. Our philosophy agrees with that of Best, who stated that *no matter how carefully a duct is explored, some calculi will be left behind.* This has been our experience, and this author is certain that anyone who has done a reasonable amount of biliary tract surgery will agree. Accepting this basic premise, our approach to the prophylaxis and treatment of residual common duct stones where the indications to be mentioned exist is to approach the papilla of Vater transduodenally and, by serial clamping, division, and suture of the common duct and duodenal walls, create a permanent noncontractile opening between the distal end of the common duct and the side of the duodenum. *The stoma must be co-equal in diameter to that of the widest portion of the supraduodenal common duct.* Such a widely patent terminal choledochoduodenostomy (sphincteroplasty)

TABLE 81–1. METHODS USED TO PREVENT RESIDUAL STONES

Technique	Author	Residual Stones (%)		
		Proven	*Probably*	*Total*
Operative cholangiography	Jolley et al	3.5	3.5	7.0
Sphincterotomy	Backer	3.9	2.6	6.5
Ampullary dilatation	Chodoff	7.0	—	7.0
Fogarty balloon	Fogarty et al	7.6	—	7.6
Choledochoscope	Shore and Shore	3.3	—	3.3
Sphincteroplasty	Present series	0	0	0

(*Source: From Jones SA, Smith LL: A reappraisal of sphincteroplasty (not sphincterotomy). Surgery 71:565, 1972, with permission.*)

should permit any overlooked stones to pass easily into the bowel. Bile stasis will be eliminated, preventing both stone reformation and cholangitis, which should not occur with a free bile flow. Hepatic duct stones that later migrate to the common duct should be able to pass harmlessly into the duodenum.

In order to produce this type of opening it is necessary to perform a transduodenal sphincteroplasty using the technique discussed in the following. This operation destroys all of the muscular sphincters affecting the distal common and pancreatic ducts as they pass through the duodenal wall. A sphincterotomy, on the contrary, divides only the sphincters of the papilla, leaving behind a substantial amount of constricting mechanism that may retain overlooked calculi.

HISTORICAL NOTE

It is remarkable to realize that in 1681 Glisson described the anatomy and physiology of the distal common duct with amazing accuracy. He stated that "all returns into the ductus communis is prevented by annular fibers which block not only the opening itself, but the whole slanting tract. Those same fibers close completely and block all passage, until some more fluid again accumulates to force an opening."

Over 300 years later our knowledge has not been greatly expanded. In Figure 81–1, showing normal anatomy, we see that the common and pancreatic ducts parallel each other as they pass obliquely through the duodenal wall. The pancreatic duct is always medial to the common duct, usually entering the latter several millimeters above the papilla. In this intramural course the common duct is reduced in caliber,

producing the distal narrowing seen in a normal cholangiogram. As the ducts pass through the bowel wall, their lumens are affected not only by contraction of the duodenal muscle per se but also by a thin sheath of specialized musculature lying in a submucosal position, as described by Boyden. Where the common duct enters the bowel, the fibers of this submucosal sheath mingle with those of the duodenal wall muscle, forming the superior sphincter of Boyden. At the termination of the duct it forms the papillary or inferior choledochal sphincter, a series of stout circular muscle trabeculae some 6 mm in length. The muscular fibers surrounding the ducts between the superior and inferior sphincters are known collectively as the submucosal sphincter of Boyden.

Anatomically, it should be clear that to eliminate the entire complex of sphincteric muscular mechanisms, *the full length of the intramural course must be divided, and therefore the incision of duodenal and common duct walls will extend through the entire thickness of the bowel.*

McBurney performed the first sphincterotomy in 1891, enabling him to extract a common duct calculus. Four years later Kocher opened the duodenum, incised the posterior wall of the duodenum and the anterior wall of the common duct *1 cm proximal to the papilla,* and removed a stone. Sphincterotomy was first used to treat recurrent pancreatitis by Archibald and later employed extensively by Doubilet and Mulholland.

Sphincteroplasty was developed in 1951 in an effort to improve upon the poor results that had been obtained with sphincterotomy in treating recurrent pancreatitis. The common channel theory was popular at that time, and as the sphincteric mechanisms described affected the

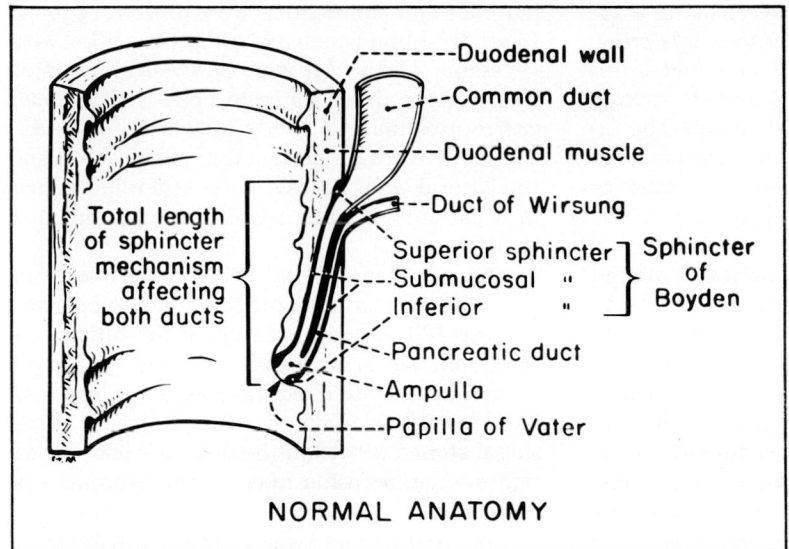

Total length
of sphincter
mechanism
affecting
both ducts

--------Duodenal wall

--Common duct

---Duodenal muscle

---Duct of Wirsung

Superior sphincter ⎤ Sphincter
----Submucosal   "   ⎬ of
Inferior   "   ⎦ Boyden

--Pancreatic duct

--Ampulla

----Papilla of Vater

NORMAL ANATOMY

Figure 81–1. The duodenal wall and the submucosal sphincter of Boyden make up the constricting mechanism affecting the distal common and pancreatic ducts.

pancreatic as well as the common duct, it was believed that complete ablation of the sphincters would eliminate this possible etiologic factor more effectively than would sphincterotomy. It was recognized early that any procedure on the distal end of the common and pancreatic ducts would be of absolutely no value in the presence of parenchymal destruction and fibrosis or intrapancreatic ductal obstruction. We were impressed by the experimental work of Lium and Maddock, who showed that pancreatitis could be produced regularly in animals by simultaneous obstruction of the duct and stimulation of the gland to secrete. In a second report we described this possible etiologic mechanism and emphasized that a pancreatic ductogram should be utilized to determine the status of the intrapancreatic ductal system before choosing the optimum surgical approach. In this same paper (1958) we reported the division of the septum between the pancreatic and common ducts in addition to sphincteroplasty in patients with recurrent pancreatitis, no gross parenchymal disease, and a ductogram that showed no intrapancreatic ductal obstruction.

As very few patients with acute recurrent pancreatitis meet these criteria, the operation has a limited although definite value in treating this disease. *It soon became apparent that the elimination of the distal sphincteric mechanism affecting the distal ducts was of great benefit in prophylaxis and treatment of residual common duct stones. At this time we consider this* *to be by far the most important indication for a transduodenal sphincteroplasty.*

INDICATIONS AND CONTRAINDICATIONS

General Considerations

There are a number of operations that may be used to produce free common duct drainage; sphincteroplasty is simply one method. These procedures should not be thought of as competitive with each other but rather as different ways to achieve the same objective. The optimum operation should be selected after evaluating the specific problem in question. This can best be illustrated by discussing some of the alternate approaches before giving our indications and contraindications for sphincteroplasty.

Lateral choledochoduodenostomy, a side-to-side anastomosis between the common duct and the first portion of the duodenum, was introduced by Riedel in 1892 and popularized in the United States by Madden and Chun's report of 1970. We have used this procedure frequently to bypass unresectable malignant disease or to treat certain benign strictures that extend up to the retroduodenal portion of the common duct. The operation can be performed easily and rapidly, an advantage in poor-risk patients.

Disadvantages of this procedure include an inability to visualize the papilla of Vater directly, which could result in overlooking a tumor. *Most important is the fact that this procedure should never be attempted on a duct of less than 20 mm diameter or subsequent obstruction may result.* In bypassing a malignancy, the tumor must not be of a size and location that would make obstruction of the duodenum or ductal anastomosis imminent. It is not our choice of procedure in the prophylaxis or treatment of residual common duct stones, as a blind distal pouch is formed and the "sump syndrome" shown in Figure 81–2 may come into play. However, in the old and severely ill patient with multiple common duct stones this operation, because of the ease and rapidity of its execution, may prove to be the procedure of choice.

The significance of the sump syndrome has been debated. There is no doubt that the duct distal to the anastomosis may become filled with vegetable debris producing anastomotic obstruction. Lord Smith of Marlow had to operate upon 25 patients sent to him after a lateral anastomosis had been performed. All had developed obstruction with cholangitis, and in addition

jaundice and pancreatitis were present in some. In all, the blind pouch or "sump" was filled with vegetable debris. All were successfully treated by a transduodenal sphincteroplasty. The upper gastrointestinal (GI) study shown in Figure 81–3 demonstrates an obstruction of the sump and the lateral anastomosis with vegetable debris in a patient we were asked to see in consultation.

The incidence of this postoperative obstruction is very debatable. Madden had no problem in over 100 patients so treated for biliary obstruction. We believe that it occurs with sufficient frequency to make the operation less than ideal for the prophylaxis and treatment of residual stones, although the patient's poor condition may on occasion make it the procedure of choice.

In treating the large multiple intrahepatic stones found in Oriental cholangiohepatitis or in the presence of a grossly enlarged ductal system packed with calculi, a Roux-Y choledochojejunostomy is preferred. This operation is also indicated in the presence of a perivaterian di-

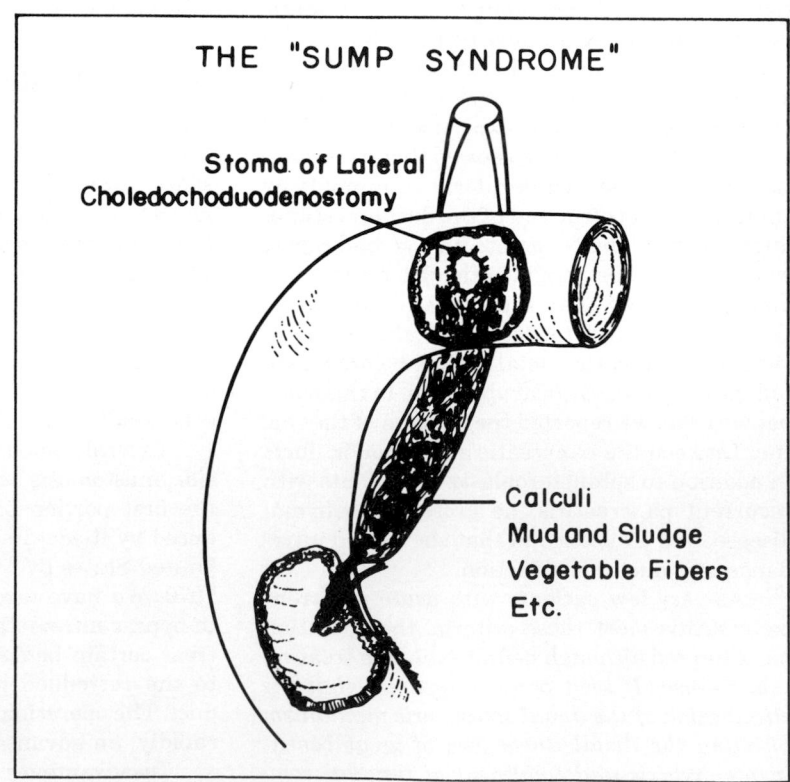

THE "SUMP SYNDROME"

Stoma of Lateral
Choledochoduodenostomy

Calculi
Mud and Sludge
Vegetable Fibers
Etc.

Figure 81–2. The normally narrowed distal common duct contributes to the formation of the "sump syndrome," which occasionally follows lateral choledochoduodenostomy.

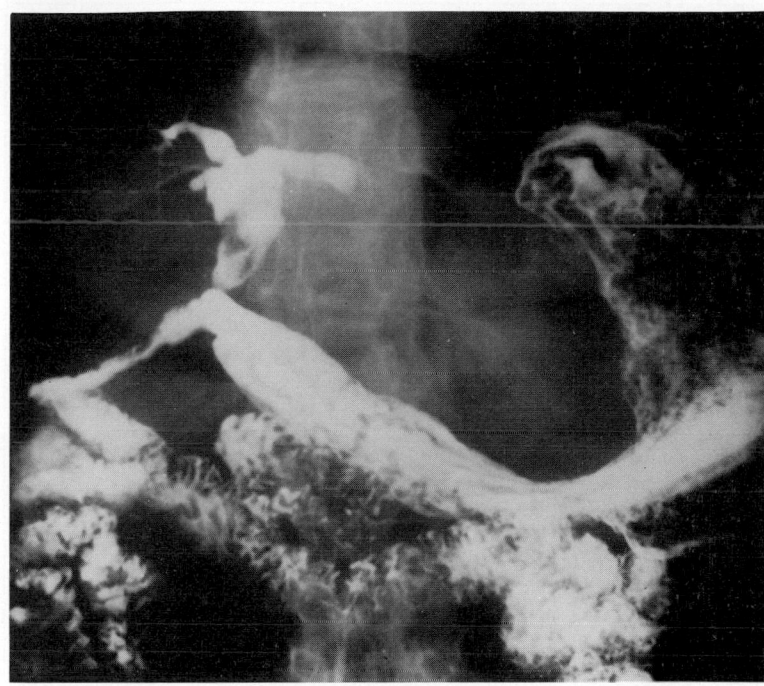

Figure 81–3. The "sump syndrome" as seen on upper GI study. Note the narrowing at the anastomosis and the dilated proximal biliary tree. This patient had severe recurrent cholangitis.

verticulum or any inflammatory disease of the distal common duct including acute pancreatitis where distal obstruction must be relieved.

When postoperative cholangiograms demonstrate a residual stone, a continuous saline irrigation through the T-tube and a course of antispasmodics are begun. This is continued for 5 to 6 days, when the cholangiogram is repeated. This long employed approach is often very successful.

Any discussion of the treatment of residual common duct stones must include the more recent methods of removal of the calculus or calculi by nonsurgical (nontransabdominal) methods. The removal of overlooked calculi by endoscopic retrograde cholangiopancreatography (ERCP) has been reported. Successful division of the papillary sphincter by a high frequency diathermy knife passed into the papilla to divide it has been described. While it is understandable that a skilled endoscopist might remove a distally lodged calculus, it is difficult to imagine how the operator could safely divide all of the sphincteric mechanisms that could trap calculi using a hot wire for the incision. A local burn should produce fibrosis and narrowing. Anatomically, if all of the sphincteric

mechanism were destroyed, the division would be outside of the duodenal wall and a leak would be inevitable. Therefore, *we must recognize that an endoscopic operation is a sphincterotomy, not a sphincteroplasty.* Indeed it is referred to in the literature as a papillotomy or sphincterotomy.

A recent report describes 59 endoscopic papillotomies. Fifty one had common duct stones. In 10 the calculi could not be removed, a retained stone percentage of 19.6. Four of these patients required surgery. Included in the 15.2 percent morbidity were 5 cases of bleeding, 3 requiring surgery for control. The overall mortality related to the procedure was 3.4 percent.

This is not mentioned to condemn ERCP. Indeed, were this author faced with the problem of an elderly poor-risk patient with a retained stone, it would probably be recommended. However, this approach can produce a sphincterotomy, not a sphincteroplasty and it is not an innocuous procedure. It took some years to demonstrate the postoperative problems associated with sphincterotomy. Similarly, after a large number of cases and a long-term evaluation, ERCP will be placed in its proper perspective.

Chemical dissolution of cholesterol stones

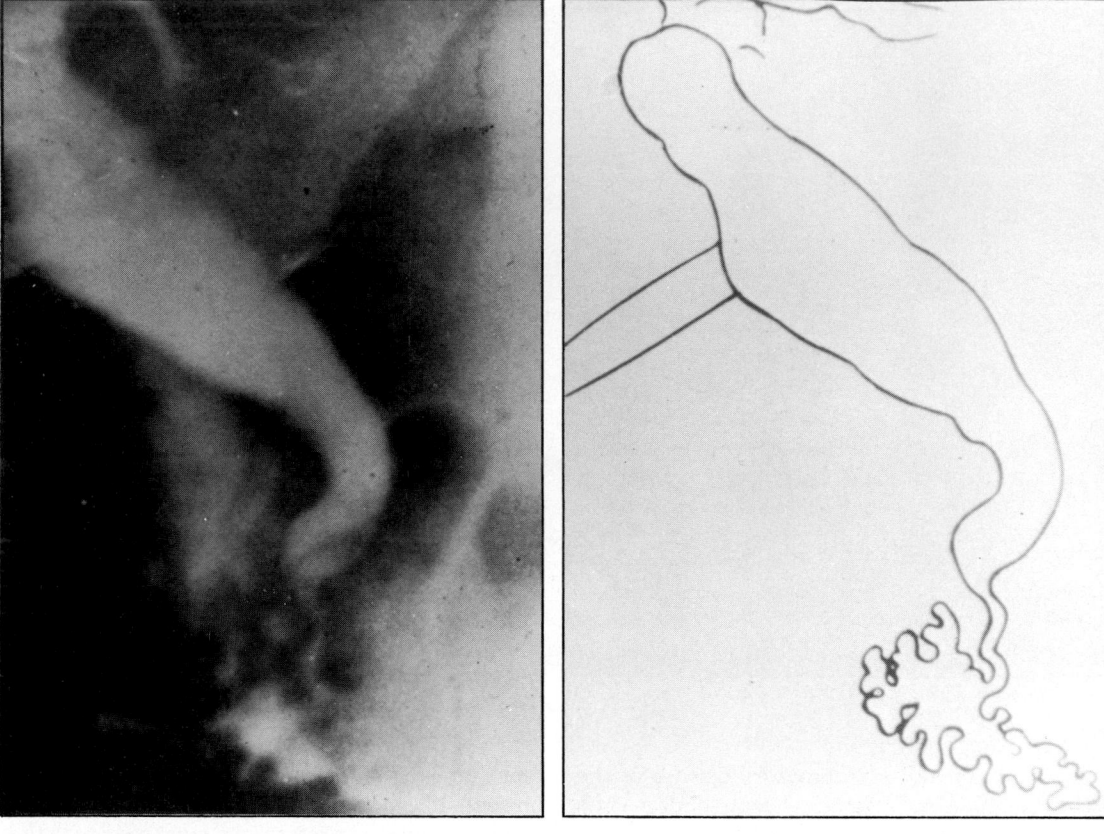

Figure 81–4. This stricture from chronic pancreatitis permitted passage of a 6 mm dilator but obstructed free bile flow, resulting in recurrent cholangitis. (*Source: Jones SA, 1978, with permission.*)

in the ducts may be successful using a solution of cholic acid in 100 mm concentration instilled through the T-tube. Way reports over 30 patients so treated, with a ⅔ dissolution rate. If successful, the stone disappears in 10 to 14 days. Stones over 1.5 cm in diameter usually do not dissolve.

Another approach to the extraction of residual common duct stones involves the passage under fluoroscopic control of a flexible forceps or a Dormia basket through the T-tube tract and into the common duct. The T-tube, which must be at least a No. 14 French, is left in position for 5 to 6 weeks after the stone or stones are demonstrated on postoperative study. The tract should then be "mature," but if it is not of sufficient size, it may be dilated gently. This approach was described in 1970 by Mazzariello who reported an 86 percent success rate in 76 patients. A more recent paper showed over 90 percent success in 220 patients. Burhenne developed a steerable catheter and obtained even better results. The success depends upon the skill and experience of the radiologist.

Should the preceding procedures fail, reoperation is usually advised, and sphincteroplasty is given strong consideration.

Indications

Primary Duct Exploration

Obstructive Biliary Tract Disease. We advise sphincteroplasty when the surgeon encounters impacted distal duct stones, stenosis of the papilla (less than 3 mm diameter when checked from above and below and from both sides of the table), short benign distal duct strictures, irremovable hepatic duct stones, mud, sludge, or stasis stones that are diagnostic of chronic distal duct obstruction, and *multiple calculi in the ducts. By the latter is meant a sufficient number of stones present to make complete clearing of the ducts doubtful.* Duca advises sphincteroplasty when a hepatic hydatid cyst ruptures into the bile ducts, as ductal stenosis may occur even after removal of the parasite.

A long distal stricture, often produced by chronic pancreatitis, can present a special problem. If the common duct above the stricture is less than 20 mm in diameter, a lateral choledochoduodenostomy is not advised. A sphincteroplasty might produce dangerous pancreatic trauma. Under these circumstances, it may be necessary to transect the common duct obliquely above the pancreas, oversewing the distal end and implanting the proximal end into a jejunal segment (loop or Roux-Y) or into the well-mobilized duodenum, the so-called transection choledochoduodenostomy. Another approach would involve the interposition of an isolated segment of jejunum between the proximal end of the common duct and the side of the duodenum.

In evaluating distal duct strictures, it is very important to realize that *the ability to pass a dilator into the duodenum is not adequate proof of free bile flow.* As an example, the operative cholangiogram in Figure 81–4 shows a distal stricture produced by chronic pancreatitis. This patient had had four biliary tract operations when first seen by us. On each occasion at common duct exploration a number 6 Bakes' dilator could be passed freely into the duodenum. However, at each operation the bile contained mud and sludge, and the proximal ducts were moderately dilated. *These findings indicated intermittent ductal obstruction, the ability to pass the dilator notwithstanding.* Manometric evaluation might have been valuable in this situation but was not done. At each operation the common duct was drained by a T-tube. Cholangitis promptly followed each T-tube withdrawal. In Figure 81–4, note that the dye filled the upper radicles of the ductal system. Figure 81–5, a cholangiogram done 9 days after sphincteroplasty, shows the elimination of the stricture and such rapid passage of the dye into the bowel that the upper biliary tree did not fill. The same response can be seen in Figure 81–6. The T-tube was withdrawn, the patient's recovery was uneventful, and he has had no further difficulty.

Acute pancreatitis has been mentioned and will not be considered further in this discussion of the prophylaxis and treatment of residual biliary tract stones.

Residual Stones

If faced with this problem, we would advise attempts at dissolution, T-tube tract, or ERCP removal. If surgery becomes necessary, our present concept of management of residual calculi differs from that which we reported some years ago. Briefly, our past approach was to do a sphincteroplasty routinely when operating for residual stones. This was based on the fact that multiple operations are frequently required in patients with residual duct calculi. In recent years, we have been selecting our cases. If there is evidence that the residual stone or stones are of gallbladder origin, the bile is clean and clear, completion x-rays and choledochoscopy reveal a clear duct, and the papilla is not stenotic, removal of the calculi alone should be adequate surgical therapy. If the indications for sphincteroplasty are present, this procedure should prevent further residual stones, either overlooked or reformed.

Sphincteroplasty is indicated when operating upon a lateral choledochoduodenostomy obstructed by the sump syndrome.

Contraindications

Sphincteroplasty is *not* advised at primary or subsequent choledocholithotomy if the bile is clear, the calculi appear to be of gallbladder origin, only a few large calculi are present, the papilla is 3 mm in diameter or larger, choledochoscopy is clear, and the completion cholangiogram is normal. It is not done in the presence of long distal duct strictures or if there is any anatomic abnormality at the lower end of the duct, such as a perivaterian diverticulum. It is contraindicated in the presence of any distal duct inflammatory disease, including acute pancreatitis.

In the presence of gross ductal dilatation, Caroli's disease or Oriental cholangiohepatitis, a Roux-Y choledochojejunostomy is a better choice. In the aged and seriously ill patient with a dilated duct and multiple calculi, lateral choledochoduodenostomy may prove to be the simplest, quickest, and safest operation.

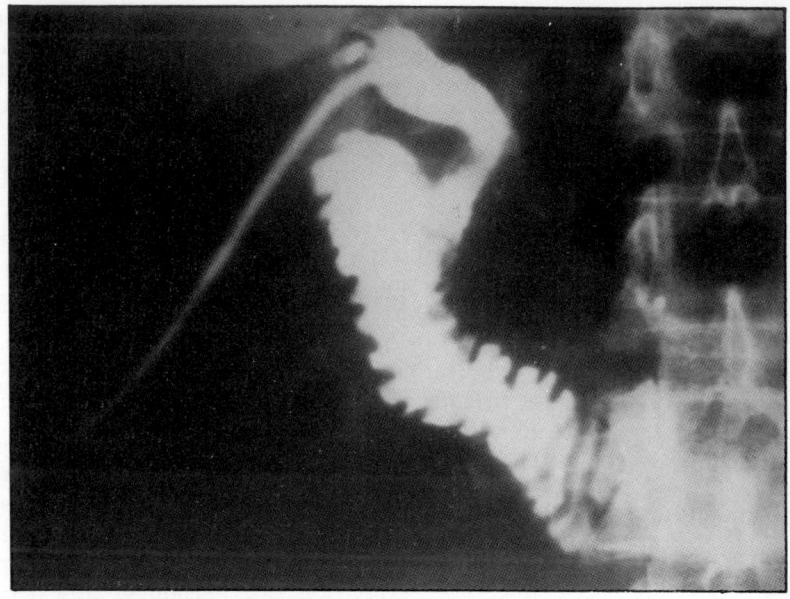

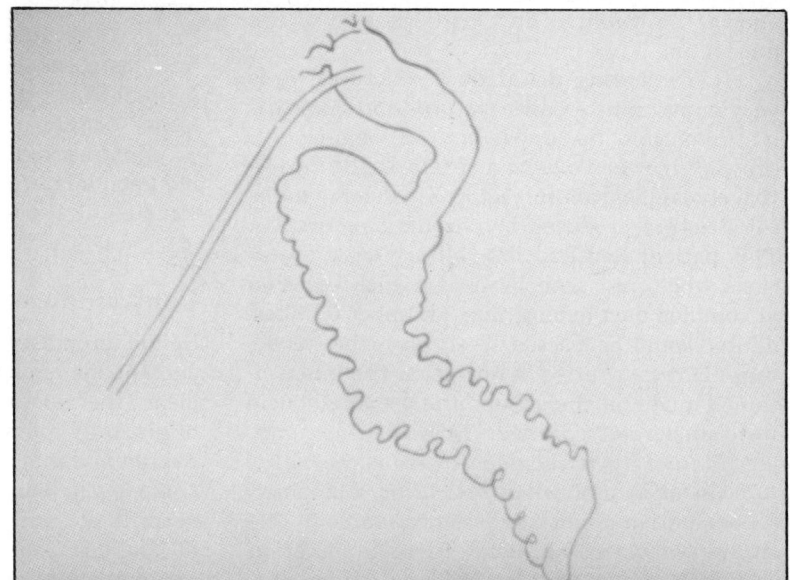

Figure 81–5. After four unsuccessful common duct explorations, the patient was relieved by sphincteroplasty. (*Source: From Jones SA, 1978, with permission.*)

TECHNIQUE OF TRANSDUODENAL SPHINCTEROPLASTY

There are numerous methods of performing sphincteroplasty. Most if not all are covered in Duca's extensive monograph on the sphincter of Oddi. The technique given here is one that we have developed and modified through the years.

We perform sphincteroplasty by approaching the papilla of Vater transduodenally and, by serial clamping, division, and suture approximation of the duodenal and common duct walls, creating a wide anastomosis between the end of the common duct and the side of the duodenum. *This opening must be equal in diameter to that of the supraduodenal common duct.* Before the procedure is described step-by-step, the

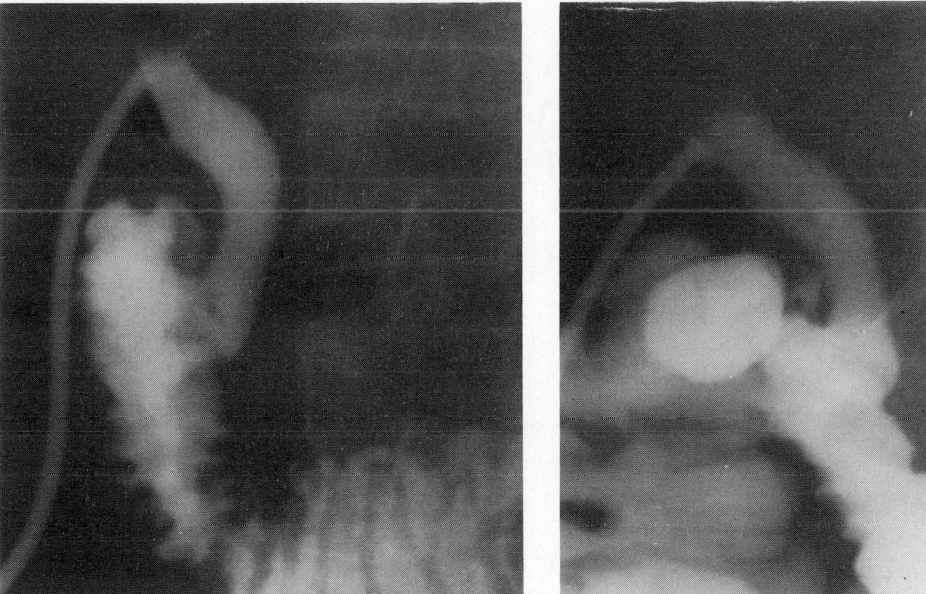

Figure 81–6. Post-sphincteroplasty T-tube cholangiograms before morphine (*left*) and after morphine (*right*). The sphincters have been destroyed, and there is no ductal constriction.

reader should refer to the following diagrams that will clarify the overall objective of the operation and emphasize the differences between sphincteroplasty and sphincterotomy.

Figure 81–7 notes that the length of the intramural course of the ducts varied from 6 to 30 mm in our and others' dissections. Therefore *the length of the incision made cannot be used as a criterion for the adequacy of a sphincteroplasty.* A 20 mm incision would be excessive in a patient whose ducts had only a 6 mm course and entirely inadequate in a subject with an oblique 30 mm intramural length. *Therefore, we disregard the length of the incision we are making in the common duct and duodenal walls and continue the serial clamping, division, and suture approximation until the stoma created equals that of the largest part of the supraduodenal common duct. This accomplished, we can feel assured that we have destroyed the sphincteric mechanism in that particular patient.* We have not relied on mucosal color change to determine the proper length of the sphincteroplasty.

Figure 81–8 diagrams the procedure from the front, as seen by the operator. The papilla is doubly clamped, the tissue between the clamps is divided or a portion is taken for biopsy,

and the clamps are oversewn, approximating common duct and duodenal walls. This process is continued upward until the opening created is co-equal to that of the supraduodenal common duct. *At the apex the operator will be outside of the duodenal wall, and a carefully placed figure-eight apex stitch placed at this point is essential to avoid a leak.*

Figure 81–9 compares a completed sphincterotomy and sphincteroplasty. Following sphincterotomy, only the distal portion of the sphincter mechanism is divided, and there is an appreciable amount of tissue left behind that can constrict the ducts. As shown, sphincteroplasty completely eliminates the sphincteric action and results in an end-to-side choledochoduodenostomy that is equal in diameter to that of the largest part of the common duct.

Transduodenal sphincteroplasty can be performed by anyone familiar with biliary tract surgery, but we urge that the points listed in the following be followed carefully.

Antibiotics. Because the majority of patients upon whom we perform sphincteroplasty have common duct calculi, distal duct obstruction with bile stasis, or both, antibiotics are advocated preoperatively, during surgery, and in

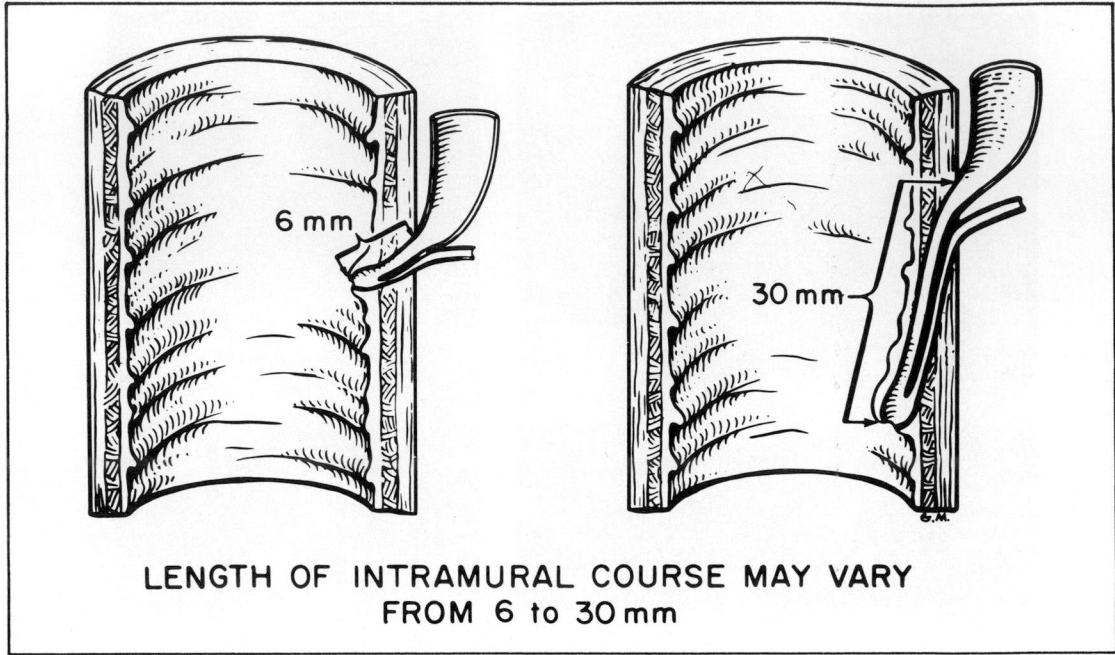

LENGTH OF INTRAMURAL COURSE MAY VARY
FROM 6 to 30 mm

Figure 81–7. The length of the intramural course shows great individual variation.

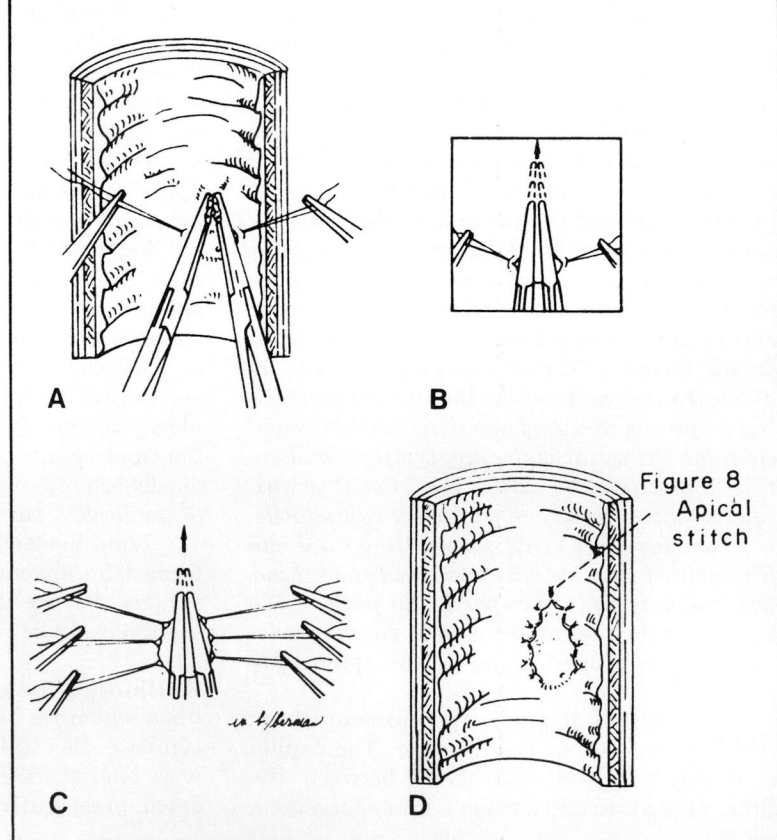

Figure 81–8. The concept of sphincteroplasty is serial clamping, division, and suture approximation of the common duct and duodenal walls until the opening created equals the largest part of the common duct.

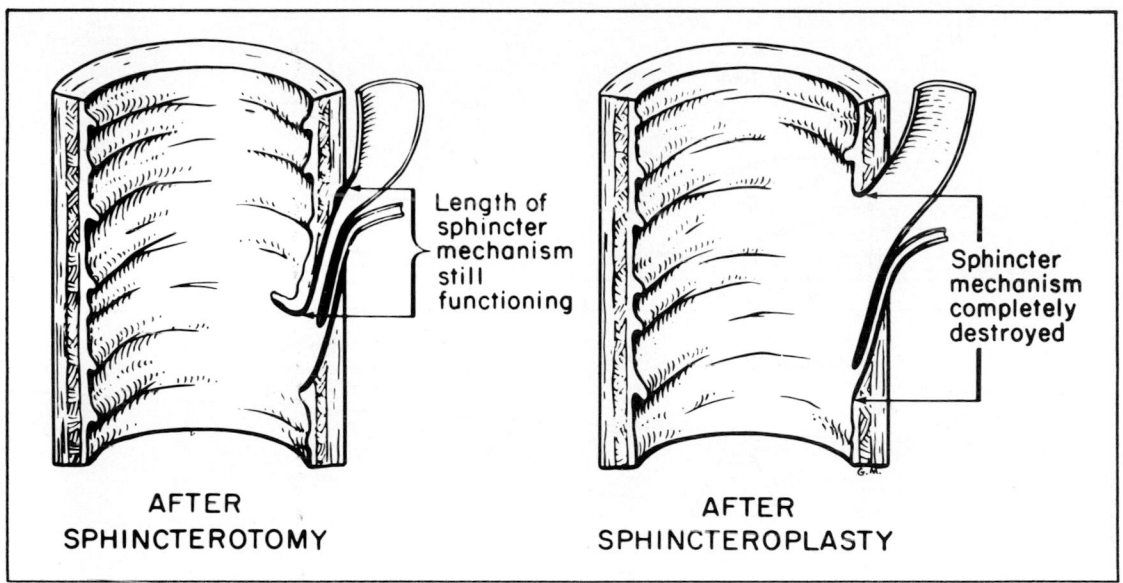

AFTER
SPHINCTEROTOMY

Length of
sphincter
mechanism
still
functioning

AFTER
SPHINCTEROPLASTY

Sphincter
mechanism
completely
destroyed

Figure 81–9. After sphincterotomy a portion of the sphincter remains. This is eliminated by sphincteroplasty.

the first 24 hours postoperatively. The antibiotics selected should be effective against aerobic gram-negative enteric coliforms, of which *Escherichia coli* predominates, and anaerobic organisms, especially *Bacteroides fragilis*. Gentamicin or kanamycin are effective against the coliforms, and *Bacteroides* is sensitive to both penicillin G and clindamycin. Specimens of bile are taken at surgery for culture and sensitivity.

Operative Position. With the table level with the floor, a wedge-shaped radiolucent pad extending from the buttocks to the scapula is used to elevate the patient's left side 25 to 30 degrees. During surgery the left side of the operating table is lowered so that the patient is directly supine. When cholangiography is performed, the table is returned to the level position, thus elevating the patient's left side. In this position the ductal system does not overlie the vertebrae and the Bucky grid is at right angles to the rays from the tube, insuring a sharp film. Following cholangiographic studies, the left side of the table is lowered as before, and the operation is completed with the patient supine (Fig. 81–10).

Incision. A right subcostal incision is employed, placing the skin incision at least three fingerbreadths below the costal margin and leaving an upper flap for retraction. A higher subcostal incision will result in undesirable pressure upon an unyielding rib cage. If necessary, exceptional exposure can be obtained by using a vertical midline extension.

Dissection of the Biliary Tree. All components are carefully isolated, and the "normal" in the individual being operated upon is determined before any structure is tied, clamped, or cut.

Cholangiography (Fig. 81–11). This is usually done through the cystic duct using a small plastic catheter with a conical tip that prevents an accidental withdrawal. The Hypaque is diluted, using a 25 percent concentration for a 1 cm duct, 15 percent for a 2 cm duct, etc. Three films are made. The first after an injection of 2 ml, a second after an additional 5 ml, and a third of larger volume varying with the caliber of the biliary tree. The films should always be checked by a radiologist. A completion cholangiogram is obtained after the ductal exploration has been done.

Television monitoring is a most valuable aid in this procedure but has not been available to us. Not only can dye be observed as it enters the ductal system and the sphincteric opening pressure noted, but the surgeon may take multi-

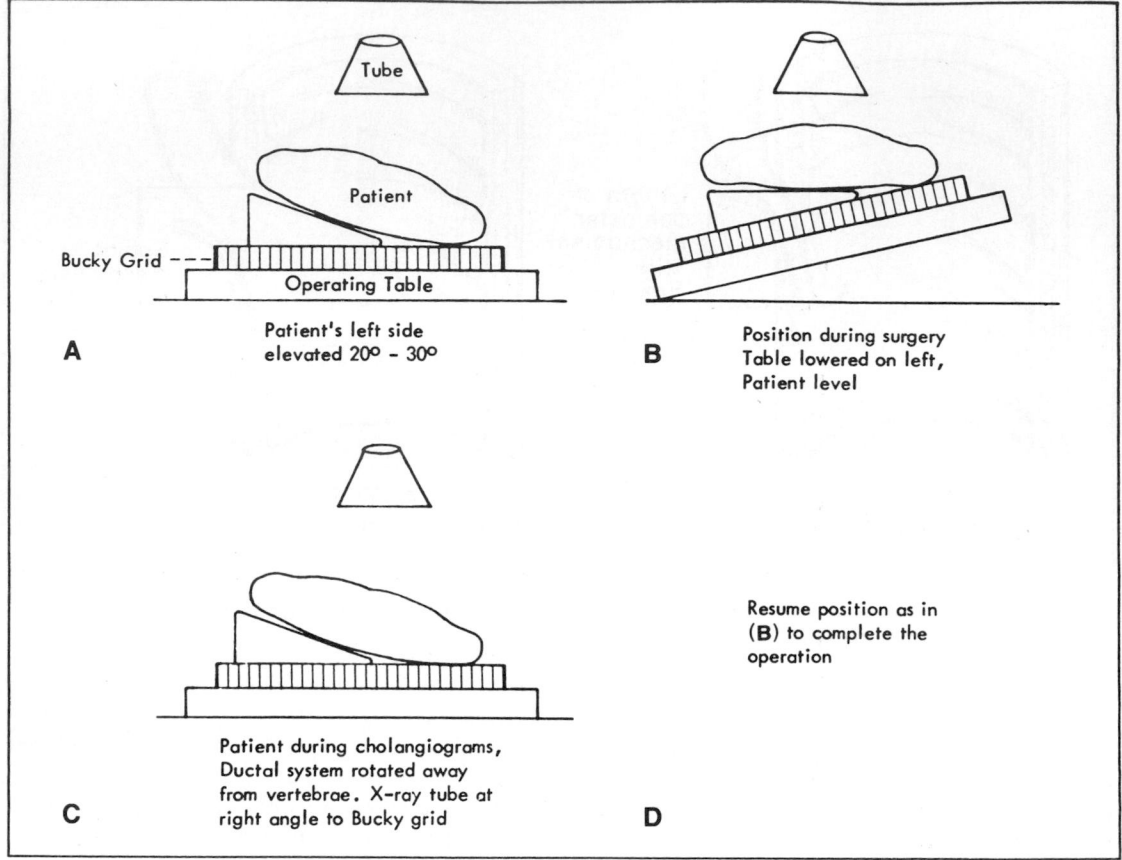

Figure 81–10. A. The patient's left side elevated 20 to 30 degrees. **B.** The position during the operation. **C.** The same position as **(A)** prevents the ductal system from overlying the vertebrae. **D.** The same position as **(B)** is used to complete the operation.

ple films during the procedure if any questionable defect is visualized.

Cholecystectomy. If the decision has been made to do a sphincteroplasty, cholecystectomy is done at this time. In the absence of distal sphincters, the gallbladder will not fill or function and can only serve as a possible site for future difficulties.

Duodenal Mobilization. The duodenum must be thoroughly mobilized by incising the peritoneum lateral to the descending second portion and including the peritoneal reflection that forms the inferior border of the foramen of Winslow.

Common Duct Exploration. The common duct is opened longitudinally between stay sutures, irrigated, and explored with finger manip-

ulation, which may yield stone recovery. Next, forceps, Fogarty catheters, and a choledochoscope are employed. When the duct appears clear, a No. 10 French (3 mm) red rubber catheter is passed downward to the papilla. With the duodenum mobilized, the finger behind the common duct palpates and guides the catheter. The point of entry into the duodenal lumen is used as the center point of the subsequent duodenotomy. We make every effort to avoid the use of metallic probes, fearing a false passage. We never dilate the papilla, as this maneuver is followed by fibrosis and subsequent ductal narrowing.

Duodenotomy. We open the duodenum longitudinally, as we are never certain of the exact level of the papilla even when a catheter has been introduced from above (Fig. 81–12). It is

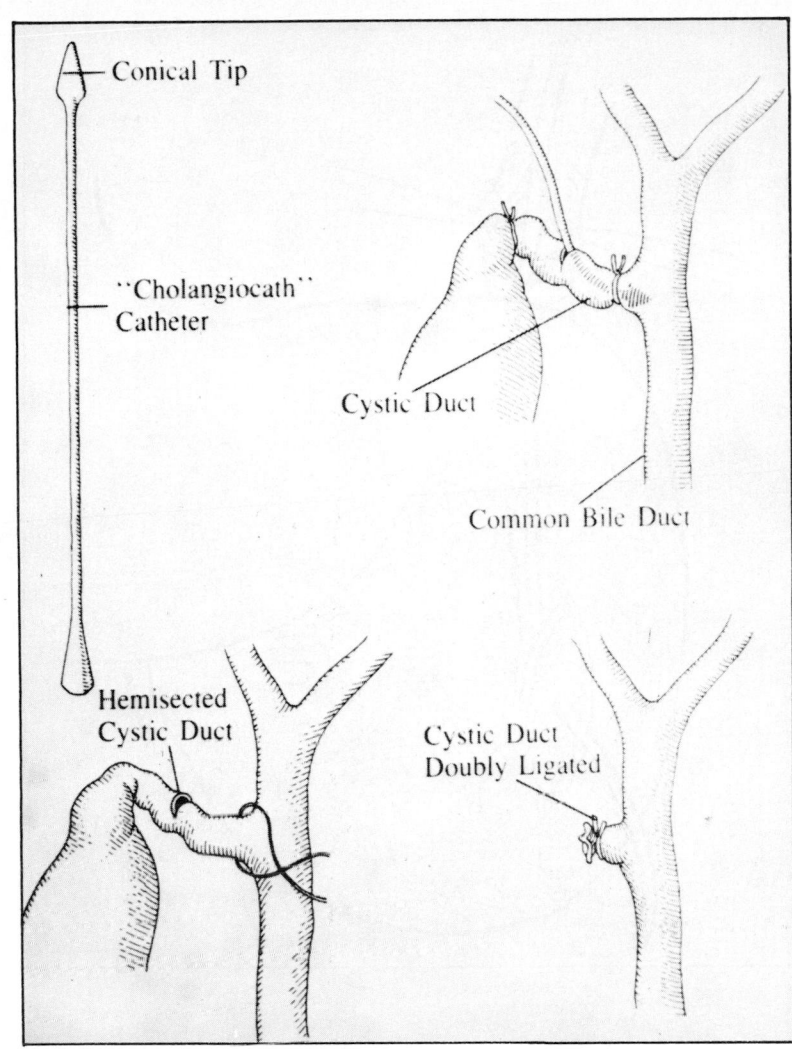

Conical Tip

"Cholangiocath" Catheter

Cystic Duct

Common Bile Duct

Hemisected Cystic Duct

Cystic Duct Doubly Ligated

Figure 81–11. The usual cystic duct cholangiography technique. (*Source: From Jones SA, 1979, with permission.*)

usually farther distal than expected, and a longitudinal incision can be extended more easily than can an oblique or transverse one. It must be recognized that while the lateral border of the duodenum can be freed by the Kocher maneuver, the medial margin cannot as it is in such intimate vascular contact with the pancreas. Hence, the principle of maintaining a large lumen by longitudinal incision and transverse closure cannot be applied in this situation, as it would result in undesirable tension on the suture line. To summarize, regardless of the axis of the duodenotomy, the incision must always be closed in the direction in which it is made.

If the duodenum is difficult to expose be-cause of previous surgery or disease, it may be visualized by incising the root of the transverse mesocolon or by the ingenious lateral extraperitoneal approach designed by Professor G.B. Ong of Hong Kong.

Locating the Papilla of Vater. If the catheter can be passed from above as described under Common Duct Exploration, this presents no problem. If this cannot be done or if previous right upper quadrant surgery has made the common duct difficult to locate, the duodenum is opened longitudinally, low in the second portion. The papilla can usually be palpated as a firm rubbery nubbin of tissue on the postero-medial mucosal wall and can be felt more read-

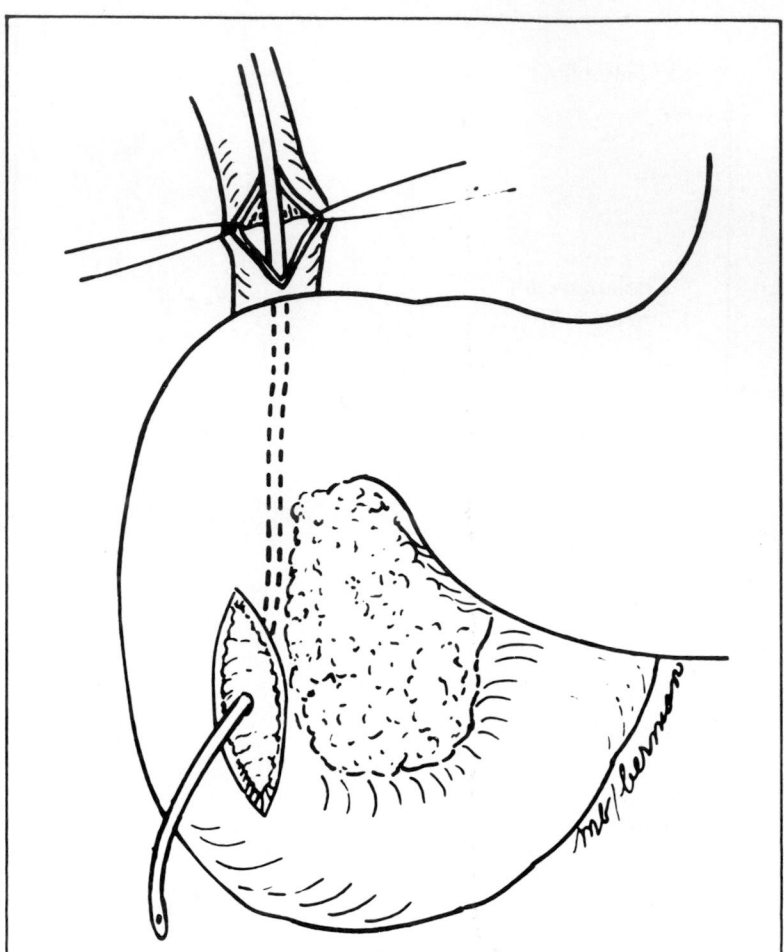

Figure 81-12. The papilla is located by the passage of a catheter downward through a choledochostomy made over the point of catheter entrance into the bowel. (*Source: From Jones SA, 1979, with permission.*)

ily than seen. Visualization of the papilla is aided by flattening the mucosal folds using a small glass circle we designed for this purpose. Careful inspection may disclose bile and/or pancreatic juice coming from the papilla. A small suction tip or repeated dabbing with small "peanut" sponges is helpful.

It is very important to recognize that exploration of the papilla from below presents the hazard of mistaking the pancreatic duct for the common duct. After the papilla is incised, the operator should gently pass a Bakes' dilator upward to make certain of the position in the common duct before proceeding.

Figure 81-13 shows the placement of a suture in the papilla at 10 o'clock. This is used as a guide for the placement of the first pair of clamps.

Initial Clamp Placement. Figure 81-14A shows the first pair of mosquito clamps placed at 10 o'clock in an anterolateral position to avoid damage to the pancreatic duct which, in our dissections, always entered on the medial side of the common duct. The tissue between this initial pair of clamps is divided, and the clamps are oversewn using 5-0 atraumatic silk. Each clamp is removed as the suture is tied. When the papilla has been opened and the pancreatic duct visualized, as in Figure 81-14B (shown at 5 o'clock), *subsequent pairs of clamps are placed directly anteriorly.* If a biopsy is desired, the handles of the clamps are separated, leaving a wedge of tissue that can be excised and removed using the suture passed through it. Figure 81-15 shows this technique employed on the third pair of clamps.

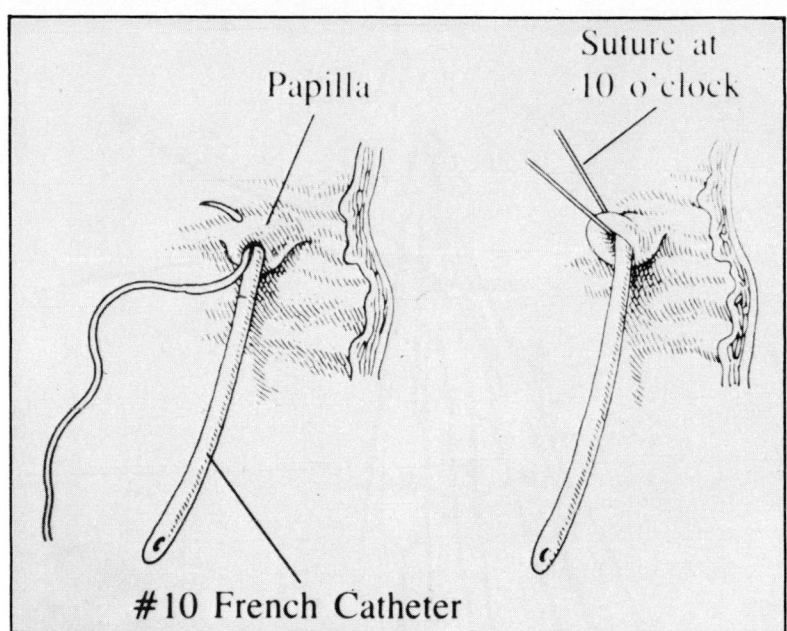

Figure 81–13. A guide stitch is placed in the papilla at 10 o'clock to act as a marker for the placement of the first pair of clamps. In this position the clamps should not produce pancreatic duct damage.

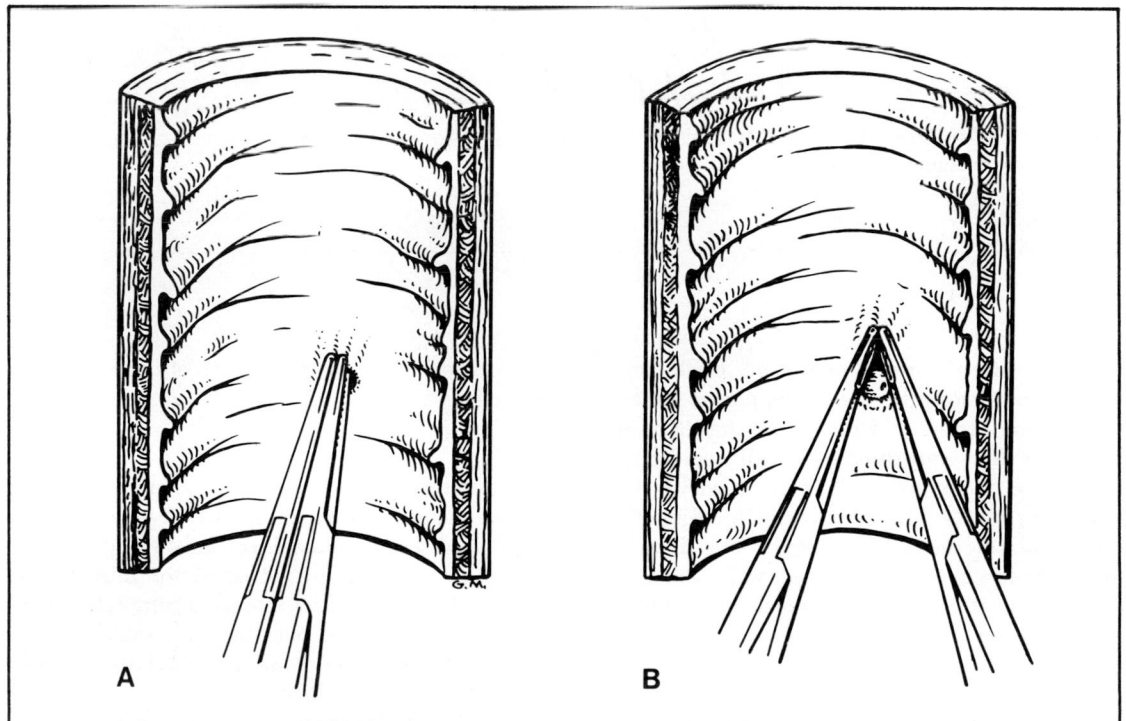

Figure 81–14. A. The first pair of clamps is placed at 10 o'clock. The tissue between them will be divided. **B.** The pancreatic duct having been visualized, successive pairs of clamps are placed directly anteriorly.

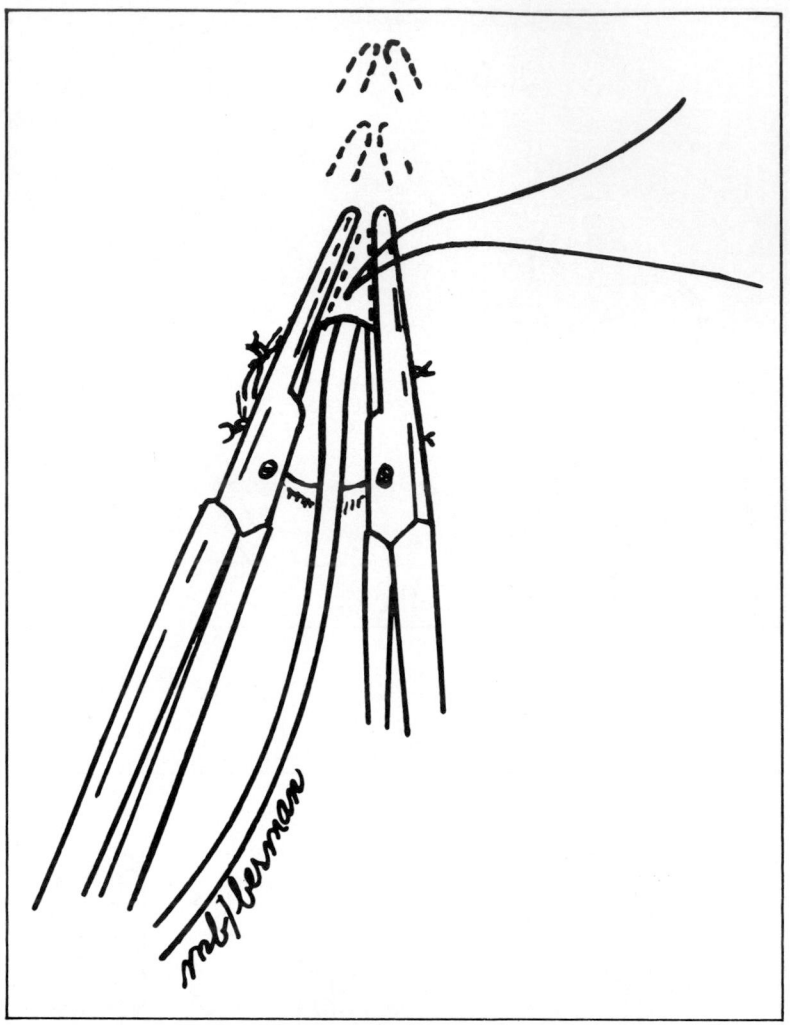

Figure 81–15. If a biopsy is desired, it may be taken between the angled clamps and the tissue removed by a previously placed suture.

Subsequent Clamp Placement. Each successive pair of mosquito clamps is placed parallel, one to the other, and not more than 3 mm of common duct and duodenal wall are included at a time. This process is continued until the diameter of the stoma is equal to that of the largest diameter of the common bile duct. The opening is carefully checked with Bakes' dilators, and if there is any question of constriction, further division is done. If the diameter is equal to that of the supraduodenal common duct we know that we have carried the incision through the duodenal wall, and suture approximation by the figure-eight apical stitch shown in Figure 81–8 is mandatory to avoid a leak. We have not relied upon mucosal color change to determine the proper length of the sphincteroplasty.

Placement of T-Tube. If the common duct has been opened, a short-limbed 14F T-tube that has been "guttered" is used. In cases where the patient has been operated upon for multiple or residual common duct stones, a completion cholangiogram can be obtained by occluding the distal common duct with a small balloon catheter inflated just prior to Hypaque injection through the T-tube.

If the sphincteroplasty is done from below without a choledochotomy, neither T-tube nor stent is employed.

Division of the Septum Separating the Common and Pancreatic Ducts. While not pertinent to a discussion on residual stones, comments on technique should include two points that are important when operating upon a patient for acute recurrent pancreatitis. As mentioned, a pancreatic ductogram is mandatory in selecting the proper surgical approach. This can often be accomplished by preoperative endoscopic retrograde cholangiopancreatography. If this approach is not available, a duodenotomy is made and a small polyethylene catheter is passed upward through the papilla. Approximately 80 percent of the time the catheter will find the way into the pancreatic duct. On the other hand, if it is necessary to do the first part of a sphincteroplasty in order to visualize the pancreatic duct, the sphincteroplasty should be completed or the remaining sphincteric mechanism may contribute to postoperative pancreatitis.

When operating for acute recurrent pancreatitis, the septum between the common and pancreatic ducts should be divided. This can usually be accomplished with simple division by fine scissors, as the septum is avascular.

Duodenal Wall Closure. The duodenum is closed in a longitudinal direction, using running 3-0 chromic in the mucosa and outer interrupted seromuscular 3-0 silk.

Drainage. A ¾-inch Penrose drain is placed in the galbladder bed. Both it and the T-tube are drawn out through small separate incisions in the abdominal wall.

PHYSIOLOGIC DIFFERENCES BETWEEN SPHINCTEROTOMY AND SPHINCTEROPLASTY

The physiologic differences between the two procedures have been presented in detail in previous reports. An outline of the methods used follows.

Postoperative T-Tube Pressure Studies. Intravenous morphine will constrict any remaining sphincteric mechanism at the lower end of the common duct. Following the administration of this drug, the postsphincterotomy patients show an abrupt rise and sustained pressure elevation, while the postsphincteroplasty group demonstrate only a transient immediate pressure elevation due to reflux of contents from the contracting duodenum followed by a rapid fall to baseline pressure (Fig. 81–16).

Postoperative T-Tube Cholangiography

ROUTINE CHOLANGIOGRAPHY. When the sphincterotomized patient is given intravenous morphine sulfate and dye is injected into the T-tube, complete occlusion of the distal common duct is demonstrable, proving that the sphincteric complex has not been eliminated (Fig. 81–17). In marked contradistinction, the postsphincteroplasty patients demonstrate a wide opening with *free flow both before and after morphine,* proving the complete ablation of the distal sphincters (Fig. 81–6).

CINERADIOGRAPHIC T-TUBE STUDIES. Postoperative cinecholangiography in the two groups verified the points that were demonstrated by standard postoperative cholangiography. In addition, discomfort occurred routinely in the postsphincterotomy patients when dye was injected following morphine, and this group also demonstrated proximal dilatation of the common duct. Neither pain nor ductal distention developed after morphine was given to patients upon whom sphincteroplasty had been performed (Table 81–2).

Postoperative Barium Reflux with Upper Gastrointestinal Studies. Reflux of barium on postoperative upper GI films was not seen after sphincterotomy. In contrast, all patients who had had a complete sphincteroplasty demonstrated free reflux of barium into the biliary tree (Fig. 81–18). We consider the absence of such reflux to be evidence of an incomplete operation.

Permanence of the Stoma Following Sphincteroplasty. While the opening produced by sphincterotomy has been shown to constrict with the passage of time, this does not occur with sphincteroplasty. Very late autopsy studies have demonstrated wide open stomas. Barium reflux has been noted following sphincteroplasty many years after the operation (Fig. 81–11). Eiseman et al have demonstrated experimentally that sphincterotomy is uniformly followed by scarring and a return to presphincterotomy caliber or less.

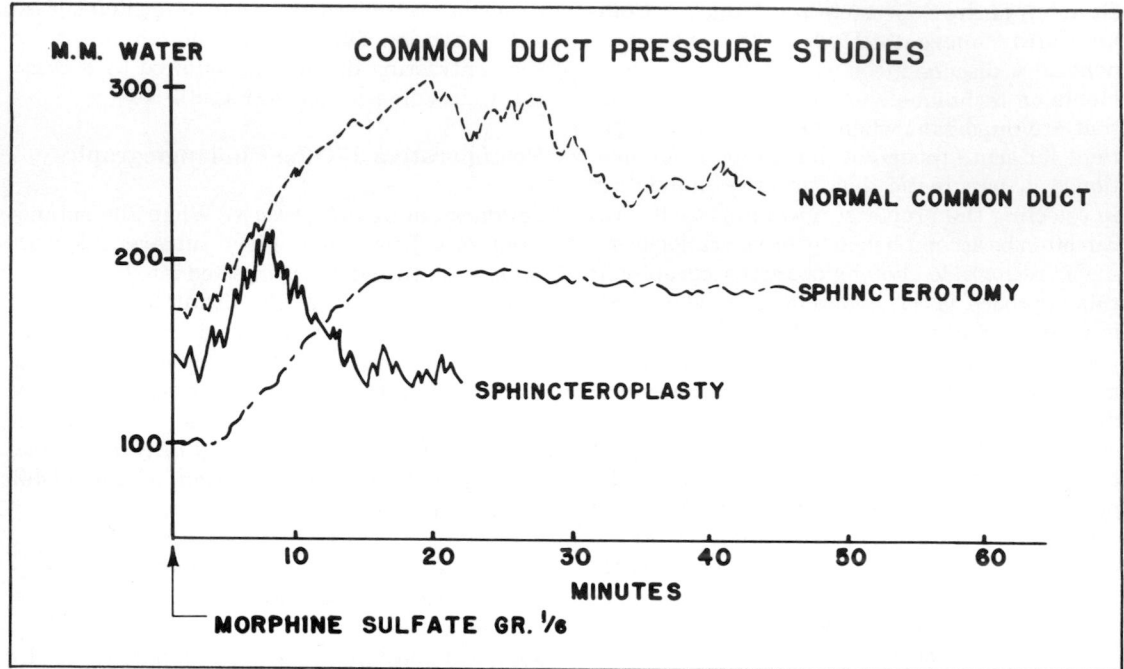

COMMON DUCT PRESSURE STUDIES

M.M. WATER

NORMAL COMMON DUCT

SPHINCTEROTOMY

SPHINCTEROPLASTY

MINUTES

MORPHINE SULFATE GR. ⅙

Figure 81–16. The sudden initial T-tube pressure rise when morphine is given after sphinctero-plasty is due to contraction of the duodenal wall and temporary reflux upward through the wide stoma. The pressure cannot be maintained as the sphincters have been eliminated.

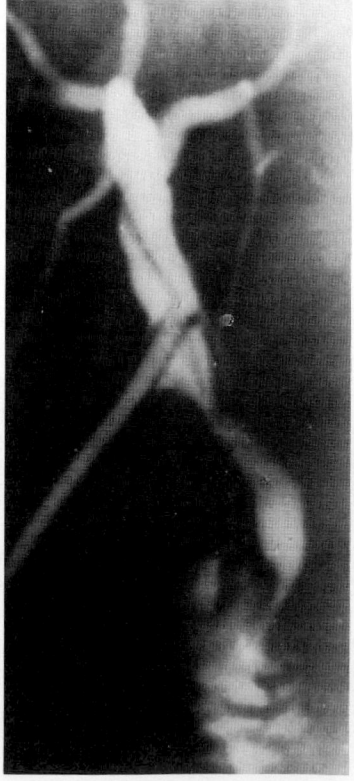 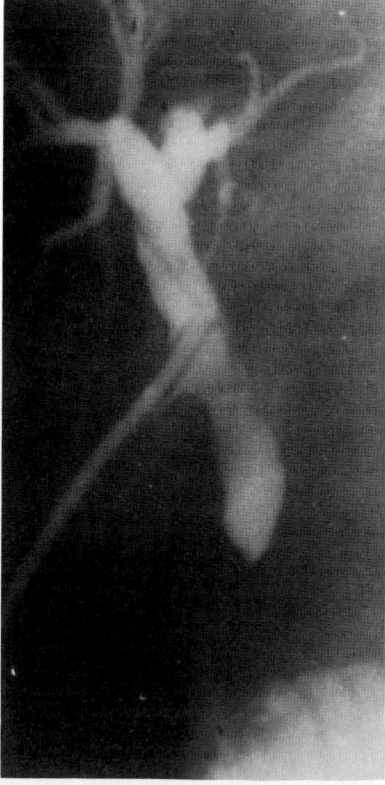

Figure 81–17. *Postsphincter-otomy T-tube cholangiograms* before morphine (*left*) and after morphine (*right*). As the sphincters are not destroyed, they can occlude the distal duct.

TABLE 81–2. POSTOPERATIVE T-TUBE CINERADIOGRAPHY

Factors for Consideration	After Sphincterotomy	After Sphincteroplasty
Position of patient	Supine	45-degree Trendelenburg
Rate of Hypaque infusion	15–30 drops/min	150 drops/min
Amount of Hypaque needed for study	30–60 ml	180–240 ml
Following intravenous morphine		
Distal duct	Occluded	Wide open
Proximal ducts	Dilated	Normal size
Pain	Marked	None
Nausea	Marked	None
Reflux from duodenum	None	In all cases

(*Source: From Jones SA, Smith LL: A reappraisal of sphincteroplasty* (*not sphincterotomy*). *Surgery 71:565, 1972, with permission.*)

We believe that the opening created by sphincteroplasty remains patent because only the anterior portion of the stoma is sutured. In contradistinction, a standard end-to-side choledochoduodenostomy requires suture closure of the entire circumference of the anastomosis and late constriction is not unusual.

RESULTS

Our conclusions are based on 314 transduodenal sphincteroplasties performed over the past 32 years. The vast majority of these were done by or under the supervision of one of four surgeons. Our criteria have been rigid, as each of us has had available a large university service as well as private patients, and the total number is small. It is emphasized that the procedure should not be used indiscriminately.

There were 3 hospital deaths in the 314 patients, an operative mortality of 0.96 percent. Two of the patients were iatrogenic (early in the series). A fourth patient developed a leak at the duodenotomy site (the only one in the series) and was reoperated upon 23 months following sphincteroplasty. This was done in another city and the patient died subsequently from what was described as postoperative peritonitis. There have been no deaths in the last 202 patients.

The morbidity of 4.7 percent includes three

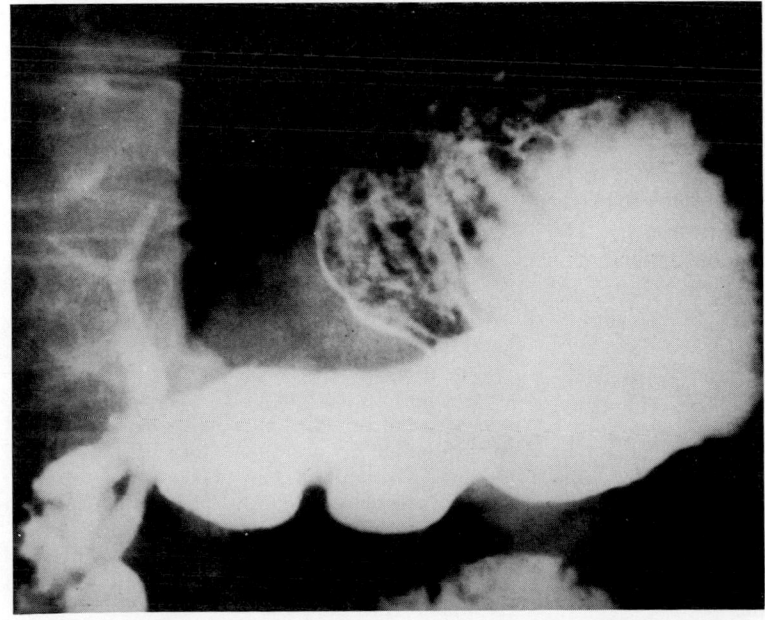

Figure 81–18. This upper GI study demonstrates two points. First, it shows the desired post-sphincteroplasty reflux. Second, it demonstrates the permanence of sphincteroplasty, as this film was taken 12.5 years after the sphincteroplasty had been done.

patients with transient postoperative pancreatitis, six wound infections, and the solitary duodenal leak described. No patient has developed cholangitis postsphincteroplasty, in spite of free reflux of barium on upper GI study. We firmly believe that in the absence of bile stasis this problem will not develop.

Of the 314 sphincteroplasties, 213 were performed for some form of biliary obstruction and 101 for acute recurrent pancreatitis. The results in this latter group are essentially identical with those we have previously reported. In the obstructive disease group, 189 had multiple common duct stones. A number of these had additional indications, such as papillary stenosis, distal duct stricture, irremovable calculi, and muddy bile filled with sludge. Irremovable hepatic duct calculi were present in 4 patients. They were followed from 2 to 7 years after sphincteroplasty and remained asymptomatic. Twenty two were sent to us with residual stones. All 213 patients were relieved of their biliary tract obstruction. *All patients had T-tube cholangiograms on the ninth postsphincteroplasty day. In 5 patients, overlooked calculi were found and immediately washed into the duodenum by saline irrigation. This author feels sure that we overlooked stones in more than 5 patients but that they had passed from the duct to the duodenum through the wide-open stoma during the interval between the sphincteroplasty and the postoperative cholangiogram. Hence, while we left stones behind, they were easily eliminated and of no clinical importance, and we have had no residual stones following sphincteroplasty.*

Our basic philosophy is that the best treatment of residual stones is prophylaxis. As shown in Table 81–1, the various standard methods of prevention presently available are not routinely successful. The results have been improved since this table was compiled but probably have reached an irreducible minimum. If a sufficiently large opening is created between the distal common duct and the duodenum, there is nothing present to prevent the passage of residual stones from the duct to the bowel. Although remarkable techniques have been developed to dissolve or remove residual calculi without operation, these procedures are not without a physical, mental, and financial strain on the patient and have definite medicolegal overtones. We believe that the objective should be to avoid the necessity for these ingenious and highly specialized approaches designed to extricate oneself from a problem.

CONCLUSIONS

Transduodenal sphincteroplasty can be done with a minimum of morbidity and mortality. While the operation should be treated with great respect, never undertaken without good indications, and performed as outlined, *it is difficult to understand why it is often referred to as a procedure carrying great risk. It has been performed by others with results comparable to ours as regards morbidity, mortality, and elimination of obstruction.*

In essence, transduodenal sphincteroplasty is only one of several ways to achieve free bile drainage. These various methods must not be considered competitive but as part of the armamentarium of the biliary surgeon so that the procedure best suited to correct the problem at hand can be selected, as each approach has its own advantages and disadvantages. We believe that if the indications listed are present and the contraindications outlined do not exist, transduodenal sphincteroplasty offers the best approach to the prevention and treatment of residual bile duct stones.

Acknowledgment. Gratitude is expressed to previous co-authors George Gregory, M.D., Louis L. Smith, M.D., and Thomas B. Keller, M.D. for permission to use their cases in compiling this chapter.

BIBLIOGRAPHY

Archibald E: The experimental production of pancreatitis in animals as the result of the resistance of the common duct sphincter. Surg Gynecol Obstet 28:529, 1919
Backer OG: Personal communication
Best RR: The incidence of liver stones associated with cholelithiasis and its clinical significance. Surg Gynecol Obstet 78:425, 1944
Boyden EA: The anatomy of the choledochal junction in man. Surg Gynecol Obstet 104:641, 1957
Burhenne HJ: Personal communication, March 1977.
Chodoff RJ: Choledocholithiasis: Failure of routine operative cholangiography to improve results. J Einstein M Ant 8:215, 1960
Classen M, Safrany L: Endoscopic papillotomy and removal of gall stones. Br Med J 4:317, 1975
Cuschieri A, Wood RAB, et al: Long-term experience with transection choledochoduodenostomy. World J Surg 7:502, 1983
Doubilet H, Mulholland JH: Recurrent acute pancreatitis: Observations on etiology and surgical treatment. Ann Surg 128:609, 1948

Doubilet H, Mulholland JH: Eight year study of pancreatitis and sphincterotomy. JAMA 160:521, 1956

Duca S: Sfincterul lui oddi, patologib si terapeutica chirugicala: Critura litera, Bucuresti, 1983

Eiseman B, Brown WH, et al: Sphincterotomy, an evaluation of its physiological rationale. Arch Surg 79:140, 1959

Fogarty TJ, Krippaehne WW, et al: Evaluation of an improved operative technique in common duct surgery. Am J Surg 116:177, 1968

Geenen JE, Hogan WJ, et al: Endoscopic electrosurgical papillotomy and manometry in biliary tract disease. JAMA 227:2075, 1977

Glisson F: In Hendrickson WF: A study of the musculature of the entire extrahepatic biliary system, including that of the duodenal portion of the common bile duct and of the sphincter. Johns Hopkins Hosp Bull 9:223, 1898

Jolley PC, Baker JW, et al: Operative cholangiography: a case for its routine use. Am Surg 168:551, 1968

Jones SA: The technique of transduodenal sphincteroplasty (not sphincterotomy). Surg Rounds 14–22, January 1979

Jones SA: The prevention and treatment of recurrent bile duct stones by transduodenal sphincteroplasty. World J Surg 2:473, 1978

Jones SA: An instrument to aid in locating the papilla of Vater. Surgery 54:480, 1963

Jones SA, Smith LL, et al: Choledochoduodenostomy to prevent residual stones. Arch Surg 86:1014, 1963

Jones SA, Smith LL, et al: Sphincteroplasty for recurrent pancreatitis: A second report. Ann Surg 147:180, 1958

Jones SA, Smith LL: Transduodenal sphincteroplasty for recurrent pancreatitis. Ann Surg 136:937, 1952

Jones SA, Steedman RA, et al: Transduodenal sphincteroplasty (not sphincterotomy) for biliary and pancreatic disease: Indications, contraindications and results. Am J Surg 118:292, 1969

Kocher T: Ein Fall von Choledochoduodenostomia interna wegen gallensteines. Korrespondenz-blatt Aerzte 7:193, 1895

Lium R, Maddock S: Etiology of acute pancreatitis: Experimental study. Surgery 24:593, 1948

Lowery BD: Personal communication

Madden JL, Chun JY, et al: Choledochoduodenostomy: An unjustly maligned surgical procedure? Am J Surg 119:45, 1970

Mazzariello R: Removal of residual biliary tract calculi without reoperation. Surgery 67:566, 1970

Mazzariello R: Review of 220 cases of residual biliary tract calculi treated without operation. Surgery 73:299, 1973

Mazzeo FT, Jordan SR, et al: Endoscopic papillotomy of recurrent common bile duct stones and papillary stenosis: A community hospital experience. Arch Surg 118,6:693, 1983

McBurney CL: Section of the intestine for the removal of a gallstone. NY State J Med 53:520, 1891

Ong GB: Personal communication

Riedel BMCL: Erfahrungen uber die gallenstein-krankheit mit und ohne icterus. Berlin: Hirschwald, 1892, p 116

Rutledge RH: Sphincteroplasty and choledochoduodenostomy for benign biliary obstructions. Ann Surg 183:476, 1976

Rutledge RH: Invited commentary. World J Surg 2:473, 1978

Shore JM, Shore E: Operative biliary endoscopy. Ann Surg 171:269, 1970

Smith R: Personal communication

Way LW: Retained common duct stones. Surg Clin North Am 53:1139, 1973

Wheeler ES, Longmire WP Jr: Repair of benign stricture of the common bile duct by jejunal interposition choledochoduodenostomy. Surg Gynecol Obstet 146:260, 1978

White TT: Invited commentary. World J Surg 2:473, 1978

Zimmon DS, Falkenstein DB, et al: Endoscopic removal of biliary stones and sludge: Preliminary experience. Gastroenterology 68:1052, 1975

82. Postoperative Strictures of the Bile Duct

John W. Braasch

Obstruction of the biliary outflow from the liver is a potentially life-threatening situation. Its consequences over the long term are biliary cirrhosis and portal hypertension. Benign biliary stricture is correctable in all patients by timely, appropriate operative procedures. The importance of this condition cannot, therefore, be overemphasized even though it is not commonly seen in surgical practice.

Adding to the importance of consideration of biliary strictures is the intrinsic usefulness of the basic questions and techniques of any procedure involving a biliary anastomosis. These basic tenets are directly applicable to anastomoses in the treatment of common duct calculi, periampullary malignant disease, sclerosing cholangitis, and choledochocyst. In the aggregate, the techniques employed in bile duct anastomosis are not uncommonly used by surgeons who care for biliary tract conditions. The gradual improvement in prevention, diagnosis, and treatment since the first biliary duct reconstruction by hepaticoduodenostomy and the first hepaticojejunostomy is described herein.

ETIOLOGY

Approximately 95 percent of all benign biliary strictures follow operative procedures on the gallbladder and bile ducts, most often cholecystectomy (Table 82–1). The exact sequence of events leading to trauma to the bile duct usually is not apparent. In only a few instances is major hemorrhage described in the operative note or recorded on the anesthesia sheet in terms of intraoperative blood transfusions. Nor is the presence of acute cholecystitis or a shrunken, fibrosed gallbladder commonly noted. It seems probable, therefore, that in most instances inattention by the operating surgeon to a careful dissection of the common hepatic duct or other structures is the causative factor. The end result is placement of a clamp across the bile duct or excision of portions of the extrahepatic biliary apparatus.

Prevention of these tragic events depends on demonstration of the common hepatic duct and its relationship to the cystic duct before any ductal structures are clamped. This demonstration is possible even in the presence of acute cholecystitis or contracted, shrunken chronic cholecystitis. When massive hemorrhage occurs, the safety maneuver of finger occlusion of the hepatic artery (Fig. 82–1) allows removal of blood from the field and the accurate placement of a clamp on the bleeding point. If the bleeding point is the side wall of the right hepatic artery or the common hepatic artery, the use of fine sutures to close the defect is indicated. If necessary, it is useful to open the distal common bile duct and pass probes retrogradely for identification of ductal structures.

Appropriate surgical technique in the treatment of acute cholecystitis can make cholecystectomy safe. However, when indicated, the use of cholecystostomy should be routine. If cholecystectomy is to be carried out, it is sometimes useful to open the gallbladder, rim the edge of the fundus with Allis clamps, and place the index finger down into the Hartmann pouch (Fig. 82–2). Using the finger as a guide to the edge of the gallbladder can protect the common hepatic duct from injury.

The common bile duct can also be injured

TABLE 82-1. CAUSE OF BENIGN BILIARY STRICTURE IN 136 PATIENTS[a]

Condition	No. of Patients
Known duct injury	70
Massive bleeding at cholecystectomy	22
Contracted difficult gallbladder	12
Probably no injury	10
Ligature on duct	8
Followed gastrectomy	7
Acute cholecystitis	6
Duct narrowed around T-tube	1
Total	136

[a] In 365 other patients in the series no ascribable cause was found.

(*Source: Adapted from Cattell RB, Braasch JW, 1959a, with permission.*)

during partial hepatectomy, gastrectomy, and closure of the duodenal stump, and in distal 95 percent pancreatectomy. Intubation of the hepatic duct or distal common duct and an awareness of its position are vital for its protection.

A number of other causes of biliary stricture that are not related to surgical trauma are responsible for only about 5 percent of cases. These include erosion of a calculus through the wall of the common bile duct, possible devascularization of the common bile duct by surgical maneuvers, stab wounds, bullet wounds, blunt trauma to the upper abdomen, the use of formaldehyde in the operative treatment of an echinococcus cyst where the cyst communicates with the biliary tree, and, finally, congenital strictures. The diagnosis and treatment of these con-

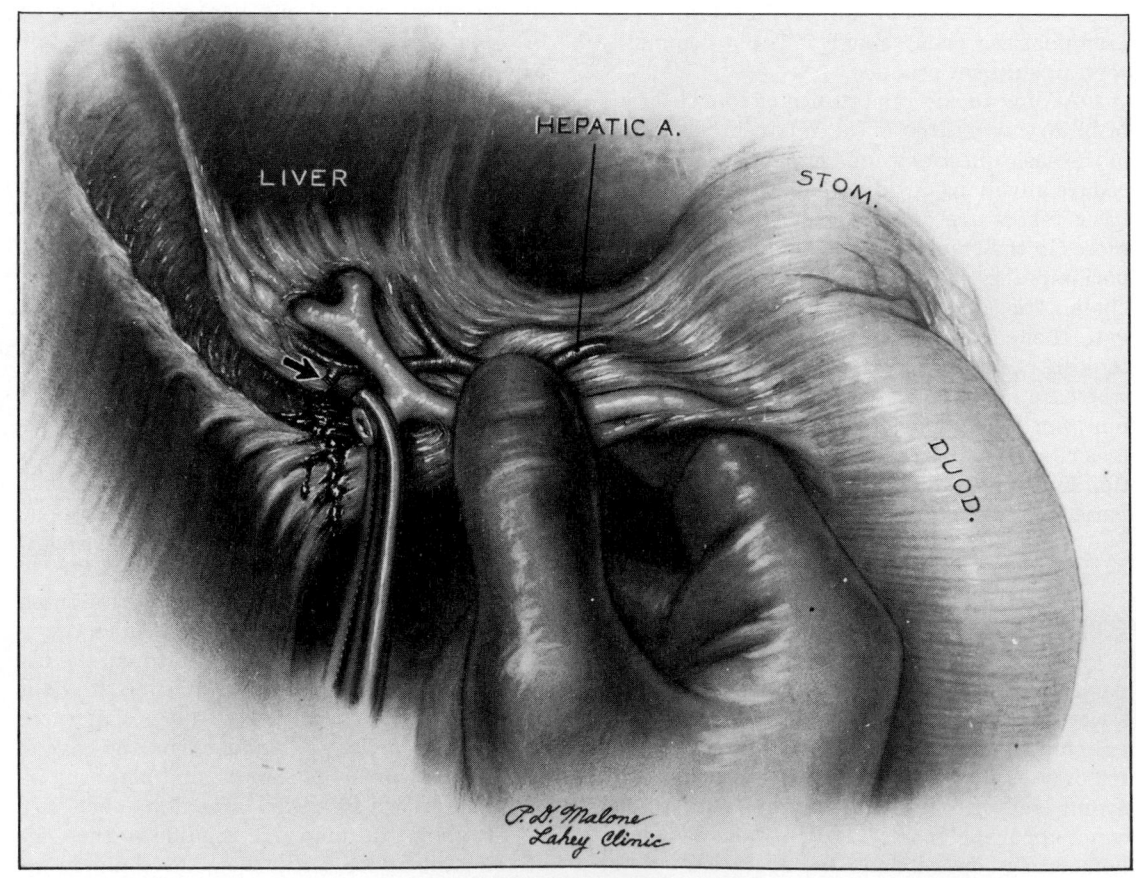

Figure 82-1. Pringle maneuver for hemorrhage during cholecystectomy. (*Source: From Cattell RB, Braasch JW: Strictures of the bile duct. Surg Clin North Am 38:647, 1958, with permission.*)

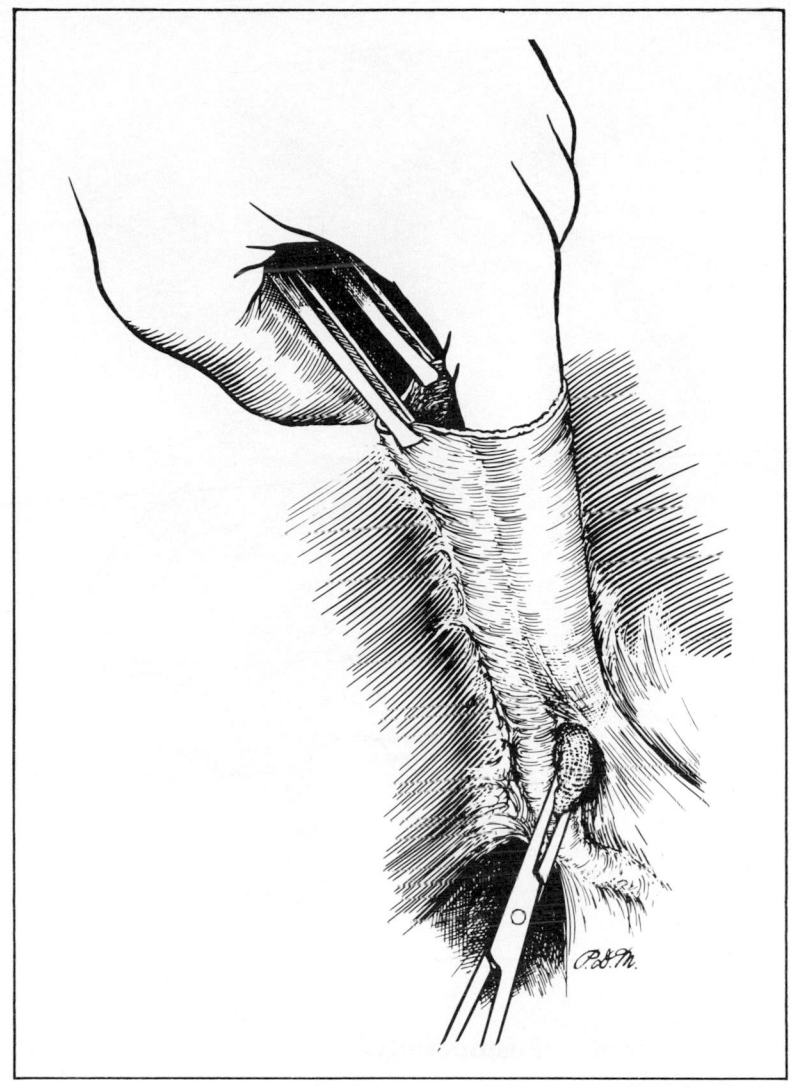

Figure 82–2. Safety maneuver during cholecystectomy for acute cholecystitis.

ditions not caused by surgical misadventure are the same as for iatrogenic strictures.

RECOGNITION

Intraoperative

A study of the operative notes of patients who had cholecystectomy that resulted in stricture is of interest since in some instances they suggest confusion on the part of the surgeon. For example, a description of a "double" cystic duct (Fig. 82–3) is included in some notes when the cystic duct probably is very short; with traction on the gallbladder both the common hepatic duct and the common bile duct are extracted from their usual locations in the duodenal hepatic ligament and may seem to the surgeon to indicate a double cystic duct. There is no evidence from dissection studies in large numbers of individuals that a double cystic duct ever exists unless a double gallbladder is present. If, therefore, in the course of cholecystectomy a "double" cystic duct is visualized, the surgeon must be especially careful that this is not just a dislocated common hepatic and common bile duct.

At times a surgical note describes a bile leak from the hilus of the liver after cholecystec-

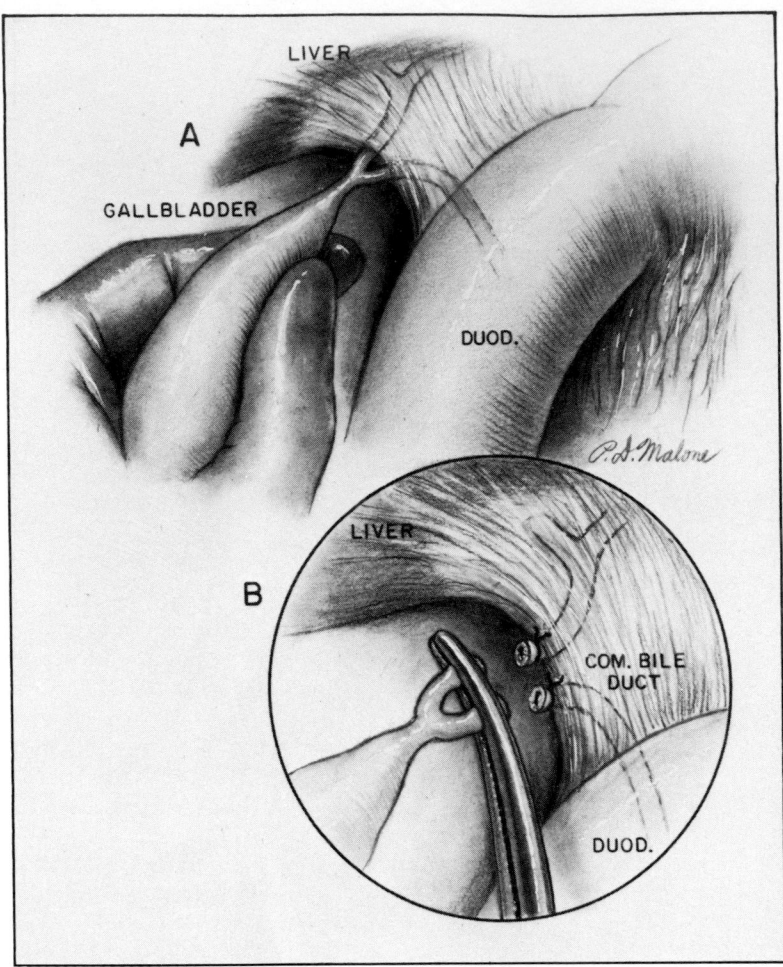

Figure 82–3. Apparent "double" cystic duct. **A.** Traction on gallbladder. **B.** "Double" duct.

tomy. This is usually ascribed to severance of a duct communicating directly to the gallbladder from the liver bed. More likely the leak is from a subsegmental or a segmental hepatic duct joining the cystic duct (Fig. 82–4) that was severed and not recognized. Subsegmental and even segmental ductal leaks have no clinical importance except that the external fistula so produced can delay convalescence. The danger exists that the bile leak might come from the common hepatic duct and be unrecognized by the surgeon. Therefore, if a bile leak is noted on inspection before closure of the incision after cholecystectomy, the surgeon must be certain of the source of the bile. This can be determined readily by operative cholangiography if the duct is large enough to accept a small catheter or needle.

Postoperative

A damaged bile duct is characterized postoperatively by any of three clinical presentations. The patient may have a bile fistula, especially one that drains over 200 ml/day. Secondly, jaundice may appear anytime, from about the second postoperative day to weeks later—an earlier onset of jaundice is more common. Lastly, bile ascites may develop, although this is not commonly seen. Patients with severed ducts can accumulate tremendous amounts of bile in the abdominal cavity without signs of toxicity or cholangitis; 4 or 5 liters is not unusual.

In the long term, cholangitis, usually intermittent, is the predominant symptom. Jaundice may be intermittent or constant. Pruritus is relatively common, but pain is infrequent. It is possible for an external bile fistula noted soon after cholecystectomy to close spontaneously, usually with the formation of an internal fistula into the duodenum.

Based on these guidelines, a reasonably accurate diagnosis of damage to the extrahepatic biliary tree or recurrent biliary stricture could be made before the era of imaging. Certainly a false-positive diagnosis was rare, and a false-negative diagnosis was correctable if cholangitis continued or recurred.

Imaging

Since the advent of percutaneous transhepatic cholangiography (Fig. 82–5) and fiberoptic endoscopic retrograde cholangiography (Fig. 82–6), determination of the exact location of the obstruction or partial obstruction is possible. The associated presence of calculi can also be recognized by these techniques. Percutaneous transhepatic cholangiography is perhaps a more useful test since it provides information about the involvement of lobes or segments as well

as the length of proximal duct available for anastomosis. However, the level of the obstructive process can be appreciated by using endoscopic retrograde cholangiography. The ultrasound examination can show dilatation of the intrahepatic bile ducts, which would support the diagnosis of biliary obstruction, and certainly indicates operative intervention. However, this test does not give accurate information about the level of the stricture. Competent, experienced surgeons do not regard this information as essential since they must find the proximal duct and must confirm that the duct drains both lobes and all segments.

Difficult Differential Diagnoses

The critical level of luminal size of the extrahepatic biliary ducts is not known. A lumen of approximately 2 mm in diameter seems adequate for normal bile flow. Anything less than this probably causes bile stasis and infection followed by cholangitis and jaundice. Only percutaneous transhepatic cholangiography can

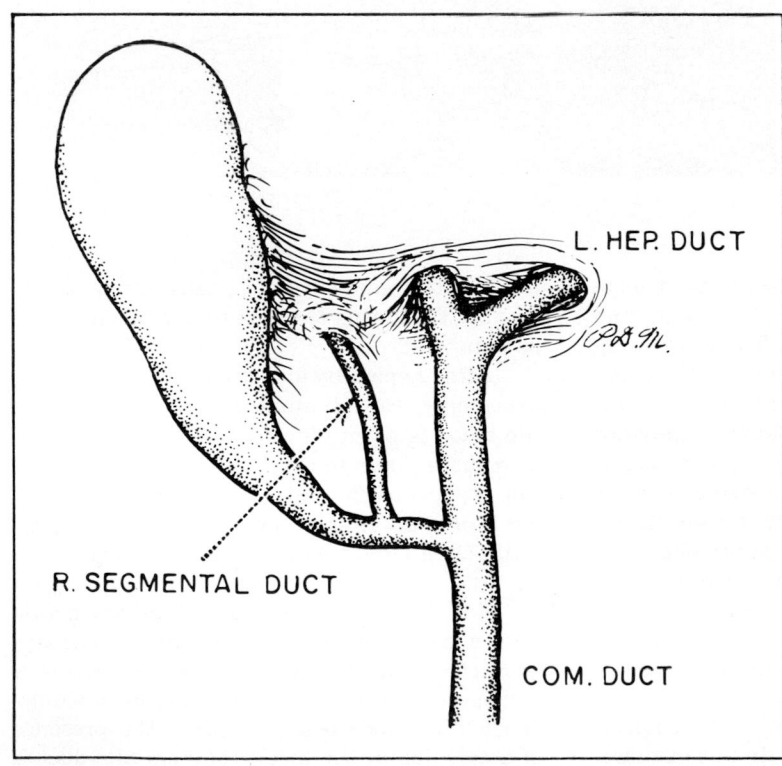

Figure 82–4. Segmental duct of right hepatic lobe traversing Calot's triangle. (*Source: From Braasch JW: Unexpected findings at surgery of the biliary tract. Probl Gen Surg 1:221, 1984, with permission.*)

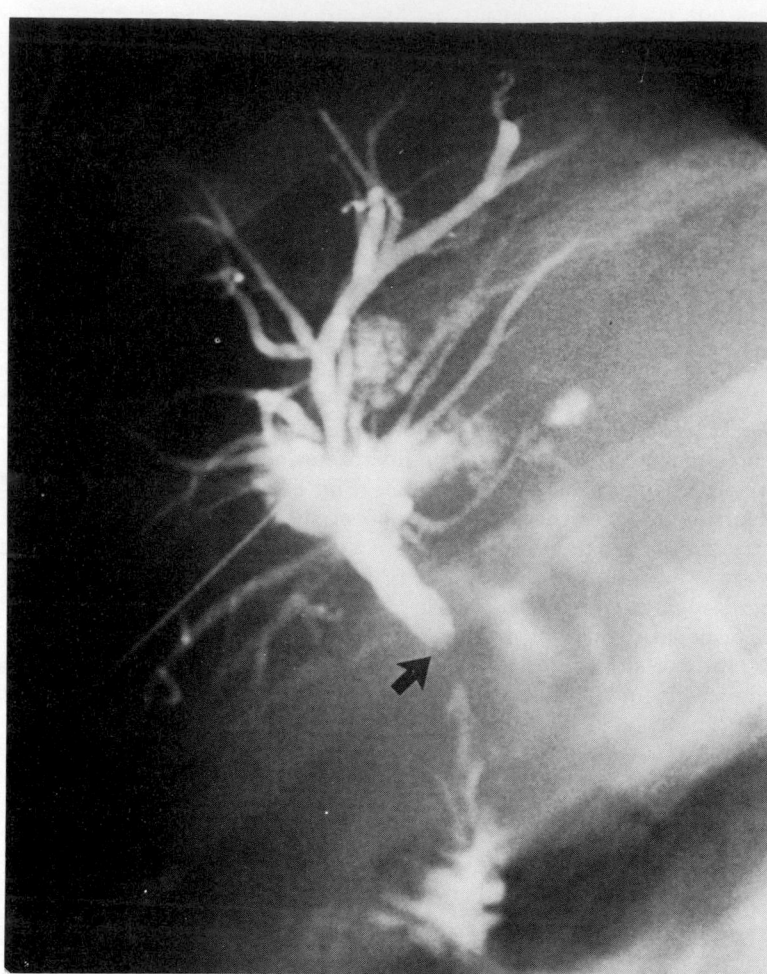

Figure 82–5. Percutaneous transhepatic cholangiogram showing obstruction (*arrow*) of common bile duct from benign stricture.

give information accurate enough to demonstrate lumens less than 2 mm in diameter and produce a measurable image. The scan using hepatobiliary iminodiacetic acid (HIDA) is not precise enough for such determinations. Likewise, neither intravenous cholangiography nor barium cholangiography, which can visualize anastomoses after hepaticoduodenostomy or loop hepaticojejunostomy, have sufficient clarity to allow luminal diameter measurement.

Differential diagnosis between biliary cirrhosis and bile duct stricture can be most difficult. Biliary cirrhosis itself can produce cholangitis with fever and jaundice and elevation of the serum alkaline phosphatase even in the presence of sufficient biliary outflow through an adequate bile duct anastomosis. In this instance, percutaneous transhepatic cholangiography is

the only technique by which an accurate assessment of the status of the patient's bile duct can be obtained.

After hepaticojejunostomy or hepaticoduodenostomy, the alkaline phosphatase level in the blood is often elevated and can rise to approximately two to three times normal values. The exact cause for this aberration is unknown, but it does not mean that the patient has a partially obstructed biliary outflow, requiring surgery.

The presence of an external biliary fistula after cholecystectomy could mean that the cystic duct ligature has slipped, causing temporary leakage of bile through the cystic duct stump. When bile leakage is prolonged, the presence of a calculus in the distal common bile duct is suspected. The bile leakage in such instances

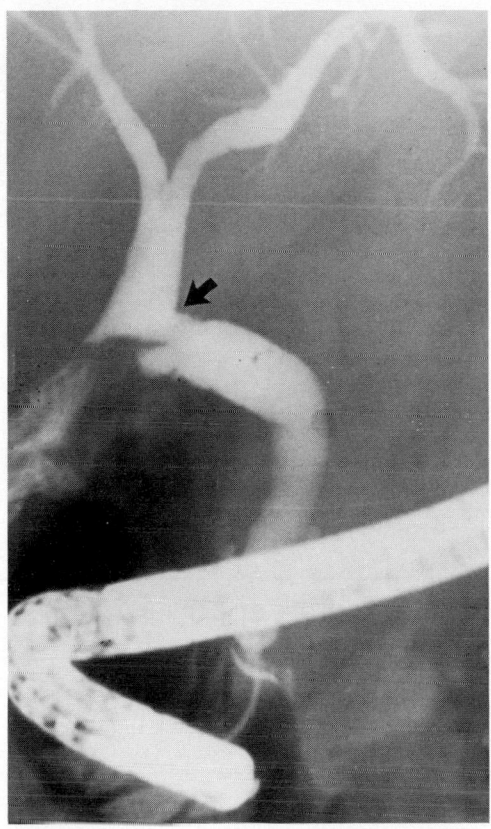

Figure 82–6. Endoscopic retrograde cholangiogram showing benign stricture (*arrow*) with partial obstruction of common hepatic duct and external fistula.

is not as great as might be expected with a transected common hepatic duct and only occasionally rises above 200 ml/day.

At times cholecystectomies are performed in patients who also have sclerosing cholangitis or carcinoma of the biliary duct that was unrecognized at the time of the cholecystectomy. These patients might become jaundiced in the postoperative period or months later, and the presence of a damaged bile duct should be considered. The proper diagnosis can be made by imaging procedures and reoperation.

GENERAL CONSIDERATIONS

The requirements for repair of biliary stricture are simple. The liver must be decompressed adequately to include both lobes and all segments.

There must be no stasis of bile, which leads to infection, cholangitis, damage to functioning liver units, and, in extreme cases, cirrhosis, obstruction of portal flow, portal hypertension, and varices. In addition, sufficient bile must be delivered to the upper small intestine to aid in digestion.

In most patients the duodenum can be mobilized by an extensive Kocher maneuver, which allows it to reach the hilus of the liver. A jejunal loop, either simple or Roux-Y, may also be apposed to the hilus of the liver. The length of the remaining bile duct is therefore not a problem. This obviates the necessity for grafts of vein, ureter, or omentum, as well as grafts of artificial materials, and avoids the burden of a second anastomosis and, in some instances, a foreign body in the biliary tree.

The loss of the function of the ampulla of Vater is not a problem because the passage of the intestinal chyme or of partially digested food into the biliary tract is not symptomatic and does not lead to long-term impairment of liver function. Therefore, neither a Roux-Y jejunal loop nor the distal bile duct is needed in the reconstruction.

The major problem in biliary tract reconstruction is subsequent stenosis of the circular anastomosis. The luminal diameter of such an anastomosis can be plotted over time (Fig. 82–7). Although the points on the time scale are not known with accuracy, it is conceivable that at some time after the construction of such an anastomosis no further scar contraction will occur. The timing of recurrences of strictures suggests that a plateau is reached at about 2.5 to 3 years postoperatively. Some controversy exists on this point, since Cattell and Braasch found that the vast majority of recurrences were evident before the 3-year mark after removal of stents. Recently, Pitt and colleagues have indicated that in their experience recurrences were possible many years after this point. Nevertheless, it is useful to think of the timing of recurrences in terms of the curve shown in Figure 82–7 in order to plan the use of stents and to prognosticate results for patients.

PRACTICAL ANATOMY

The blood supply to the common bile duct has recently been demonstrated by Northover and Terblanche and Terblanche and associates us-

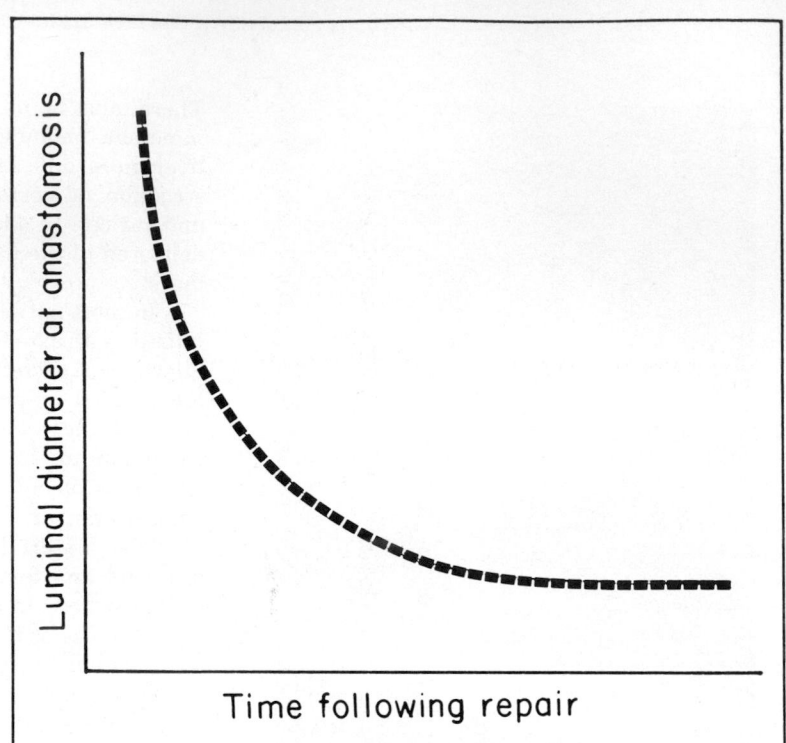

Figure 82–7. Plot of luminal diameter versus time after circular suture in stricture repair. (*Source: From Bolton JS, Braasch JW, et al: Management of benign biliary stricture. Surg Clin North Am 60:330, 1980, with permission.*)

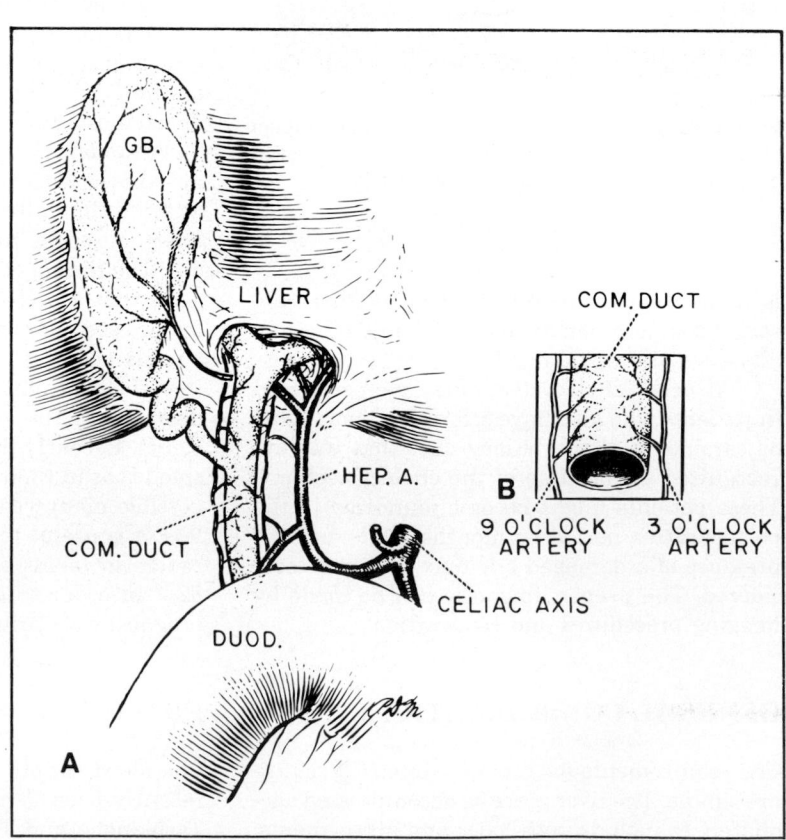

Figure 82–8. Arterial blood supply of common bile duct. **A.** Hepatic artery sources. **B.** Close-up of arterial syncytium. (*Source: From Bolton JS, Braasch JW, et al: Management of benign biliary stricture. Surg Clin North Am 60:323, 1980, with permission.*)

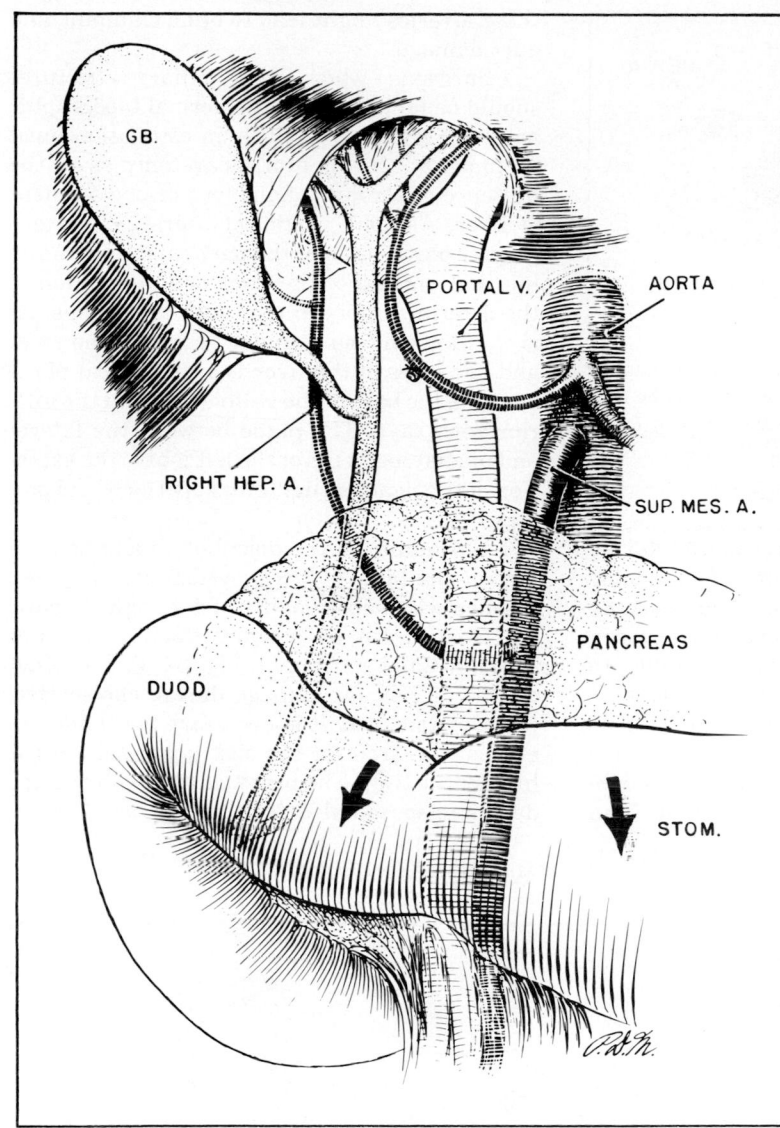

Figure 82–9. Anteroposterior view. Course of replaced right hepatic artery relative to bile duct. (*Source: From Braasch JW, Gray BN: Technique of radical pancreatoduodenectomy: With consideration of hepatic arterial relationships. Surg Clin North Am 56:644, 1976, with permission.*)

ing injection corrosion techniques. Their work showed that arterioles form a plexus in the submucosal layer of the duct, and these in turn are fed by small branches from longitudinal arteries, one on each side of the duct (Fig. 82–8). In general, blood supply to the lower duct is by way of the gastroduodenal artery and to the upper three quarters of the duct by way of the common hepatic or the right and left hepatic arteries. The practical application of this arterial arrangement is that ischemia of the duct is entirely possible if the periductal tissues are dissected for too great a distance. Presumably,

ischemia might lead to necrosis of tissue, which in turn might lead to scar formation and recurrence of stricture at the anastomosis. This means that only a short segment of the proximal duct should be freed in preparation for the anastomotic procedure and that possibly the anastomosis should be in the common hepatic duct since there are more feeding arterial twigs in this area.

Variations of the course(s) of the hepatic arteries are well known. At times the right hepatic artery may ascend to the liver posterior or lateral to the common bile duct (Figs. 82–9

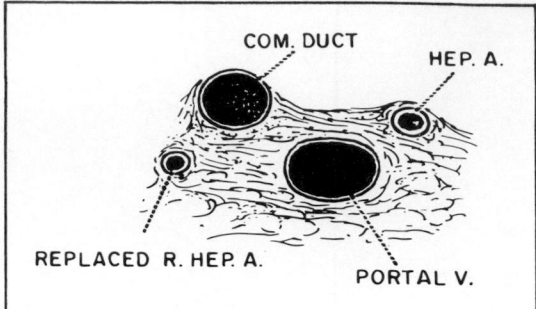

Figure 82–10. Cross-sectional view of duodenohepatic ligament. (*Source: From Braasch JW: Unexpected findings at surgery of the biliary tract. Probl Gen Surg 1:223, 1984, with permission.*)

these arteries might lead to blind clamping and duct damage.

Surgeons who repair biliary strictures should be familiar with the normal topographic anatomy of the liver since an estimation must be made at the time of laparotomy as to the presence of atrophy of one lobe or one segment of liver. Atrophy would, of course, indicate a chronic obstruction of the particular duct draining that portion of the liver or interruption of the arterial supply to that segment or lobe. As is well known, the boundary between the right and left lobes of the liver is a theoretical plane between the base of the gallbladder and the inferior vena cava. The plane between the lateral and medial segments of the left lobe is the extension of the ligamentum teres superiorly and posteriorly.

Variability in the distribution and branchings of the biliary ductal system can be great. Segments or subsegments of the right hepatic lobe may drain by a small duct that passes through Calot's triangle (Fig. 82–4). This duct can be at risk for damage during cholecystectomy. If damaged, it is necessary to conduct an extensive search for the obstructed duct in the hilus of the liver. The presence of this obstructed duct is also signaled by the lack of filling of

and 82–10) and thereby be in jeopardy during dissection of the duct, a situation that renders reconstruction most difficult in some cases. By careful dissection, however, such an artery can be removed from the proximity of the duct to allow an accurate sutured anastomosis. It is entirely possible that the proportion of patients with hepatic arteries at risk because of anomalous positions might be higher in those with biliary stricture, since sudden hemorrhage from

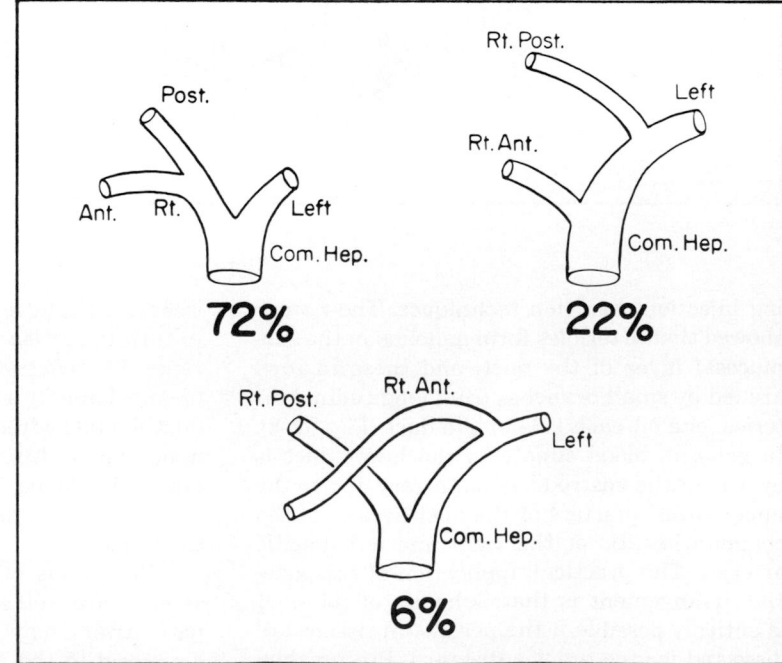

Figure 82–11. Configurations of intrahepatic bile ducts. (*Source: From Braasch JW: Segmental surgical disease of the liver. Ann Surg 168:115, 1968, with permission.*)

segments or subsegments of the right lobe on cholangiography.

The drainage pattern of the segmental ducts of the right lobe may vary intrahepatically (Fig. 82–11). In 22 percent of patients the right posterior segmental duct drains within the liver into the left hepatic duct; in 6 percent of patients the right anterior segmental duct crosses over in a similar fashion. Thus, damage to the extrahepatic right hepatic duct might only deprive a portion of the right lobe of free drainage of bile.

When the proximal bile duct cannot be located, it is important to know that just under or lateral to the ligamentum teres on the undersurface of the left lobe of the liver a large tributary of the left hepatic duct can frequently be located by needling and dissection. Less commonly, a longitudinal duct deep to the gallbladder bed may be found. Needle localization and dissection of these ducts for bypass anastomosis can be useful for palliation of obstruction.

PREOPERATIVE PREPARATION

Among the supportive ancillary procedures the preoperative preparation of the patient ranks high in importance. It is sometimes necessary or desirable to perform the reconstruction in two stages, the first stage being that of external bile drainage to relieve obstruction of the liver cells and to improve liver function before the major definitive operation. At other times the local situation in the hilus of the liver is not suitable for an anastomosis at the time of the first operation. In the first instance, percutaneous transhepatic insertion of catheters into the intrahepatic obstructed biliary system can relieve obstruction of the liver and improve liver function as well as clotting, resistance to infection, and possibly wound healing. The evidence for these benefits of preoperative drainage is not clear-cut; in a prospective study Hatfield and colleagues found no difference in the results between patients who were externally drained as a first-stage procedure and those who were operated on primarily for relief of obstructive jaundice. It is interesting to note that only a few patients had very deep jaundice, above 20 mg/dl, in that series. The work of Denning and others supports this hypothesis. It is probably best to reserve external drainage as the initial step in a two-stage procedure for those patients

with definite liver dysfunction and with blood bilirubin levels in excess of 20 mg/dl.

In some patients with bile duct destruction caused by external trauma, such as that which occurs with stab wounds, bullet wounds, or blunt trauma, the proximal duct might not be suitable for anastomosis at that time. In such instances a straight catheter may be inserted into the proximal duct as an external hepaticostomy to allow time for the patient's general condition to improve and for the proximal duct wall

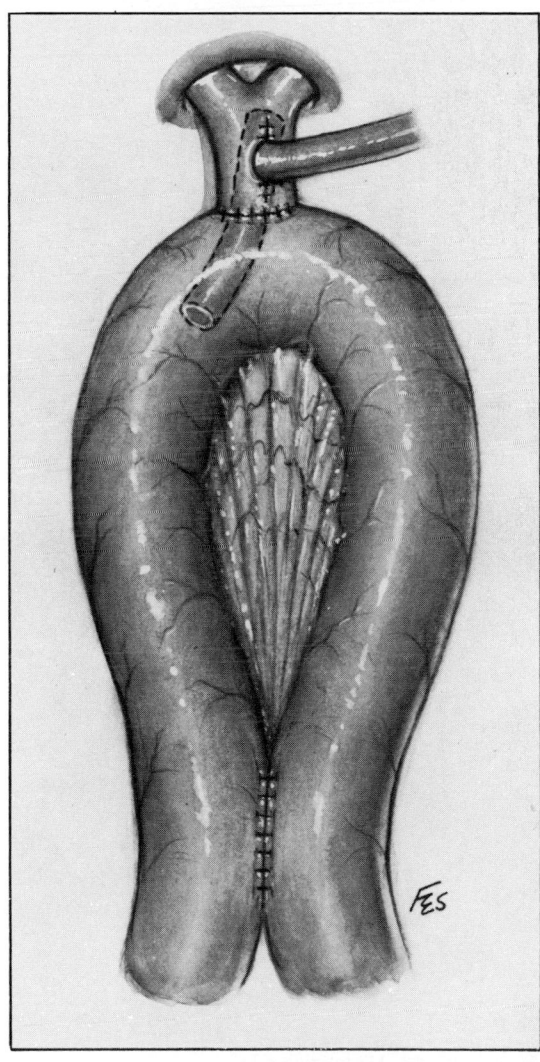

Figure 82–12. Hepaticojejunostomy using simple jejunal loop with enteroenterostomy. (*Source: From Rossi RL, Gordon M, et al, 1980, with permission.*)

to thicken and become more suitable for suturing.

The development of biliary cirrhosis leading to portal hypertension in long-standing strictures of the bile duct is seen less often now. In these instances extensive collateral formation can occur in the abdominal wall and around the adhesions in the right upper quadrant. Operative procedures in these patients are carried out with great difficulty because of massive blood loss. As has been reported by Sedgwick and Hume, it is advisable in some instances to perform a portal shunt as a first-stage procedure in biliary stricture repair. Fortunately, portal

hypertension complicating biliary stricture is becoming much less common than it was formerly.

The use of antibiotics preoperatively, during the procedure, and for several days postoperatively is strongly recommended. The most serious complications of biliary reconstruction and stricture repair are septicemia and subphrenic or subhepatic abscesses. The organisms most commonly encountered are gram-negative, and appropriate antibiotics to cover these organisms are indicated.

In some instances of long-standing obstruction the clotting mechanism is deranged be-

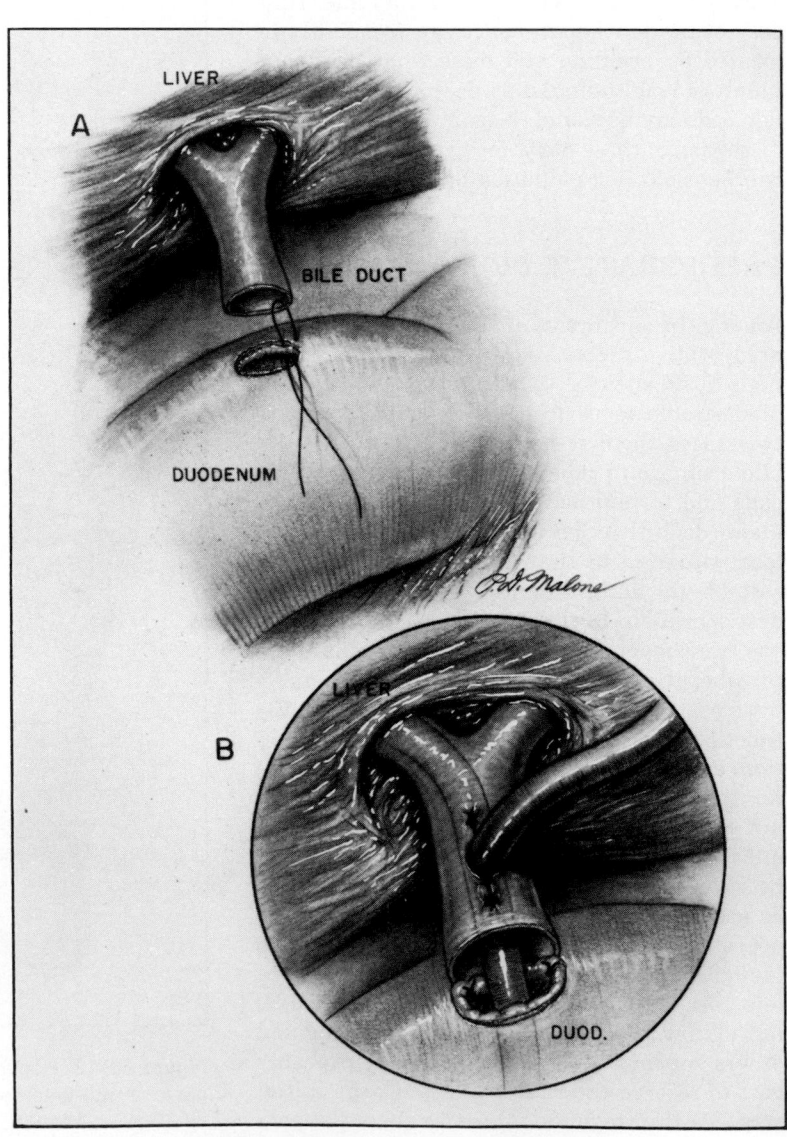

Figure 82–13. Hepaticoduodenostomy. **A.** Placement of first suture. **B.** Posterior row completed.

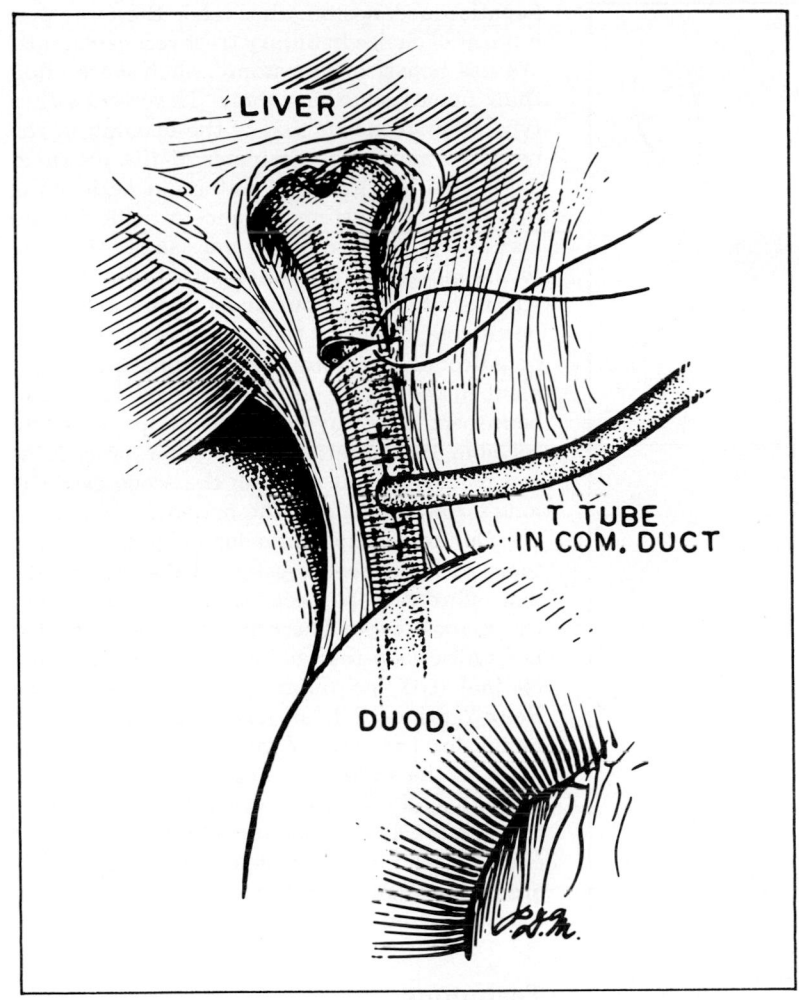

Figure 82–14. End-to-end repair with T-tube stent. (*Source: From Bolton JS, Braasch JW, et al: Management of benign biliary stricture. Surg Clin North Am 60:327, 1980, with permission.*)

cause of a deficiency of vitamin K. This vitamin should therefore be given parenterally to patients who are jaundiced preoperatively, whether or not measurable deficiencies are evident in the prothrombin time. It is possible for the peripheral clotting mechanism to be normal when tested while a bleeding diathesis exists.

RECONSTRUCTION

The four basic types of biliary reconstructive anastomoses are hepaticojejunostomy (Fig. 82–12) or hepaticoduodenostomy (Fig. 82–13), end-to-end anastomosis (Fig. 82–14), plastic or Heineke–Mikulicz procedures (Fig. 82–15), and dilatations (Fig. 82–16) of strictures of the right hepatic duct. Each has its particular usefulness in certain situations.

Dilatation of strictures should not be carried out unless the stricture involves the right hepatic duct and is of minimal significance with a lumen through it of at least 2 mm. Strictures of the common hepatic duct should not be dilated, but the duct should be reconstructed in all instances. Past results of operative dilatation of strictures of the common hepatic or common bile duct have been exceptionally poor.

The usefulness of plastic procedures or the Heineke–Mikulicz type of repair is limited, and this technique is effective only in minimal stricturing of the common hepatic duct. Only a short stricture should be present for this type of repair to succeed. End-to-end anastomosis of the

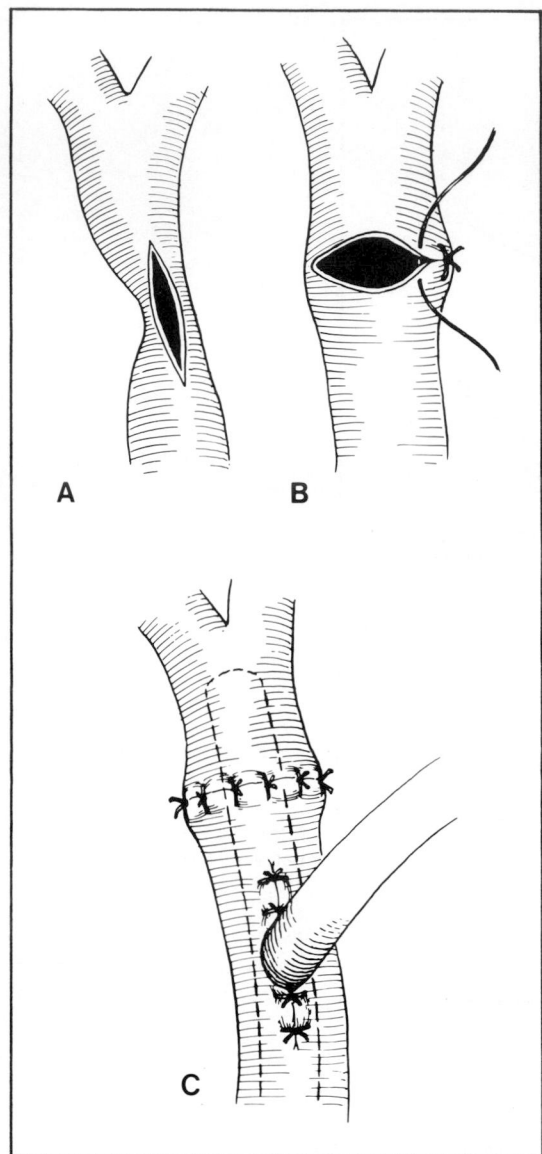

Figure 82–15. Heineke–Mikulicz plastic repair. **A.** Longitudinal incision. **B,C.** Closure. (*Source: From Braasch JW: Part II. Reconstruction of the biliary tract, in Nora PF (ed): Operative Surgery: Principles and Techniques, 2 edt. Philadelphia: Lea & Febiger, 1980, p 578, with permission.*)

severed common duct is also of limited usefulness and is indicated only for the immediate repair of a sectioned or clamped duct if the two ends are suitable. We do not use this particular repair for a secondary procedure.

The usefulness of hepaticojejunostomy or hepaticoduodenostomy has made these the procedures of choice in biliary tract reconstruction. We use hepaticojejunostomy much more often than hepaticoduodenostomy. However, either type allows construction of the opening in the bowel to match the diameter of the proximal duct. This is a great advantage in performing a leak-proof anastomosis and in achieving an accurate apposition of the mucosa of the bowel to the mucosa of the biliary tract (Fig. 82–17). At present, more of our anastomoses are of the hepaticojejunostomy type, but it is possible that hepaticoduodenostomies will become more prevalent in the future, since this anastomosis can be inspected by way of the fiberscope. It is conceivable that dilatations or other procedures can be carried out through the scope over the long-term follow-up of the patient.

Our preference is for loop hepaticojejunostomy with enteroenterostomy between afferent and efferent loops because it is simpler than the Roux-Y type. There is no evidence that a peristaltic loop inserted between the gastrointestinal (GI) and biliary tracts by use of the Roux-Y principle is an advantage. One use remains for the Roux-Y configuration: In some patients the simple jejunal loop will not reach the hilus of the liver even if it is brought through the mesocolon, and a Roux-Y loop gives extra length for hepaticojejunostomy. This preference is not universally accepted, however, and today most biliary surgeons use Roux-Y loops.

Technique

The technique to be described will be that for chronic strictures seen late after the causative event. The repair of acute damage to the biliary tract will be considered under the section on special situations. The incision best suited for biliary tract reconstruction is a right upper rectus muscle-splitting incision, the superior aspect of which should extend to the angle between the xiphoid process and the costal margin. It should at least extend to the umbilicus and be of whatever length is necessary for ease and adequacy of exposure. The peritoneum is best entered at the upper end of the incision where the round ligament protects the small intestine, which might be adherent to the undersurface of the scar. If previous repairs have been made, adhesions of the omentum to the previous incision are almost always present. The hepatic flexure of the colon is usually adherent to the

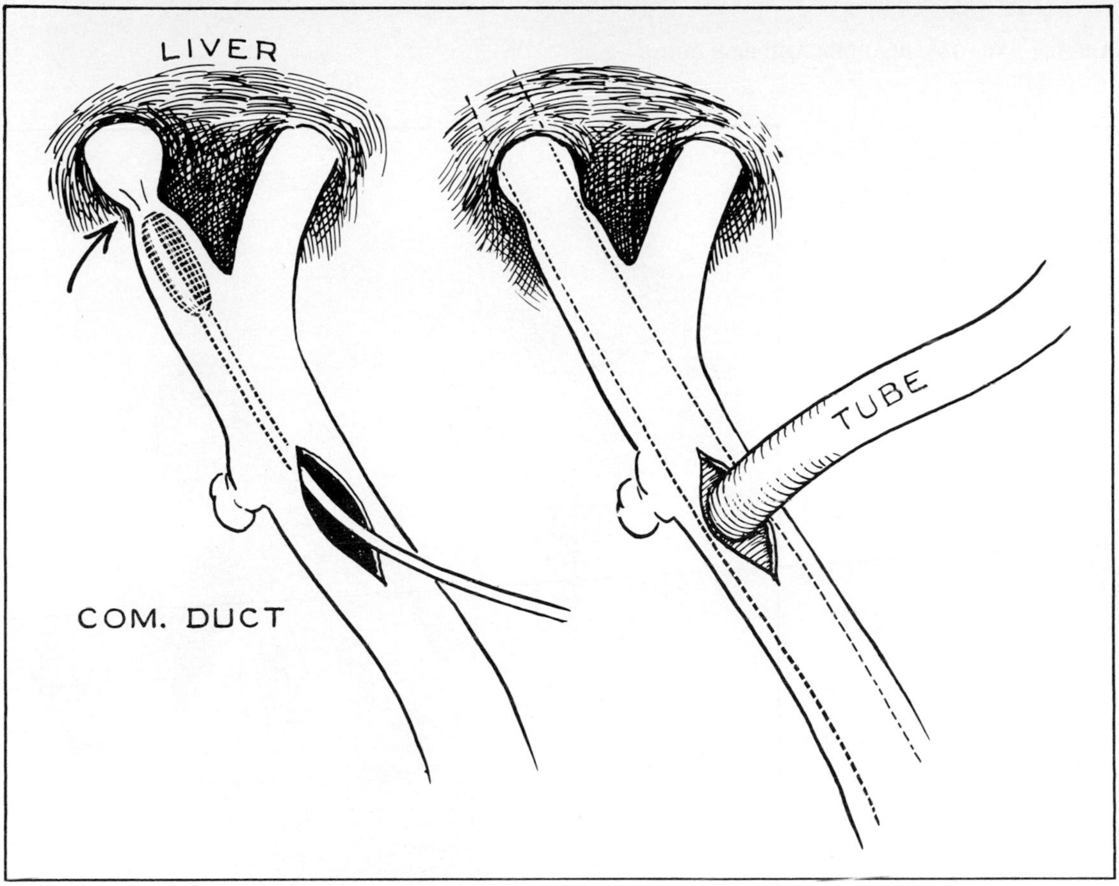

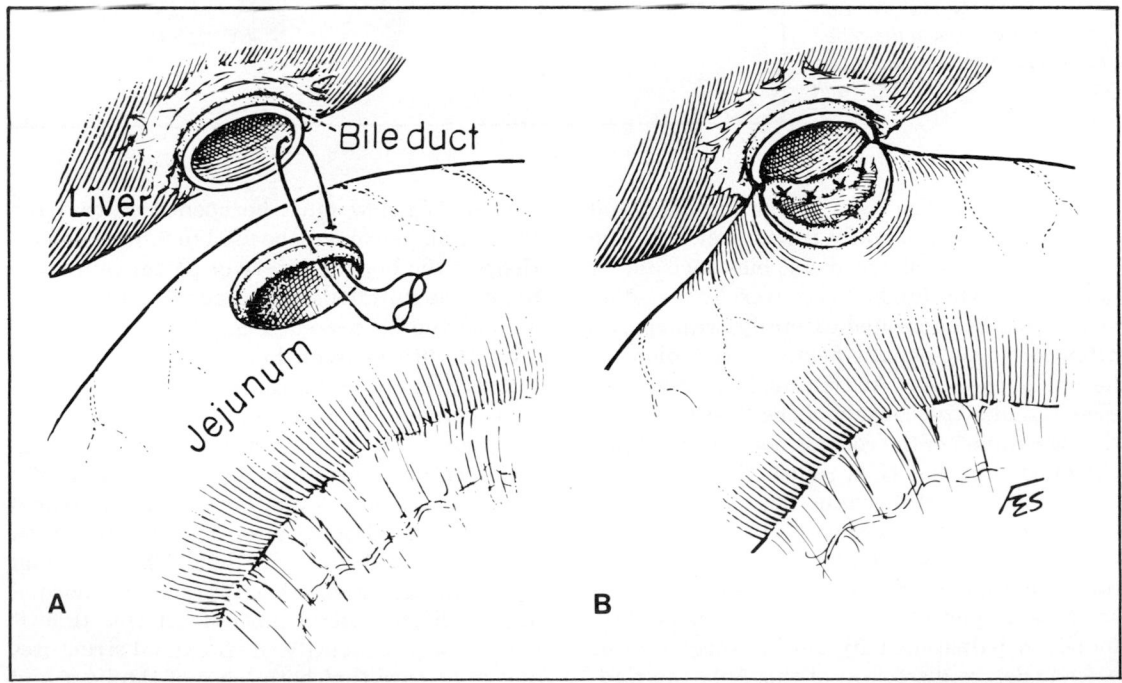

Figure 82–16. Dilatation of right hepatic duct. (*Source: From Cattell RB, Braasch JW, 1960, with permission of Surgery, Gynecology & Obstetrics.*)

Figure 82–17. Mucosal suture technique. **A.** Placement of first suture. **B.** Posterior row completed.

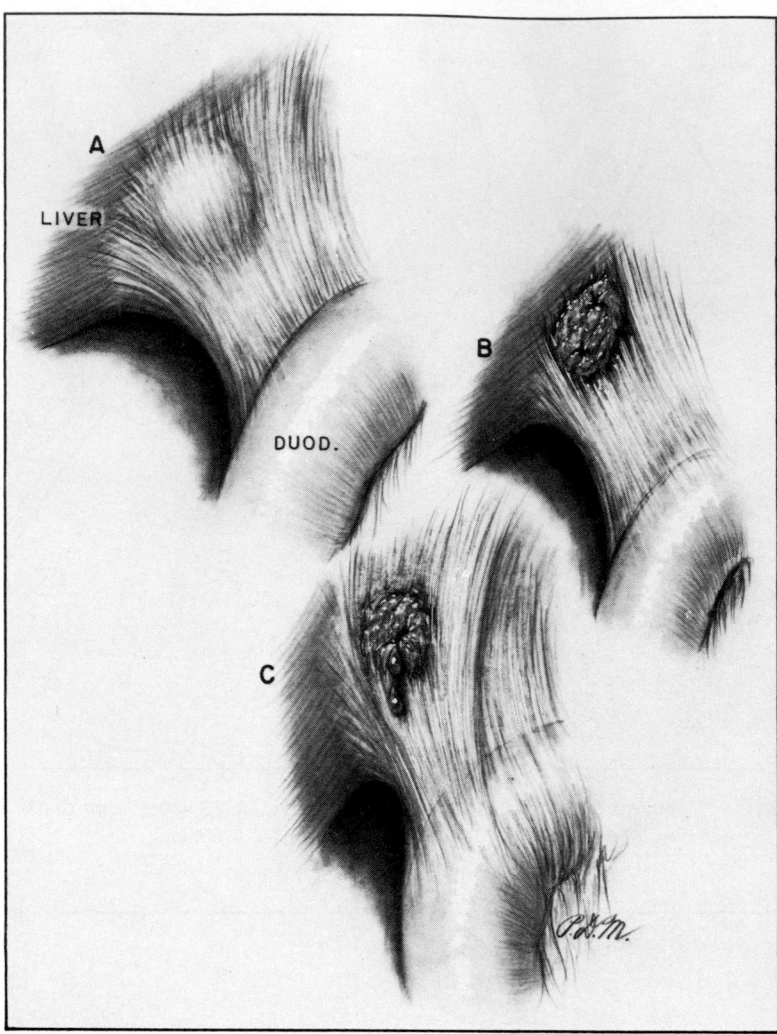

Figure 82–18. Possible appearances of strictured proximal hepatic duct after dissection of hilus of liver. **A.** Bulging duct. **B.** Sutured scar. **C.** Bile leak. (*Source: From Braasch JW: Current considerations in the repair of bile duct strictures. Surg Clin North Am 53:427, 1973, with permission.*)

undersurface of the right lobe of the liver, and the duodenum is usually rolled over onto the anterior surface of the distal bile duct and is adherent to the hilus of the liver. These adhesions must be separated carefully, with special attention to the hepatic flexure of the colon adherent to the liver. At times it is necessary to dissect under the capsule of the liver to ensure that the lumen of the colon is not entered. After the duodenum has been rolled off the anterior surface of the distal common bile duct and frequently off the damaged portion of the common hepatic duct, the proximal ductal structures must be located. Figure 82–18 shows that a stitch, a droplet of bile, or a hard scarred area found on palpation may aid in recognition of a duct. Before dissection of this area the fora-

men of Winslow must be opened so that the Pringle maneuver can be used to control hemorrhage if the hepatic artery or portal vein is entered. The initial dissection at this point should be into the hard area (Fig. 82–19) or into the area of sutures; soon bile should be observed coming from a small opening into the proximal ductal system. Samples of bile are taken for culture and sensitivity, and dissection of the proximal ductal system is begun. One must be careful to dissect up only 1 mm or so of the proximal duct (Fig. 82–20) since more extensive dissection might devascularize the duct. The proximal duct must be sectioned back to relatively normal duct wall and ductal mucosa. At this time it is necessary to identify the proximal structures and to be sure that both lobes of the liver and

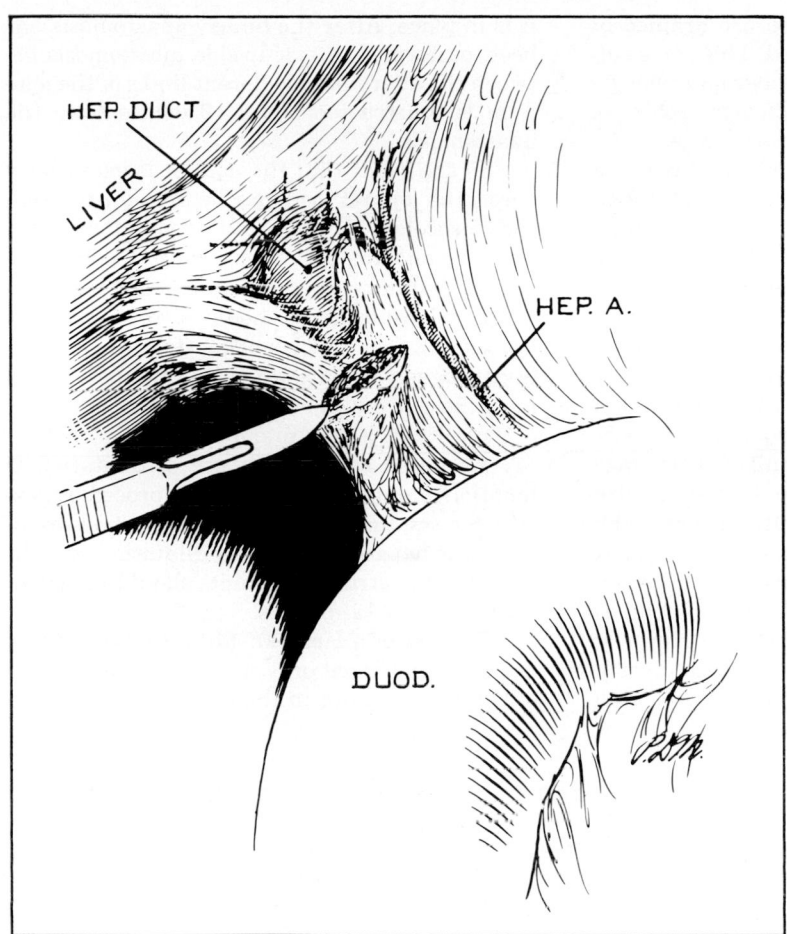

Figure 82–19. Incision of scar in mid-duct. (*Source: From Braasch JW: Part II. Reconstruction of the biliary tract, in Nora PF (ed): Operative Surgery: Principles and Techniques, 2 edt. Philadelphia: Lea & Febiger, 1980, p 577, with permission.*)

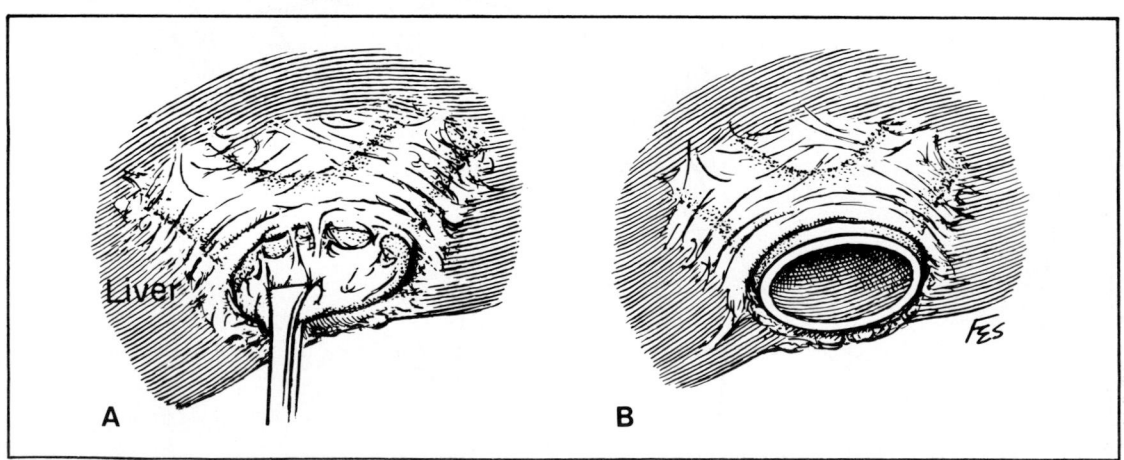

Figure 82–20. Dissection of proximal duct. **A.** Traction on covering scar. **B.** Dissection completed.

all segments of the right lobe are drained by the ductal structure discovered. This can easily be done by operative cholangiography using a No. 8 Foley catheter or by judicious probing or inspection through the choledochoscope.

A decision is made at this time as to the type of anastomosis to be constructed. Hepaticojejunostomy, end-to-side to a loop of jejunum, is our preferred anastomosis. A suitable loop of proximal jejunum is selected that will allow the serosa of this loop to reach the proximal bile duct so isolated. An incision that is about half the diameter of the proximal bile duct is made in the antimesenteric wall of the jejunum. This will stretch with subsequent manipulations and should be kept small at this stage. This opening in the jejunum is then anastomosed with interrupted fine sutures, preferably 3-0 chromic catgut. If the sutures are placed properly, a leakproof anastomosis can be constructed with a single layer. We recommend using a stent, which serves to aid the surgeon in constructing the anastomosis and also possibly prevents contraction of the anastomosis while

it is in place. After the biliary anastomosis has been performed, a side-to-side anastomosis between the afferent and efferent limbs of the jejunum is constructed about 12 inches from the anastomosis.

In the event that the patient is excessively obese, the jejunal loop may be brought through the mesocolon. If even this does not allow a tension-free anastomosis, then a Roux-Y configuration of jejunum may give an extra 2 inches of length. Consideration should also be given to the use of a hepaticoduodenostomy or even a hepaticogastrostomy, which in one instance in my experience was necessary because of a lack of mobility of jejunum and duodenum.

As noted earlier, the use of dilatation is mentioned only to condemn this procedure, except for the unusual situation of a stricture of the right hepatic duct. After dilatation of right hepatic duct strictures, stents should be left in place for 6 to 12 months.

The use of a Heineke–Mikulicz type of procedure is indicated only in minimal narrowing of the duct and not in the usual stricture. This

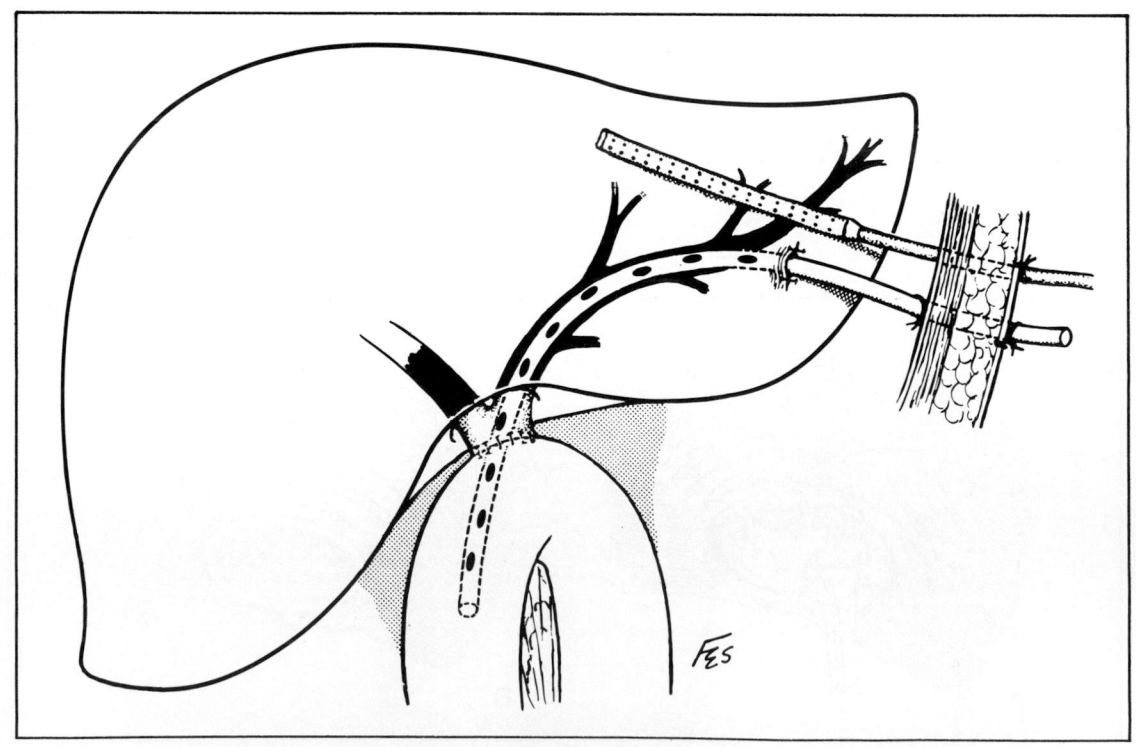

Figure 82–21. Transhepatic tube in hepaticojejunostomy. (*Source: From Rossi RL, Gordon M, et al, 1980, p 304, with permission.*)

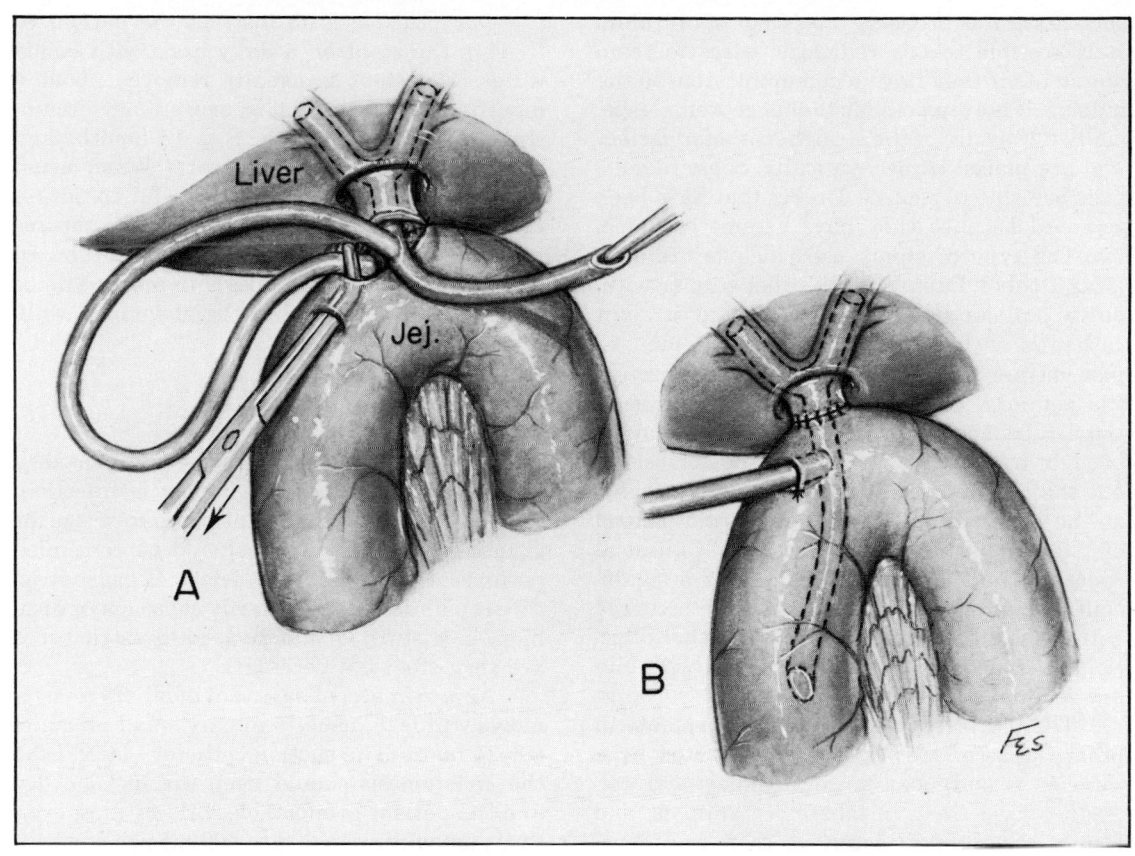

Figure 82–22. Y-tube hepaticojejunostomy. **A.** Insertion of tube. **B.** Completed anastomosis. (*Source: From Rossi RL, Gordon M, et al, 1980, with permission.*)

latter technique is simply a vertical incision across the strictured area of the duct and a horizontal closure with interrupted sutures. This should be stented as usual.

Drainage of the operative area is most important because at times these anastomoses will leak. A sump type of drain, which is placed under the anastomosis down to the inferior portion of the subhepatic space, is preferable. These drains are brought out the upper angle of the incision for simplicity and for ease of function. If a transhepatic tube is used, subphrenic drains of the same variety should also be employed (Fig. 82–21).

Stenting

The evidence for or against the use of stents within biliary tract anastomoses is not clear. No proper data are available with which to eval-

uate this point. An earlier Lahey Clinic series described by Cattell and Braasch and a recent series reported by Pitt and co-workers give only sketchy information. The earlier series was comprised of a small group of patients in whom the stent was removed accidentally soon after the operative repair. The recurrence rate in these patients was extraordinarily high. In the series reported by Pitt and co-workers the recurrence rate in those patients in whom the stent was removed early was higher than that for the rest of the group. In any case no good evidence suggests that stents within the biliary tract do harm.

The full usefulness of stents is impaired because they tend to become occluded with biliary detritus after about 6 months in situ. The use of daily irrigations to prevent this phenomenon is of questionable value. The material that occludes the tubes is insoluble to any of the known solvents and is probably a polymer of bilirubin. It is possible to use radiologic wires to ream out stents if they have a communication to the outside. It is even possible to change stents, especially if they are of the straight catheter variety and are placed transhepatically. Some radiologists are able to replace T-tubes that have been removed because they have become occluded.

The type of stents used include ordinary latex T-tubes, latex Y-tubes either with or without a pull-out limb (Fig. 82–22), and straight catheters of latex or Silastic, which may be placed transhepatically or brought out through the jejunum. Perhaps the most useful tube is the T-tube, the external limb of which may be brought out above or below the anastomosis or out the left hepatic duct if the anastomosis is at the bifurcation. The use of Silastic instead of latex stents is open to question. Kolff et al reported that in comparison to latex a significant foreign body reaction to Silastic occurred within the biliary system of dogs and that Silastic as well as latex became encrusted with biliary sediment.

The use of transhepatic tubes as stents in biliary anastomoses has been advocated by a number of surgeons since Grindlay and colleagues used them in laboratory animals, and Muñoz and Praderi described their use in patients. Cameron and associates have championed their use in stricture repair and are in the practice of changing percutaneous transhepatic Silastic stents frequently, leaving a stent in place for 2 years or longer. In this author's experience transhepatic tubes are not well accepted by patients because jejunal juice leaks around the tubes, causing skin irritation. They tend to emerge from positions in the abdominal or thoracic wall that are uncomfortable to the patient, and, in the short term, their use carries a higher incidence of subphrenic and subhepatic abscesses. Occasionally, however, an anastomosis will require a percutaneous transhepatic stent, and in that case this author uses a uterine sound passed retrogradely up the duct and out through the liver capsule as far anterior as is allowable. The stent is attached to this tube and is withdrawn down through the liver and through the anastomosis into the jejunum. One must be careful to have good drainage of the subphrenic space and to avoid use of the tube in liver cirrhosis since fatal hemorrhage from the liver has occurred after passage of a transhepatic tube.

Our practice is to instruct the patient to irrigate the stent on a daily basis with boiled water. The stent is usually removed about 6 months after placement. In exceptional circumstances it may be left for 6 to 12 months and then replaced over a guidewire. When using straight tubes, one must be careful to suture them to the abdominal wall with nylon sutures placed deeply and tied securely to the tube. In general, T-tubes and Y-tubes with pull-out limbs do not require fixation to the abdominal wall.

POSTOPERATIVE CARE

As the major cause of morbidity and mortality in patients with stricture repair is infection, preoperatively instituted antibiotic coverage for gram-negative organisms should be continued postoperatively for at least 4 days. Because stricture repair does not ordinarily cause major disability or disturb GI function, nasogastric tubes are very often not necessary.

Approximately 20 percent of biliary anastomoses will leak, usually in only small amounts per 24 hours. The suction catheter placed near the anastomosis should keep the incision dry and the patient comfortable. Bile fistulas, even those amounting to 300 to 400 ml per day, will close spontaneously almost without exception. Usually by postoperation day 21, fistulas have dried up, and the patient is able to be discharged. If the fistula persists beyond the 3-week postoperative interval, it is still not worthwhile to reoperate since closure can be expected. If suction drains are appropriately placed, one need not fear a subhepatic abscess in patients in whom fistulas have developed.

Any postoperative fever of major importance is caused by septicemia, a subphrenic abscess, or a subhepatic abscess, especially if it occurs after the fourth or fifth postoperative day. It is generally not important to survey the patient for abscess until about 10 to 16 days postoperatively, because the abscess will not be ready for drainage until that time. Plain upright films of the abdomen may show air–fluid levels, or computed tomographic (CT) scans may disclose collections in the subphrenic or subhepatic spaces. It is conceivable that collections of fluid can be drained by needle, especially if a second needle is placed for counterdrainage. This should be tried before resorting to open operative intervention.

TABLE 82–2. RESULTS OF BILE DUCT STRICTURE REPAIR

Author (Year)	Years Reported	No. of Operations	Follow-up (Years)	Satisfactory Outcome (%)
Cole et al (1948)	1938–1948	46	0–10	67
Walters (1953)	1924–1952	297	1–4	53
Cattell & Braasch (1959)	1940–1955	447[a]	3+	46[b]
Hermann (1975)	1951–1971	79[a]	2–20	84
Smith (1979)	1946–1977	< 1500	2–31	85[b]
Way et al (1981)	1968–1981	59	Mean 3.8	92
Braasch et al (1981)	1971–1975	37[a]	3+	86[b]
Pitt et al (1982)	1955–1980	138[a]	3+ (93%)	77[b]

[a] Unsatisfactory follow-up excluded.
[b] Those who died of disease or died postoperatively were counted as unsatisfactory result.

With extended periods of preoperative jaundice, the postoperative concentration of bilirubin in the blood may increase before it slowly decreases to normal within 1 to 2 months. With short periods of acute obstruction, a prompt fall in the blood bilirubin level can confidently be expected. Pruritus present before operation is almost always relieved within 24 to 48 hours after the operation. This phenomenon is of interest relative to the pathogenesis of pruritus and is unexplainable at this time.

RESULTS

In evaluating the reported results of stricture repair in any series, close attention must be paid to the method, length of recovery, and completeness of follow-up. As mentioned earlier, controversy exists as to the adequate length of time necessary to accumulate almost all of the recurrences. In our experience, the great majority of recurrences will happen within 3 years after removal of the stent. Recently, Pitt et al have indicated that an appreciable number of recurrences can take place years after the 3-year span has passed.

Earlier reports of stricture repair in the 1950s and 1960s indicated a recurrence rate of approximately 40 percent. Since that time the results have gradually improved, so that now many centers report satisfactory results in approximately 85 percent of patients (Table 82–2). This improvement is probably multifactorial. Clearly, patients are referred to the biliary tract surgeon earlier. Major technical advances have been made, resulting in fewer leaking anastomoses. Less dissection of the proximal duct reduces the incidence of ischematic necrosis at the suture line and recurrent stricture.

The postoperative mortality in large series has also declined precipitously and is now about 2 percent. This is also a reflection of earlier referral and improved surgical techniques.

ALTERNATIVE RECONSTRUCTION

A major figure in biliary tract reconstruction has been Lord Smith, formerly a surgeon at St. George's Hospital, London. He developed and championed a technique of anastomosis called the mucosal graft technique, which he has applied to a vast number of patients with biliary tract obstruction (Fig. 82–23). His results indicate a very satisfactory outcome in approximately 85 percent of patients. The main features of his technique are minimal dissection of the proximal hepatic duct and a "pull-through" type of procedure using a Roux-Y loop of jejunum from which a large amount of mucosa protrudes. This loop with protruding mucosa is drawn into the open end of the proximal duct with a transhepatic straight catheter. A few simple sutures tack the Roux-Y limb to the biliary serosa. Smith believes that the jejunal mucosa, which is apposed to the biliary epithelium, retards scar formation and lowers the incidence of recurrent stricture. His procedure is simple in that it avoids direct placement of sutures to bring jejunal to biliary mucosa. No long-term follow-up studies have yet been performed on series of patients treated by this method in other institutions.

The long-term use of transhepatic Silastic tubes as stents through Roux-Y hepaticojejunos-

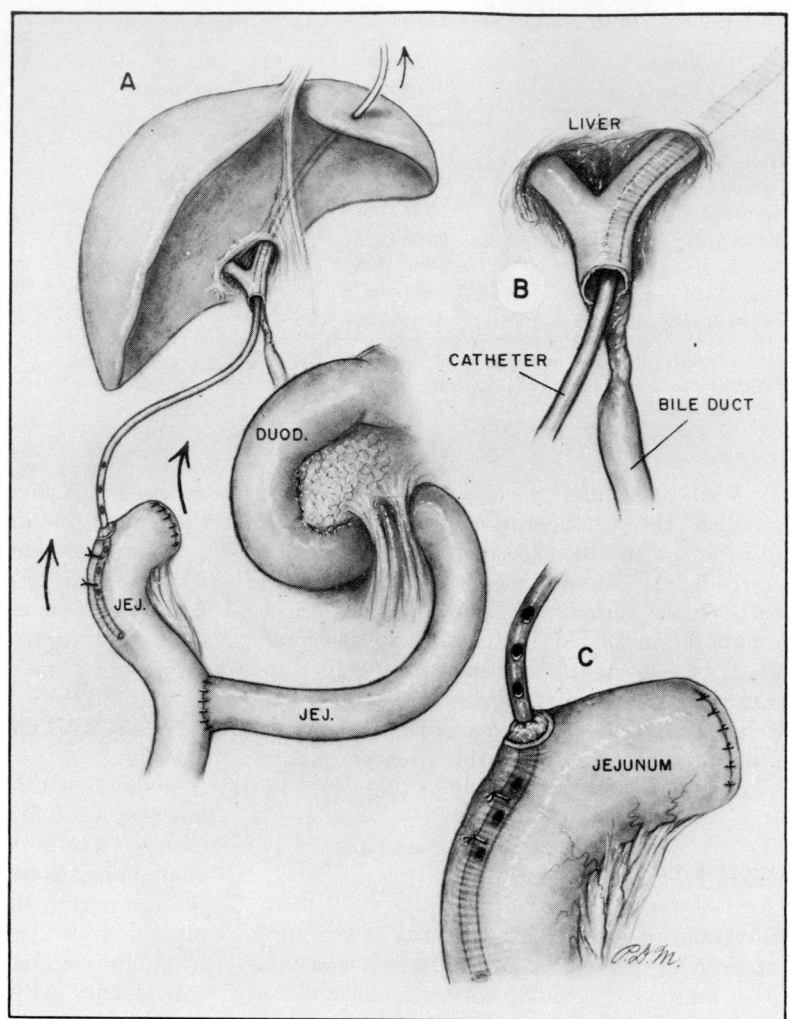

Figure 82–23. A through **E.** Smith's mucosal graft hepaticojejunostomy. **A,B,C.** Preparation for pulling mucosa into proximal duct.

tomies has been reported by Cameron and colleagues. As noted earlier, the Silastic tubes are replaced after being in place for several months. Cameron reported excellent results in the large majority of a small series of patients; however, a later report indicated that the incidence of hepatic abscess may be increased.

Wheeler and Longmire have reported another variation in which an isoperistaltic jejunal interposition of at least 15 cm is placed between proximal duct and duodenum (Fig. 82–24). In their experience a relatively high incidence of duodenal ulceration follows traditional

hepaticojejunostomy. This technique delivers alkaline juices to the duodenum and prevents duodenal contents from reaching the biliary tract. Experience with this method is not extensive.

The use of percutaneous transhepatic intubation of the biliary tree has led to an extension of this procedure in which dilators may be passed percutaneously through the liver and through recurrent strictures. This technique has a certain appeal since it avoids an operative procedure; on the other hand, it implies the long-term use of a transhepatic tube and re-

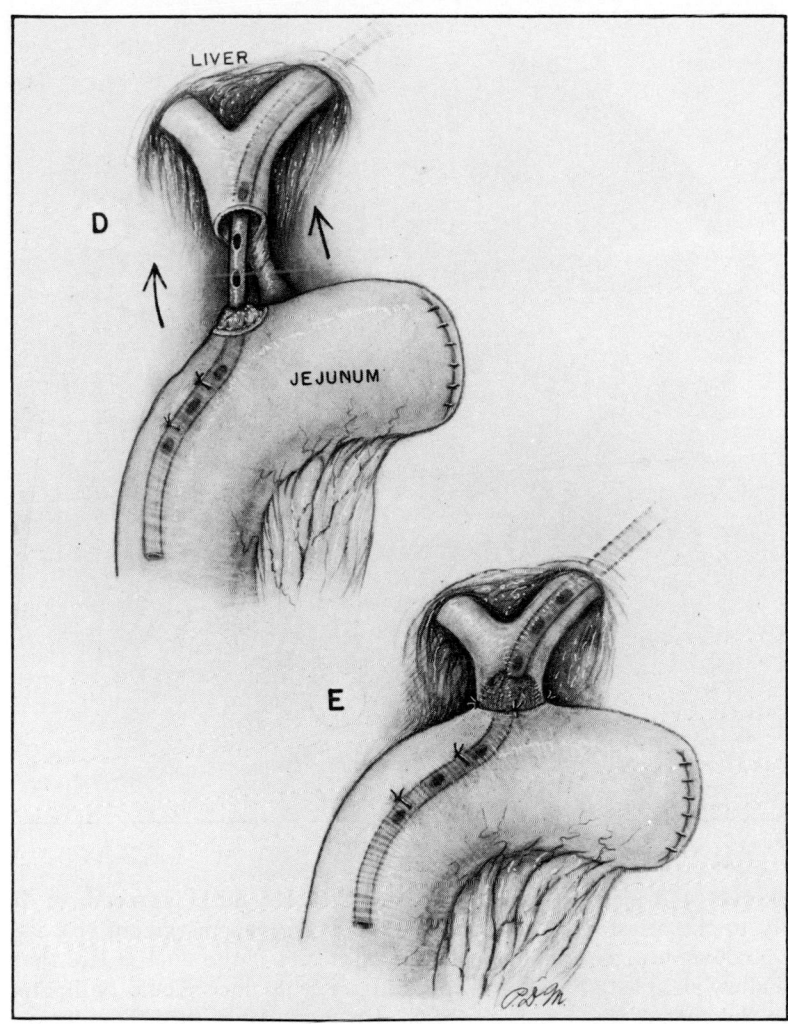

Figure 82–23. D,E. Anastomosis. (*Source: From Braasch JW: Liver, gallbladder, biliary tract, pancreas, and spleen, in Beahrs OH (ed): Therapy Update Service: General Surgery. Boston: Houghton Mifflin, 1978, p 6, with permission.*)

peated dilatations. Our experience with operative dilatation of strictures and the use of stents has not been happy.

SPECIAL SITUATIONS

Repair at Time of Damage

Four types of damage are possible at the time of cholecystectomy. The common hepatic or common bile duct can be clamped, tied, or excised, and a segmental or subsegmental duct from the right lobe can be severed. Fortunately, no one surgeon has had much experience with repair of acute bile duct damage, but the principles that follow seem valid.

With just a simple ligature around the bile duct it is advisable to deligate the duct and pass a T-tube of the largest possible size through the area formerly ligated. This tube should be left in place for at least 6 months; one can expect no further trouble from this situation.

If a clamping injury of the duct has occurred, it is probably wise to excise the area clamped, with care taken not to free up the prox-

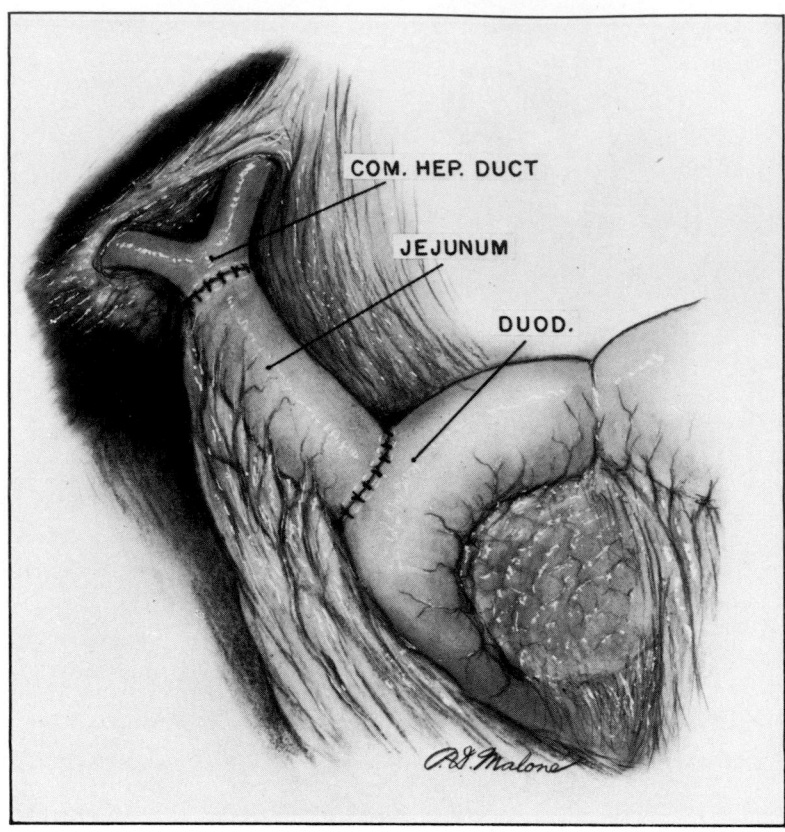

Figure 82–24. Longmire's jejunal interposition.

imal or distal segments of the duct and in so doing destroy the blood supply to the anastomotic area. A wide Kocher maneuver can be carried out, which will usually allow an anastomosis to be performed between the ends of the duct without tension. Again, fine interrupted sutures in one layer are advisable for the repair. A T-tube brought out through the duct at a distance from the anastomosis should be used as a stent and left in place for 6 months.

If a segment of duct has been excised, either hepaticojejunostomy or hepaticoduodenostomy performed with the techniques described for the repair of chronic stricture seems advisable. Again, this anastomosis should be stented in the usual fashion.

At times a low hepatic duct insertion of a segmental or subsegmental duct drains a portion of the right lobe of the liver. Since this insertion may be into the cystic duct or into the common bile duct at Calot's triangle, these ducts are subject to damage during cholecystectomy. With use of appropriate dissection or operative cholangiography, the drainage area of

the duct in question should be ascertained. In general, if it drains only a subsegment or a segment on the right and if the duct is less than 3 mm in diameter, this duct should be ligated simply with a permanent suture. For ducts 3 to 4 mm in diameter an anastomosis should be made to a loop of jejunum. Subsegments of the liver can be obstructed totally by permanent ligature without expecting symptoms of cholangitis. If an external bile fistula develops after ligature of such a duct, watchful waiting is the best policy because in all likelihood the fistula will close spontaneously without further difficulty.

High Obstructions

Most often direct suture anastomosis can be accomplished with segmental or lobar ducts. At times the obstructed liver enlarges over the common hepatic duct bifurcation. With persistence, however, 1 to 1.5 inches of duct structure can be dissected out of the hilus of the liver, provided that the liver is mobilized so that with suitable retraction the hilus can be tipped to face anteriorly.

One maneuver that is useful for extremely high intrahepatic strictures is to dissect a plane between the right and left lobes of the liver down to the common hepatic duct bifurcation. This is a substitute maneuver for the hilar extraction of the duct described previously. In patients with destruction of the common hepatic duct, crushing the septum between the right and left ducts (Fig. 82–25) sometimes recreates the common hepatic duct for a single anastomosis.

In certain cases of lobar obstruction with atrophy and infection of the obstructed lobe, hepatic lobectomy should be considered to remove the septic area. This is a rare situation but one that deserves consideration.

Longmire and Sanford have suggested a procedure of left hepaticojejunostomy for patients in whom hilar dissection is exceptionally difficult or impossible. Their technique involves excision of a portion of the left lateral segment of the liver, locating the left hepatic duct distally, and performing an anastomosis between the duct at that point and the jejunum. Other modifications of this procedure have been suggested that involve methods of locating the left hepatic duct by cannulation of small superficial ducts and cutdown on the larger structure within the left lobe, but basically the techniques are similar. Blumgart uses a dissection technique modified from the method of Champeau and Pineau to explore the base of the ligamentum teres to locate the left hepatic duct for anastomosis without resection of liver tissue. These types of procedures are desperate maneuvers attempted when hilar dissection and major duct anastomosis cannot be performed.

Lobar or Segmental Obstruction

The response in humans to lobar obstruction or segmental obstruction is variable. At times

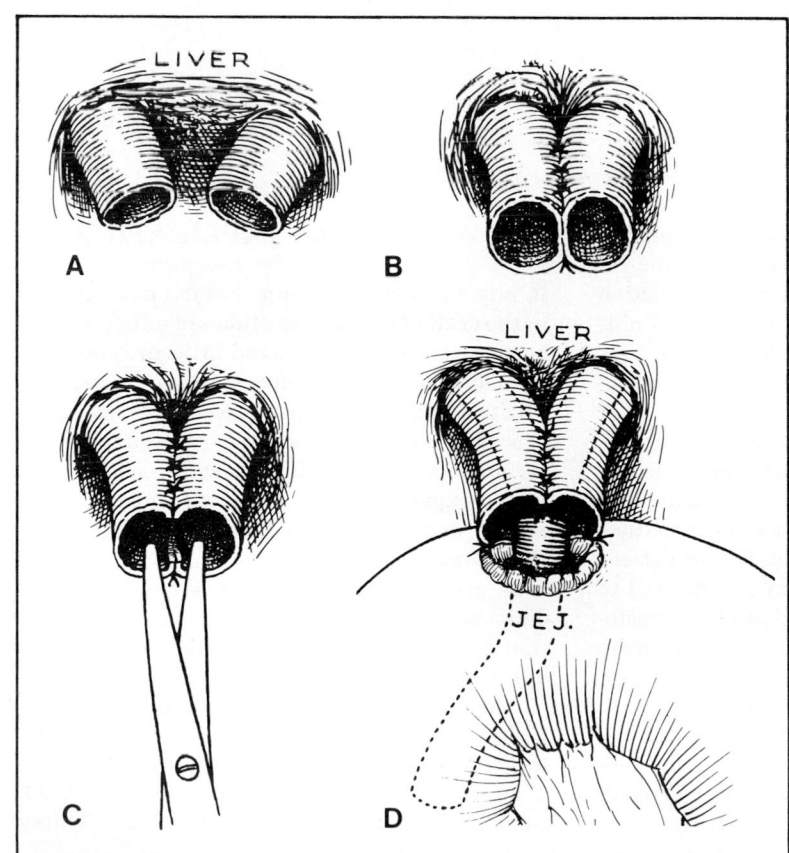

Figure 82–25. Formation **(A,B)** and crushing **(C,D)** of septum between right and left hepatic ducts in high stricture to create a new common hepatic duct. (*Source: From Cattell RB, Braasch JW, 1960, with permission of Surgery, Gynecology & Obstetrics.*)

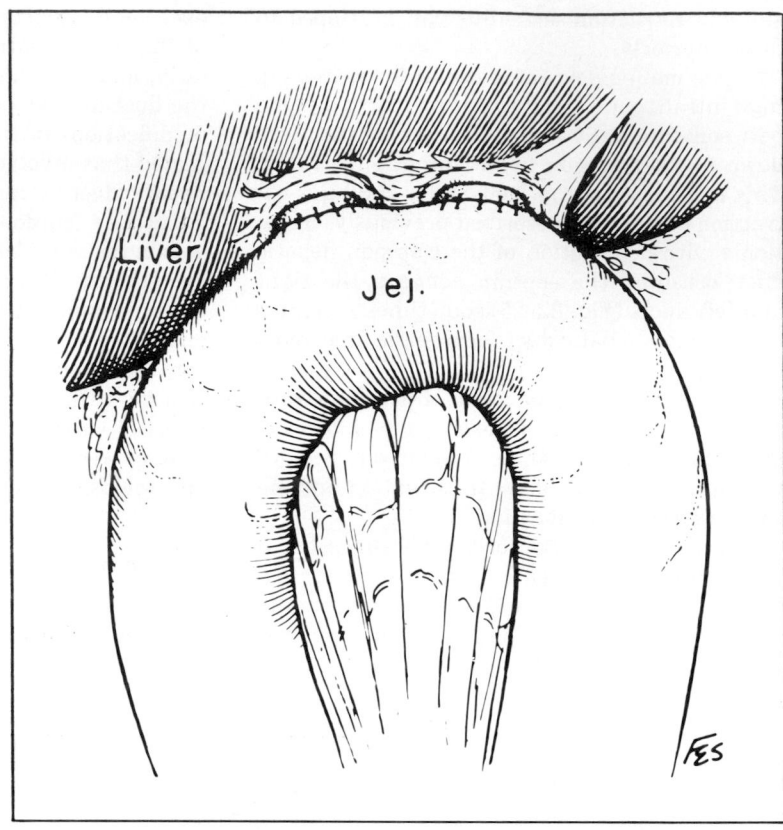

Figure 82–26. Double hepaticojejunostomy.

low-grade jaundice with or without cholangitis results if the obstructed segments become infected. At other times even a lobar obstruction will cause no clinical problem. In both animals and humans the obstructed segment or lobe eventually undergoes atrophy, and other segments and lobes of the liver hypertrophy. If at the time of laparotomy for stricture an atrophied right lobe is seen, the surgeon generally must only be certain that the left lobar duct is not obstructed and only a single left hepaticojejunostomy need be performed. In the patient is experiencing fever, dissection is indicated to try to find the right hepatic duct, and an anastomosis must be carried out to give free drainage to the atrophied lobe. Operative cholangiography is of great importance in the recognition of obstructed, atrophic, or otherwise altered segments and lobes of the liver. A solution for double duct obstruction can be double hepaticojejunostomy (Fig. 82–26).

MEDICAL–LEGAL IMPLICATIONS

In any endeavor involving manual dexterity, as in the craft of surgery, mistakes of either mental or manual nature are bound to occur. The price of mistakes during cholecystectomy is high, as illustrated in this chapter. Recurrent operative procedures and even death from biliary cirrhosis are possible should reparative efforts fail. In the experience of the Lahey Clinic, approximately one third of patients eventually died of their stricture 30 to 40 years ago. Since that time great improvements have been made in diagnosis, technique of repair, and follow-up so that death is now uncommon, and the likelihood of a successful first repair is high.

There is no solution, however, to the dilemma of balancing the possibility of damage to the common hepatic duct by even the best of surgeons against the expectation of each patient that mistakes will not be made. Thirty years ago it was a rare occurrence for a case of stricture of the bile duct to find its way into the law courts for adjudication of culpability and assuagement of pain and suffering with monetary payments. This has now changed because in the last few years in the United States almost every case receives the attention of the legal profession.

The problem for the courts is proof of culpability, as in the majority of cases no definite misadventure is recorded. This is compounded by the fact that in at least 5 percent of cases the likelihood of surgical damage to the duct is extremely remote. The nub of this matter is a situation where honesty and accuracy in the recording of the operative note leads to great emotional and mental turmoil as the legal process proceeds.

BIBLIOGRAPHY

Black HC, Hawk JC Jr, et al: Long-term intubation of the biliary tract with Silastic catheters. Am Surg 37:198, 1971

Blumgart LH: Personal communication, 1983

Braasch JW, Bolton JS, et al: A technique of biliary tract reconstruction with complete follow-up in 44 consecutive cases. Ann Surg 194:635, 1981

Braasch JW, Whitcomb FF Jr, et al: Segmental obstruction of the bile duct. Surg Gynecol Obstet 134:915, 1972

Cameron JL, Gayler BW, et al: The use of Silastic transhepatic stents in benign and malignant biliary strictures. Ann Surg 188:552, 1978

Cameron JL, Skinner DB, et al: Long term transhepatic intubation for hilar hepatic duct strictures. Ann Surg 183:488, 1976

Cattell RB, Braasch JW: Long-term follow-up after repair of bile duct strictures. Lahey Clin Bull 10:194, 1958

Cattell RB, Braasch JW: General considerations in the management of benign strictures of the bile duct. N Engl J Med 261:929, 1959a

Cattell RB, Braasch JW: Primary repair of benign strictures of the bile duct. Surg Gynecol Obstet 109:531, 1959b

Cattell RB, Braasch JW: Two stage repairs of benign strictures of the bile duct. Surg Gynecol Obstet 109:691, 1959c

Cattell RB, Braasch JW: Repair of benign strictures of the bile duct involving both or single hepatic ducts. Surg Gynecol Obstet 110:55, 1960

Champeau M, Pineau P: Voie d'abord élargie transhé-patique du canal hépatique gauche: possibilité de découverte totale du canal. Mem Acad Chir (Paris) 90:602, 1964

Cole WH, Reynolds JT, et al: Strictures of the common duct. Ann Surg 128:332, 1948

Denning DA, Ellison EC, et al: Preoperative percutaneous transhepatic biliary decompression lowers operative morbidity in patients with obstructive jaundice. Am J Surg 141:61, 1981

Grindlay JH, Eberle J, et al: Technique for external drainage of the biliary tract which leaves ducts intact: An experimental study. Arch Surg 67:289, 1953

Hatfield ARW, Tobias R, et al: Preoperative external biliary drainage in obstructive jaundice: A prospective controlled clinical trial. Lancet 2:896, 1982

Hermann RE: Diagnosis and management of bile duct strictures. Am J Surg 130:519, 1975

Kolff J, Hoeltge G, et al: Silastic T-tube splints for biliary repair. Am J Surg 129:236, 1975

Longmire WP Jr, Sanford MC: Intrahepatic cholangiojejunostomy for biliary obstruction—further studies; report of 4 cases. Ann Surg 130:455, 1949

Longmire WP Jr, Tompkins RK: Lesions of the segmental and lobar hepatic ducts. Ann Surg 182:478, 1975

Mayo WJ: Some remarks on cases involving operative loss of continuity of the common bile duct. With the report of a case of anastomosis between the hepatic duct and the duodenum. Ann Surg 42:90, 1905

Michels NA: Blood Supply and Anatomy of the Upper Abdominal Organs with a Descriptive Atlas. Philadelphia: JB Lippincott, 1955

Molnar W, Stockum AE: Transhepatic dilatation of choledochoenterostomy strictures. Radiology 129:59, 1978

Monprofit A: Du remplacement du choledoque et de l'hépatique par une anse jéjunale. Cong de Chir 21:206, 1908

Muñoz R: Reconstruction of the bile ducts: Biliointestinal anastomosis with transhepatic insertion of a T tube. Rev Invest Clin 11:217, 1959

Northover JMA, Terblanche J: A new look at the arterial supply of the bile duct in man and its surgical implications. Br J Surg 66:379, 1979

Pennington L, Kaufman S, et al: Intrahepatic abscess as a complication of long-term percutaneous internal biliary drainage. Surgery 91:642, 1982

Pitt HA, Miyamoto T, et al: Factors influencing outcome in patients with postoperative biliary strictures. Am J Surg 144:14, 1982

Praderi R: El drenaje biliar externo o interno por el hepático izquierdo. Rev Ass Med Brasil 9:401, 1963

Rossi RL, Gordon M, et al: Intubation techniques in biliary tract surgery. Surg Clin North Am 60:297, 1980

Sedgwick CE, Hume A: Management of bile duct strictures with associated portal hypertension. Surg Gynecol Obstet 108:627, 1959

Smith R: Obstructions of the bile duct. Br J Surg 66:69, 1979

Stone RM, Cohen Z, et al: Bile duct injury: Results of repair using a changeable stent. Am J Surg 125:253, 1973

Templeton JY III, Dodd GD: Anatomical separation of the right and left lobes of the liver for intrahepatic anastomosis of the biliary ducts. Ann Surg 157:287, 1963

Teplick SK, Wolferth CC Jr, et al: Balloon dilatation of benign postsurgical biliary-enteric anastomotic strictures. Gastrointest Radiol 7:307, 1982

Terblanche J, Allison HF, et al: An ischemic basis for biliary strictures. Surgery 94:52, 1983

Waddell WR, Taubman J: Mechanical and chemical methods of opening occluded T-tubes. Surgery 71:91, 1972

Walters W: Physiologic studies in cases of stricture of the common bile duct: A twenty-eight-year survey with data on 254 patients. Ann Surg 138:609, 1953

Way LW, Bernhoft RA, et al: Biliary stricture. Surg Clin North Am 61:963, 1981

Wheeler ES, Longmire WP Jr: Repair of benign stricture of the common bile duct by jejunal interposition choledochoduodenostomy. Surg Gynecol Obstet 146:260, 1978

83. Sclerosing Cholangitis

Alfred Cuschieri

INTRODUCTION

Sclerosing cholangitis remains a poorly defined syndrome of uncertain aetiology resulting in a progressive inflammatory and fibrotic obliteration of the biliary tract. First described by Delbert in 1924, the disease is generally regarded as a rare condition. However, it is diagnosed more often today, largely due to the introduction of endoscopic retrograde cholangiography, (Wiesner and LaRusso, 1980), but there is no firm evidence of a true rise in its incidence over the past two decades. Controversy exists concerning its aetiology, classification, and management. Although the disorder has well-recognised histologic, radiologic, and clinical features, there are no pathognomonic findings that reliably differentiate sclerosing cholangitis from other hepatobiliary disorders.

Although considered a medical disorder in the first instance, there is no proof of any effective medical therapy and the condition usually progresses to biliary cirrhosis and premature death from end-stage liver disease or bleeding oesophageal varices. Surgical intervention designed to enhance or promote bile drainage into the gastrointestinal (GI) tract is often required at some stage during the natural history of the disease, and properly designed surgical management often results in dramatic symptomatic relief and not infrequently in long-term improvement in the patency of the biliary tract.

Primary and Secondary Forms

The insistence on distinguishing between primary and secondary sclerosing cholangitis is both confusing and unwarranted, especially since the more recent attempts at this separation include cases associated with inflammatory bowel disease within the primary (idiopathic) group. Furthermore ductal calculi and sludge invariably occur as a sequel to bona fide cases of "primary cholangitis" and the insistence that biliary calculi must be absent is unacceptable on pathologic grounds. The causes of so-called secondary sclerosing cholangitis (common duct calculi, iatrogenic bile duct injury/stricture, cholangiocarcinoma and congenital anomalies) produce distinctive disorders that may simulate sclerosing cholangitis but that, excepting cholangiocarcinoma, can usually be differentiated from this condition.

AETIOLOGY

The various hypotheses concerning the aetiology of sclerosing cholangitis postulate a ductal injury of infective, immunologic, or toxic origin. The frequent association with ulcerative colitis, the demonstration of bacteria in the portal venous blood in patients during surgery for inflammatory bowel disease (Brooke and Slaney, 1958), and the reported beneficial effect of tetracycline therapy for pericholangitis complicating ulcerative colitis (Rankin et al, 1969) has been interpreted as evidence for a bacterial infection. Although the suggestion has been repeatedly dismissed with statements that the majority of patients with sclerosing cholangitis have no demonstrable bacteria in the bile, the evidence for this viewpoint in the reported literature is scanty. In the author's series, all patients undergoing surgical treatment have had infected bile at operation and positive blood cultures have been obtained during episodes of cholangitis in 75 percent of patients before surgery. The organisms cultured have always included gram-negative aerobes. Anaerobic organisms (*Bactero-*

ides fragilis, Clostridium welchii) have been-encountered in mixed infections only. On the other hand, there is little or no correlation between the histologic appearances of the liver biopsy and the presence of either positive bile or blood cultures. Thus, the bacterial infection may well be a secondary phenomenon.

The condition is often regarded as an immune-complex disorder involving antigenic substances such as endotoxin. It is postulated that an excess of endotoxin–antibody complexes may overwhelm hepatocyte clearance and thereby enter the systemic circulation (Thomas and Vaez-Zadeh, 1974). Indeed such immune complexes have been demonstrated in the peripheral blood of patients with inflammatory bowel disease (Hodgson et al, 1977), but the incidence is no higher in patients with extraintestinal manifestations, including sclerosing cholangitis, than in patients without. Further evidence for a primary immunologically induced bile duct injury is the reported inhibition of leucocyte migration in the presence of an antigen derived from bile duct epithelium (Waldram et al, 1975). In addition, sclerosing cholangitis may occur in association with disorders of obscure but probable immunologic nature such as mediastinal and retroperitoneal fibrosis, pernicious anaemia, Riedel's (lymphocytic) thyroiditis, orbital pseudotumour, Peyronie's disease, recticulum-cell lymphoma, and familial immunodeficiency syndrome (Record et al, 1973).

There is some experimental evidence that sclerosing cholangitis may be due to a chemically induced bile duct injury by an agent secreted in the bile. Thus administration of 1,4 phenylene-disothiocyanate and saccharated ferric oxide in rodents results in cholangitis (Selye and Szabo, 1972) and drug ingestion, particularly sulphonamides, has been implicated in the human (Stauffer et al, 1965).

GROSS PATHOLOGY

Liver. During the early stages of the disease the liver, though somewhat enlarged, appears normal at laparotomy even in the presence of marked cholangiographic abnormalities affecting the intrahepatic biliary tree and abnormal liver histology. In late cases, secondary biliary cirrhosis with obvious varices, ascites, and splenomegaly are encountered.

TABLE 83–1. SCLEROSING CHOLANGITIS

Extent of Involvement	Incidence (%)
Total diffuse	50
Localised hilar	25
Diffuse extrahepatic	10
Diffuse intrahepatic	10
Localised distal CBD	5

Extrahepatic Biliary Tract. The gallbladder is frequently abnormal, with a thickened fibrous wall, although calculi are rare and, when present, co-exist with ductal calcium bilirubinate concretions and sludge. When the disease affects the extrahepatic ductal system, the findings in the hepatoduodenal areas are distinctive. The region appears thickened and fleshy with oedema and enlarged lymph nodes, the histology of which shows nonspecific hyperplasia. The identification of the bile duct is often difficult and is best traced from below after complete mobilisation of the duodenum and head of pancreas. When exposed, the bile duct is seen to be grossly and irregularly thickened by dense fibrosis, which often extends outside the confines of the bile duct into the surrounding tissues. Often the strictured lumen is difficult to find.

Surgical Types. The most useful classification is that described at the Lahey Clinic (Warren et al, 1966) because, in the author's experience, this forms a rational basis for the surgical management of the individual case (Table 83–1). Diffuse involvement of both the intra- and extrahepatic biliary tract is encountered in 50 percent of patients. Localised disease usually affects the hilar region at the junction of the right and left hepatic ducts (25 percent) and less commonly the lower end of the common bile duct (5 percent).

HISTOLOGY

The histologic appearances are suggestive but not pathognomonic of the condition. Considerable confusion has emanated by interpreting the pathology of sclerosing cholangitis from hepatic biopsies. As a general consideration, these often represent the morphologic response of the hepatic parenchyma to bile duct obstruction and exhibit nonspecific changes of cholestasis.

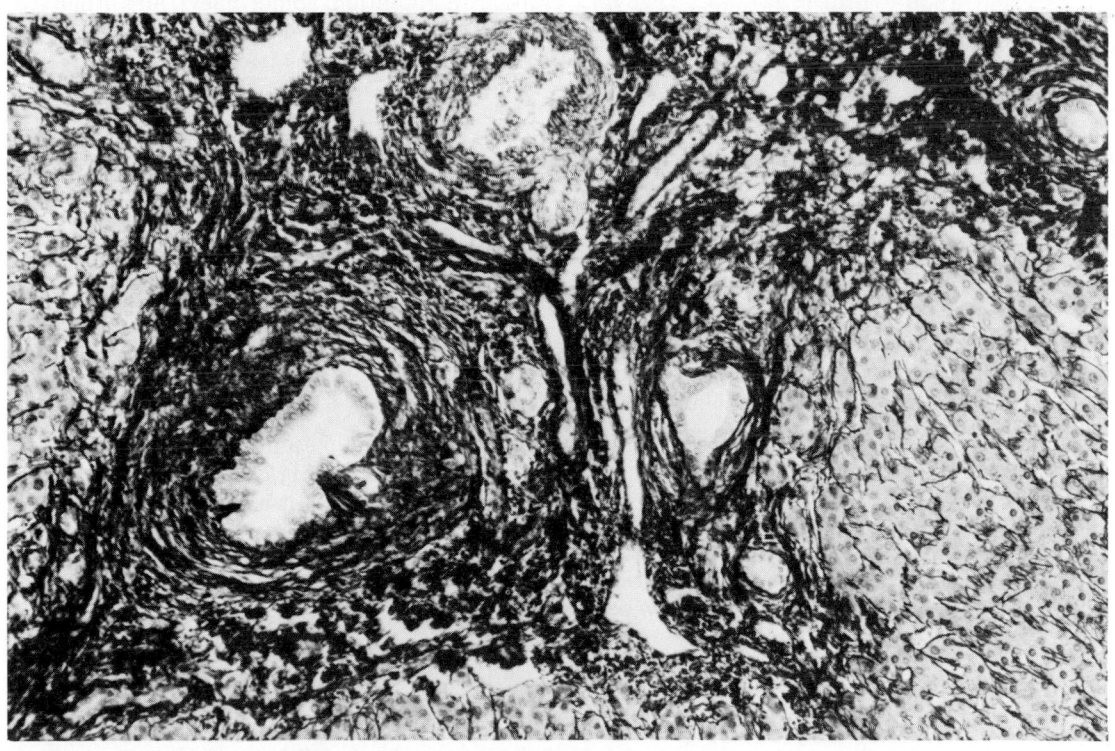

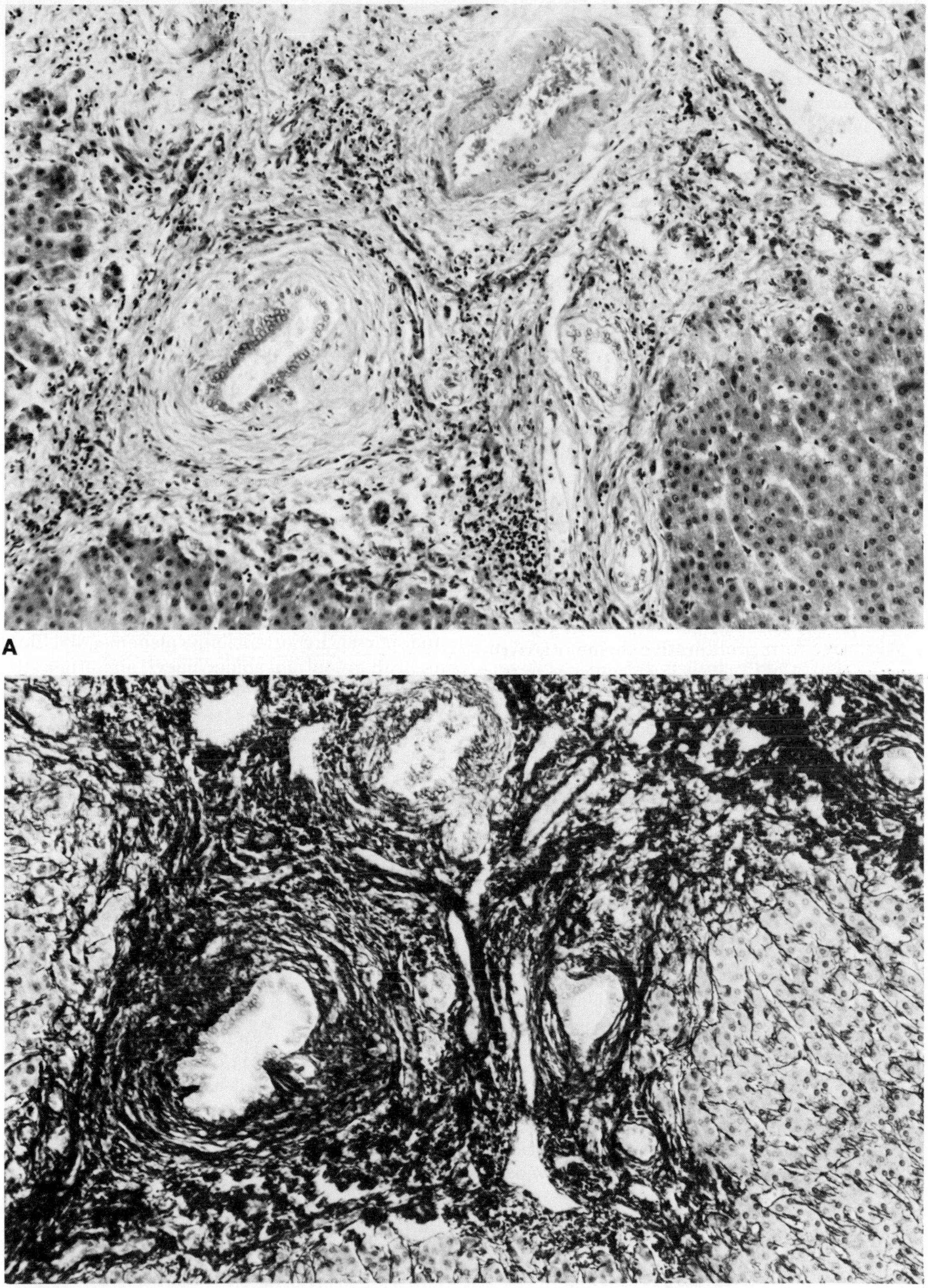

Figure 83–1. A. Histology showing concentric periductal fibrosis with patchy chronic inflammatory infiltrate. **B.** Reticulin stain demonstrating the periductal (onion shell) disposition of the fibrosis in sclerosing cholangitis.

Liver. The changes include periductal fibrosis and inflammation with accumulation of plasma cells, lymphocytes, and polymorphs, portal oedema, and fibrosis with infiltration by lymphocytes and histiocytes, focal proliferation of bile ductules, obliteration, and loss of intrahepatic ducts, cholestasis, and copper deposition.

Bile Ducts. The appearances are dominated by extensive fibrosis that extends beyond the confines of the duct wall. Characteristically the fibrosis is concentric (onion shell), with patchy chronic inflammatory infiltrate (mononuclear cells and polymorphs) (Fig. 83–1A,B.) The gross fibrotic thickening results in considerable narrowing of the lumen. Although the ductal epithelium is frequently normal, it may be ulcerated and exhibit saccule formation. Furthermore, areas of glandular hyperplasia may be present (Thompson and Read, 1981). More recently, cases showing a proliferative mucosal histology and saccule formation have been reported as a previously unrecognised condition and referred to as proliferative cholangitis (Krukowski et al, 1983). There is no evidence in this publication to prove that the six cases reported in this series constitute an entity that can be distinguished from sclerosing cholangitis.

The electron microscopic features of the biliary epithelial cells in sclerosing cholangitis are similar to those of primary biliary cirrhosis, with swollen mitochondria and larger than normal lysosomal elements (residual bodies). The basement membrane is intact.

Relation to Pericholangitis. There is increasing evidence from biopsy studies and cholangiographic surveys that sclerosing cholangitis and the more common condition of pericholangitis represent parts of the same spectrum of hepatobiliary disorders that frequently complicate inflammatory bowel disease (Blackstone and Memchunsky, 1978; Rohrmann et al, 1978) and instances of apparent progression from pericholangitis to sclerosing cholangitis have now been reported.

CLINICAL MANIFESTATIONS

The disease is more commonly found in males with a sex ratio of 3:2 and usually presents in the fifth decade, although diagnosis is often delayed for up to 2 years from onset of symptoms. Jaundice with pale stools and dark urine dominates the clinical picture. Frequent accompaniments include vague ill health, weight loss, anorexia, malaise, and pruritus. Pain in the right hypochondrium is encountered in 70 percent of patients. Episodes of cholangitis with rigors and pyrexia occur and are of variable severity. Often the patients become accustomed to these attacks and self-administer antibiotics prescribed by their general practitioner. This may account for the high incidence of negative blood cultures during these attacks reported in the literature. In the author's experience, 76 percent of blood cultures taken within 6 hours of the onset of an attack of cholangitis are positive.

During the early stages of the disease the physical signs include jaundice, hepatomegaly, and liver tenderness. The nutritional state is usually well preserved. In patients with inflammatory bowel disease, extracolonic manifestations of ulcerative colitis may be present. With the development of secondary biliary cirrhosis and portal hypertension, splenomegaly, fluid and salt retention, spider naevi, and other stigmata of end-stage liver disease are encountered. Bleeding from oesophageal varices carries a particulary bad prognosis in these patients.

Association with Inflammatory Bowel Disease

In the author's series of 13 cases, 10 had ulcerative colitis (total involvement) and one patient had Crohn's disease of the colon and ileum. In the literature ulcerative colitis is reported to be present in 30 to 70 percent of patients with sclerosing cholangitis (Schrumpf et al, 1980; La Russo et al, 1983; Tobias et al, 1983). Overall, some 3 percent of patients with ulcerative colitis will develop sclerosing cholangitis. Usually the inflammatory bowel disease is active and severe with total involvement, and long standing, although cases have been described where the sclerosing cholangitis developed years after proctocolectomy. Rarely, the biliary tract disorder may antedate the development of ulcerative colitis. The association with Crohn's disease is less well established but there are now a few well-documented cases and one endoscopic retrograde cholangiopancreatography (ERCP) study demonstrated the presence of sclerosing cholangitis in 3 out of 164 patients with Crohn's disease (Tobias et al, 1983).

DIAGNOSTIC STUDIES

There is no one single pathognomonic feature. A firm diagnosis can only be made on the basis of the appropriate clinical picture, a cholestatic jaundice, essentially negative serology, demonstration of radiologic abnormalities by cholangiography, liver and/or bile duct biopsy, and a minimum period of three years follow-up (to exclude intrahepatic cholangiocarcinoma).

Radiologic Findings. The procedure that is used in the first instance is ERCP. In patients with dense hilar strictures, the intrahepatic biliary tree may not be well defined by this proce-

dure and fine needle percutaneous transhepatic cholangiography may be required. Both investigations require antibiotic cover with a cephalosporin. The most common ERCP findings include irregular and diffuse narrowing of entire biliary tree, resulting in diminished branching and eventual pruning of the intrahepatic system (Fig. 83–2). At times the stenotic areas are associated with ectatic segments, resulting in a beaded appearance (Fig. 83–3). Less frequently sacculation is seen in the intrahepatic biliary tree. The most common extrahepatic type consists of a tight stricture affecting the junction of the right and left hepatic ducts, giving a radiologic appearance that is virtually indistin-

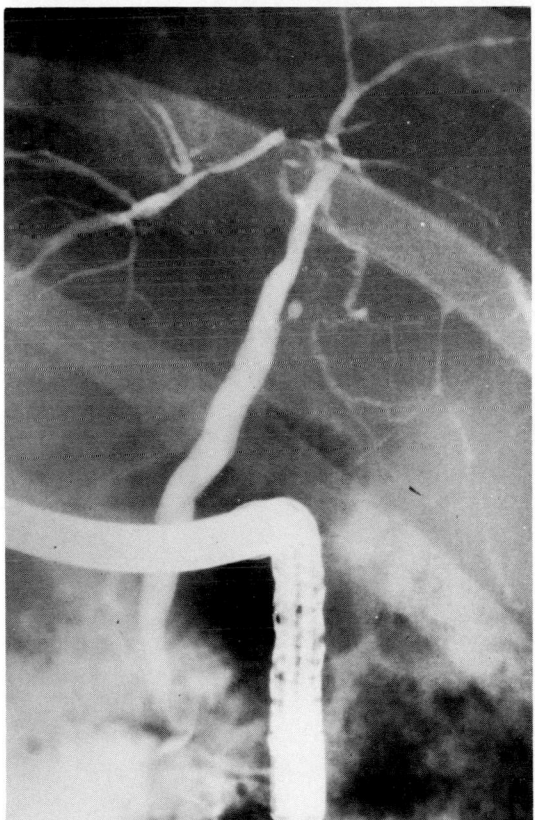

A

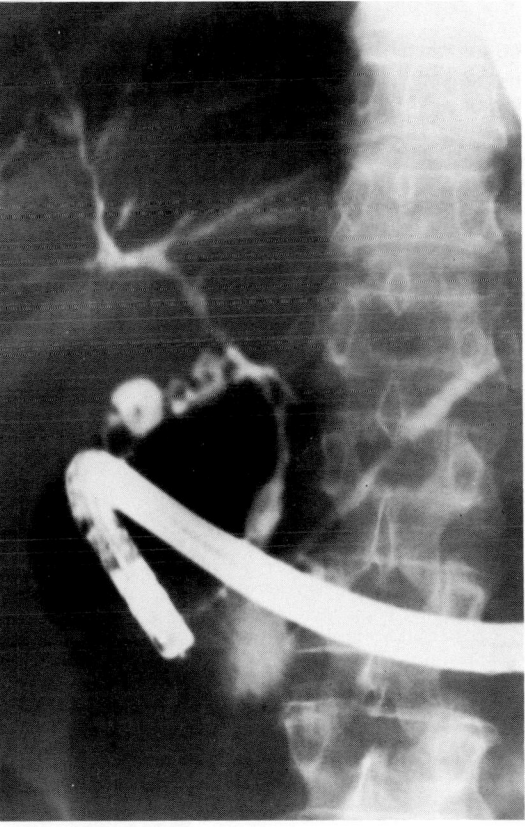

B

Figure 83–2. A. Endoscopic retrograde cholangiogram in a 40-year-old male with sclerosing cholangitis not associated with inflammatory bowel disease. The disorder affects predominantly the intrahepatic duct system with multiple strictures. Although diseased, the common bile duct is not markedly involved. **B.** Total extensive sclerosing cholangitis in a 35-year-old female with ulcerative colitis of 9 years' duration. There is irregular narrowing of the extrahepatic duct system and extensive pruning of the intrahepatic system.

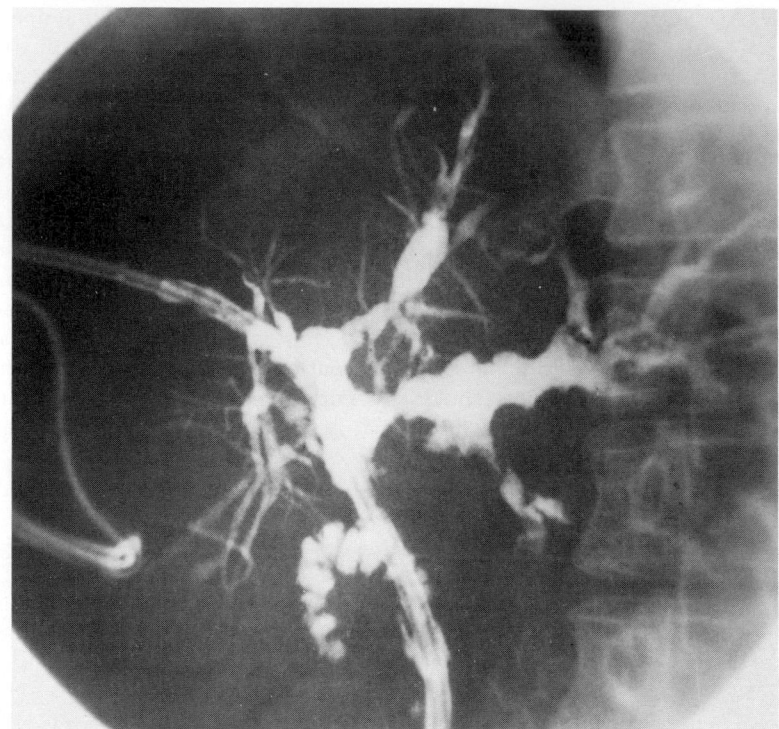

Figure 83-3. Total involvement of the entire biliary tract with sclerosing cholangitis. In this instance there is an admixture of stenotic and ectatic/saccular segments.

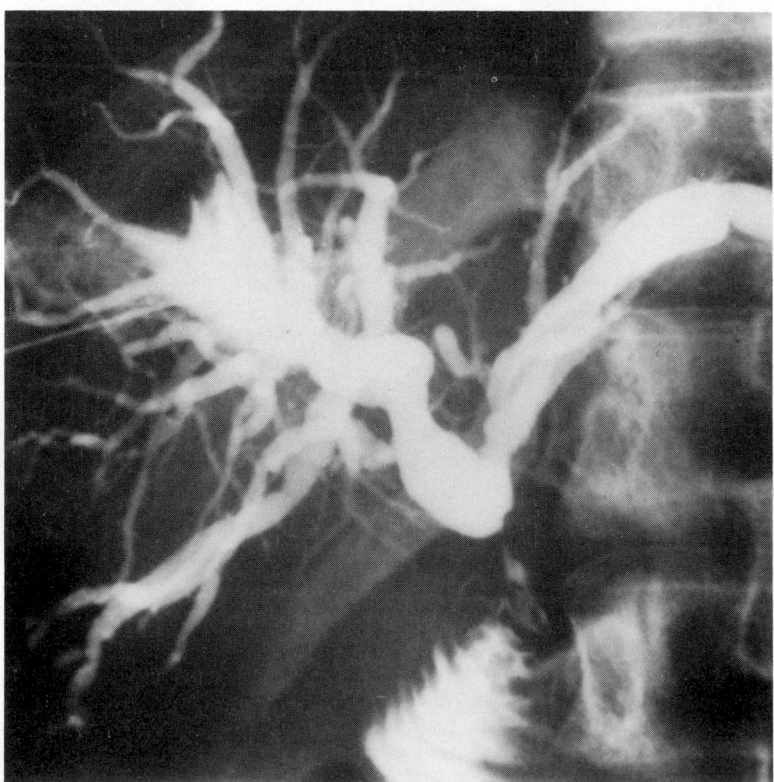

Figure 83-4. A. Localised sclerosing cholangitis affecting the hilar region with considerable dilatation of the intrahepatic biliary tree.

A

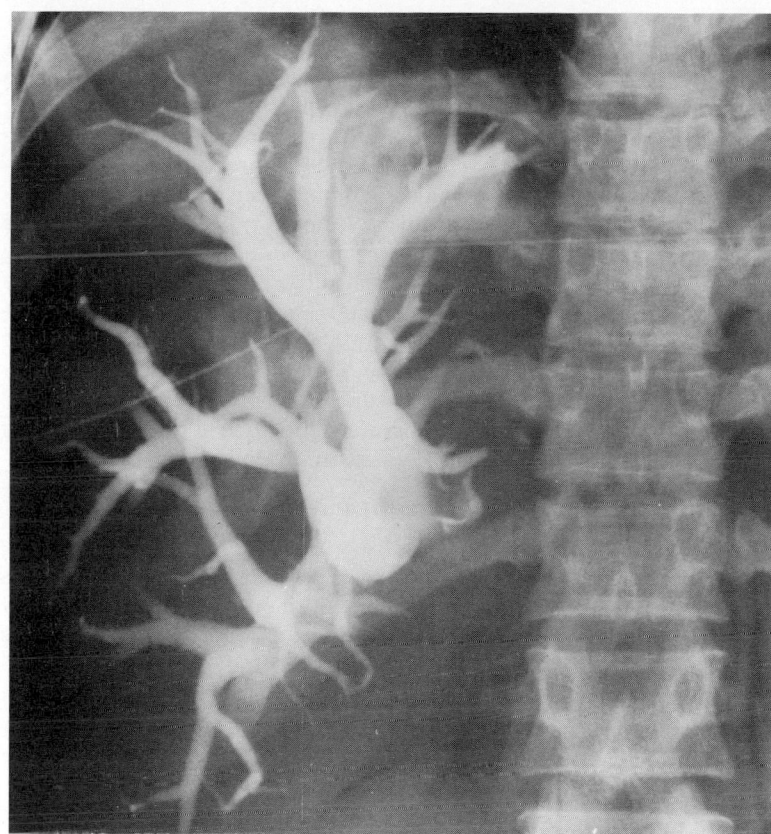

Figure 83–4. B. Hilar cholangiocarcinoma. The radiologic appearances are virtually indistinguishable from those of hilar sclerosing cholangitis. Differentiation between the two conditions may at times be impossible even after histologic examination of relevant biopsy material.

B

guishable from hilar cholangiocarcinoma (Fig. 83–4A,B). In the diffuse disease, dilatation proximal to strictured areas is minimal but intrahepatic dilatation is encountered in localised disease.

Biochemical Findings. The liver function tests demonstrate a cholestatic jaundice with an elevated serum bilirubin, raised alkaline phosphatase, and γ-glutamyl transpeptidase. The serum transaminases are marginally elevated. The majority of patients are HBs Ag negative. Antimitochondrial, antismooth muscle, and antinuclear antibodies are absent and the LE test is negative. Some patients exhibit moderate elevation of the serum IgM levels.

MANAGEMENT

Medical Treatment

There is no effective drug therapy. Contrary to initial reports (Myers et al, 1970), corticosteroids do not alter the natural history of the disease. Treatment with D-penicillamine (cupruretic agent) has been recommended in view of its proven efficacy in primary biliary cirrhosis (Dickson et al, 1982). The pruritus is often well controlled with cholestyramine. Episodes of cholangitis are managed with antibiotic therapy. There have not been any studies on the efficacy of long-term antibiotic treatment in this disorder.

Surgical Treatment

Timely surgical intervention can result in dramatic relief of jaundice, recurrent cholangitis, and liver pain. In some patients considerable and sustained radiologic improvement in the condition of the biliary tract can be obtained (Wood and Cuschieri, 1980). However, the timing of surgical intervention is crucial. The decision when to operate is often difficult and requires a refined clinical judgement. Despite an alarming radiologic appearance, there is no indication for operation if the patient is fairly symptom free and in reasonable health. On the

**TABLE 83–2. INDICATIONS AND
CONTRAINDICATIONS FOR SURGICAL
INTERVENTION IN SCLEROSING CHOLANGITIS**

I. *Indications*
   Progressive jaundice
   Recurrent cholangitis
   Localised disease
   Chronic ill health

II. *Contraindications*
   Adequate control with medical R_x
   Established secondary biliary cirrhosis

other hand, the results of surgical treatment are poor and the operative mortality is high in patients with established biliary cirrhosis. Table 83–2 lists the indications and contraindications for surgical intervention. It reflects the author's experience and current management policy. It should be stressed, however, that the treatment is not standardised and needs tailoring to the individual case. In patients with active ulcerative colitis, colonic resection is per-

formed by the author at the time of biliary intervention. Although there is no evidence that the colectomy alters the natural history of the disease, the removal of a diseased colon as an additional source of ill health, anaemia, and portal bacteraemia makes practical sense. Nevertheless this remains a controversial issue.

The objectives of surgical intervention are to relieve obstruction and to eradicate any infections within the biliary tract. The procedures available include transhepatic stenting with silicone tubes, dilatation of strictures, patching of the common bile duct (autologous vein or gallbladder flap), and bilioenteric bypass. More often than not, more than one of these procedures are necessary in the individual patient.

Diffuse Involvement (Intra- and Extrahepatic)

Initially the common bile duct is explored. As the lumen of the common bile duct is invariably narrowed, needling for identification purposes is often unsuccessful and should not be attempted repeatedly, as this exercise often

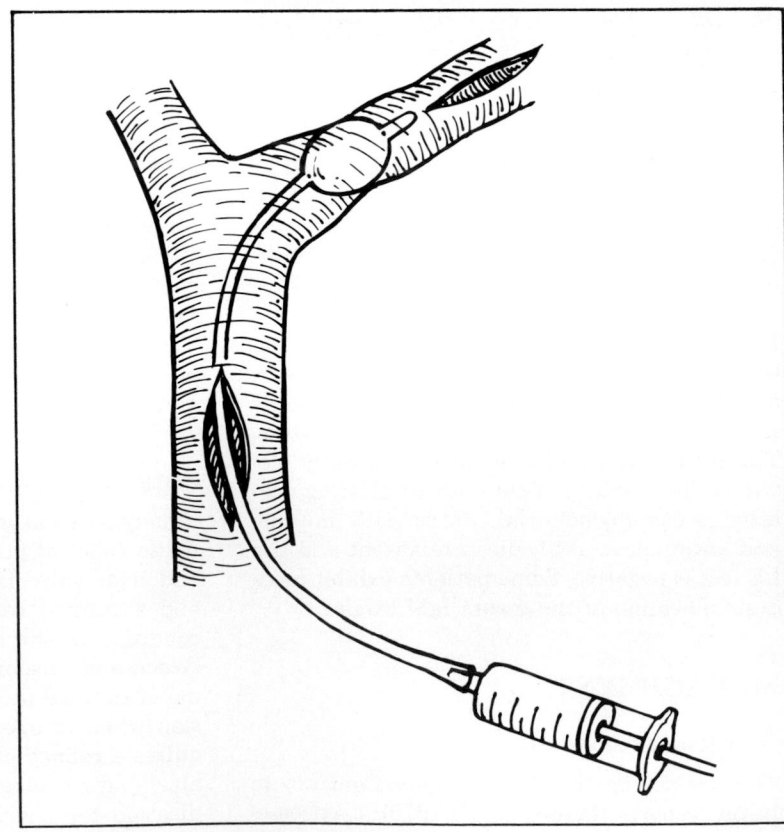

Figure 83–5. Balloon dilatation of main ductal stricture. Initially a way through the stenosed area is negotiated by means of copper flexible probes. If a stricture in either main duct is impassable, the hepatic parenchyma is divided down to it and the stricture incised along the longitudinal axis of the duct.

shreds the already diseased duct. After insertion of stay sutures into the thickened cord-like duct, a 1-cm scalpel incision is made in the midline and is progressively deepened until the lumen is entered. The bile often contains calcium bilirubinate stones or sludge. A specimen is obtained and sent for both aerobic and anaerobic cultures. The CBD is then dilated with graded copper malleable probes distally and proximally. Not infrequently, extension of the choledochotomy wound from splitting is witnessed during the CBD dilatation. This is inevitable but of little consequence provided that it occurs along the axis of the duct. The object is to dilate the duct to approximately 0.7 to 1.0 cm. If available, a choledochoscope should then be inserted, and the proximal bile duct and hilar bifurcation visualised. Biopsies of the duct are best obtained through the choledochoscope. A

biliary balloon catheter (2.0 ml) is then passed into the right ductal system. At each site of hold up the balloon is inflated forcibly. This is then followed by insertion of a 0.5-cm copper malleable probe into the right ductal system until its tip can be felt through the hepatic parenchyma by means of the left hand placed on the superior surface of the right lobe. The probe is then withdrawn. The identical procedure is repeated on the left ductal system. If a stricture in either main duct is impassable, the hepatic parenchyma is divided down to it and the stricture incised along the longitudinal axis of the duct. Forcible dilatation with the biliary balloon can then be performed via the opened common bile duct (Fig. 83–5).

A 90-cm length of medical grade silicone tubing (internal diameter of 0.5 cm) is used for the transhepatic stenting (Fig. 83–6). The entire

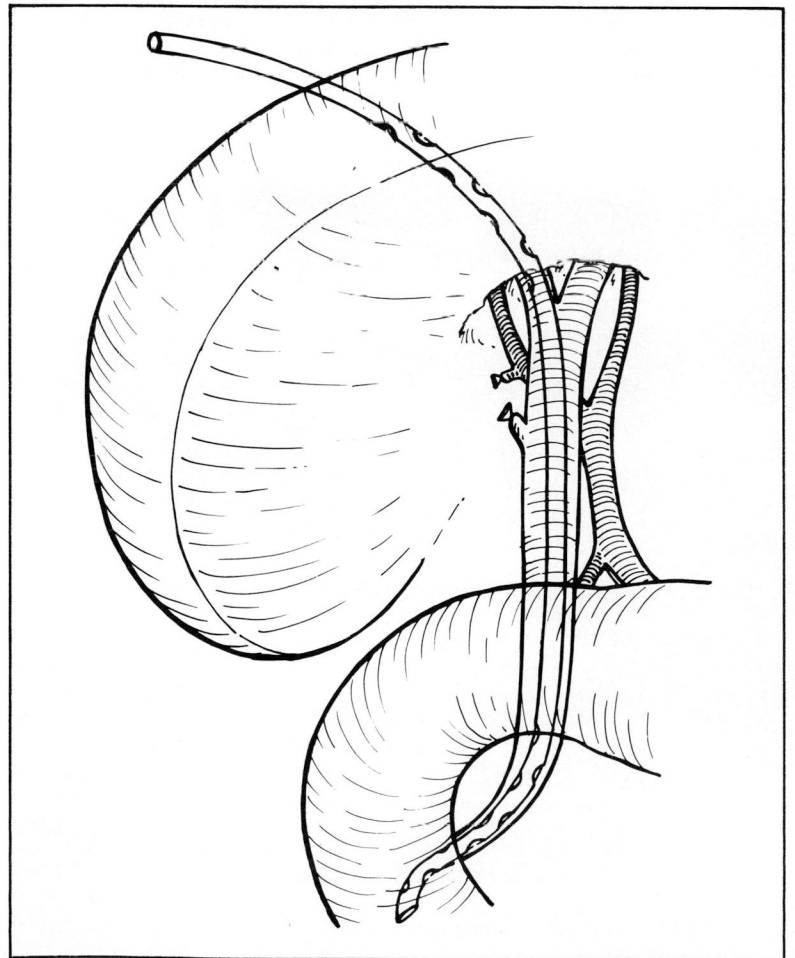

Figure 83–6. Transhepatic silicone stenting for total diffuse sclerosing cholangitis.

biliary tract is irrigated with antibiotic solution (750 mg of cefuroxime in 1 L of isotonic saline) by means of soft rubber catheters introduced proximally and distally. The copper malleable probe is then inserted via the choledochotomy wound into the right intrahepatic ductal system. With the left hand on the superior surface of the right lobe for counterpressure, the probe is forced through the hepatic substance to emerge on the superior surface of the right lobe. The emergent probe is gradually bent forward as it is pushed cephalad from below until it emerges beneath the costal margin. The silicone tubing is then fitted on the end of the probe and tied securely over its terminal groove. The probe is then gradually withdrawn back through the hepatic parenchyma out of the choledochotomy railroading the silicone stent (Fig. 83–7). A temporary marking black silk ligature is tied around the stent some 40 cm from the proximal end above the liver (Fig. 83–8). The stent is then gradually withdrawn until this ligature just disappears into the hepatic substance. A small haemostat is then inserted on

the stent as it emerges from the choledochotomy. The stent is then gradually withdrawn further until the black silk ligature is encountered. To ensure that the proximal end of the silicone tube does not slip into the hepatic parenchyma, another haemostat is affixed on the tube above the liver. Spirally disposed side holes at distances of 1 cm are cut out starting 2 cm distal to the black silk ligature, with the last one situated 1 cm proximal to the distal haemostat. The latter is then removed and by applying traction on the suprahepatic haemostat, the stent is withdrawn until the black silk suture has reached the superior surface of the right lobe. The copper probe, still attached to the distal end of the stent, is reintroduced into the CBD and guided distally until its tip can be felt tenting the anterior duodenal wall. A small stab wound is made in the anterior duodenal wall over the tented area, and the probe exteriorised and withdrawn, bringing with it the silicone tube. It is then cut off obliquely and the end replaced into the duodenum such that it lies unkinked in the second part of the duodenal

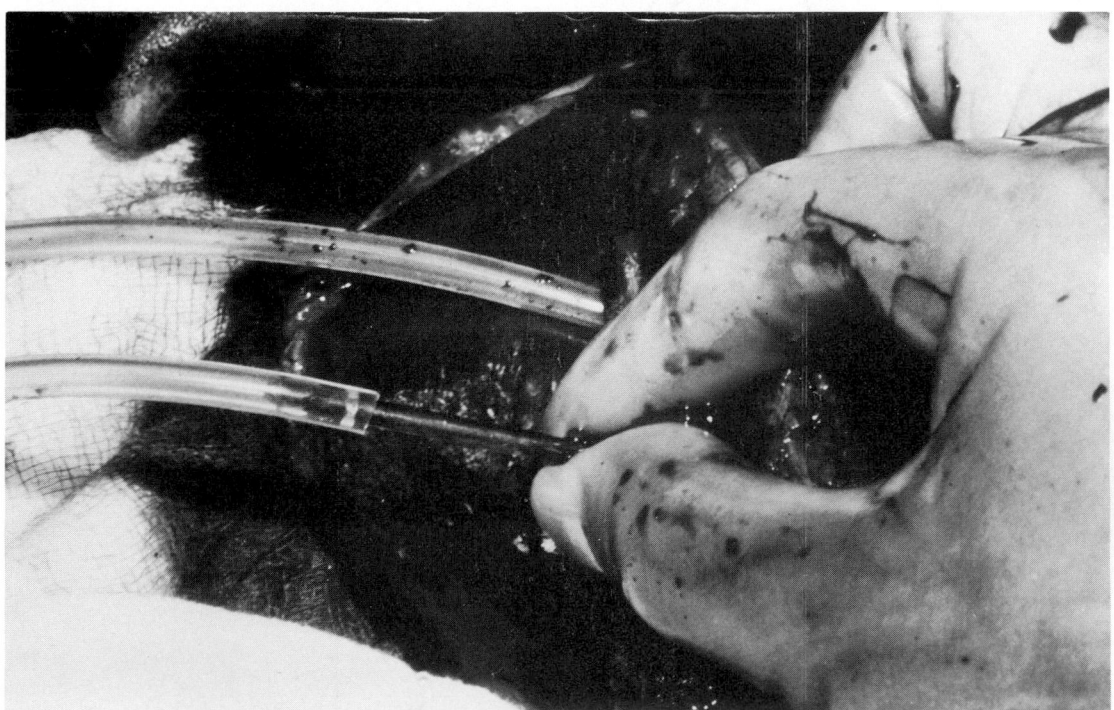

Figure 83–7. The silicone stent has been introduced through the hepatic parenchyma.

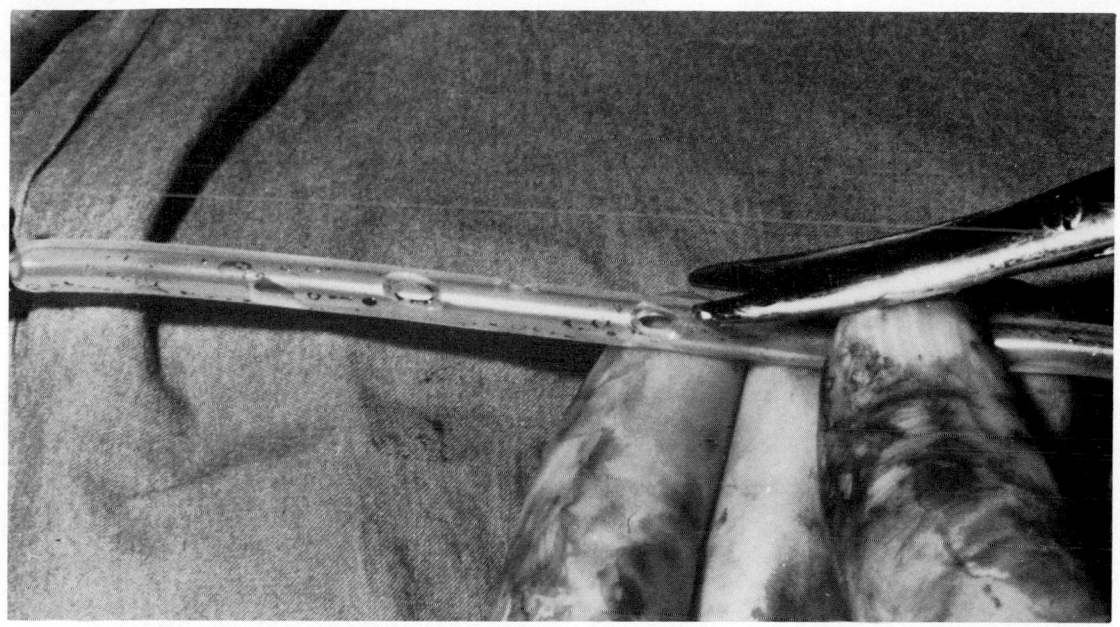

Figure 83–8. A temporary black silk ligature has been tied round the suprahepatic portion of the stent. This marks the exit point of the stent from the superior surface of the liver. Spirally disposed side holes at distances of 1 cm are cut starting 2 cm distal to the black silk ligature.

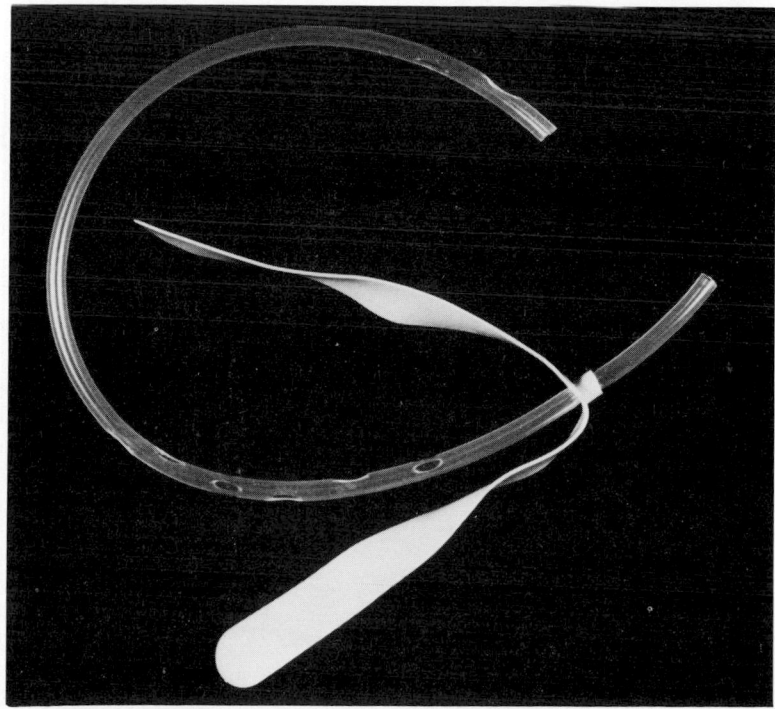

Figure 83–9. Flange used to secure the stent to the chest wall.

lumen. The small stab wound in the duodenum is closed with 3/0 black silk sutures.

The transhepatic stent is anchored and exteriorised through the ninth/tenth right costal interspace along the anterior axillary line. A flange obtained from a No. 14 Gibbon catheter is used to secure the stent to the skin of the chest wall (Fig. 83–9).

Closure of the choledochotomy is effected with interrupted fine sutures (5/0 Prolene). Often approximation of the choledochotomy

wound edges to cover the stent is not possible. In this situation a patch of autologous vein (Ellis and Hoile, 1980; Cuschieri et al, 1983) or a gallbladder patch (Fig. 83–10A,B,C) is used to effect cover. The gallbladder is otherwise removed.

Localised Disease

Hilar Stricture. The best results are obtained by excision of the stricture with a hepatojejunostomy-Y. As the disease usually involves the common hepatic duct and adjacent right and left

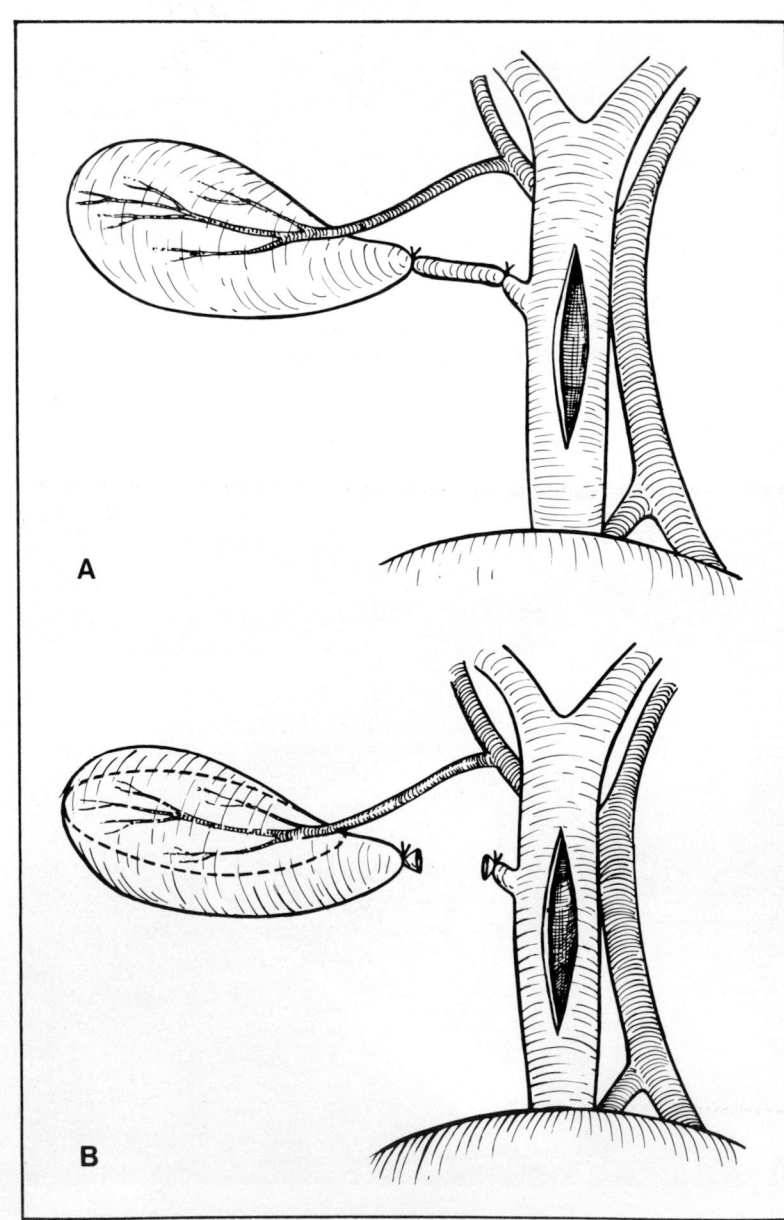

Figure 83–10. A through **C. A.** Technique of creating a vascularised gallbladder flap for patching of narrowed common bile duct. The cystic artery and duct are fully mobilised. The cystic duct is doubly ligated and divided. **B.** An oval, full-thickness patch of gallbladder wall centered on the cystic artery is mapped out. The gallbladder is emptied by suction and opened longitudinally on the opposite aspect. The gallbladder flap is then trimmed to size.

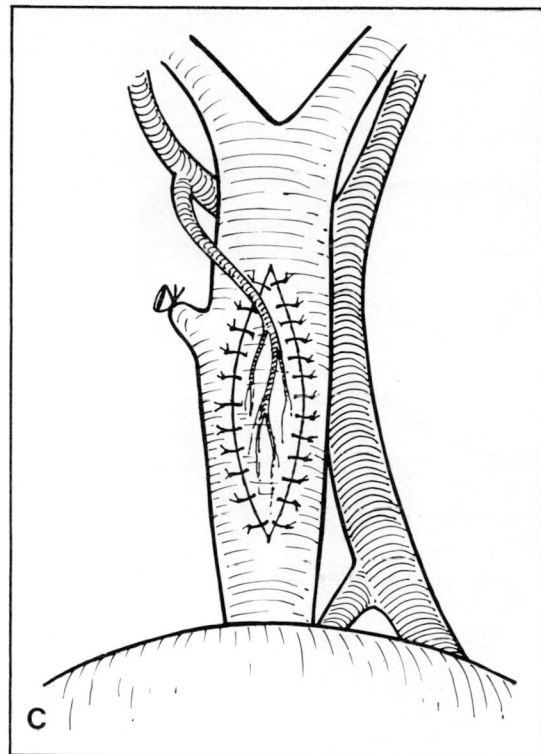

Figure 83-10. C. The gallbladder flap is then swung medially and sutured to the edges of the choledochotomy wound by means of 5/0 interrupted Prolene sutures.

hepatic ducts, an anterior segmentectomy IV (Bismuth et al, 1982) is required for access. This consists of resection of the anterior half of the quadrate lobe from the medial edge of the gallbladder fossa to the falciform ligament. A block of liver parenchyma is thus removed from in front of the hilum of the liver. The only large vessel encountered is a branch of the middle hepatic vein on the posterior wall of the hepatic resection line. This requires suture ligation. A Roux-Y loop (50 cm) is fashioned and brought up through the transverse mesocolon. Anastomosis is carried out with both the right and left hepatic ducts (Fig. 83-11). Often the two ducts proximal to the resection line are juxtaposed with an intervening septum. After insertion of two interrupted 4/0 chromic catgut sutures at either end of the septum, a wedge resection of this structure is performed (Fig. 83-12). Thereafter an apical 4/0 catgut suture is performed. This procedure results in a common

channel that is then anastomosed to the Roux loop. The bilioenteric anastomosis is carried out with 5/0 Prolene using a running stitch for the posterior wall and interrupted sutures (with the knots tied on the outside) anteriorly (Fig. 83-13).

Distal Stricture. This is best managed by mobilisation of the duct, which is then transected above the strictured area. After obtaining a full thickness biopsy, the distal end is closed with a running black silk suture. The proximal end is then implanted either in the duodenum, after complete mobilisation of the latter (Fig. 83-14A,B), or into a Roux-Y loop. Again, the anastomosis is performed with 5/0 Prolene using the technique described above.

In both hilar and distal strictures, the bilioenteric anastomosis is stented using a transhepatic stent as previously described.

Care of the Stent

The silicone stent is spigoted for the first 48 hours. Thereafter, irrigation with 50 ml of heparinised saline is performed twice daily using an aseptic technique. Appropriate antibiotic therapy is continued until bile cultures are negative and restarted if, at any stage, bile cultures become positive.

Despite daily irrigation, encrustation of the stent with calcium bilirubinate is encountered in all the patients (Fig. 83-15). Stent renewal is therefore mandatory at 2- to 3-monthly intervals. This procedure must be performed under radiologic control. With the proper set-up, renewal is fairly straightforward because a smooth fibrous track forms round the stent. A guide wire is first inserted and the stent then withdrawn. An identical tube (with matching side holes) is then introduced over the guide wire. Stent renewal must be covered with systemic antibiotic therapy because of the risk of septicaemia.

Follow-up radiologic investigations of the biliary tract are performed by injecting 30 to 40 ml of 20 percent Hypaque (Nadiatrizoate) via the stent. The procedure should be performed just prior to stent replacement.

In patients with localised disease (hilar or distal) the transhepatic stent is removed at 2 to 4 months. In patients with diffuse disease the period of transhepatic stenting is determined by radiologic assessment. When encountered, radiologic improvement is evidenced over

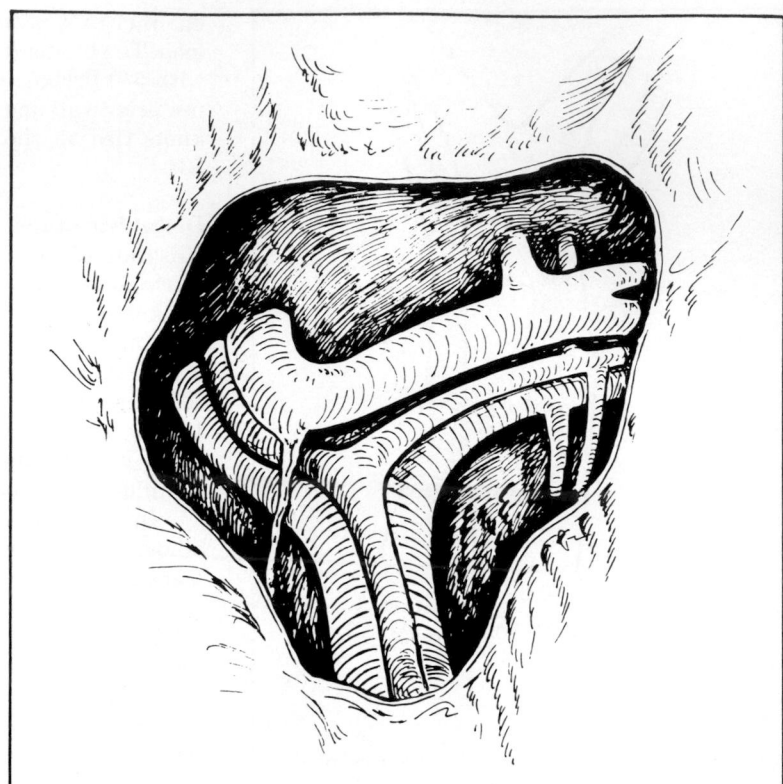

Figure 83–11. Exposure of the hilar bifurcation after resection of the anterior portion of segment IV (quadrate lobe). If the process involves the right hepatic duct, the intrahepatic bilioenteric anastomosis is carried out with the long axis of the left hepatic duct.

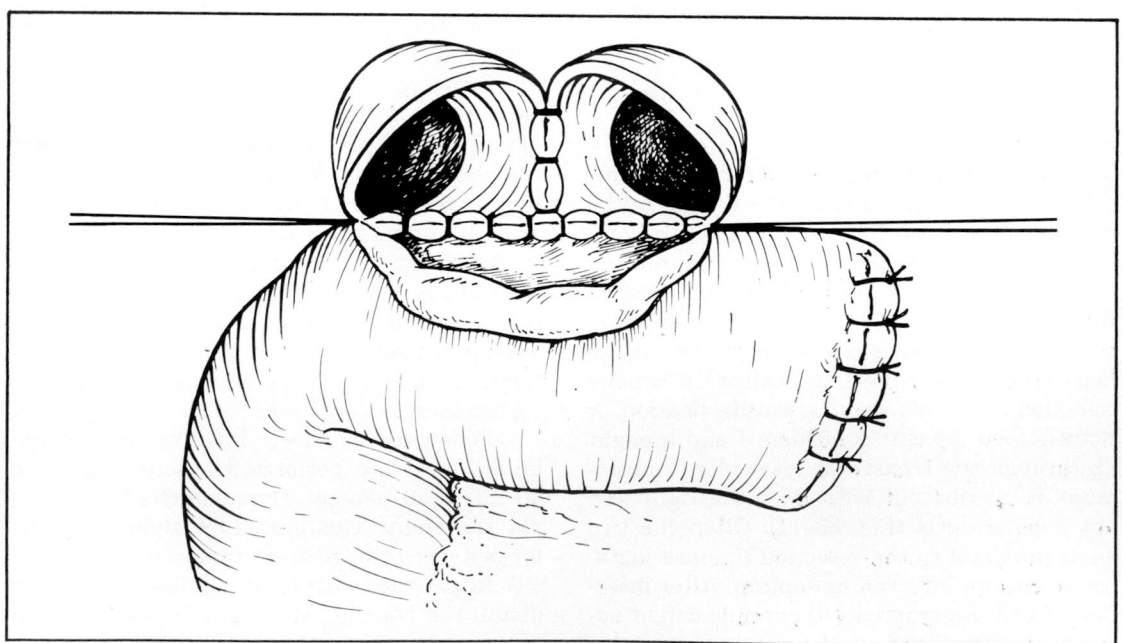

Figure 83–12. The septum between the right and left hepatic ducts has been divided after the insertion of fine interrupted catgut sutures. This procedure results in a common channel that is then anastomosed to the Roux loop. The bilioenteric anastomosis is carried out with 5/0 Prolene, using a running stitch for the posterior wall and interrupted sutures anteriorly.

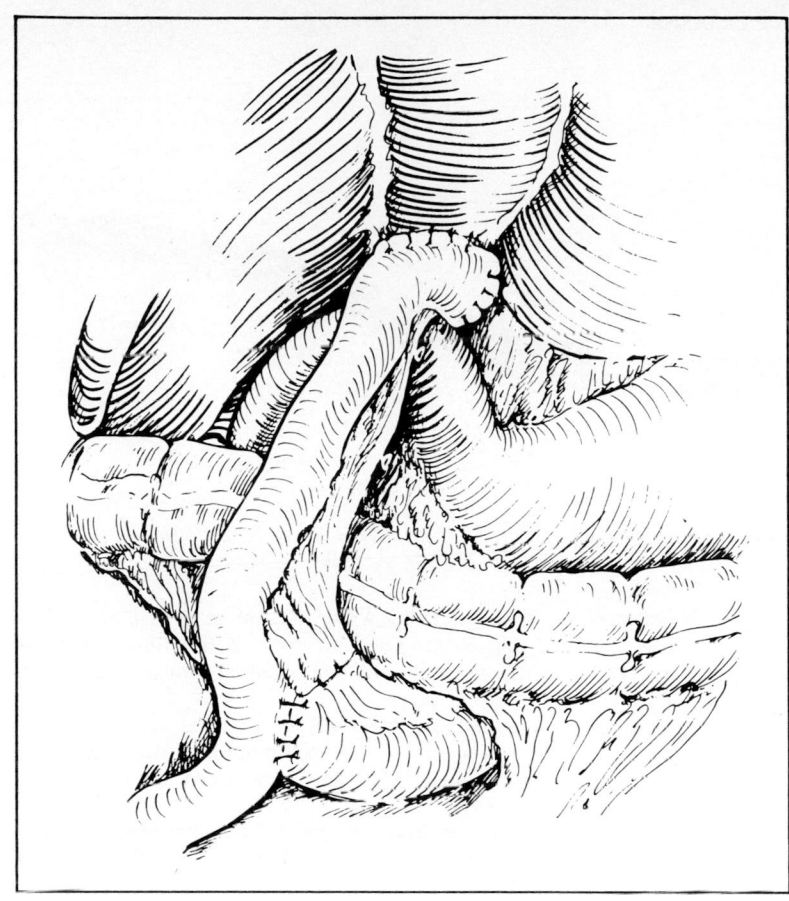

Figure 83–13. Completed hepatojejunostomy. The Roux loop is brought up ante- or retrocolically.

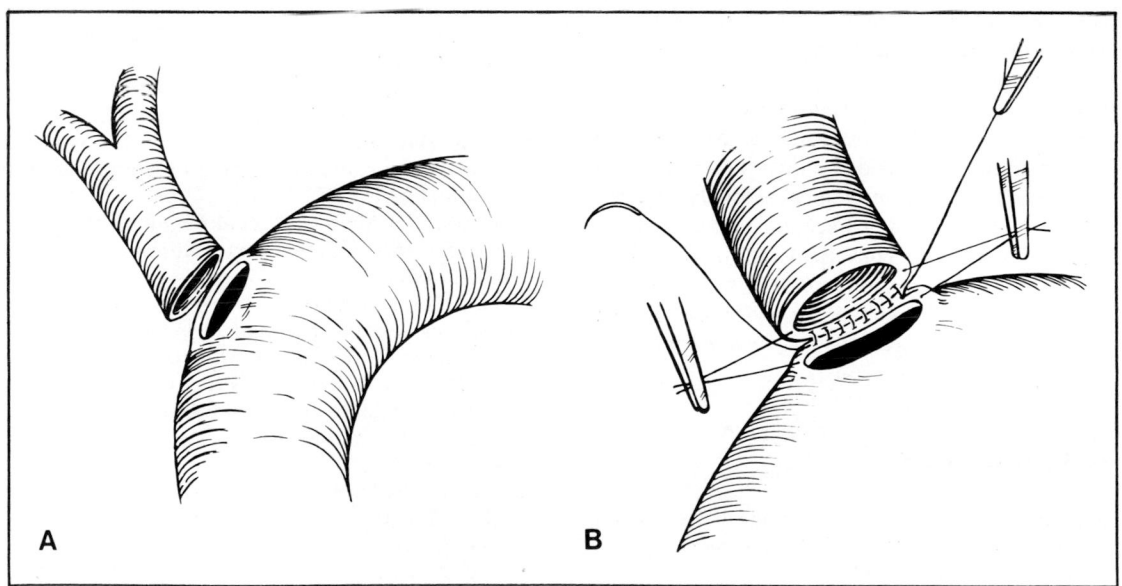

A   B

Figure 83–14. A. The common bile duct is mobilised proximal to the diseased distal segment and then transected. A full-thickness duct biopsy is performed. **B.** After complete mobilisation of the second and third parts of the duodenum, the transected bile duct is implanted at the junction of the first with the second part of the duodenum. A single-layer technique with 5/0 Prolene is performed with a continous stitch for the back wall of the anastomosis and interrupted sutures anteriorly.

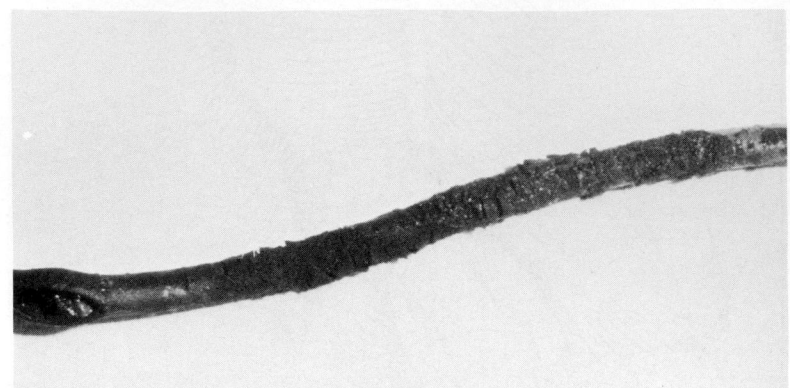

Figure 83–15. Encrustation of transhepatic stent with calcium bilirubinate complexed with sulphated glycoprotein. This stent had been in place for 9 weeks.

several months up to a year from time of surgery. Once a static situation is reached, as judged by radiology and liver function tests, the stent is withdrawn. The interval of transhepatic stenting in patients with diffuse disease has averaged 12 months.

PROGNOSIS

Overall, the disease carries a poor prognosis although long-term survival is possible with adequate surgical management. Two patients in the author's series have developed, and died of, intrahepatic cholangiocarcinoma (5 and 7 years after diagnosis). The association between sclerosing cholangitis and the development of cholangiocarcinoma has been previously reported (Ritchie et al, 1974; Chapman et al, 1980). In the absence of this complication, the disease ultimately progresses to secondary biliary cirrhosis and portal hypertension, with death from chronic end-stage liver disease or variceal haemorrhage.

BIBLIOGRAPHY

Bismuth H, Houssin D, et al: Major and minor segmentectomies "Reglées" in liver surgery. World J Surg 6:10, 1982

Blackstone HO, Memchausky BA: Cholangiographic abnormalities in ulcerative colitis associated pericholangitis which resemble sclerosing cholangitis. Am J Dig Dis 23:379, 1978

Brooke BR, Slaney G: Portal bacteraemia in ulcerative colitis. Lancet i:1206, 1958

Chapman RWG, Arborgh BAM, et al: Primary sclerosing cholangitis: A review of its clinical features, cholangiography and hepatic histology. Gut 21:870, 1980

Cuschieri A, Baker PR, et al: Total and subtotal replacement of the common bile duct: Effect of transhepatic silicone tube stenting. Gut 24:756, 1983

Delbert P: Rétrécissement du choledoque:cholecystoduodénostomie. Bull Mém Soc Nat Chir 50:1144, 1924

Dickson ER, Weisner RH, et al: D-penicillamine improves survival and retards histologic progression in primary biliary cirrhosis. Gastroenterology 82:1225, 1982

Ellis H, Hoile RW: Vein patch repair of the common bile duct. J R Soc Med 73:635, 1980

Hodgson HJF, Potter BJ, et al: Immune complexes in ulcerative colitis and Crohn's disease. Clin Exp Immunol 29:187, 1977

Krukowski ZH, McPhie JL, et al: Proliferative cholangitis (cholangitis glandularis proliferans). Br J Surg 70:155, 1983

LaRusso NF, Russell H, et al: Recent advances in the diagnosis and management of primary sclerosing cholangitis. Curr Concepts Gastroenterol 2:2, 1983

Myers RN, Cooper JH, et al: Primary sclerosing cholangitis: Complete gross and histologic reversal after long term steroid therapy. Am J Gastroenterol 53:527, 1970

Rankin JG, Boden RW, et al: The liver in ulcerative colitis. Treatment of pericholangitis with tetracycline. Lancet ii:1110, 1969

Record CO, Eddleston ALWF, et al: Intrahepatic sclerosing cholangitis associated with a familial immunodeficiency syndrome. Lancet ii:18, 1973

Ritchie JK, Allan RN, et al: Biliary tract carcinoma associated with ulcerative colitis. Q J Med 170:263, 1974

Rohrmann CA, Ansel HJ, et al: Cholangiographic abnormalities in patients with inflammatory bowel disease. Radiology 127:635, 1978

Schrumpf E, Elgjo K, et al: Sclerosing cholangitis in ulcerative colitis. Scand J Gastroenterol 15:689, 1980

Schrumpf E, Fausa O, et al: Sclerosing cholangitis in ulcerative colitis: a follow-up study. Scand J Gastroenterol 17:33, 1982

Selye H, Szabo S: Experimental production of cholangitis by 1,4 phenylene-diisothiocyanate. Arch Pathol 94:486, 1972

Stauffer MH, Sauer WG, et al: The spectrum of cholestatic hepatic disease. JAMA 191:829, 1965

Thomas HC, Vaez-Zadeh F: A homeostatic mechanism for the removal of antigen from the portal circulation. Immunology 26:375, 1974

Thompson BW, Read R: Sclerosing cholangitis and other intraabdominal fibrosis. Am J Surg 128:777, 1974

Tobias R, Wright JP, et al: Primary sclerosing cholangitis associated with inflammatory bowel disease in Cape Town 1975–1981. S Afr Med J 63:229, 1983

Waldram R, Kopelman H, et al: Chronic pancreatitis, sclerosing cholangitis and sicca complex in two siblings. Lancet i:550, 1975

Warren KW, Athanassiades S, et al: Primary sclerosing cholangitis: A study of 42 cases. Am J Surg 111:23, 1966

Wiesner RH, La Russo NF: Clinicopathologic features of the syndrome of primary sclerosing cholangitis. Gastroenterology 79:200, 1980

Wood RAB, Cuschieri A: Is sclerosing cholangitis complicating ulcerative colitis a reversible condition? Lancet ii:716, 1980

84. Recurrent Pyogenic Cholangitis

John Wong

INTRODUCTION

Recurrent pyogenic cholangitis (RPC) is characterized by repeated attacks of bacterial infection of the biliary tract. This name was introduced by Cook in 1954 to describe a disease that is prevalent in Hong Kong (and other parts of Southeast Asia) in which cholangitis occurred primarily in the bile ducts with subsequent pigment stone and stricture formation, in contrast to the cholangitis seen in Western countries where it is secondary to stones passing from the gallbladder, iatrogenic strictures, and tumor obstruction.

Although rarely seen outside Southeast Asia in the past, ease of travel and migration have meant that this condition is now encountered in Western countries more regularly. Unlike gallstone disease seen in Western countries, which affects well-nourished females in their 40s and 50s, RPC afflicts a younger group of patients, with a peak age of 20 to 40 years; males and females are equally susceptible and those of the lower socioeconomic class are more at risk. A decline in the incidence of this disease over the last decade has been noted in the more developed countries of this region.

The exact etiology of RPC is not yet defined, but the pathogenesis and pathology are now fairly well documented, and careful studies of its clinical course have allowed a more rational approach to the surgical treatment of this difficult problem.

ETIOLOGY

Many hypotheses have been advanced for the cause of RPC; most are difficult if not impossible to prove. The balance of available evidence firmly indicates that the initiating process is the establishment of bowel organisms, via the portal venous system, in the intrahepatic biliary radicals. The reasons for the breakdown of normal host defense mechanisms may be: (1) the organisms are particularly virulent, (2) the bowel wall is injured (e.g., by enteric infection), thus allowing a larger than normal load of organisms of ordinary virulence to enter the bloodstream, (3) the metabolic activities of the hepatocytes have been altered (e.g., by malnutrition) to produce bile that lacks or is reduced in bactericidal properties, or that is increased in lithogenicity, and (4) the biliary tree is damaged by the presence of parasites (e.g., *Clonorchis sinensis, Ascaris lumbricoides*) to increase its susceptibility to infection. There are little data to support the first possibility, and RPC is found in countries where parasitic infestation is not endemic. Even in countries where both RPC and infestation are present, only the minority of patients (<25 percent) with RPC show infestation. Therefore, the most likely cause is the establishment of bowel organisms (of ordinary virulence and perhaps in greater dose) in the liver and biliary tract of a compromised host. However, this theory does not explain one of the main pathologic features of RPC, i.e., the significant preponderance of left lobe involvement. Thus it is likely that anatomic factors, such as the size, angulation, and branching of the intrahepatic ducts, which may have functional consequences such as changes in flow rate and physicochemical properties, are also important determinants of the pattern of the disease.

PATHOGENESIS

Once the organisms are established in the liver, an intense acute inflammatory reaction is set up in the liver parenchyma (as evidenced by

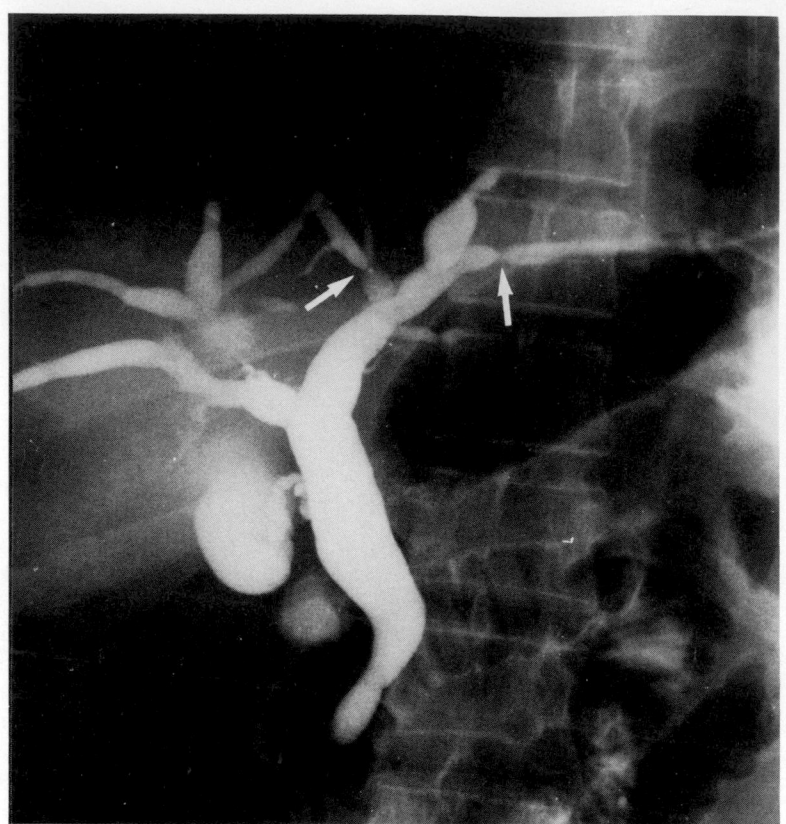

Figure 84–1. Early RPC changes. Left hepatic duct showing mild dilatation with intrahepatic strictures (*arrows*). Stones are absent in the bile ducts and gallbladder. The ampulla of Vater is patulous.

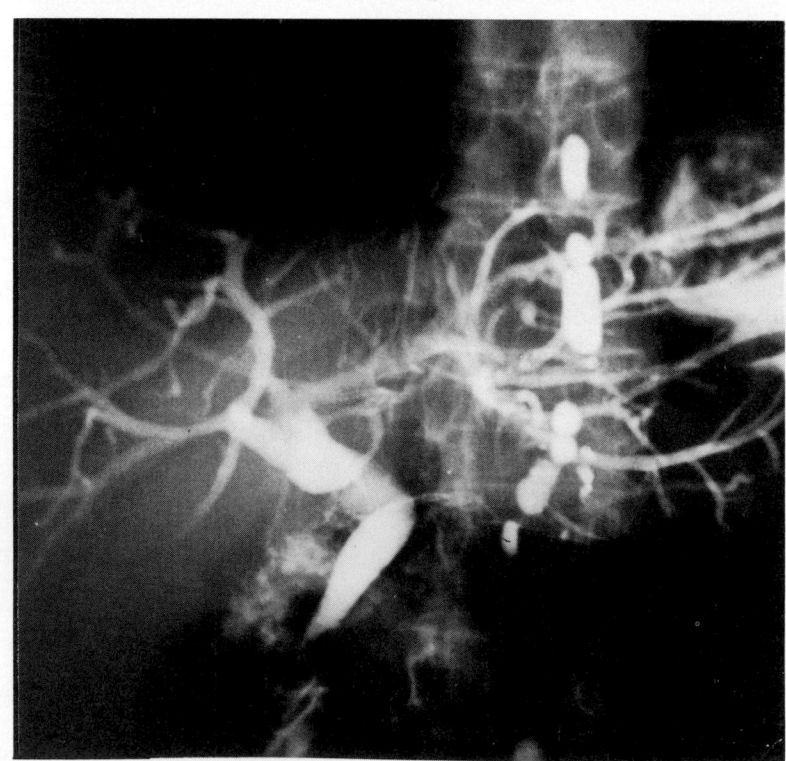

Figure 84–2. Extensive branching of left intrahepatic bile ducts in early RPC changes. Previous myelogram is noted.

neutrophil infiltration in the sinusoids of the lobules) and in the portal triad. Infection probably then spreads from the cholangioles to the larger ducts as the process continues. The bile components are altered by infection (deconjugation of bilirubin diglucuronide by β-glucuronidase) which leads to the formation of microcalculi, which may be discharged through the sphincter of Oddi into the duodenal lumen. However, if the attack does not resolve quickly, or if there are frequent and recurrent attacks, then the microcalculi become niduses (in addition to live or dead parasites) for large stones to form, which may fail to pass downward, especially if strictures are also present. Strictures are probably formed by the perpetuation of the normal healing process excited by transmural

ductal injury from infection, the presence of stones that stimulate continual tissue overgrowth, and the destruction of liver parenchyma, resulting in loss of external support. In some patients, the stricture is a relative one; the diameter of the narrowed part is not smaller than a normal duct of corresponding level, but the proximal ducts are grossly dilated (often containing stones) and thus give the appearance of obstruction. This relative or functional obstruction has the same pathologic outcome, resulting in stagnation, inadequate drainage, stone formation, and cholangitis, regardless of the absolute size of the narrowed segment. The most common organisms isolated from blood and bile cultures are *Escherichia coli, Klebsiella, Bacteroides,* and *Clostridium.* Mixed in-

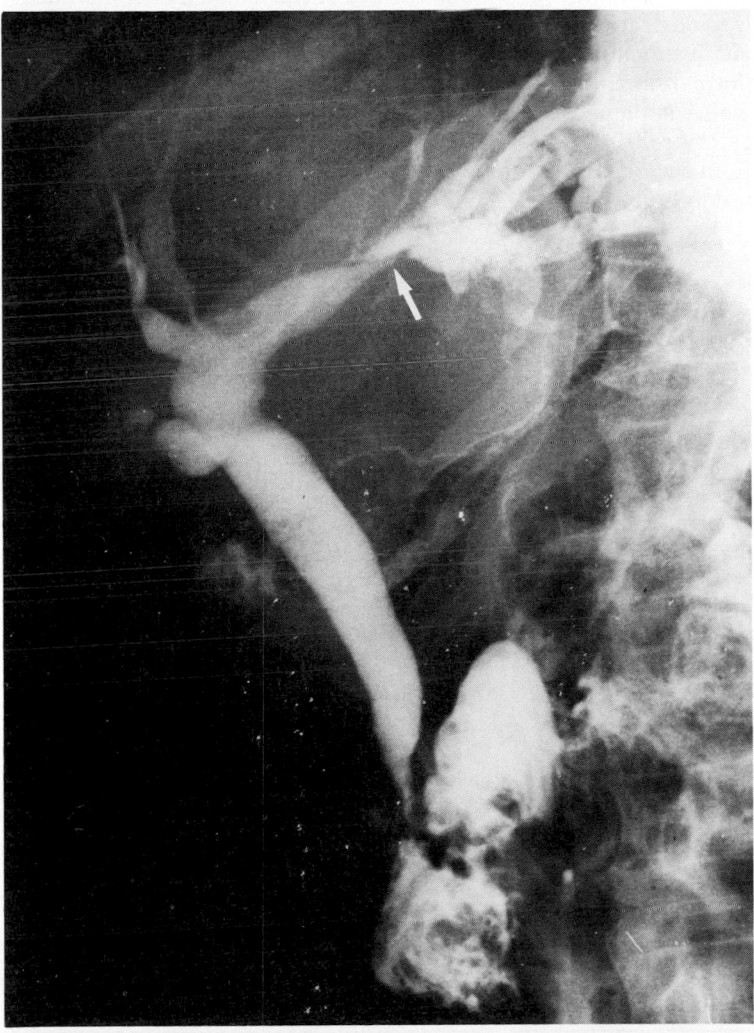

Figure 84–3. Intrahepatic stones are seen in the left intrahepatic duct proximal to a tubular stricture (*arrow*). The right duct is only minimally affected.

fections, including uncommon organisms, are also frequently encountered.

PATHOLOGY

Biopsy specimens of the liver taken at emergency operation shows infiltration of hepatic sinusoids by neutrophils. Since neutrophils are rarely seen in sinusoids in cholangitis secondary to tumor or gallstone obstruction, this finding lends support to the hypothesis that the pathogenic organisms arrive by the hematogenous route. The hepatocyte and Kupffer cells usually appear normal, but in severe cases toxic vacuolation is seen in the hepatocytes, and the Kupffer cells are stained with bile pigments.

In the acute stage neutrophils infiltrate the portal triad and are also found in the small bile ducts. Continuing infection leads to destruction of these small ducts and adjacent liver parenchyma, leading to microabscess formation. Subsidence of the infective process is accompanied by fibrosis and chronic inflammatory cell infiltration of the portal tract, which, in severe and persistent cases, results in bridging fibrous bands developing between portal tracts and ultimately biliary cirrhosis.

The early ductal changes in RPC have been documented by endoscopic retrograde cholangiopancreatography (ERCP). There is excessive branching, "arrow head" formation or abrupt termination of the proximal ducts, loss of parallelism of the walls of the larger ducts, and dilatation of the first and second order hepatic duct (Figs. 84–1 through 84–3). Stricture formation is not a feature in the early stages of the disease, but becomes the sine qua non in established disease.

Examination of the resected liver shows thickened and dilated ducts which contain many pigmented stones (Fig. 84–4). Sometimes the stones and thick biliary mud form a cast of the biliary tree.

The surface of the affected duct has patchy, congested, or hemorrhagic areas, and mucosa lining may be incomplete. Strictures have a predilection for the origin of the left hepatic duct but may also be present in the second or third order ducts, more often at the confluence of ducts (Fig. 84–5). The right duct origin is rarely the only site of stricture. Most strictures in the

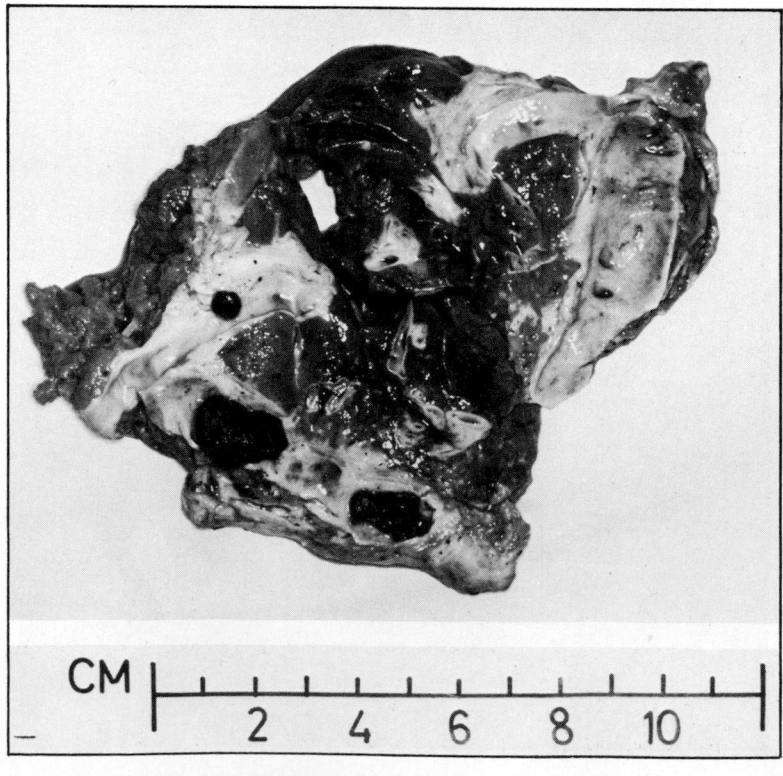

Figure 84–4. Specimen of a resected left lobe of liver affected by RPC. The intrahepatic ducts are thickened and dilated, and some are filled with pigmented stones. There is still residual liver parenchyma which is traversed with fibrotic bands.

CM

2   4   6   8   10

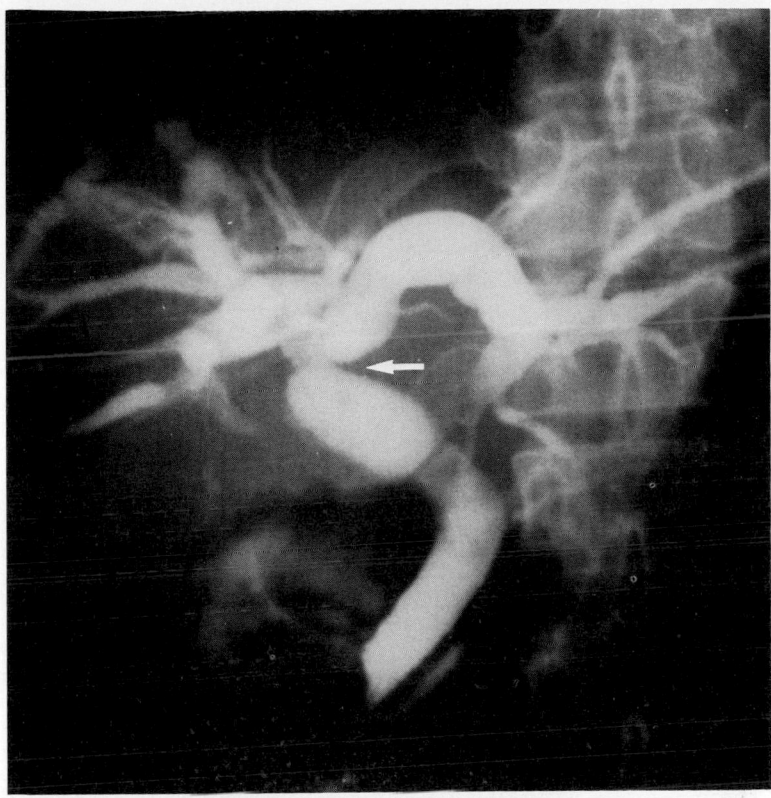

Figure 84–5. Moderate RPC changes. Strictures are present at the junction of both hepatic ducts with the common hepatic duct (*arrow*), with dilatation, excessive branching, and "arrowhead" formation of the intrahepatic ducts. Stones are present in the intra- and extrahepatic ducts. There is also a stricture in the common bile duct.

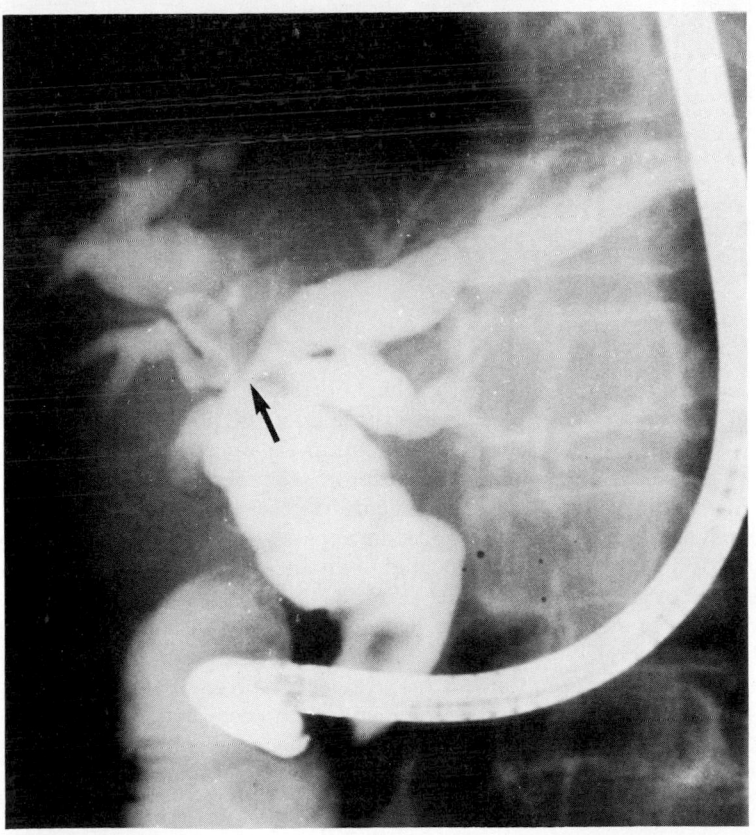

Figure 84–6. Severe RPC changes. Tight strictures are seen in the confluences of the right and left hepatic ducts (*arrow*), with dilatation of the intrahepatic ducts. Stones are present in the right duct and in the common bile duct.

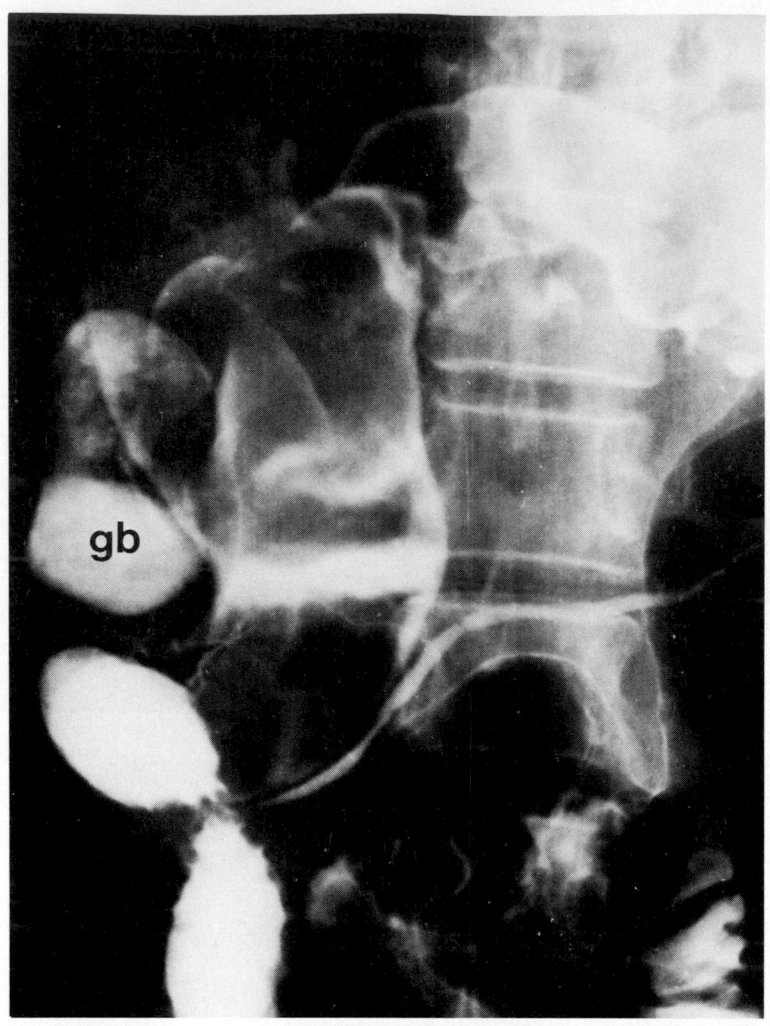

Figure 84–7. Severe RPC changes. The grossly dilated extrahepatic duct is completely filled with soft stones and thick biliary mud. The intrahepatic ducts are dilated and contain similar debris. The gallbladder (gb) was found to be normal at operation.

larger ducts are localized over a short distance; in the smaller ducts the strictures may be tubular (Fig. 84–3).

When the disease process is severe, liver parenchyma is destroyed and the left lobe of the liver is little more than a fibrous sac containing dilated ducts and stones (Fig. 84–6). In these circumstances there is compensatory hypertrophy of the right lobe, which may be to such an extent as to distort normal anatomic relationships. When stones are present, the common hepatic and bile ducts may become grossly thickened and dilated (up to 10 cm; average 2 to 3 cm); thus even when the mud and stones have been completely removed, the ducts do not

return to their normal size (Figs. 84–7 and 84–8). Because these ducts do not drain effectively they act as a sump that predisposes to further stone formation. Strictures may also occur in the extrahepatic ducts; they are usually diaphragmatic in appearance and are more likely to be located near the lower end of the common bile duct (Figs. 84–9 and 84–10A).

The sphincter of Oddi is usually patulous and large dilators pass through without resistance. Pressure necrosis from a stone impacted at the lower end of the common bile duct may lead to a spontaneous choledochoduodenostomy and allow air to enter the biliary tree.

Stones are found in 90 percent of patients

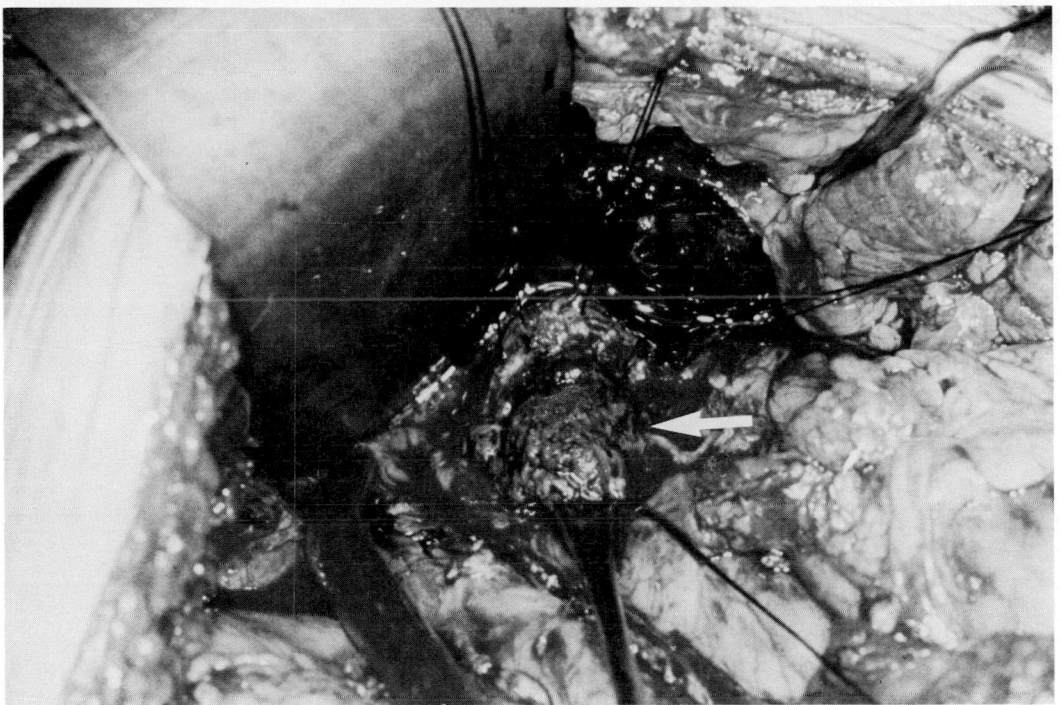

A

B

Figure 84–8. **A.** Operative finding of patient whose cholangiogram is seen in Figure 84–7. The common bile duct is opened and a scoop is used to evacuate the thick biliary mud through the choledothotomy (*arrow*). **B.** After mud, debris, and soft stones have been removed from the thickened and dilated common bile duct, a retractor is placed in the duct to allow direct visual inspection and digital examination. A choledochojejunostomy is the operation of choice.

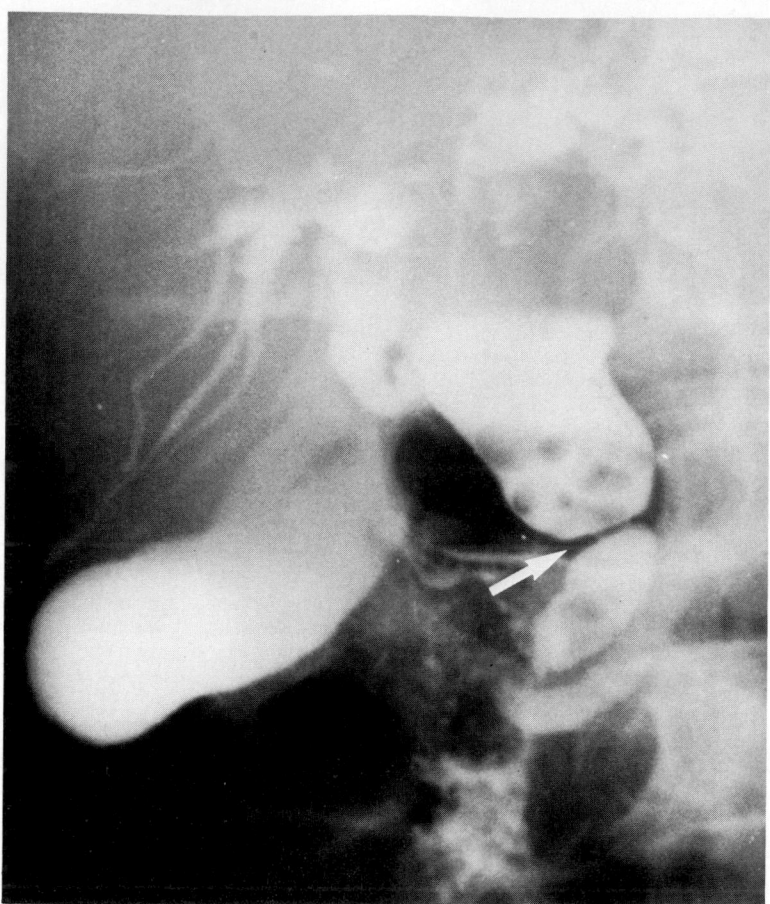

Figure 84–9. A diaphragmatic stricture (*arrow*) in the intrapancreatic portion of the common bile duct with stones above and below the stricture. The ducts proximal to the stricture are dilated, and the gallbladder is free of stones.

with RPC, and the most common site of occurrence is in the common hepatic or bile ducts (50 percent). In 25 percent of all patients with RPC, stones are found only in the intrahepatic ducts, with a 4 to 1 preponderance of left to right duct. Thus, if stones are present in the right duct, they are very likely to be found in the left duct as well. Even when stones are present in both ducts, the left is usually more severely affected. Only 15 percent of patients with RPC have stones in the gallbladder, all of whom have stones elsewhere in the biliary tree also.

The stones found in RPC are pigmented and faceted; they have a brown earthy appearance and are soft and friable. Inside, the color is usually yellow or orange (Fig. 84–10B). When stone forceps are gently applied, the stones fragment. The pigment is bilirubinate, and layers of this pigment are deposited on top of each other over a central nidus, which may be a dead parasite,

such as *Clonorchis sinensis* or *Ascaris lumbricoides,* desquamated epithelium, or inspissated bile, mucus, or pus (Fig. 84–11). The laminated nature of some stones bears testimony to the recurrent nature of this condition. Chemical analysis reveals the constituents of stones to be bilirubin 24.7 percent, cholesterol 5.9 percent, and calcium 0.5 percent (the rest being insoluble residue), thus accounting for their radiolucency. An abscess in the left lobe may rupture into the peritoneal cavity, or into the pericardium leading to cardiac tamponade. A right lobe abscess may rupture through the diaphragm and cause empyema thoracis, or if it ruptures into the lung, result in bronchobiliary fistula. A chronic abscess may render distinction from a tumor difficult (Fig. 84–12).

Thrombophlebitis of the hepatic veins may rarely give rise to pulmonary emboli and pulmonary hypertension.

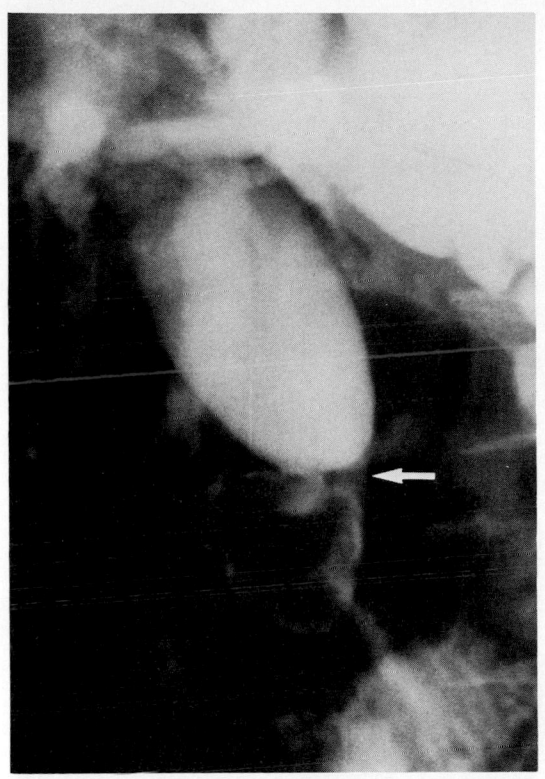

A

Figure 84–10. A. A stricture (*arrow*) in the intrapancreatic portion of the common bile duct is seen above a large stone, which fills the distal bile duct completely. **B.** At operation, a soft pigmented stone, measuring 2.5 cm in length, is removed after a large sphincteroplasty is performed; the edges of the sphincteroplasty are indicated by the stay sutures.

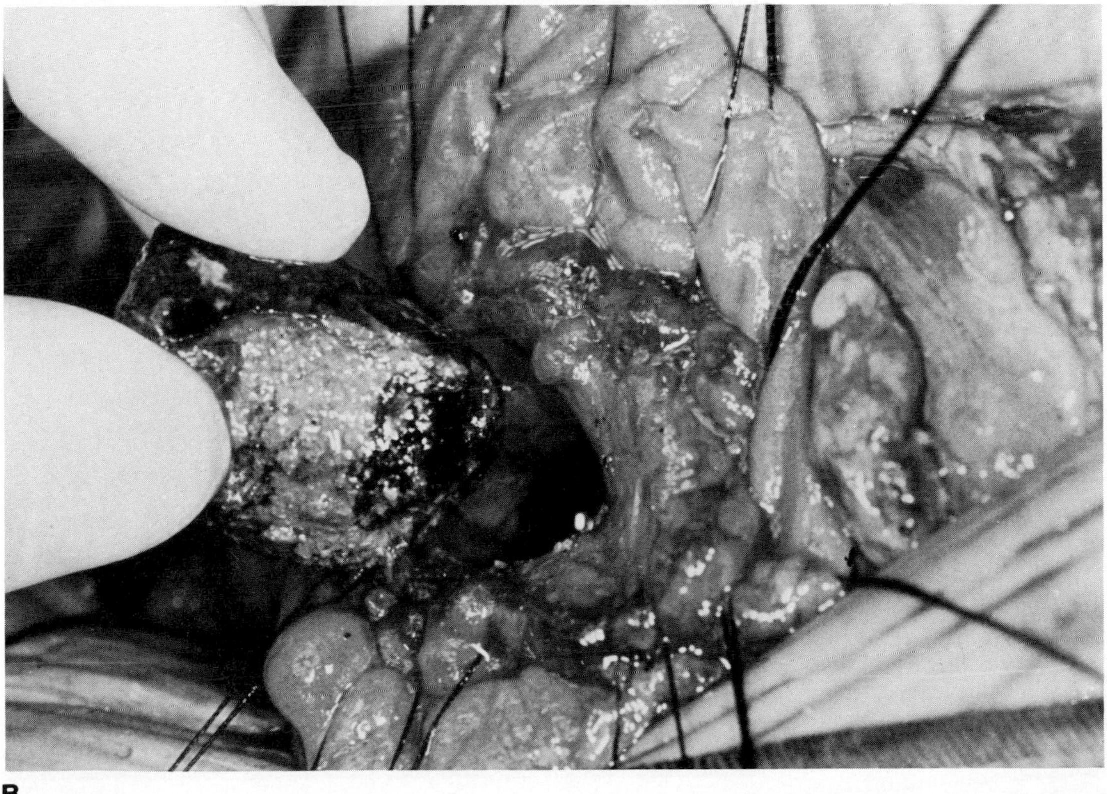

B

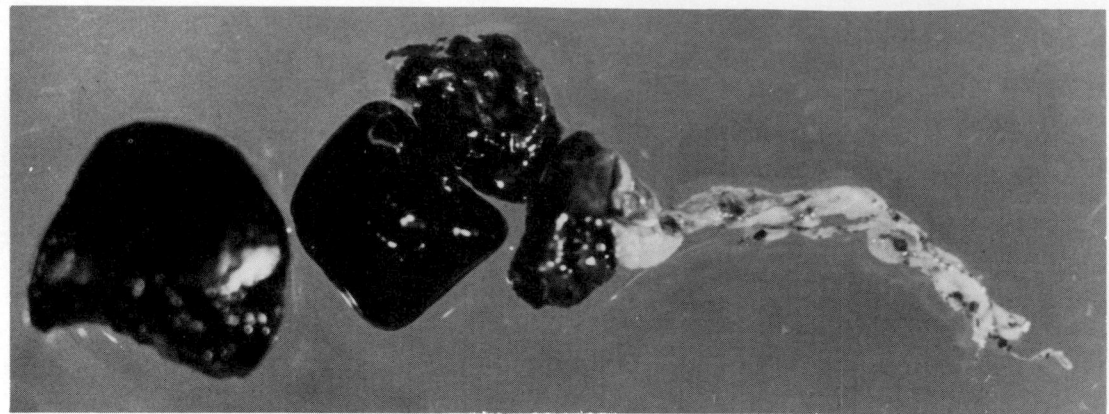

Figure 84–11. A dead *Ascaris lumbricoides* in the bile duct is the nidus for the development of stones. (*Courtesy of C.A. Arcilla.*)

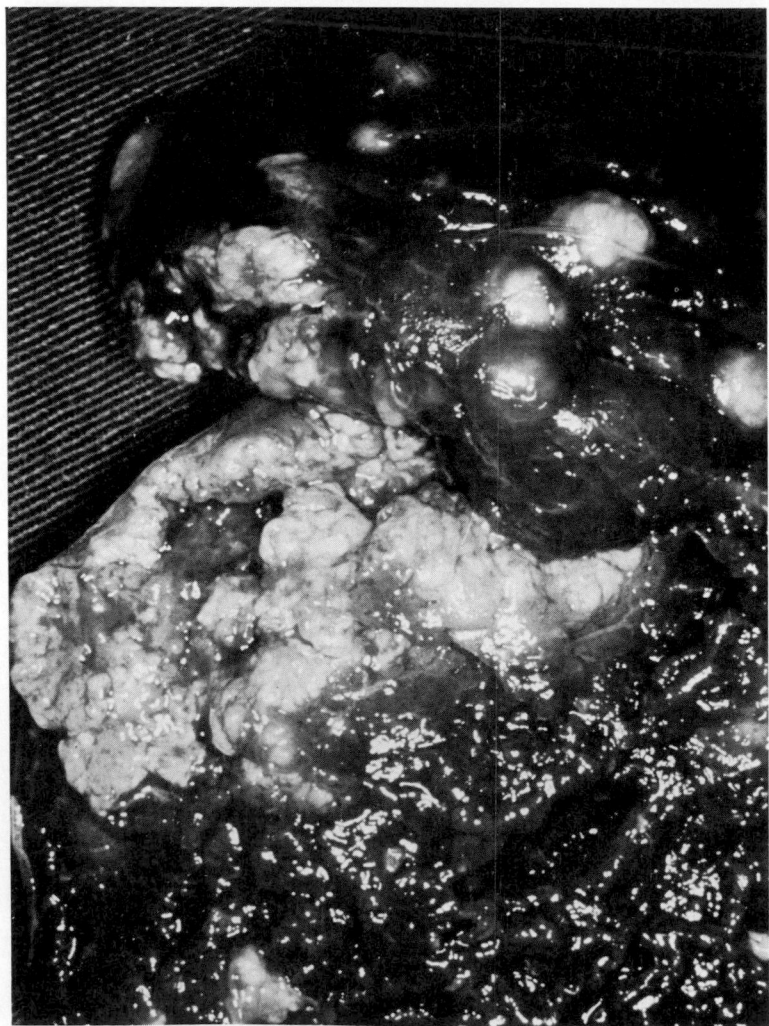

Figure 84–12. Chronic liver abscesses in a cholangitic liver. Resection is the only method to eradicate this persistent source of infection, or to differentiate from a tumor.

CLINICAL FEATURES

Patients are usually young, thin, and sometimes malnourished. Most have had previous episodes of cholangitis. Typically the frequency and severity of attacks increases with the passage of time.

The chief complaints are right upper quadrant or epigastric pain, fever, and passing tea-colored urine. The pain is described as distending, sharp, cutting, or gnawing and often radiates to the back and right shoulder; this pain may last for hours or days and is usually unremitting. Only rarely is the pain colicky. Fever is continuous and is between 38.0°C and 39.5°C but is seldom above 40°C and suggests septicemia. Often the fever is associated with chills and is ushered in by rigors. Nausea is present with pain but vomiting is not a dominant feature.

Jaundice is mild and just perceptible clinically, as biliary obstruction is incomplete. For this reason the stool is not pale and pruritis is not a complaint. More characteristically the patient notices that the urine is tea-colored.

Physical examination shows a restless patient who not infrequently bears the scars of previous surgery (20 percent). There is tenderness in the right upper quadrant or epigastrium. If the latter is marked, a left lobe abscess must be suspected. However, in 14 percent of patients tenderness is absent; these patients are usually old and jaundiced and may not have fever or chills.

The liver is enlarged in 60 percent of patients, but this finding may be masked by abdominal guarding; the gallbladder is palpable in 30 percent, and the spleen in 25 percent. Acute pancreatitis is associated with RPC in 12 percent. Signs of generalized peritonitis are present in 5 percent of patients and this may be caused by rupture of a diseased gallbladder or liver abscess, or because of severe acute pancreatitis. These complications are associated with shock, which becomes rapidly fatal unless surgery is immediately undertaken.

LABORATORY FINDINGS

Routine laboratory tests do not show any diagnostic pattern specific to RPC, and the findings are those expected in obstructive jaundice and infection. Thus there is a leukocytosis with a left shift, an elevated serum alkaline phosphatase and γGTP (the level depending on the severity and duration of obstruction), and an elevation of serum transaminases if there is associated hepatocellular damage. As the biliary obstruction is incomplete, urinary urobilinogen is present in addition to bile pigments. Blood cultures for aerobic and anaerobic organisms are taken for all patients in an acute attack.

Serum amylase is elevated in about 20 percent of patients and in half of them it exceeds 700 Somogyi units/L. In these patients, a stone impacted at the lower end of the common bile duct must be suspected. Stool examination for parasites should be performed. Although the incidence of infestation in RPC is not different from other hospital patients, treatment is given to those with positive results.

INVESTIGATIONS

The diagnosis of RPC is usually not in doubt because the clinical features are quite typical. Investigations are therefore used for confirmation in doubtful cases, and to define the location, extent, and severity of the disease in patients with known disease.

Ultrasonography and computed tomography (CT) scans are noninvasive investigations and are of particular value in providing objective evidence during an acute attack, especially when surgical intervention is likely. Ultrasonography of the upper abdomen will show features of biliary obstruction (with dilated intra- and extrahepatic ducts and gallbladder), stones in the biliary system, the presence or absence of liver abscesses of concomitant pancreatitis. A CT scan may also provide similar information, with the advantage of being less subjected to interference by surgical scars and observer bias. However, these tests do not offer the scope or precision of information that surgeons would prefer to have before embarking on exploration in the elective situation.

Although intravenous cholangiogram has been the mainstay of biliary imaging of RPC in the past, it has now been completely replaced by ERCP and percutaneous transhepatic cholangiography (PTC). We have favored ERCP because, in our experience, it is safer and provides a more complete outline of the whole biliary system. The characteristic features of different stages of RPC have now been defined and have been validated by the severity of clinical findings and the need for surgery. These studies have also allowed a more exact construction of the pathogenetic mechanism.

On rare occasions a chronic abscess develops for which further specific investigations by radionuclide scanning and hepatic arteriography is required to distinguish it from a tumor, or other mass lesions. Peritoneoscopy may also provide additional information in the unusual patient with RPC who presents a diagnostic dilemma. When it is not possible to exclude a liver tumor, exploration and usually resection will be required.

MANAGEMENT

Initial Treatment

After admission to hospital the clinical course exhibited by most patients is that of resolution on conservative therapy, which involves intravenous fluid replacement, administration of broad-spectrum antibiotics, nasogastric aspiration, and relief of pain with adequately potent analgesics.

However, even though the majority respond favorably, this period of treatment should be regarded as a phase of energetic preoperative preparation, as 25 percent of patients will fail to improve and emergency surgery is required. Such a patient will show increasing abdominal tenderness, spreading peritonitis, and rising fever. A rise in pulse rate associated with a transient increase in blood pressure is a prelude to rapid deterioration. These findings indicate impending septic shock, which may rapidly become irreversible if surgical intervention is not immediately instituted.

The principle of emergency exploration is to decompress the obstructed bile duct containing infected bile under pressure by a limited exploration of the bile duct and insertion of a T-tube. Stones that can be easily extracted are removed, and irrigation should not be vigorous as infected material may be forced into the bloodstream, thus exacerbating the septicemic state. Any tight strictures in the left or right hepatic duct should be dilated until there is free egress of infected bile from these ducts. Residual stones and co-existing ductal pathology should be dealt with at a subsequent operation. A stone impacted at the end of the common bile duct in itself does not require removal, but if acute pancreatitis is present the stone must be taken out to relieve pancreatic duct obstruction even if a sphincteroplasty is required. Any abscesses in the liver should be drained directly to the exterior. The gallbladder is left alone unless it is very distended or is the seat of empyema, when a cholecystostomy is performed. On some occasions, when the condition of the patient permits, definitive surgery may be carried out. Percutaneous or endoscopic biliary drainage in the acute attack, which may be successful in patients with cholesterol or mixed stone, is unlikely to be effective in RPC because the bile is thick with mud and debris and would quickly block a small drainage tube.

Definitive Surgery

The principle of definitive surgery in the elective situation comprises: (1) the complete removal of intra- and extrahepatic stones and (2) the establishment of satisfactory drainage of the affected segment of the biliary tree.

Removal of stones in the extrahepatic ducts is usually straightforward, as these stones can be approached directly. On the other hand, complete removal of intrahepatic stones presents the following technical difficulties: (1) there are strictures within the intrahepatic ducts that frustrate attempts to gain access through the extrahepatic duct, (2) branching of the intrahepatic ducts increases their angulation and decreases their caliber so that complete removal of stones in these far reaches, even with fiberoptic choledoscopic guidance, is virtually impossible, (3) a direct approach to the stones by hepatotomy, especially when there is still a good bulk of overlying liver parenchyma, may cause excessive bleeding and may damage major liver vasculature, and (4) even when all the stones are removed, the presence or recurrence of strictures in the intrahepatic ducts will lead to further stone formation. Therefore, when intrahepatic stones are localized to a segment of the liver, and that segment is scarred and atrophic, and where the liver reserve of the residual liver is good, hepatic resection offers the only definitive solution to the problem of intrahepatic stones to date. Hopes that chemical and/or physicochemical methods, applied systematically or locally, may dissolve pigmented stones remain unrealized.

The procedures selected in definitive surgical treatment of RPC are determined by the location of stones and ductal pathology. For stones and strictures in the extrahepatic system, conventional and well-established biliary tract operations can be expected to achieve good long-term results. These operations include exploration of common bile duct, transduodenal sphincteroplasty, choledochojejunostomy, and cholecystectomy. Supraduodenal side-to-side choledochoduodenostomy, though simple and safe, is probably not as effective.

For stones and strictures in the intrahepatic ducts, there are no established methods of conservative surgical procedures that have been shown to be durably efficacious. These conservative measures include dilatation of strictures and removal of stones via a choledochotomy, transhepatic intubation and irrigation, plastic repair of localized strictures in larger ducts, hepatotomy, and intrahepaticodochojejunostomy, with a cutaneous jejunostomy to allow repeated endoscopic examination and stone extraction of the intrahepatic duct.

When, as is the common finding, both intra- and extrahepatic pathology is present, then any of the above procedures, singly or in combination, may be required, and their selection will depend on the preponderance, severity, and exact location of the disease.

The operation(s) selected therefore depends on a subjective evaluation of the pattern of disease, but it should be clearly recognized that an extrahepatic procedure, however technically perfect, may be inappropriate when stones reside behind a tight stricture in the intrahepatic duct. In this case, recurrence of symptoms and progression of disease is inevitable. Therefore,

for early disease with minimal ductal pathology, and for purely extrahepatic disease, surgery offers excellent results. For patients with a combination of intra- and extrahepatic disease, the relative contribution of each will determine the degree and duration of relief of symptoms after surgery; those with predominantly extrahepatic disease may expect a good outcome from drainage surgery, while for those with mainly intrahepatic pathology recurrent symptoms are likely to continue following conservative surgery. For localized intrahepatic disease, eradication of the pathologic focus mandates hepatic resection. To this extent, long-term results are dependent more on the pathology than on the technical performance of the procedure.

Rarely, through a combination of progression of disease and technical failure, patients may develop biliary cirrhosis, portal hypertension with bleeding varices, and liver failure.

Although the peak age of presentation is between 20 and 40 years, the median age of definitive surgery is between 40 and 60 years, reflecting a more advanced stage of disease as the process continues in certain patients.

A summary of the long-term results of sphincteroplasty, choledochojejunostomy, and operations for intrahepatic stones is shown in Table 84–1; the causes of failure following these procedures is presented in Table 84–2.

Extrahepatic Disease

Exploration of Common Bile Duct. This is the most common procedure performed as an elective or emergency operation. In instances when early disease is encountered this alone is adequate and patients may expect lasting relief following this simple intervention, together

TABLE 84–1. RESULTS OF DEFINITIVE SURGERY

	Sphincteroplasty	Choledochojejunostomy	Procedures for Intrahepatic Stones	Total
Number of patients[a]	271	106	91	468
Results				
Good (Asymptomatic)	226 (83.4%)	78 (73.6%)	66 (72.5%)	370 (79.1%)
Fair (Mild symptoms controlled conservatively)	23 (8.5%)	14 (13.2%)	5 (5.5%)	42 (9.0%)
Poor (Severe symptoms requiring reoperation)	22 (8.1%)	14 (13.2%)	20 (22.0%)	56 (11.9%)

[a] At risk at least 7 years after operation.

TABLE 84–2. FAILURE OF DEFINITIVE SURGERY REQUIRING REOPERATION

	Sphincteroplasty	Choledochojejunostomy	Procedures for Intrahepatic Stones	Total
Number of patients[a]	271	106	91	468
Causes				
Recurrence of stones	8	5	16	29
Intrahepatic	3	3	14	20
Extrahepatic	3	2	2	7
Both	2	0	0	2
Anastomotic stricture	4	4	4	12
Liver abscess	2	2	0	4
Infected bile only	1	2	0	3
Empyema of gallbladder	2	0	0	2
Total	17[b]	13[c]	20	53[d] (11.3%)

[a] At risk at least 7 years after operation.
[b] Five of the original 22 patients with poor results refused surgery.
[c] One of the original 14 patients with poor results refused surgery.
[d] Hospital mortality of re-operated group: 4/53 (7.5%); patients requiring further re-operation: 6/53 (11.3%)

with removal of identifiable stones. The rationale for the success of this operation is not obvious, as after the T-tube is removed the underlying pathophysiology is apparently not reversed.

The common bile duct is often of sufficient size for digital exploration to be performed. Although a postexploratory cholangiogram was routinely performed in the past, rigid or flexible choledochoscopy is now carried out instead. A large T-tube is inserted so that retained stones may be subsequently removed via the T-tube tract; this is required in 25 percent of RPC patients. The choledochotomy is closed with continuous fine absorbable sutures.

Sphincteroplasty. Sphincteroplasty is indicated when: (1) a stone is found impacted at the lower end of the common bile duct, (2) the duct is thickened and dilated up to the sphincter of Oddi; (3) periampullary stricture is present, and (4) there is associated pancreatitis. This operation can be performed transabdominally or, in patients who had undergone previous biliary surgery, extraperitoneally. The extraperitoneal approach is conducted through a right-flank incision and it is important to avoid mistaking the colon for the duodenum by first identifying the kidney posteriorly and visualizing the head of the pancreas medially. Using either approach the second part of the duodenum is exposed and

opened vertically, and the sphincter of Oddi is divided at the 11 o'clock position. The division is extended to the most dilated part of the common duct, which may be 2 cm or more from the ampullary opening. The edge of the common bile duct and the duodenum is then approximated with fine silk sutures (Fig. 84–10). After complete removal of stones, the duodenum is closed longitudinally with an inner layer of continuous fine absorbable sutures and an outer layer of interrupted silk sutures.

The limitation of extraperitoneal approach is that the common bile duct cannot be explored through a separate choledochotomy and other additional intraperitoneal procedures cannot be carried out; the indications and versatility are therefore more confined. In the intraperitoneal approach a choledochotomy is usually made to facilitate the sphincteroplasty.

The complication rate in 324 operated patients was 9.4 percent, of which half resulted in deaths, a mortality rate of 4.8 percent. The mortality of emergency operation is three times that of an elective one (12.9 percent versus 3.9 percent). The common postoperative complications are septicemia, pancreatitis, and bronchopneumonia; all patients who developed the first two complications died.

Long-term follow-up (7 years and 4 months after operation) showed that 83.4 percent of patients had good results and were cured of their symptoms; 8.5 percent had fair results, i.e., mild symptoms of cholangitis requiring hospitalization but no operation; and 8.1 percent had poor results, i.e., severe symptoms of cholangitis requiring reoperation (Table 84–1). The common reasons for failure are recurrence of stones or mud (in the presence of a patent sphincteroplasty), and sphincteroplasty stricture, followed by liver abscesses, and empyema of gallbladder. These problems are dealt with by further exploration of common duct and removal of recurrent stones, liver resection, conversion of the sphincteroplasty into a choledochojejunostomy, drainage of abscess, and cholecystectomy (Table 84–2).

RPC was the cause of acute pancreatitis is 40.8 percent of patients in Hong Kong. Of 127 patients whose pancreatitis was caused by RPC, all of whom underwent emergency operation, a sphincteroplasty was performed in 19 to remove a stone impacted at the lower end of the common bile duct with no mortality. Therefore even in the presence of acute pancreatitis, sphincteroplasty can be safely performed, and should be carried out in these instances.

With the established place of endoscopic papillotomy and removal of residual stones through a T-tube tract, the question of whether a sphincteroplasty by operation is still indicated is inevitably raised. While these nonoperative procedures have been shown to be effective in removing cholesterol and mixed stones, their ability to deal with the soft pigmented intrahepatic stones of RPC with similar success has not been demonstrated. Since the sphincter of Oddi is already patulous in most patients with RPC, a modest enlargement by papillotomy is a questionable gain. However, in elderly, high-risk patients these procedures should be attempted first; if found to be unsuccessful, a formal exploration of common bile duct and sphincteroplasty should then be undertaken. In young, fit patients, definitive surgery is still recommended.

A supraduodenal, or side-to-side, choledochoduodenostomy has not been favored by us because in circumstances where this operation is indicated a choledochojejunostomy offers greater protection, and in circumstances where a successful outcome may be in doubt, a sphincteroplasty would be more appropriate. Furthermore, there is the added (though uncommon) risk of the sump syndrome resulting from stones and debris collected at the lower end of the common bile duct, and the greater likelihood of repeated attacks of cholangitis.

Sphincteroplasty is a safe and effective way of treating RPC when appropriate indications are present; failures are few when selection of patients has been judicious.

Choledochojejunostomy. Choledochojejunostomy is indicated when: (1) the common bile duct is extremely dilated and fibrotic, (2) there is a stricture or stenosis at the lower end of the common bile duct occurring above the level of the duodenum or extending supraduodenally from below, and (3) previous biliary–enteric anastomosis has failed (Fig. 84–8). This operation is usually performed in patients who had undergone previous emergency or elective biliary tract surgery. In a series of 128 patients, 97 had undergone previous surgery and 49 had the choledochojejunostomy carried out as a primary procedure. The majority of the previous procedure had been exploration of the common bile duct, and a few had prior sphincteroplasty.

Choledochojejunostomy is constructed by a Roux-Y, end-to-end method using a long 40-cm loop; the anastomosis is effected by one layer of interrupted fine absorbable sutures. The loop is usually placed in the retrocolic position, and intestinal continuity is restored with an end-to-side jejunojejunostomy. A transanastomotic stent is brought out either through the jejunal loop or through the left lobe of the liver.

The mortality rate of this operation is 2.3 to 4.3 percent for emergency and 1.9 percent for elective operations. Complications occurred in 12 out of 128 patients (10.6 percent). The causes of death were stress ulcer, hemobilia, and septicemia. Complications include subphrenic abscesses, biliary fistulas, and pancreatitis, none of which led to death. Choledochojejunostomy was performed on 23 patients as an emergency procedure, with 1 death.

With a mean follow-up of 8 years, 73.6 percent of patients had good results and were asymptomatic, 13.2 percent had some residual low-grade cholangitis that was resolved with conservative treatment, and 13.2 percent had poor results, with severe symptoms of cholangitis requiring further surgical treatment (Table 84–1). In the last group of 13 patients who underwent surgery, 5 had stone recurrence in the intra- or extrahepatic duct with a patent anastomosis and 4 had stenosis of the choledochojenostomy. Two further patients had neither stones nor stricture and underwent exploration of common bile duct from which *E. coli* was cultured from the bile; of the remaining patients two had liver abscesses. Anastomotic strictures were revised, hepatic lithiasis were dealt with by hepatic resection, and abscesses were drained (Table 84–2).

Like sphincteroplasty, choledochojejunostomy, when performed with proper indications, is a safe procedure and confers lasting protection for patients with RPC. There are few long-term problems; the two most common causes being recurrence of stones and anastomotic stricture.

Cholecystectomy. As the gallbladder is not frequently affected in RPC, cholecystectomy is performed only when conventional indications are present, such as evidence of chronic cholecystitis or presence of stones. Although there is a small risk of subsequent acute complication, we consider the unnecessary removal of a normal gallbladder in the majority of RPC patients unwarranted (Table 84–2).

Intrahepatic Disease

Unlike extrahepatic stones, intrahepatic stones do present a serious threat to the well-being of patients suffering from RPC and are a challenge to the ingenuity and technical skills of surgeons. The essence of this difficulty is that there is no effective method to deal with strictures of the intrahepatic ducts, apart from hepatic resection. Thus even when the stones can be completely removed by one of an increasing number of innovative procedures, unless the intrahepatic ductal stricture can be enlarged and prevented from restenosis, redevelopment of stricture will inevitably lead to a recurrence of stones and perpetuation of cholangitis.

The traditional methods available to deal with intrahepatic stones are: (1) common duct exploration, dilatation of strictures, and removal of intrahepatic stones through a high choledochotomy, (2) transhepatic intubation and irrigation, (3) hepatotomy, and (4) hepatic resection. With the availability of small fiberoptic instruments, visualization and extraction of stones may be attempted via T-tube or transhepatic tube tracts. Per oral choledochoscopy (after endoscopic papillotomy) also allows manipulation within the intrahepatic duct. To facilitate the use of these endoscopic methods repeatedly,

a side-to-side intrahepaticodocho-jejunostomy with a Roux-Y loop is used, with the end of the jejunal loop brought out to the exterior as a cutaneous stoma.

Plastic repair of the stricture duct may be performed for a short segment stricture, which may be excised and reanastomosed. This can be carried out either through a hepatotomy for an intrahepatic stricture, or by a combined intra- and extrahepatic approach when the stricture lies at the interface. For strictures of the left or right hepatic duct just outside the liver, a side-to-side anastomosis, similar in principle to the Finney pyloroplasty, may be employed. When the stricture is located at the confluence of the left and right hepatic ducts, a Y-V plasty is also an alternative. Whenever possible, if there is sufficient hepatic duct outside the liver, a hepaticojejunostomy would be the drainage operation of choice.

Hepatic resection is indicated when substantial liver parenchyma has been destroyed and the ducts are fibrous sacs containing numerous pigment stones. Usually a left lateral segmental resection is carried out, but a left lobectomy is required when the medial segment is also affected. Hepatotomy is performed when there is still a good amount of normal liver tissue remaining. Transhepatic intubation and irrigation is a simple and safe procedure but the stone recurrence rate is high. Reconstruction of a strictured intrahepatic duct is a difficult procedure to perform and our limited experience indicates that recurrence is the rule. A plastic procedure in the extrahepatic segment of the hepatic ducts also has an unsatisfactory outcome. The reason for failure in direct repair of diseased duct is the same as for iatrogenic strictures, i.e., approximation of devitalized, denuded duct edges will heal by scarring. Fresh mucosal-lined tissues, such as the jejunum, is thus required if better long-term result is expected.

Of 115 patients treated by one of the four conventional methods cited earlier, 5 patients died (4.3 percent), the causes being massive bleeding from stress ulceration, septicemia from cholangitis, pancreatitis, and volvulus of small bowel. Complications include subphrenic abscesses, abdominal dehiscences and bronchopneumonia. In 91 patients (followed up for a median period of 7 years and 8 months) only hepatic resection has an acceptably low failure rate (4.2 percent, or 1 out of 24). Failure rates for the other three methods ranged from 23.6 to 75 percent. For the whole group good results were obtained in 72 percent (66 out of 91) and poor results, i.e., those requiring operation, in 22 percent (Table 84–1). The main reason for failure was recurrence of intrahepatic stones (16/20); the other 4 patients had late complications of drainage procedure (Table 84–2).

CONCLUSION

Recurrent pyogenic cholantitis exhibits a clinical syndrome that is characteristic and the diagnosis is seldom in doubt. Although most patients can expect a favorable outcome from appropriate treatment in the acute attack and also after definitive surgical treatment, a few may develop life-threatening complications in the emergency situation and in the long term. The conventional surgical repertoire can deal with extrahepatic disease safely and adequately. Failures are due primarily to recurrence of stones, particularly in the intrahepatic site. Anastomotic stricture accounts for the next most frequent cause of failure.

The major residual therapeutic problem in the surgical management of RPC is intrahepatic ductal stricture. Technologic advances in fiberoptic instrumentation have enabled these ducts to be examined and allowed stones contained therein to be removed on repeated occasions without operative intervention, but their inability to deal definitively with these strictures means that they offer only a solution to the consequences of ductal strictures. For these patients, hepatic resection offers the only cure. Successful conservative methods are still awaited.

BIBLIOGRAPHY

Choi TK, Wong J, et al: Late result of sphincteroplasty in the treatment of primary cholangitis. Arch Surg 116:1173, 1981

Choi TK, Wong J, et al: The surgical management of primary intrahepatic stones. Br J Surg 69:86, 1982

Choi TK, Wong J, et al: Choledochojejunostomy in the treatment of primary cholangitis. Surg Gynecol Obstet 115:43, 1982

Choi TK, Lee NW, et al: Extraperitoneal sphincteroplasty for residual common bile duct stones—an update. Ann Surg 196:26, 1982

Cook J, Hou PC, et al: Recurrent pyogenic cholangitis. Br J Surg 42:188, 1954

Digby KH: Common-duct stones of liver origin. Br J Surg 17:578, 1930

Fung J: Liver fluke infestation and cholangio-hepatitis. Br J Surg, 48:404, 1961

Lam SK, Wong KP, et al: Recurrent pyogenic cholangitis: A study by endoscopic retrograde cholangiography. Gastroenterology 74:1196, 1978

Ong GB: A study of recurrent pyogenic cholangitis. Arch Surg 84:63, 1962

Ong GB, Adisehiah M, et al: Acute pancreatitis associated with recurrent pyogenic cholangitis. Br J Surg 58:891, 1971

Ong GB, Lam KH, et al: Acute pancreatitis in Hong Kong. Br J Surg 66:398, 1979

Teoh TB: A study of gall-stones and included worms in recurrent pyogenic cholangitis. J Path Bact 86:123, 1963

Wong J: Recurrent pyogenic cholangitis, in Okuda (ed): International Association for the Study of the Liver/Asian Pacific Association for the Study of the Liver—Postgraduate Course. Hong Kong, 1982

Wong J, Choi TK: Pigment gallstones and hepatolithiasis, in Okuda K, Nakayama F, et al (eds): Progress in Clinical and Biological Research. Hong Kong, 1983 Kunio

85. Tumours of the Gallbladder and Bile Ducts

Leslie H. Blumgart

Malignant bile duct stricture is a major challenge in biliary surgery and may result either from primary cancer of the ducts or as a result of tumours involving them by extension from the liver, the gallbladder, the pancreas, the papilla of Vater, or the duodenum.

This chapter discusses the diagnosis and management of tumours of the gallbladder and cystic duct and primary tumours affecting the bile ducts. Major emphasis is placed on cholangiocarcinoma at the confluence of the hepatic ducts.

PATHOPHYSIOLOGIC EFFECTS

Malignant strictures of the biliary tree produce a degree of biliary tract obstruction. The obstruction is not necessarily complete and jaundice may not be present initially. In addition, segmental obstruction is important, particularly in high biliary carcinoma, which may occlude one or more branches of the intrahepatic biliary tree. Thus the early phases of the disease may pass unrecognised, especially where the biochemical evidence of biliary obstruction may be masked by the mass of adequately functioning nonobstructed liver. However, the alkaline phosphatase is elevated even with minor or intermittent degrees of obstruction. Indeed, the finding of an isolated raised level of liver alkaline phosphatase should always lead to imaging investigations of the biliary tree in an attempt to display a possible obstructing lesion. A proportion of such patients will be found to be harbouring an early cholangiocarcinoma.

Although serum albumin levels are often reduced in patients with biliary tract obstruc-tion, it is important to realise that this may not necessarily reflect impaired hepatic synthesis but is often related to a complex of other factors.

Systemic endotoxaemia occurs in jaundiced patients before, during, and after surgery, in contrast to nonjaundiced patients with disease of comparable severity. This is important since endotoxaemia is associated with postoperative renal failure in jaundiced patients.

Liver Atrophy. Distribution of liver mass amongst the various segments of the liver is regulated by a complex balance in which bile flow, portal venous flow, and hepatic venous flow are the principal factors. Uniform liver atrophy will occur in the presence of total or of partial occlusion of the main stem of the portal vein. Both the quality and quantity of portal venous inflow are important in maintenance of liver cell size and mass. Segmental or lobar atrophy results from a reduction of portal venous flow, or bile duct occlusion to that area of liver tissue. The left lobe of the liver appears more susceptible to atrophy than the right. Unilobar atrophy is usually associated with hypertrophy of the contralateral lobe and this may present diagnostic difficulty because the large palpable liver felt is not a mass but an indicator of pathology principally affecting the contralateral lobe of the liver. Changes of this nature are frequently found in hilar cholangiocarcinoma (Fig. 85–1) and arise through a gradual process of asymmetric and asynchronous cancerous involvement of the lobar hepatic ducts, sometimes involving the portal vessels. Appreciation of gross atrophy is important because it may have a significant impact on the planning of therapy. Drainage

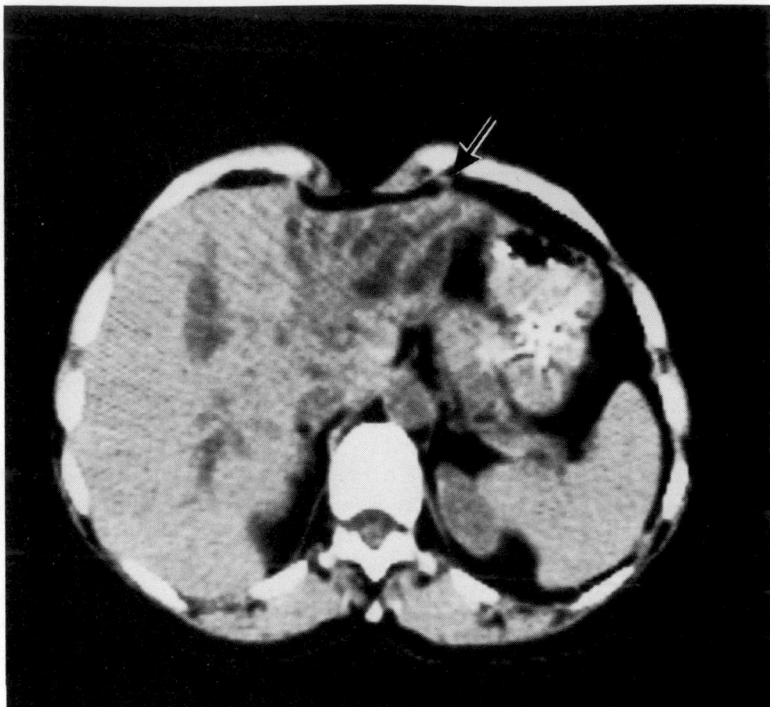

Figure 85–1. CT scan in a patient with hilar cholangiocarcinoma. The right lobe is of normal size. There are markedly dilated bile ducts throughout but crowded together in a shrunken left lobe (*arrow*). Atrophy of the left lobe confirmed at subsequent surgery. Percutaneous transhepatic cholangiography in this case confirmed the hilar lesion and also demonstrated the crowded left lobe ducts.

of dilated ducts within an atrophic segment may not be effective in relieving obstruction, and resection of liver tissue that leaves an atrophic remnant is dangerous and associated with liver failure in the postoperative period.

Infection. The normal biliary tract is sterile. However, in cases of primary malignant obstruction there is a high incidence of infection. Keighley, in 1977, reported a biliary bacterial contamination rate of 36 percent, and in 1982 McPherson et al have shown a positive bile culture rate at initial percutaneous transhepatic cholangiography (PTC) of 32 percent for patients with obstruction due to cholangiocarcinoma. Previous operation increases the risk of infection. Multiple previous operations or the presence of indwelling tubes are invariably associated with infection, and this group of patients also have the highest incidence of anaerobic biliary contaminants.

Although many patients have episodes of cholangitis, bacterial contamination of the biliary tract is not always clinically apparent. Infection does, however, assume considerable clinical importance at the time of surgery, since invasive sepsis constitutes a major risk factor

and is responsible for the majority of postoperative complications and mortality.

The most common infecting organisms are *Escherichia coli* and *Streptococcus faecalis*. Anaerobic bacteria are rare as a primary finding. Following radiologic intubation or surgical interference the spectrum of bacteria changes and there is a danger of acquisition of exogenous organisms.

CARCINOMA OF THE GALLBLADDER

Carcinoma of the gallbladder has always had a bad reputation, with a median survival of 5.2 months from diagnosis and a 5-year survival of 1 to 6 percent.

Although often considered a rare condition, it has been claimed that gallbladder carcinoma represents almost 20 percent of all gastrointesinal (GI) carcinomas. There are, however, some racial and ethnic differences in the incidence of gallbladder cancer, Caucasians in the United States having an incidence of gallbladder cancer 50 percent higher than that of blacks. Similarly the rate of gallbladder cancer in the southwest of America is particularly high in American Indians as compared to Caucasians.

The tumour is more common in women and has a peak incidence in the 70 to 75-year-old group and a female-to-male ratio of approximately 3:1. There is a close association with cholelithiasis and more than 90 percent of patients with gallbladder cancer have gallstones.

No human carcinogen has been identified that might be responsible for gallbladder cancer. It is possible that some endogenous carcinogen, resulting from bacterial degradation of bile salts, might act on a susceptible mucosa possibly damaged by long-standing cholelithiasis.

Histologically 75 to 90 percent of these lesions are well-differentiated mucin-secreting adenocarcinomas, while 5 percent are squamous cell lesions and approximately 10 percent are anaplastic. The mode of spread of carcinoma of the gallbladder is mainly by the lymphatics along the cystic duct and thence to the common bile duct or by direct extension into the adjacent liver.

The gallbladder lies in its fossa between the right and quadrate lobes of the liver so that as the tumour spreads it will involve Segment IV and Segment V (Fig. 85–2). The common hepatic duct is frequently involved by direct extension and presentation is then with painless progressive jaundice, differential diagnosis being from cholangiocarcinoma at the confluence of the bile ducts. This mode of spread through Cal-

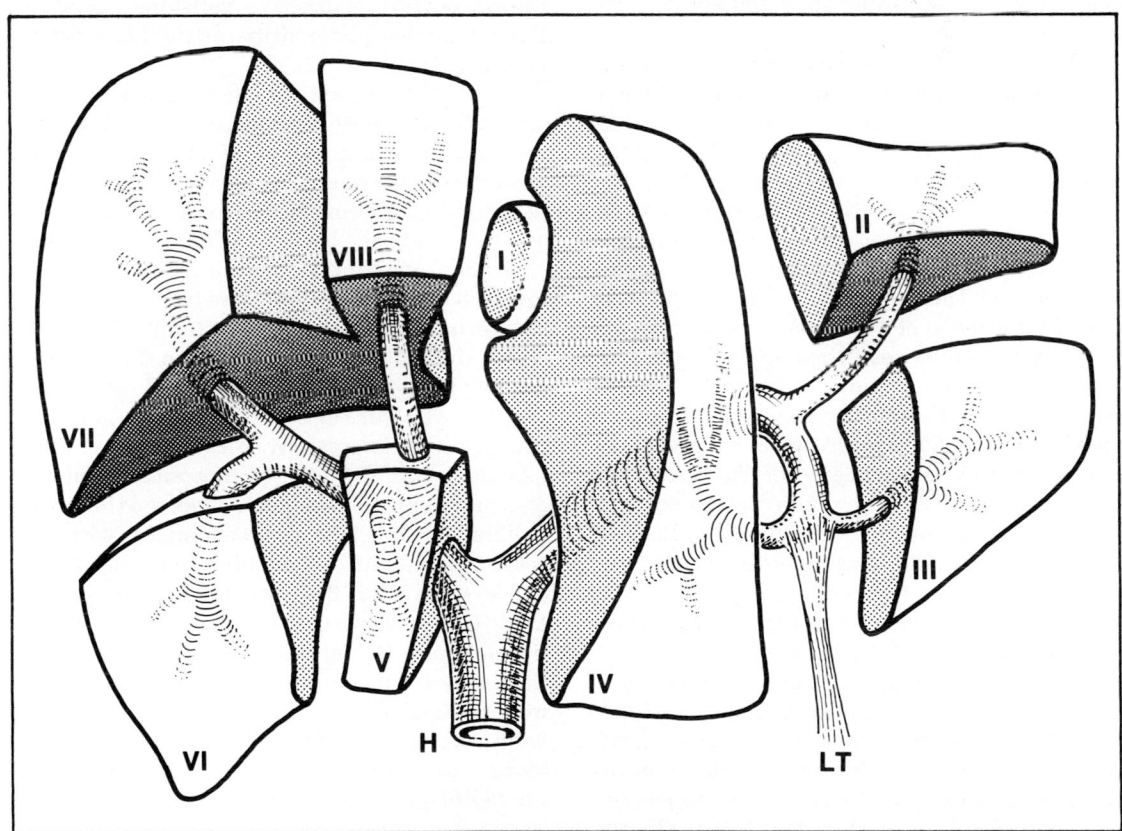

Figure 85–2. Anatomic segments of the liver as described by Couinaud. The portal triads are represented as a single trunk. Note the hilar area, the right system being distributed to the right side of the liver (Segments V, VI, VII and VIII) and the left triads to the left liver (Segments II, III and IV). Segment I is the caudate lobe. Important anatomic features in relation to biliary enteric bypass for gallbladder cancer and hilar cholangiocarcinoma are that the left hepatic duct has a long extrahepatic course beneath the quadrate lobe and then turns forward and caudally in the umbilical fissure receiving here tributaries from Segments II and III. LT = ligamentum teres. H = liver hilus. (*Source: From Blumgart LH, Kelley CJ, 1984, with permission.*)

ot's triangle to the common hepatic duct is frequent with tumours that arise in the region of the neck of the gallbladder or Hartmann's pouch, but less so with tumours growing close to the fundus of the gallbladder, where the duct to the anteroinferior segment of the liver may be involved early. Indeed, selective involvement of ducts and vessels in the anteroinferior part of the right lobe of the liver on cholangiography/angiography, particularly in the presence of obstructive jaundice, should arouse suspicion of gallbladder cancer. Occasionally, endoscopic retrograde choledochopancreatography reveals an irregular filling defect within the gallbladder or obstruction of the common hepatic duct or cystic duct, but an apparently normal study does not exclude early disease. Computed tomography (CT) scanning may sometimes suggest the diagnosis.

However, preoperative diagnosis is uncommon and although many patients may have a history of biliary disease extending over 1 year in duration, 50 percent will have no such history and present with obstructive jaundice. The majority of patients are still diagnosed either as an incidental finding at elective biliary surgery or during laparotomy for suspected cholangiocarcinoma at the confluence of the duct. In a recent experience of 115 cases of carcinoma affecting the confluence of the bile ducts at a specialist hepatobiliary clinic and seen over a period of 5 years, the author has encountered 17 cases of gallbladder cancer. A correct preoperative diagnosis was considered in five cases, this being significantly higher than the 8.6 percent preoperative diagnostic rate recorded by Piehler and Crichlow in 1978. This high yield of preoperative diagnosis has been dependent upon a high index of clinical suspicion and critical appraisal of percutaneous cholangiograms.

A proportion of patients are, of course, submitted to cholecystectomy for cholelithiasis and found to have either frank carcinoma evident in the gallbladder at the time of operation or to have carcinoma discovered microscopically after removal of the gallbladder. These patients are clearly at an early stage of the disease, but the tendency for cancer of the gallbladder to be locally invasive and to present with widespread disease is well known.

Treatment

Most gallbladder cancers have extensively involved the liver and structures in the porta hepatis by the time operation is performed so that only biopsy or palliative bypass are possible.

The results of excisional treatment are in general poor. However, where cholecystectomy has been carried out for cancer that has only microscopically involved the gallbladder, the results are better. Early diagnosis in general is only made at operation, and prompt cholecystectomy for cholelithiasis may account for increased salvage in some more recent series. It should be noted, however, that the risk of dying after cholecystectomy is probably very similar to that of developing a cancer of the gallbladder. As pointed out by Tompkins (1982), it is hard to justify cholecystectomy for the prevention of cancer, but more support can be found for the recommendation of early cholecystectomy for the prevention of possible gallstone complications (jaundice, pancreatitis, acute cholecystitis, perforation).

At cholecystectomy the surgeon should open the gallbladder and inspect the lining. Frozen section examination of suspicious areas should be performed. If an early cancer is identified, immediate consideration should be given to a more radical excision, including lymph node clearance. It is much more difficult to recommend reoperation several days later in a patient recovering from cholecystectomy. Bergdahl (1980) studied 32 patients in whom the gallbladder had been removed for presumed benign disease but who were discovered to have a gallbladder cancer at microscopy. Eleven of these cases had cancer confined to the mucosa and submucosa and in 21 the carcinoma involved the entire gallbladder wall. The group of patients with mucosal and submucosal involvement only had a 5-year survival of 63.6 percent (7 patients) and a 10-year survival of 45.5 percent (5 patients). By contrast, the group of patients with full-thickness involvement of the gallbladder wall were all dead within 2 years and 5 months. Bergdahl recommends that patients with microscopic carcinoma discovered after removal of the gallbladder for presumed benign disease be reoperated and a wedge resection of approximately 5 cm of normal liver tissue and dissection of the regional lymph nodes be carried out. A similar suggestion for improvement of results is made by Nevin et al in 1976 who found that 6 of 7 patients who only had intramucosal involvement lived 5 years or more. These authors suggest that simple cholecystectomy be employed for lesions involving the mucosa or the muscularis mucosae alone, but prefer a radical cholecystectomy for more advanced cases. Moossa et al in 1975 examined retrospectively a 30-year experience at the University of Chicago in the management of 82 cases with gallbladder cancer. Only 4 patients survived 5 years (4.9 percent). However, they pointed out that only 42 patients were treated; when this is taken into account the 5-year survival increases to 9.5 percent. Further, when only the 28 patients who underwent cholecystectomy are considered the 5-year survival rises to 14.3 percent. Others have not been able to demonstrate improved results by the use of radical procedures for cancer of the gallbladder. Nevertheless, it does seem that the only possibility of cure lies in those patients discovered early or in a more radical operation for selected cases.

Tompkins (1982) also recommends radical cholecystectomy (removal of the gallbladder with adjacent wedge of liver tissue and regional lymphatics) in those cases where the tumour is small and appears localised to the gallbladder. In more advanced lesions palliative decompression is recommended and radiotheraphy and chemotherapy considered. However, since the gallbladder lies in the anatomic plane separating the right from the left liver, involvement of the quadrate lobe (Segment IV) is early. The recommendation for wedge resection with a reasonable clearance is not easily performed, and extended right hepatic lobectomy may be required. The minimum and safest procedure likely to produce tumour clearance is dissection of the extrahepatic bile duct from duodenum to the confluence with clearance of nodes and resection of Segments IV, V, and VI with the attached gallbladder. The technique for such resections have been well described by Bismuth (1982).

This author has no record of a 5-year survival in any treated case of gallbladder cancer, but excellent palliation can usually be obtained by a biliary enteric bypass utilising the left hepatic ductal system approach via the umbilical fissure. This allows anastomosis to be carried out, usually to a dilated ductal system at a good distance from the primary lesion; the anastomosis tends to be involved by tumour extension only late in the disease. This surgical approach, based on the anatomic features of the fetal circulation, was first described by Soupault and Couinaud (1957) and has been extensively used in France and recently in the US and the United Kingdom. An understanding of the anatomic features of the left hepatic ductal system and vasculature is a necessary preliminary to a description of the procedure.

Technique of Biliary Enteric Bypass

The following anatomic description is based on the segmental nature of the liver as described by Couinad (1954) (Fig. 85–2). The left hepatic duct *always* has an extrahepatic course and traverses (together with the left branch of the portal vein) within a peritoneal reflection of the gastrohepatic ligament which is lightly fused with Glisson's capsule on the undersurface of the quadrate lobe (Segment IV). The vessels (including the left branch of the hepatic artery) and the accompanying duct enter the umbilical fissure of the liver, at the limits of which division to and from the left lobe (Segments II and III) and the quadrate lobe (Segment IV) occur (Fig. 85–2). Thus, the left lobe lateral to the ligamentum teres is divided into a posterior and anterior segment (Segments II and III). The left hepatic duct receives a major branch from each of these segments, these branches converging in the depths of the umbilical fissure above and behind the left portal vein. Branches to the quadrate lobe (Segment IV) also originate from the left ducts and vessels, and recurve to supply the quadrate lobe (Fig. 85–2).

The ligamentum teres in the lower edge of the falciform ligament traverses the umbilical fissure of the liver which is usually, but not always, bridged in its lowermost part by a tongue of liver tissue joining the left lobe lateral to the ligamentum teres to the base of the quadrate lobe. The ligamentum joins the umbilical portion of the left portal vein close to its division into its Segments II and III branches, and at its base on its upper surface splays somewhat in the manner of a goose's foot, the prolongations containing portal vessels recurving and traversing over the bile ducts (see the following).

The surgical approach to be described is modified from the report of Soupault and Couinaud and depends on display of the left hepatic ducts by opening the umbilical fissure at the base of the ligamentum teres (ligamentum teres approach).

An important feature is early division of the ligamentum teres and freeing of the falciform ligament from the abdominal wall right back to the diaphragm. The liver is elevated so as to display its undersurface. The bridge of tissue (if present) connecting the left lateral segment of the liver to the quadrate lobe is now divided (Fig. 85–3). While the liver is then held

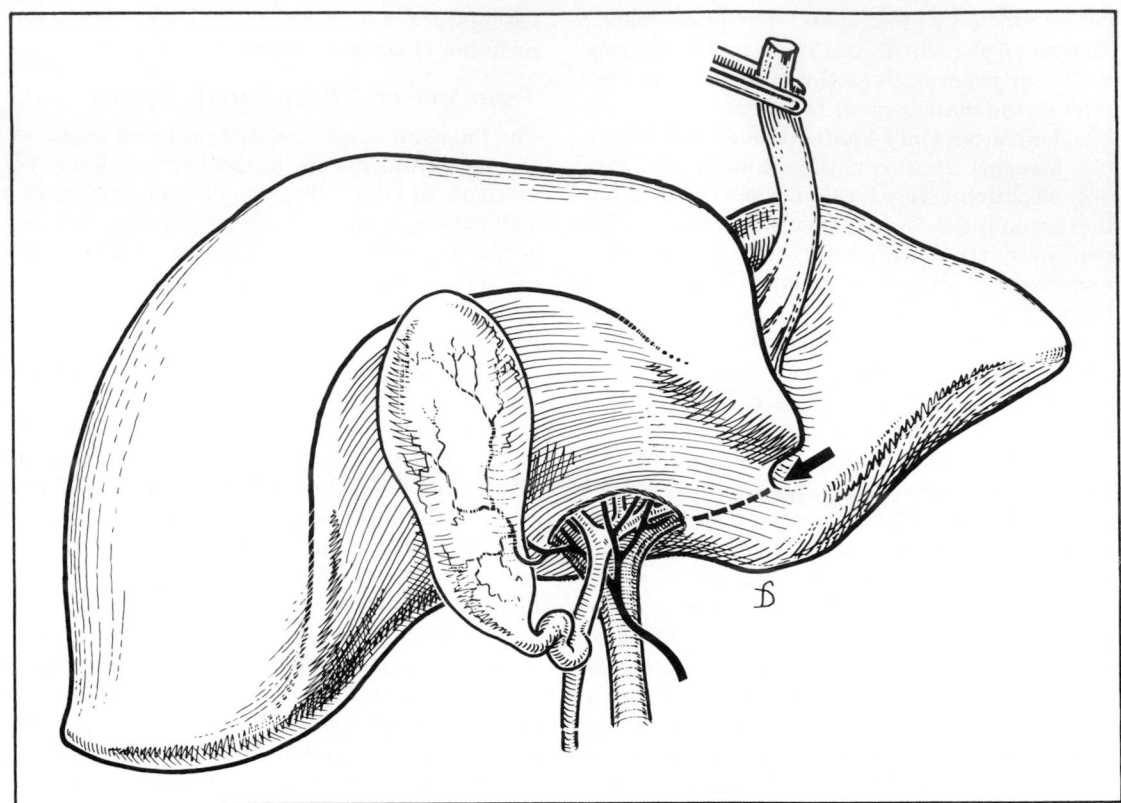

Figure 85–3. The liver is held up together with the ligamentum teres. There is a bridge of tissue, very frequently bridging the base of the umbilical fissure and this is divided (*arrow*). The base of the umbilical fissure is thus exposed, the ligamentum teres running down to its junction with the portal vein. (*Source: From Blumgart LH, Kelley CJ, 1984, with permission.*)

up so that its inferior surface can be seen, the ligamentum teres is pulled downward (Fig. 85–4). When this is done and the upper surface of the ligament is dissected, the small extensions passing into the liver at its base are exposed. These extensions are individually dissected and divided between ligatures. The use of a small aneurysm needle facilitates ligation. If exposure is inadequate then a small "split" of the liver substance can be made by dividing the liver substance just to the left of the falciform ligament.

Downward traction is continued on the ligamentum teres and the tissue above it and overlying the duct is cleared. Needle aspiration may assist identification of the bile duct. The duct is then opened longitudinally at or just proximal to the point of its division into the Segment III and Segment II ducts (Fig. 85–5). If dissection is commenced to the left of the base of the liga-

mentum teres then the Segment III duct itself is exposed early in the procedure.

The duct is incised and initial stay sutures are put in place. A Roux-Y loop of jejunum, 70 cm in length, is prepared and brought up for subsequent side-to-side anastomosis, performed using the technique described by Voyles and Blumgart (1982) and by Blumgart and Kelley (1984). An important point is early placement of the anterior layer of sutures prior to any attempt to place the posterior row. These sutures are serially introduced through the bile duct wall and the needles are left on each suture, so that the row thus placed can subsequently be elevated to allow exposure of the lower margin of the duct (Fig. 85–6). This manoeuvre not only allows precise placement of the anterior row of sutures, which may be difficult if the posterior layer is inserted first and tied, but also

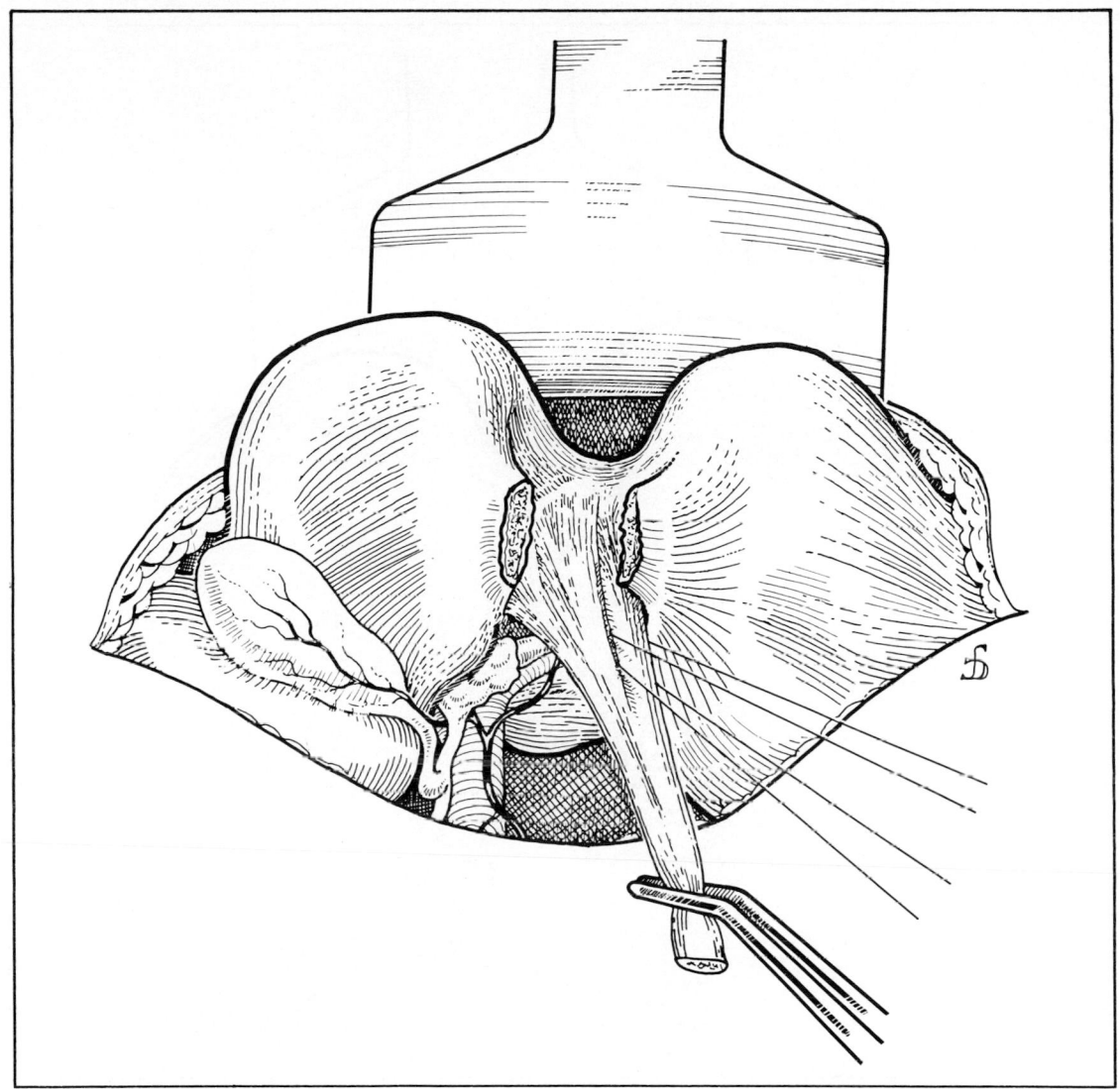

Figure 85–4. The ligamentum teres is now pulled downward and dissected free so that the upper surface of its base can be displayed. Here there are a number of radiating folds of peritoneum covering branches of the portal vein issuing to Segments III and IV. The prolongations are dissected and divided between ligatures working mainly on the left side and close to the medial portion of Segment III. The bile duct lies just above and behind the portal vein, and as these ligamentous extensions are divided the ligamentum teres pulls the vein downward and the duct is exposed (see Fig. 85–5). (*Source: From Blumgart LH, Kelley CJ, 1984, with permission.*)

facilitates placement of the posterior layer, which is introduced through the jejunum and the bile duct wall and held taut, the jejunal limb then being "railroaded" upward. The posterior sutures are then tied serially on the inside.

The previously placed anterior row of sutures is now completed by picking up the needles and passing them through the jejunal wall from outside inward. The entire layer may be so placed and again held and serially tied.

Since this author has adopted these ap-

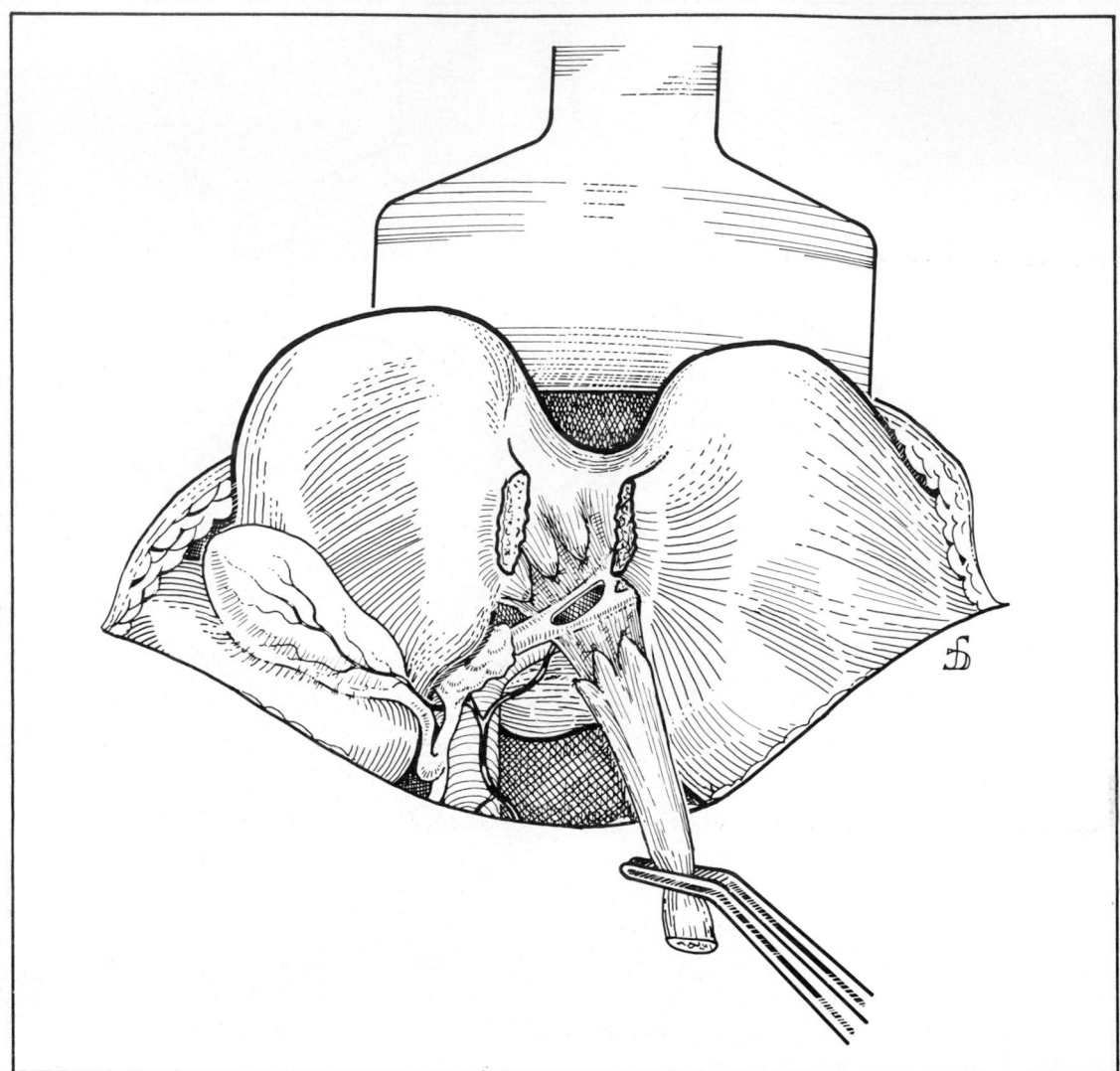

Figure 85–5. The Segment III duct is exposed close to its junction with the left hepatic duct and the junction of the Segment II duct. A wide choledochotomy can be made in a dilated duct. The procedure is more difficult if the ducts are not grossly dilated or if the liver tissue is fibrous and there is a degree of hypertrophy of the left lobe. Usually only the left side of the ligamentous prolongations need be divided. (*Source: From Blumgart LH, Kelley CJ, 1984, with permission.*)

proaches to the left duct, 40 malignant bile duct strictures at the confluence of the bile ducts have been approached for biliary–enteric anastomosis. There need be no continuity of left and right ducts at the hilus and prolonged and valuable palliation can yet be achieved by anastomosis to the left duct only (Fig. 85–7). The procedure is not useful if there is left lobar atrophy and not necessary if the confluence is not involved by tumour and can be approached directly.

As demonstrated by Bismuth and Corlette in 1956, biliary–enteric anastomosis leaves the patient free of tubes in the postoperative period and the incidence of cholangitis is reduced.

The more extensive liver split procedure, whereby an hepatectomy is employed to expose high strictures, should not be employed if ap-

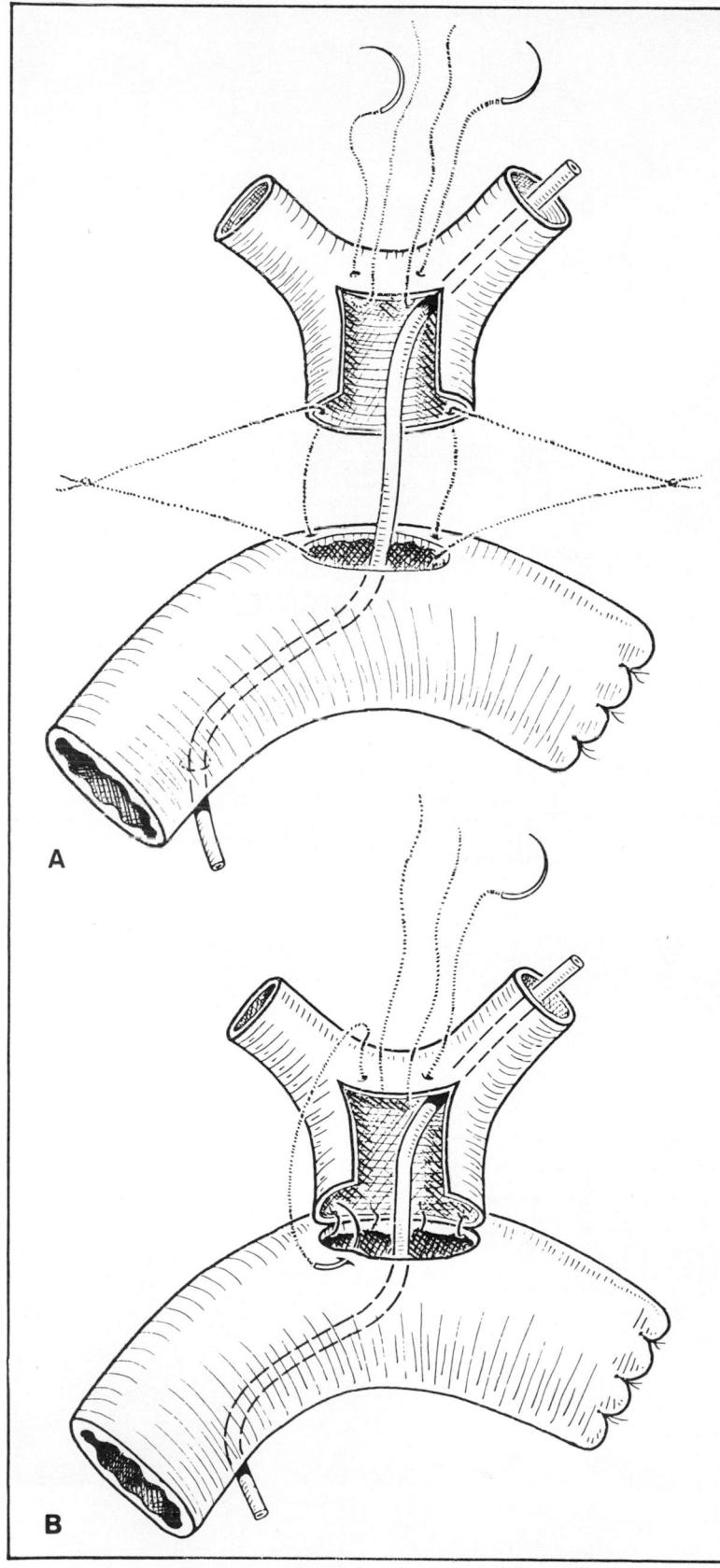

Figure 85–6. Suture techniques. **A.** For high biliary enteric anastomoses stay sutures are placed and then sutures (3/0 Vicryl) are inserted on the upper edge of the choledochotomy first. The needles are passed from within outward and are held on the sutures serially in order to elevate the upper duct wall. **B.** This facilitates placement of the posterior layer of sutures between the enterotomy and choledochotomy, which are also serially placed, the gut then being railroaded upward and the posterior layer tied before completion of the anterior row of sutures. This is completed by passing the needles through the gut from outside in, right across the anastomosis, and then tying these sutures serially.

If there are multiple anastomoses to be made, closely adjacent exposed ducts at the hilus may be joined. If this is not possible, the anterior layer of sutures on all the separated ducts are made first. Following this all posterior sutures are placed and tied before final completion of the anterior suture lines. It is not possible to complete each anastomosis individually and accurately, but readily possible if anastomoses are made in the manner indicated. (*Source: From Voyles CR, Blumgart LH: A technique for the construction of high biliary enteric anastomoses. Surg Gynecol Obstet 154:885, 1982, with permission.*)

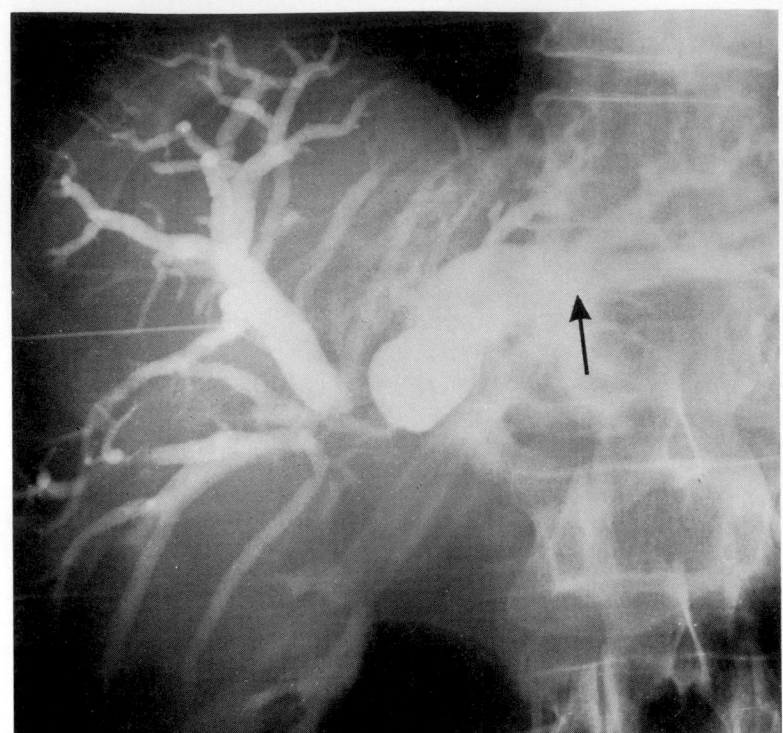

Figure 85–7. A. PTC in a patient with gallbladder carcinoma involving the hilar biliary structures. Separate punctures have been made so as to outline both the right and left ductal system. The arrow indicates the area of the Segment III duct for anastomosis. Note the distance between this duct and the area of the carcinoma.

A

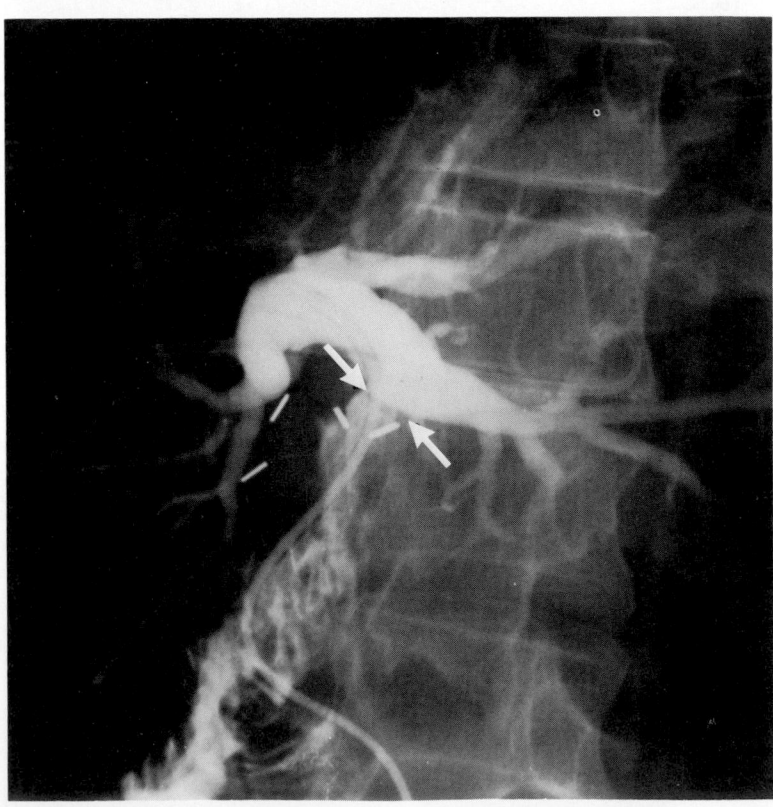

Figure 85–7. B. Roux-Y intrahepatic biliary enteric anastomosis to Segment III duct, demonstrated by means of tubography performed through a transanastomotic tube, which was removed before the patient left hospital. The exposure is oblique. The arrows indicate the wide anastomosis obtainable in such circumstances. Prolonged palliation from symptoms (18 months) was achieved without the presence of any tubal stents.

B

proaches to the left hepatic duct are possible. Nevertheless, it can occasionally be useful in allowing exposure at the hilus. Similarly, the left hepaticojejunostomy described by Longmire and Sandford in 1949 is a more difficult procedure, associated with greater blood loss and a less adequate anastomosis than the left duct approach already described.

Despite the fact that palliative measures are all that is possible in most cases, it would seem that early diagnosis and adequate treatment can have an effect on survival and that some patients may be curable.

CARCINOMA OF THE CYSTIC DUCT

This is an extremely rare lesion and usually only found at incidental operation for obstruction of the gallbladder or in the specimen removed at cholecystectomy. This author has only seen one such case and in this patient it was not clear whether total removal had been effected at initial operation. The patient was submitted to reexploration, during which the common bile duct and the common hepatic duct were excised together with adjacent lymphatic tissues and reconstruction carried out by means of hepaticojejunostomy.

In the advanced stages the disease is indistinguishable from cancer arising in the midportion of the bile ducts or the gallbladder. Nishimura et al (1975) reviewed 25 cases and recommend operative removal of the gallbladder, the entire cystic duct, and periductal lymphatics for localised lesions. If the adjacent common bile duct is involved, radical resection of the duct from the hilus to the pancreas is indicated with reconstruction by Roux-Y hepaticojejunostomy.

BENIGN TUMOURS OF THE BILE DUCTS

Nonmalignant tumours of the bile ducts are very uncommon. However, the exact incidence is not known since many are probably asymptomatic and never discovered.

The pathologic presentation of epithelial benign tumours of the bile duct are of two varieties.

A papilloma is the most common and is usually situated in the region of the papilla of Vater. The tumours, polypoid in character, are rarely larger than 2 cm in diameter and are covered by columnar cells with a minimum of associated subepithelial inflammatory change. These tumours may have a malignant potential.

Multiple papillomatosis presenting as diffuse intrahepatic and extrahepatic biliary papillomas are extremely rare. Most patients with intrahepatic papillomatosis present with obstructive jaundice, frequently intermittent and often complicated by cholangitis. This complication is a result of partial and intermittent obstruction of the bile duct by fragments from the villous tumour. In some patients, however, the only symptom has been abdominal pain. The history may extend for more than 20 years and be associated with anaemia as a result of bleeding. In only two cases has there been associated cholelithiasis and choledocholithiasis has not been reported.

Preoperative diagnosis is made radiologically and may be made more frequently now because of the widespread availability of percutaneous, retrograde, and operative cholangiography. Nonetheless, the filling defects seen have in the past been attributed to air bubbles or intrabiliary blood clots.

Although many authors have suggested that these tumours have malignant potential, histologic evidence of malignancy has been confidently described in only two cases and the author has one case of this nature occurring in association with congenital cystic disease of the liver. This is in direct contrast to the described relationship between benign papillomas and carcinoma of the ampulla of Vater referred to previously. In addition to frank carcinomatous change, areas of premalignant epithelial atypia have also been described. Recently, Gouma et al described in 1983 a case of intrahepatic bile duct papilloma associated with changes of nuclear atypia in a young man. Their review of previous publications suggests that it is reasonable to regard these lesions as of low-grade malignant potential.

Treatment of this uncommon tumour is difficult. Most patients reported have been treated by palliative surgical techniques, generally consisting of cholecystectomy, curettage, and an internal surgical drainage procedure or even T-tube drainage. However, the majority of patients have had recurrence associated with jaundice and cholangitis. Of 14 cases reviewed by Gouma et al (1983) proven recurrence occurred in 79 percent of patients in whom adequate follow-up data was available.

Attempted radical curative surgery by means of hepatic lobectomy has been reported in only five cases. One of these patients who was operated upon at the Royal Postgraduate Medical School is alive and well without recurrent tumour 1.5 years after surgery and one was reported alive 6 months after surgery with no evidence of recurrence. One patient died 6 years after resection with diffuse malignant tumours in the right lobe of the liver after initial left hepatic lobectomy. The remaining two patients had multiple papillomatosis apparently localised to the left hepatic duct at operation, but both had recurrence in the common and right hepatic duct 6 months and 3 years after lobectomy and died 5 and 6 years, respectively, after the first operation. It seems clear therefore that even major resectional surgery for this lesion has a high recurrence rate, and indeed in 12 patients for whom adequate follow-up figures were available (mean age 54 years) the mean survival was 28 months. It should be noted, however, that although no patient survived more than 6 years, the only 5-year survivals were in 3 cases submitted to radical surgery.

A reasonable approach to this rare condition includes preoperative and operative cholangiographic diagnosis, early choledochotomy, and assessment of the intrahepatic biliary tree by choledochoscopy. If the tumour is bulky, then curettage may be necessary in order to identify the sites of origin within the bile duct. Care must be taken to perform choledochoscopy of all accessible intrahepatic ducts. When the papillomatosis appears to be confined to one lobe, it seems reasonable to perform radical resection consisting of partial hepatectomy, including excision of the involved ducts. Although this does not guarantee freedom from recurrence, it offers good palliation and carries the best possibility of long-term cure in a young patient. In cases of papillomatosis involving both the right and left ducts, radical surgery is not applicable. It seems best to avoid long-term external drainage as a primary palliative manoeuvre and curettage or internal bypass is indicated. However, the prognosis should be regarded as poor if the complete removal of the tumour is impossible.

CARCINOMA OF THE BILE DUCTS

Cancer arising from the bile ducts has proved a frustrating and difficult lesion, not only in diagnosis but in management. Although the outlook in most cases is very poor, a significant number of long-term survivors after treatment have now been reported. Adenocarcinoma of the bile duct is of three main types.

The *papillary* lesion grows within the lumen of the duct and there is a tendency to produce a field change with multiple tumour sites. The *nodular* type of tumour forms a small well-localised mass involving a portion of the ductal system. In the *diffuse* variety the wall of the duct is thickened over an extensive area, the lumen narrowed, and the surrounding tissues of the hepatoduodenal ligament often inflamed. This type of lesion is very difficult to differentiate from sclerosing cholangitis.

Histologically the great majority of tumours of the bile ducts are adenocarcinomas of variable types and most are well differentiated and mucin secreting. Although fibrosis characterises the tumour, which is usually schirrhous, some have a papillary pattern. Importantly, Weinbren and Mutum (1983) have demonstrated that intracellular and extracellular mucin, identified by the Alcian blue diastase PAS procedure, is almost invariably present and helps distinguish carcinoma from the reactive fibrosis and glandular hyperplasia frequently seen in chronic benign biliary obstruction.

Natural History. The majority of patients with bile duct cancer die within 3 to 6 months of diagnosis, death being related to the effects of biliary obstruction and cholangitis, which leads to liver failure. The prognosis is worst for lesions affecting the confluence of the bile ducts and best for lesions close to the papilla.

Incidence. The incidence of bile duct tumours in large autopsy series varies from 0.01 to 0.2 percent and may constitute about 2 percent of all cancers found at autopsy. Although still a relatively rare form of cancer, 4500 new cases per annum may be expected in the United States, an incidence similar to that of carcinoma of the tongue. Indeed, there is some evidence that the incidence of the disease is increasing. However, it is also true that the advent of new diagnostic methods applicable in obstructive jaundice has led to the preoperative discovery of many more of these lesions, almost certainly misdiagnosed in the past. Thus, at the Royal Postgraduate Medical School 94 cases of cancer of the confluence at the ducts have been recorded over a 4-year period. Most tumours occur in the age group 50 to 70 years, the median age of the patients studied being 56 years. The tumour has been reported in very young patients. Males are more frequently affected than females.

Aetiology. Aetiology is unknown and there is no convincing link with the presence of gallstones. However, coincident stones are not uncommon and occurred in 33 of 94 cases seen by the author. There may be a relationship between ulcerative colitis and cholangiocarcinoma, though the number of documented patients with this combination is small. The disease may present some years after proctocolectomy. The bile duct lesion may, however, be the presenting feature, ulcerative colitis only being discovered during subsequent investigation. Roberts-Thomson et al (1973) found 29 patients with cholangiocarcinoma and ulcerative colitis and considered there was a definite consequential relationship between the two diseases. It has been suggested by others that infection and bile stasis may be important in the genesis of bile duct cancer, and a relationship has been demonstrated between congenital hepatic fibrosis or polycystic disease and the presence of these tumours. Long-standing, poorly drained choledochal cysts may also undergo neoplastic change. Infestation with *Clonorchis sinensis* is found more frequently in patients with intrahepatic cholangiocarcinoma in Southeast Asia than in control subjects.

A 1979 study by Welton et al reports that chronic typhoid carriers in New York died of hepatobiliary cancer six times more often between 1922 and 1975 than matched controls and they propose that bacterial degradation of bile salts might be the aetiologic factor.

Location. It has been suggested that cancer of the extrahepatic biliary system may be classified into three anatomic areas: the upper third, comprising the common hepatic duct and the confluence of the hepatic ducts; the middle third, comprising the common bile duct between the cystic duct and the upper border of the duodenum; and the lower third, between the upper border of the duodenum and the papilla of Vater. Diagnosis, prognosis, and treatment of these tumours varies and in this chapter the difficult group of lesions affecting the upper third of the biliary ductal system, and in particular the confluence of the bile ducts, is examined

in detail. This group presents the greatest challenge in preoperative diagnosis and, in acquisition of histologic material for confirmation of diagnosis, has the worst prognosis and is the most difficult in which to effect palliative or curative treatment.

Cholangiocarcinoma at the Confluence of the Bile Ducts

Ever since the first descriptions of adenocarcinoma at the bifurcation of the bile ducts by Altemeier et al in 1957 and Klatskin in 1965, there has been pessimism about these tumours. A number of concepts have been generally accepted:

1. The lesion is rare.
2. Preoperative diagnosis is frequently not possible.
3. Histologic confirmation is difficult to obtain.
4. Excisional therapy for cure is rarely possible.
5. Biliary–enteric anastomosis is very difficult for palliation and intubation is preferable.

Over the last 5 years, however, in a concentrated experience of high bile duct cancers, a policy of detailed preoperative investigation to define the extent of the lesion, an aggressive surgical approach directed at excision whenever possible and an appraisal of tubal drainage compared with cholangio–enteric anastomoses have been performed. The results of this study have allowed challenge of these assumptions. It is possible now to say that:

1. Preoperative diagnosis is nearly always possible, the only real difficulty arising in relation to differentiation from localised or diffuse sclerosing cholangitis and rarely from localised benign stricture associated with gallstone disease.
2. Histologic and/or cytologic material is usually obtainable for diagnosis.
3. Preoperative cholangiography combined with angiography gives an excellent guide to the extent of tumour and to irresectability.
4. Resection can be accomplished with an acceptable postoperative mortality in about 20 percent of cases.
5. Biliary–enteric anastomosis is often possible and is probably preferable to intubational methods.

These points are discussed in the following.

Diagnosis. There are no characteristic early symptoms and initial complaints are insidious.

Upper abdominal discomfort or pain, pruritus, anorexia, malaise, and weight loss are frequent and may precede the onset of jaundice by weeks or months. Jaundice, once it occurs, is usually unremitting and is the usual feature leading to investigation, although in cases affecting one or the other hepatic duct jaundice may be a late feature, the presence of the disease being reflected only by a raised serum alkaline phosphatase. Cholangitis and abscess formation may occur in obstructed segments of the liver. Unilateral lobar atrophy may be found, especially if the tumour invades the portal blood supply to the obstructed segment. The gallbladder is never palpable and is found collapsed and empty at operation.

The diagnosis of hilar cholangiocarcinoma is frequently not made in patients submitted to laparotomy for obstructive jaundice. Thus, in 9 of 13 cases recorded by Klatskin (1965) and in 8 of 25 cases reported by Longmire (1977), the true nature of the obstruction was not identified at initial operative biliary exploration for obstructive jaundice. Similarly of 37 patients referred to the Royal Postgraduate Medical School, London, between January 1980 and May 1981, 5 had been explored elsewhere and no diagnosis reached. By contrast, the diagnosis was made in 21 of these patients in whom PTC was undertaken as an initial procedure. Indeed, the dramatic advance in accurate preoperative diagnosis of obstructive jaundice that has occurred since the early 1970s has led to a situation where laparotomy should not be carried out without preoperative cholangiographic delineation of the site, nature and extent of any obstructing lesion. An ordered use of ultrasonography, fine-needle PTC, and endoscopic retrograde cholangiopancreatography (ERCP) should be successful in imaging the obstructive lesion in nearly all cases. In particular, fine-needle PTC is successful in 100 percent of cases with dilated ducts and is the most useful and accurate technique in hilar cholangiocarcinoma (Figs. 85–8A,B). It is important, however, not to accept a simple cholangiographic diagnosis, but to pursue the examination until the entire intrahepatic biliary tree on both left and right sides has been outlined, since this gives a valuable guide to resectability and to later operative approaches. The extent of ductal disease and multicentricity may be revealed by intraoperative choledochoscopic examination, which is desirable in all cases, although this may not be

possible in sclerosing and nodular high bile duct lesions, which occlude the duct and make passage of the choledochoscope difficult.

The major diagnostic problem is the differential diagnosis between cholangiocarcinoma and sclerosing cholangitis. It might be thought that real diagnostic difficulty only exists in differentiating sclerosing cholangitis from cholangiocarcinoma in its diffuse form. However, in four recent cases appearances at the hilus of the liver were those of malignant obstruction, with a stricture localised to the confluence of the ducts without diffuse involvement, either of the common bile duct or intrahepatic ducts. Radical excision of the obstructing lesion was carried out and at histology proved to represent a benign sclerosing lesion. One of these patients subsequently developed further benign strictures within the left and right hepatic ductal systems, proximal to the original cholangio–enteric anastomosis, and required further operation. Thus, the newer diagnostic means available may now detect cases of benign stricture localised to a small area of the biliary tree and closely resembling the focal type of cholangiocarcinoma. Similarly, localised benign strictures may occur in association with cholelithiasis and may present difficulty. Primary biliary cirrhosis may also be associated with narrowing of ducts at the hilus of the liver, but this is usually of a more tapering nature when seen at cholangiography than the common abrupt lesion seen in carcinoma.

Aspiration cytology is now being employed in an attempt to obtain preoperative cytologic diagnosis. A fine needle is passed into the suspect area under radiologic control. For small hilar lesions it is preferable to use the PTC as a guide, but ultrasonography can also be successful in directing the needle. A combination of cytology and histology of specimens obtained at operation has yielded a positive diagnosis in 91 of 94 recent cases at the Royal Postgraduate Medical School.

Assessment of the Extent of Tumour. Although it has been recognised that cholangiocarcinomas at the hilus are small and apparently well localised, few authors have remarked on the involvement of adjacent blood vessels and the extent of spread along the ducts into the hepatic parenchyma. These factors compromise complete excision of the tumour without extensive resection of the liver and its blood supply.

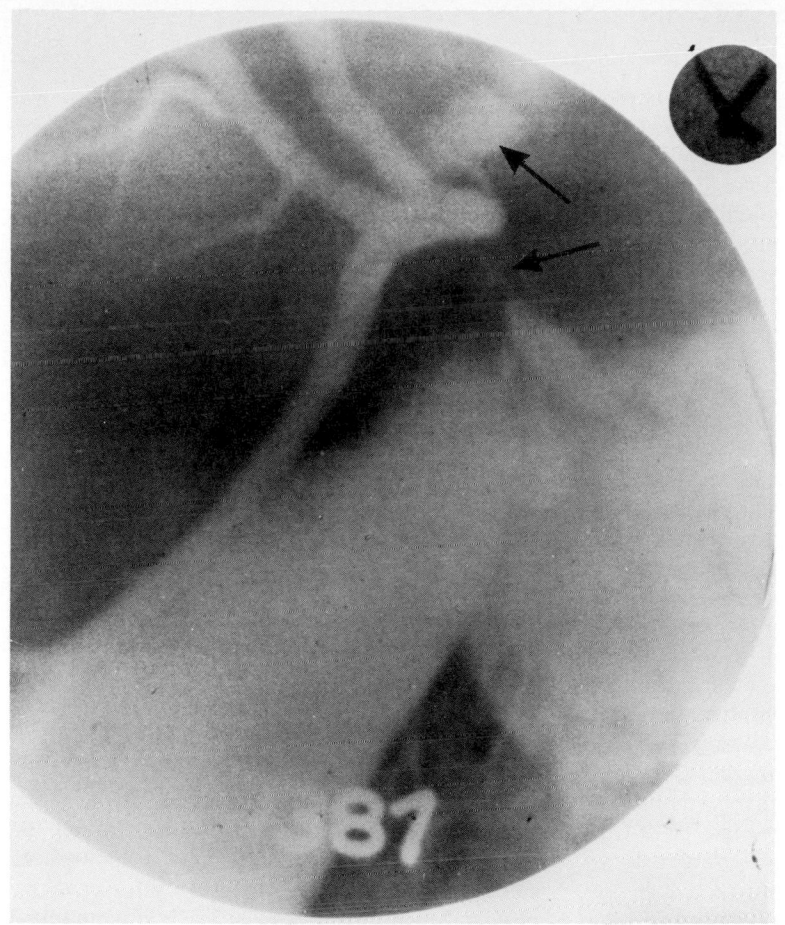

A

Figure 85–8. **A.** Cholangiogram showing ducts at the hilus of the liver obtained after endoscopic retrograde injection. Film sent with the patient referred for possible resection of cholangiocarcinoma. Note the apparently localised small stricture at the confluence (*arrows*).

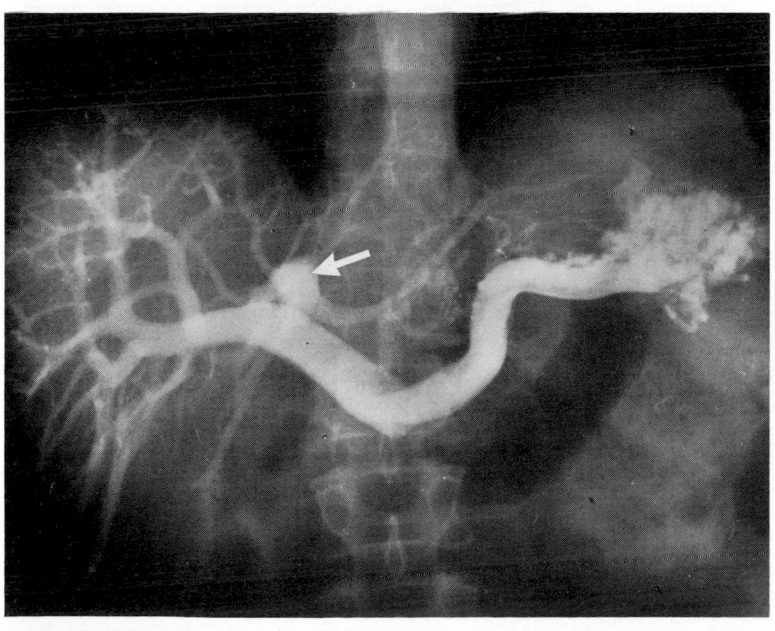

B

Figure 85–8. **B.** Splenovenogram in the same patient reveals involvement of the left branch of the portal vein. Thus an apparently small tumour is accompanied by extensive vascular involvement. There was also involvement of the right branch of the hepatic artery. Tumour was not resected.

Because of the low propensity for distant spread and because it is very difficult to be sure at surgery of the extent of the involvement of vessels, an approach aimed at full radiologic diagnosis and an effort to correlate radiologic findings with subsequent findings and procedures at operation has been made.

In an initial study, arteriographic and venographic changes in *a variety* of intrahepatic tumours and tumours affecting the confluence of the bile ducts, were examined. Involvement of the main stem portal vein *or* contralateral involvement of the hepatic artery to one side of the liver and the portal vein to the other were always associated with irresectability. Unilateral involvement of the artery or the vein or both were compatible with resection. During this study several cases with apparently extensive stricture shown at cholangiography that proved resectable for potential cure were encountered (Figs. 85–8A,B). One such patient is alive 5 years after surgery, symptom free, and without known recurrence. Conversely, patients with small strictures on cholangiography who had quite extensive vascular involvement precluding resection were found (Figs. 85–9A,B). Thus the length of the biliary stricture is an insufficient guide to resectability. More recently, 37 consecutive patients treated in London over a 17-month period have been studied by Voyles et al in 1982. Detailed cholangiographic studies have been related to selective hepatic arteriography and portal venography. PTC was performed using the fine-needle technique and frequently separate punctures were necessary to fill segmentally occluded ducts and display the entire biliary tree. Main stem aortography with selective coeliac and superior mesenteric studies were obtained and the venous phase of the splenic arteriogram was used to provide indirect portography. In a few patients direct percutaneous splenic portography was performed. With the exception of three with terminal disease, all patients underwent subsequent laparotomy, and an assessment of resectability was made on the basis of the operative and radiologic findings.

In all, 13 of 37 patients were assessed to be potentially resectable after cholangiography and angiography. Of these 13, 5 were resected with histologically free margins. Resection was technically feasible in three additional patients, who were considered unfit for hepatic resection on the grounds of age and general medical condi-tion, and a palliative drainage procedure was performed. In the remaining five patients, resection was precluded by the laparotomy findings of extensive liver involvement including the inferior vena cava in two and distant metastases in three (omentum, 1; nodes, 2).

These studies have allowed judgement of *irresectability* at preoperative investigation by the following criteria:

1. Cholangiographic display of bilateral intrahepatic bile duct spread of the disease so extensive as to preclude resection (or multifocal disease)
2. Involvement of the main trunk of the portal vein
3. Involvement of both branches of the portal vein or bilateral involvement of the hepatic artery and portal vein
4. A combination of vascular involvement to one side of the liver with extensive ductal involvement on the other, so that it is impossible to excise the tumour and preserve a vascularised remnant of liver

Inaccuracies in this approach include the fact that lymph node metastases are not detected and that the caudate lobe is not well visualised. Furthermore, inferior vena cavography is difficult to assess, since involvement of the vena cava, although unusual, tends to be anterior in the region of the caudate lobe and may not show on x-ray. CT scanning may improve assessment in the future.

In addition, in three recent cases it has been possible to carry out extensive hepatic resection of the right or left liver with excision of hilar tumour involving the bifurcation of the portal vein. Cholangiography on its own has one further important advantage in allowing assessment of the possibilities for palliative treatment. We have increasingly employed biliary–enteric anastomosis rather than tubal drainage, and found cholangiography extremely valuable in demonstrating preoperatively the likely ducts available for anastomosis (see the following).

Treatment Options. The place of resection for attempted cure of tumours at the confluence of the bile duct is strongly debated, as are resectability and mortality rates. Experience with resection of hilar cholangiocarcinoma is small. Most surgeons, even in specialist centres, have found the majority to be irresectable. Thus,

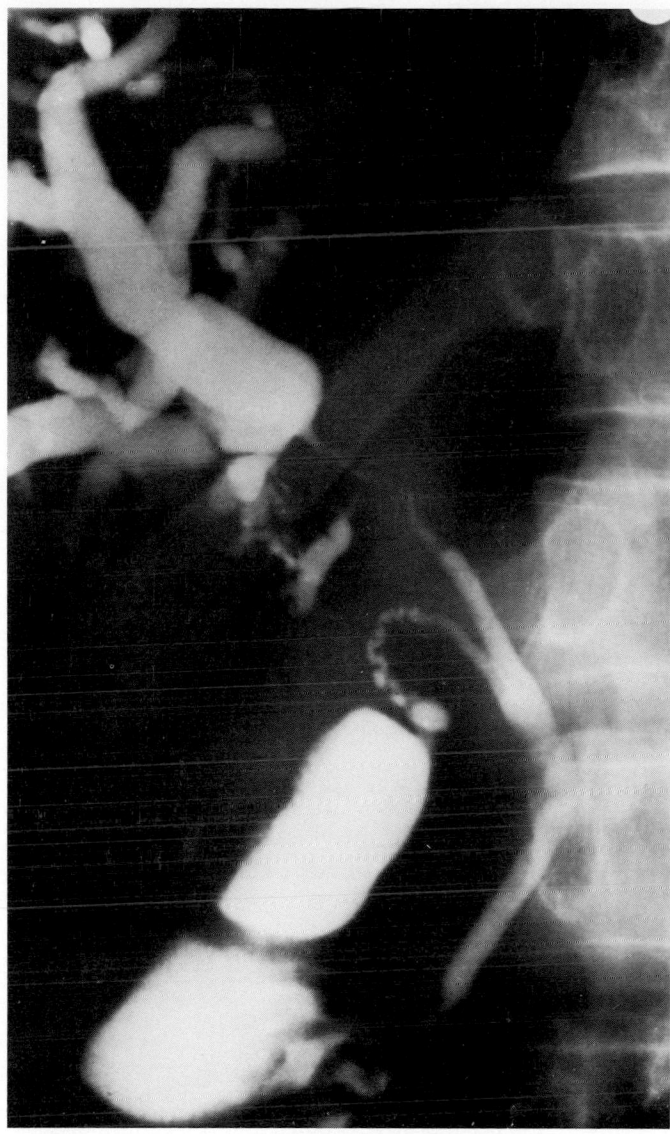

Figure 85–9. A. Percutaneous transhepatic cholangiogram reveals extensive tumour at the confluence of the bile ducts and extending into the right hepatic duct. The left hepatic duct was later shown to be not involved except at the confluence.

A

Longmire was only able to resect 6 of 33 lesions and tumour excision was combined with hepatic resection in but two of these. Similarly Smith (1981) treated 33 cases in 33 years and excised only 5. In none of these was hepatic resection stated to be a part of the procedure. Tompkins and colleagues (1981) have reported 47 cases seen over 24 years in whom resection was only possible in 22 (hepatic resection being part of the procedure in 5). The resectability rate of 47 percent in this latter series falls within the reported range for hilar tumours, figures vary-

ing from 5 to 58 percent. Operative mortality rates range from 0 to 50 percent. The author has analysed 1406 cases of hilar cholangiocarcinoma in 47 reports; 258 cases were resected, with an operative mortality of 18.3 percent. However, some series contain a high proportion of patients with simple excision of the tumour, as opposed to excision of the tumour combined with hepatic resection. In addition, it should be clearly appreciated that the risk of drainage operations in the treatment of biliary tract obstruction is high, with a reported operative mor-

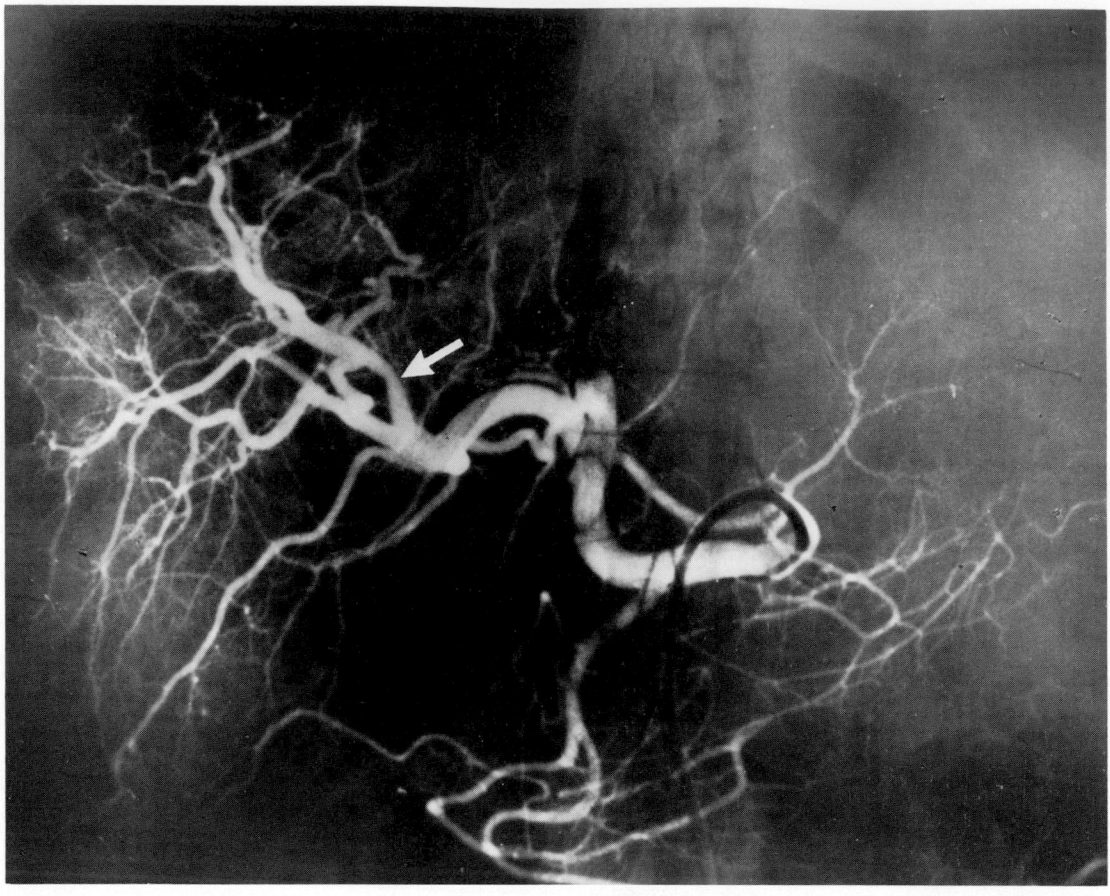

B

Figure 85–9. B. Selective hepatic arteriogram revealing involvement of the right hepatic artery (*arrow*). The left branch of the portal vein was not compromised. Treatment was by means of extended right hepatic lobectomy (same case as Fig. 85–11B).

tality of 20 percent or more. Indeed even nonoperative endoscopic or percutaneous intubational methods for the relief of obstructive jaundice are associated with a significant morbidity and a 30-day hospital mortality of 20 to 53 percent (Table 85–1).

Longmire (1973), in an anatomic and clinical study, recognised that involvement of the vessels was the limiting factor to resection in many instances. He postulated several methods for resection with vascular reconstruction and reported a case. Encouraged by reports of success for resection, patients have been approached in the Hepatobiliary Unit at the Royal Postgraduate Medical School with the objective of resection whenever possible as indicated by the preoperative studies and the general status of the patient.

In this author's experience of 94 patients (median age 56.5 years) resection has been carried out in 18 (20 percent). In six patients submitted to local excision of the tumour there was no mortality. Twelve patients required major liver resection to achieve tumour clearance. In nine patients extended right hepatic lobectomy and in three patients left hepatic lobectomy were carried out. Of the patients submitted to hepatic resection, nine had involvement of the portal vein and in three of these complete excision of the bifurcation was carried out with subsequent direct anastomosis of the main trunk of the portal vein to its own left branch.

TABLE 85–1. PERCUTANEOUS AND
ENDOSCOPIC DRAINAGE OF MALIGNANT
BILE DUCT OBSTRUCTION

	30-Day Mortality (%)
Percutaneous:	
Dooley et al (1981)	34
Burcharth et al (1981)	30
Mueller et al (1982)	33
Lorelius et al (1982)	52
Endoscopic:	
Cotton (1982)	20
Hagenmüller et al (1982)	53
Tytgat et al (1983)	24 [a]

[a] Hilar tumours.

Techniques of Resection

The liver should be fully exposed, usually through a bilateral subcostal incision. The ligamentum teres is held on a suture and the umbilical fissure of the liver defined. Since the key dissection behind the bile duct cannot be carried out until the bile duct is divided, the first step in the procedure is mobilisation of the duodenum and identification and transection of the bile duct in the immediate supraduodenal region. The lower bile duct is closed with a catgut suture; the whole common bile duct is turned upward with a wide clearance from the underlying vessels and mobilisation of the supraduodenal and cystic lymph nodes. As the dissection proceeds, the gallbladder is mobilised from its fossa and turned medially and upward together with the common bile duct and common hepatic duct, serially exposing the tissues lying behind the duct and working immediately in front of the portal vein and hepatic artery (Fig. 85–10A). By this means the tumour can be approached from below and clearance established from the underlying vessels and particularly from the portal vein.

The hilar plate is incised and the left bile duct and hilus lowered from the undersurface of the liver. This allows identification of the right and left ductal system and local resection. Reconstruction is by means of hepaticojejunostomy Roux-Y using the techniques described by Voyles and Blumgart in 1982 and Blumgart and Kelley in 1983.

If there is portal venous involvement either of the right branch or left branch of the portal vein then the vein is identified above and below the involved portion and clamps are applied. This allows excision of the right or left lobe of the liver together with the involved portion of the portal vein. Reconstruction is by means of end-to-end anastomosis between the main trunk of the portal vein and its own right or left branch (Figs. 85–10A,B). Once this has been done and the specimen removed using standard techniques of hepatic resection, hepaticojejunostomy is performed to the remnant (Figs. 85–11A,B).

Results. Two of the 12 patients submitted to hepatic resection died of uncontrolled sepsis and its sequelae within 30 days of surgery and a third patient died 9 weeks after surgery, also of sepsis. Two of these three patients had been submitted to percutaneous transhepatic drainage procedures previously and both died of infection due to organisms acquired during drainage. The overall 30-day hospital mortality for patients submitted to radical excision for cure was 11 percent, there being no mortality for local resection and a 16.5 percent mortality rate for those patients in whom major liver resection was required (Table 85–2). Eleven of the 18 patients submitted to resection had no previous surgery or percutaneous drainage or evidence of infected bile. Of these, six of whom had major hepatic resection including excision and reconstruction of the bifurcation of the portal vein in two cases, only one died in hospital (mortality 9 percent). On the other hand, of the seven patients who had been submitted to previous surgery or percutaneous drainage, two (28.5 percent) died as a result of infection from organisms acquired during the period of previous percutaneous decompression.

Long-term results cannot yet be reported. However, of the 18 patients who underwent potentially curative resection, 15 left the hospital, the mean survival for the entire group being 17 months. Eight patients died at intervals ranging from 6 to 28 months, with a mean survival of 13 months. Two of these patients died at 7 and 9 months of causes unrelated to cholangiocarcinoma, but the remainder died of the effects of recurrent tumour. Seven patients submitted to resection are alive, with a mean survival of 22.2 months (range 9 to 58 months). The longest survivor in this group had a tumour that was involving the right branch of the portal vein and was submitted to excision of the tumour with extended right hepatic lobectomy

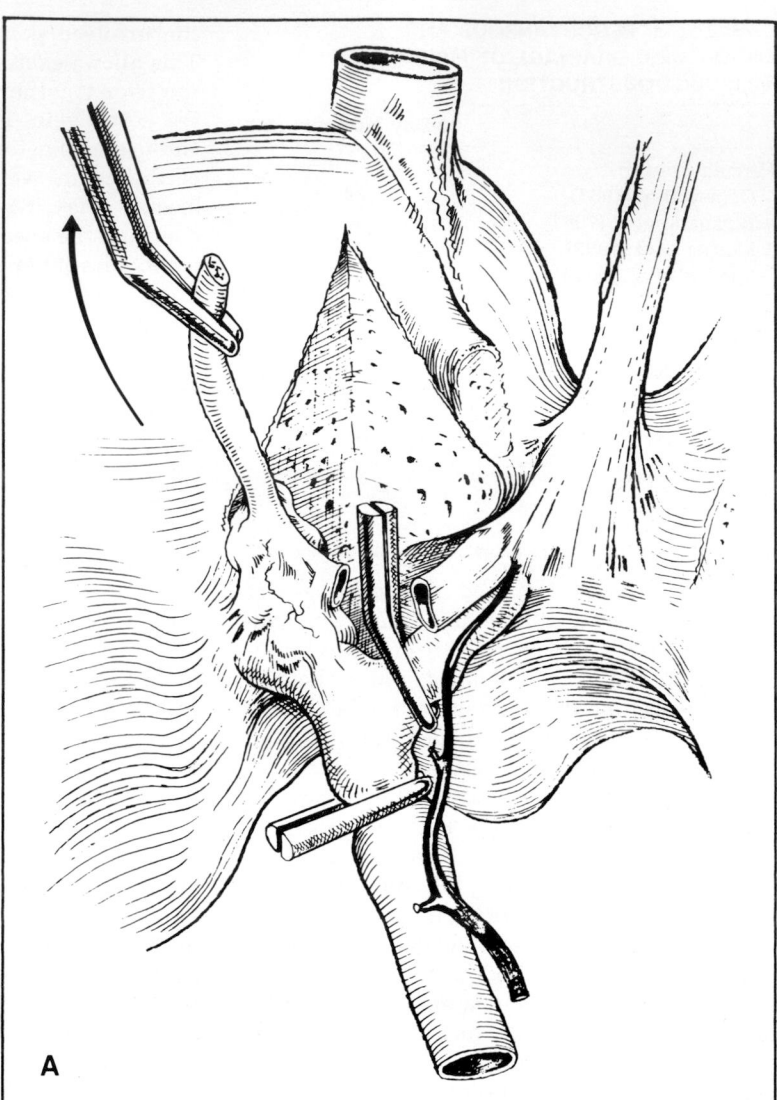

Figure 85–10. A. Tumour is shown involving the portal vein close to the bifurcation. The common bile duct has been dissected above the duodenum and turned up so as to allow an approach to the vessels behind the ducts. Clamps can be applied in this situation, which illustrates a stage of extended right hepatic lobectomy together with removal of the bifurcation of the portal vein.

A

and reconstruction by hepaticojejunostomy to the liver remnant.

In the future it is likely that more cases will be diagnosed primarily and not be submitted to unnecessary initial operative procedures. Better preoperative preparation, possibly using percutaneous transhepatic drainage, and an ordered operative strategy will allow better selection of patients for resectional surgery and results should improve. Few others have pursued a policy of radical excision of hilar cholangiocarcinoma but some, and in particular workers in Sweden and France, agree with the concept and make a case for tumour excision,

either for potential cure or for palliation. Thus, Launois (1979) reports 11 patients in whom tumour resection was carried out, followed by reconstruction of the biliary tree. All were adenocarcinomas affecting the hilus. Four of these 11 had simple hepatic duct resection, but in the others some form of hepatic lobectomy was necessary. There were two postoperative deaths. The mean survival time for the remaining nine patients was 1.5 years, but 5 were alive at intervals up to 3.25 years. Launois found these results to be superior to his own earlier experience, during which palliative decompression was carried out. Similarly, Bengmark's group

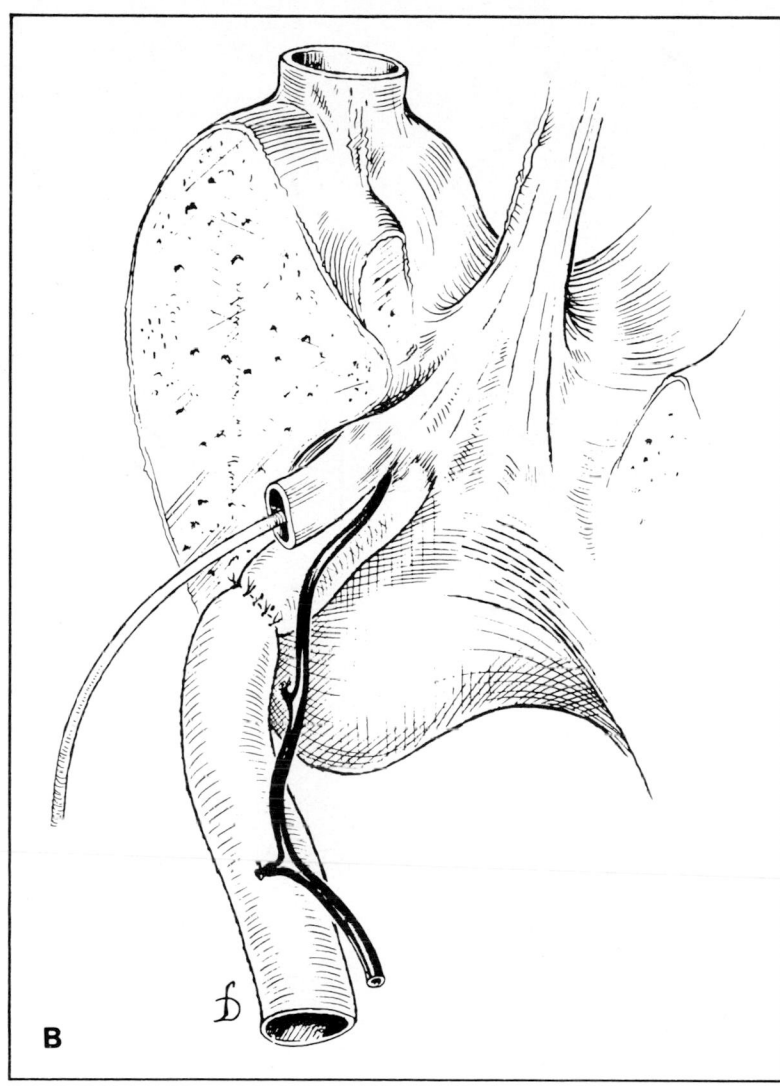

B

Figure 85–10. B. Direct end-to-end anastomosis of the portal vein. The specimen has been removed. Left hepatic duct exposed for anastomosis.

in Lund (1980) records 16 of 34 hilar tumours resected. The extent of the lesions in this study was apparently less than that in the French report or in this author's series, and local invasion of the hepatic artery or portal vein was regarded as excluding radical surgery. Nevertheless, the results in terms of quality of life and survival were better for patients submitted to resection than for bypass. Similar results are reported by Skoog and Thoren (1982). Clearly, it is very difficult to compare patients submitted to resection with those submitted to palliative operation only, since the extent of tumour is almost certainly less in the former group, and the general status of the patients almost certainly better. Indeed there are no controlled studies of resection as opposed to palliative bypass or intubation. However, Beazley et al (1983) at the Royal Postgraduate Medical School compared a series of 16 patients submitted to resection, with 15 cases subjected to palliative bypass or intubation. The patients were matched for age, and extent of local disease, but patients in the palliated group were not subjected to resection on the grounds of positive nodes or metastases found at laparotomy, because the combination of angiographic and cholangiographic features rendered them irresectable or because it was judged that the extent of surgery required to affect clearance involved too great a risk in

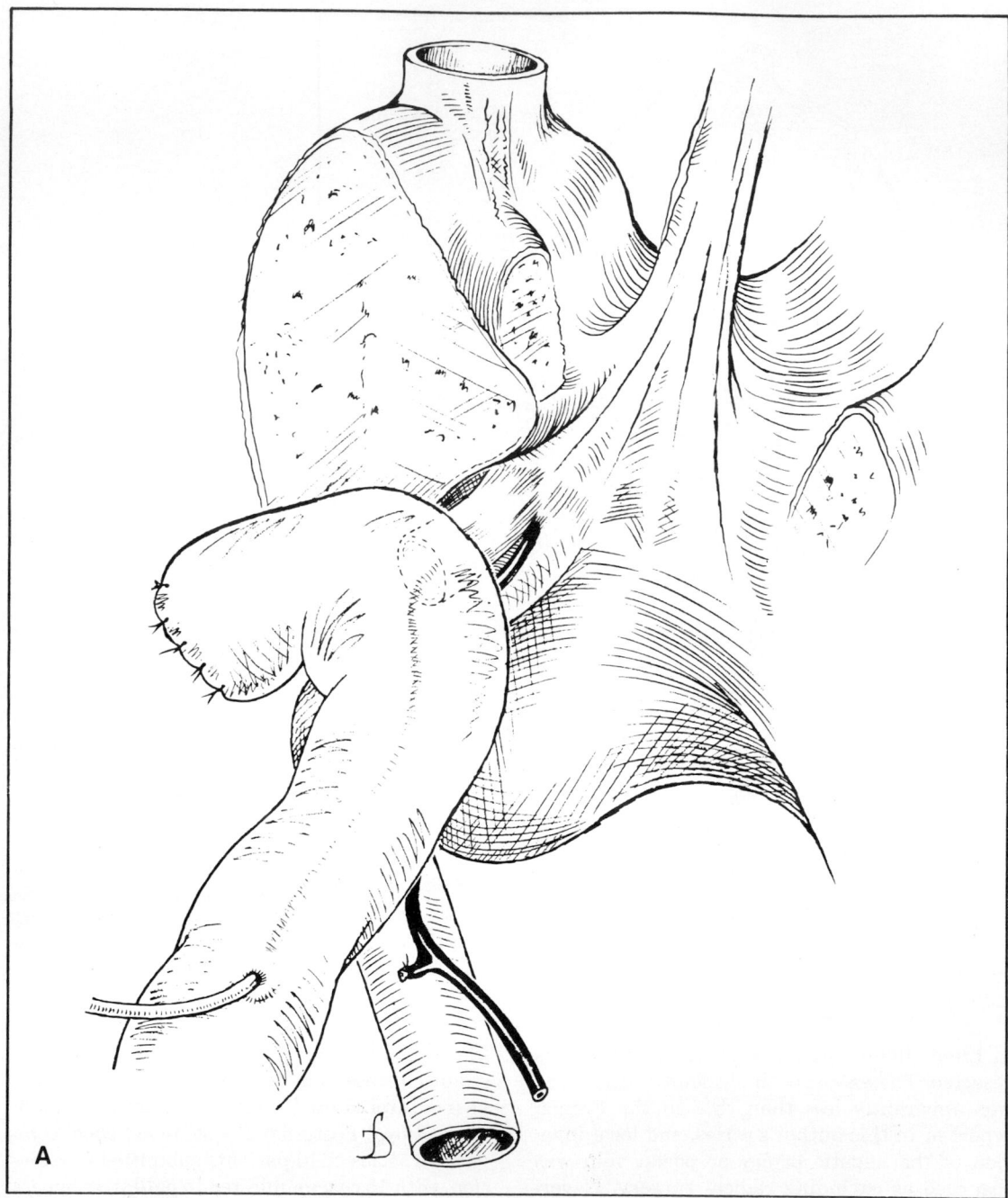

A

Figure 85–11. A. Reconstruction by means of hepaticojejunostomy Roux-Y over a transanastomotic tube which is removed soon after operation. The sketch illustrates an anastomosis similar to that shown in Figure 85–11B.

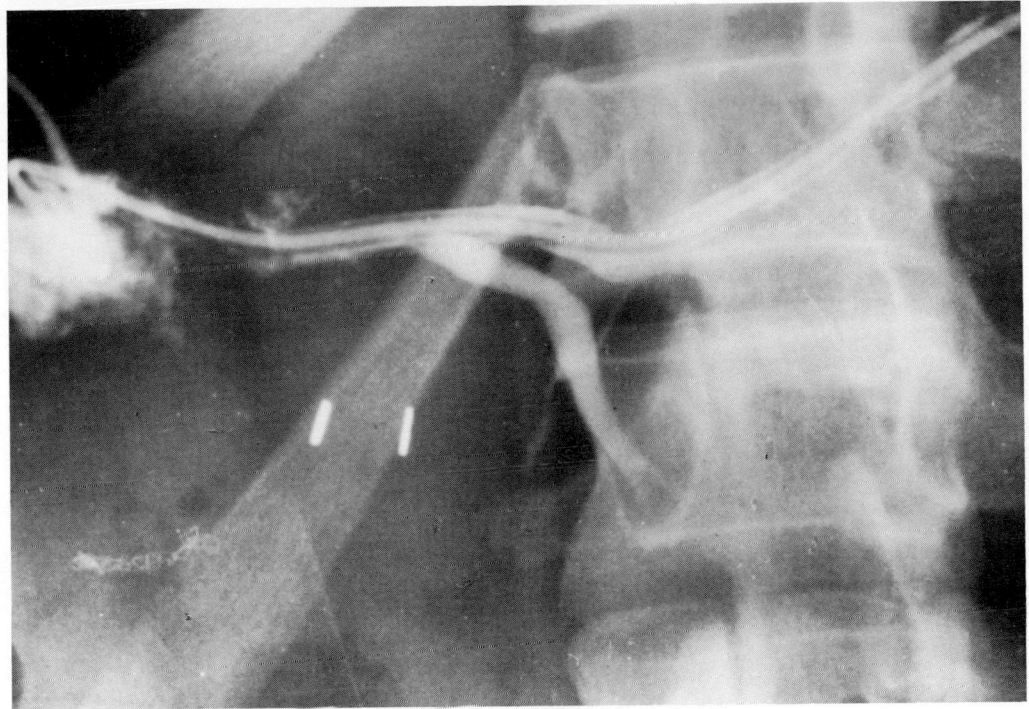

B

Figure 85–11. B. Tubogram showing hepaticojejunostomy to left hepatic duct at the point of origin of Segments II and III ducts. Excellent results were achieved with a symptom-free survival at five years (same case as Figs. 85–9A,B).

some cases. The resected group fared better than the palliated group in every respect, the operative (30-day hospital) mortality, quality of life and survival being superior for resection.

It should be noted that these results have been achieved even though major hepatic resection was necessary in a high proportion of patients, and that many had been submitted to previous surgery or intubation, which has been shown to influence the outcome adversely. This is important and there should be caution in pro-

TABLE 85–2. RADICAL RESECTION FOR HILAR CHOLANGIOCARCINOMA: 30-DAY MORTALITY

	No. of Patients	Died	(%)
Local resection	6	0	0
Major liver resection	12	2	16.5
Total	18	2	11

(*Source: Adapted from Blumgart et al, 1984, with permission.*)

ceeding to surgical, endoscopic, or percutaneous intubational approaches in patients who may be resectable, since such methods may compromise the results of subsequent attempts at curative or palliative bypass surgery. Claims as to the beneficial effects of intubation prior to surgery in order to ameliorate the adverse pathophysiologic effects of jaundice have also not been substantiated. A controlled clinical trial is presently in progress at Hammersmith Hospital and does not lend support to such an approach.

It is important not to deny a patient who can tolerate operation the possibility of cure or the best possible palliation, and not simply resort to surgical intubational methods or bypass as a panacea.

Other Forms of Treatment

The majority of patients with hilar cholangiocarcinoma will not be suitable for resection and many will be old or have coincident disease. The options open in the management of this group of patients are either no treatment at all or some form of biliary decompression, either by means of biliary–enteric anastomosis or by the use of a transtumour tube allowing relief of biliary obstruction. Bypass or intubation may be combined with radiotherapeutic approaches.

Assessment of the results of such palliative methods is no less difficult than for resection. A major problem is that many series of patients submitted to surgical decompression contain some patients who might have been suitable for resection, and therefore constitute a better risk group, and others possibly too ill to tolerate any form of treatment at all. In many series histologic confirmation of the nature of the stricture has not been available or indeed has often not been sought. More recently, percutaneous transhepatic and endoscopic intubational techniques have allowed biliary decompression without laparotomy, and these methods are being used for definitive treatment in some cases without due consideration as to the possibility of resection, or indeed as to whether biliary–enteric bypass might provide a better form of palliation.

The "U"-tube technique described by Praderi (1963, 1964, 1971) and popularised by Terblanche (1972, 1973) has been utilised by many. A long tube with appropriately placed side holes is passed through the tumour into the intrahepatic ducts, out through the liver parenchyma, and then out through the anterior abdominal wall to the exterior. The lower end of the tube

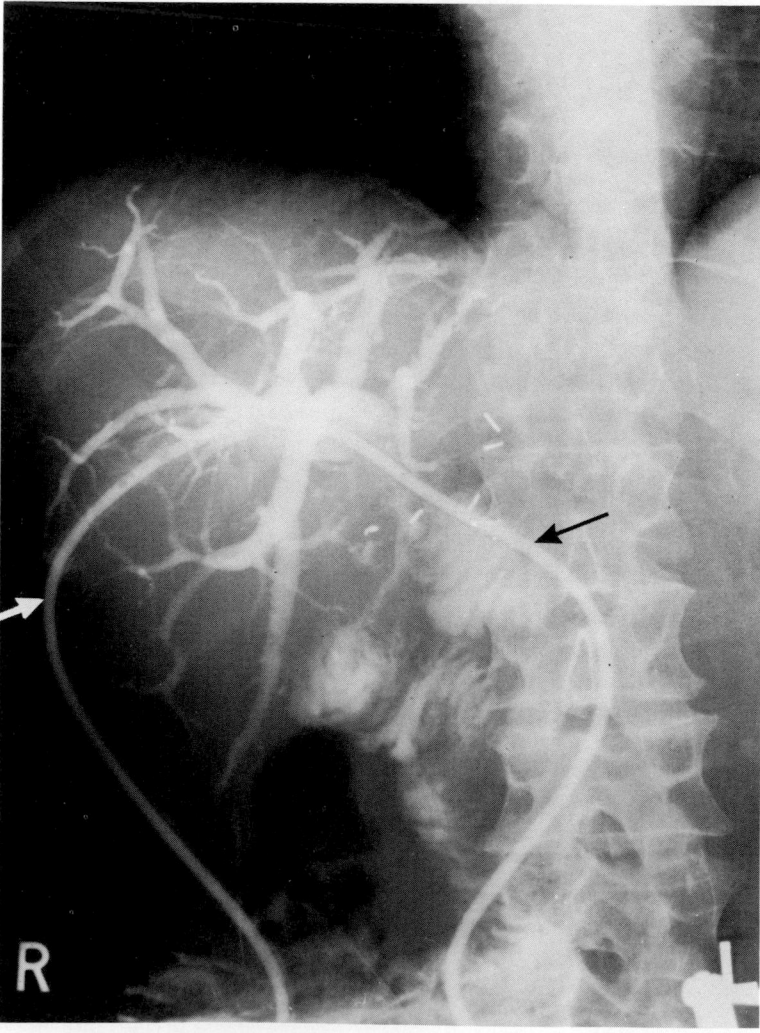

Figure 85–12. Tubogram obtained in the postoperative period to illustrate U-tube passing across inoperable carcinoma at the confluence of the bile ducts. The tube passes from the skin and then upward through the dome of the liver (*white arrow*) in a transhepatic fashion, traverses the bile ducts where there are holes to provide drainage, passes across the tumour and then down, in this instance into a Roux-Y loop where further holes allow egress of bile (*black arrow*). The tube then continues and is delivered transjejunally to the skin surface, thus forming a complete loop or U-tube. This tube can be replaced readily (see text).

is also delivered at the skin. The tube thus traverses the tumour and allows drainage of bile into the gut (Fig. 85–12). The tube can be readily washed out and can be replaced by attaching another tube to one end and pulling it through the established sinus track. The procedure may be combined with a hepaticojejunostomy Roux-Y rather than bringing the lower end out through the common bile duct. This is a preferable approach, particularly if bilateral tubes are to be employed, since the bile ducts are seldom big enough to harbour two such tubes. There is no doubt that the method does give palliation, sometimes for several years, in a proportion of patients. Thus Longmire (1977) reports relief of jaundice in 15 patients, partial relief in 9, but no relief at all in 6. One patient lived 4.5 years after operation but it is not stated that histologic confirmation was obtained. Terblanche (1979) has stated disbelief that resection should not be done for carcinoma in the area of the confluence of the bile duct; intubation of these tumours and treatment with radiotherapy is recommended. In a recent update (1981) he reported that 2 of 15 patients treated by this method survived 8 and 10 years and of the 13 who died the longest survivor was 5 years. However, there is doubt that these were biopsy-proven carcinoma of the bile ducts and, indeed, Terblanche (1983) has recently indicated that the two longest survivors in his series did not have tissue diagnosis. It is important that care is taken to prove the diagnosis before claims of long survival after intubation can be accepted. Unfortunately, not only is histologic confirmation of tumour lacking in many series, but, as pointed out earlier in this chapter, benign localised strictures do occur. There are also other difficulties in the use of the U-tube that require consideration.

Firstly, they are not always easy to place, and this is particularly true in the patient with a lesion extending for some distance into the biliary tree, where it is easy to create a false passage during dilatation of the narrow track through the tumour. This is unfortunate because this is also precisely the type of case in which biliary–enteric anastomosis may not be possible.

Secondly, there may be difficulty in bringing the lower end of the U-tube through the bile duct distal to the tumour, especially if the duct is small, or if bilateral tubes are inserted. This may be overcome by combined use of a hepaticojejunostomy Roux-Y with a transhepatic tube, as described above.

Thirdly, there is a significant incidence of postoperative fistula formation along the tube track that may be troublesome in some patients.

Finally, and most importantly, despite efforts to maintain sterility these tubes invariably become infected, and recurrent, low-grade cholangitis and progressive liver damage is the fate of nearly all the patients. Alternative methods of tubal drainage, such as the placement of a transhepatic endoprosthesis introduced peroperatively or the more recently introduced percutaneous transhepatic drainage or endoprosthesis, have similar disadvantages and carry with them the potential for serious infection and for the latter procedures a 30-day hospital mortality of at least 20 percent (Table 85–1). Endoscopically-placed endoprostheses can now be used to afford biliary decompression, and although they are successfully placed in a high proportion of cases with low lesions they are not yet widely applicable to lesions at the confluence, where the success rate for relief of jaundice is no greater than 70 percent of cases and the operative and 30-day hospital mortality high (Table 85–1). Evander and colleagues (1980), in a series of 53 palliatively treated patients, submitted 40 to some form of biliary drainage, the majority by a percutaneous transhepatic technique. The median survival time was only 2.5 months. It is clear that the results of nonoperative techniques for biliary decompression in biliary cancer have yet to show improvement over those obtained by surgical approaches. At Hammersmith Hospital this author's results for operative relief of biliary obstruction due to hilar cholangiocarcinoma by means of tubal drainage (usually U-tube) or biliary–enteric anastomosis have also been disappointing. In a series of 49 patients (median age 59 years) submitted to operative biliary–enteric or tubal drainage we had a hospital mortality of 33 percent accompanied by a significant morbidity in the form of immediate postoperative fistula formation and cholangitis, and a mean survival time of 8.5 months. Launois (1979) surveyed the collected results of 12 reports of palliative biliary–jejunal anastomoses, including his own patient, and found that the postoperative death rate was 40 percent and the mean survival only 7 months. Biliary fistulation and cholangitis were the most frequent complications and cholangitis the most lethal. It is important to note that included within this survey were satisfactory results from three centres. Like Launois, this author has been unable to obtain good results, especially in the older patient with extensive lesions.

However, more recently, with liberal use of the round ligament approach (Figs. 85–3 through 85–7), 28 patients have been operated, with a mortality of 21 percent and, indeed, if the patients who were never submitted to surgery or nonsurgical intubation before referral are studied the mortality is only 18 percent.

A new method for "exoendoprosthesis" has been recently developed, the proximal end of a transhepatic tube being buried beneath the skin where it can be readily recovered if necessary at a later time for washing or drainage. This may avoid the potential avenue for exogenous infection that exists with externally placed tubes.

A number of authors have used external irradiation in conjunction with tubal placement, and some long-term survivors have been reported. Our own experience has been similar and we have had one survivor for 2 years after external beam irradiation and tubal placement in a histologically proven bile duct carcinoma at the hilus of the liver. However, we have encountered severe complications, including duodenal stenosis and severe irradiation duodenitis with intractable GI bleeding in three patients. More recently a small group of patients at King's College Hospital, London, have been treated by Fletcher and colleagues (1981) by means of an iridium-192 wire passed down a U-tube. This gives the advantage of high-dose local irradiation without the side effects mentioned above. Six of eight patients so managed were alive up to 23 months after treatment, but as with all tubal drainage systems maintenance of drainage was a problem and tubes required changing in several patients. In two, bile drainage was not achieved with both patients dying at 6 and 22 months from a combination of cholangitis and tumour extension. Tumour recurrence causing further biliary obstruction occurred in one patient. Two patients are alive and well nearly 2 years after treatment. The authors point out that cholangitis is likely to remain a problem in patients so treated and this is in keeping with other experiences with tubal drainage.

Elderly patients with extensive tumours have poor results regardless of the method of treatment and certainly a short period of life

complicated by an external tube, whether passed preoperatively or percutaneously, with a high risk of infection, seems hardly worthwhile. It may well be that full cholangiographic studies to delineate the tumour extent and possibly no treatment at all would be the best approach for some elderly infirm patients. The use of percutaneously placed endoprostheses appears a more attractive option in such cases, but in the management of obstructive jaundice even this procedure carries a high mortality.

In conclusion, hilar cholangiocarcinoma continues to pose major problems, but recent advances in the use of diagnostic methods should allow preoperative diagnosis in most cases. An ordered use of cholangiography combined with angiographic techniques will give an excellent index of irresectability and of the anatomic possibilities for biliary–enteric anastomosis, which is almost certainly superior to any form of tubal drainage. Transhepatic intubational techniques may allow preparation of some patients for resectional surgery, but the true benefits of such preoperative decompression await the results of controlled studies. Local irradiation may have a place in the management of these tumours.

Perhaps the most important points to emphasize are that resection may be carried out in up to 20 percent of patients with an acceptable operative mortality. Patients should not be submitted to intubational methods of decompression, whether operative or percutaneous, and thus denied a chance for cure, without careful studies to define their selection. The well-tried surgical dictum that in malignant disease of the GI tract it is better to remove tumour with restoration of continuity as the best form of palliation and possible cure seems to hold true for cholangiocarcinoma at the hilum of the liver and claims for other approaches that leave tumour in situ require substantiation.

Tumours in the Mid- and Low Common Bile Duct

Some 40 percent of bile duct cancers occur in the mid- or low bile duct. These tumours are best managed by surgical excision and this is possible in many such cases.

Occasionally if a tumour is involving the midportion of the bile duct, local resection with anastomosis or reconstruction by means of a Roux-Y loop is sufficient, but most such lesions, if resectable, require wide excision, including the head of the pancreas. Those tumours arising in the immediate supraduodenal portion of the bile duct, its intrapancreatic portion, or in direct relation to the papilla are conveniently considered along with true ampullary tumours.

It is not clearly understood that the presentation of these lesions may be with intermittent or indeed sometimes with only one attack of jaundice, that the pain may be of a dyspeptic nature, and that the patient may present with haematemesis or melaena. Even in a specialised unit there is misdiagnosis of periampullary lesions at operation in 10 percent of patients. Finally there remains a belief that the mortality for resection or surgery is prohibitive and that the outcome of resection is uniformly poor. None of these statements are true. Pessimism is not warranted provided precise diagnosis is used and operation performed by an experienced surgeon. Thus Tompkins (1982) reported 28 of 42 middle and low bile duct cancers resected with a mortality of 8 percent and a significantly better survival (30 percent cumulative survival at 9 years) than for palliative procedures.

Pancreaticoduodenectomy, originally introduced as a two-stage procedure, is now frequently performed in centres specialising in this type of surgery with a mortality less than 16 percent. Even in large series when the patients are drawn from multiple hospitals and not treated by specialist surgeons, the overall hospital mortality for *all types of tumour* in the peripapillary area is no higher than 21 percent. Resectability rates vary with the origin of the tumour, being over 70 percent for ampullary carcinoma but falling sharply for carcinoma of the head of the pancreas to approximately 10 percent. For bile duct cancer the resectability is approximately 27 percent. The mortality rate also varies with the origin of the tumour. Ampullary carcinoma has the lowest mortality within one month of surgery, and bile duct cancer a better outlook than pancreatic lesions.

The majority of low bile duct cancers are well differentiated but local extension to the pancreas, duodenum, and lymph nodes is present in almost half. The lesion may be very difficult and sometimes impossible to differentiate from small carcinomata of the head of the pancreas, although involvement of both the pancreatic and biliary ductal system at ERCP is highly suggestive of pancreatic tumour rather than a lesion of bile duct origin, and occasionally ERCP clearly shows the biliary origin of the lesion. The hospital mortality for pancreaticoduodenectomy carried out for bile duct cancer ranges from 8 to 22 percent. Five-year survival figures up to 25 percent are less good than those for duodenal and ampullary cancer, but some have achieved better results. Curative surgery should be attempted provided it can be carried out with an acceptable mortality rate. Although the results of endoscopic or percutaneous intubation for palliation in mid- and low bile duct tumour are better than for high lesions (Table 85–1) they are still unsatisfactory with a significant mortality, often in excess of that for resection and as high as recorded for surgical bypass. Furthermore, a greater proportion of such patients will be found resectable than those with high lesions. It is therefore most important that diagnosis is accurate and that resection is carefully considered before resorting to palliative intubation. In addition, palliative biliary–enteric bypass for low or mid-bile duct cancer has a mortality rate no greater than that recorded for nonoperative intubation. Although it may be argued that patients submitted to endoscopic or percutaneous decompression are poor-risk cases, this is not evident in publications concerning these techniques, many reports apparently reflecting an unselected approach. It is perhaps important to remember that intubation does not treat the disease, offers no chance of cure, and leaves the patient with a tube in place that inevitably results in infection, may become blocked or dislodged, or may require replacement. None of these disadvantages follows adequate surgical biliary–enteric bypass. Finally, suggestions that preliminary percutaneous drainage may improve the results of surgery does not appear substantiated by recent studies.

Bile duct cancer continues to pose formidable problems to the surgeon, but recent advances in the management of the jaundiced patient and in surgical approaches should improve the outlook in the future.

BIBLIOGRAPHY

Altemeier WA, Gall EA, et al: Sclerosing carcinoma of the major intrahepatic bile ducts. Arch Surg 75:450, 1957

Beazley RM, Hadjis N, et al: Clinicopathological aspects of high bile duct cancer: Experience with resection and bypass surgical treatments. Ann Surg (in press)

Bergdahl L: Gallbladder carcinoma first diagnosed at microscopic examination of gallbladders removed for presumed benign disease. Ann Surg 191:19, 1980

Bismuth H, Corlette MB: Intahepatic cholangioenteric anastomosis in carcinoma of the hilus of the liver. Surg Gynecol Obstet 140:170, 1975

Bismuth H: Surgical anatomy and anatomical surgery of the liver. World J Surg 6:3, 1982

Blumgart LH, Kelley CJ: Hepaticojejunostomy in benign and malignant high bile duct stricture: Approaches to the left hepatic ducts. Br J Surg 71:257, 1984

Burcharth F, Eisen F, et al: Nonsurgical internal biliary drainage by endoprosthesis. Surg Gynecol Obstet 153:857, 1981

Cotton PB: Duodenoscopic placement of biliary prostheses to relieve malignant obstructive jaundice. Br J Surg 69:501, 1982

Couinaud C: Lobes et segments hepatique, nots sur l'architecture anatomique et chirurgicale du foie. La Presse Medicale 62:709, 1954

Dooley S, Dick R, et al: Relief of bile duct obstruction by the percutaneous transhepatic insertion of an endoprosthesis. Clin Radiol 32:163, 1981

Evander A, Fredlund P, et al: Evaluation of aggressive surgery for carcinoma of the extrahepatic bile ducts. Ann Surg 191:23, 1980

Fletcher MS, Dawson JL, et al: Treatment of high bile duct carcinoma by internal radiotherapy with Iridium 192 wire. Lancet ii:172, 1981

Gouma DJ, Mutum SS, et al: Intrahepatic biliary papillomatosis. Br J Surg (in press)

Hagenmüller F, Classen M: Therapeutic endoscopic and percutaneous procedures for biliary disorders, in Popper H, Schaffer F (eds): Progress in Liver Disease, vol. VII. New York: Grune & Stratton, 1982, p 299

Keighley MRB: Microorganisms in the bile: A preventable cause of sepsis after biliary surgery. Ann R Coll Surg Engl 59:328, 1977

Klatskin G: Adenocarcinoma of the hepatic duct at its bifurcation within the porta hepatis. Am J Med 38:241, 1965

Launois B, Campion J-P, et al: Carcinoma of the hepatic hilus. Surgical management and the case for resection. Ann Surg 190:151, 1979

Longmire WP: The diverse causes of biliary obstruction and their remedies. Current Problems in Surgery XIV, vol 7. Chicago: Year Book, 1977, p 29

Longmire WP Jr, McArthur MS, et al: Carcinoma of the extrahepatic biliary tract. Ann Surg 178:333, 1973

Longmire WP Jr, Sandford MC: Intrahepatic cholangiojejunostomy for biliary obstruction—further studies. Report of 4 cases. Ann Surg 130:455, 1949

Lorelius LE, Jacobson G, et al: Endoprosthesis as an internal biliary drainage in inoperable patients with biliary obstruction. Acta Chir Scand 148:613, 1982

McPherson GAD, Blenkharn JI, et al: Significance of bacteria in external biliary drainage systems: A possible role for antisepsis. J Clin Surg 1:22, 1982

Moossa AR, Anagnost M, et al: The continuing challenge of gallbladder cancer. Survey of thirty years experience at the University of Chicago. Am J Surg 130:57, 1975

Mueller PR, van Sonnenberg E, et al: Percutaneous biliary drainage: Technical and catheter-related problems in 200 procedures. AJR 138:17, 1982

Nevin JE, Moran TJ, et al: Carcinoma of the gallbladder. Cancer 37:141, 1976

Nishimura A, Mayama S, et al: Carcinoma of the cystic duct: Case report. Jpn J Surg 5:109, 1976

Piehler JM, Crichlow RW: Primary carcinoma of the gallbladder. Surg Gynecol Obstet 147:929, 1978

Praderi R: El drenaje biliar externo o interno per el hepatico izquierdo. Rev Ass Med Brasil 9:401, 1963

Praderi R: Obstruction neoplasia de las hepaticos. Rev Argent Cir 20:115, 1971

Praderi R, Parodi H, et al: Tratamiento de las obstrucciones neoplasicas de la via biliar supra pancreatica. An Fac Med Montevideo 49:221, 1964

Roberts-Thompson IC, Strickland RJ, et al: Bile duct carcinoma in chronic ulcerative colitis. Aust NZ J Med 3:264, 1973

Skoog V, Thoren L: Carcinoma of the junction of the main hepatic ducts. Acta Chir Scand 148:411, 1982

Smith R: Carcinoma of the gallbladder and of the common hepatic duct, in Smith R, Sherlock S (eds): Surgery of the Gallbladder and Bile Ducts, 2 edt. London: Butterworths, 1981, p 393

Soupault R, Couinaud CL: Sur un procede nouveau de derivation biliaire intra-hepatique. Les cholangio-jejunostomies gauches sans sacrifice hepatique. La Presse Medicale 65:1157, 1957

Terblanche J: Carcinoma of the proximal extrahepatic biliary tree—definitive and palliative treatment. Surg Annu 11:249, 1979

Terblanche J: In discussion of Tompkins RK, et al: Prognostic factors in bile duct carcinoma. Ann Surg 194:447, 1981

Terblanche J, Louw JH: "U"-tube drainage in the palliative therapy of carcinoma of the main hepatic duct system. Surg Clin North Am 53:1245, 1973

Terblanche J, Saunders SG, et al: Prolonged palliation in carcinoma of the main hepatic duct junction. Surgery 71:720, 1972

Terblanche J: Cholangiocarcinoma: Bypass Discussion. British Society of Gastroenterology Second International Teaching Day, London, 20 April, 1983

Tompkins RK: Carcinoma of the gallbladder and biliary ducts, in Blumgart LH (ed): The Biliary Tract, vol 5. Edinburgh: Churchill Livingstone, 1982, p 183

Tompkins RK, Thomas D, et al: Prognostic factors in bile duct carcinoma. Ann Surg 194:477, 1981

Tytgat GNJ, Huibregtse K: Transpapillary introduction of large bore biliary endoprothesis in malignant bile duct obstruction—experience in 300 patients. 3rd International Symposium of Digestive Surgery and Endoscopy, Rome, 26–29, April, 1983

Voyles CR, Bowley NJ, et al: Carcinoma of the proximal extrahepatic biliary tree. Radiological assessment and therapeutic alternatives. Ann Surg 197:188, 1983

Weinbren K, Mutum SS: Pathological aspects of cholangiocarcinoma. J Pathol 139:217, 1983

Welton JC, Marr JS, et al: Association between hepatobiliary cancer and typhoid carrier state. Lancet i:791, 1979

Additional Reading

Akwari OE, Kelly KA: Surgical treatment of hilar adenocarcinomas. Arch Surg 114:22, 1979

Benjamin IS, Blumgart LH: Biliary bypass and reconstruction, in Wright R, Alberti KGMM, et al (eds): Liver and Biliary Disease: Pathophysiology, Diagnosis, Management. London: Saunders, 1979, chap 54

Berquist TH, May GR, et al: Percutaneous biliary decompression internal and external drainage in 50 patients. AJR 136:901, 1981

Bloustein PA: Association of carcinoma with congenital cystic conditions of the liver and bile ducts. Am J Gastroenterol 67:40, 1977

Blumgart LH, Hadjis NS, et al: Surgical approaches to cholangiocarcinoma at the confluence of the hepatic duct. Lancet, 1:66, 1984

Blumgart LH, Voyles CR, et al: Exo-endoprosthesis for relief of obstructive jaundice. Lancet ii:306, 1981

Buckwalter JA, Lawton RL, et al: Bypass operations for neoplastic biliary tract obstruction. Am J Surg 109:100, 1965

Cady B, Fortner JG: Surgical resection of intrahepatic bile duct cancer. Am J Surg 118:104, 1969

Cattell RB, Braasch JW, et al: Polypoid epithelial tumors of the bile ducts. N Engl J Med 266:57, 1962

Caroli J. Disease of the intrahepatic biliary tree. Clin Gastroenterol 2:147, 1973

Diehl AK: Epidemiology of gallbladder cancer: A synthesis of recent data. J Natl Cancer Inst 65:1209, 1980

Donaldson LA, Busutill A: A clinico-pathological review of 68 carcinomas of the gallbladder. Br J Surg 62:26, 1975

Fortner JG, Kallum BO, et al: Surgical management of carcinoma of the junction of the main hepatic ducts. Ann Surg 184:68, 1976

Ham J: Partial and complete atrophy affecting hepatic segments and lobes. Br J Surg 66:333, 1979

Harbin WP, Mueller PR, et al: Transhepatic cholangiography: Complications and use patterns of the fine needle technique. Radiology 135:15, 1980

Hatfield ARW, Tobias R, et al: Preoperative external biliary drainage in obstructive jaundice. A prospective controlled trial. Lancet ii:896, 1982

Howard JM: Pancreatico-duodenostomy. 41 consecutive Whipple resections without an operative mortality. Ann Surg 168:629, 1968

Hunt DR, Allison MEM, et al: Endotoxaemia, disturbance of coagulation and obstructive jaundice. Am J Surg 144:325, 1982

Iwasaki Y, Ohto M, et al: Treatment of carcinoma of the biliary system. Surg Gynecol Obstet 144:219, 1977

Kirschbaum JD, Kozoll DC: Carcinoma of the gallbladder and extrahepatic bile ducts. Surg Gynecol Obstet 73:740, 1941

Krain LS: Gallbladder and extrahepatic bile duct carcinoma. Analysis of 1808 cases. Geriatrics 27:111, 1972

Kuwayti E, Baggenstoss AH, et al: Carcinoma of the major intrahepatic and the extrahepatic bile ducts exclusive of the papilla of Vater. Surg Gynecol Obstet 104:357, 1957

Longmire WP Jr: Tumours of the extrahepatic biliary radicals, in Hickey RC (ed): Curr Probl Cancer. Chicago: Year Book, 1976

Longmire WP, Shaffy OA: Certain factors influencing survival after pancreatico-duodenal resection for carcinoma. Am J Surg 111:8, 1966

Malt RA, Warshaw AL, et al: Left intrahepatic cholangiojejunostomy for proximal obstruction of the biliary tract. Surg Gynecol Obstet 150:193, 1980

McPherson GAD, Benjamin IS, et al: Percutaneous transhepatic drainage in obstructive jaundice: Advantages and problems. Br J Surg 69:261, 1982

Nakase A, Mautsumoto Y, et al: Surgical treatment of cancer of the pancreas and periampullary region: Cumulative results in Japan. Ann Surg 185:52, 1977

Nakayama T, Ikeda A, et al: Percutaneous transhepatic drainage of the biliary tract. Gastroenterology 74:554, 1978

Ross AP, Braasch JW, et al: Carcinoma of the proximal bile ducts. Surg Gynecol Obstet 135:928, 1973

Sako S, Seitzinger GL, et al: Carcinoma of the extrahepatic bile ducts. Review of the literature and report of six cases. Surgery 41:416, 1957

Smadja C, Bowley N, et al: Idiopathic localized bile duct strictures. Relationship to primary sclerosing cholangitis. Am J Surg 146:404, 1983

Tompkins RK, Johnson J, et al: Operative endoscopy in the management of biliary tract neoplasm. Am J Surg 132:174, 1976

Tsuzuki T, Hoshimo Y, et al: Compensatory hypertrophy of the lateral quadrant of the left hepatic lobe due to atropy of the rest of the liver appearing as a mass in the left upper quadrant of the abdomen. Am J Surg 177:406, 1972

Warren KW, Choe DS, et al: Results of radical resection for periampullary cancer. Ann Surg 181:534, 1975

Warren KW, Jefferson MF: Carcinoma of the exocrine pancreas, in Carey LC (ed): The Pancreas. St. Louis: CV Mosby, 1973, p 243

Warren KW, Mountain JC, et al: Malignant tumours of the bile ducts. Br J Surg 59:501, 1972

Warren KW, Veidenheimer MC, et al: Pancreatico-duodenostomy for periampullary cancer. Surg Clin North Am 47:639, 1967

Whipple AO, Parsons WB, et al: Treatment of carcinoma of ampulla of Vater. Ann Surg 102:763, 1935

Wheeler PG, Dawson JL, et al: Newer techniques in the diagnosis and treatment of proximal bile duct carcinoma—an analysis of 41 consecutive cases. Q J Med 50:247, 1981

Williamson BW, Blumgart LH, et al: Management of tumours of the liver. Combined use of arteriography and venography in the assessment of resectability especially in hilar tumours. Am J Surg 139:210, 1980

SECTION XIII
Pancreas

86. Injuries to the Pancreas

A.R. Moossa
Michael H. Scott

INTRODUCTION

Pancreatic injuries occur relatively infrequently in patients with abdominal trauma, the incidence ranging from 1 to 12 percent, and a single surgeon seldom gains extensive personal experience in their management. The rarity of pancreatic injuries following abdominal trauma may be accounted for by the relatively "protected" position of the gland in the retroperitoneum beneath the thoracic cage. The intimacy of the organ with major blood vessels may lead to the early death of some critically injured patients from hemorrhage prior to the recognition of a pancreatic injury.

Pancreatic trauma may be inflicted by blunt or penetrating injuries. Although the pancreatic injury itself rarely, if ever, accounts for the early death of a patient, it adds significantly to the morbidity and late mortality, especially if it is recognized late or improperly managed.

Injuries to the pancreas are being encountered more frequently today than 30 years ago. This may be attributed to the increasing incidence of automobile accidents and civilian violence. It is plausible that the increasing and often compulsory use of seat belts may further increase the incidence of blunt pancreatic trauma since the gland may be ruptured by its sudden compression against the lumbar spine.

It is fortunate that the incidence of pancreatic trauma is low, since the mortality and morbidity of such injuries can be devastating. In a recent series by Northup and Simmons the mortality rate was about 20 percent. Stab wounds had a mortality rate of 8 percent, gunshot wounds 25 percent, and shotgun wounds 60 percent. Mortality following blunt trauma from steering wheel injuries was approximately 50 percent. One third of all pancreatic injuries were secondary to blunt trauma, and two thirds were due to penetrating trauma. Most of the early deaths result from massive hemorrhage and shock due to associated injuries to major vascular structures. Sepsis is the second most frequent cause of death and is the agent most responsible for late mortality.

Historically, the first recorded case of blunt trauma to the pancreas was described by Travers in the *Lancet* in 1827. The case report describes a lady who was struck down by a stagecoach while intoxicated. At a postmortem examination, the patient was found to have a transverse laceration of the pancreas and an extensive liver injury, the latter being the cause of death.

Otis, editor of the medical and surgical history of the American Civil War (published in 1876), noted seven patients with pancreatic injuries. In three instances, following stabbing injuries, the pancreas protruded from the wound. All three patients survived following excision of the portion of protruding gland, thus setting a precedent for the value of distal pancreatectomy in pancreatic injury. However, the accepted treatment of the time was conservatism and, although a small number of surgical pioneers tried to advocate operative management, this did not become fully accepted until World War II, when the importance of associated injuries, particularly those to major vessels, was recognized as a significant factor.

DIAGNOSIS

It should always be remembered that in less than 10 percent of patients with pancreatic trauma the pancreas is the only injured organ.

2045

Conversely, this means that over 90 percent of patients will have further internal injuries. The pancreatic injury is unlikely to be the potential cause of death, or a cause of symptoms and signs. Therefore, a high index of suspicion for pancreatic injuries must always be borne in mind both preoperatively and intraoperatively.

Pancreatic injury may result from either penetrating or blunt trauma.

Patients with definite evidence of an injured intraabdominal viscus and/or intraabdominal hemorrhage following penetrating or blunt trauma to the abdomen are in need of an emergency laparotomy and should not be investigated further for evidence of pancreatic trauma. The diagnosis is made intraoperatively. Initial emphasis is placed on adequate resuscitation rather than an elaborate, time-consuming and often unrewarding investigation.

Patients with doubtful evidence of intraabdominal injury should be observed and carefully investigated as dictated by clinical circumstances. They are the group of patients in whom an isolated pancreatic injury may easily be missed.

Penetrating Injury

It is difficult to imagine a situation in which there would be isolated pancreatic damage in a penetrating abdominal injury. The possibility of a pancreatic injury should always be considered whenever a penetrating object passes in the vicinity of the pancreas. The point of entry for such a missile can be abdomen, lower chest, or either flank.

The clinical picture usually seen with a penetrating abdominal injury makes exploration essential and thus the diagnosis of the pancreatic injury should be made at operation.

Stab wounds are the least morbid of the pancreatic injuries. Death is usually secondary to associated vascular damage. Gunshot wounds, however, may cause devastating pancreatic injury, particularly if from high velocity weapons or shotguns.

Blunt Injuries

The main diagnostic problem to the clinician is recognition of a pancreatic injury secondary to blunt abdominal trauma. Clinical signs and symptoms are notoriously unreliable or minimal as a result of retroperitoneal containment of blood and pancreatic juice, and abdominal findings may be limited to deep tenderness in the region of the epigastrium.

The most important factors are probably a knowledge of the history of the injury and a high index of suspicion. Injury to the pancreas may result from direct impact, deceleration, rotary forces, and shear forces. The latter three play only a minor role, with direct impact being the most common cause of blunt pancreatic injury. This, in turn, is most often due to steering wheel impact, but may be caused by a kick or punch to the abdomen. Children, whose rib cages offer less protection to the pancreas than in the adult, may suffer pancreatic injury by merely falling against an object, for example, the handlebar of a bicycle.

Whether the head, body, or tail of the pancreas is injured in a particular accident depends on the angle from which the impinging force crushes the pancreas, which is wrapped about the anterior half of the rigid vertebral column. If the patient is struck on the left side, the tail of the pancreas is compressed between the impinging object and the vertebral column; if the patient is struck head on, the neck or body of the pancreas may be divided between the impinging force and the vertebral column; or if the patient is struck from the right, the head of the pancreas, duodenum, and common bile duct are at risk of injury.

In cases where there has been blunt abdominal trauma and there are no obvious reasons for exploratory operation, but the index of suspicion for pancreatic injury is high, there are a few diagnostic aids that can be used, but none can be considered to be completely reliable:

1. Serum amylase
2. Urinary amylase
3. Peritoneal lavage and/or estimation of peritoneal fluid amylase content
4. Radiology, including computed tomography (CT)

Amylase Determination. Since Ellman noted in 1929 that serum amylase values become elevated when a major pancreatic duct is obstructed or injured, this has been a mainstay of diagnosis for pancreatic disease. Unfortunately, with all blunt injuries, the amylase test has been disappointing with regard to its accuracy.

Elevated levels of serum amylase may reflect ductal obstruction associated with pancreatic injury, but may also result from elevations of salivary amylase due to parotid injury, the administration of narcotics, or perforation of a hollow viscus in the absence of pancreatic injury. Moreover, upper gastrointestinal (GI) perforations release pancreatic enzymes into the peritoneal cavity, where they may be absorbed by the abdominal lymphatics and in time elevate serum levels of amylase. Some closed head injuries may occasionally be associated with spurious elevation of serum amalyase. Therefore, elevation of serum amylase on a single determination is not useful in assessing whether or not the patient is a candidate for operation.

In the absence of clinical indication for operation, serial amylase levels may be helpful in following the patient suspected of having a pancreatic injury. A progressive increase or persistent elevation in serum or urine values of amylase over three or five successive determinations, obtained every 3 or 4 hours, is an acceptable reason to explore the pancreas and duodenum in the absence of other signs. Conversely, if in the absence of other indications for operation, the serum or urine amylase level falls after an initial elevation, there is no indication for operation.

On the other hand, the possibility of pancreatic injury cannot be eliminated on the basis of an initially low amylase determination. In some patients observed by Bach and Frey in whom the pancreatic duct was completely fractured, the serum amylase did not rise until as long as 24 to 48 hours after injury.

Radiologic Studies. Plain abdominal x-ray is not useful in evaluating pancreatic injuries although, occasionally, obliteration of the psoas shadow or retroperitoneal air is observed and suggests the diagnosis. In selected nonemergency circumstances, visceral angiography has been of diagnostic value; it will delineate the presence of associated splenic vein thrombosis and left-sided portal hypertension, which has a high incidence of gastric variceal hemorrhage. Endoscopic retrograde cholangiopancreatography (ERCP) can be employed to diagnose a major ductal injury following blunt abdominal trauma. This technique is recommended only in selected cases, provided injuries to other intraabdominal organs have been excluded, and if the suspicion of a major ductal injury still exists.

The role of ultrasonography is very limited in the early, acute situation, but it has a definite place in monitoring the development and course of a subsequent pseudocyst or pancreatic abscess.

CT is emerging as the best initial investigation for evaluating a suspected pancreatic injury. CT is capable of visualizing early pseudocysts, pancreatic contusions, lacerations, and fractures with a high degree of accuracy.

In examinations conducted in the few hours following injury, pancreatic features and other CT findings of pancreatic trauma may be quite subtle. Unexplained thickening of the anterior renal fascia should alert the radiologist to a possible pancreatic injury.

Meticulous attention to the scanning technique is important to avoid a false-positive diagnosis. This requires adequate bowel opacification with the contrast material, gastric decompression, sedation of the patient, and repeat scans if the initial images are not satisfactory. Emergency ERCP may be required to investigate pancreatic injuries when CT findings are equivocal or when the scans are technically inadequate. CT is noninvasive, and images of the pancreas can be obtained rapidly. Thus CT would seem uniquely suited as a diagnostic method for the evaluation of pancreatic trauma.

TREATMENT

The surgical management of pancreatic injuries is based on five principles:

1. Arresting hemorrhage
2. Controlling contamination from GI content
3. Selective pancreatic debridement, if indicated
4. Securing adequate drainage
5. Controlling pancreatic secretions

Adequate exposure through a generous midline abdominal incision cannot be overemphasized. Surgeons should always be prepared to extend the midline incision up to the sternum or into the left or right chest if necessary. The chest, therefore, should be prepared prior to surgical exploration, along with the abdomen. The initial operative efforts must be directed at arresting all major bleeding. The intimacy of the pancreas to major intraabdominal blood vessels and the vascularity of the gland makes significant hemorrhage following pancreatic injury a frequent problem. The surgeon must be prepared to mobilize adjacent structures expeditiously to gain access to and control the major blood vessels. Significant injuries to the gland may be overlooked in this emergency setting and a thorough examination of the pancreas is mandatory. Any upper retroperitoneal or peripancreatic hematoma must be considered presumptive evidence of pancreatic injury and explored.

The blind application of clamps to bleeding joints and the insertion of deep mass ligatures must be avoided. Hemorrhage should be controlled by precise application of multiple suture ligatures of fine nonabsorbable material without the prior application of hemostatic clips.

Major intraabdominal hemorrhage may also occur at sites remote from the pancreatic bed, such as in the liver or renal parenchyma, and should be handled according to established principles. This often takes precedence over the pancreatic injury, especially if a partial hepatectomy or nephrectomy is necessary to control exsanguinating hemorrhage.

Once bleeding has been controlled and continuous contamination from bowel content stopped by the application of clamps or sutures, the extent of the pancreatic injury must be assessed.

The lesser sac should be widely opened by dividing the gastrocolic omentum to visualize and palpate the ventral surface of the whole gland (Fig. 86–1). The tail of the pancreas may be mobilized by dividing the lienorenal ligament and freeing the spleen and tail of the pancreas by blunt dissection to examine the undersurface of the gland. An extensive Kocher maneuver should be performed to thoroughly examine the dorsal surface of the head of the pancreas and the first and second parts of the duodenum. Since pancreatic and duodenal injuries often co-

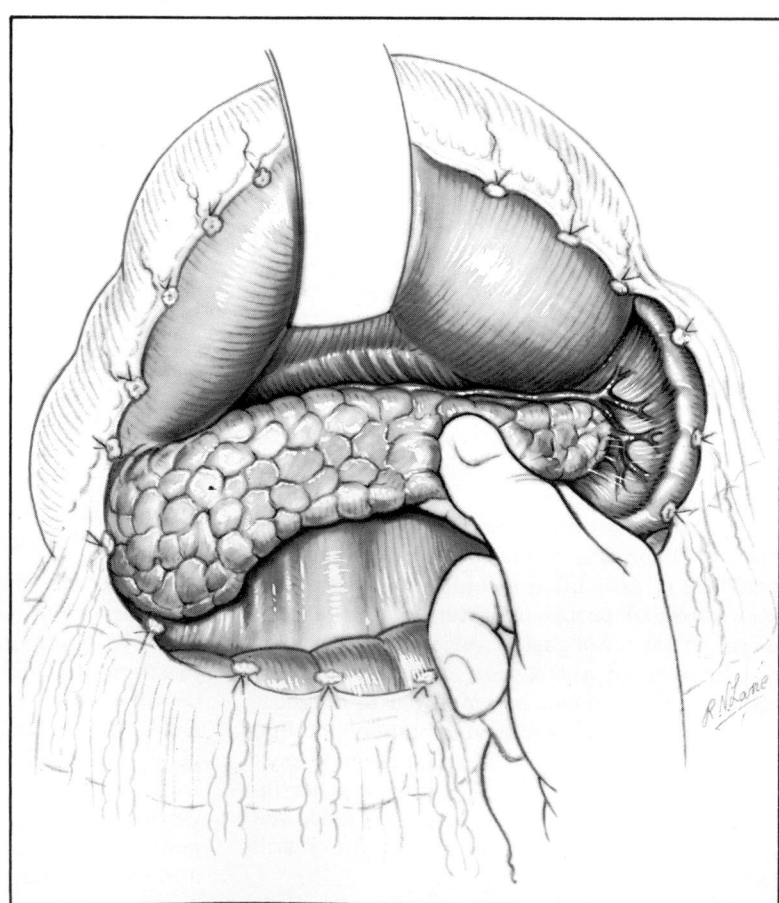

Figure 86–1. Exposure of the pancreas in cases of penetrating and nonpenetrating wounds.

Nonductal Injuries

Patients who have a simple contusion without capsular tear, hematoma formation, or devitalization of pancreatic tissue can be managed by adequate external drainage alone. If the "capsule" is torn it may be repaired by fine interrupted nonabsorbable sutures and external drainage established. All pancreatic hematomas should be explored to identify possible ductal injuries, devitalized tissue should be debrided, and the area drained externally.

Even with the closest scrutiny, minor lacerations of the pancreatic "capsule" and ductules may be overlooked at operation. Fluid collections are frequent and pancreatic fistulae often develop from the traumatized gland. These usually close spontaneously. Inadequate drainage, however, will result in pancreatic pseudocysts or abscesses which are potentially devastating complications and require reoperation.

Adequate drainage implies a combination of sump suction and Penrose drains. The former should be left in place for 7 to 10 days and then removed to avoid erosion into adjacent blood vessels; the latter should be left in place for a minimum of 2 weeks or longer if drainage of amylase-containing fluid persists.

Major Ductal Disruption

The significance of pancreatic injury depends on whether the major pancreatic duct remains intact. If the duct is ruptured, there is an increase in both morbidity and mortality. This factor was recognized by Gooch in the late eighteenth century when he declared that "Wounds of the pancreas are to be concluded mortal if its ducts or blood vessels are injured, whence the succus pancreaticus or blood may be discharged into the cavity of the abdomen and there putrifying, cause inevitable death."

Injury to the Left of Superior Mesenteric Vessels

A disruption of the major pancreatic duct to the left of the superior mesenteric vessels is best managed by distal pancreatectomy and splenectomy and external drainage of the pancreatic bed. The cut distal end of the pancreatic remnant can usually be oversewn with nonabsorbable sutures. The duct should always be closed separately with a single nonabsorbable transfixion stitch (Figs. 86–3 and 86–4).

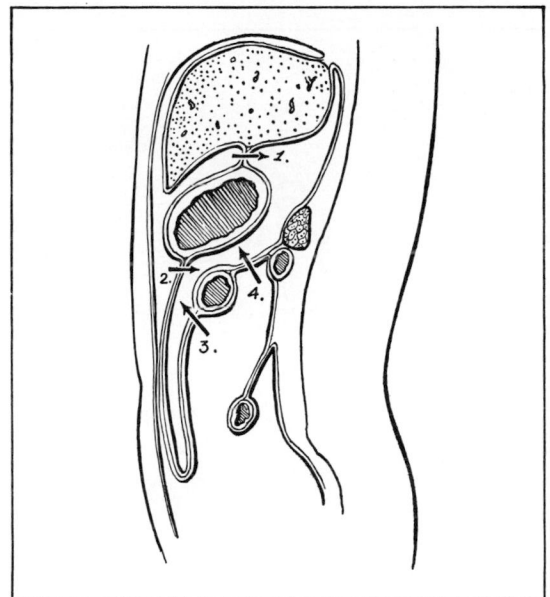

Figure 86–2. Routes for approaching the pancreas: (1) through the gastrohepatic omentum, (2) through the gastrocolic omentum, (3) by detaching the great omentum from the transverse colon, and (4) through the mesocolon.

exist, other parts of the duodenum must also be thoroughly examined. Division of the ligament of Treitz, mobilization of the right colon and small bowel, along with their mesentery from their retroperitoneal attachments will facilitate thorough inspection of the third and fourth parts of the duodenum. The routes for approaching the pancreas are shown in Figure 86–2.

Particular attention must be given to the tail of the pancreas in patients with hilar injuries to the spleen. Often, the tail of the pancreas will extend well into the hilum of the spleen. There may be an associated injury to the tail of the pancreas which, if left untreated or undrained, may lead to serious postoperative sequelae.

In general, pancreatic injuries may be classified as follows:

1. Simple contusion
2. Parenchymatous tear without major ductal disruption
3. Major ductal disruption
4. Combined pancreaticoduodenal injury

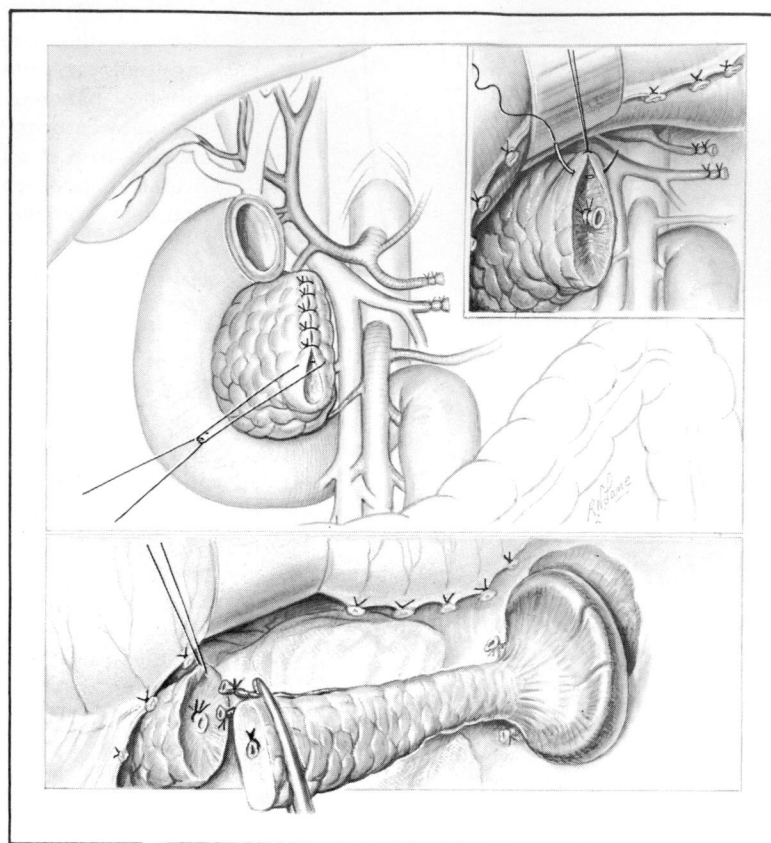

Figure 86–3. A buffer accident causing transection of the neck of the pancreas. Distal subtotal resection of the pancreas with splenectomy; methods of dealing with the duct of Wirsung and the margins of the head of the pancreas.

A splenectomy is almost always necessary while accomplishing a distal pancreatectomy, but if possible it should be preserved, especially in pediatric patients. If in a case requiring a distal pancreatectomy there is any question of injury to the head and neck area of pancreatic tissue with possible periampullary obstruction, the distal cut end of the pancreatic remnant may be drained internally via a Roux-Y jejunostomy (Fig. 86–5) to avoid fistula formation, or even via a gastrostomy. Direct repair of the injured main pancreatic duct with stenting has been recommended from time to time. This difficult technical procedure under emergency conditions should be condemned since the incidence of postoperative complications is too high.

Injury to the Right of Superior Mesenteric Vessels

Injuries to the head of the pancreas are potentially more serious than those of the body and tail, for a fistula in the head will result in a larger volume of secretion than if the injury

were in the body or tail, because of the greater mass of acinar tissue distal to the fracture.

Although exocrine and endocrine insufficiency is a rare consequence of distal pancreatectomy, it may follow extensive resection of the body and tail, especially when more than 80 percent of the gland has been resected. This hazard has prompted many surgeons to conserve pancreatic tissue, especially when the ductal injury lies well to the right of the superior mesenteric vessels.

For most proximal pancreatic ductal fractures, there is a much favored alternative to the 80 to 90 percent distal resection, which is to preserve the body and tail of the pancreas by oversewing the proximal severed end of the pancreas with nonabsorbable interrupted mattress sutures and anastomosing the distal cut end of the pancreas with a Roux-Y limb of jejunum. This, of course, is only possible if there has not been extensive trauma to the remaining gland. In the past, others have advocated anastamosing both the proximal and distal pan-

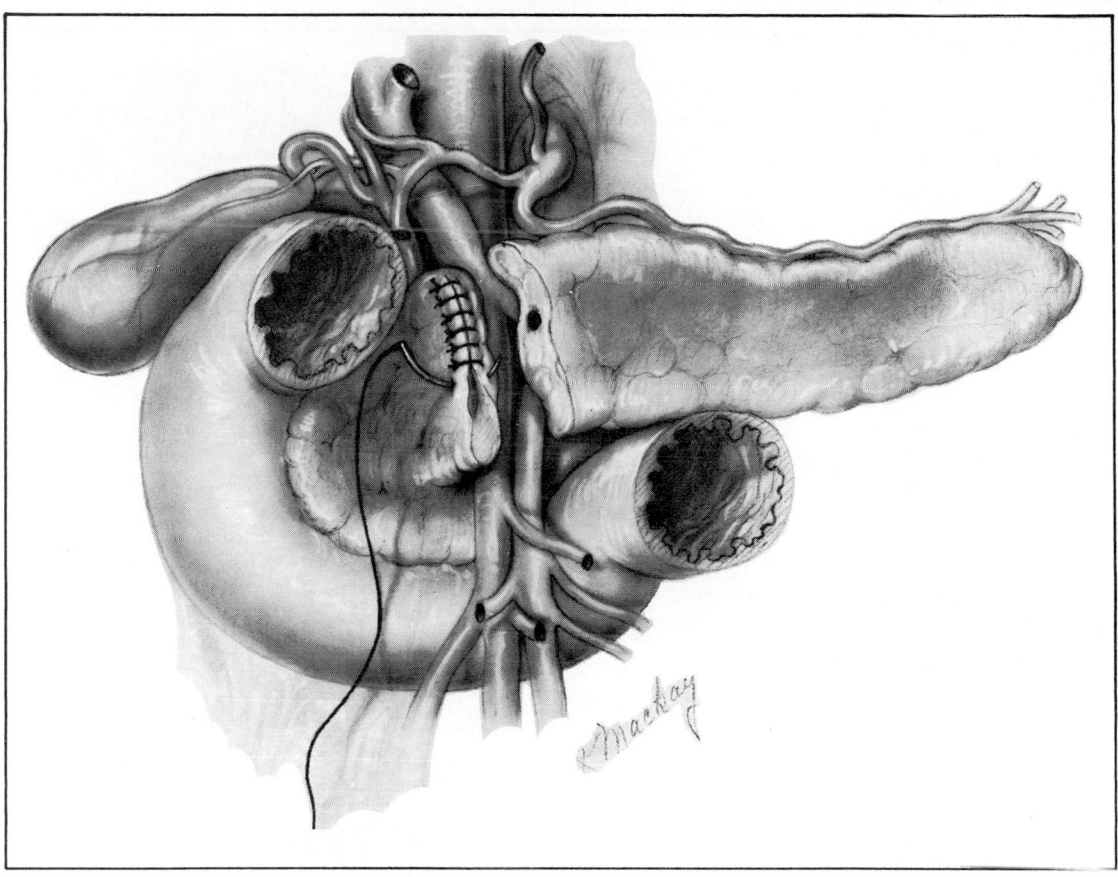

Figure 86–4. Complete rupture of the pancreas. Almost identical findings in two patients operated on by Drs. Letton and Wilson: Pancreas completely divided and ends retracted, with exposure of superior mesenteric vein and splenic vessels intact. (*Source: From Letton AH, Wilson JP, by permission of Surgery, Gynecology & Obstetrics.*)

creatic fragments into a Roux-Y loop, although this technique is now passing out of favor as being unnecessary and hazardous. The safety of performing one or more pancreatic anastomoses under emergency situations, often by an inexperienced team, must be seriously questioned. The decision to conserve pancreatic tissue and to perform an initial pancreatoenteric anastomosis should be based also upon the presence and magnitude of associated injuries, the general condition of the patient, the degree of contamination with bowel contents, and the surgeon's expertise with pancreatic surgery. An anastomotic leak is potentially lethal whereas pancreatic glandular insufficiency can always be controlled with enzyme and insulin therapy.

Injuries to the head of the pancreas may present formidable problems, both of a decisive and of a technical nature. Their management has to be individualized and a great deal of surgical judgment needs to be exercised. An emergency pancreatoduodenectomy is never indicated for a major pancreatic duct injury to the head of the gland if the common bile duct and duodenum are intact. An isolated fracture of the pancreatic head without concomitant damage to the duodenum, pancreatic duct, or intrapancreatic bile duct may be treated by drainage alone. An operative cholangiogram and/or pancreatogram may occasionally be necessary to confirm major ductal continuity. The postoperative course is invariably complicated by fistula formation with prolonged drainage of pancreatic juice. With judicious application of total parenteral nutrition, these patients may be maintained in a positive nitrogen balance for

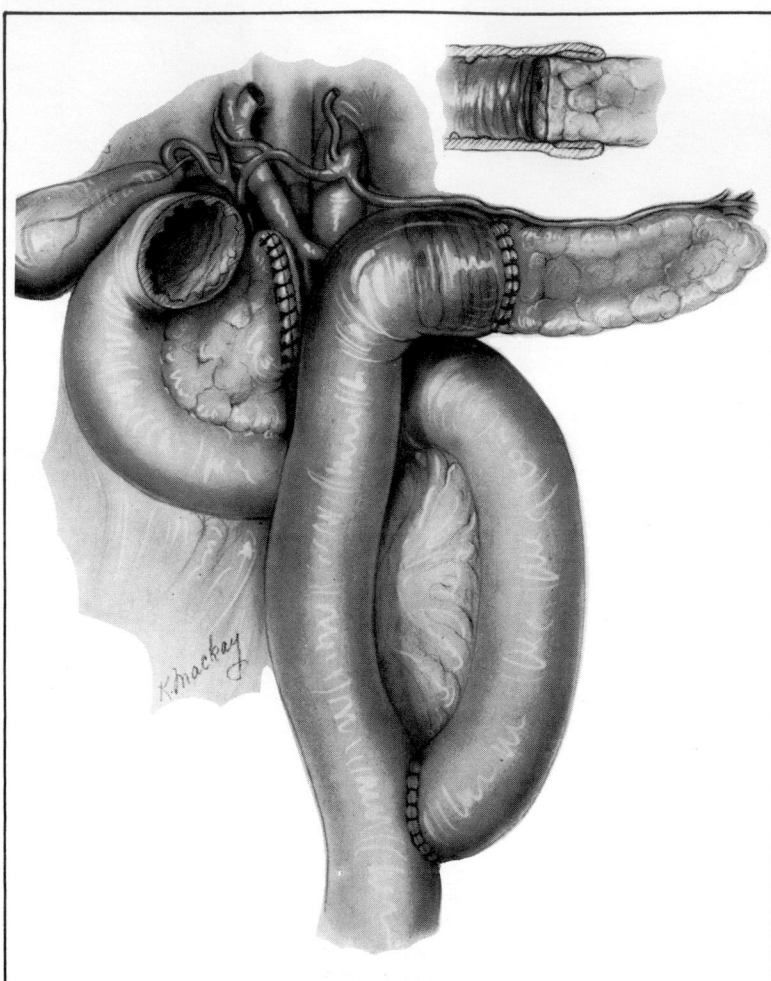

Figure 86–5. Complete rupture of body of pancreas and technique adapted by Drs. Letton and Wilson. Roux-Y type of pancreatojejunostomy has been made with caudal portion of pancreas and defunctionalized jejunum. The raw surface in the head of pancreas has been closed with interrupted silk sutures. Inset shows technique of anastomosis. (*Source: From Letton AH, Wilson JP, by permission of Surgery, Gynecology & Obstetrics.*)

months and the fistulous tract usually closes spontaneously. Otherwise, the tract may be implanted into a Roux-Y loop of jejunum at a second operation.

Combined Pancreaticoduodenal Injury

The morbidity and mortality for combined pancreaticoduodenal injuries are considerably higher than for pancreatic or duodenal injuries alone.

This group of patients can be further subdivided into:

1. Duodenal injury associated with "nonductal" pancreatic head injury
2. Duodenal injury associated with major ductal pancreatic head injury

Duodenum and Nonductal Injury

If tissue destruction is limited, a duodenorrhaphy and external drainage is sufficient. When more extensive wounds are encountered the integrity of the duodenal repair may be in question and exclusion of the duodenum from the normal gastrointestinal stream may be necessary (Fig. 86–6). Both the "pyloric exclusion" and "duodenal diverticulization" operations have been advocated to protect the duodenal repair during the period when breakdown usually occurs.

Pyloric Exclusion. This procedure entails suturing of the duodenal and pancreatic defects, and closure of the pylorus with a continuous absorbable suture through an antral gastrot-

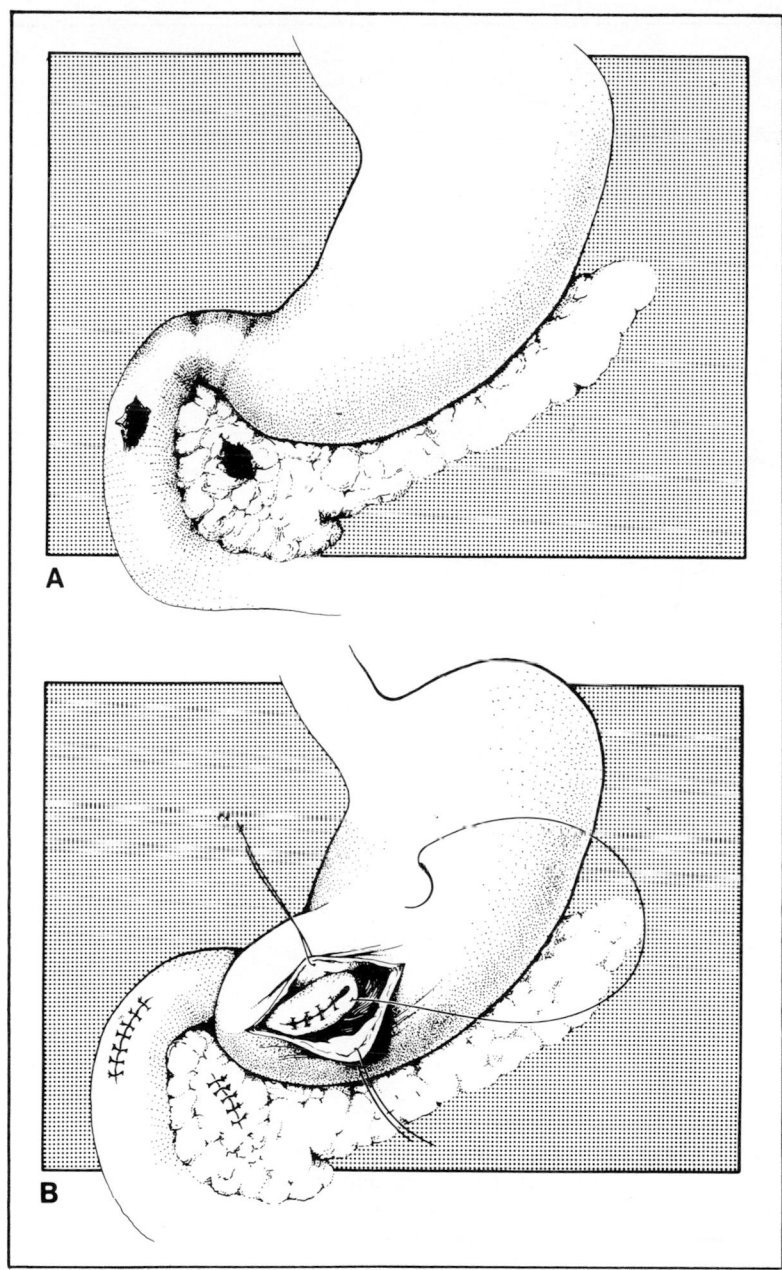

Figure 86–6. Duodenal and pancreatic injury, methods of repair, and temporary pyloric exclusion.

omy that is then anastomosed to the upper jejunum (Fig. 86–7). The area of the duodenal head is externally drained.

Duodenal Diverticulization. This procedure, championed by Berne, is more extensive and consists of an antrectomy with anticolic end-to-side gastrojejunostomy, tube duodenostomy, T-tube drainage of the common bile duct, and sump external drainage (Fig. 86–8).

Although both of these procedures are originally recommended for extensive combined pancreaticoduodenal injury, including major pancreatic duct injury, neither operation provides for the management of the major pancreatic duct disruption except by sump and/or Penrose drainage.

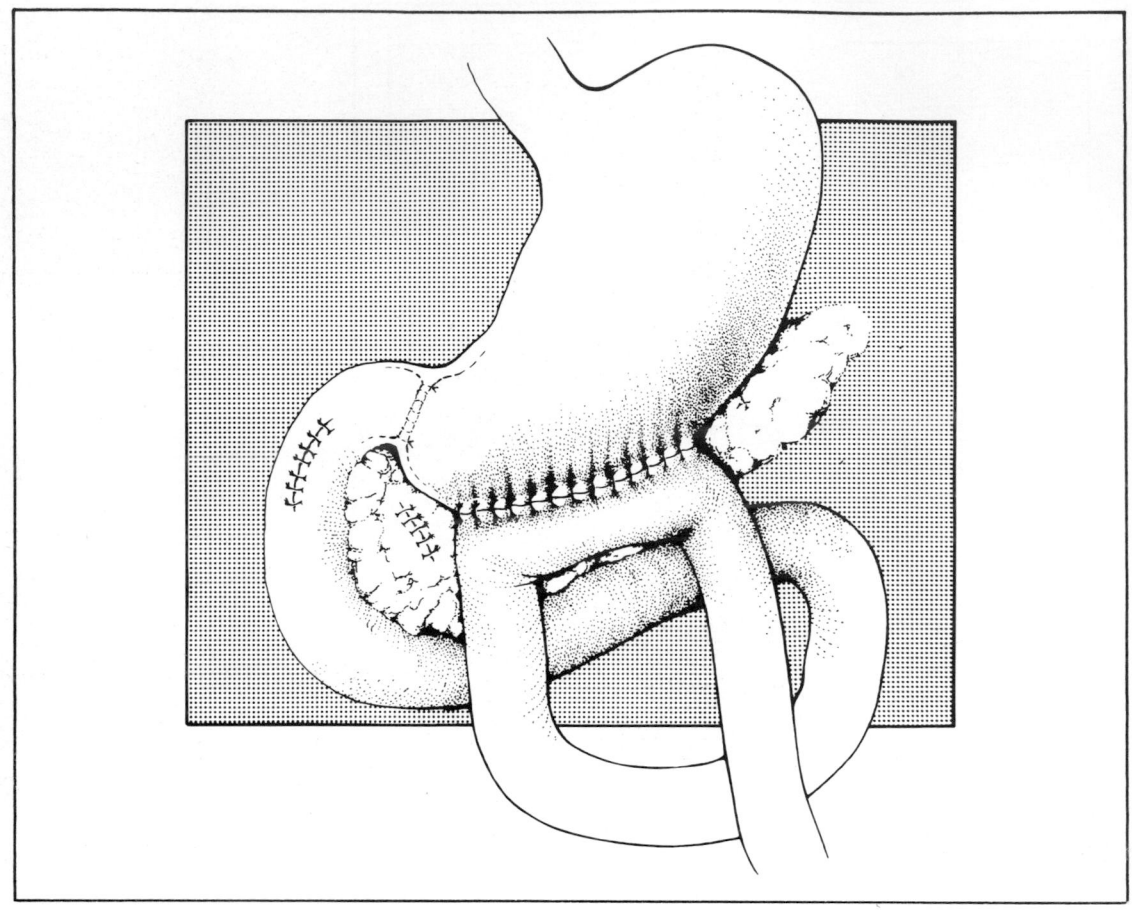

Figure 86–7. Completed duodenal diversion with addition of antral gastrojejunostomy.

More extensive injuries to the duodenum have been managed with partial resection of the injured segment with primary reanastomosis or with Roux-Y duodenojejunostomy (serosal patch) reconstruction.

Duodenal and Major Ductal Injury

As previously mentioned, there are some schools of thought that recommend the duodenal exclusion type of operation for these injuries.

Extensive injuries to the head of the pancreas with devitalization of pancreatic and duodenal tissue, avulsion of the common duct, or uncontrolled hemorrhage may be an indication for emergency pancreaticoduodenectomy even though the operation carries a high mortality under these circumstances. Although the antrum of the stomach is resected in pancreaticoduodenectomy for cancer, it is not necessary in trauma, and, as Longmire has shown, the pylorus can be preserved. Care should be taken to preserve as much length of common bile duct as feasible to facilitate the choledochojejunal anastomosis, which can be technically difficult if the common duct is small. Biliary and pancreatic anastomoses should always be splinted in such circumstances.

COMPLICATIONS

The complications of pancreatic and duodenal injury include pancreatic and duodenal fistulas, pancreatic abscesses, pancreatic pseudocyst formation, vascular necrosis within the vicinity of the gland with hemorrhage, both acute and chronic pancreatitis, and intraperitoneal sepsis.

The complication most commonly associ-

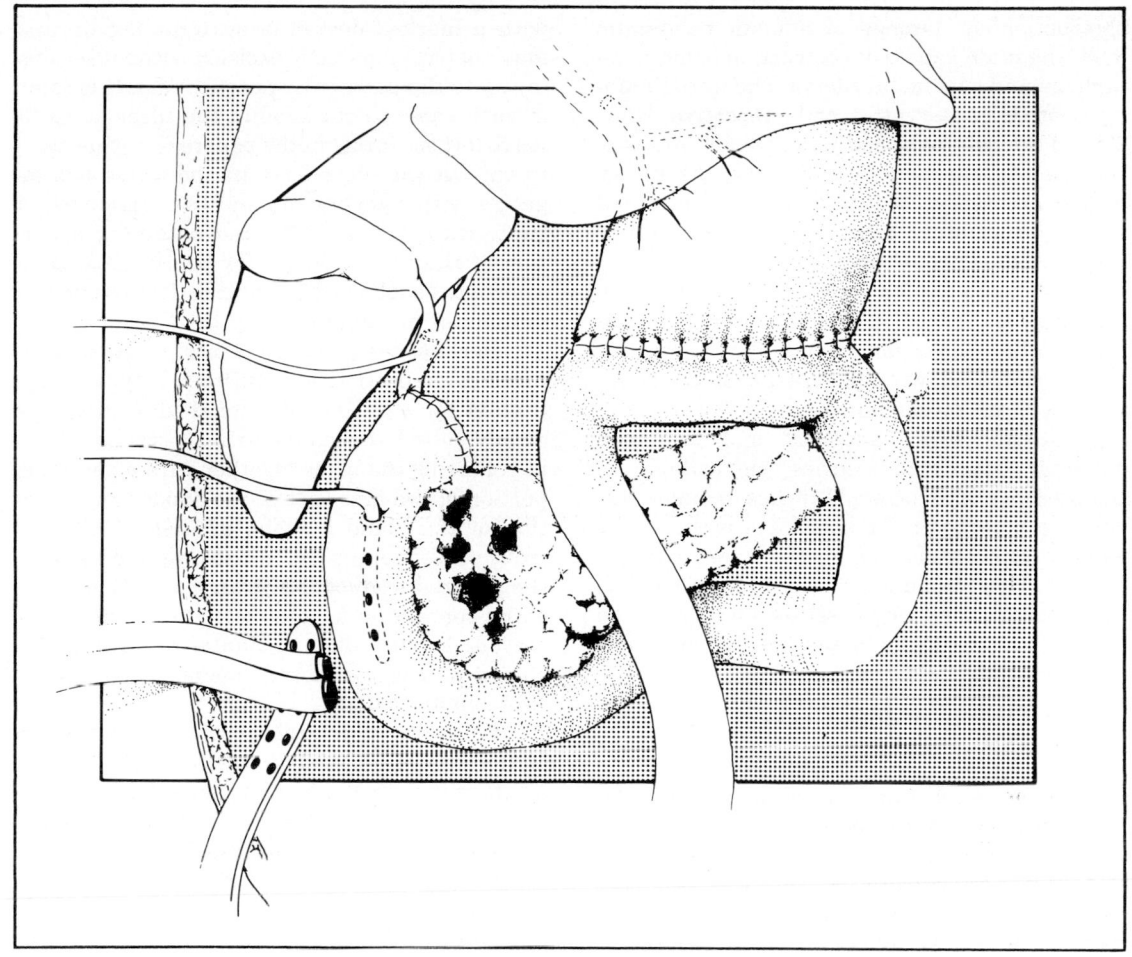

Figure 86–8. The essential components of duodenal diverticulization including gastric antrectomy, tube duodenostomy, gastrojejunostomy, and drainage. Truncal vagotomy and drainage of the biliary tract may be advisable.

ated with an isolated pancreatic injury is pancreatic fistula, occurring in up to 35 percent of cases, and usually following blunt trauma. Presumably, this is due to unrecognized injury of a major pancreatic duct. However, most pancreatic fistulas are minor and close in less than 4 weeks. Major pancreatic fistulas have been arbitrarily defined as those that persist in excess of 1 month. Almost all pancreatic fistulas will eventually close spontaneously, thus their treatment is usually conservative. Vigorous fluid replacement and total parenteral nutrition with close electrolyte control are strongly indicated.

A pancreatic pseudocyst following trauma is usually associated with blunt injury and results from the accumulation and walling off of undrained pancreatic fluids secreted from the distal portion of the severed gland. Persistent ileus in the absence of overt sepsis often signals the development of a pseudocyst. Pancreatic pseudocyst should now be a rare complication of pancreatic trauma if the pancreas is explored and drained adequately. The majority of pseudocysts resolve by the sixth week; failure to do so necessitates further intervention.

Shock secondary to major hemorrhage, when present on the patient's admission to the emergency room, predisposes to the development of abscess and sepsis, as do colon injuries. Pancreatic abscesses, per se, have a high mortality rate and it is essential that they are recognized and treated early.

Pancreatitis following trauma is an avoidable complication. It results from unrecognized obstruction or damage to a main pancreatic duct, the main causes of obstruction being hemorrhage and periductal edema. The initial management is conservative and supportive. However, if the patient's condition does not improve, resection of the pancreas distal to the injury may be necessary. Some patients with untreated or inappropriately treated pancreatic injury may develop chronic pancreatitis.

The complication rate and mortality are markedly increased in pancreatic or duodenal injury when the common bile duct is also injured, compared with pancreatic or duodenal injuries alone or combined.

Patients with pancreatic and combined pancreaticoduodenal injuries, particularly in the presence of associated injuries to major vascular structures or the colon, are prone to develop complications seen in other types of major trauma. These include respiratory insufficiency, renal failure, and major sepsis, and should be managed aggressively in an intensive care unit.

IATROGENIC PANCREATIC INJURIES

It must be emphasized at the outset that all iatrogenic pancreatic injuries are preventable by the application of proper operative judgment and technique. Operations on the stomach, duodenum, gallbladder, spleen, colon, and pancreas itself may all, in certain instances, result in injury to the pancreatic tissue (Fig. 86–9). The injury may have no ill effect, but occasionally will result in acute pancreatitis, pseudocyst or fistula formation, subphrenic abscess, hemorrhage from the pancreas, or even necrosis of the gland. Schmieden and Sebening collected a series of pancreatic injuries caused during operations on the upper abdominal viscera. The incidences are as shown:

Operation	Injuries to Pancreas
Stomach	91
Biliary tract	38
Spleen	7
Diagnostic biopsy of pancreas	4
Others	5
Total	145

Gastric and Duodenal Procedures

Gastric and duodenal ulcers that deeply penetrate the pancreas and that are often associated with a marked degree of surrounding fibrosis may not be amenable to excision without serious injury to the pancreatic parenchyma. It is safer in such cases to cut around the ulcer so as to leave its base intact in the pancreas, rather than to cut out the ulcer from its indurated bed together with a portion of pancreatic tissue. Even cauterization, curettage, and obtaining a portion of the ulcer margin for biopsy have been known to be followed by pancreatitis, fistula formation, or an inflammatory pseudocyst.

Perhaps the pancreas is most frequently injured in connection with Billroth II types of operation for a chronic duodenal ulcer that has deeply pitted the pancreatic substance. Here, in removing the ulcer together with a generous portion of the first part of the duodenum a portion of the gland may be excised with disastrous consequences. In transfixing and ligating the pancreaticoduodenal artery, a portion of the gland containing a small segment of the accessory pancreatic duct of Santorini may be included in a ligature, and this may give rise to subsequent trouble.

Following wide excision of the first portion of the duodenum and inversion of the stump, a suture may pick up and occlude the accessory duct or include a portion of pancreatic tissue, producing pancreatitis, localized necrosis, or an external pancreatic fistula. Excessive inversion of a duodenal stump during the performance of a Billroth II operation may be a cause of obstruction to the pancreatic ducts and of the terminal end of the common bile duct.

Attempts at radical excision of gastric carcinoma provide more possible sources of danger. In attempting to carry the dissection well beyond a suspicious infiltrating area, it may be necessary to include a portion of the pancreas in the resected mass. In cases of carcinoma of the stomach where the growth is adherent to the body or tail of the pancreas it is advisable to perform radical subtotal or total gastrectomy with distal pancreatectomy, rather than trying to excise some of the pancreatic parenchyma and almost certainly damaging the ductal system.

Biliary Procedures

Pancreatitis may follow transduodenal sphincterotomy or exploration of the common bile duct or ERCP. Severe pancreatic injury may result from injudicious and forceful "dilatation" of the sphincter of Oddi during common bile duct ex-

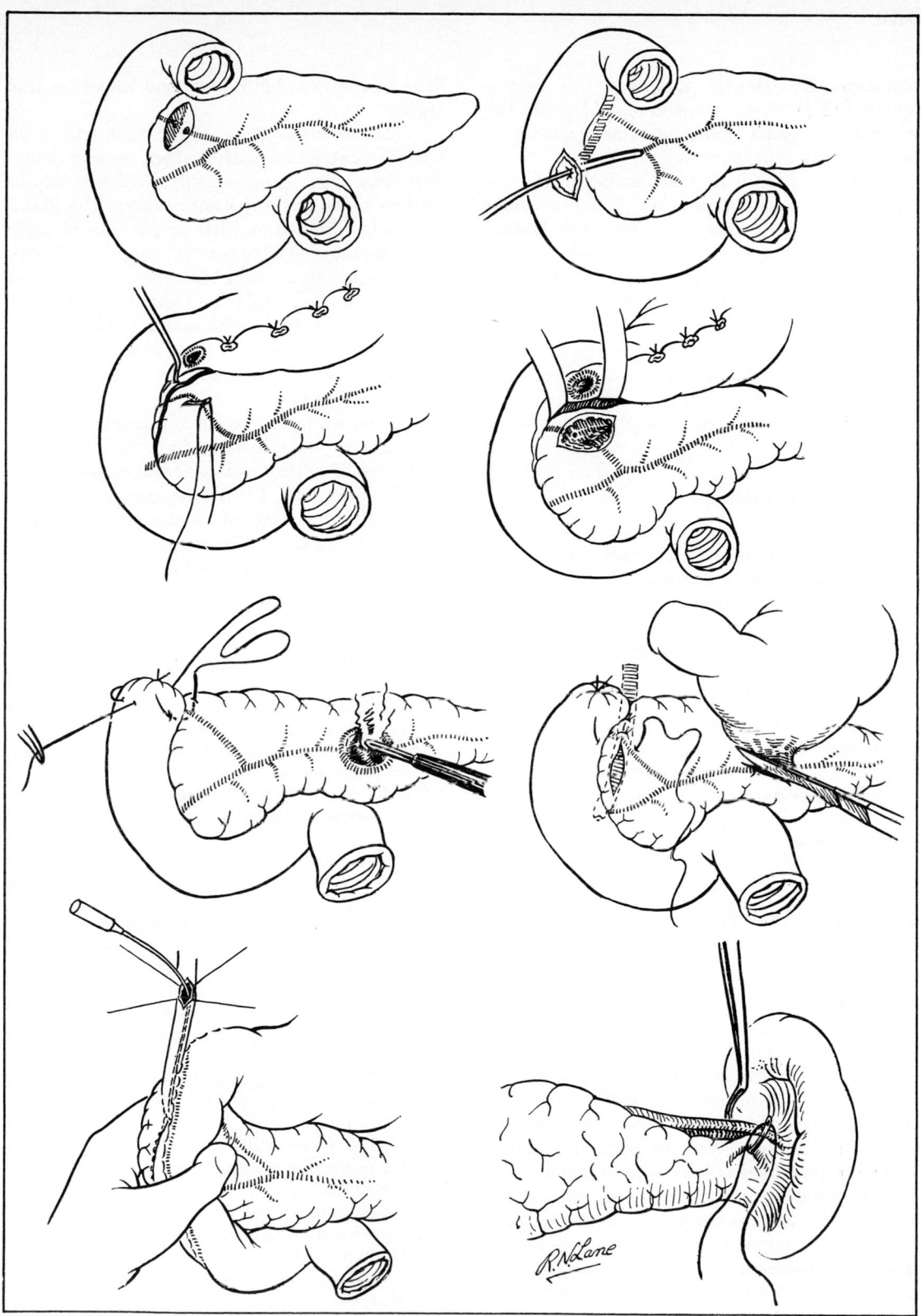

Figure 86–9. Operative injuries of the pancreas. (*Source: Adapted from Wright LT, Prigot A, et al: Traumatic subcutaneous injuries to the pancreas. Am J Surg 80:170, 1950, with permission.*)

ploration. Dr. Robert Zollinger has recommended that "every surgeon should dilate the common bile duct with the same temerity as he would his own urethra."

Following the Kocher mobilization, an overly vigorous manipulation of the terminal portion of the common bile duct in palpating a stone or a suspected stone has been known to be followed by severe inflammatory reaction of the head of the gland. A number of cases of acute pancreatitis have been reported following the use of a long-limbed T-tube for biliary tract disease, the descending limb of the tube being passed through the ampulla into the duodenum. This practice should be strongly discouraged.

Splenic Operations

Splenectomy is another operation in which the pancreas may be injured. The tail of the gland may be clamped with hemostats and ligated as the pedicle is being secured, particularly in the emergency situation of a traumatized spleen. As a result, a fistula or pseudocyst may subsequently occur.

During the performance of a distal splenorenal shunt operation for the correction of portal hypertension it is necessary to dissect the splenic vein from the body and tail of the pancreas. The gland in this situation is often fibrotic and the dissection is difficult; damage may occur to the pancreas.

Pancreatic Procedures

It can be exceedingly difficult in some cases to determine whether a hard craggy mass in the head of the pancreas is a cancer or a localized area of chronic pancreatitis, and the temptation for some surgeons to excise a small portion of the gland as a "wedge" biopsy is a very real one. This should be resisted. With the advent of ultrasonography, CT scanning, ERCP, and cytology, most doubtful cases are sorted out preoperatively. The surgeon may elect to perform one or two needle biopsies of the mass, but it must be remembered that truly representative biopsies of the pancreas may be hard to obtain because of sampling error and confusion between tumor and associated histologic pancreatitis. It is essential that the patient is not "biopsied to death," and a pancreaticoduodenal resection may in the end be necessary because of the in-

flicted trauma to both ducts and vessels in this region.

The pancreas is an organ that has to be treated gently and with respect, as any deviation from this standard will almost certainly lead to some form of complication. The gland should be handled as little as possible; clamps, hemostats and electrocautery should not be applied to the gland; and bleeding points should be ligated accurately and singly. The duct should be transfixed with a single nonabsorbable suture, and there is little excuse for using a stapling gun in the gland, as this inflicts unnecessary trauma.

When an injury to the pancreatic duct occurs, and remains unrecognized, the grave complications of peritonitis, pancreatic abscess, external pancreatic fistula, or pseudocyst may follow. Prompt surgical treatment should improve the prognosis of acute postoperative pancreatitis, which up to now has been very poor.

BIBLIOGRAPHY

Babb J, Harmon H: Diagnosis and management of pancreatic trauma. Am Surg 42:390, 1976

Bach RD, Frey CF: Diagnosis and treatment of pancreatic trauma. Am J Surg 121:20, 1971

Baker RJ, Dippel WF, et al: The surgical significance of trauma to the pancreas. Arch Surg 86:1038, 1963

Baker RJ, Bass RT, et al: External pancreatic fistula following abdominal injury. Arch Surg 95:556, 1967

Balasegaram M: Surgical management of pancreatic trauma. Am J Surg 131:536, 1976

Berne CJ, Donovan AJ, et al: Duodenal diverticulization for duodenal and pancreatic injury. Am J Surg 127:503, 1974

Bozymski EM, Orlando RC, et al: Traumatic disruption of the pancreatic duct demonstrated by endoscopic retrograde pancreatography. J Trauma 21:244, 1981

Cogbill TH, Moore EE, et al: Changing trends in the management of pancreatic trauma. Arch Surg 117:722, 1982

Corley RD, Norcross WJ, et al: Traumatic injuries to the duodenum, a report of 98 patients. Ann Surg 181:92, 1975

Crass RA, Trunkey DD: Pancreatic trauma in pancreatic disease, diagnosis and therapy, in Dent TL, Eckhauser FE, et al (eds): Pancreatic Disease, Diagnosis and Therapy. New York: Grune & Stratton, 1981, p 221

Doublier L, Garren A: Les plaies duodeno pancreatoques par projectiles. Lyons Chir 65:842, 1969

Federle MP, Goldberg HI, et al: Evaluation of abdominal trauma by computed tomography. Radiology 138:637, 1981

Fraser CG: Handlebar injury of the pancreas. J Pediatr Surg 4:216, 1969

Frey CT: Trauma of the pancreas, in Brooks JR (ed): Surgery of the Pancreas. Philadelphia: WB Saunders, 1983, p 396

Graham JM, Mattox KL, et al: Combined pancreatoduodenal injuries. J Trauma 19:340, 1979

Grosfield JL, Cooney DR: Pancreatic and gastrointestinal trauma in children. Pediatr Clin North Am 22:365, 1975

Heitsch RC, Knutson CO, et al: Delineation of critical factors in the treatment of pancreatic trauma. Surgery 80:523, 1976

Henarejos A, Cohen DM, et al: Management of pancreatic trauma. Ann R Coll Surg Engl 65:297, 1983

Jeffrey RB Jr, Federle MP, et al: Computed tomography of pancreatic trauma. Radiology 147:491, 1983

Jones RC: Management of pancreatic trauma. Ann Surg 187:555, 1978

Karl HW, Chandler JG: Mortality and morbidity of pancreatic injury. Am J Surg 134:549, 1977

Kaude JV, McInnis AN, et al: Pancreatic ultrasound following blunt abdominal trauma. Gastrointest Radiol 7:53, 1982

Lucas CE: Diagnosis and management of pancreatic injury. Ann Emerg Med 10:172, 1981

Maingot R: Injuries of the pancreas, in Maingot R (ed). Abdominal Operations, 7 edt. New York: Appleton-Century-Crofts, 1980, p 785

Matthewson C Jr, Halter BL: Traumatic pancreatitis with and without associated injuries. Am J Surg 83:409, 1952

Moossa AR: Pancreatic cancer. Approach to diagnosis, selection for surgery and choice of operation. Cancer 50:2689, 1982

Mortez JA, Campbell DP, et al: Significance of serum amylase level in evaluating pancreatic trauma. Am J Surg 130:739, 1975

Northrup WF, Simmons RL: Pancreatic trauma: A

review. Surgery 71:27, 1972

Otis GA: Penetrating wounds of the abdomen, in Otis GA (ed): The Medical and Surgical History of the War of the Rebellion, part 2, vol 2. Washington, D.C.: Government Printing Office, 1876

Parrish RA, Humphries AL, et al: Massive pancreatic ascites. Arch Surg 96:887, 1968

Poole LH: Wounds of the pancreas (62 casualties), in Surgical History of World War II, Office of the Surgeon General. Washington, D.C.: Government Printing Office, 1945

Sheldon GF, Cohn LH, et al: Surgical treatment of pancreatic trauma. J Trauma 10:795, 1970

Shires GT, Jones RC: Pancreatic trauma, in Carey LC (ed): The Pancreas. St. Louis: CV Mosby, 1973, p 335

Sims EH, Lou MA, Schlater T, et al: Surgical management of pancreatic trauma. Am J Surg 145:278, 1983

Steele M, Sheldon GF, et al: Pancreatic injuries. Arch Surg 106:544, 1973

Stone HH, Fabian TC: Management of duodenal wounds. J Trauma 19:334, 1979

Thomassen B, Linna MJ, et al: Blunt pancreatic trauma. Acta Chir Scand 139:48, 1973

Toombs BD, Lester RG, et al: Computed tomography in blunt abdominal trauma. Radiol Clin North Am 19:17, 1981

Travers B: Rupture of the pancreas. Lancet 12:384, 1827

Weitzman JJ, Rothschild PD: The surgical management of traumatic rupture of the pancreas due to blunt trauma. Surg Clin North Am 48:1347, 1968

Werschky LR, Jordan GL: Surgical management of traumatic injuries to the pancreas. Am J Surg 116:768, 1968

White PH, Benfield JR: Amylase in the management of pancreatic trauma. Arch Surg 105:158, 1972

Wilson RF, Tagett JP, et al: Pancreatic trauma. J Trauma 7:643, 1967

Yellin AE, Vecchione TR, et al: Distal pancreatectomy for pancreatic trauma. Am J Surg 124:135, 1972

87. Acute Pancreatitis

John H.C. Ranson

INTRODUCTION

Acute pancreatitis has been defined as pancreatic inflammation that may be followed by clinical and biologic restitution of the gland if the primary cause is eliminated. It includes a spectrum of clinical illness that ranges from mild self-limiting symptoms to rapid deterioration and death. The initiating etiologic factors are multiple and diverse and the pathologic findings may range from pancreatic edema to hemorrhagic infarction. Therefore, although acute pancreatic inflammation of all types has certain common features, it is important to recognize that multiple disease entities are included in this term and the management of patients must be highly individualized.

ETIOLOGY

Etiologic associations of acute pancreatitis have been identified primarily on the basis of epidemiologic evidence. Approximately 80 percent of patients either have gallstones or a history of sustained alcohol abuse. The relative frequency of these two associations depends on the prevalence of alcoholism in the population studied. Other factors that have been implicated in the etiology of acute pancreatitis are listed in Table 87-1.

Metabolic Factors

Alcohol. Clinical pancreatitis is recognized in 0.9 to 9.5 percent of alcoholic patients. Symptoms are usually first noted only after a 6- to 10-year period of heavy alcohol ingestion. Studies by Sarles have shown that chronic alcohol administration leads to changes in pancreatic exocrine secretion, with development of precipitates within the pancreatic ducts. It is postulated that these precipitates may lead to ductal obstruction and inflammation.

Other. Pancreatitis is associated with hyperlipoproteinemia, especially Frederickson Types I, IV, or V, with hypercalcemia and with the bite of the black scorpion of Trinidad. In addition, a causal relationship is generally accepted between the administration of adrenal corticosteroids, thiazide diuretics, estrogens, azothioprine, and furosemide and the occurrence of pancreatitis. It may also occur as an unexplained familial illness.

Mechanical Factors

Cholelithiasis. Gallstones are present in approximately 60 percent of nonalcoholic patients with acute pancreatitis. Their causative role is further indicated by the finding that, if stones are allowed to persist, 36 to 63 percent of patients will develop recurrent acute pancreatitis. This risk can be reduced to 2 to 8 percent by surgical correction of biliary lithiasis. Studies of the stool of patients recovering from gallstone pancreatitis have demonstrated gallstones in 85 to 94 percent of cases. It has been proposed that obstruction of a common biliary and pancreatic channel at the ampulla of Vater may lead to reflux of bile into the pancreas and the initiation of pancreatitis. Although reflux of dye into the pancreatic duct during cholangiography is more frequent in patients with pancreatitis, it is not clear whether pancreatitis is secondary to reflux or to simple calculous obstruction of the pancreatic duct.

Postoperative Pancreatitis. Acute pancreatitis has been recognized following 0.8 to 17 percent of surgical operations on the stomach and 0.7 to 9.3 percent of biliary operations. In these patients, it is probable that direct injury to the

TABLE 87–1. ETIOLOGIC FACTORS IN ACUTE PANCREATITIS

Metabolic:	• Alcohol • Hyperlipoproteinemia • Hypercalcemia • Drugs • Scorpion venom • Genetic
Mechanical:	• Cholelithiasis • Postoperative (gastric, biliary) • Posttraumatic • Retrograde pancreatography • Pancreatic duct obstruction: Pancreatic tumor, Ascaris infestation • Duodenal obstruction
Vascular:	• Postoperative (cardiopulmonary bypass) • Periarteritis nodosa • Atheroembolism
Infection:	• Mumps • Coxsackie virus

pancreas or to its blood supply or obstruction of the pancreatic duct at the duodenum is responsible. Acute pancreatitis also occurs in patients following cardiopulmonary bypass or major vascular surgery and ischemic injury to the pancreas is probably a major factor in this setting.

Other Mechanical Factors. Acute pancreatitis occurs in approximately 6 percent of patients who sustain blunt or penetrating injuries to the pancreas. The injection of dye into the pancreatic duct during endoscopic retrograde pancreatography is followed by clinically obvious pancreatitis in about 1 percent of such studies. Finally, obstruction of the pancreatic duct due to tumor or parasitic infestation occasionally leads to pancreatitis.

Vascular Factors

Pancreatitis has been demonstrated in association with atheromatous emboli to the pancreatic vessels and in patients with periarteritic nodosa. It also occurs following periods of profound hypoperfusion.

Infectious Factors

Viral infection of the pancreas has been implicated in the pathogenesis of pancreatitis observed during mumps or Coxsackie viral infections.

PATHOLOGY AND PATHOPHYSIOLOGY

The mildest pathologic change observed in the pancreas during acute pancreatitis consists of edema of the gland. This may be accompanied by infiltration of the intralobular septa by inflammatory cells. Microscopic examination may also show areas of fat necrosis in the pancreas and in surrounding tissues. If such necrosis is more extensive, it becomes grossly recognizable as characteristic whitish-yellow plaques. Finally, vascular thrombosis or disruption may result in pancreatic necrosis or gross hemorrhagic infarction. Increased levels of active pancreatic enzymes have been observed within the pancreas, in the peritoneal exudate, and in the bloodstream of patients with pancreatitis and are usually implicated in the multiple systemic and local complications of this disease.

Fluid and Electrolyte Changes

Circulating blood volume is frequently markedly reduced due to losses from the intravascular space, primarily of plasma. These losses occur both systemically and into the retroperitoneum. Additional fluid and electrolyte losses occur secondary to vomiting or nasogastric suction. Hypocalcemia and hypomanganesemia are frequent. In many instances, decreased total calcium levels are a reflection of hypoalbuminemia but decreases in ionized calcium levels also occur and are usually attributed to binding of calcium in areas of fat necrosis.

Cardiovascular Failure

Hypotension, tachycardia, increased total peripheral resistance, and decreased cardiac output are well-recognized sequelae of hypovolemia and are observed frequently in patients with acute pancreatitis. In some patients, hypotension persists despite restoration of the functional intravascular volume. The occurrence of such hypotension has been attributed to kinin formation by pancreatic proteolytic enzymes.

Respiratory Complications

Arterial hypoxemia is a frequent early feature of acute pancreatitis and arterial oxygen tensions less than 66 mm Hg are observed in 38 percent of patients during the initial 48 hours of treatment. Early pulmonary function studies have shown decreases in inspiratory lung volume, with decreased pulmonary compliance and decreased diffusing capacity. Early pathologic changes in the lung are increased lung weight, with pulmonary congestion, microatelectasis, and infarction.

Early respiratory failure often resolves as pancreatitis subsides, but patients with severe or unresolving pancreatitis may develop progressive pulmonary insufficiency, infiltrates, and pleural effusions. Factors that have been implicated in the pathogenesis of pulmonary complications in acute pancreatitis include abdominal distention and elevation of the diaphragm, alteration in the lecithin of pulmonary surfactant by circulating pancreatic lecithinase, pulmonary thromboembolism, circulating free fatty acids, and circulating products of the proteolytic cleavage of complement.

Renal Failure

In the past, impaired renal function was a major factor in deaths from pancreatitis. In most instances renal failure was due principally to hypovolemia. Nonetheless, renal impairment occurs in normovolemic patients and histologic studies have shown deposits of fibrin and fibrinogen within the glomeruli.

Other Systemic Features

Abnormal liver function with elevations of serum bilirubin, alkaline phosphatase and transaminase levels occur and have been attributed to biliary obstruction, hepatic parenchymal necrosis, and pericholangitis.

Early intravascular thrombosis with decreased platelet counts, and fibrinogen levels are well documented and are usually attributed to the effects of pancreatic proteolytic enzymes. Early changes may be followed by marked thrombocytosis and hyperfibrinogenemia.

Local Sequelae

The intraabdominal complications of acute pancreatitis include paralytic ileus and duodenal or biliary obstruction. In most patients these are attributable to pancreatic inflammation and enlargement. Release of pancreatic enzymes may also lead to enzyme-rich peripancreatic fluid collections and to destruction of tissues adjacent to the pancreas. The accumulation of fluid in the general peritoneal cavity and in the tissues around the pancreas is common. It is rarely associated with demonstrable gross disruption of the pancreatic ductal system and is usually self-limited. In approximately 1 percent of patients with acute pancreatitis, a persistent chronic pseudocyst may evolve. In severe acute pancreatitis, extensive destruction of tissues in and around the pancreas may become secondarily infected. Infected pancreatic abscesses occur in 1 to 9 percent of patients and the organisms involved are usually enteric. Extension of local necrosis to involve the colonic wall occurs in about 1 percent of patients. It leads to colonic perforation, usually in the left transverse colon or splenic flexure.

CLINICAL MANIFESTATIONS AND DIAGNOSIS

The initial symptoms and signs of acute pancreatitis are varied and may closely mimic those of acute myocardial or other intraabdominal disease. Nonetheless, in most patients, diagnosis depends primarily on careful clinical evaluation. Abdominal pain is usually the dominant initial complaint and is present in 85 to 100 percent of cases. Characteristically, the pain is upper abdominal and constant. It radiates to the back in approximately 50 percent of patients and may be severe. The pain often starts after a heavy meal or during a drinking binge. It increases rapidly in intensity but its onset is less sudden than that of the pain due to perforated ulcer.

The second most prominent symptoms are nausea and vomiting, which are noted in up to 92 percent of patients. Vomiting may be repeated but usually is not copious in volume. The vomitus is primarily gastric and duodenal contents and is not feculent.

The findings on physical examination are variable. The patient may be restless, with a rapid pulse and respiratory rate. Arterial hypotension may be present but transient hypertension also occurs. The abdomen usually is moderately distended and may exhibit a characteristic epigastric fullness. Tenderness may be generalized, but is usually most marked over the upper abdomen. Moderate muscle spasm is usual but true rigidity is infrequent. Grey Turner sign or a grey-green discoloration of the flank may be present in patients with peripancreatic hemorrhage.

Laboratory Findings

Determination of serum amylase level is the most widely used laboratory test for the diagnosis of pancreatic disease. Elevated levels are observed at hospital admission in 95 percent of patients with acute pancreatitis and only 5 percent of patients with other acute intraabdominal conditions. The most common nonpancreatic intraabdominal conditions associated with elevated serum amylase levels are perforated peptic ulcer, biliary lithiasis, intestinal obstruction, and mesenteric infarction. Clearly a normal initial serum amylase level does not exclude acute pancreatitis and this is particularly true in patients with hypertriglyceridemia and lactescent serum. Routine determination of serum amylase in these patients often yields normal results and dilution of the serum is necessary to demonstrate hyperamylasemia. It has been suggested that the diagnostic specificity of amylase measurements may be increased by determination of the urinary amylase-to-creatinine clearance ratio. This ratio is normally less than 4 percent and is often elevated in acute pancreatitis. The value of this measurement is, however, controversial.

Elevated serum lipase levels are also observed in acute pancreatitis. They appear to be somewhat more specific than amylase levels but are more difficult to measure. Hyperglycemia or glycosuria may occur in patients with acute pancreatitis but is nonspecific. Hypocalcemia is a well-recognized feature of acute pancreatitis but may also occur in patients with perforated peptic ulcer.

Radiographic Findings

Plain radiographs of the chest and abdomen demonstrate findings that may support a diagnosis of acute pancreatitis in 79 percent of patients. The most common findings are segmental small bowel ileus or a "sentinel loop" in the left upper quadrant, dilatation of the transverse colon, increased epigastric soft tissue density, and obscured psoas margins. Although these findings are nonspecific, they may be valuable in the overall clinical evaluation. When simpler studies are equivocal, radiographic evaluation of the upper gastrointestinal (GI) tract using water-soluble contrast media may be helpful. Occasionally, duodenal edema or pancreatic enlargement may be demonstrated, but even when positive evidence of pancreatitis is absent, such studies help to reduce the possibility of overlooked upper GI obstruction or perforation. In the rare patient in whom life-threatening obstructive biliary disease must be excluded, per-

cutaneous transhepatic cholangiography is a valuable method for demonstrating biliary anatomy.

Abdominal ultrasonography is helpful in evaluating the presence or absence of associated cholelithiasis but early demonstration of the pancreas is often incomplete in patients with acute pancreatitis due to gas within the GI tract. Computed tomography (CT) provides better definition of pancreatic anatomy but may show little abnormality in the early phase of acute pancreatitis.

Paracentesis

The character of the peritoneal fluid in patients with pancreatitis is variable and, unless clear evidence of GI perforation or infarction is found, paracentesis has not proved to be a reliable method for differentiating acute pancreatitis from conditions requiring urgent surgical correction.

Diagnostic Laparotomy

In most patients, careful clinical, radiographic, and biochemical evaluation combined with observation of the response to treatment permits differentiation of acute pancreatitis from other acute intraabdominal diseases. Life-threatening extrapancreatic pathology cannot, however, always be excluded by nonoperative measures and approximately 5 percent of patients require early laparotomy to exclude or treat possible mesenteric infarction, gangrenous cholecystitis, or other conditions requiring urgent surgical correction.

Prognostic Assessment

The spectrum of clinical acute pancreatitis ranges from a mild, self-limiting disease to a catastrophic, rapidly lethal illness that appears refractory to every treatment. Because the natural history of this disease is so varied, a rational approach to treatment requires the early identification of those patients who have a high risk of developing life-threatening complications. Clearly, treatment that itself has little risk or morbidity can be applied to all patients with pancreatitis. However, many of the monitoring and therapeutic measures that may be helpful to patients with severe pancreatitis are associated with risks and morbidity that make them inappropriate or unduly hazardous for patients with mild disease. In the past, identifica-

TABLE 87–2. EARLY OBJECTIVE PROGNOSTIC SIGNS THAT CORRELATE WITH THE RISK OF MAJOR COMPLICATIONS OR DEATH IN ACUTE PANCREATITIS

At admission or diagnosis:
- Age over 55 years
- White blood cell count over 16,000/μl
- Blood glucose level over 200 mg/dl
- Serum lactic dehydrogenase concentration over 350 IU/L
- Serum glutamic oxaloacetic transaminase over 250 sigma-Frankel units/dl

During initial 48 hours:
- Hematocrit decrease greater than 10 percentage points
- Blood urea nitrogen increase more than 5 mg/dl
- Serum calcium level below 8 mg/dl
- Arterial Po_2 below 60 mm Hg
- Base deficit greater than 4 mEq/L
- Estimated fluid sequestration more than 6000 ml

tion of "severe" pancreatitis has usually been based upon findings such as failure to respond to treatment, the severity of abdominal signs, or the appearance of the pancreas at operation. Most of these findings are impossible to quantify and are therefore influenced by observer variation.

Statistical analysis of multiple early laboratory and clinical measurements in patients with

pancreatitis have led to the identification of the eleven early prognostic signs shown in Table 87–2. Figure 87–1 shows the relationship between the number of these signs that were present in individual patients and the risk of death or complications requiring more than 1 week of treatment in an intensive care unit. Clearly not every patient with three, four, or even five positive signs has severe pancreatitis. The signs serve only to identify groups of patients with increased risk of major complications.

Other objective measurements of reported prognostic value include serum levels of methemalbumin, albumin, and ribonuclease. It has also been reported by McMahon that prognostic classification can be made on the basis of the volume and color of fluid obtained from the peritoneal cavity by paracentesis and peritoneal lavage. The accuracy of most of these measurements has not yet been evaluated by large prospective trials.

TREATMENT

Nonoperative Therapy

Measures that have been proposed for the treatment of patients with acute pancreatitis may be classified as those that are intended to limit

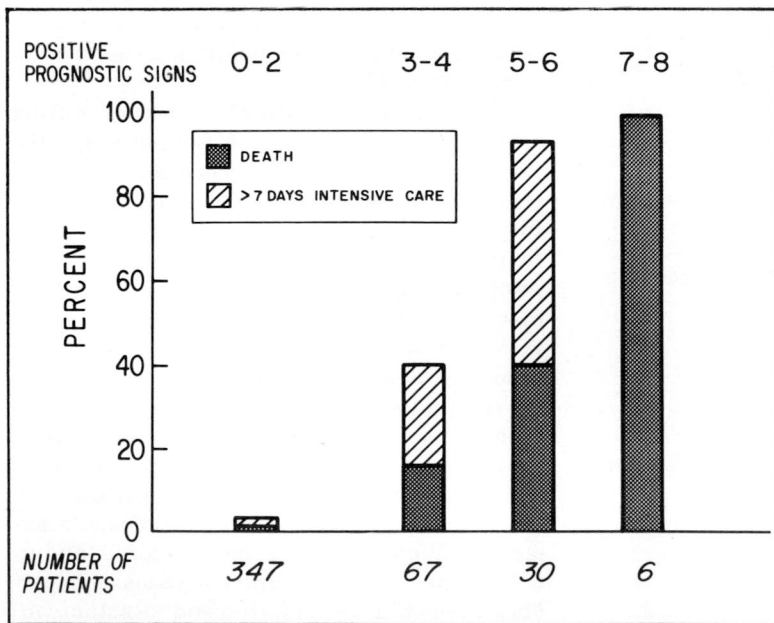

Figure 87–1. The relationship between the number of positive early prognostic signs recorded and the morbidity and mortality in 450 patients with acute pancreatitis. (*Source: From Ranson JHC: The role of peritoneal lavage in acute pancreatitis. Ann Surg 187:566, 1978, with permission.*)

the severity of pancreatic inflammation or to interrupt the pathogenesis of complications and those that are intended to support the patients and treat specific sequelae (Table 87–3).

Nasogastric suction is usually initiated to reduce vomiting and abdominal distention. It has also been suggested that aspiration of gastric acid may reduce pancreatic exocrine secretion by reducing secretin release. Small unstratified controlled clinical trials have failed to demonstrate significant improvement in the course of mild acute pancreatitis by nasogastric suction. We continue, however, to recommend nasogastric suction in most patients because of the symptomatic improvement that often follows and the occasional reduction in pancreatic inflammation, which is apparent. Although the role of nasogastric suction is controversial, it has been clearly shown that early oral feedings may increase the severity of pancreatic inflammation and it is important that such feedings be withheld until abdominal pain and tenderness, fever, and leukocytosis have all subsided. This is an average of 8 days in patients with mild pancreatitis (less than three positive prognostic signs) and 16 days in those with more severe disease.

Attempts to inhibit pancreatic secretion by a variety of drugs, hypothermia, or pancreatic irradiation have been recommended on the basis of experimental studies or anecdoctal clinical experience. The administration of anticholinergic drugs, Glucagon, cimetidine, and calcitonin have been evaluated in prospective clinical studies, and, with the exception of possible benefit from calcitonin, all have been found ineffective in reducing morbidity.

The inhibition of pancreatic enzymes has been proposed, but the only agent that has been extensively studied is aprotinin, an extract of bovine parotid glands that inhibits trypsin and kallikrein. Large trials have failed to demonstrate clinical benefit from this drug.

Adrenal corticosteroids have been recommended because of their antiinflammatory effects, but there is no clinical evidence to support their administration.

Controlled clinical studies have shown no benefit from the administration of ampicillin to patients with mild, alcoholic pancreatitis. The efficacy of antibiotics in patients with gallstone-associated or severe pancreatitis is not known, but we continue to give broad-spectrum antibiotics to these groups.

GI bleeding from gastroduodenal ulceration is a frequent complication of severe pancreatitis. It may be greatly reduced by monitoring of gastric pH and administration of antacids to maintain a pH greater than 5. In some patients, cimetidine may help to maintain a satisfactory intragastric pH.

Intravascular coagulation occurs during acute pancreatitis and it has been suggested that administration of anticoagulants may be beneficial. Experimental evaluation of the efficacy of heparin has led to variable results. Our limited clinical experience has, however, indicated that heparin administration during the first few days of pancreatitis may be associated with extensive retroperitoneal hemorrhage and should be avoided whenever possible. Although the early administration of heparin may be hazardous, marked hypercoagulability occurs after the first week of treatment of some patients with severe pancreatitis. Pulmonary emboli are a frequent problem in these patients. Coagulation factors should, therefore, be monitored, and in patients with marked thrombocytosis or hyperfibrinogenemia, we recommend constant in-

TABLE 87–3. NONOPERATIVE MEASURES PROPOSED FOR THE TREATMENT OF ACUTE PANCREATITIS

A. *To limit the severity of pancreatic inflammation*
   1. Inhibition of pancreatic secretion
      a. Nasogastric suction
      b. Pharmacologic: anticholinergics, Glucagon, 5-fluorouracil, acetazolamide, cimetidine, calcitonin, somatostatin
      c. Hypothermia
      d. Pancreatic irradiation
   2. Inhibition of pancreatic enzymes
      a. Aprotinin, ε-aminocaproic acid, soybean trypsin inhibitor, insulin, snake antivenom
   3. Corticosteroids
B. *To interrupt the pathogenesis of complications*
   1. Antibiotics
   2. Antacids, cimetidine
   3. Heparin
   4. Low-molecular-weight dextran
   5. Vasopressin
C. *To support the patient and treat complications*
   1. Restoration and maintenance of intravascular volume
   2. Electrolyte replacement
   3. Respiratory support
   4. Nutritional support
   5. Heparin

travenous administration of heparin, 750 to 1000 units per hour, depending on the partial thromboplastin time. Heparin administration is begun only after the first 2 weeks of treatment.

Intravascular Volume Management

Assessment of intravascular volume and cardiovascular function depends upon regular measurements of pulse rate and blood pressure. In most patients, a central venous catheter should be introduced and an indwelling urethral catheter placed for monitoring of central venous pressure, venous blood gases, and hourly urine output. Further monitoring of pulmonary arterial pressures by a Swan–Ganz catheter may be essential in those patients with associated cardiovascular disease, massive fluid requirements, or respiratory failure.

In most patients, intravascular volume can be satisfactorily restored and maintained using crystalloid solutions. Blood transfusion may be required to maintain a satisfactory hematocrit, and albumin given to correct early hypoalbuminemia.

Electrolyte Management

Hypokalemia is frequent and potassium administration is usually required once adequate urinary output has been established. The intravenous administration of calcium and magnesium has been recommended. In many patients, decreased calcium levels in acute pancreatitis are related to hypoalbuminemia, with normal circulating levels of ionized calcium. Since hypercalcemia has been implicated in the genesis of pancreatitis, calcium administration should be cautious.

Renal Failure

Renal failure is a well-recognized complication of severe acute pancreatitis, but it is usually secondary to hypovolemia and hypoperfusion. It may be largely prevented by adequate restoration and maintenance of the intravascular volume and cardiovascular function. In those patients in whom renal function does not respond to these measures, dramatic improvement may sometimes be observed following the introduction of peritoneal lavage.

Respiratory Monitoring and Support

Since early respiratory failure occurs in patients who do not have severe disease by the usual clinical criteria and who may not have any obvious clinical evidence of pulmonary insufficiency, it is essential that arterial blood gas values be determined at diagnosis and at intervals of not less than 12 hours for the initial 48 to 72 hours of treatment in every patient.

In most patients with early arterial hypoxemia, the only necessary management is close monitoring and administration of oxygen. In patients with progressive respiratory failure, the volume of fluid administered intravenously should be decreased and the urinary output maintained or increased by the administration of diuretic drugs. There is usually no clinical or radiographic evidence of fluid overload in these patients, but improvement of respiratory function is often observed following such management. In those patients with severe pulmonary insufficiency, endotracheal intubation and postive-end-expiratory pressure ventilation should be instituted early.

Analgesia

The pain associated with acute pancreatitis may be extremely severe. It is traditional to administer meperidine rather than morphine because of the spasm of the ampulla of Vater that is associated with the latter drug. Splanchnic block or continuous epidural anesthesia have been recommended because they do not cause ampullary spasm and may increase pancreatic blood flow. They have not, however, been widely used.

Nutritional Support

Marked nutritional depletion has been well documented in patients with severe acute pancreatitis. In those with mild pancreatitis, oral feedings can usually be resumed after a shord time. Patients with severe pancreatitis cannot accept oral feedings for substantial periods and intravenous alimentation should be instituted in this group as soon as practical.

Operative Management

Surgical intervention in patients with acute pancreatitis may be required for diagnostic, therapeutic, or preventive reasons (Table 87–4).

Diagnosis

In the majority of patients, a reasonably certain diagnosis of acute pancreatitis can be reached on the basis of careful clinical, laboratory, and

TABLE 87–4. OPERATIVE MEASURES PROPOSED FOR THE MANAGEMENT OF ACUTE PANCREATITIS

A. *Diagnostic laparotomy*
B. *To limit the severity of pancreatic inflammation*
   1. Biliary operations
C. *To interrupt the pathogenesis of complications*
   1. Pancreatic drainage
   2. Pancreatic resection
   3. Thoracic duct drainage
   4. Peritoneal lavage
D. *To support the patient and treat complications*
   1. Drainage of pancreatic abscesses
   2. Feeding jejunostomy
E. *To prevent recurrent pancreatitis*

radiographic evaluation. However, a small proportion of patients require surgical exploration of the abdominal cavity to exclude or treat acute extrapancreatic pathology. In this regard, it is important to remember that nonpancreatic disease may closely mimic acute pancreatitis and also can occasionally occur coincidentally with pancreatitis. Thus the presence of strong evidence of pancreatitis does not exclude the possibility of co-existent gangrenous cholecystitis, mesenteric infarction, or other intraabdominal catastrophe.

When diagnostic laparotomy is undertaken, abdominal exploration must be complete and thorough. If uncomplicated acute pancreatitis is found, the choice of surgical procedure should be determined by specific therapeutic goals. If cholelithiasis is present and pancreatitis is very mild, definitive correction of biliary disease may usually be undertaken to prevent subsequent episodes of pancreatitis. Early biliary surgery does not, however, reduce the morbidity of the acute episode of pancreatitis and it may be hazardous in the presence of severe pancreatitis. If, therefore, severe gallstone pancreatitis is found at diagnostic laparotomy or if the severity of pancreatitis is unclear, it is our present practice to limit biliary surgery to cholecystostomy and cholangiography. There is no evidence that cholecystostomy improves the course of these patients. However, severe pancreatitis is often associated with high fevers and jaundice and the subsequent management is simplified by the presence of established biliary drainage and access to the biliary tree for radiographic study.

Peritoneal lavage appears to ameliorate the early complications of acute pancreatitis, and, therefore, soft Silastic catheters may be placed into the lesser omental sac and pelvis for postoperative lavage. More extensive procedures such as pancreatic debridement or resection should be avoided at this time. Furthermore, soft rubber or sump drains in the area of the pancreas are, in our experience, associated with a substantially increased incidence of late pancreatic sepsis and should not be placed.

Early Therapeutic Operations

Biliary Operations. In patients with acute pancreatitis associated with gallstones, it has been suggested that early biliary surgery may ameliorate the severity of pancreatic inflammation. Operative recommendations have included cholecystostomy, common duct drainage and cholecystectomy. Recently, Acosta has advocated early cholecystectomy, common bile duct exploration, and, when indicated, transduodenal sphincterotomy in patients with acute pancreatitis and cholelithiasis when symptoms are of less than 48 hours' duration.

Evaluation of the efficacy of early biliary surgery in ameliorating acute pancreatitis has been confused by difficulty in determining the diagnosis and estimating the severity of pancreatitis. Up to 75 percent of patients with acute abdominal pain, gallstones, and elevated serum amylase levels have no gross evidence of significant pancreatitis at early operation or autopsy. In such patients, early definitive treatment of biliary disease may usually be undertaken safely, with biliary symptoms promptly subsiding. Among patients who have clear evidence of pancreatitis, approximately 80 percent have mild disease; in this group, early biliary surgery can often be undertaken safely but does not ameliorate the course of pancreatitis. However, in patients with severe gallstone pancreatitis, early intraabdominal surgery has, in our experience, been associated with a higher mortality than early nonoperative treatment and should be avoided if gangrenous cholecystitis or obstructive cholangitis can be excluded.

It has been reported that early endoscopic papillotomy may ameliorate the course of gallstone pancreatitis, but the efficacy of this measure has not been determined.

Pancreatic Drainage. Early operative drainage of the pancreas was recommended at the beginning of this century and has recently received renewed attention. A small controlled trial of early sump drainage of the pancreas in patients with severe pancreatitis demonstrated a marked increase in frequency of intraabdominal sepsis and in severity of respiratory complications in those patients who underwent early operation.

Pancreatic Resection. There has been extensive interest in the possibility that early removal of part or all of the pancreas may reduce the devastating sequelae of severe acute pancreatitis. In clinical reports of resection, it is usually difficult to evaluate the severity of pancreatitis treated. However, in a review of 124 patients treated by primary resection, overall survival was 60 percent. The mortality after total pancreatectomy was 67 percent; pancreatoduodenectomy, 43 percent; distal subtotal pancreatectomy, 50 percent; and distal pancreatectomy, 41 percent. In 65 patients treated by resection of necrotic tissue alone, mortality was 29 percent.

Our own experience with early pancreatic resection for severe acute pancreatitis includes only five patients. All had severe pancreatic hemorrhage or frank pancreatic necrosis and the average number of positive prognostic signs was five. All underwent distal subtotal pancreatectomy within 48 hours of diagnosis. Unfortunately, their course was similar to that of other patients with pancreatitis of comparable severity. It was marked by severe respiratory failure, intraabdominal sepsis, and death in each case.

It has been our overall experience that early intraabdominal surgery, whether a biliary procedure, pancreatic drainage, or pancreatic resection, does not ameliorate the morbidity and mortality of acute pancreatitis in any group of patients. Occasionally, operation is followed by a dramatic improvement in cardiovascular function. This improvement is unfortunately greatly outweighed by increased respiratory complications and late pancreatic sepsis (Fig. 87–2).

Thoracic Duct Drainage. Since pancreatic enzymes may reach the bloodstream by lymphatic channels, it has been proposed that diversion of thoracic duct lymph by construction of a thoracic duct fistula may benefit patients with acute pancreatitis. Reported clinical experience has been too limited to allow any conclusions regarding the efficacy of this measure.

Peritoneal Lavage. By contrast with formal intraabdominal operations, peritoneal lavage by catheters introduced percutaneously appears to be associated with immediate clinical improve-

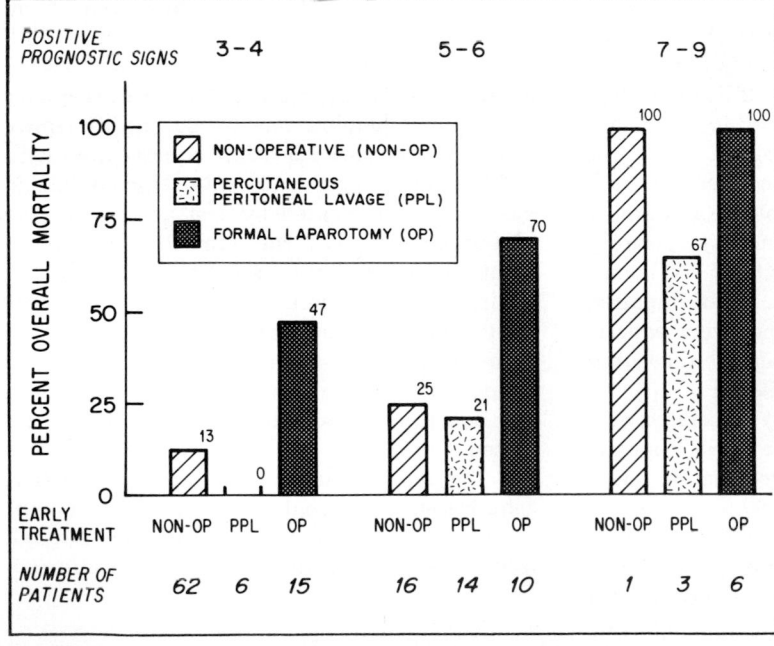

Figure 87–2. The overall hospital mortality rate related to early treatment (days 0 to 7) in patients with acute pancreatitis and three or more positive prognostic signs. The three early treatment groups are: NON-OP = conventional nonoperative measures, PPL = percutaneous peritoneal lavage under local anesthesia, OP = formal early laparotomy. (*Source: From Ranson JHC: Conservative surgical treatment of acute pancreatitis. World J Surg 5:353, 1981, with permission.*)

ment without increased respiratory or septic complications.

We consider any patient experiencing a first or second episode of acute pancreatitis and who has three or more positive prognostic signs to be a candidate for lavage. Because bowel distention is common in severe pancreatitis, the lavage catheter should be introduced through an open incision about 4 to 5 cm in length, with direct visualization of the peritoneum to reduce the risk of visceral injury. The incision is placed in the midline below the umbilicus, using full sterile technique and local infiltration anesthesia. In patients with previous abdominal incisions, an area remote from these incisions is selected. Our preferred lavage catheter is a soft but noncollapsible Silastic tubing. The incision is closed tightly about the catheter.

The lavage fluid is an approximately isotonic, balanced electrolyte solution containing 15 g/L of dextrose (Dianeal). Potassium (4 mEq), heparin (500 USP units), and a broad-spectrum antibiotic are usually added to each liter of lavage fluid. In general, 2 liters of fluid are run into the peritoneal cavity under gravity over about 15 minutes, remain intraperitoneally for about 30 minutes, and then are drained out by gravity. This cycle is repeated hourly. Lavage should be instituted during the initial 48 hours of treatment and continued for 48 hours to 7 days, depending upon the patient's clinical course.

In addition to the risk of visceral injury, there are two important hazards of peritoneal lavage. First, respiratory failure is frequent in severe pancreatitis and adding 2 liters of fluid to the peritoneal cavity may lead to significant decrease in ventilation. Respiratory status must, therefore, be closely monitored, and it is often necessary to reduce the volume and timing of the lavage cycle to avoid undue respiratory impairment. Second, the tonicity of the lavage fluid is maintained with glucose. Since impaired glucose tolerance is a feature of severe pancreatitis, serum glucose levels must be measured and insulin administered as needed.

Peritoneal lavage is usually associated with a marked improvement in the early systemic manifestations of severe pancreatitis. In nonlavaged patients, approximately 40 percent of all deaths occur during the first 10 days of treatment and are primarily due to respiratory and cardiovascular failure. Peritoneal lavage has been an extremely effective adjunct to the management of these complications and has been associated with almost complete prevention of early deaths.

Since hemodialysis is not associated with significant reduction in mortality from acute pancreatitis, it is usually presumed that the efficacy of lavage is due to removal of toxic factors present in the peritoneal exudate rather than to improvement in fluid and electrolyte status or removal of dialyzable substances from the blood.

As shown in Table 87–4, peritoneal lavage has also been associated with some improvement in overall mortality, but this improvement is disappointingly small. The reason for this is that lavage does not appear to be effective in preventing the occurrence of late pancreatic sepsis.

Operative Management of Local Complications

The most common local sequelae of acute pancreatitis are paralytic ileus, acute sterile peripancreatic fluid collection, and duodenal or biliary obstruction. These complications usually resolve as pancreatitis subsidies and they rarely require specific treatment. Chronic pseudocysts occur in approximately 1 percent of patients. Peripancreatic fluid collections that do not decrease in size 4 to 6 weeks after acute pancreatitis has subsided and that are more than 5 cm in diameter should be drained surgically. Failure to provide drainage is associated with significant risk of intraperitoneal rupture, secondary infection, or hemorrhage. Percutaneous aspiration has been described but is associated with a 70 percent recurrence rate. Uncomplicated cysts are best treated by cyst gastrostomy or cyst duodenostomy if the stomach or duodenum form part of the cyst wall. Other cysts should be drained into a defunctionalized jejunal loop. Cysts that are complicated by infection or that do not have a well-formed wall are usually best treated by external drainage. Most cysts with significant intracystic hemorrhage should be resected.

The most common local complication that requires surgical treatment is the development of infection in peripancreatic fluid and devitalized tissues, leading to pancreatic abscess formation.

PANCREATIC ABSCESS

Incidence

Pancreatic abscesses occur in up to 9 percent of patients but their frequency is related to the severity of the underlying pancreatitis. They occur in 2.7 percent of patients with less than three positive early prognostic signs and in 34 percent of those with more severe disease. Pancreatic sepsis occurs in 3.6 percent or 6.6 percent of patients with alcoholic or gallstone-associated pancreatitis and 14.8 percent of those with other etiologies. It is much more common in patients in whom postoperative pancreatitis is diagnosed, occurring in 39 percent of this group. Finally, pancreatic infection is increased in patients who undergo early laparotomy and should be anticipated in this group.

Clinical Diagnosis

Peripancreatic sepsis may occur at any time during the course of acute pancreatitis, but it is most commonly recognized after the first 2 weeks of treatment. The clinical and laboratory features are listed in Table 87–5. The cardinal clinical features are persistent or recurrent fever and leukocytosis, usually with abdominal distention and a palpable mass, after 14 to 21 days of treatment. The occurrence of positive blood cultures without another source is also strong evidence for pancreatic infection.

Radiographic Diagnosis

Plain radiographic examination of the abdomen is rarely helpful in the diagnosis of pancreatic abscesses. However, when contrast studies of the upper GI tract are possible, they demonstrate displacement of the stomach or duode-

TABLE 87–5. PERCENT INCIDENCE OF CLINICAL AND LABORATORY FEATURES IN PATIENTS WITH INFECTED PANCREATIC ABSCESSES

Fever > 101°F	100
Abdominal distention	94
Abdominal mass	71
Hypotension (BP < 90 mm Hg)	39
Pneumonia or effusion	89
Renal failure	39
Coma	28
Elevated serum amylase	28
Leukocytosis (> 10,000/mm³)	78

num in 76 percent of cases. Unfortunately, similar displacement may occur secondary to uninfected peripancreatic fluid or pancreatic enlargement. Radiographic demonstration of gas outside the GI tract provides clear evidence of sepsis and was documented in 16 percent of our patients.

Abdominal ultrasonography has, in our experience, been of limited value in the diagnosis of pancreatic abscess, possibly due to the presence of marked intestinal gaseous distention in these patients. Computerized tomography has been far more accurate, demonstrating a peripancreatic fluid collection in 85 percent of our patients (Fig. 87–3). When, however, a cystic mass can be demonstrated, the presence or absence of infection is not established unless gas is identified within the abscess.

Treatment

As indicated in Table 87–5, patients with pancreatic abscesses are usually critically ill. This is due not only to the infection but also to the fact that abscesses occur in patients with severe underlying pancreatitis. Supportive management must therefore be vigorous. This includes antibiotic administration and meticulous attention to respiratory care, nutritional support, and prevention of GI hemorrhage. The most essential feature of treatment is, however, to provide adequate drainage of the infection.

Percutaneous drainage by catheters placed under radiographic control has been described by Gerzof. In most cases, however, contents of the abscess include semisolid infected tissue that cannot be evacuated except by surgical debridement and placement of large drains.

Since these patients are severely ill, there is a tendency to limit the surgical procedure to identification of the most obvious abscess and provision of external drainage. It is estimated that this approach is associated with a 30 percent incidence of recurrent abscesses, and the frequent need for repeated surgical intervention is usually stressed. To decrease this need, Bradley has described debridement and open packing of pancreatic abscesses. These patients are returned to the operating room every 2 to 3 days for further debridement and repacking. Encouraging results have been reported by these authors.

We have preferred to follow an approach of systematic exploration of the whole peripan-

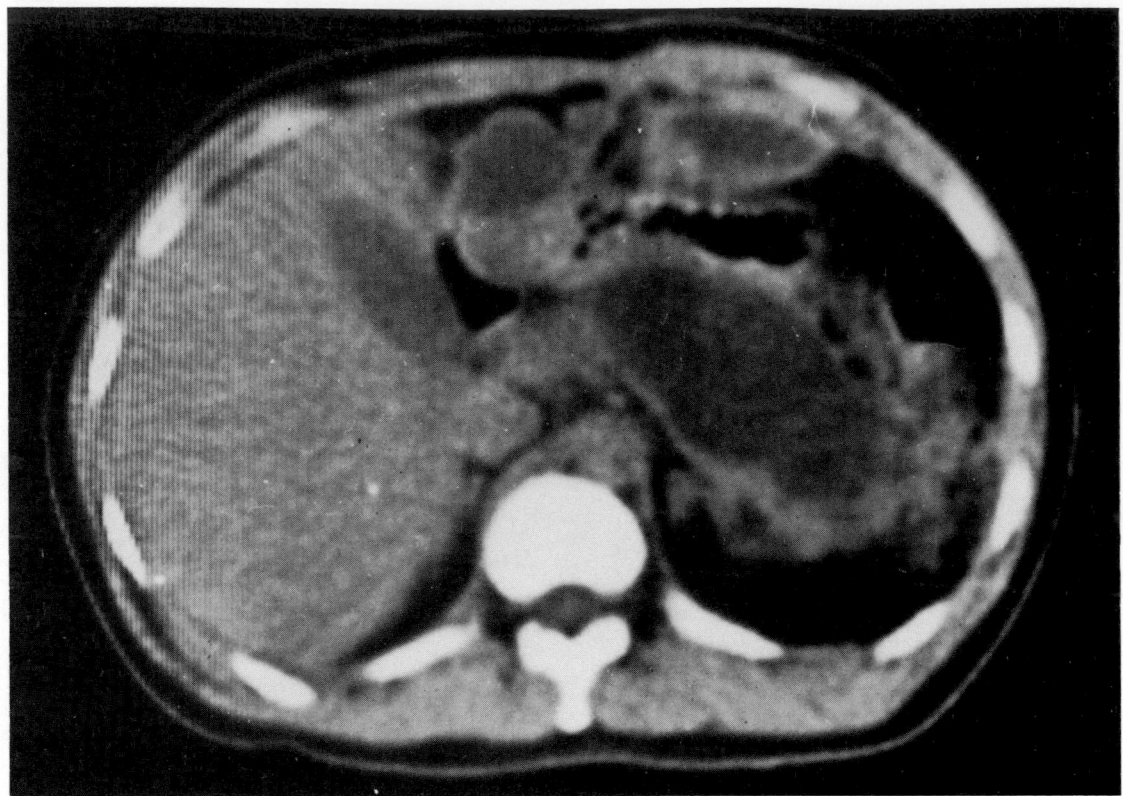

Figure 87–3. CT scan showing an abscess involving the pancreatic tail. (*Source: Ranson JHC: Necrosis and abscess, in Bradley E* (*ed*): *Complications of Pancreatitis, Philadelphia: WB Saunders, 1982, p 83, with permission.*)

creatic retroperitoneum and institution of prolonged sump drainage, as diagrammed in Figure 87–4. The patient is placed supine with the left side elevated approximately 20 degrees. A long, bilateral subcostal incision is made, extending from the anterior axilliary line on the right to the midaxilliary line on the left. The lesser omental sac is opened widely by dividing the gastrocolic omentum and the entire anterior surface of the pancreas is exposed, including the pancreatic head. It is important to open the fat covering the anterior surface of the pancreas and expose the pancreas itself. The duodenum is mobilized and the area posterior to the pancreatic head is explored. The area posterior to the tail of the pancreas is examined by exploration carried posteriorly at the inferior margin of the distal one third of the pancreas. The areas posterior to the descending and ascending colon are explored, and the root of the small intestinal

mesentery is examined closely. As much devitalized tissue as possible is debrided.

Penrose drains and soft, sump catheters are placed anterior and posterior to the head of the pancreas, along the body of the pancreas and anterior and posterior to the tail of the gland. Additional sump drains are placed into any large abscess cavity identified. Drains are brought through separate incisions as far posteriorly as possible. A feeding jejunostomy is constructed and a cholecystostomy is added if gallstones are detected.

To minimize visceral injury, it is essential that the drains be soft. We have used the sump catheter illustrated in Figure 87–5. Continuous suction and irrigation of the drains are maintained, and they have been left in place for an average of 25 days in surviving patients. These drains have many shortcomings. They are cumbersome, difficult to maintain, and require me-

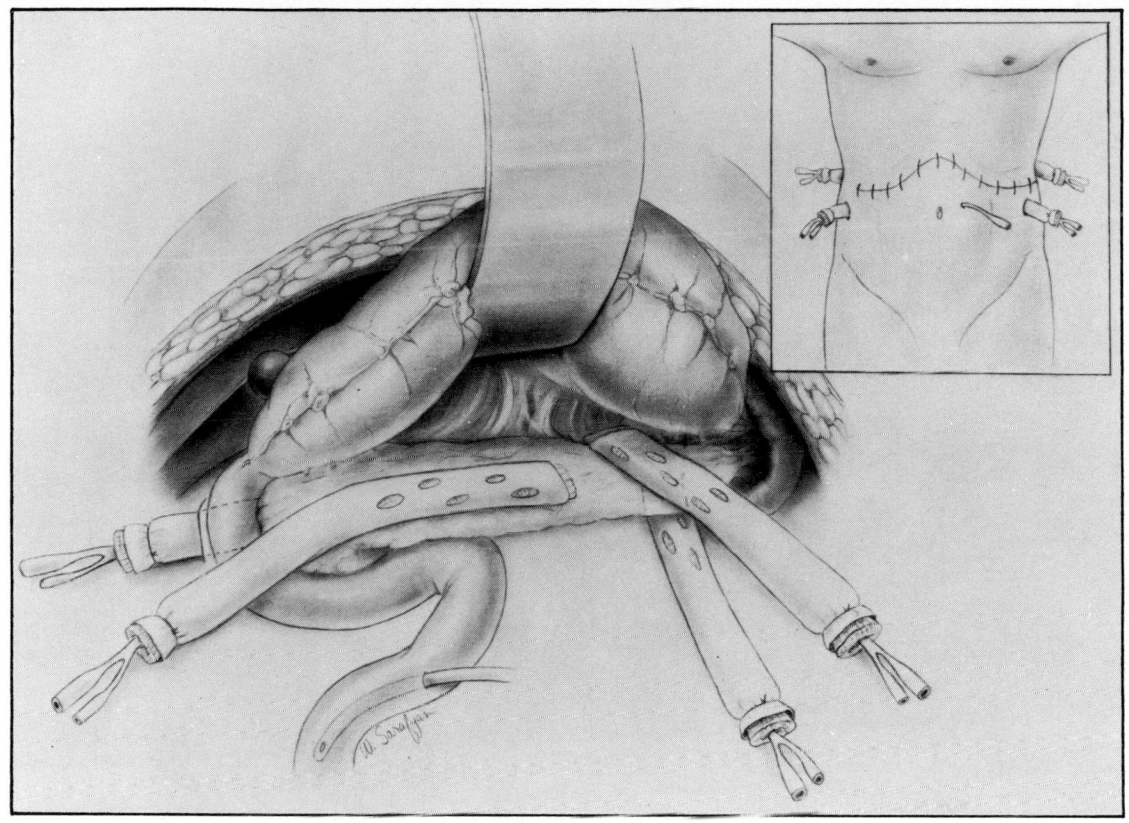

Figure 87-4. The technique of wide sump drainage of the peripancreatic retroperitoneum in patients with infected pancreatic abscesses. (*Source: From Ranson JHC: Necrosis and abscess, in Bradley E (ed): Complications of Pancreatitis, Philadelphia: WB Saunders, 1982, p 88, with permission.*)

ticulous nursing care to minimize further contamination of the abscess cavity from the outside. They do, however, permit evacuation of thick material for which smaller drains are inadequate.

Prognosis

The overall reported mortality of pancreatic abscesses is high. Our own experience is summarized in Figure 87–6. This shows that the mortality is related to the severity of the underlying acute pancreatitis as estimated by early prognostic signs. Furthermore, the efficacy of "wide" sump drainage as described above is compared to that of conventional "local" drainage. In patients with the most mild or the most severe pancreatitis, the type of surgical drainage did not affect the outcome. In the largest group, those with "moderately severe" pancreatitis,

wide sump drainage was associated with a dramatic improvement in overall survival compared to conventional local drainage. It has also been striking that no surviving patient treated by wide sump drainage has required reexploration for recurrent abscess.

Other Local Complications

Severe peripancreatic necrosis may extend to involve the colon and small bowel. Colonic necrosis is best treated by resection of the involved bowel, with colostomy and mucous fistula formation. Massive hemorrhage may occur due to necrosis of major blood vessels or their erosion by drains placed during drainage of pancreatic abscesses. Bleeding may be extremely rapid; however, immediate surgical intervention will usually lead to control.

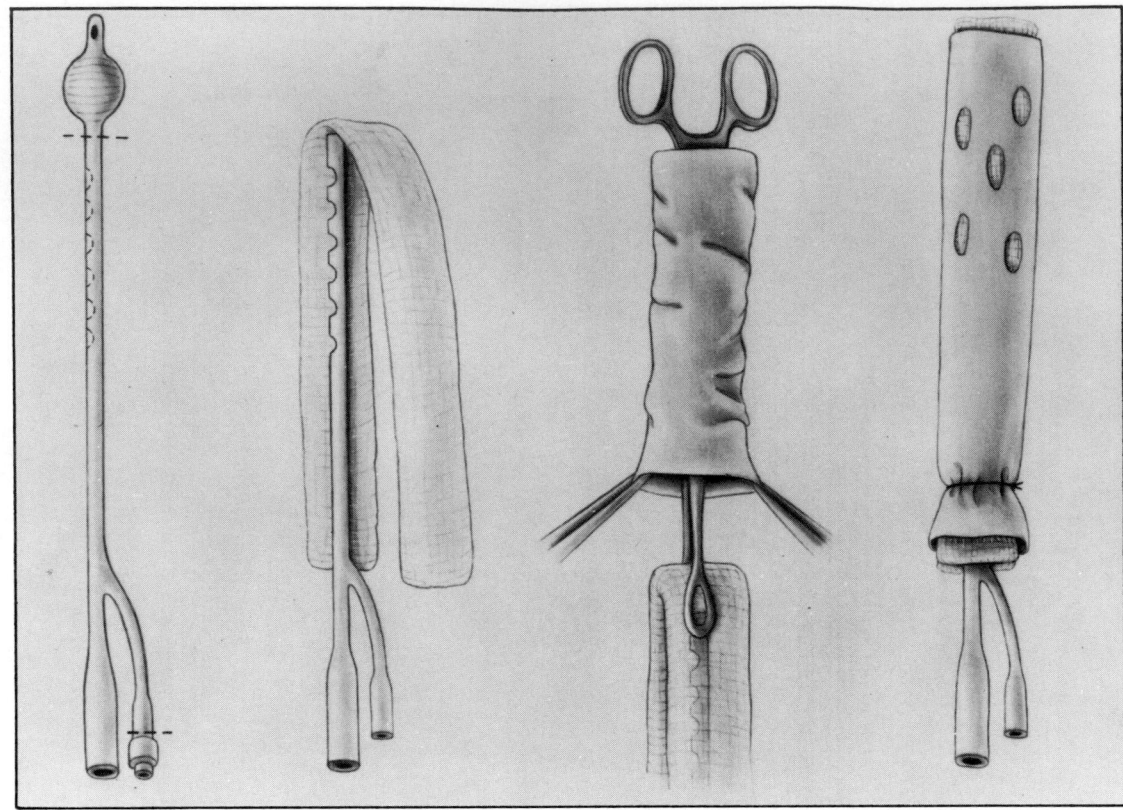

Figure 87–5. Method of construction of a large soft catheter used for drainage of pancreatic abscesses. No. 24 Foley catheter is covered by two to three layers of sympathectomy packing and placed in a 1½-inch Penrose drain. (*Source: From Ranson JHC: Necrosis and abscess, in Bradley E (ed): Complications of Pancreatitis, Philadelphia: WB Saunders, 1982, p 88, with permission.*)

Protracted Pancreatitis

In a small group of patients, acute pancreatitis does not subside completely with nonoperative management. These patients usually do not have evidence of severe pancreatitis and respond well initially to nonoperative measures. However, when attempts are made to reintroduce oral feedings, pain, fever, and hyperamylasemia recur. These findings resolve with the reintroduction of nasogastric suction but recur when oral feedings are reinstituted. When this course repeats itself over several weeks, a mechanical local cause must be sought, by exploratory operation if necessary. The most common cause, in our experience, has been biliary calculi that were too small to visualize with current cholangiographic techniques. Small pseudocysts or pancreatic ductal obstruction may also cause

this clinical picture. It should be emphasized that this group forms less than 2 percent of patients.

Prevention of Recurrent Pancreatitis

In patients who survive one episode of acute pancreatitis, every effort must be made to prevent recurrent disease. This involves the identification and correction of remediable etiologic associations such as hyperlipoproteinemia or cholelithiasis. Patients in whom gallstones are demonstrated radiographically have traditionally been advised to wait 4 to 6 weeks before undergoing correction of cholelithiasis. For most patients, this delay is unnecessary and exposes them to the risk of recurring bouts of pancreatitis. There is no evidence that the risk of definitive biliary surgery is increased once acute

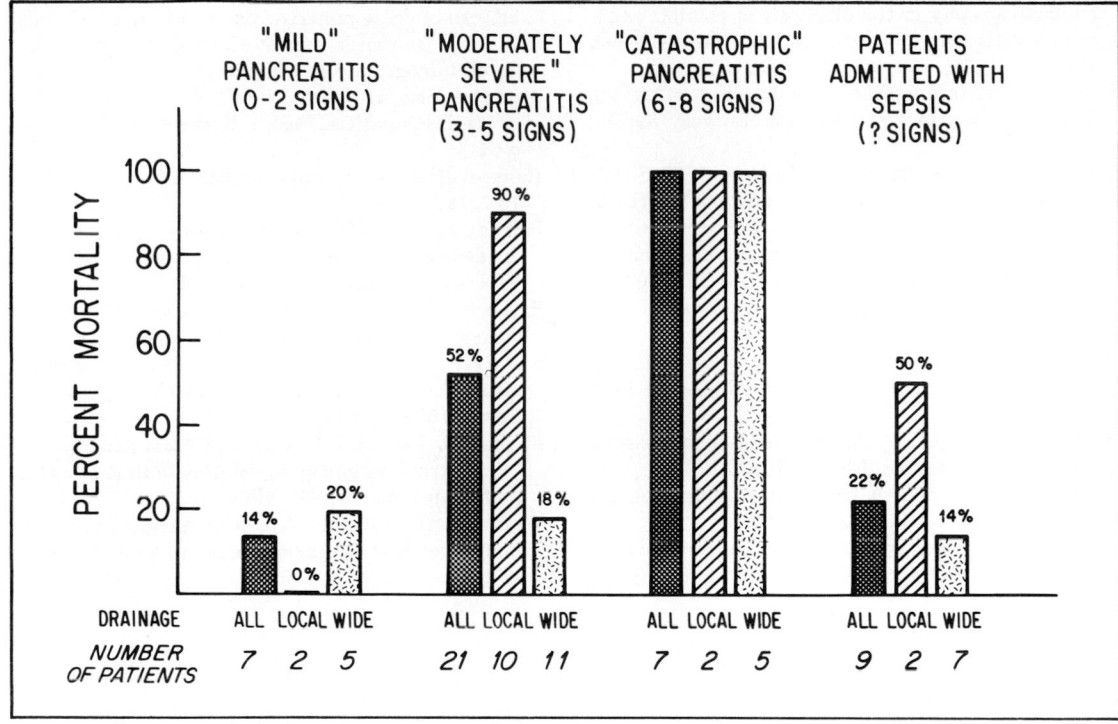

Figure 87–6. Percent mortality following pancreatic sepsis related to severity of underlying pancreatitis and to type of surgical drainage. (*Source: Ranson JHC, 1979, with permission.*)

pancreatitis has subsided. It is, therefore, our usual practice to correct cholelithiasis during the same hospitalization as soon as signs of pancreatitis have subsided. In the occasional patient who has a large pancreatic phlegmon, it is advisable to postpone surgery for a further period.

TABLE 87–6. SUMMARY OF CURRENT MANAGEMENT OF ACUTE PANCREATITIS

All patients:
- Nasogastric suction
- No oral feedings until pancreatitis subsides
- Monitoring and maintenance of intravascular volume
- Respiratory monitoring and support: measure Po_2, diuretics, PEEP
- Antibiotics (selective)
- Early laparotomy: only for diagnosis
- Estimate prognosis by early signs

If 3 or more positive prognostic signs:
- Peritoneal lavage
- Nutritional support
- Suspect and treat pancreatic sepsis at 14 to 21 days
- Late heparin (after 14 days) if hypercoagulable

CURRENT MANAGEMENT

The major features of our current treatment of patients with acute pancreatitis are summarized in Table 87–6. Since no single therapeutic measure has been clearly demonstrated to limit the severity of pancreatitis itself, management is directed primarily at avoiding pancreatic stimulation and support of the patient. Nonetheless, the approach described is associated with an overall survival of 95 percent.

BIBLIOGRAPHY

Acosta JM, Pellegrini CA, et al: Etiology and pathogenesis of acute biliary pancreatitis. Surgery 88:118, 1980

Balldin G, Ohlsson K: Demonstration of pancreatic protease–antiprotease complexes in the peritoneal fluid of patients with acute pancreatitis. Surgery 85:451, 1979

Banks PA: Pancreatitis. New York: Plenum, 1979

Bradley EL (ed): Complications of Pancreatitis. Philadelphia: WB Saunders, 1982

Coppa GF, LeFleur R, et al: The role of Chiba-needle

cholangiography in the diagnosis of possible acute pancreatitis with cholelithiasis. Ann Surg 193:393, 1981

Davidson ED, Bradley EL: "Marsupialization" in the treatment of pancreatic abscess. Surgery 89:252, 1981

Durr GH-K: Acute pancreatitis, in Howat HT, Sarles H (eds): The Exocrine Pancreas. London: WB Saunders, 1979

Edelmann G, Boutelier P: Le traitement des pancreatites aigues necrosantes par l'ablation chirurgicale precoce des portions necrosees. Chirurgie 100:155, 1974

Gerzof SG, Robbins AH, et al: Percutaneous catheter drainage of abdominal abscesses. N Engl J Med 305:653, 1981

Imrie CW, Ferguson JC, et al: Arterial hypoxia in acute pancreatitis. Br J Surg 64:185, 1977

Imrie CW, Whyte AS: A prospective study of acute pancreatitis. Br J Surg 62:490, 1975

McMahon MJ, Playforth MJ, et al: A comparative study of methods for the prediction of severity of attacks of acute pancreatitis. Br J Surg 67:22, 1980

Pringot J, Dardenne AN, et al: Contribution of computed tomography in the diagnosis of severe acute pancreatitis, in Hollender LF (ed): Controversies in Acute Pancreatitis. Berlin: Springer-Verlag, 1982, p 64

Ranson JHC: Acute pancreatitis. Curr Probl Surg 16:1, 1979

Safrany L, Cotton PB: A preliminary report: Urgent duodenoscopic sphincterotomy for acute gallstone pancreatitis. Surgery 89:424, 1981

Sarles H: Chronic calcifying pancreatitis—Chronic alcoholic pancreatitis. Gastroenterology 66:604, 1974

Stone HH, Fabian TC: Peritoneal dialysis in the treatment of acute alcoholic pancreatitis. Surg Gynecol Obstet 150:878, 1980

Stone HH, Fabian TC, et al: Gallstone pancreatitis: Biliary tract pathology in relation to time of operation. Ann Surg 194:305, 1981

Warshaw AL, Imbembo AL, et al: Surgical intervention in acute necrotizing pancreatitis. Am J Surg 127:484, 1974

88. Pancreatic Cysts, Pseudocysts, Fistulas, and Pancreas Divisum

A.R. Moossa
Richard H. Bell, Jr.

INTRODUCTION

Cysts of the pancreas were considered to be rare as recently as twenty years ago. With the advent of improved imaging methods, pancreatic fluid collections are being recognized with increasing frequency. Cysts of the pancreas are of several varieties, but, in general, fall in two basic categories: (1) true cysts, which are lined by epithelium, and (2) pseudocysts, which consist of a collection of fluid in the lesser sac and/or retroperitoneum. Such a fluid collection may resolve spontaneously (acute pseudocyst) or may lead to the development of a fibrous nonepithelialized capsule (chronic pseudocyst). A clear distinction between true cysts and pseudocysts is not always possible since epithelial cysts, particularly those associated with chronic pancreatitis, may lose some of their epithelial lining with progressive enlargement, hemorrhage, or secondary infection. Nevertheless, the general distinction is useful provided that the functional behavior of these fluid collections is investigated and characterized before appropriate management of the patient is entertained.

The symptomatology and clinical presentation of pancreatic cysts vary greatly depending on several factors: (1) location of the cyst, (2) size of the cyst—of particular importance is whether the amount of fluid is increasing, decreasing, or remaining constant, (3) involvement of adjacent structures, and (4) development of complications such as hemorrhage, infection, rupture, or neoplastic change. Most pancreatic cysts, especially those less than 5 cm in diameter, are asymptomatic and are diagnosed incidentally during investigation or laparotomy for other suspected abdominal conditions, or at necropsy. About 80 percent of patients with a pancreatic cyst have upper abdominal pain of varying type and severity; 50 percent will complain of nausea and vomiting; weight loss is a feature in about 40 percent of instances.

The widespread and indiscriminate routine use of standard radiologic procedures (such as plain film of the abdomen and contrast studies of the gastrointestinal (GI) tract) for the diagnosis and evaluation of pancreatic masses, cystic or solid, should be strongly discouraged. Radionuclide scans of the liver or pancreas are also inaccurate and not cost effective and should be abandoned in this setting. At present, our diagnostic armamentarium for evaluating the pancreas include computed tomography (CT), ultrasonography, endoscopic retrograde cholangiopancreatography (ERCP), and celiac and superior mesenteric anteriography.

Pancreatic fistulas and pancreatic ascites are frequently associated with pancreatic pseudocysts and, for that reason, are included in this chapter. Pancreas divisum is discussed here purely for convenience.

PANCREATIC CYSTS (TABLE 88–1)

True Cysts

True pancreatic cysts, which are lined by epithelium, can be divided into congenital and acquired varieties.

TABLE 88–1. CLASSIFICATION OF PANCREATIC CYSTS

A. *True cysts of the pancreas*
1. Simple (congenital) cysts—usually single
2. Retention (acquired) cysts—single or multiple
3. Polycystic disease of the pancreas
4. Dermoid cysts
5. Parasitic cysts

B. *Pseudocysts of the pancreas*
1. Acute pseudocyst
2. Chronic pseudocyst

C. *Cystic tumors of the pancreas*
1. Cystadenoma
2. Cystadenocarcinoma
3. Secondary cavitation of cystic tumors
   a. Lymphoma
   b. Leiomyosarcoma
   c. Adenocarcinoma

Congenital True Pancreatic Cysts

Simple Cysts. Isolated congenital pancreatic cysts are very rare. Jordan reported two cases seen during life, one in an infant and one in an adult. In addition, he reported three cases discovered incidentally at autopsy. Miles reviewed the eight reported cases in infants, most of whom presented with an unexplained abdominal mass in the first year of life. These cysts are lined by cuboidal epithelium, presumably of ductal origin. In most instances, there is no demonstrable communication with the main pancreatic ductal system. Excision of the cyst is usually possible and is the treatment of choice.

Pilcher recently described the second reported case of enterogenous (duplication) cyst of the pancreas.

Polycystic Disease of the Pancreas. Multiple cysts of the pancreas may be seen in association with cysts of the liver and kidneys. The pancreatic cysts are ordinarily small, multiple, and lined by cuboidal epithelium. Nygaard and Smith reported an unusually large single pancreatic cyst associated with cysts in the liver. Multiple pancreatic cysts also occur in approximately one half of patients with cerebellar and retinal hemangioblastomas (von Hippel–Lindau's syndrome). Polycystic disease of the pancreas rarely causes any pancreatic problem requiring surgical treatment.

Fibrocystic Disease of the Pancreas. Fibrocystic disease (mucoviscidosis) is the most common cause of pancreatic insufficiency in children in the Western world. The disease is characterized by generalized disturbance of fluid secretion throughout the body. It is inherited as an autosomal recessive and is estimated to occur in one out of every 2000 live births. The greatest morbidity and mortality associated with cystic fibrosis is due to the development of chronic pulmonary insufficiency and intercurrent pulmonary infection. In the past, most patients died in early childhood, but at the present time 80 percent survive beyond the age of 20 years.

Park and Grand have recently reviewed the GI and pancreatic manifestations of cystic fibrosis. Approximately 90 percent of the patients demonstrate pancreatic exocrine insufficiency. In fact, until the development of the sweat electrolyte test by di Sant'Agnese and associates in 1973, pancreatic function tests were employed to make the diagnosis of cystic fibrosis.

Fat and protein malabsorption are very common in cystic fibrosis, and pancreatic enzyme replacement is usually prescribed. Pancreatic secretion is markedly diminished in volume; many patients do not respond to the pancreozymin–secretin stimulation. Histologic examination of the pancreas demonstrates chronic inflammation, fibrosis, and atrophy of the gland. Multiple cystic spaces filled with inspissated secretions are present due to widespread obstruction of the pancreatic ducts.

Although pancreatic insufficiency is nearly universal in cystic fibrosis and the disease may also be characterized by recurrent pancreatitis, the pancreatic component of the disease fortunately is rarely associated with the need for surgical intervention.

Dermoid Cysts. Teratatomous cysts of the pancreas are occasionally reported. A pancreatic dermoid, such as the one reported by De Courcy, contains the usual elements such as sebum, hair, and teeth.

Acquired True Pancreatic Cysts

Retention Cysts. Retention cysts of the pancreas are associated with diseases that lead to chronic obstruction of the pancreatic ducts, such as chronic pancreatitis or pancreatic cancer. These cysts, which form by progressive dilation of pancreatic ducts beyond the obstruction, are lined by epithelium, although continued increased pressure within the cysts or secondary inflammation may lead to flattening or obliteration of the epithelial lining to the extent that it is no longer recognizable on microscopic examination. The pathogenesis of this lesion thus differs from that of the pancreatic pseudocyst that follows an attack of acute pancreatitis, although the two conditions cannot always be distinguished on clinical grounds and it may be difficult to separate them even on microscopic examination.

Sarles found that one fourth of his patients with chronic calcific pancreatitis had retention cysts. The majority of the patients were males suffering from chronic alcoholism. In patients with chronic pancreatitis, retention cysts may present with new abdominal pain, with persistent elevation of serum level of pancreatic enzymes, with obstructive jaundice, or simply as an abdominal mass. On many occasions, asymptomatic retention cysts are now being discovered during pancreatic imaging.

Retention cysts may be single or multiple. They are found in all parts of the gland. More than half communicate with the duct of Wirsung when examined by ERCP, in keeping with the fact that most retention cysts contain high levels of pancreatic enzymes. Pathologic examination of the cyst wall reveals fibrosis and a lining of cuboidal epithelial cells. As indicated previously, the epithelial lining may be incomplete.

The appropriate surgical approach to retention cysts depends on the severity of the symptoms associated with the underlying chronic pancreatitis. In those cases in which the pancreatitis is severe enough to warrant resection, the cyst should be excised in continuity. Warren has reported that approximately 25 percent of his patients undergoing resection for chronic pancreatitis had retention cysts, which were also excised. Good results were obtained in 80 percent of the patients in whom the cyst was included in the resection. In those situations in which the underlying pancreatitis is relatively quiescent, internal drainage of the retention cyst employing the methods described below for pseudocysts is probably the most reasonable approach.

Retention cysts occasionally form behind a malignant obstruction of the pancreatic duct, although this is a relatively rare presentation of pancreatic cancer. Warren has reported his experience with ten such cases. Treatment of the cyst is dependent on the resectability of the underlying carcinoma. If the tumor can be excised, the cyst may be removed along with it. When the tumor is not resectable and the cyst is large, internal drainage of the cyst may be appropriate for palliative reasons. The prognosis in all such cases is very poor.

Nardi has described eight patients with chronic epigastric pain who had small retention cysts in the head of the pancreas, which he attributed to isolated fibrotic obstructions of the papilla of Vater. Six of the patients improved after sphincteroplasty of the major papilla which was extended along the duct of Wirsung far enough to partially unroof the cyst. Such cases are undoubtedly distinctly unusual; in most patients with retention cysts, which are associated with diffuse pancreatic disease, sphincteroplasty is not considered to be adequate therapy.

Neoplastic Cysts

Cystadenomas and cystadenocarcinomas of the pancreas are acquired neoplastic cysts, which together account for approximately 10 percent of pancreatic cysts. These tumors are rare, and few institutions have acquired experience with a substantial number of cases.

Cystadenoma. According to Strodel and Eckhauser, approximately 325 cases of cystadenoma has been reported in the literature as of 1981. An increased appreciation of these lesions in the past few years is reflected in the fact that Jordan found only 88 documented cases in his review in 1960.

Cystadenomas have been reported in patients varying in age from 16 to 90 years. There is a strong female predominance, the sex ratio being about 6 to 1. Soloway noted a frequent association with benign and malignant tumors or other organs, although such a relationship has not been observed by other authorities. Cystadenomas range in size from 1 to 25 cm; 10 cm is a typical diameter at the time of diagnosis.

Approximately two thirds of reported cystadenomas are discovered during life; the remainder are unexpectedly encountered at necropsy. Of the clinical cases, about 70 percent are symptomatic, the remainder being discovered incidentally during physical examination or radiologic studies. The most common presenting symptoms are pain, which is present in half of the cases, or a palpable abdominal mass, usually noted by the patient. On physical examination, a mass is usually palpable in about two thirds of the patients. A few individuals present with jaundice due to obstruction of the common bile duct, or with GI bleeding, which may be the result of direct extension into a neighboring viscus or to splenic vein thrombosis with resulting left-sided portal hypertension and gastric variceal formation. About 20 percent of the cases are associated with diabetes mellitus.

In the past, the diagnosis of cystadenoma was rarely made definitively prior to abdominal exploration. The reason was that the diagnosis was based on inadequate and insensitive radiologic examination. For example, plain films of the abdomen will demonstrate calcification in the cyst wall in only 10 percent of cases. Barium upper GI series may demonstrate forward displacement of the stomach in only two thirds of the cases, according to Becker. Both findings are nonspecific. CT and ultrasonography are the best methods to demonstrate the cystic lesion in the pancreas and, if the clinical picture is taken into consideration, will often distinguish between a cystadenoma and other pancreatic cysts (Fig. 88–1). Splenic angiography is a very useful preoperative investigation. The usual findings are displacement of pancreatic arteries around the mass, the presence of large feeding vessels, and, occasionally, a tumor blush in the venous phase. It is worth remembering that 27 percent of the Mayo Clinic patients had gallstones.

Cystadenomas occur in all parts of the pancreas. The gross and microscopic pathology of these tumors has been carefully reviewed by Hodgkinson and associates, by Campbell and Cruickshank, and by Compagno and Oertel. Characteristically, cystadenomas are of two varieties. The serous cystadenoma is a uniloculated tumor or multiloculated tumor composed of innumerable small (1 cm or less) cysts giving a honeycomb appearance in cut section. The cys-

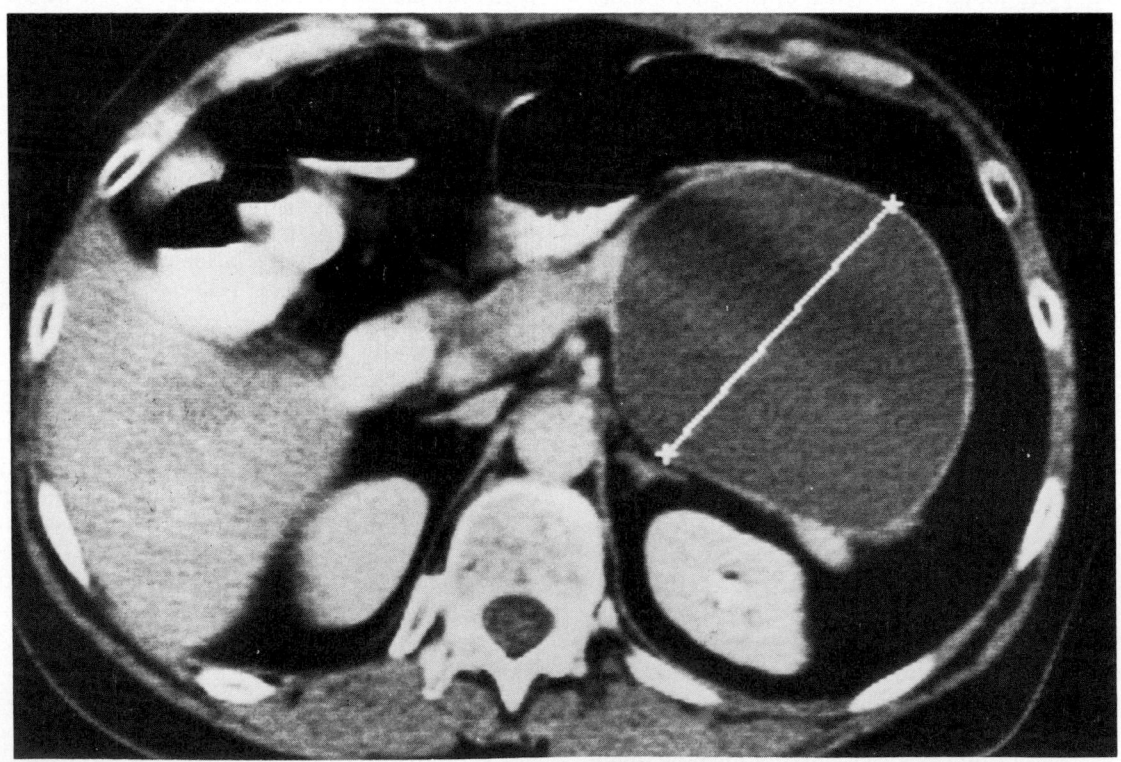

Figure 88–1. CT appearance of cystadenoma of the pancreatic tail in a 62-year-old woman. There was no history of pancreatitis or alcoholism. Note that the pancreatic head, neck, and body are normal.

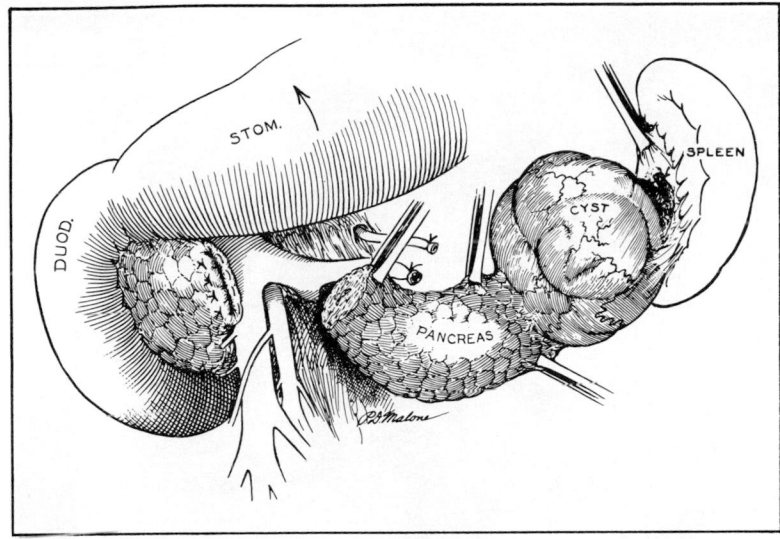

Figure 88–2. Splenectomy and distal pancreatectomy for cystadenoma of the tail of the pancreas. (*Illustration courtesy of K.W. Warren.*)

tic spaces are lined by cuboidal epithelial cells with clear cytoplasm that stains strongly for glycogen but not for mucin. These cells resemble fetal centroacinar cells. The cyst spaces contain largely serous fluid. The second type of cystadenoma is the mucinous variety, which contains large cystic spaces that may measure several centimeters in diameter. These spaces are lined by tall columnar epithelium and abundant goblet cells. The epithelium is often thrown into folds and may be characterized by papillary projections which are large enough to be observed grossly within the cyst. The cystic spaces themselves contain mucous. The importance of distinguishing between these two types of lesions lies in the fact that the serous cystadenomas have little malignant potential while the mucinous cystadenomas, however, frequently undergo malignant degeneration and are considered to be the precursor of cystadenocarcinoma. Thus, it is important for the surgeon to be familiar with the gross and microscopic characteristics of cystadenoma and be able to intelligently advise the consulting pathologist. In the cases reviewed by Compagno and Oertel, the initial histologic diagnosis was incorrect one third of the time, probably reflecting the lack of familiarity with these relatively rare lesions. It should also be emphasized that the distinction between the two types of cystadenomas cannot be made with 100 percent accuracy because intermediate types containing both serous and mucinous components may occur.

The optimum treatment for cystadenoma of the pancreas is total excision including a margin of normal pancreatic tissue. This may entail an extensive distal pancreatic resection with splenectomy for a tumor in the usual location of the body and tail of the pancreas (Fig. 88–2). If the mass is in the head of the gland, it may be necessary to perform a Whipple procedure. Tumors that are very extensive and reach across most of the surface of the gland may occasionally need a total pancreatoduodenectomy for their complete removal. After total surgical resection, the recurrence rate is less than 2 percent. Unfortunately, about one fourth of the tumors cannot be totally excised, usually because of intimate adherence of the growth to the superior mesenteric vessels. This is one of the few instances when careful and aggressive "debulking" of the tumor is indicated. Survival for many years has been reported after simple biopsy or after partial excision of cystadenomas. Internal or external drainage of cystadenoma is not effective and is rarely, if ever, indicated. There are reports of malignant tumor spread along the drainage tract after external drainage of mucinous cystadenomas.

Cystadenocarcinoma of the Pancreas. This is believed to arise from malignant degeneration of mucinous and, rarely, serous cystadenomas. They account for about 1 percent of all malignant pancreatic tumors and are about one third to one half as common as benign cystadenomas.

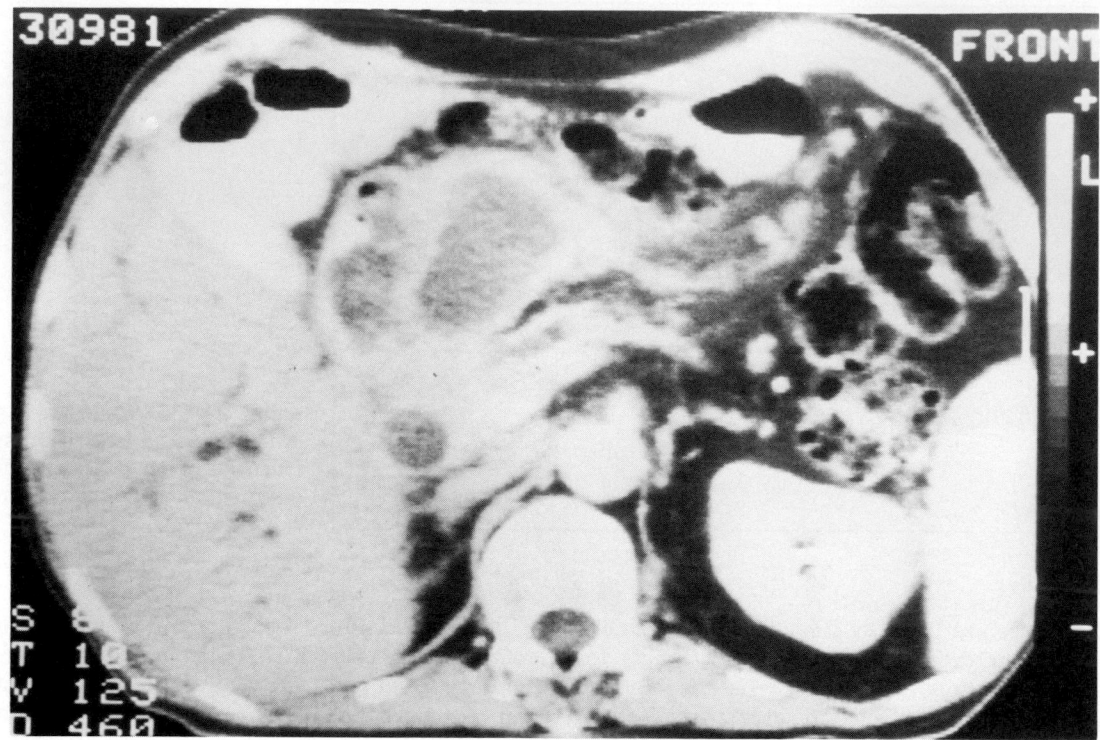

Figure 88–3. CT appearance of a multiloculated cystadenocarcinoma of the head of the pancreas causing obstructive jaundice and portal vein occlusion.

In reviewing 41 cases of mucinous cystic tumors of the pancreas, Campagno and Oertel found on an histologic examination that 19 cases were frankly malignant, 8 cases were completely benign, and 14 contained areas of premalignant atypia. They regard all mucinous tumors of the pancreas as potentially malignant.

As with cystadenoma, females appear to be more susceptible in a ratio of approximately only 3 to 1. The average age of onset is 60 years. The presenting complaint is pain in 80 percent of cases; cystadenocarcinomas are less often asymptomatic than cystadenomas. Weight loss is present in 40 percent of the cases. Some patients present with jaundice or GI bleeding. An abdominal mass is palpable in 60 to 75 percent of the patients. Distant metastases are occasionally present at the time of diagnosis. CT (Fig. 88–3) and angiography are again essential diagnostic tests.

In reviews by Compagno and Oertel and by Hodgkinson and colleagues, only two thirds of cystadenocarcinomas were found to be resect-able. Total extirpation of the tumor is the only satisfactory treatment and, depending on the location of the tumor, may again require distal pancreatectomy with splenectomy, pancreatoduodenectomy of the Whipple type, or even a total pancreatectomy. Under favorable conditions, even the presence of metastases is not a contraindication to resection, and excision of the isolated liver metastases may even be indicated. In the Mayo Clinic series, 5-year survival after total resection for cystadenocarcinoma was 68 percent. No patient survived 5 years in the absence of complete extirpation.

PSEUDOCYSTS OF THE PANCREAS

Etiology

Pancreatic pseudocyst is by far the most common fluid-filled lesion associated with the pancreas. Several years ago, when the diagnosis of pseudocyst could only be made on clinical grounds backed by contrast studies of the upper GI tract, the lesion was considered to be a relatively rare entity. However, with improvement in pancreatic imaging techniques over the past decade, pseudocysts are now recognized with regularity on most medical and surgical wards.

Pseudocysts are distinguished from true cysts of the pancreas by their lack of an epithelial lining. They consist of a rim of fibrotic, inflammatory, or granulation tissue surrounding a collection of extravasated pancreatic juice, serum, and blood in the peripancreatic tissues and/or lesser peritoneal sac. These collections of fluid follow an attack of acute pancreatitis in 70 to 80 percent of cases and can now be labeled an acute pseudocyst. Approximately one fourth of the cases are secondary to blunt abdominal trauma or operative injury to the pancreas. In a small number of patients with pseudocysts, no prior history of pancreatic disease or trauma can be elicited.

Pseudocysts develop in approximately 10 percent of patients who suffer an attack of acute pancreatitis. They are more commonly associated with alcoholic pancreatitis than with biliary disease. Some authorities believe that pseudocysts are more commonly seen in patients with recurrent bouts of acute pancreatitis than after a single attack.

Pseudocysts appear to develop as a consequence of the extravasation of pancreatic juice through the pancreatic ductal system into the peripancreatic tissues. This leaking pancreatic juice, along with blood and devitalized peripancreatic tissues, incites an inflammatory response that seals the fluid within a fibrous capsule, thus walling off the collection from the general peritoneal cavity. According to Sugawa and Walt the pseudocyst cavity remains in communication with the pancreatic ductal system in over 90 percent of the cases. Thus the fluid within the pseudocyst ordinarily contains high levels of pancreatic enzymes.

The development of a pseudocyst after pancreatic trauma presumably is due to the leakage of pancreatic juice from a disrupted pancreatic duct system. Posttraumatic pancreatic pseudocysts tend to occur in the body and tail of the pancreas, reflecting the fact that most ductal injuries occur in the body of the pancreas as it crosses the vertebral column. Blunt abdominal trauma is the most common cause of pseudocysts in children. Injury to the pancreas during surgical procedures and subsequent pseudocyst

formation may occur after a variety of operations, including pancreatic resection, gastrectomy, operations on the periampullary area, splenectomy, and splenorenal shunt for portal hypertension.

Natural History

Whenever a patient is labeled as having a pseudocyst, ambiguity still persists in the precise definition of the condition. The term pseudocyst may imply an acute and often transient accumulation of fluid in the lesser sac and peripancreatic tissues (acute pseudocyst) that may be poorly defined anatomically. This cannot always be differentiated from pancreatic and peripancreatic edema even by modern imaging methods. The current temptation to aspirate such collections should be avoided. Serial ultrasonographic and CT studies are necessary to document if a chronic pseudocyst is developing. Thus, the functional or dynamic behavior of an acute pseudocyst needs to be assessed and the following questions should be posed:

- Is the size of the cyst (amount of fluid) remaining constant, decreasing, or increasing over a period of days?
- Is the patient symptomatic or not?
- Is the general condition of the patient improving or deteriorating?
- Has a complication, such as infection, hemorrhage, or rupture, supervened?

Serial studies and continuous monitoring over a period of days or a few weeks may be necessary to answer all of these questions and only then can established therapeutic guidelines be advised and implemented.

Another common misconception is to confuse an infected pseudocyst with a pancreatic abscess. A pancreatic abscess consists mainly of pancreatic and retroperitoneal necrosis with secondary infection. Substantial pancreatic and retroperitoneal debridement (which often needs to be repeated) and wide drainage are essential. The mortality and morbidity in such cases are prohibitive. On the other hand, an infected pseudocyst can essentially be cured with acceptable risks by external drainage with minimal or no debridement.

In the first few weeks of their development, pseudocysts typically have only a thin fibrous capsule and the borders of the collection may be indistinct. There follows a period of matura-

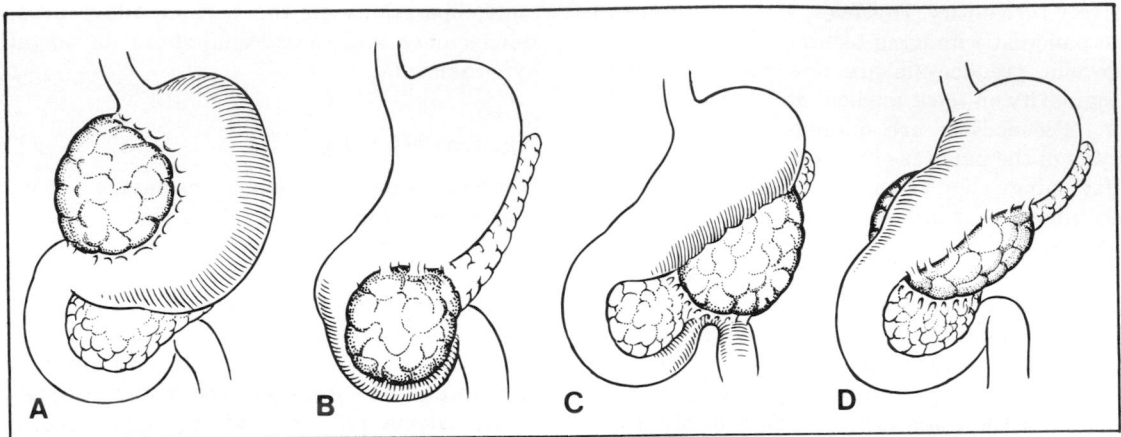

Figure 88–4. Pseudocyst of the pancreas may **(A)** push the stomach over to the left, **(B)** compress the duodenal C loop and cause obstruction, **(C)** block the duodenojejunal flexure, and **(D)** displace the stomach forward.

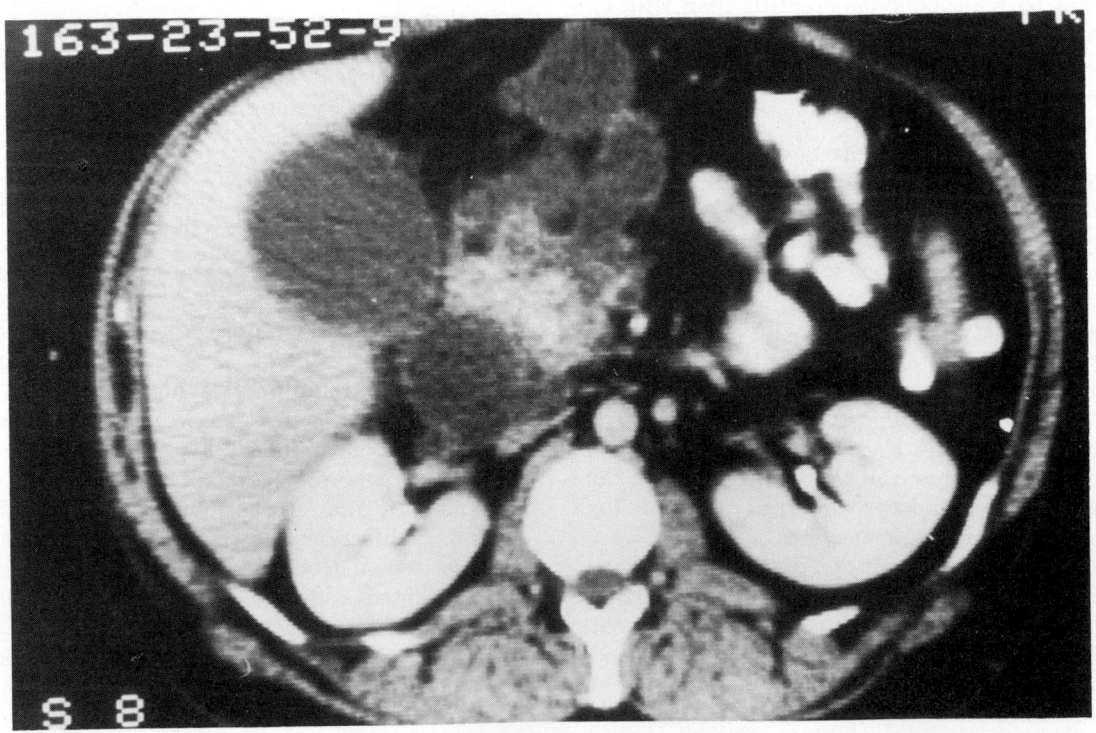

Figure 88–5. CT appearance of acute multiloculated pseudocyst in a patient with acute pancreatitis. The pseudocyst resolved spontaneously on conservative management.

tion in which the capsule of the cyst thickens and its margins become distinct. This process typically occurs approximately 4 to 6 weeks after the initial formation of the cyst. Once the mature (chronic) pseudocyst is formed, it may remain relatively stable in size, it may continue to grow slowly within a confined space (Fig. 88–4), or it may begin to spread along retroperitoneal tissue planes, insinuating itself into such locations as the splenic hilum or between the leaves of the colonic or intestinal mesentery. Pseudocysts may even spread to distant areas such as the mediastinum or even the inguinal regions.

Twenty years ago it was believed that pseudocysts rarely resolve spontaneously. In fact, it is still true that mature (chronic) pseudocysts almost always persist. However, since the advent of ultrasonography and CT scanning, it has become clear that it is not unusual for immature (acute) pseudocysts to disappear spontaneously (Fig. 88–5). Bradley and colleagues studied 54 patients with pseudocysts by serial ultrasonography. In patients with a pseudocyst of less than 6 weeks' duration, there was a 40 percent incidence of spontaneous resolution. Aranha and colleagues noted a 29 percent incidence of resolution in a similar study. Most of the cysts that disappeared did so within the first 6 weeks. Smaller pseudocysts (less than 5 cm in diameter) appeared to be more likely to resolve spontaneously.

The cause of spontaneous resolution of pseudocysts is unknown. Presumably, the peritoneum of the lesser sac is capable of resorbing the fluid in some patients. In other cases it is suspected, though unproven, that the pseudocyst drains back into the pancreatic ductal system. Finally, some pseudocysts drain by the formation of a fistula into an adjacent organ such as the stomach, duodenum, or colon. These spontaneous fistulas are observed from time to time when a pseudocyst is incidentally filled with contrast medium during ERCP or a GI series.

The natural history of posttraumatic pseudocysts is not as well studied as in the case of postpancreatitis cysts. Although it is likely that some pseudocysts resolve spontaneously after pancreatic injury, it is more commonly observed that posttraumatic cysts are much less likely to do so than those that follow an attack of acute pancreatitis. This difference in behavior can be probably explained by the fact that most posttraumatic cysts are not suspected for weeks after the injury, and therefore more likely to be mature (chronic) at the time of diagnosis. In addition, it is possible that leakage from a main pancreatic duct is more likely to be extensive after injury than after an attack of acute pancreatitis.

Diagnosis

Pseudocysts of the pancreas should be considered in all patients who have protracted symptoms after an attack of acute pancreatitis or following abdominal trauma. Abdominal pain is the most common complaint and was present in 90 percent of 104 patients reviewed by Becker. The pain associated with pancreatic pseudocysts is usually located in the epigastrium or left upper quadrant and frequently radiates to the back. Sixty percent of patients complain of nausea or vomiting and 40 percent experience weight loss. According to Becker et al, Gilman and associates, and Shatney and Lillihei, an abdominal mass is palpable in 60 to 70 percent of patients with pseudocysts. It is usually located in the left upper quadrant or in the epigastric region. The mass is ordinarily rounded and relatively immobile. Some tenderness on palpation is present in approximately 60 percent of cases, but it is rarely marked. It should also be emphasized that even a large pseudocyst can remain hidden under the costal margin. Thus, failure to palpate a mass does not exclude the presence of a pseudocyst.

Low grade fever is a relatively common finding. High spiking fever suggests secondary infection in a pseudocyst or a pancreatic abscess rather than an uncomplicated cyst. Mild jaundice is present on admission in about 10 percent of cases and is ordinarily due to distal common bile duct obstruction by the pseudocyst or by the associated pancreatic inflammation. Pleural effusion or pancreatic ascites (discussed in the following) are present in approximately 5 percent of the patients.

Blood studies on admission may reveal a variable but usually mild leukocytosis. The serum amylase is significantly elevated in about 50 percent of cases, according to Donaldson and colleagues. In fact, persistent hyperamylasemia after an attack of acute pancreatitis is highly suggestive of the development of a pseudocyst. Hyperglycemia is present in approximately one third of the patients. In cases associated with pleural effusion or ascites, the amylase levels

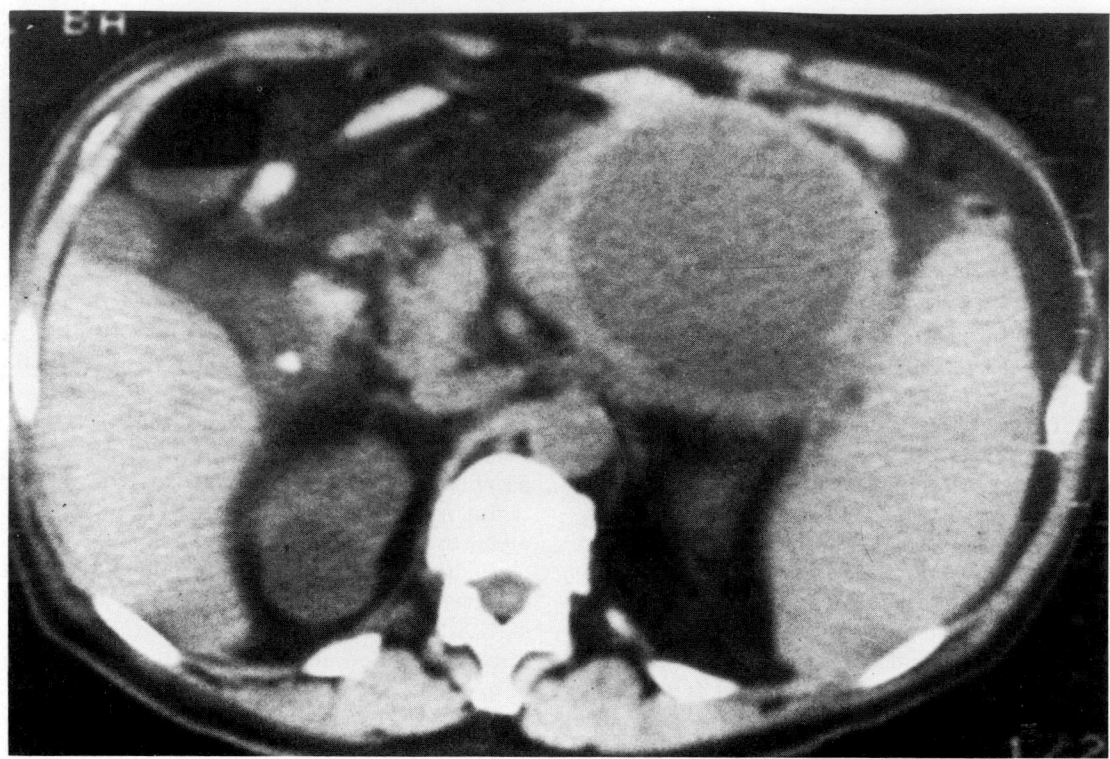

Figure 88–6. CT appearance of chronic pseudocyst. The thickened irregular wall suggests
the presence of hemorrhage and/or infection in the cyst. The splenomegaly is indicative of
splenic vein thrombosis and left-sided portal hypertension.

will be increased in the aspirated pleural or
peritoneal fluid.

The imaging techniques that are most
useful in the initial diagnosis of pancreatic
pseudocysts are ultrasonography and CT. On
ultrasonic examination, a pseudocyst is
characterized by an anechoic "cystic" center,
a strongly echoic rim, and good through transmission of sound. Approximately one third of
patients suspected of harboring a pseudocyst
will have a technically unsatisfactory ultrasonic
examination, usually because of gas-filled loops
of bowel, which interfere with transmission. In
the remaining patients, however, sonography
has a diagnostic accuracy of 75 to 90 percent,
according to Bradley et al and to Willford and
associates. CT (Fig. 88–6) has an overall accuracy rate of over 90 percent, with a technical
failure rate of about 1 percent. With this technique, pseudocysts appear as nonenhancing
fluid densities with distinct margination. The
anatomic detail of CT scanning is much better
than with ultrasound. In particular, CT scans
are superior to sonography in delineating extension of the pseudocysts into areas of the retroperitoneum beyond the peripancreatic region.
For the initial study of a pseudocyst, CT scan
is probably the investigation of choice. Ultrasonography, on the other hand, is particularly useful for serial studies of pseudocyst size, since
it is somewhat more convenient, is less expensive, and does not carry the hazard of repeated
radiation doses.

CT scan and ultrasonography have totally
supplanted the upper GI series in the diagnosis
and follow-up of a pancreatic pseudocyst. All
the necessary information, including gastric
outlet obstruction, can be provided by CT. The
presence of splenomegaly is suggestive of
splenic vein occlusion and is an absolute indication for angiography. Celiac and superior mesenteric arteriography is essential in this setting
to confirm the presence of portal or splenic vein
thrombosis with left-sided portal hypertension

and gastric varices. Upper GI barium study will demonstrate some abnormality only in about 60 percent of patients with pancreatic pseudocysts and hence should be abandoned.

Patients with pancreatic pseudocysts occasionally present with symptoms of colonic obstruction. In these circumstances, barium enema may demonstrate an extrinsic mass effect causing narrowing of the transverse colon or splenic flexure. At times, the findings may be misinterpreted as representing a carcinoma or other primary colon pathology.

ERCP is an invasive technique that has, in many instances, been underutilized in the evaluation of pancreatic pseudocysts. Sugawa and Walt report an 89 percent diagnostic accuracy rate. ERCP is probably not indicated in every case of pancreatic pseudocyst, but it provides essential information in certain situations. It is touted as the best method for the diagnosis of small (2 cm or less) pseudocysts, especially when they are multiple, but whether these small lesions are true pseudocysts or pancreatic duct ectasia is probably a matter of semantics. ERCP is mandatory in the evaluation of pancreatic ascites, since it usually demonstrates both the associated pseudocyst and the area of ductal disruption. ERCP is also useful in cases in which a resection of a distal pseudocyst is entertained, since it demonstrates whether proximal ductal disease will require retrograde drainage of the tail of the pancreas into an intestinal loop. ERCP is also usually recommended in the evaluation of pseudocysts which recur after operation.

The role of splanchnicarteriography in the evaluation of pancreatic pseudocysts is controversial. Although some authorities rarely employ it, angiography may provide important information and ought to be performed whenever there is a history of associated GI bleeding or signs suggestive of portal hypertension. It is well known that pseudocysts may cause life-threatening hemorrhage by direct erosion of the splenic, pancreaticoduodenal, gastroduodenal, or gastroepiploic vessels. Angiography may demonstrate extravasation from these vessels with or without pseudoaneurysm formation, in which case resection of the pseudocyst along with the abnormal vessel should be strongly considered, as discussed below. Angiography may also demonstrate thrombosis of the splenic or portal vein and the formation of gastric varices, in which case splenectomy with resection

or internal drainage of the cyst is probably the treatment of choice. In a study of nine patients with major hemorrhage associated with pseudocysts, Stanley and associates found that arteriography demonstrated the probable site of bleeding in eight of the nine cases. Selective catheterization and angiographic embolization should be considered whenever the risk of operative intervention appears prohibitive. Direct surgical attack can then be postponed until the general condition of the patient becomes optimal.

Finally, in patients with a pancreatic pseudocyst who present with extrahepatic biliary obstruction, study of the common bile duct either by ERCP or by percutaneous transhepatic cholangiography is useful in demonstrating whether the obstruction is due to the pseudocyst itself (and thus likely to resolve after drainage of the cyst) or is due to a fibrotic stricture secondary to chronic pancreatitis (in which case biliary diversion will be required).

Complications

According to Becker et al, 42 percent of patients with pancreatic pseudocysts experience a major complication. These complications include obstruction, infection, hemorrhage, and rupture (free perforation or fistula formation).

Obstruction of the common bile duct and duodenum have already been mentioned and are encountered in approximately 10 percent of patients with pseudocysts.

Infection is the most common complication of pancreatic pseudocysts. It is most likely to occur in the early stages of pseudocyst formation. The onset of infection is heralded by the appearance of high fever, tachycardia, tachypnea, and increasing abdominal pain. A variety of bacteria have been isolated from the infected pseudocyst, although coliforms are the most common. Often multiple strains of enteric organisms are cultured.

Hemorrhage associated with pancreatic pseudocysts may be gastrointestinal, intraperitoneal, or intracystic. Although the bleeding may be mild and chronic, it is often sudden, major, and catastrophic. Cogbill reports an overall mortality of 56 percent.

GI bleeding due to mucosal disease such as peptic ulceration or stress ulceration are largely preventable by the routine administration of cimetidine and/or antacids in all patients with severe acute pancreatitis. Of more ominous significance is hemorrhage into the GI tract, which results from direct erosion into the bowel lumen or from gastric varices secondary to splenic vein thrombosis. Intracystic or intraperitoneal hemorrhage is usually due to direct erosion into one of the arteries of the gland. The splenic artery or one of its branches is most commonly involved.

Perforation of a pseudocyst may occur into the free peritoneal cavity or into an adjacent viscus such as the stomach, duodenum, or transverse colon. In a review of 45 reported cases, Hanna found them equally divided between free perforations into the peritoneal cavity and fistulation into the GI tract. Free perforation is usually a catastrophic event, leading to shock and peritonitis. The reported mortality rate is approximately 50 percent. Perforation into a viscus, on the other hand, is not always clinically obvious and may be discovered only at ERCP when the fistula is demonstrated. In some patients, perforation of a pseudocyst into the GI tract is signaled by an episode of GI hemorrhage, which may be major and may be the main source of danger in the formation of an internal fistula.

Surgical Treatment

Because of the high rate of complications associated with mature (chronic) pseudocysts, the presence of a persistent pseudocyst is an indication for operation. In addition, surgical treatment is required in essentially all pseudocysts when a complication occurs. Chronic pseudocysts cannot be adequately drained percutaneously by aspiration under ultrasonographic or CT guidance, nor can they be adequately drained internally through the endoscope. Inadequate drainage, hemorrhage, infection, and persistence of the cyst are the rule rather than the exception when nonoperative methods are attempted.

Modern surgical therapy for pancreatic pseudocysts offers three operative options:

1. External drainage
2. Internal drainage, which includes cystogastrostomy, cystoduodenostomy, or cystojejunostomy Roux-Y
3. Resection of the portion of the pancreas containing the pseudocyst

Each of these procedures has its own advantages and disadvantages. Preoperative assessment and operative judgment are thus essential. The choice of operation depends on several factors, such as maturity of the pseudocyst, its size, its anatomic location, and whether or not a complication has occurred. In order to achieve the best results in the treatment of pancreatic pseudocysts, it is essential to choose the operation which is best suited to the individual patient.

The Timing of Operation. In general, pseudocysts that are less than 6 weeks old have a thin capsule that precludes internal drainage. Polk and associates have described the danger subsequent to the anastomosis of a thin friable cyst wall to the GI tract. Cerilli and Faris have likewise demonstrated a high mortality associated with internal drainage of immature (acute) pseudocysts. Thus, most authorities advocate a waiting period of about 6 weeks before definitive operation. The wisdom of this approach is supported by the observations of Bradley and associates: that catastrophic complications of pseudocysts rarely occur during the first 6 weeks of observation and that pseudocysts that resolve spontaneously usually do so within the first 6 weeks after diagnosis. When surgical intervention becomes necessary during the first 6 weeks, it is usually because infection or rupture has supervened. Under these circumstances, there is unanimous agreement that external drainage of the pseudocyst is the operation of choice.

External Drainage

External drainage is indicated in the treatment of pseudocysts with immature capsules and in the presence of obvious infection. The technique is standardized. After aspirating fluid to confirm the location of the cyst and for bacterial culture and sensitivity, an opening is made in the cyst wall. The cavity is thoroughly irrigated and any loculi broken down. Gentle debridement of the inside of the cavity is performed with the index finger as is deemed necessary. A soft rubber catheter such as a Malecot or de Pezzer catheter, or a soft sump suction drain is passed into the cavity (Fig. 88–7). If possible, the cyst wall is secured around the catheter with silk sutures. The catheter is brought out of the abdomen through a separate stab incision and is secured to the skin. Low-grade continuous suction should be applied to the catheter.

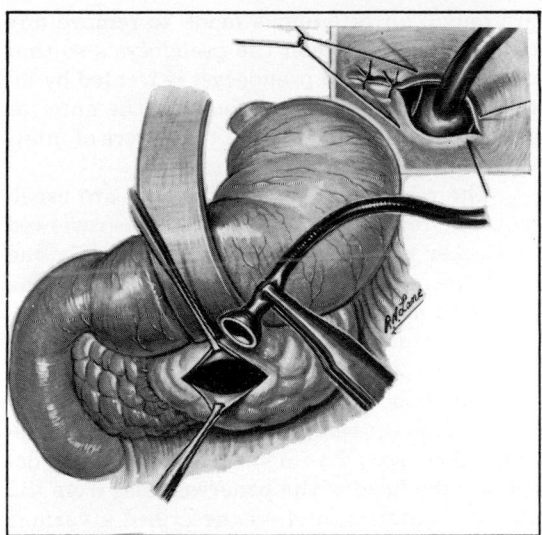

Figure 88-7. Simple drainage of a pancreatic pseudo-cyst with a de Pezzer catheter. (*Source: From Cattell RB, Warren KW: Surgery of the Pancreas. Philadelphia: WB Saunders, 1953, with permission.*)

In infected pseudocysts that are thick walled and are firmly adherent to the posterior gastric wall, Smith's technique of transgastric external drainage may be employed. Through an appropriately placed anterior gastrotomy incision, a large trocar-cannula is passed through

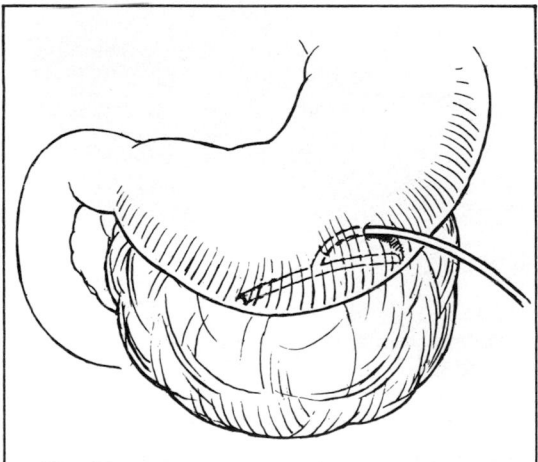

Figure 88-8. Transgastric T-tube drainage of an infected pancreatic cyst. (*Source: From Smith R, 1965, with permission.*)

the back wall of the stomach and the pseudocyst wall to evacuate the contents of the cyst. After aspirating some of the material for culture and sensitivity, the cystogastrotomy hole is gently enlarged to allow the index finger to pass through it into the cyst cavity. Again, gentle debridement and breaking of loculi are performed and a suitable drainage tube (usually a Foley catheter or a large T-tube) is inserted into the cyst and then brought out through stab wounds in the anterior stomach wall and the anterior abdominal wall (Fig. 88–8). The gastrotomy incision is closed in two layers, and the puncture wound in the stomach through which the drainage catheter exists is invaginated with a purse string and then secured to the peritoneum of the anterior abdominal wall with interrupted 3-0 silk sutures. The drainage catheter is secured to the skin and low-grade continuous suction is applied.

External drainage of pancreatic pseudocysts is an effective operation. The operative mortality is approximately 5 percent, reflecting the fact that the procedure is usually reserved for patients in dire circumstances. The major disadvantages of external drainage are recurrence of the pseudocyst, which occurs in about 20 percent of cases, and pancreatic fistula, which usually subside spontaneously on total parenteral alimentation, but which may persist for months before finally closing (Fig. 88–9). For the above reasons, external drainage, of all the operations for pseudocysts, is associated with the highest likelihood of a subsequent operation. In Becker's review, 25 percent of patients treated by external drainage required at least one further procedure. This fact, however, does not detract from the usefulness of external drainage. In most cases, external drainage can be a life-saving procedure that gives the patient some time to improve for a definitive operation if needed.

Internal Drainage

Internal drainage is, in general, the operation of choice for mature, uncomplicated pancreatic pseudocysts. The specific choice of procedure, namely, cystogastrostomy, cystoduodenostomy, or cystojejunostomy Roux-Y, is dictated mainly by the anatomic location of the cyst.

Transgastric cystogastrostomy (Fig. 88–10), usually attributed to Jurasz, was first performed by Jedlicka in 1921. It is the most frequently

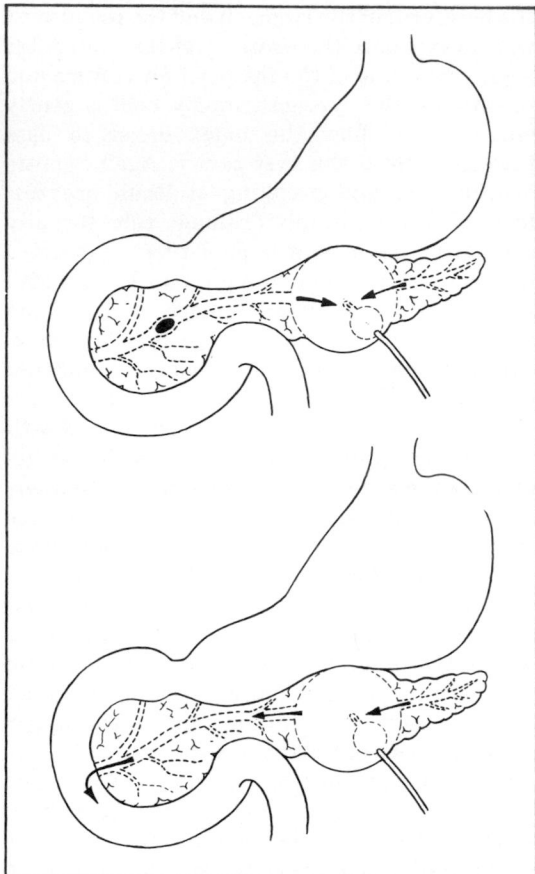

Figure 88–9. External drainage of a pancreatic pseudocyst involving the body of the pancreas. Closure of the fistula is unlikely if there is an obstruction in the proximal portion of the duct of Wirsung.

performed operation but has often received bad connotation because of its indiscriminate application for pseudocysts that are not suitable for the operation. It takes advantage of the fact that many mature pseudocysts are densely adherent to the posterior wall of the stomach. Through a long vertical epigastric incision, a long anterior gastrotomy is made, and an opening is made in the anterior wall of the stomach over the cyst. An ellipse of joint stomach and cyst wall measuring about 3 to 4 cm in length is excised and hemostasis in the cyst wall and the posterior gastric wall is maintained with interrupted nonabsorbable sutures. The finger is placed into the cavity and gentle debridement is performed. If several contiguous pseudocysts

are found, an attempt is made to remove any common wall between the pseudocysts so that the newly enlarged pseudocyst is treated by internal drainage into the stomach. The anterior gastrotomy is then closed in two layers of interrupted nonabsorbable sutures.

The results of cystogastrostomy are excellent. The recurrence rate in 220 cases reviewed by Becker was 2.3 percent, approximately one tenth the rate seen after external drainage. The operative mortality was 3.6 percent.

Transduodenal cystoduodenostomy (Fig. 88–11) for pseudocysts located in the head of the pancreas in close contact with the duodenum follows the same principles as cystogastrostomy. Anderson has noted that some pseudocysts of the head of the pancreas arise from the duct of Santorini, and has described a variant of cystoduodenostomy that incorporates transduodenal sphincteroplasty of the minor papilla. These patients invariably have a pancreas divisum.

Cystojejunostomy Roux-Y (Fig. 88–12) is reserved for those situations in which the anatomic location of the cyst makes transgastric or transduodenal drainage technically impossible. These cysts usually enlarge inferiorly

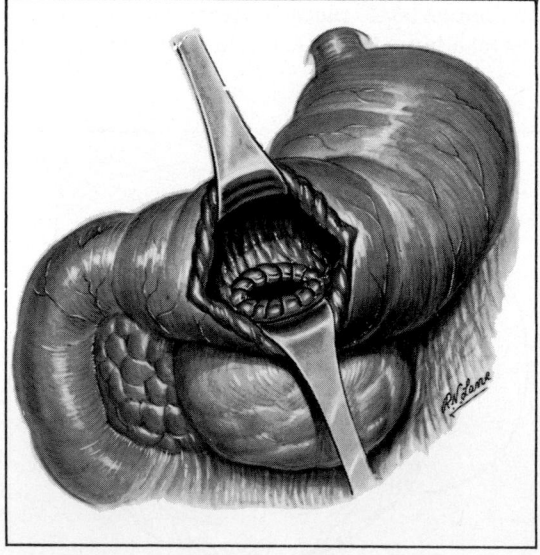

Figure 88–10. Transgastric cystogastrostomy. This is the most popular operation for a chronic pseudocyst that is firmly adherent to the posterior wall of the stomach. (*Source: Adapted from Cattell RB, Warren KW: Surgery of the Pancreas. Philadelphia: WB Saunders, 1953, with permission.*)

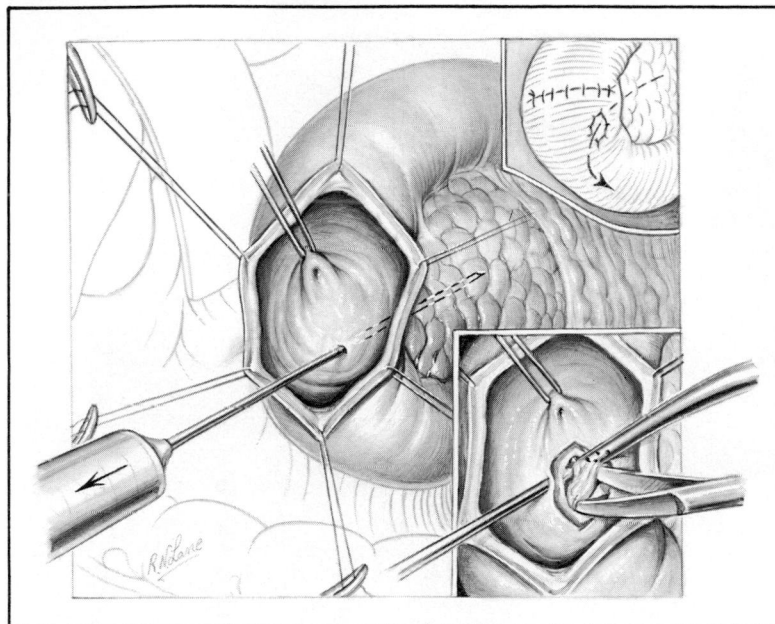

Figure 88–11. Transduodenal cystoduodenostomy for a pseudocyst of the head of the pancreas. After the firmly adherent portion of the pseudocyst wall is excised, the fibrous margins of the cyst wall are sutured to the oval "defect" in the posterior wall of the second portion of the duodenum with a series of closely applied sutures of fine silk or Merselene. Note the position of the papilla of Vater.

through the transverse mesocolon. The jejunum is divided 20 cm or so below the ligament of Treitz, and the distal jejunal limb is anastomosed to the cyst wall at the level of the transverse mesocolon in two layers using either side-to-side or end-to-side technique. The proximal jejunal limb is then sutured end-to-side to the small bowel 40 cm below the cystojejunostomy.

Resection

Occasionally, a pseudocyst is encountered that may be excised by enucleation, with sacrifice of minimal adjacent pancreatic tissue. This is, however, a very rare situation. Misguided attempts at simple excision of the cyst may lead to life-threatening complications such as hemorrhage, pancreatic fistula, or sepsis. In virtually all reported series, excision of the cyst was accompanied by a higher operative mortality than any other procedure.

The question of whether to resect the tail or the head of the pancreas when it contains a pseudocyst is a difficult one. Resectional therapy results in the lowest recurrence rate but is accompanied by an operative mortality of almost 10 percent in collected series. Resection is generally recommended for posttraumatic pseudocysts, which are reputed to have a high incidence of recurrence. Pseudocysts that invade the splenic substance or that have led to splenic vein thrombosis are probably best treated by distal pancreatectomy and splenectomy, as recommended by Haff and colleagues. Resection is also the optimal treatment for pseudocysts associated with major arterial hemorrhage. If resection is not possible, the alternative is the considerably less satisfactory operation of internal drainage with ligation of the feeding vessel and direct oversewing of the bleeding point. Finally, resection is usually recommended for pseudocysts that recur after internal drainage or that are associated with pancreatic ascites.

Resection of the head of the pancreas is a formidable procedure in the presence of a pseudocyst and is rarely, if ever, indicated as a primary procedure.

Complications of Operation

Three major complications that may occur after operations on pancreatic pseudocysts are pancreatic fistula, recurrence of the pseudocyst, and postoperative hemorrhage.

Pancreatic fistulas occur after external drainage of pseudocysts in approximately 25 percent of cases. The majority of these fistulas will close spontaneously in a period ranging from a few days to several months. The management of pancreatic fistulas is further discussed below.

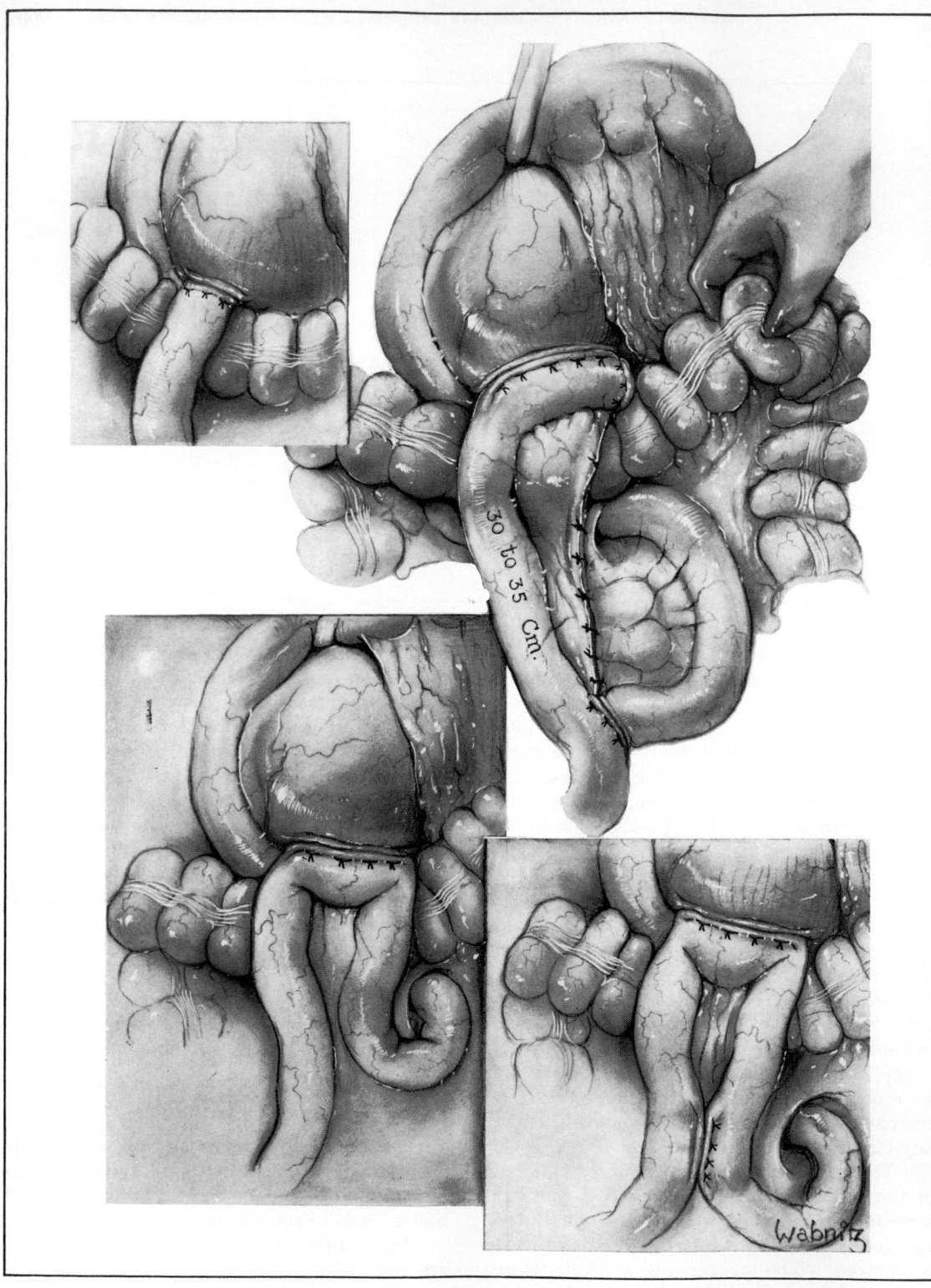

Figure 88–12. Cystojejunostomy for a pancreatic pseudocyst illustrating Roux-Y method and the simple loop method with or without enteroanastomosis. (*Source: From Madden J: Atlas of Technics in Surgery, 2 edt. New York: Appleton-Century-Crofts, 1964, with permission.*)

Recurrence of pancreatic pseudocysts is most common after external drainage; a 20 percent recurrence rate is expected under these circumstances. Reappearance of the cyst is much less common after internal drainage (4 percent) or resection (2 percent).

Bleeding from a pseudocyst after external or internal drainage is a particularly difficult problem. It occurs in approximately 10 percent of patients after transgastric cystogastrostomy. The etiology of postoperative hemorrhage after cystogastrostomy is unclear. Hudson and associates have attributed bleeding to the practice of placing a continuous suture around the rim of the cystogastrostomy. They believe that this maneuver prevents the gastric and cyst walls from coapting and allows a reflux of acid into the cyst. Other authorities take the opposite point of view and recommend a continuous hemostatic suture of the cystogastric anastomosis to avoid hemorrhage from this junction. A more rational evaluation of hemorrhage in this setting implies an understanding of the site of the bleeding:

1. Bleeding from the cystogastrostomy suture line is invariably due to inadequate hemostasis by suture ligation with interrupted nonabsorbable mattress sutures of the edges of the cyst wall and the gastric wall. Unrecognized left-sided portal hypertension due to splenic vein thrombosis is often a contributory factor.

2. Bleeding from the gastric mucosa is invariably due to undetected left-sided portal hypertension and gastric varices.
3. Bleeding originating in the depth of the pseudocyst cavity is always due to unrecognized pseudoaneurysm involving the pancreatic or peripancreatic vessels.

Thus, postoperative hemorrhage following cystogastrostomy can largely be avoided by a more liberal use of preoperative angiography to identify those patients at risk who might be better treated by resection than by drainage, who might be better treated by splenectomy as well as cystogastrostomy, and, finally, by careful attention to hemostasis at the cystogastrostomy suture line.

PANCREATIC ASCITES

Pancreatic ascites is a condition in which the peritoneal cavity fills with pancreatic juice emanating from a disruption in the pancreatic ductal system. Most of the cases are associated with alcoholic pancreatitis; a few follow pancreatic trauma. The onset may be gradual or abrupt. An associated pseudocyst is present in the majority of cases. Presumably, pancreatic ascites results from a noncatastrophic leak of the pseudocyst into the general peritoneal cavity. Approximately 15 percent of the cases are associated with a pleural effusion, usually on the left

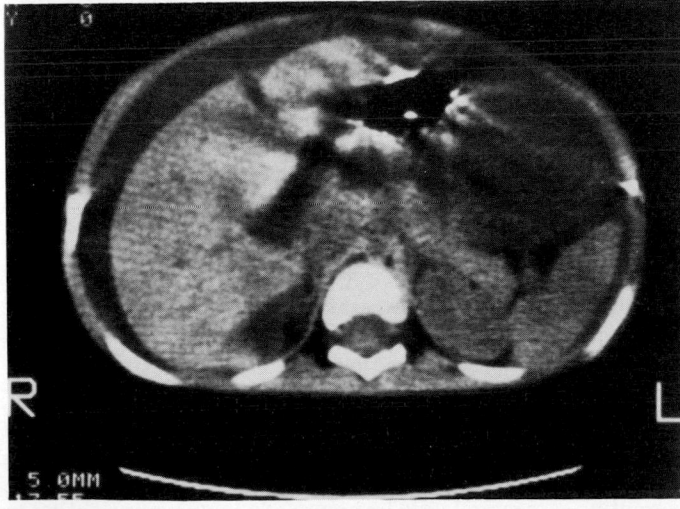

Figure 88–13. CT showing pancreatic ascites due to a leaking pseudocyst in a 2½-year-old child. The etiology is probably blunt trauma.

side, but sometimes on the right side or bilateral. Occasionally, chest symptoms are predominant in the presentation. Zuidema and Cameron have made the interesting observation that there is often a modest or absent history of pancreatitis in patients with pancreatic ascites. For this reason, pancreatic ascites may be erroneously assumed to be of the more common hepatic variety. The diagnosis of pancreatic ascites is made by first thinking of it as a possibility. It is confirmed by demonstrating a high amylase and high protein content in the peritoneal fluid, both of these findings distinguishing pancreatic from cirrhotic ascites. Donowitz and associates report an average amylase content of 20,000 SU in pancreatic ascites. The serum amylase level is also usually elevated. CT (Fig. 88–13) is the best initial test to delineate the presence or absence of a pseudocyst, to confirm the presence of ascites and/or pleural effusions. The most useful further procedure in diagnosis is ERCP, which will demonstrate the area of ductal disruption, outline the associated pseudocysts further, and reveal extravasation of dye into the peritoneal cavity. ERCP is also helpful in demonstrating whether the abnormality in the ductal system is localized or diffuse. The importance of ERCP in guiding the treatment of pancreatic ascites is suggested by the experience of Sankaran and Walt, who reported that the incidence of failed surgical treatment was reduced from 53 to 0 percent after the introduction of routine preoperative ERCP.

The optimal treatment for pancreatic ascites is a matter of some controversy. Sankaran and Walt have advocated early operation in all cases. On the other hand, Zuidema and Cameron advocate an initial trial of medical therapy consisting of paracentesis, nasogastric suction, and intravenous total hyperalimentation. They report that 7 of 17 patients thus treated had permanent resolution of their ascites without operative intervention. However, if medical therapy fails over a period of 2 to 3 weeks, operation becomes mandatory.

The choice of an operative procedure should be dictated by the ductal anatomy, as demonstrated by pancreatography and by the gross findings at laparotomy. The ideal procedure for a small pseudocyst situated in the tail of the pancreas is a distal pancreatectomy and splenectomy. If the pancreatogram had demonstrated no proximal duct disease, the pancreatic remnant can be oversewn. If proximal obstruc-

tive duct disease is present, the pancreatic remnant should be drained by retrograde pancreatojejunostomy using a Roux-Y jejunal loop. If the pseudocyst is large, or is located proximally in the head of the pancreas, drainage by cystogastrostomy or cystojejunostomy Roux-Y is indicated. External drainage of the pseudocyst has been associated with a very high recurrence rate and a high incidence of persistent pancreatic fistula and is therefore not recommended. In about 10 percent of cases a direct duct leak is demonstrated without any pseudocyst. The recommended or preferred treatment in this situation is an anastomosis between the ruptured duct and the Roux-Y jejunal loop.

PANCREATIC FISTULAS

Pancreatic fistulas ordinarily result from operations on the pancreas and neighboring organs. External drainage of a pancreatic pseudocyst is the most common cause of a postoperative pancreatic fistula. Other operations associated with fistula formation include distal pancreatectomy, pancreatoduodenectomy of the Whipple type, gastrectomy for penetrating peptic ulcer, splenectomy, and splenorenal shunts for portal hypertension. Blunt and penetrating abdominal trauma account for the remainder of pancreatic fistulas.

Approximately two thirds of postoperative pancreatic fistulas ultimately close spontaneously. The period of drainage ranges from a few days to 2 years or longer. In the early management of pancreatic fistulas, attention should be directed to providing fluid and electrolyte replacement, maintaining adequate nutrition, diminishing pancreatic secretion, and caring for the skin around the fistula tract, which may be severely excoriated by pancreatic enzymes. Dimunition of pancreatic secretion is best accomplished by passing a nasogastric tube and prohibiting oral intake. In rare instances of high output fistula a few days treatment with Glucagon or somatostatin to further suppress pancreatic exocrine secretion may be occasionally helpful. Nutritional needs are met by instituting total parenteral nutrition through a central venous catheter. An excellent alternative is total enteral nutrition through a feeding jejunostomy tube if one is already in place. Thus, the prophylactic insertion of a jejunostomy catheter should always be considered during complicated pancreatic and peripancreatic operations in which the surgeon feels that there is a possibility of a postoperative pancreatic fistula.

Serum electrolyte levels should be measured at intervals and the alimentation fluids adjusted accordingly. Occasionally, massive bicarbonate replacement may be necessary in patients with high output fistulas.

Care of the skin around the fistula is usually not a problem after catheter drainage of a pseudocyst but may present serious difficulties when unexpected pancreaticocutaneous fistulas develop. If possible, a soft sump drainage catheter should be passed into the fistulous tract and attached to low-grade suction. To protect the skin from pancreatic juices that may escape around the catheter, the area around the fistula may be protected by the commercially available plastic skin barriers, over which an ostomy drainage bag may be attached to collect the secretions. The involvement of an enterostomal therapist in the management of patients with pancreatic fistulas is often invaluable.

Like all fistulas, pancreatic fistulas are unlikely to heal in the presence of continued infection or if an obstruction exists in the main pancreatic duct between the fistula and the duodenum. If peripancreatic infection is suggested by continuing tenderness, fever, and hyperamylasemia, further operation, to drain and debride areas of necrosis and abscess formation, may be necessary before the fistula will heal. The presence of pancreatic duct obstruction is best diagnosed by ERCP, fistulography, or both. If dye passes from the fistula into the duodenum without obstruction, the likelihood is high that the fistula will heal spontaneously. On the other hand, a high-grade obstruction in the pancreatic duct will prevent healing and will necessitate further operation which should not be needlessly delayed. The ideal surgical treatment for pancreatic fistula consists of resection of the portion of the pancreas from which the fistula originates, along with the area of ductal obstruction. Such a procedure is usually possible in fistulas that arise from the body and tail of the pancreas. Pancreatogastrostomy with T-tube drainage has been used in this situation (Fig. 88–14). For fistulas that arise in the pancreatic head, resection carries greater risks; as an alternative to resection, it is occasionally possible to excise the fistulous tract down to the pancreatic duct and to perform a side-to-side anastomosis between the duct and a defunctionalized

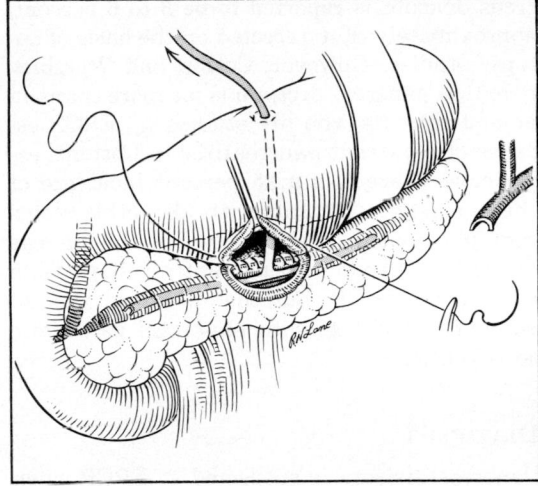

Figure 88–14. Pancreatogastrostomy with T-tube drainage for a chronic pancreatic fistula involving the duct of Wirsung. *Inset:* Maingot's guttered T-tube. Note the position of the posterior suture.

Roux-Y jejunal loop. When the head of the pancreas is the site of chronic pancreatitis and multiple areas of ductal obstruction, a total pancreatectomy may be the only method of effecting a cure.

PANCREAS DIVISUM

The condition referred to as pancreas divisum results from the failure of the dorsal and ventral pancreatic primordia to fuse. As a result, the usual anastomosis between the dorsal and ventral ducts does not take place, with the result that the dorsal duct (duct of Santorini) becomes the dominant duct draining the body and tail of the gland. The ventral duct (duct of Wirsung) remains short and rudimentary, draining only the lower portion of the pancreatic head and the uncinate process that arise from the ventral anlage.

Pancreas divisum is not a rare anomaly and has a documented incidence of 5 percent in cadaver pancreatic specimens in which the duct system was injected with vinyl acetate. The reported incidence at autopsy is 5 to 8 percent. The condition has been recognized for many years but has received additional attention since the advent of ERCP. In large series of patients undergoing ERCP, the incidence of pancreas divisum is reported to be 3 to 6 percent, approximately that expected on the basis of autopsy studies. However, Cotton and Warshaw note that pancreas divisum is far more common among patients who are studied by ERCP because of recurrent pancreatitis; in Cotton's experience, there was a 25 percent incidence of the anomaly in patients with idiopathic recurrent pancreatitis. Rosch found that pancreas divisum occurred in 6 percent of all patients undergoing ERCP, but the incidence was 20 percent in patients with abnormal pancreatic secretion tests.

Diagnosis

Pancreas divisum is suspected at ERCP when the duct of Wirsung fails to visualize after injection of the major papilla or when it is attenuated and rudimentary. If pancreas divisum is suspected after injection of the papilla of Vater, an attempt should be made to cannulate the minor papilla, although this is possible in less than half of the cases because of the small size of the minor papilla and the difficult angle of entrance. If the minor papilla can be entered, injection of dye will demonstrate that the duct of Santorini is the dominant duct and extends the length of the body and tail of the pancreas. On occasion, the duct of Santorini will demonstrate dilation, irregularity, or stricture suggestive of chronic pancreatitis, but in the majority of cases, it will appear to be normal.

To prove that pancreas divisum is causally related to the development of pancreatitis is difficult. It is hard to understand why some patients with the anomaly develop symptoms, but the vast majority do not. Even among patients with symptoms suggesting pancreatitis who are found to have pancreas divisum at ERCP, many do not demonstrate ductal changes, impaired pancreatic secretion, or even elevation of the serum amylase. Moossa, among others, has questioned the clinical relevance of pancreas divisum even in symptomatic patients. The usual explanation for the development of pancreatitis in patients with pancreas divisum is that the minor papilla acts as a point of relative obstruction to the flow of pancreatic juice since its small size is unable to accommodate the bulk of pancreatic secretion. No firm evidence to support this theory is forthcoming as yet, and the usual lack of dilation of the duct of Santorini seems to argue against it. Nevertheless, the occasional reports of histologic evidence of pancreatitis in the dorsal gland in the absence of ductal changes on ERCP and the even rarer reports of histologic pancreatitis affecting the dorsal gland but sparing the ventral gland suggest that divided pancreas may have a significant relationship to pancreatitis in some patients.

Prior to considering operations in patients with pancreas divisum, an exhaustive search for other causes of pancreatitis should be undertaken. If any of the more usual explanations for pancreatitis is found, it should be treated first. In the absence of any explanation for the patient's symptoms other than pancreas divisum, we believe that operative intervention should be considered only in patients with some objective evidence of pancreatitis, such as elevation of the serum amylase or ductal changes demonstrated by ERCP.

Treatment

Based on the belief that pancreatitis associated with pancreas divisum is due to obstruction at the minor papilla, therapy has been directed at enlarging the outflow tract of the duct of Santorini. Cotton tried endoscopic minor papillotomy in two patients, but in both cases, restenosis occurred in a matter of weeks.

Warshaw, Spiro, and Cooperman et al have reported a small experience with surgical sphincteroplasty of the minor papilla. The operation is analogous to the more commonly performed sphincteroplasty of the papilla of Vater, and is performed through a longitudinal duodenostomy. The administration of secretin intravenously may assist in locating the minor papilla. In Warshaw's cases, sphincteroplasty of the major papilla and cholecystectomy have been performed in addition to division of the minor papilla. The rationale for this triple procedure is unclear.

The results of minor sphincteroplasty have been variable. Most patients are reported improved but follow-up is still short in the few reported cases. Warshaw has noted that patients with chronic abdominal pain have not improved, whereas those with intermittent acute pain have responded well.

In patients with chronic pancreatitis and pancreatic insufficiency who have pancreas divisum, surgical therapy to relieve pain is based on the same considerations as apply to chronic pancreatitis in general. Longitudinal pancreaticojejunostomy has been employed in a few cases in which the dorsal duct was dilated. In patients without ductal dilation, subtotal resection of the pancreas may be indicated on rare occasions.

Rational surgical therapy for pancreatitis associated with pancreas divisum awaits a clearer demonstration of the mechanism involved in the production of symptoms and a method for determining whether operations such as minor sphincteroplasty result in objective improvement in the pancreas.

BIBLIOGRAPHY

Anderson MC: Pseudocyst of the head of the pancreas—Relationship to the duct of Santorini. Ann Surg 190:719, 1979

Aranha GV, Prinz RA, et al: The nature and course of cystic pancreatic lesions diagnosed by ultrasound. Arch Surg 118:486, 1983

Becker WF, Pratt HS, et al: Pseudocysts of the pancreas. Surg Gynecol Obstet 127:744, 1968

Becker WF, Welsh RA, et al: Cystadenoma and cystadenocarcinoma of the pancreas. Ann Surg 161:845, 1965

Bradley EL, Clements JL, et al: The natural history of pancreatic pseudocysts—A unified concept of management. Am J Surg 137:135, 1979

Campbell J, Cruickshank A: Cystadenoma and cystadenocarcinoma of the pancreas. J Clin Pathol 15:432, 1962

Cogbill DL: Hemorrhage in pancreatic pseudocysts. Review of literature and report of two cases. Ann Surg 167:112, 1968

Compagno J, Oertel J: Microcystic adenomas of the pancreas (glycogen rich cystadenomas). A clinicopathologic study of 34 cases. Am J Clin Pathol 69:289, 1978

Compagno J, Oertel J: Mucinous cystic neoplasms of the pancreas with overt and latent malignancy (cystadenocarcinoma and cystadenoma). Am J Clin Pathol 69:573, 1978

Cooperman M, Ferrara JJ, et al: Surgical management of pancreas divisum. Am J Surg 143:107, 1982

Cotton PB, Kizu M: Malfusion of dorsal and ventral pancreas; A cause of pancreatitis? Br Soc Gastroenterol 18:A400, 1977

Cotton PH: Progress report: ERCP. Gut 18:316, 1977

Cotton PH: Congenital anomaly of pancreas divisum as cause of obstructive pain and pancreatitis. Gut 21:105, 1980

DeCourcy JL: Dermoid cyst of pancreas. A case report. Ann Surg 118:394, 1943

di Sant'Agnese PA, Darling RC, et al: Abnormal electrolyte composition of sweat in cystic fibrosis of the pancreas. Clinical significance and relationship to the disease. Pediatrics 12:549, 1953

Donaldson LA, Joffe SN, et al: Serial serum amylase levels in patients with pancreatic pseudocysts. Scot Med J 24:13, 1979

Donowitz M, Kerstein MD, et al: Pancreatic ascites. Medicine 53:183, 1974

Gilman PK, Gibbons JC, et al: Unusual diagnostic aspects and current management of pancreatic pseudocysts. Am Surg 40:326, 1974

Gregg JA: Pancreas divisum: Its association with pancreatitis. Am J Surg 134:539, 1977

Haff RC, Page CP, et al: Splenectomy. Its place in operations for inflammatory disease of the pancreas. Am J Surg 134:555, 1977

Hanna W: Rupture of pancreatic cysts. Report of a case and review of the literature. Brit J Surg 47:495, 1960

Hodgkinson D, ReMine W, et al: Pancreatic cystadenoma. A clinicopathologic study of 45 cases. Arch Surg 113:512, 1978

Hodgkinson D, ReMine W, et al: A clinicopathologic study of 21 cases of pancreatic cystadenocarcinoma. Ann Surg 188:679, 1978

Hutson DG, Zeppa R, et al: Prevention of postoperative hemorrhage after pancreatic cystogastrostomy. Ann Surg 177:689, 1973

Jedlicka: Eine neue Operations methode der Pankreascyten Pankreatogastrostomie. Zentralbl Chir 50:132, 1923.

Jordan GL: Surgical diseases of the pancreas, in Howard JM, Jordan GL (eds): Philadelphia: JB Lippincott, 1960, p 283

Jurasz A: Zur Frage der operativen Behandlung der Pankreascysten. Arch Klin Chir 164:272, 1931

Miles RM: Pancreatic cyst in the newborn. A case report. Ann Surg 149:576, 1959

Moossa AR: Pancreatic pseudocysts in children. J R Coll Surg Edinb 19:149, 1974

Nardi GL, Lyon DC, et al: Solitary occult retention cysts of the pancreas. N Engl J Med 280:11, 1969

Nygaard KK, Stacy LJ: Solitary congenital (dysontogenetic) cyst of the pancreas. Arch Surg 45:206, 1942

Park RW, Grand RJ: Gastrointestinal manifestations of cystic fibrosis: A review. Gastroenterol 81:1143, 1981

Pilcher CS, Bradley EL, et al: Enterogenous cyst of the pancreas. Am J Gastroenterol 77:576, 1982

Polk HC, Zeppa R, et al: Surgical significance of differentiation between acute and chronic pancreatic collections. Ann Surg 169:444, 1969

Rösch W, Koch H, et al: The clinical significance of pancreas divisum. Gastrointest Endosc 22:206, 1976

Sankaran S, Walt AJ: Pancreatic ascites. Recognition and management. Arch Surg 111:430, 1976

Sarles JC, Sahel J, et al: Cysts and pseudocysts of the pancreas, Howat HT and Sarles H (eds): Exocrine Pancreas. London: WB Saunders 1979, p 463

Shapiro R, Richter J, et al: Surgical management of pancreas divisum. (Discussion). Am J Surg 143:111, 1982

Shatney CH, Lillehei RC: Surgical treatment of pancreatic pseudocysts. Analysis of 119 cases. Ann Surg 189:386, 1979

Smith R: Transluminal T-tube drainage in pancreatobiliary surgery. A way out of difficulty. Lancet 2:1063, 1965

Soloway H: Constitutional abnormalities associated with pancreatic cystadenomas. Cancer 18:1297, 1965

Stanley JC, Frey CF, et al: Major arterial hemorrhage. A complication of pancreatic pseudocysts and chronic pancreatitis. Arch Surg 111:435, 1976

Strodel WE, Eckhauser FE: Cystic neoplasms of the pancreas, in Dent TL, Eckhauser FE, et al (eds): Pancreatic Disease, Diagnosis and Therapy. New York: Grune & Stratton, 1981, p 363

Sugawa C, Walt A: Endoscopic retrograde pancreatography in the surgery of pancreatic pseudocysts. Surgery 86:639, 1979

Warren KW, Athanassiades S, et al: Surgical treatment of pancreatic cysts. Review of 183 cases. Ann Surg 163:886, 1966

Williford ME, Foster WL, et al: Pancreatic pseudocyst. Comparative evaluation by sonography and computed tomography. AJR 140:53, 1983

Zuidema GD, Cameron JL: Pancreatic ascites and pancreatic pleural effusions, in Dent TL, Eckhauser FE, et al (eds): Pancreatic Disease, Diagnosis and Therapy. New York: Grune & Stratton, 1981, p 285

89. Chronic Relapsing Pancreatitis

Kenneth W. Warren

Chronic relapsing pancreatitis is an accurate descriptive title for a syndrome that is otherwise surrounded by illusions and that is treated surgically by an unbecoming array of inappropriate procedures. The disease is chronic, inflammatory, and relapsing.

Chronic relapsing pancreatitis is characterized by recurrent attacks of upper abdominal pain associated with varying degrees of exocrine and endocrine pancreatic dysfunction. The disease produces a wide variety of progressive and irreversible structural changes in the pancreas. At present, the most controversial aspect of the disease is the choice of an appropriate surgical procedure.

The disease is difficult to diagnose preoperatively and is resistant to medical management. Furthermore, it is associated with a diversity of antecedent conditions and is complicated by numerous mechanical, physiologic, and metabolic consequences. Since no single cause and no consistent lesion can be found, no surgical procedure is ideal. Even when the appropriate operation is chosen for a particular patient, the nature of the disease hinders the prospects for excellent results.

CLASSIFICATION

Pancreatitis may assume one of several forms; these forms of pancreatitis often overlap. A simple but arbitrary classification is acute pancreatitis, relapsing pancreatitis, and chronic pancreatitis.

Acute Pancreatitis. Acute pancreatitis is, by far, the most common type. It may be edematous or hemorrhagic or a combination of both. It is commonly associated with cholecystitis and gallstones, abdominal trauma, acute alcohol poisoning, or systemic infection (for example, mumps).

Relapsing Pancreatitis. This form of chronic pancreatitis is associated with recurrent episodes of acute pancreatitis. It may be related to infections of the gallbladder, choledocholithiasis, sclerosing papillitis, or stenosis of the sphincter of Oddi. The relationship of this form of pancreatitis to alcohol is controversial.

Chronic Pancreatitis. Chronic pancreatitis is a progressive disorder leading to sclerosis of the gland and many distressing complications. It is commonly associated with alcoholism and, less frequently, hyperparathyroidism, familial hyperlipemia, severe protein-deficiency states, and metabolic disturbances. Alcohol poisoning, hyperparathyroidism, and the hereditary forms of pancreatitis are important factors in pancreatolithiasis and calcification of the gland. Pancreatolithiasis, however, may occur in the absence of any of these factors.

A diagnosis that differentiates acute pancreatitis and chronic pancreatitis can be made with assurance, but the distinction between recurrent acute and chronic pancreatitis may be and often is difficult to make. Nevertheless, it should be possible in most instances to distinguish between these two types of chronic pancreatitis provided that the clinician is prepared to undertake an elaborate and searching study of the clinical findings, laboratory investigations, and radiologic studies. For example, during the period of remission, patients with relapsing pancreatitis may regain their health and strength. Their appetite may improve and they gain weight.

Patients who have chronic pancreatitis present a different picture. They continue to complain of indigestion, nausea, anorexia, flatulence, and loss of weight. Steatorrhea, severe epigastric pain, backache, and other objective evidence of pancreatic insufficiency may occur. They usually do not respond to medical treatment. As the disease progresses, patients may increase their consumption of alcohol and narcotics. The alcohol abuse usually precedes the onset of the disease, and narcotic addiction is a consequence of this progressive illness. As the disease worsens, weight loss becomes more pronounced. In many of these patients, diabetes mellitus, severe steatorrhea, obstruction of the duct of Wirsung, parenchymal cystic collections, and pancreatolithiasis develop. Duodenal ulcers are not uncommon; pulmonary tuberculosis is rare.

Sarles et al have stated that repeated attacks of acute pancreatitis do not invariably result in chronic pancreatitis; in fact, advanced chronic pancreatitis may, and often does, occur in the absence of a clinical history of acute pancreatitis. The author has not found that this observation fits his clinical experience.

INCIDENCE

Sex. According to Bockus the sex distribution depends on the relative number of cases attributed to alcohol versus biliary tract disease. In his series of 44 men and 34 women there was a preponderance of "alcohol pancreatitis" among men and of "biliary pancreatitis" in women. The preponderance of biliary pancreatitis evidently explains the high ratio of women to men in the series of Siler and Wulsin (59 percent women) and Pollock (71 percent women, of whom 75 percent had abnormal gallbladders).

Age. Chronic relapsing pancreatitis may occur at any age. In the hereditary form and in most patients, the attacks begin in childhood or early adult life. The majority of patients, however, are admitted to the hospital when they are between the ages of 40 and 60 years; the average age at onset is 45 years.

The chronicity of the disease is indicated by the period that elapses between the onset of symptoms and abdominal exploration. Gross et al discussed the subject of chronic relapsing pancreatitis occurring in infancy and childhood. Hendren et al reported that 12 of 15 children who underwent operation for chronic recurrent or chronic progressive pancreatitis were greatly improved, although 1 had minor symptoms.

Vernon et al, in discussing the incidence of chronic relapsing pancreatitis in childhood, reported four patients who were successfully treated by operation. They confirmed that this disease is rare in infancy and childhood but must be considered in young patients having recurrent attacks of abdominal pain, nausea, vomiting, weight loss, and steatorrhea. Most of these patients enjoyed long periods of complete freedom from any symptoms.

ETIOLOGY

The causes of chronic relapsing pancreatitis are unknown. Many factors have been implicated; alcohol abuse and gallstones are the most frequently cited offenders. Other factors that have been implicated: obstructing lesions of the ampulla of Vater; trauma—nonpenetrating, penetrating, and operative injuries; hyperparathyroidism; certain systemic diseases, such as mumps, scarlet fever, and viral and parasitic infections; familial hyperlipemia; protein-deficiency states; benign and malignant tumors of the pancreas; pseudocysts, duodenal and gastric ulcers, and vascular disease; such metabolic disturbances as resulting from chemotoxic agents; hyperplasia and metaplasia of the pancreatic ductal epithelium; and idiopathic factors. In 35 to 40 percent of patients, no etiologic antecedents are apparent to explain the presence of chronic relapsing pancreatitis.

In young children the most common causative factors are systemic infection, congenital anomalies, and trauma.

Biliary Tract Disease

In the author's series, cholelithiasis was an associated finding in 28 percent of patients operated on for chronic relapsing pancreatitis. In some of these patients it was impossible to ascertain whether cholelithiasis was present before or after the onset of chronic relapsing pancreatitis. In many patients with gallstones, the gallstones definitely preceded the pancreatic disease, but in another group cholelithiasis appeared after the diagnosis of chronic relapsing pancreatitis had been established.

Cholelithiasis is such a common disease that one would assume that acute and chronic relapsing pancreatitis would also be common diseases if gallstones were a prime consideration in the cause. It is a well-known fact, as shown

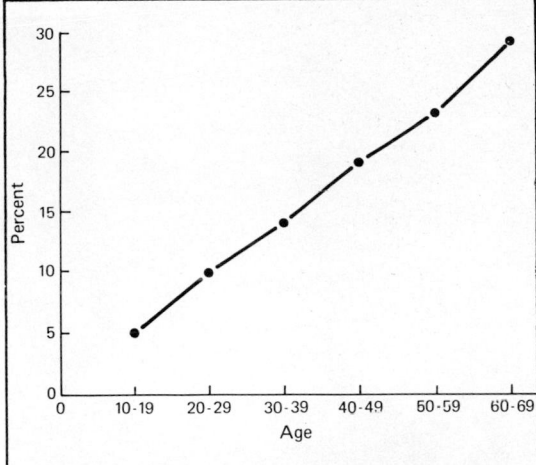

Figure 89–1. Graft depicting the increasing incidence of gallstones with advancing age. At age sixty five, approximately 30 percent of the population has gallstones. (*Source: From Warren KW: Surgical management of chronic relapsing pancreatitis. Am J Surg 117:25, 1969, with permission.*)

in Figure 89–1, that the incidence of gallstones increases with advancing age. Approximately one third of persons over 65 years of age have gallstones. Although the incidence of cholelithiasis increases with advancing age, the incidence of acute and chronic pancreatitis reaches a peak between the fourth and fifth decades and then diminishes rapidly, as shown in Figure 89–2.

Since cholelithiasis is so common, choledocholithiasis is relatively uncommon, and acute

and chronic pancreatitis are rare, it appears best to consider that cholelithiasis is an antecedent or a concomitant factor or that both cholelithiasis and pancreatitis have a common etiologic background.

Many clinicians, including Maingot, believe that biliary tract disease is a much more direct and common cause of both acute and chronic pancreatitis. Maingot stated that the important etiologic factors are cholecystitis, calculous cholecystitis, choledocholithiasis, stricture of the lower end of the choledochus, papillitis, dysfunction or fibrosis of the sphincter of Oddi, and benign and malignant growths of the ampulla of Vater or periampullary region. He believed that they were responsible for 50 percent of cases of acute and chronic relapsing pancreatitis. More impressive as a causative factor in acute pancreatitis than in the chronic forms is the presence of gallstones.

Alcohol

The relationship of alcohol to the etiology and pathology of pancreatitis is poorly understood. Considerable basic research at many centers is currently under way in an attempt to elucidate this relationship. The association of alcohol with chronic pancreatitis in the Western world is estimated to vary from 30 to 40 percent. The relationship between the consumption of alcohol and the development of pancreatitis is discussed in considerable detail by Strum and Spiro and by White. In their opinion, alcohol is associated with approximately 75 percent of all cases of chronic pancreatitis in the United States.

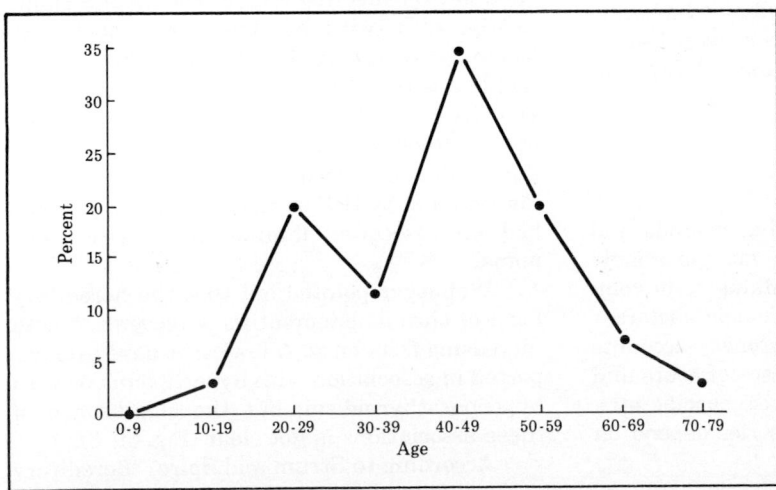

Figure 89–2. Graph indicating the incidence of pancreatitis according to age. The incidence of pancreatitis peaks between the ages of 20 and 30 years, and then reaches the highest incidence between 40 and 50 years. Thereafter it drops dramatically. Pancreatitis rarely appears in the elderly. (*Source: From Warren KW: Surgical management of chronic relapsing pancreatitis. Am J Surg 117:25, 1969, with permission.*)

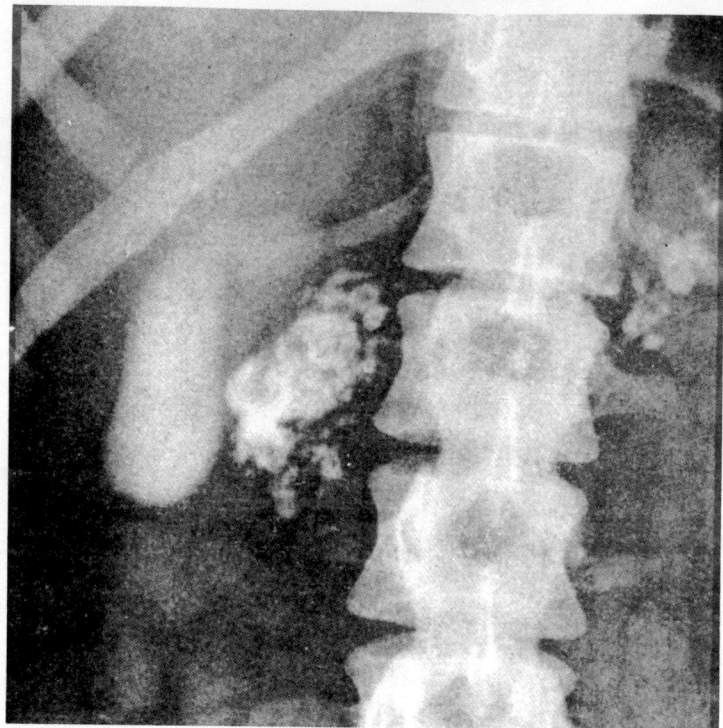

Figure 89–3. Cholecystogram showing normal gallbladder. Advanced calcification of the pancreas is present. The patient was a 14-year-old girl suffering from congenital hyperlipemia. Her main symptoms were severe epigastric pain and bouts of steatorrhea. Transabdominal coeliac and superior mesenteric ganglionectomy failed to relieve her symptoms.

Calcification of the pancreas is more common in patients with chronic pancreatitis who suffer from alcohol abuse. Although steatorrhea is observed in some 30 percent, chronic peptic ulcer is an added complication in about 20 percent of these patients.

In the author's experience, 10 percent of patients operated on for chronic pancreatitis use alcohol to excess and also have gallstones. In patients with pancreatolithiasis, 18 percent are or have been alcoholics and also have concomitant gallstones. In a large collected series from India of patients with pancreatolithiasis, only 2 percent used alcohol to excess.

Trauma

Penetrating and nonpenetrating wounds and operative injuries account for an appreciable number of cases. According to Maingot, the combination of three specific etiologic factors—trauma, alcoholism, and gallstones—accounts for more than 90 percent of cases of acute and chronic pancreatitis. The precise specific etiologic factors in any reported series depend on the patient population.

Hyperparathyroidism

On occasion, pancreatitis may be a secondary manifestation of adenoma, carcinoma, or hyperplasia of a parathyroid gland or glands.

Hereditary Pancreatitis

Hyperlipemia. Gross stated that Comfort and Steinberg reported an occurrence of relapsing pancreatitis affecting four members of a single family, with two other members probably affected. Gross reported on two well-documented families with a high incidence of pancreatitis, and Gross et al reported subsequent studies on five kindreds from the Mayo Clinic. Several similar familial occurrences have been reported by Poulsen and by Bell et al. One of these patients had an associated familial parathyroid adenoma.

Wollaeger pointed out that the hereditary form of chronic pancreatitis is recognized with increasing frequency. A few cases have been reported in association with hyperlipemia or with hyperparathyroidism, but the significance of these associations is not clear (Fig. 89–3).

According to Strum and Spiro, "hereditary

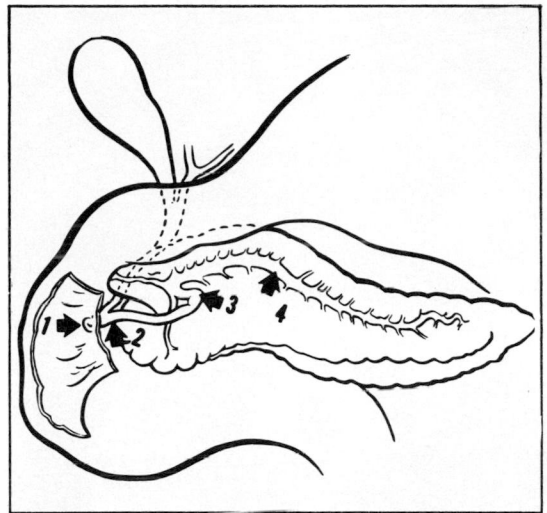

Figure 89–4. Common sites of obstruction of the main pancreatic duct.

pancreatitis appears to be inherited as non-sex-linked Mendelian dominant, but incomplete recessiveness and poor penetrance of the gene have not been excluded." The disorder is not associated with gallstones, alcohol, or any other specific cause of pancreatitis in any more than the usual frequency. The operative and necropsy findings suggest that the inherited defect might well be muscular hypertrophy of the sphincter of Oddi. Calcification of the gland was noted in most patients before operation.

The Common Channel Theory

Opie stressed the importance of the common channel, which is present in some 50 percent of patients. At autopsy on a patient with acute hemorrhagic pancreatitis, Opie found an impacted calculus at the ampulla of Vater and was able to express bile into the main pancreatic duct by applying pressure to the gallbladder. From this observation arose the concept of the common channel mechanism for the development of acute pancreatitis. Currently, much controversy exists regarding the importance of the common channel in the spectrum of chronic pancreatitis.

Obstruction to the Outflow of Pancreatic Juice

Intrapancreatic obstruction, partial or complete, involving the duct of Wirsung or the duct

of Santorini or both, is often responsible for continuing or recurrent attacks of pancreatitis. In many patients with chronic relapsing pancreatitis, multiple points of obstruction have been demonstrated at operation or at autopsy (Figs. 89–4 and 89–5). Consequently, surgeons have attempted to detect and to eliminate intrapancreatic obstruction. Partial or complete obstruction to the outflow of pancreatic juice may be caused by hyperplasia of the mucosa of the duct of Wirsung, by edema or inflammatory stricture, or by a benign polyp, annular pancreas, and fibrosis of the sphincter of Oddi.

The importance of intrapancreatic obstruction in the pathology of recurrent pancreatitis has been emphasized. Investigations of Rich and Duff, and Appleby support this view.

Peptic Ulcer and Other Factors

Peptic ulcer may be a cause of or the result of chronic pancreatitis in 10 to 20 percent of cases. Strum and Spiro found 10 patients who had chronic peptic ulceration in their series of 50 patients with chronic pancreatitis. Recurrent peptic ulcer is a relatively common complication after operative procedures on the pancreas.

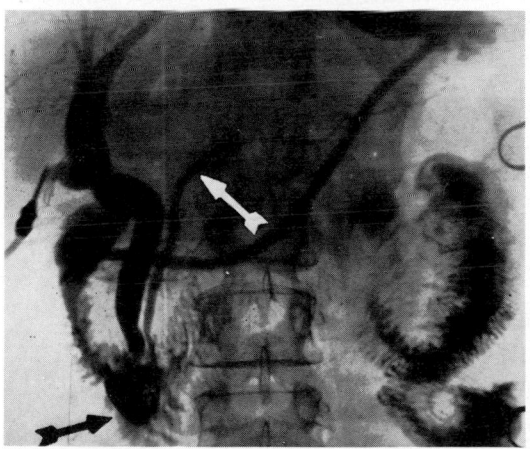

Figure 89–5. Operative cholangiogram demonstrating common passageway. While radiopaque solution was being injected, spasm of the sphincter of Oddi was produced by injection of N/10 hydrochloric acid through a Rehfuss tube with a metal tip positioned against the papilla (*black arrow*). Consequent reflux resulted in visualization of the whole duct of Wirsung (*white arrow*). (*Courtesy of Dr. H. Doubilet and the Royal Society of Medicine.*)

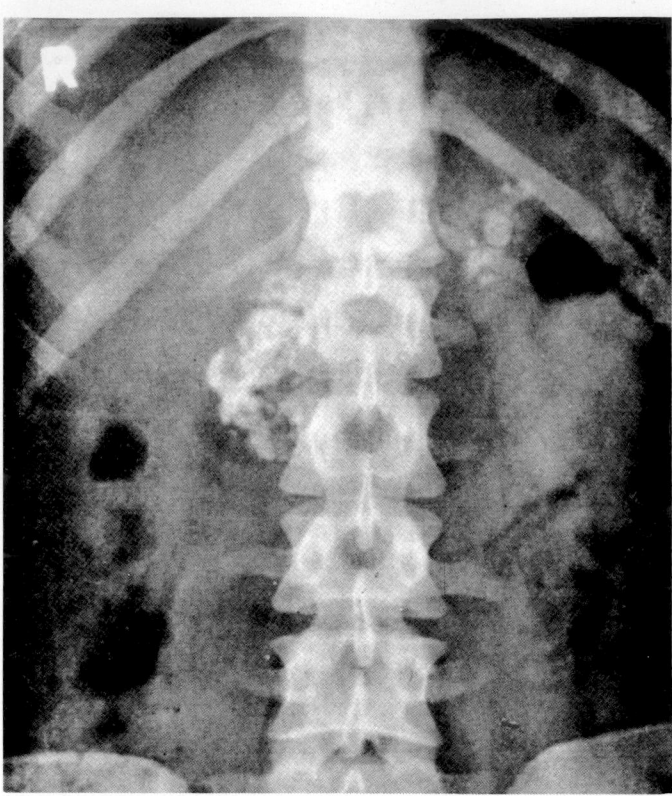

Figure 89–6. Calcification of the pancreas. The patient was a 53-year-old chronic alcoholic male. Considerable relief of his symptoms was afforded by total pancreatectomy.

Trauma to the gland and previous pancreatic surgery are etiologic antecedents in 3 and 0.4 percent, respectively.

Frey believed that in 10 to 25 percent of patients with chronic relapsing pancreatitis no clear cause could be found. Mountain and Warren found no etiologic antecedent with chronic relapsing pancreatitis in approximately 30 percent of their series.

DIAGNOSIS

Clinical Manifestations

Clinical experience has taught that the patient who has had one attack of pancreatitis will usually have other frequent and similar attacks. The clinical syndrome may be divided into two stages: an early stage characterized by repeated attacks of acute or subacute pancreatitis without obvious evidence of permanent damage to the pancreas and a late stage during which, in addition to the painful seizures, permanent functional impairment of the gland occurs. This impairment may lead to diabetes mellitus, steatorrhea, and severe malnutrition. Pancreatolithiasis or calcinosis may be evident on radiographic studies.

The painful episodes in both stages are similar to those that occur in acute pancreatitis and may last for a few days or even weeks. Between these acute attacks the patient may be free of symptoms. The attacks recur at varying intervals, with remissions that may last for some years. During the second stage of the disease, the acute exacerbations increase in frequency and severity. However, a number of patients with chronic pancreatitis suffer from the effects of pancreatic insufficiency, steatorrhea, weight loss, and diabetes mellitus in the absence of epigastric pain or discomfort. It is probable that the absence of pain is caused by destruction of the pancreatic acini. In some patients pain may be constant and unrelenting; in fact, its devastating effects frequently lead to narcotic addiction. Approximately 20 percent of patients have a history of transient obstructive jaundice.

During the early phase of the disease, the diagnosis is usually established if the patient is examined during one of the painful seizures when the serum amylase and lipase and blood sugar levels are greatly elevated. It is important to recognize that low serum amylase levels do not exclude acute pancreatitis. Scout films of the abdomen, ultrasonography, endoscopic retrograde cholangiopancreatography (ERCP), computed tomography (CT) scans, and contrast studies of the stomach and duodenum often prove helpful in diagnosis.

In the late stage of the disease the clinical features and radiographic findings permit a precise diagnosis, even in the intervals between acute attacks.

Pancreatic calculi or calcification of the parenchyma of the gland was present in 40 percent of patients in one study, which is in accord with the 48 percent reported by Comfort and Gambill in a series of 29 patients. At present, as patients with relapsing pancreatitis are diagnosed at an earlier stage in the disease, the incidence of pancreatolithiasis is rarely higher than 30 percent (Fig. 89–6). Calcification is seen less frequently in pancreatitis secondary to biliary tract disease.

The disease must be differentiated from biliary colic, calculous cholecystitis, choledocholithiasis, periampullary carcinoma, cancer of the head, body, or tail of the pancreas, malignant disease of the stomach, penetrating gastric and duodenal ulcers, aortic aneurysm, atherosclerosis of the superior mesenteric artery, retroperitoneal sarcoma, subacute attacks of high intestinal obstruction, coronary artery insufficiency, nontropical sprue, and Whipple's disease.

Diagnostic Procedures

Routine Laboratory Tests. Important aids to diagnosis include a complete blood cell count, liver function tests, serum bilirubin, amylase, and lipase, urinary amylase and lipase, blood calcium, and blood glucose. Some investigators are enthusiastic about the serum pancreatozymin-secretin test, and others depend on an estimation of the concentration of fat and proteolytic enzymes in the stool.

Radiologic Examinations. Plain films of the abdomen may display radiopaque gallstones,

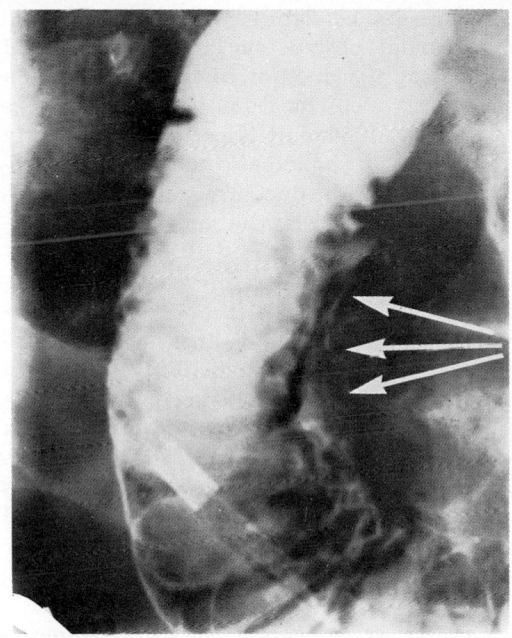

Figure 89–7. Duodenogram showing extrinsic pressure effect caused by chronic pancreatitis with a smooth inner margin (*arrows*).

pancreatic calculi, or calcinosis of the gland. Barium meal examination may show the presence or absence of concomitant peptic ulcer or demonstrate the presence of an unresolved pancreatic mass or pseudocyst. Irregularity of the duodenal curve may suggest involvement of the head of the pancreas. Hypotonic duodenography may better detail the mucosal pattern of the duodenum (Fig. 89–7).

Cholecystography and Intravenous Cholangiography. These tests formerly were of the greatest value. Today, ultrasonography, CT, and ERCP are superior.

Endoscopic and Retrograde Cholangiography. Retrograde pancreatography with the fiberoptic duodenoscope has made major contributions to the diagnosis and, to a lesser degree, to the pathologic features of chronic pancreatitis. Endoscopists who specialize in the use of this instrument are able to cannulate the main pancreatic duct in 90 to 95 percent of patients. Retrograde injection of the contrast medium into the duct of Wirsung may reveal normal ductal size and configuration, anomalous variations, partial obstruction at one or several points along the duct, or complete obstruction near the sphincter of Oddi. Complete obstruction near the duodenum is seen most frequently in patients with pancreatic calculus that completely occludes the duct. The author has previously described this as the sentinel stone.

Ultrasonography. Ultrasonography is another recent technique that is proving extremely valuable in the diagnosis of some pancreatic diseases. It is particularly helpful in distinguishing between solid and cystic enlargements of the pancreas. It is also of benefit in identifying calculi in the gallbladder and, less frequently, in the common duct. Ultrasound is a safe and simple noninvasive procedure and should be considered complementary to other diagnostic tests.

CT. The latest model of whole body scanner is proving remarkably rewarding in the study of some pancreatic pathology, including chronic relapsing pancreatitis.

PATHOLOGY

A basic consideration in the choice of a surgical procedure as a treatment for any disease should be the pathologic manifestations accompanying that disease. In addition, any and all surgical maneuvers should be designed to remove the pathologic condition or to alter those factors that will reverse the pathologic process. In many instances, it is obvious that the disease cannot be removed entirely, and in other instances no surgical maneuver will accomplish the secondary design of restoring the normal anatomic and physiologic function of a particular organ. Yet, despite these practical limitations of this approach to surgery of chronic relapsing pancreatitis, it is remarkable to what small degree fundamental considerations of the pathologic anatomy of the disease play in initial attempts to correct this condition surgically. The author and colleagues have emphasized on several occasions some aspects of the morbid pathology of chronic relapsing pancreatitis in discussing the choice of surgical procedure in the management of this disease.

Review of the operative findings and examination of excised specimens reveal the extreme variability of the pathologic changes in chronic pancreatitis. The structural alterations in the pancreas range from edema and induration of the gland to atrophy, fibrosis, necrosis, abscesses, cysts, and pancreatolithiasis. All of these changes occasionally have been observed in the same specimen. These pathologic lesions may involve the entire organ or one part only, such as the head or body of the gland. Changes in the character and severity of these lesions may continue throughout the course of the disease, especially during alterations in the severity of the inflammation.

Partial or complete intrapancreatic duct obstruction in one or many sites was observed repeatedly. Although multiple points of duct obstruction are present in most patients with advanced chronic pancreatitis, obstruction presumably is the result rather than the cause of pancreatitis. Once a stricture is formed, however, it seems to cause progression of the disease and recurrent attacks of pancreatitis.

Pancreatolithiasis, varying in severity, was present in 22 percent of the author's series. Pancreatic calculi represent a phase in the course of certain types of chronic pancreatitis, and they are almost always associated with far-advanced disease. The precise mode of formation of these calculi is not known. The author has repeatedly observed that the first calculus usually forms just distal to the most proximal intraductal stricture and that subsequent calculi, which are usually smaller, appear distal to this point. This large proximal stone is the sentinel stone because it indicates the most proximal point of intraductal obstruction. When two or more major points of obstruction are present, pancreatolithiasis is often extensive, involving the primary and secondary pancreatic ducts throughout the gland.

TREATMENT

Medical Treatment

The medical measures directed toward prevention of acute attacks and toward halting the progression of disease are indeed few and of limited value; however, a reasonable attempt with careful medical management should be pursued before surgical intervention is undertaken. Exceptions to this rule are made when cholelithiasis has been demonstrated and when a reasonable suspicion of carcinoma of the pancreas is entertained.

Medical measures include a bland, low-fat diet. Alcohol should not be used in any form. Antispasmodics and mild sedatives may be helpful. Codeine or Demerol is preferable to morphine but should be used only during severe attacks. Control of diabetes mellitus is important and usually requires the administration of insulin. Steatorrhea is treated with pancreatin (Viokase) tablets, four or five with each meal, pancrelipase (Cotazym), or enteric-coated Pancrease. Cimetidine (Tagamet), 300 mg three times a day with meals and at bedtime, is the drug of choice to reduce gastric hyperacidity.

Operative Treatment*

The selection of one or more operative procedures that will be appropriate in any given patient may prove quite difficult both before and at the time of operation. Lord Smith has emphasized that the only indications for surgery are pain, recurrent, severe exacerbations of subacute pancreatitis, such major surgical complications as pancreatic cyst, pancreatic fistula, and portal vein obstruction, and suspicions of a superimposed malignant condition.

The surgical methods applicable to the treatment of chronic relapsing pancreatitis can be classified as follows:

I. Indirect
  A. Biliary tract procedures
    1. Cholecystectomy and choledochostomy
    2. Biliary–intestinal anastomosis
    3. Transduodenal sphincteroplasty
  B. Gastrointestinal (GI) diversion
    1. Gastroenterostomy
    2. Pyloric exclusion
    3. Partial gastrectomy with or without vagotomy
  C. Nerve interruption
    1. Sympathectomy
      a. Thoracolumbar
      b. Splanchnicectomy

---

* Much of the material in this section has been taken from a previous chapter in the Sixth Edition of *Abdominal Operations* written by the editor, Rodney Maingot, who, in turn, has drawn on the valuable publications of other surgeons to whom credit was and will be given in this section.

II. Direct
  A. Drainage of cyst
  B. Anastomosis
    1. Longitudinal pancreaticojejunostomy
    2. Diversion after distal pancreatectomy
  C. Resection
    1. Radical distal pancreatectomy (95 percent)
      a. Distal pancreatectomy alone when the disease is limited to the tail of the gland
      b. Distal pancreatectomy followed by anastomosis of the pancreatic duct to the proximal jejunum, employing the Roux-Y (DuVal and Leger) or by using the simple loop method combined with enteroanastomosis
      c. Distal pancreatectomy followed by pancreaticogastrostomy
    2. Pancreatoduodenectomy
    3. Total pancreatectomy
    4. Autotransplantation of body and tail of the pancreas

Indirect Surgical Procedures

Cholecystectomy and Choledochostomy. Gallstones are associated with chronic pancreatitis in approximately one third of patients. Cholecystectomy must be performed when gallstones are present. Reports in the literature attest to the existence of a type of pancreatitis caused by gallstones and that an excellent result is obtained after removal of the gallstones. This depends primarily on the severity of the pancreatitis. If the degree of pancreatitis is moderate or advanced, results are poor. Poor results were also obtained in 10 of 70 of the author's patients with far-advanced pancreatitis, as judged by the presence of pancreatic cysts or pancreatic calculi.

In most instances, the common bile duct should be explored. Operative cholangiography should be obtained before choledochostomy. This study may reveal the presence of common duct calculi or narrowing of the intrapancreatic portion of the duct. The sphincter of Oddi is calibrated with graduated Bakes' dilators.

In some instances a 3- to 4-mm Bakes' dilator cannot be passed through the ampulla of Vater into the duodenum owing to the presence of stenosis of the sphincter of Oddi or an impacted calculus. The dilator should be held in situ, as it will act as a useful guide to the position of the papilla. Transduodenal sphinctero-

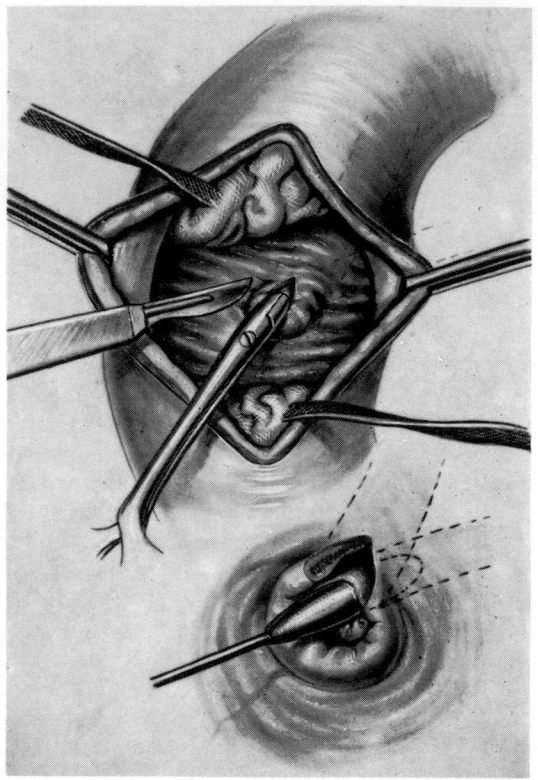

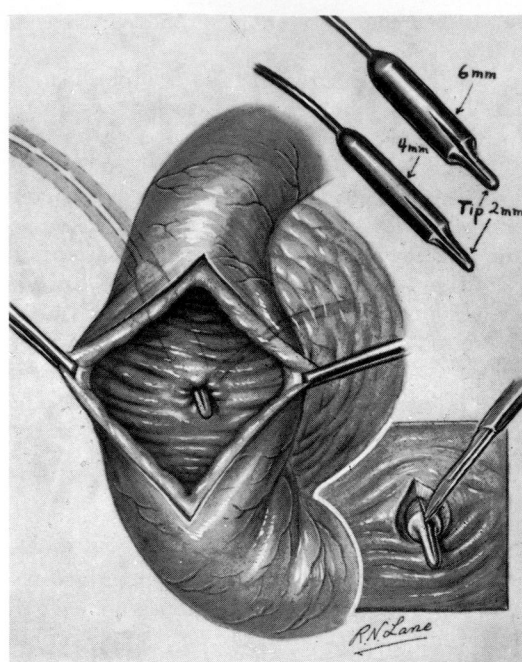

Figure 89–9. Transduodenal sphincterotomy (R. Smith's technique).

Figure 89–8. Transduodenal choledochal sphincterotomy, as practiced by many surgeons. *Inset:* The duct of Wirsung is being dilated with a Bakes' dilator. (*Source: Adapted from Cattell RB, Warren KW: Surgery of the Pancreas. Philadelphia: WB Saunders, 1954, with permission.*)

plasty should then be performed and should be of sufficient length to assure permanent patency.

Biliary–Intestinal Anastomosis. Bowers and Greenfield have advocated biliary–intestinal diversional anastomosis. The common bile duct is transected below the orifice of the cystic duct and the ascending Roux-Y limb of the jejunum is anastomosed to the cut end of the choledochus. The proximal limb of the jejunum is anastomosed to the ascending limb of the jejunum, 40 to 45 cm distal to the choledochojejunostomy. In some instances, the common bile duct has been anastomosed (side-to-side) to the first portion of the duodenum and especially in the presence of chronic pancreatitis associated with severe obstructive jaundice.

This operation has proved to be unsatisfactory, as reflected in the reports of poor results in the literature, except for the relief of jaundice.

Transduodenal Sphincteroplasty. The opening of the duct of Wirsung is identified and a lacrimal duct probe is inserted. The portion of the septum between the common bile duct and the duct of Wirsung is excised, thus enlarging the opening of the main pancreatic duct. Retrograde pancreatography is obtained to determine the size and configuration of the pancreatic duct. If no point of obstruction within the ductal system is observed, the duodenotomy is closed with a single layer of interrupted fine silk sutures. A short-limb T-tube of appropriate size is inserted into the common bile duct.

Frequently, the author performs transduodenal sphincteroplasty and excision of a portion of the septum between the common bile duct and the duct of Wirsung without a choledochostomy.*

---

* Maingot, again in the Sixth Edition, has detailed the evaluation of sphincterotomy, which has subsequently been modified to sphincteroplasty. I am including his description.

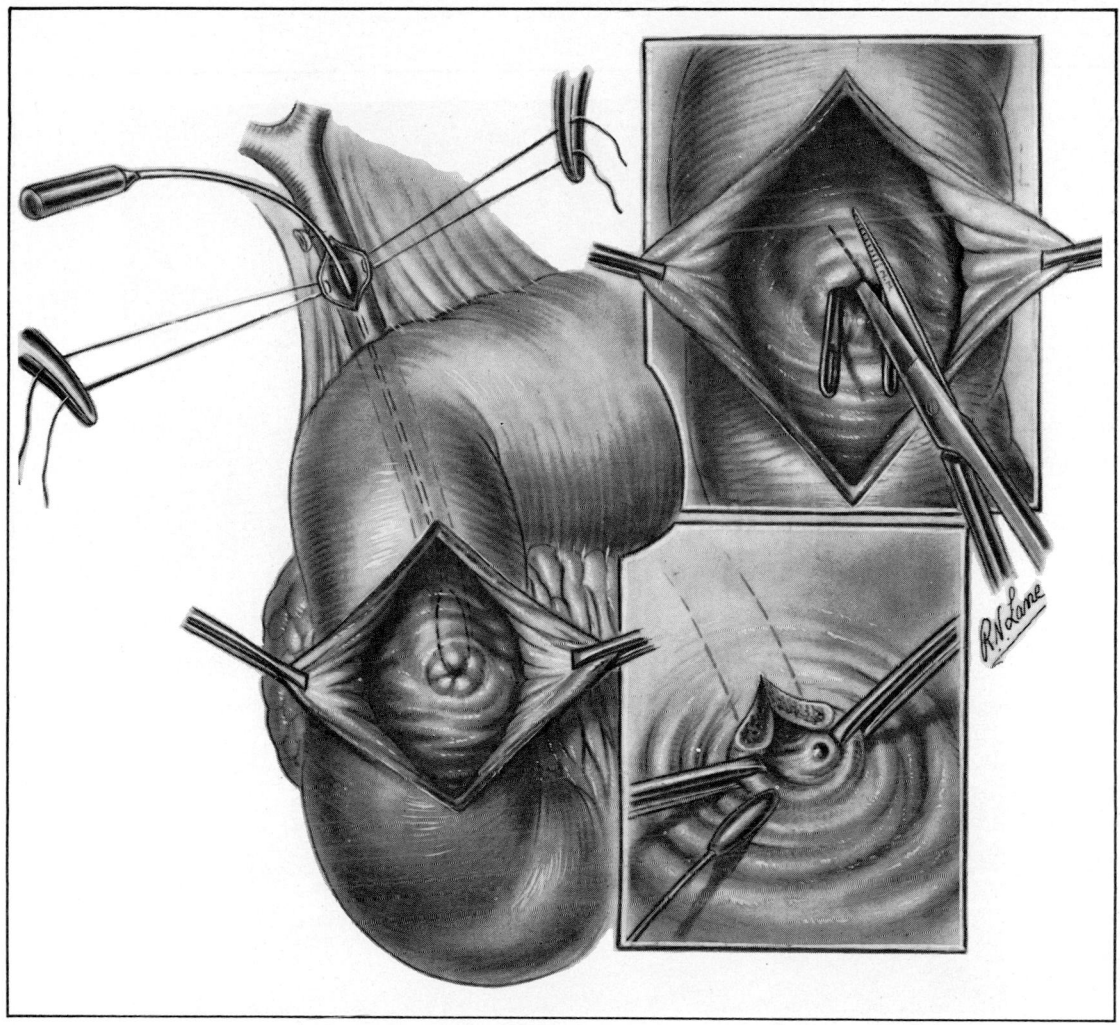

Figure 89–10. Maingot's method of performing a transduodenal sphincterotomy after exploration of the common bile duct.

This operation was originally sponsored by Archibald, but during a period of 25 years, it was cogently advocated by Doubilet and Mulholland (Figs. 89–8 through 89–12). These surgeons have recommended sphincterotomy as a definitive treatment of chronic pancreatitis and have claimed good results in 89 percent of their patients (500 patients with chronic pancreatitis were treated by sphincterotomy up to May 1957).

Doubilet stated that the concept that pancreatitis results from reflux of bile into the pancreatic duct must be based on three premises: The bile and pancreatic ducts join above the papilla of Vater, increased tonicity of the sphincter of Oddi converts these ducts into a common duct, and section of the sphincter of Oddi, by preventing further entry of bile into the pancreatic duct, will halt progress of the disease.

Jones et al reported that after sphincterotomy in 25 patients, 76 percent experienced no further attacks of pancreatitis. According to Waugh, the operations of sphincterotomy and sphincteroplasty had not appeared to be effective in more than 65 percent of patients.

The author and associates performed sphincterotomy as a definitive procedure in 39

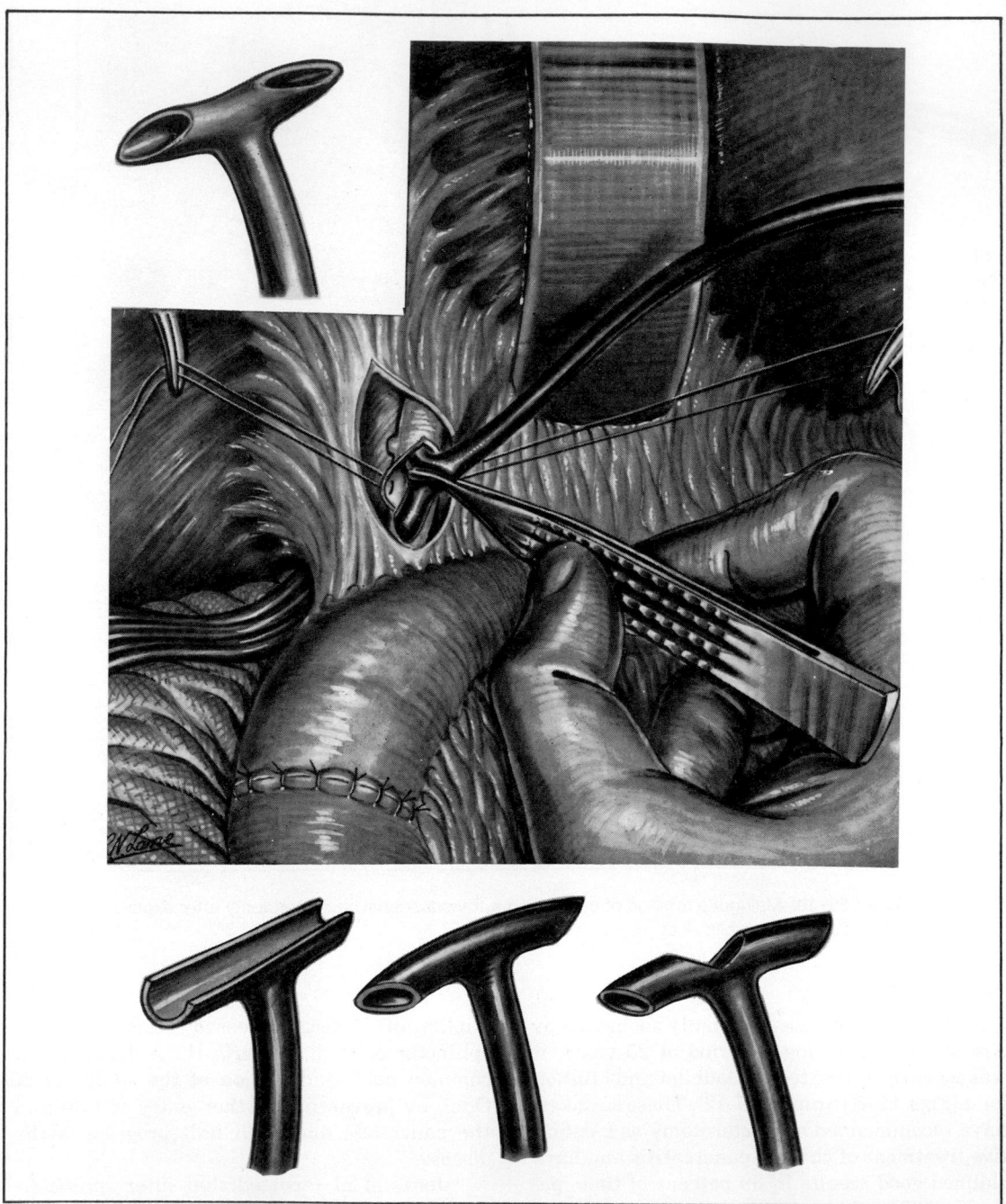

Figure 89–11. Short T-tube drainage following sphincterotomy. The operation is nearly completed. A short T-tube is being inserted into the choledochus, and the incision will be sutured around the issuing limb of the T-tube. *Inset:* Various types of T-tubes in common use. Maingot's guttered T-tube has proved invaluable.

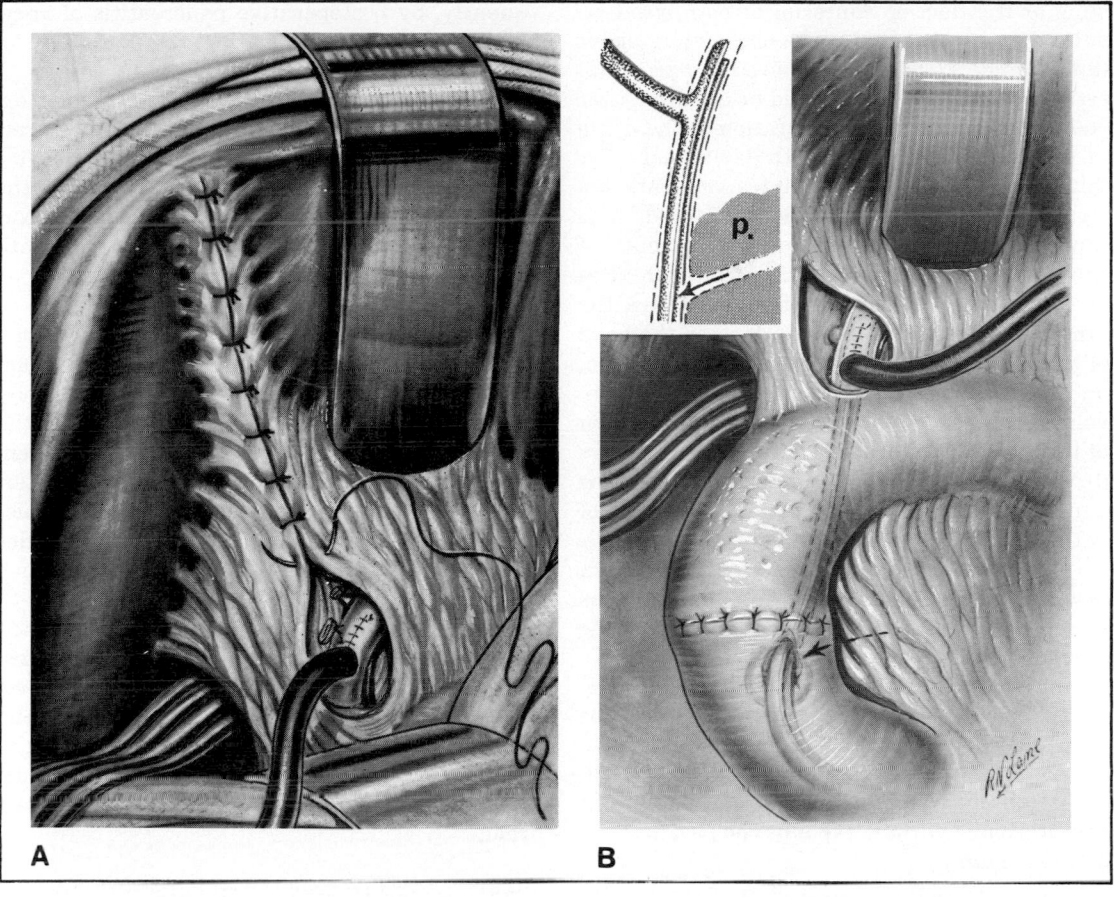

Figure 89–12. A. Cholecystectomy, exploration of the bile ducts, dilation of the ampulla of Vater with graduated Bakes' dilators, and T-tube choledochostomy. **B.** Chronic pancreatitis associated with fibrosis of the sphincter of Oddi. Transduodenal sphincterotomy combined with cholecystectomy and long T-tube choledochostomy and duodenostomy, employing Maingot's guttered T-tube.

patients. This operation was performed on patients with moderate degrees of pancreatitis, although the disease was severe in two instances. The results were good in 49 percent, although 3 of 39 patients died of pancreatitis after operation. Since the previously mentioned report, the author has performed a large number of sphincteroplasties with better results and with lower morbidity and only rare mortality. Despite this improvement, the author believes sphincteroplasty has a limited and highly selective place in the surgical management of patients with chronic pancreatitis.

Thistelthwaite and Smith collected 23 cases in which sphincterotomy was performed for chronic pancreatitis. All were caused by alcohol-

ism. More than 70 percent of patients failed to be relieved of their symptoms (Fig. 89–11).

Sphincterotomy or sphincteroplasty is also indicated for fibrosis or stenosis of the sphincter of Oddi, for calculi impacted in the ampulla of Vater or the distal portions of the common bile duct (Fig. 89–12), and for overlooked or recurrent calculi in the biliary passages.

Sphincterotomy as a definitive procedure combined with cholecystectomy—when the gallbladder is present and normal—and T-tube choledochostomy will relieve about 40 percent of patients who have the milder forms of relapsing pancreatitis. When sphincterotomy is combined with direct procedures on the pancreatic ducts, such as retrograde dilatation of the duct of Wirsung or the duct of Santorini or both, good results may be expected if the obstructing agent (for example, calculus) is removed or a proximal stricture is adequately dilated or divided. After routine transduodenal exploration of the ducts of Wirsung and Santorini with Bakes' and other dilators, varying degrees of intrapancreatic obstruction have often been demonstrated. It is unusual to find an obstruction at the mouth of the duct of Wirsung. The most common sites of obstruction, in order of frequency, are the junction of the two pancreatic ducts in the head of the gland and then the body and tail. When, on the other hand, the duct of Santorini is involved, the point of obstruction is at the ostium of the minor papilla itself or a few millimeters further on. The duct of Santorini is the major pancreatic duct in approximately 3 percent of patients.

Recently, considerable attention has been given to this anomaly in several publications under the heading of pancreas divisum. The tenor of these articles implies that pancreas divisum is a frequent cause of recurrent pancreatitis. The author thinks that this concept has been overemphasized. If structural changes characteristic of recurrent or chronic pancreatitis are absent at laparotomy, it is unlikely that this anatomic variant explains the patient's abdominal pain.

The ostium of the duct of Wirsung is situated at the summit of the papilla of Vater in about 12 percent of patients. Retrograde dilatation of the main duct should be performed in selected patients, and when combined with pancreatography this will frequently confirm that partial or complete ductal obstruction is a common event. It is exactly in patients with multiple ductal obstruction that Puestow's operation should be entertained.

The author's current opinion is that sphincteroplasty has a limited place in the treatment of chronic relapsing pancreatitis. It is most effective in treating recurrent acute pancreatitis. The ultimate result will depend on careful selection of patients and excision of a segment of the septum between the common duct and the duct of Wirsung. The author frequently intubates the main pancreatic duct with an appropriate size ureteric catheter exteriorized through the duodenum and anterior abdominal wall, and this is left in place for 3 to 4 months. This operation is frequently followed by elevation of the serum amylase level and, less fre-

quently, by postoperative pancreatitis of varying severity.

GI Diversion. Gastroenterostomy, pyloric exclusion, and partial gastrectomy have been recommended for the management of certain aspects of chronic relapsing pancreatitis. For the most part, these operations are designed to correct certain complications of chronic pancreatitis.

GASTROENTEROSTOMY. Gastroenterostomy may be indicated when a patient has partial or complete obstruction of the duodenum. This may occur during the phase of pancreatitis when the duodenum is compressed over the greatly enlarged head of the pancreas. When gastroenterostomy is performed, proper consideration must be given to the addition of vagotomy in order to minimize or to prevent marginal ulcer.

PYLORIC EXCLUSION. Pyloric exclusion, which obviously must be attended by some gastrointestinal procedure, is rarely indicated. It is advocated by some in the hope that diverting the gastric contents from the duodenum and the papilla of Vater will minimize pancreatic secretion. However, this is more theoretic than real.

PARTIAL GASTRECTOMY. Partial gastrectomy may have a definite place in the management of chronic pancreatitis. First, it may be necessary in patients who have duodenal ulcer and phlegmon of the pancreas in whom gastroenterostomy with or without vagotomy would be a less than desirable operation. Furthermore, partial gastrectomy with a Billroth II gastrojejunostomy completely diverts the gastric contents from the duodenum and, if properly performed, minimizes gastric secretion and probably reduces the Glucagon effect.

Nerve Interruption. A number of operations have been directed toward the interruption of portions of the sympathetic nervous system: unilateral or bilateral thoracolumbar sympathectomy and splanchnicectomy, transabdominal celiac and superior mesenteric ganglionectomy or transthoracic splanchnicectomy, and total neurectomy of the head of the pancreas. It is claimed that such nerve interruption procedures may not only relieve pain, which is the most prominent symptom in chronic pancreatitis, but may also have a beneficial effect on the diseased gland by markedly increasing its blood supply. These nerve interruption operations for the treatment of patients with chronic relapsing pancreatitis give poor results.

Direct Pancreatic Drainage Procedures

Drainage of Cysts. Pancreatic cysts are a common complication of chronic pancreatitis. These cysts may be pseudocysts, retention cysts, or a combination of pseudocysts and retention cysts. They may appear at any anatomic location in or around the pancreas.

Pseudocysts associated with chronic pancreatitis should be drained either internally to the stomach or the upper portion of the jejunum or externally. External drainage is indicated primarily when the patient has an infected cyst or a cyst that is not anatomically appropriate for internal drainage. Internal drainage by cystogastrostomy or cystojejunostomy is a more effective operation in the sense that it results in the lowest incidence of recurrence.

Other chronic cysts occurring in the distal portion of the pancreas are best treated by distal pancreatectomy and splenectomy. Multiple cysts in the head of the pancreas associated with diffuse derangement of the entire architecture of the ducts and parenchyma may require a Whipple procedure.

Distal Pancreatectomy with Pancreaticojejunostomy by the Methods of DuVal and Leger. Cattell was the first to suggest performance of lateral or side-to-side anastomosis of the duct of Wirsung to an antecolic loop of proximal jejunum to relieve proximal obstruction of the main pancreatic duct for irremovable carcinoma of the head of the pancreas or the periampullary zone. The additional operative procedures included cholecystojejunostomy combined with anastomosis of the afferent and efferent limbs of the jejunum to shunt the pent-up bile in the gallbladder and biliary tree into the intestine and thereby overcome (for a few months at least) jaundice and its effects.

By Cattell's method, pancreatic juice and bile were restored to the alimentary tract with the result that icterus was allayed and weight gain was assured for about 5 to 7 months. Again, if the diagnosis proves to be incorrect, the combined procedures would afford considerable mit-

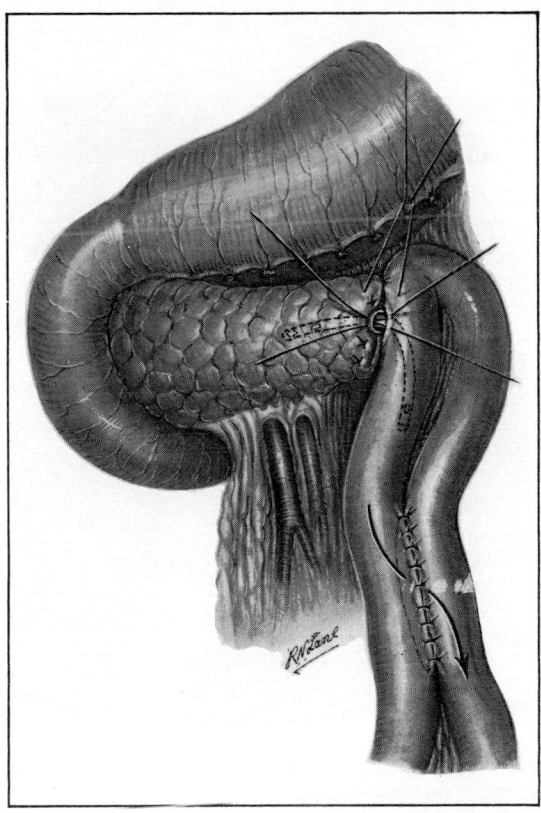

Figure 89–13. Pancreatojejunostomy and enteroanastomosis. DuVal usually performs this operation employing a Roux-Y loop of proximal jejunum.

igation of some of the manifestations of chronic pancreatitis.

Pancreaticojejunostomy may be performed by the Roux-Y plan or by uniting the duct of Wirsung to the apex of a loop of proximal jejunum. When the latter operation is selected, a supplementary enteroanastomosis should be performed to divert the irritating GI contents away from the pancreaticojejunal stoma (Fig. 89–13). In certain instances and especially when the main pancreatic duct is small, the stoma may be splinted with an inlying radiopaque latex tube.

DuVal advocated caudal pancreatectomy with end-to-side pancreaticojejunostomy, based on the Roux-Y plan, when chronic relapsing pancreatitis is associated with irremovable ductal obstruction in the head of the gland. The primary point of the stricturing almost invariably occurs at a point approximately 4 cm above the sphincter of Oddi in the pancreatic duct,

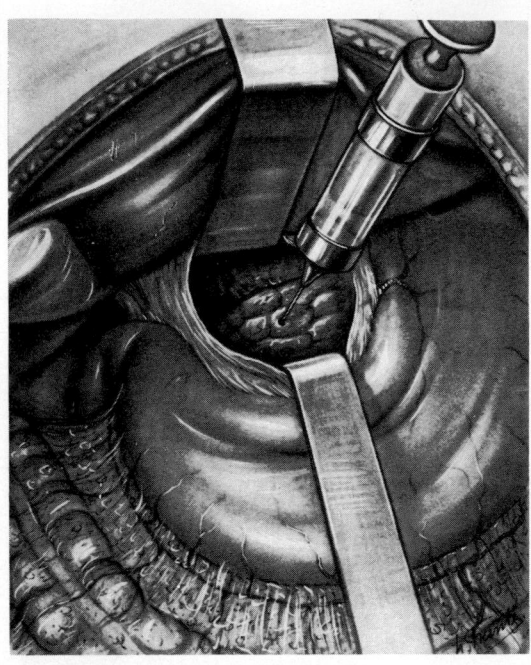

Figure 89–14. Leger's technique. (*Source: From Leger L, 1958, with permission.*)

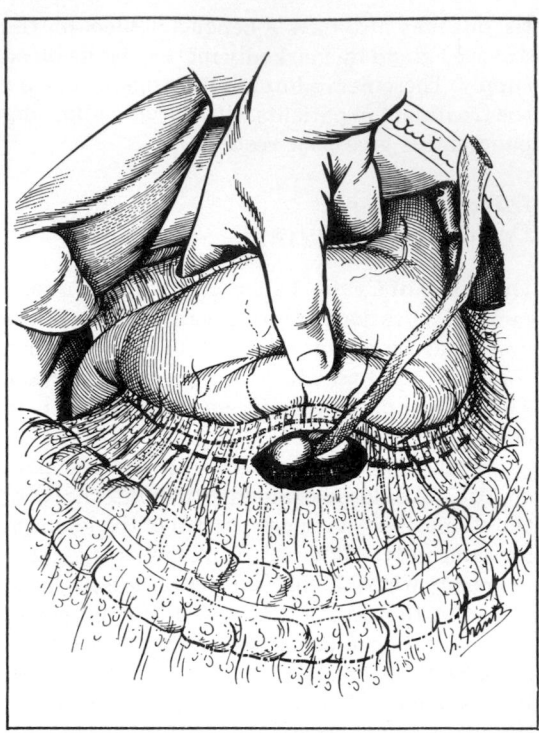

Figure 89–15. Leger's technique. (*Source: From Leger L, 1958, with permission.*)

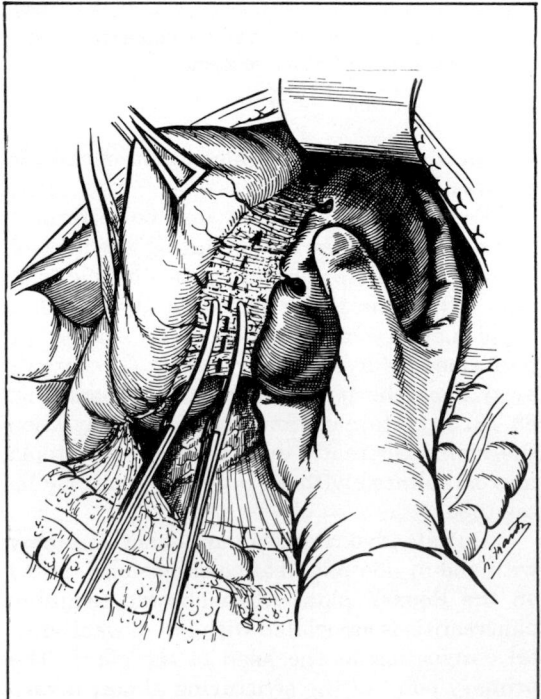

Figure 89–16. Leger's technique. (*Source: From Leger L, 1958, with permission.*)

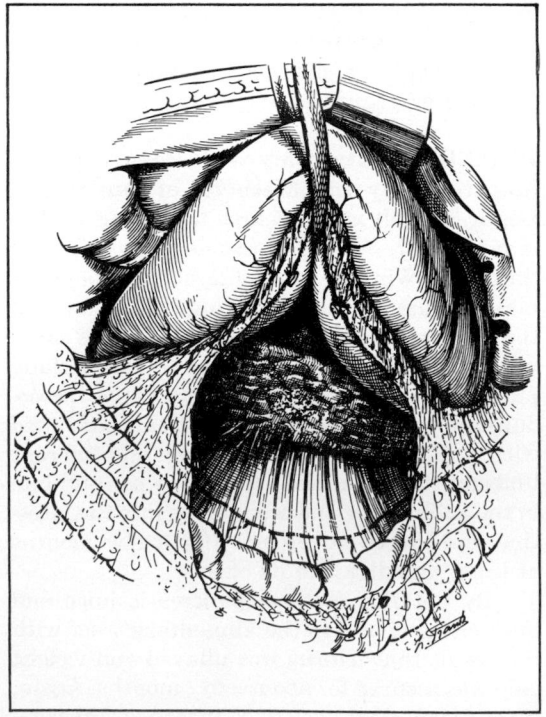

Figure 89–17. Leger's technique. (*Source: From Leger L, 1958, with permission.*)

Leger has presented a good account of this operation based on the Roux-Y principle. He submits a number of well-executed illustrations depicting the important steps in this technique (Figs. 89–14 through 89–24). The long-term results of this operation have been less rewarding than early reports indicated. Failures presumably result from stenosis of the anastomosis. The stoma is more likely to remain patent if the pancreatic duct is considerably dilated.

When obstruction in the proximal portion of the main pancreatic duct is irremovable, better results may be anticipated by anastomosing the duct in the proximal end of the tail of the divided pancreas to the posterior wall of the stomach (pancreaticogastrostomy by Smith's technique).

Pancreaticogastrostomy (The Smith Technique). The initial steps of this operation are as follows: liberation of the gastrocolic ligament from the entire length of the greater curvature of the stomach to obtain an excellent view of the anterior surface of the pancreas; ligation and division of the vasa brevia; mobilization of the tail of the pancreas together with the spleen; isolation, ligation, and division of the splenic blood vessels in the hilus of the spleen; transection of the neck of the pancreas; and removal of the spleen together with the body and tail of the pancreas. Two transfixion sutures are inserted and tied in the substance of the superior and inferior surfaces of the pancreas to control bleeding and to act as tractors during the early stages of pancreaticogastrostomy. After transection of the gland, the proximal end of the duct is gently dilated, irrigated with warm saline solution, and any debris or calculi are removed. A French No. 3 or 4 catheter is passed down the duct toward the duodenum, and a pancreatogram is taken to illuminate the ductal system. If any obstruction is detected in the head of the gland, the surgeon should proceed with performance of intraluminal pancreaticogastrostomy.

The technical steps of this procedure are illustrated in Figures 89–25 through 89–29. The mucosa of the pancreatic duct is sutured to the mucosa of the stomach with a few interrupted sutures of 4-0 silk or Merselene. This ensures a mucosa-to-mucosa approximation that mitigates the tendency to formation of stricture at the small stoma.

The polyethylene tube is brought through the abdominal wall to the exterior, and the gap

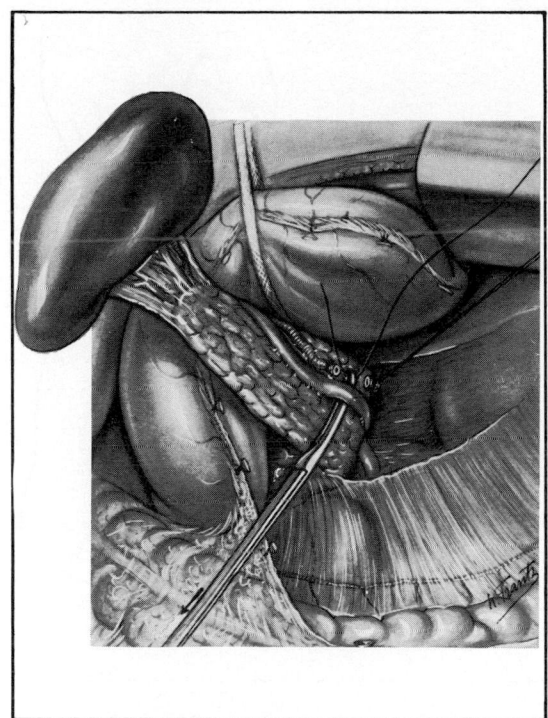

Figure 89–18. Leger's technique. (*Source: From Leger L, 1958, with permission.*)

that is, in the neck of the gland, where it crosses the vertebral bodies.

The object of this operation is to produce relief of this blockage by permitting retrograde flow of pancreatic secretion into a loop of proximal jejunum. The technical steps include splenectomy with resection of the tail (and, on occasion, a portion of the body) of the pancreas, end-to-side anastomosis of the duct of Wirsung to a loop of proximal jejunum, and an adequate side-to-side anastomosis between the afferent and efferent limbs of the jejunum.

Pancreaticojejunal anastomosis is accomplished with a series of interrupted sutures of fine silk through all coats, the mucosa of the duct is approximated to the mucosa of the jejunum, and the stoma is splinted with a polyethylene or latex tube, which subsequently is passed into the small intestine by means of jejunal peristalsis. The author frequently splints the stoma with a ureteral catheter. These splints should be brought through the opposite side of the jejunum and the abdominal wall. This maneuver permits measurement of the volume of pancreatic secretion, allows pancreatography, and enables the surgeon to determine timing of removal of the splint.

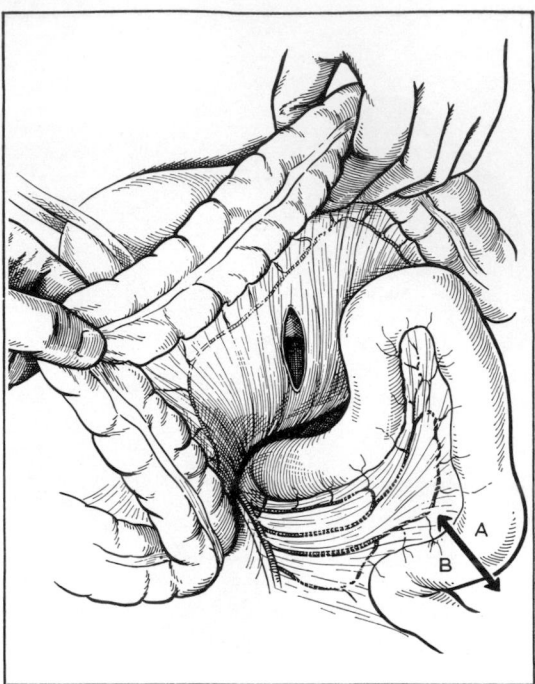

Figure 89–20. Leger's technique. (*Source: From Leger L, 1958, with permission.*)

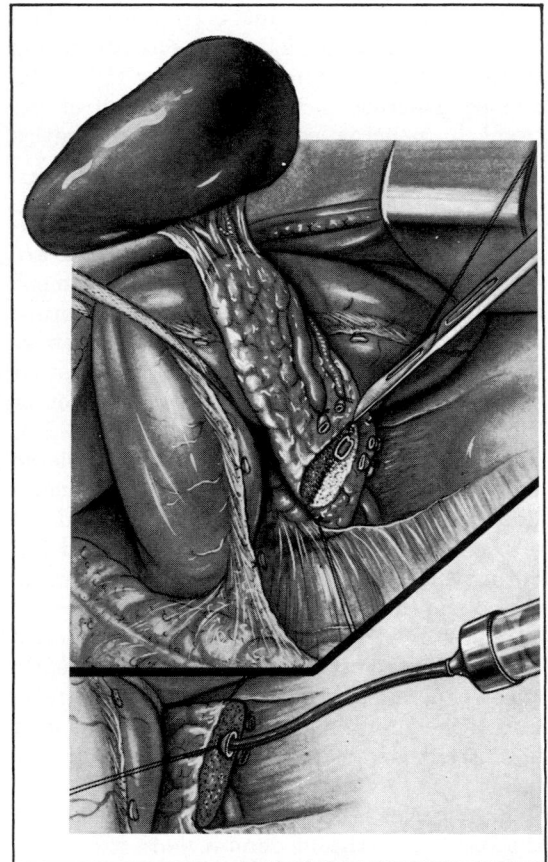

Figure 89–19. Leger's technique. (*Source: From Leger L, 1958, with permission.*)

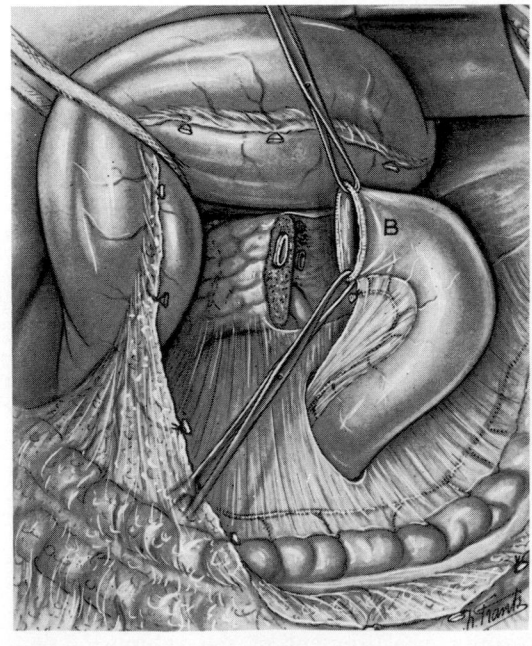

Figure 89–21. Leger's technique. (*Source: From Leger L, 1958, with permission.*)

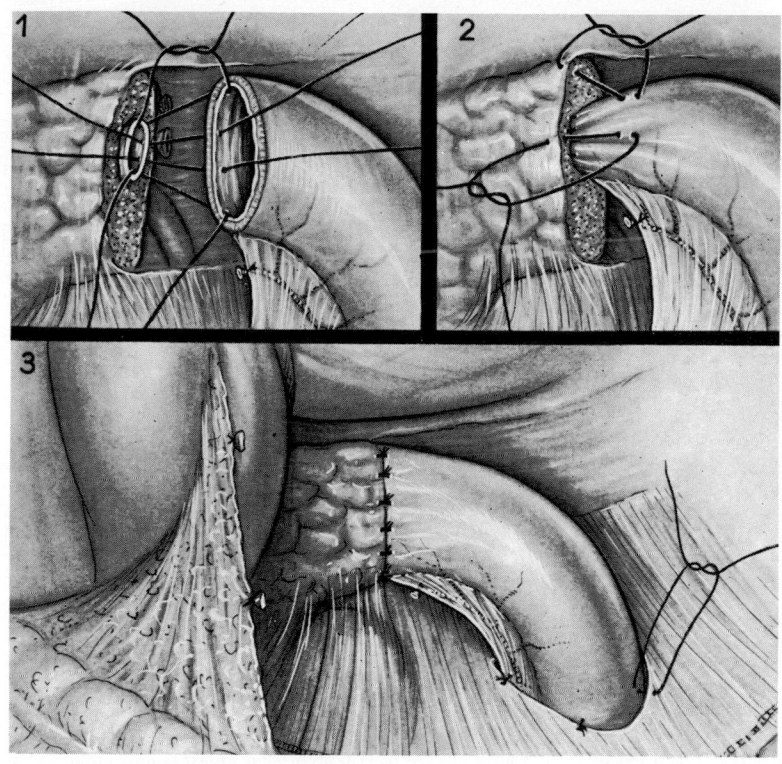

Figure 89–22. Leger's technique. (*Source: From Leger L, 1958, with permission.*)

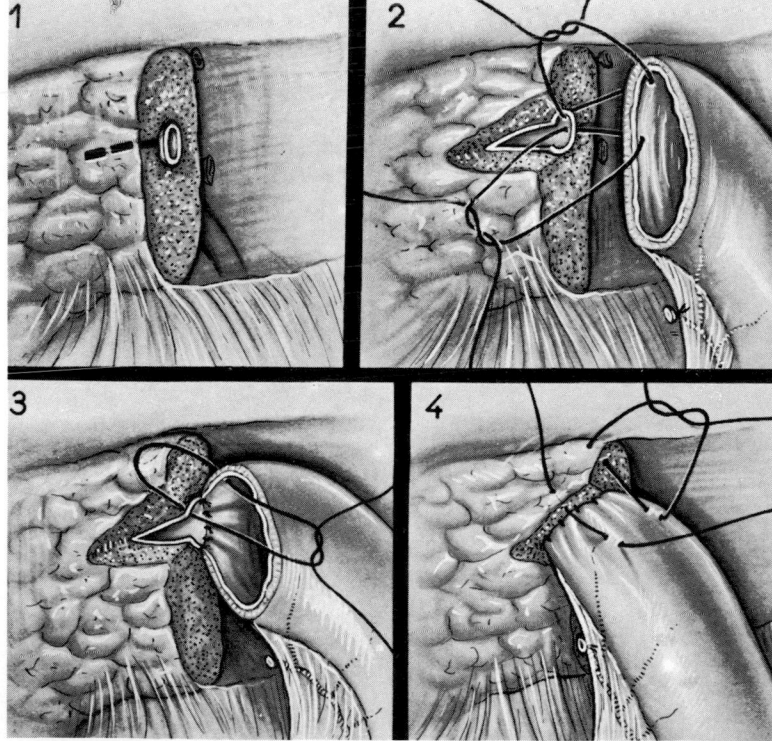

Figure 89–23. Leger's technique. (*Source: From Leger L, 1958, with permission.*)

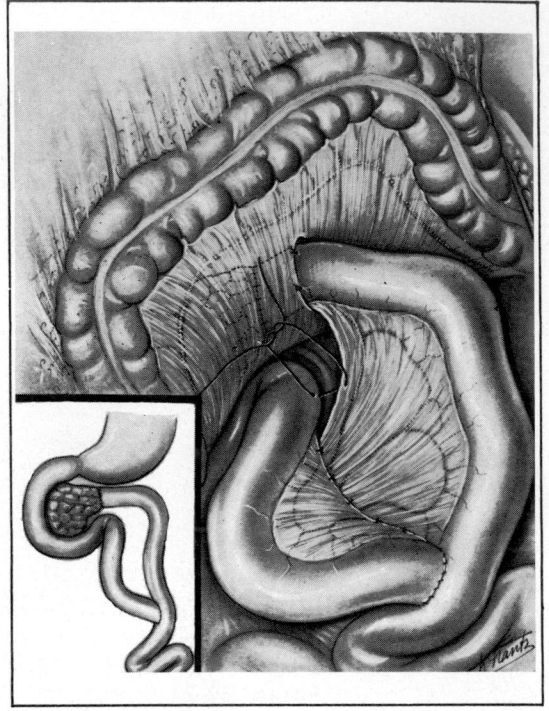

Figure 89–24. Leger's technique. (*Source: From Leger L, 1958, with permission.*)

between the anterior wall of the stomach and the parietes is closed with two interrupted sutures of catgut. The end of the tube is fastened to the abdominal wall with strips of Micropore, and the excess of the tubing is cut away. The tube drains pancreatic juice into a Uri-bag or bottle for 7 to 10 days; after a final pancreatogram, it is removed. The author has performed this operation many times and currently uses a ureteral catheter instead of polyethylene.

Pancreaticogastrostomy is, unquestionably, one of the most efficient retrograde duct drainage procedures practiced at the present time. It yields approximately 75 percent good results.

Longitudinal Pancreaticojejunostomy.* According to Puestow, adequate drainage can be established by incising the anterior wall of the pancreas and the duct of Wirsung from the tail through the body and head until the final, and generally largest, pocket is opened close to the

---

* The material in this section was written by the late Charles B. Puestow, for the Sixth Edition of *Abdominal Operations.* I have altered it with additional information from my own experience.

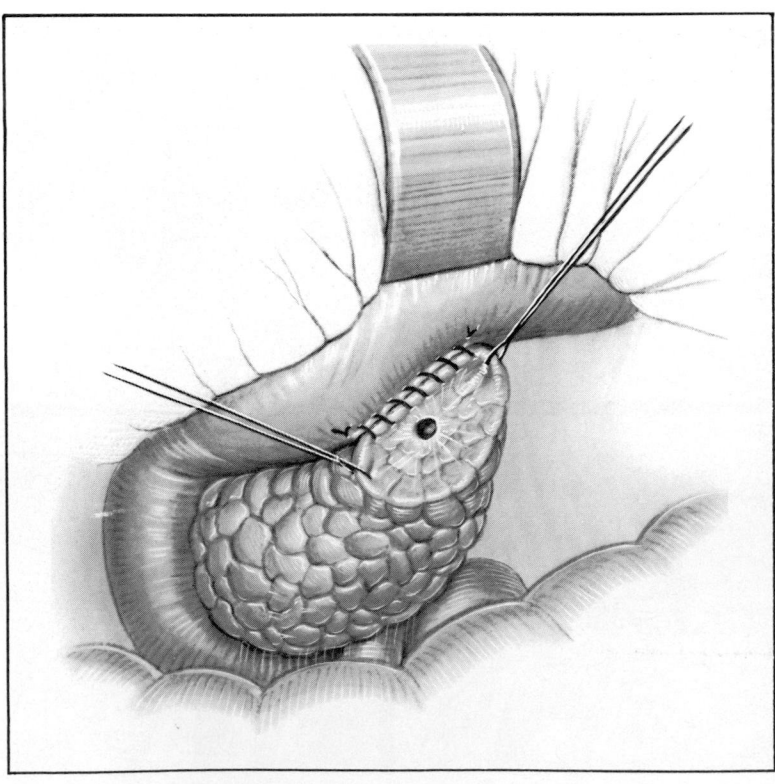

Figure 89–25. Pancreatogastrostomy. An anastomosis of the main duct in the transected pancreas to the posterior aspect of the stomach is begun using silk sutures. (*Source: From Maingot R: Stenosis of the sphincter of Oddi, in Smith R, Sherlock S (eds): Surgery of the Gallbladder and Bile Ducts. London: Butterworths, 1964, p 184, with permission.*)

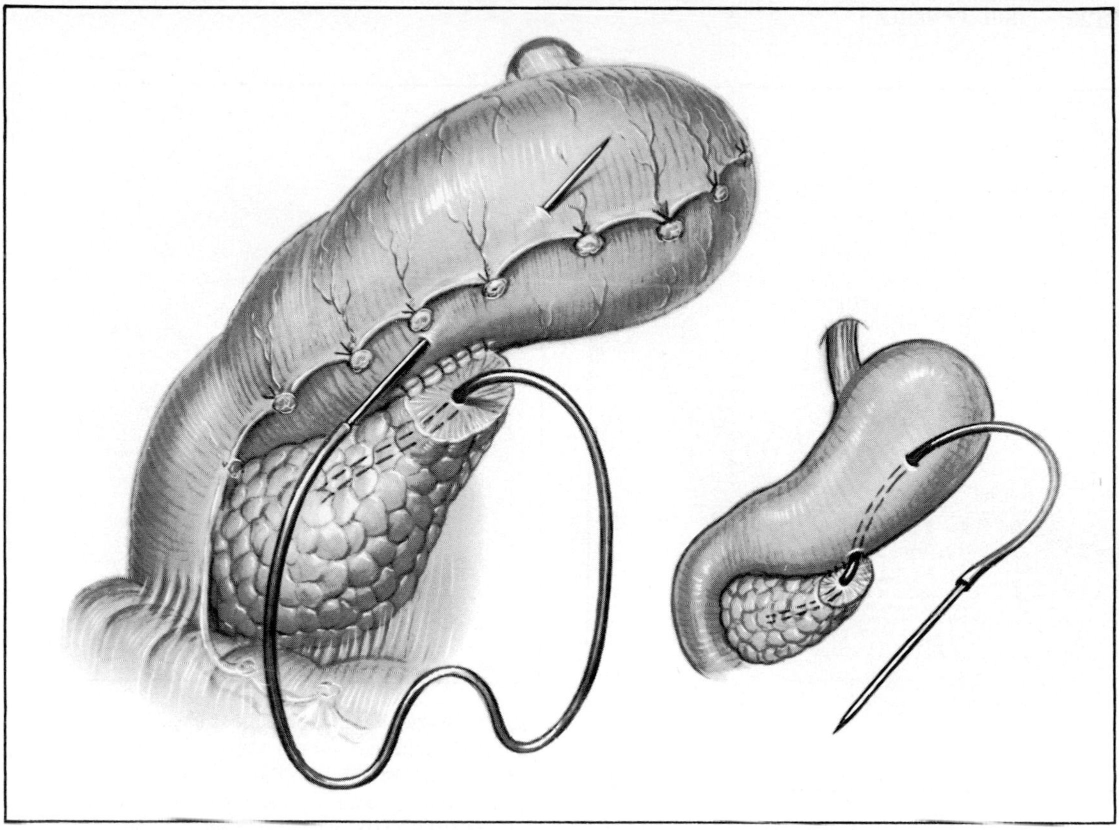

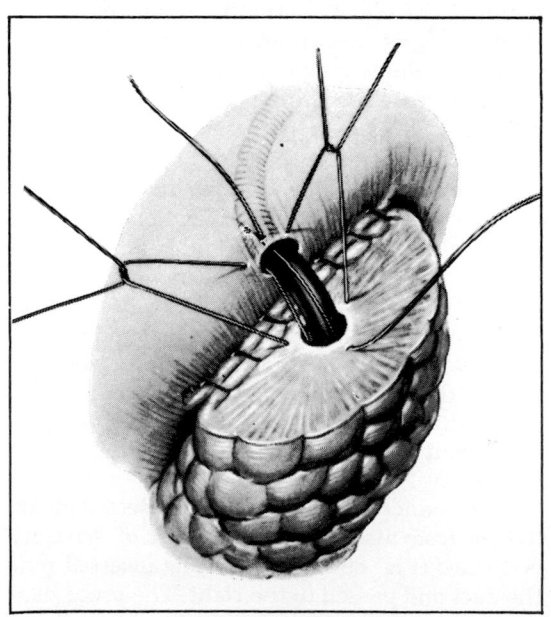

Figure 89–26. Pancreatogastrostomy—Smith's technique. With half the anastomosis completed, a long polyethylene tube is inserted into the pancreatic duct and the other end brought out through the stomach as illustrated. (*Source: From Maingot R: Stenosis of the sphincter of Oddi, in Smith R, Sherlock S (eds): Surgery of the Gallbladder and Bile Ducts. London: Butterworths, 1964, p 184, with permission.*)

Figure 89–27. Distal pancreatectomy. The posterior half of the anastomosis between the pancreas and the back of the stomach has been completed. Note the insertion of fine silk sutures to obtain an approximation of the mucosa of the stomach to the mucosa of the pancreatic duct. (*Source: From Smith R: Operations on the pancreas, in Rob C, Smith R: Operative Surgery, 2 edt, vol 4. London: Butterworths, 1964, p 308, with permission.*)

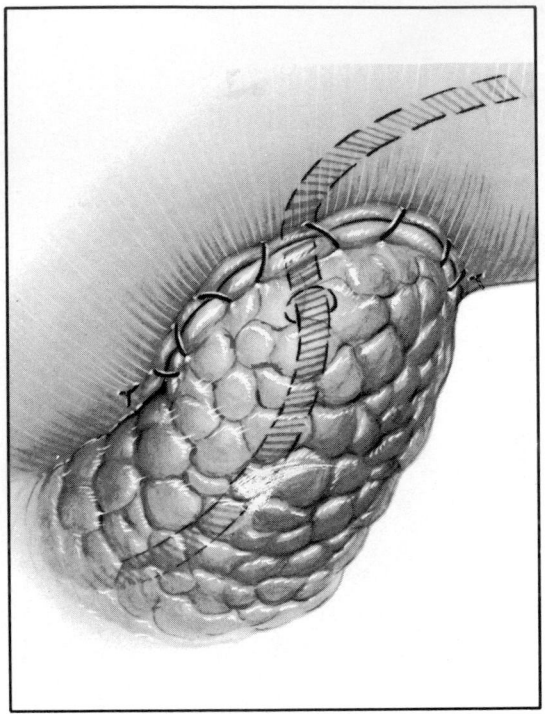

Figure 89–28. Pancreatogastrostomy. An indwelling tube anastomosis of the pancreas to the stomach is completed. (*Source: From Maingot R: Stenosis of the sphincter of Oddi, in Smith R, Sherlock S (eds): Surgery of the Gallbladder and Bile Ducts. London: Butterworths, 1964, p 185, with permission.*)

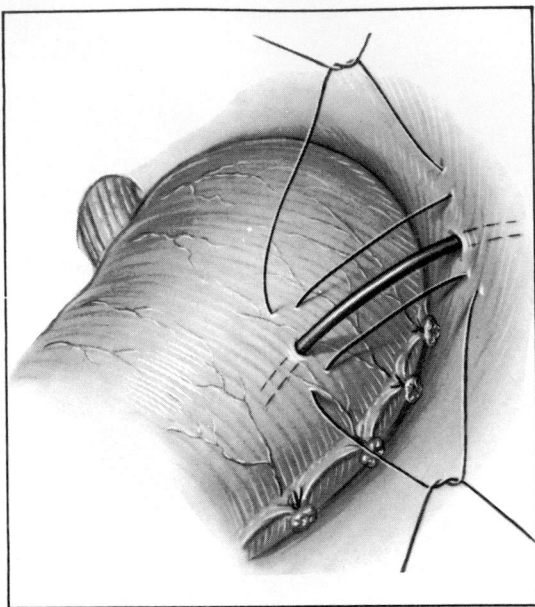

Figure 89–29. Pancreatogastrostomy. A polyethylene tube is brought through the abdominal wall to the exterior, and the gap between the anterior wall of the stomach and the parietes is closed with two interrupted sutures of catgut. The tube will drain into the bottle for 7 to 10 days; after the final pancreatogram it will be removed. (*Source: From Maingot R: Stenosis of the sphincter of Oddi, in Smith R, Sherlock S (eds): Surgery of the Gallbladder and Bile Ducts. London: Butterworths, 1964, p 185, with permission.*)

duodenal wall. It is not necessary to incise the long proximal strictures if no pockets are overlooked. A defunctionalized limb of jejunum is anastomosed to the pancreas, and intestinal continuity is reestablished by a Roux-Y jejunojejunostomy. Puestow used two techniques: in one, the pancreas is inserted into the divided end of the jejunum; in the other, a side-to-side longitudinal pancreaticojejunostomy is performed.

PANCREATICOJEJUNOSTOMY WITH SPLENECTOMY. The abdomen is opened through a long, high, left paramedian incision. If the surgeon desires, a long transverse incision may be approximately 5 cm above the umbilicus. The anterior surface of the pancreas is exposed by division of the gastrocolic omentum (Fig. 89–30). The pancreas may be aspirated with a syringe and needle in an effort to locate the pockets. The pancreas is then mobilized from its bed, beginning at its inferior margin. Because of

minimal vascularity in this anatomic region, little bleeding is encountered. In chronic pancreatitis the splenic vessels are densely adherent to or incorporated within the pancreas. For this reason, it is usually necessary to remove the spleen. The spleen is mobilized by dividing the splenorenal and splenophrenic ligaments and dividing the gastrosplenic ligament with its vasa brevia and the splenocolic ligament. This permits the spleen and left portion of the pancreas to be elevated from the abdominal cavity. The splenic vessels are then divided and ligated (Fig. 89–31). Mobilization of the posterior surface of the pancreas is continued to the right until the superior mesenteric vessels are reached. It is well to religate the splenic vessels at this level.

The pancreas is vertically transected about 0.5 cm from its tip until the duct of Wirsung is divided (Fig. 89–32). A probe is inserted into the duct and passed to the right. The probe usually encounters a stricture in from 2 to 3 cm

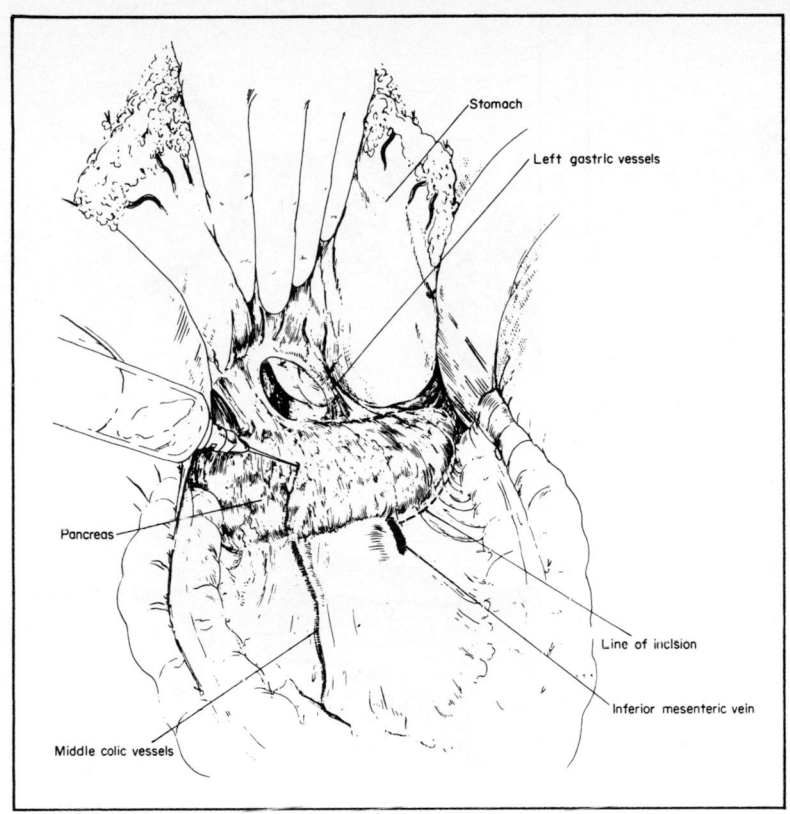

Stomach

Left gastric vessels

Pancreas

Line of inclsion

Inferior mesenteric vein

Middle colic vessels

Figure 89–30. Exposure of the anterior surface of the pancreas by division of the gasrtrocolic omentum. Aspiration of the pancreas to locate a pocket.

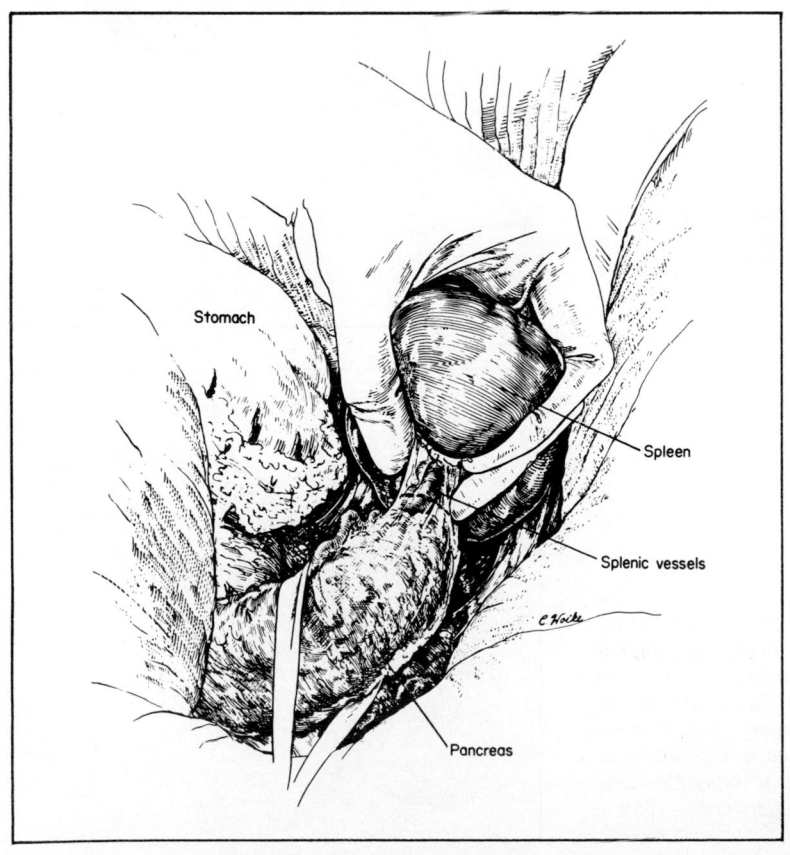

Stomach

Spleen

Splenic vessels

Pancreas

Figure 89–31. Mobilization of the distal pancreas and spleen, and subsequent splenectomy.

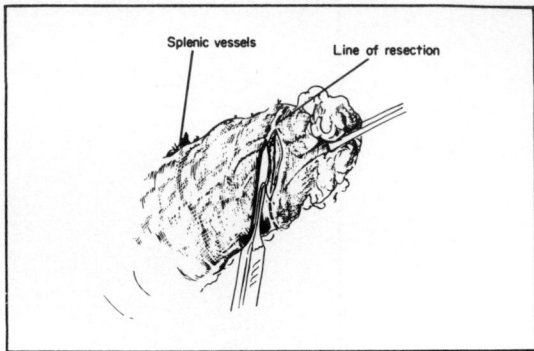

Figure 89–32. Transection of the tip of the pancreatic tail to locate the duct of Wirsung.

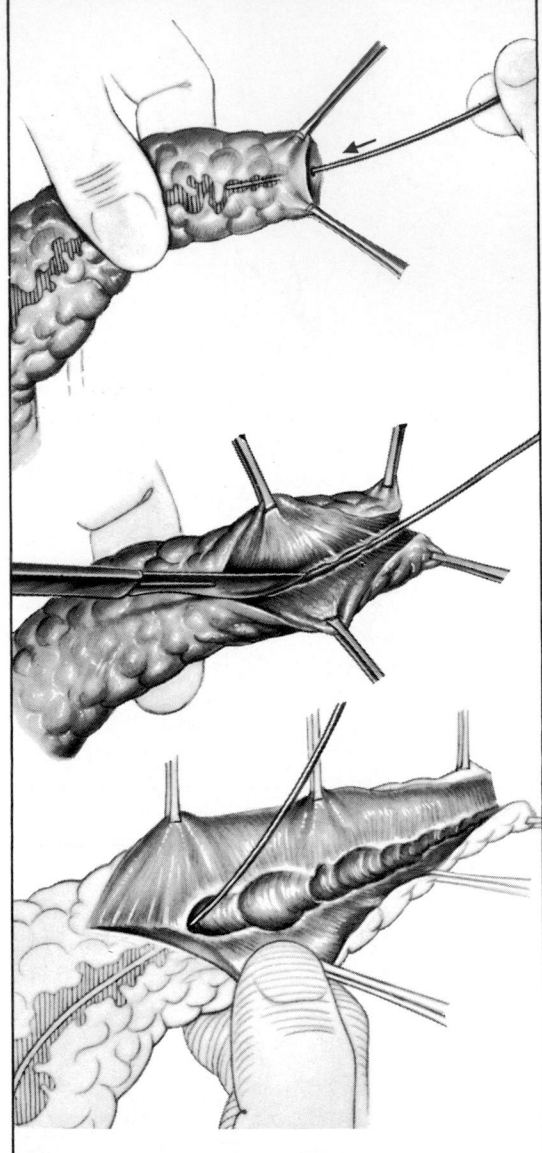

Figure 89–33. Probing of the pancreatic duct to locate the most distal stricture. (*Source: From Smith R: Operations on the pancreas, in Rob C, Smith R, et al (eds): Operative Surgery, 2 edt, vol 4. London: Butterworths, 1969, p 315, with permission.*)

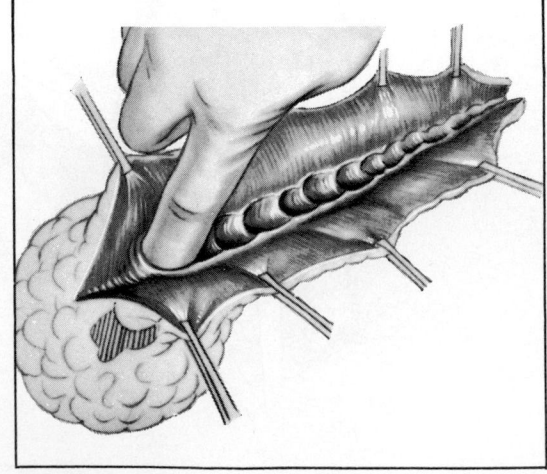

Figure 89–34. Using the probe as an indication of the site of the anterior surface of the duct, the pancreas is split in order to open up the pancreatic duct. This proceeds from the tail end of the gland right up into the neck and head, every pocket being opened, in the manner shown. (*Source: From Smith R: Operations on the pancreas, in Rob C, Smith R, et al (eds): Operative Surgery, 2 edt, vol 4. London: Butterworths, 1969, p 315, with permission.*)

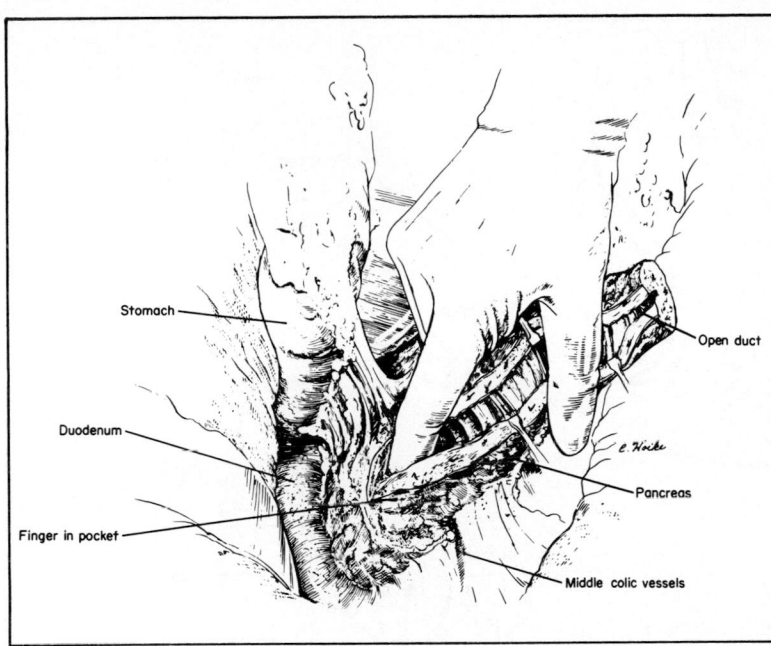

Stomach

Duodenum

Finger in pocket

Open duct

Pancreas

Middle colic vessels

Figure 89–35. Completion of dissection of the pancreas to open all pockets including the final one in the head of the gland.

from its introduction (Fig. 89–33). By sharp dissection, the anterior portion of the pancreas and the anterior wall of the duct of Wirsung are divided, the dissection continuing to and through the first stricture. Beyond this stricture, the duct is usually considerably dilated, permitting further section of the pancreas and anterior duct wall to be performed with scissors, one blade being within the duct and the other outside the pancreas (Fig. 89–34). The dissection is carried toward the duodenal wall into the head of the pancreas. A large pocket is usually encountered in the head of the gland and is of sufficient size to admit the surgeon's finger (Fig. 89–35). This pocket must not be overlooked. It is usually necessary to carry the incision to within 0.5 to 1 cm of the duodenum.

The jejunum is then divided about 25 cm below the ligament of Treitz, the site being selected by the vascular arcades to permit free mobility of the distal limb. The distal limb of the jejunum is brought through a rent in the transverse mesocolon. The jejunum is placed beside the pancreas in order to measure the site at which the transfixion sutures will be brought through the bowel wall (Fig. 89–36). One or two traction sutures are placed through the tail of the pancreas and tied (Fig. 89–37). With the needle reversed in the needle holder, it is passed into the lumen of the bowel for the desired distance and then brought through the bowel wall

(Fig. 89–38). These sutures aid in pulling the pancreas into the bowel. When the pancreas is properly positioned, the traction sutures are tied. They hold the pancreas in position and take tension off the suture line between the end of the bowel and the outer surface of the pancreas. Anteriorly, the anastomosis must go to the right of the incision in the pancreas; posteriorly, the suture line cannot go beyond the superior mesenteric vessels (Fig. 89–39).

The opening in the transverse mesocolon is closed snugly around the jejunal limb. The proximal limb of the divided jejunum is anastomosed to the distal limb by a Roux-Y anastomosis approximately 25 cm below the pancreaticojejunostomy (Fig. 89–40).

PANCREATICOJEJUNOSTOMY WITHOUT SPLENECTOMY. This technique exposes the anterior surface of the pancreas in a manner similar to the preceding operation. The pancreas, however, is not mobilized from its bed. After its anterior wall is completely exposed, the pancreas is aspirated to identify a pocket (Fig. 89–41). When a pocket is encountered, the needle is left in place as a guide, and an incision is made into the pocket by sharp dissection (Fig. 89–42). The duct is then incised to the right and to the left until all pockets have been opened. Any calculi within the ducts are removed (Fig. 89–43).

The jejunum is divided about 25 cm below

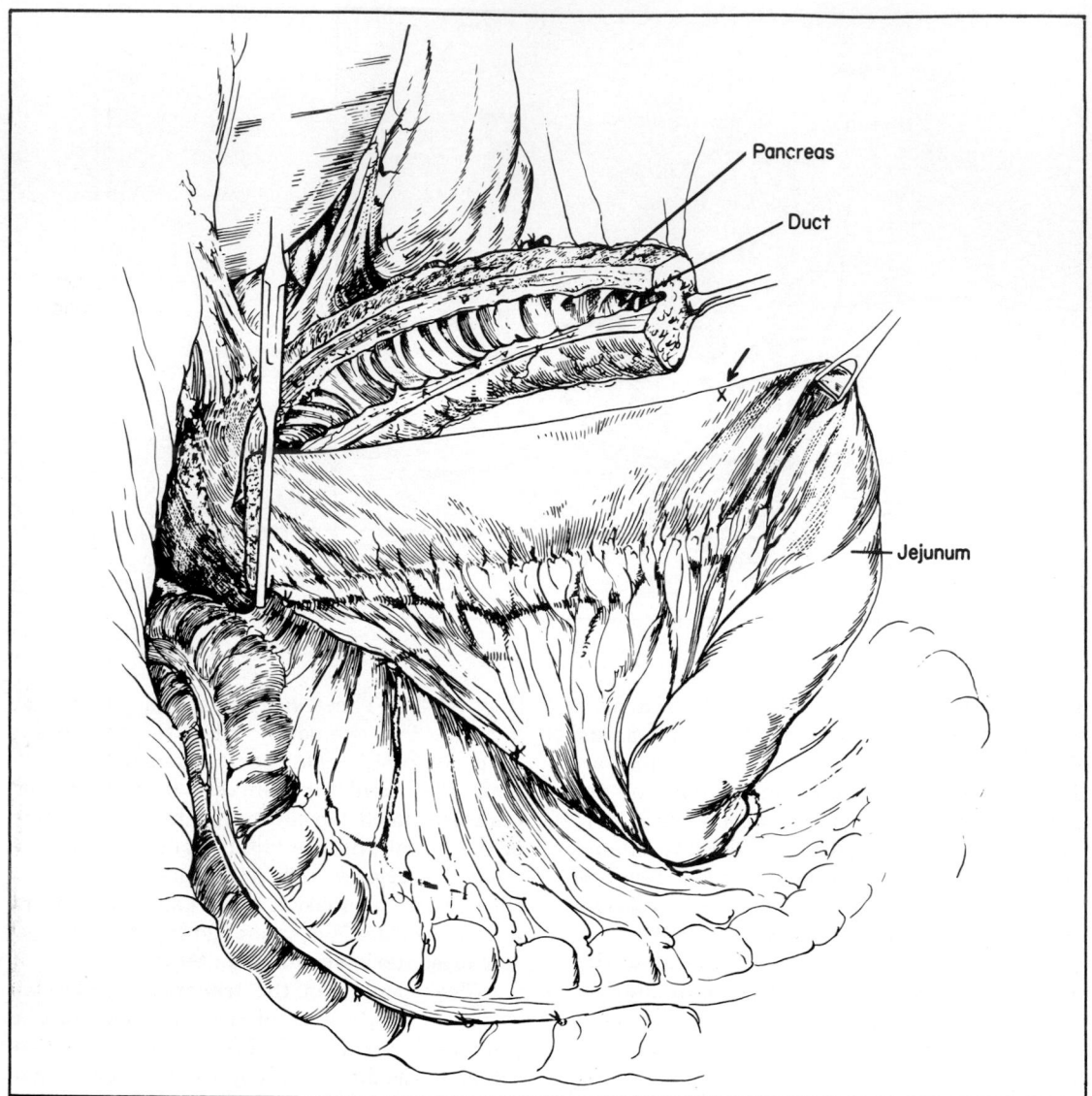

Figure 89–36. Measurement of the distal limb of the jejunum to determine the length necessary to cover the incised portion of the pancreas completely.

the ligament of Treitz and the distal end brought through an opening in the transverse mesocolon. The antimesenteric border is crushed and incised for a sufficient distance to give a lumen somewhat larger than the opening in the pancreas. The serosa of the bowel is sutured to the anterior surface of the pancreas around the opening (Figs. 89–44 through 89–46). The sutures should be placed at least 5 mm beyond the cut edges of the pancreas. One should not attempt a mucosa-to-ductal anastomosis nor should sutures be placed in the cut surface of the gland. By placing the sutures well beyond

the margin, all divided ducts will drain freely into the bowel. Intestinal continuity is then reestablished by performing a Roux-Y jejunojejunostomy about 25 cm below the pancreaticojejunostomy.

This technique is of value when the size of the pancreas prevents it from being introduced into the lumen of the bowel. It also obviates the need for splenectomy. Both techniques are equally effective, and the selection depends on the desires of the surgeon.

A few cardinal principles in the performance of longitudinal pancreaticojejunostomy

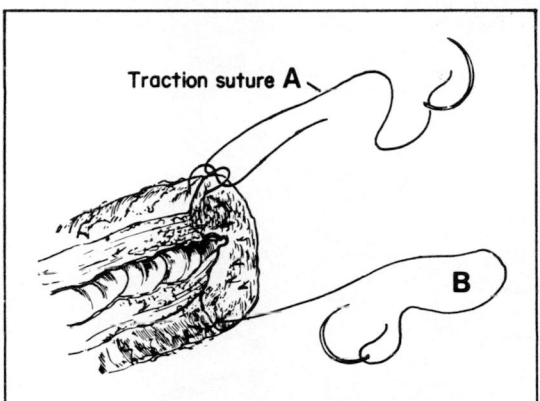

Figure 89–37. Traction sutures placed in the tail of the pancreas.

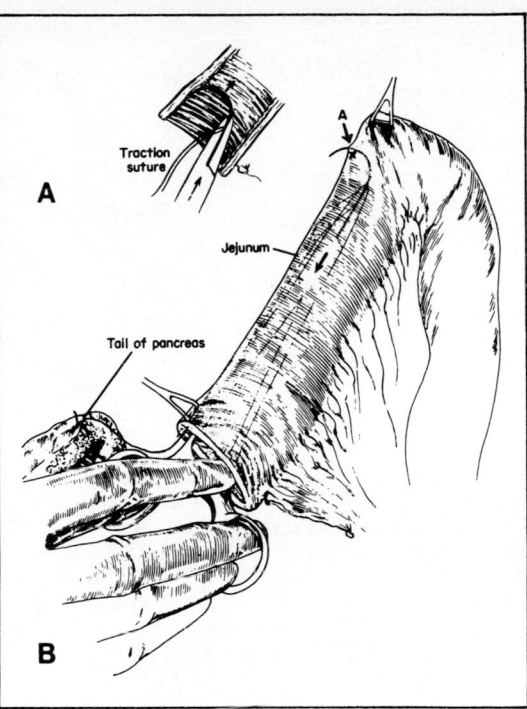

Figure 89–38. Traction sutures inserted in the lumen distal of the jejunum and brought out through the serosa surface.

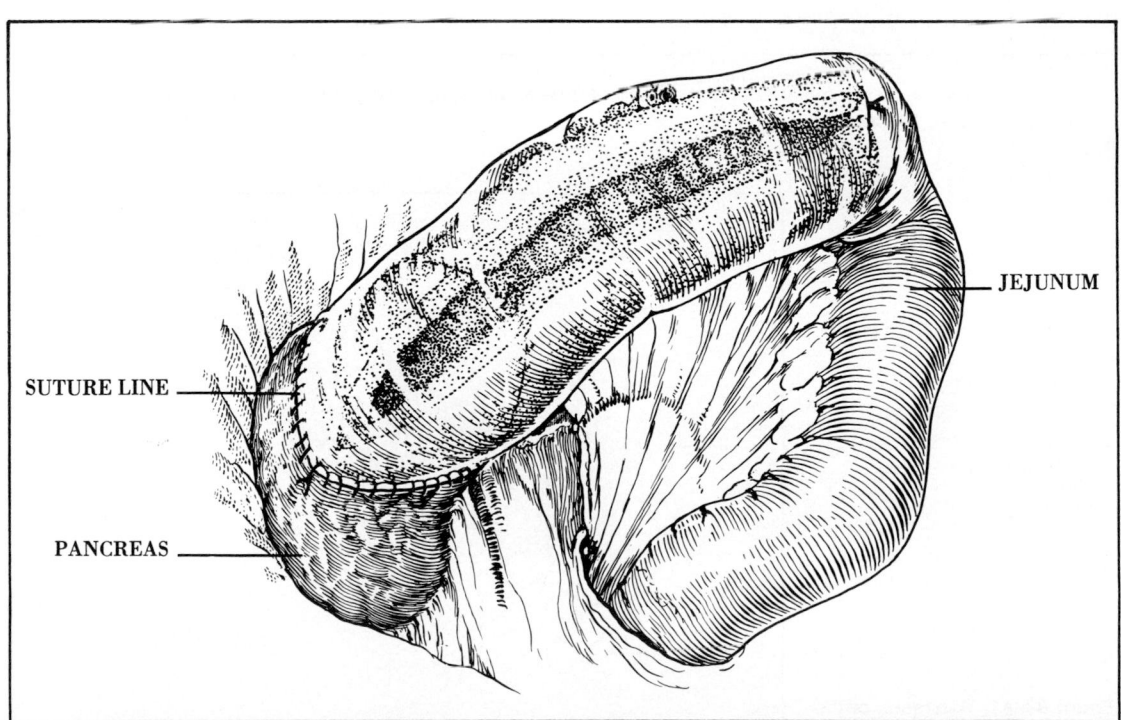

Figure 89–39. Completion of an anastomosis between the distal limb of the jejunum and the outer surface of the pancreas.

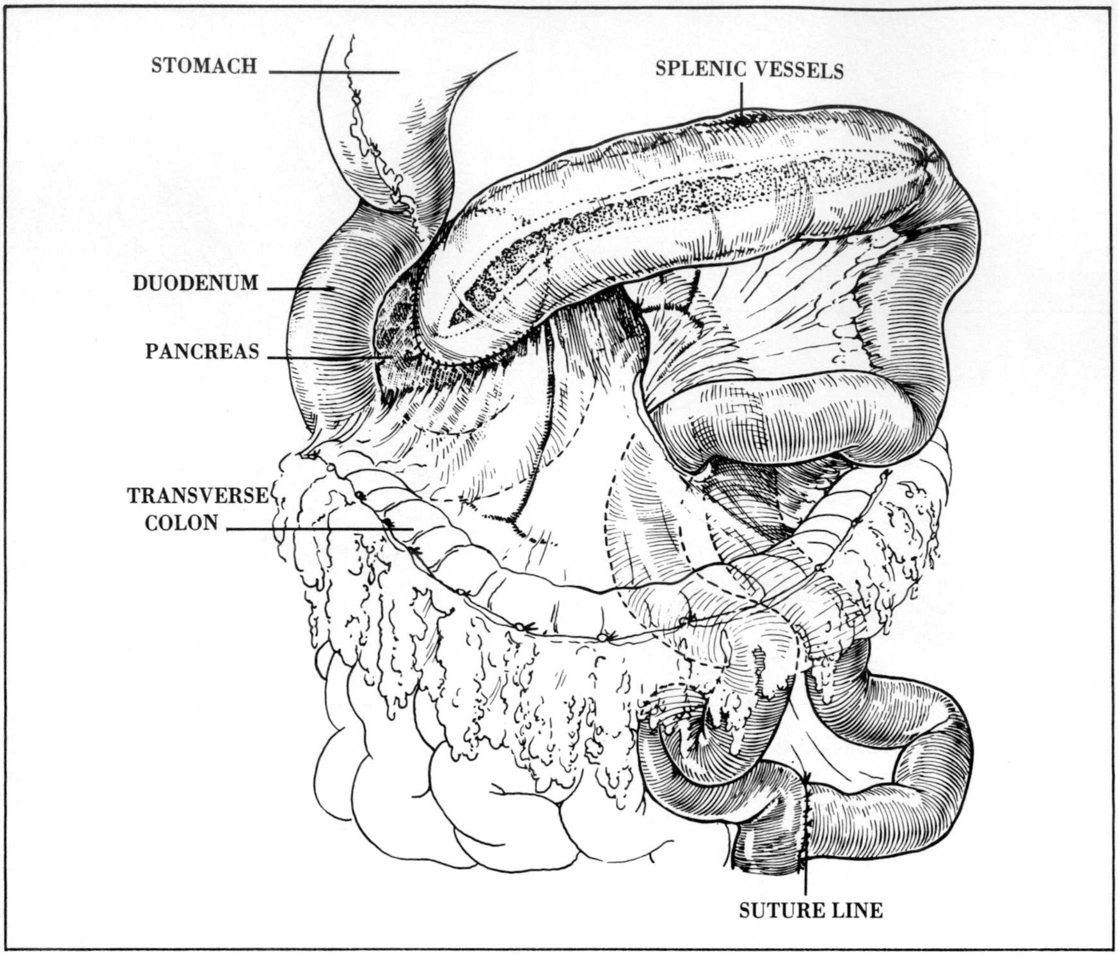

STOMACH — SPLENIC VESSELS

DUODENUM —

PANCREAS —

TRANSVERSE
COLON —

SUTURE LINE

Figure 89–40. Completed operation showing pancreatojejunostomy and enteroanastomosis. (*Source: From Warner-Chilcott.*)

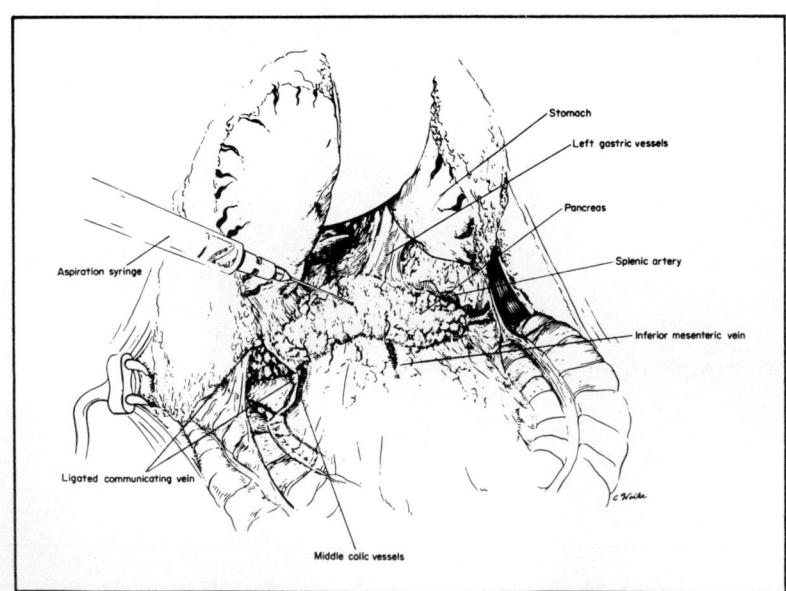

Stomach

Left gastric vessels

Pancreas

Splenic artery

Aspiration syringe

Inferior mesenteric vein

Ligated communicating vein

Middle colic vessels

Figure 89–41. Aspiration of the exposed anterior surface of the pancreas with the spleen intact.

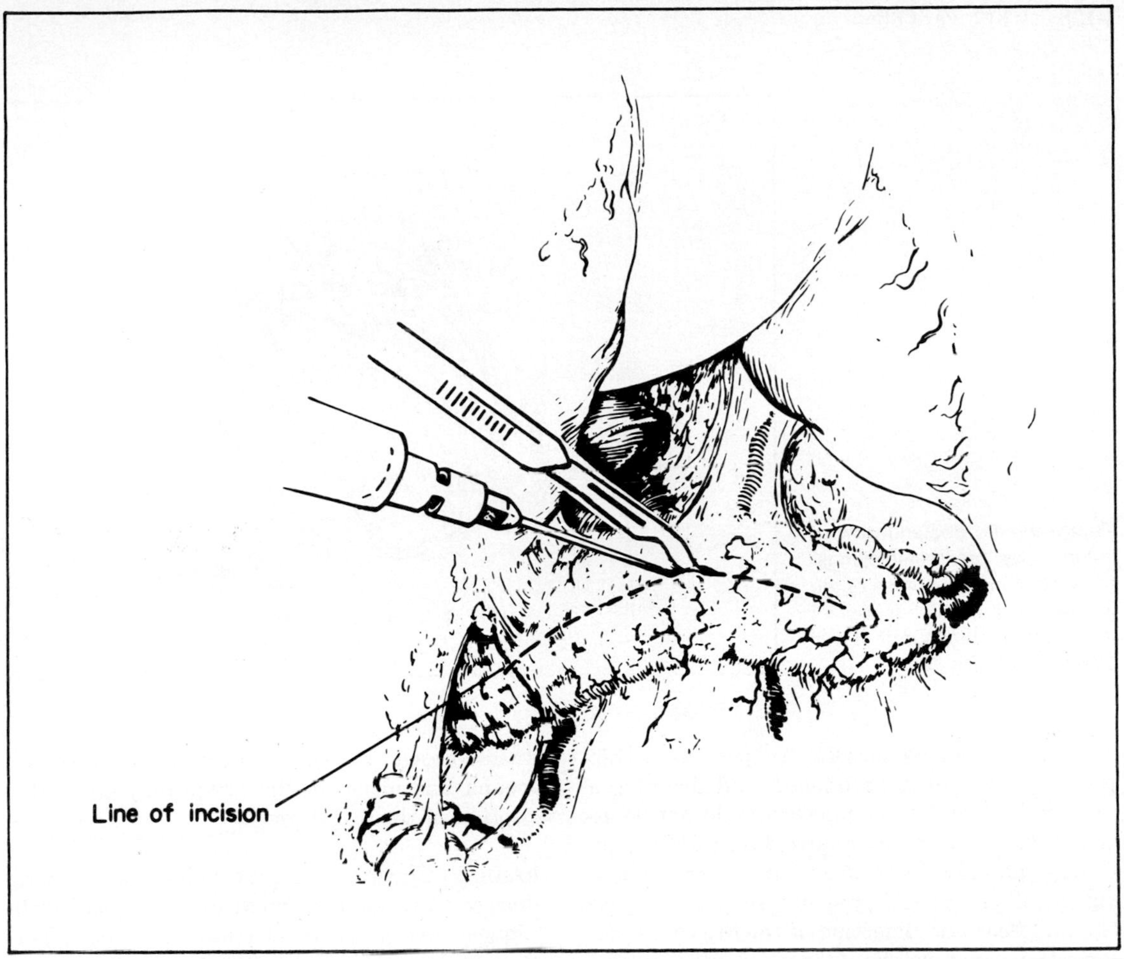

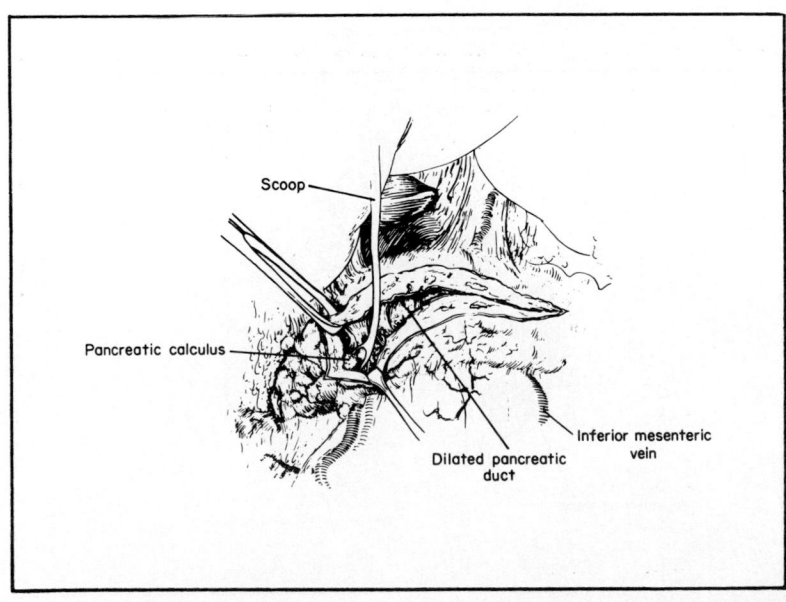

Figure 89–42. Incision of the anterior wall of the pancreas using a needle as a guide. (*Source: From Hines.*)

Scoop

Pancreatic calculus

Dilated pancreatic
duct

Inferior mesenteric
vein

Figure 89–43. Completed incision of the anterior wall of the pancreas and duct. Removal of calculi.

Line of incision

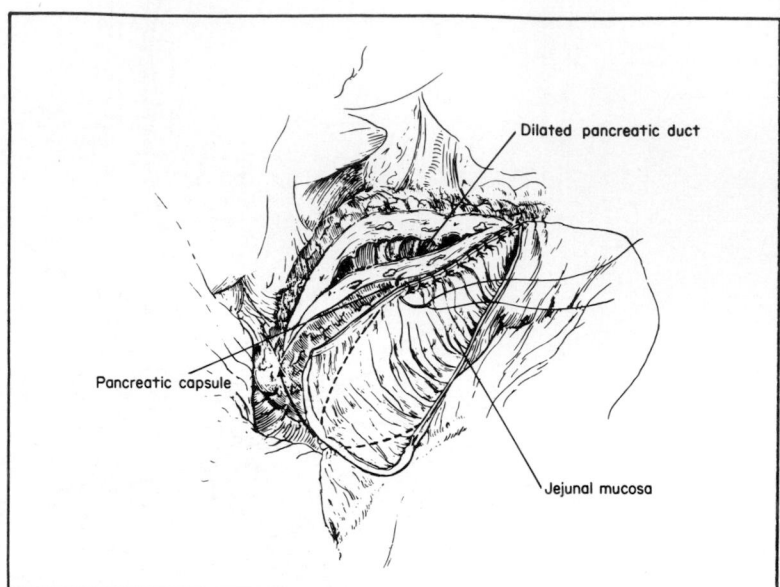

Figure 89–44. Posterior row of sutures for pancreatojejunostomy. Suturing the serosa of the jejunum to the anterior wall of the pancreas. (*Source: From Warner-Chilcott.*)

are essential to its success: All pockets within the pancreas must be opened and drained, a mucosa-to-ductal anastomosis should not be attempted, and a defunctionalized limb of the jejunum should always be used. This prevents activation of pancreatic enzymes in proximity to the pancreas and digestion of the organ. Therefore, the pancreas should not be anastomosed to the small bowel in continuity. Finally, the distal jejunal limb should be brought to the pancreas in a retrocolic manner. If the jejunum is

anastomosed to the pancreas by antecolic means, distention of the bowel may cause disruption of the anastomosis.

RESULTS. Chronic pancreatitis is a discouraging disease to treat. Few medical or surgical techniques have given good results. We have performed approximately 120 longitudinal pancreaticojejunostomies, with 3 hospital deaths. Many of these patients have been poor-risk candidates who have had from one to five previous

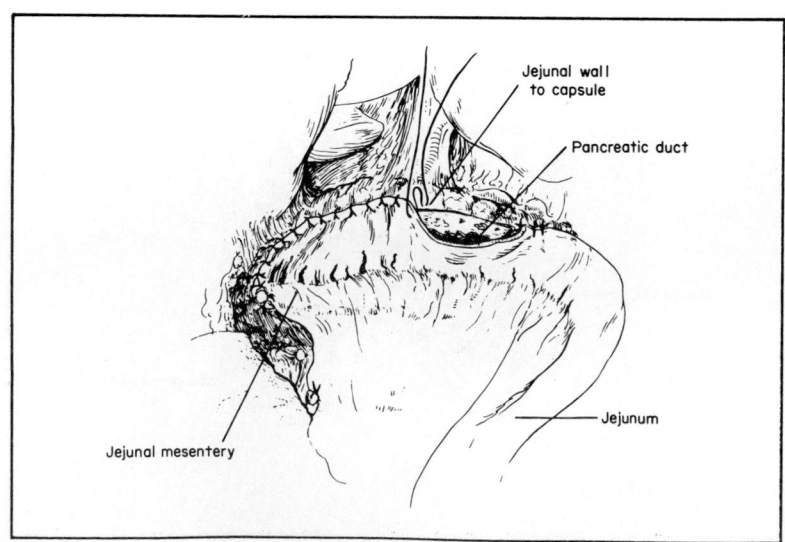

Figure 89–45. Continuation of pancreatojejunostomy inserting anterior superior row of sutures. (*Source: From Warner-Chilcott.*)

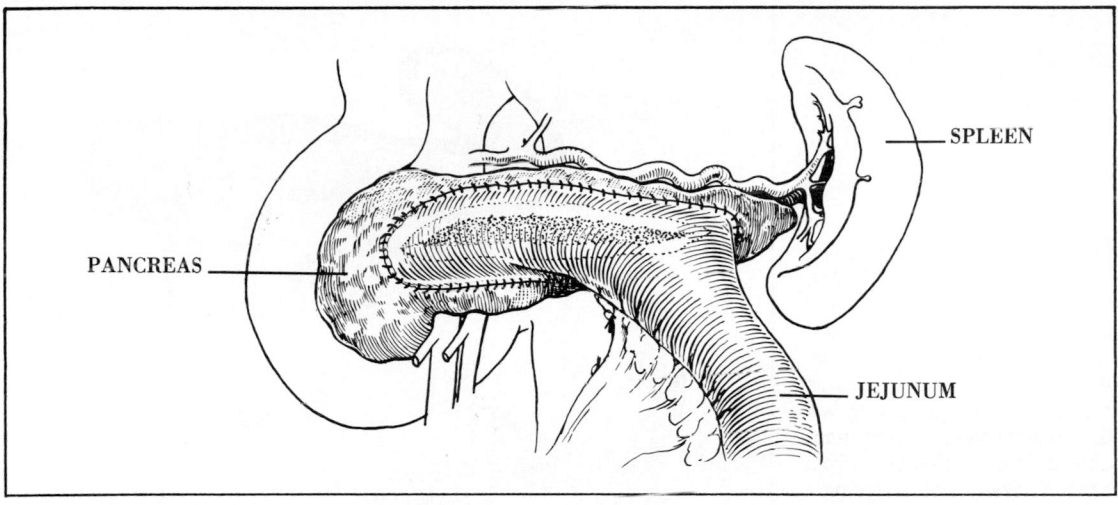

Figure 89–46. Completed pancreatojejunostomy with spleen intact. (*Source: From Warner-Chilcott.*)

operations of various kinds for pancreatitis. Seventy five percent of the patients have been relieved of pain, have regained their normal weight, and have had a return to normal pancreatic digestion. Ten percent of the patients have not benefited; most of these patients were severe alcoholics and narcotic addicts who returned to their drinking and drug habit and generally had an inadequate diet. The remainder benefited but had an occasional recurrence of pancreatic pain, usually associated with excesses of alcohol.

Puestow's contribution to longitudinal pancreaticojejunostomy is primarily his insistence that a moderately large opening be made into the pancreatic duct and that points of obstruction, especially in the midportion of the distal part of the pancreatic duct, be overcome. The author's major disagreement with Puestow's technique is two-fold. First, it is not necessary to expose the entire length of the pancreatic duct. It is possible to make a generous opening in the neck and body of the pancreatic duct by calibrating, dilating, and removing points of obstruction that are commonly caused by the presence of intraductal calculi. The pancreatic duct is cleared adequately to permit the longitudinal pancreaticojejunostomy. The pictorial demonstration describes precisely how the author performs this operation. It delineates the second and the most important difference between the

author's technique and that of Puestow. The author emphasizes that the anastomosis between the pancreatic duct and the jejunum should be precise. It is the author's belief that neither the intussusception technique, which Puestow first described, nor the on-lay technique, in which the jejunum is not precisely anastomosed to the pancreatic duct, is less likely to remain patent than if a precise anastomosis is performed.

The author has also found that splinting the anastomosis with a T-tube in place for a minimum of 4 months assures patency of the anastomosis. The author has recently adopted the technique of leaving the transverse limb of the T-tube in the pancreatic duct and inserting the vertical limb of the T-tube into the jejunum. When this technique is employed, the T-tube is anchored with silk because it is intended to be permanent, thus assuring patency. The author's willingness to perform this technique is based on the observation that when a T-tube is removed from the pancreatic duct, it is not encrusted and appears similar to when it was originally placed into the duct.

When multiple cysts are present in the head of the pancreas and when they can be converted into a single cavity, it is possible to anastomose the converted cystic cavity and the duct of Wirsung to the side of a Roux-Y limb of jejunum, thus obviating the need for multiple anas-

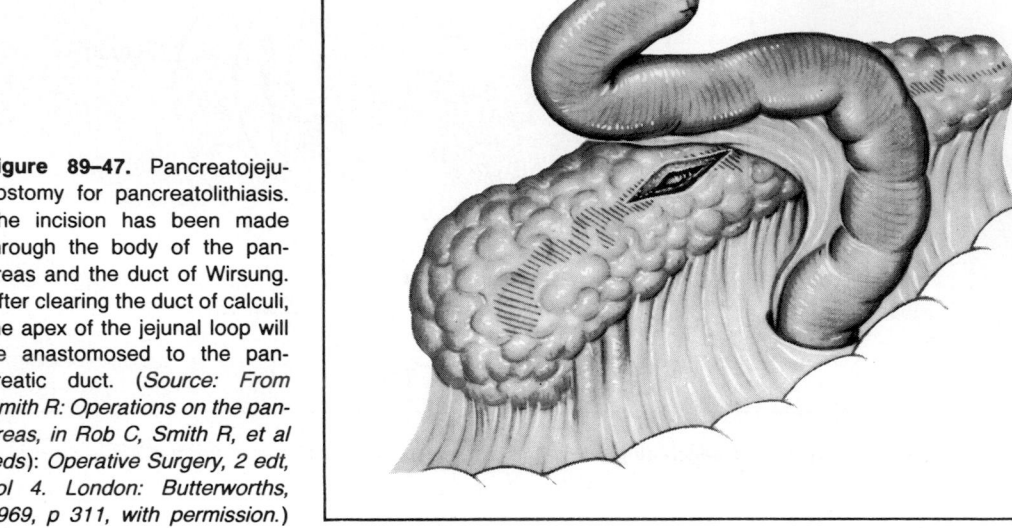

Figure 89–47. Pancreatojejunostomy for pancreatolithiasis. The incision has been made through the body of the pancreas and the duct of Wirsung. After clearing the duct of calculi, the apex of the jejunal loop will be anastomosed to the pancreatic duct. (*Source: From Smith R: Operations on the pancreas, in Rob C, Smith R, et al (eds): Operative Surgery, 2 edt, vol 4. London: Butterworths, 1969, p 311, with permission.*)

tomoses. In chronic pancreatitis, with cysts that do not communicate with the duct of Wirsung, external drainage will suffice.

Side-to-Side Pancreaticojejunostomy (Mucosal Graft Technique). Lord Smith has described side-to-side pancreaticojejunostomy. This procedure is preferred to any other if there is a generalized wide dilatation of the duct of Wirsung without strictures and if the main pancreatic duct can be cleared of calculi from head to tail. A minimal degree of peripheral calcifica-

tion (nearly always being, in fact, tiny calculi in the peripheral ducts rather than parenchymatous calcification) can be ignored and, provided that there is free drainage of the main pancreatic duct, it may not result in continuing symptoms.

Anastomosis of the pancreatic duct to a Roux-Y loop of jejunum is effected by using the mucosal graft method. This technique is shown in Figures 89–47 through 89–51.

This preference arises from the following reasons: It is a simple procedure and technically

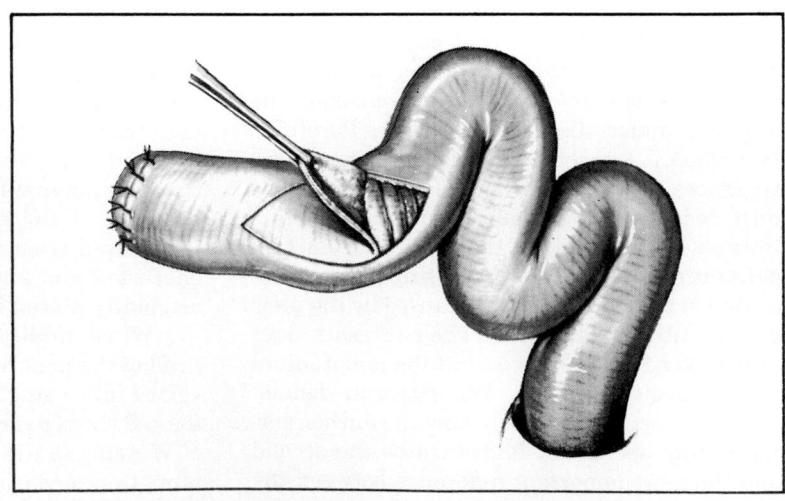

Figure 89–48. The plan is to line the tract through the pancreatic substance into the duct with jejunal mucosa. An oval segment is excised exposing the mucosa. (*Source: From Smith R: Operations on the pancreas, in Rob C, Smith R, et al (eds): Operative Surgery, 2 edt, vol 4. London: Butterworths, 1969, p 312, with permission.*)

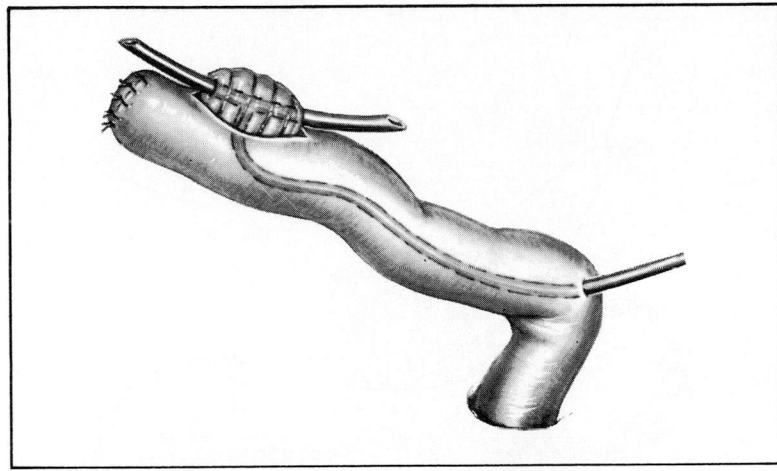

Figure 89–49. Placing the latex rubber T-tube in position. (*Source: From Smith R: Operations on the pancreas, in Rob C, Smith R, et al (eds): Operative Surgery, 2 edt, vol 4. London: Butterworths, 1969, p 312, with permission.*)

easy to perform; it is practically without hazard during the operation and free from postoperative complications; it has a high success rate; and even if, after a period of relief, symptoms recur, a further operation, for example, distal pancreatectomy, is not made more difficult.

The dilated duct is already opened in the most accessible part of the body. All calculi are extracted with scoops of various sizes and a dilator passed in both directions to be sure that the duct is empty from head to tail (Figs. 89–47 through 89–51). A latex T-tube is then placed in the duct, and an operative pancreatogram is used to confirm filling of the whole of the duct without strictures or residual calculi.

A corrugated rubber drain is placed in the lesser sac through a separate stab incision, and the abdomen is closed. Postoperatively, the cor-

rugated drain is removed after 48 hours if, as is usually the case, there is no drainage. The T-tube is allowed to drain freely into a plastic bag for 7 to 10 days, until the pancreatic juice is seen to be clear and free of debris. The tube is then spigotted and washed out once daily with sterile water. The patient is taught to do this and is discharged from the hospital with the tube in situ. T-tube drainage into the jejunum is continued for 3 months, and the tube is then removed.

T-Tube Drainage of the Duct of Wirsung. In rare instances the moderately or greatly dilated duct of Wirsung may have a narrow stricture near the ampulla of Vater. When this situation is present, it is possible to dilate the strictured portion of the duct with graduated

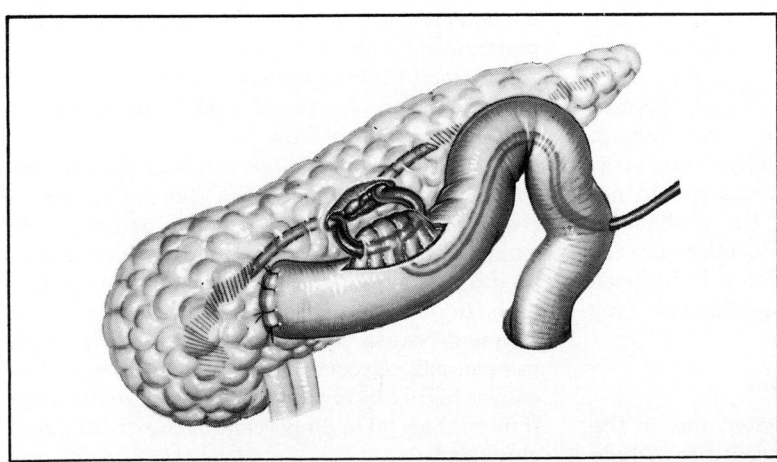

Figure 89–50. The two limbs of the T-tube are now inserted into the duct so that when pressed home the T-tube will carry the jejunal mucosal graft with it into the duct. (*Source: From Smith R: Operations on the pancreas, in Rob C, Smith R, et al (eds): Operative Surgery, 2 edt, vol 4. London: Butterworths, 1969, p 312, with permission.*)

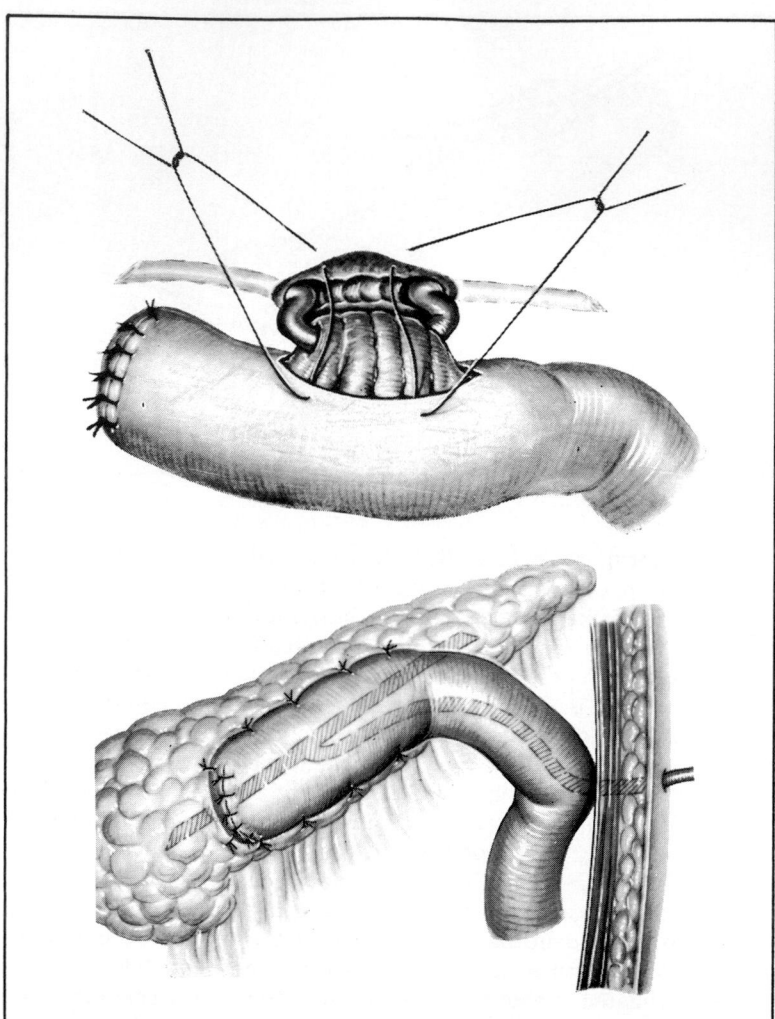

Figure 89–51. Fixing the jejunum to the pancreas. The jejunal loop is now sewn to the front of the pancreatic substance and the long limb of the T-tube is brought through the abdominal wall to the exterior. (*Source: From Smith R: Operations on the pancreas, in Rob C, Smith R, et al (eds): Operative Surgery, 2 edt, vol 4. London: Butterworths, 1969, p 313, with permission.*)

Bakes' dilators and then to insert a long-limb T-tube traversing the ampulla of Vater, with a short limb of the T-tube extending into the distal portion of the pancreatic duct. If this maneuver is employed, the T-tube should remain in place for a minimum of 4 months. Long strictures in the head of the pancreas should not be dilated forcibly because of the probability of creating a false passage. If a false passage is made and the long-limb T-tube is inserted through the false passage, the opening will close when the T-tube is removed.

Partial Pancreatic Resections

Indications for subtotal pancreatectomy in the management of chronic pancreatitis include normal-sized ductal systems, pain, and chronic pancreatitis and dilated ducts in patients in whom longitudinal pancreaticojejunostomy or decompression of a pseudocyst failed to relieve the pain of pancreatitis.

Other indications for subtotal pancreatectomy include pseudocysts in the uncinate process that cannot be internally drained, multiple small pseudocysts, or pseudoaneurysms associated with the pseudocyst. Frey stated that hemorrhage from pseudoaneurysm is the most frequent cause of death in patients with pseudocysts. Exocrine and endocrine insufficiency is highly likely after distal pancreatectomy if more than 80 to 85 percent of the distal gland is excised.

Limited Distal Pancreatectomy. Distal or caudal pancreatectomy alone is indicated when chronic pancreatitis is limited to the body and tail of the pancreas, the remainder of the organ being normal in every other respect. This type of pancreatitis is rare, but it is prone to occur after nonpenetrating abdominal injuries. After transection, the proximal end of the pancreatic duct is found, transfixed at two sites, and then elevated with two stay sutures. A French No. 3 or 4 ureteric catheter is cautiously passed along its lumen and directed toward the pancreatic mouth and lumen of the duodenum. If any obstacle, such as a fibrous stricture, is encountered, pancreatography becomes a mandatory procedure. When the catheter passes without restraint into the duodenum, the end of the duct is elevated and carefully sutured with a series of closely applied sutures of fine silk. This method is more secure than transfixion-ligation of the ductal stump. The operation is completed by snugly suturing the anterior and posterior margins of the gland together without tension. If, on the other hand, it is evident that the main duct is obstructed, for example, at a point where it traverses the head of the pancreas, retrograde drainage—pancreaticojejunostomy or pancreaticogastrostomy—must be performed (Fig. 89–52).

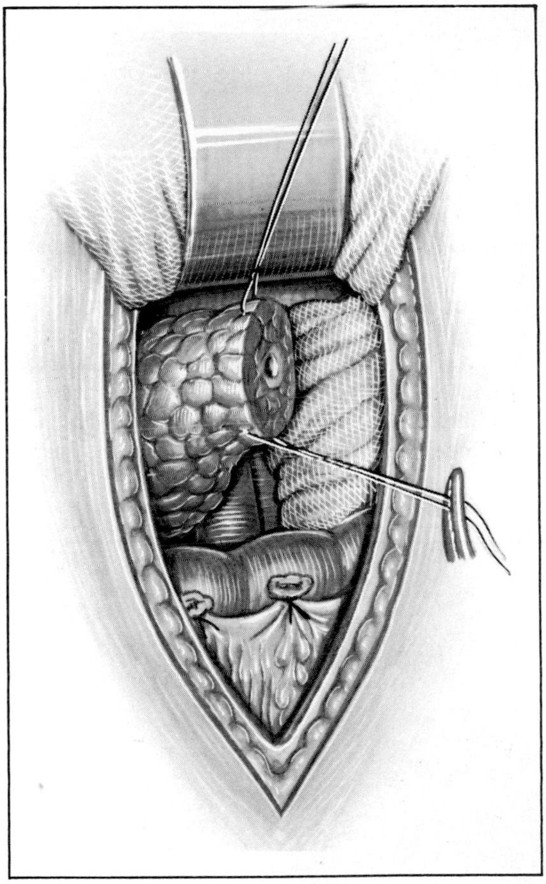

Radical Distal Pancreatectomy. Radical distal pancreatectomy (95 percent pancreatectomy) entails removal of the spleen and 95 percent of the distal pancreas (Figs. 89–53 through

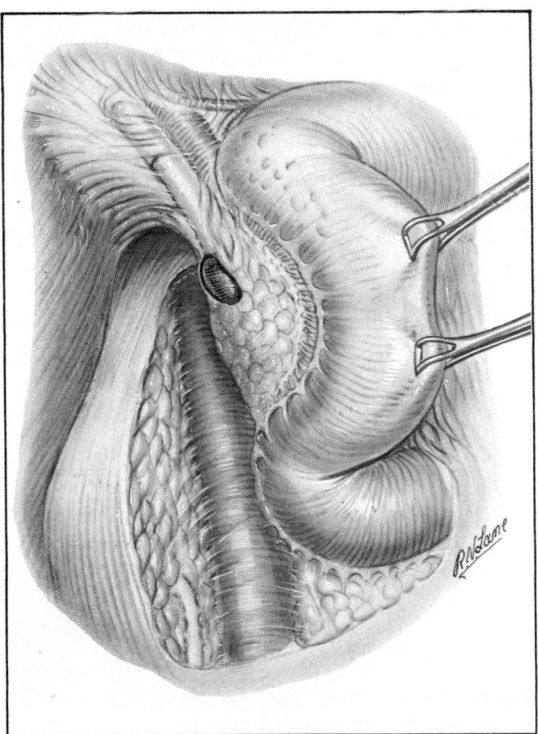

Figure 89–52. Distal pancreatectomy with pancreatojejunostomy or pancreatogastrostomy. The pancreas has been transected at its neck, and the body and the tail of the gland have been removed. The duct of Wirsung is cleared of stones and debris. At this stage, a pancreatogram may be taken. (*Source: From Maingot R: Stenosis of the sphincter of Oddi, in Smith R, Sherlock S (eds): Surgery of the Gallbladder and Bile Ducts. London: Butterworths, 1964, p 183, with permission.*)

Figure 89–53. Exposure of the head of the pancreas and the choledochus by Kocher's method. The common duct lymph node, the inferior vena cava, and the right ureter are also displayed. A good view of the posterolateral aspects of the duodenum (second part) and the head of the pancreas is obtained.

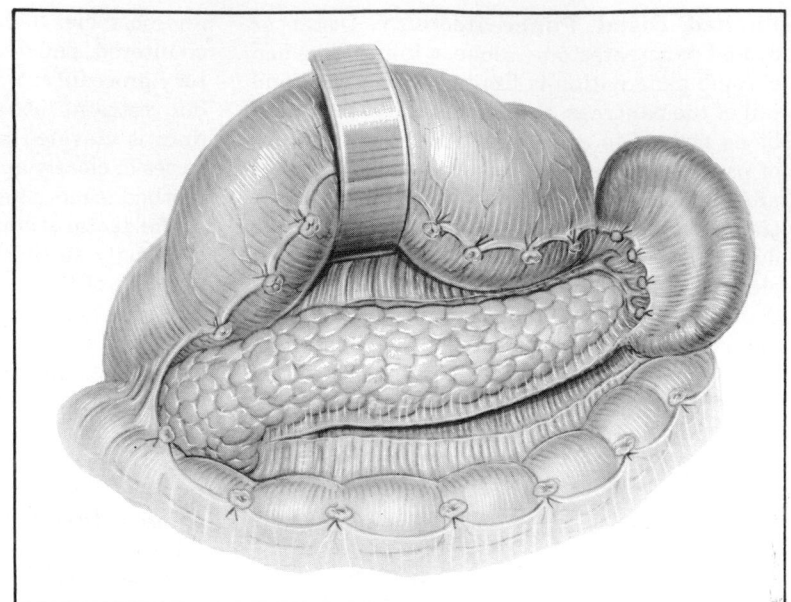

Figure 89–54. Exposure of the pancreas and the hilus of the spleen. The peritoneum on the posterior wall just inferior and superior to the pancreas is incised to allow a ready manipulation of the organ prior to the performance of 95 percent pancreatectomy.

89–55). At the completion of the operation, all that remains is a small cuff of pancreas lying within the lesser curvature of the duodenum. The duct of Wirsung is ligated, hemostasis of the raw surface of the pancreas is obtained by means of transfixion sutures, and the normal choledochoduodenal relationships are maintained. In most cases, exocrine substitution therapy is required. (Good accounts of the operation are given by Child and Fry, Fry and Child, and Child et al.)

TECHNIQUE. An oblique incision extending from the left costal margin to the right flank provides adequate exposure for proximal or distal pancreatic resection (Fig. 89–56). The gastrocolic

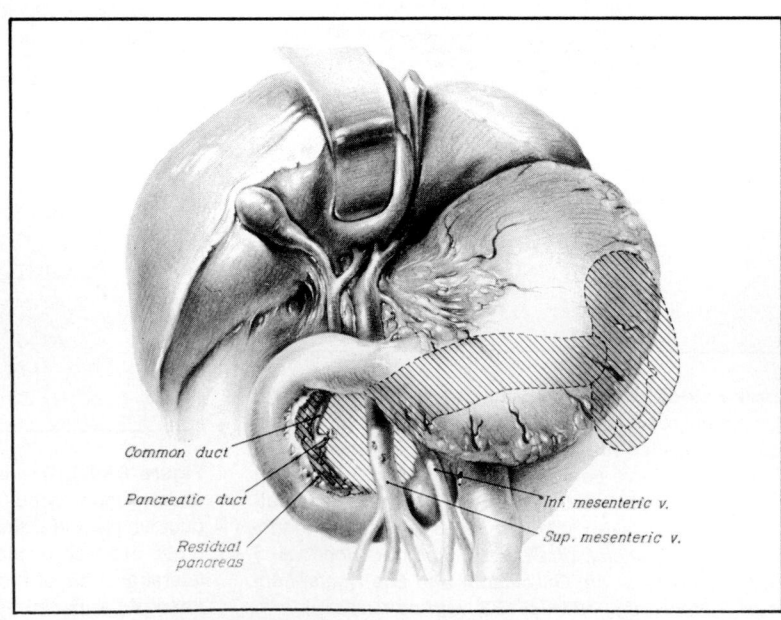

Figure 89–55. A 95 percent pancreatectomy for relapsing or chronic progressive pancreatitis. (*Source: From Child CG III, Frey CF, et al: A reappraisal of removal of ninety five percent of the distal portion of the pancreas. Surg Gynecol Obstet 129:49, 1969, with permission.*)

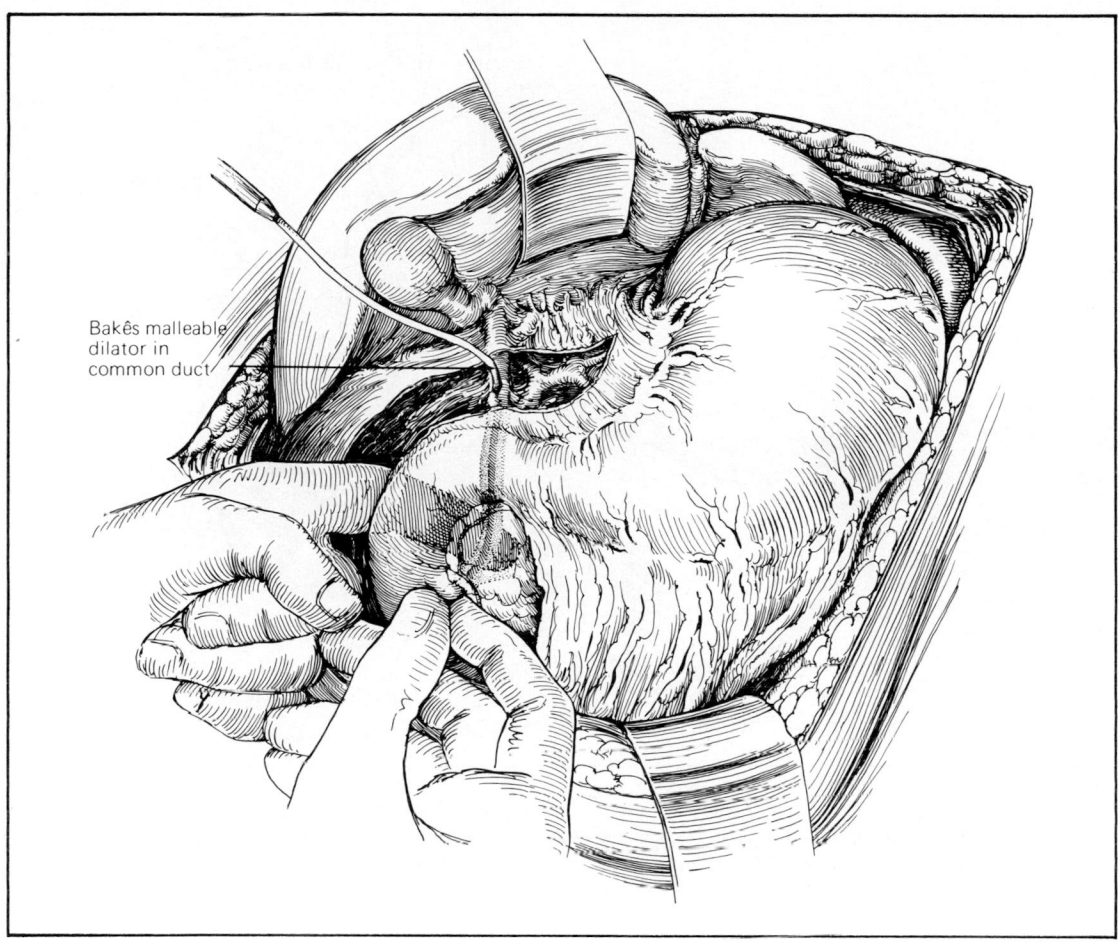

Figure 89–56. Exposure of the pancreas. (*Source: From Frey CF: Distal subtotal pancreatectomy, in Malt R (ed): Surgical Techniques Illustrated, Surgery for Chronic Pancreatitis, vol 2. Boston: Little, Brown, 1977, with permission.*)

Bakês malleable dilator in common duct

and colosplenic ligaments are divided, and a Kocher maneuver is performed to visualize and palpate the body and tail of the pancreas and the head of the gland for evidence of small pseudocysts and chronic pancreatitis.

The common bile duct is exposed, and the anterior wall is incised longitudinally to insert a French No. 2 or 3 metal bougie. By palpating the metal bougie in the common duct between the thumb and index finger, the duct can be located and injury to it avoided.

The superior mesenteric vein is identified by tracing the middle colic vein to its entry point into the superior mesenteric vein. Mobilization of the body and tail of the pancreas is begun by separating the inferior border and undersur-

face of the pancreas from the retroperitoneal tissues. This dissection, which is usually bloodless, is carried from the superior mesenteric vein to the splenic hilum. The splenic artery is traced by palpation from its origin from the celiac axis to the superior border of the pancreas where it is isolated and divided (Fig. 89–57).

The spleen is freed from its attachments to the diaphragm, and the hilum of the spleen is exposed by carefully clamping, ligating, and dividing the short gastric and left gastroepiploic vessels. The spleen and tail of the pancreas can then be elevated to the patient's right, providing access to the splenic vein and artery on the undersurface of the pancreas (Fig. 89–58). The inferior mesenteric and coronary veins may termi-

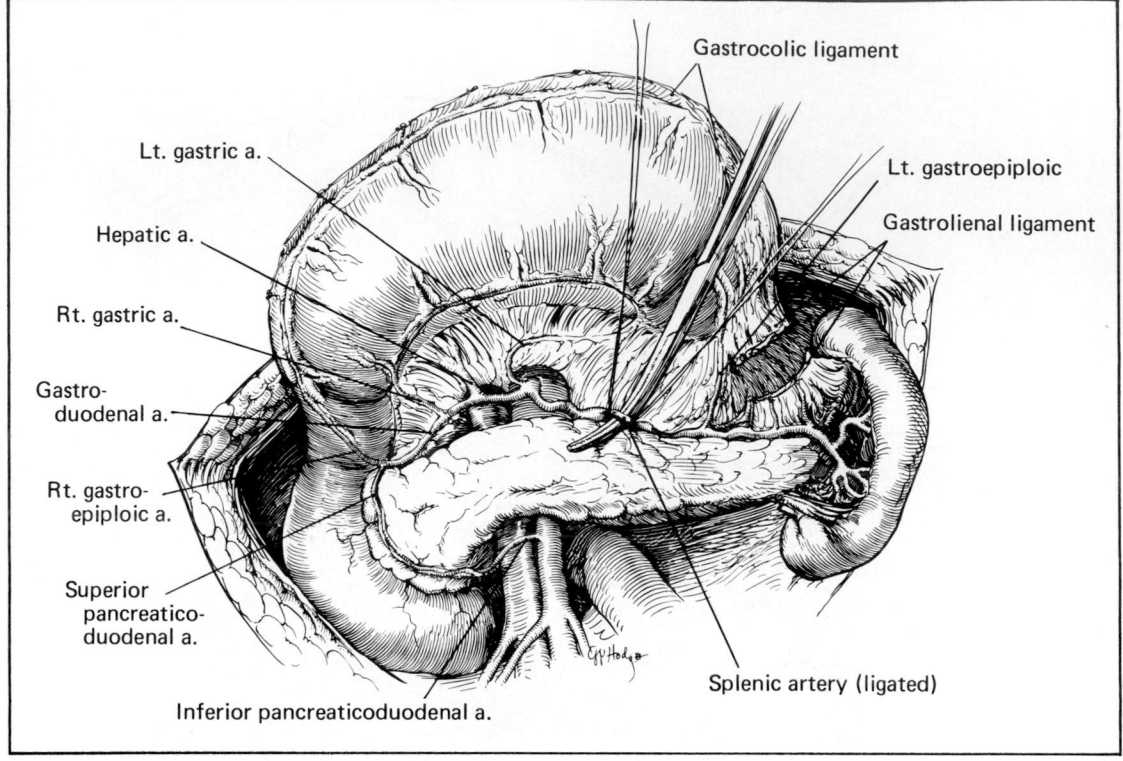

Figure 89–57. Division of the splenic artery. (*Source: From Frey CF: Distal subtotal pancreatectomy, in Malt R (ed): Surgical Techniques Illustrated, Surgery for Chronic Pancreatitis, vol 2. Boston: Little, Brown, 1977, with permission.*)

nate in the splenic vein. Should this happen, the splenic veins should be ligated distal to their entry.

With the splenic pedicle left intact, the dissection is carried from left to right along the superior border of the pancreas to ligate the splenic artery if this maneuver has not been performed previously. The splenic vein is traced to its entry into the superior mesenteric vein and ligated and divided.

The uncinate process is freed from the portal and superior mesenteric veins. When the pancreas is markedly inflamed, the surgeon can feel thankful to have obtained superior mesenteric and celiac angiography preoperatively. Forewarning of a totally replaced hepatic artery coming off the superior mesenteric, as occurred in two of our patients, reduces the risk of vascular injury. The small branches of the superior mesenteric artery and vein supplying the uncinate process should be doubly ligated and divided in continuity. The superior mesenteric

vein should be retracted to the left to expose three vessels.

A cuff of pancreas must be left along the superior part of the third portion of duodenum to preserve intact the superior and inferior pancreatic duodenal artery, which maintains the blood supply and viability of the duodenum. The major portion of the head of the pancreas is removed after returning the pancreas and spleen to their usual positions. A curvilinear incision is then made in the pancreatic head along the inner aspect of the duodenal C (Fig. 89–59). During this incision, it is essential that the surgeon avoid injury to the common duct by identifying the course of the duct by palpating the metal bougie contained within it.

The specimen can then be removed, leaving a cuff of pancreatic tissue containing the common duct and duodenal blood supply through the inferior and superior pancreatic duodenal arcades. Patency of the remaining pancreatic duct can be probed, following which it is ligated

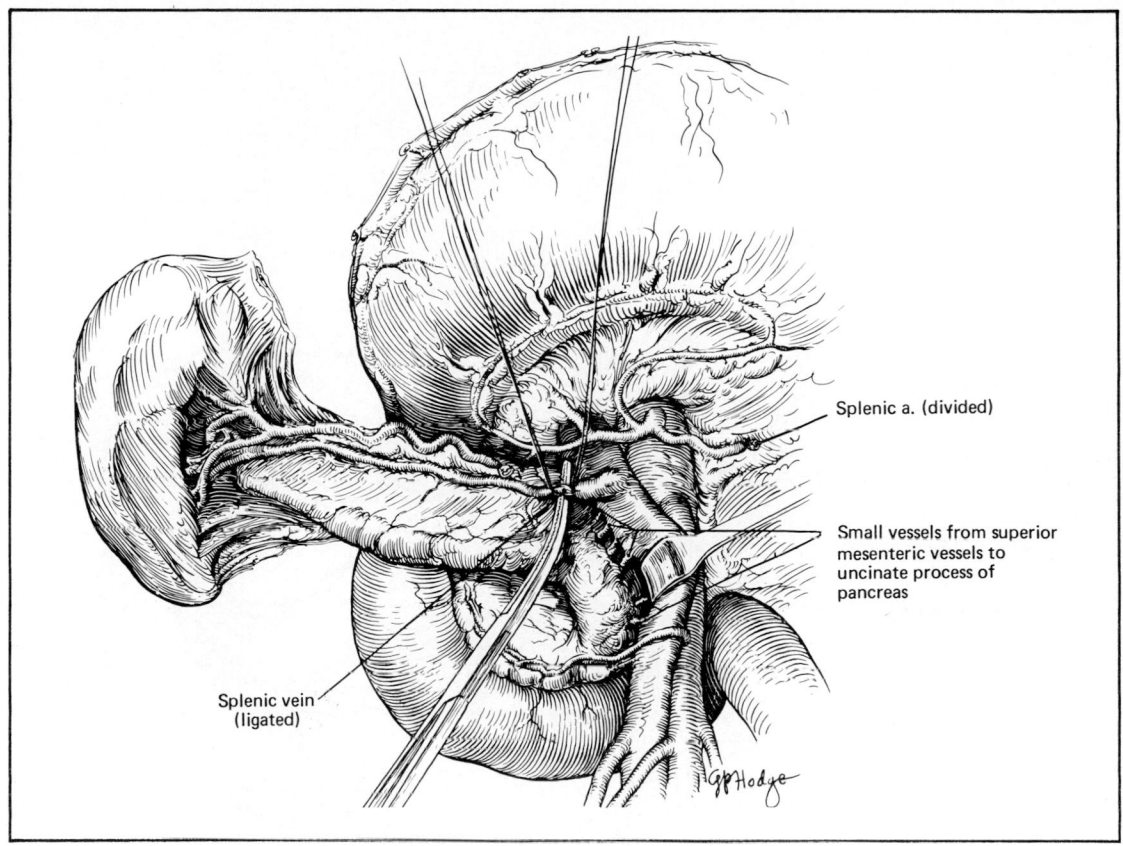

Figure 89–58. Exposing and ligating the splenic vein. (*Source: From Frey CF: Distal subtotal pancreatectomy, in Malt R (ed): Surgical Techniques Illustrated, Surgery for Chronic Pancreatitis, vol 2. Boston: Little, Brown, 1977, with permission.*)

distally. Vagotomy and pyloroplasty should be performed on patients with evidence of a peptic ulcer diathesis.

The splenic bed and head of the pancreas are drained separately through stab incisions. A T-tube is placed in the common duct and brought out through a separate stab incision. The incision is closed in layers with No. 30 wire or 0 monofilament polypropylene.

Pancreatoduodenectomy

GENERAL CONSIDERATIONS. Pancreatitis produces such a wide variety of progressive and irreversible structural changes that we choose the method of treatment on the basis of these changes in each patient rather than on any etiologic classification. The pathologic changes of chronic relapsing pancreatitis range from swell-ing and mild induration of the gland to fibrosis, atrophy, patchy or widespread necrosis, cystic change, and pancreatolithiasis. Several of these alterations may be seen in the same gland, and different phases in the progression of the disease may be observed in the same patient. For example, the head of the pancreas may be normal macroscopically, while far-advanced disease is present in its body and tail. The core of these observations is that partial or complete intra-pancreatic obstruction is apparently responsible for recurrent attacks of pancreatitis, and the treatment, therefore, depends on relief of this obstruction.

Our increased understanding of these obstructions has shown the futility of dealing with pancreatitis by procedures directed to the biliary tract, stomach, or pancreatic autonomic nerves. Unquestionably, associated biliary tract

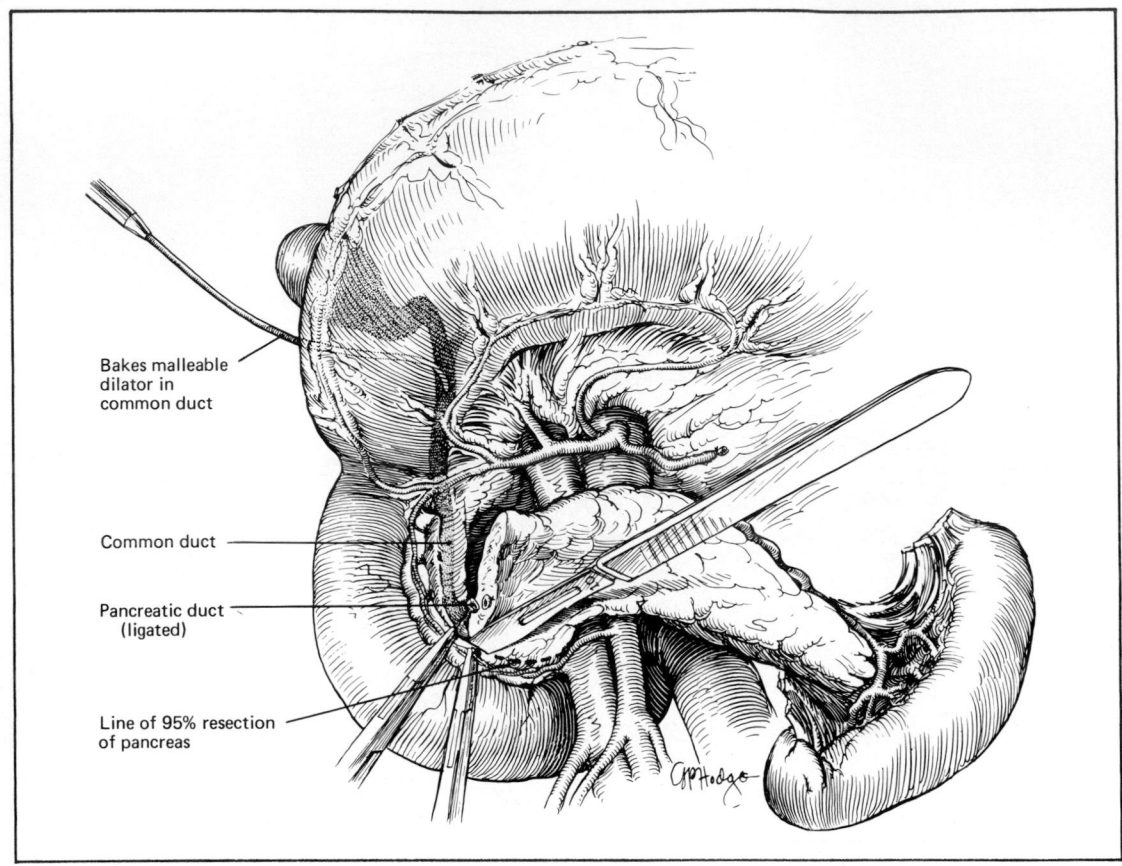

Bakes malleable
dilator in
common duct

Common duct

Pancreatic duct
(ligated)

Line of 95% resection
of pancreas

Figure 89–59. Line of resection in 95 percent distal pancreatectomy. (*Source: From Frey CF: Distal subtotal pancreatectomy, in Malt R (ed): Surgical Techniques Illustrated, Surgery for Chronic Pancreatitis, vol 2. Boston: Little, Brown, 1977, with permission.*)

disease should be corrected; however, our extensive experience in the surgical management of patients with severe pathologic alterations proves that the most effective methods of treatment involve direct pancreatic ductal decompression or resection.

The method of decompression or the extent of resection is dictated by the specific pathologic changes found at laparotomy. Our choice is pancreatoduodenectomy if many points of obstruction are found in the head of the pancreas, and in the presence of long-standing advanced pancreatic disease, pancreatolithiasis, where the distribution of the pancreatic calculi is associated with complete anatomic disorganization of the head of the pancreas, or failure of lesser operations. It is a technically difficult procedure, involving sacrifice of a considerable portion of the pancreas; thus, we use it only if we believe

that the pathologic alterations are too advanced to be dealt with by less radical measures.

Regardless of whether the pathologic changes are minimal or advanced, caution should be the watchword in surgical manipulation of an inflamed and edematous pancreas because of the risk of postoperative acute pancreatitis. In contrast, the pancreas, which is fibrotic and calcific, tolerates surgical manipulation with less postoperative reaction.

Table 89–1, which shows the clinical features of our patients who have had pancreatoduodenectomy, indicates the chronicity and severity of the disease in this group. Of these patients, 81 percent have had one or more operations for pancreatitis, and 33 percent have had sphincterotomy before registering at the Lahey Clinic or with the author. We have performed 185 pancreatoduodenectomies, including 34 to-

TABLE 89–1. CLINICAL FEATURES IN 148 PATIENTS WHO HAD PANCREATODUODENECTOMY FOR CHRONIC RELAPSING PANCREATITIS

Clinical Features	(%)
Pain	100
Weight loss	79
Previous operation	81
Pancreatolithiasis	66
Alcoholism	61
Diabetes	50
Narcotic addiction	43
Cysts	39
Jaundice	29
Peptic ulcer	17

tal pancreatectomies. Intractable pain was the principal reason for operation. Almost 80 percent had a marked weight loss. Alcoholism and narcotic addiction were prominent features, although the exact incidence is difficult to determine because many persons deny having these problems.

Pancreatic calculi, which were present in two thirds of our patients who had pancreatoduodenectomy, are probably a phase in the natural course of chronic pancreatitis. Usually they are associated with far-advanced disease. The precise mode of formation of these calculi is unknown, but we have observed repeatedly that the first calculus usually forms just distal to the most proximal intraductal stricture, and that subsequent calculi, which are usually smaller, appear distal to this point (the sentinel stone). When two or more major points of obstruction are present, pancreatolithiasis is often extensive, involving the primary and secondary pancreatic ducts throughout the gland.

Geevarghese has reported 400 patients with pancreatolithiasis observed in India; only 2 percent were alcoholics. His series now numbers more than 1200 cases. Dietary habits, unknown genetic factors, and other metabolic aberrations must play a definite, if subtle, role in the onset or progression of pancreatitis and pancreatolithiasis.

In a previous discussion* of pancreatolithia-

---

* Much of the following section is taken from Lord Smith's previous chapter on pancreatolithiasis, written for the Seventh Edition of this text.

sis by Lord Smith, he emphasized that the mere presence of pancreatic calculi is no indication that an operation should be performed, and some patients have considerable collections of calculi with relatively minor symptoms while others have symptoms of pancreatic insufficiency that call for medical care, such as diabetes mellitus or steatorrhea. Pain is the main indication for operation and occurs because of the presence of pancreatolithiasis and chronic pancreatitis. This must always be taken into account in planning an operation. In Lord Smith's view, the only indications for surgery are pain, recurrent severe exacerbations of subacute pancreatitis, major surgical complications, such as pancreatic cyst, pancreatic fistula, or portal vein obstruction, and suspicions of a superimposed malignant condition (for example, a short history of increasing pancreatic pain with marked weight loss).

PREOPERATIVE CARE. Because of the variety and severity of nutritional and metabolic changes associated with far-advanced pancreatitis, particular attention must be directed toward assessment and correction of such deficiencies. Restoration of blood volume by appropriate transfusions of whole blood and by administration of albumin is urgent. Severe protein deficiency may require forced feeding or intravenous hyperalimentation. If the patient can ingest an adequate amount, we prescribe a high-carbohydrate, high-protein, and low-fat diet supplemented with vitamins. If the patient is diabetic, the dose of insulin is increased to cover the increased amount of food. Diabetes mellitus is common in advanced chronic relapsing pancreatitis, although it may be so mild that a fasting blood sugar determination will fail to detect it. A blood sugar value determined 2 hours after a meal is much more reliable.

The status of calcium metabolism must be determined, since hypocalcemia or, more rarely, hypercalcemia secondary to a parathyroid adenoma may be present. Adequate replacement therapy when hypocalcemia is detected is most efficiently managed by intravenous administration of appropriate amounts of calcium gluconate. If a parathyroid adenoma is present, it should be removed before pancreatic surgery is attempted.

In addition to the previously mentioned studies, we routinely perform liver and pancreatic function tests. Barium contrast studies of the stomach and duodenum are also helpful.

Selective celiac angiography is yielding increasing information regarding the pancreas, and it outlines the origin and course of major and even the smaller arteries to the pancreas and the liver. An understanding of these may be helpful during the operation. Increasing experience with the flexible fiberoptic duodenoscope has provided much useful data when the pancreatic duct and bile ducts have been cannulated and studied by radiographic contrast techniques. Ultrasonography and computerized scans have been increasingly valuable in assessing pancreatic pathology.

TECHNIQUE. The operation is usually performed through a long, right paramedian incision extending superiorly to the costal margin near the xiphoid. If the patient is obese, a transverse incision may be preferred. Lysis of extensive adhesions is usually necessary. The extent of the operation and the structures to be removed are indicated in Figure 89–60.

The operation is performed in the following order—mobilization of the head of the pancreas and duodenum, elevation of the neck of the pancreas from the superior mesenteric and portal veins, mobilization of the distal segment of the common bile duct, division of the stomach or duodenum, mobilization and division of the proximal jejunum, division of the neck of the pancreas and common bile duct, removal of the specimen by division of the blood supply to the uncinate process of the pancreas and duodenum and division of the uncinate process, and reconstruction of the digestive tract by anastomosis of the pancreatic duct, common bile duct, and stomach to the jejunum.

Mobilization of Head of Pancreas and Duodenum. After thorough examination of the

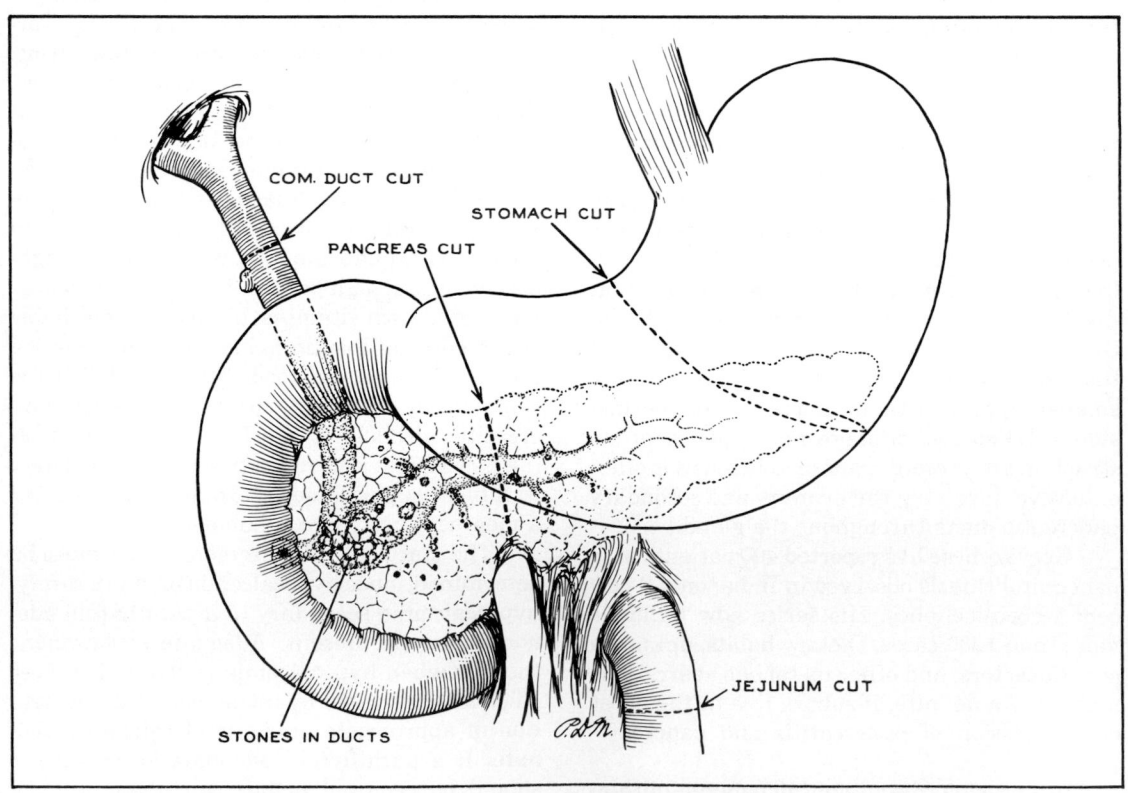

Figure 89–60. The extent of the resection is indicated. Note that approximately 65 percent of the stomach is removed. The common duct is divided above its junction with the cystic duct. The jejunum is divided approximately 5 cm distal to the ligament of Treitz. The pancreas is divided at its neck, where it crosses the superior mesenteric and portal veins.

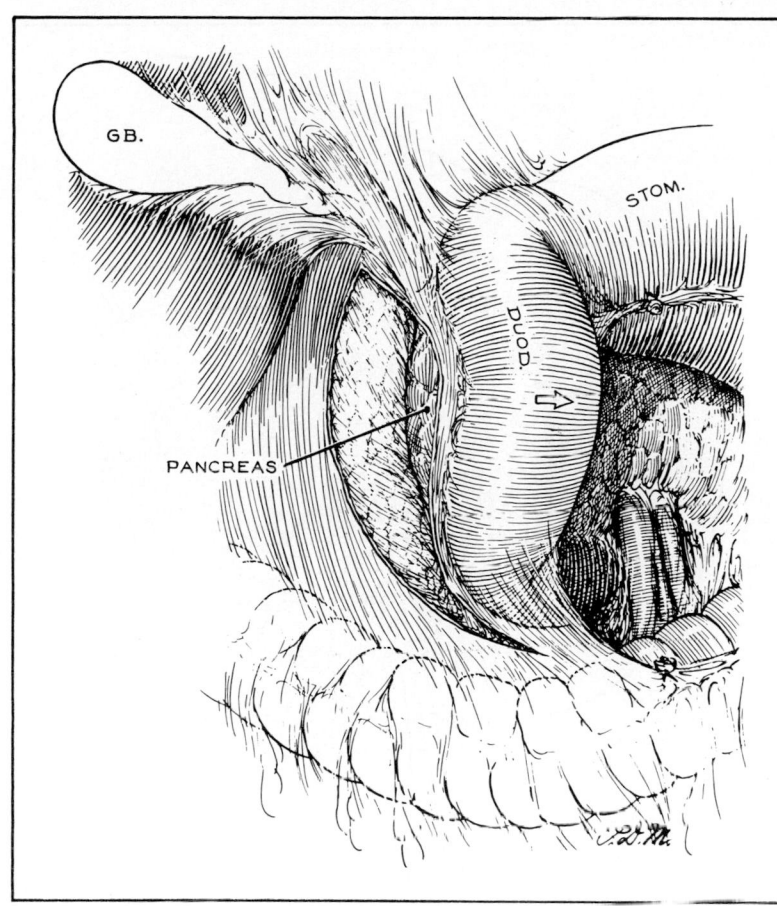

GB.

STOM.

DUOD.

PANCREAS

Figure 89–61. The peritoneum lateral to the descending portion of the duodenum has been incised. A hepatic flexure of the colon has been displaced downward. The duodenum and head of the pancreas have been completely mobilized. This mobilization is extended from right to left beyond the inferior vena cava and the abdominal aorta. Superiorly, the dissection extends to the common bile duct.

pancreas and the abdominal and pelvic structures, the peritoneum is incised along the lateral aspect of the descending duodenum (Fig. 89–61). With Babcock forceps elevating the duodenum, the head of the pancreas is dissected from the posterior abdominal wall. This will expose, in turn, the right spermatic or ovarian vein, the inferior vena cava, the aorta, and approximately 5 cm of the left renal vein.

Elevation of Neck of Pancreas from Superior Mesenteric and Portal Veins. The lesser omental sac is entered through the anterior layers of the gastrocolic omentum at the extreme right margin of the bursa. The ventral peritoneal leaflet of the transverse mesocolon is then displaced downward, displaying the middle colic vessels in the transverse mesocolon. The peritoneal incision is continued to the right, freeing the hepatic flexure and the right half of the transverse colon. A moist abdominal pad is placed over the

hepatic flexure of the colon and retracted downward.

The peritoneum is incised along the inferior border of the pancreatic neck and body, exposing the superior mesenteric vein inferior to the neck of the pancreas. The superior pancreatic lymph node will be used as a guide to the cleavage plane where the portal vein emerges from beneath the neck of the pancreas. The superior mesenteric artery can then be palpated and identified, and the inferior pancreaticoduodenal artery can be ligated and divided.

With use of a small wad of gauze in a right-angle clamp and beginning from below, the neck of the pancreas is elevated from the anterior surface of the superior mesenteric vein (Fig. 89–62). A small Penrose drain is passed around the neck of the gland (Fig. 89–63). It is used for subsequent manipulation and provides a helpful anatomic landmark throughout the operation.

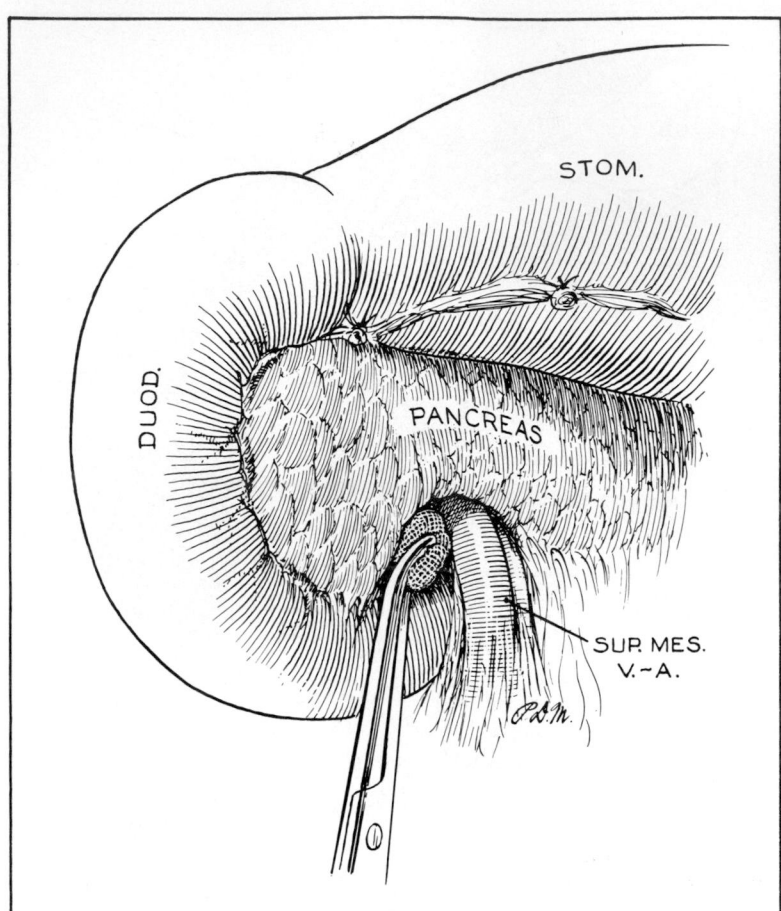

Figure 89–62. The neck of the pancreas is being elevated from the superior mesenteric vein following incision of the peritoneum. A small pledget of gauze, secured by a right angle clamp, is used for this delicate dissection, which will be carried out completely under the neck of the pancreas.

Mobilization of Distal Segment of Common Bile Duct. The common bile duct is usually slightly distended in advanced chronic pancreatitis, but it is thickened and pale. The common bile duct is freed from the portal vein medially and posteriorly, preferably at a site above the entrance of the cystic duct. The segment of mobilized duct is encircled with a Penrose drain to facilitate future mobilization (Fig. 89–64). If present, the gallbladder is removed.

Division of Stomach. Once resectability has been determined, the right lateral half of the gastrohepatic omentum is incised, and the right gastric artery is divided and ligated. The course of the hepatic artery is then determined (Fig. 89–65). It is important to know whether this artery arises from the celiac axis (as usual) or from the superior mesenteric artery.

The gastroduodenal artery is identified where it joins the hepatic artery. It has an ex-

tremely short trunk and then divides into four branches, allowing about 1 cm to be dissected and divided between ligatures. The stomach is pulled downward and to the right to allow the main trunk of the left gastric artery to be identified, divided, and ligated.

Suitable clamps are applied along the line of division for a 65 percent gastrectomy. If less of the stomach is resected, bilateral subdiaphragmatic vagotomy is performed to prevent jejunal ulceration.

Stimulated by the work of Longmire and associates, we have performed several pancreatoduodenectomies in which the entire stomach was preserved. It is imperative, when using this technique, to preserve the marginal artery along the lesser curvature of the antrum and pylorus.

Mobilization and Division of Proximal Jejunum. With the Penrose drain encircling the

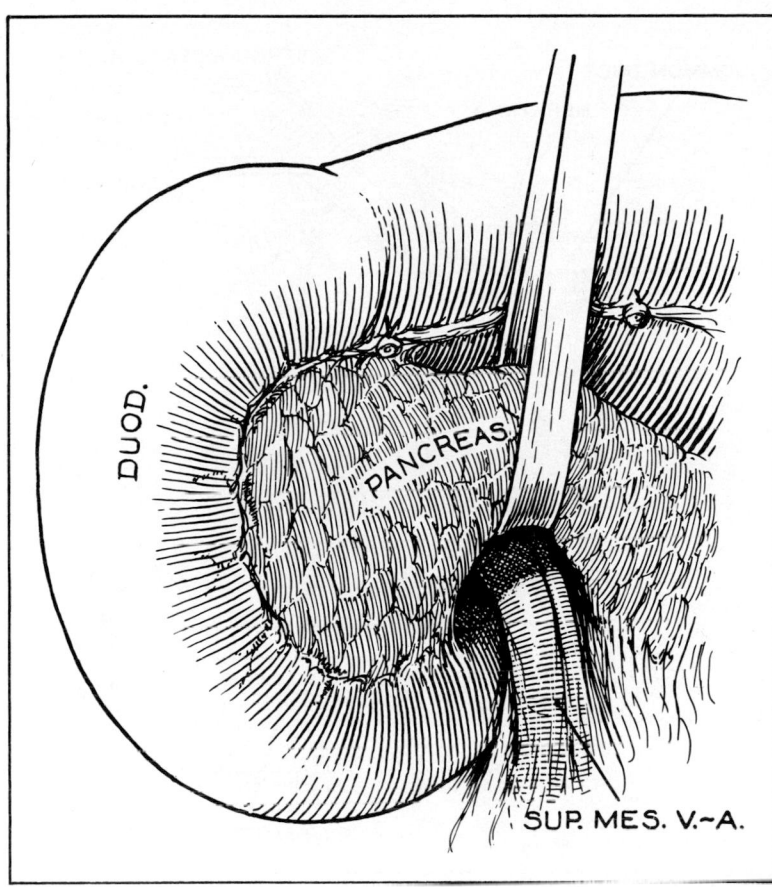

Figure 89–63. The neck of the pancreas has been completely mobilized from the superior mesenteric and portal veins, and a small Penrose drain has been passed beneath it. The drain will be used subsequently for manipulation of this structure.

neck of the pancreas and serving as a landmark, the ligament of Treitz is incised to the right of the superior mesenteric vessels, exposing the fourth portion of the duodenum and the proximal jejunum. The mesentery of the proximal jejunum is divided, and the vessels are ligated. The proximal jejunum is drawn to the right and beneath the superior mesenteric vessels and divided between two Kocher clamps (Fig. 89–66). The stump of the proximal jejunum is inverted by an inner row of continuous chromic catgut sutures reinforced by a row of interrupted fine silk sutures. The peritoneum is closed at the ligament of Treitz.

Division of Neck of Pancreas and Common Bile Duct. Four nonabsorbable hemostatic ligatures are placed, two superiorly and two inferiorly, into the neck of the pancreas, about 1 cm deep, to control the longitudinal pancreatic arteries (Fig. 89–67A). A right-angle artery clamp is placed for protection beneath the neck of the

pancreas on the anterior surface of the superior mesenteric and portal veins. The neck of the pancreas is divided with a scalpel. During this procedure, the duct of Wirsung is identified and left to project from the cut surface of the distal pancreas. As the duct is divided, a fine silk suture is placed in each quadrant. Bleeding from the proximal portion of the neck is controlled by a series of silk mattress sutures (Fig. 89–67B).

After any small calculi are scooped from the duct of Wirsung, the distal pancreas is closed with interrupted mattress sutures of silk, leaving the duct open for the pancreaticojejunostomy (Fig. 89–67C). After the neck of the pancreas has been divided, the portal vein and the junction of its tributaries—the superior mesenteric and splenic veins—are exposed. The common bile duct is divided between paired clamps above its junction with the cystic duct.

Division of Blood Supply to Uncinate Process of Pancreas and Duodenum. Elevation of

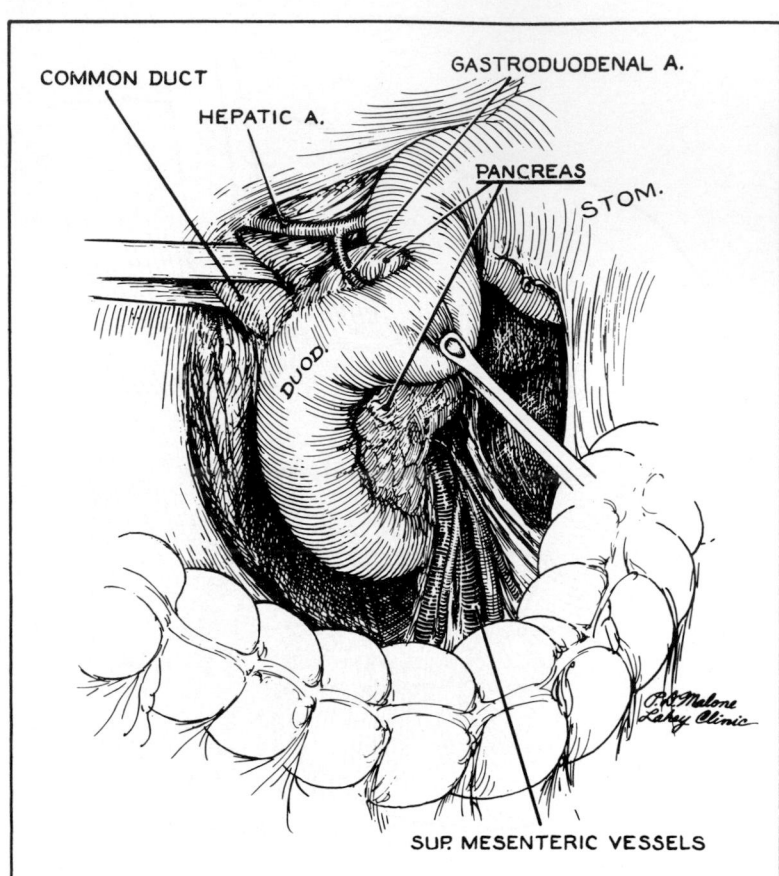

COMMON DUCT

HEPATIC A.

GASTRODUODENAL A.

PANCREAS

STOM.

DUOD.

SUP. MESENTERIC VESSELS

Figure 89–64. Completed mobilization of the distal portion of the common bile duct, the course of the hepatic artery, and a segment of the gastroduodenal artery. The gastroduodenal artery will be divided approximately 1 or 2 cm from its junction with the hepatic artery.

the duodenum and head of the pancreas allows the uncinate process to be freed posteriorly. The dissection permits visualization of the medial aspect of the uncinate process. Following the plane between the right lateral wall of the portal vein superior to the neck of the pancreas, the areolar tissue between the portal vein and the common duct is divided. This division permits further mobilization of the neck of the pancreas as it is apposed to the right lateral wall of the superior mesenteric and portal veins. One major and several small venous branches emerge from the posterior aspect of the neck of the pancreas and enter the portal or superior mesenteric vein. These veins are carefully isolated, divided between clamps, and ligated. This dissection facilitates visualization of the medial aspect of the uncinate process.

When gentle traction is applied to the divided segment of the distal common duct superi-

orly and the divided jejunum inferiorly, the uncinate process is further elevated and separated from the superior mesenteric and portal veins. The uncinate process is divided between paired clamps near the superior mesenteric artery (Fig. 89–68). The entire specimen is then removed. This can be the most difficult part of the procedure. The tributaries of the superior mesenteric artery and vein are so short that great care must be exercised while they are being clamped, divided, and ligated.

Reconstruction of Digestive Tract—Pancreaticojejunostomy. With use of interrupted silk sutures, the dorsal surface of the neck of the pancreas is sutured to the proximal jejunum. A small opening is made in the jejunum to permit precise mucosa-to-mucosa anastomosis between it and the duct of Wirsung (Fig. 89–69). A rubber catheter of appropriate size is inserted and anchored with a catgut suture

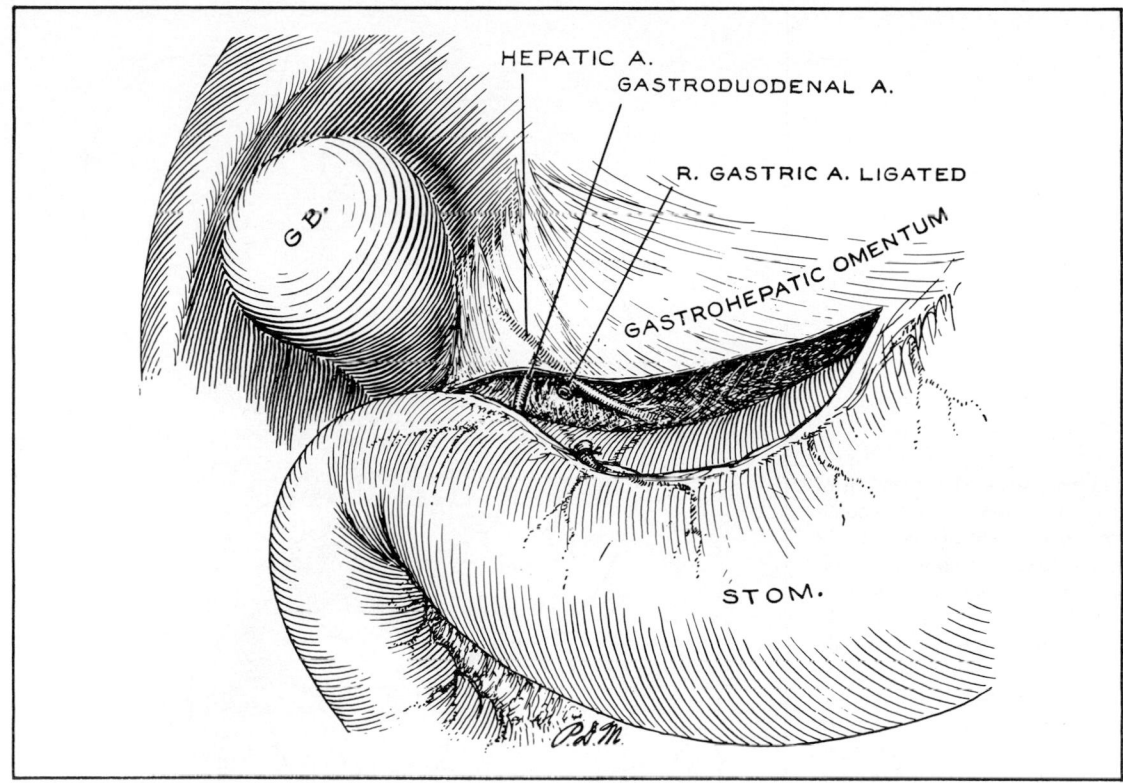

Figure 89–65. The distal 60 percent of the gastrohepatic omentum has been divided. The right gastric artery has been divided and ligated, exposing the courses of the hepatic and gastroduodenal arteries.

to the posterior wall of the divided duct of Wirsung. With the four sutures previously placed in the duct of Wirsung, the duct is precisely anastomosed to the opening made in the jejunum. The other end of the catheter previously placed in the pancreatic duct is brought out through an opening in the jejunum and exteriorized before the anterior ductal suture is tied. The anastomosis is completed by inserting a series of transverse silk mattress sutures, which approximates the anterior wall of the jejunum to the anterior surface of the neck of the pancreas.

Hepaticojejunostomy. After the posterior wall of the hepatic duct is apposed to the jejunum with interrupted silk sutures approximately 9 cm distal to the pancreaticojejunostomy, an opening is made in the anterior wall of the hepatic duct about 2 cm proximal to the anastomotic line. A T-tube, threaded on a

Bakes' dilator or grasped with a right-angle arterial clamp to facilitate its passage, is passed through the opening into the distal segment of the hepatic duct to splint the hepaticojejunostomy. The two-layer mucosa-to-mucosa anastomosis is completed in the same manner as pancreaticojejunostomy.

Gastrojejunostomy. The jejunum, 40 cm distal to the hepaticojejunostomy, is approximated to the posterior wall of the stomach with a layer of seromuscular sutures of fine silk. A longitudinal opening is made in the jejunum. The posterior–interior layers of jejunum and stomach are approximated with continuous interlocking suture of medium chromic catgut. This suture is continued anteriorly after the manner of Connell, approximating the anterior walls of the jejunum and stomach. This is reinforced with sutures of fine silk. The completed reconstruction of the digestive tract is shown in Figure

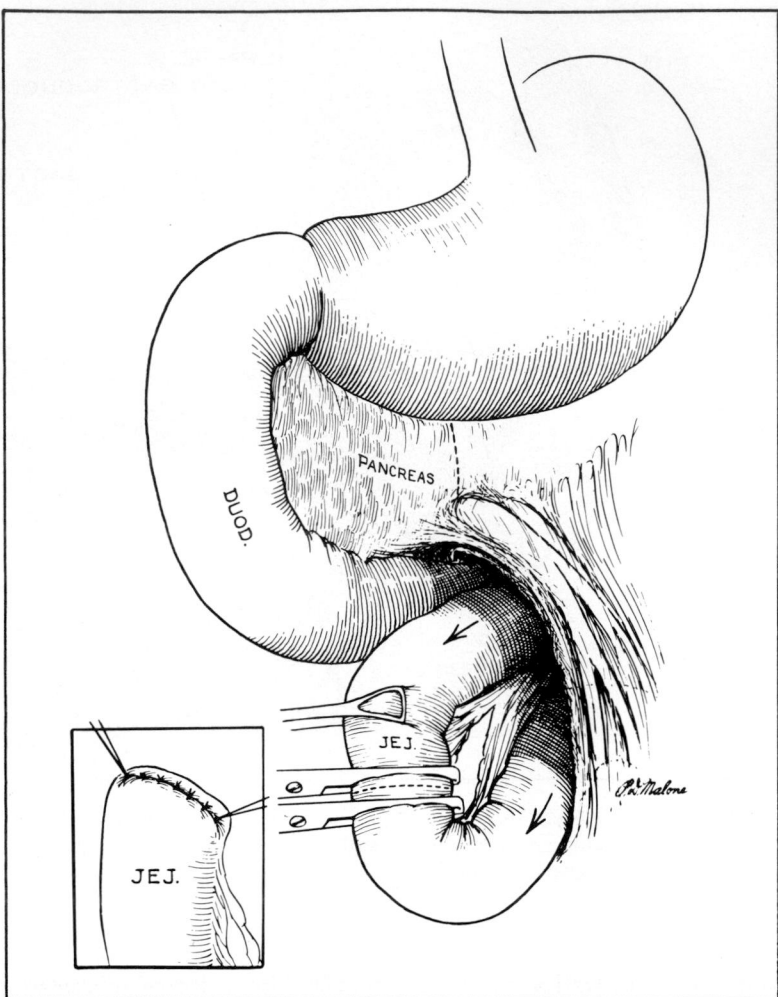

Figure 89–66. The ligament of Treitz has been incised beneath and to the right of the superior mesenteric artery and vein. The ventral and dorsal leaflets of Treitz have been incised superiorly to the uncinate process. The proximal jejunum has been drawn underneath the mesenteric vessels. Two branches of mesenteric vessels supplying the proximal jejunum have been divided and ligated. The jejunum is then divided between paired clamps. *Inset:* Distal stump of divided jejunum inverted. This inversion is accomplished with a continuous suture of fine catgut reinforced with interrupted sutures of fine silk.

89–70. Two sump drains and two Penrose drains are placed in Morison's pouch, and the sump drains are connected to wall suction.

POSTOPERATIVE CARE

Decompression. The stomach is decompressed by gastric suction, which is not discontinued immediately after normal peristalsis returns because continued decompression eliminates the gastric phase of pancreatic secretion. We find it expedient to continue nasogastric suction for approximately 5 to 7 days. The T-tube and pancreatic catheter drain dependently. Wound suction by way of sump drains is maintained for 5 to 7 days, and if biliary or pancreatic fistula occurs, wound suction is continued until the fistula is closed.

Fluid and Electrolyte Balance. During gastric drainage and until adequate oral intake is permissible, the fluid, nutritional, and electrolyte requirements are met by administration of appropriate quantities of glucose, saline, and amino acid solutions, supplemented by potassium chloride as required. Because of the preceding protein deficiency, it is wise not to give too much saline solution. We prefer to keep the serum chloride on the low side of normal. A feeding jejunostomy tube (T-tube) is inserted 40 cm distal to the gastrojejunostomy in the severely protein-depleted patient. The presence of this feeding tube is particularly valuable if emptying of the stomach is delayed or if a major biliary fistula occurs. A continuous infusion pump delivers a prepared formula at a constant

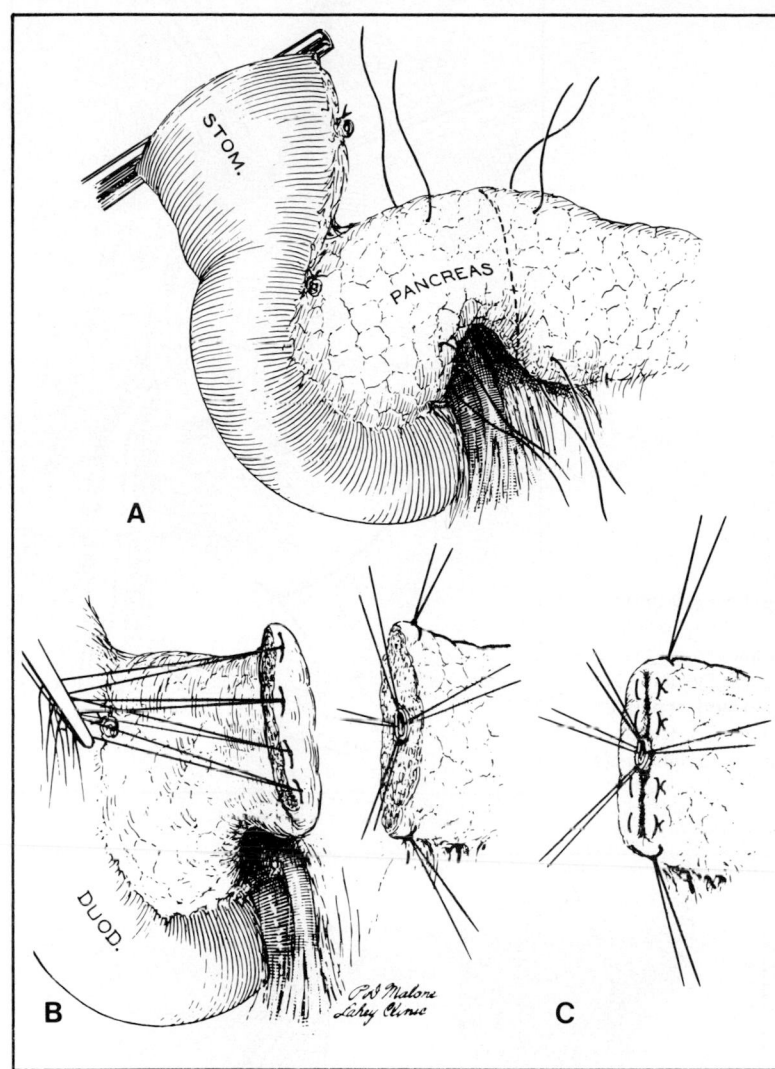

Figure 89–67. A. The superior and inferior longitudinal pancreatic arteries have been encircled with transfixion sutures of medium silk proximal and distal to the point where the pancreas will be divided. **B.** The neck of the pancreas has been divided. Four fine silk sutures have been placed one in each quadrant of the duct of Wirsung. The proximal divided end of the neck of the pancreas has been secured with four interrupted sutures of medium silk held in a single clamp for future traction. **C.** The cut surface of the pancreatic remnant is shown with four previously placed fine silk sutures in the duct of Wirsung. The divided end of the pancreatic remnant with the exception of the duct of Wirsung is compressed with several mattress sutures of medium silk.

rate. The formula contains 1.5 calories in each cubic centimeter. Intravenous hyperalimentation is frequently employed.

Blood Transfusions. As acute pancreatitis may be precipitated by operative trauma, the serum amylase, hemoglobin, and hematocrit are measured 4 and 24 hours after operation. The rate and strength of the pulse are carefully assessed. If the serum amylase is elevated significantly or if the pulse is rapid and weak, there is frequently excessive fluid loss into the peritoneal cavity, and 1 or 2 units of Plasmanate is given. The value of frequent blood transfusions in maintaining the occasional patient who will

have delayed opening of the GI stoma cannot be overemphasized.

Insulin. In the presence of diabetes mellitus, appropriate amounts of insulin are administered. Rarely, an apparently mild or latent preoperative diabetic state will become temporarily severe after excision of a large mass of pancreatic tissue. Diabetes may occur months or years after pancreatoduodenectomy.

Nutrition. When gastric decompression is discontinued, a liquid diet is given, and selected solid foods are added gradually. Replacement of exocrine pancreatic enzymes is frequently necessary and frequently neglected. Pancreatic

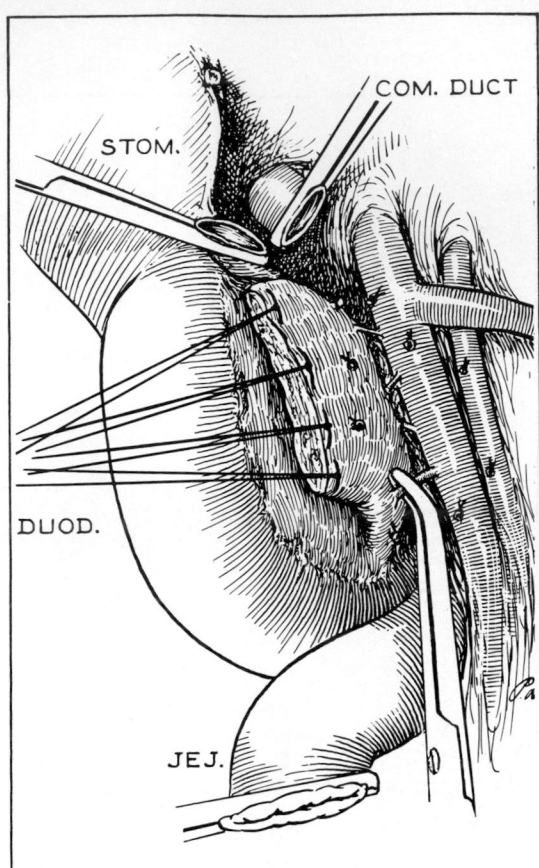

Figure 89–68. Small vessels entering the superior mesenteric and portal veins from the head of the pancreas have been divided and ligated. With traction on the divided common duct above and the divided jejunum below, the uncinate process is elevated and separated from the superior mesenteric and portal veins. The uncinate process will be divided between paired right angle clamps.

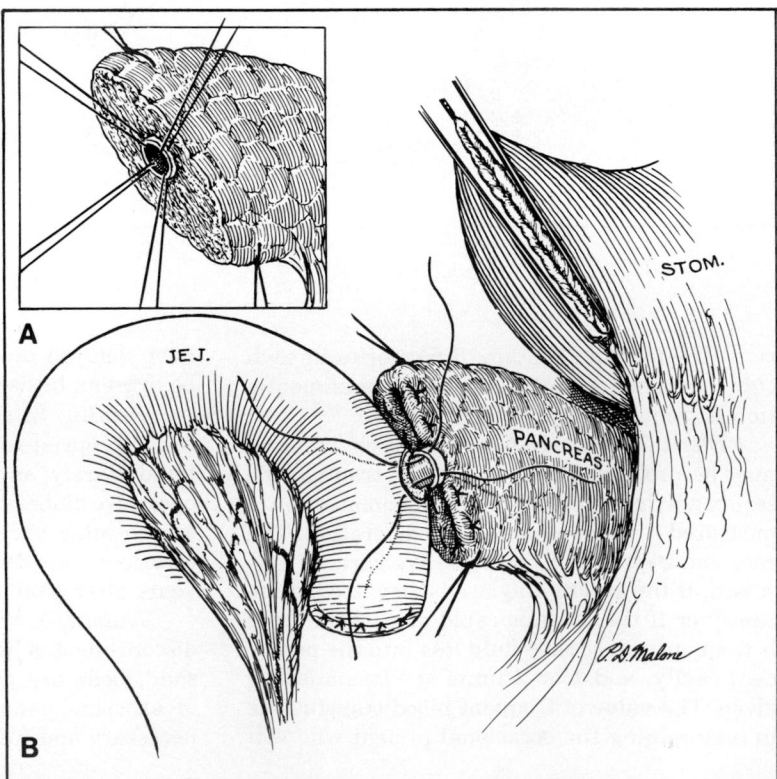

Figure 89–69. The proximal jejunum has been apposed to the posterior surface of the pancreatic remnant with interrupted medium silk sutures. An opening approximately the size of the caliber of the divided duct of Wirsung has been made in the jejunum. Precise mucosa-to-mucosa anastomosis of the duct of Wirsung to the jejunum is made with previously placed interrupted fine silk sutures. A segment of rubber catheter is usually used as stent in this anastomosis.

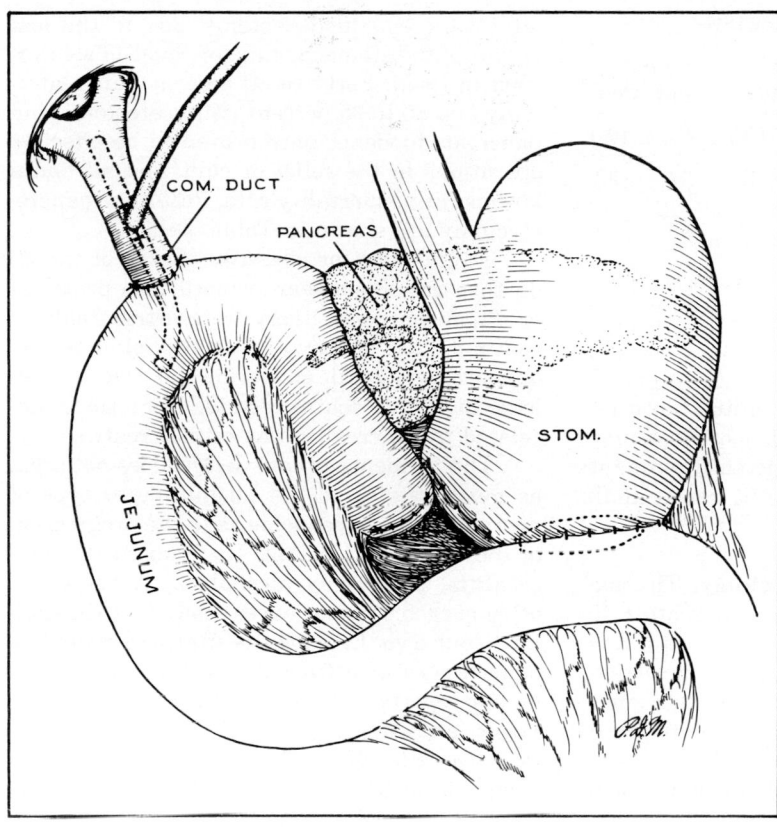

Figure 89–70. Completed reconstruction of the digestive tract. Note that the end-to-side pancreatojejunostomy is proximal to other anastomoses. The anterior wall of the jejunum has been approximated to the anterior surface of the pancreas with interrupted fine silk sutures. End-to-side hepaticojejunostomy has been constructed using a T-tube to splint the anastomosis. Hofmeister's gastrojejunostomy has been performed 40 cm distal to hepaticojejunostomy.

diarrhea is best controlled by allowing a moderate intake of fat and by the administration of pancreatin (Viokase or Pancrease), 15 to 20 g (900 to 1200 mg), with each meal. Vitamin K is administered as necessary. In severe degrees of malnutrition associated with excessive diarrhea, a typical sprue syndrome occurs and is treated with strict gluten-free diet. Dramatic results have been observed.

Antibiotics. An appropriate broad-spectrum antibiotic is administered.

Complications of Partial Pancreatectomy. Complications after proximal or distal pancreatic resection were common, the most frequent of which were intraabdominal abscess and short-lived pancreatic fistulas, which occurred in 25 percent and 11 percent of patients, respectively. Most abscesses were localized collections associated with the drain tract. There was no mortality associated with these collections, which seemed to represent the penalty associated with prolonged use of drains to deal with the frequently encountered transient leak-

age of pancreatic juice from the cut end of an obstructed ductal system. The incidence of peptic ulcer diathesis was highest after 80 to 95 percent distal resection of the pancreas. Vagotomy and pyloroplasty are recommended in association with 80 to 95 percent distal resection if a history of peptic ulcer diathesis or hypersecretion is evident during preoperative evaluation.

COMPLICATIONS OF PANCREATICODUODENECTOMY
Fistula. Leakage of the pancreaticojejunostomy causing a pancreatic fistula was the most common serious complication. Now, a pancreatic fistula is a rare complication. The essential requirement in the management of such a fistula is constant suction until the drainage ceases. Biliary fistula occurs when there is leakage at the choledochojejunal anastomosis. Continued suction drainage will allow this to heal.

Hemorrhage. Severe hemorrhage may occur at any time in the postoperative period, either through the drainage tracts or into the intestinal tract, causing hematemesis or melena.

TABLE 89–2. INCIDENCE OF DIABETES

Operation	Pre-operative No.	Pre-operative (%)	Post-operative No.	Post-operative (%)
40–80 percent distal resection	9	17	17	32
80–95 percent distal resection	22	28	56	72
Pancreatoduodenectomy	3	15	5	26

If the bleeding continues after initial blood replacement, surgical control of hemorrhage may be required. Removal of the pancreatic remnant for the control of hemorrhage is rarely indicated.

Results of Partial Pancreatectomy. The major difference in postoperative results after 40 to 80 percent distal resection of the pancreas in 53 patients and 80 to 95 percent resection in 77 patients was the much higher incidence and severity of diabetes in patients undergoing 80 to 95 percent distal resection (Table 89–2). Clinically troublesome steatorrhea was common

after pancreatoduodenectomy, due to the loss of half of the stomach, a major cause of steatorrhea in itself. Forty to 80 percent pancreatectomy and 80 to 95 percent pancreatectomy and pancreatoduodenectomy proved to be effective operations in the relief of pain, and all had a low operative mortality rate. Results of pancreatectomy are shown in Table 89–3.

Twenty two, or over two thirds, of the 30 deaths occurring a year or more after proximal or distal pancreatectomy were attributable to continued use of narcotics or alcohol or the sequelae of pancreatic endocrine and exocrine deficits. Eight late deaths resulted from causes unrelated to pancreatectomy or pancreatitis.

The incidence of late deaths does not seem as much related to the magnitude or type of operation and its sequelae as to the progression of the underlying disease that caused the pancreatitis, principally alcoholism. A review of other surgeons' experiences showed it to be similar to our own. Late deaths after pancreatoduodenectomy range from 22 to 50 percent based on our reports and those of Warren, Guillemin, Leger, and Mercadier et al. The incidence of late deaths for 80 to 95 percent distal resection ranges from 22 to 50 percent based on reports

TABLE 89–3. RESULTS OF PANCREATECTOMY

Result	Pancreato-duodenectomy (19 Patients) No.	Pancreato-duodenectomy (19 Patients) (%)	40–80% Distal Resection (55 Patients) No.	40–80% Distal Resection (55 Patients) (%)	80–95% Distal Resection (77 Patients) No.	80–95% Distal Resection (77 Patients) (%)
Alive						
Working well	9	47.4	29	54.7	38	49.4
Not working well	2	10.5	1	1.9	5	6.5
Not working—pain	—	—	1	1.9	1	1.3
Working—pain	—	—	—	—	1	1.3
Institutionalized (brain damage)	—	—	1	1.9	3	3.8
Converted to pancreatectomy	—	—	—	—	4	5.2
Lost to follow-up	5	26.3	12	22.6	4	5.2
Working well	—	—	10	18.9	3	4.0
Not working well	—	—	1	1.9	—	—
Not working—pain	—	—	—	—	1	1.0
Institutionalized	—	—	1	1.9	—	—
Operative deaths	1	5.3	1	1.9	1	1.3
Late deaths						
Not related to pancreatitis	1	5.3	4	7.5	9	11.7
In part due to pancreatitis	—	—	4	7.5	10	13.0
Institutionalized	1	5.3	—	—	—	—
Due to pancreatitis	—	—	—	—	1	1.3

from Frey, Weiland, and Leger, and the incidence of late deaths after longitudinal pancreaticojejunostomy ranges from 25 to 43 percent according to Leger, Way et al, Sato et al, and Prinz et al and 22 percent for distal pancreaticojejunostomy of DuVal. Much of the variation in the incidence of late deaths cited in these reports may, in part, be the result of differences in length of follow-up study.

In evaluating the results of operation for the relief of pain associated with chronic pancreatitis, relief of pain and a low operative mortality are goals that both proximal and distal pancreatectomy satisfy. However, particularly in the alcoholic patient, prevention of exocrine and endocrine insufficiency, if not already present (70 to 80 percent), deserves a high priority. To satisfy this precedence, all available diagnostic techniques should be used to localize the disease so that a decision can be made at operation as to whether it is most appropriate to excise the proximal or the distal pancreas. Eighty to 95 percent distal resection of the pancreas should be reserved for patients whose entire gland is diseased from head to tail. When the head or uncinate process is clearly more involved, pancreatoduodenectomy is preferable to 80 to 95 percent pancreatectomy in both removing the primary focus of disease and conserving pancreatic tissue. Although the importance of preserving pancreatic tissue and consequently pancreatic exocrine and endocrine function is emphasized, no proof exists that life is prolonged for the alcoholic even after longitudinal pancreaticojejunostomy in which tissue mass and function are not altered. In fact, despite the greater technical difficulty of performing 80 to 95 percent distal resection of the pancreas and the greater likelihood of making more patients diabetic and dependent on enzyme replacement after 80 to 95 percent distal resection than after longitudinal pancreaticojejunostomy, the operative mortality and incidence of late deaths are similar for both operations according to recent reports.

The observed differences in longevity between patients subjected to 80 to 95 percent distal pancreatectomy and longitudinal pancreaticojejunostomy may be observed due to unequal periods of follow-up, failure to use life tables, and the adequacy of follow-up care patients receive or permit.

Surgeons who embark on the operative management of patients with chronic pancreatitis should be prepared preoperatively to evaluate the emotional health of the patient as well as the structural changes present in the pancreas. The technical expertise of the operator is immediately important to the patient's survival, but the surgeon must also be committed to following up these patients for a period of years during which time emotional support and assistance to the patient in the management of diabetes, alcoholism, and any nutritional deficiencies may be required.

We had performed pancreatoduodenectomy in 148 patients before 1968, including 20 patients who had total pancreatectomy performed in one or two stages. Four patients died in the postoperative period (2.7 percent). No operative deaths occurred among the patients who had total pancreatectomy.

Of these 148 patients, 90 were operated on before June 1965; 82 had pancreatoduodenectomy and 8 had total pancreatectomy. Good or excellent results were obtained in approximately two thirds of patients treated with pancreatoduodenectomy, as shown in Table 89–4. Since 1968 an additional 27 pancreatoduodenectomies and 15 total pancreatectomies have been performed.

These figures show a low mortality rate and an improved rate of success in comparison with other operations advocated for the treatment of this devastating disease. Eighty one percent of our patients had previous unsuccessful operations for chronic relapsing pancreatitis; one third had sphincterotomy. Many of the patients who had unsatisfactory results after pancreatoduodenectomy were narcotic or alcohol addicts.

Therefore, we emphasize total care of the patient after pancreatic resection, including intensive and prolonged therapy for these addiction problems, either of which may be the determining factor in success or failure of surgery. In addition, we prescribe a proper diet, vitamins,

TABLE 89–4. RESULTS OF PANCREATODUODENECTOMY (148 PATIENTS)

Results	(%)
Excellent	35.4
Good	32.9
Poor	26.8
Hospital deaths	2.7
Unable to evaluate	2.4

and exocrine pancreatic enzymes and insulin, if necessary.

Total Pancreatectomy

We have performed 35 total pancreatectomies for end-stage chronic pancreatitis. Total pancreatectomy is a difficult technical procedure when performed for advanced chronic pancreatitis because of the extent of the acute and chronic inflammation. Despite the tedious dissection, only 1 death occurred in these 35 patients.

Although the mortality rate is acceptably low, the postoperative complications are numerous and frequently serious. Twenty six of these patients have been reported in a previous communication. The author has reported on life after total pancreatectomy for chronic pancreatitis and emphasized that this operation was feasible but was indicated only for far-advanced pancreatitis when other measures had failed and when there was no prospect of helping these patients with less extensive surgery.

In these 26 patients, only 3 had had no previous operative procedure for pancreatitis. The other 23 patients had had a total of 62 operations. Interestingly, 36 of these previous procedures were extrapancreatic, directed primarily at the biliary tract. The complications are listed in Table 89–5; delayed complications requiring readmission to the hospital are listed in Table 89–6. These complications are related primarily to the extent of the operation and the severity of the disease, but some are related to the pa-

TABLE 89–5. INHOSPITAL COMPLICATIONS AFTER PANCREATECTOMY (14 PATIENTS)

Complications	No.
Biliary fistula (1 patient reoperated)	4
Heart failure, ischemia, or arrhythmia	3
Pneumonia	2
Pulmonary insufficiency	2
Intraabdominal abscess	2
Urinary tract infection	2
Lower GI tract bleeding	1
Hypoglycemia and rib fracture	1
Skin wound infection	1
Ulnar neuropathy	1
Intraperitoneal hemorrhage	1
Septic phlebitis	1
Total	21

TABLE 89–6. REASONS FOR ADDITIONAL HOSPITALIZATIONS (24 PATIENTS)

Reason for Admission	No.
Control of diabetes	14
Upper GI tract bleeding	
Marginal ulcer	2
Esophagitis	1
Unknown	3
Abdominal pain	5
Myocardial infarction	4
Intraabdominal sepsis	4
Malabsorption, cachexia	4
Viral pneumonia	3
Depression	3
Wound hernia, suture abscess	3
Penetrating marginal ulcer	2
Thrombophlebitis	2
Stricture of choledochojejunostomy	1
Constipation	1
Rectal bleeding	1
Small bowel obstruction	1
Bile gastritis	1
Total	55

tient population. Many of these patients have been, or still are, chronic alcoholics. Practically all of them have been addicted to narcotics. As a result, they are not a well-disciplined group of persons.

Recently, we have made improvements in the care of these patients, particularly in terms of the control of their diabetes and their exocrine insufficiency. Twelve of the 26 patients have died. Four of the deaths were the result of related causes, and two were the result of possibly related causes.

Postoperative management of these patients, once they have resumed a reasonable caloric intake and are increasingly active, requires a bland diet. Patients tolerate midchain triglycerides better than fat. They require large doses of Viokase or Pancrease. The most important feature in the management of their diabetes is to avoid insulin reactions. It is much safer for these patients to register a blood sugar level of 150 mg/dl than it is to experience an insulin reaction.

Although total pancreatectomy for chronic relapsing pancreatitis can be performed with a low mortality rate, the operation is followed by serious complications. Therefore, it should be reserved for end-stage pancreatitis when other direct operations on the pancreas have failed.

Segmental Pancreatic Autotransplantation for Chronic Pancreatitis

In a recent personal communication, Rossi of the Lahey Clinic gave a brief summary of his and his colleagues' experiences with extensive (60 to 95 percent) distal pancreatectomy and segmental autotransplantation to the left femoral vessels. His informal description follows.

In seven of nine patients the operation was accomplished successfully, with "take" of the transplant. Follow-up varied from 2 weeks to 2.5 years. None of the seven patients with successful operations require insulin. Thrombosis of the graft in two patients necessitated removal of the graft. The patient who had 95 percent resection became an insulin-dependent diabetic, whereas the second patient had only a 60 percent (distal) resection and has not required any insulin.

Graft patency has been demonstrated in all patients by arteriography, and the production of insulin by the grafts was demonstrated by percutaneous selective venous assays that confirmed higher concentrations of insulin in the iliac vein of the transplanted side compared to that of the nontransplanted side. Although graft biopsies obtained during the late postoperative period (as long as 1 year) have shown fibrosis, many islet cells were seen in the biopsy specimen. We still do not know how long these grafts will function, but for the time being we believe we have prevented or delayed the onset of diabetes in these patients. Further studies are required to evaluate the long-term function of these grafts and to determine the functional characteristics of a heterotopically placed and denervated pancreas.

The procedure is not free of complications. Of the nine patients, five have had pancreatic graft fistulas in the groin despite administration of neoprene. In four of the five patients, these have been transient, with the problem lasting less than 1 month. In one patient small amounts drained intermittently for about 8.5 months. In one of the successful transplants, a groin infection during the early postoperative period was drained under local anesthesia. In one of the two patients whose transplants failed, infection and bleeding occurred in the early postoperative

period, requiring removal of the graft, angioplasty of the femoral artery, and rotation of the sartorius muscle to cover the angioplasty. We now routinely perform arteriography in all patients between the third and the fifth postoperative day, and if the graft has thrombosed we remove it before any complication, such as infection or bleeding, occurs.

When deterioration of the function of the graft because of fibrosis is seen during follow-up study of these patients, we may consider placing the graft in the iliac fossa, anastomosing it to the iliac vessels and leaving the pancreatic duct open and anastomosed to a Roux-Y loop.

BIBLIOGRAPHY

Appleby LH: Nonmalignant intrinsic stricture of pancreatic duct: Report of case. Arch Surg 63:115, 1951

Archibald E: Further data concerning the experimental production of pancreatitis. Ann Surg 74:426, 1921

Beall JII Jr, Bell JW, et al: Fatal acute hemorrhagic pancreatitis occurring simultaneously in identical twins. Gastroenterology 39:215, 1960

Brooks JR: Surgery of the Pancreas. Philadelphia: WB Saunders, 1983, p 182

Bockus HL (ed): Gastroenterology, vol 3. Philadelphia: WB Saunders, 1966

Bowers RF: Surgical therapy for chronic pancreatitis. Surgery 30:116, 1951

Bowers RF, Greenfield J: Choledochojejunostomy: Its role in treatment of chronic pancreatitis. Ann Surg 134:99, 1951

Cattell RB: Anastomosis of duct of Wirsung: Its use in palliative operations for cancer of head of pancreas. Surg Clin North Am 27:636, 1947

Cattell RB, Warren KW: Choice of therapeutic measures in management of chronic relapsing pancreatitis and pancreatolithiasis. Gastroenterology 20:1, 1952

Cattell RB, Warren KW: Surgery of the Pancreas. Philadelphia: WB Saunders, 1953

Child CG III, Fry WJ: Current status of pancreatectomies. Surg Clin North Am 42:1353, 1962

Child CG III, Frey CF, et al: A reappraisal of removal of ninety-five per cent of the distal portion of the pancreas. Surg Gynecol Obstet 129:49, 1969

Comfort MW, Steinberg AG: Pedigree of a family with hereditary chronic relapsing pancreatitis. Gastroenterology 21:54, 1952

Comfort MW, Gambill EE, et al: Chronic relapsing pancreatitis: A study of twenty-nine cases without associated disease of the biliary or gastro-intestinal tract. Gastroenterology 6:239, 376, 1946

Dean RH, Scott HW Jr, et al: Chronic relapsing pancreatitis in childhood: Case report and review of the literature. Ann Surg 173:443, 1971

Doubilet H: Treatment of recurrent pancreatitis by sphincterotomy, in Mulholland JH, Ellison EH, et al (eds): Current Surgical Management. Philadelphia: WB Saunders, 1957, p 35

Doubilet H: Sphincterotomy in the treatment of pancreatic pseudocysts, in Mulholland JH, Ellison EH, et al (eds): Current Surgical Management. Philadelphia: WB Saunders, 1957, p 43

Doubilet H, Mulholland JH: Recurrent acute pancreatitis: Observations on etiology and surgical treatment. Ann Surg 128:609, 1948

Doubilet H, Mulholland JH: Some observations on the treatment of trauma to the pancreas. Am J Surg 105:741, 1963

DuVal MK: Caudal pancreatico-jejunostomy for chronic relapsing pancreatitis. Ann Surg 140:775, 1954

DuVal MK: Discussion in Bartlett MK: Chronic pancreatitis. Am J Surg 109:113, 1965

DuVal MK, Enquist IF: The surgical treatment of chronic pancreatitis by pancreaticojejunostomy: An 8-year reappraisal. Surgery 50:965, 1961

Frey CF: The operative treatment of pancreatitis. Arch Surg 98:406, 1969

Frey CF: Personal communication, 1972

Frey CF: 95% pancreatectomy, in Carey L (ed): The Pancreas. St. Louis: CV Mosby, 1973

Frey CF: Distal subtotal pancreatectomy, in Malt RA (ed): Surgical Techniques Illustrated, vol 2. Boston: Little, Brown, 1977, p 75

Frey CF: Pancreatic pseudocyst—operative strategy. Ann Surg 188:652, 1978

Frey CF, Child CG 3d, et al: Pancreatectomy for chronic pancreatitis. Ann Surg 184:403, 1976

Fry WJ, Child CG 3rd: Ninety-five percent distal pancreatectomy for chronic pancreatitis. Ann Surg 162:543, 1965

Geevarghese PJ: Pancreatic Diabetes: A Clinico-Pathologic Study of Growth Onset Diabetes with Pancreatic Calculi. Bombay: Popular Prakashan, 1968, p 29

Gillesby WJ, Puestow CB: Surgery for chronic recurrent pancreatitis. Surg Clin North Am 41:83, 1961

Gillesby WJ, Puestow CB: Pancreaticojejunostomy for chronic relapsing pancreatitis: An evaluation. Surgery 50:859, 1961

Gross JB: Some recent developments pertaining to pancreatitis. Ann Intern Med 49:796, 1958

Gross JB, Comfort MW, et al: Abnormalities of serum and urinary amino acids in hereditary and nonhereditary pancreatitis. Trans Assoc Phys 70:127, 1957

Gross JB, Gambill EE, et al: Hereditary pancreatitis: Description of a fifth kindred and summary of clinical features. Am J Med 33:358, 1962

Hendren WH, Greep JM, et al: Pancreatitis in childhood: Experience with 15 cases. Arch Dis Child 40:132, 1965

Jones SA, Smith LL, et al: Sphincteroplasty for recurrent pancreatitis: A second report. Ann Surg 147:180, 1958

Leger L: Technique de la pancréato-jéjunostomie après pancréatectomie gauche pour pancréatite chronique. J Chir (Paris) 76:93, 1958

Maingot R: The recognition of and operations for chronic relapsing pancreatitis, in Maingot R (ed): Abdominal Operations, 6 edt. New York: Appleton-Century-Crofts, 1974, p 792

Mallet-Guy P, deBeaujeu MJ: Treatment of chronic pancreatitis by unilateral splanchnicectomy. Arch Surg 60:233, 1950

Mercadier M, Clot JP, et al: La triple dérivation dans les pancréatites chroniques. Ann Chir 28:473, 1974

Mixter CG Jr, Keynes WM, et al: Further experience with pancreatitis as a diagnostic clue to hyperparathyroidism. N Engl J Med 266:265, 1962

Nardi GL: Pancreatitis. N Engl J Med 268:1065, 1963

Opie EL: The relation of cholelithiasis to disease of the pancreas and to fat necrosis. Am J Med Sci 121:27, 1901

Priesel A: Beiträge zur Pathologie der Bauchspeicheldrüse mit besonderer Berücksichtigung adenomatöser Geschwulstbildungen, sowie der Autonomie der Langerhansschen Inseln. Frankfurt Ztschr f Path 26:453, 1921–1922

Prinz RA, Kaufman BH, et al: Pancreaticojejunostomy for chronic pancreatitis: Two- to 21-year follow-up. Arch Surg 113:520, 1978

Puestow CB: Chronic pancreatitis: Technique and results of longitudinal pancreatojejunostomy. Comptes Rendus XXI Congres de la Societe Internationale de Chirurgie, Bruxelles, 1965

Puestow CB: Chronic pancreatitis: Medical and surgical management. II. Surgical treatment by pancreaticojejunostomy. Hosp Pract 5:58, 1970

Puestow CB: Surgery of the Biliary Tract, Pancreas and Spleen, 4 edt. Chicago: Year Book, 1970, p 257

Puestow CB, Gillesby WJ: Longitudinal pancreatojejunostomy, in Ellison E, Friesen S, et al (eds): Current Surgical Management, vol 3. Philadelphia: WB Saunders, 1965, p 183

Rich AR, Duff GL: Experimental and pathological studies on pathogenesis of acute haemorrhagic pancreatitis. Bull Johns Hopkins Hosp 58:212, 1936

Rob C, Smith R (eds): Operative Surgery, 2 edt. London: Butterworths, 1969

Rousselot LM, Sanchez-Ubeda R, et al: Choledochoenterostomy in chronic relapsing pancreatitis: A study of five cases with prolonged follow-up observation. N Engl J Med 250:267, 1954

Sarles H, Sarles JC, et al: Chronic inflammatory sclerosis of the pancreas—an autonomous pancreatic disease. Am J Dig Dis 6:688, 1961

Sato T, Saitoh Y, et al: Appraisal of operative treatment for chronic pancreatitis: With special reference to side to side pancreaticojejunostomy. Am J Surg 129:621, 1975

Sensenig DM, Bowers RF: Retrograde pancreaticoenterostomy in experimental pancreatitis. Surgery 38:113, 1955

Smith R: Pancreatic resection for severe chronic pancreatitis. Acta Gastroenterol Belg 23:1031, 1960

Smith R: Basic Science and Pancreatic Surgery. Lettsonian Lecture. Transactions Med Soc London 84, 1968

Smith R: Strictures of the bile ducts. Proc R Soc Med 62:131, 1969

Smith R: Strictures of the bile ducts, in Badenoch J, Brooke BN (eds): Recent Advances in Gastroenterology, 2 edt. Baltimore: Williams & Wilkins, 1972, p 331

Smith R: Progress in the surgical treatment of pancreatic disease. Am J Surg 125:143, 1973

Stanley JC, Frey CF, et al: Major arterial hemorrhage: A complication of pancreatic pseudocysts and chronic pancreatitis. Arch Surg 111:435, 1976

Strum WB, Spiro HM: Chronic pancreatitis. Ann Intern Med 74:264, 1971

Thistlethwaite JR, Smith DF: Evaluation of sphincterotomy for the treatment of chronic recurrent pancreatitis. Ann Surg 158:226, 1963

Vernon JK, Stening F, et al: Chronic relapsing pancreatitis in childhood: A report of 3 cases. Br J Surg 57:906, 1970

Warren KW: The surgical exposure in the differential diagnosis of pancreatic disorders at operation. Surg Clin North Am 38:799, 1958

Warren KW: Pathologic considerations as a guide to the choice of surgical procedures in the management of chronic relapsing pancreatitis. Gastroenterology 36:224, 1959

Warren KW: Surgery of Pancreatic Disease. Modern Trends in Gastro-enterology. London: Butterworths, 1961, p 264

Warren KW: The management of chronic relapsing pancreatitis. Henry Ford Hosp Med Bull 14:143, 1966

Warren KW: Surgical management of chronic relapsing pancreatitis. Am J Surg 117:24, 1969

Warren KW, Cattell RD: Pancreatic surgery. N Engl J Med 261:280, 333, 387, 1959

Warren KW, Garabedian M: Surgical management of chronic relapsing pancreatitis. Hosp Pract 9:72, 1974

Warren KW, Mountain JC: Comprehensive management of chronic relapsing pancreatitis. Surg Clin North Am 51:693, 1971

Warren KW, Veidenheimer MC: Pathological considerations in the choice of operation for chronic relapsing pancreatitis. N Engl J Med 266:323, 1962

Warren KW, Poulantzas JK, et al: Life after total pancreatectomy for chronic pancreatitis: Clinical study of eight cases. Ann Surg 164:830, 1966

Way LW, Gadacz T, et al: Surgical treatment of chronic pancreatitis. Am J Surg 127:202, 1974

White TT: Pancreatitis. London: Edward Arnold, 1966

White TT, Keith RG: Long term follow-up study of fifty patients with pancreaticojejunostomy. Surg Gynecol Obstet 136:353, 1973

Wittingen J, Frey CF: Islet concentration in the head, body, tail and uncinate process of the pancreas. Ann Surg 179:412, 1974

90. Insulin Tumors and Apudomas

Stanley R. Friesen

INTRODUCTION

A general characteristic of endocrine tumors is that they produce systemic effects in patients because of humoral elaboration of hormones even from small hyperfunctioning tumors. The resulting syndromes may be recognized clinically, especially if the presentation is fulminant; in other instances the clinical picture may be obscure or even silent, often attributed to "nonfunctioning" endocrinopathies.

Pathologic Features of Endocrinopathies

The dysplasias of neuroendocrine cells that hypersecrete humoral agents include hyperplasia and neoplasia, benign and malignant. In addition, neoplasms that have the histologic appearance of carcinoid tumors are also known to elaborate humoral substances. Other features of endocrinopathies include the cytologic presence of cytoplasmic secretory granules, the proximity of the cells to a capillary membrane into the circulating blood stream by emiocytosis, and an affinity of the secreted hormone or transmitter to specific receptors on end-organ target cells where a specific biologic activity is set in motion. Either interruption or accentuation at any point in the above sequence of events may alter normal physiologic balance or the clinical presentation of patients having hyperfunctioning dysplasias. The implication of such alterations in the chain of endocrine events on diagnosis is evident with the use of stimulation and suppression tests; the implication for therapy is obvious with the use of inhibitors of hormone release and receptor blockade.

Because of the role of neuroendocrine cells in the control and regulation of physiologic homeostasis, it is important to note that pathologic hyperplasias that hyperfunction still generally respond to their environment (stimulation or suppression) in a normal fashion; contrarily, hyperfunctioning neoplasias either function autonomously of their milieu or respond in a paradoxical manner. An insulinoma, for instance, autonomously hypersecretes insulin and fails to demonstrate suppression of insulin output in response to a falling blood glucose level on fasting. An example of a paradoxical response to stimulation is observed when a tumor gastrinoma responds to secretin stimulation by increased release of gastrin, instead of a diminished gastrin response of normal antral gastrin cells. Endocrine tumors usually cannot be judged to be benign or malignant on histologic examination, except for the presence or absence of invasion or metastases. Neuroendocrine characteristics can be identified by the demonstration of secretory granules by electron microscopy; their functional capabilities can be demonstrated pathologically by histochemical immunoperoxidase studies and by immunofluorescent techniques. Malignant tumors often contain multiple peptides and have the potential for multihormonal activity.

Endocrine tumors may occur sporadically or may be instigated by genetic abnormalities. Sporadic tumors usually occur singly without pattern; genetically-induced tumors are often multiple, being characterized by the presence of multiple cells in multiple tumors (or hyperplasias) in multiple organ systems in multiple members of affected families. In the instance of the genetic multiple endocrine adenopathy syndrome, type I (MEA I), the organs predictably involved are the pituitary, parathyroids, and pancreas.

Functional Features of Endocrinopathies

Hyperfunctioning tumors have been found in almost every organ of the body, but of course they are preponderant in neuroendocrine tissues and organs. The tumors are considered to function entopically if they are located in the organ that normally secretes the hormone in question. Hence, an insulinoma of the pancreas is considered to function entopically because the normal pancreas secretes insulin from its β-cells. On the other hand, a neoplasm of the pancreatic islets is considered to be functioning ectopically, if it is elaborating hormones that are not native to that organ, for example the abnormal secretion of gastrin. Tumors that function in an ectopic manner are usually, but not always, malignant; insulinomas are usually, but not always, benign. The entopic tumors of the pancreas are insulinoma, glucagonoma, somatostatinoma, pancreatic polypeptidoma, and the carcinoid tumor. Islet cell tumors that function ectopically include those that elaborate gastrin, corticotrophin, melanocyte-stimulating-hormone, a parathyroid-like peptide, vasoactive intestinal peptide, growth hormone, or potentially any of the other polypeptide hormones.

Neuroendocrine tumors secrete three types of hormones: steroids, polypeptides, and amines. The steroid-secreting tumors are found in tissues originating in the embryonic mesoderm. The protein-secreting tumors that elaborate the polypeptides and the amines originate in cells that have the same cytochemical characteristics of neuroectodermal cells. The common cytochemical characteristics shared by neuroendocrine cells of brain and gut have given rise to an acronym (APUD) denoting their capability for Amine Precursor Uptake and Decarboxylation. Normal neuroendocrine cells and tumor cells demonstrating these characteristics are called APUD cells and APUDomas; the conceptual understanding of their potentialities is often referred to as the APUD concept.

There is a controversy regarding the embryologic origin of neuroendocrine cells that have APUD function. There is good experimental evidence both for and against the origin or migration of these cells from the neuroectoderm to the entoderm, e.g., lungs and gut, but the embryologic question is moot because it is apparent that APUD cells, irrespective of their habitat in endocrine, neural, or epithelial tissues, have cytochemical characteristics in common; they function by elaborating protein hormones or transmitters and affect target cells by endocrine, paracrine, or neurocrine stimulation. Moreover, tumor cells of the APUD system, including islet cell tumors, pheochromocytomas and oat-cell tumors of the lung, contain an enzyme, neuron-specific enolase, a finding not demonstrable in non-neuroectodermal tissues. There are recent reports of epithelial tumors not in endocrine organs that have developed endocrine function and contain cells with APUD characteristics; it has been suggested that the malignant cells in such instances have dedifferentiated to stem cells that have adopted neuroendocrine function. Another physiologic concept that is clinically useful is to understand that most hormonal polypeptides are paired, having antithetical functions. For instance, insulin and Glucagon have opposite effects on carbohydrate metabolism, and as an added homeostatic safeguard, glucose metabolism is further regulated by another islet polypeptide, somatostatin, which inhibits, by paracrine activity, the release of both insulin and glucagon.

Finally, the function of tumors can be qualitatively determined by appropriate bioassays and more importantly, their degree of hyperfunction may be quantitatively measured by radioimmunoassay as peptide concentrations in tissues and in plasma. Sophistication of diagnostic function can be enhanced by the use of provocation tests that demonstrate abnormal stimulation and suppression of peptide release.

INSULIN-SECRETING TUMORS

History

The majority of cells that secrete polypeptides are located in the gastroenteropancreatic (GEP) system. This diffuse distribution of clear cells was first described by Feyrter in 1938 and this system constitutes the largest neuroendocrine conglomerate in the body. The pancreatic component consists of clumps of islet cells described as islands by Langerhans in 1869 in his inaugural anatomic dissertation as a student. The relationship of the islets to glucose metabolism was suggested by Minkowski in 1889 from his observations of sweet glucose in the urine of dogs after pancreatectomy. However, actual humoral products from this area in the GEP were not postulated until 1902 and 1905 when Bayliss, Starling, and then Edkins demonstrated duodenal secretin and antral gastric secretin (gastrin) as secretogogues. Single adenomas of the pancreas were observed by Neve and by Nichols in 1891 and 1902, respectively, and multiple islet adenomas were described by Lang in 1925. Laidlaw documented nesidioblastosis of the pancreas in 1938.

As is often the case, the clinical picture associated with hypoglycemia as possibly related to islet tumors was not recognized until after the discovery of insulin by Banting et al in 1922 when overdosage of insulin was observed in early clinical trials. Harris, in 1924, suggested the possibility of a clinical syndrome from the excess production of insulin; this was substantiated by Wilder et al in 1925 in a patient with a malignant islet cell tumor, operated upon by W.J. Mayo. The first successful operation for the removal of a benign insulinoma was done by Roscoe Graham, reported by Howland in 1929. The classic Whipple's triad for the clinical diagnosis was based on a study of 35 patients operated on in 1935. Twenty years later, the first instances of a causal relationship between islet cell adenomas and another syndrome, the ulcerogenic gastrinoma syndrome, was reported by Zollinger and Ellison; this clinical observation was made 50 years after Edkins postulated gastrin from the antrum. The islet tumor source of gastrin was soon recognized as an ectopic phenomenon; an entopic antral source of hypergastrinemia has since been described as Pseudo-Zollinger–Ellison syndrome. Clinical observations, past and present, have prompted a virtual explosion of investigations within the basic sciences.

Among these fundamental revelations, a most important technique for the quantitative measurement of circulating plasma immunoreactive insulin was developed by Yalow and Berson. This seminal event led to similar techniques for other polypeptides and for their identification in normal and abnormal tissues, such as McGuigan's studies for gastrin cells in the antral mucosa and in gastrinomas. The characterization of gastrin molecules by Gregory and Tracy led to similar identification of other peptides. Finally, it was the development of the

APUD concept by Pearse that led to a better understanding of neuroendocrinopathies.

Pathology

There are no known precursor states leading to the sporadic development of insulinomas; the less common familial pattern of genetic instigation is observed as an autosomal dominant trait in MEA, type I (Wermer's syndrome). The penetrance is variable, however, so that islet cell involvement in MEA I more commonly surfaces as a gastrinoma than as an insulinoma or a pancreatic polypeptide apudoma.

In contrast to other islet cell dysplasias, the pathologic lesion associated with organic hyperinsulinism is preponderantly (at least 75 percent) a benign, single adenoma. The usually small (1 to 2 cm) insulinoma functions entopically and may occur in any part of the pancreas; the location of the insulinomas is evenly distributed throughout the gland. Occasionally an insulinoma is found in an aberrant location, such as in the hilus of the spleen. Ectopically functioning tumors that secrete insulin or insulin-like substances are exceedingly rare, reported only in the adrenal, liver, lung, kidney, ovary, cervix, gastrointestinal (GI) tract, and in mesodermal tissues. The latter tumors, which include large fibrous mesotheliomas and fibrosarcomas, are more frequent than the former. Extraction of these tumors has been shown to demonstrate an insulin-like activity on bioassay, but not on immunoassay; the humoral substance is probably a somatomedin and not insulin.

Multiple sites of islet hypersecretion of insulin may take the form of metastatic islet cell carcinomas, multiple adenomas, microadenomas, islet cell hyperplasia, and nesidioblastosis in decreasing incidence. The hypoglycemia of infancy is usually due to diffuse islet cell hyperplasia; adenomas occur most frequently in the second to fourth decades of life and malignancies in older patients. Microadenomas and nesidioblastosis are often described in patients affected with MEA I, but the frequency of these diagnoses may depend also on the experience and bias of the pathologist.

The functional potential of these β-cell dysplasias can be recognized as insulin secretors by usual techniques: electron microscopy demonstrates irregular shaped secretory granules; histochemical and immunochemical techniques illustrate the affinity for antiinsulin antibody, and tissue extracts demonstrate insulin concentration by radioimmunoassay and hypoglycemic effects by bioassay. Malignant insulin-secreting tumors secrete a higher proportion of proinsulin than do benign insulinomas.

Clinical Manifestations

The symptoms and signs related to the autonomous secretion of insulin by any of the β-cell dysplasias are triggered by hypoglycemia. Hypoglycemia sufficient to initiate symptoms in these patients occurs in the fasting state, usually before breakfast or when a meal is missed, and it may be provoked by exertion when glucose is catabolized. Whipple's diagnostic triad is usually, but not always, present and consists of symptoms associated with a blood sugar value of less than 50 mg/dl relieved by the ingestion of carbohydrates.

Two mechanisms for the production of symptoms exist, depending upon the rapidity of the fall in blood sugar. When the fall in blood sugar is slow, the symptomatology is due to cerebral dysfunction (disorientation, "black-out spells," proceeding even to coma) and is related to neuroglucopenia; the brain is dependent upon glucose for its energy requirements. When the fall in blood sugar is more rapid, the second mechanism comes into play. In this instance the hypoglycemic stimulation of catecholamine release from the autonomic nervous system produces symptoms of trembling, sweating, palpitations, nervousness, and hunger. The catecholamine release also stimulates glycogenolysis which tends to raise the blood sugar level in a compensatory manner and may even terminate the attack spontaneously. Patients soon learn that attacks can be ameliorated or aborted by frequent eating, which not infrequently proceeds to the development of obesity. On the other hand, prolonged and repeated attacks with unconsciousness, if untreated, may eventually result in brain damage.

Diagnostic Studies

The symptoms that are provoked by "organic hypoglycemia" and inappropriate hyperinsulinism must be differentiated diagnostically from

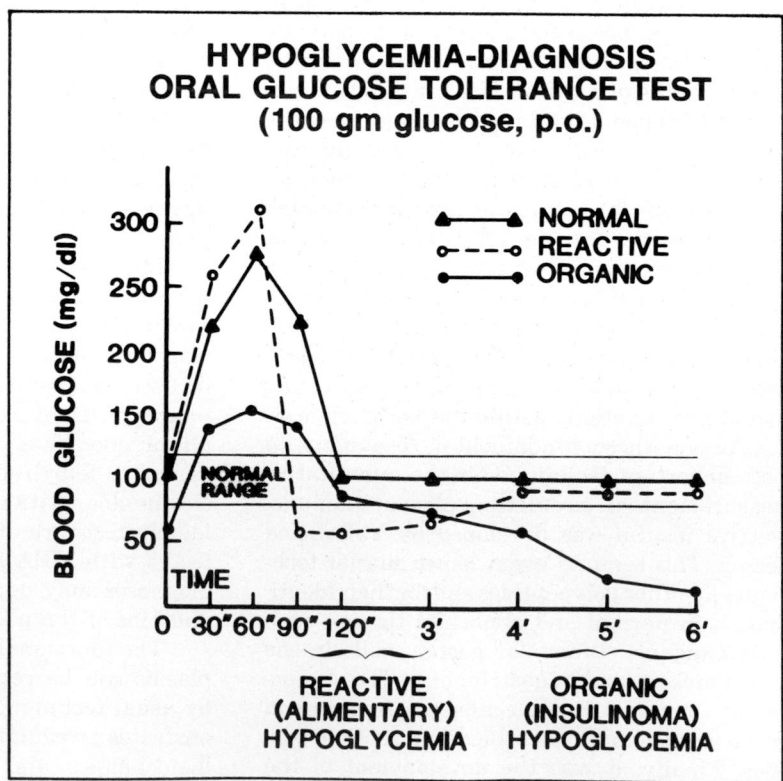

Figure 90–1. Reactive hypoglycemia can usually be differentiated from organic hypoglycemia by noting that the symptoms with moderate reactive hypoglycemia occur early (within 90 minutes after ingestion of carbohydrates) as contrasted to the late (5 to 6 hour) nadir of severe hypoglycemia in patients with an insulinoma.

other causes of hypoglycemia. The most common type of hypoglycemia that requires consideration is called reactive or alimentary hypoglycemia. Such patients have a highly sensitive insulin response reacting to the normal hyperglycemia after eating (or after glucose administration in an oral glucose tolerance test). This reactive type of hypoglycemia is accentuated in patients who have rapid gastric emptying after operations that destroy the pylorus. The characteristic clinical feature of reactive hypoglycemia is that symptoms and moderate hypoglycemia occur approximately 1 to 3 hours after ingestion, rather than at 5 to 6 hours in the fasting state of organic hypoglycemia (Fig. 90–1). These hypoglycemic symptoms should not be confused with the dumping syndrome in which symptoms characteristic of hypovolemia occur within 20 minutes after the ingestion of a hyperosmolar meal (Fig. 90–2). Another misleading diagnosis

to be ruled out is factitious or iatrogenic hyperinsulinism in which hidden injection equipment should be searched for; additionally, studies to demonstrate the absence of bovine insulin antibodies (from prior injections) and the presence of C-chain insulin molecules, tend to rule out the factitious etiology. Diagnoses of intoxication with alcohol or barbiturates, which mimic hypoglycemic symptoms, are sometimes made erroneously in patients who have insulin tumors. Organic causes of hypoglycemia, other than insulin-secreting tumors, include severe liver disease, hypofunction of the anterior pituitary or adrenal gland, and large mesenchymal tumors, as mentioned above. Physical examination and routine x-rays may assist in ruling out other causes of hypoglycemia, but they rarely are helpful in the diagnosis of an insulin-secreting tumor unless hepatic metastases from an insulin-secreting malignancy are detected.

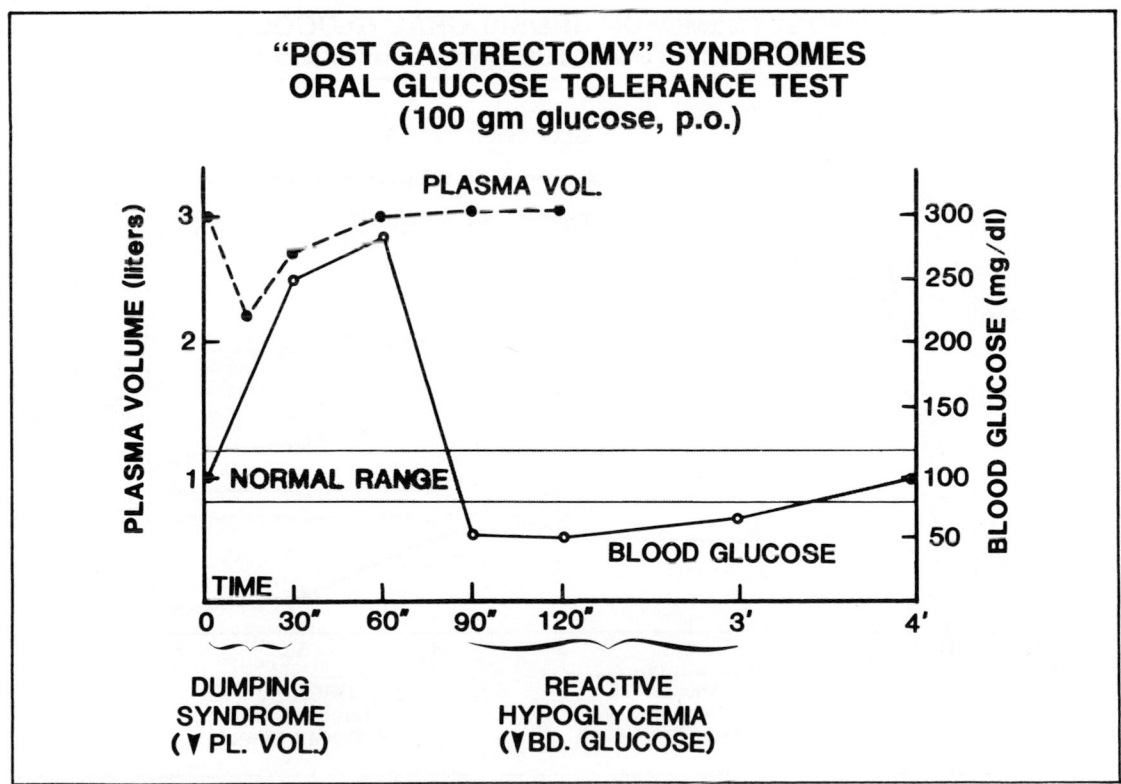

Figure 90–2. The symptoms of reactive hypoglycemia that usually occur about 90 minutes after ingestion of carbohydrates can be differentiated from the symptoms due to relative hypovolemia of the dumping syndrome which occur without hypoglycemia within 20 minutes after ingesting hyperosmolar carbohydrates in patients after distal gastrectomy or pyloroplasty.

Diagnostic Confirmation

When other causes of hypoglycemia are ruled out, it is necessary to confirm a diagnosis of organic hyperinsulinism before treatment is instituted. An oral glucose tolerance test is of little value in establishing a diagnosis unless it is a 6-hour test that demonstrates a late 5th or 6th hour glucose nadir associated with measured hyperinsulinism (Fig. 90–3). Whether or not a glucose tolerance test is performed, simultaneous measurements, preferably at the time of symptoms, of blood glucose and plasma immunoreactive insulin (IRI) are important. Usually these determinations are performed during a prolonged 24- to 48-hour fast which constitutes the best provocative confirmatory test for an insulinoma. Blood is drawn simultaneously for glucose and IRI at 6-hour intervals and especially at the time when symptoms are definitely

present, after which the test is terminated by the administration of glucose. The test is based on observations of departures from normal physiologic responses to fasting hypoglycemia. The normal β-cell is responsive to its intracellular glucose concentration. An increased glucose concentration stimulates insulin release and a decreased concentration suppresses it. During fasting, even in a normal individual, glucose is continually being used by the brain, erythrocytes, and other tissues during physical activity; the resulting fall in blood sugar suppresses β-cell secretion of insulin so that plasma IRI also falls normally and may become undetectable. In patients with an autonomously secreting insulinoma, the normal suppression of insulin secretion is not observed; the insulin level remains inappropriately high for the concurrent hypoglycemia of values often less than 40 mg/dl (Fig. 90–4). A reliably diagnostic feature is an inap-

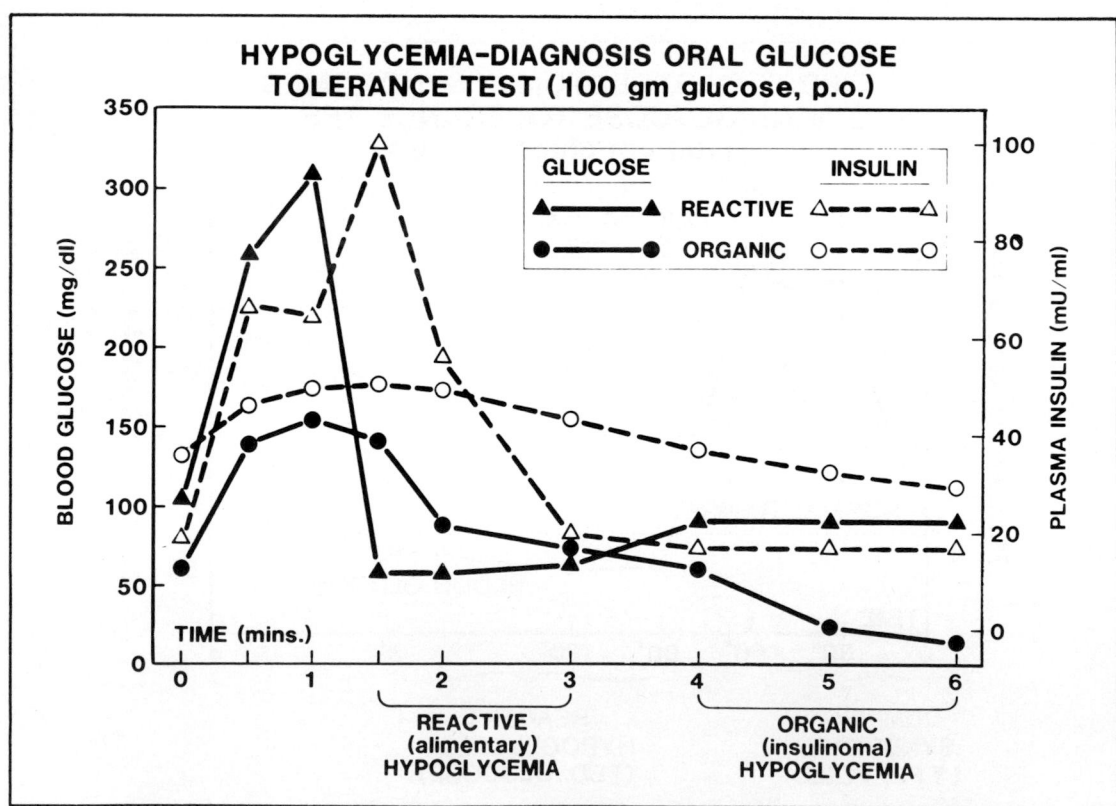

Figure 90–3. The simultaneous measurements of blood glucose and immunoreactive insulin further differentiate reactive from organic hypoglycemia. In addition to the late nadir of blood glucose in a 6-hour oral glucose tolerance test, an inappropriately high level of insulin is observed in patients with insulinoma.

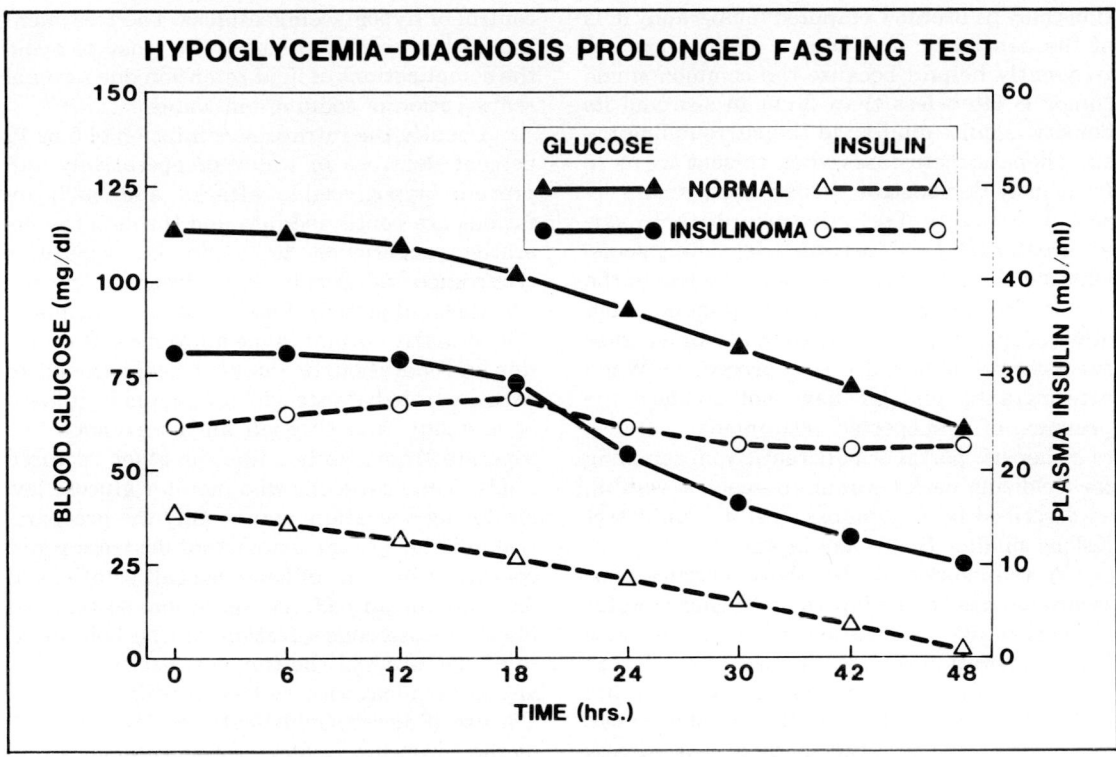

Figure 90–4. The prolonged fast with simultaneous determinations of blood glucose and immunoreactive insulin is the most reliable provocative test for insulinoma. The normal response to fasting is that of a decreasing blood glucose level without severe hypoglycemia during which insulin secretion is suppressed to almost undetectable levels. This response is contrasted to that usually observed in patients with an autonomously secreting insulinoma in whom the insulin level remains inappropriately elevated in the presence of progressive hypoglycemia with concurrent development of symptoms. The ratio of the numerical values of insulin to glucose concentrations that exceeds 0.3 is diagnostic of insulinoma.

propriately high ratio (> 0.3) of plasma IRI (in microunits per milliliter) to blood glucose (in milligrams per deciliter) during prolonged fasting. Most insulinoma patients will develop symptoms within the 24-hour fast, but occasionally it is necessary to prolong the test for 48 or even 72 hours.

Because of the apparent proclivity for calcium to enhance emiocytosis and/or secretion of polypeptides from APUD cell tumors, Kaplan et al have described its use as a provocative test for insulinomas. Stimulation by intravenous calcium gluconate produced hypoglycemia and an increase in IRI in nine of ten patients with tumors, but not in those without tumors. Other diagnostic tests for insulinoma, such as the tolbutamide and arginine tests, have not proved to be uniformly helpful. However, it is useful to determine preoperatively whether insulin secretion from an insulinoma or its malignant counterpart is suppressible by the administration of diazoxide. If it is determined that diazoxide will suppress insulin and elevate blood sugar in the patient, it can then be available for subsequent use therapeutically if it becomes necessary in the event of nonresectability of the tumor.

Tumor Localization

Extensive preoperative localization studies are not universally employed unless surgical exploration has failed to identify the insulinoma. In such patients or in those unoperated patients in whom there are additional reasons for confirmation of a tumor diagnosis, further investigations may be useful. Computed tomography (CT) of the pancreatic and hepatic regions are not frequently helpful because the common single tumor is often less than 2 cm in size and its density is quite similar to the surrounding tissues; hepatic metastases when present are more frequently demonstrated than the primary lesion. The success of selective arteriography varies greatly (16 to 95 percent), depending somewhat on the technique used and the size of the tumor. Insulinomas are more vascular than other islet tumors and this accounts for a higher success rate of this invasive procedure. When arteriography and CT have not divulged the presence of a suspected insulinoma, selective transhepatic portal or pancreatic vein sampling for localizing peaks of immunoreactive insulin, as described by Ingemansson et al, can detect lesions smaller than 1 cm in size.

A refinement of the above percutaneous technique has been adapted by Turner et al for intraoperative localization of occult tumors. During operation venous samples from different areas draining the pancreas are obtained and the insulin concentration in the samples is measured by a special rapid method. The success of this method (localization of seven of eight insulin tumors) is obviously dependent upon the ready availability of the rapid method and its use has further implications for the intraoperative detection of second or multiple tumors after excision of one.

Management

The definitive treatment of insulin-secreting islet cell tumors is surgical excision when possible, as is the case with most endocrinopathies. The clinical and laboratory diagnosis of a possible insulinoma should be secure before operation. Both the patient and the surgeon must have an awareness of the possible pathologic entities and proposed options of treatment for each.

Preoperative Care. Depending on the condition of the patient, ease of preoperative control of hypoglycemic attacks, and the presence or absence of associated diseases that require clarification, the preparation of the patient may involve short-term treatment with diazoxide. The initial dosage is 15 mg every 8 hours, but in some patients it may be necessary to increase the dosage to as much as 500 mg/day to obtain

control of hypoglycemic attacks. The treatment should be monitored closely in order to avoid the complications of fluid retention due to renal reabsorption of sodium and water.

Usually the intravenous infusion of 5 or 10 percent dextrose in water preoperatively will prevent hypoglycemic attacks and such infusions are continued into and through the operative experience to avoid intraoperative occurrence of occult hypoglycemia in the anesthetized patient. Blood glucose levels maintained in the normal range allow for safe induction and operation. In order to better accomplish carbohydrate balance, glucose should be infused at a steady rate through an intravenous line separate from another line for other required fluids. Some surgeons who monitor glucose levels during operation, may modify the preoperative infusions to the extent that dextrose is discontinued in favor of balanced salt solutions at 6:00 AM (for an 8:00 AM operation) so that the blood glucose concentration can be held at 60 to 80 mg/dl until the tumor is excised so that any subsequent rise will be readily apparent. The use of newer sophisticated equipment, such as the Biostator system,* for continuous monitoring now allows safer control at normal glucose concentrations.

Intraoperative Management

It is agreed that safe conduct of the operation is enhanced by close monitoring of glucose levels for dextrose or insulin requirements. However, there is no universal agreement as to the reliability of glucose monitoring for accurate indications of complete removal of hypersecretory tumors. It is generally believed that following removal of an insulinoma, a prompt rise in the blood glucose level indicates that the tumor is a solitary one, successfully removed. It should be realized, however, that a prompt rise does not always occur. Harrison et al have shown that there may be no demonstrable difference in the rate of the rise of blood glucose whether or not occult hyperfunctioning tissue remains in the patient. According to Tutt et al, a lack of hyperglycemic rebound within 90 minutes after excision of an insulinoma should not be used as a criterion to proceed further with blind distal pancreatectomy.

Because the goal of operation is to search for, locate, and remove all hyperfunctioning in-

---

* Biostator system, Miles Laboratories, Elkhart, Indiana.

sulin tissue that often is small in size, every effort should be made to expedite exposure with an adequate incision. Excessive time and trauma during operation tend to disrupt carbohydrate–insulin balance in these patients; for these reasons, a generous upper midline abdominal incision is favored over the more traditional bilateral "bucket handle" transverse incision. Early in the exploration of the peritoneal cavity particular attention is given to rule out retroperitoneal mesotheliomas and metastatic deposits in the liver.

Initial inspection of the left anterior pancreas can be done easily by dividing the thin gastrohepatic membrane. Also, quick inspection of the inferior margin of the body of the pancreas can be made from the inferior colic approach, but the thorough exploration that is eventually necessary anyway, is made via the gastrocolic omentum. Most surgeons prefer to enter the lesser omental sac by dividing the gastrocolic omentum just inferior to the gastroepiploic vessels (Fig. 90–5). Care should be taken to maintain the blood supply to the omentum from each of the lateral margins. If the omentum is large and bulky in these patients who tend to be obese, an alternative approach to the lesser sac is to separate the omentum from the transverse colon at its avascular attachment.

Inspection of the anterior surface of the entire pancreas is now possible. The color of insulinomas ranges from reddish brown to pink or light tan; they may not be visible on the surface at all. However, insulinomas are almost always discernable on palpation by the experienced surgeon who provides additional exposure of both the anterior and posterior aspects of the pancreas. For the head of the pancreas, the Kocher

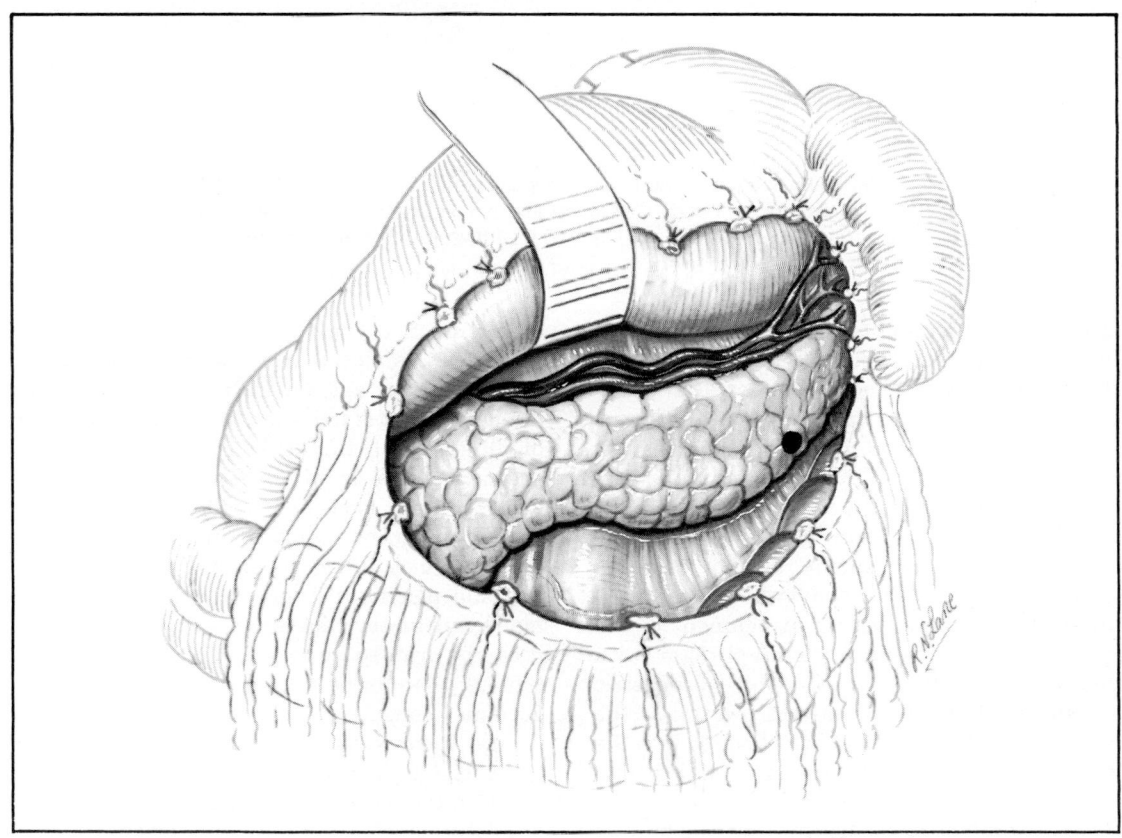

Figure 90–5. Good exposure of the anterior surface of the body and tail of the pancreas is accomplished through the gastrocolic omentum, care being taken to preserve the blood supply to the omentum at its lateral attachments to the gastroepiploic vessels. (Drawing done during operation, R. Maingot's patient.) (*Source: From LeQuesne LP, 1980, with permission.*)

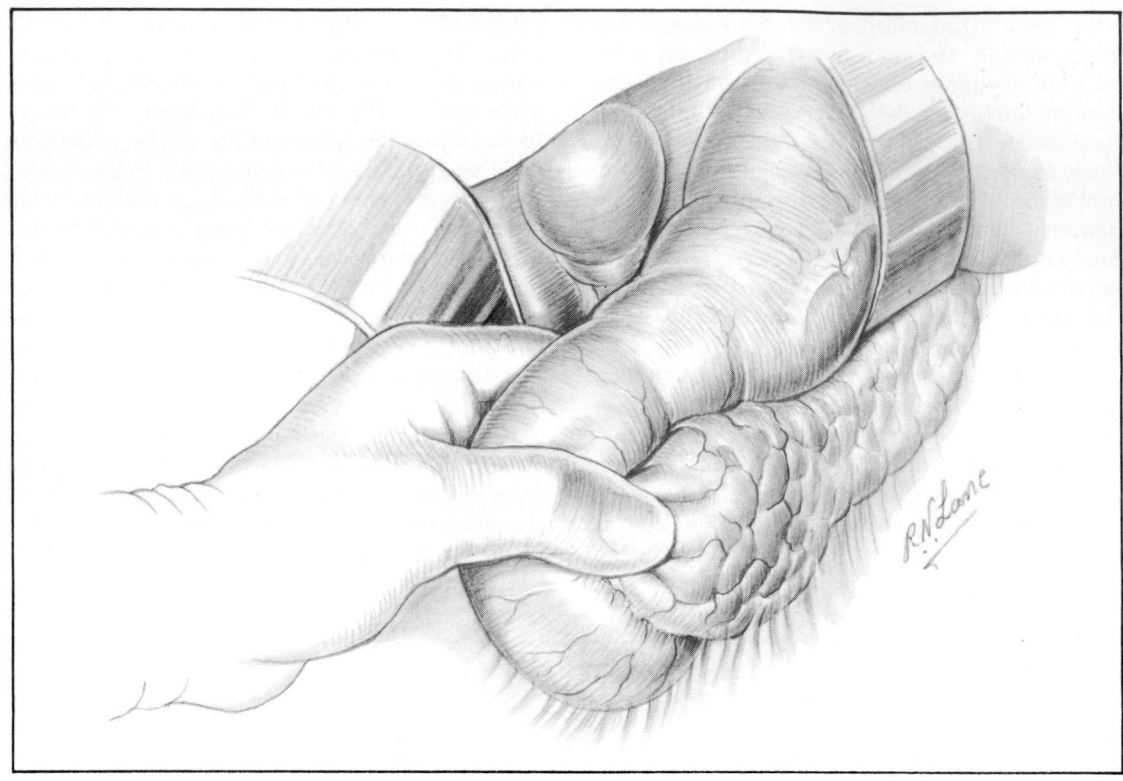

Figure 90–6. Bidigital palpation of the head of the pancreas is accomplished by the Kocher maneuver with mobilization of the duodenum so that the fingers can be placed between the gland and the aorta and vena cava. (*Source: From LeQuesne LP, 1980, with permission.*)

maneuver of dividing the lateral peritoneal attachments of the duodenum is necessary so that the fingers can be placed between the aorta–caval area and the pancreas (Fig. 90–6). For palpation of the body and tail of the pancreas, the peritoneal reflection of the avascular transverse mesocolon just above the inferior margin of the pancreas, can be incised (Fig. 90–7).

If the suspected tumor has not been detected by this time, it is advisable to carefully incise the posterior lateral attachment of the spleen to the kidney and the diaphragm (with division and ligation of a few of the short gastric vessels) so that the spleen and the tail of the pancreas can be mobilized and elevated into the wound for closer inspection and palpation (Fig. 90–8). The hilus of the spleen should then be closely examined since aberrant lesions may be present there.

Most insulinomas, even larger ones, can be excised simply by complete enucleation with care being taken to avoid injury to the pan-

creatic duct. If the tumor is on the surface, a suture can be placed into it with slight traction to assist in its extraction by blunt and sharp dissection. If it is palpated within the substance of the gland an incision with coagulation diathermy is made over it for its exposure and enucleation. After excision, the bleeding or leaking canaliculi can be sealed by diathermy and the area sealed by suturing the omentum to the defect and placing a drain near the area. If the main pancreatic duct is injured in the process it can be drained by an anastomosis to the contiguous jejunum or stomach; however, the surgeon may consider that it may be safer and necessary to carry out a distal pancreatectomy if the defect is in the left part of the pancreas.

If, after thorough exploration, a tumor has not been detected in patients in whom the preoperative diagnosis is firm, it is important to rule out islet cell hyperplasia, nesidioblastosis, and microadenomatosis. The tip of the tail of the pancreas or a small piece of the inferior

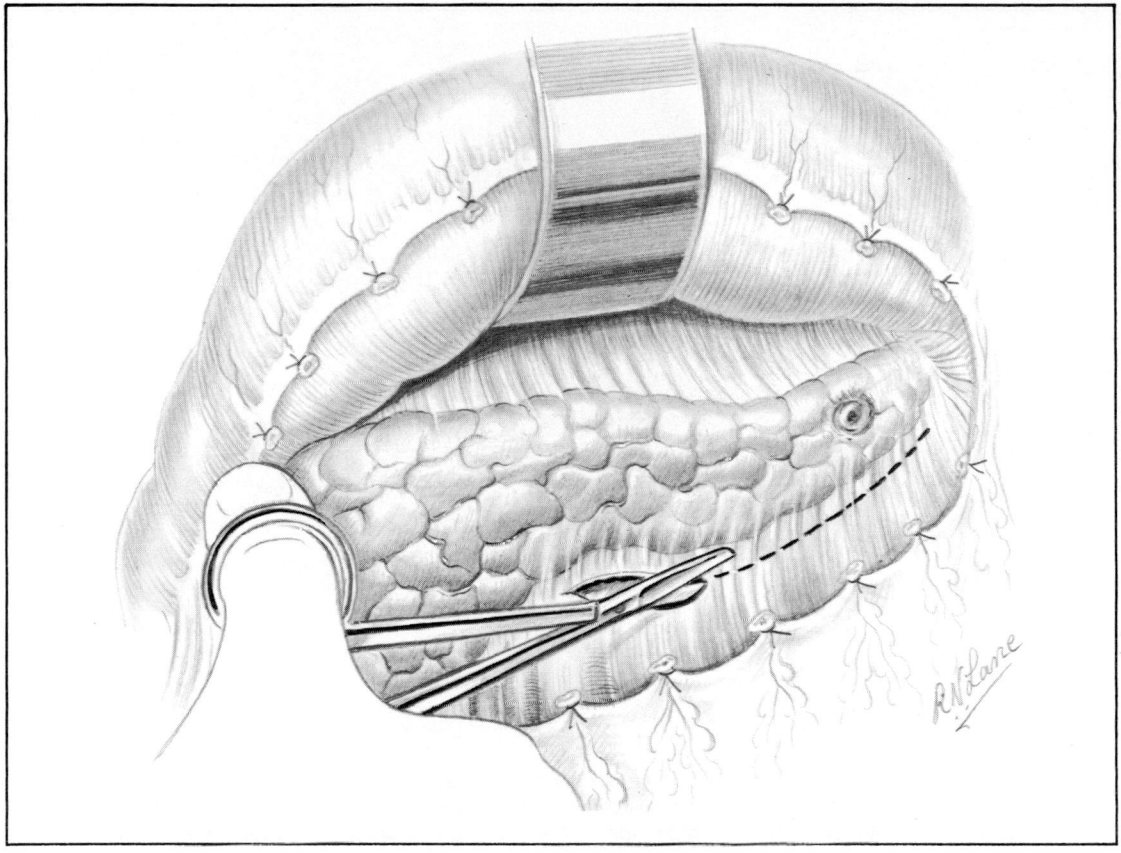

Figure 90–7. Palpation of the anterior and posterior surfaces of the body and tail of the pancreas can be accomplished by incising the peritoneal reflection along the inferior margin of the pancreas from the inferior mesenteric vein to the splenic hilus. (*Source: From LeQuesne LP, Thomson JPS: Operations of the pancreas for insulinoma, in Rob C, Smith R (eds): Operative Surgery, 3 edt. London: Butterworths, 1977, p 305, with permission.*)

margin of the pancreas should be excised between stay sutures for frozen section and microscopic examination by a competent surgical pathologist. If there is evidence of diffuse involvement, which more often occurs in the "hypoglycemia of infancy" than in adults, a subtotal distal pancreatectomy to the right of the superior mesenteric vessels is indicated. The only other indication for extensive pancreatic resection in patients with hypoglycemia is the presence of a large resectable malignancy.

"Blind" distal resections are no longer universally recommended when the surgeon does not detect an insulinoma. Several reasons have been proposed for this reluctance to perform "blind" resections. Because the location of insulinomas is evenly distributed throughout the

gland, as illustrated by Harrison et al, a distal hemipancreatectomy has only a 50 percent chance of successful disclosure and excision of an occult adenoma. If the surgeon has access to intraoperative sonography or to rapid (30 minute) assays for insulin from intraoperative selective venous aspirations, as reported by Turner et al, the search may continue, of course. Failing those special techniques, alternative considerations are appropriate to each patient. With continuing improvements in localizing techniques, particularly if sophisticated selective venous assays were not obtained preoperatively, surgeons may prefer to discontinue the operative search and resume radiologic investigations at a later time. There are, however, particular circumstances, such as failure of medical

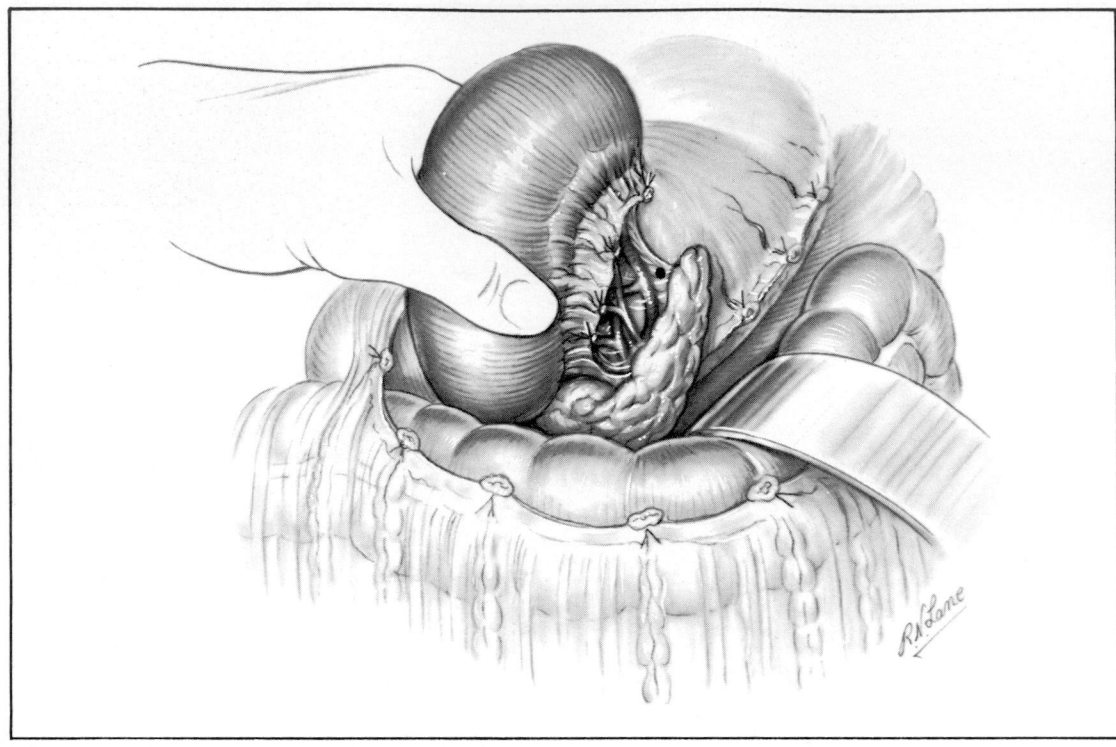

Figure 90–8. Further exposure for thorough palpation and inspection of the body and tail of the pancreas and the hilus of the spleen can be accomplished by careful division of the posterior peritoneal attachments of the spleen. (*Source: From LeQuesne LP, 1980, with permission.*)

control or noncompliance that may tilt the decision toward "blind" resection of a suspicious area with the realization that hemipancreatectomy may be only 50 percent successful. To aid in this decision it is useful to know beforehand if insulin hypersecretion can be suppressed by diazoxide administration, which can provide added time for future attempts at radiologic localization and surgical reexploration.

After the enucleation of one insulinoma, the decision to desist from further search for the 10 percent incidence of multiple adenomas is made easier if the surgeon has carefully monitored blood glucose concentrations throughout the operation and a rising glucose level occurs which, with the use of a Biostator, "trips off" the automatic administration of insulin. Patients who have the palliative distal pancreatectomy for malignancy and unresected hepatic metastases, are candidates for the intraoperative placement of a catheter into the hepatic artery, via the right gastric artery, for postoper-

ative intraarterial administration of chemotherapeutic agents.

Postoperative Care. The success or failure of the operation is usually evident within a few days. After excision of an insulinoma, continuing determinations of blood glucose levels every 6 hours and once a day at a time when dextrose is not being given intravenously usually indicates the outcome. Insulin can be given on a sliding scale based on the degree of glucosuria and ketonuria. When the patient has fully recovered from the operation, it may be wise to measure the insulin and glucose concentrations simultaneously after a 24-hour fast to confirm that the condition is cured. If, on the other hand, symptoms or evidence of hypoglycemia persist after intravenous infusions have been discontinued, the administration of dextrose and the cautious use of diazoxide is indicated. If insulin-secreting hepatic metastases remain in the patient with persistent hypoglycemia, selective percutaneous transfemoral intraarterial administration, or repeated intravenous injections of streptozocin can produce response rates of approximately 50 percent. Mithramycin, an inhibitor of DNA synthesis, has been reported to reverse the clinical course of hypoglycemia temporarily and to reduce the high serum proinsulin levels in metastatic insulin malignancies. Hydrocortisone may be symptomatically effective but it causes Cushing's syndrome. In rare emergencies, administration of Glucagon or somatostatin may be necessary to control severe hypoglycemic attacks. However, frequent eating and intravenous dextrose infusions usually prevent such occurrences.

Prognosis

After successful removal of a solitary insulinoma, the prognosis is excellent in that recurrent hypoglycemia rarely occurs. A 25-year follow-up by Markowitz et al, of the 6 patients first described by Whipple and Frantz, interestingly revealed the occurrence of GI bleeding and mental aberrations long after the hypoglycemia had been surgically cured. In a later study of 41 "cured" patients, he found a 36 percent incidence of peptic ulceration and a 28 percent incidence of neuropsychiatric disorders. In view of the fact that some patients who are considered to have sporadic insulinomas may actually be members of families affected with the MEA I, continuing follow-up with intermittent screening is probably advisable.

BIBLIOGRAPHY

Baylin SB, Mendelsohn G: Ectopic (inappropriate) hormone production by tumors: Mechanisms involved and the biological and clinical implications. Endocr Rev 1:45, 1980

Bhattacharya SK, Sealy WC: Paraneoplastic syndromes resulting from elaboration of ectopic hormones, antigens and bizarre toxins. Curr Probl Surg (May):1, 1972

Broder LE, Carter SK: Pancreatic islet cell carcinoma. II. Results of therapy with streptozotocin in 52 patients. Ann Intern Med 79:108, 1973

Conn JW, Pek S: On spontaneous hypoglycemia, current concepts. Kalamazoo, Michigan: The Upjohn Co, 1970

Duncan WE, Duncan TG, et al: Artificial pancreas as an aid during insulinoma resection. Am J Surg 142:523, 1981

Edis AJ, McIlrath DC, et al: Insulinoma—Current diagnosis and surgical management. Curr Probl Surg 13:1, 1976

Feyrter F: Uber die Pathologie peripherer vegetativer Regulationen am Beispiel des Karzinoids und des Karzinoidsyndrom. Hanbuch der Allgemainen Pathologie, vol 8, part 2. Berlin: Springer-Verlag, 1966, p 344

Friesen SR: APUD tumors of the gastrointestinal tract. Curr Probl Cancer 1:1, 1976

Friesen SR (ed), Bolinger RE (ed cons): Surgical Endocrinology: Clinical Syndromes. Philadelphia: JB Lippincott, 1978

Friesen SR, Kimmel JR, et al: Pancreatic polypeptide as a screening marker for pancreatic polypeptide apudomas in multiple endocrinopathies. Am J Surg 139:61, 1980

Friesen SR, Tomita T: Pseudo-Zollinger–Ellison syndrome: Hypergastrinemia, hyperchlorhydria without tumor. Ann Surg 194:481, 1981

Friesen SR: Tumors of the endocrine pancreas. N Engl J Med 306:580, 1982

Galbut DL, Markowitz AM: Insulinoma: Diagnosis, surgical management and long-term follow-up. Review of 41 cases. Am J Surg 139:683, 1980

Gordon P, Hendricks CM: Hypoglycemia associated with non-islet-cell tumor and insulin-like growth factors. N Engl J Med 305:1453, 1981

Gregory RA, Tracy HJ: Constitution and properties of two gastrins extracted from hog antral mucosa. J Physiol (Lond) 169:18, 1963

Harrison TS, Child CG III, et al: Current surgical management of functioning islet cell tumors of the pancreas. Ann Surg 178:485, 1973

Hirsch HJ, Loo S, et al: Hypoglycemia of infancy and nesidioblastosis: Studies with somatostatin. N Engl J Med 296:1323, 1977

Ingemansson S, Kuhl C, et al: Localization of insulinomas and islet cell hyperplasias by pancreatic vein catheterization and insulin assay. Surg Gynecol Obstet 146:725, 1978

Kaplan EL, Rubenstein AH, et al: Calcium infusion: A new provocative test for insulinomas. Ann Surg 190:501, 1979

Kiang DT, Frenning DH, et al: Mithramycin for hypoglycemia in malignant insulinoma. N Engl J Med 299:134, 1978

Laidlaw GF: Nesidioblastoma, the islet tumor of the pancreas. Am J Pathol 14:125, 1938

LeQuesne LP: Insulin tumours, in Maingot R (ed): Abdominal Operations, 7 edt. New York: Appleton-Century-Crofts, 1980, p 905

Lips CJM, van der Sluys Veer J, et al: Common precursor molecule as origin for the ectopic-hormone-producing-tumour syndrome. Lancet 1:16, 1978

Markowtiz AM, Slanetz CA Jr, et al: Functioning islet cell tumors of the pancreas: 25-year follow-up. Ann Surg 154:877, 1961

McGuigan JE: Gastric mucosal intracellular localization of gastrin by immunofluorescence. Gastroenterology 55:315, 1968

Mengoli L, LeQuesne P: Blind pancreatic resection for suspected insulinoma: A review of the problem. Br J Surg 54:749, 1967

Miller DR, Bolinger RE, et al: Hypoglycemia due to nonpancreatic mesodermal tumors: Report of two cases. Ann Surg 150:684, 1959

Pearse AGE: Common cytochemical and ultrastructural characteristics of cells producing polypeptide hormones (the APUD series) and their relevance to thyroid ultimobranchial C cells and calcitonin. Proc R Soc Lond 170:71, 1968

Pearse AGE: The diffuse neuroendocrine system and the APUD concept: Related "endocrine" peptides in brain, intestine, pituitary, placenta, and anuran cutaneous glands. Med Biol 55:115, 1977

Schwartz SS, Horwitz DL, et al: Continuous monitoring and control of plasma glucose during operation for removal of insulinomas. Surgery 85:702, 1979

Shetty MR, Boghossian HM, et al: Tumor-induced hypoglycemia. A result of ectopic insulin production. Cancer 49:1920, 1982

Sigel B, Duarte B, et al: Localization of insulinomas of the pancreas at operation by real-time ultrasound scanning. Surg Gynecol Obstet 156:145, 1983

Smith LH: Ectopic hormone production. Surg Gynecol Obstet 141:443, 1975

Tapia FJ, Polak JM, et al: Neuron-specific enolase is produced by neuroendocrine tumours. Lancet 1:808, 1981

Turner RC, Lee ECG, et al: Localisation of insulinomas. Lancet 1:515, 1978

Tutt GO Jr, Edis AJ, et al: Plasma glucose monitoring during operation for insulinoma: A critical reappraisal. Surgery 88:351, 1980

Wermer P: Genetic aspects of adenomatosis of endocrine glands. Am J Med 16:363, 1954

Whipple AO, Frantz VK: Adenoma of islet cells with hyperinsulinism. Ann Surg 101:1299, 1935

Yalow RS, Berson SA: Assay of plasma insulin in human subjects by immunological methods. Nature 184:1648, 1959

Zollinger RM, Ellison EH: Primary peptic ulcerations of the jejunum associated with islet cell tumors of the pancreas. Ann Surg 142:709, 1955

91. Ulcerogenic Tumors of the Pancreas and the Vipoma Syndrome

Robert M. Zollinger
Robert M. Zollinger, Jr.

ULCEROGENIC TUMORS OF THE PANCREAS

Introduction

The gastrinoma syndrome, or the Zollinger–Ellison syndrome, associated with the presence of an ulcerogenic islet cell tumor of the pancreas was first described in 1955 and is now recognized to be second in frequency to the insulinoma syndrome. Additional clinical syndromes associated with islet cell tumors of the pancreas have been recognized in recent years, and the suspected presence of these functioning pancreatic tumors is usually confirmed by specific radioimmunoassays. As the incidence of peptic ulceration has decreased, the importance of the identification and treatment of the gastrinoma causing gastric hypersecretion has become more urgent.

The original description of the gastrinoma was based on a study of two patients operated on between 1952 and 1954. In retrospect, it is evident that such a tumor had been resected by hemipancreatectomy with vagotomy and pyloroplasty in an earlier patient in 1947, but the significance of the dramatic fall in the volume of gastric juice rich in hydrochloric acid following that procedure had not been appreciated.

The gastrinoma triad was initially proposed in the fashion of the Whipple triad and it included: (1) primary peptic ulceration in unusual locations such as the second or third portions of the duodenum or the upper jejunum beyond the ligament of Treitz, or recurrent marginal ulcers following any gastric surgical procedure short of total gastrectomy, (2) marked gastric hypersection despite adequate, intensive medi-

cal or surgical therapy, and (3) identification of a non-beta islet cell tumor of the pancreas. During the years that have followed, approximately one fourth of patients have been shown to have other associated endocrine tumors, especially in the parathyroid glands. Some have suggested that clinical symptoms and findings may be quite similar to those of a patient with duodenal ulcer. However, in other patients without proof of gastric or duodenal ulceration, it has become apparent that diarrhea (steatorrhea) from the irritating effects of massive gastric hypersecretion should be considered a symptom of gastrinoma.

Clinical acceptance of the proposed syndrome was relatively slow for a decade, because of general belief that the only hormone the pancreas produced was insulin. However, the concept was affirmed in 1960 when Gregory et al proved that the secretagogue produced by the islet cell tumors and their metastases was gastrin, in amounts 35 times greater than those produced by similar weights of porcine antrum. Proof of the presence of these pancreatic tumors was established by a sensitive radioimmunoassay that measures gastrin concentrations in serum which was developed by McGuigan and Trudeau in 1968.

Diagnosis

Clinical Symptoms. All too frequently, the presence of a gastrin-producing pancreatic tumor is not suspected until a catastrophic occurrence takes place. Indeed, the symptoms are variable and may mimic those of a duodenal ulcer, or they may become manifested gradually because of the slow growth of the tumor so that early diagnosis may be understandably delayed. However, among the findings which should suggest the presence of a gastrinoma are recurrence of a marginal ulcer after a standard ulcer operation or the development of a complication such as perforation or hemorrhage in a patient on intensive antacid medication. Gastrinoma should be suspected also when symptoms of an ulcer appear in very young patients under 15 years of age or in elderly patients who have not previously had ulcer symptoms.

Other conditions that suggest gastrinoma are the presence of a fulminating ulcer that fails to respond to intensive medical therapy, a complicated ulcer that follows immediately postpartum after a pregnancy, or a persistently high gastric juice output with high acid values after vagotomy and gastric resection. However, the most dramatic and precisely diagnostic indication of gastrinoma is the presence of an ulcer just beyond the ligament of Treitz. Both of the original patients had either perforation or a massive recurrent hemorrhage from jejunal ulcerations near the ligament of Treitz, although neither had had previous gastric surgery.

Diarrhea is not an uncommon symptom, but can delay the accurate diagnosis of a gastrinoma, especially when no ulcerations are noted in x-ray studies of the stomach or duodenum.

Radiologic Signs. Before gastrin radioimmunoassay became available, the roentgenologist was often the first to suspect the presence of a gastrinoma. Characteristic of these patients was a large amount of fluid in an unobstructed stomach and the presence of prominent mucosal folds (Fig. 91–1). Christoforidis and Nelson described in 1966 the classic radiologic criteria for the diagnosis of gastrinoma from barium studies of the gastrointestinal (GI) tract. Pyloric obstruction or gastric ulceration were not common, and an enlarged duodenum often had a "cobblestone" appearance, due to hyperplasia of Brunner glands. An ulceration was frequently present in unusual locations such as the second or third portion of the duodenum or beyond the ligament of Treitz. When no ulceration was present, the diagnosis was likely to be delayed because diarrhea due to exaggerated gastric hypersecretion was the only GI complaint. Additionally, gastrinomas tend to be small and usually do not produce detectable compression deformities of the stomach or duodenum on barium studies.

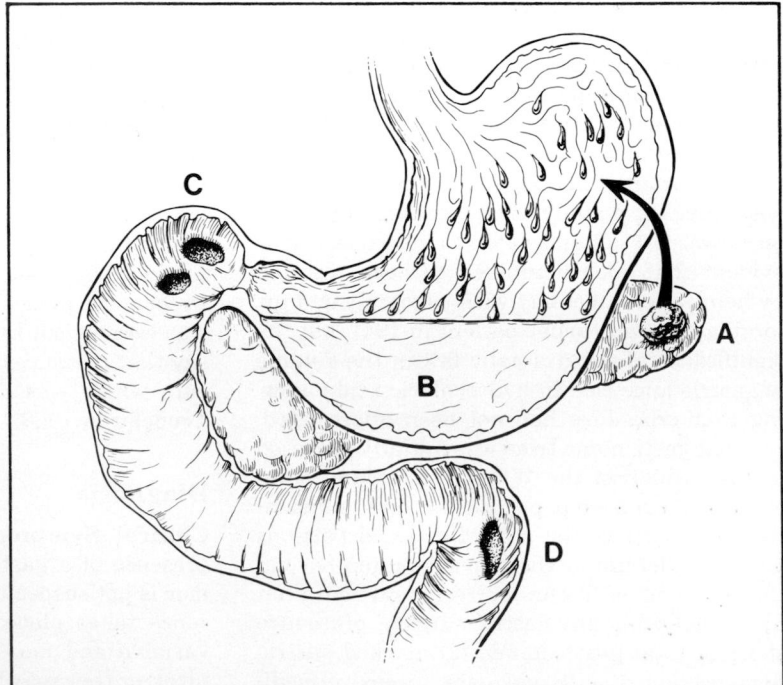

Figure 91–1. The non-beta islet cell tumor **(A)** produces gastrin which is a potent gastric secretagogue **(B)**. The gastrinoma is characterized by multiple ulcers **(C)** in an enlarged shaggy duodenum, and ulcers in unusual location, i.e., just beyond the ligament of Treitz **(D)**.

Gastric Analysis. Although gastric analysis is less commonly performed than it used to be, it is a very important procedure not only to establish the diagnosis of gastrinoma, but to monitor the effectiveness of medical therapy. A prolonged gastric aspiration of several days while on variable medications has been used to determine effective medical control. The dose of H_2-receptor antagonist is increased until the hourly output of hydrochloric acid remains below 10 mEq. Furthermore, the presence of hydrochloric acid rules out achlorhydria which can be associated with elevated serum gastrin levels. In the untreated patient, an output of at least 100 ml/hr with hydrochloric acid exceeding 10 mEq/hr is common from an unobstructed stomach. Tremendous volumes of gastric juice, exceeding 4000 to 5000 ml in a 12-hour overnight aspiration have not been uncommon. Concurrently, the patient's symptoms, including diarrhea, are relieved by constant aspiration of excess gastric juice rich in hydrochloric acid. Similarly the finding of an increased volume of gastric juice with high acid values in a patient who has already undergone gastric surgery for duodenal ulcer should be viewed with suspicion, especially if vagotomy and antrectomy have been performed.

Laboratory Procedures. Basal serum gastrin levels, normally 100 to 150 ng/ml, are elevated in patients with a gastrin-producing tumor as well as in those with achlorhydria associated with pernicious anemia or gastric carcinoma. Serum gastrin may also be elevated in the presence of atrophic gastritis, renal failure, progressive obstruction of the ureters by carcinoma, retained gastric antrum following a gastric resection, or antral G-cell hyperplasia, but these levels will be depressed within 30 seconds following the infusion of 2 clinical units of secretin per kilogram of body weight.

In contrast, gastrin levels will be elevated to at least 200 ng/ml above fasting levels within 30 seconds in a patient with a gastrinoma following the intravenous administration of 2 clinical units of secretin per kilogram of body weight. This secretin "push" is particularly useful when fasting gastrin levels are high normal or near borderline diagnostic levels such as 250 to 500 ng/ml. However, over the years of follow-up, the same secretin "push" is most useful in measuring the increasing activity of these slowly growing tumors or their functioning metastases.

Endocrine Survey. The presence of a gastrinoma is a clear indication to search for other endocrine tumors, especially those involving the parathyroid glands. Approximately one fourth of the patients with gastrinoma will also have parathyroid adenomas, and the association of these two entities is termed the multiple endocrine adenopathy syndrome, type I (MEA I). Because of a strong tendency toward familial occurrence, symptomatic relatives and the children of such patients require a close survey.

Additional endocrine studies may be undertaken with safety since the H_2-receptor antagonists introduced in 1976 make it possible to control the dangerous gastric hypersecretion that accompanies a gastrinoma. Calcium, parathormone, and phosphorus levels should be measured. Many patients with hypercalcemia have kidney stones, and pyelograms and kidney function studies are essential. Roentgenograms of the skull, teeth, and clavicle may confirm bone changes that support the diagnosis of hyperparathyroidism. One or more parathyroid glands may be sufficiently enlarged to be palpable. Computed tomography (CT) scans, radionuclide scans, or angiograms with digital subtraction of the neck along with localized venous sampling may be required to confirm the diagnosis of hyperparathyroidism or to localize parathyroid adenoma. This is especially true in patients who have undergone previous explorations of the thyroid area or in those suspected of having a mediastinal lesion.

In addition to studies of the parathyroid glands, it is essential to evaluate the pituitary gland. Serum prolactin levels should be routinely measured in all patients with a gastrinoma, especially those with an associated MEA I syndrome. Scans of the pituitary fossa should be undertaken when prolactin levels are found to be modestly elevated. Elevated prolactin levels may be lowered by bromocriptine as eye fields are evaluated, along with the findings of other scans. The effects of certain medications and other causes for elevated prolactin levels must be evaluated before surgical exploration of the sella turcica is advised.

Although pheochromocytomas are considered to be part of the MEA II syndrome, they are not uncommon in patients with gastrinoma and hyperparathyroidism, or MEA I. Catecholamines should be measured and scans of both adrenal glands performed as, unfortunately, endocrine tumors do not follow a predictable, fixed pattern.

Summary of Diagnostic Procedures

For nearly 30 years, the growing awareness of the clinical syndrome of gastrinoma and the availability and accuracy of the gastrin radioimmunoassay have made the diagnosis of this pancreatic gastrin-producing tumor so routine that it is no longer considered a clinical novelty. However, many physicians may never encounter a patient with such a tumor.

Therefore, it must be emphasized that serum gastrin levels should be measured in every patient who has recurrent symptoms after a standard ulcer operation. Reexploration should not be undertaken until the results of the secretin "push" have been determined. Although incomplete vagotomy, especially with failure to divide the posterior vagus nerve, is by far the most common cause of persistent or recurrent symptoms after an ulcer operation, there are other causes. These include inadequate drainage of the antrum, inadequate gastric resection (less than hemigastrectomy), or a retained antrum. The secretin "push" test is not positive in the presence of a retained antrum or antral G-cell hyperplasia. The operative notes of the previous operation should always be reviewed in a search for a possible cause for recurrence before a second operation for recurrent ulcer is performed. An incomplete operation or an unphysiologic procedure is more likely to be the cause of recurrent ulceration than is a gastrinoma.

Among the most challenging patients are those with digestive complaints and evidence of increased gastric hypersecretion with only modest elevations in serum gastrin levels. The patient may have eaten before the serum sample was taken or may have a very small gastrinoma in the submucosa of the first portion of the duodenum. The validity of these evaluations depends on a complete gastric analysis that has shown the presence of hydrochloric acid and the absence of failing kidneys. Extensive investigation for a gastrinoma because of elevated gastrin levels not infrequently precedes the finding of achlorhydria by a delayed gastric analysis. It is in these patients that the secretin "push" test is so important. An alternative test, preferred by some, is the rapid infusion of calcium glucornate (2 mg Ca^{++}/kg administered over 1 min) followed immediately by a bolus injection of secretin (2 mg/kg). This combination is a potent gastric secretagogue.

An exceptional patient may have symptoms and gastrin levels consistent with the diagnosis of gastrinoma but may fail to show gastrin elevation in response to secretin infusion. Antral biopsies by gastroscopy will show hyperplasia of the antral G cells. Vagotomy and antrectomy should control symptoms in these rare patients.

Treatment

The introduction in 1976 of the effective H_2-receptor antagonist, cimetidine, rekindled the debates over medical versus surgical therapy of gastric hypersecretion. Administration of 300 to 600 mg of the drug four times a day controls the gastric hypersecretion and the symptoms in the majority of patients with gastrinoma, and the effectiveness of this therapy convinced many physicians that medical therapy ought to be chosen over surgical treatment. The early preferred treatment of total gastrectomy with aggressive removal of as much tumor as was safely possible as well as the metastasis to lymph nodes and liver, presented grave surgical risks and possible long-term nutritional problems. Patients readily accepted the alternative of medical therapy. However, the fact remained that the gastrin-producing tumor was usually malignant, was usually metastatic, and was usually continuing to grow intraabdominally as the medical treatment provided relief of pain.

Although the H_2-receptor antagonists were generally well tolerated, it was to be expected that as the gastrinoma grew in size and the gastrin-producing metastases developed, there would be a need to increase the medication. As the dosage was increased to ensure that gastric acidity was maintained below 10 mEq/hr, side effects became more pronounced. Hypospermia, impotence, and tender gynecomastia were reported in as many as 50 percent of young men. In addition, the hepatic effects of the drug increased the risks of concurrent medications of such drugs as warfarin, diazepam, and propanolol. It often became necessary to reduce dosages by one half in the elderly and in those who required other medications.

Although many patients did well for some years, a few did not respond to the H_2-receptor antagonist and others failed to comply with the rigid requirements of regular medication at stated times. Some substituted other medications because of the expense. After several years of experience, the disadvantages of indefinitely prolonged or increasing medication, failure of the medication to control symptoms, unacceptable side effects, and the development of complications made operation necessary in growing numbers of patients. Despite the hope of some physicians that newer drugs might be more effective at a lower dosage without side effects or liver toxicity, a trend back to earlier operation became apparent.

However, as the opposition to radical surgery softened, a trend toward less than total gastrectomy gained support. Resection of a solitary tumor was increasingly advocated, although experience showed this was rarely possible. Some advocated the performance of a highly selective vagotomy rather than total gastrectomy if no tumor could be found, with the presumption that vagotomy would decrease the acid output by approximately 50 percent, thereby increasing the effectiveness of the H_2-receptor antagonist in controlling the symptoms.

The gastrinoma remains the only pancreatic tumor about which such debate persists, i.e., not only when operation should be performed but the extent of it. This is due, in part, to the emphasis on the control of gastric hypersecretion by medication and on the fears concerning the morbidity and mortality of total gastrectomy and pancreatic resection. Because the gastrinoma is relatively uncommon, few surgeons have had extensive experience with these patients. They hesitate to carry out the extensive surgery that may be required and therefore yield to the recommendations for a conservative procedure. The surgeon who accepts the responsibility of treating patients with gastrinoma should be familiar with the malignant potential and the endocrinologic complications of these tumors. The surgeon should be resolute in allaying the fears of those who favor long-term palliative therapy because of anxiety about the results of radical surgical treatment.

The surgeon must be certain of the diagnosis preoperatively and must be well informed of the results of studies done in a search for other endocrine involvement, especially hyperparathyroidism which should be corrected before abdominal exploration is undertaken. At least three and one half parathyroid glands

should be removed because of the recurrence tendency, especially in patients with MEA I. Some surgeons, however, prefer radical parathyroidectomy with transplantation of an aliquot of parathyroid tissue into the muscles of the forearm. After parathyroidectomy, the blood calcium should return to normal levels, and gastrin levels are lowered. Patients respond more effectively to the H_2-receptor antagonists for a time, but the untreated malignant gastrinoma will continue to grow.

At abdominal exploration, decisions concerning the extent of the procedure may be influenced by several factors. If no tumor is found or if what appears to be a solitary tumor can be resected, the surgeon may be tempted to avoid total gastrectomy. However, the patient's history of compliance with medication regimes and the effectiveness of the medication to keep the hourly output of acid gastric juice below 10 mEq/hr of hydrochloric acid must be considered. These factors may reinforce the indications for removal of all acid-secreting surface by total gastrectomy.

Preoperative Preparation

The surgeon must take the time to discuss fully with the patient and family the various procedures that may be performed. Patients need reassurance that after total gastrectomy they can eventually eat three regular meals a day.

The postoperative nutrition of patients undergoing total gastrectomy tends to relate to their preoperative nutritional status. The majority sustain a satisfactory weight, which is a much better record than that following total gastrectomy for other reasons. They need to be reassured that diabetes does not necessarily follow removal of a portion of the pancreas. Although no one can predict the future course of the patient with gastrinoma, almost 50 percent will be living 10 years after operation. Obviously, the patient must be informed concerning the malignant potential of the tumor and the fact that total removal of the tumor at the time of exploration, with the likelihood of a return of the gastrin levels to a sustained normal, is relatively small, although it is apparently improved each year by surgeons experienced in the surgical treatment of gastrinoma.

Excessive losses of fluids, which may amount to 3 or 4 L, and electrolyte losses from gastric aspiration or diarrhea must be corrected immediately before operation. The patient's weight and electrolytes should be monitored morning and evening, with special emphasis on the morning of operation. Blood volume and nutritional deficits should be replaced. Preoperative antibiotics should be given the night before operation and immediately before operation because of the tendency of ulcers to penetrate the GI wall into adjacent tissue, and occasionally the colon. Previously typed and cross-matched blood should be available for possibly three or four transfusions. The inlying nasal gastric tube should remain in place, and any changes in the volume output noted after the removal of a questionably solitary tumor, and after vagotomy. A decided intraoperative decrease in the output of gastric juice can be useful evidence that a solitary tumor has been resected.

Operative Technique

Under general intratracheal anesthesia, the patient is placed in a moderate reverse Trendelenburg position to enhance the exposure of the gastroesophageal area. A long midline incision is made, extending up over the xyphoid and down to the left and well below the umbilicus. Previous incisions may dictate the placement of the upper abdominal incisions. The inflammatory appearance of the tissues and the increased vascularity of the stomach is apparent. Inflammatory masses from a penetrating ulcer may be encountered, especially if the patient has undergone previous gastric operations. Occasionally a gastrojejunocolic fistula is found.

The liver should be carefully inspected for evidence of grey metastatic nodules. Occasionally a frosted appearance due to tumor metastasis is observed under the capsule. Superficial metastatic nodules should be excised, and the specimen sent to the pathologist for verification. Even in the presence of hepatic metastases, a total gastrectomy should be considered in good risk patients, since 10-year survival is not unusual.

The stomach feels spongy, the blood vessels appear engorged, and the duodenum is enlarged and thickened. Evidence of an active duodenal ulcer may or may not be present. The area on either side of the pylorus is palpated in a careful search for a small carcinoid-like gastrinoma located within the wall, especially of the first part of the duodenum. These tumors may be easy to find, or may be smaller than a pea. Their presence can be detected only by actual visual-ization combined with repeated digital palpation.

The region of the jejunum beyond the ligament of Treitz should be carefully inspected and palpated. Any evidence of ulceration in this area should be considered pathognomonic of an ulcerogenic tumor of the pancreas.

The entire pancreas must be visualized, as well as bimanually palpated. The greater omentum is freed from the transverse colon, including both the hepatic and splenic flexures. Any adhesions between the stomach and the anterior surface of the pancreas are divided, and the stomach is retracted upward. The visual inspection should extend all the way to the tail of the pancreas, which may ultimately be attached to the hilus of the spleen. In addition to exploring the body and tail of the pancreas, it is very important to thoroughly explore the region of the head of the gland.

Stabile et al have emphasized the operative implications of the gastrinoma triangle because of the frequency of tumor in this area. They observed that a high proportion of tumors was found in an anatomic triangle outlined by the junction of the cystic and common ducts superiorly, the junction of the neck and the body of the pancreas medially, and the second and third portions of the duodenum inferiorly. Following an extensive Kocher maneuver, the head of the pancreas is completely mobilized. All enlarged or suspicious lymph nodes are excised and frozen sections are performed. In general, solitary tumors within the head of the pancreas were locally enucleated and pancreaticoduodenectomy was avoided in their series.

The body and tail of the pancreas should be mobilized to ensure adequate visual and digital examination. The peritoneum along the inferior surface of the body of the pancreas is incised, as well as the peritoneum above the splenic vessels. Blunt finger dissection is used to free the posterior aspects of the pancreas. This permits palpation between the thumb and index finger. If the exposure of the tail of the pancreas is difficult, it may be wise to mobilize the spleen after division of the gastrosplenic vessels. The spleen and the entire left side of the pancreas can be mobilized into the wound and the posterior surface more effectively inspected. A small portable ultrasound scanner may be used to search the pancreas more accurately for tumor masses. If no tumor is found on multiple biopsies, the pylorus is divided, and a search is made for a small tumor in the submucosa of the wall of the first portion of the duodenum. It may be difficult to identify such a small tumor mass because hyperplasia of the Brunner glands may give the duodenal mucosa a "cobblestone" appearance. If tumor is found, it is excised with the surrounding full thickness of duodenal wall. Although the removal of a duodenal gastrinoma may return the gastrin levels to normal in the majority of patients, other tumors or metastases will be present in most and will eventually result in reelevation of the gastrin levels.

When no tumor is found, a small biopsy is taken from the inferior margin of the left side of the pancreas to verify the status of the pancreatic islets (Fig. 91–2).

Occasionally a discrete tumor nodule, which can be easily enucleated, is found in the body or head of the pancreas. Sometimes the tumor is found in what appears to be a pedunculated lymph node with an attached blood supply.

In general, it is difficult to be certain what percentage of patients will sustain a long-term normal gastrin level after aggressive surgical therapy that includes a meticulous search of the entire pancreas. The percentage of patients with normal postoperative gastrin levels has ranged from 7 to 43 percent, and this may be related more to the type of patients in each series than to the aggressiveness of the surgical procedure.

Although there is no uniform agreement even after 30 years, most surgeons with experience in the treatment of gastrinoma favor surgical exploration with an effort to cure the patient by an aggressive search and removal of any tumor or metastases. The most common surgical procedure on the stomach is total gastrectomy (Fig. 91–3). When no tumor is found or when the patient is elderly and a poor risk, or when it is believed all tumor has been removed, a vagotomy may be performed and a total gastrec-

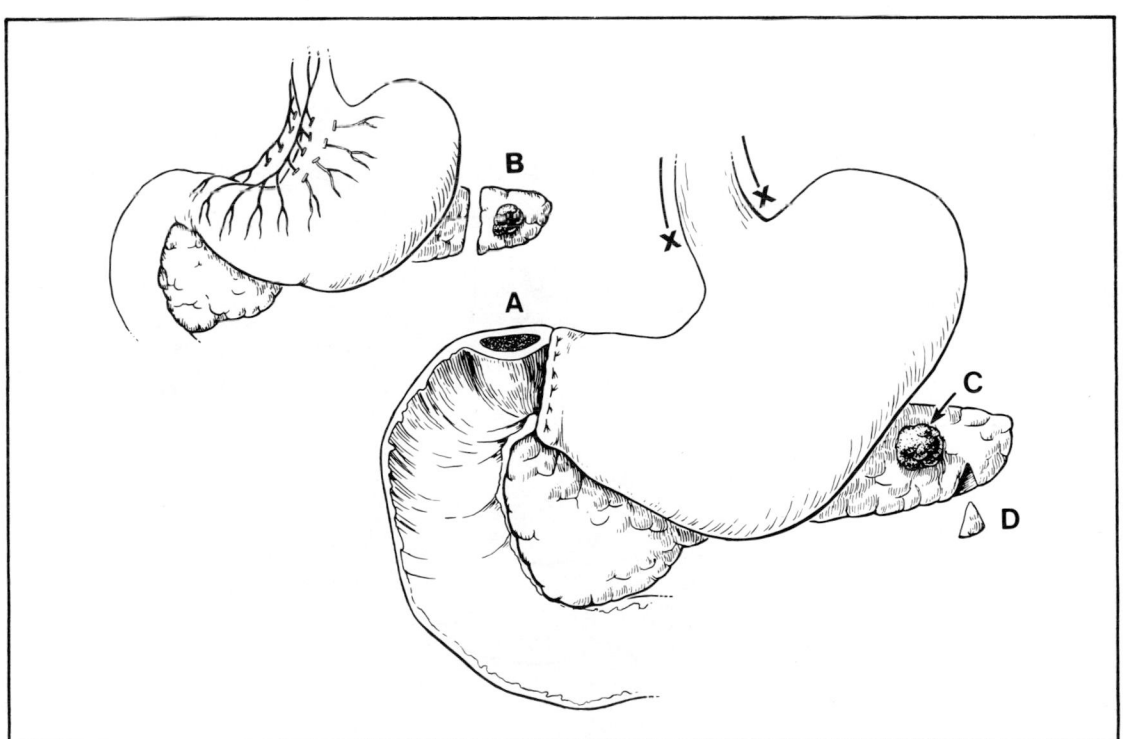

Figure 91–2. Truncal vagotomy and pyloroplasty may occasionally be considered when localized and resectable tumor is found in the duodenum **(A)**, or pancreas **(C)**. Biopsy of the pancreas should be included for evaluation of the islets of Langerhans **(D)**. Highly selective vagotomy without pyloroplasty **(B)** has been advocated for the same indications, including failure to verify gross tumor.

tomy avoided. Some prefer a highly selective vagotomy without pylorplasty, whereas others support truncal vagotomy with pylorotomy in order to search more effectively for a possible carcinoid gastrinoma in the submucosa in that area (Fig. 91–2).

Total gastrectomy should continue to be the operation of choice in the majority of patients, including those who have failed to respond to medical therapy, the very young, those in whom tumor obviously remains despite aggressive attempts to remove it, and in patients with the MEA I syndrome because of the probability of multitumor involvement.

Total Gastrectomy. The success of total gastrectomy (Fig. 91–3) depends in large measure on a good exposure of the esophageal hiatus opening. The removal of the elongated xyphoid, a modest reverse Trendelenburg position, and mobilization of the left lobe of the liver are important in providing good exposure. If the patient has had a previous vagotomy, great care must be exercised to avoid fraying the muscular wall of the esophagus. The nasogastric tube must remain in place during this procedure. After the duodenum has been divided and closed with two layers of silk, the left gastric artery is doubly ligated, both vagus nerves, and all gastrosplenic vessels are divided and tied. The esophagus can now be pulled gently downward into the peritoneal cavity for 5 or 6 cm and anchored to the margins of the hiatus with three or four interrupted silk sutures. This prevents retraction of the esophagus when it is divided from the stomach. It is important that all gastric-secreting surface be removed. A noncrushing vascular clamp is useful to apply to the esophagus when the Levin tube has been withdrawn upward into the upper portion of

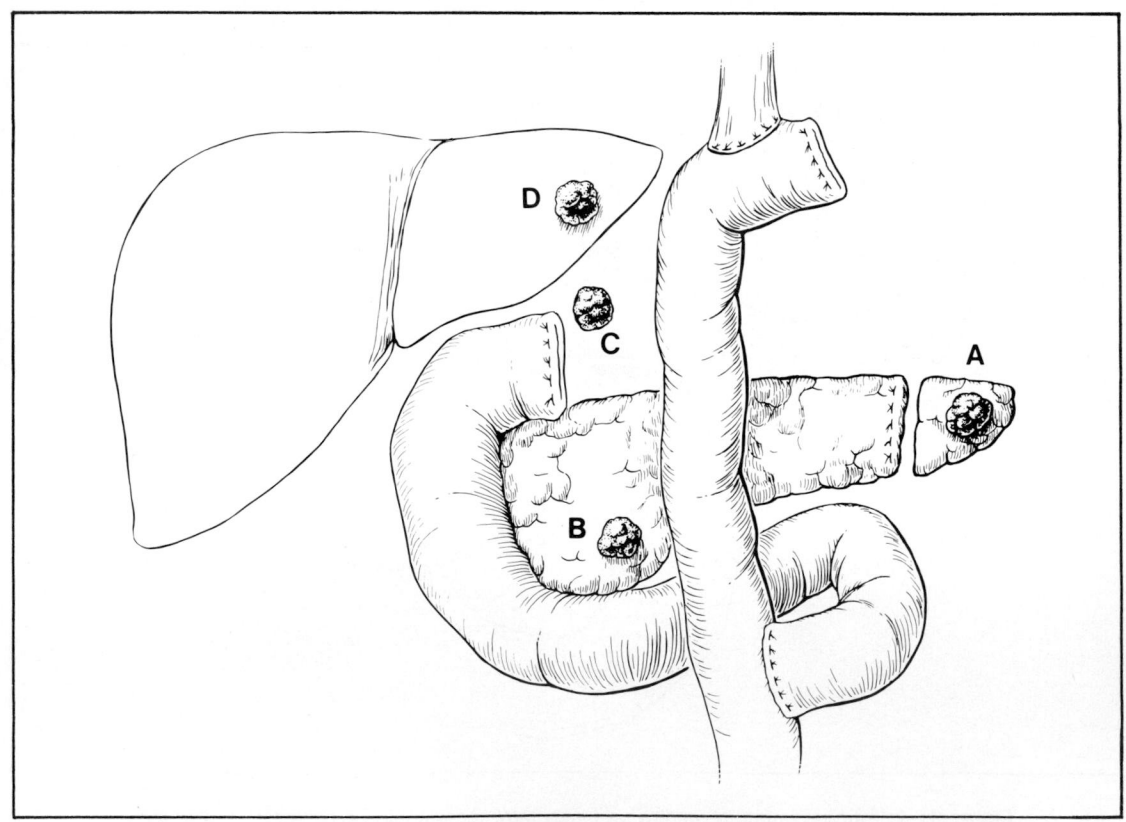

Figure 91–3. The Roux-Y reconstruction after total gastrectomy. Improved 10-year survival follows total gastrectomy combined with aggressive resection **(A)** or enucleation of pancreatic tumors **(B)**, combined with excision of lymph node metastases **(C)**, and surface liver metastases **(D)**.

the esophagus. Technically it is helpful to place a few through-and-through mattress sutures in the end of the esophagus to prevent fraying and to provide a cuff for the subsequent anastomosis with the Roux-Y arm of jejunum. Interrupted sutures of silk have been used to anchor the jejunal limb to the diaphragm posterior to the esophagus, followed by a two-layer anastomosis. The closure of the anterior layer is facilitated if a larger stomach tube is passed down the esophagus alongside the Levin tube to ensure an adequate stoma and to facilitate the inversion of the anterior mucosal layer. The jejunal limb is anchored to the diaphragm anteriorly as well as posteriorly. The larger tube is removed, and the Levin tube is directed around into the region of the duodenal stump.

Some surgeons prefer to use a stapling device for the anastomosis with supplemental interrupted sutures for the angles. The construction of pouches is not essential to ensure adequate nutrition postoperatively.

Postoperative Care

The postoperative care of the patient with gastrinoma must continue indefinitely. The patient's weight and eating habits should be evaluated at regular intervals, such as at 3, 6, 12 weeks, and so forth. Some may experience difficulty at first in swallowing dry bread or tough steak. They must be instructed to keep a record of monthly vitamin B_{12} injections and to record weight trends.

Of major importance in the follow-up of these patients is the necessity to remain alert for evidence of other endocrine tumors, especially a recurrence of hyperparathyroidism. Patients with MEA I tend to have recurrence of hyperparathyroidism unless three and one half glands have been removed. Elevated prolactin levels in a few patients may indicate the need for a transphenoidal attack on the pituitary. Pheochromocytoma is not uncommonly found in the MEA I group. Additional endocrine tumors developing late in the follow-up period may present more problems than the gastrinoma.

The children of these patients should have an endocrine survey in a search for endocrine tumors, including gastrinoma. The latter tends to become apparent later in life, although hyperparathyroidism seems to be found at an earlier age.

During the follow-up period, patients may exhibit symptoms that should not be routinely attributed to recurrent tumor. A few may be the result of a small esophagojejunal stoma which requires repeated dilations. Gallstones, a not uncommon late finding, can be managed effectively by cholecystectomy. Renal calculi recur in patients who have had hyperparathyroidism as well in those who have elevated serum calcium levels. An increase in kidney stones has also been observed in patients whose major symptom of gastric hypersecretion was diarrhea. Rarely, the expanding tumor will encroach on the lumen of the upper GI tract. Chemotherapy or, more uncommonly, a bypass around the obstructing lesion may be necessary. A few patients with mounting serum gastrin levels have had angiograms that suggested a localized tumor, which has been successfully removed by a "second-look" procedure. However, angiography has not been as rewarding in demonstrating the gastrinoma as it has been in showing other types of pancreatic islet cell tumors.

Chemotherapy. The role of chemotherapy in the postoperative treatment of the patient with gastrinoma, either prophylactically or when there is evidence of extensive involvement, has not been crystallized. Streptozotocin or chlorozotocin have been used either alone or in combination with other drugs such as 5-fluorouracil. The responses have been varied, and at times there has been considerable delay before a beneficial effect became apparent. Chemotherapy should be considered when the gastrin levels are persistently elevated in the presence of hepatic metastases or palpable abdominal masses, or the development of gastrointestinal complaints due to encroachment on the lumen by tumor.

Summary

The gastrinoma remains a challenging tumor that fails to provide consistent guidelines as to its rate of growth or malignant potential. Although dramatic advances have been made in the medical control of its secretagogue effect on the stomach, the fact remains that this tumor should always be considered a menacing malignant lesion. The diagnosis of gastrinoma should be considered an indication for surgery as soon as a complete endocrine survey has been performed and maximum benefit from the H_2-receptor medication is attained. The benefits of early diagnosis should not be lost by prolonged delays in surgical management.

THE VIPOMA SYNDROME

Introduction

Shortly after the gastrinoma syndrome was first described, Priest and Alexander reported a patient with an islet cell tumor who had intractable watery diarrhea with extreme potassium depletion, but no ulceration. Verner and Morrison reported two cases and added others from the literature and, as a result, the symptoms associated with this particular islet cell tumor have been termed, the Verner–Morrison syndrome. Murray et al, in 1961, documented the presence of achlorhydria in a patient with watery diarrhea and severe potassium depletion. This syndrome has come to be known by several additional terms: pancreatic cholera, or the WDHA syndrome, an acronym for watery diarrhea, hypokalemia, and achlorhydria, which are the major clinical symptoms.

Although secretin was suspected to be the hormone produced by these islet cell tumors, there is now general agreement that vasoactive polypeptide (VIP) is responsible for the clinical syndrome. The term, vipoma, has become the generally accepted designation for this particular islet cell tumor, which is being recognized more frequently, but occurs more rarely than either the gastrinoma or the insulinoma.

Diagnosis

Because there are so many causes of diarrhea, it is understandable that the diagnosis of vipoma is often delayed. The classic syndrome consists of watery diarrhea of 5 to 6 L/day. A clue to the diagnosis is the extreme hypokalemia which exceeds that observed in patients with a large villous adenoma of the colon. The heavy loss of potassium can result in severe abdominal distention, suggesting small bowel obstruction. These symptoms promptly subside when adequate fluid and electrolyte replacements are given, but death can result from hypokalemic nephrosis. The achlorhydria, or low acid values, may be overcome by the augmented histamine test. Hypercalcemia is present in more than one half of these patients and is more pronounced during the period of fulminating di-

arrhea, but the calcium levels tend to return to normal following the removal of the islet cell tumor. This is in contrast to the hypercalcemia caused by the hyperparathyroidism that accompanies gastrinoma. Interestingly, diabetes mellitus is present in approximately 40 percent of the patients with vipoma.

Laboratory Studies. These tumors tend to be much larger than the ulcerogenic gastrinoma and are therefore more likely to be localized by appropriate scans or an angiogram. They may reach sufficient size to demonstrate encroachment on the stomach or transverse colon on barium studies. The gallbladder was observed by Zollinger et al to be definitely enlarged, and this clinical observation has been recorded by Longmire and others.

The vasoactive intestinal polypeptide stimulates the production of the juices in the small intestine with the development of marked hypokalemia. There is an increase in the output of hepatic glucose. It inhibits gastric acid secretion and relaxes the gallbladder. These responses are closely related to those anticipated from stimulation by secretin.

Persistent or recurrent watery diarrhea in the absence of infection and the failure to establish disease of the GI tract by roentgenography and other studies should suggest investigation for a vasoactive intestinal polypeptide-producing islet cell tumor. In addition to calcium and glucose studies, repeated determinations should be made of the VIP levels. In contrast to the normal value of 150 pg/ml, very high levels may be found. The potassium loss is so great that electrolyte levels, including kidney function studies, may be required more than once a day. Intravenous administration of 300 mEq of potassium or more may be required daily. Scans and an angiogram are more likely to show these tumors than a gastrinoma.

Treatment

Local excision of a solitary tumor results in dramatic clinical improvement. More than one tumor may be present in the pancreas, and unfortunately hepatic metastases are common. Along with the subsidence of the diarrhea, hypercalcemia also abates. Free acid returns in the gastric juice and may increase, especially if the patient has received steroid therapy. The diabetes requires frequent and careful monitoring.

Other endocrine tumors may occur in association with the vipoma, making a general endocrine survey important as soon as the patient's condition warrants. Both adrenal glands should be carefully visualized and inspected at the time of the removal of the vipoma.

As in patients with other islet cell tumors, it is difficult to establish a reliable prognosis based on the usual microscopic studies of the tumor unless hepatic metastases are found. Recurrence of tumor is signaled by a return of the watery diarrhea and by dangerously low serum potassium levels. The control of symptoms associated with extensive metastases may require frequent administration of large doses of steroids. Prostaglandin and indomethacin have been given. Potassium levels and kidney function must be frequently monitored. Chemotherapy using streptozotocin, either alone or in combination with one or more of the newer anticarcinogenic drugs, should be considered. These tumors sometimes improve dramatically on chemotherapy. A "second-look" procedure to resect solitary hepatic masses may prolong life in some patients.

The more widespread use and availability of the vasoactive intestinal polypeptide immunoassay in the investigation of watery diarrhea should increase the accuracy of early diagnosis and improve the outcome in patients with this tumor.

BIBLIOGRAPHY

Bonfils S, Mignon M, et al: Cimetidine treatment of acute and chronic Zollinger–Ellison syndrome. World J Surg 3:597, 1979

Christoforidis AJ, Nelson SW: Radiological manifestations of the ulcerogenic tumors of the pancreas. JAMA 198:511, 1966

Desmond PV, Patwardhan RV, et al: Cimetidine impairs elimination of chlordiazepozide (Librium) in man. Ann Intern Med 93:266, 1980

Deveney CL, Deveney KS, et al: Use of calcium and secretin in the diagnosis of gastrinoma. Ann Intern Med 87:680, 1977

Gregory RA, Tracy HJ, et al: Extraction of a gastrin-like substance from a pancreatic tumor in a case of Zollinger–Ellison syndrome. Lancet 1:1045, 1960

Longmire WP Jr: Discussion of Zollinger RM, Tompkins RK, et al: Identification of the diarrheogenic hormone associated with non-beta islet cell tumors of the pancreas. Ann Surg 168:521, 1968

McGuigan JE, Trudeau WL: Immunochemical measurement of elevated levels of gastrin in the serum of patients with pancreatic tumors of the Zollinger–Ellison variety. N Engl J Med 278:1308, 1968

Murray JS, Paton RR, et al: Pancreatic tumor associated with flushing and diarrhea. N Engl J Med 264:436, 1961

Passaro EP Jr, Basso N, et al: Newer studies in the Zollinger–Ellison syndrome. Am J Surg 120:138, 1970

Priest WM, Alexander MK: Islet cell tumor of the pancreas with peptic ulceration, diarrhea and hypokalemia. Lancet 2:1145, 1957

Richardson CT, Feldman M, et al: Tiotidine, a new long-acting H_2-receptor antagonist: Comparison with cimetidine. Gastroenterology 80:301, 1981

Romanus ME, Neal JA, et al: Comparison of four provocative tests for the diagnosis of gastrinoma. Ann Surg 197:608, 1983

Stabile BE, Morrow DJ, et al: The gastrinoma triangle: Operative implications. Am J Surg 147:25, 1984

Tompkins RK, Kraft AR, et al: Secretin-like choleresis produced by a diarrheogenic non-beta islet cell tumor of the pancreas. Surgery 66:131, 1969

Van Thiel DH, Gavaler JS, et al: Hypothalamic-pituitary-gonadal dysfunction in men using cimetidine. N Engl J Med 300:1012, 1979

Verner JV, Morrison AB: Islet cell tumor and a syndrome of refractory watery diarrhea and hypokalemia. Am J Med 25:374, 1958

Way LW, Golman L, et al: Zollinger–Ellison syndrome. An analysis of twenty-five cases. Am J Surg 116:293, 1968

Wermer P: Genetic aspects of adenomatosis of endocrine glands. Am J Med 16:363, 1954

Zollinger RM, Ellison EC, et al: Primary peptic ulceration of the jejunum associated with islet cell tumors: Twenty-five-year appraisal. Ann Surg 192:422, 1980

Zollinger RM, Ellison EH: Primary peptic ulcerations of the jejunum associated with islet cell tumors of the pancreas. Ann Surg 142:709, 1955

Zollinger RM, Tompkins RK, et al: Identification of the diarrheogenic hormone associated with non-beta islet cell tumors of the pancreas. Ann Surg 168:502, 1968

92. Pancreatic and Periampullary Carcinoma

Avram M. Cooperman

INTRODUCTION

The mystique, respect, and pessimism that accompany pancreatic tumors and surgery is easily understood. Cloaked and obscured by viscera and peritoneum, access to the pancreas has been limited because of indirect tests of imaging. In that last decade, newer diagnostic tests, an appreciation of optimal timing for surgery, and a choice of nonoperative and operative procedures for palliation and cure have significantly altered and improved the diagnostic accuracy and immediate results of the surgical treatment of periampullary tumors and pancreatic cancer. Although the outlook remains discouraging for many periampullary cancers, continued investigation into etiology, and a quest for "early presentation," may improve survival rates. This chapter reviews the histopathology, etiology, clinical features, diagnostic tests, operative approaches, and results of surgery for pancreatic tumors and periampullary cancer. (Functioning endocrine tumors are discussed separately in Chapter 90.)

INCIDENCE

The incidence of pancreatic and periampullary cancer is increasing at an alarming rate. In the United States, 11,000 cases of periampullary cancer were diagnosed in 1978, but by 1982 the number had increased to more than 23,000. The increase is worldwide. In England and Wales, the incidence has doubled in the last two decades, whereas in Japan it has increased four-fold. In Sweden and Finland, it is also increasing and is presently the ninth most common cause of cancer-related deaths. As a cause of cancer deaths, pancreatic cancer ranks fourth in the United States. The 5-year survival rate is 2 percent or less, and more than 20,000 people die annually of this disease. Most discouraging is the fact that the percentage of cases where pancreatic cancer remains confined to the gland is unchanged over the past 30 years.

Etiology

The epidemiology of pancreatic cancer has been studied. Since this tumor accounts for 80 to 90 percent of all periampullary malignancies and has such a bleak prognosis, any insight into its cause may provide clues to much-needed therapy. Industrial, dietary, and environmental hazards have been investigated and reviewed by Morgan and Wormsley. Cigarette smoking increases the risk of pancreatic cancer two-fold, with the risk directly proportional to the number of cigarettes smoked. Some cite an inverse relationship between smoking and pancreatic cancer because smokers have an increased mortality from other diseases. The carcinogen is either present in smoke itself or acts by altering blood lipid levels. Both pipe and cigar smoking have been incriminated, but fewer subjects have been studied. If noninhalation of smoke can cause pancreatic cancer, then this carcinogen must be very potent.

In countries with increased dietary fat and protein, pancreatic cancer has also increased. Adapting a Western diet in Japan may be responsible for the four-fold increase in pancreatic cancer since 1950. Coffee consumption in the West, and perhaps tea in the East, may be other risk factors, particularly in males. One study on coffee consumption and pancreatic cancer in the United States has aroused much concern (but probably not altered habits), since it disclosed a significant risk of pancreatic cancer with increased coffee consumption. Whether the diet or coffee contains the carcinogen, or whether enzymes are stimulated causing cellular changes in the pancreatic ducts and acini is unclear.

The incidence of pancreatic cancer in diabetics is twice that of the general population. No other malignancy is increased with diabetes. In one study, the abrupt onset of diabetes mellitus after age 40, particularly unstable diabetes, was a clue to the diagnosis of pancreatic cancer. Presumably the cancer and diabetes co-exist, but this relationship is not causal and has not been emphasized by others.

Chronic pancreatitis and cancer may co-exist, and a pancreatic duct obscured by cancer may present as or mimic pancreatitis. Any association between chronic pancreatitis and cancer is serendipitous, although a suggestion that cellular hyperplasia and duct changes precede pancreatic cancer was published in 1894. Pancreatic cancer, carcinoma in situ, and hyperplasia of the pancreatic duct may co-exist, indicating a spectrum and perhaps sequence of pathologic changes in the same gland. Chemical and industrial carcinogens and cancer have also been studied. Nitrosamines and their metabolites have been implicated as potent carcinogens. These chemical toxins must reach the bloodstream, and/or pancreatic duct, and exert a direct toxic effect, or are converted from a procarcinogen. The toxin is then concentrated in the acinar cells or secreted by ductal epithelium. A higher incidence of pancreatic carcinoma in chemical workers is strong but presumptive evidence for this association.

An association between polyposis of the colon, Gardner's syndrome, and periampullary malignancy has been noted. The increase in periampullary malignancy may be 100 to 200 times that of the normal population with these polyposis syndromes. Preexisting adenomatous polyps of the duodenum or ampulla may also predispose to cancer, and benign areas co-exist in most patients with polypoid ampullary cancers.

Histopathology

The histopathology of periampullary tumors is varied and impressive. Unfortunately, malig-

nant tumors far outnumber benign lesions and pancreatic cancer accounts for 90 percent of all periampullary tumors. A suggested classification for pancreatic cancer is presented in Table 92–1.

Duct cell adenocarcinoma accounts for 75 to 85 percent of pancreatic cancers. Mucin is the diagnostic histologic feature of this cancer. Since mucin is produced only by primary and secondary pancreatic ducts, it is the hallmark of duct cell carcinoma. Atypical hyperplasia and carcinoma in situ may co-exist in one fourth of patients with duct cell carcinoma. Perineural and lymph node involvement occur in more than 90 percent of cases.

Adenosquamous cancer (adenoacanthoma) implies a mixture of glandular and squamous cells. Although found in other organs, adenosquamous cancers are rare in the pancreas. Twenty tumors were reviewed, and they had equal elements of squamous and epithelial cells. Perineural invasion is characteristic of these tumors, as are metastases to lymph nodes, liver, and peritoneum.

The term microadenocarcinoma implies small glands, smaller than those found in duct cell carcinoma. They center in sheets or solid foci of cells, and resemble carcinoid cells. Mucin is common in the cytoplasm of these glands. Microadenocarcinomas are an uncommon tumor and most patients are so ill that only palliative treatment can be given.

Mucinous adenocarcinoma is a well-recognized but uncommon pancreatic tumor. These tumors are larger and softer than other pancreatic cancers, as excessive amounts of mucin are secreted. The term mucinous adenocarcinoma is a gross description.

Cystadenocarcinomas are uncommon tumors that typically occur in young females (less than 50 years). Fewer than 400 have been re-

TABLE 92–1. PATHOLOGIC CLASSIFICATION OF CANCER OF THE PANCREAS (NONENDOCRINE)

I. Primary (93%)
  Duct Cell Origin (90%): duct cell adenocarcinoma, mucinous carcinoma, cystadenocarcinoma
  Acinar Cell Origin (1%): acinar cell carcinoma, cystadenocarcinoma (acinar cell)
  Uncertain Histogenesis (9%): pancreatoblastoma, papillary and cystic neoplasm, mixed tumor
  Connective Tissue Origin (1%): malignant fibrous histiocytoma, osteogenic sarcoma, leimyosarcoma, hemangiopericytoma

II. Metastatic (7%)

ported. They are large and primarily arise in the body and tail of the pancreas (85 percent). Nearly 90 percent of cases have occurred in Caucasians and only 5 percent of tumors involve the head of the pancreas. These tumors may be mucinous, serous, or have mixed elements. Mucin production predominates in 55 percent of patients. The outlook is significantly better than with type ordinaire pancreatic cancer, as most are resectable, so that survival rates are better. Campagno and Oertel noted 20 of 41 patients were alive (mean survival 6.7 years) after surgery.

Acinar cell carcinoma accounts for fewer than 10 percent of pancreatic cancers. This lesion can occur at any location within the pancreas and is characterized by the presence of zymogen granules within the tumor.

Pancreaticoblastomas are very rare tumors that occur in young children. Too few have been reported to characterize their course or features definitely.

Papillary and cystic neoplasm denote a relatively rare tumor of which 74 have been recently reviewed. Nearly all occur in young black females. These are large tumors and metastases are uncommon. The tumor is nearly always resectable, although total pancreatectomy may be required. Recurrence, if any, tends to be local. The prognosis is excellent.

Anaplastic carcinoma refers to a group of tumors that do not exhibit any specific patterns of the above cell types, are rarely resectable, and have a very poor prognosis.

Sarcomas of the pancreas arise from connective tissue, as blood vessel walls, fibrous tissue, smooth muscle, or nerve endings, and generally are included as isolated case reports of each unusual tumor.

Metastatic cancer involving the pancreas is seen in approximately 10 to 13 percent of autopsied patients. In decreasing incidence, the primary tumors are breast, lung, malignant lymphoma, malignant melanoma, leukemia, stomach, and colon. Metastatic tumors to the pancreas are therefore uncommon and the 10 to 13 percent may be unduly high and reflect disseminated disease in autopsy studies at tertiary neoplastic disease centers.

CLINICAL MANIFESTATIONS

Malignant neoplasms of the periampullary area include cancer of the ampulla of Vater, of the descending duodenum, of the distal common bile duct, and of the head of the pancreas. They are discussed together for several reasons: They occur within a short distance of each other, they have similar, if not indistinguishable features of presentation, and they are treated by similar operations.

It is unfortunate that these neoplasms do not occur with equal frequency. Cancer of the head of the pancreas accounts for 85 percent of all tumors and has a significantly worse prognosis than all of the other lesions.

Both benign and malignant periampullary tumors have varied presentations. Since malignant lesions are discovered late, it is unfortunate that these tumors are asymptomatic until a local or systematic complication develops. These complications include obstruction of the bile duct (jaundice, pruritus), duodenum, or stomach (gastric outlet obstruction), ulceration (gastrointestinal (GI) hemorrhage), and infiltration of peripancreatic nerve roots (pain). Symptoms are intermittent and mild with benign tumors, but are insidious and progressive with malignancy. About one third of benign tumors are asymptomatic. Nonspecific "tumor" symptoms include malaise, early satiety, anorexia, and mild postprandial pain. These may antedate the actual diagnosis of a tumor by 6 to 18 months. These symptoms are so prevalent in the general population that early attention or suspicion is not directed to the periampullary area. Evidence suggests that an increase in bile duct or pancreatic duct pressure present with benign or malignant obstruction may account for some of these nonspecific symptoms, as they have been relieved with endoscopic stents. At any rate, patients are generally not referred to surgeons at this stage in the diagnosis, and when specific symptoms do appear, the tumor is in its later stages.

Not surprisingly, an early diagnosis of a periampullary tumor was a rare event usually obtained by serendipity. An occasional tumor found at laparotomy done for another disease was rare for the surgeon and probably signaled good fortune for the patient. With the liberal use of endoscopy and ultrasound for nonspecific upper GI symptoms, a number of asymptomatic patients with smaller neoplasms have been discovered. These events happen too infrequently to alter the survival statistics of these diseases but provide encouragement and optimism for patients and physicians.

Regardless of the publication or time period, jaundice, pain, weight loss, and pruritus remain the most common presenting symptoms of periampullary cancers. Jaundice depends on the proximity of the tumor to the common bile duct and is detected in 50 to 90 percent of cases. The level of serum bilirubin is of diagnostic importance; levels greater than 10 mg/dl are often more associated with malignancy than benign disease. Continued bile duct obstruction from malignancy is much more common than from benign disease, and jaundice from malignant obstruction tends to be progressive, insidious, and, if untreated, complete. Jaundice from benign disease (common duct stones or strictures) is abrupt, incomplete, and usually transient. In malignant obstruction, the gallbladder is nearly always enlarged, although it is palpable in fewer than half of the patients. There is no difference in distensibility of the gallbladder wall in patients with chronic cholecystitis or periampullary cancers, and a dilated, palpable gallbladder therefore represents long-standing obstruction from a malignant tumor below the cystic duct. Abdominal pain is common, and although it may be caused by retroperitoneal extension of a neoplasm, it is often due to distention of an obstructed pancreatic or bile duct. Pain per se does not mean a late stage or incurable or unresectable tumor. The pain is usually postprandial, and in the epigastrum. When it is deep seated, in the upper back, and present at night, it denotes retroperitoneal extension of the tumor, an ominous sign.

Anorexia and weight loss that exceeds 10 percent of the body weight is common, even in the absence of metastases. There are several explanations: diabetes and/or pancreatic insufficiency (an obstructed pancreatic duct or diseased acini), biliary obstruction, obstructed pancreatic duct or diseased acini, bile salt malabsorption, and anorexia (hepatocellular dysfunction). Although insulin has been cited in the malnutrition and catabolism of malignancy, insulin secretion and pancreatic cancer have not been investigated. When hepatocellular dysfunction is corrected, after biliary decompression, weight gain and appetite often improve markedly even if the tumor is not resected.

Physical findings tend to be nonspecific, and if lymph nodes are palpable in the supraclavicular (Virchow's node) region or periumbilical region (Sister Joseph's sign), advanced carcinoma is present. Hepatomegaly may be secondary to an obstructed bile duct or metastatic carcinoma.

Laboratory Studies

Differentiation between periampullary tumors is not possible by laboratory tests, nor is it possible to distinguish benign from malignant diseases by laboratory tests alone. Elevations in serum alkaline phosphatase and serum bilirubin are the most common abnormalities. Alkaline phosphatase is a nonspecific, six-phosphate ester that is secreted by the bile canaliculus and is the first enzyme to rise, and fall, after obstruction and correction of bile duct obstruction. Alkaline phosphatase levels may rise to six or seven times normal before there is an increase in bilirubin. Pruritus, secondary to bile salt deposition in the skin, may precede clinical jaundice by 18 months. The level of serum bilirubin varies, depending on the proximity of the lesion to the bile duct and the completeness of obstruction.

Anemia, if present, is due to mucosal ulceration by a periampullary tumor or varices secondary to obstruction of the portal or splenic veins. Silver stools (acholic stools mixed with blood) are thought to be pathognomonic of an ampullary cancer, but this is an unusual sign and has been reported in English literature on only three occasions, although probably seen more often.

Special laboratory tests, including hormone and tumor markers (oncofetal antigen, carcinoembryonic antigen), have held great promise but are less accurate and have not been of great value or importance. Their major use is in serial determinations pre- and postoperatively. A rise is an additional concern that metastases are present.

Routine radiologic diagnosis consisting of flat and upright abdominal films and barium roentgenograms are of help in nearly half of the patients. They suggest, but do not diagnose, a specific neoplasm. Extrinsic compression on the duodenal wall, the presence of a duodenal mass, and a large duodenal ulceration are suggestive, but not pathognomonic, of malignancy (Fig. 92–1).

SPECIAL DIAGNOSTIC STUDIES

Significant advances in pancreatic and periampullary cancers have been directly related to improved techniques that provide imaging of the hepatobiliary and pancreatic ducts and pa-

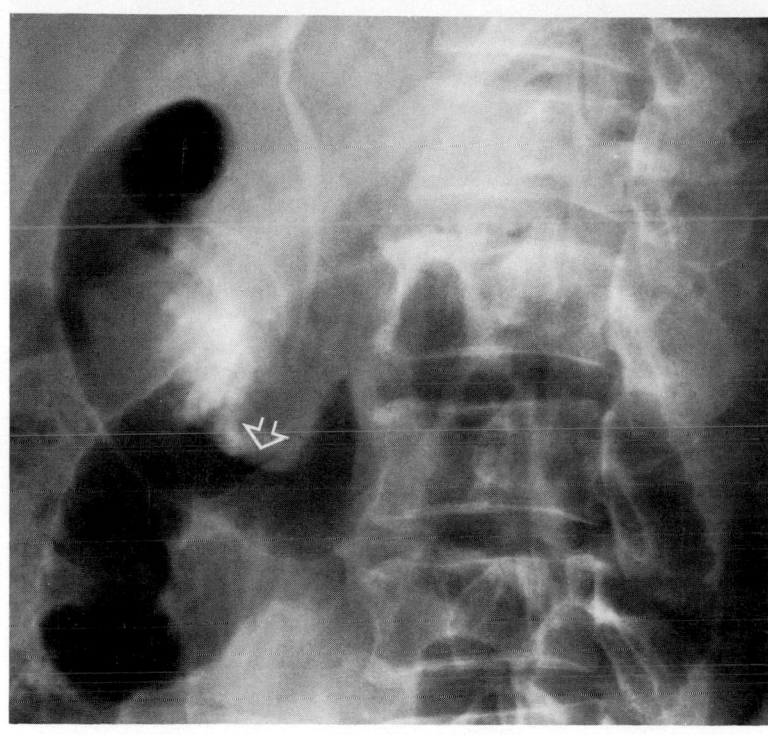

Figure 92–1. Extrinsic compression of the medial duodenal wall, caused by a pancreatic cancer (*arrow*), seen during an intravenous pyelogram.

renchyma by endoscopic retrograde studies (ER), angiography, computed tomography (CT), ultrasonography (US), and most recently nuclear magnetic resonance (NMR). Until these tests were developed, the differential diagnosis of jaundice included debatable decisions and indirect tests that relied on dye excreted by liver parenchyma and occasionally an abdominal exploration. The problem has been simplified by these new measures. As exciting as the diagnostic use of these tests is their therapeutic application. The order and place for each of the mentioned tests is unclear. The necessity and priority of each is altered as technical expertise and new equipment is developed.

It is important to emphasize that these diagnostic tests are very much dependent on individual expertise. The technical and interpretive skills available to an institution are more important than any authoritative recommendations in the literature to determine the order and priority of each. Reports comparing the value and accuracy of each procedure, whether the studies are prospective or retrospective, must be interpreted with caution. The following order of tests reflects the expertise available today and presupposes that each is available and well done at an institution.

Ultrasonography and Computed Tomography. An imaging test of the biliary tree and pancreas such as US or CT has much to offer as an initial diagnostic procedure in a jaundiced patient. They each will demonstrate dilated bile ducts, stones in the gallbladder, metastases in the liver, and, by outlining the head of the pancreas, a tumor, if present. US will infrequently show an ampullary or bile duct tumor. US has theoretical and practical advantages over computed tomography. There is no radiation exposure or rise, it separates fluid and solid interfaces, and it is one third to one half the cost of CT. CT is popular because of the excellent images it provides, fewer artefactual errors, and enhancement by contrast agents. The higher cost and machine repair time are practical disadvantages. NMR is even newer than CT and its role is still to be determined. The impression at the present time is that it offers little that CT does not provide (Figs. 92–2 and 92–3).

Endoscopy. An endoscopic examination of the stomach and duodenum is done next. Visualization and biopsy of an ampullary or duodenal tumor is easily accomplished. This saves time and concern preoperatively and avoids a duode-

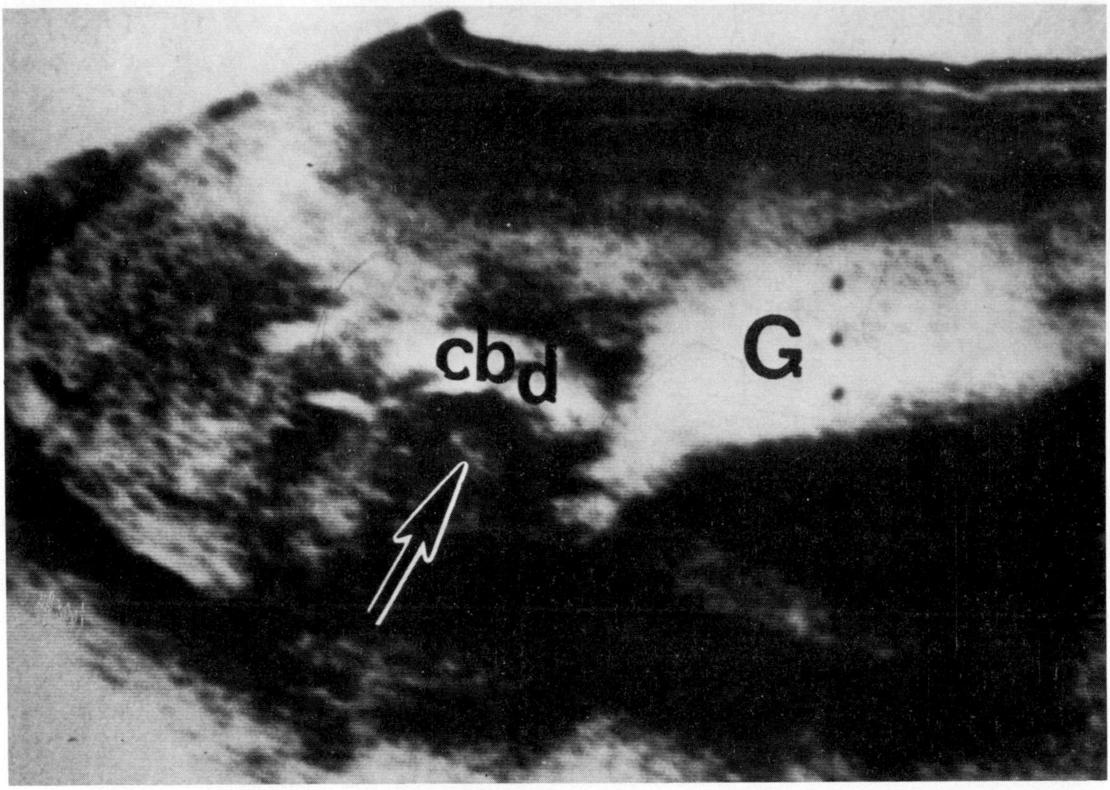

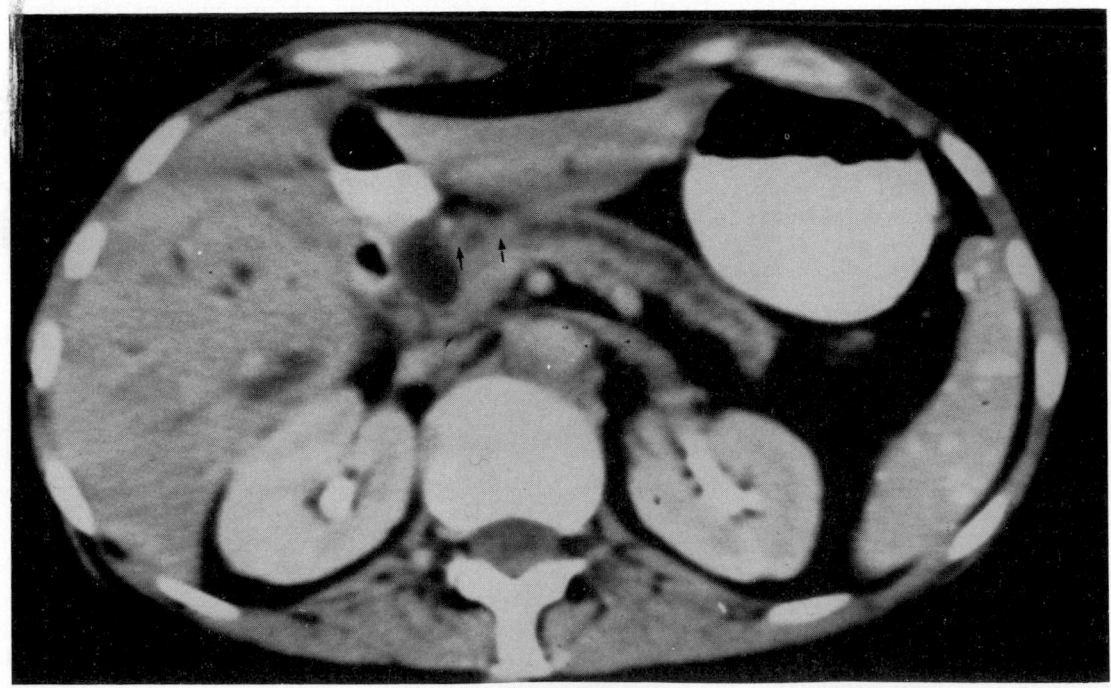

Figures 92–2 and **3.** An ultrasound (2) and CT (3) both show a mass in the head of the pancreas. A dilated gallbladder and bile duct are also seen on the CT scan. Two obstructions are seen on CT scan, which in this instance are due to a multicentric cancer of the pancreas.

Figure 92–3.

notomy and the theoretical possibility of implanting tumor cells intraoperatively. Encroachment on the medial duodenal wall by a pancreatic tumor is often suggested. With expertise, a retrograde study of the bile and pancreatic ducts is done simultaneously. The site of biliary and/or pancreatic obstruction is precisely defined, and by the radiologic pattern a diagnosis is made with a high degree of certainty. Since pancreatic ductal carcinoma accounts for 90 percent of pancreatic malignancies, complete pancreatic duct obstruction is almost always diagnostic of pancreatic cancer. Ten percent of pancreatic cancers arise from acini, and a normal pancreatogram is possible although this happens in only 5 to 10 percent of cases. ER allows for the collection of pancreatic juice and cytologic analysis, which has an accuracy of 30 to 80 percent. When positive, it is diagnostic.

At the same endoscopy, a therapeutic endoscopic stent may be placed to decompress an obstructed liver and bile duct (Fig. 92–4). This author believes this to be state of the art and the coming wave at institutions where it is not presently available. It is safe, and successful in more than 90 percent of attempts.

Percutaneous Cholangiography (PTC). Percutaneous transhepatic cholangiography is a safe, rapid means to decompress and localize the site of obstruction in the biliary tree. Initially introduced as a diagnostic procedure it has now been extended to provide internal drainage in patients with obstructive jaundice by advancing the catheters beyond the obstruction into the duodenum (Fig. 92–5A). Technical modifications and newer catheters have permitted internal drainage in more than 90 percent of patients. The complications of PTC and internal stenting are few but include sepsis (catheters may puncture the bile duct and hepatic vein), bleeding, subcapsular hematomas, and transient fever. Complication rates range from 10 to 25 percent (Fig. 92–5B) but the complications are generally transient. Surgery may be required in 1 to 2 percent of these cases. Not all percutaneous stents successfully decompress obstructed bile ducts. Injecting a stent with contrast material nearly always shows good emptying and flow of contrast into the duodenum, but at least 5 to 10 percent of stented patients develop cholangitis. At first, we changed stents frequently, often increasing their diameter. This is usually not the solution. HIDA scans

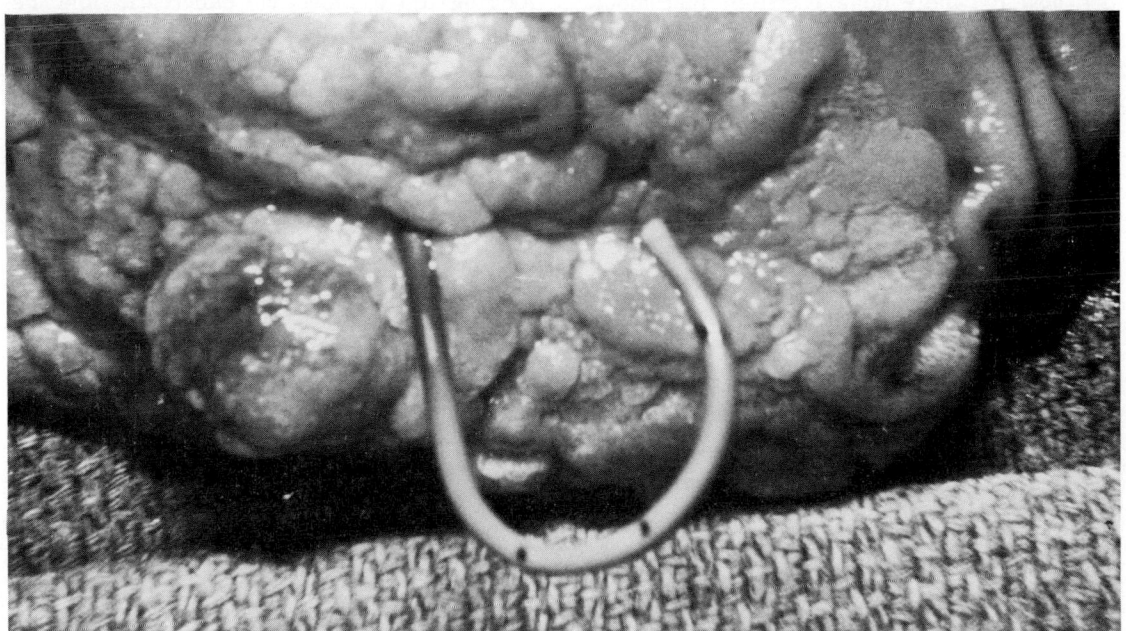

Figure 92–4. An endoscopic stent passed through a villous tumor that had obstructed the bile duct.

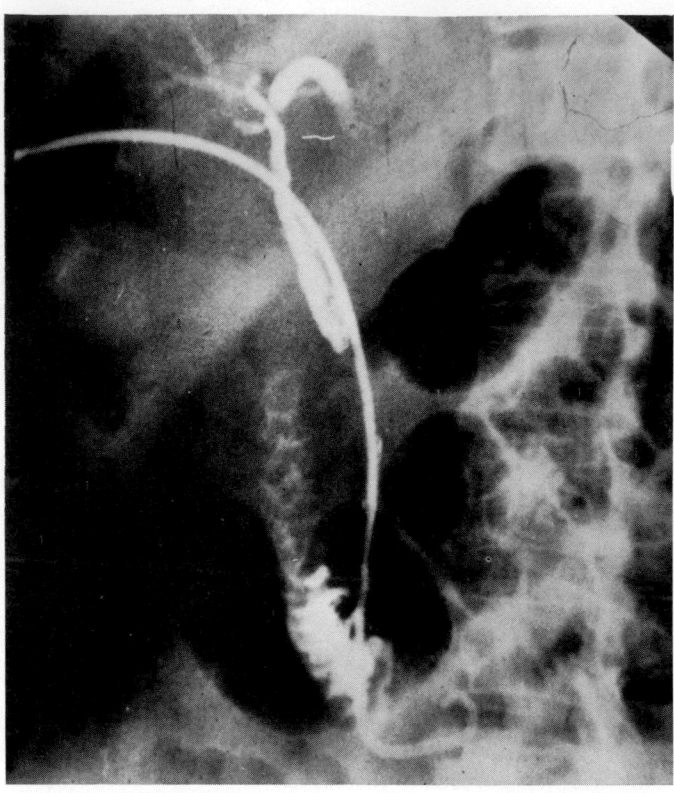

Figure 92–5. A. A percutaneous transhepatic stent placed through an obstructed bile duct.

A

are now routinely done poststent placement. This will demonstrate bile flow and determine if surgery will be necessary to decompress bile ducts if a stent does not provide adequate decompression.

Angiography. Selective pancreatic and hepatic angiography as a routine preoperative test for periampullary cancer has its advocates. Until recently, angiography was considered an option. There was little choice but to operate to

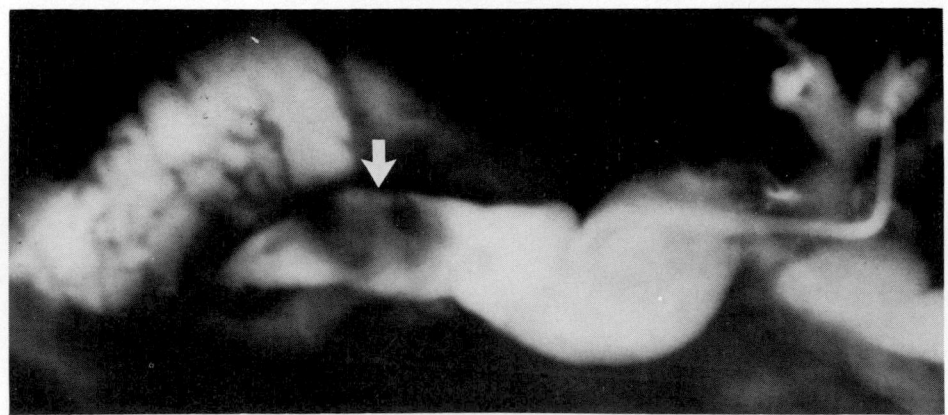

B

Figure 92–5. B. Clots in the bile duct (hemobilia), a complication of percutaneous stenting. Since bile contains fibrinolysins, when the bleeding stops, the clots will clear.

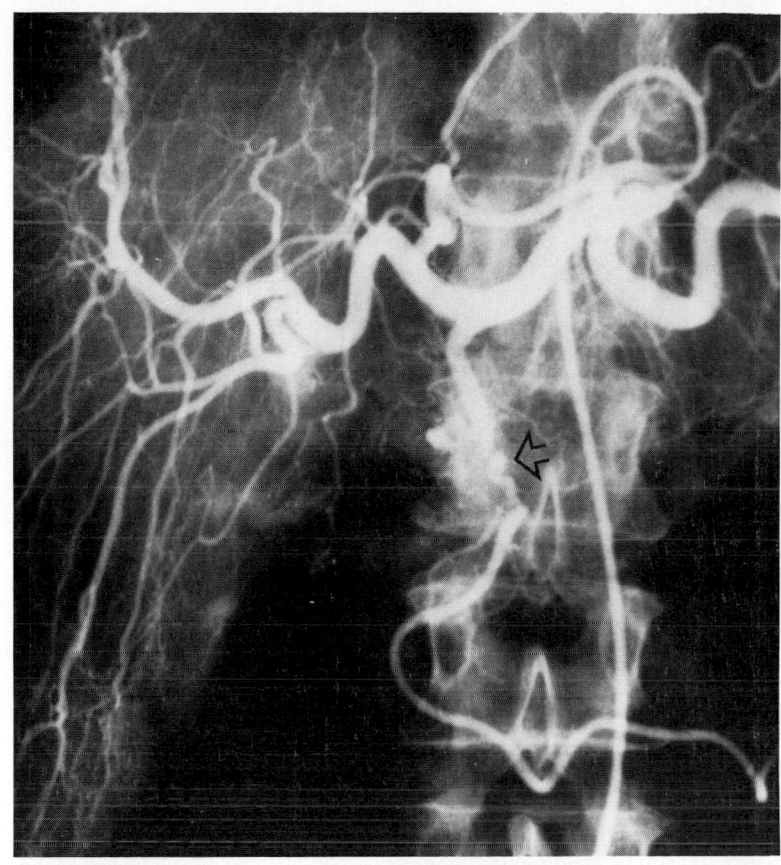

Figure 92–6. An encased gastroduodenal artery (*arrow*) in the field of pancreatic resection.

decompress an obstructed liver, and surgeons familiar with periampullary anatomy and vascular anomalies believed angiography was of ancilliary benefit. With the advent of nonoperative biliary decompression, palliation by nonoperative means plays an increasing role in treatment. Preoperative angiography is important when pancreatic tumors involve the head of the pancreas.

Angiography has a particular value preoperatively to demonstrate proximity or invasion of a pancreatic tumor to the mesenteric vein and artery. Encasement of vessels in the "field of resection" does not mean unresectability, although encasement of the mesenteric vein effectively denotes incurability (Figs. 92–6 through 92–9). The occasional surprise finding of a hypervascular lesion implies an islet cell or carcinoid tumor and is an additional benefit of angiography.

Although angiography has a diagnostic accuracy of 70 to 90 percent, other tests for diagnosing a pancreatic mass are as accurate and less invasive. Angiography has a definite place when symptoms suggest pancreatic cancer, particularly of the body and tail, and when other imaging tests are negative.

With cost containment and hospital admissions closely reviewed today, the entire workup and staging of a periampullary tumor can usually be accomplished in one morning. An ultrasound followed by an angiogram, and then by endoscopy and ER (angiography is done before ER because the contrast material with ER will pool in the intestine and obscure the angiogram) provides rapid, accurate, diagnostic and therapeutic benefit. If jaundice is severe, there is a danger that the contrast material injected with an angiogram will adversely affect renal function. In this circumstance angiography is deferred and the patient allowed to recover at home while liver function shows signs of improvement. The angiogram is done prior to a planned operation if the lesion is a pancreatic

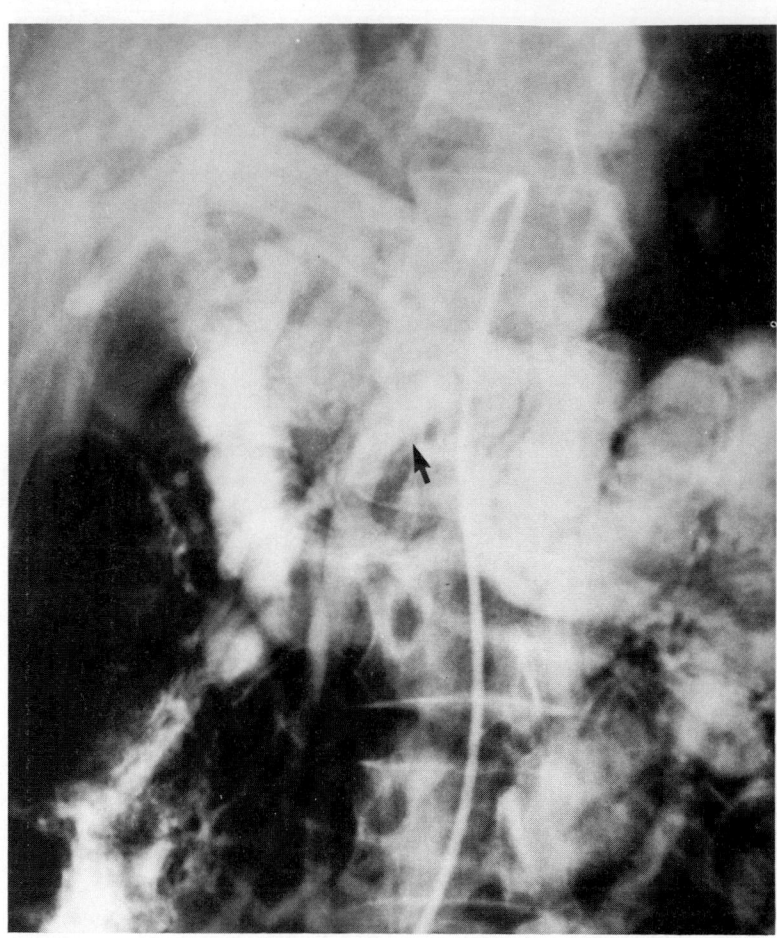

Figure 92–7. High entry of the ileocolic vein into the mesenteric vein under the neck of the pancreas.

cancer. There is less necessity for angiography when the primary cancer is ampullary since the resectability rate exceeds 80 percent.

THERAPY

General Considerations

The surgical priorities and timing of treatment have changed significantly since the last edition of this text. Today, surgeons need not operate to decompress the liver to diagnose a malignant lesion or palliate jaundice. Surgery should be done with the intent to resect a lesion for cure, and not to palliate. There have always been adverse effects of doing surgery in the presence of jaundice and there was wisdom in doing staged operations whereby the gallbladder and liver were decompressed prior to resecting a

pancreatic cancer. These effects include poor wound healing, decreased renal function and glomerular filtration rate, reticuloendothelial (RE) cell function, and cell-mediated immunity, and failure of the liver to remove endotoxins from the portal vein.

It is sometimes difficult to separate the theoretical from the clinical circumstance. For example, poor wound healing and jaundice in the clinical situation often co-exist with malnutrition and chronic illness, which are common with periampullary tumors. In the experimental animal, however, when the bile duct was ligated and a wound produced elsewhere, there was poor wound healing. The defect in poor healing is in collagen synthesis, which is presumably due to a deficit in proliferation of fibroblasts. The liver is abundant with RE cells, and jaundiced patients have depressed immune responses and a greater incidence of sepsis. Many

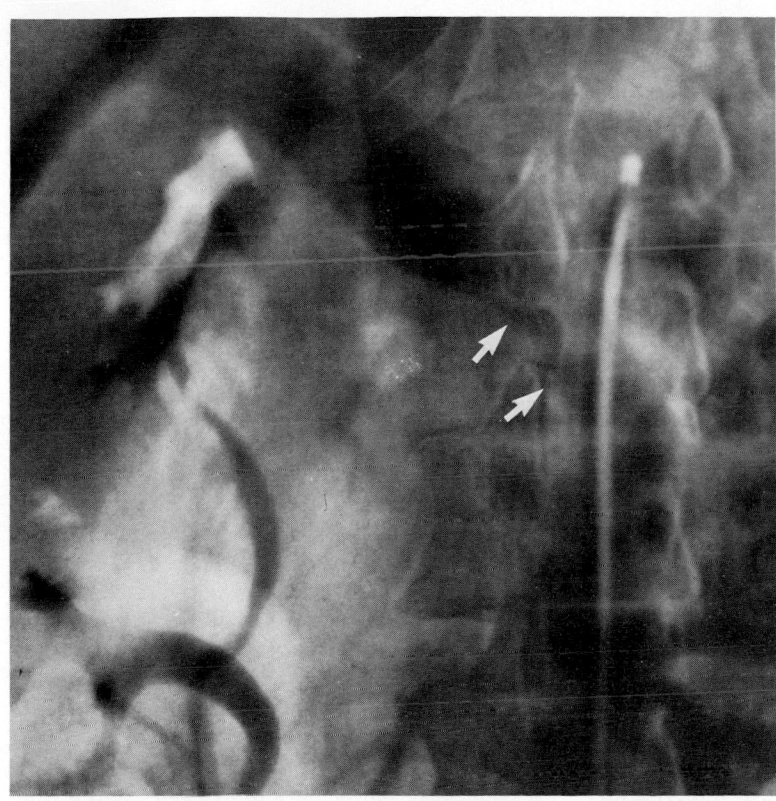

Figure 92–8. Extrinsic compression of the mesenteric vein by a large pancreatic cancer. This was not encased and the tumor was resectable.

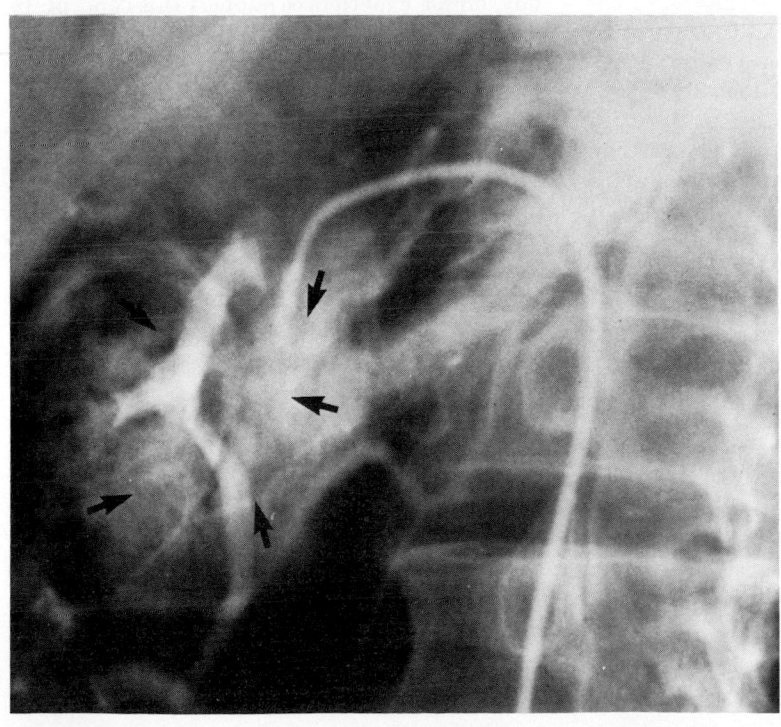

Figure 92–9. The cancer of the head of the pancreas was vascular but resectable.

of these deficiencies can be corrected by decompression of the liver and bile duct preoperatively. In some circumstances, these may exist with bile duct obstruction without jaundice. The role of stenting in these circumstances is less defined.

The new methodology is reflected in recent surgical studies. Pitt and associates summarized risk factors in 155 patients undergoing biliary surgery. Of 15 factors analyzed, 8 were associated with increased operative risk. These were malignancy, leukocytosis, age greater than 60, hematocrit less than 30 percent, and elevation in creatinine, alkaline phosphatase, and bilirubin. When seven signs were present and an operation was done, the mortality was close to 100 percent, whereas no deaths occurred in patients with two or fewer risk factors. Ten of twelve deaths occurred in patients with five or more signs. Benign causes of bile duct obstruction were incomplete and transient. Therefore, multiple signs denote the presence of malignancy, and risk may be decreased if these are corrected preoperatively.

A second nonrandomized study, by Denning and associates, summarized the course of 57 icteric patients, 48 of whom had a malignancy. Thirty two were decompressed preoperatively and 25 were not. The postoperative morbidity was twice as great in the nondecompressed patients (56 versus 29 percent) and the operative mortality was higher (25 percent versus 16 percent), although this was not statistically significant.

We reported 80 patients with malignancy who underwent preoperative transhepatic biliary drainage for jaundice (Table 92–2). Of 46 patients with periampullary malignancy, 32 had pancreatic carcinoma. The patients were classified into three groups. In the first group (29 patients, or 63 percent), the serum bilirubin returned to a normal level after stenting. The average survival was 198 days and the 30-day mortality was 10 percent. The second group, consisting of 9 patients (20 percent), had a 50 percent decline in serum bilirubin, i.e., a mean fall from 18 to 9 mg/dl. These patients survived only an average of 72 days, with a 30-day mortality of 33 percent. The third group, consisting of 8 patients (17 percent) who did not differ physically from the other two groups, had no change in serum bilirubin, despite good catheter positioning. Their average survival was only 12 days, and the 30-day mortality was 88 percent. Regardless of the fall in serum bilirubin, when liver metastases were present, the 30-day mortality was 47 percent and the average survival was less than 50 days. This study showed a prognostic significance to nonoperative biliary drainage and may help explain the varying mortality with bypass operations for hepatic decompression, which ranges from 5 to 33 percent. The varying mortality after operative bypass reflects a poor selection of patients rather than a difficult technical procedure. Although these recent studies reflect on the technical advances of today, ample experiences support this concept. In one large study the morbidity (bleeding, sepsis, renal failure) and mortality in 279 pancreaticoduodenal resections were very significant when the bilirubin was greater than 20 mg/dl (Table 92–3).

Not all surgeons agree that preoperative decompression is necessary. In a retrospective

TABLE 92–2. PROGNOSTIC VALUE OF PREOPERATIVE DECOMPRESSION IN MALIGNANT JAUNDICE

Group	Bilirubin Response	No. of Patients	Average Survival (Days)	30-Day Mortality
I (Good Response)	Return to normal (Average 17 to 2 mg/dl)	29 (63%)	198	10%
II (Intermediate Response)	50% decline (Average 18 to 9 mg/dl)	9 (20%)	72	33%
III (Poor Response)	No change (Average 18 to 17 mg/dl)	8 (17%)	12	88%
Total		46	141	28%

(*Source: From Neff, RA, Fankuchen EI, et al: The radiologic management of malignant biliary obstruction. Clin Radiol 34:143, 1983, with permission.*)

TABLE 92–3. INCIDENCE OF COMPLICATIONS AFTER WHIPPLE PROCEDURE: CORRELATION WITH SERUM BILIRUBIN LEVEL

Serum Bilirubin (mg/dl)	No. of Cases	Renal Failure (%)	Wound Hemorrhage (%)	Wound Sepsis (%)	Mortality
1.0	92	2.6	6.5	22.1	13.0
1– 9.9	111	2.6	15.0	20.4	9.7
10–19.9	48	775	10.0	20.0	12.5
20–30+	28	9.0	22.0	26.0	22.0

(*Source: From Braasch JL, Gray BN, 1977, with permission.*)

study comparing preoperative biliary decompression with early surgery, 109 consecutive patients (90 with malignancy) who underwent percutaneous transhepatic decompression were compared to 65 patients (42 with malignancy) with obstruction of the biliary tree who underwent immediate surgery after cholangiography. Eight of 44 decompressed patients (18 percent) with malignancy died and 14 of 42 nondecompressed patients (33 percent) with malignancy died. All deaths in the decompressed group had no fall in serum bilirubin after decompression. Although the authors indicate there was no advantage to preoperative decompression, all deaths in the preoperatively drained group occurred in patients whose bilirubin did not fall after decompression. Avoiding surgery in these patients would have reduced the operative mortality to 0 percent, a highly statistical difference.

Anergy. Cell-mediated immunity has been examined in pancreatic and periampullary cancer. Most patients have at least one abnormality, with lymphocyte function depressed in most patients. The correlation between immune function, prognosis, and tumor resectability is poor, but most patients with pancreatic cancer have unresectable and incurable tumors.

The role of anergy and skin testing in surgical patients, particularly its correlation with nutritional assessment, has been extensively studied. Preoperative correction of nutritional deficits may decrease postoperative morbidity and mortality. The role of preoperative nutritional correction in diseases where less than 10 percent of cancers are resectable is unclear but should be selectively applied. A small personal experience in nonjaundiced patients with elevated alkaline phosphatase levels and minimal weight loss indicated anergy was present in 30 percent of cases. This improved with endoscopic stenting preoperatively.

Ampullary Carcinoma

Cancer of the ampulla of Vater is certainly more favorable than pancreatic cancer. Whether this reflects a biologic innocence, an earlier onset of symptoms, more favorable histopathology (low-stage tumors), or less frequent metastases is unclear. Patients with ampullary cancer ideally undergo pancreaticoduodenal resection as the preferred treatment.

There is a definite malignant potential of adenomatous, duodenal, and ampullary polyps. Benign adenomatous tissue on the periphery of an ampullary cancer was found in 18 of 21 (82 percent) ampullary cancers. The analogy with colon polyps as a precursor of cancer is well founded.

Colonic polyposis, soft-tissue tumors, and bone tumors (Gardner's syndrome) are associated with duodenal, ampullary, and gastric cancers. This is an autosomal dominant disorder with a high degree of penetrance. The risk of periampullary cancer in this disease is 100 to 200 times the normal population. In one extreme case, 256 duodenal adenomas, 91 gastric antral polyps, and a periampullary cancer were described in the same patient. At least 29 cases of periampullary cancer and 21 gastric cancers with polyposis syndromes have been reported.

Endoscopy and endoscopic biopsy or brushing should be very accurate in establishing a preoperative diagnosis of ampullary cancer. Since most lesions are soft and polypoid, endoscopic sphincterotomy or stenting has been utilized for decompression of an obstructed liver or palliation in isolated instances. Three operative procedures are employed: resection, bypass, or local excision with or without a bypass. Ideally, patients with ampullary cancer should be

TABLE 92–4. OUTCOME OF 38 CASES OF AMPULLARY CANCER BY TREATMENT GROUP

	Pancreaticoduodenal Resection	Bypass with Excision	Bypass Only
Number of patients	23	9	7
Operative deaths	2 (8.6%)	1 (12.5%)	1 (14%)
Subsequent deaths	14	7	5
Due to metastases	12	5	5
Mean survival (months)	28	32	23
Range	7–78	3–82	6–54
Mean survival without metastases	55	42	42
Mean survival with metastases	23	13.5	6
Number alive (follow-up, months)	7 (12–216)	0	1

resected by local means or pancreaticoduodenectomy. Less favorable tumors or patients with severe co-existing medical diseases that preclude resection undergo less extensive procedures. The bias of selection must always favor the resected patient. Survival should be better after resection for this reason alone. It is necessary to review numerous reports, since most studies involve small numbers of patients and valid conclusions may reflect a referral pattern or selection bias. We retrospectively reviewed 38 patients with ampullary cancer (Table 92–4) and noted better 5-year survival, with papillary tumors (six times better than with ulcerating tumors), and negative nodes (26 percent versus 11 percent 5-year survival in patients with positive nodes). More patients survive 5 and 10 years after pancreatoduodenal resection than do "bypass patients" but selection may play as important a role as the operation itself. These findings are reflected in other studies. Table 92–5 is a compilation of reports which summarize the results of pancreaticoduodenal resection in 900 patients with ampullary cancer. In some select studies, lesser operations have been followed by a similar mean survival. An additional and crucial factor is the histopathologic review. We subsequently noted that 10 percent of ampullary carcinomas were benign papillary adenomas with foci of atypia when reviewed and reclassi-

TABLE 92–5. RECENT RESULTS OF MAJOR RESECTIONS FOR AMPULLARY CANCER

	No.	No. Resected	Operative Mortality (%)	5-Year Survival (%)	10-Year Survival (%)
Nakase et al (1977)	459	331	16.5	6	1
Akwari et al (1977)		87	11.5	34	20
Stephenson et al (1977)	13	9	22	33	
Braasch et al (1977)		61	67		
Treadwell et al (1978)	31	19	16	32	
Makipor et al (1979)	38	23	9	24	
Williams et al (1979)	33	26	11	27	
Langer et al (1979)	24	24	6	6	
Ta-Cheng (1980)	44	34	15	17	
Smith (1981)		140	2.7	35	
McRussell et al (1982)	18	9	10	33	10+
Cooperman et al (1982)	40	38	10	26	10+
Cohen et al (1982)		22	24	30	
Walsh et al (1982)	51	44	16	11	
Barton et al (1983)	56	44	2	31	10

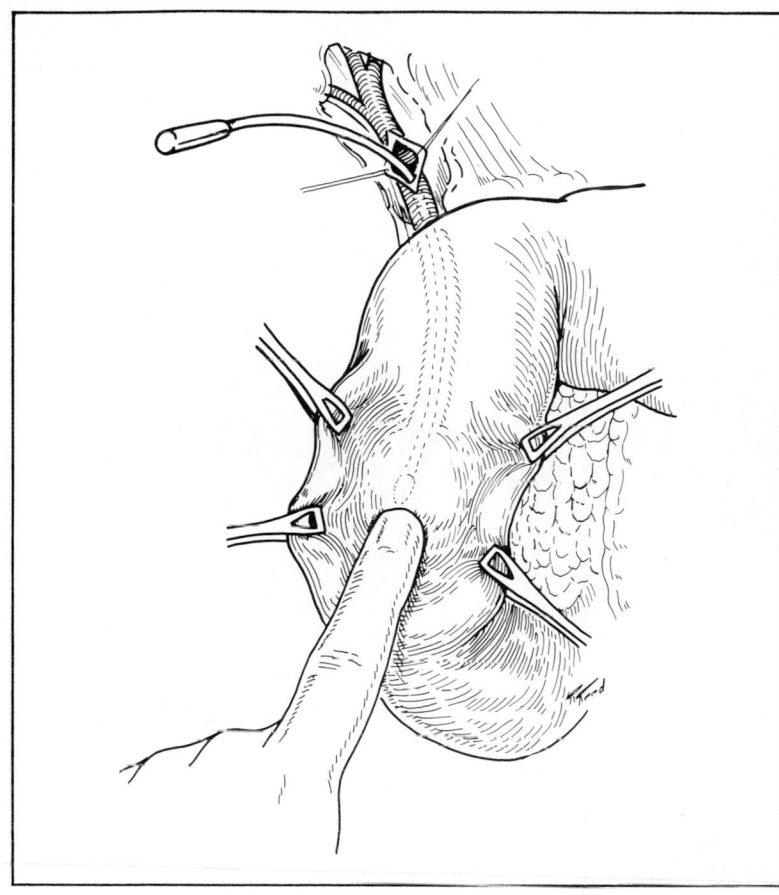

Figure 92–10.

Figures 92–10, 11, and 12. Palpation of a polypoid ampullary tumor. Four traction sutures or Babcock clamps facilitate initial exposure. A Kocher maneuver will deliver the duodenum anteriorly. The common duct may be opened and a probe or catheter introduced to the ampulla if a lesion cannot be palpated through the duodenum. The duodenum may be opened longitudinally, transversely, or obliquely.

fied. This factor will greatly alter the prognosis and improve survival statistics for any operation.

Local resection for polypoid ampullary cancers was first described by Halsted in 1899. The operation is employed selectively for elderly patients with co-existing severe medical diseases. Isolated reports involving few patients indicate some 5-year survivors. A recent report of 13 cases noted only a 17 percent 5-year survival. More than 150 local excisions have been reported for ampullary cancers with 40 surviving 2 to 22 years. The operative technique is detailed in Figures 92–10 through 92–17. A resected tumor is shown in Figure 92–18.

Carcinoma of the Lower Bile Duct

Carcinoma of the lower third of the bile duct has a better survival rate than carcinoma of the middle or upper third of the bile duct but is an uncommon lesion. This may be because the lower third of the duct is surrounded by parenchymal pancreatic tissue, whereas middle- and upper-third lesions invade hepatic artery and portal vein directly. Ten or more years ago survival with any bile duct cancer was limited and uncommon. Lesions in the terminal third of the bile duct tend to obstruct the duct early, but they also tend to ulcerate and infiltrate the surrounding pancreas. In a collected review from Japan, Nakase and associates reported 300 patients with cancer in the distal bile duct, 161 of whom underwent a pancreaticoduodenal resection. The resectability rate was 52 percent, the operative mortality was 21 percent. The mean survival was 17.5 months. The 5-year survival was only 5 percent, and the 10-year survival was 1 percent.

Other studies involving fewer patients indicate a 5-year survival rate for lower-third bile duct cancers that range from 25 to 40 percent. The difficulty in drawing firm conclusions from

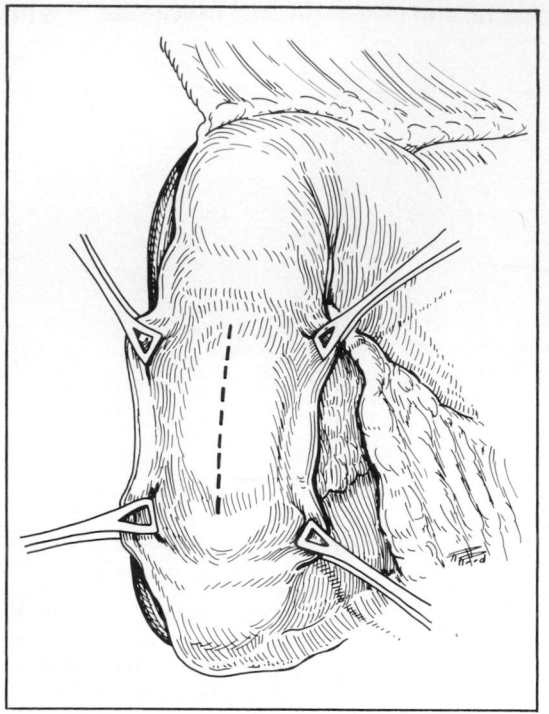

Figure 92–11.

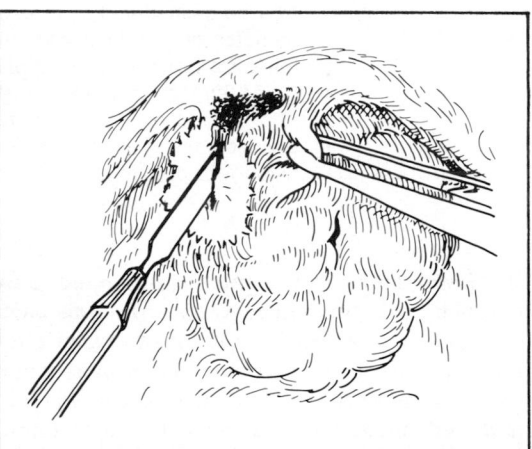

Figure 92–13. A cautery unit (our preference) facilitates hemostasis and submucosal removal of the lesion.

Figure 92–12.

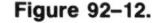

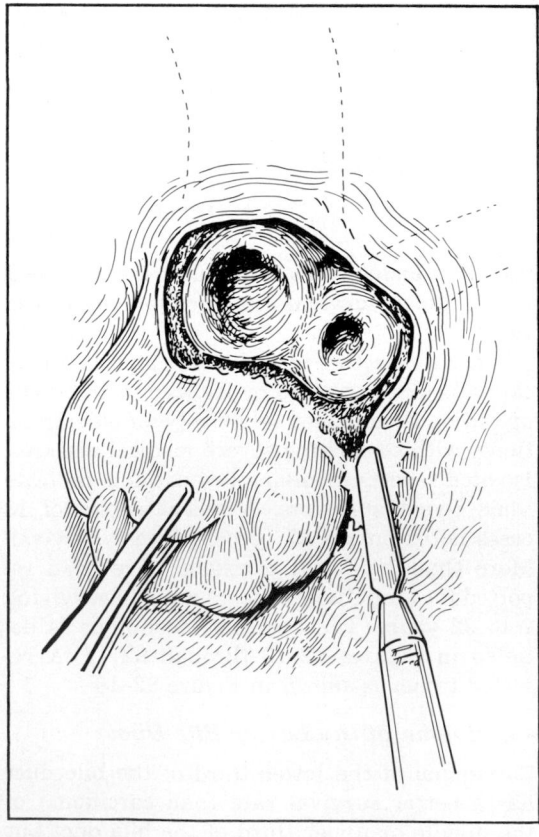

Figure 92–14. As the tumor is excised, the orifices of the common bile duct and pancreatic duct are visualized.

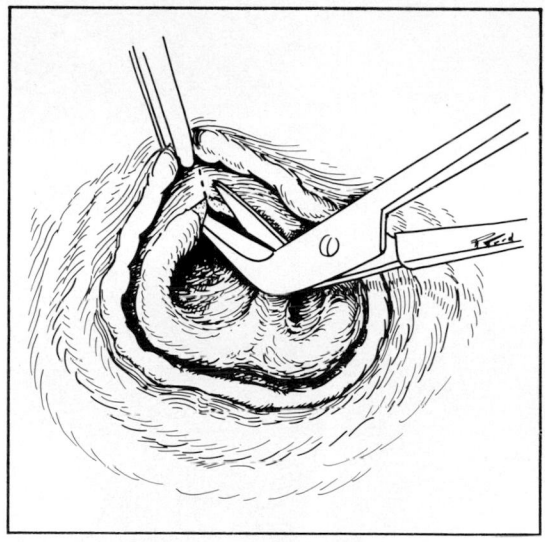

Figure 92–15. A sphincteroplasty in the common bile duct is made by excision of a wedge of anterior common bile duct wall. This procedure may prevent a distal duct stricture from developing. I utilize it when the orifices of the bile duct and pancreatic duct are small (< 7mm).

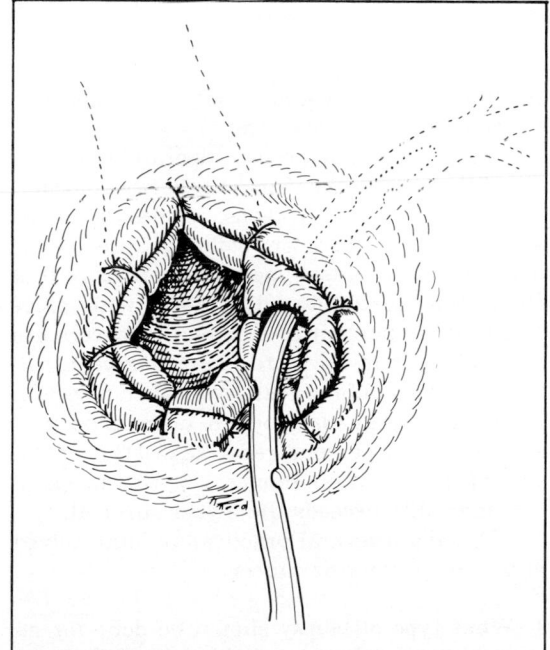

Figure 92–16. It is even less clear how to deal with the pancreatic duct. If the duct is dilated, nothing is done. If the duct is of normal size, a short sphincteroplasty is performed or a small nonobstructing catheter is inserted, with the expectation that the catheter will pass spontaneously in weeks or months. The duct is sutured to the mucosa with fine, interrupted absorbable sutures.

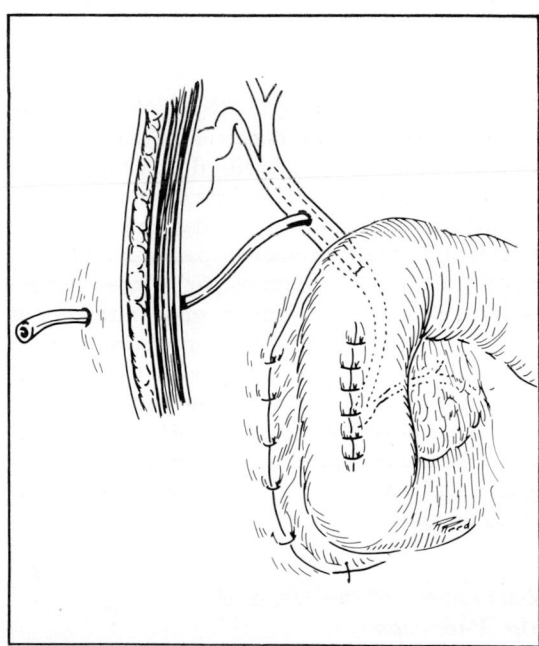

Figure 92–17. Longitudinal closure of the duodenum (rather than tranverse closure) is probably easiest, but care must be taken to avoid excessive inversion. Either an inner layer of chromic catgut and an outer layer of silk sutures or a single carefully placed layer of nonabsorbable sutures will suffice. A T-tube may be placed in the common bile duct prior to closure of the abdomen. This is done when the duct is explored or to decompress the distal duct.

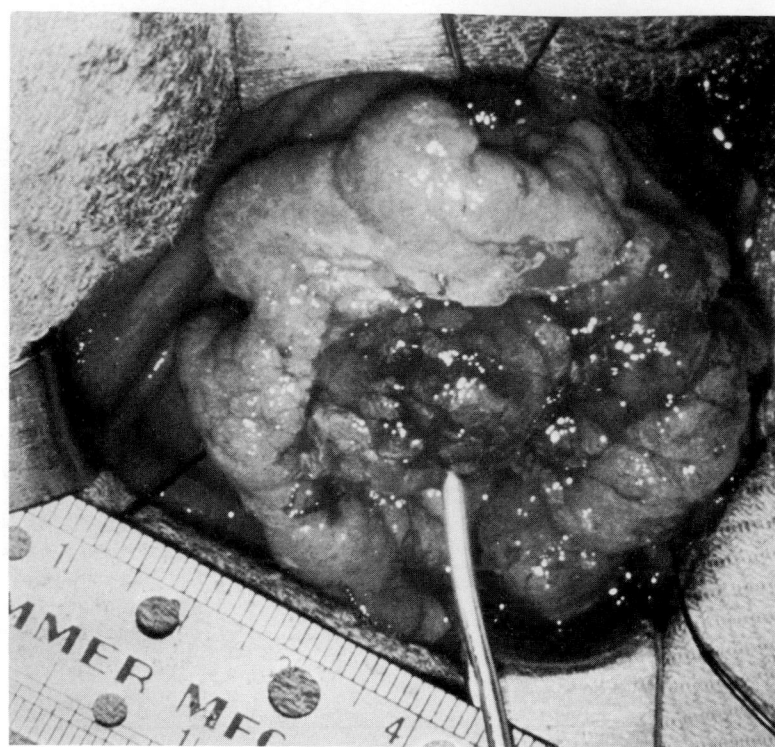

Figure 92–18. A polypoid ampullary tumor excised.

isolated reports is illustrated by Bjorck and associates, who reported a 33 percent 5-year survival rate for resected distal bile duct cancer with or without positive nodes. The seeming contradiction about the status of nodes and prognosis reflected a small number of patients and indicated that node metastases per se were not an adverse prognostic factor in small numbers of patients. The limitations of predicting cancer survival in individual patients on the basis of local pathologic findings is shown by this study.

In a collective review of 181 resected patients with choledochal cancer, the 5-year survival rate was 15 percent but ranged from 6 to 33 percent.

Carcinoma of the Head of the Pancreas

Although some optimism is expressed by all who treat periampullary malignancy, good results are clouded by the increasing number of patients with carcinoma of the head of the pancreas, a disease characterized by a very modest survival. Despite continued technical modifications and "rationale" operations, advances in pancreatic cancer must be directed at eliminat-

ing the as yet undefined factor(s) responsible for the increased incidence.

The "correct or proper" operation for cancer of the head of the pancreas creates considerable debate among surgeons, as does the necessity for tissue diagnosis before a resection is done. From the outset one must emphasize that these issues pertain to only a few patients, since less than 10 percent of pancreatic cancers are resectable. Thus, for more than 90 percent, palliation is the realistic goal. Even when resection is possible, 5-year survivors are uncommon, usually less than 5 percent, regardless of the magnitude of the operation. In most reports the operative mortality exceeds the 5-year survival.

There are several practical and unresolved issues for pancreatic cancer:

1. What type of biopsy should be done for an undiagnosed lesion in the head of the pancreas? Is it necessary to have a tissue diagnosis before resection?
2. What should the extent of resection be (total pancreatectomy, Whipple operation, or bypass)?
3. Is adjuvant therapy (radiation or chemotherapy) of benefit?

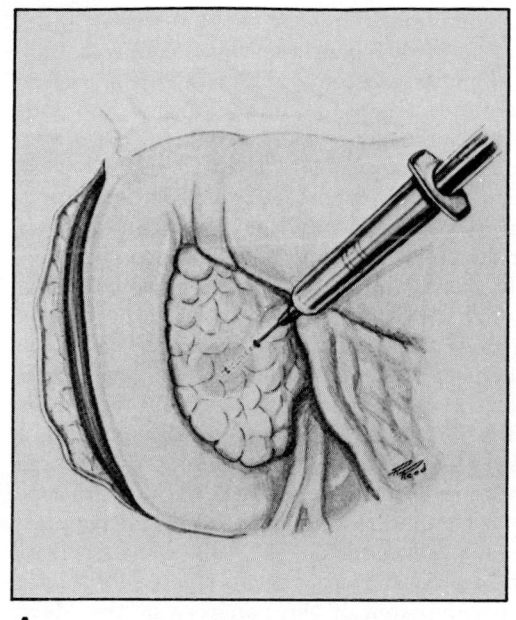

A

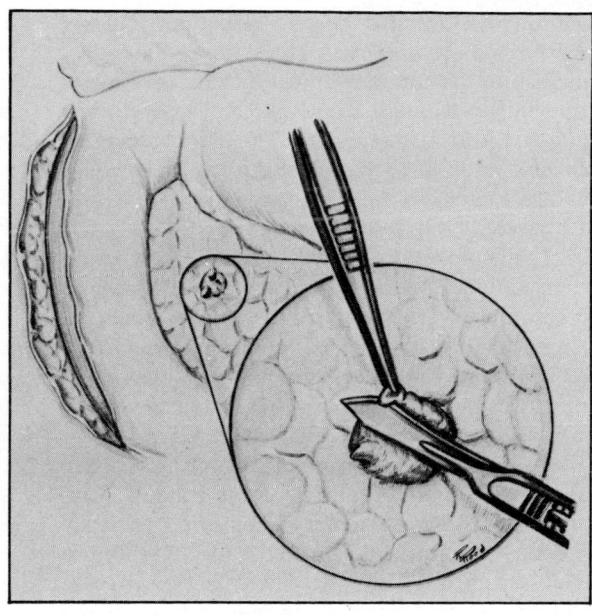

B

Figure 92–19. A. Direct fine needle (No. 23 gauge) aspiration biopsy of pancreatic cancer. The aspirate is placed on a glass slide, fixed, and then read. **B.** Direct shave biopsy of a protruding pancreatic cancer that has penetrated the anterior surface.

These issues are important because the mortality and morbidity continue to be significant after pancreatic resection for cancer, and the limited survival statistics remain unchanged.

Pancreatic biopsy has been controversial. Enthusiasts are generally surgeons who have had positive tissue diagnoses and few complications, whereas those who have toiled for many frustrating moments attempting to establish a diagnosis with several biopsies, or have had significant complications, understandably react differently. There are three types of pancreatic biopsies: "shave," large needle, or thin needle cytologic. When a pancreatic mass presents through the capsule of the gland, a shave biopsy using a knife held parallel to the pancreas is safe and accurate. It should not be directed deeply into the pancreas (Fig. 92–19A,B).

Large needle biopsies, usually with a Vim Silverman or TruCut needle, have been most popular. They are directed into the tumor mass through the duodenum or directly into the pancreas. By removing a core of the tissue they provide a satisfactory sample for the pathologist. They may also puncture blood vessels, pancreatic ducts, or miss the tumor itself. In a review of more than 2000 large needle biopsies,

the average error in diagnosis was 15 percent (range 4 to 50 percent), and the complication rate was 5 percent (0 to 20 percent). Hemorrhage, pancreatitis, and death have been reported after large needle biopsy.

Cytologic aspiration biopsy of the pancreas was first reported by Christoffersen and Poll in 1970, who correctly diagnosed pancreatic cancer in 66 of 68 cases by cytologic studies. A thin-gauge (21 to 25 French) needle is used to puncture a pancreatic tumor and cells are aspirated into the hub of the needle or barrel of the syringe. This is the safest biopsy, essentially free of complications. The diagnostic accuracy ranges from 76 to 100 percent. The sensitivity, specificity, and predictive value of cytologic biopsy is higher than with other biopsy techniques, whether done intraoperatively or percutaneously guided by ultrasonography.

In some cases a positive tissue diagnosis cannot be established. This is less of a problem today since a thorough preoperative evaluation, including ERCP, will suggest a correct diagnosis in more than 90 percent of cases. In this era, patients are intimately involved in their care and the problems of obtaining a positive diagnosis can be candidly discussed preoperatively. Resection (including a gastric resection). Nearly section can be done without a tissue diagnosis, providing the surgeon's mortality rate for resection is less than 5 to 10 percent and clinical diagnostic accuracy is high. The error in diagnosis of a mass in the head of the pancreas based on assessment in the operating room is less than 10 percent in experienced hands.

Nowhere is the issue of magnitude of operation as debatable as for carcinoma of the pancreatic head. The standard procedure, practiced since 1935, has been a pancreaticoduodenal re-50 years after its introduction, its role is unsettled because of a varying operative mortality (5 to 30 percent) and a limited survival.

Assessing series and comparing procedures of surgery for pancreatic cancer is difficult. Randomization has not been done; when possible, "better" tumors are removed and "less favorable" ones are left in situ. The selection process should always favor the resected patient. Some reports that tout better survival after a specific operation include other more favorable periampullary tumors; others compare mean survival today with resections done 15 or 20 years ago. Both of these would make a "bias" very significant.

In 1975, Shapiro thoughtfully analyzed 17 series of pancreaticoduodenal resection for pancreatic cancer (some included islet cell and cyst adenocarcinoma) published between 1964 and 1974. A total of 496 patients were reviewed and 20 (4 percent) 5-year survivors noted. The operative mortality averaged 21 percent and the mean survival was 13.9 months. Shapiro additionally reported 48 patients with pancreatic cancer (24 resected, 24 bypassed). Twelve of the bypassed patients had regional extension of the disease, and 12 had small cancers confined to the pancreas. Sixteen of the bypassed patients were not biopsied, a valid objection to this comparative study. Since only one of these patients survived 2 years, the operative assessment of malignancy was probably correct. The mean survival was 10.6 months after resection and 8.1 months after bypass.

Limited survival with pancreatic cancer was vividly shown in a cumulative series from 57 major institutions in Japan. Over a 26-year period, 1819 patients with carcinoma of the head of the pancreas were reviewed. Only 18 percent had resectable lesions. The operative mortality was 25 percent and the 5-year survival only 3 percent after pancreatic resection.

Poor survival and significant mortality and morbidity make it easy to understand disenchantment with pancreaticoduodenal resection. Total pancreatectomy (TP) was introduced as a genuine attempt to improve survival and limit morbidity. Its genesis was two-fold: to deal with multicentric foci of cancer that might be left in the remaining unresected pancreas after a Whipple operation and to avoid fistulas from the pancreaticojejunal anastomosis. The theoretic basis was sound. Carcinoma extending throughout the duct or into the gland beyond the line of resection with a Whipple operation is seen in 5 to 31 percent of TP cases. Ten reports of 334 patients who underwent TP for cancer of the head of the pancreas indicate at most twenty 5-year survivors (5.9 percent). Two large series are of interest because these institutions had been important in establishing the popularity and rationale for TP. Edis and associates reviewed 51 TP patients, all treated for ductal adenocarcinoma of the pancreas at the Mayo Clinic. Multicentric disease was found in 16 patients (31 percent) and positive nodes in 25 (49 percent) specimens. The average postoperative hospitalization was 26 days and the mortality was 16 percent. This mortality rate was similar for both TP and pancreaticoduodenal resection, but the mortality was unchanged after TP. Only one patient survived 5 years after TP (1.9 percent), and died at 80 months, of metastases. Two patients (4 percent) died of hypoglycemia. In comparison, 146 patients who underwent a standard pancreaticoduodenectomy for many diseases were evaluated. Fifty three patients had adenocarcinoma of the head of the pancreas; 5.2 percent survived 5 or more years.

We reviewed the experience with pancreatic resection from the Columbia-Presbyterian Medical Center. Seventy patients with ductal adenocarcinoma were studied. Twenty seven underwent pancreaticoduodenectomy and 43 TP. The operative mortality was 3 of 27 (11 percent) after pancreaticoduodoenal resection, and a similar percentage survived 5 years. in contrast, of 43 TPs there were 12 postoperative deaths (28 percent) and only 1 patient (2 percent) survived 5 years. Multicentric cancer was found in 5 percent of TP specimens. In both the Mayo and Columbia-Presbyterian series, survival was independent of nodal status or histologic grade of the lesion.

Since results of total pancreatectomy and pancreaticoduodenal resection have been so disappointing, two other approaches have been suggested. A more aggressive approach designed to encompass a wider tissue margin and all lymphatics had been suggested. By resecting more regional tissue, that is, portal vein, superior mesenteric vein and artery, and hepatic artery, the associated morbidity and mortality are significantly higher. Of 40 patients undergoing this extensive surgery, only 22 had carcinoma of the pancreas. Five-year survivors have not been reported. It is unlikely that this approach will become popular or improve survival statistics. The length of the operation, blood loss, and morbidity reflect the magnitude of this approach.

A smaller resection that preserves both distal pancreas and the entire stomach (pylorus-preserving resection) was introduced by Traverso and Longmire. Encouraged by specimen analyses that revealed no metastases on either curvature of the stomach, this operation has been adopted for malignancy. This author has employed it in more than 30 malignancies. Survival statistics should not be improved or worsened by this operation, but postgastrectomy sequelae have been abolished. Aside from delayed gastric emptying (4 of 30 patients) and marginal ulcer (3 of 30 patients), none of whom required operation, the procedure has physiologic merit.

The management of diabetes, which is purported to be "easy to control" after TP, certainly adds to the immediate postoperative convalescence. In most reports, little is said about diabetes and hypoglycemia after TP. As mentioned, there were more deaths from hypoglycemia in the Mayo series (4 percent) than 5-year survivors after TP (2 percent). Ihse and associates reported three deaths from hypoglycemia after total pancreatectomy, one which occurred in the hospital. Most survivors of pancreaticoduodenal resection are not diabetic, even though insulin and Glucagon levels are altered by resection. Functional reserves of the pancreas are great and histologic changes in the distal gland are rarely of functional significance.

Multicentricity is less of a practical issue than reported. For most patients an area between tumor and normal pancreas is easily discerned. A frozen section of the transected pancreas will ensure that microscopic tumor does not extend to the line of resection. This improved mean survival from 13 months (when positive) to 20 months (when negative) in one series, but was less important in another. When firm areas are present in the pancreas distal to the resection, they should be biopsied and, if suspicious or positive for cancer, then a TP should be done. There is some disagreement about multicentricity and microscopic cancer. Most patients succumb from hematogenous metastases, disseminated before the gross tumor has been removed and before residual microscopic disease in the pancreas could ever become a problem. The same inference may apply to lymph nodes. More nodes are removed during TP than pancreaticoduodenal resection, but this does not affect prognosis. As with breast and colon cancers, involved nodes may mean systemic disease is already present.

Palliation. On the basis of the poor survival statistics for pancreatic resection and morbidity *and limited survival* after resection, bypass alone has been advocated. Crile, in a retrospective matched pair analysis, showed no difference in mean survival in bypassed or resected patients. A review of 151 biliary bypass procedures for ductal adenocarcinoma of the pancreas reported an operative mortality of 6.9 percent, a median survival of 6.0 months, and a 3-year survival of 2 percent. A similar mean survival (6.0 months) was found after bypass in 172 patients, as contrasted to 9 months after TP and 14 months after Whipple operation from the same institutions.

The benefits of palliative surgery in more than 8000 patients (between 1965 and 1980) with carcinoma of the pancreas have been reviewed. The mean survival was 5 to 6 months whether common duct or gallbladder was used to bypass the biliary obstruction. The question of adding an anticipatory gastrojejunostomy when there is no outlet obstruction should be a "nonissue" today. Since survival patterns in individual patients with pancreatic cancer are to some extent unpredictable and 10 to 15 percent of patients will develop gastric outlet obstruction, a complementary gastrojejunostomy is advocated. This, of course, holds for patients with unresectable regional disease. When liver metastases are present, individual judgments should apply. If tumor is encroaching on the second or third portion of the duodenum, and the antrum is free, then the first part of the duodenum may be utilized.

Carcinoma of the Body and Tail of the Pancreas

Malignant tumors of the body and tail of the pancreas are particularly ominous. Since these tumors gradually obstruct the pancreatic duct, they remain asymptomatic until very late. The most common symptom is back pain, mild at first, but then progressive, severe and unrelenting. Weight loss is the second most common symptom. By the time the diagnosis is suspected, the lesion is incurable because of retroperitoneal involvement and liver metastases. The acute onset of diabetes mellitus, particularly if unstable, in patients past 40 years of age, may be a clue to cancer of the body and tail of the pancreas. This author has, however, not found a resectable lesion with this presentation. Should a cancer acutely obstruct the pancreatic duct, then a pseudocyst may develop. We have recently seen four instances of pseudocysts developing behind a pancreatic cancer; only one was resectable (but the patient died within 7 months). The cumulative Japanese experience included 268 cancers arising from the body and tail of the pancreas. Two hundred forty were resected. The operative mortality was 10 percent; the mean survival 3.1 months, and no patient survived more than 1 year. Lord Smith reported 110 such cancers, only 8 of which were resectable. There were no operative mortalities, but mean survival was 5 months without resection and 7 months with resection.

Since the outlook is so bleak and so few tumors are resectable, a diligent search for metastases by ultrasound, CT, angiography, or laparoscopy should be done. If a solid mass in the body or tail of the pancreas is seen by ultrasound or CT, then a percutaneously guided biopsy may provide a diagnosis. Laparoscopy has an increasingly important role, since the liver and pancreas can be examined simultaneously and biopsied. The presence of liver metastases, documented by laparoscopy and biopsy will avoid an unnecessary laparotomy. The diligent search for metastases is necessary before surgery since cancer of the body and tail of the pancreas is so infrequently resectable and rarely cured.

Adjuvant Therapy

Disappointments with resection, for all pancreatic cancers, have encouraged radiotherapy and chemotherapy to be utilized for pancreatic cancer, either as adjuvant or palliative therapy.

Radiation (6000 to 7000 rads) was given to 44 patients with histologically confirmed unresectable pancreatic cancer. Pain was relieved in 69 percent. Twelve patients also had chemotherapy which increased mean survival to 15 months. One patient survived 69 months.

When 5-FU was given as a radiation sensitizer intravenously with radiation therapy the mean survival was significantly better—10 months versus 6 months—in two trials. Radiation may provide local benefit but will not alter metastatic disease, and should not significantly alter survival statistics.

Chemotherapy with single or multiple agents has been the subject of several studies. Response rates of 20 to 43 percent have been recorded. The median survival is prolonged by weeks to months, but the inexorable course of the disease is generally not altered.

More recently a study of resected head of the pancreas cancers compared adjuvant chemotherapy and radiation therapy to resection alone. The 2-year survival was significantly prolonged with adjuvant therapy. Resection implantation of radioactive seeds into the head of the pancreas for locally unresectable cancer has provided local control for some patients and may find further application. Finally, control of back pain can be provided for nearly all patients by a splanchnic block with alcohol, done percutaneously.

Technique of Pancreaticoduodenectomy

History of Pancreatic Resection

The history of pancreatic resection dates to at least 1898, when Codivilla resected an adenocarcinoma of the head of the pancreas. Reconstruction of the gastrointestinal tract was with a Roux-Y gastroenterostomy and cholecystojejunostomy. The pancreatic duct was oversewn. The patient survived 24 days. Further technical modifications were suggested by Suave 10 years later in cadaver dissections.

Technical advances and further attempts at resection were limited because of poor results, the lack of blood transfusions, antibiotics, and nutritional support.

The modern era of pancreatic surgery dates to 1935 when Whipple and associates performed a two-stage pancreaticoduodenectomy for an ampullary cancer. A cholecystogastrostomy was done initially to relieve hepatobiliary obstruction. At the second stage, the duodenum, between the pylorus and its ascending portion, and a wedge of pancreas were excised. The pancreas was reapproximated, the distal duodenum and pylorus oversewn, and a side-to-side gastrojejunostomy made.

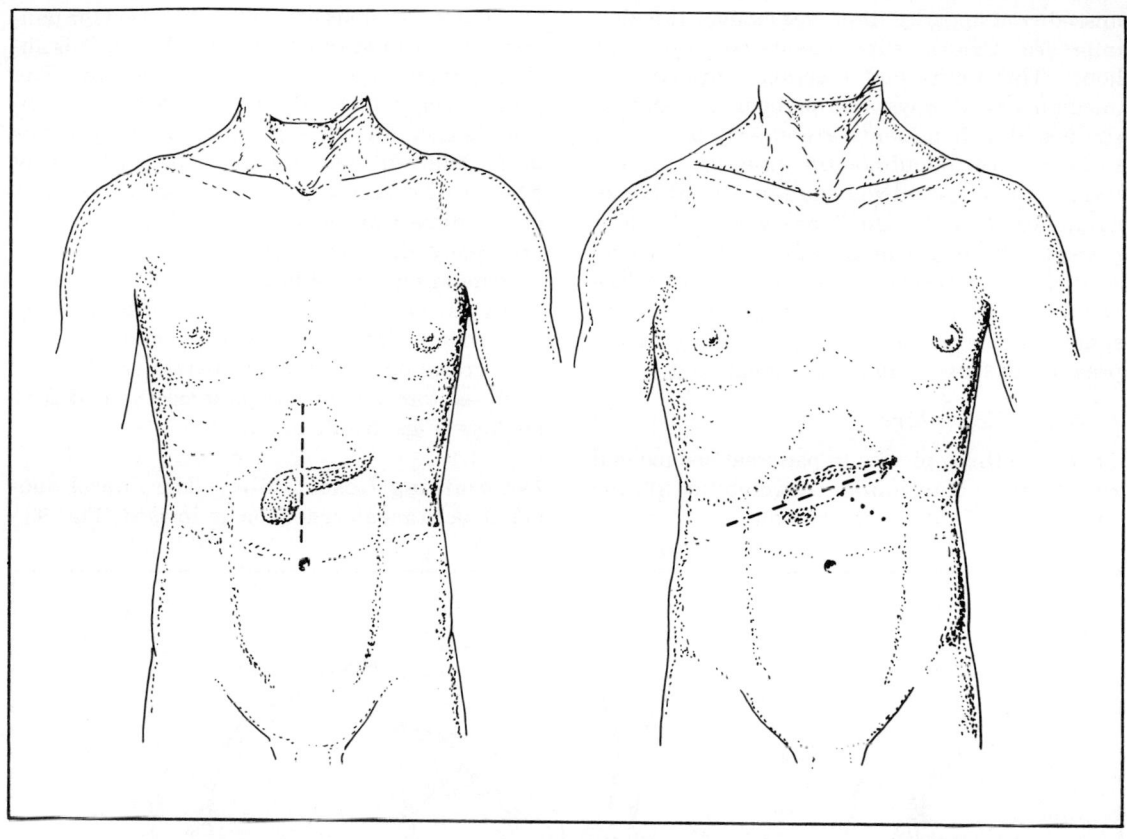

Figure 92–20. Three incisions commonly used for pancreaticoduodenal resection. Most often the upper midline incision is used. The right upper abdominal oblique or subcostal incision is used for obese patients: When a wide costal arch is present, the incision may be enlarged to the left as shown by the dotted line. (*Source: From Cooperman AM, Hoerr S: Surgery of the Pancreas. St. Louis: CV Mosby, 1978, with permission.*)

Brunschwig performed a one-stage resection for a pancreatic cancer on February 11, 1937. The pancreatic stump was oversewn. The patient survived only 2.5 months before succumbing to metastases. Whipple and associates accomplished a one-stage pancreaticoduodenal resection in 1940. The tumor was an islet cell carcinoma. A choledochojejunostomy and gastrojejunostomy were fashioned and the pancreas oversewn. Liver metastases developed and the patient died 9 years after surgery. In 1942 the operation was modified to include a pancreaticojejunal anastomosis to prevent a pancreatic fistula. When we reviewed the results of pancreatic surgery at Columbia, it was a testimony to Whipple and associates that mortality and fistula rates were not significantly different from today.

Preoperative Assessment

The most common indication for pancreaticoduodenal resection is a malignant tumor. Jaundice, anemia, and weight loss are frequent associated findings. Since preoperative preparation is essential, it would be ideal to correct all of those abnormalities prior to surgery. On the other hand, since palliative procedures will be done in 50 to 90 percent of patients, prolonged hospitalization has practical disadvantages and shortens the home stay with family members.

This author's policy is to correct anemia before surgery. Most nutritional deficiencies improve after correction of jaundice. Personal sentiments and reasoning regarding the importance of preoperative stenting have been expressed. After stenting, patients are dismissed, and appetite improves as liver function improves. Caloric supplements are given at home. This limits postresection convalescence (median 7 to 10 days) and preoperative stay in the hospital. If patients are elderly or have a history of cardiopulmonary disease, a Swan–Ganz catheter is utilized and the patient hemodynamically "optimized" preoperatively. If a patient is cachectic or the tumor clearly unresectable, or metastases present, and gastroduodenal obstruction not evident, surgery can be spared, and nonoperative hepatobiliary decompression utilized as palliative treatment.

Surgical Procedure

There are three phases to pancreaticoduodenal resection: (1) determining resectability, (2) the resection, and (3) reconstruction.

Three incisions are commonly used for pancreaticoduodenal resection (Fig. 92–20). This author prefers the upper-midline incision. The right upper abdominal oblique, or subcostal incision, is used for obese patients. Some surgeons prefer bilateral subcostal incisions, particularly when a wide costal arch is present. Since most of the dissection is in the midline, nearly all are easily done through a midline approach or extending the oblique incision across the midline. Self-retaining retractors (Smith Ring, Bookwalter Retractor) allow for one assistant and unequaled, stationary exposure. A thorough exploration of the pancreas should first be done (Figs. 92–21 and 92–22).

Determining Resectability. The lateral duodenal peritoneal reflection is incised (Fig. 92–

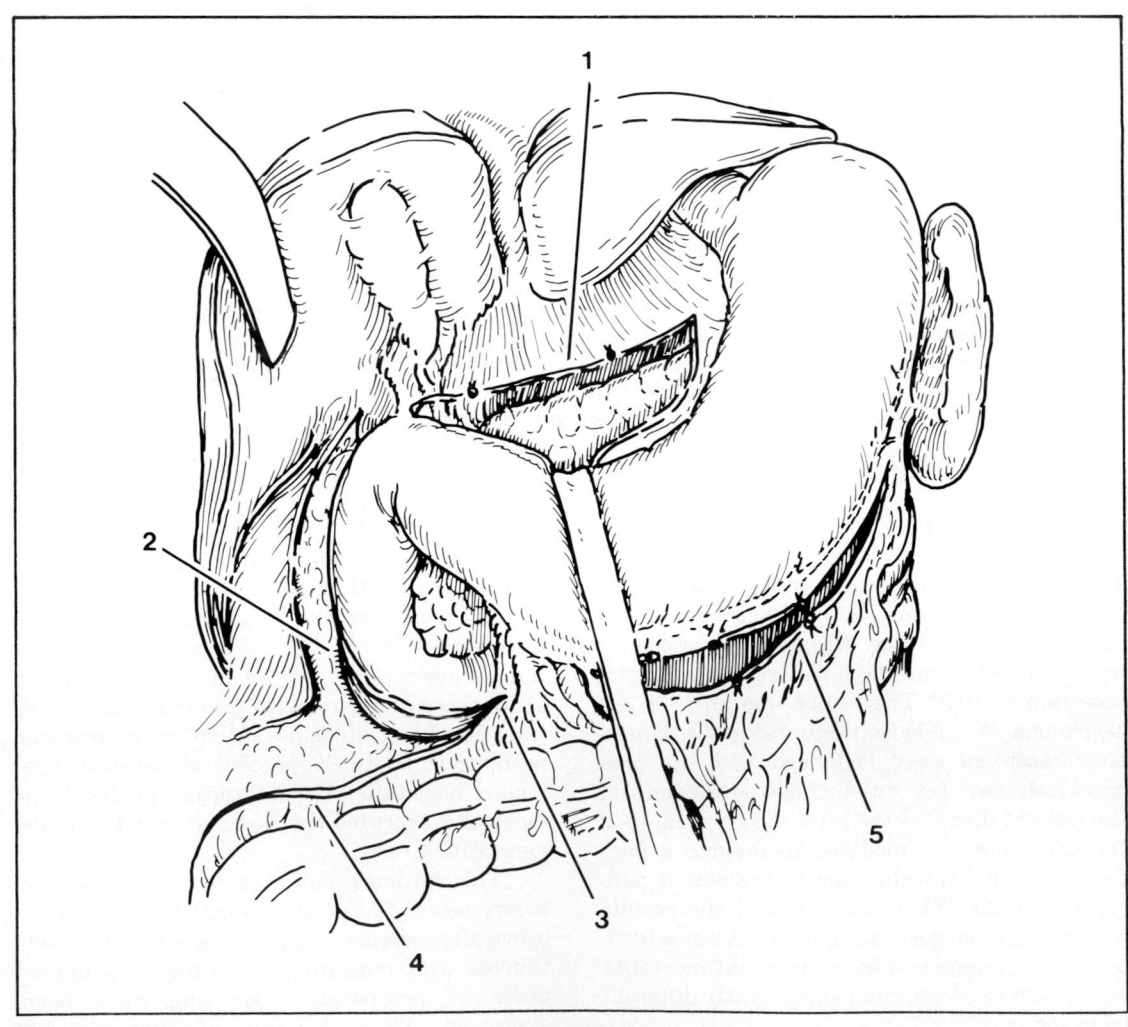

Figure 92–21.

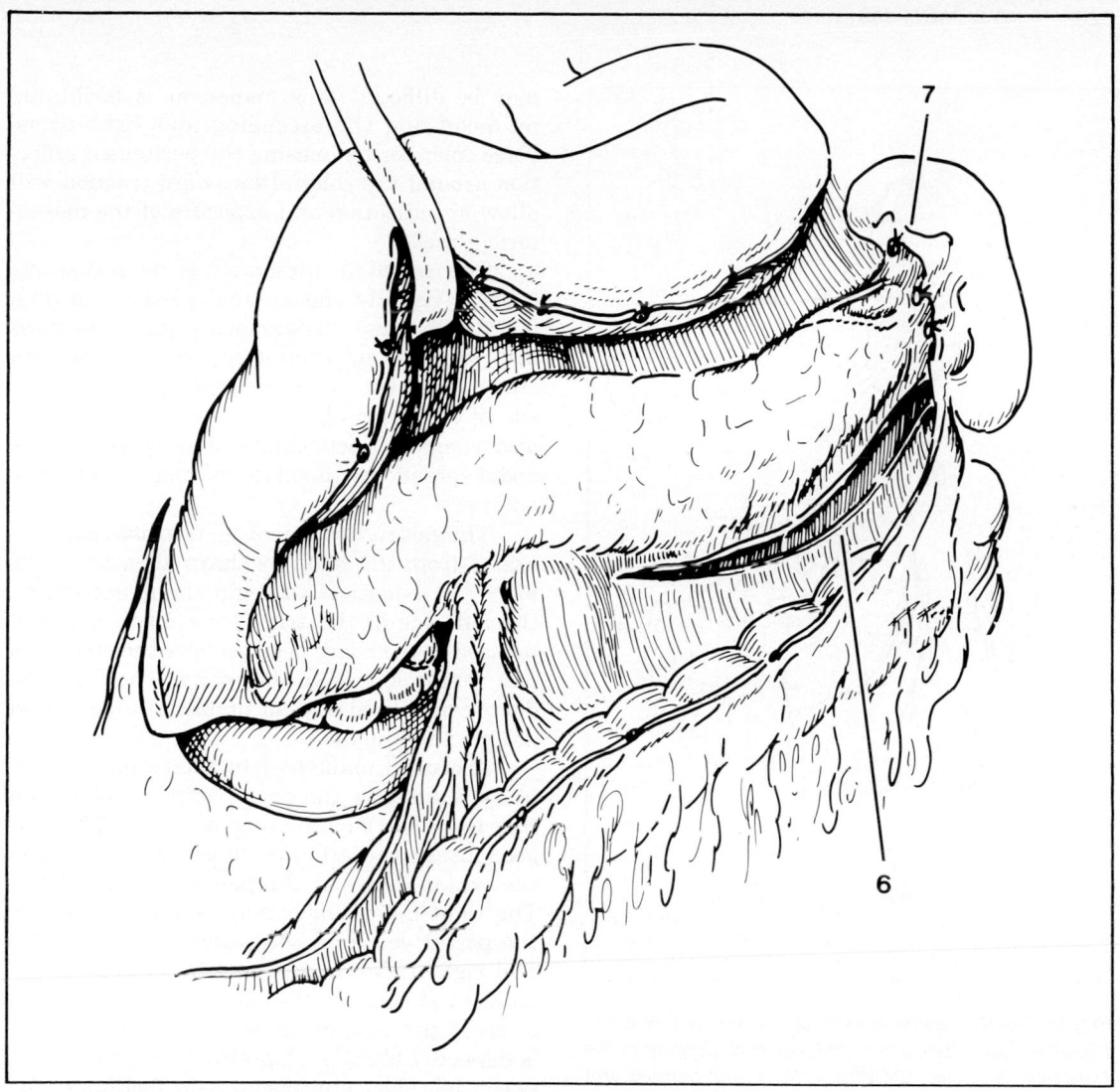

Figure 92–22.

Figures 92–21 and **22.** 1. With traction on the stomach displacing it downward and to the left, the gastrohepatic omentum is incised lateral to the left gastric vein and the nerves of Latarjet. This allows visualization and palpation of the neck and body of the gland. 2, 3. The duodenum is next pulled to the left and the peritoneum over the descending duodenum incised. The dissection can be carried to the mesenteric vessels below and allows visualization of the inferior vena cava medially. 4. If the patient is obese or exposure of the third portion of the duodenum incomplete, an important maneuver is to incise the peritoneum overlying the right and transverse colon and reflect the ascending and right transverse colon downward. Complete exposure of the third portion of the duodenum is thereby obtained. 5. The gastrocolic omentum is next incised. This tissue plane is easier to enter toward the left, where the tissue is thinner and avascular and where the mesocolon and middle colic artery are less easily injured. The opening is widened and the stomach retracted upward by a malleable retractor or a drain placed around the stomach. This then allows complete visualization of the neck, body, and tail of the gland. 6. The avascular plane of tissue beneath the inferior portion of the pancreas is incised to permit bimanual palpation of the gland. 7. Finally, if it is difficult to develop a tissue plane beneath the pancreas because of inflammation or scarring, medial rotation of the spleen delivers the tail of the gland into a more accessible location. Planned splenectomy is generally unnecessary.

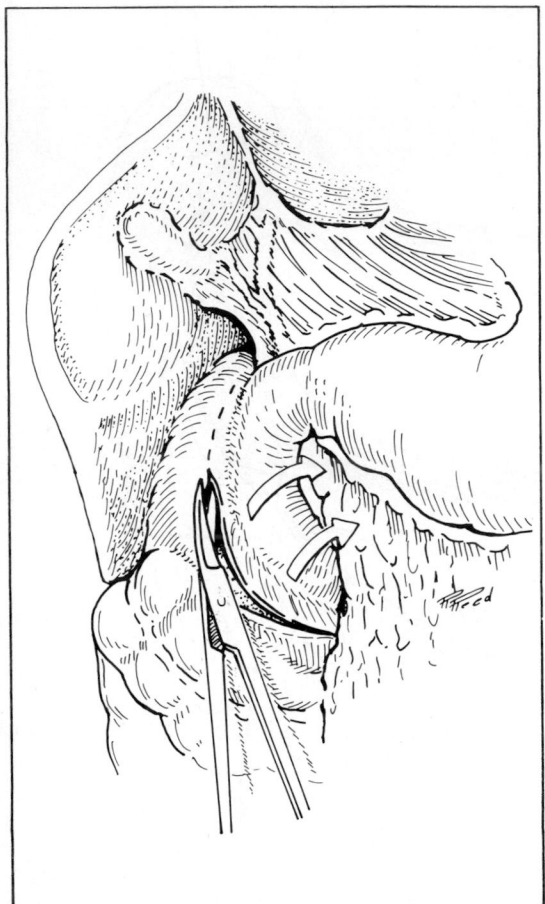

Figure 92–23. Lateral duodenal peritoneal reflection. (*Source: From Cooperman AM, Hoerr S: Surgery of the Pancreas. St. Louis: CV Mosby, 1978, with permission.*)

23). The incision may be extended to the mesenteric vessels and superiorly to the porta hepatis. The duodenum must be mobilized as far as the vena cava medially to allow complete examination of the head of the pancreas (Fig. 92–24). Careful bimanual palpation of the head of the pancreas is then done.

The porta hepatis and the regional lymph nodes are examined next (Fig. 92–25). Suspicious or enlarged nodes are removed for frozen section examination. Many surgeons regard a metastatic node as evidence of incurability but, as mentioned, survival with pancreatic cancer is so uncommon that it may be independent of nodal metastases. In obese patients, mobilization of the descending and ascending duodenum

may be difficult. This maneuver is facilitated by mobilizing the ascending and right transverse colon, or by incising the peritoneal reflection around the colon. Downward traction will allow visualization and exposure of the mesenteric vessels.

The root of the mesentery of the transverse colon is visually and manually examined (Fig. 92–26). Obvious or suspicious nodal metastases are removed and submitted for frozen section study. The root of the mesentery is often the site of extension of the primary growth, which also connotes incurability. Rarely retrograde nodal spread may involve the small bowel mesentery.

The gastrocolic omentum is incised and separated from the colon by sharp dissection (Fig. 92–27). It is easiest to begin the dissection on the left side of the transverse mesocolon and proceed to the right, because here the omentum and mesocolon separate easily. The common duct is mobilized and an umbilical tape passed around the bile duct.

A crucial maneuver to determine resectability is whether the portal vein is mobile and free from the surrounding pancreas. The surgeon inserts the left index finger placed between the portal vein and the pancreas (Fig. 92–28). The right index finger may be placed between the portal vein and the pancreas (Fig. 92–28). The right index finger may be placed on the anterior surface of the mesenteric vein below to meet the advancing left finger. This plane is dissected bluntly. Exposing the interface between bile duct and portal vein facilitates the dissection. At times this can be facilitated by dividing the bile duct early in the operation. If the lesion is unresectable the proximal duct may be used for a bypass. Since the plane is avascular (with the exception of anamalous vessels), any resistance encountered is likely from neoplasm or from pancreatitis. Tumor invasion of the mesenteric vein, or extension behind the vein and mesenteric artery, is an ominous prognostic sign and for practical purposes denotes incurability. Even though segments of vein may be resected, added survival benefit is dubious.

The relationship of the pancreas to the superior mesenteric vein is shown in cross-section in Figure 92–29. The vessels from the uncinate process enter the right lateral side of the vein. The ventral surface should be free of tumor and the dissection done on this surface.

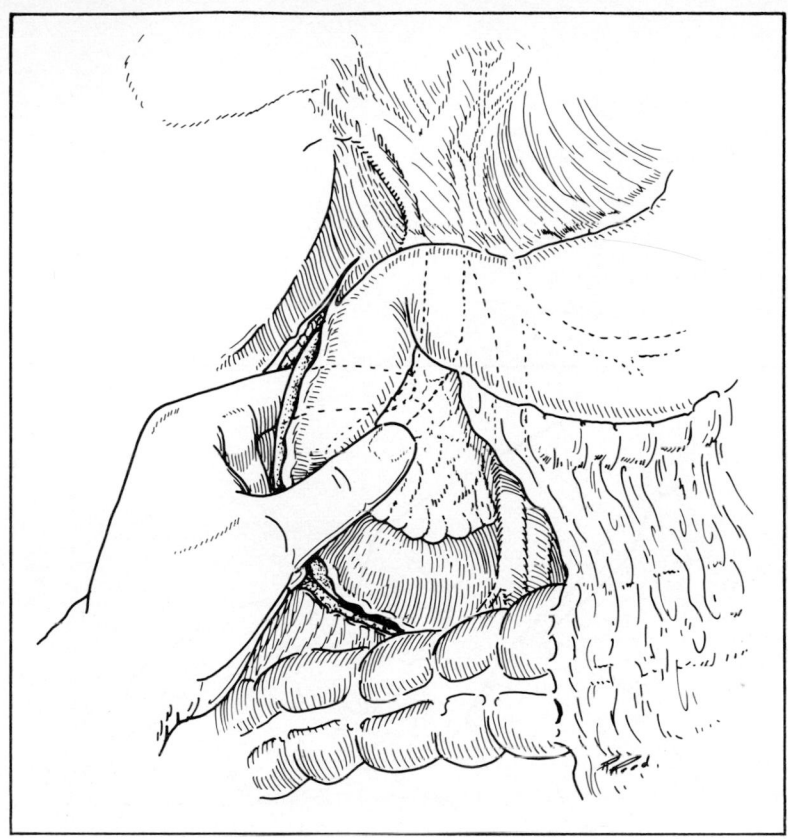

Figure 92–24. Bimanual palpation of the head of the pancreas. (*Source: From Cooperman AM, Hoerr S: Surgery of the Pancreas. St. Louis: CV Mosby, 1978, with permission.*)

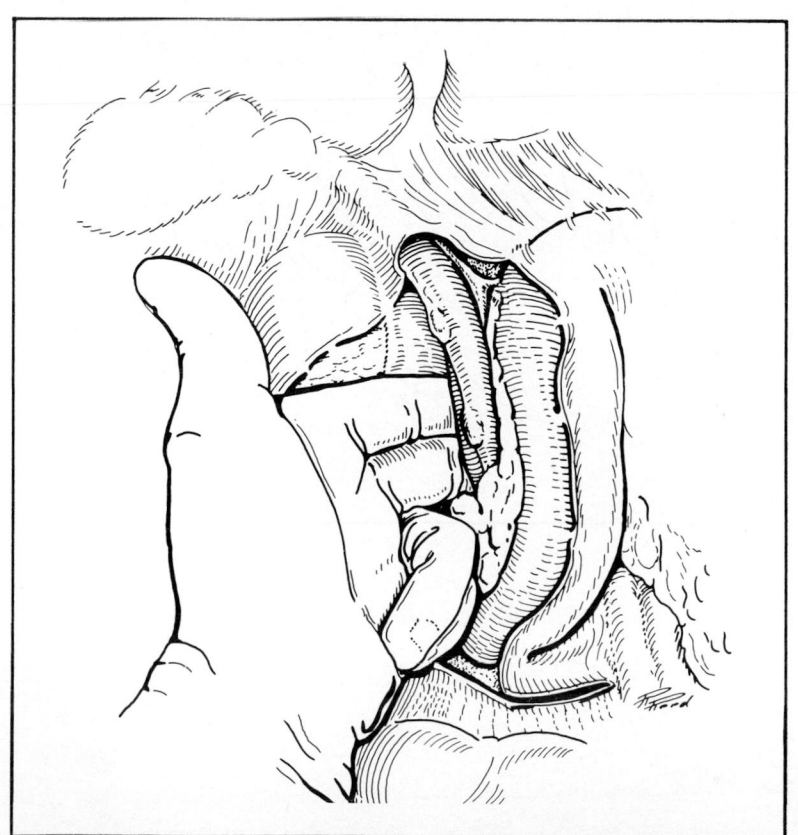

Figure 92–25. Examination of the porta hepatis and the regional lymph nodes. (*Source: From Cooperman AM, Hoerr S: Surgery of the Pancreas. St. Louis: CV Mosby, 1978, with permission.*)

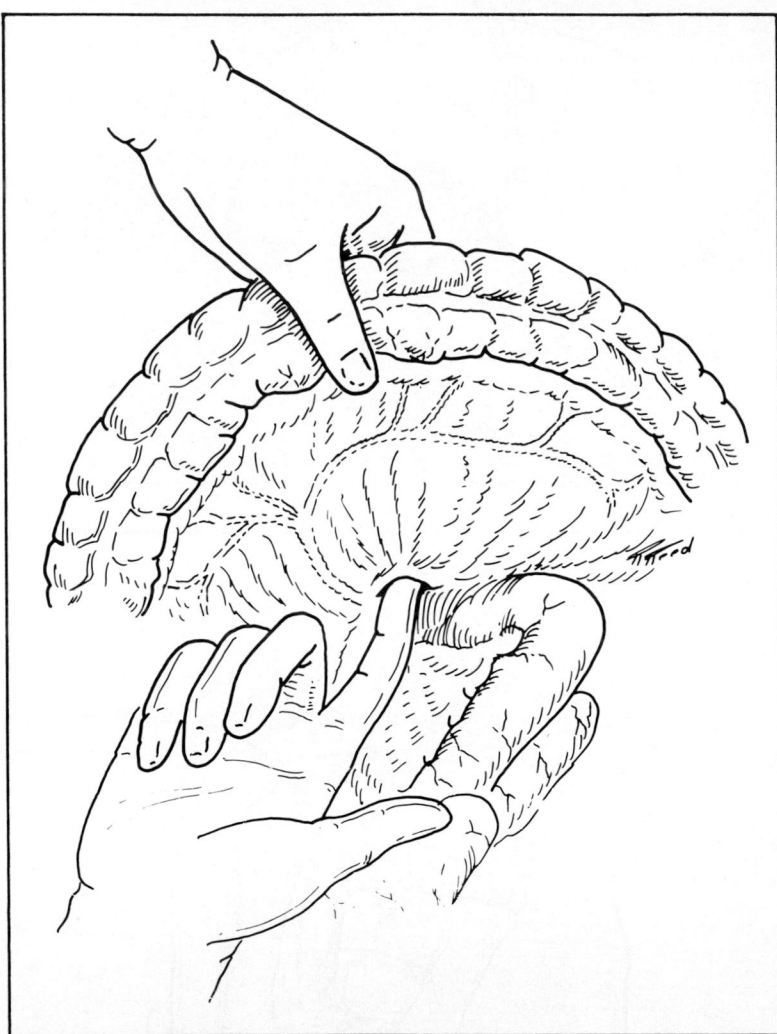

Figure 92–26. Examination of the root of the mesentery of the transverse colon. (*Source: From Cooperman AM, Hoerr S: Surgery of the Pancreas. St. Louis: CV Mosby, 1978, with permission.*)

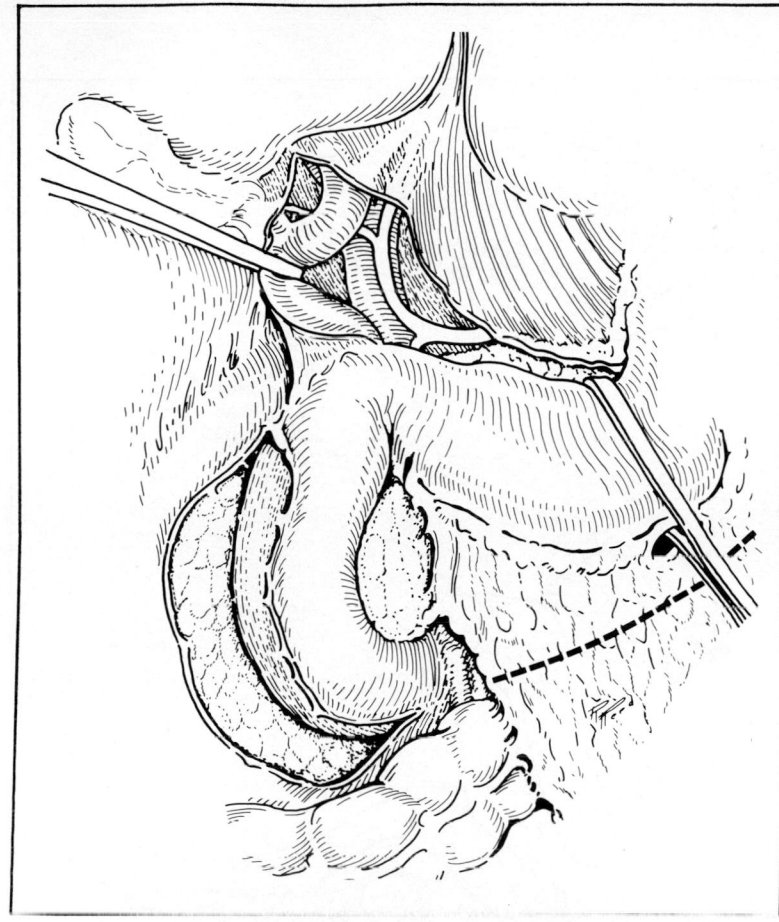

Figure 92–27. Incision and separation of the gastrocolic omentum. (*Source: From Cooperman AM, Hoerr S: Surgery of the Pancreas. St. Louis: CV Mosby, 1978, with permission.*)

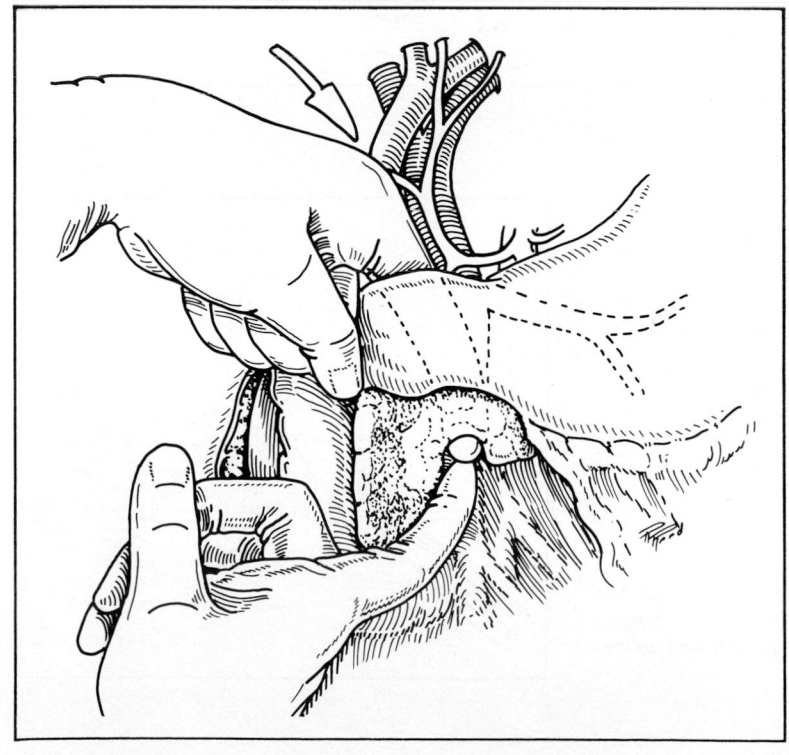

Figure 92–28. Determination of status of portal vein. (*Source: From Cooperman AM, Hoerr S: Surgery of the Pancreas. St. Louis: CV Mosby, 1978, with permission.*)

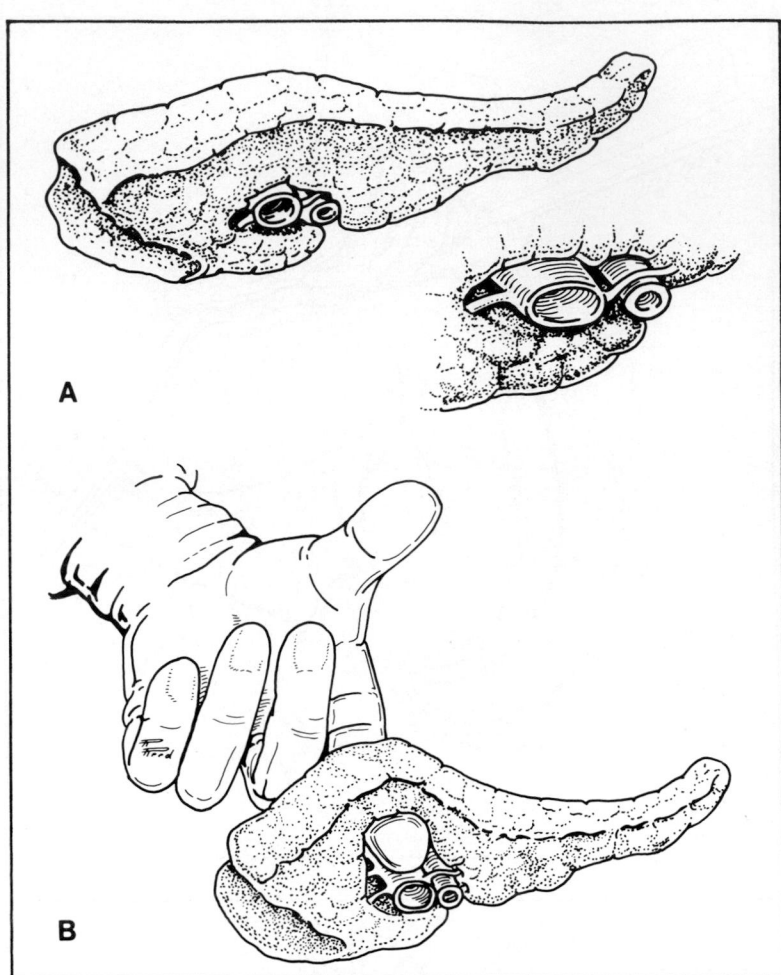

Figure 92–29. A. Relationship of the pancreas to the superior mesenteric vein as shown in cross section. **B.** Dissection of ventral surface of vein. (*Source: From Cooperman AM, Hoerr S: Surgery of the Pancreas. St. Louis: CV Mosby, 1978, with permission.*)

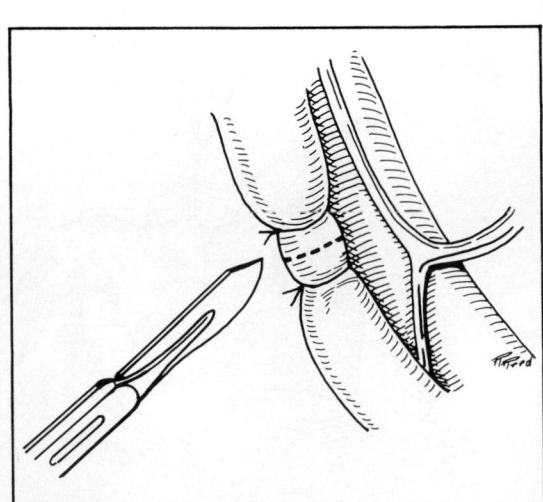

Figure 92–30. Ligation and division of common bile duct. (*Source: From Cooperman AM, Hoerr S: Surgery of the Pancreas. St. Louis: CV Mosby, 1978, with permission.*)

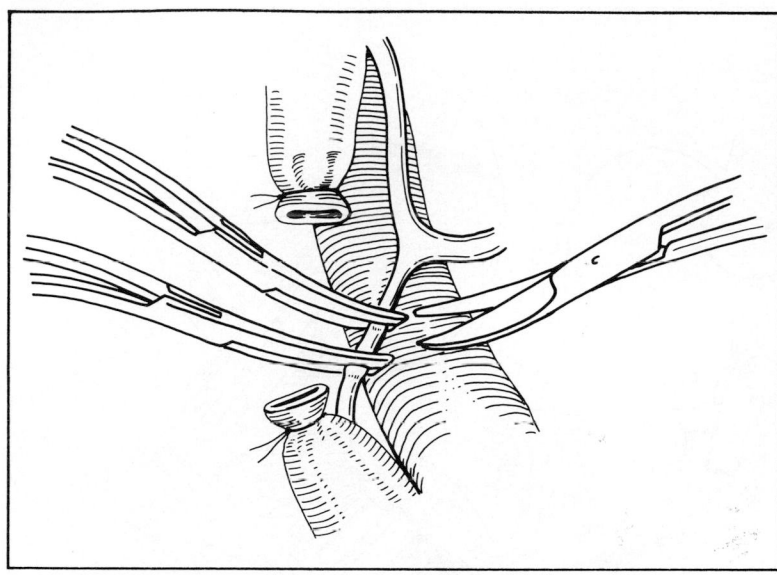

Figure 92–31. Division of gastroduodenal artery. (*Source: From Cooperman AM, Hoerr S: Surgery of the Pancreas. St. Louis: CV Mosby, 1978, with permission.*)

Resection. The common bile duct is ligated and divided between ties (to prevent bile leak during surgery) (Fig. 92–30); the gastroduodenal artery is then ligated near its origin from the hepatic artery and divided (Fig. 92–31). The junction with hepatic artery should be accurately visualized to preclude accidental ligation of the hepatic artery.

Should a distal gastric resection be necessary, the stomach may be divided in a number of ways (using clamps, staples, or sutures) (Fig. 92–32). If the pylorus is to be preserved, the duodenum is transected.

Before transecting the pancreas, it is helpful to place four traction sutures or large hemoclips on the upper and lower borders of the gland (Fig. 92–33). This helps control bleeding from the transverse pancreatic vessels. Overlapping mattress sutures near the line of resection are another means of ensuring hemostasis. The pancreas is then divided. To protect the superior mesenteric vein from injury, the pancreas may be divided over a finger, a malleable retractor, or a clamp. Should the wrong tissue place be entered and venous bleeding develop, a small pack placed alongside the mesenteric vein will control bleeding from the uncinate branches or the vein compressed between the duodenum below and the pancreas above. If the mesenteric vein is injured, the surgeon can facilitate direct repair by dividing the pancreas, permitting exposure of the entire anterior and lateral surface of the mesenteric vein. Although nonfatal ligation of the vein has been reported, it is hazardous and not advised. In the rare circumstances when it must be contemplated, improved exposure and lengthening of the mesenteric vein can be accomplished by mobilizing the root of the mesentery and hepatic and splenic flexures. An additional alternative is to use the splenic vein swung down to the distal mesenteric vein.

To free the uncinate process from the mesenteric vein (Fig. 92–34), the surgeon retracts the head of the pancreas to the patient's right and the mesenteric vein gently to the left. A vein retractor is useful here. The vessels from the uncinate process are then accurately identified. They may be divided between hemoclips or sutures. When inflammation obscures these vessels, this author prefers to leave some of the uncinate process, dividing it between large hemoclips placed parallel with the mesenteric vein. This method is safer and there is much less bleeding.

When division of the uncinate process is complete, the duodenum is transected. An automatic stapling and cutting instrument facilitates this (Fig. 92–35). The division can be done on either side of the mesocolon. The specimen is then removed.

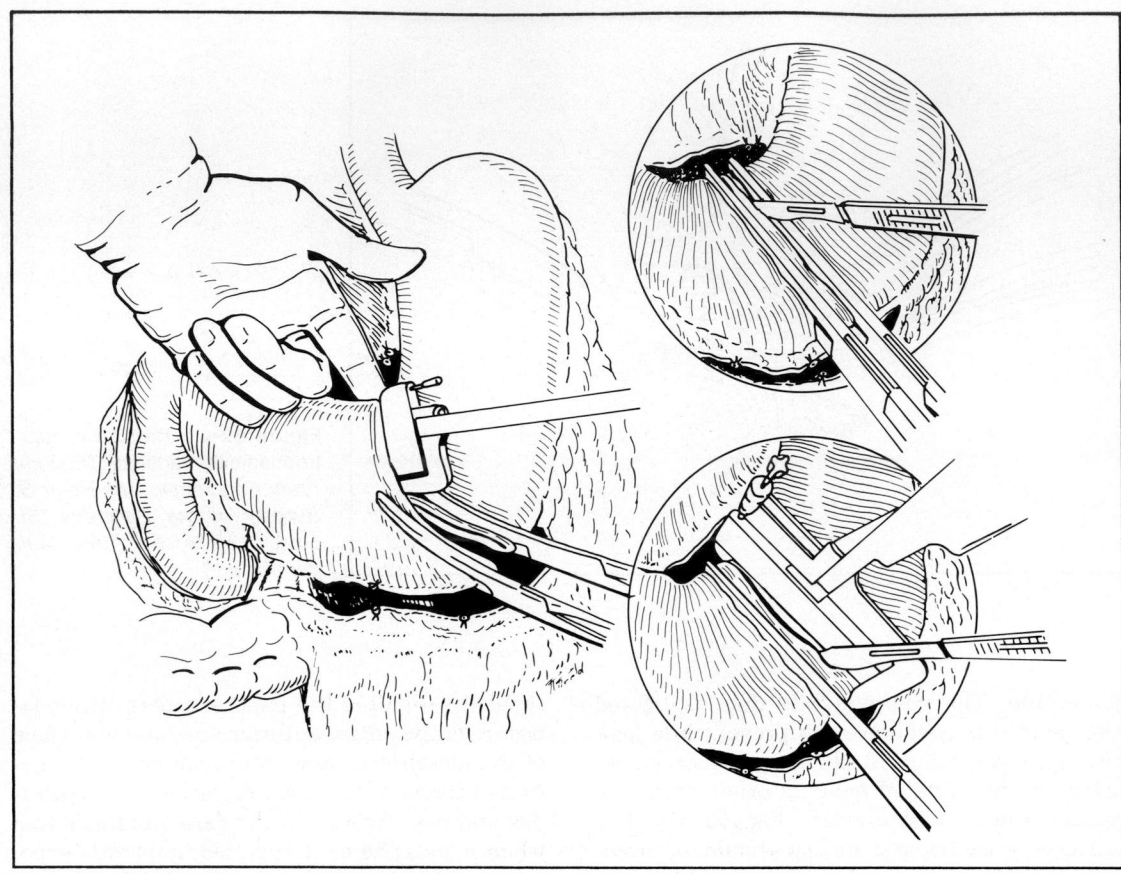

Figure 92–32. Transection of stomach. (*Source: From Cooperman AM, Hoerr S: Surgery of the Pancreas. St. Louis: CV Mosby, 1978, with permission.*)

Figure 92–34. Freeing the uncinate process from the mesenteric vein. (*Source: From Cooperman AM, Hoerr S: Surgery of the Pancreas. St. Louis: CV Mosby, 1978, with permission.*)

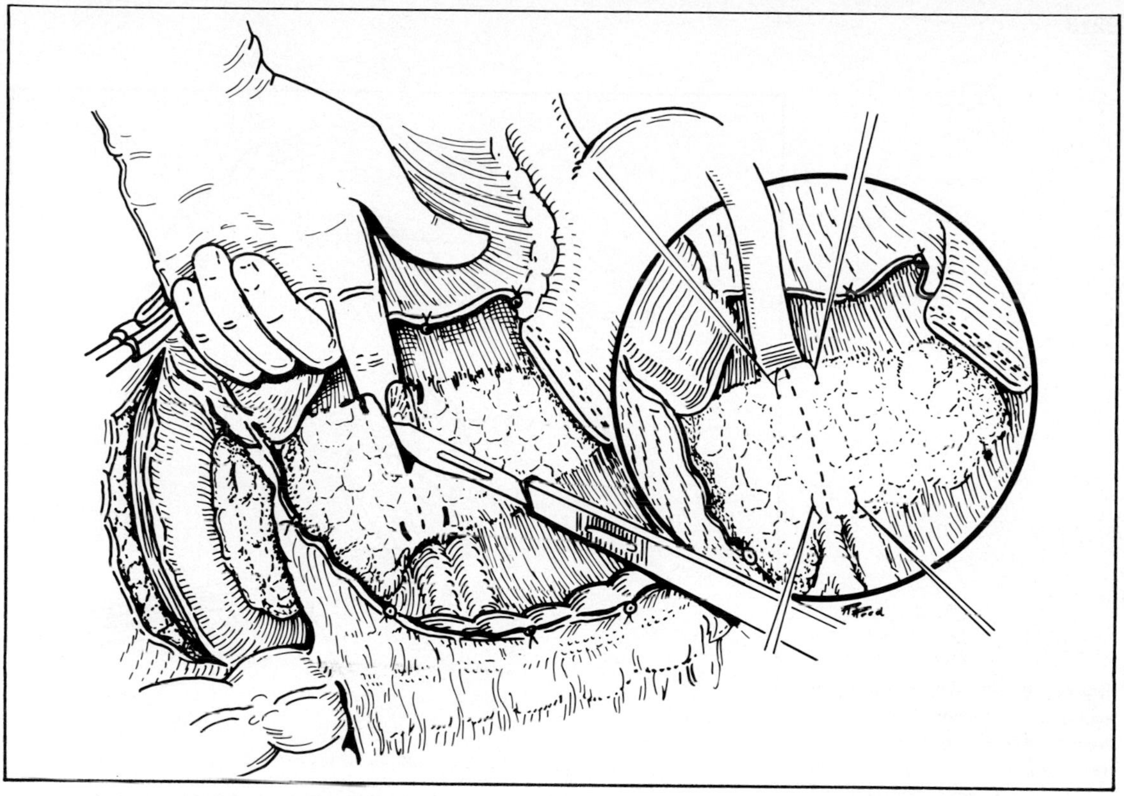

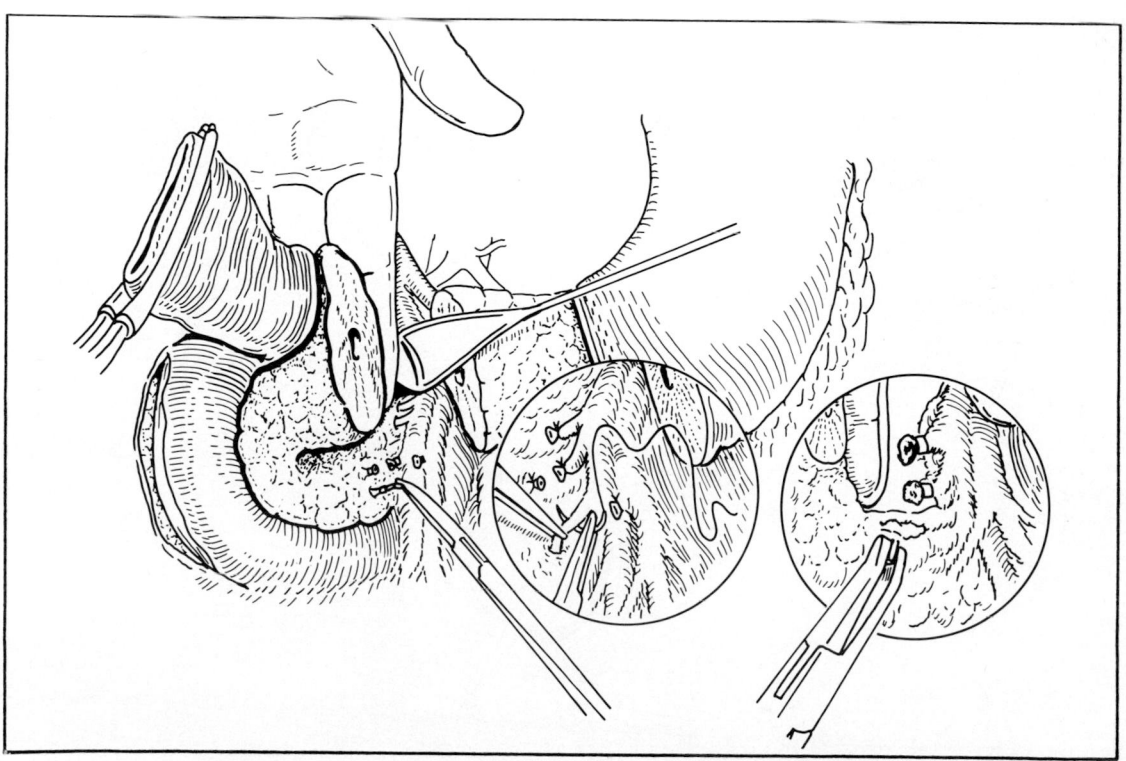

Figure 92–33. Transection of pancreas. (*Source: From Cooperman AM, Hoerr S: Surgery of the Pancreas. St. Louis: CV Mosby, 1978, with permission.*)

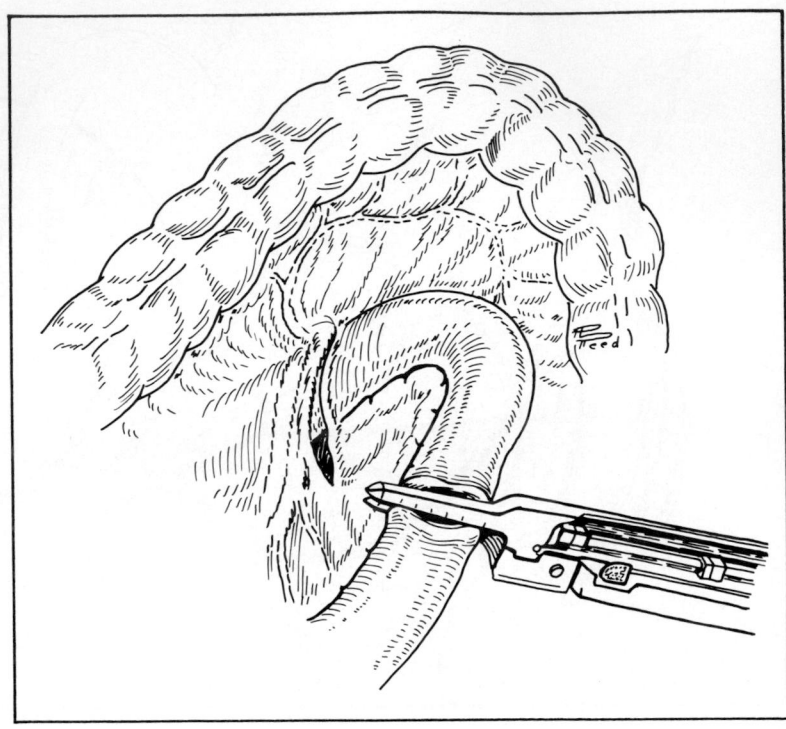

Figure 92–35. Transection of jejunum. (*Source: From Cooperman AM, Hoerr S: Surgery of the Pancreas. St. Louis: CV Mosby, 1978, with permission.*)

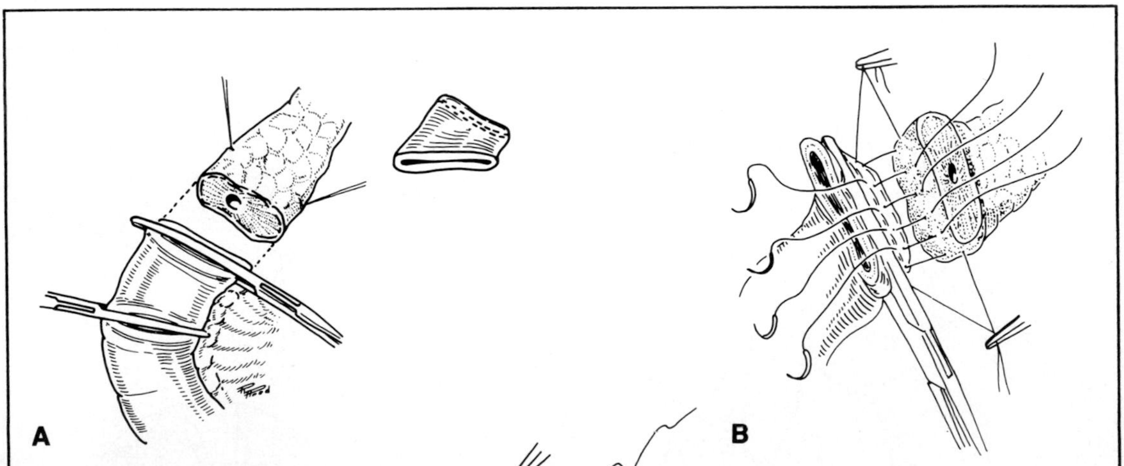

A

B

C

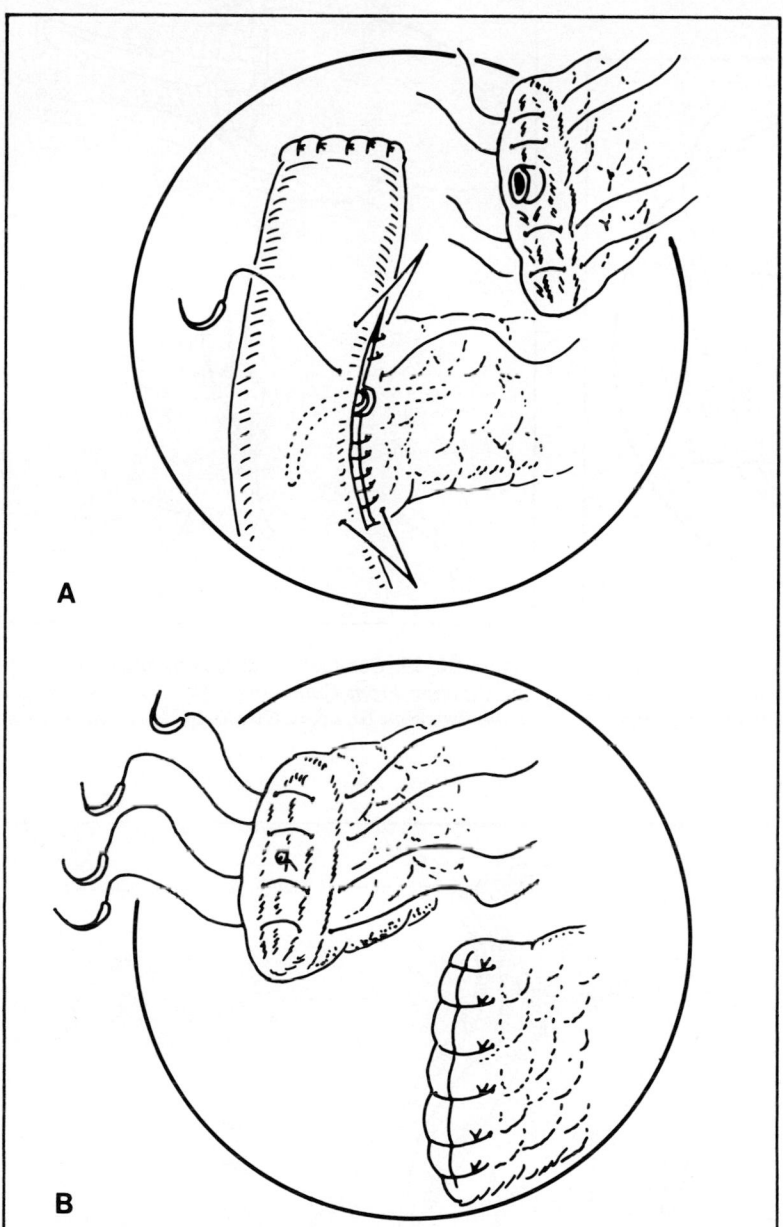

Figure 92–37. A. End-to-side anastomosis between pancreatic duct and jejunum. **B.** Simple closure of pancreas without implantation into jejunum. (*Source: From Cooperman AM, Hoerr S: Surgery of the Pancreas. St. Louis: CV Mosby, 1978, with permission.*)

Figure 92–36. End-to-end pancreaticojejunostomy. (*Source: Adapted from Cooperman AM, Hoerr S: Surgery of the Pancreas. St. Louis: CV Mosby, 1978, with permission.*)

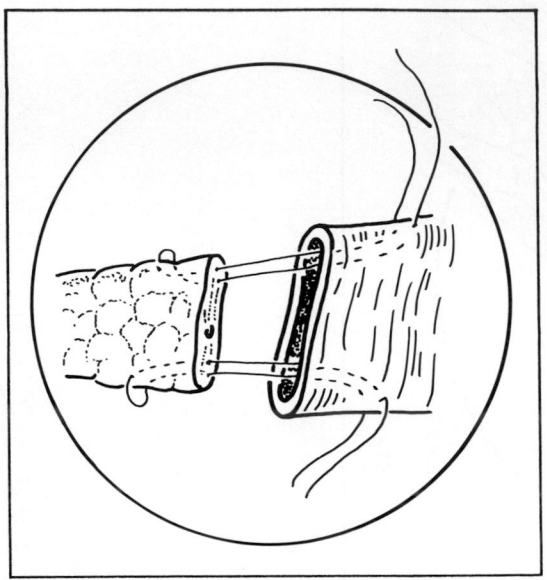

Figure 92–38. Invagination of pancreas into jejunum. (*Source: From Cooperman AM, Hoerr S: Surgery of the Pancreas. St. Louis: CV Mosby, 1978, with permission.*)

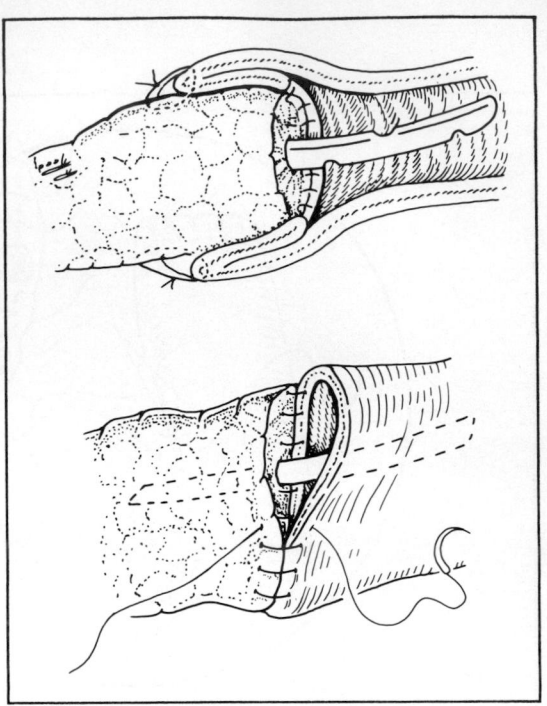

Figure 92–39. Completed pancreatojejunal anastomosis. (*Source: From Cooperman AM, Hoerr S: Surgery of the Pancreas. St. Louis: CV Mosby, 1978, with permission.*)

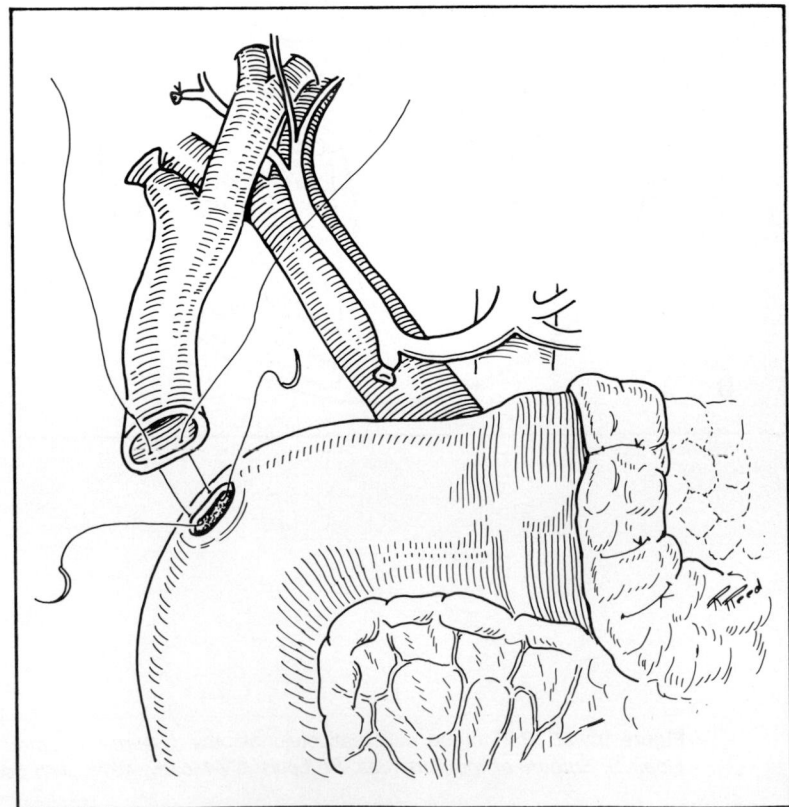

Figure 92–40. The beginning of hepaticodochojejunostomy. (*Source: From Cooperman AM, Hoerr S: Surgery of the Pancreas. St. Louis: CV Mosby, 1978, with permission.*)

Reconstruction. When the distal pancreas is firm and not edematous, an end-to-end pancreaticojejunostomy is made (Fig. 92–36A). The surgeon can facilitate the procedure by measuring the width of the pancreas against the end of the jejunum to minimize spillage. An inner posterior row of continuous or interrupted nonabsorbable sutures is placed and continued anteriorly (Fig. 92–36B,C). If the pancreatic duct is close to the ventral surface of the gland, a small nonobstructing plastic catheter may be placed to protect the duct from an inaccurately placed suture. Sutures of fine (5-0, 6-0) Prolene are then placed between the pancreatic duct and the jejunal mucosa. This precise anastomosis will maintain exocrine function in 90 percent of patients. An alternate method may be used when the pancreatic duct is dilated. The capsule of the pancreas is closed with interrupted silk sutures (if it approximates easily) and an end-to-end anastomosis is established between the duct and the side of the jejunum (Fig. 92–37A). At times the pancreas is edematous and an anastomosis may be unsafe. In these instances the pancreatic duct is ligated (with nonabsorbable sutures) and the

capsule oversewn with nonabsorbable sutures. The technique illustrated (Fig. 92–37B) (anterior and posterior capsular sutures, with some of the central tissue removed as a wedge) is particularly good when the pancreas is firm. A third alternative is to pull the glandular remnant into the jejunum by a mattress suture and fasten the capsule to the jejunum (Fig. 92–38). A fourth alternative, pancreatogastronomy, has also been used. This author has no experience with this procedure, but its advocates have found it safe and easy to perform. My preference is to always suture the pancreatic duct to the jejunal mucosa, with precise interrupted sutures. A stent is placed if the duct is less than 8 mm. The jejunum is then sutured to the pancreatic capsule. Exocrine pancreatic function is maintained in more than 90 percent of patients who remain tumor free.

A completed pancreatojejunal anastomosis is illustrated (Fig. 92–39). The anterior surface of the gland has been imbricated with interrupted sutures of nonabsorbable suture. A catheter has been placed in the pancreatic duct to ensure its patency. As stated, jejunal mucosa

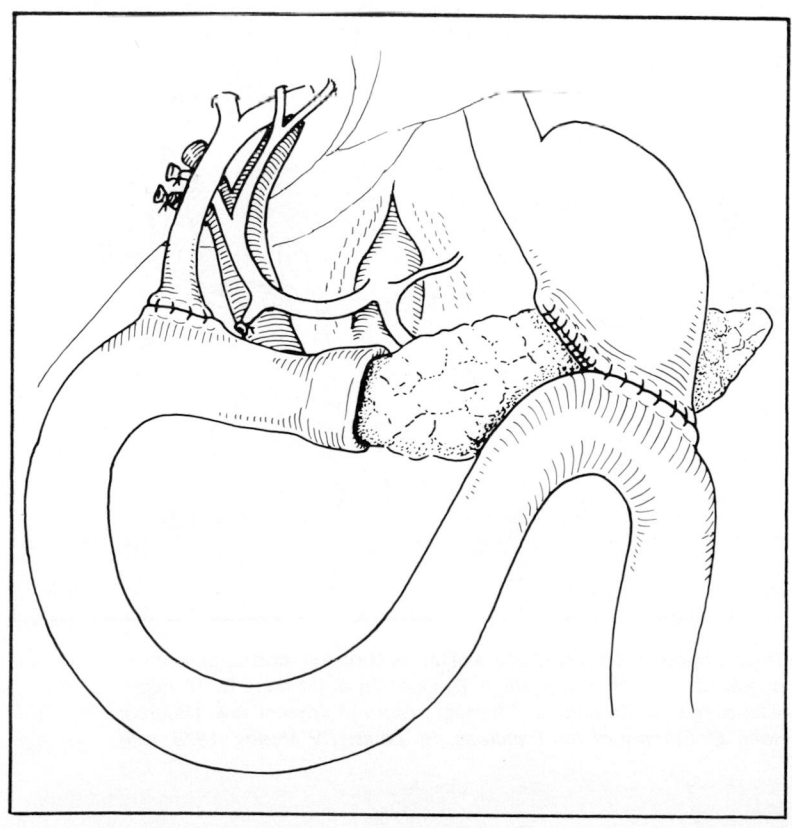

Figure 92–41. Completed hepaticodochojejunostomy. (*Source: From Cooperman AM, Hoerr S: Surgery of the Pancreas. St. Louis: CV Mosby, 1978, with permission.*)

2220

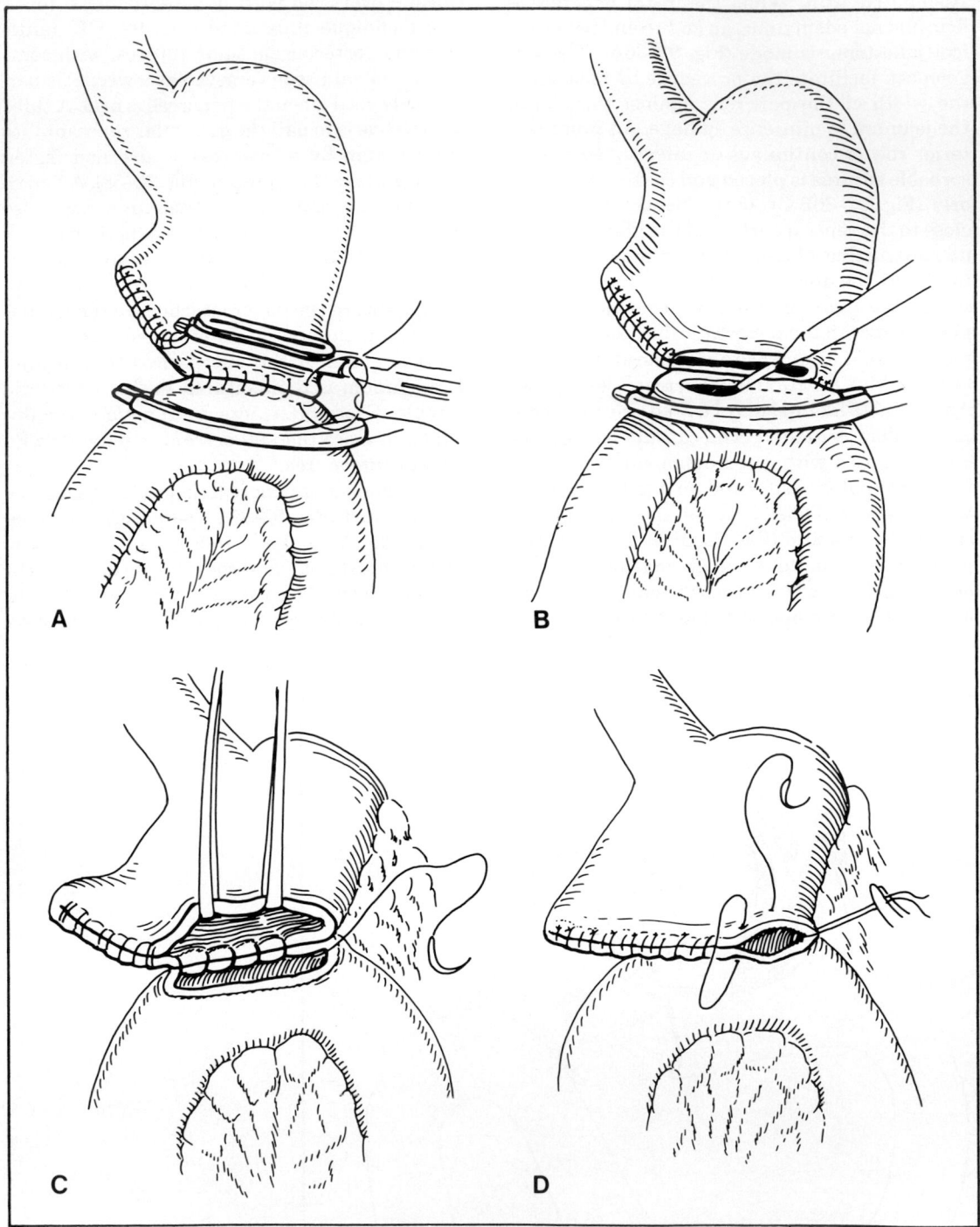

Figure 92–42. End-to-side gastrojejunostomy. **A.** Closure of lesser curvature and seromuscular approximation of posterior row of stomach and jejunum. **B.** Opening of jejunum. **C.** Through-and-through suture of posterior row. **D.** Through-and-through suture of anterior row. (*Source: From Cooperman AM, Hoerr S: Surgery of the Pancreas. St. Louis: CV Mosby, 1978, with permission.*)

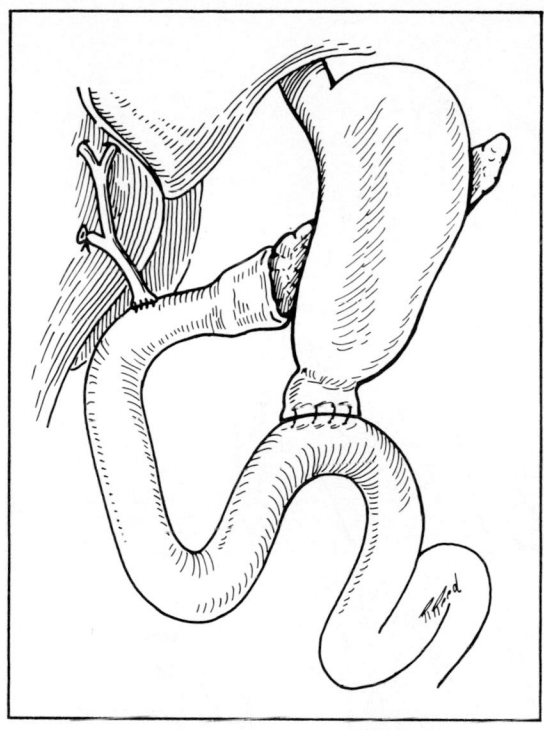

Figure 92–43. End-to-side duodenojejunostomy. (*Source: From Cooperman AM, Hoerr S: Surgery of the Pancreas. St. Louis: CV Mosby, 1978, with permission.*)

should be sutured to the duct.

Omentum from the stomach is mobilized and wrapped around the pancreatic anastomosis, if available. A hepaticojejunostomy is constructed distal to this (Fig. 92–40). Technical factors determine the site of the anastomosis. The opening in the jejunum is made smaller than the lumen of the duct, since it invariably enlarges as the anastomosis is completed (Fig. 92–41). Corner traction sutures are first placed, but not tied. The hepaticojejunal anastomosis is completed in one or two layers: the inner layer (which approximates the mucosa) is made with absorbable suture. A stent is not used if the diameter of the duct is wide (greater than 1 cm) or thick walled. An objection to preoperative duct decompression is that a dilated duct will become narrow and more difficult to suture with malignancy. The duct becomes thicker from chronic obstruction and this facilitates suturing.

An end-to-side gastrojejunostomy is made with an outer layer of nonabsorbable suture and inner layer of absorbable suture (Fig. 92–42). Sump drains are placed around the pancreatojejunal union. As mentioned, the alternative to gastric resection when the first part of the

duodenum is "free" is to divide the duodenum distal to the pylorus and establish an end-to-side duodenojejunostomy (Fig. 92–43). This avoids a gastric resection and vagotomy. A liver biopsy is taken prior to closure.

Postoperative Management

General postoperative measures apply to these patients. The use of incentive spirometry to decrease pulmonary complications is inexpensive and theoretically desirable. Nearly all patients tolerate ambulation within 24 hours. Intravenous fluids and parenteral nutrition administered before operation are continued until the surgeon and patient are comfortable that anastomotic healing is satisfactory and appetite adequate. Soft sumps are connected to a closed, continuous suction system to maintain sterility. The nasogastric tube is usually removed the evening of or morning after the operation unless delayed emptying develops.

If vagotomy and gastric resection are done, the nasogastric tube is left for at least 24 hours to determine if gastric retention develops. Antibiotics may be given three times at 8-hour intervals prior to, during, and after surgery to cover enteric flora and decrease the chance of wound

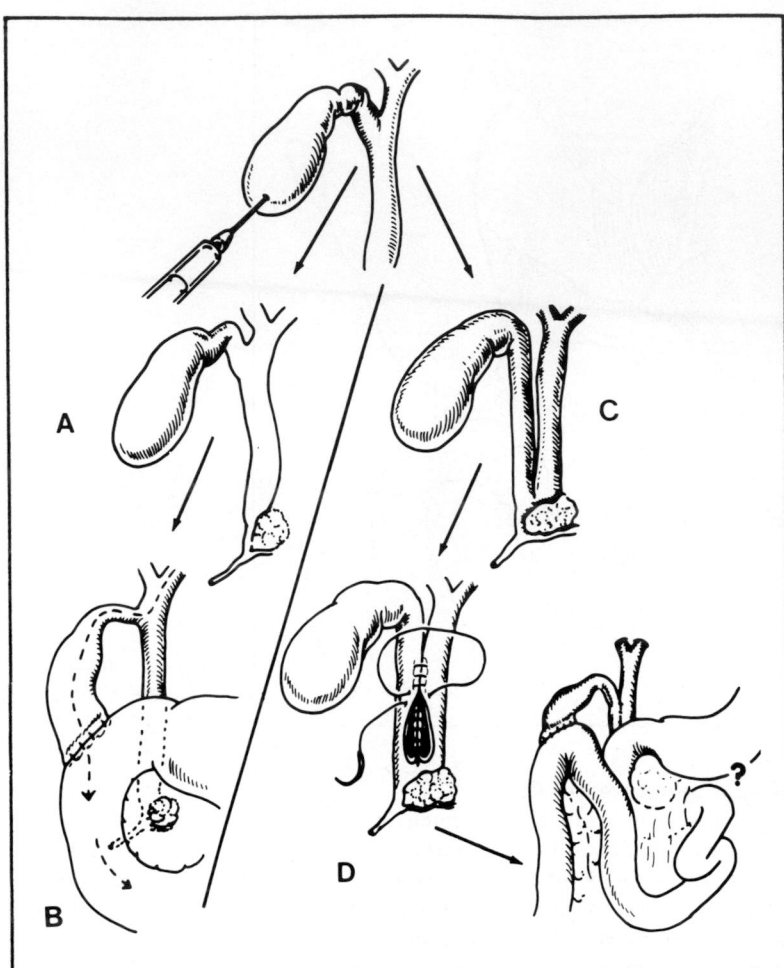

Figure 92–44. Palliative procedure. **A,B.** Cholecystoduodenostomy in the face of normal insertion of cystic duct into common bile duct. **C,D.** Method for handling low insertion of cystic duct into common bile duct. (*Source: From Cooperman AM, Hoerr S: Surgery of the Pancreas. St. Louis: CV Mosby, 1978, with permission.*)

infection. Wound dressings are removed within 24 hours of surgery and the subcuticular incision is left exposed. Hemorrhage is uncommon and may develop early (within hours of surgery) or late (5 to 10 days). Slippage of a tie is the usual cause of early hemorrhage and surgery may be necessary to correct this. Late bleeding is associated with fistula formation.

Specific Complications. Since three suture lines are placed, fear of an anastomotic leak is genuine. The duodenojejunal or gastrojejunal anastomosis should not cause problems. The choledochojejunal anastomosis leaks infrequently, and if it does it is usually transient. The real issue with this operation is the pancreatojejunal anastomosis. Fistula and sepsis from

the anastomosis have caused some surgeons to abandon it and favor total pancreatectomy. This author does not agree with this position; our unpublished institutional experience (Cleveland Clinic) with 75 pancreatoduodenal resections shows that no deaths were caused by leakage of the pancreatic anastomoses, nor has there been mortality in at least 30 additional resections from leakage of this anatomosis. With precise suture technique, facilitated by magnification, the anastomotic leak rate is less than 5 percent. We believe that improper timing of surgery and errors in exercising available options to treat the distal pancreas account for the disappointing results mentioned by some surgeons. Since a 100 percent watertight pancreaticojejunal anastomosis has yet to be devised, fistulas develop in some patients, but with closed drain-

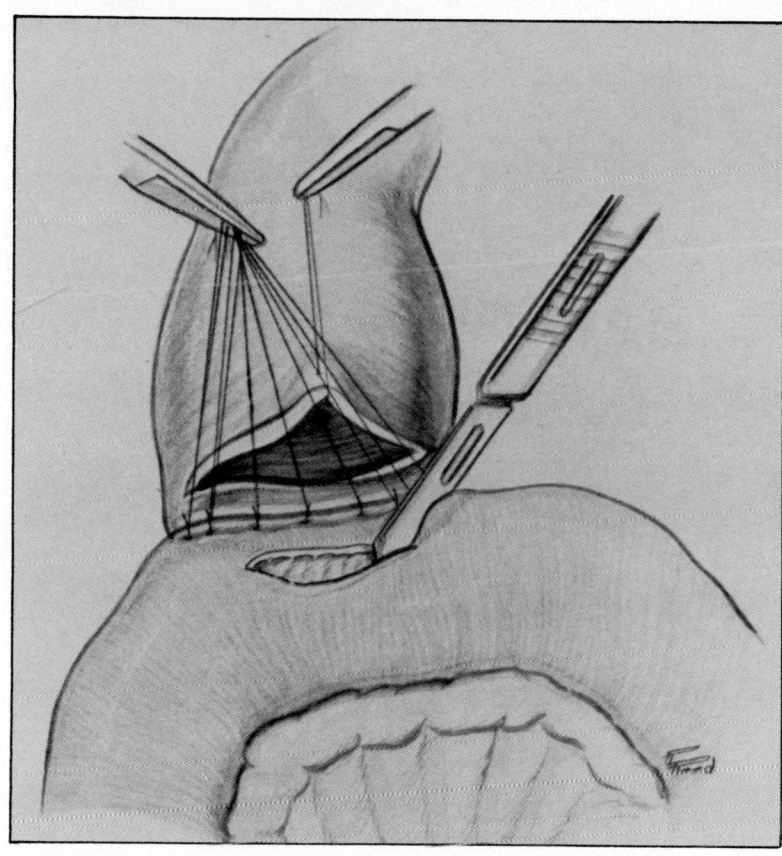

A

Figure 92–45. Cholecystojejunostomy. **A.** Posterior row using nonabsorbable suture material approximates seromuscular layers.

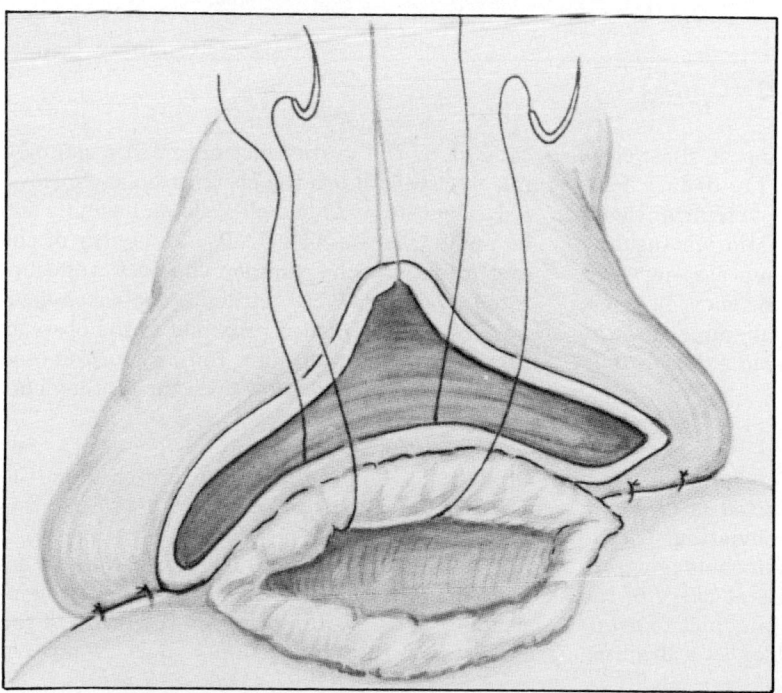

Figure 92–45. B. Inner row of absorbable catgut sutures.

B

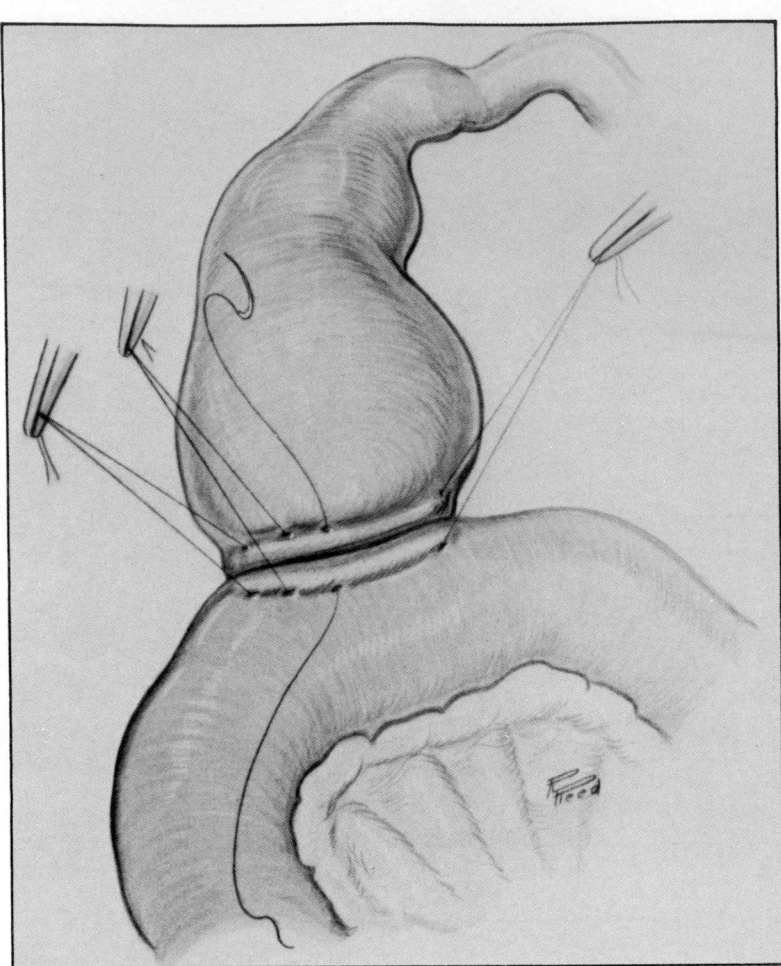

Figure 92–45. C. Completion of anterior row using nonabsorbable sutures placed seromuscularly. (*Source: From Cooperman AM, Hoerr S: Surgery of the Pancreas. St. Louis: CV Mosby, 1978, with permission.*)

C

age systems and nutritional support, these close spontaneously, usually within 7 to 10 days. Pancreatic insufficiency secondary to truncal vagotomy or strictures of the pancreatic duct (usually when it is not sewn mucosa-to-mucosa) may lead to exocrine pancreatic insufficiency in some long-term survivors with malignant disease. Should this develop, pancreatic extracts may be given.

Palliative Operations

Palliative procedures are directed at relieving jaundice and correcting, or obviating, gastric outlet obstruction. A cholecystocholangiogram is obtained to identify the site of entry of the cystic duct into the common bile duct to determine the use of the gallbladder as a draining

conduit. If the cystic duct enters the common bile duct well above the obstruction, a cholecystoduodenostomy or a cholecystojejunostomy can be made (Fig. 92–44A,B). If a low entry of the cystic duct into the common bile duct is encountered (Fig. 92–44C,D), either a choledochojejunostomy is established proximal to the obstruction, or the common duct can be anastomosed to the cystic duct to allow for a functioning cholecystoenteric anastomosis.

The gastrojejunostomy is generally performed for large masses encountered in the head of the pancreas in order to avoid subsequent gastric outlet obstruction.

In most instances, the simplest way to decompress the biliary tree is by cholecystojejunostomy (Fig. 92–45), provided the entry of the cystic duct into the common duct is not ob-

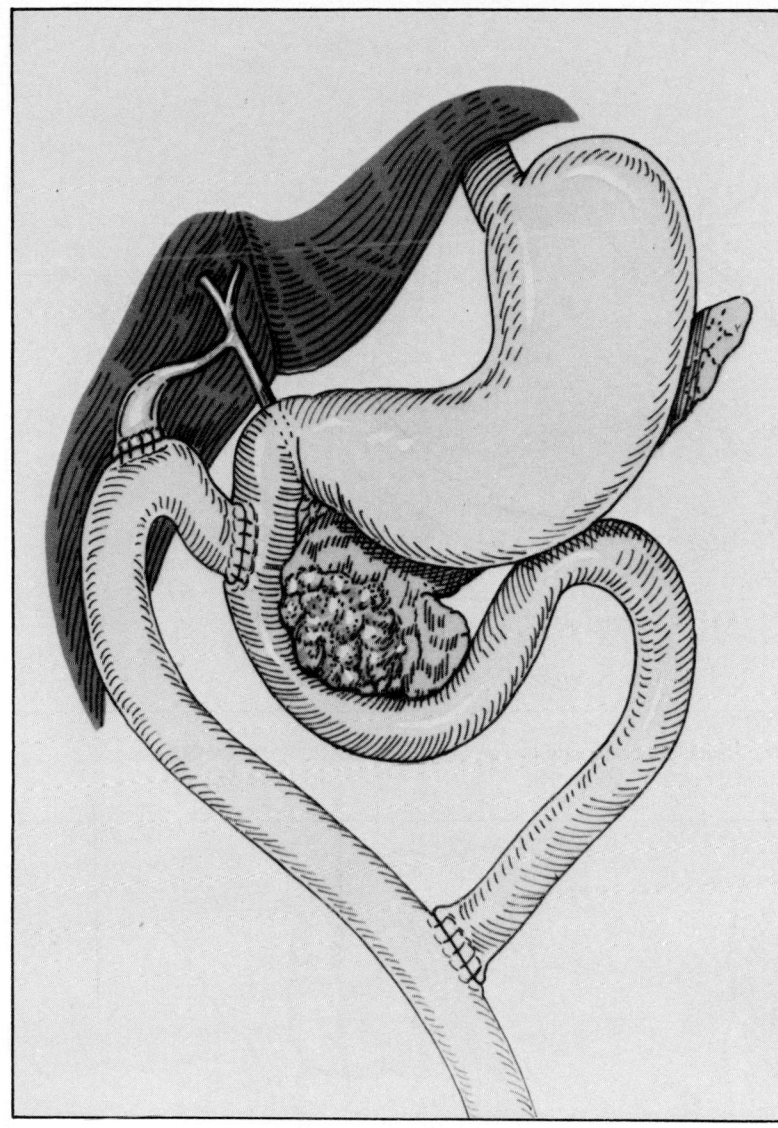

Figure 92–46. An alternative to gastric bypass using duodenojejunostomy Roux-Y limb. (*Source: From Cooperman AM, Hoerr S: Surgery of the Pancreas. St. Louis: CV Mosby, 1978, with permission.*)

structed by tumor. Either a one- or two-layer anastomosis is constructed, using an outer layer of interrupted nonabsorbable sutures and an inner layer of absorbable sutures. An alternative to gastric bypass is duodenojejunostomy (Fig. 92–46), made above the tumor using the same Roux-Y limb that decompressed the biliary tree.

Excision of Distal Pancreatic Lesions

Tumors of the tail and distal body of the pancreas are excised by entering the lesser sac through the gastrocolic omentum (Fig. 92–47).

The stomach is retracted superiorly, and the colon inferiorly. The spleen and distal pancreas are mobilized anteriorly out of their retroperitoneal position. Blunt dissection behind the pancreas carries mobilization of the gland to the right until an area of normal pancreas is encountered. At this point, the splenic artery and vein are individually ligated. After hemostasis is secured by ligature or suture of the fine blood vessels within the pancreatic parenchyma, the pancreatic duct is ligated separately. The divided end of the gland is then beveled to permit closure and is oversewn with interrupted su-

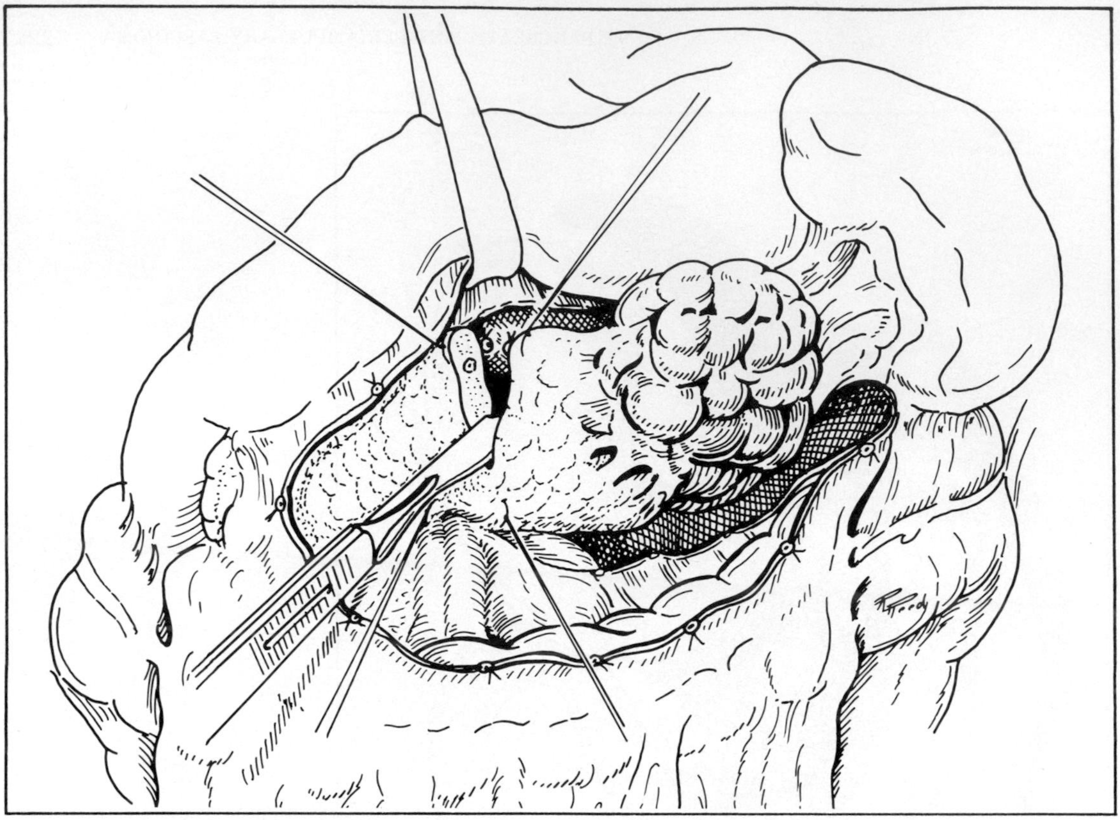

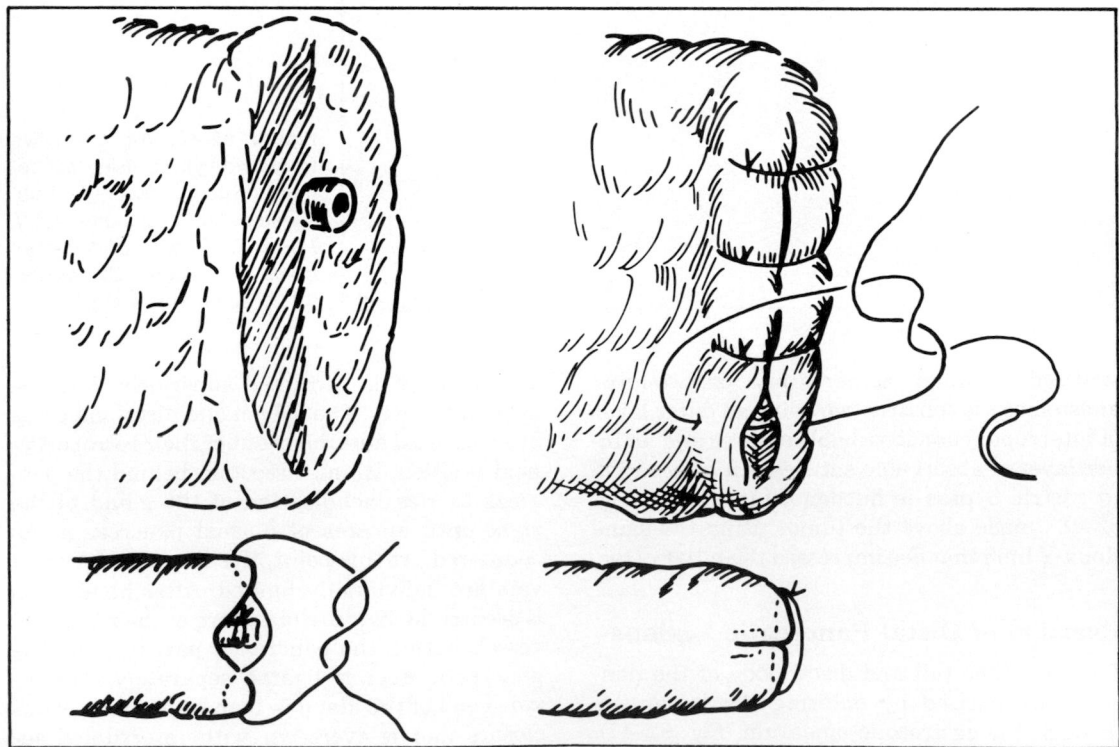

Figure 92–47. Dissection of distal pancreas and lesser sac. The divided pancreatic duct can be seen in the upper central gland.

Figure 92–48. Management of divided pancreas showing isolation and ligation of pancreatic duct and closure of the cut surface of the gland.

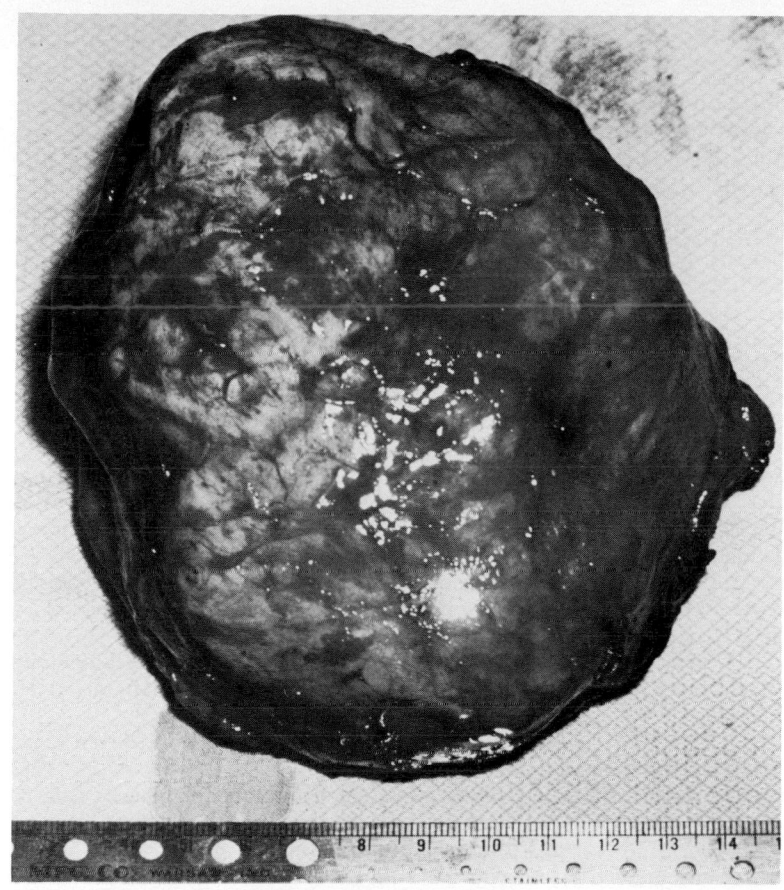

Figure 92–49. Cystadenoma of the pancreas. **A.** External surface. **B.** Specimen showing unilocular cystic nature.

A

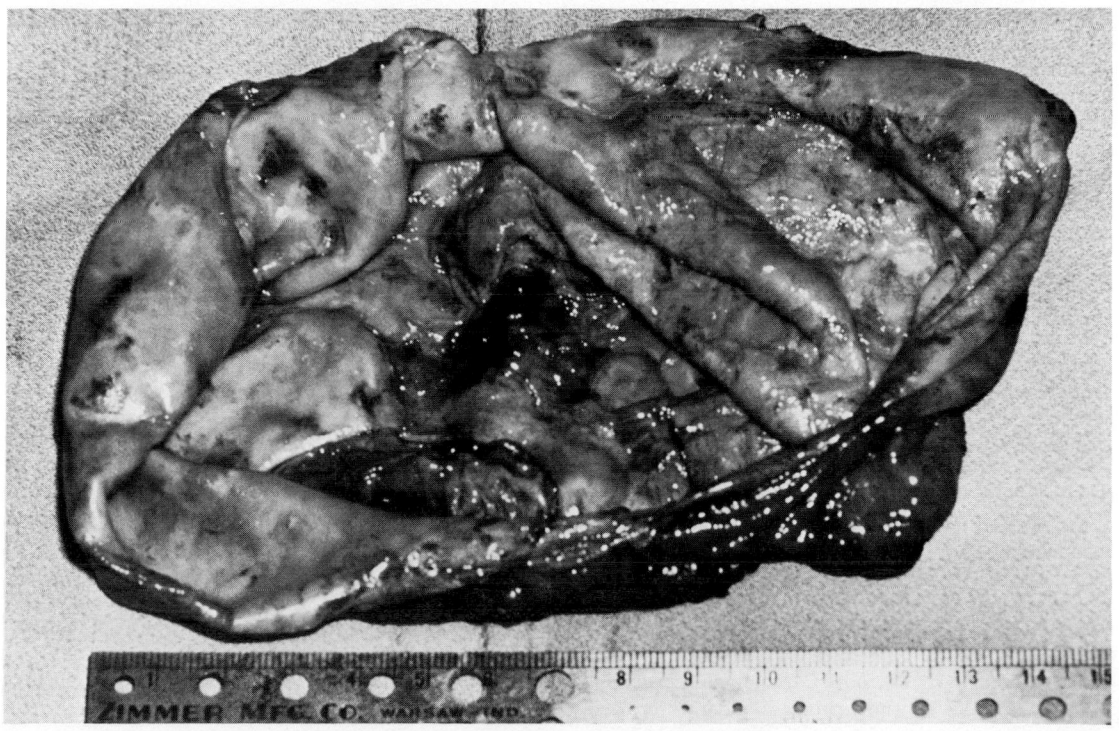

B

tures of 3-0 silk (Fig. 92–48). A Penrose drain is usually left for several days after the operation. An example of an excised cystadenoma of the tail of the pancreas is shown in Figure 92–49.

BIBLIOGRAPHY

Al Bahranj Z, Hamid AB, et al: Carcinoma of the pancreas in Iraq. Oncology 19:353, 1982

Alderson D, Lavelle MI, et al: Endoscopic sphincterotomy before pancreaticoduodenectomy for ampullary carcinoma. Br Med J (Clin Res) 282:1109, 1981

Allison MEM, Prentice CRM, et al: Renal function and other factors in obstructive jaundice. Br J Surg 66:392, 1979

Arnaud J, Humber W, et al: Effect of obstructive jaundice on wound healing. Am J Surg 141:593, 1981

Akwari O, VanHeerden HA, et al: Radical pancreatoduodenectomy for cancer of the papilla of Vater. Arch Surg 112:451, 1977

Bailey ME: Endotoxin, bile salts and renal function in obstructive jaundice. Br J Surg 63:744, 1976

Bancou O, Bersey J, et al: New oncofetal antigen for human pancreas. Lancet 1:643, 1973

Barkin J, Vinning D, et al: Computerized tomography, diagnostic ultrasound, and radionuclide scanning: Comparison of efficacy in diagnosis of pancreatic carcinoma. JAMA 238:2040, 1977

Barton RM, Copeland EM III: Carcinoma of the ampulla of Vater. Surg Gynecol Obstet 156:287, 1983

Beazley RM: Needle biopsy diagnosis of pancreatic cancer. Cancer 47:1685, 1981

Best EWR: A Canadian study of smoking and health. Department of National Health and Welfare, Ottawa, 1966, p 65

Bjorck S, Svensson JO, et al: Cancer of the head of the pancreas and choledochoduodenal junction: A clinical study of 88 Whipple resections. Acta Chir Scand 147:153, 1981

Blackstone MO, Cockerhan L, et al: Intraductal aspiration for cystodiagnosis in pancreatic malignancy. Gastrointest Endosc 23:1545, 1977

Braasch JL, Gray BN: Considerations that lower pancreatoduodenectomy mortality. Am J Surg 133:480, 1977

Brunschwig A: Resection of the head of the pancreas and duodenum for carcinoma and pancreaticoduodenectomy. Surg Gynecol Obstet 65:681, 1937

Burchapth F: A new endoprosthesis for nonoperative intubation of the biliary tract in malignant obstructive jaundice. Surg Gynecol Obstet 146:76, 1978

Cancer, Journal for Clinicians 32:1982

Capps WF Jr, Lewis MI, et al: Carcinoma of the colon, ampulla of Vater and urinary bladder associated with familial multiple polyposis: A case report. Dis Colon Rectum 11:198, 1968

Christou N: Anergy testing in surgical patients. Infections in Surgery 2:692, 1983

Christoffersen P, Poll P: Preoperative pancreas aspiration. Acta Pathol Microbiol Scand (suppl)212:28, 1970

Chung RS: Pathogenesis of the "Courvoisier gallbladder." Dig Dis Sci 28:33, 1983

Clarke CC, Mitchell P: Diabetes mellitus and primary carcinoma of the pancreas. Br Med J 2:1259, 1961

Clarke DN, Norman JN, et al: Pancreatitis and duodenal obstruction due to periampullary carcinoma associated with familial polyposis coli. Postgrad Med J 54:418, 1978

Clement A, Zimmon D: Personal communication

Cohen JR, Kuchta N, et al: Pancreaticoduodenectomy, a 40-year experience. Ann Surg 195:608, 1982

Compagno J, Oertel JE: Mucinous cystic neoplasms of the pancreas: A clinicopathological study of 34 cases. Am J Clin Pathol 69:289, 1978

Cooperman AM: Cancer of the ampulla of Vater, bile duct and duodenum. Surg Clin North Am 61:99, 1981

Cooperman AM: Periampullary cancer. Semin Liver Dis 3:181, 1983

Cooperman AM: The management of pancreatitis, in Irving M, Beart R (eds): Gastroenterologic Surgery. London: Butterworths, 1982, p 117

Cooperman AM: Treatment dilemma in pancreatic cancer. Surg Clin North Am 61:106, 1981

Cooperman AM, Herter FP, et al: Pancreaticoduodenal resection: An institutional review. Surgery 70:707, 1981

Crile G Jr: The advantages of bypass operations over radical pancreatoduodenectomy in the treatment of pancreatic carcinoma. Surg Gynecol Obstet 130:1049, 1970

Cubilla A, Fitzgerald PJ, et al: Cancer (non-endocrine) of the pancreas: A suggested classification, in Fitzgerald PJ, Morrison AB (eds): The Pancreas. Baltimore: Williams and Wilkins, 1980, p 82

Cuschieri A: Laparoscopy in general surgery and gastroenterology. Br J Hosp Med 24:252, 1980

Denning D, Ellison EC, et al: Preoperative percutaneous transhepatic biliary decompression lowers operative morbidity in patients with obstructive jaundice. Am J Surg 141:61, 1981

DiMagno EP, Malegelada JR, et al: Prospective evaluation of the pancreatic secretion of imuno-reactive carcinoembryonic antigen, enzyme and bicarbonate in patients suspected of having pancreatic cancer. Gastroenterology 73:457, 1977

DiMagno EP, Malagelada JR, et al: The relationship between pancreatic ductal obstruction and pancreatic secretion in man. Mayo Clin Proc 54:157, 1979

Dobelbower R: The radiotherapy of pancreatic cancer. Semin Oncol 6:378, 1979

Edis AJ, Kiernan PD, et al: Attempted curative resection of ductal carcinoma of the pancreas. Review of Mayo Clinic Experience 1951–1975. Mayo Clin Proc 55:531, 1980

Endo Y, Morii T, et al: Cytodiagnosis of pancreatic malignant tumors by aspiration under direct vision using a duodenal fiberoscope. Gastroenterology 67:944, 1974

Fitzgerald PJ, Fortner JG, et al: The value of diagnostic aids in detecting pancreatic cancer. Cancer 41:868, 1978

Fortner JG: Surgical principles for pancreatic cancer: Regional, total and subtotal pancreatectomy. Cancer 47:1712, 1981

Fortner JG, Kim DK, et al: Immunologic function in patients with carcinoma of the pancreas. Surg Gynecol Obstet 150:215, 1980

Friedman S, Lichtman J, et al: Solid and papillary epithelial neoplasms. South Gastroint Radiol (Abstracts), 1983

Gastrointestinal Tumor Study Group: Comparative therapeutic trial of radiation with or without chemotherapy in pancreatic carcinoma. Int J Radiat Biol 5:1643, 1979

Gelder R, Reese C, et al: Studies on a pancreatic oncofetal antigen (POA). Cancer Res 43 (suppl 3):1635, 1978

Gianni I, DiPadova F, et al: Bile acid induced inhibition of the lymphoproliferative responses to phytohemoglutinin and poke weed mitogen: An in vitro study. Gastroenterology 78:231, 1980

Haaga JR: Personal communication

Haaga JR, Alfidi RJ, et al: Definitive role of CT scanning of the pancreas. The second year's experience. Radiology 124:723, 1977

Halsted WS: Contributions to the surgery of the bile passages, especially the common bile duct. Boston Med Surg J 141:641, 1899

Hammond EC: Smoking in relation to the death rates of one million men and women. Natl Cancer Inst Mono 19:127, 1966

Herlinger H, Finlay DB: Evaluation and follow up of pancreatic arteriograms. A new role for angiography in the diagnosis of carcinoma of the pancreas. Clin Radiol 29:277, 1978

Hermann RE: Manual of Surgery of the Gallbladder, Bile Duct and Exocrine Pancreas. New York: Springer-Verlag, 1979

Herter FP, Cooperman AM, et al: Antinoric: Surgical experience with pancreatic and periampullary cancer. Ann Surg 195:274, 1982

Hirayama T: Smoking in relation to the death rates of 295,118 men and women in Japan. National Cancer Center, Research Inst 14, 1967

Hus Y-H, Guzman LG: Carcinoma of the pancreas: Diagnosis and treatment. South Med J 75:972, 1982

Ihse I, Lilja P, et al: Total pancreatectomy for cancer—An appraisal of 65 cases. Ann Surg 186:675, 1977

Isakasson G, Ihse A, et al: Local excision for ampullary carcinoma—An alternative treatment for patients unfit for pancreatectomy. Acta Chir Scand 148:163, 1981

Kessler II: Cancer mortality among diabetics. J Natl Cancer Inst 44:673, 1970

Kozuka S, Tsubon E, et al: Adenomatous residue in cancerous papilla of Vater. Gut 22:1031, 1981

Langer B, Lipson R, et al: Periampullary tumors: Advances in diagnosis and surgical treatment. Can J Surg 22:34, 1979

Levin B, Remine WH, et al: Panel. Cancer of the pancreas. Am J Surg 135:85, 1978

Longmire WP Jr, Traverso W: The Whipple procedure and other standard operative approaches to pancreatic cancer. Cancer 47:1706, 1981

Lord Smith of Marlow: Surgery of carcinoma of the pancreas. Can J Surg 24:176, 1981

MacMahon B, Yen S, et al: Coffee and cancer of the pancreas. N Engl J Med 304:630, 1982

Makipour H, Cooperman AM, et al: Carcinoma of the ampulla of Vater. Review of 38 cases with emphasis on treatment and prognostic factors. Ann Surg 183:341, 1976

Mirkin KR, Rossin R: Long-term palliation of ampullary carcinoma using endoscopic papillotomy. Conn Med 46:4, 1982

Miyata M, Hamaji M, et al: An appraisal of radical pancreaticoduodenectomy based on glucagon secretion. Ann Surg 191:282, 1980

Moertel C, Childs D, et al: Combined fluorouracil and supervoltage radiation therapy of locally unresectable gastrointestinal cancer. Lancet 2:865, 1969

Moley JF, Morrison S, et al: Effects of exogenous insulin administration on food intake, body weight change and tumor doubling time. Surg Forum 34:91, 1983

Molnar W, Stockman AE: Relief of obstructive jaundice through percutaneous transhepatic catheter: A new therapeutic method. Am J Roentgenol 122:356, 1974

Morgan RGH, Wormsley KG: Cancer of the pancreas—Progress report. Gut 18:580, 1977

Mueller PR, vanSonenberg E, et al.: Percutaneous biliary drainage: Technical and catheter related problems in 200 procedures. AJR 138:17, 1982

Nakase A, Matsumoto Y, et al: Surgical treatment of cancer of the pancreas in the periampullary region. Cumulative results in 57 institutions in Japan. Ann Surg 185:57, 1976

Norlander A, Kalin B, et al: Effect of percutaneous transhepatic drainage upon liver function and postoperative mortality. Surg Gynecol Obstet 155:151, 1982

Neff RA, Fankuchen EI, et al: The radiological management of malignant biliary obstruction. Clin Radiol 34:143, 1983

Office of Population Censuses and Surveys. Cancer Mortality, England and Wales, 1911–1970. Studies on Medical and Population Subject, No. 29, London, HMSO, 1975

Ong V, Pintauro WM: Silver stools. JAMA 242:2433, 1979

Pauli M, Pauli E, et al: Gardner syndrome and periampullary malignancy. Am J Med Gene 108:205, 1980

Piotrowski RJ, Blievernicht SW, et al: Pancreatic and periampullary cancer. Am J Surg 143:100, 1982

Pitt HA, Cameron JL, et al: Factors affecting mortality in biliary tract surgery. Am J Surg 141:66, 1981

Russell D, Roberts-Thomson IC, et al: Carcinoma of the papilla of Vater. Aust N Z J Surg 52:44, 1981

Sanfey H, Mendelsohn G, et al: Solid and papillary neoplasm of the pancreas: A potentially curable lesion. Ann Surg 197:272, 1983

Sauve L: Des pancreatectomies et special ement de la pancreatectomie cephalique. Res Chir 37:335, 1908

Schein PS, Kisner D, et al: Cachexia of malignancy: Potential role of insulin in nutritional management. Cancer 43:2070, 1979

Shapiro TM: Adenocarcinoma of the pancreas: A statistical analysis of biliary bypass versus Whipple resection in good risk patients. Ann Surg 182:715, 1975

Sheedy DF II, Stephens DH, et al: Computerized tomography in the evaluation of patients with suspected carcinoma of the pancreas. Radiology 124:731, 1977

Silverberg E: Cancer statistics. Cancer 27:26, 1978

Sobol S, Cooperman AM: Villous adenoma of the ampulla of Vater, an unusual cause of biliary colic and obstructive jaundice. Gastroenterology 75:107, 1978

Stephenson LW, Blackstone EH, et al: Radical resection for periampullary carcinomas—Results in 53 patients. Arch Surg 112:245, 1977

Stocks P: Cancer mortality in relation to national consumption of cigarettes, solid fuel, tea, and coffee. Br J Cancer 24:215, 1970

Sugihara K, Muto T, et al: Associated with periampullary carcinoma, duodenal and gastric adenomatosis—Report of a case. Dis Colon Rectum 25:766, 1982

Tetsuichiro M, Konishi F, et al: Gardner's syndrome associated with periampullary carcinoma, duodenal and gastric adenomatosis—Report of a case. Dis Colon Rectum 25:766, 1982

Traverso LW, Longmire WP Jr: Preservation of the pylorus in pancreaticoduodenectomy. Surg Gynecol Obstet 146:959, 1978

Treadwell TA, Jimenez-Chapa JF, et al: Carcinoma of the ampulla of Vater. South Med J 71:365, 1978

VanHeerden JA, Edis JA, et al: Total pancreatectomy for ductal adenocarcinoma of the pancreas. Mayo Clinic experience. Am Surg 142:308, 1981

VanHeerden JA, Heath PM, et al: Biliary bypass for ductal adenocarcinoma of the pancreas. Mayo Clinic Proc 55:537, 1980

Walsh DB, Eckhauser FE, et al: Adenocarcinoma of the ampulla of Vater—Diagnosis and treatment. Ann Surg 195:152, 1982

Warren KW, Choi OS, et al: Results of radical resection for periampullary cancer. Ann Surg 181, 1975

Wei T, Hsu S: Pancreatoduodenectomy for periampullary cancer. J Formosan Med Assoc 79:1038, 1980

Weir JM, Dunn JE: Smoking and mortality: A prospective study. Cancer 25:105, 1970

Whipple AO: The rationale of radical surgery for cancer of the pancreas and ampullary region. Ann Surg 114:612, 1941

Williams JA, Cubilla A, et al: Twenty-two year experience with periampullary carcinoma at Memorial Sloan-Kettering Cancer Center. Am J Surg 138:662, 1979

Wise L, Pizzimbono C, et al: Periampullary cancer. A clinicopathological study of 62 patients. Am Surg 131:141, 1976

World Health Organization. World Health Statistics Report 27, 1974, p 393

Wynder EL, Mabuchi K, et al: Epidemiology of cancer of the pancreas. J Natl Cancer Institute 50:645, 1973

Wynder EL, Mabuchi M, et al: A case control of cancer of the pancreas. Cancer 31:641, 1973

93. Total Pancreatectomy

A.R. Moossa

INTRODUCTION

As recently as 60 years ago, complete removal of the pancreas was considered to be a virtually impossible technical exercise. The resulting physiologic state was also, in a sense, incompatible with continued normal life. Since that time it has become apparent that the operation is both possible and safe to perform, but it has acquired a bad reputation largely for two reasons: (1) Most surgeons felt that the operation was not affecting the usually hopeless prognosis of the disease (namely, pancreatic adenocarcinoma) for which it was being carried out. (2) The operation is still often attempted by surgeons inexperienced in the operation and with inadequate preoperative preparation and postoperative care. This has resulted in frequent reports of a prohibitive morbidity and mortality.

In these respects, the development of total pancreatectomy has much historical resemblance to that of total gastrectomy. Current belief is that the operation can be safely performed provided meticulous attention is paid to details. With improved operative technique, pre- and postoperative management, and methods of anesthesia, the indications for total pancreatectomy have broadened, and the merits of the operation per se can be appraised. In many ways, the pancreas is more difficult to manage surgically than other viscera. It is situated at a complex anatomic crossroad where its central position provides lymphatic drainage radially along several major routes (splenic, hepatic, and superior mesenteric vessels). This makes it hard to design an adequate cancer operation that in an orderly manner removes primary, secondary, and tertiary nodal basins. Moreover, the intimate association of the pancreas with the major vessels of the epigastrium at once limits the extent of the procedure and dictates what must be removed. Thus, when a tumor spreads a short distance to involve the portal vein or superior mesenteric artery, it usually becomes incurable. Similarly, if the gland is removed in a radical fashion, the need to excise the vessels and lymph nodes that go with it makes removal of the spleen, duodenum, gallbladder, common bile duct, upper jejunum, and a large portion of the stomach necessary (Fig. 93–1).

When any part of the pancreas is removed or even if the gland is incised, safe management of any draining of pancreatic juice becomes a matter of primary importance, since the enzymes, if allowed to remain in the peritoneal cavity, may cause havoc. A first principle of pancreatic surgery therefore is the provision of adequate drainage. Similarly, the exudation and accumulation of serum, lymph, and blood following a total pancreatectomy need to be drained. Second, since catgut is a protein substance that is readily digested by trypsin, it cannot be trusted as a ligature on major vessels, or as a suture material for anastomosis, or for closing the abdomen. Silk, cotton, wire, nylon, or Prolene are much safer.

INDICATIONS

Most surgeons reserve total pancreatectomy for what they believe to be resectable tumors of the pancreas. The criteria for resectability are clearly defined in the following. The indications for total pancreatectomy can be extended to cover the following:

1. Resectable and localized adenocarcinoma of the head, body, or tail of the exocrine pancreas
2. Other rarer primary malignant tumors of the pancreas such as cystadenocarcinomas, apudomas, sarcomas, etc.
3. Hyperinsulinism in the adult for which no discrete tumor can be identified at the time of operation and on pathologic examination of a blind partial pancreatectomy specimen
4. Hyperinsulinism in infants and children (nesidioblastosis, infantile islet cell hyperplasia) that has failed to respond to a 90 to 95 percent pancreatectomy
5. Selected cases of end-stage chronic relapsing pancreatitis (with substantial loss of endocrine and exocrine function) when the ducts are so damaged as to preclude a Puestow-like procedure
6. Failure of a Puestow-like procedure or a partial pancreatectomy to control pain in patients with chronic relapsing pancreatitis

7. Selected cases of major abdominal trauma involving the disruption of large areas of the pancreas and its major blood supply
8. Selected patients with acute fulminant pancreatitis, leading to total pancreatic necrosis, who fail to improve under conservative management
9. Failure to construct a technically sound pancreatojejunal anastomosis following a Whipple resection

KEY INVESTIGATIONS

Over the past ten years, four investigative tools have come to the forefront of pancreatic research and they provide the surgeon with vital information preoperatively and obviate the need for many time-consuming ancillary maneuvers on the operating table. Computed tomography (CT) and/or ultrasonography of the pancreas provide clues to the presence of any

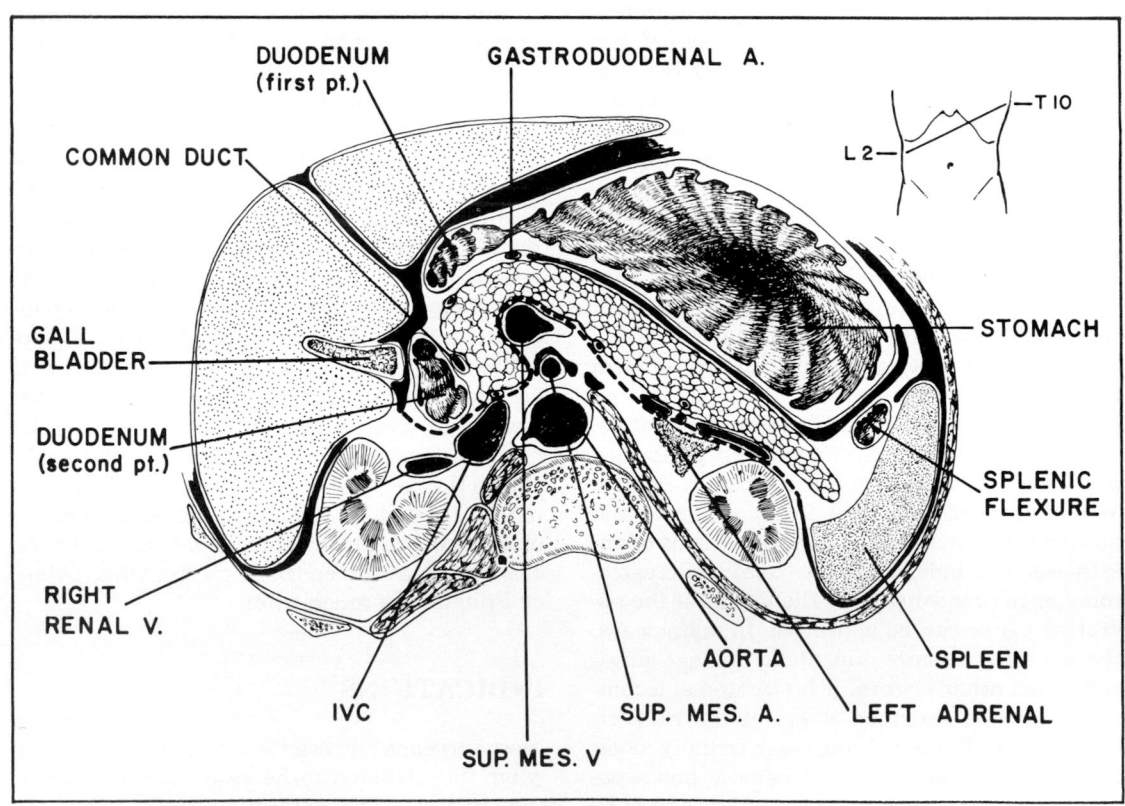

Figure 93–1. Oblique transverse cross-section of the upper abdomen along the long axis of the pancreas (corresponding approximately to levels indicated on inset) viewed from below. Dotted line indicates posterior plane of dissection.

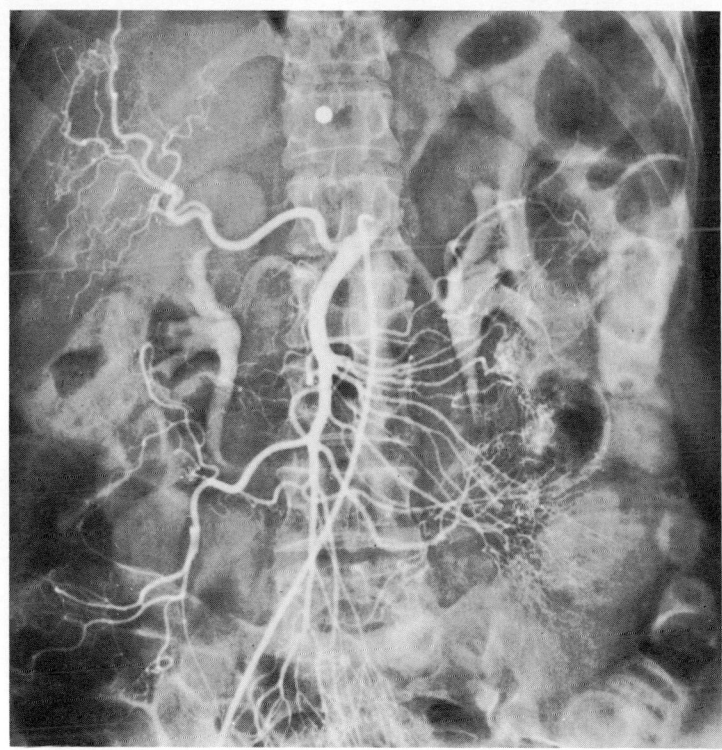

Figure 93–2. Selective superior mesenteric arteriogram obtained preoperatively in a patient who underwent total pancreatectomy for carcinoma of the head of the pancreas. The right hepatic artery is shown arising from the superior mesenteric artery.

mass in the gland, dilatation of the extrahepatic biliary tree, and the presence of liver metastases. Endoscopic retrograde colangiopancreatography (ERCP) for contrast radiology and cytology delineates the state of the main pancreatic duct and/or the common bile duct. The degree of obstruction and proximal dilation of the two main ducts can thus be established. Most importantly, a positive cytology from the papillary aspirate confirms the suspicion of cancer. In cases where ERCP technically fails or is not available, duodenal drainage studies following secretin administration is an alternative method for obtaining material for cytologic examination.

Celiac and superior mesenteric angiography outlines anomalies in the foregut vasculature and can warn the surgeon about portal and splenic vein involvement and the presence of subclinical portal hypertension that will intensify intraoperative hemorrhage. Major arterial (hepatic, splenic, or superior mesenteric) encasement or major venous (portal, superior mesenteric, or splenic) occlusion usually indicates unresectability of the cancer. Previously emphasized was that a major anatomic anomaly of the foregut vasculature is demonstrated in

at least 25 to 30 percent of angiographic studies. Damage to the hepatic blood supply, especially likely when it originates from the superior mesenteric artery (Fig. 93–2) and is not easily palpable behind and to the right of the common bile duct, will lead to fatal hepatic necrosis in the jaundiced patient.

PREOPERATIVE PREPARATION

Although the essential investigations are under way, meticulous attention must be paid to the preoperative preparation of the patient for pancreatic resection. Emphasis must be placed on the following aspects of preoperative care.

Hydration and Nutrition. Since starvation for long hours is mandatory prior to many tests, the patient must be kept well hydrated by supplemental intravenous fluid given as necessary. Renal failure due to hypovolemia is a tremendous hazard in the jaundiced patient; a continuous diuresis must therefore be ensured at all times.

The patient must be given by mouth an elemental diet (Vivonex, Precision, Ensure, Sustacal) with multivitamin supplements. A short period of total parenteral nutrition both before and after the operation may be of additional benefit. However, if the patient is already in optimum condition, little is gained by prolonged and exhaustive preparations.

Correction of Blood Deficiencies. Anemia is corrected by blood transfusion as required. Since hemorrhage is the most common single complication of pancreatectomy, especially in the jaundiced patient, the author insists on a preoperative hematocrit of about 40 percent. All jaundiced patients must receive daily injections of vitamin K, preferably for 5 days prior to operation, regardless of whether the prothrombin index is normal or not. Six units of fresh frozen plasma, 6 units of platelets, and at least 6 units of packed red blood cells are made available in the operating room.

Cardiopulmonary Function. Assessment of cardiopulmonary function by pulmonary function tests, chest x-ray, and electrocardiogram

is followed by intensive pulmonary physiotherapy and physical activity, including leg exercises. Smoking is prohibited. The question of prophylactic digitalization and diuretic therapy is considered in individual patients to achieve maximum cardiac compensation.

Bowel Preparation. Mechanical bowel preparation, consisting of an elemental diet with clear liquids and appropriate amounts of laxatives and saline enemas given twice daily, is maintained for 4 to 5 days preoperatively. Oral kanamycin (500 mg every 6 hours for 2 days) is also given. This part of the preoperative care is important because in selected patients the transverse mesocolon, and hence the transverse colon, may have to be removed with the pancreas.

Prophylactic Systemic Antibiotics. Intravenous broad-spectrum antibiotics such as penicillin (one million units every 6 hours) and chloromycetin (500 mg every 6 hours) are given for 4 days starting 6 hours prior to operation to all patients with biliary tract obstruction and

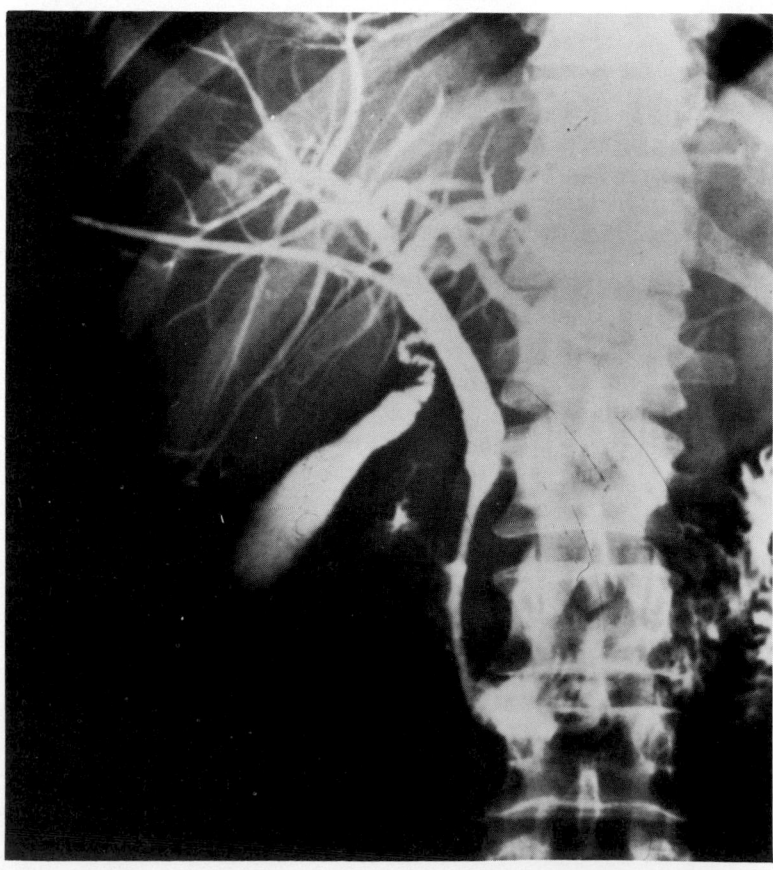

Figure 93–3. Percutaneous transhepatic biliary decompression (external and internal) in patient with cancer of the head of pancreas.

in selected cases where the surgeon suspects that operative contamination may occur.

Percutaneous Transhepatic Biliary Decompression (Fig. 93–3). This maneuver is strongly advocated preoperatively in the following situations:

1. Patients with a highly elevated serum bilirubin, exceeding 20 mg/dl.
2. Severely jaundiced patients with a reversible disease, such as pneumonia, which needs to be treated before embarking on a major operation under general anesthesia.
3. Patients who are grossly malnourished who would benefit from a few days of intravenous feeding prior to operation.

CONTRAINDICATIONS

Except under the most unusual circumstances, a major pancreatic resection should not be undertaken in the elderly (older than 70 years). Frail patients with multiple systemic disorders who are unlikely to tolerate a major operation and those individuals with an estimated life expectancy of less than 3 years should also be excluded. The nonreformed nondiabetic alcoholic or drug addict with chronic relapsing pancreatitis must not be subjected to a total pancreatectomy until suitably rehabilitated. Conversion of a nonreformed alcoholic or drug addict into an insulin-requiring diabetic by total pancreatectomy can be lethal.

The operation should not be undertaken by the registrar or resident in training without adequate supervision and assistance. It should not be performed in the district or community hospital where there is inadequate expertise, experience, facilities, and commitment to care of such difficult problems.

TECHNIQUE

Incision

The operation is usually done through an oblique upper abdominal incision along the long axis of the pancreas (Fig. 93–4). The incision is virtually transverse in its right extension and provides easy access to the lateral part of the duodenum and the biliary tract, whereas its left-sided extension over the left costal margin provides good exposure of the spleen, the tail of the pancreas, the upper part of the stomach,

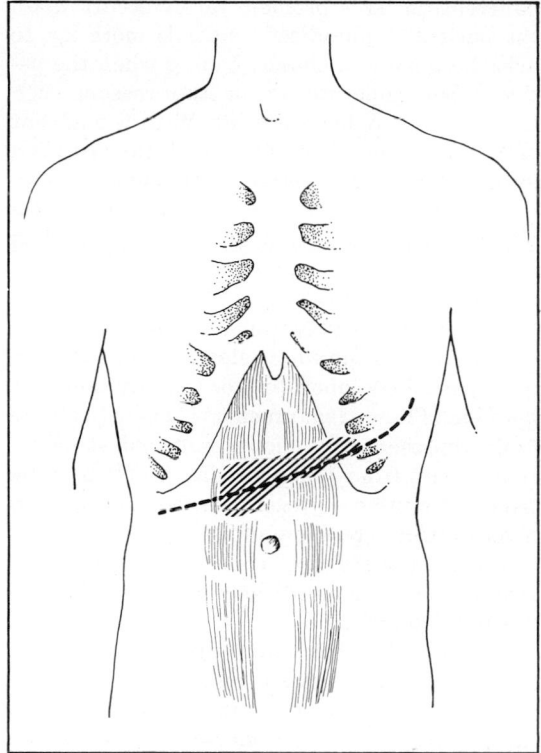

Figure 93–4. Diagram showing the abdominal wall incision used for pancreatic resection. Access to the spleen and tail of the pancreas may be improved by extending the abdominal incision over the left costal margin.

and the celiac axis. In individuals with an unusually narrow costal angle, a long midline vertical incision starting at the xiphisternum and ending near the pubic symphysis is recommended instead.

Transverse incisions are performed in most patients because they provide easy access to the whole pancreas and are least apt to be complicated by weakness postoperatively. In making this type of transverse incision, it is well to keep two fingers' breadth below the right costal margin, as this provides greater postoperative comfort and consequently better ventilation of the lungs than would be obtained otherwise.

The account that follows deals with total pancreatectomy with regional lymphadenectomy for a cancer in the head of the pancreas.

Diagnosis in the Operating Room

One of the most advertised dilemmas in abdominal surgery is the differentiation between carcinoma of the head of the pancreas and chronic pancreatitis. This problem rarely occurs when the patient is jaundiced, but it is more apt to arise because of a chance finding when the patient is being operated on for other reasons, such as a routine cholecystectomy. With the advent of ERCP and cytology, most doubtful cases can be sorted out preoperatively. Occasionally, a tumor is small and hidden in the midst of a virtually ligneous gland that is totally involved in fibrotic and calcific pancreatitis. In such instances, unless positive cytology has been obtained preoperatively, the diagnosis may elude discovery until the whole gland reaches the surgical pathology laboratory or autopsy table, regardless of how great an effort is made to obtain truly representative biopsy material at operation. Apart from this sampling problem, some pancreatic tumors present the pathologist with a very difficult problem of identification on frozen section histology. The diffuse infiltrating type of cancer is most likely to cause this diagnostic dilemma.

It is well to remember the old adage that, in the absence of acute inflammation and/or gallstones, solid, hard, noncystic masses in the head of the pancreas associated with obstructive jaundice and dilation of the common bile duct are rarely due to pancreatitis and are usually carcinoma. Conversely, hard, noncystic masses involving a major part of the retroampullary part of the gland and unassociated with jaundice and dilation of the biliary tree are usually pancreatitis. Small areas of induration in the head of the pancreas are usually benign and, because they are small, they are more amenable to precisely placed biopsies (needle or knife) than larger masses.

Obviously these generalizations, although helpful, will not serve to differentiate all carcinomas from chronic pancreatitis. The surgeon must, in such situations, decide whether to try to establish a diagnosis by frozen section biopsies prior to assessing resectability of the mass. Each operator will be quite properly influenced by individual philosophies and the pathologist's experience in this field as well as by the clinical situation.

The author's general policy relative to pancreatic biopsy can be stated as follows:

1. The operative strategy is planned *preoperatively* and is fully discussed with the patient and the relatives. The issues, uncertainties, limitations, and dangers of pancreatic biop-

sies, the operative risks, and potential benefits are all explained in simple terms by the surgeon (not the resident). Emphasis is placed on the fact that a major resection may be needed in spite of a negative biopsy.

2. In about 80 percent of all pancreatic cancer cases, we rely on a positive cytology obtained preoperatively at ERCP. All masses in the head of the pancreas are first assessed for resectability, and if conditions are favorable, they may be resected without a preliminary biopsy. In other words, primary intrapancreatic growths are rarely subjected to biopsy when resectable. (This does not necessarily apply when cystic tumors are present.)

3. All unresectable tumors are diagnosed before the surgeon leaves the operating room, even if the job is time consuming. This takes the matter out of the realm of doubt—an especially important point when a palliative procedure restores the patient to relatively good health for a long period and doubt is raised as to the diagnosis. A known positive biopsy for carcinoma will then prevent a fruitless second laparotomy. All biopsies of a mass in the head of the pancreas are performed by the transduodenal approach, without a duodenotomy, using a disposable Travenol Tru-Cut needle after an adequate Kocher maneuver. A useful, less traumatic alternative is to employ a long No. 21 needle, pushed in similar fashion through the duodenum and attached to a 10-ml syringe for aspiration in order to provide a smear for cytology.

4. Frozen sections may be made of lymph nodes adjacent or peripheral to the proposed specimen if unresectability and/or the presence of liver metastasis has been established. The presence of a positive regional node per se is *not* an absolute criterion of unresectability if the node is part of the total pancreatectomy specimen. The author has several patients with involved lymph nodes who underwent total pancreatectomy and have survived longer than 3 years and 2 patients who have survived longer than 5 years.

The arguments supporting these policies include the following:

1. Truly representative biopsies of the pancreas are often hard to obtain because of sampling error and confusion between tumor and surrounding pancreatitis. The earlier the tumor

the more difficult it is to obtain a positive diagnosis.

2. Errors in interpretation of frozen section biopsy specimens of the pancreas may be made because some desmoplastic carcinomas closely resemble chronic pancreatitis. Fortunately, however, such errors are rarely made by an experienced histopathologist.

3. The establishment of diagnosis by means of frozen section biopsy specimens is sometimes time consuming and traumatic. The surgeon should not "biopsy the patient to death" because, in the end, a pancreatoduodenal resection may be needed because of the inflicted trauma to, and hemorrhage in, the pancreatoduodenal area.

When a pancreatic biopsy is done, the operator should make great efforts to avoid major pancreatic ducts and vessels, the typical anatomy of which must be well known. A good Kocher maneuver enables the surgeon to palpate the head of the pancreas between the fingers and thumb of the left hand and to guide the needle biopsy through the duodenum into the appropriate suspicious area of the pancreas. Hemorrhage, when encountered, can be controlled by pressure. Silk mattress sutures are occasionally needed and are much more preferable to clamping and tying. Chromic catgut should not be used, since it may be rapidly digested in the presence of trypsin spilled by the gland. The surgeon must beware of biopsying any part of the pancreas behind an obstructed duct, as this is likely to produce a pancreatic fistula.

Assessment of Operability and Choice of Procedure

It should be emphasized that full abdominal exploration through a generous abdominal incision is mandatory to visualize and palpate the whole peritoneal cavity. A lesion in the head of the pancreas is considered unresectable if there are distant metastases, invasion of major vessels (especially the portal vein, the hepatic artery, or the superior mesenteric vessels), or any extension beyond the area of the usual total pancreatectomy specimen. Thus, special care should be taken to look for liver metastases, peritoneal seeding deposits, and involvement of the root of the mesentery, the transverse mesocolon, and the ligament of Treitz. Positive nodes in areas to be included in the pancreatectomy

specimen are no contraindication to a resection. It is therefore a waste of time to biopsy suspicious nodes in these locations for examination by frozen section histology. Large, rubbery, greenish nodes at the porta hepatis are frequently seen and are less apt to reveal metastases than are smaller, harder nodes from the area under discussion.

In assessing resectability, a thorough mobilization of the duodenum and pancreatic head is continued (Kocher maneuver), exposing in turn the right kidney, the right renal vein, the inferior vena cava and gonadal vessels, the left renal vein, and the abdominal aorta (Figs. 93–5 and 93–6). For a proven or suspected cancer of the head of the pancreas, the right renal fascia and aortocaval nodes are also mobilized anteriorly and to the left, freeing them from the adventitia of these major vessels. This maneuver not only reveals any existing invasion of the lumbar gutter structures but also facilitates examination of the portal vein and the superior mesenteric artery, thus identifying their relationship to the tumor. The artery can be felt with the fingers behind the gland. If the tumor invades it or completely surrounds it posteriorly, the case is probably incurable. The portal vein cannot be felt, but it lies anteriorly and to the right of the artery, i.e., closer to the operator. Hence, if this area is involved in tumor, it is better to check the vein more carefully. This is done from the anterior aspect of the gland.

The lesser sac is entered by dividing the avascular portion of the gastrocolic omentum close to the transverse colon. The greater curvature of the stomach and its attached omentum are elevated anteriorly and superiorly and the transverse mesocolon is followed down to the region of the pancreas (Fig. 93–7). The superior mesenteric vein is identified, just above the reflection of the mesocolon posteriorly, where it ducks beneath the pancreatic neck (Fig. 93–7). It can be rapidly located by following the middle colic vein to the point where it enters the superior mesenteric vein. As soon as it goes beneath the pancreas, the superior mesenteric is joined by the splenic to form the portal vein, which emerges behind the superior border of the pancreatic neck.

Often, the inferior mesenteric vein joins this right-angled bifurcation to form the tripod portal vein of Douglas. There is seldom any tributary to the anterior surface of these two major veins behind the neck of the pancreas,

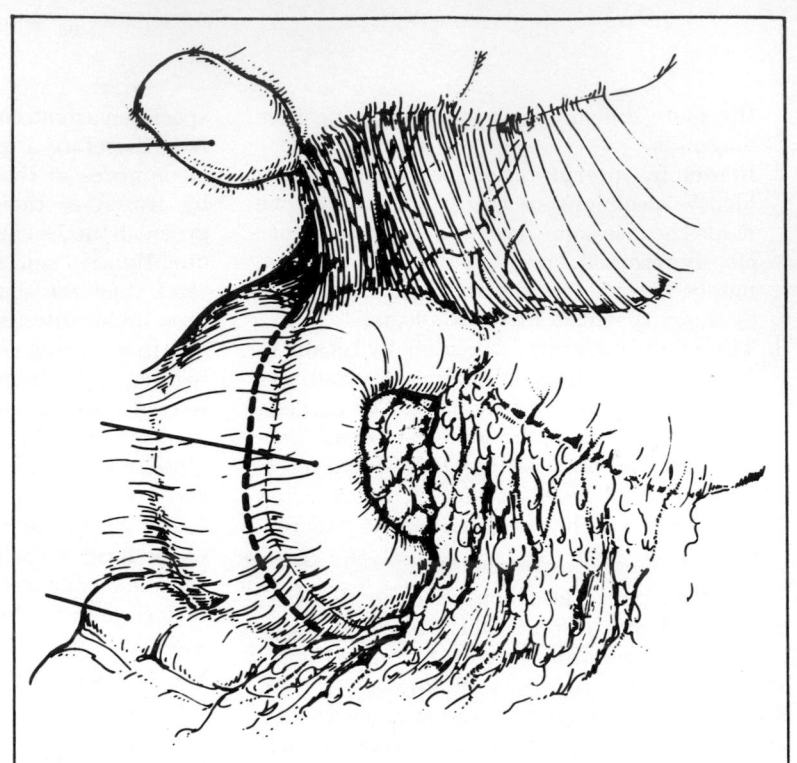

Figure 93–5. Start of the Kocher maneuver. The dotted line depicts the incision in the peritoneum lateral to the second part of the duodenum.

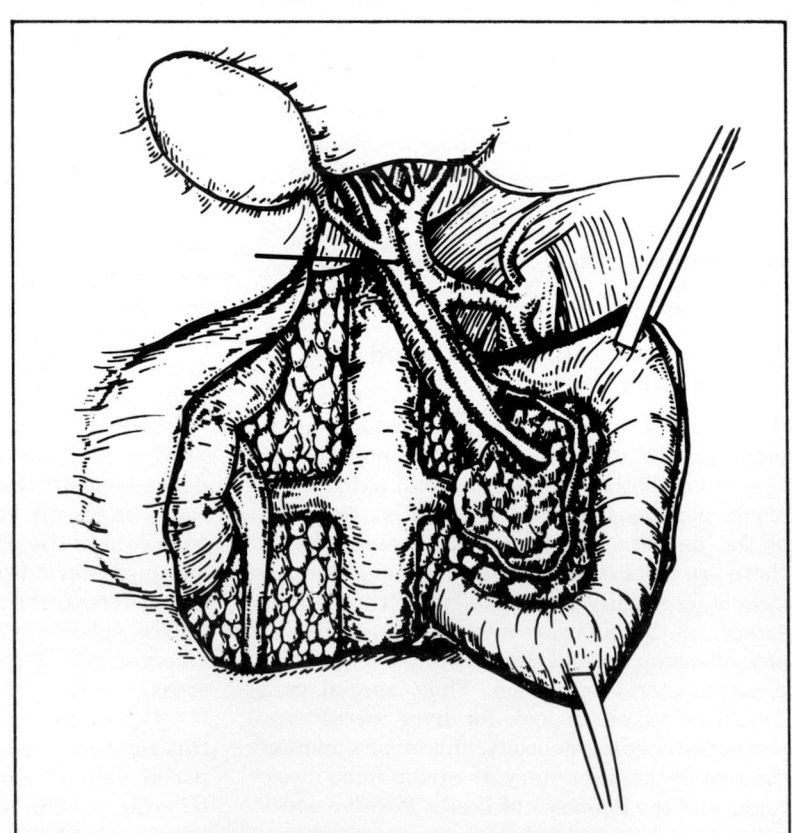

Figure 93–6. Completion of the Kocher maneuver. The cava and left renal vein are visualized.

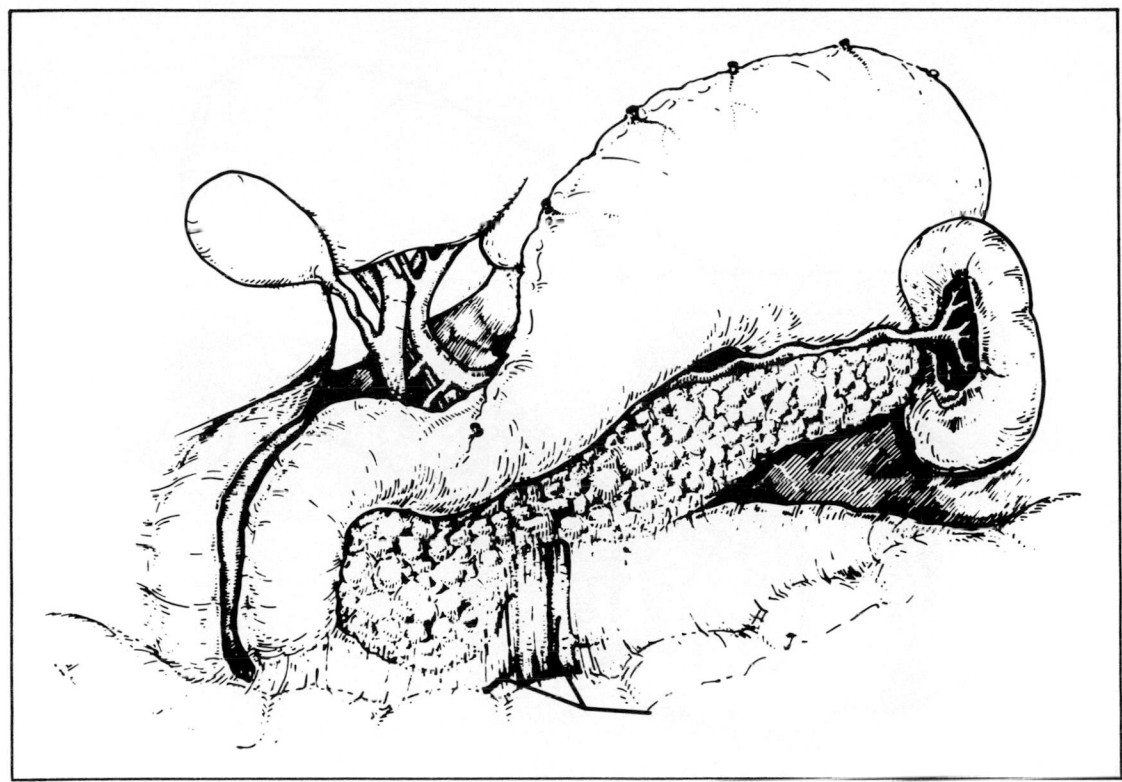

Figure 93–7. The lesser sac has been widely opened, the stomach elevated, the transverse colon retracted inferiorly, to expose the anterior surface of the pancreas. The greater omentum is omitted for clarity.

and instruments or fingers can be gently inserted from below, anterior to the portal vein, in order to assess tumor invasion. Some surgeons prefer to enter this plane from above; if this is done, ligation and division of the gastroduodenal artery and/or the right gastric artery at their origin from the hepatic artery should be done to facilitate this approach (Figs. 93–8 and 93–9).

If the portal vein is invaded, the case is incurable. Resectable tumors in the pancreas, whatever their cell type or location in the gland, are treated by total pancreatectomy. Resectable tumors confined to the duodenum, ampulla of Vater, or distal common bile duct can be adequately treated by a pancreatoduodenectomy of the extended "Whipple type," leaving behind the body and tail of the pancreas intact.

A study of cases of carcinoma of the exocrine pancreas has brought to light some facts, all of which are interpreted as reason for doing a total pancreatectomy:

1. Over 90 percent of all malignant tumors of the head of the pancreas are ductal adenocarcinoma, which is potentially multifocal in origin. Scattered microscopic foci of carcinoma have been found in the tail and body of the gland after total resection for a carcinoma of the head of the pancreas.
2. Microscopic intraglandular strands of tumor have often been cut through at the time of partial resection. In the author's experience, such histologic tumor spread at or behind the line of resection has sometimes been missed by frozen section histology of the cut margin.
3. A cancer of the head of the pancreas often exfoliates malignant cells down the dilated main pancreatic duct behind the obstruction and, if the gland is divided, may be a source of seeding for recurrence.
4. Lymphatic interchange exists between the head and body of the pancreas and an adequate regional lymphadenectomy can best be

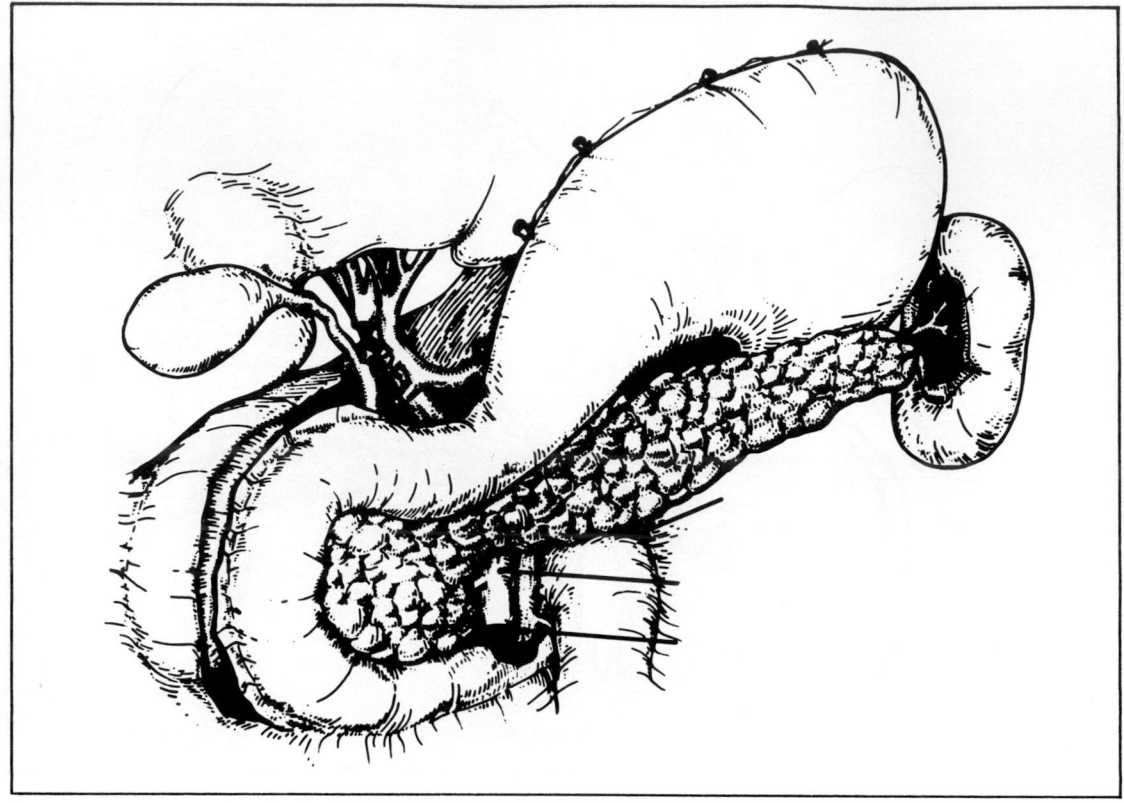

Figure 93–8. The gallbladder has been taken down, the common hepatic duct transected, and the gastroduodenal artery divided to expose the portal vein.

performed as part of a total, as opposed to a partial, pancreatectomy.

5. Removal of the entire pancreas eliminates the risks of postoperative pancreatitis and also obviates the need for a pancreatojejunostomy, which, even in the best of hands, has a small risk of leakage.

6. Preservation of endocrine or exocrine function is not sufficient justification for leaving part of the pancreas behind because about 81 percent of all patients with cancer of the head of the pancreas have chemical or clinically overt diabetes at the time of presentation. Further, late postoperative stenosis of the pancreatojejunal anastomosis often occurs after a variable period of time and leads to insufficiency of pancreatic enzyme flow.

To these six reasons can be added the author's admitted prejudice against partially resecting a gland harboring a lethal cancer.

Resection

Following an adequate Kocher maneuver, the gastrocolic omentum is dissected from the transverse colon through the relatively avascular plane as described. Thus, the greater omentum and the stomach can be elevated superiorly and anteriorly to open the lesser sac widely and to provide a full view of the anterior aspect of the head, neck, and body of the pancreas. The gastroduodenal artery is doubly ligated and divided at its origin from the hepatic artery. The hepatic arterial blood supply, as delineated by arteriography, should be clearly identified to prevent its inadvertent damage and consequent hepatic ischemia. The gallbladder is taken down from the liver bed starting at the fundus moving toward the triangle of Calot. The cystic artery is defined, doubly ligated, and divided. The common hepatic duct is isolated both from the portal vein posteriorly and the hepatic artery (usu-

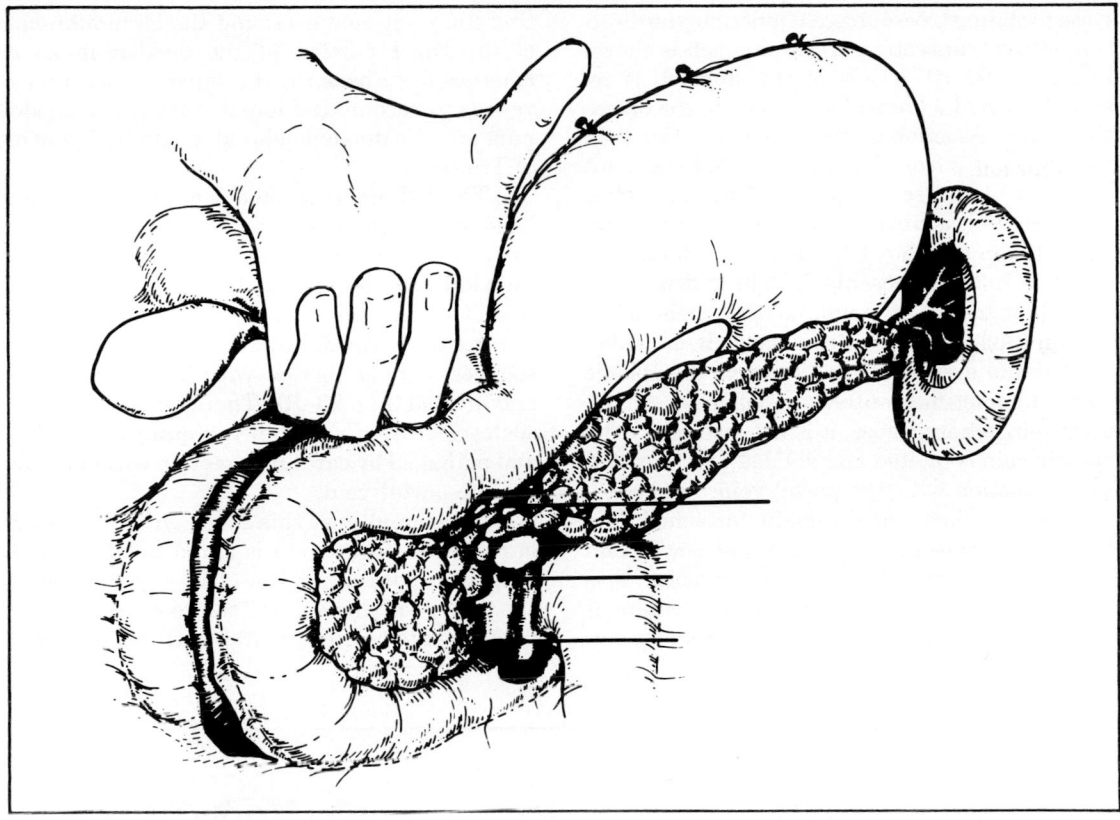

Figure 93–9. Assess freedom of the neck of the pancreas from the anterior aspect of the portal vein from above.

ally medially) by blunt dissection, and it is transected just above the entrance of the cystic duct. The distal end of the transected duct is suture-ligated, and traction on the suture provides access to the anterior aspect of the portal vein (Fig. 93–9). The proximal end of the divided common hepatic duct may be occluded with a small light bulldog clamp if constant spilling of bile into the field of dissection is troublesome. The porta hepatis lymph nodes are cleaned away inferiorly along the hepatic artery and portal vein. The dissection is continued until the hepatic artery has been followed to its origin from the celiac axis or the superior mesenteric artery. A superior pancreatoduodenal vein often enters the portal vein high up and can easily be identified at this stage, doubly ligated, and divided.

The spleen is next mobilized from its posterolateral attachment by tensing the dome of the spleen toward the right iliac fossa and by divid-ing the posterior leaf of the lienorenal ligament. In this way, the spleen, tail of pancreas, and fundus of the stomach are mobilized anteriorly and toward the right. The uppermost two or three short gastric vessels are doubly ligated and divided. This provides an appropriate site at the junction of the gastric fundus and body on the greater curvature where the stomach can be divided. At this stage, it is usually better to transect the stomach to improve exposure for subsequent pancreatic mobilization. Resection of the antrum and part or all of the pancreas removes a major source of alkali to the intestinal tract and predisposes to marginal ulceration in long-term survivors. For this reason, it is preferable to remove at least 75 percent of the stomach. The left gastric artery, having been "skeletonized" from the celiac axis, is ligated and divided at an appropriate point, care being taken to preserve its esophageal branches. The lesser curvature of the stomach is divided close to the gastroesophageal junction; the direction of the transection of the stomach is shown in Figure 93–10. If less of the stomach is resected, we add a truncal vagotomy to the operation. The dissection of the pancreatic tail then moves rapidly from left to right, and the point of origin of the splenic artery from the celiac axis is found, doubly ligated, and divided, care being taken to protect the hepatic artery.

The inferior mesenteric vein is dealt with according to the anatomic arrangement of its termination, which varies widely. It is doubly ligated and divided where it enters the splenic vein. It sometimes enters the superior mesenteric vein; when it does, it is not disturbed. The splenic vein is ligated and divided just proximal to its junction with the portal vein.

The specimen now remains attached only by the uncinate process, the small bowel, and their vascular attachments. At this point, it is better to free the bowel completely where it passes through the transverse mesocolon by cut-

ting the peritoneum around the circumference of the third portion of the duodenum as it emerges from beneath the superior mesenteric vessels to become the fourth part of the duodenum and the duodenojejunal junction (ligament of Treitz).

The left hand is then placed beneath the head of the pancreas, and the specimen is folded to the patient's right and held by the operator's left thumb in front. The major tributaries from the uncinate process to the portal vein are gently "wiped into view" with "peanut" sponges, doubly ligated with 4-0 silk sutures, and divided (Fig. 93–10). There are usually four such tributaries, and they can easily be isolated and managed by careful dissection without tearing the portal vein.

Occasionally, at this stage, with all bridges burned, the portal vein is found to be invaded. In this circumstance, we elect to cut through the tumor to "shave it off" the vein—such cases, in our opinion, being incurable. On six occasions

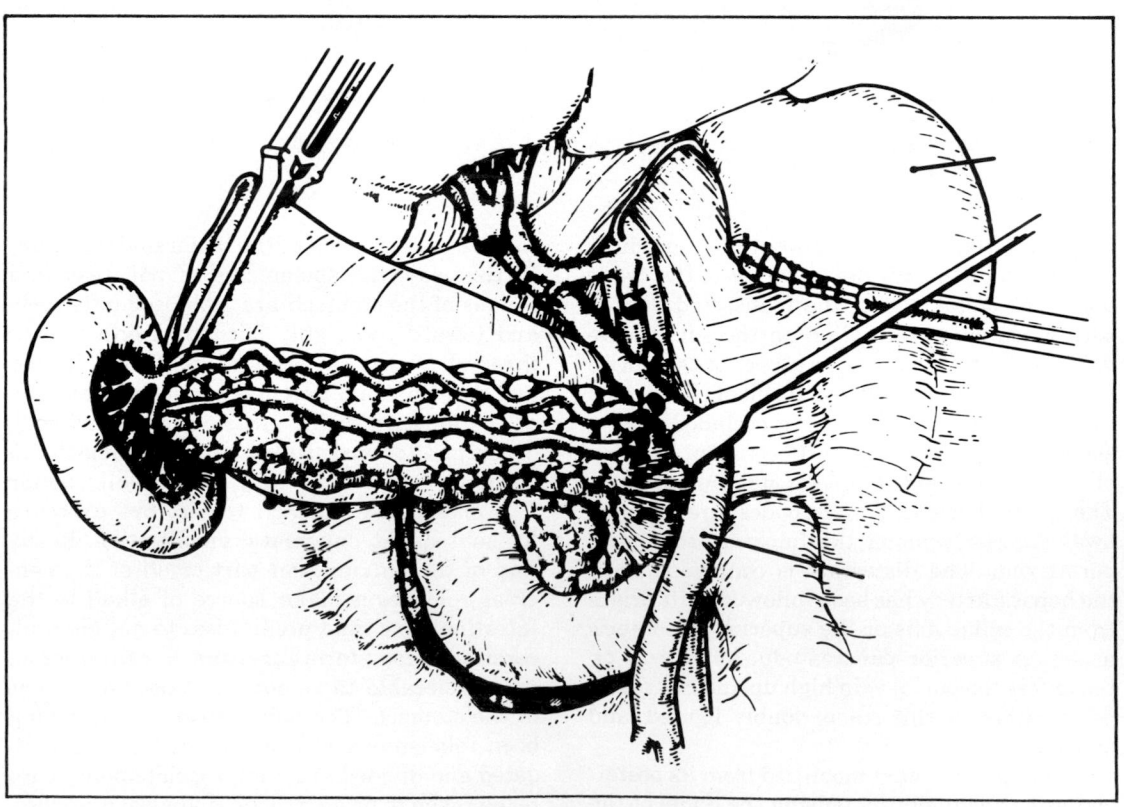

Figure 93–10. The portal vein is retracted and the uncinate process is being detached from the superior mesenteric artery and the portal and superior mesenteric veins.

when the author personally encountered this situation, he elected to resect 1 to 3 cm of the portal vein with the specimen, repairing the vessels by end-to-end anastomosis. In two of these patients, the adherence of the pancreas to the portal vein was due to severe pancreatitis; both patients survived more than 3 years following operation. The remaining four patients had histologically confirmed tumor involvement of the vein and they all died from 9 to 19 months later with metastatic disease. Porter reported resection of the portal vein in five such patients. The vein ends were simply ligated and no anastomosis or shunt was done. One patient died postoperatively and was found at autopsy to have a thrombosed hepatic artery. The other four had uncomplicated postoperative courses but died later of metastases. We feel strongly that it is poor judgment to embark on a portacaval shunt at this point.

The portal vein is retracted to the left with a vein retractor, and the dissection drops down one level to the bridge of tissue between the uncinate process and the superior mesenteric artery, which is defined by the left thumb anteriorly and the left forefinger behind the pancreas. Unlike the venous connections of the area, the arteries are not all easily demonstrated. At this stage, it is easier and faster to stay on the adventitia of the superior mesenteric artery and, using fine right-angled Lahey clamps, doubly ligate and divide the fibrofatty isthmus in serial fashion. At the beginning of this step, the location of the superior mesenteric artery is constantly checked by palpation using the left thumb and forefinger; this prevents damage to the vessel, which, although palpable, is not usually clearly visible at the start. Figure 93–1 shows the anatomy of this area on cross-section. The author prefers not to have hemostats in this field, since they can be inadvertently pulled, damaging the vulnerable vascular structures.

When the inferior pancreaticoduodenal artery has been tied and divided, a bridge of tissue remains that binds the upper jejunum to the superior mesenteric vessels. This is best defined by herniating some of the upper jejunum into the right upper quadrant beneath the mesenteric vessels. When the uppermost few vessels of the jejunal mesentery are ligated and divided, the bowel slides easily into the right subhepatic space, where it can be divided to free the specimen (Fig. 93–11).

The whole operative area is next carefully irrigated with warm saline while looking for small bleeders that need to be ligated.

Regional Pancreatectomy

The term *regional pancreatectomy* was coined by Fortner in 1973 to indicate a "super radical" pancreatectomy whereby routine removal of the pancreatic segment of the portal vein is advocated in addition to the procedure just described (type I). En bloc excision of the celiac axis and/or superior mesenteric artery with the pancreas is a further additional procedure recommended for the type II regional pancreatectomy. In the author's opinion, patients needing such a surgical *tour de force* to have their primary tumor removed invariably have overt or occult metastatic disease and are incurable. However, in selected cases, when the transverse mesocolon is adherent to the tumor mass, the middle colic vessels are ligated and divided flush with the superior mesenteric vessels, and an appropriate V-shaped area of the mesocolon and middle colic vessels is removed with the specimen. If the transverse colon appears to be nonviable as a result of this devascularization, it is resected and the two flexures are mobilized and anastomosed in two layers of interrupted 3-0 silk sutures.

Reconstruction

The sequence of the anastomosis from proximal to distal varies according to the surgeon's personal preference and the patient's anatomy. The author usually closes the upper end of the jejunum in two layers of interrupted 3-0 silk. A new lesser curve of the stomach is constructed using 3-0 interrupted silk in two layers, and the free lower border of the divided gastric stump, measuring 5 to 6 cm in length, is anastomosed in two layers of interrupted 3-0 silk to the upper jejunum as shown in Figure 93–12. The upper jejunum may be further supported with multiple sutures to the new lesser curve as is necessary. The common hepatic duct is implanted into the side of the jejunum distal to the gastrojejunostomy in end-to-side fashion. The arrangement is not technically difficult, and for the hepaticojejunostomy, 4-0 arterial sutures are used in interrupted fashion, the anastomosis being performed in one layer, taking care to achieve mucosa-to-mucosa apposition. Following placement of the posterior row of sutures, a small

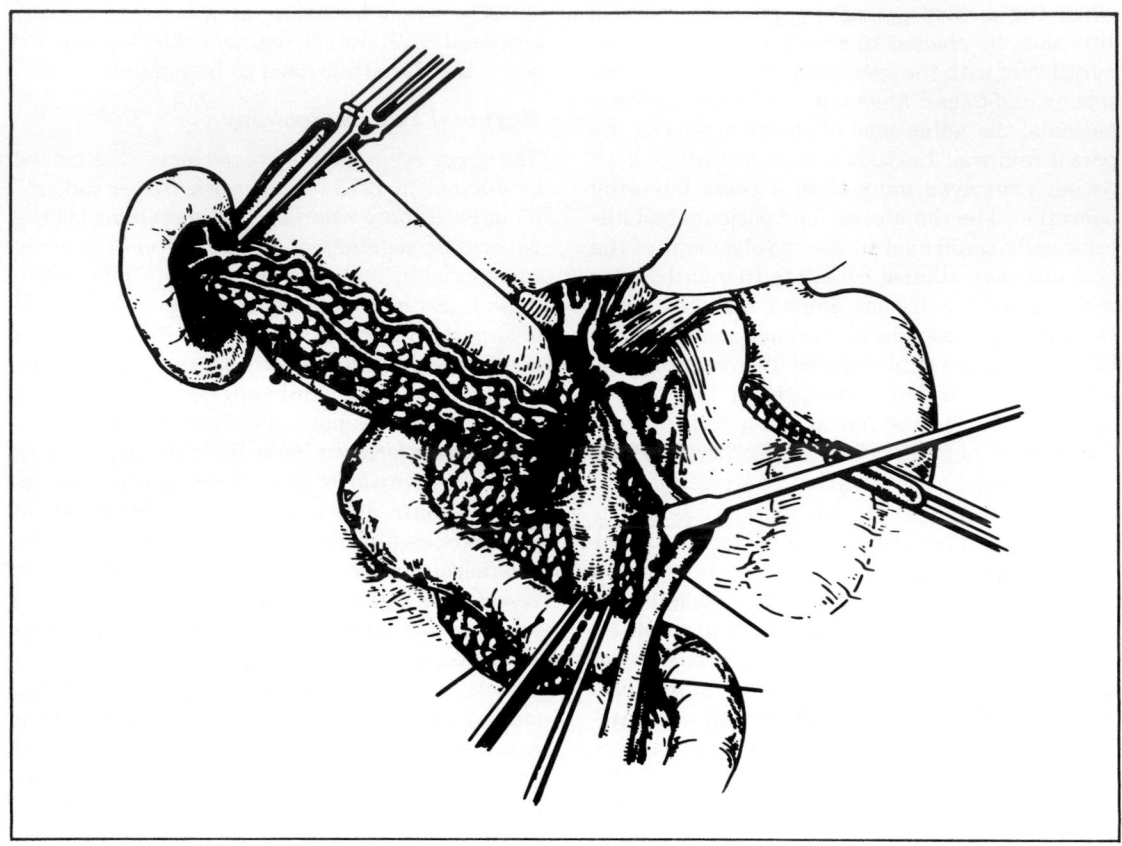

Figure 93–11. Transection of the upper jejunum frees the whole specimen and completes the resection.

(No. 8 or 10) T-tube is carefully placed across the anastomosis, the transverse limb of the T being brought out proximal to the suture line through the anterior wall of the common hepatic duct. T-tube splints are not always used, but in situations in which the duct is small or the tissues unusually friable, a T-tube splint is helpful. Stenosis of the anastomosis should not occur unless recurrent tumor occludes the duct.

Some surgeons do not pull the intestine up behind the mesenteric vessels but prefer to take the closed end of jejunum directly through the transverse mesocolon, or in front of it, to reach the stomach and the common hepatic duct. However, the more direct route recommended here seems to provide a very satisfactory rearrangement. The jejunum on either side of the hepaticojejunostomy is supported by 3-0 silk sutures to the gallbladder bed and the falsiform

ligament. The jejunum distal to this anastomosis is arranged to create a new C-loop and it is tacked on to the residual lateral peritoneum in front of the right renal capsule. The defect in the mesocolon in the region of the original duodenojejunal flexure is closed with interrupted 3-0 silk around the descending jejunum to prevent the possibility of an internal herniation. Although reflux of gastric contents into the biliary tree can easily be demonstrated radiographically, cholangitis does not occur unless there is obstruction of the distal small bowel or of the anastomotic site.

The area of the biliary anastomosis (subhepatic space) is drained, as is the left posterior subdiaphragmatic space. Two large Jackson–Pratt or similar suction drains are placed in each area and brought out through separate stab incisions; they are connected to low-grade continuous suction. A nasogastric tube is passed

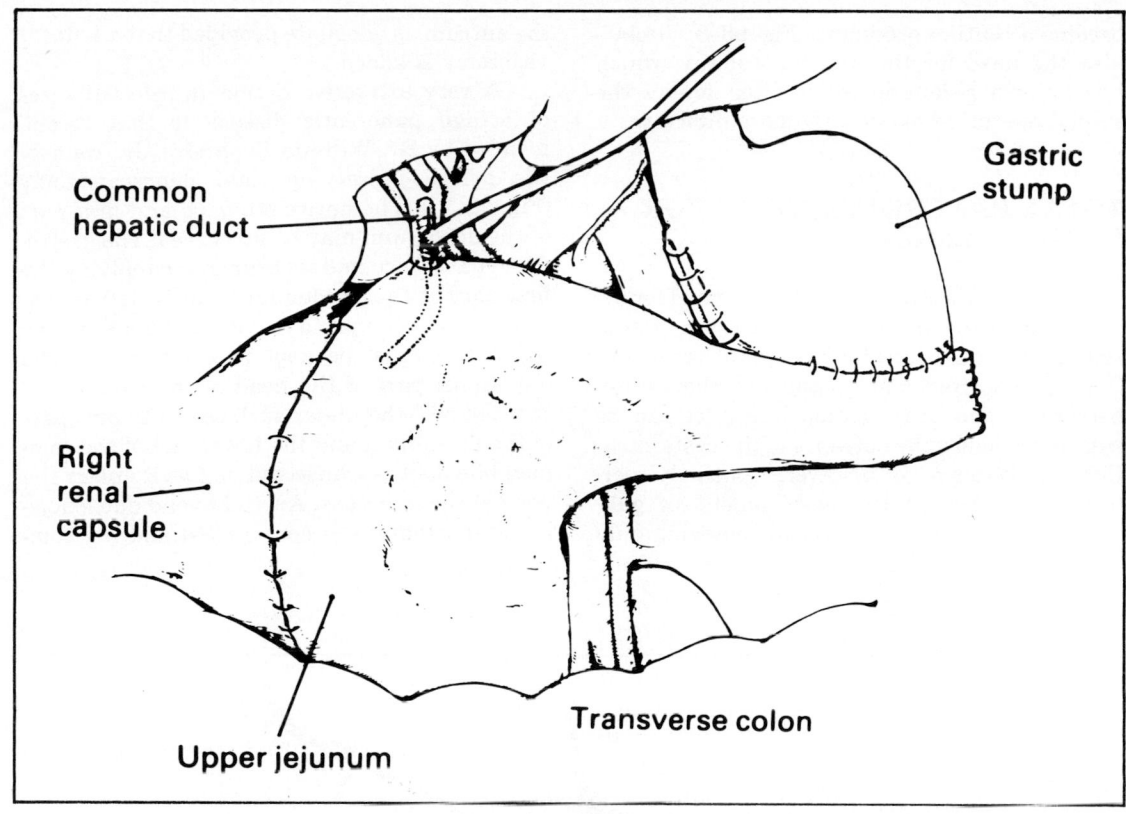

Figure 93–12. The reconstruction after total pancreatoduodenectomy with regional lymphadenectomy for cancer of the head of the pancreas.

through the gastric stump into the upper jejunum and is connected to low-grade intermittent suction.

Throughout the operation, the team of surgeons and anesthesiologists monitor the patient's blood loss, fluid replacement, pulse, blood pressure, central venous pressure, ECG, urine output, and blood sugar level. Once again, the abdominal cavity is carefully irrigated with warm saline, and the T-tube is brought out through a separate stab wound on the right side of the abdomen. We prefer to close the abdomen with interrupted 3-0 stainless steel wire in one or two layers. The skin is approximated with either Steri-Strip or nylon sutures.

Immediate Postoperative Care. All patients undergoing total pancreatectomy are transferred to the surgical intensive unit, where experienced nursing and sophisticated mointoring

techniques are available. They may require respiratory assistance for the first 12 to 24 hours.

TWO-STAGE TOTAL PANCREATECTOMY

Occasionally, one encounters a critically ill patient with impending liver failure, sepsis, and a serum bilirubin greater than 200 mg/dl. In this clinical setting, a case should be made for an initial biliary decompression (internal or external) followed, within 2 to 3 weeks, by a total pancreatectomy. In the past, this first stage necessitated a laparotomy for cholecystostomy, T-tube drainage of the common bile duct, or a biliary–enteric anastomosis. This "two-operations" approach is now outdated. Percutaneous transhepatic cholangiogram followed by external and/or internal biliary decompression has become a routine procedure (Fig. 93–3). It obviates the need for the first laparotomy, which has its own risks and which often makes the second operation technically more difficult.

TOTAL PANCREATECTOMY FOR BENIGN LESIONS

When total pancreatectomy is performed for benign lesions, the dissection need not be as extensive as that described for malignant tumors of the pancreas. Regional lymphadenectomy is unnecessary, and the common bile duct can be transected below the entrance of the cystic duct. Cholecystectomy is, however, routinely performed to prevent the development of gallstones. A low gastric resection, removing only the antrum, is adequate provided that a truncal vagotomy is added.

A very attractive option in selected cases of benign pancreatic disease is that recommended by Dr. William Longmire, Jr., namely the pylorus-preserving total pancreatectomy (Fig. 93–13). The entire stomach and first part of the duodenum may be preserved. The gastroduodenal artery and its branches supplying the first part of the duodenum must be left intact. Dissection at the porta hepatis and supraduodenal region must be kept to a minimum. The uppermost part of the head of the pancreas is "shaved off" the under surface of the first part of the duodenum and the lower end of the common bile duct is transected just as it enters the head of the pancreas. An end-to-end duodenojejunal anastomosis is constructed and the com-

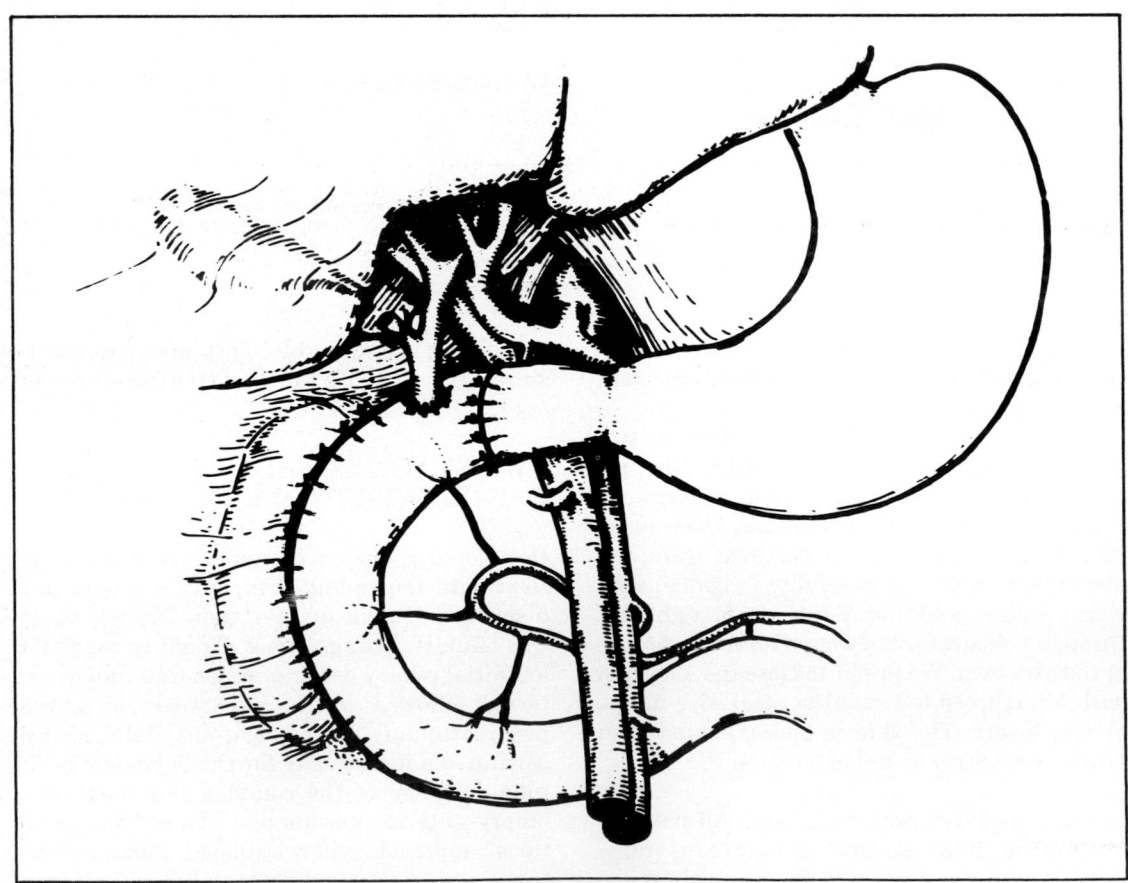

Figure 93–13. The reconstruction after pylorus-preserving total pancreatectomy for benign disease.

mon bile duct is reimplanted into the upper jejunum just distal to it. A cholecystectomy is routinely performed. The advantage of this operation is that the patient can eat a normal size meal without dumping. The long-term results are as yet unknown. The operation should not be performed in patients with malignant disease of the head of the pancreas or of the distal common bile duct since it may compromise their chance of cure by not providing adequately wide margins of excision of the tumor.

Pylorus-preserving pancreatectomy may also be performed as part of a Whipple operation for selected localized tumor of the distal duodenum or at the ampulla of Vater.

The choice between a partial and a total pancreatectomy may present a dilemma to the surgeon exploring a patient with hyperinsulinism. The recommended procedure is based on the following premises:

1. A careful preoperative diagnostic workup including provocation tests and measurement of blood glucose, insulin, and proinsulin levels has been performed to the surgeon's entire satisfaction.
2. Selective celiac and superior mesenteric angiogram has been carried out, and good filling of the hepatic, superior mesenteric, and splenic branches to the pancreas has been obtained, as well as good visualization of the venous drainage of the gland.
3. Careful mobilization, visualization, and palpation of the whole pancreas has been carried out by an experienced surgeon.

With care, most insulinomas can be enucleated from the pancreas. Adenomas greater than 3 cm in diameter or those that are deeply embedded in the substance of the gland are better treated by partial pancreatectomy.

If the insulinoma is occult (i.e., no tumor can be seen or palpated) we recommend a blind 75 percent distal pancreatectomy (Fig. 93–14) transecting the neck of the gland just to the right of the superior mesenteric vein, followed by immediate serial frozen section histology and blood sugar monitoring. If the lesion is not found in the resected gland and no hyperglycemic rebound occurs, we recommend a total pancreatectomy at the same operation, provided the patient is a good operative risk and all the issues had been discussed with the patient and relatives prior to operation. In the author's experience, subtotal (85 to 90 percent) distal pancrea-

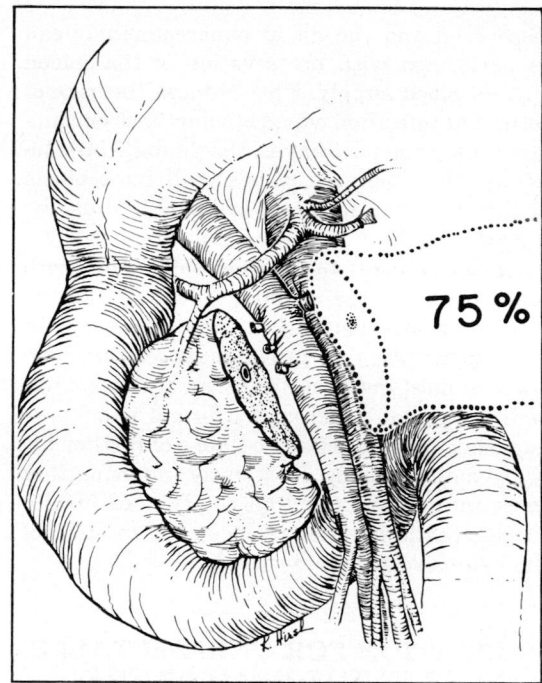

Figure 93–14. Seventy five percent distal pancreatectomy. The splenic vessels have been ligated and divided near their origins. The neck of the pancreas has been dissected from the portomesenteric venous trunk with ligation and division of small veins draining to the right side of the venous trunk.

tectomy in such a situation has a 30 percent chance of missing a nonpalpable lesion, the tumor usually being found later, at autopsy or reexploration, embedded somewhere between the duodenal wall and the head of the pancreas.

Some surgeons terminate the operation after a distal 60 to 75 percent pancreatectomy even if intraoperative evidence suggests that the tumor has not been removed. This is justifiable only under extreme circumstances of a seriously ill, poor-risk patient. It is not often appreciated that the second-stage pancreatectomy, weeks or even months later, is a technically difficult and hazardous operation. Further, we believe that the continued hypoglycemia and its complications usually outweigh the morbidity and mortality associated with a total pancreatectomy.

Surgical considerations in infants and children with suspected islet cell hyperplasia are somewhat different. An adenoma is not usually discovered and the distal pancreatectomy can be performed with preservation of the spleen and its blood supply. This reduces the risk of recurrent infection, which is sometimes encountered after splenectomy in the young. Unfortunately, the diagnosis of islet cell hyperplasia by frozen section histology is difficult. Thus, the surgeon, in these situations, is committed to a 90 to 95 percent distal pancreatectomy, with preservation of the common bile duct and the duodenum together with a rim of pancreas. In our experience, this provides successful treatment in most instances. Only rarely is removal of the residual pancreas by formal pancreatoduodenectomy necessary because of further hypoglycemic episodes. It is always amazing that these infants and children rarely need insulin or pancreatic enzyme replacement in spite of the extensive pancreatectomy.

PALLIATION FOR UNRESECTABLE CANCER IN THE HEAD OF THE PANCREAS

It is widely accepted that pancreatic resection of any type is too formidable a procedure to be employed for palliative purposes. The author never knowingly performs a total pancreatectomy for palliation, although this is often all that may be achieved. If cure is impossible, jaundice, intractable pruritus, and impending cholangitis must be palliated by cholecystojejunostomy (side-to-side anastomosis with a distal jejunojejunostomy or as a Roux-Y, to prevent regurgitation of food into the biliary tree), provided the gallbladder is dilated and the cystic duct is in wide open communication with the dilated proximal biliary tree. When the gallbladder is diseased or the cystic duct is long, narrow, and enters the common bile duct low down near the tumor, a cholecystectomy should be performed and a hepaticojejunostomy constructed.

It is a tragic and unhappy situation when, several weeks or months after having decompressed a biliary tree, it is necessary to reoperate for duodenal obstruction. It is much wiser to anticipate the need and to provide the solution at the first operation by a gastrojejunostomy. If the patient is relatively young and fit and is likely to live more than a few months, a truncal vagatomy should be added.

Pain, especially the characteristic backache of advanced pancreatic cancer, can be controlled by open chemical splanchnicectomy using a 20-gauge spinal needle and a syringe containing 15 to 20 ml of 6 percent phenol. The abdominal aorta is identified by palpation with the left index finger, and the phenol is then injected into the region between the splanchnic nerves and the celiac ganglia. The site of the injection is retroperitoneal and slightly lateral, posterior, and superior to the origin of the celiac artery. Intermittent aspiration prevents inadvertent injection of chemical into the vascular system. Analgesics, starting with high doses of aspirin and codeine and ending with the stronger narcotic drugs such as morphine and Demerol, are often need postoperatively. Since most of these patients have complete obstruction of alkaline pancreatic juice, they are prone to develop benign peptic ulceration of the duodenum, which may even lead to hemorrhage. For this reason, and especially because epigastric distress is difficult to interpret in such patients, intravenous cimetidine is used in the immediate postoperative period, after which oral antacids are recommended for an indefinite period.

Percutaneous celiac ganglion blockade is unlikely to help if the operative blockade fails. Smith's technique of decompressing a dilated pancreatic ductal system into the back wall of the stomach using a T-tube is occasionally useful.

CANCER OF THE BODY AND TAIL OF THE PANCREAS

One is rarely called upon to resect a carcinoma that has arisen in the body or tail of the gland since such tumors are virtually always incurable by the time they reach the surgeon. The author has resected only two such cancers and neither patient survived longer than 1 year. As far as we know, there has not been a reported long-term survivor following resection of a ductal adenocarcinoma of the body or tail of the pancreas. It must, however, be emphasized that often the operative recognition of the exact cellular origin of the body or tail of the pancreas is not precise even if it is "substantiated" by frozen section histology. For this reason, such lesions should always be resected either by a formal total pancreatectomy under favorable circumstances or as a distal pancreatectomy and splenectomy. Occasionally, the patient and the surgeon will have the pleasant surprise of finding that the tumor is of islet cell origin and has a much better prognosis than was anticipated.

As far as palliation is concerned, the relief of pain is even more important than for cancer of the head of the pancreas. Chemical splanchnicectomy is mandatory. The tumor mass should be outlined with silver clips to help in the planning of radiation ports postoperatively. If the tumor is invading into the duodenojejunal junction at the ligament of Treitz, a palliative gastrojejunostomy is indicated. In selected young patients who are likely to survive an appreciable amount of time, splenectomy should be considered if there is splenic vein thrombosis with left-sided portal hypertension to eliminate the risk of gastric variceal hemorrhage.

POSTOPERATIVE PROBLEMS

Hemorrhage

Hemorrhage is the most common intraoperative and postoperative complication encountered with total pancreatectomy. Meticulous preoperative preparation and adequate replacement of blood and clotting factors during the operation are essential.

All vessels must be carefully ligated. It is vital to check all vascular areas for hemostasis before closing the abdomen. In spite of these precautions, blood may ooze at a fairly alarming rate from the drainage sites during the first 24 hours. This is especially so in the severely jaundiced patient. Reoperation is mandatory when there is reason to suspect a major bleeding site or when clot accumulation in the abdomen causes distention and tamponade and/or when a consumption coagulopathy is recognized. In most situations one never finds a discrete bleeding point at reoperation. The clots are gently evacuated and the whole abdomen irrigated prior to reclosure with drainage.

Hemobilia

When a biliary tree that has been completely obstructed for many weeks is suddenly decompressed, it is usually found to contain light yellow, watery bile. Within a few minutes it may become somewhat sanguinous in appearance or even grossly bloody. Occasionally, the fluid that runs from the common bile duct or gallbladder may seem to contain more blood than bile, and sometimes the hemorrhage may reach alarming proportions. It has, in our experience, always stopped. The discharge seems to be analogous to the bleeding from the kidneys that occurs when long-standing urinary obstruction is suddenly relieved. The release of the dammed-up bile produces oozing from the walls of the bile passages. When this occurs, jaundice may also fail to improve or may even deepen temporarily; within 4 to 5 days, steady improvement is noticed. Fortunately, this complication is usually mild; it may occur after palliative cholecystojejunostomy as well as after pancreatic resection. We have not felt it necessary to try to arrange for a slow release of the bile pressure.

During the period of continuing hemorrhage, the patient must be kept normovolemic by adequate blood and fluid replacement, and a continuous diuresis must be insured. Intermittent doses of furosemide may be given as necessary. Hepatorenal failure is the most common sequence of events leading to postoperative death.

Diabetes Mellitus Following Total Pancreatectomy

Total pancreatectomy leaves the patient with a relatively mild type of diabetes mellitus that, in the average case, requires about 30 to 40 units of regular insulin a day for adequate control. Provided the patient and the relatives are properly instructed, management of a totally pancreatectomized patient is like the management of a mild diabetic who has had a gastrectomy. Hyperglycemia during operation is best managed by an "artificial B-cell" system, which monitors the blood sugar level and infuses the appropriate amount of regular insulin with minimum inconvenience to the anesthesiologist. If this is not available, blood sugar monitoring every 2 hours with infusion of the appropriate amount of intravenous insulin (5 to 10 units) is usually adequate.

In the immediate (first 3 to 4 days) postoperative period, the patient's blood sugar is checked every 3 to 4 hours, and small doses of regular insulin (2 to 10 units every hour) are given intravenously as boluses. Alternatively, a continuous intravenous infusion of insulin can be given. It is desirable to maintain the blood sugar between 100 and 200 mg/dl at all times. During this early postoperative period, when fluid shifts are in a prominent phase and absorption is unpredictable, subcutaneous or intramuscular administration of drugs or insulin should be discouraged.

Once the major arterial and intravenous lines have been dismantled, the urine can be examined every 6 hours and regular insulin given subcutaneously as indicated. A constant intravenous infusion of glucose (5 g/hr = 100 ml/hr of a 5 percent dextrose solution) is maintained for 7 to 10 days. After this, oral feeding is sufficient, and intermediate (NPH or Lente) insulin is given daily, the usual dose being half the daily requirement of the previous 5 days. It is important to start teaching the patient and at least one relative to administer the insulin and to measure the urine fractionals as soon as the patient is returned to the ward so that confidence and independence occurs by the end of the second week when discharged from the hospital. At this time, small amounts of intermediate insulin (NPH or Lente), approximately 10 to 15 units a day, is all that is required in the vast majority of cases. The patient should be reminded that the diabetes is different from most in that hypoglycemia is a relatively common occurrence, probably due to the absence of pancreatic Glucagon. This can be avoided by increasing the intake of food slightly and decreasing the insulin dose, especially when physical activity is increased.

Pancreatic Exocrine Function Replacement

The totally pancreatectomized patient should take a low-fat diet and frequent regular small meals. Two to three pancreatin tablets (Viokase, Pancrease) must be taken with each main meal. More may be required if steatorrhea develops. Most patients have had a fairly high gastric resection and produce insufficient gastric acid and pepsin to inactivate the ingested enzyme. The patient who has had a pylorus-preserving operation may benefit from supplementary cimetidine or antacid therapy.

Late Recurrence of Jaundice

Recurrent jaundice with or without cholangitis may be seen after total pancreatectomy. This may be due to recurrent tumor or to partial distal small bowel obstruction. In the latter situation, nausea, vomiting and abdominal cramps are usually prominent features. The small-bowel obstruction may itself be due to recurrent tumor or simply to adhesions. Laparotomy may be indicated to establish the diagnosis and to see what can be done to alleviate the problem.

Monitoring of Recurrence and Response to Postoperative Adjuvant Therapy

There is currently no efficacious chemotherapy regimen for patients with metastatic pancreatic cancer. Following total pancreatectomy and examination of the specimen, those patients who are found to have regional nodal spread and/or extrapancreatic invasion on histologic examination seem to benefit from a combination of radiation therapy and 5-fluorouracil given postoperatively. For patients with locally unresectable disease, surgical implantation of radionuclides such as iodine-125 have given disappointing results with unacceptable complication rates. Intraoperative electron beam irradiation as a means of delivering high dosage to the direct area of the tumor as a supplement to external beam irradiation postoperatively is being tried in several centers with encouraging early results.

Serial monitoring of serum pancreatic oncofetal antigen (POA) or carcinoembryonic antigen (CEA) is occasionally useful in confirming the completeness of surgical excision and in the detection of recurrent pancreatic cancer. Unfortunately, few patients with pancreatic cancer have an elevated POA level and most patients with high elevations of CEA levels have unresectable lesions. We have previously demonstrated that in patients who have elevated preoperative POA values and resectable tumors, the serum levels of POA fell to within normal range following total pancreatectomy. In several of these cases, the levels of POA rose again in parallel with recurrence.

All functioning malignant islet cell tumors that are unresectable or associated with metastases are best treated by "debulking" of the main tumor mass to remove as much of the lesions as possible if this can be performed safely. Postoperative adjuvant therapy with streptozotocin can be of benefit to relieve the symptoms of these tumors, which are usually slow growing compared to pancreatic exocrine cancer. Serial measurements of the appropriate peptide markers (e.g., insulin, Glucagon, gastrin, gastric inhibitory polypeptide, vasoactive intestinal peptide, etc.) may be helpful in mointoring the response to therapy.

MORTALITY AND PROGNOSIS

Selection of patient and meticulous attention to detail are essential to obtain the best results. It is difficult to compare survival data between groups and to draw meaningful conclusions from the literature. This is in part due to the small number of cases involved with early cancer, to differing statistical manipulation and interpretation of results, and also to our inability to ascertain the number of surgeons involved and their expertise and experience. As usual, the surgeon's judgment is paramount in the determination of relative indications and contraindications. The operative mortality should never exceed 10 percent and should be nearer 5 percent. The intelligent patient, if actively selected, educated, and supported by his physician and relatives, can lead a normal active life following total pancreatectomy. At our last analysis, the cumulative 3- and 5-year survivals for total pancreatectomy in patients with ductal adenocarcinoma of the head of the pancreas were 51 and 21 percent, respectively, with an operative mortality of 7 percent.

Centralization of Care to Specialized Regional Centers. It has become clear to the author that major pancreatic resections should be performed by an experienced surgeon in conjunction with an appropriate back-up team in a specialty center where there is a major commitment to pancreatic disorders. It should not be attempted by the registrar-resident in training or by the "occasional" pancreatic surgeon in a district-community hospital. Too many reports deal in a retrospective fashion with poor results obtained by various surgeons with varying expertise in several hospitals with a low percentage of tissue diagnosis in nonresected patients. In many such cases, the cause of death is not even confirmed by autopsy.

Consider the inexperienced surgeon in the small district or community hospital who, unexpectedly, finds a mass in the head of the pancreas during the course of a laparotomy for some other procedure, for example, a cholecystectomy? Unless the surgeon is prepared (rarely, if ever, is this so) to proceed with an immediate pancreatic resection if the biopsy is positive for cancer, no biopsy should be performed at that time. A negative biopsy does not help and the inflicted trauma to the pancreatoduodenal area will make interpretation of postoperative evaluation, by CT and other studies, exceedingly difficult. In addition, the surgeon should refrain from mobilizing and assessing resectability at that operation. Such unnecessary manipulation and dissection will also undoubtedly make interpretation by subsequent investigations exceedingly difficult and will render a second laparotomy even more dangerous. If the patient is jaundiced with a dilated gallbladder, a tube cholecystostomy or a T-tube placed in the common bile duct may be an acceptable temporizing procedure. Alternatively, one can make a strong case for the dictum that a surgeon should not operate on a patient with obstructive jaundice unless prepared to perform a pancreatoduodenal resection. This somewhat controversial view can be highlighted by the following personal data: Reexploration of 17 selected patients referred over an 8-year period after a diagnosis of inoperable pancreatic cancer was made at laparotomy revealed that only 3 had metastatic disease and another 3 had locally unresectable pancreatic cancer. Two of the patients did not have cancer, and the remaining 9 patients had total pancreatectomy with mean survival of 3.6 years (range 1 to 6 years). Thus, in experienced hands, a small but meaningful number of patients with pancreatic cancer can be salvaged by an appropriate total pancreatectomy. It should be reemphasized that major pancreatic resections should be planned well in advance and proper informed consent obtained from the patients and the relatives to avert the many medicolegal problems that are cropping up around the country.

BIBLIOGRAPHY

Blackstone MO, Cockerham L, et al: Intraductal aspiration for cytodiagnosis in pancreatic cancer. Gastrointest Endosc 23:145, 1977

Brooks JR: Surgery of the Pancreas, 1st edt. Philadelphia: WB Saunders, 1983

Cooper MJ, Moossa DE, et al: The place of duodenal drainage studies in the diagnosis of pancreatic disease. Surgery 84:457, 1978

Fortner JG: Regional resection of cancer of the pancreas: A new surgical approach. Surgery 73:307, 1973

Gelder FB, Reese CJ, et al: Purification, partial characterization and clinical application of a pancreatic oncofetal antigen. Cancer Res 38:313, 1978

Hall TJ, Blackstone MO, et al: Prospective evaluation of endoscopic retrograde cholangiopancreatography in the diagnosis of periampullary tumors. Ann Surg 187:313, 1978

Longmire WP, Traverso LW: The Whipple procedure and other standard operative approaches to pancreatic cancer. Cancer 47:1706, 1981

Mackie CR, Bowie J, et al: Prospective evaluation of gray scale ultrasonography in the diagnosis of pancreas cancer. Am J Surg 136:575, 1978

Mackie CR, Lu CT, et al: Prospective evaluation of angiography in the diagnosis and management of patients suspected of having pancreatic cancer. Ann Surg 189:11, 1979

Moossa AR: Investigative approaches to the problem of pancreatic cancer—Hunterian lecture. Ann R Coll Surg Engl 136:575, 1978

Moossa AR: Re-operation for pancreatic cancer. Arch Surg 114:490, 1979

Moossa AR: Tumors of the Pancreas, 1 edt. Baltimore: Williams and Wilkins, 1980

Moossa AR: Pancreatic cancer-approach to diagnosis, selection for surgery and choice of operation. Cancer 50:2689, 1982

Moossa AR, Altorki N: Pancreatic biopsy. Surg Clin N Am 63:1706, 1981

Moossa AR, Dawson P: The diagnosis of pancreatic cancer. Pathol Annu II:229, 1981

Porter M: In Rodney Maingot (ed): Abdominal Operations, 6 edt. New York: Appleton-Century-Crofts, 1976

ReMine W, Priestly JT, et al: Total pancreatectomy. Ann Surg 172:595, 1970

Schwartz SS, Ziedler A, et al: A prospective study of glucose tolerance, insulin, C-peptide and glucagon responses in patients with pancreatic cancer. Am J Dig Dis 23:1107, 1978

Schwartz SS, Horwitz DC, et al: Use of a glucose controlled insulin infusion system (artifical B-cell) to control diabetes during surgery. Diabetologia 16:157, 1979

Smith R: Progress in the surgical treatment of pancreatic disease. Am J Surg 125:143, 1973

Smith R: Cancer of the pancreas. J R Coll Surg Edinb 23:133, 1978

Wood RAB, Moossa AR: The prospective evaluation of tumour-associated antigens for early diagnosis of pancreatic cancer. Br J Surg 64:718, 1977

SECTION XIV
Spleen

94. The Spleen
Seymour I. Schwartz

HISTORICAL BACKGROUND

The spleen was regarded by Galen as "an organ of mystery," by Aristotle as unnecessary, by Pliny as an organ that might hinder the speed of runners and also as an organ that produced laughter and mirth, a concept reasserted in the Babylonian Talmud. The first recorded splenectomy was performed for splenomegaly on a 24-year-old Neapolitan woman in 1549 by Adrian Zacarelli. The first successful partial splenectomy for trauma was reported by Franciscus Rosetti in 1590. Thus, partial splenectomy for trauma antedated total splenectomy for trauma, first performed by Nicolaus Matthias in 1678 in Capetown, South Africa, on a patient whose spleen protruded through a flank wound. The first splenectomy for trauma in the United States was reported by O'Brien, a Royal Navy surgeon, in 1816. In 1866, Sir Thomas Spencer Wells gave an account of the first successful splenectomy in England.

Although Billroth, reporting on an autopsy in 1881, felt that a splenic injury might have healed spontaneously, as recently as 1927 Hamilton Bailey asserted that "surgical aid is always needed." During the first two decades of the twentieth century, however, proponents began to appear championing the use of judicious tamponade of the organ and suture repair was reported to be successful. Zikoff, in Russia, is credited with the first successful repair of a lacerated spleen in 1895. The first successful partial splenectomy for trauma in modern times was reported by Campos Christo in 1962.

The role of the spleen in relation to infection has been considered for many years. Countering early experiments that showed no adverse effects of splenectomy on infection, Morris and Bullock, conducting controlled experiments with rat plague bacillus in 1919, concluded that removal of the spleen "robs the body of its resistance." Until relatively recently, however, most physicians and surgeons have felt that splenectomy did not compromise the host defense against infection. The first of the recent reports was that of King and Shumacker in 1952, chronicling an increased susceptibility to infection in children following splenectomy for hematologic disorders. In 1973, Singer's review of the literature emphasized the increase in postsplenectomy sepsis in infants and childen.

ANATOMY

The spleen arises by mesenchymal differentiation along the left side of the dorsal mesogastrium in juxtaposition to the anlage of the left gonad in the 8-mm embryo. In the healthy adult, the weight of the spleen ranges between 75 and 100 g. It resides in the posterior portion of the left upper quadrant lying deep to the ninth, tenth, and eleventh ribs, with its long axis corresponding to that of the tenth rib. Its convex, superior, and lateral surfaces are immediately adjacent to the undersurface of the left leaf of the diaphragm. The configuration of the concave, medial surface of the spleen is a consequence of impressions made by the stomach, pancreas, kidney, and splenic flexure of the colon (Fig. 94–1).

The position of the spleen is, in part, maintained by several suspensory ligaments including the gastrosplenic, splenophrenic, splenocolic, and splenorenal ligaments (Figs. 94–2 and 94–3). The gastrosplenic ligament contains the short gastric vessels that course to the splenic hilum from the greater curvature while the remaining ligaments are generally avascular, except in patients with portal hypertension and/or myeloproliferative disorders.

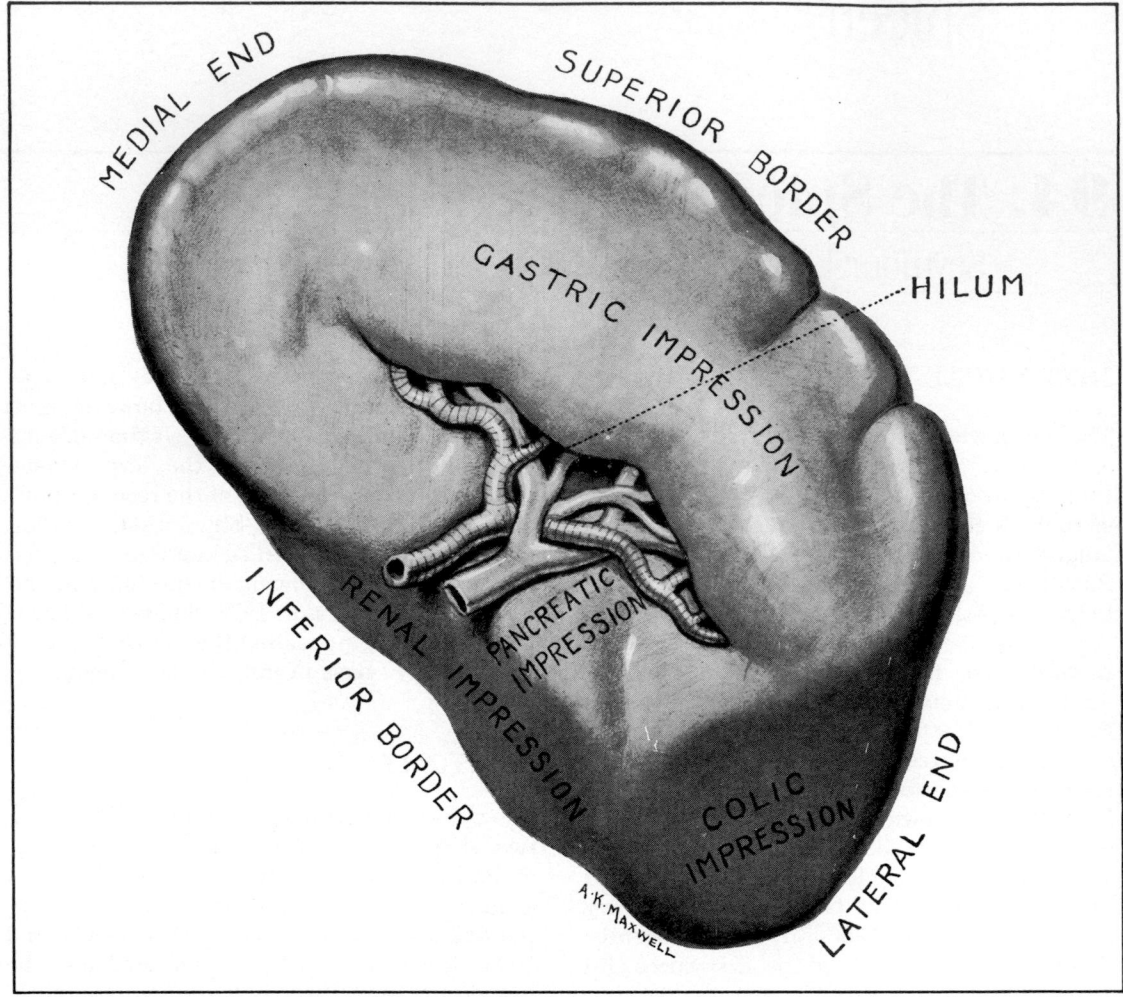

Figure 94–1. Gross anatomy of the spleen.

The splenic artery, a branch of the celiac artery, provides the spleen with arterial blood. A varying degree of branching occurs proximal to the hilus. Frequently a branch to the inferior pole originates centrally. The major venous drainage flows through the splenic vein, which usually receives the inferior mesenteric vein centrally, and then joins the superior mesenteric vein to form the portal vein.

Accessory spleens, made of blood, sinuses, and malpighian bodies, have been classified into two types: (1) the more uncommon is a constricted part of the main organ to which it is bound by fibrous tissue, and (2) the more common distinct, separate mass. The latter has been reported in 14 to 35 percent of patients; a higher

incidence of this has been reported in patients with hematologic disorders. These accessory organs that receive their blood supply from the splenic artery are present in decreasing order of frequency in the hilus of the spleen, the gastrosplenic and the splenocolic ligaments, the gastrosplenic ligament, the splenorenal ligament, and the greater omentum (Fig. 94–4). Accessory spleens may also occur in the pelvis of the female, either in the presacral region or adjacent to the left ovary, and in the scrotum in juxtaposition to the left testicle.

The spleen is made up of a capsule that is normally 1 to 2 mm thick, and trabeculae that surround and invaginate the pulp. The parenchyma (Fig. 94–5) is made up of "white pulp"

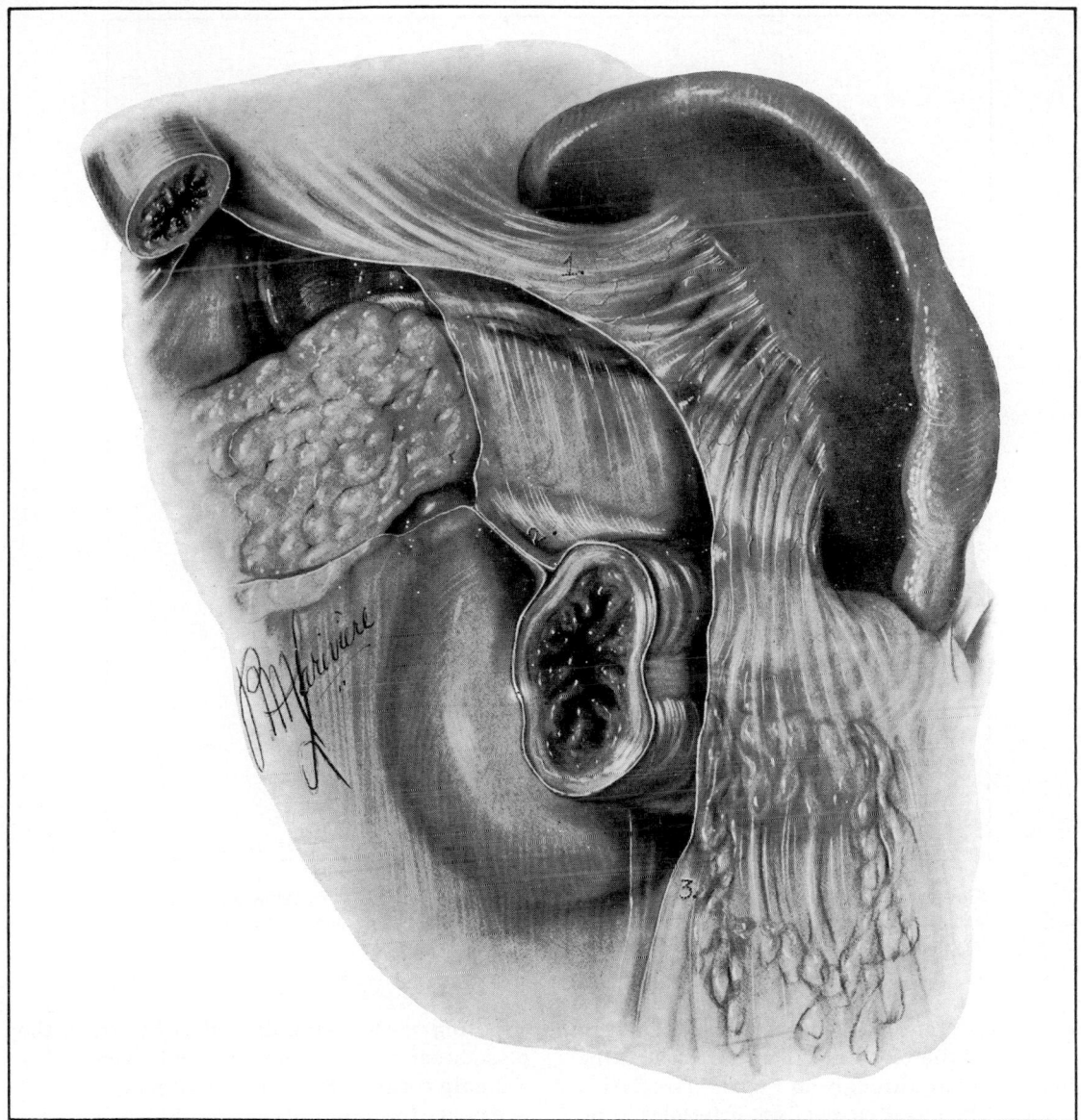

Figure 94–2. Anatomy of the spleen showing complicated peritoneal reflections in the region of the hilus.

that functions as an immunologic organ, "red pulp" that phagocytizes particulate matter from the blood, and a marginal zone. The white pulp, which is central and surrounds a central artery, is made of lymphatic nodules with germinal centers and periarterial lymphatic sheaths that constitute a reticular network filled with lymphocytes and macrophages. Peripheral to the white pulp is the marginal zone that contains end arteries arising from the central artery and from peripheral penicillar arteries. The marginal zone contains lymphocytes and macrophages and some red blood cells that have exited from terminal arteries. The marginal zone also contains the marginal sinus that filters material from the centrally located white pulp. Locally produced immunoglobulins enter the marginal zone, eventually coursing to the bloodstream.

Peripheral to the marginal zone is the red pulp. This pulp consists of cords and sinuses

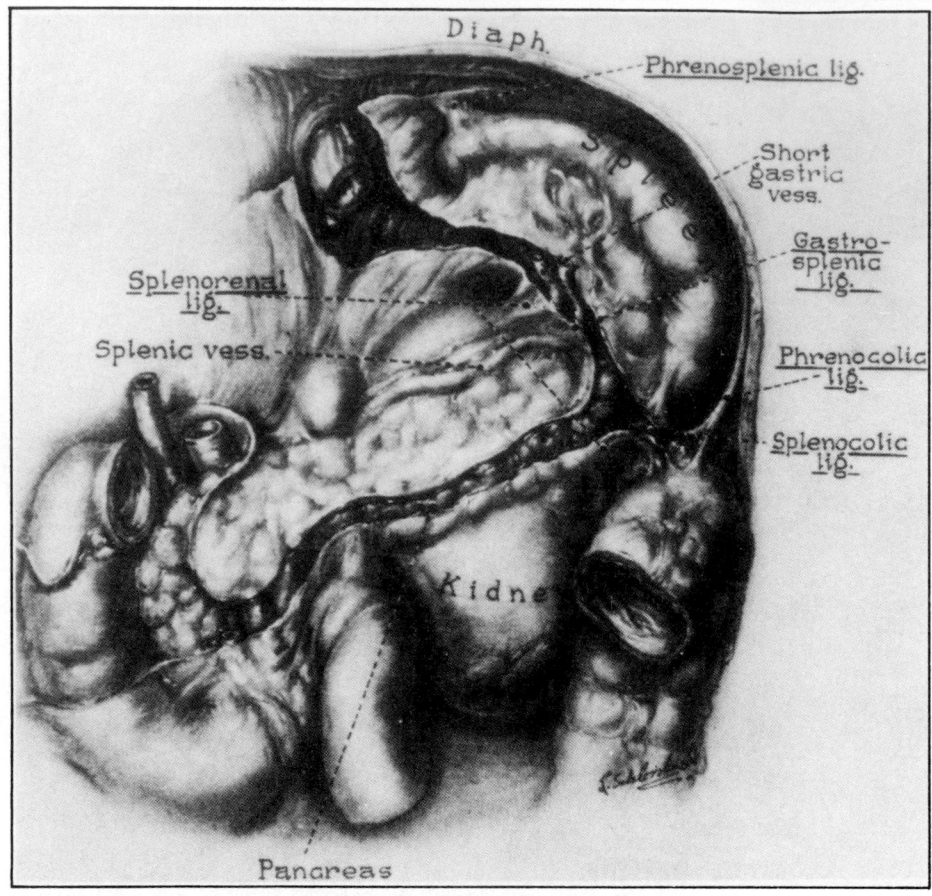

Figure 94–3. Ligaments of the spleen. (*Source: Schwartz SI: Spleen, in Schwartz SI, Shires GT, et al (eds.): Principles of Surgery, 4 edt. New York: McGraw-Hill, 1984, p 1373, with permission.*)

that contain cellular elements of blood in transit. Most of the blood flow passing through the spleen courses through an "open" circulation in which the blood passes from arterioles to reticular cell-lined networks of the splenic cords and thence to the sinuses. In addition, there is a "closed" circulation with direct arterial venous connections.

The vascular supply of the spleen enters along the trabeculae. The intrasplenic arteries first pass through the white pulp where branches come off almost perpendicularly, con-

tributing to the skimming effect by which the plasma exits, while most red cells pass to the red pulp cords. It is in the red pulp at the point of passage from cords to sinuses that deformability and flexibility is demanded of the red cells so that they can squeeze through. The normally biconcave discs elongate and become thinner. Almost 90 percent of cells slowly make their way through "open" circulation, whereas 10 percent pass more rapidly through direct arterial venous conduits. The resultant cumulative flow through the spleen averages 300 ml/min.

Figure 94–4. A. The more common locations of accessory spleens. Accessory spleens are also found in the left ovary, in the left testicle along the course of the left ureter, and in the lesser sac and greater omentum. **B.** Locations of accessory spleens. Note position of presacral and paraureteric spleniculi.

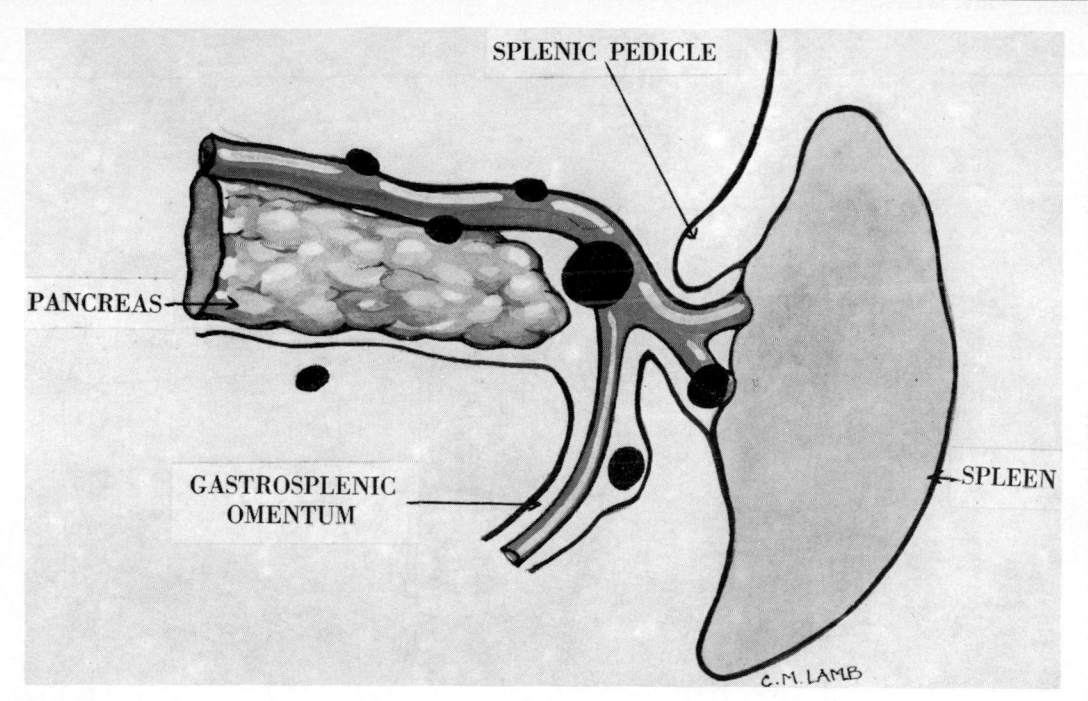

SPLENIC PEDICLE

PANCREAS

GASTROSPLENIC
OMENTUM

SPLEEN

C.M. LAMB

A

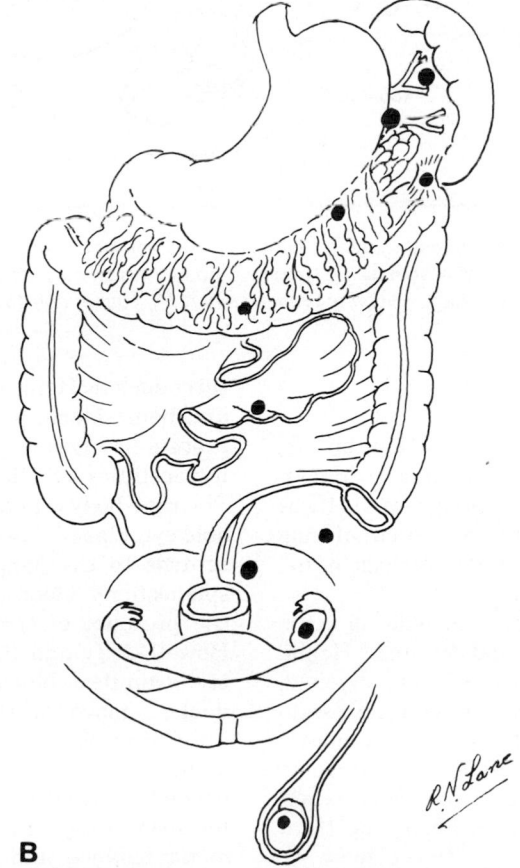

R.N.Lane

B

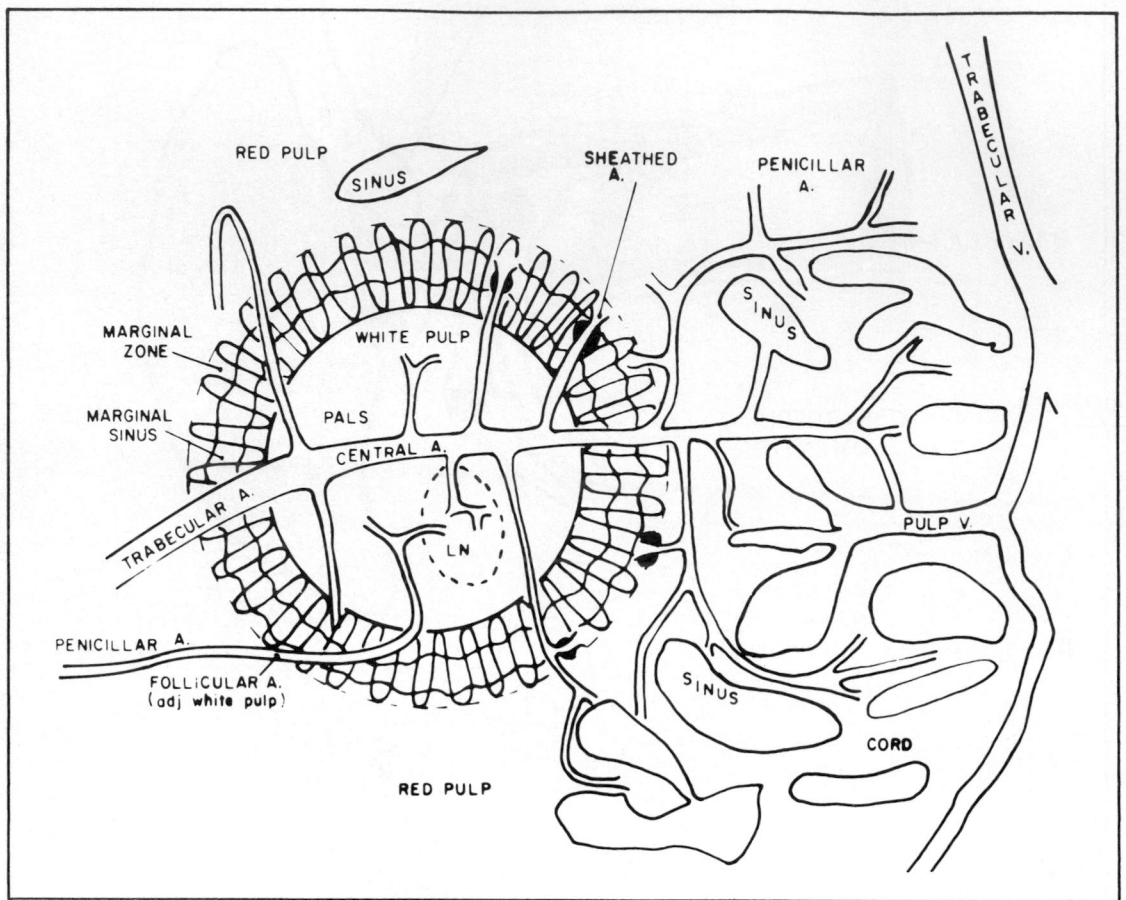

Figure 94–5. Diagram illustrating splenic compartments and potential vascular supply routes. A = artery or arteriole, V = vein, LN = lymphatic nodule which may include germinal center, PALS = periarterial lymphatic. (*Source: From Barnhart MI, Lusher JM, 1979, with permission.*)

PHYSIOLOGY

Although the spleen is not necessary for life, it performs important functions that are generally divided into two major categories: (1) those related to cellular elements in the circulating blood and (2) those that are immunologic in nature.

The cellular functions include hematopoiesis, storage, "pitting," and "culling." Hematopoiesis, which supplies erythroid, myeloid, lymphoid cells, and platelets in fetal life, essentially ceases by the seventh intrauterine month. In human beings the spleen does not serve as an important reservoir for blood cells except platelets. At any given time, about one third of the total platelet mass is in the spleen.

Pitting refers to the removal of rigid structures such as Heinz bodies, Howell–Jolly bodies, and hemosiderin granules from red cells. The process involves the removal of nondeformable intracellular substances from deformable cells. The rigid body is phagocytized while the deformable cytoplasmic mass passes into the sinus and returns to the general circulation. The postsplenectomy blood smear is characterized by the presence of circulating erythrocytes with Howell–Jolly and Pappenheimer bodies (siderotic granules). Nucleated cells also have their nuclei removed in the same fashion.

Culling is the term applied to the spleen's ability to remove red cells that are aged or abnormal. Normally, as the red cell ages after a life-span of approximately 120 days, it loses osmotic balance and membrane integrity, and therefore deformability. When these cells lose their deformability they are phagocytized by native macrophages. The spleen does not represent the only site for red cell destruction, and there is no difference in red cell survival following splenectomy. Naturally deformed cells and red cells that are affected by disease states are also removed by phagocytosis. In those circumstances in which there is a superabundance of reticulocyte formation, these cells are remodeled in the spleen and exit as mature cells. In the normal adult, the spleen is the most important site of selective erythrocyte sequestration and during its 120-day life cycle, the red cell spends an estimated minimum of 2 days within the spleen which, when normal, contains about 25 ml red blood cells.

The neutrophil has a half-life of about 6 hours; hence 85 percent of neutrophils either emigrate at random into tissues or are destroyed within 24 hours. Although the role of the spleen in the destruction of neutrophils under normal conditions is not well quantified, in some hypersplenic states the spleen's role is augmented, with resulting neutropenia. This augmented removal can occur because of splenic enlargement and accelerated sequestration of granulocytes or because of enhanced splenic removal of altered granulocytes, as seen in immune neutropenias.

There is significant interaction between the platelets and splenic cells. Normally about one third of the platelet mass is pooled in the spleen, and this pool exchanges freely with the circulating platelets that have a life-span of about 10 days. With splenomegaly, a large proportion of platelets is sequestered in the spleen (up to 80 percent) and this, coupled with accelerated platelet destruction in the spleen, accounts for thrombocytopenia. Splenic phagocytosis of platelets occurs in normal states but in pathologic states, such as immune thrombocytopenia (ITP), it is greatly accelerated.

In addition to the phagocytosis of antibody-coated cells, the immunologic functions of the spleen include antibody synthesis (especially IgM), generation of lymphocytes, and production of tuftsin, opsonins, properdin, and interferon.

The Asplenic State

The spleen plays a role in the phagocytic clearance of bacteria, especially encapsulated bacteria such as pneumococci and *Hemophilus influ-*

enzae, particularly if the host has deficient concentrations of opsonizing antibodies. The spleen also produces specific IgM antibody to blood-borne bacteria. It is generally felt that if sufficient opsonins are present and the reticuloendothelial (RE) system is normal, the spleen probably plays a relatively small role in the clearance of blood-borne organisms. Any dysfunction of the RE system, such as hematologic disease, or immunosuppressive therapy, increases the likelihood of sepsis.

In a series reported by Albrechtsen and Ly of 221 patients with hematologic disease, late postsplenectomy pulmonary infection was seen in 8 patients. All but one was either on immunosuppressive therapy or had advanced malignancy. No neutrophil defect or impairment of serum opsonin or chemotactic activity could be demonstrated after incidental or traumatic splenectomy in the study by Deitch and O'Neal of 24 healthy adult patients. Also, screening for complement activation by classic and alternative pathways did not reveal any defects resulting from splenectomy in 12 patients who underwent incidental splenectomy. A recent study by Schwartz et al of 93 adult patients subjected to splenectomy revealed only 2 cases of fulminant sepsis documented during 1090 person-years of follow-up. The incidence of any type of serious infection was 7 per 100 person years. Patients undergoing splenectomy in association with a malignant lesion had higher subsequent infection rates, and patients receiving immunosuppressive or radiation therapy were also at higher risk.

Children who have undergone splenectomy should be protected with pneumococcus vaccine and they should receive penicillin until age 18. Pneumococcus vaccine should also be administered to splenectomized adult patients. Patients with diseases associated with high infection rates such as thalassemia, sickle cell anemia, and autoimmune hemolytic anemia and thrombocytopenia should not be denied splenectomy but should be under close surveillance.

RUPTURE OF THE SPLEEN

Etiology. The causes of splenic rupture, in which the organ's parenchyma and/or capsule is disrupted, include penetrating trauma, non-penetrating or blunt trauma, operative trauma, and, rarely, a spontaneous event. Rupture of the spleen may be caused by puncture wounds due to stabbings or missiles. The trajectory of the penetrating wound may pass through the anterior abdominal wall, the posterior abdominal wall, the flank, or transthoracically, piercing the pleural space and diaphragm. Isolated splenic injury may be present, or organs in juxtaposition may be involved; this would include the stomach, left kidney, pancreas, and root of the mesentery. Nonpenetrating or blunt trauma represents an increasing etiologic factor in splenic rupture. The spleen, alone or in combination with other viscera, is the most frequently injured organ, following blunt trauma to the abdomen or lower thoracic cage. In this circumstance, splenic trauma is an isolated event in only 30 percent of patients. Other organs that may be injured, in decreasing order of frequency, include: (1) chest (rib fracture), (2) kidney, (3) spinal cord, (4) liver, (5) lung, (6) craniocerebral structures, (7) small intestine, (8) large intestine, and (9) pancreas, and (10) stomach.

Operative trauma to the spleen most commonly occurs during operation on adjacent viscera. The spleen has been injured in approximately 2 percent of patients whose operations involved viscera in the left upper quadrant. Subtotal gastrectomy and abdominal repair of a diaphragmatic hernia are high on the list of operations associated with splenic trauma. In these situations, injury usually results from retractors placed against the organ in order to obtain exposure.

Although spontaneous rupture of the normal spleen has been reported in approximately two dozen cases, it is a much more common event when the spleen is involved with a hematologic disorder. Spontaneous rupture, or rupture associated with minor trauma, is the most common cause of death for patients with infectious mononucleosis; this is second only to malaria as a cause of spontaneous splenic rupture. The complication of splenic rupture occurs most frequently in the second to fourth weeks in the patient with infectious mononucleosis. Splenic rupture has also been reported in patients with sarcoidosis, acute and chronic leukemia, hemolytic anemia, congestive splenomegaly, and polycythemia vera.

Pathology. The spectrum of lesions associated with trauma to the spleen include linear and stellate lacerations, capsular tears, puncture wounds, subcapsular intrasplenic hematomas, avulsion of the organ from its vascular pedicle, and laceration of the short gastric vessels within the gastrosplenic omentum. The spleen is an extremely friable, vascular organ, and even minor trauma may result in significant bleeding, particularly if the spleen is enlarged or diseased. Most injuries result in transverse ruptures as a consequence of the internal architecture of the spleen, which is arranged on a transverse plane. Injuries through this plane usually do not cross any major segmental arteries. Experimentally it has been shown that injuries coursing along the blood supply heal by primary intention, while those traversing segmental vessels are attended by infarction of the involved segment, but persistent viability of the remainder of the organ.

The vascular anatomy of the spleen favors spontaneous cessation of bleeding following trauma. Large and small arteriovenous anastomoses permit segments of the organ to be bypassed, particularly in states of shock. The complex arterial–capillary venous circulation and arterial–capillary sinus circulations result in a meshwork that facilitates platelet aggregation and clot formation. When lacerations occur along the horizontal axis, control of the arterial supply to individual segments is technically feasible.

Splenic rupture may be acute, delayed, or occult. Acute rupture, which is attended by immediate intraperitoneal bleeding, occurs in over 90 percent of cases of blunt trauma to the spleen. Delayed rupture, with an interval of days or weeks between the injury and intraperitoneal bleeding, has been reported in approximately 10 percent of cases of blunt trauma. The quiescent period referred to as the "latent period of Baudet" persists for less than 7 days in half of these patients, and less than 2 weeks in three quarters of them. Occult rupture is a term applied to traumatic pseudocysts of the spleen when injury to the organ previously had not been diagnosed. This is an extremely rare event.

Another pathologic lesion related to splenic trauma is splenosis; this is the result of autotransplantation of fragments of the traumatized spleen onto the peritoneal surface. Patients with splenosis are generally asymptomatic, but the lesion may stimulate the formation of adhesions, which, in turn, may lead to intestinal obstruction. It is not known whether splenosis protects against the infection that has been associated with the asplenic state. At least two deaths, caused by overwhelming infection following traumatic rupture of the spleen, have been reported in patients who were proven to have splenosis.

Clinical Manifestations. The signs and symptoms produced by splenic rupture vary according to the severity and rapidity of intraabdominal hemorrhage, the presence of other organ injuries, and the interval between the injury and the examination. Most patients present with some degree of hypovolemia and therefore have tachycardia and hypotension. This can be accentuated by raising the head of the bed. Usually, there is generalized abdominal pain, which, in one third of cases, is localized in the left upper quadrant. Pain at the tip of the shoulder (Kehr sign) is evidence of diaphragmatic irritation, but occurs in less than one half the patients. This may be produced by placing the patient in a Trendelenburg position. Tenderness in the left upper quadrant is a frequent physical sign, and a mass or a percussible area of fixed dullness in this region (Ballance sign) has been described but is rarely detected.

Diagnostic Studies. Serial determinations of the hematocrit may suggest continued intraperitoneal bleeding. Increases in the white blood count to levels frequently greater than 15,000/ mm³ are to be anticipated. Routine abdominal radiographs may demonstrate fractured ribs, which should arouse suspicion of injury to the spleen. More specific findings, which may be noted on abdominal films include: (1) elevated, immobile left diaphragm, (2) enlarged splenic shadow, (3) medial displacement of the gastric shadow with serration of the greater curvature due to dissection of blood into the gastrosplenic omentum, and (4) widening of the space between the splenic flexure and the properitoneal fat pad. Ultrasonography may define blood in the peritoneum, and has been shown to be sensitive to as little as 300 ml accumulation. Computed tomography (CT) scanning may demonstrate a splenic rupture; the same may be effected by splenic radionuclide scan, but in both instances false-positives may be caused by congenital clefts (Fig. 94–6). The diagnosis may be established angiographically by visualization of: (1) disruption of the parenchyma, (2) radiopacity in the peritoneal cavity, and (3) early filling of the splenic vein (Fig. 94–7).

Treatment. Spontaneous rupture of a diseased organ usually requires splenectomy. By contrast, iatrogenic lacerations that are detected intraoperatively generally can be repaired. Concern with the risk of asplenic sepsis has led to an altered approach to penetrating and blunt splenic trauma. Many recent series have reported that observation, without operative intervention, is possible in over half the cases of

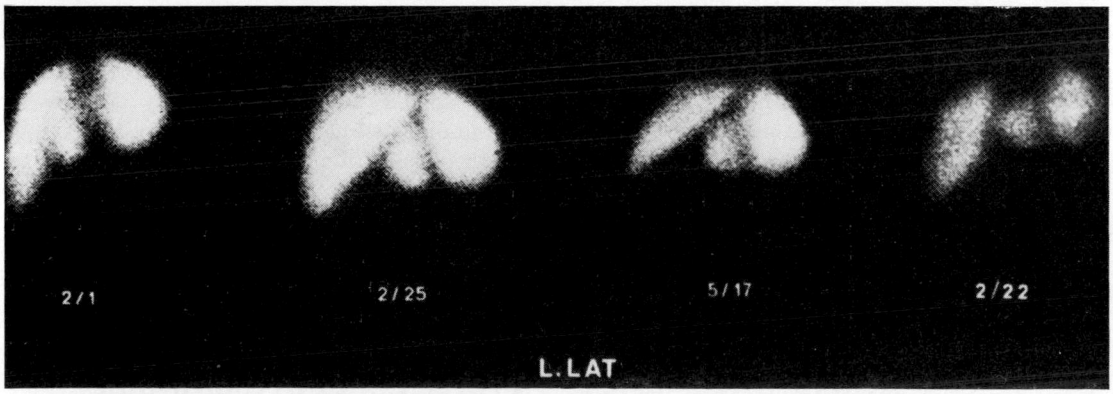

Figure 94–6. Initial left lateral scan (2/1) in patient who fell on stairs shows a wide band of decreased activity through spleen. Subsequent scans show that the band persists, with only minor narrowing. (*Source: From Fischer KC, Eraklis A, et al: Scintigraphy in follow-up of pediatric splenic trauma treated without surgery. J Nucl Med 19:3, 1978, with permission.*)

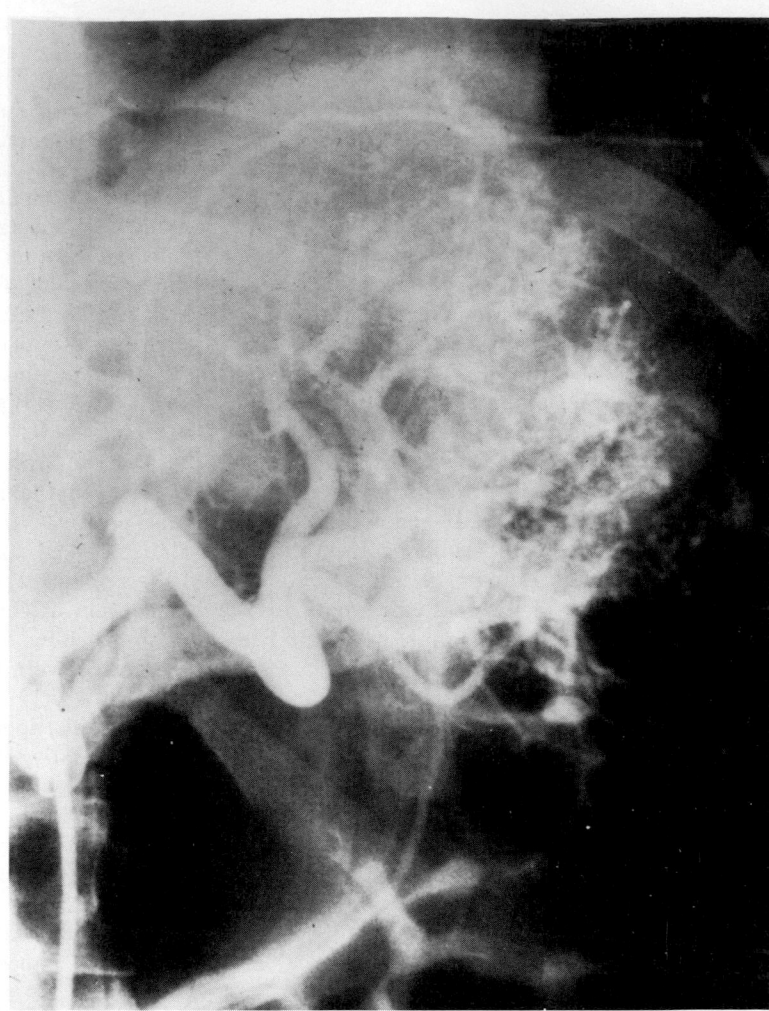

Figure 94–7. Splenic angiogram showing early filling of splenic vein diagnostic of parenchymal rupture.

splenic rupture in children. These cases are observed for 7 to 14 days and delayed rupture rarely occurs. Operation is mandated if there is suggestion of injury of other intraabdominal organs. In adult series, approximately one third of the spleens have been salvaged. Although splenectomy as a lifesaving procedure is the standard in many cases, splenic repair can be successfully effected for the majority of parenchymal injuries.

A midline incision is recommended for the management of splenic trauma, and the chest should be prepared at the same time to permit extension of the incision. A clot is usually detected in the left upper quadrant, and if this is not apparent, the spleen should be exposed gently to avoid inadvertent trauma. If there is

no apparent active bleeding from the traumatized spleen, no further therapy is indicated. If minor bleeding is noted, it may be managed by the application of micronized collagen or oxidized cellulose, absorbable sutures passed through the capsule, or suturing the omentum to the area of laceration to effect tamponade. The techniques of splenorrhaphy and splenic preservation are discussed later.

LOCAL SPLENIC DISORDERS

Aneurysms of the Splenic Artery

The lesion was first mentioned by Baussier in 1770. St. Leger Brockman described one of the first surgical cases in 1930. The first radiologic diagnosis was made by Lindboe 2 years later.

The splenic artery is the most common site of an intraabdominal aneurysm when the abdominal aorta is excluded. The incidence in autopsy series ranges between 0.02 and 0.16 percent. The lesion occurs most frequently in women, usually as a consequent of atherosclerosis. In a series of 125 cases collected by Sherlock and Learmonth, the average diameter of the aneurysmal sac was 3.4 cm and the largest was 15 cm. The main splenic artery was involved in 81 percent of the cases, while 26 percent were multiple. Eighty seven percent of splenic artery aneurysms occurred in women, and 92 percent of the women had been pregnant an average of 4.5 times.

A splenic artery aneurysm usually is discovered in the sixth decade as an incidental finding. Eighty three percent of patients are asymptomatic at the time of diagnosis. The remainder present with epigastric, left upper quadrant, or flank pain. The pain usually cannot be attributed conclusively to the lesion. The physical examination is usually normal, and a bruit is detectable in less than 10 percent of cases. A calcified lesion is noted on plain film of the abdomen in 70 percent of the patients (Fig. 94–8).

Rupture is usually manifested by sudden abdominal pain. In 12.5 percent a warning hemorrhage occurs, with temporary cessation of bleeding. Rupture into the colon, stomach, and intestine may take place, but intraperitoneal rupture is by far the most common presentation. The risk of rupture in a calcified aneurysm is small, occurring in only 1 of 34 patients, followed for 1 to 19 years and that aneurysm was 7 cm in diameter. When rupture occurs in the nonpregnant female, it is usually contained in the lesser sac, resulting in a patient mortality rate of less than 5 percent. Rupture in the pregnant female, however, has been associated with a 70 percent maternal and a 95 percent fetal mortality. Sixty nine percent of the ruptures during pregnancy occur during the third trimester.

Criteria for operation are not firm, but it is generally felt that removal is not required for the asymptomatic lesion that is less than 2 cm detected on a radiograph. Symptomatic aneurysms, and those that are greater than 2 cm in diameter, should be removed if the patient is a reasonable risk. An aneurysm detected in a female who anticipates pregnancy should be removed; one detected early in pregnancy should be resected prior to the third trimester. Lesions proximal to the hilus of the spleen can be managed by proximal and distal ligation, with resection of the involved segment, if possible. Distal lesions and multiple lesions generally necessitate splenectomy. Proximal ligation is reasonable, since the spleen will not become ischemic following central ligation of the main splenic artery.

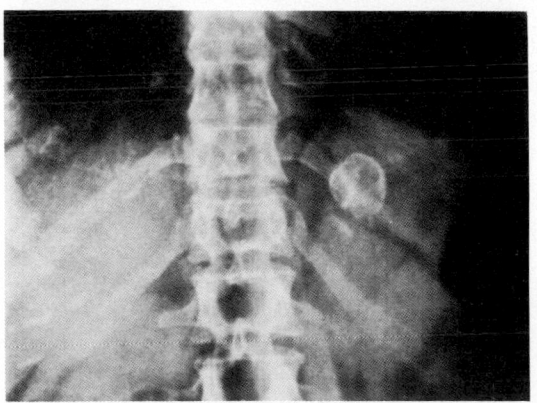
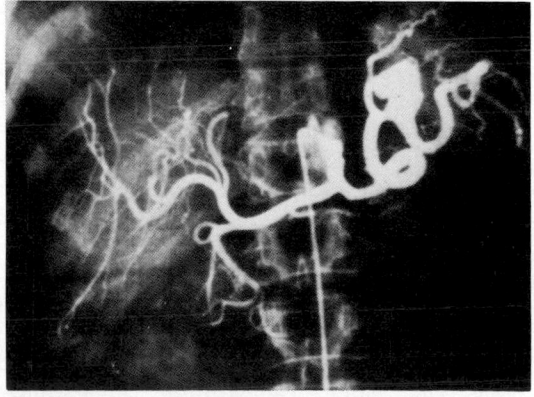

A   **B**

Figure 94–8. A. Plain abdominal roentgenogram demonstrating "signet-ring" pattern of calcification in left upper quadrant. Diameter is 3.0 cm. **B.** Selective celiac artery arteriogram of same patient demonstrating saccular splenic artery aneurysm. (*Source: From Trastek VF, Pairolero PC, et al, 1982, with permission.*)

Cysts

In 1929, Andral first described a splenic cyst; this was a dermoid found at autopsy. Pean performed the first recorded splenectomy for cyst in 1867. Cysts are generally subdivided into those of nonparasitic etiology and those that are caused by echinococcus.

Nonparasitic Cysts

This category is made up of cysts devoid of cellular lining (pseudocysts), simple cysts, epidermoid cysts, and dermoid cysts.

Pseudocysts comprise 70 to 80 percent of nonparasitic cysts of the spleen; most result from trauma and represent the resolution of a subcapsular or intraparenchymal hematoma. Malaria, infectious mononucleosis, tuberculosis, and syphilis are all predisposing factors. The pseudocysts vary in size, can reach large proportions, and contain as much as 3 L of a dark, turbid fluid. In over 80 percent of the cases the lesion is unilocular (Fig. 94–9); the cyst wall is dense and smooth. Microscopically the wall consists of fibrous tissue without an internal epithelial lining.

Pseudocysts occur more frequently in women, and in children and young adults. Many patients recall a history of trauma. One third of the patients are asymptomatic. The most frequent complaint is left upper quadrant pain radiating to the left shoulder or chest. Symptoms related to pressure on the stomach occur less frequently. Physical examination usually reveals a smooth mass in the left upper quadrant that can be seen on routine abdominal films (Fig. 94–10). A focal calcification may be noted. Ultrasonography, CT, and arteriography will define the cystic nature of the lesion. Splenectomy is curative, and cases also have been managed by unroofing and draining the area, preserving the bulk of splenic parenchyma.

Simple congenital cysts, lined by flattened or cuboidal cells, may originate from infolding of peritoneal mesethelium during splenic development. These lesions are usually small and asymptomatic. Large simple cysts present with the same manifestations as pseudocysts and have the same radiographic appearance. Smaller lesions found incidentally do not require excision; larger lesions are removed by total or partial splenectomy.

About 10 percent of cystic lesions are lined

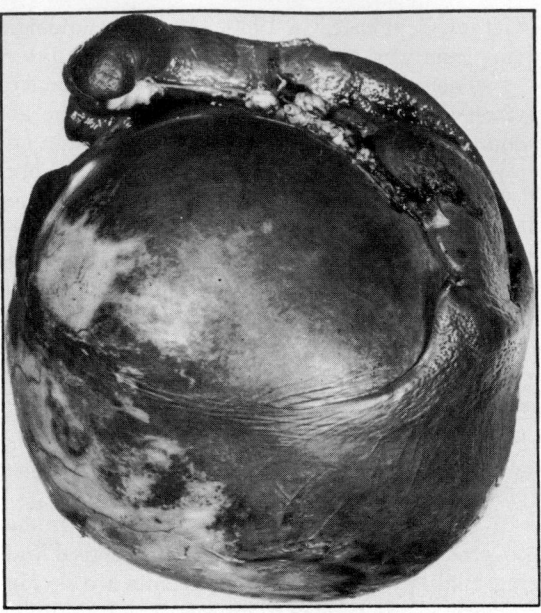

Figure 94–9. Pseudocyst of the spleen. The patient was a girl aged 11 years. Splenectomy was successfully performed. (*Courtesy of Dr. R. Dick, Royal Free Hospital, London.*)

by squamous epithelium; less than 100 cases of this lesion have been reported. These cysts are usually round and unilocular, and may be very large. They are filled with yellow or brown turbid fluid. The cyst is dense and the diagnosis is established by microscopic definition of the stratified squamous lining. Examination of multiple cuts may be required to demonstrate the pathology.

Epidermoid cysts of the spleen occur in children and in young adults in 75 percent of the cases. About two thirds of the patients have been female. The clinical manifestations are dependent upon the size and are similar to those of the pseudocysts, as are the radiologic findings. Splenectomy, or partial splenectomy, effects a cure.

True dermoid cysts of the spleen are exceedingly rare; fewer than ten cases have met the pathologic criteria of a squamous epithelium with dermal appendages such as hair follicles and sweat glands. Splenectomy is indicated.

Echinococcal Cysts

Hydatid disease occurs epidemically in south central Europe, South America, Australia, and

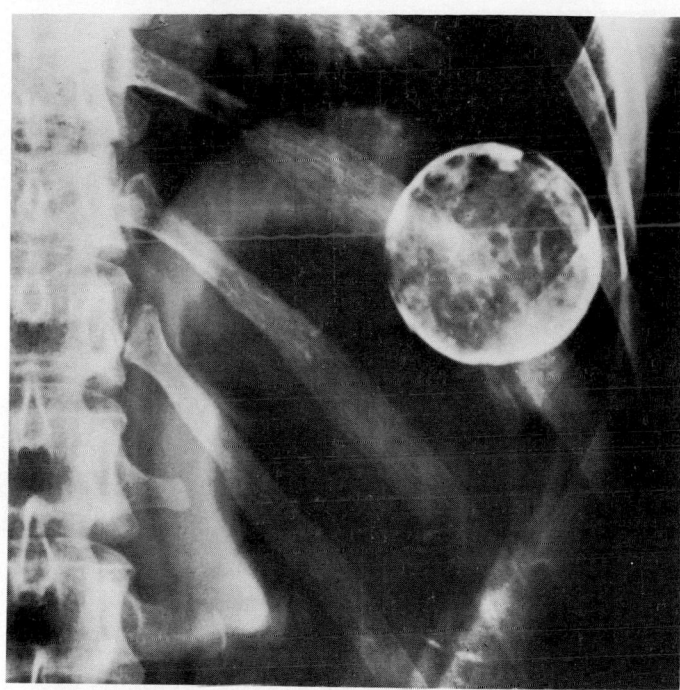

Figure 94–10. Calcified splenic cyst, confirmed at operation to be nonparasitic. (*Courtesy of Dr. R. Dick, Royal Free Hospital, London.*)

Alaska. Two thirds or more of the splenic cysts are caused by echinococci. The parasitology of echinococcal disease is presented in the section on liver disease. *E. granulosus,* the most commonly implicated species, usually results in a unilocular cyst composed of an inner germinal layer (endocyst) and an outer, laminated layer (ectocyst) surrounded by a fibrous capsule. Unlike the nonparsitic cysts, these are filled with fluid under positive pressure, and also contain daughter cysts and infective scolices.

Echinococcal cysts are usually asymptomatic unless they reach a size causing pressure symptoms or they become secondarily infected or rupture.

As a diagnostic tool the Casoni skin test is sensitive but not specific. The passive hemoglutination test provides the best diagnostic specificity and sensitivity and is preferable to flocculation and complement fixation tests. The abdominal film may show a partially calcified mass in the left upper quadrant. Ultrasound and CT scan may demonstrate a cystic mass that is septated and contains daughter cysts.

Splenectomy is the treatment of choice since there is no effective medical therapy. Care should be taken to avoid spilling the contents of the cyst. The lesions can be sterilized by instilling a 3 percent sodium chloride solution. If intraperitoneal spillage occurs during the course of dissection, an anaphylactic hypotension may occur and require intravenous epinephrine to treat the shock.

Splenic Abscesses

Splenic abscesses occur more frequently in the tropics, where there is a higher incidence of sickle cell anemia, with associated thrombosis of parenchymal vessels and consequent infarction. In North America and the European countries, intrasplenic abscess is usually a consequence of bacteria associated with endocarditis or postoperative infection, frequently in a patient with a hematologic disorder. Seventy five percent of splenic abscesses are caused by bacteremia; 15 percent are secondary to trauma, and 10 percent represent direct extension from a neighboring process. The organisms most frequently implicated are *S. aureus,* streptococci, and gram-negative bacilli.

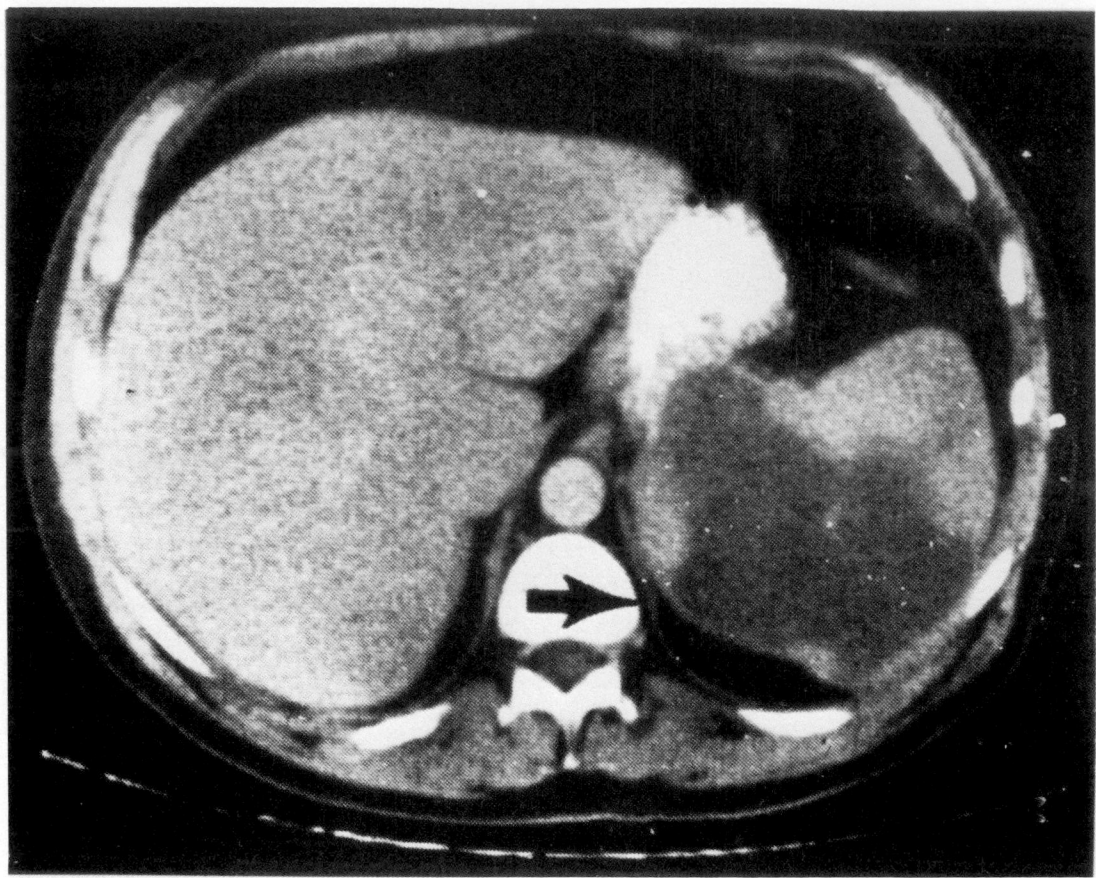

Figure 94–11. CT scan of abdomen with oral medium, demonstrating splenic abscess. (*Source: From Linos DA, Nagorney DM, et al, 1983, with permission.*)

Patients present with asthenia, weight loss, high fever, and rigors. Pain is most pronounced in the left upper quadrant, and there may be restriction of respiratory excursions. Spread, or transdiaphragmatic rupture may result in empyema. The diagnosis may be established by sonogram (Fig. 94–11) or by CT scan.

Splenectomy should be performed if feasible. Frequently, however, the extent of the perisplenic inflammatory process compromises removal of the organ, in which case splenotomy and drainage is indicated. Percutaneous ultrasonographically-directed insertion of a pigtail catheter for drainage represents an alternative approach. With drainage and appropriate antibiotics, recent mortality rates of less than 10 percent have been reported.

Benign Neoplasms

Hemangioma is the most common, benign neoplasm of the spleen, but fewer than 100 cases have been reported. The lesion may be focal, multiple, or involve the entire organ. Marked enlargement resulting in a splenic weight of 13,000 g has been reported. The vast majority of lesions are the cavernous type. Most splenic hemangiomas remain asymptomatic; they cause symptoms when they reach sufficient size to encroach on adjacent organs. Spontaneous rupture may occur, and has been reported in 25 percent of Husni's series of 56 cases.

There may be pancytopenia or isolated thrombocytopenia caused by platelet trapping in the cavernous spaces of the lesion. X-ray may reveal a soft tumor mass with anterior displacement of the stomach and downward displacement of the kidney and splenic flexure of the colon. CT scan demonstrates an enlarged spleen. The diagnosis can be established by angiography which demonstrates the "laking" effect in the capillary phase. This is identical to that noted for hepatic hemangiomas. The "laking" effect is often accompanied by early filling of the splenic vein, characteristic of an arteriovenous shunt.

Surgical intervention is not indicated for small, asymptomatic, incidentally detected hemangiomas. The treatment is splenectomy for the larger and symptomatic hemangiomas, including those that have ruptured intraperitoneally. In one series of cases complicated by rupture, 79 percent survived splenectomy and were cured, 14 percent died preoperatively, and 7 percent died postoperatively.

Lymphangioma of the spleen is made up of a malformation of lymphatics, and occurs much less frequently than hemangioma. The lesion may be part of a generalized lymphangiomatosis. Cystic spaces of varying sizes, containing clear gelatinous fluid may account for a splenic weight of 2000 to 3000 g. Microscopically, endothelial lined spaces constitute the major portion of the lesion.

Symptoms, when present, are related to the size of the tumor. CT scan reveals a lesion with a density approximating that of water. Angiography demonstrates splaying of the blood vessels and the absence of "lakes," characteristic of hemangiomas. Splenectomy is indicated for symptomatic lesions.

Other benign tumors that have rarely required splenectomy include hamartoma, with fewer than 50 reported cases, and an occasional case of lipoma and fibroma.

Primary Malignant Tumors

In previous editions of this text, primary lymphoma was considered the most common primary malignant tumor of the spleen. Approximately 150 cases were included in reviews, representing 1 percent of all cases of lymphoma. It is now agreed that it is more appropriate to classify these cases in the general category of *lymphoma,* with primary involvement of the spleen. Primary *hemangiosarcoma,* although rare, is now regarded as the most frequent primary, malignant tumor of the spleen. Less than 100 cases have been reported. The tumor arises from endothelial or primitive mesenchymal cells. The average weight of the spleen in one series was 1700 g. The lesions grow rapidly and metastasize to regional lymph nodes, marrow, liver, and lungs. Most patients are middle aged, and symptoms are related to the mass effect of the lesion, in addition to general weight loss and cachexia, ascites, and pleural effusions. Angiographic findings are similar to those noted for hemangiomas. Splenectomy is indicated, but is rarely curative. Four cases of fibrosarcoma of the spleen have also been reported.

Metastatic Tumors

Recent autopsy series have refuted the concept that metastases to the spleen are rare. Metastatic involvement of the spleen was present in 9 percent of autopsy patients with epithelial malignancies. Laparotomy for undiagnosed splenomegaly, however, rarely reveals metastatic deposits in the absence of known, generalized metastases. Rarely, spontaneous rupture of the spleen with consequent intraperitoneal hemorrhage may be due to metastatic deposits. It is only in this situation that splenectomy may be indicated.

HEMATOLOGIC DISORDERS

The role of splenectomy in the management of hematologic disorders has greatly increased in recent years. In general, removal of the spleen in these disorders affects its role in cellular sequestration and destruction and also its role as an immunologic organ. In 1887 Sir Thomas Spencer Wells, the renowned gynecologist, performed a therapeutic splenectomy in a patient with what subsequently proved to be hereditary spherocytosis. The first splenectomy for autoimmune hemolytic anemia was performed in 1911 by Micheli; 6 years later Schloffer, responding to the suggestion of a fourth year medical student, Kaznelson, removed a spleen for idiopathic thrombocytopenic purpura.

Anemias

The two major categories of anemia that benefit from splenectomy are (1) intracellular defects including membrane abnormalities, enzyme defects, and hemoglobinopathy, and (2) extracellular defects, particularly autoimmune hemolytic anemia.

Hereditary Spherocytosis

Hereditary spherocytosis is a hemolytic anemia caused by an inherited disorder of the red cell membrane; this category also includes hereditary elliptocytosis (ovalocytosis) and stomatocytosis. The disorder is a prime example of a loss of cellular deformity, based on an inherited defect of the red cell membrane resulting in an excessive splenic trapping and consequent hemolysis. In addition to the fundamental abnormality found in the erythrocyte membrane, the cells also demonstrate an increased osmotic fragility, i.e., lysis occurs at a higher than normal concentration of sodium chloride.

The role of the spleen in this disorder is related to the inability of the spherocytes to pass through the splenic pulp. The cells that escape from the spleen are more susceptible to trapping and disintegration during each successive passage. The red cells entering the circulation from the bone marrow in patients with hereditary spherocytosis are normal; they become spherical within the circulation and the spleen further conditions them by means of its unique environment, making them more spheroidal and susceptible to destruction in subsequent passages through the organ.

Hereditary spherocytosis is transmitted as an autosomal dominant trait, and is the most common of the symptomatic, familial hemolytic anemias. In rare instances the disease occurs in patients whose parents appear to be unaffected. Hereditary spherocytosis primarily affects people of European origin and is rare in the black population. The salient clinical features are anemia, jaundice, and an enlarged spleen. The symptoms and findings may vary greatly in severity, but it is unusual for the anemia to be extremely severe. The jaundice usually parallels the severity of anemia, and generally is not intense; it is related to an increased red cell destruction, with the production of amounts of bile pigments that cannot be cleared totally by the liver, and regardless of intensity, is unaccompanied by pruritus or bradycardia. Bile pigment is not present in the urine unless there is associated biliary obstruction by pigmented gallstones or hepatic damage following severe hemolytic crises.

Periodic and sudden increases in the intensity of anemia and jaundice may occur, and this circumstance may be accompanied by abdominal pain, pyrexia, vomiting, and tachycardia. These so-called minor crises often follow intercurrent infections, emotional stress, fatigue, or exposure to cold and may last for a few hours to several days. Occasionally there may be a sudden, sometimes fatal, acute illness representing a major crisis. This usually follows an acute viral infection. The crises are characterized by a marked increase in the severity of the anemia, thrombocytopenia, leukopenia, and increased jaundice. Cholelithiasis has been reported in 60 percent of patients with hereditary spherocytosis but is unusual in children under the age of 10. Gallstones usually are of the pigment variety, presumably developing as a result of an increased bilirubin concentration within the bile. Splenomegaly is almost invariable, and it may be the cause of pressure symptoms within the abdomen. Chronic leg ulcers represent an unusual complication; although their pathogenesis has not been defined, but they tend to heal quickly after splenectomy.

The diagnosis can be established by an evaluation of a peripheral bloodstream that demonstrates small, spherocytic-shaped erythrocytes that appear thick. The degree of spherocytosis varies from case to case, but usually more than 80 percent of the red cells demonstrate this characteristic. In most patients, the hematocrit is in the range of 30 percent, and the reticulocyte count is usually increased to levels between 5 and 20 percent. The serum bilirubin is rarely greater than 5 mg/dl, and most of it is unconjugated. The red blood cell survival in these patients, as in all patients with hemolytic anemia, is reduced. The normal half-life of the red cell is 25 to 30 days, whereas a half-life of less than 20 days is indicative of increased hemolysis.

In 1922 Gansslen reported clinical cure following splenectomy in nine patients; his results led to the establishment of this procedure as the principal method of treatment. The results of removal of the spleen in almost all series have been uniformly good and associated with a low operative mortality and morbidity. Within a few days following removal of the spleen, the erythrocytes achieve a normal life-span and the intensity of jaundice, if present, is reduced. The morphology of the red cell is not altered as the inherent membrane abnormality persists. An established diagnosis of hereditary spherocytosis is now generally accepted as an indication for splenectomy. Even if the hemolytic process is compensated, the longer it is allowed to continue, the greater the potential for complications such as crises or gallstone formation. There have been differences of opinion regarding the timing of operation, and it is now generally recommended that the procedure be delayed until the fourth year of life. It is appropriate to perform an ultrasound prior to splenectomy, and the gallbladder should always be examined at the time of operation. If gallstones are present, the gallbladder should be removed at the time of splenectomy. It is also important to search for accessory spleens since this may be the cause of failure to respond to splenectomy in this disease.

Hereditary Elliptocytosis and Other Membrane Defects

Hereditary elliptocytosis (ovalocytosis) is transmitted as a simple Mendelian trait on a gene linked to the Rh blood type. It occurs in approximately 0.04 percent of the population. Oval erythrocytes constitute up to 25 percent of the total red cell population in many patients with macrocytic and hyprochromic microcytic anemia, and it is also seen in patients with sickle cell anemia, thalassemia, and hemoglobin-C disease. In patients with hereditary elliptocytosis, however, the oval and rod shaped forms constitute about 80 to 90 percent of the red cell population.

This disorder usually exists as a harmless trait, but in about 12 percent of the cases there is an active, variably compensated hemolytic anemia. The presence of hemolysis often is a familial characteristic, and it has been suggested that excessive hemolysis occurs only when the gene for elliptocytosis is present in the homozygous form, or is modified in some other way.

The majority of patients with hereditary elliptocytosis are Caucasians and the signs and symptoms are directly related to the severity of the hemolysis. Occasionally an acute hemolytic episode may be precipitated by infection. The clinical syndrome is indistinguishable from that described for hereditary spherocytosis. Gallstones are frequent, and chronic leg ulcers have been reported. The spleen is usually palpably enlarged in symptomatic cases. Diagnosis is established by the smear; Cr-51 studies in symptomatic cases demonstrate decreased red cell survival coupled with splenic sequestration.

A reticulocytosis of 20 percent or higher occurs in patients with overt hemolysis.

Splenectomy is indicated in all symptomatic patients, since removal of the organ is almost always followed by lasting effects of decreased hemolysis and corrected anemia, although the morphologic abnormality of the red blood cell remains unchanged. Associated cholelithiasis should be managed as in hereditary spherocytosis.

Hereditary stomatocytosis does not respond as well to splenectomy.

Hereditary Hemolytic Anemia with Red Cell Enzyme Deficiency

This disorder also has been referred to as hereditary nonspherocytic hemolytic anemia. On the basis of autohemolysis studies, two forms termed Type I and Type II have been defined. Type I has been shown to be due to a red cell deficiency of glucose-6-phosphate dehydrogenase (G-6-PD), whereas Type II is due to a deficiency of pyruvate-kinase (PK). As a consequence of these enzyme deficiencies, the red cells are unable to utilize glucose at a normal rate, resulting in a disturbed metabolism that renders the cells susceptible to increased hemolysis. Cr-51-tagged red cell studies have demonstrated that the spleen serves as a major site for hemolysis, particularly in patients with PK deficiency.

G-6-PD deficient hereditary nonspherocytic hemolytic anemia is transmitted as a sex-linked, incompletely dominant factor. PK deficiency is transmitted as a recessive factor affecting both sexes equally, and without racial predominance. Clinically, the two types cannot be differentiated and are usually detected in children who are investigated because of jaundice and anemia. The spleen is rarely enlarged in patients with G-6-PD deficiency, whereas enlargement occurs more frequently with PK deficiency. The survival time of erythrocytes in PK deficiency is reduced to a mean life-span averaging approximately half normal, and sometimes the reticulocyte count may be as high as 70 percent. The reticulocyte count is not increased to the same extent in patients with G-6-PD deficiency. Pigmented gallstones may be associated with both disorders.

Differentiation of the two disorders is important to define therapy. In the G-6-PD deficiency, the rate of hemolysis occurring on incubation of red cells is similar to that of normal cells, and, like normal cells, is diminished when glucose is added. With PK deficiency autohemolysis is greater than normal and is unaffected by the addition of glucose. There are specific screening tests available in most laboratories.

The majority of patients who maintain a hemoglobin greater than 8 g/dl are asymptomatic and do not require therapy. With significant anemia, and increasing transfusion requirements, splenectomy should be considered in patients with PK deficiency. The role of splenectomy is not predictable in a given case, and radiolabeled red cell sequestration studies are not accurately predictive of results. Postoperative thrombocytosis may occur if the hemolytic rate is unabated after splenectomy. In some cases this represents a serious sequela that may lead to hepatic, portal, and even caval thrombosis. Thus, the risk–benefit ratio of splenectomy is considerably higher in these disorders than in hereditary membrane disorders.

Heinz Body Hemolytic Anemias (Thalassemia)

The development of intracellular hemoglobin precipitates (Heinz bodies) that damage red cells and contribute to their premature destruction can occur because of thalassemia, unstable hemoglobins, or enzyme deficiencies in the pentose phosphate pathway.

Thalassemia (Mediterranean anemia) is a congenital disorder transmitted as a dominant trait in which the anemia is due primarily to a defect in hemoglobin synthesis. It has been referred to as Cooley's anemia, erythroblastic anemia, and target cell anemia. As a consequence of the defect, there are intracellular precipitates (Heinz bodies) that contribute to premature red cell destruction. The hemoglobin deficient red cells are small, thin, misshapen, and have a characteristic resistance to osmotic lysis.

The disease is classified as alpha, beta, and gamma types, determined by the specific defect in the synthesis rate of the peptide chain. In the United States, most patients suffer from beta thalassemia, and there is a quantitative reduction in the rate of beta chain synthesis, resulting in a decrease in the hemoglobin A. Gradations of the disease range from heterozygous thalassemia minor to severe homozygous thalassemia major. The latter is manifested by chronic anemia, jaundice, and splenomegaly. Patients with homozygous thalassemia ma-

jor usually present with clinical manifestations in the first year of life. In addition to the anemia and consequent pallor, there is usually retarded body growth and enlargement of the head. Intractable leg ulcers may be noted, and intercurrent infections are particularly common. Some patients present with repeated episodes of left upper quadrant pain related to splenic infarction. Cardiac dilatation occurs and in advance stages there is subcutaneous edema and effusion into the serous cavities. Intercurrent infections occur frequently, often leading to death in the more severe cases. These infections may be associated with aplastic crises. Gallstones have been reported in up to 24 percent of cases.

Therapy is directed only at symptomatic patients, i.e., those having thalassemia major or intermedia. In these patients transfusions are usually required at regular intervals. Since most children with thalassemia major accommodate to low hemoglobin levels, transfusions are given when the hemoglobin is less than 6 g/dl. Although splenectomy does not influence the basic hematologic disorder, it may eliminate or reduce the hemolytic process responsible for accelerated destruction of normal donor red cells within the patient's circulation, and thus reduce transfusion requirements. In general the best results associated with splenectomy have been obtained in older children and in young adults with large spleens in whom excessive splenic sequestration of red cells has been demonstrated. Occasionally, splenectomy may be indicated because of mechanical symptoms associated with marked splenomegaly or repeated episodes of abdominal pain due to splenic infarction.

Patients with homozygous beta thalassemia have an overall increased susceptibility to bacterial infection, but the immunoglobulin levels cannot be demonstrated as consistently abnormal. It is difficult to evaluate the effect of splenectomy per se on the risk of infection in these patients. A review of 130 splenectomized thalassemic patients, in whom the incidence of infection was assessed, revealed that 21 patients developed severe infection following splenectomy, seven of these within 2 years of the operation, and most in a 5- to 10-year period. The majority of studies indicate that there is no difference in the risk of infection before or after operation, and the overall benefit–risk ratio seems to favor the performance of splenectomy when appropriate indications are present.

Sickle Cell Disease

Sickle cell anemia is a hereditary hemolytic anemia, seen predominantly in blacks, and characterized by the presence of crescent-shaped erythrocytes which, because of a lack of deformity, are trapped in the splenic cords. In this disorder the normal hemoglobin A is replaced by hemoglobin S. Under conditions of reduced oxygen tension, hemoglobin S molecules undergo crystallization within the cell; this, in turn, elongates and distorts the cell. The sickle cells themselves increase the blood viscosity and circulatory stasis, thus establishing a vicious cycle. Sickling occurs so rapidly that blood flow through both the fast and slow compartments of the spleen is obstructed, and, as a consequence, a series of microinfarcts develop. In most adult patients only a fibrous area of the spleen remains, but autosplenectomy is preceded by splenomegaly in about 75 percent of patients.

In addition to serving as the site of destruction for damage of nondeformable erythrocytes, there are other splenic functional abnormalities in sickle cell anemia. These include: (1) an abnormal role that the spleen plays as a red cell reservoir in these patients, (2) a reduced antibody production by the spleen, and (3) reduction in the spleen's ability to filter bacteria, especially streptococcal pneumonia.

There are two situations in sickle cell anemia where the spleen is a pathologic red cell reservoir. The first is a form of chronic hypersplenism that usually occurs in childhood or adolescence, and is manifested by reduced red cell survival, leukopenia, and thrombocytopenia. In these patients, for some unknown reason, there is a failure to undergo autosplenectomy, and in this rare circumstance splenectomy will correct the leukopenia and thrombocytopenia and also will decrease the rate of red cell survival. The second abnormality has been termed acute splenic sequestration and is marked by sudden splenic enlargement associated with worsening anemia and profound hypotension. It usually occurs in the first five years of life in an SS child; streptococcal pneumonia infection may act as a precipitating event in these patients. The acute splenic sequestration is usually effectively treated with packed red cell transfusion. If there is a propensity for recurrence, splenectomy may be indicated.

Although the sickle cell trait occurs in approximately 9 percent of the black population, the majority of patients are asymptomatic. Sickle cell anemia is observed in 0.3 to 1.3 percent of blacks. Depending upon the vessels affected by vascular occlusion, the patients may have bone or joint pain, priapism, neurologic manifestations, or skin ulcers. Abdominal pain and cramps due to visceral stasis are frequent. Rarely, thrombosis of the splenic vessels may result in the complication of splenic abscess manifested by splenomegaly, splenic pain, and spiking fever.

For most patients with sickle cell anemia, only palliative therapy is available. Recent studies have shown that sodium cyanate will prevent sickling of hemoglobin S. Adequate hydration and partial exchange transfusion may help the crisis. In the circumstance of splenic abscess, incision and drainage of the abscess cavity may be required. Splenectomy is of benefit in only a few patients in whom excessive splenic sequestration of red cells, leukocytes, and/or platelets can be demonstrated.

Anemias Due to Extracellular Defects

These include fragmentation hemolytic diseases and immune hemolytic anemia. The most frequent cause of fragmentation hemolysis is associated with a regurgitant stream through and around a heart valve prosthesis. Aortic valves are more common sites than mitral valves. Fragmentation can also be due to microangiopathic disease. In this circumstance, hemolytic anemia results from red cell fragmentation in small blood vessels. Heterogeneous disorders such as disseminated carcinoma, collagen vascular disease, disseminated intravascular coagulation as associated with abruptio placentae and purpura fulminans, giant hemangiomas, and thrombotic thrombocytopenic purpura all have sufficient vascular damage to lead to red cell fragmentation within these vessels.

Immune Hemolytic Anemia

This is a disorder in which the life-span of presumably normal erythrocytes shorten when exposed to an endogenous hemolytic mechanism. The first description of the disease is credited to Chauffard and Troisier who, in 1908, demonstrated autohemolysins in the serum of several patients with acute hemolytic anemia. Three years later Micheli performed the first planned, successful splenectomy, thus stimulating the application of splenectomy for hematologic disease in general.

The etiology of the disorder has not been defined, but an immune mechanism seems to be fundamental. There is an antibody coating of blood cells that predisposes them to increased phagocytosis by reticuloendolethial cells in the spleen and other organs. IgG antibodies bind to the red cell, and complement becomes fixed. Phagocytosis occurs primarily in the spleen and is initiated by the binding of the Fc portion of the IgG molecule to the corresponding macrophage surface Fc receptor. In this process, phagocytosis may be partial and remove only a portion of the red cell membrane, but it results in spherocytes that have increased rigidity and are more sensitive to destruction in the splenic microcirculation.

The diagnosis of immune hemolytic anemia is made in a patient with anemia and reticulocytosis, who has a positive antiglobulin test. The direct antiglobulin reaction (Coombs' test) is characteristically positive, but recently Coombs' negative cases have been reported. Both warm and cold antibodies have been described. Warm antibodies, which react best at 37°C, occur more frequently. They are "incomplete" antibodies because they produce agglutination of normal erythrocytes when exposed to antiglobulin serum but do not cause agglutination in a saline medium. Cold antibodies are potentiated by temperatures below 37°C and act as "complete" agglutinating antibodies.

Although immune hemolytic anemia may occur or be encountered at any age, it is more frequent after the age of 50 and occurs twice as often in females. The onset may be insidious, and the course of the disease may be chronic. The disease, however, may develop abruptly and be fulminant; chills, fever, backache, and other symptoms of rapid blood destruction may occur. The acute cases occasionally develop as a complication of viral illnesses.

Symptoms and signs vary with the severity of the hemolytic process, and mild jaundice is often present. The spleen is palpably enlarged in half the cases and gallstones are demonstrated in one quarter of the cases. The most severe cases may have hemoglobinuria followed by renal tubular necrosis. The diagnosis of hemolysis is made by demonstrating anemia and reticulocytosis, accompanied by increased products of red cell destruction in the blood, urine, and stool. The distinguishing feature of the disease is the demonstration by direct and indirect Coombs' test of an autoantibody on the patient's own red cells, in the patient's serum, or in both. Platelets are usually normal, but occasionally autoimmune hemolytic anemia and idiopathic thrombocytopenic purpura occur together (Evans' syndrome).

In some patients the disorder tends to run an acute, self-limited course. Steroids constitute the first approach to patients requiring therapy. In the "warm" antibody immune hemolytic anemias, splenectomy should be considered: (1) if the steroids have been ineffective, (2) if excessive doses of steroids are required to maintain remission, (3) if toxic manifestations of steroids become apparent, and (4) if steroids are contraindicated for other reasons. A favorable response to splenectomy is anticipated in about 80 percent of selected splenectomized patients. The demonstration of excessive splenic sequestration of Cr-51-tagged red cells offers a guide to the selection of patients who may respond to splenectomy. More important than splenic sequestration alone is the ratio of spleen–liver sequestration; ratios greater than 2:1 and preferably 3:1 usually indicate a favorable response to splenectomy. Using these criteria, improvement following splenectomy has risen to approximately 80 percent. Splenectomy is rarely beneficial in diseases associated with cold antibodies.

Purpuras

Idiopathic Thrombocytopenic Purpura

Idiopathic thrombocytopenic purpura (immune thrombocytopenic purpura) (ITP), is the most common hematologic indication for splenectomy, is an acquired disorder, characterized by destruction of platelets exposed to circulating IgG antiplatelet factors. It is known that the spleen is the source of IgG specific for platelets; following splenectomy in these patients there is a normalization of platelet associated IgG levels. In ITP the spleen is also an important organ for platelet destruction by macrophagic phagocytosis. The fact that 30 percent of circulating platelets are in the spleen at all times provides a high concentration upon which a high antiplatelet antibody concentration of the spleen can act.

Female patients outnumber males 3:1. The most common presenting signs are petechiae and/or ecchymosis; bleeding gums, vaginal bleeding, mild gastrointestinal (GI) bleeding, and hematuria may also occur. In some patients, the purpuric manifestations take an almost cyclic course with exacerbations occurring at the time of the onset of menses. The incidence of central nervous system bleeding ranges between 2 and 4 percent and usually occurs early in the course of disease. The spleen is rarely palpable.

The platelet count is generally less than 50,000/mm³ and at times approaches 0. With markedly reduced platelet counts the bleeding time may be prolonged, but the clotting time remains normal. There is usually no significant anemia or leukopenia with the exception of the uncommon circumstance in which there is combined autoimmune hemolytic anemia. Bone marrow reveals a normal or increased number of megakaryocytes.

Idiopathic thrombocytopenic purpura in children has an excellent prognosis and rarely requires surgical intervention. In adults the disease is usually more persistent and a sustained response to steroid therapy occurs in only about 15 percent of cases. Between 75 and 80 percent of patients subjected to splenectomy, however, respond permanently and require no further steroid therapy. In most patients the platelet count rises to over 10,000/mm³ in 7 days. Rarely, return to normal can take months. A positive effect of splenectomy is noted even in those patients in whom the platelet count does not return to normal because recurrent bleeding rarely takes place.

Steroids constitute the initial form of therapy. Splenectomy should be performed in patients who have not responded to gluticocorticoid treatment within 6 weeks or who have responded to gluticocorticoids and then have become thrombocytopenic when the dosage is reduced. Rarely, either intracranial bleeding or profound GI hemorrhage may require intensive intravenous corticoid treatment and emergency splenectomy.

Some studies have suggested that patients who respond to gluticocorticoids with an elevation in platelet count are more likely to respond to splenectomy. Failure to respond to gluticocorticoids does not indicate that splenectomy will be unsuccessful and should not dissuade one from performing splenectomy. Radioactive chromium-labeled platelet sequestration studies are of little practical value in selecting patients. Platelet transfusions are never given preoperatively and are reserved for an occasional patient who continues to bleed diffusely following removal of the spleen. In patients undergoing splenectomy for ITP, a careful search should be made for accessory spleens, present in 18 to 30 percent of these patients.

Either ITP or immune hemolytic disease may proceed to or be concomitant with the manifestations of systemic lupus erythematosus. The indications for splenectomy in these patients are the same as in the idiopathic diseases. The majority of patients with systemic lupus erythematosus who are operated on specifically for thrombocytopenia respond with elevation of platelet counts.

Thrombotic Thrombocytopenic Purpura

Thrombotic thrombocytopenic purpura (TTP) is a disease of the arterioles or capillaries that undergo widespread, subintimal hylanization and consequent occlusion. It is associated with marked trapping of platelets, particularly in the spleen (Fig. 94–12). The etiology has not been defined precisely, but immune mechanisms have been suggested. Approximately 5 percent of reported cases occur during pregnancy.

A pentad of clinical features present in virtually all cases consists of fever, purpura, hemolytic anemia, varied neurologic manifestations, and signs of renal disease. In our own experience none of the patients had splenomegaly, although this has been reported in approximately 20 percent of cases. Pertinent laboratory findings include anemia, reticulocytosis, thrombocytopenia, leukocytosis, elevated serum bilirubin, proteinuria, hematuria, and azotemia. The peripheral blood smear reveals pleomorphic normochromic red cells that are fragmented and distorted and may include triangular cells, helmet cells, schistocytes, and polychromatic macrocytes. The degree of thrombocytopenia varies during the course of the illness, with a profound decrease in platelets often developing within hours of onset.

The majority of patients with this disease experience a rapid onset and fulminant course. Recovery has been reported for patients treated with heparin, exchange transfusions, fresh blood, dextran, antimetabolites, and massive doses of steroids. The combination of steroid therapy and splenectomy has achieved the highest degree of success (Fig. 94–13).

Other Hypersplenic Disorders

Primary Idiopathic Hypersplenism

Enlarged spleen and either neutropenia or pancytopenia in the presence of a normal or hyper-

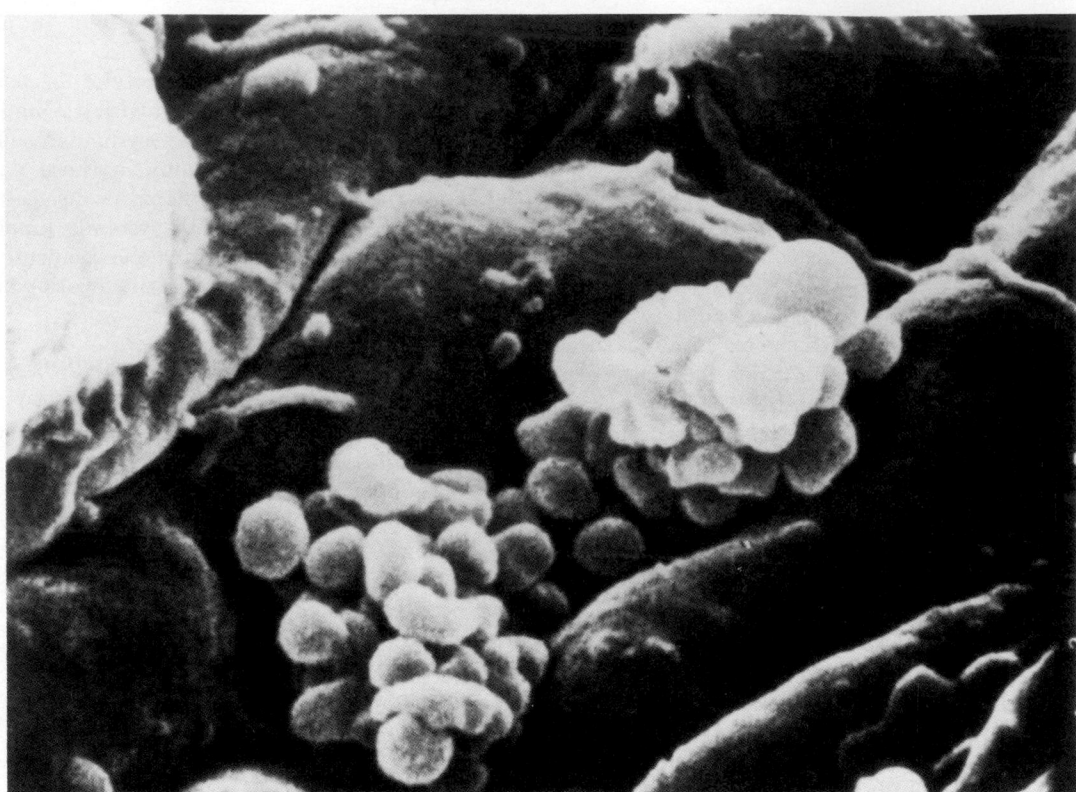

Figure 94–12. Electron microscopic scan of spleen removed from patient with ITP. Note clumping of platelets. (*Source: From Schwartz SI, Hoepp LM, et al, 1980, with permission.*)

cellular marrow, without evidence of an underlying disease, has been reported. Women constitute about 80 percent of cases of primary splenic neutropenia; over 50 percent of the patients with primary pancytopenia are men. The clinical manifestations are related, to some extent, to the cell type that is depressed. With neutropenia, fever, frequent recurring infections, and oral ulcerations may be noted. There may be hepatomegaly but none of the stigmata of cirrhosis are present. The lymph nodes are not enlarged. The total white blood count is below 4000/mm³, and in one third of cases below 1000/mm³. Anemia is common, but severe anemia is rare. The peripheral blood smear is devoid of any diagnostic features of leukemia or myeloproliferative disorders. The bone marrow reveals a pancellular hyperplasia.

Corticosteroids rarely affect the disease process. Once the diagnosis is suspected, splenectomy is indicated in view of excellent reported results. Sustained hematologic improvement is noted in almost all patients. Some patients, over the course of years develop lymphosarcoma or histiocytic lymphoma.

Secondary Hypersplenism

Pancytopenia may be a consequence of portal hypertension. Thrombocytopenia is present in approximately one third of patients with portal hypertension, secondary to schistosomiasis, and one quarter of patients with portal hypertension secondary to nutritional cirrhosis. The portal hypertension results in delayed passage and engorgement of the vascular spaces within the spleen which, in turn, leads to accelerated destruction of the circulating cells as they course through the organ.

Hypersplenism per se is rarely an indication for operative intervention in patients with portal hypertension. Splenectomy alone generally will not permanently reduce portal hypertension in patients in whom the primary disorder is cirrhosis. Splenectomy, however, may be curative of portal hypertension in patients with

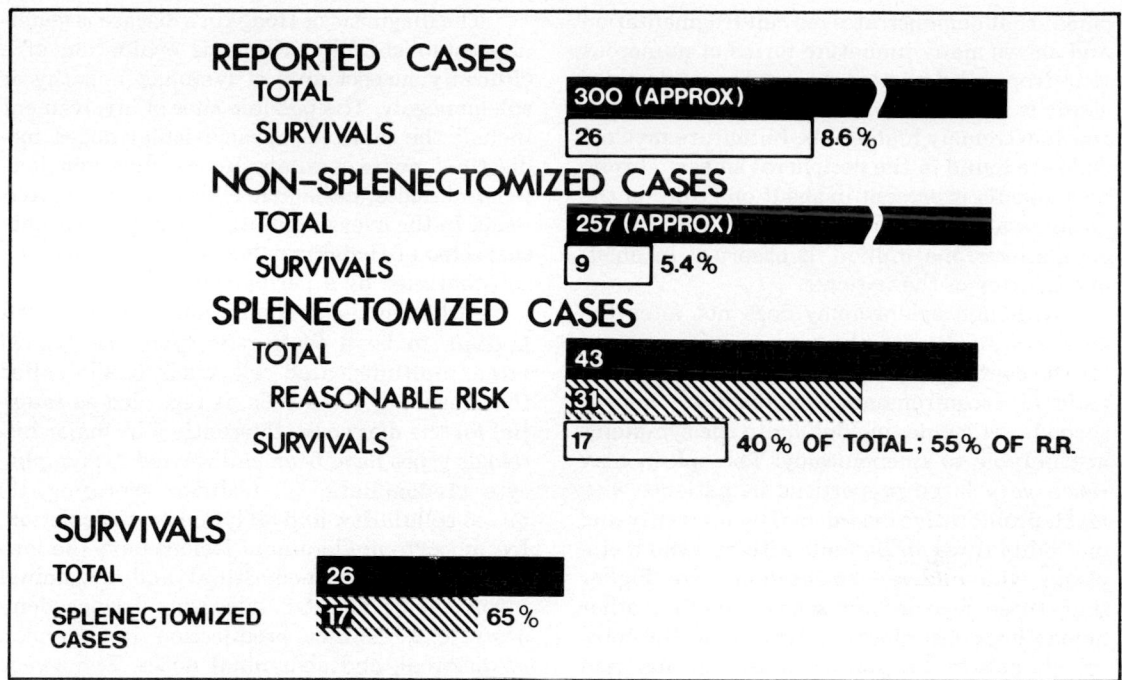

Figure 94–13. Thrombotic thrombocytopenic purpura. Effect of splenectomy on survival. (*Source: From Schwartz SI, Adams JT, et al, 1971, with permission.*)

isolated splenic vein thrombosis or myeloid metaplasia. In patients who undergo a decompressive procedure for bleeding esophagogastric varices, regardless of the procedure performed, the hypersplenism is usually corrected.

In patients with lymphomas and chronic lymphocytic leukemia, splenectomy is carried out when the organ is sufficiently enlarged to cause symptoms, or when cytopenia is severe while the marrow is apparently adequate. In patients with very large spleens and chronic lymphocytic leukemia, improvement may be substantive even with reduced numbers of hematopoietic cells in the marrow. In these patients, the hematologic response is favorable in the majority of patients subjected to splenectomy. In most patients the neutropenia and thrombocytopenia are improved, and the hemolytic response is controlled. There is no correlation between the response to steroids and the hematologic remission following splenectomy. There is little evidence that splenectomy alters the course of chronic myelogenous leukemia, but it may be applicable in an occasional patient whose platelet count is markedly reduced.

Splenectomy offers significant increase in the neutrophil count in neutropenic patients with Felty's syndrome and is particularly applicable if there is a history of recurrent infection. The arthralgia is not affected. Similarly, although splenectomy does not alter the course of the disease in sarcoidosis or Gaucher's disease, it may play a palliative role for patients with symptomatic splenomegaly and may be indicated for control of secondary hypersplenism.

Myeloproliferative Disorders

The myeloproliferative disorders, including myeloid metaplasia and myelofibrosis, represent panproliferative processes manifested by increased connective tissue proliferation of the bone marrow, liver, spleen, and lymph nodes and a simultaneous proliferation of hematopoietic elements in the liver, spleen, and long bones. In the past, splenectomy was regarded as contraindicated in these disorders, suggesting that the procedure removed an important organ of production of cellular elements of blood. This is no longer believed and it is extremely rare for splenectomy to result in an adverse hematologic effect due to the removal of an hematopoietic organ.

The laboratory hallmark is a peripheral

smear that demonstrates red cell fragmentation and shows many immature forms of numerous tear-drop and elongated shapes. The white blood count is in the range of 50,000/mm³ and may reach extremely high levels. Immature myeloid cells are found in the peripheral smear. Thrombocytopenia is present in about one third of the patients and thrombocytosis, with white blood counts over one million, is observed in about one quarter of the patients.

Although splenectomy does not alter the course of the disease, the procedure is indicated for the control of anemia, and increasing transfusional requirements, leukopenia, and/or thrombocytopenia, in addition to the symptoms attributable to splenomegaly. The spleen may reach very large proportions in patients with myeloproliferative disorders. The mortality and morbidity rates for patients with myeloid metaplasia who undergo splenectomy are higher than those reported for splenectomy for other hematologic disorders. Postoperative thrombocytosis and/or thrombosis of the splenic vein extending to the portal and mesenteric veins occurs more commonly in these patients. The incidence of this complication can be reduced by using alkylating agents preoperatively and employing drugs to prevent platelet aggregation and thrombosis during the perioperative period.

Portal hypertension has been described, due either to hepatic involvement of sufficient degree to be obstructive to the portal circulation, or due to an increased forward blood flow through the splenoportal system. In the latter circumstance splenectomy alone effects a significant reduction in portal hypertension and has resulted in disappearance of varices. In this group of patients, it is appropriate to measure pressure in an omental vein prior to splenectomy; if portal hypertension is defined, the pressure should be measured once again subsequent to removal of the organ, in order to define the etiology of portal hypertension, i.e., hepatic sinusoidal obstruction or increased afferent flow.

Hodgkin's Disease

In addition to the role that splenectomy plays in the palliation of patients with Hodgkin's disease who have symptomatic splenomegaly or hypersplenism, removal of the spleen as part of a diagnostic laparotomy functions significantly in the definition of the extent of Hodgkin's disease.

The diagnosis of Hodgkin's disease is generally established by histologic evaluation of a clinically suspect area of lymphadenopathy or splenomegaly. The possible sites of involvement include the cervical supraclavicular nodes, mediastinal nodes, axillary nodes, iliac and ileofemoral nodes, periaortic nodes, and the spleen itself. In the overwhelming majority of patients suspected of Hodgkin's disease, the diagnosis is substantiated by a peripheral node biopsy.

Although the predominant neoplastic cell appears to be a histiocytic type, the typical large, multinucleated cell, traditionally called the Sternberg–Reed cells, is regarded as essential for the diagnosis. Currently four major histologic types have been categorized: (1) lymphocyte predominant, (2) nodular sclerosing, (3) mixed cellularity, and (4) lymphocyte depletion. Lymphocyte predominant lesions have the lowest incidence of mediastinal and abdominal involvement; nodular sclerosing lesions demonstrate a distinct predilection for cervical, mediastinal, and abdominal nodes. The 5-year survival rate for patients with lymphocyte predominance approaches 90 percent; those with lymphocyte depletion and a mixed cellularity have a 5-year survival of 40 percent. Nodular sclerosing lesions are associated with an intermediate survival time.

The application of laparotomy, splenectomy, liver biopsy, retroperitoneal and hepatoduodenal node biopsy, in addition to marrow biopsy, as diagnostic tools for Hodgkin's disease is based on several considerations. The first is that the lesion usually begins as a single focus and spreads in a predictable manner along adjacent lymphoid channels. The second is that therapy may be dictated by the stage. The third, and most important, is that previous methods of evaluating the stage, including physical examination, laboratory studies, and radiologic studies, have significant indices of inaccuracy.

Stage I Hodgkin's disease is limited to one anatomic area, either one lymph node region, or a localized extralymphatic organ or site. Stage II is involvement of two or more lymph node regions on the same side of the diaphragm, or solitary involvement of an extralymphatic organ or site, and one or more lymph node regions on the same side of the diaphragm. Stage III is involvement of lymph node regions on both sides of the diaphragm, which may also be accompanied by involvement of the spleen (IIIs). Stage IV is diffuse or disseminated involvement of one or more extralymphatic organs or tissues, with or without associated lymph node involvement. Each stage is divided into two groups: A, based on the absence of specific symptoms, and B, based on the presence of fever, night sweats, or weight loss greater than 10 percent of normal body weight.

The definition of intraabdominal areas involved by Hodgkin's disease is difficult, as clinical appraisal of this region is, at best, imprecise. Neither periaortic nor iliac nodes are generally palpable, and the palpability of both the liver and spleen is related, to a large extent, to the habitus of the patient as well as to the organ size. More important, it is now well established that both splenic and hepatic involvement may occur in the absence of specific organomegaly. Liver function tests and scintillation scanning procedures only infrequently provide unequivocal evidence of hepatic involvement. Inferior venacavography, CT, and lymphangiography have been applied to define infradiaphragmatic nodal involvement.

Surgical staging was introduced in 1968 at the Stanford University Medical Center. Since that time there have been several studies demonstrating a lack of correlation between clinical assessment and subsequent operative and histopathologic findings. Preoperative determinations of splenic involvement based on palpability and/or radiographic and isotopic splenomegaly have proved to be imprecise. There has been approximately 30 percent error relying on these indices; spleens that had been adjudged clinically normal proved to have involvement with Hodgkin's disease. Conversely, spleens that were thought to be abnormal failed to demonstrate involvement with Hodgkin's histologically in approximately 38 percent of cases. Forty percent of patients thought to have hepatic involvement, based on hepatomegaly or abnormal liver function tests, proved to have no evidence of Hodgkin's disease in the organ, while approximately 4 percent of patients whose livers were normal clinically, based on function studies, had Hodgkin's involvement. The preoperative assessment of lymphatic involvement by computed tomography or lymphangiography has an index of error of approximately 15 percent with normal preoperative studies, and 30 percent of those lymph nodes thought to be involved proved to have no involvement. Overall, operative staging of Hodgkin's disease has altered the stage in 42 percent of cases, increasing

it in approximately 28 percent of cases and decreasing it in 14 percent (Fig. 94–14).

There is disagreement regarding the applicability of operative staging for Hodgkin's disease. The consensus is presently that with lymphocyte predominant lesions and no evidence of mediastinal involvement, staging is not applicable. With nodular sclerosing lesions that are clinically staged IA and IIA, surgical staging is considered appropriate.

In reference to the routine staging for non-Hodgkin's lymphoma, a difference of opinion also pertains. Veronesi and associates conclude that diagnostic laparotomy and staging should be carried out in centers in which the information can be translated into aggressive treatment but feel that it should not have the wide adoption that Hodgkin's staging has had. Chabner et al reported that percutaneous and peritoneoscopically directed biopsies were reasonable alternatives to staging for non-Hodgkin's lymphoma and that the presence or absence of subdiaphragmatic disease could be established in over 80 percent of the patients by nonsurgical procedures, including lymphangiography, marrow biopsy, and percutaneous liver biopsy. The yield of staging procedures was highest in patients with nodular lymphomas and lowest in patients with histiocytic lymphomas.

Surgical Staging

A variety of incisions may be used. Generally, a long, subcostal incision approximately two fingerbreadths below the left costal margin, extending from a point just to the right of the midline to a point above the anterior iliac crest, will facilitate dissection of the lower periaortic and iliac nodes. A midline incision is preferable when oophoropexy to preserve ovarian function is performed. The iliac crest marrow biopsy is taken through a separate incision using an osteotome.

After the peritoneal cavity is entered the liver is first assessed for grossly apparent lesions, and a wedge biopsy is performed in both the left and right lobes. We no longer do needle biopsies in addition to the wedge biopsy since we have never experienced a case in which a needle biopsy was positive in the face of a negative wedge biopsy. Both wedge biopsies should be carried out prior to general abdominal exploration and before retractors are placed on the liver in order to avoid confusion of histologic

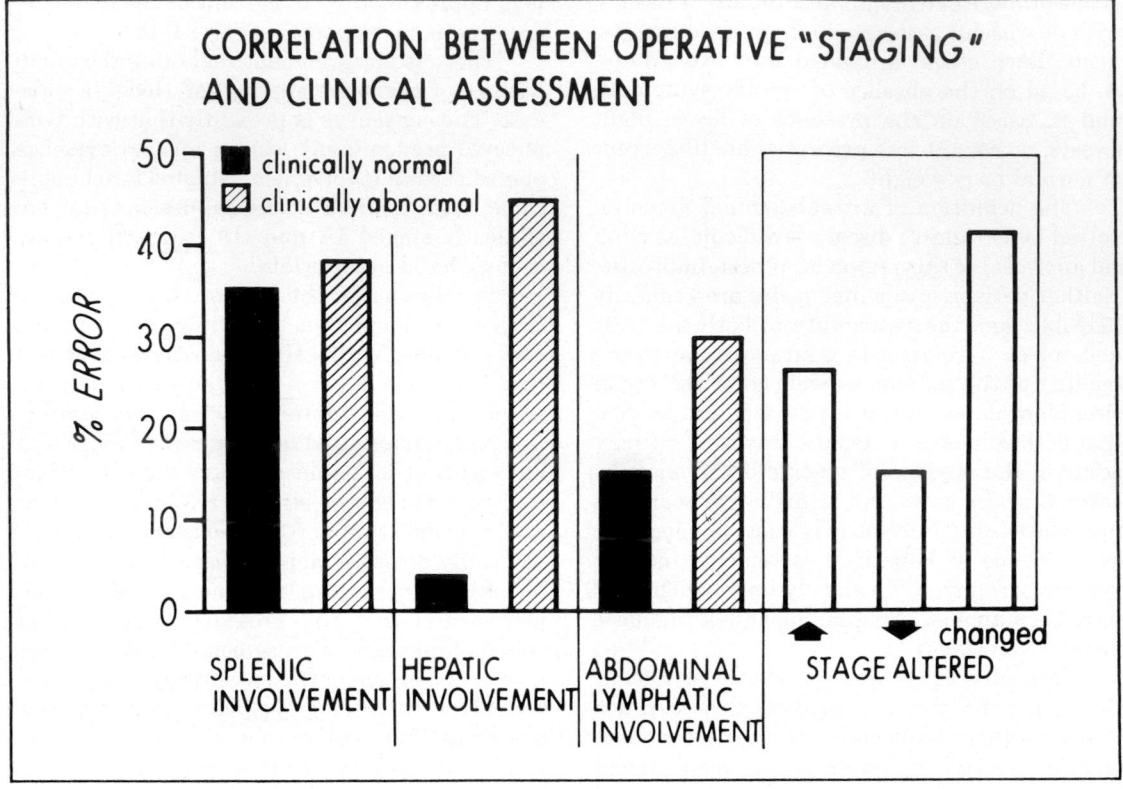

Figure 94–14. Correlation between operative "staging" and clinical assessment. (*Source: From Schwartz SI, Cooper RA Jr, 1972, with permission.*)

evaluation because prolonged application of the retractor rapidly results in cellular infiltration.

Attention is next directed to removing the spleen. The splenectomy is carried out in the fashion described later. In most instances lesions can be defined on gross examination. If marked adenopathy limits the dissection of hilar vessels, it may be expeditious to enter the lesser sac through the gastrocolic omentum and to ligate the vessels more centrally as they course along the superior surface of the pancreas.

The biopsy sites for periaortic nodes may be selected by palpation at laparotomy or based on the finding of CT or lymphangiography. Representative nodes from areas that either look or feel suspicious should be removed, and these areas should be marked with clips. The nodes should be sent for pathologic study separately, with their locations indicated. This can be facilitated by drawing a map on a piece of paper

and submitting the nodes positioned on the map to the pathologist (Fig. 94–15). Since the greatest yield is from the region of the twelfth thoracic and first lumbar vertebra, the colon is retracted craniad in all instances and the ligament of Treitz transected to provide ready access to the upper retroperitoneum (Fig. 94–16). The retroperitoneal incision is carried down to the bifurcation of the iliac vessels and may be extended into the pelvis if nodes are palpable in that region. Representative mesenteric nodes are also biopsied. It is imperative that a representative node be removed from the hepatoduodenal ligament because cases have been recorded in which nodes in this region were involved in the absence of other nodal involvement.

In young females, oophoropexy by suturing the ovaries to one another in the midline, posterior to the uterus, preserves ovarian function by obviating subsequent radiation damage to these organs.

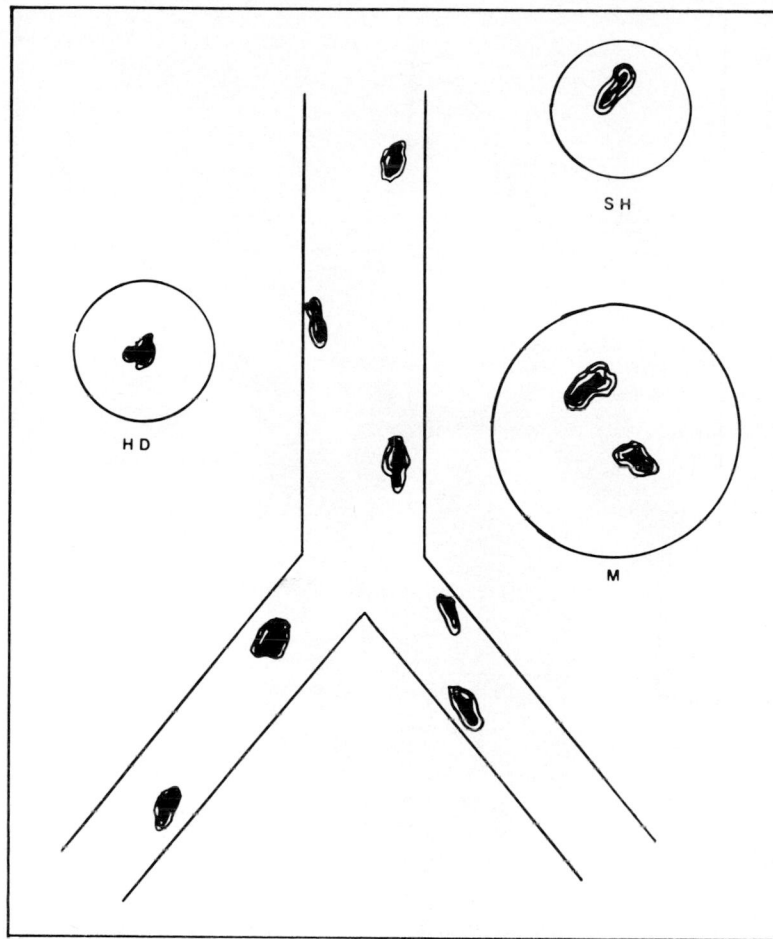

Figure 94–15. Mapping of nodes excised during Hodgkin's staging. HD = hepatoduodenal ligament, SH = splenic hilus, M = mesentery.

SPLENECTOMY

Preoperative Preparation. In most instances, there is no specific treatment required for the preoperative management of patients undergoing splenectomy. Patients with a past history of multiple transfusions and those with autoimmune hemolytic anemia may require a longer preoperative stay because of difficulties in blood typing and cross-matching. Platelets should not be administered preoperatively to patients with idiopathic thrombocytopenic purpura, since these cells will not survive. It is even more important that platelets not be given to patients with thrombotic thrombocytopenic purpura because the thrombotic process may be accelerated. In those patients with myeloproliferative disorders who have a tendency to develop thrombosis, it is beneficial to medicate the pa-

tient with low-dose heparin, 5000 units twice daily, and aspirin on the day prior to surgery, and to continue this regimen for 5 days postoperatively. In elective cases, the pneumovax is administered approximately 10 days to 2 weeks prior to operation, and in emergency cases it is given immediately preoperatively. A nasogastric tube is used during the operation to decompress the stomach and to facilitate ligation of the short gastric veins. The tube can be inserted intraoperatively and removed immediately at the end of the procedure.

Operative Technique. A variety of incisions may be used, depending upon the nature of the disease and the personal preference of the surgeon. They include upper midline incision, left paramedian incision, and left oblique subcostal incision, which may be extended to the right

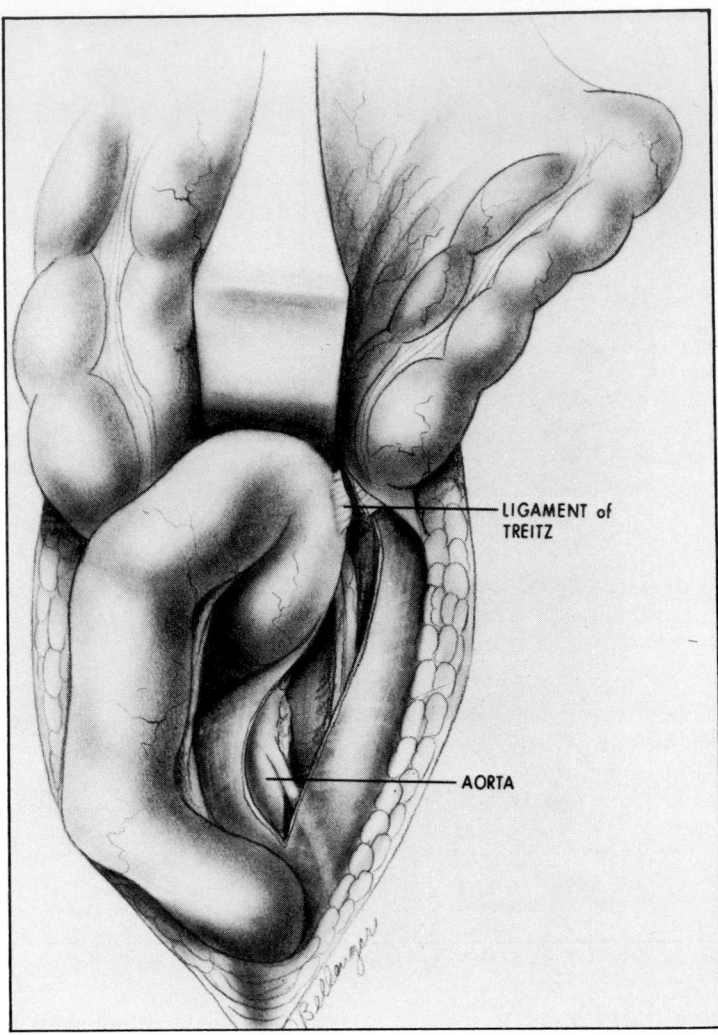

Figure 94–16. Retroperitoneal node dissection. The ligament of Treitz has been transected to permit exposure of T-12 and L-1 area, which provides the highest yield of suspicious nodes. (*Source: From Schwartz SI, Cooper RA Jr, 1972, with permission.*)

upper quadrant as a "hockey stick" and a combined abdominothoracic approach.

The midline incision is the one most applicable in cases of suspected rupture of the spleen because it is made rapidly, and affords satisfactory access to the spleen and other viscera that may have been traumatized. This incision is generally preferred when splenectomy is performed as part of a staging procedure in order to facilitate dissection of the lower paraaortic and iliac nodes and oophoropexy.

The left paramedian incision is preferred by many surgeons. The left rectus muscle is retracted laterally. The incision should reach to, or extend beyond, the costal margin craniad and about 5 cm below the umbilicus caudad. A variant of this incision is the left vertical muscle splitting incision, which divides the inner portion of the left rectus muscle in a vertical plane, starting at the costal margin itself and extending down below the level of the umbilicus.

This author's preference is the left oblique subcostal incision, which should begin to the right of the midline and proceed obliquely outward and downward about two finger breadths below the costal margin. In the case of patients with ITP and small spleens, the oblique muscles do not have to be divided. With larger spleens, the oblique muscles are divided in the course of their fibers laterally, and if additional exposure is required, a "hockey stick" extension is used transecting the right rectus muscle.

In the case of marked splenomegaly with significant diaphragmatic adhesions, some surgeons have advised a thoracocabdominal incision with the patient's left side elevated between 45 and 60 degrees. The incision represents an extension from a transverse left upper quadrant incision into the eighth intercostal space transecting the eighth costal cartilage and dividing the diaphragm. It is this author's opinion that this incision should be avoided because it is associated with a higher incidence of morbidity. We have been able to remove spleens as large as 17 pounds through a left subcostal incision extended into the right upper quadrant.

Usually splenectomy is performed by a technique of mobilization and dissection down to an ultimate pedicle of splenic artery and vein. Exploration with the right hand, following the convex surface of the organ, will define the extent of ligamentous attachments. In the case of splenic trauma, a hematoma frequently has

dissected these attachments and rapid delivery of the organ into the wound is facilitated. In the case of elective splenectomy, the first step is transection of the ligamentous attachments (Fig. 94–17). This includes the splenophrenic ligament at the superior pole and the splenocolic and splenorenal ligaments at the inferior pole posteriorly. Once the splenophrenic ligament has been completely transected, the spleen can be sufficiently mobilized to identify, and to permit interruption of, two or three short gastric veins that run from the spleen to the greater curvature of the stomach (Fig. 94–18). It is important not to incorporate the gastric wall in these ligations, and should there be any question of this circumstance, a Lembert suture should be placed in the gastric wall to cover the area with serosa and to avoid the complication of gastric fistulization.

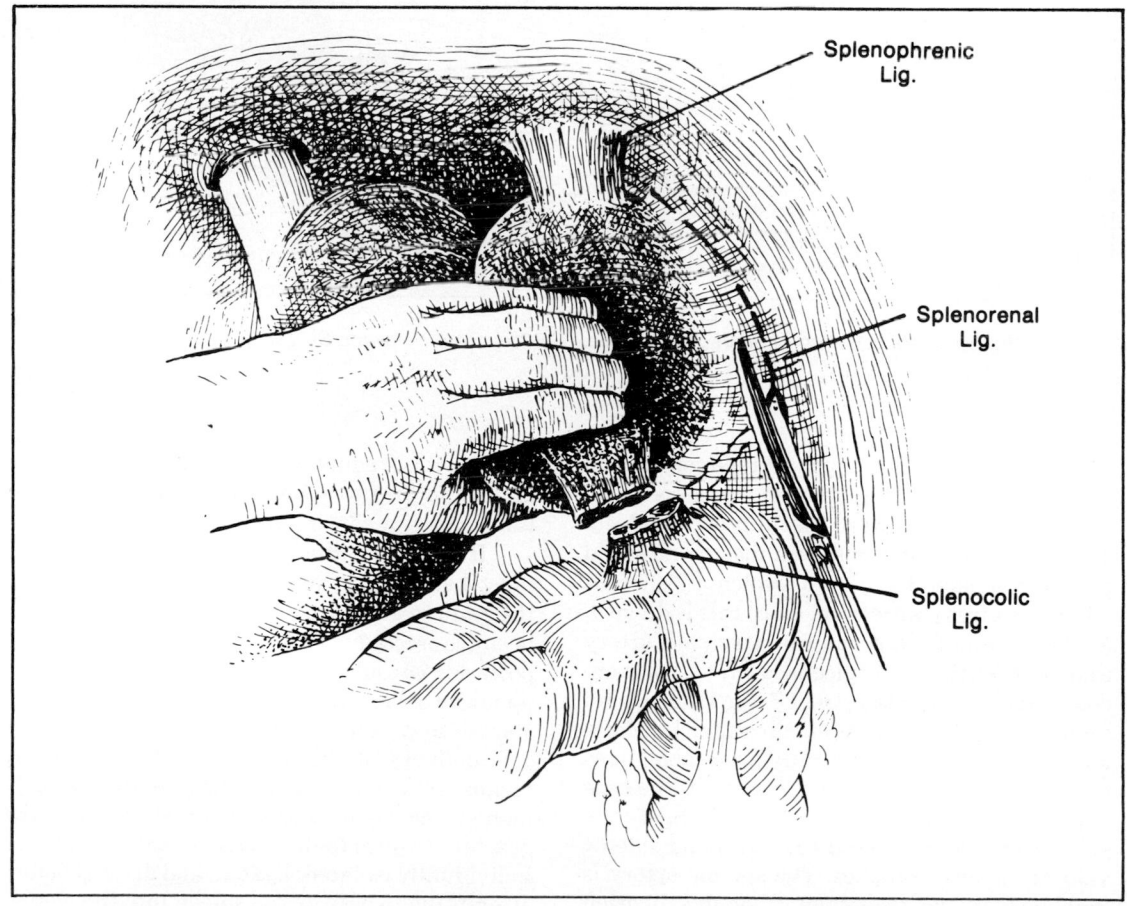

Figure 94–17. Transection of ligamentous attachments. (*Source: From Schwartz SI, 1980, with permission.*)

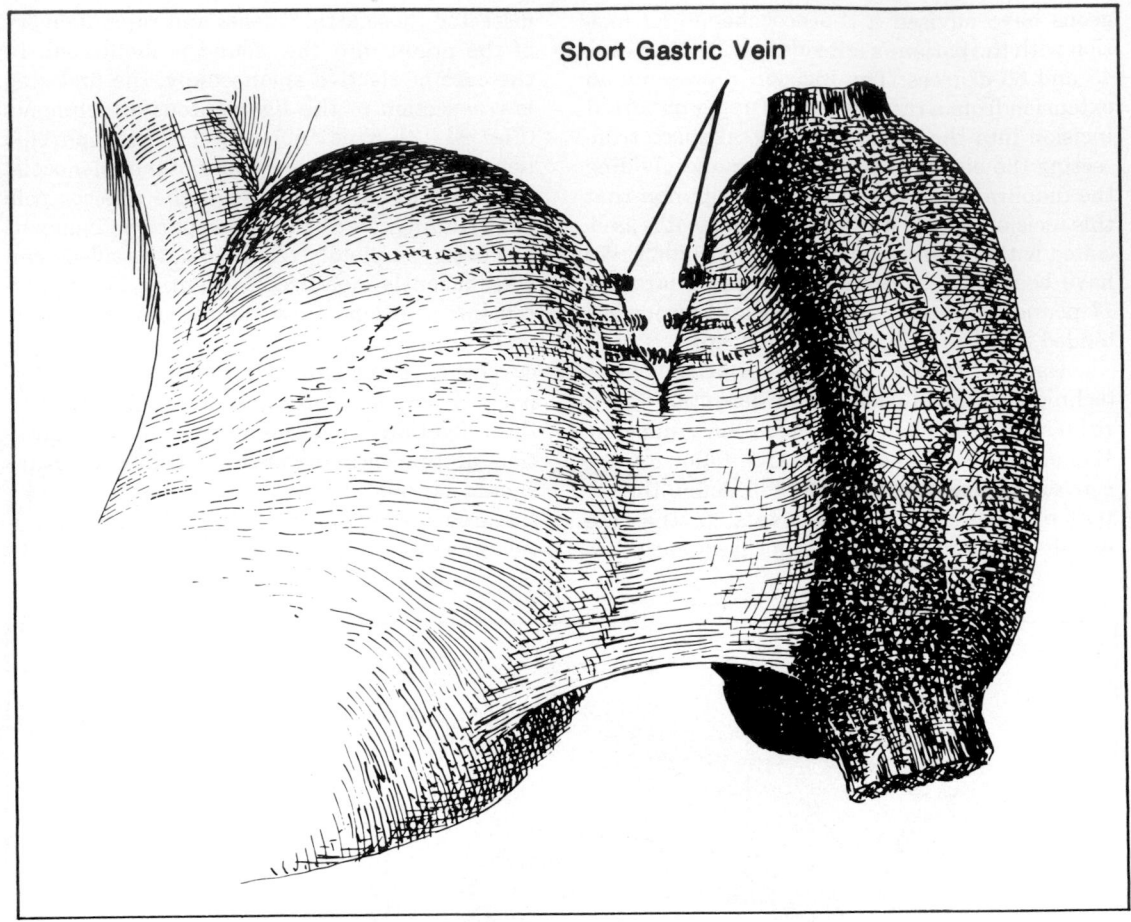

Short Gastric Vein

Figure 94–18. Ligation of short gastric veins. (*Source: From Schwartz SI, 1980, with permission.*)

After the ligamentous attachments and short gastric vessels have been transected, dissection is directed toward the hilus of the spleen. The inferior pole of the spleen may be attached to the stomach by a gastrosplenic ligament which requires transection. Once this is divided, all that remains are the main splenic artery and vein. With small spleens, such as those encountered in patients with ITP, the three-clamp method of Federoff has been advocated by Maingot (Fig. 94–19). It is generally preferable, however, in all instances, and certainly in the case of an enlarged spleen, to individually ligate the splenic artery or arterial branches and splenic vein or venous branches. The splenic artery is managed by the technique of double ligation and suture ligature (Fig. 94–20). In the case of myeloid metaplasia, with markedly enlarged

spleens, it is frequently necessary to use a vascular clamp on the splenic vein and to close the lumen with a continuous vascular suture.

It is during the hilar dissection that care must be taken to avoid damage to the tail of the pancreas. If the tail of the pancreas has been transected inadvertently, the anterior and posterior capsule should be approximated with nonabsorbable suture material. In rare circumstances in which adhesions apparently preclude safe delivery of the spleen into the wound by means of transecting the ligamentous attachments, the lesser sac is entered through the greater omental fold, and the splenic vessels are individually isolated, ligated, and divided before attempting to deliver the spleen into the wound (Fig. 94–21).

Following removal of the spleen hemostasis

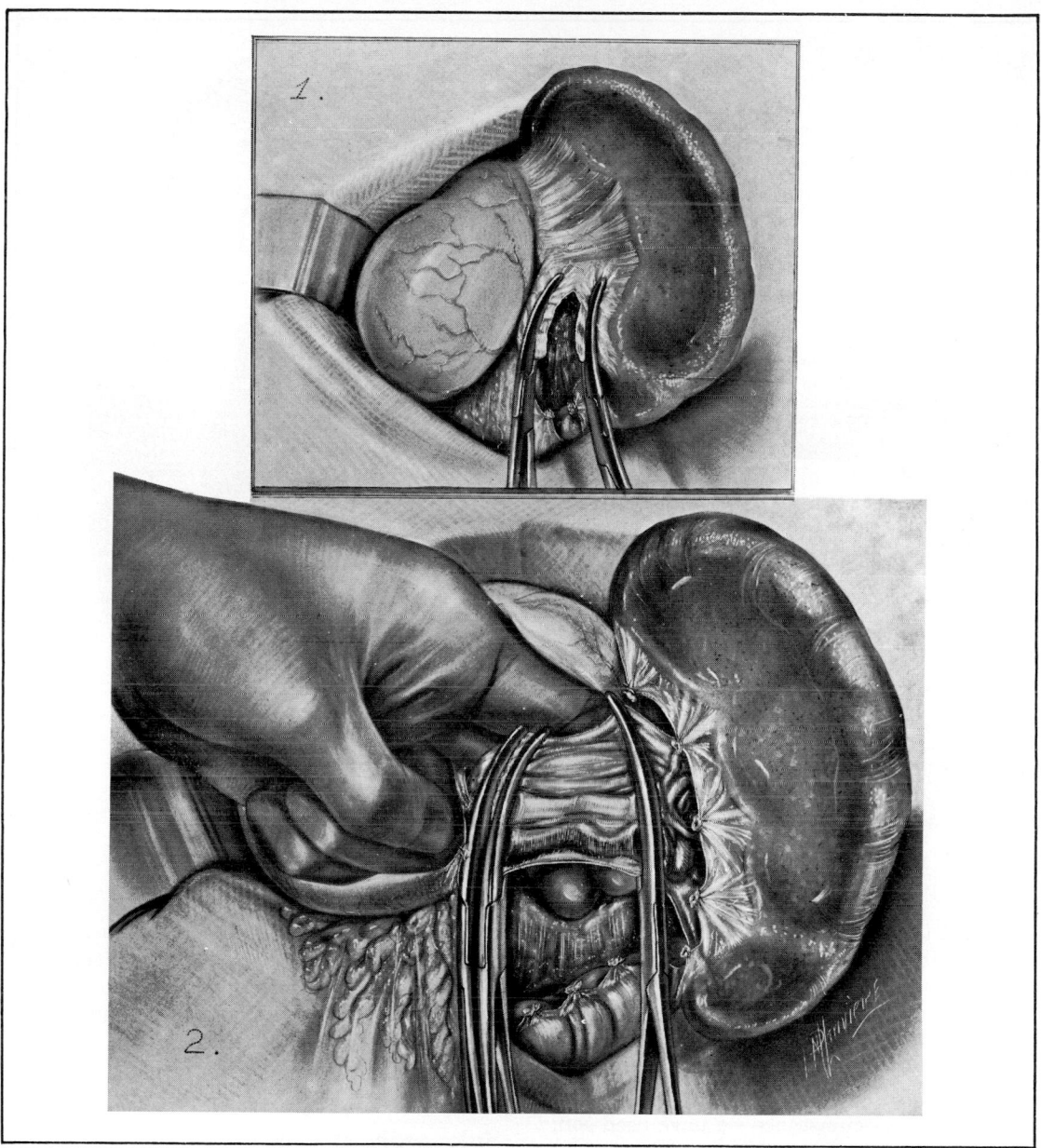

Figure 94–19. Splenectomy by the three-clamp method of Federoff. 1. Division of the gastrosplenic omentum. 2. Three-clamp method. Note the position of the fingers guarding the tail of the pancreas while the clamps are being applied.

is checked in three major areas: the inferior surface of the diaphragm, the greater curvature of the stomach in the region of the short gastric vessels, and the region of the hilus. This is readily accomplished, inserting two Mikulicz pads into the left upper quadrant and first exerting downward and medial traction on the stomach and hilar region. This permits visualization of the undersurface of the diaphragm. The pads are then moved caudad to permit visualization of the greater curvature of the stomach and the short gastric vessels that have been divided. The final step is uncovering the hilar dissection to determine any evidence of bleeding.

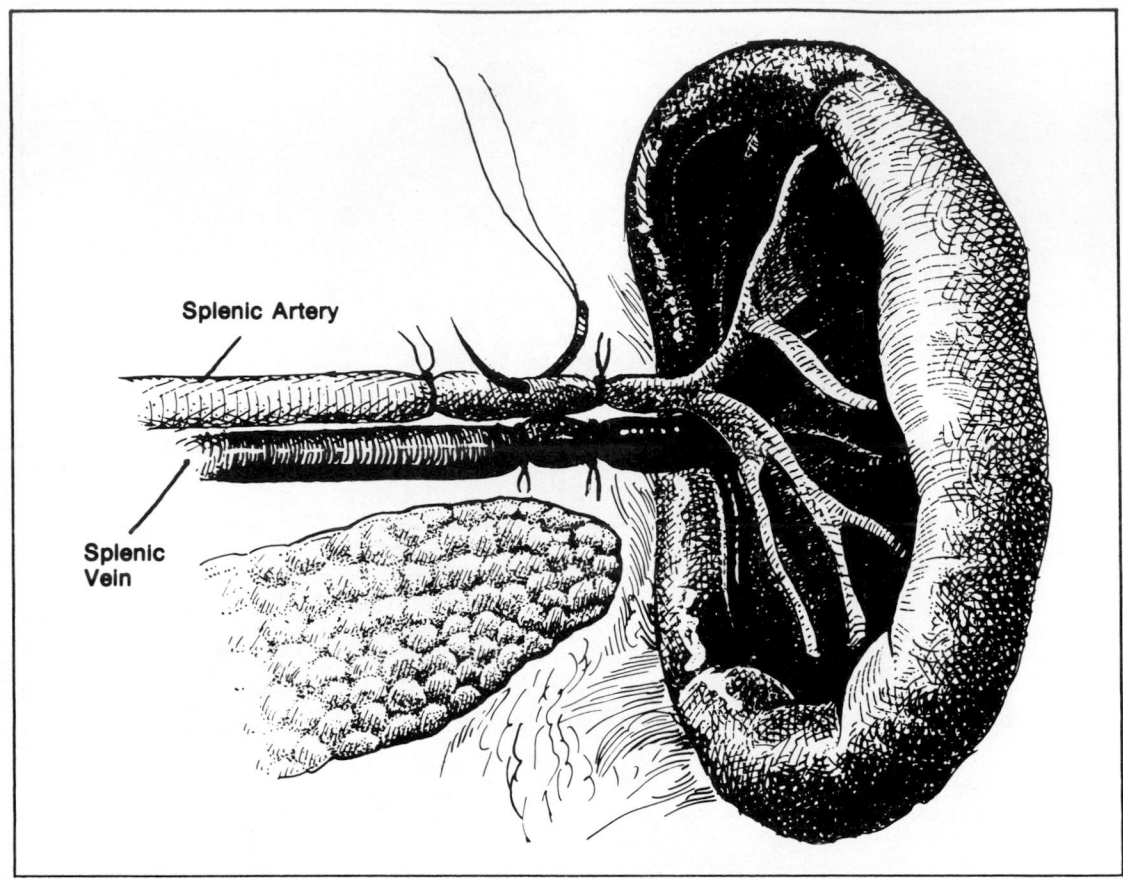

Figure 94–20. Management of hilus. (*Source: From Schwartz SI, 1980, with permission.*)

If the tail of the pancreas has not been injured, drainage is not performed on a routine basis. It has been our policy to drain the subphrenic region in patients with myeloproliferative disorders and markedly enlarged spleens accompanied by evidence of portal hypertension and collateralization of the ligamentous attachment. In this circumstance we have used soft, rubber drains exiting through a stab wound into a closed system Hollister bag. If the tail of the pancreas has been inadvertently injured, a sump drain is brought out through a stab wound.

An integral part of the procedure of splenectomy for hematologic disease consists of a thorough laparotomy to identify accessory spleens which must be removed. These are present in 18 to 30 percent of patients with hematologic disease. The more common locations of the accessory spleens are in the region of the hilus and the gastrosplenic ligament, gastrocolic liga-

ment, and the greater omentum, mesentery, and presacral space. Accessory spleens have been found in juxtaposition to the left ovary and left testicle. The overwhelming majority of accessory spleens are located in the region of the splenic hilus (Fig. 94–4).

Splenorrhaphy and Autotransplantation

The techniques to preserve splenic tissue and function are dictated by the extent of damage. Small lacerations can be managed by compression and the application of a hemostatic agent, such as oxydized cellulose, or micronized collagen (Fig. 94–22.) Hemostasis associated with significant disruptions of the splenic capsule and parenchyma can generally be managed with absorbable sutures that traverse the capsule and incorporate the parenchyma. In this circumstance, the horizontal mattress suture is advan-

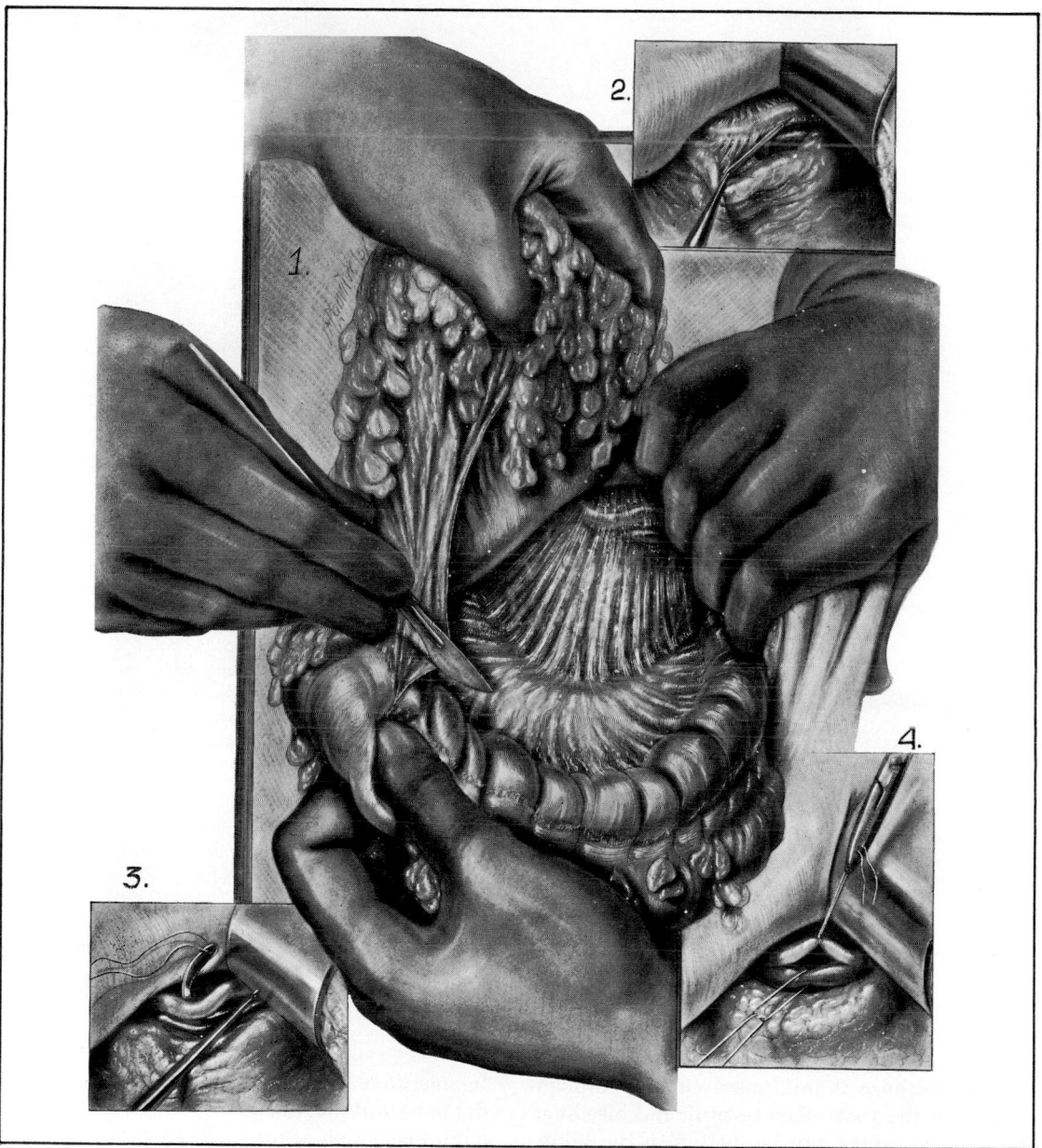

Figure 94–21. In some cases of splenomegaly where the spleen is firmly attached to the diaphragm by numerous adhesions, this approach through the omental bursa to the splenic artery and vein (above the superior border of the pancreas) is sometimes selected. The splenic artery and vein should be cautiously dissected free from their bed before applying silk ligatures proximally and distally to them (firmly but not too tightly) and then dividing each vessel between the ligatures. Following this procedure the bulky tethered spleen is carefully mobilized from the diaphragm, tail of the pancreas, stomach, and colon before ligating its pedicle once again and removing the organ.

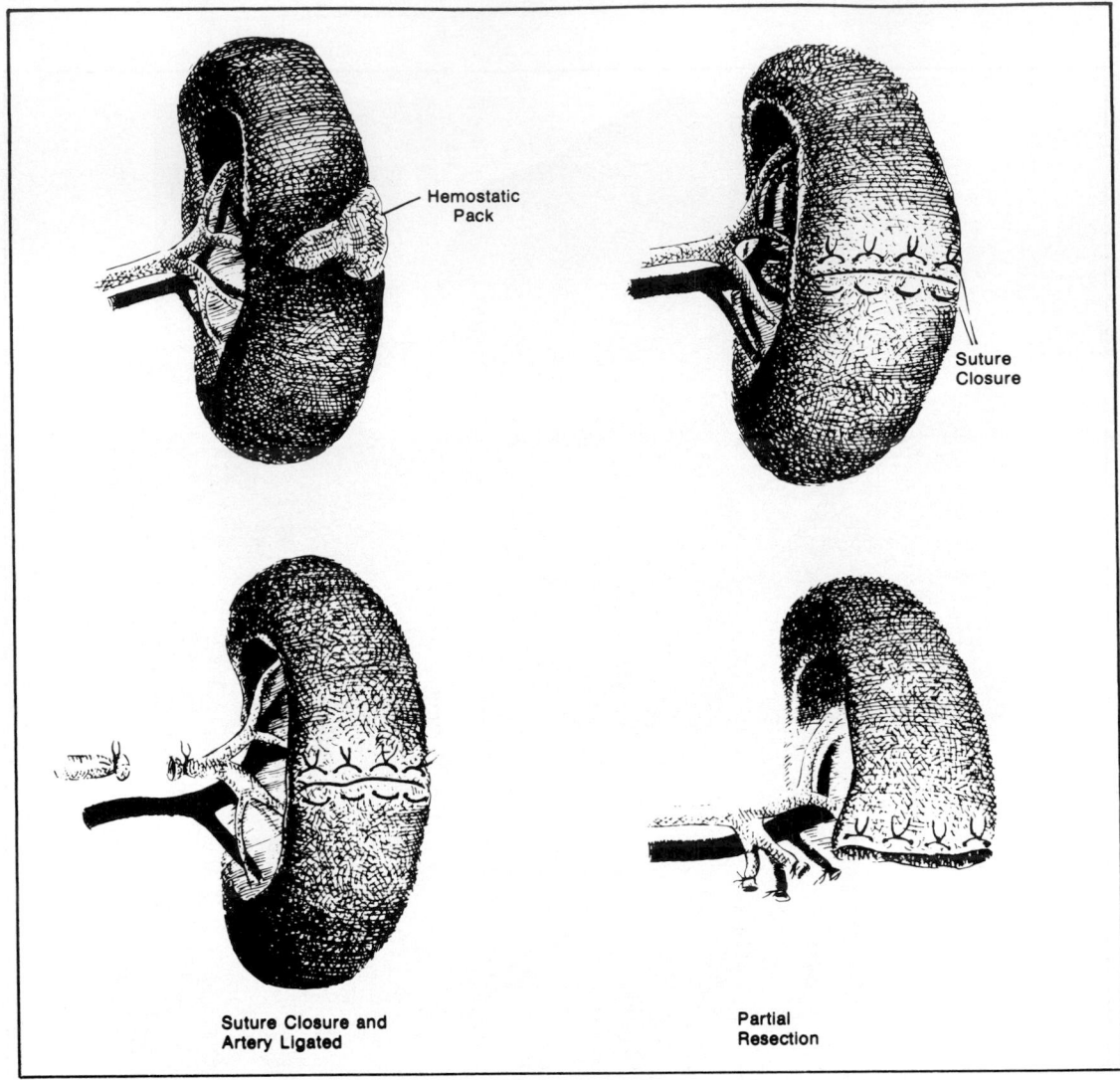

Figure 94–22. Preservation of traumatized spleen. (*Source: From Schwartz SI, 1980, with permission.*)

tageous because it minimizes cutting through tissue. In the case of more profound bleeding, the splenic artery can be ligated in the hilus, following which the transcapsular suture is inserted and tied. If trauma is localized to one pole of the spleen, this area should be resected and the edges approximated with a series of mattress sutures. The omentum may be used to fill large defects, or to suture over the injury site to provide tamponade.

In order to determine which of these techniques is applicable, and to effect the splenic repair and preservation, it is essential that the ligamentous attachments are transected in order to permit mobilization of the organ and thorough inspection of all surfaces.

In the event of trauma sufficient to require splenectomy some investigators have reported salutory effect with implantation. The spleen is cut into slices that are approximately 0.5 cm in diameter, and these slices are then placed in an omental pocket so that there is drainage into the portal venous system. Viability of these implants has been demonstrated, and the tuftsin, opsonin complement, and IgM levels have all returned to normal. There is an argument about whether sufficient splenic material results to permit phagocytosis of encapsulated bacteria.

Complications. Early postoperative bleeding must be closely monitored, particularly in patients with thrombocytopenia and/or myeloproliferative disorders. In these patients it is an error to indict hematologic abnormalities as the cause of bleeding, and it is generally safer to reexplore the patients early and to evacuate a hematoma to reduce the incidence of subphrenic abscess. Left lower lobe atelectasis is another complication; it occurs more frequently following splenectomy than other abdominal procedures. Much has been written about the incidence of deep venous thrombosis following splenectomy, but most large series have not substantiated this finding. In unusual cases, the platelet count may rise to very high levels, at times greater than 2,000,000/mm³, but no specific therapy other than hydration is generally indicated. If medical therapy is thought to be appropriate, a drug that inhibits platelet aggregation, such as acetylsalicylic acid or dipyridamole, can be used. Thrombosis of the splenic vein with extension into the portal vein and superior vein is an extremely rare complication, occurring mostly in patients with myeloproliferative disorders or in those with sepsis as a consequence of intraabdominal abscess.

The increased incidence of fulminant sepsis related to pneumococcus or to hemophilus influenza following splenectomy is an established fact, but it occurs more commonly in patients who are immunosuppressed or have diseases with a propensity for infection. All patients subjected to splenectomy should be treated with pneumovax, and younger patients should receive long-term antibiotic prophylaxis against *H. influenza* sepsis until they reach adulthood.

BIBLIOGRAPHY

Abrams HL, Spiro R, et al: Metastases in carcinoma. Cancer 3:74, 1950

Albrechtsen D, Ly B: Complications after therapeutic splenectomy for hematologic disease in adults. Acta Chir Scand 146:577, 1980

Babb RR: Aneurysm of the splenic artery. Arch Surg 111:924, 1976

Bailey H: Traumatic rupture of the normal spleen. Br J Surg 15:40, 1927

Barnhart M, Baechler CA, et al: Arteriovenous shunts in human spleen. Am J Hematol 1:105, 1976

Barnhart MI, Lusher JM: Structural physiology of the human spleen. Am J Pediatr Hematol Oncol 1:311, 1979

Barnhart MI, Lusher JM: The human spleen as revealed by scanning electron microscopy. Am J Hematol 1:243, 1976

Bernard RP, Bauman AW, et al: Splenectomy for thrombotic thrombocytopenic purpura. Ann Surg 169:616, 1969

Boxer MA, Braun J, et al: Thromboembolic risk of postsplenectomy thrombocytosis. Arch Surg 113:808, 1978

Broe PJ, Conley CL, et al: Thrombosis of the portal vein following splenectomy for myeloid metaplasia. Surg Gynecol Obstet 152:488, 1981

Buntain WL, Lynn HB: Splenorrhaphy: Changing concepts for the traumatized spleen. Surgery 86:748, 1979

Buchanan JG, DeGruchy GC: Splenectomy in chronic lymphocytic leukaemia and lymphosarcoma. Med J Aust ii:6, 1967

Cannon WB, Nelson TS: Staging of Hodgkin's disease: A surgical perspective. Am J Surg 132:224, 1976

Carter BN: The combined thoracoabdominal approach with particular reference to its employment in splenectomy. Surg Gynecol Obstet 84:1019, 1947

Chabner BA, Johnson RE, et al: Sequential nonsurgical and surgical staging of non-Hodgkin's lymphoma. Ann Intern Med 85:149, 1976

Chen LT: Microcirculation of the spleen: An open or closed circulation? Science 201:157, 1978

Christo MC: Segmental resections of the spleen: Report on the first eight cases operated on. Hospital (Rio) 62:575, 1962

Chulay JD, Lankerani MR: Splenic abscess: Report of 10 cases and review of literature. Am J Med 61:513, 1976

Coon WW, Liepman MK: Splenectomy for agnogenic myeloid metaplasia. Surg Gynecol Obstet 154:561, 1982

Dacie JV, Brain MC, et al: Nontropical idiopathic splenomegaly (primary hypersplenism): Review of 10 cases and their relationship to malignant lymphomas. Br J Haematol 17:317, 1969

Deitch EA, O'Neal B: Neutrophil function in adults after traumatic splenectomy. J Surg Res 33:98, 1982

Doan CA: The spleen: Its structure and functions. Postgrad Med 43:126, 1968

Ein SH, Shandling B, et al: The morbidity and mortality of splenectomy in children. Ann Surg 185:307, 1977

Engelhard D, Ciridalli G, et al: Splenectomy in homozygous beta thalassemia: A retrospective study of 30 patients. Br J Haematol 31:391, 1975

Fabri PJ, Metz EN, et al: A quarter century with splenectomy: Changing concepts. Arch Surg 108:569, 1974

Flye MW, Silver D: The role of surgery in sickle cell disease. Surg Gynecol Obstet 137:115, 1973

Fowler RH: Nonparasitic benign cystic tumors of the spleen. Int Abst Surg 96:209, 1953

Gadacz T, Way LW, et al: Changing clinical spectrum of splenic abscess. Am J Surg 128:182, 1974

Gill PG, Souter RG, et al: Splenectomy for hypersplenism in malignant lymphomas. Br J Surg 68:29, 1981

Glatstein E, Guernsey JM, et al: The value of laparotomy and splenectomy in the staging of Hodgkin's disease. Cancer 24:709, 1969

Glatstein E, Vosti KL, et al: Serious bacterial infections in pediatric Hodgkin's disease: Relative risks of radiotherapy, chemotherapy and splenectomy. Proc Am Soc Clin Oncol 17:252, 1976

Grant E, Mertens MA, et al: Splenic abscess: Comparison of four imaging methods. AJR 132:465, 1979

Golumb HM, Catovsky D, et al: Hairy cell leukemia: Clinical review based on 71 cases. Ann Intern Med 89 (pt 1):677, 1978

Gordon DH, Schaffner D, et al: Postsplenectomy thrombocytosis: Its association with mesenteric, portal, and/or renal thrombosis in patients with myeloproliferative disorders. Arch Surg 113:713, 1978

Hirsch J, Dacie JV: Persistent postsplenectomy thrombocytosis and thromboembolism: A consequence of continuing anemia. Br J Haematol 12:45, 1966

Husni EA: The clinical course of splenic hemangioma. Arch Surg 83:681, 1961

King H, Shumacker HB Jr: Splenic studies: I. Susceptibility to infection after splenectomy performed in infancy. Ann Surg 136:239, 1952

Lawthorne TW Jr, Zuidema GD: Splenic abscess. Surgery 79:686, 1976

Liebowitz HR: Splenomegaly and hypersplenism pre- and post-portacaval shunt. NY J Med 63:2631, 1963

Linos DA, Nagorney DM: Splenic abscess—the importance of early diagnosis. Mayo Clin Proc 58:261, 1983

Martin JK, Clark SC, et al: Staging laparotomy in Hodgkin's disease. Arch Surg 117:586, 1982

Martin JW: Congenital splenic cysts. Am J Surg 96:302, 1958

Montanaro A, Patton R: Primary splenic malignant lymphoma, histiocytic type, with sclerosis. Cancer 38:1625, 1976

Meakins JL: Splenectomy for rupture of the spleen: A reappraisal. Can Med Assoc J 121:11, 1979

Moore RA, Brunner CM, et al: Felty's syndrome: Long term follow-up after splenectomy. Ann Intern Med 75:381, 1971

Necheles TF, Allen DM, et al: The many forms of thalassemia: Definition and classification of thalassemia syndromes. Ann NY Acad Sci 165 (Art 1):5, 1969

Necheles TF, Finkel HE, et al: Red cell pyruvate kinase deficiency. The effect of splenectomy. Arch Intern Med 118:75, 1966

O'Brien E: Case of removal of the human spleen, without injury or derangement of the animal economy. Med Chir J Rev Lond 1:8, 1816

O'Grady JP, Day EJ, et al: Splenic artery aneurysm rupture in pregnancy. Obstet Gynecol 50:627, 1977

Olsen WR, Beaudoin DE: Increased incidence of accessory spleens in hematologic disease. Arch Surg 98:762, 1969

O'Neill JA Jr, Scott HW Jr, et al: The role of splenectomy in Felty's syndrome. Ann Surg 167:81, 1968

Owens JC, Coffey RJ: Collective review: Aneurysm of the splenic artery, including a report of 6 additional cases. Surg Gynecol Obstet: Int Abstr Surg 97:313, 1953

Patel J, Williams JS, et al: Preservation of splenic function by autotransplantation of traumatized spleen in man. Surgery 90:683, 1981

Romero-Torres R, Campbell JR: An interpretive review of the surgical treatment of hydatid disease. Surg Gynecol Obstet 121:851, 1965

Ross ME, Ellwood R, et al: Epidermoid splenic cysts. Arch Surg 112:596, 1977

Salky BA, Kreel I, et al: Splenectomy for thrombotic thrombocytopenic purpura. Mt Sinai J Med 50:56, 1983

Sasser WD, Golden GT, et al: Posttraumatic splenic cyst. Va Med Mon 103:125, 1976

Schwartz PE, Sterioff S, et al: Postsplenectomy sepsis and mortality in adults. JAMA 248:2279, 1982

Schwartz SI: Myeloproliferative disorders. Ann Surg 182:464, 1975

Schwartz SI: Splenectomy and splenorrhaphy, in Modern Technics in Surgery. Mt. Kisco, New York: Futura Publishing Company, 1980

Schwartz SI, Adams JT, et al: Splenectomy for hematologic disorders. Current Problems in Surgery. Chicago: Year Book, 1971

Schwartz SI, Cooper RA Jr: Surgery in the diagnosis and treatment of Hodgkin's disease, in Advances in Surgery, vol 6. Chicago: Year Book, 1972

Schwartz SI, Hoepp LM, et al: Splenectomy for thrombocytopenia. Surgery 88:497, 1980

Schwartz SI, Lichtman MA: Surgical considerations in hematologic patients, in Lichtman MA (ed): Hematology for Practitioners. Boston: Little, Brown, 1978, p 421

Sherlock PV, Learmonth JR: Aneurysm of the splenic artery: With an account of an example complicating Gaucher's disease. Br J Surg 30:151, 1952

Sherman R: Perspectives in management of trauma to the spleen: 1979 Presidential Address, American Association for the Surgery of Trauma. J Trauma 20:1, 1980

Silverstein MN, ReMine WH: Sex, splenectomy, and myeloid metaplasia. J Am Med Assoc 227:424, 1974

Singer DB: Postsplenectomy sepsis. Perspect Pediatr Pathol 1:285, 1973

Sirinek KR, Evans WE: Nonparasitic splenic cysts. Am J Surg 126:8, 1973

Stanley JC, Fry WJ: Pathogenesis and clinical significance of splenic artery aneurysms. Surgery 76:898, 1974

Trastek VF, Pairolero PC, et al: Splenic artery aneurysms. Surgery 91:694, 1982

VerHeyden CN, Beart RW, et al: Accessory splenectomy in management of recurrent idiopathic thrombocytopenic purpura. Mayo Clin Proc 53:442, 1978

Veronesi U, Musumeci R, et al: Value of staging laparotomy in non-Hodgkin's lymphomas (with emphasis on the histiocytic type). Cancer 33:446, 1974

von Ronnen JR: The Roentgen diagnosis of calcified aneurysms of the splenic and renal arteries. Acta Radiol (Stockh) 39:385, 1953

Wright FW, Williams EW: Large post-traumatic splenic cyst diagnosed by radiology, isotope scintigraphy and ultrasound. Br J Radiol 47:454, 1974

Index